To my family: Both the family at home who makes work meaningful
and to the extended family at the office, laboratory, clinic,
and operating theater who makes work productive and fun.

WEG, Jr.

To Mac and Louise for every opportunity,
Fritz for the direction,
Sara, Trevor, and Katy for the reason.

DTK

Contents

Contributing Authors

James R. Andrews, MD
Clinical Professor
Department of Orthopaedic Surgery
University of Kentucky Medical Center;
Clinical Professor of Orthopaedics and Sports Medicine
University of Virginia Medical School;
Clinical Professor of Surgery
Division of Orthopaedic Surgery
University of Alabama at Birmingham School of Medicine
Orthopaedic Surgeon
Alabama Sports Medicine & Orthopaedic Center
1201 11th Avenue South, Suite 200;
Medical Director
American Sports Medicine Institute
1313 13th Street South
Birmingham, Alabama 35205

Greg Atkinson, PhD
Senior Lecturer
Research Institute for Sport and Exercise Sciences
Liverpool John Moores University
Trueman Building, Webster Street
Liverpool L3 2ET
England

David W. Bacharach, PhD
Professor, Department of Health, Physical Education, Recreation, and Sport Science
Director, Human Performance Laboratory
St. Cloud State University
720 4th Avenue South
St. Cloud, Minnesota 56301

Jens Bangsbo, PhD
Associate Professor
Institute of Exercise and Sport Sciences
Department of Human Physiology
University of Copenhagen
13, Universitetsparken
Copenhagen DK-2100
Denmark

William R. Barfield, PhD
Assistant Professor
College of Charleston;
Adjunct Professor
Department of Orthopaedic Surgery
Medical University of South Carolina
96 Jonathan Lucas Street, Suite 708
Charleston, South Carolina 29425

M. Janet Barger-Lux, MS
Senior Research Associate
Department of Medicine
Creighton University
Osteoporosis Research Center
601 North 30th Street, Suite 5766;
Omaha, Nebraska 68131

Coen van den Berg, PhD
Researcher
Faculty of Human Movement Sciences
Vrije Universiteit Amsterdam
9, van der Boechorststraat
Amsterdam 1081 BT
The Netherlands

Bernard Bilodeau, PhD
Sports Science and Technology Division,
United States Olympic Committee
421 Old Military Road
Lake Placid, New York 12946

Richard A. Boileau, PhD
Departments of Kinesiology and Nutritional Science & Internal Medicine
University of Illinois
906 South Goodwin Avenue
Urbana, Illinois 61801

Frank W. Booth, PhD
Professor
Department of Integrative Biology, Pharmacology and Physiology
University of Texas Medical School
6431 Fannin Street
Houston, Texas 77030

J. David Branch, PhD
Assistant Professor of Exercise Science
Department of Exercise Science, Physical Education, and Recreation
Old Dominion University
Norfolk, Virginia 23529-0196

Fred Brouns, PhD
Sandoz Nutrition
PO Box 1250
Maastricht 6201 BT
The Netherlands

Dale D. Brown, PhD, FACSM
Associate Professor of Exercise Physiology
Department of Health, Physical Education and Recreation
Illinois State University
Campus Box 5120
Normal, Illinois 61790-5120

Robert-Jan M. Brummer, MD, PhD
Associate Professor
Nutrition and Toxicology Research Institute
Maastricht University
50, Universiteitssingel
NL-6200 MD Maastricht;
Gastroenterologist and Head of GI Motility Laboratory
Department of Gastroenterology and Hepatology
University Hospital Maastricht
P.O. Box 5800
NL-6202 AZ Maastricht
The Netherlands

Edmund R. Burke, PhD
Professor
Department of Biology
University of Colorado at Colorado Springs
1420 Austin Bluffs Parkway
Colorado Springs, Colorado 80933

James A. Carson, PhD
Department of Exercise Science
South Carolina University
Columbia, South Carolina 29208

T. Jeff Chandler, EdD, CSCS, FACSM
Associate Professor
Department of Exercise Science, Sports, and Recreation
Marshall University
400 Hal Morris Blvd.
Huntington, West Virginia 25755-2450

Robert F. Chapman, PhD
Adjunct Professor
Human Performance Laboratory
Indiana University
1001 East 17th Street
Bloomington, Indiana 47408

Teri Ciapponi
Department of Exercise Science
University of Georgia
300 River Road
Athens, Georgia 30602-6554

Philip S. Clifford, PhD
Professor
Sports Performance and Technology Laboratory
Departments of Anesthesiology and Physiology
The Medical College of Wisconsin
8701 Watertown Plank Road;
Research Physiologist
Department of Anesthesia Research
Veterans Affairs Medical Center
5000 West National Avenue
Milwaukee, Wisconsin 53295

Bernd Coen
Exercise Physiologist
Institute of Sports and Preventive Medicine
University of Saarland
Im Stadtwald
Saarbrücken 66041;
Olympic Training Centre
Saarbrücken 66123
Germany

Victor A. Convertino, PhD
U.S. Army Institute of Surgical Research
3400 Rawley E. Chambers Avenue
Building 3611
Fort Sam Houston, Texas 78234-6315

Diane M. Cullen, PhD
Associate Professor
Department of Medicine
Creighton University
Osteoporosis Research Center
601 North 30th Street, Suite 4820
Omaha, Nebraska 68131

Lynn A. Darby, PhD
Assistant Professor
Kinesiology Division, School of Human Movement, Sport and Leisure Studies
Bowling Green University
215 Eppler South
Bowling Green, Ohio 43403

Charles J. Dillman, PhD
Group Vice President for Research and Development
Orthofix International Inc.
10115 Kincey Avenue
Suite 250, Storrs Building
Huntersville, North Carolina 28078

Brendon Downey
Performance Lab
Berkenhead, Auckland
New Zealand

Serge P. von Duvillard, PhD
Professor, Department of Physical Education and Exercise Science
Director, Human Performance Laboratory
University of North Dakota
P.O. Box 8235
Grand Forks, North Dakota 58202-8235

Rafael F. Escamilla, PhD, CSCS
Research Assistant Professor
Department of Surgery
Duke University Medical Center
P. O. Box 3435
Durham, North Carolina 27710

William J. Evans, PhD
Director
Nutrition, Metabolism, and Exercise Laboratory
Veterans Affairs Medical Center
North Little Rock, Arkansas 72114

Mark O. Farber, MD
Department of Medicine
Indiana University
1481 West 10th Street
Veterans Administration Medical Center
Indianapolis, Indiana 46202

Glenn S. Fleisig, PhD
Adjunct Professor
Biomedical Engineering
University of Alabama at Birmingham School of Medicine
1075 13th Street South;
Smith & Nephew Chair of Research
Department of Research
American Sports Medicine Institute
1313 13th Street South
Birmingham, Alabama 35205

Lawrence J. Folinsbee, PhD
Adjunct Associate Professor
Department of Medicine
University of North Carolina
Chapel Hill;
Chief, Environmental Media Assessment Branch
National Center for Environmental Assessment
U.S. Environmental Protection Agency
Mail Drop 52
Research Triangle Park, North Carolina 27711

Carl Foster, PhD
Associate Professor
Department of Exercise and Sport Science
University of Wisconsin—LaCrosse
132 Mitchell Hall
1725 State Street
LaCrosse, Wisconsin 54601

Barry A. Franklin, PhD
Professor of Physiology
School of Medicine
Wayne State University
Scott Hall
540 East Canfield
Detroit 48201;
Director, Cardiac Rehabilitation and Exercise Laboratories
Cardiology Department
William Beaumont Hospital
3601 West 13 Mile Road
Royal Oak 48073;
Beaumont Rehabilitation and Health Center
Cardiac Rehabilitation Department
746 Purdy Street
Birmingham, Michigan 48009

John Garhammer, PhD
Professor
Department of Kinesiology & Physical Education
California State University, Long Beach
1250 Bellflower Blvd.
Long Beach, California 90840

Steven E. Gaskill, MS
School of Kinesiology and Leisure Studies
University of Minnesota
Minneapolis, Minnesota 55455

Gilbert W. Gleim, PhD, FACSM, FACN
Director, Research Institute
Mission St. Joseph's Hospital
509 Biltmore Avenue
Asheville, North Carolina 28801;
Adjunct Associate Professor
Department of Physiology
New York Medical College
Valhalla, New York 10458

Lincoln A. Gotshalk, MS
College of Osteopathic Medicine
Ohio University
Grosvenor Hall 056
Athens, Ohio 45701

Robert J. Gregor, PhD
Professor and Head
Department of Health and Performance Sciences;
Director, Center for Human Movement Studies
The Georgia Institute of Technology
Atlanta, Georgia 30332-0110

Anthony C. Hackney, PhD
Professor
Department of Physical Education, Exercise, and Sport Science
University of North Carolina
CB #8700
Chapel Hill, North Carolina 27599

Fredrick C. Hagerman, PhD
Professor of Physiology
Department of Biomedical Sciences
Ohio University
Irvine Hall 001
Athens, Ohio 45701

Gene R. Hagerman, PhD
Sportsmedicine Consultant
Topper Sportsmedicine
P. O. Box 1374
Edwards, Colorado 81632

Mark Hargreaves, PhD
Professor of Exercise Physiology
School of Health Sciences
Deakin University
Burwood, Victoria 3125
Australia

Robert A. Hintermeister, PhD
P. O. Box 504
2030 Wildridge Road, #3
Avon, Colorado 81620

Robert S. Hikida
Department of Biomedical Sciences
College of Osteopathic Medicine
Ohio University
Irvine Hall
Athens, Ohio 45701

Jay R. Hoffman, PhD
Knoll Pharmaceutical Company
Mt. Olive, New Jersey 07828

Martin D. Hoffman, MD
Professor
Sports Performance and Technology Laboratory
Department of Physical Medicine and Rehabilitation
Medical College of Wisconsin
9200 West Wisconsin Avenue
Milwaukee, Wisconsin 53226

A. Peter de Hollander, PhD
Professor in Exercise Physiology
Department of Kinesiology
Faculty of Human Movement Sciences
Vrije Universiteit
9, van der Boechorststraat
Amsterdam 1081 BT
The Netherlands

Sue L. Hooper, PhD
Department of Human Movement Studies
The University of Queensland
Brisbane, Queensland 4072
Australia

Craig A. Horswill, PhD
Senior Research Scientist
Department of Research and Development
Gatorade Exercise Physiology Laboratory
The Quaker Oats Company
617 West Main Street
Barrington, Illinois 60010

Urszula T. Iwaniec
Creighton University
Osteoporosis Research Center
601 North 30th Street
Omaha, Nebraska 68131

Kevin Allen Jacobs, MA
Sport and Exercise Science Section
School of Physical Activity and Educational Services
The Ohio State University
344 Larkins Hall, 337 West 17th Avenue
Columbus, Ohio 43210

Eugene G. Jameson, MA
Coordinator of Clinical Biomechanics
American Sports Medicine Institute
1313 13th Street South
Birmingham, Alabama 35205

Li Li Ji, PhD
Professor
Departments of Kinesiology and Nutritional Science
University of Wisconsin—Madison
2000 Observatory Drive
Madison, Wisconsin 53706

Jay T. Kearney, PhD
Senior Sports Physiologist
Sport Science and Technology Division
United States Olympic Committee
One Olympic Plaza
Colorado Springs, Colorado 80909

Dean L. Kellogg, Jr., MD, PhD
Assistant Professor
Division of Geriatrics and Gerontology
Department of Medicine
University of Texas Health Science Center at San Antonio
7703 Floyd Curl Drive;
Staff Physician
Department of Geriatrics and Extended Care
Audie L. Murphy Memorial Veterans Administration Hospital
7400 Merton Minter Boulevard
San Antonio, Texas 78284

Wilfried Kindermann, MD, PhD
Professor
Chief, Faculty of Medicine
Institute of Sports and Preventive Medicine
University of Saarland
Im Stadtwald
Saarbrücken 66041
Germany

Donald T. Kirkendall, PhD
Clinical Assistant Professor
Department of Orthopaedics
University of North Carolina
252 Burnett-Womack Building
Chapel Hill, North Carolina 27549-7055

Kenton B. Kirksey
Department of Exercise Science
Appalachian State University
530 River Street
Boone, North Carolina 28608

Pieter Kollen
Indiana/World Skating Academy
Indianapolis, Indiana 46202

Jos J. deKoning, PhD
Assistant Professor
Faculty of Human Movement Sciences
Vrije Universiteit
9, van der Boechorstraat
Amsterdam 1081 BT
The Netherlands

William J. Kraemer, PhD
The John and Janice Fisher Chair in Exercise Physiology
Professor, Physical Education, Biology, and Health Science
Director, The Human Performance Laboratory
Director, Graduate and Undergraduate Programs in Exercise Science
Ball State University
Muncie, Indiana 47306

Jeffrey E. Lander, PhD, FACSM
Assistant Professor
Department of Sport Health Science
Life University
1269 Barclay Circle
Marietta, Georgia 30060

John B. Leiper, PhD
Research Fellow
Department of Biomedical Sciences
University of Aberdeen
Foresterhill, Aberdeen AB25 2ZD
Scotland

Peter W. R. Lemon, PhD
Professor and Weider Chair, Exercise Nutrition
Department of Health Sciences
University of Western Ontario
2212 3M Centre
London, Ontario N6A 3K7
Canada

Benjamin Levine, PhD
Presbyterian Hospital of Dallas
Institute for Exercise and Environmental Medicine
7332 Greenville Avenue
Dallas, Texas 75231

Donald C. McKenzie
Allan McGaivin Sports Medicine Center
University of British Columbia
Vancouver, British Columbia
Canada

Laurel T. Mackinnon, PhD
Associate Professor
Department of Human Movement Studies
The University of Queensland
Brisbane, Queensland 4072
Australia

Robert G. McMurray, PhD
Professor
Department of Physical Education, Exercise and Sport Science
University of North Carolina
CB #8700
Chapel Hill, North Carolina 27599-8700

Robert M. Malina, PhD, FACSM
Institute for the Study of Youth Sports
Michigan State University
213 IM Sports Circle
East Lansing, Michigan 48824-1049

Edward T. Mannix, PhD
Associate Scientist
Department of Medicine
Indiana University;
Roudebush VA Medical Center
Pulmonary/Critical Care Section
1481 West 10th Street;
Associate Director of Research
The National Institute for Fitness and Sport
250 University Boulevard
Indianapolis, Indiana 46202

Carl M. Maresh, PhD
Professor and Department Head
Department of Kinesiology
University of Connecticut
2095 Hillside Road
Storrs, Connecticut 06269-1110

Philip E. Martin, PhD
Professor
Department of Exercise Science and Physical Education
Arizona State University
Tempe, Arizona 85287-0404

Ronald J. Maughan, PhD
Department of Biomedical Sciences
University of Aberdeen
Foresterhill, Aberdeen AB25 2ZD
Scotland

Mary P. Miles
Department of Health and Human Development
Montana State University
Bozeman, Montana 59717

David L. Montgomery
Professor
Department of Physical Education
McGill University
475 Pine Avenue West
Montreal, Quebec H2W 1S4
Canada

Stephen D. Murphy, MSc
Department of Kinesiology
Faculty of Applied Health Sciences
University of Waterloo
200 University Avenue West
Waterloo, Ontario N2L 3G1
Canada

David C. Nieman, DrPH, FACSM
Department of Health, Leisure, and Exercise Science
Appalachian State University
530 River Street
Boone, North Carolina 28608

Michiel A. van Nieuwenhoven, PhD
Departments of Human Biology and Gastroenterology
Maastricht University
50, Universiteitssingel
Maastricht 6229 ER
The Netherlands

David Richard Paul
Sport and Exercise Science Section
School of Physical Activity and Educational Services
The Ohio State University
344 Larkins Hall, 337 West 17th Avenue
Columbus, Ohio 43210

David J. Pearsall, PhD
Assistant Professor
Department of Physical Education
McGill University
475 Pine Avenue West
Montreal, Quebec H2W 1S4
Canada

Pablo Pérgola, MD, PhD
Assistant Professor
Division of Geriatrics and Gerontology
Department of Medicine
University of Texas Health Science Center at San Antonio
7703 Floyd Curl Drive
San Antonio, Texas 78284

Thomas Reilly, PhD, DSc
Director
Research Institute for Sport and Exercise Sciences
Liverpool John Moores University
Trueman Building, Webster Street
Liverpool L3 2ET
England

David G. Rowbottom, PhD
Lecturer
School of Human Movement Studies
Queensland University of Technology
Victoria Park Road
Kelvin Grove, Queensland 4059
Australia

Thomas W. Rowland, MD
Professor
Department of Pediatrics
Tufts University School of Medicine
Boston;
Director of Pediatric Cardiology
Department of Pediatrics
Baystate Medical Center
Springfield, Massachusetts 01199

David S. Rowlands, BSc
School of Physical Education
University of Otago
P.O. Box 56
Dunedin 9015
New Zealand

Kenneth W. Rundell, PhD
Sport Physiologist
Sports Science and Technology Division
United States Olympic Committee
421 Old Military Road
Lake Placid, New York 12946

David J. Sanderson, PhD
Associate Professor
School of Human Kinetics
University of British Columbia
210-6081 University Boulevard
Vancouver, British Columbia V6T 1Z1
Canada

Michael N. Sawka, PhD
U.S. Army Research Institute of Environmental Medicine
Thermal & Mountain Medicine Division
Natick, Massachusetts 01760-5007

Rick L. Sharp, PhD
Associate Professor
Department of Health and Human Performance
Iowa State University
250 Barbara E. Forker Building
Ames, Iowa 50011

W. Michael Sherman, PhD
Sport and Exercise Science Section
School of Physical Activity and Educational Services
The Ohio State University
344 Larkins Hall, 337 West 17th Street
Columbus, Ohio 43210

Susan M. Shirreffs, PhD
Lecturer
Department of Biomedical Sciences
University of Aberdeen
Foresterhill, Aberdeen AB25 2ZD
Scotland

Kathy J. Simpson, PhD
Associate Professor
Department of Exercise Science
University of Georgia
300 River Road
Athens, Georgia 30602-6554

Lucille L. Smith, PhD
Department of Health, Leisure, and Exercise Science
Appalachian State University
530 River Street
Boone, North Carolina 28608

Ann C. Snyder, PhD
Professor
Department of Human Kinetics
University of Wisconsin—Milwaukee
2400 East Hartford Avenue
Milwaukee, Wisconsin 53201

Robert S. Staron, PhD
Associate Professor
Department of Biomedical Sciences
College of Osteopathic Medicine
Ohio University
Irvine Hall
Athens, Ohio 45701

Michael H. Stone, PhD
Professor
Department of Sports Science
Edinburgh University
Edinburgh, Scotland

Huub M. Toussaint
Associate Professor
Department of Kinesiology
Faculty of Human Movement Sciences
Vrije Universiteit
9, van der Boechorststraat
Amsterdam 1081 BT
The Netherlands

René A. Turcotte, PhD
Associate Professor
Department of Physical Education
McGill University
475 Pine Avenue West
Montreal, Quebec H2W 1S4
Canada

Axel Urhausen, MD, PhD
Professor and Substitute of Medical Director
Institute of Sports and Preventive Medicine
University of Saarland
Im Stadtwald
Saarbrücken
Germany

Atko Viru, DSc
Professor Emeritus
Institute of Exercise Biology
University of Tartu
18, Ülikooli Street
Tartu 51014
Estonia

Mehis Viru
Senior Researcher
Institute of Exercise Biology
University of Tartu
18, Ülikooli Street
Tartu 51014
Estonia

Jeff S. Volek, PhD, RD
Assistant Professor
The Human Performance Laboratory
Ball State University
Muncie, Indiana 47306

Andrei R. Vorontsov, PhD
Associate Professor
Department of Sport Swimming
Russian State Academy of Physical Education
Moscow, Russia;
British Coach/Sport Science Specialist
National Performance Center Bath
Bath University
Claverton Down
Bath, Somerset BA2 7AY
England

He Wang, MS
Department of Exercise Science
University of Georgia
300 River Road
Athens, Georgia 30602

Jim Waterhouse
Senior Lecturer
Research Institute for Sport and Exercise Sciences
Liverpool John Moores University
Trueman Building, Webster Street
Liverpool L3 2ET
England

Randall L. Wilber, PhD
Sports Physiologist
Sport Science and Technology Division
United States Olympic Committee
One Olympic Plaza
Colorado Springs, Colorado 80909

Kevin E. Wilk, PT
Rehabilitation Consultant
Tampa Bay Devil Rays Baseball Club
St. Petersburg, Florida 33705;
Adjunct Assistant Professor
Physical Therapy Programs
Marquette University
Milwaukee, Wisconsin 33201;
National Director of Research and Clinical Education
Healthsouth Rehabilitation Corporation
1201 11th Avenue South, Suite 100
Birmingham, Alabama 35205

Melvin H. Williams, PhD, FACSM
Department of Exercise Science, Physical Education, and Recreation
Old Dominion University
Norfolk, Virginia 23529-0196

Andrew J. Young, PhD
Research Physiologist
U.S. Army Research Institute of Environmental Medicine
Thermal & Mountain Medicine Division
Natick, Massachusetts 01760

Preface

Exercise and Sport Science is the basic science component of a three-volume series on sports medicine. Although the subject matter is complex and the audience is diverse, including exercise physiologists, biomechanists, and sports medicine physicians, we hope that the text will serve as the definitive reference for all serious students of sport medicine.

Perhaps the simplest component of sports medicine is the study of "performance" as applied to exercise of athletic participation. All of the basic science of sports medicine builds from that component. For exercise physiologists, the study of sports medicine has led to investigations of the responses to exercise and the adaptations to training of those individuals with acute or chronic diseases, normal or untrained persons, and competitive athletes. Biomechanists have defined the mechanics of both the specific skills required in each sport and the injuries that can occur in that sport, and they have also described cellular and tissue biomechanics.

Our goal in this book was to cover the most basic aspect of exercise—energy production—and then cover some general topics of the physiology of exercise. Because exercise is a whole-body commitment, the entire body must respond and adapt. Therefore, we recruited authorities to address the various systems of the body. From there, we examined the primary specialty topics of exercise physiology; the unique features of exercise in children and the elderly; and the effects of the environment, overtraining, chronobiology, and microgravity. Next, we felt that it was imperative that the biomechanics of sporting activities be addressed because, in order to understand how injuries happen, we need to know how sports skills are supposed to occur. Finally, each sport has its own unique characteristics. Our authors for this final section are all individuals actively investigating their chosen sport. They report on the current standards of practice with respect to the physical requirements of their sport and subsequent training.

We hope that this volume will be useful to not only the basic scientists involved in the study of sports medicine but to all other experts in the discipline, because the understanding of these topics will form the basis of future developments in sports medicine. In future volumes, we will cover primary care and musculoskeletal aspects of sports medicine.

All of us involved in this project are indebted to the staff at Lippincott Williams & Wilkins: Darlene Cook and Fran Klass who helped us get this project underway and Danette Knopp, Tanya Lazar, Sonya Seigafuse, and Sally Scott, whose continued patience throughout this project must be commended. The guidance of Lottie Applewhite, author's editor, and the efforts of Marsha Dohrmann, medical illustrator, cannot be overstated. Without the help of these people, we still would be way over our heads and still struggling to complete our work.

William E. Garrett, Jr., MD
Donald T. Kirkendall, PhD

Exercise and Sport Science

PART I

Energy Metabolism

Exercise and Sport Science,
edited by William E. Garrett, Jr., and Donald T. Kirkendall.
Lippincott Williams & Wilkins, Philadelphia © 2000.

CHAPTER 1

Carbohydrate Metabolism and Exercise

Mark Hargreaves

Carbohydrate is the preferred fuel for contracting skeletal muscle during strenuous exercise, and depletion of endogenous carbohydrate reserves is often associated with impaired exercise performance. Since the endogenous carbohydrate stores are relatively limited, dietary carbohydrate intake is important for ensuring adequate carbohydrate availability before, during, and after exercise, and there has been great interest over the years in nutritional strategies that optimize carbohydrate delivery to contracting skeletal muscle. This chapter briefly summarizes aspects of carbohydrate metabolism at rest and during exercise.

CARBOHYDRATE RESERVES

Ingested carbohydrate enters the bloodstream primarily as glucose after digestion by gastrointestinal enzymes and transport across the luminal and basolateral membranes of the intestinal epithelium by the sodium-linked and facilitative (GLUT-2) glucose transporters, respectively (1). In animal tissues, carbohydrate is stored as glycogen, a branched polymer of glucose with a mixture of α-1,4 and 1,6 linkages between glucose units. The liver has the highest concentration of glycogen (approximately 250 mmol·kg^{-1}), but because of the size of the skeletal muscle mass (40% of body mass) this tissue contains the largest glycogen reserve (Table 1–1).

The magnitude of both the liver and muscle glycogen reserves is very much influenced by the levels of exercise and dietary carbohydrate intake. Following an overnight fast or prolonged severe exercise, the liver can be completely emptied of glycogen, whereas the liver glycogen can be as high as 500 mmol·kg^{-1} following carbohydrate refeeding. Similarly, muscle glycogen levels may range from close to zero up to 200 mmol·kg^{-1}, depending on the interactions among exercise intensity and duration, training status, and dietary carbohydrate intake.

TABLE 1–1. *Sites and amount of carbohydrate (CHO) stored in a rested, moderately active, 70-kg man with 40% of body mass as skeletal muscle*

Tissue	Weight or volume (kg or l*)	Concentration (mmol · kg^{-1} or l^{-1}*)	CHO store (g)
Liver	1.8	250 (0–500)	80 (0–160)
ECF	10*	5*	9
Muscle	28	100 (0–200)	500 (300–700)

Numbers in parentheses represent potential range of values with extremes of exercise, training, and diet. ECF, extracellular fluid; *, concentrations are expressed as liters rather than as kilograms.

CARBOHYDRATE METABOLISM UNDER RESTING CONDITIONS

Net muscle glycogen utilization under resting conditions is negligible, and the muscle glycogen store is preserved for use during times of increased skeletal muscle activity. Although muscle glycogenolysis cannot contribute directly to maintenance of blood glucose, the release of lactate from active and inactive skeletal muscle during and after exercise (2,3) can provide a gluconeogenic precursor for the liver. In contrast, the principal role of the liver glycogen store is to maintain blood glucose levels between meals, thereby ensuring adequate substrate supply to those organs dependent on glucose, such as brain, central nervous system (CNS), blood cells, and kidneys. These tissues account for about 75% of glucose utilization under resting conditions, whereas skeletal muscle accounts for about 15% to 20% (Fig. 1–1). Most (about 75%) of the liver glucose output at rest is due to glycogenolysis, but there is also a contribution from gluconeogenesis (4).

M. Hargreaves: School of Health Sciences, Deakin University, Burwood, Australia.

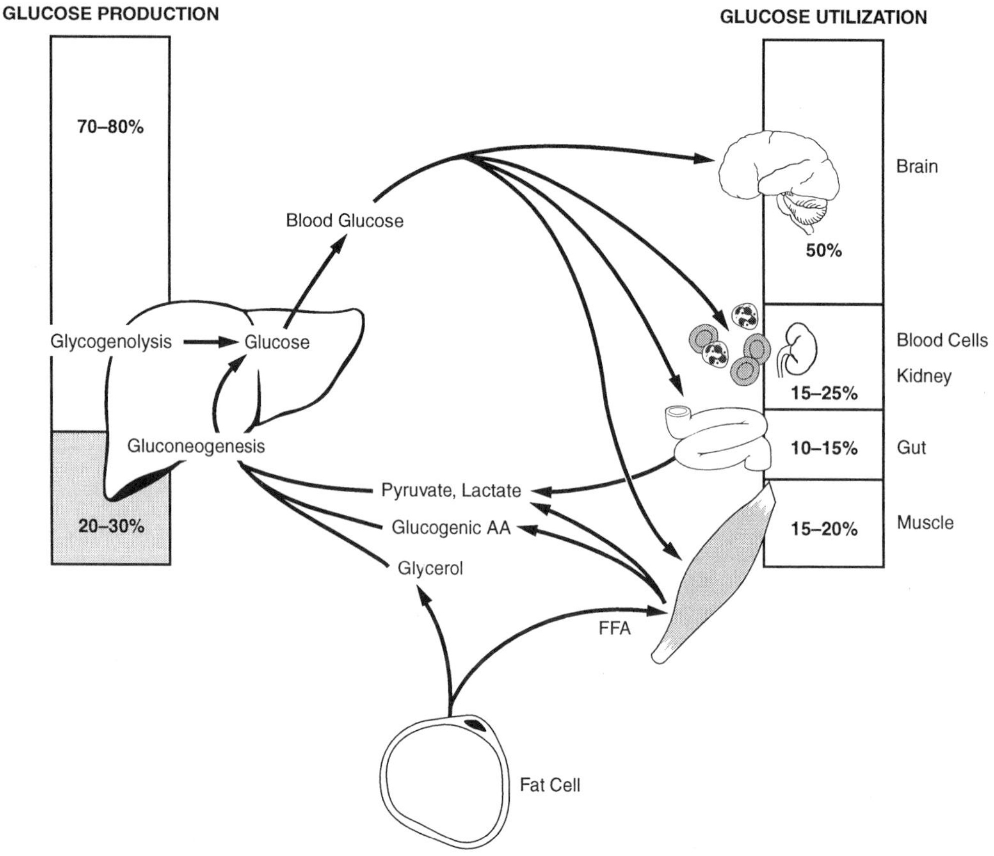

FIG. 1–1. Whole-body glucose metabolism in the basal, overnight-fasted state in normal human. (From ref. 4, with permission.)

CARBOHYDRATE METABOLISM DURING EXERCISE

During prolonged strenuous exercise, muscle glycogen and blood-borne glucose, derived from liver glycogenolysis and gluconeogenesis [and the gastrointestinal (GI) tract when glucose is ingested], are important substrates for contracting skeletal muscle. Fatigue during such exercise is often associated with depletion of these carbohydrate reserves (5). Increased muscle glycogen availability prior to exercise and carbohydrate ingestion during exercise have been shown to enhance endurance exercise performance (5,6), and it is generally believed that this is due to a maintenance of carbohydrate availability and oxidation during exercise.

Muscle Glycogenolysis

Muscle glycogen degradation during exercise is primarily dependent on exercise intensity and is most rapid during the early stages of exercise (7,8). As exercise at a given intensity continues, the rate of muscle glycogenolysis declines as a function of reduced glycogen levels and glycogen phosphorylase activity and of increased blood-borne substrate availability. The increase in glycogenolysis during exercise occurs due to activation of glycogen phosphorylase, which exists in two forms: a less active *b* form and the more active *a* form. Phosphorylase *b* to *a* transformation occurs in response to increased sarcoplasmic [Ca^{2+}] with muscle contractions and hormonal stimulation by adrenaline, mediated via the β-adrenergic receptor and the intracellular second messenger 3′,5′-cyclic adenosine monophosphate (cyclic AMP) (9,10). In addition, allosteric modulators such as AMP and inosine monophosphate (IMP), as well as the substrates inorganic phosphate (Pi) and glycogen itself, influence glycogen phosphorylase activity. This complex regulation of glycogen phosphorylase activity ensures that the rate of muscle glycogenolysis is closely coupled to the adenosine triphosphate (ATP) demand.

Increased muscle glycogen availability results in a greater rate of glycogenolysis during submaximal (11), but not maximal (12), exercise. Despite the increase in muscle glycogen utilization, increased preexercise muscle glycogen availability is associated with enhanced endurance exercise performance (6). Blood glucose availability appears to have little effect on net muscle glycogen degradation, at least during prolonged cycling exercise (5,13). In contrast, alterations in plasma free fatty acid (FFA) levels influence muscle glycogen metabolism. Inhibition of FFA mobilization by nicotinic acid lowers plasma [FFA] and increases muscle glycogen use, whereas an increase in plasma [FFA] has been shown to reduce net muscle glycogen utilization during exercise (14–16). This observation has led to interest in the potential ergogenic benefits of caffeine ingestion, which increases plasma FFA availability, reduces muscle glycogen use, and enhances endurance exercise performance (17).

Muscle Glucose Uptake

Exercise is a potent stimulus for skeletal muscle glucose uptake, with the increase during muscle contraction being greater than that elicited by maximal insulin stimulation (18). The magnitude of the exercise-induced increase in muscle glucose uptake is related to both the intensity and duration of exercise. At higher exercise intensities, an increase in intramuscular free glucose suggests a decrease in glucose utilization as muscle glycogen degradation is enhanced (19). As exercise duration increases at a given exercise intensity, there is an increase in muscle glucose uptake. This is the result of a progressive increase in sarcolemmal glucose transport (Fig. 1–2) (20) and an increase in glucose metabolism due to a lower [glucose-6-phosphate] as the rate of muscle glycogenolysis decreases with continued exercise (21).

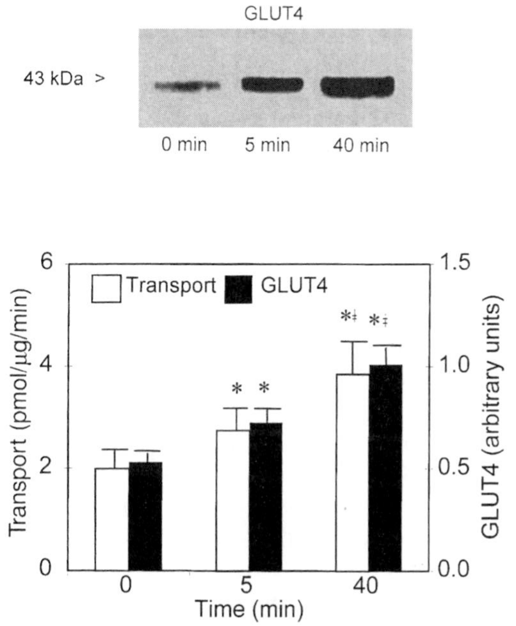

FIG. 1–2. A representative immunoblot of GLUT-4 (*top*) and the mean GLUT-4 protein content and glucose transport (*bottom*) in sarcolemmal vesicles produced from human skeletal muscle samples obtained before and after 5 and 40 minutes of exercise. Values are means + standard error of the mean from nine subjects. (From ref. 20, with permission.)

The delivery of glucose and insulin to contracting skeletal muscle is increased during exercise as a consequence of the large increase in muscle blood flow, but it cannot fully explain the exercise-induced increase in muscle glucose uptake. Thus, local factors within the muscle play the major role (22). These include increased sarcolemmal transport of glucose and activation of the glycolytic and oxidative enzymes responsible for glucose metabolism. Sarcolemmal glucose transport occurs by facilitated diffusion, with the GLUT-4 isoform being responsible for contraction and insulin-stimulated glucose transport. GLUT-4 is one member of a family of facilitative glucose transporters (23) (Table 1–2).

GLUT-4 translocation from an intracellular storage site to the plasma membrane is the major mechanism responsible for the increase in sarcolemmal glucose transport during exercise. This has been demonstrated in both rat (24,25) and human (Fig. 1–2) (20,26) skeletal muscle. The intracellular distribution of GLUT-1, the isoform responsible for basal glucose transport, is unaltered by exercise (24,26). The increase in muscle glucose uptake and GLUT-4 translocation can occur in the absence of insulin (27,28). This is consistent with observations that contractions stimulate muscle glucose uptake via a mechanism that is different from insulin stimulation (25,29), and that the effects of contractions and insulin are additive. Despite these observations, the prevailing plasma insulin level has an important influence on skeletal muscle glucose uptake during exercise (30).

Substrate availability also influences muscle glucose uptake during exercise. In general, there is an inverse relationship between muscle glycogen availability and muscle glucose transport and metabolism (13). Increased blood [glucose] results in enhanced glucose uptake and disposal during exercise (31,32), whereas a decline in arterial blood [glucose] may limit muscle glucose uptake during the latter stages of prolonged exercise (2,33). There are conflicting reports in the literature on the effect of elevated plasma [FFA] on muscle glucose uptake—the so-called glucose fatty acid cycle (13). Despite this, it is tempting to speculate that the increase in plasma FFA may limit muscle glucose uptake at a

TABLE 1–2. *The facilitative glucose transporters*

Isoform	Function
GLUT-1	Basal glucose transport in most tissues
GLUT-2	Glucose transport in liver, kidney, small intestine, and β cells of pancreas
GLUT-3	Glucose transport into central nervous system
GLUT-4	Insulin-stimulated transport into adipose tissue and cardiac and skeletal muscle; contraction-stimulated glucose transport

time when muscle glycogen and arterial blood glucose levels are low.

Liver Glucose Output

Accompanying the increase in muscle glucose uptake is an increase in liver glucose output, so that blood glucose levels stay at or slightly above resting levels. During intense exercise, a greatly increased liver glucose output results in hyperglycemia; in contrast, during prolonged moderate-intensity exercise, peripheral glucose uptake may exceed liver glucose output, resulting in hypoglycemia. The magnitude of increase in liver glucose output during exercise is determined by both exercise intensity and duration. The majority of liver glucose output is derived from liver glycogenolysis; the decline in liver glycogen availability during prolonged, strenuous exercise results in a reduced liver glucose output since gluconeogenesis, although increasing due to increased liver gluconeogenic enzyme activity and precursor availability, is unable to compensate fully for the decrease in liver glycogenolysis.

The regulation of liver glucose output during exercise is complex and far from being completely understood. During low-intensity exercise it is thought that alterations in the plasma levels of the pancreatic hormones insulin and glucagon and their molar ratio are crucial for the increase in liver glucose output. Even in the absence of large changes in the systemic plasma levels of these hormones, it is possible that small fluctuations in the portal vein exert a major effect on liver metabolism. Glucagon is likely to be most important during prolonged exercise and is known to stimulate liver gluconeogenesis. At higher exercise intensities, increased plasma adrenaline and sympathetic activity play a greater role but cannot fully account for the increased liver glucose output that is observed (34,35). For many years it was thought that liver glucose output responded to a fall in blood glucose during the early stages of exercise (classic feedback regulation). It is now apparent that stimulation of the liver may occur in parallel with activation of the contracting skeletal muscles, the cardiorespiratory responses, and the neuroendocrine centers that modulate many metabolic processes, such that there is "feed-forward" stimulation of the liver, particularly at higher exercise intensities. This does not diminish the importance of feedback regulation. Indeed, increased blood glucose availability can inhibit (32) or completely abolish (36) the exercise-induced rise in liver glucose output. In addition, afferent feedback from contracting skeletal muscle may also influence liver glucose output during exercise (37). It has also been suggested that a "factor" released from contracting skeletal muscle may act to stimulate liver glucose output in proportion to the intensity of muscle contraction. Finally, there is evidence that the liver glycogen level may influence liver glucose output in much the same way that the preexercise muscle glycogen level determines its subsequent rate of utilization. The complex and redundant nature of the regulation of liver glucose output only serves to emphasize the crucial role of the liver in glucose homeostasis during exercise. Nevertheless, during prolonged strenuous exercise liver glucose output can fall behind peripheral glucose uptake, resulting in the development of a relative hypoglycemia, which may contribute to fatigue. Under such exercise conditions, ingestion of carbohydrate has been shown to be an effective strategy to enhance endurance performance by maintaining blood glucose availability and a high rate of carbohydrate oxidation at a time when muscle glycogen stores are low (5).

POSTEXERCISE CARBOHYDRATE METABOLISM

Following exercise that results in significant depletion of the endogenous carbohydrate reserves, restoration of muscle glycogen is a priority. In the absence of carbohydrate ingestion, there is minimal resynthesis of glycogen, and maximal rates are achieved with ingestion of relatively large amounts of carbohydrate soon after the cessation of exercise. The protein primer glycogenin forms a backbone upon which glucose residues are added to initiate synthesis of proglycogen; this is then converted to macroglycogen by glycogen synthase (38). The existence of these two forms of glycogen has been known for many years and their relative abundance was recently quantified in human skeletal muscle (39). The two forms of glycogen are synthesized at different rates following exercise and are both sensitive to dietary carbohydrate; the large increase in muscle glycogen levels observed following ingestion of a high carbohydrate diet results from a greater synthesis of macroglycogen (40).

The rate-limiting steps in the resynthesis of muscle glycogen are transport of glucose across the sarcolemma, mediated by GLUT-4, and the activity of glycogen synthase. Postexercise muscle glycogen storage is significantly correlated with skeletal muscle GLUT-4 (41,42) and glycogen synthase activity (42). Overexpression of GLUT-4 (43) and glycogen synthase (44) in skeletal muscles of transgenic mice results in enhanced glycogen storage. The initial muscle glycogen resynthesis in the early postexercise period is insulin independent and the result of a higher sarcolemmal GLUT-4 content and activation of glycogen synthase by glycogen depletion (45,46). The extent of activation is directly related to the magnitude of glycogen depletion, which is thought to be linked to enhanced protein phosphatase-1 activity and greater dephosphorylation of glycogen synthase (47). Higher plasma insulin levels following carbohydrate ingestion result in insulin-stimulated GLUT-4 translocation and further activation of glycogen synthase. The plasma glucose and insulin responses following carbohydrate ingestion can account for a large proportion of the variance in postexercise muscle glycogen storage (48) and are determined by the type and amount of carbohydrate ingested.

In the early postexercise period (<6 hours), ingestion of glucose or sucrose results in higher rates of muscle glycogen storage than from fructose ingestion (49), which is consistent with the observation that ingestion of carbohydrate foods with a high glycemic response promotes a greater muscle glycogen storage than low glycemic, carbohydrate foods (50). Furthermore, addition of protein to a carbohydrate supplement, thereby enhancing the plasma insulin response, increases postexercise muscle glycogen storage (51). Ingestion of carbohydrate at a rate of 0.7 to 1 $g \cdot kg^{-1} \cdot 2\ h^{-1}$ results in rates of muscle glycogen synthesis of 5 to 8 $mmol \cdot kg^{-1} \cdot h^{-1}$ (49,52), which can be increased to as high as 10 $mmol \cdot kg^{-1} \cdot h^{-1}$ over a 4-hour period by ingesting carbohydrate at 1.6 $g \cdot kg^{-1} \cdot h^{-1}$ (48). There may not be much advantage in consuming more than 600 g of carbohydrate over a 24-hour period, and in our studies increasing 24-hour carbohydrate intake from 520 g (7 $g \cdot kg^{-1}$) to 870 g (11.8 $g \cdot kg^{-1}$) did not result in additional muscle glycogen storage (53).

Another aspect of postexercise carbohydrate metabolism worthy of mention is the relatively long-lasting increase in whole-body insulin sensitivity that occurs following glycogen-depleting exercise (54). This is predominantly caused by local factors within the active muscle (55), and glycogen depletion is a prime candidate. Indeed, in rat skeletal muscle the reversal of the exercise-induced increase in insulin sensitivity is closely correlated with the restoration of muscle glycogen stores. It has been speculated that glycogen depletion causes liberation of GLUT-4 vesicles, which are then available for translocation to the sarcolemma in response to insulin stimulation, and activation of glycogen synthase (47). In addition, increased hexokinase activity (56) may contribute to enhanced rates of insulin-stimulated glucose disposal. Regardless of the underlying mechanisms, the increase in insulin sensitivity in skeletal muscle is likely to explain the beneficial effects of acute and chronic exercise on whole-body insulin action in insulin-resistant states (57).

CONCLUSION

Muscle glycogen and blood glucose, derived from liver glycogenolysis and gluconeogenesis, are major substrates for contracting skeletal muscle during strenuous exercise, and fatigue is often associated with depletion of these carbohydrate reserves. The rates of muscle glycogen utilization, muscle glucose uptake, and liver glucose output are determined primarily by exercise intensity and duration, but they can be modified by the preceding diet and training status. Important regulatory mechanisms include local control by intramuscular levels of calcium and metabolic intermediates, alterations in substrate availability, and neural and hormonal regulation. In the postexercise period, restoration of muscle glycogen stores is a priority and is dependent on the ingestion of carbohydrate. Alterations in skeletal muscle carbohydrate metabolism following exercise contribute to the enhanced insulin action following exercise and are likely to account for the beneficial effects of acute and chronic exercise in insulin-resistant states.

REFERENCES

1. Lenzte MJ. Molecular and cellular aspects of hydrolysis and absorption. *Am J Clin Nutr* 1995;61:946S–951S.
2. Ahlborg G, Felig P. Lactate and glucose exchange across the forearm, legs, and splanchnic bed during and after prolonged leg exercise. *J Clin Invest* 1982;69:45–54.
3. Ahlborg G, Felig P, Wahren J. Splanchnic and peripheral glucose and lactate metabolism during and after prolonged arm exercise. *J Clin Invest* 1986;77:690–699.
4. Björkman O, Wahren J. Glucose homeostasis during and after exercise. In: Horton ES, Terjung RL, eds. *Exercise, nutrition, and energy metabolism.* New York: Macmillan, 1988:101.
5. Coyle EF, Coggan AR, Hemmert MK, Ivy JL. Muscle glycogen utilization during prolonged strenuous exercise when fed carbohydrate. *J Appl Physiol* 1986;61:165–172.
6. Hawley JA, Schabort EJ, Noakes TD, Dennis SC. Carbohydrate-loading and exercise performance: an update. *Sports Med* 1997;24:73–81.
7. Gollnick PD, Piehl K, Saltin B. Selective glycogen depletion pattern in human muscle fibres after exercise of varying intensity and at varying pedalling rates. *J Physiol* 1974;241:45–57.
8. Vøllestad NK, Blom PCS. Effect of varying exercise intensity on glycogen depletion in human muscle fibres. *Acta Physiol Scand* 1985;125:395–405.
9. Johnson LN. Glycogen phosphorylase: control by phosphorylation and allosteric effectors. *FASEB J* 1992;6:2274–2282.
10. Richter E, Ruderman NB, Gavras H, Belur ER, Galbo H. Muscle glycogenolysis during exercise: dual control by epinephrine and contractions. *Am J Physiol* 1982;242:E25–E32.
11. Hargreaves M, McConell G, Proietto J. Influence of muscle glycogen on glycogenolysis and glucose uptake during exercise. *J Appl Physiol* 1995;78:288–292.
12. Hargreaves M, Finn JP, Withers RT, et al. Effect of muscle glycogen availability on maximal exercise performance. *Eur J Appl Physiol* 1997;75:188–192.
13. Hargreaves M. Interactions between muscle glycogen and blood glucose during exercise. *Exerc Sports Sci Rev* 1997;25:21–39.
14. Costill DL, Coyle E, Dalsky G, Evans W, Fink W, Hoopes D. Effects of elevated plasma FFA and insulin on muscle glycogen usage during exercise. *J Appl Physiol* 1977;43:695–699.
15. Dyck DJ, Peters SJ, Wendling PS, Chesley A, Hultman E, Spriet LL. Regulation of muscle glycogen phosphorylase activity during intense aerobic cycling with elevated FFA. *Am J Physiol* 1996;270:E116–E125.
16. Vukovich MD, Costill DL, Hickey MS, Trappe SW, Cole KJ, Fink WJ. Effect of fat emulsion infusion and fat feeding on muscle glycogen utilization during cycle exercise. *J Appl Physiol* 1993;75:1513–1518.
17. Spriet LL, MacLean DA, Dyck DJ, Hultman E, Cederblad G, Graham TE. Caffeine ingestion and muscle metabolism during prolonged exercise in humans. *Am J Physiol* 1992;262:E891–E898.
18. James DE, Kraegen EW, Chisholm DJ. Muscle glucose metabolism in exercising rats: comparison with insulin stimulation. *Am J Physiol* 1985;248:E575–E580.
19. Katz A, Broberg S, Sahlin K, Wahren J. Leg glucose uptake

during maximal dynamic exercise in humans. *Am J Physiol* 1986;251:E65–E70.
20. Kristiansen S, Hargreaves M, Richter EA. Progressive increase in glucose transport and GLUT-4 in human sarcolemmal vesicles during moderate exercise. *Am J Physiol* 1997;272:E385–E389.
21. Katz A, Sahlin K, Broberg S. Regulation of glucose utilization in human skeletal muscle during moderate dynamic exercise. *Am J Physiol* 1991;260:E411–E415.
22. Zinker BA, Lacy DB, Bracy DP, Wasserman DH. Role of glucose and insulin loads to the exercising limb in increasing glucose uptake and metabolism. *J Appl Physiol* 1993;74:2915–2921.
23. Mueckler M. Facilitative glucose transporters. *Eur J Biochem* 1994;219:713–725.
24. Goodyear LJ, Hirshman MF, Horton ES. Exercise-induced translocation of skeletal muscle glucose transporters. *Am J Physiol* 1991;261:E795–E799.
25. Lund S, Holman GD, Schmitz O, Pedersen O. Contraction stimulates translocation of the glucose transporter GLUT4 in skeletal muscle through a mechanism distinct from that of insulin. *Proc Nat Acad Sci USA* 1995;92:5817–5821.
26. Kristiansen S, Hargreaves M, Richter EA. Exercise-induced increase in glucose transport, GLUT-4 and VAMP-2 in plasma membrane from human muscle. *Am J Physiol* 1996;270:E197–E201.
27. Gao J, Ren J, Gulve E, Holloszy JO. Additive effect of contractions and insulin on GLUT-4 translocation into the sarcolemma. *J Appl Physiol* 1994;77:1597–1601.
28. Ploug T, Galbo H, Richter EA. Increased muscle glucose uptake during contractions: no need for insulin. *Am J Physiol* 1984; 247:E726–E731.
29. Lee AD, Hansen PA, Holloszy JO. Wortmannin inhibits insulin-stimulated but not contraction-stimulated glucose transport activity in skeletal muscle. *FEBS Lett* 1995;361:51–54.
30. Wasserman DH, Geer RJ, Rice DE, et al. Interaction of exercise and insulin action in humans. *Am J Physiol* 1991;260:E37–E45.
31. Ahlborg G, Felig P. Influence of glucose ingestion on fuel-hormone response during prolonged exercise. *J Appl Physiol* 1976;41:683–688.
32. McConell G, Fabris S, Proietto J, Hargreaves M. Effect of carbohydrate ingestion on glucose kinetics during exercise. *J Appl Physiol* 1994;77:1537–1577.
33. Ahlborg G, Felig P, Hagenfeldt L, Hendler R, Wahren J. Substrate turnover during prolonged exercise in man: splanchnic and leg metabolism of glucose, free fatty acids, and amino acids. *J Clin Invest* 1974;53:1080–1090.
34. Coggan AR, Raguso CA, Gastaldelli A, Williams BD, Wolfe RR. Regulation of glucose production during exercise at 80% VO_2 peak in untrained humans. *Am J Physiol* 1997;273:E348–E354.
35. Kjær M, Engfred K, Fernandes A, Secher NH, Galbo H. Regulation of hepatic glucose production during exercise in humans: role of sympatho-adrenergic activity. *Am J Physiol* 1993;265:E275–E283.
36. Howlett K, Angus D, Proietto J, Hargreaves M. Effect of increased blood glucose availability on glucose kinetics during exercise. *J Appl Physiol* 1998;84:1413–1417.
37. Kjær M, Secher NH, Bangsbo J, et al. Hormonal and metabolic responses to electrically induced cycling during epidural anesthesia in humans. *J Appl Physiol* 1996;80:2156–2162.
38. Alonso MD, Lomako J, Lomako WM, Whelan WJ. A new look at the biogenesis of glycogen. *FASEB J* 1995;9:1126–1135.
39. Adamo KB, Graham TE. Comparison of traditional measurements with macroglycogen and proglycogen analysis of muscle glycogen. *J Appl Physiol* 1998;84:908–913.
40. Adamo KB, Tarnopolsky MA, Graham TE. Dietary carbohydrate and postexercise synthesis of proglycogen and macroglycogen in human skeletal muscle. *Am J Physiol* 1998;275:E229–E234.
41. Hickner RC, Fisher JS, Hansen PA, et al. Muscle glycogen accumulation after endurance exercise in trained and untrained individuals. *J Appl Physiol* 1997;83:897–903.
42. McCoy M, Proietto J, Hargreaves M. Skeletal muscle GLUT-4 and postexercise muscle glycogen storage in humans. *J Appl Physiol* 1996;80:411–415.
43. Hansen PA, Gulve EA, Marshall BA, et al. Skeletal muscle glucose transport and metabolism are enhanced in transgenic mice overexpressing the GLUT-4 transporter. *J Biol Chem* 1995; 270:1679–1684.
44. Manchester J, Skurat AV, Roach P, Hauschka SD, Lawrence JC. Increased glycogen accumulation in transgenic mice overexpressing glycogen synthase in skeletal muscle. *Proc Natl Acad Sci USA* 1996;93:10707–10711.
45. Bak JF, Pedersen O. Exercise-enhanced activation of glycogen synthase in human skeletal muscle. *Am J Physiol* 1990;258:E957–E963.
46. Zachwieja JJ, Costill DL, Pascoe DD, Robergs RA, Fink WJ. Influence of muscle glycogen depletion on the rate of resynthesis. *Med Sci Sports Exerc* 1991;23:44–48.
47. Ivy JL, Kuo C-H. Regulation of GLUT4 protein and glycogen synthase during muscle glycogen synthesis after exercise. *Acta Physiol Scand* 1998;162:295–304.
48. Doyle JA, Sherman WM, Strauss RL. Effects of eccentric and concentric exercise on muscle glycogen replenishment. *J Appl Physiol* 1993;74:1848–1855.
49. Blom PCS, Høstmark AT, Vaage O, Kardel KR, Mæhlum S. Effect of different post-exercise sugar diets on the rate of muscle glycogen synthesis. *Med Sci Sports Exerc* 1987;19:491–496.
50. Burke LM, Collier GR, Hargreaves M. Muscle glycogen storage after prolonged exercise: effect of the glycemic index of carbohydrate feedings. *J Appl Physiol* 1993;75:1019–1023.
51. Zawadzki KM, Yaspelkis BB, Ivy JL. Carbohydrate-protein complex increases the rate of muscle glycogen storage after exercise. *J Appl Physiol* 1992;72:1854–1859.
52. Ivy JL, Lee MC, Brozinick JT, Reed MJ. Muscle glycogen storage after different amounts of carbohydrate ingestion. *J Appl Physiol* 1988;65:2018–2023.
53. Burke L, Collier GR, Beasley SK, et al. Effect of co-ingestion of fat and protein with carbohydrate feedings on muscle glycogen storage. *J Appl Physiol* 1995;78:2187–2192.
54. Bogardus C, Thuillez P, Ravussin E, Vasquez B, Narimiga M, Azhar S. Effect of muscle glycogen depletion on in vivo insulin action in man. *J Clin Invest* 1983;72:1605–1610.
55. Richter EA, Mikines KJ, Galbo H, Kiens B. Effect of exercise on insulin action in human skeletal muscle. *J Appl Physiol* 1989;66:876–885.
56. Koval JA, DeFronzo RA, O'Doherty RM, et al. Regulation of hexokinase II activity and expression in human muscle by moderate exercise. *Am J Physiol* 1998;274:E304–E308.
57. Perseghin G, Price TB, Petersen KF, et al. Increased glucose transport-phosphorylation and muscle glycogen synthesis after exercise training in insulin-resistant subjects. *N Engl J Med* 1996;335:1357–1362.

Exercise and Sport Science,
edited by William E. Garrett, Jr., and Donald T. Kirkendall.
Lippincott Williams & Wilkins, Philadelphia © 2000.

CHAPTER 2

Fat Metabolism

Kevin Allen Jacobs, David Richard Paul, and W. Michael Sherman

Fat is a nearly limitless energy source that plays an integral role in metabolism at rest and during exercise. This chapter reviews fat digestion, absorption, and metabolism. It begins by describing the digestion and absorption of exogenous fat, which, due to its insoluble nature, is a more prolonged and complex process than that of carbohydrate and protein. The endogenous fat stores are then characterized, followed by a description of the anabolic and catabolic pathways that constitute fat metabolism. The remote location of a majority of endogenous fat stores requires unique modes of transport in the bloodstream and across cell membranes. Finally, the interplay of these unique processes at rest and during exercise is discussed.

EXOGENOUS FAT DIGESTION AND ABSORPTION

Digestion

The digestive process in the stomach and small intestine takes place in an aqueous environment where dietary fats have a tendency to separate into an oily film. Therefore, the water-soluble lipolytic enzymes of the stomach and small intestine have access only to the surface of the large insoluble fat droplets, effectively reducing the surface area for enzymes to act upon. To counteract the insolubility of dietary fat, the body emulsifies the large lipid droplets with the combined actions of bile and a series of contractions in the stomach. Bile is an emulsifying agent that contains bile acids, cholesterol, lecithin, and bile pigments, and it is produced in the liver and stored in the gallbladder. Contractions in the stomach and the process of forcing fat through the pyloric sphincter produce strong shear forces. These combined processes sufficiently decrease the size of the lipid droplets, increasing the exposed surface area of the lipid droplets thousands of times to facilitate the actions of digestive enzymes.

The digestion of dietary triglyceride (TG) occurs in the stomach and upper small intestine. A class of lipolytic enzymes referred to as *preduodenal lipases* begin the limited digestion of fat in the stomach. Glands lying beneath the lining of the tongue secrete the enzyme lingual lipase, while gland cells lining the stomach secrete the enzyme gastric lipase. Most lipid hydrolysis, however, occurs in the small intestine by a group of enzymes secreted by the pancreas. These lipolytic enzymes are pancreatic lipase, colipase, cholesterol esterase, and phospholipase A_2. Pancreatic lipase is considered the major enzyme of dietary lipid digestion, because it acts specifically upon TG and is secreted in large volumes.

Absorption

The products of the digestive process, mainly combinations of monoglycerides, lysolecithin, cholesterol, fatty acids, and bile, form particles called *micelles.* The water-soluble micelles cross the unstirred water layer that covers the intestinal mucosal cells, and are absorbed at the brush border of these cells. The lipid contents of the micelles, in turn, diffuse into the intestinal mucosal cells by moving down a concentration gradient.

Upon absorption into the intestinal mucosal cells, the lipid products are reesterified into TG, phosphatidylcholine, and cholesterol esters. Long-chain fatty acids (LCFAs) (≥16 carbons) that are reesterified in the intestinal mucosal cells are subsequently combined with fat-soluble vitamins to form large fat particles. Due to the

K. A. Jacobs, D. R. Paul, and W. M. Sherman: Sport and Exercise Science Section, School of Physical Activity and Educational Services, The Ohio State University, Columbus, Ohio 43210.

low solubility of these particles, transport in the liquid environment of plasma becomes problematic. These lipid droplets can be transported, however, if they are packaged with a soluble coating of phospholipids, cholesterol, and protein. These molecules made up of an insoluble core (TG and cholesterol esters) and a soluble coating (phospholipids, cholesterol, and protein) are referred to as *lipoproteins.* The class of lipoproteins that carry the reesterified LCFAs and cholesterol esters from the gastrointestinal tract to the plasma are referred to as *chylomicrons.*

Once lipid particles have been packaged in the form of chylomicrons, they must first travel through the lymphatic circulation. Upon appearance in the bloodstream, chylomicrons undergo intravascular hydrolysis at different tissues throughout the body. This hydrolysis is catalyzed by the enzyme lipoprotein lipase (LPL), which exists on the endothelial surface of small blood vessels and capillaries within adipose and skeletal muscle. LPL acts extracellularly and releases free fatty acids (FFAs) and diglycerides that are absorbed by different tissues.

The entry of chylomicrons into the bloodstream from the lymphatic circulation can continue for approximately 14 hours after the consumption of a high-fat meal and prevents drastic changes in the plasma lipid content. Approximately 80% of the TG released from chylomicrons is taken up by adipose, heart, and skeletal muscle, while the remaining 20% is taken up by the liver (1). Chylomicrons are usually cleared from the bloodstream within 1 hour of a fatty meal.

After hydrolysis and the release of approximately 90% of the TG carried by chylomicrons, the chylomicrons decrease in size and increase in relative composition of cholesterol and cholesterol esters. The resulting lipoproteins are referred to as *chylomicron remnants.* The chylomicron remnants are then taken up by the liver and the remaining cholesterol esters and TG are hydrolyzed and metabolized.

The absorption of the smaller and more soluble short-chain fatty acids (SCFAs) (2 to 4 carbons) and medium-chain fatty acids (MCFAs) (6 to 14 carbons) differs from that of LCFAs. SCFAs and MCFAs follow the same route of intestinal absorption as monosaccharides and amino acids. They are directly absorbed by the small intestine and passed on to the liver by the portal circulation bound to albumin. This direct route of absorption means that SCFAs and MCFAs appear in the bloodstream and can function as a substrate more rapidly than LCFAs. Massicotte and colleagues (2) found that MCFAs consumed 1 hour before exercise are oxidized within the first 30 minutes of exercise.

ENDOGENOUS FAT STORES

Endogenous fat represents 90,000 to 100,000 kcals of energy or 70% to 80% of the body's total energy stores (3). Only 2% to 3% of endogenous fat is stored within skeletal muscle fibers as intramuscular TG (IMTG) (4). Intramuscular TG is important for endurance exercise because it is the only immediately available fat source to skeletal muscle. Nearly all endogenous fat is stored in adipose tissue as TG.

FAT METABOLISM

Lipogenesis

In humans, it is possible to synthesize fat from both FFA sources and non-FFA sources. Tissues such as the liver, kidney, brain, lung, mammary gland, and adipose can convert acetylcoenzyme A (acetyl-CoA) (from sources such as glucose) into palmitate in the cytosol of the cell. The liver and adipose tissue are considered the primary sites of lipogenesis in humans (5). In addition, the liver endoplasmic reticulum can perform fatty acid elongation, which converts acetate into LCFAs (6). Insulin is the primary promoter of lipogenesis, while glucagon and epinephrine inhibit this process.

The occurrence of lipogenesis is dependent on the nutritional state of the individual. According to Acheson and colleagues (7), nonobese men who consumed a 500-g meal containing mostly carbohydrate converted only a minor portion of that meal (1% to 2%) into fat. Hellerstein and colleagues (8) confirmed these findings in a similar population that received a 260- to 380-g meal of mostly carbohydrate over a 9-hour period. Aarsland and colleagues (5), however, demonstrated significant lipogenesis after a 4-day hyperenergetic diet (about 2.5 times caloric expenditure) containing 15 g carbohydrate·kg body weight^{-1}.

It is reasonable to assume that, under normal conditions, the conversion of dietary carbohydrate to fat is limited. However, significant amounts of fat can be synthesized from carbohydrate if bodily glycogen stores are saturated and the individual continues to consume carbohydrate in amounts that are exceptionally high (approximately 15 g·kg body weight^{-1}) and in excess of caloric expenditure.

Mobilization and Transport

Lipolysis is the process by which TG is broken down into fatty acids and glycerol. This process is responsible for the mobilization of fatty acids in a variety of tissues including skeletal muscle, liver, and adipose. Lipolysis occurs both intracellularly and extracellularly. Triglycerides that travel bound to very-low-density lipoprotein (VLDL) and chylomicrons are acted upon by LPL outside of the cell, and the FFA can be taken up by adipose tissue, skeletal muscle, and the liver. Intracellularly, stored TGs are acted on by hormone sensitive TG lipase. Fatty acids from adipose tissue may be released into the bloodstream but they must be circulated bound to albumin in the plasma due to the insoluble nature of fatty acids. Circulating fatty acids are referred to as FFAs. The term *free fatty acid* must be interpreted with caution since fatty acids that remain completely unbound compose less than 0.01% of the total plasma pool. Fatty acids mobilized from IMTG do not require transport in the bloodstream.

Glycerol released from lipolysis is also transported into the bloodstream, where it is converted to glycerol-3-phosphate and glucose in the liver. The enzyme glycerol kinase is required for the conversion of glycerol to glycerol-3-phosphate and glucose, but the activity of this enzyme in tissues other than the liver and kidneys is low in animals (9). Since glycerol cannot be reesterified by skeletal muscle or adipose tissue and must be released into the bloodstream to be transported into the liver, regardless of the site of lipolysis, the appearance of glycerol in the blood may serve as a marker of whole-body lipolysis. Romijn and colleagues (10) confirmed this hypothesis using stable isotope tracer techniques during exercise.

Several different processes regulate lipolysis. The most potent inhibitor of lipolysis is insulin, but other factors such as adenosine, ketone bodies, and changes in blood flow may also have an effect (11). Catecholamines serve as the most potent activators of lipolysis. These hormones likely act on α-adrenergic receptors at rest, and β-adrenergic receptors during exercise (12). Other factors that stimulate lipolysis include growth hormone and glucocorticoids (11).

Not all of the fatty acids mobilized from adipose tissue are released into the circulation. Fatty acids may remain in the adipocyte and be reesterified into TG. The glycerol backbone for the reesterification of TG is supplied by the conversion of glucose to glycerol-3-phosphate. The mobilization of TG and subsequent reesterification is referred to as the *triglyceride–fatty acid cycle* (Fig. 2–1). Reesterification may occur in adipose tissue or circulating FFA can be reesterified in other tissues such as the liver and is regulated by blood flow, albumin-binding capacity, and the rates of lipolysis and fatty acid oxidation (13). The triglyceride–fatty acid cycle provides a mechanism for rapidly altering plasma FFA availability to match metabolic demand. Wolfe and colleagues (13) demonstrated that in conditions of reduced availability, the release of FFA into the bloodstream is increased due to a decrease in the rate of reesterification. At rest, approximately 70% of fatty acids released were reesterified, but during exercise at 40% maximal oxygen consumption ($\dot{V}O_2max$), the rate dropped to 25% with a concomitant increase in FFA release. This resulted in a sixfold increase in FFA availability.

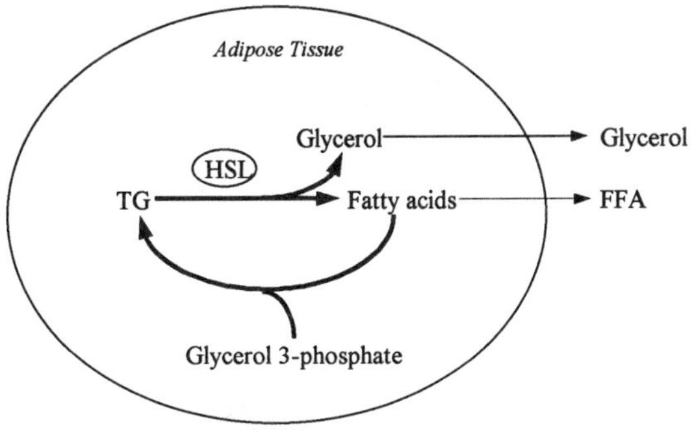

FIG. 2–1. The triglyceride-fatty acid cycle. *TG,* triglyceride; *HSL,* hormone sensitive lipase; *FFA,* free fatty acid.

Peripheral Uptake: Adipose Tissue and Skeletal Muscle

Triglycerides that travel bound to lipoproteins and/or albumin cannot be incorporated into the muscle. The FFA must be released in the vascular space prior to incorporation into the cell. Traditionally, it was thought that the uptake of plasma FFA into muscle cells and adipocytes occurred via passive diffusion (14,15), so that the uptake was directly proportional to the plasma FFA concentration. Plasma FFA uptake demonstrates saturation kinetics, however, which means that there is a plasma FFA concentration beyond which uptake ceases to increase (16). It is currently thought that there may be a system of carrier proteins that transfer plasma FFA from the vascular space into the cell, and eventually into the mitochondria (16–19). Once inside the cell, fatty acids can be oxidized in the mitochondria, used to replenish IMTG stores, or used to synthesize phospholipids.

β-Oxidation

Fatty acids from plasma or IMTG are oxidized in the same manner. Fatty acids of any chain length must move inside mitochondria to be oxidized. However, while SCFA and MCFA can diffuse into mitochondria freely, LCFA must be transported from the cytosol into the mitochondria by two bound enzymes, carnitine palmitoyl-transferase I and II (CAT I and II).

Once inside the mitochondria, fatty acids of any chain length undergo a process referred to as *β-oxidation.* The end product of β-oxidation is acetyl-CoA, which may be utilized three different ways: first, it may enter the tricarboxylic acid (TCA) cycle and be oxidized completely to carbon dioxide and water; second, it may serve as a source of carbon atoms in cholesterol and/or steroid synthesis; and third, it may be converted to ketone bodies in the liver.

Fat oxidation by skeletal muscle at rest and during exercise is ultimately dependent on mitochondrial transport. Mitochondrial transport of LCFA is regulated by malonyl CoA, a product of lipogenesis that inhibits CAT I. Malonyl CoA concentration may be high in the postabsorptive state when insulin is elevated and lipogenesis is stimulated. Malonyl CoA concentration may also be elevated during high rates of glycolytic flux and carbohydrate oxidation that may occur with exercise (20).

FAT TURNOVER AT REST

Postprandial State

In the resting postprandial and postabsorptive states, fat supplies a majority of the energy used by the body (21). Most of this fat is in the form of plasma FFA. The high insulin/glucagon ratio in the postprandial state drives the metabolic systems toward storage of fat and lipogenesis while inhibiting lipolysis and β-oxidation. A majority of the plasma FFA taken up by the periphery is reesterified into TG droplets while the remainder is oxidized.

Postabsorptive State

In the postabsorptive state, the lowering of the insulin/glucagon ratio increases the mobilization of fatty acids from adipose tissue due to the attenuated inhibition of lipolysis. Fatty acid mobilization may be further enhanced by the strong counterregulatory response to the decrease in plasma glucose characterized by increases in epinephrine, norepinephrine, cortisol, and growth hormone. As the postabsorptive state continues, plasma FFA concentration may rise to more than 10 times the normal resting concentration (0.10 to 1.40 mmol/L). The increase in plasma FFA concentration produces an increase in skeletal muscle FFA uptake and oxidation, eventually leading to the formation of ketone bodies (acetoacetone, β-hydroxybutyrate, and acetone) by the liver. The plasma concentration of β-hydroxybutyrate may triple after a 12-hour fast and increase nearly 50-fold after 3 days (22). With hypoglycemia likely during a prolonged fast, ketone bodies provide an alternative fuel source for peripheral tissue including the brain and skeletal muscle (23).

Body Weight Status

Beyond changes in the fed state, resting fat turnover is influenced by body weight status. The set-point theory of body weight hypothesizes that body weight is regulated by controlling energy intake and expenditure (24). Thus, weight loss is counteracted by increased energy intake and decreased expenditure, while weight gain is balanced by decreased energy intake and increased expenditure. Although studies in this area have concentrated on total energy expenditure, fat expenditure specifically is likely to follow the same pattern.

FAT TURNOVER DURING EXERCISE

Influence of Intensity, Duration, and Substrate Availability

The oxidation of fat during exercise is influenced by intensity, duration, plasma FFA availability, and carbohydrate availability. Romijn and co-workers (10) performed the most extensive examination of the influence of both exercise intensity and duration on fat metabolism. Trained cyclists exercised for 120 minutes at 25% and 65% $\dot{V}O_2max$ and 30 minutes at 85% $\dot{V}O_2max$ on separate days in random order. Whole-body fat oxidation, plasma FFA oxidation, IMTG oxidation, the rate of appearance (Ra) of plasma FFA, as well as the rates of both peripheral (adipose tissue) lipolysis and IMTG lipolysis were quantified through the combined use of indirect calorimetry and stable isotope tracer techniques. The Ra of glycerol was used as the marker of whole-body lipolysis.

While glycerol Ra increased for all three conditions indicating increased whole-body lipolysis, plasma FFA concentration only increased at 25% and 65% $\dot{V}O_2max$ to 1.0–1.2 mM. The decrease in plasma FFA concentration from 1.0 to 0.5 mM at 85% $\dot{V}O_2max$ in spite of an increased rate of lipolysis indicated that fatty acid mobilization was impaired. While fatty acids were liberated by lipolysis, they were not being transported from the adipose tissue at a rate that matched that of lipolysis. This was confirmed by the failure of FFA Ra to increase above resting values at 85% $\dot{V}O_2max$. Thus, basal plasma FFA Ra coupled with increased skeletal muscle FFA uptake produced a decrease in plasma FFA concentration at 85% $\dot{V}O_2max$.

The rates of whole-body lipolysis were greater for the 65% and 85% $\dot{V}O_2max$ conditions. This was due to greater IMTG lipolysis because peripheral lipolysis was equivalent for each exercise intensity. Whole-body fat oxidation was greater than could be accounted for by plasma FFA uptake and oxidation at 65% and 85% $\dot{V}O_2max$, suggesting that IMTG provided the additional source of fat oxidation at these intensities.

At 25% $\dot{V}O_2max$, fat provided 86% of the energy expended; nearly all of this was accounted for by plasma FFA oxidation. IMTG oxidation occurred only at the two higher intensities of exercise. At 65% $\dot{V}O_2max$, both plasma FFA and IMTG contributed 30% of the total energy expenditure, and this decreased to 13% each at 85% $\dot{V}O_2max$. This study indicated that fat is the major substrate for low and moderate exercise intensities below 65% $\dot{V}O_2max$. The decreased contribution of plasma FFA between 25% and 65% $\dot{V}O_2max$ was partially compensated by the increased oxidation of IMTG.

The effects of exercise duration on fat oxidation could be examined only at 25% and 65% $\dot{V}O_2max$ because these work loads were maintained for 2 hours. There were no significant fluctuations in substrate use at 25%

$\dot{V}O_2max$ from 30 minutes to the end of the test. At 65% $\dot{V}O_2max$ there was a progressive increase in plasma FFA and glucose oxidation, while total fat and carbohydrate oxidation did not change. Therefore, it was concluded that there was a progressive reduction in the use of IMTG and muscle glycogen as these stores became depleted. This was compensated for by the increased metabolism of plasma FFA and glucose. It was estimated that the contribution of plasma FFA to total energy expenditure rose from 30% during the first 30 minutes to 49% by the end of the test. On the other hand, the contribution of IMTG decreased from 27% to 16%.

The effect of exercise duration on plasma FFA utilization can also be viewed as the effect of intramuscular substrate depletion on plasma FFA utilization. Evidence that contradicts the findings above was presented by Turcotte and colleagues (25). This study compared the uptake and oxidation of the FFA palmitate in contracting perfused rat skeletal muscle that was either glycogen depleted or supercompensated by prior exercise and dietary manipulations. Muscle glycogen concentration of the depleted rats was approximately 50% lower than that of the supercompensated rats while IMTG content was similar. Palmitate uptake and oxidation at rest and during electrically stimulated contractions were the same in both conditions. In contrast, glucose uptake was increased in the glycogen-depleted condition at rest and during contractions. The authors suggested that the regulation of the pathways of carbohydrate metabolism took precedence over the regulation of the pathways between fat and carbohydrate metabolism. As IMTG content was similar between the two conditions, however, there is the possibility that plasma FFA uptake and oxidation are also influenced by the availability of IMTG.

The availability of plasma FFA is thought to influence its uptake by skeletal muscle both at rest and during exercise. The minimal contribution of plasma FFA to energy expenditure during high-intensity exercise is thought to be related to the fact that the mobilization, transport, and uptake of plasma FFA are simply too slow to support high rates of metabolism. Romijn and colleagues (10) indicated that the plasma FFA concentration decreased by 50% at 85% $\dot{V}O_2max$ and coincided with a lower rate of fat oxidation than at 65% $\dot{V}O_2max$. There is the possibility that part of the reason for the decrease in fat oxidation was decreased plasma FFA availability. This was examined by Romijn and associates (26) by exercising trained subjects for 20 to 30 minutes at 85% $\dot{V}O_2max$ under control conditions when plasma FFA was low or when plasma FFA was maintained between 1.0 and 2.0 mM by the infusion of Intralipid and heparin. Total fat oxidation was measured by indirect calorimetry, and plasma FFA Ra was measured by stable isotope tracer techniques. Increasing plasma FFA availability increased total fat oxidation by 27% compared to control. However, the increased rate of fat oxidation was still lower than that measured at 65% $\dot{V}O_2max$. Therefore, it seems that part of the reason for lower fat oxidation rates during high-intensity exercise is due to the failure to increase fatty acid mobilization following lipolysis. The other factors responsible for the decreased rate of fat oxidation were not clear from this study but could involve the attenuation of the normal decline in malonyl CoA, an inhibitor of LCFA transport into mitochondria.

Finally, fat oxidation during exercise may be directly regulated by carbohydrate availability (20). Compared to an overnight fast, glucose ingestion before 40 minutes of exercise at 50% $\dot{V}O_2max$ elevated plasma glucose and insulin concentrations and reduced fat oxidation by 34%. Stable isotope tracer techniques revealed that LCFA oxidation was reduced while MCFA oxidation was unchanged. These results indicate that increases in glycolytic flux due to elevated plasma glucose and insulin concentrations during exercise selectively inhibit LCFA oxidation, possibly due to increases in malonyl CoA. MCFA oxidation is not affected, however, due to its unregulated mitochondrial transport.

Acute Fat Supplementation

Why would one want to supplement plasma FFA levels when fat stores are virtually limitless? The idea is based on the work of Randle and colleagues (27) that hypothesizes that a glucose–fatty acid cycle exists by which increased muscle citrate and acetyl-CoA from increased fat oxidation inhibit phosphofructokinase (PFK) and pyruvate dehydrogenase (PDH), respectively (Fig. 2–2). PFK is a regulatory enzyme of glycolysis, while PDH regulates the entry of pyruvate into the TCA cycle. Inhibition of these enzymes would in turn slow the rate of carbohydrate oxidation, "sparing" both plasma glucose and muscle glycogen.

If the glucose–fatty acid cycle existed, the effectiveness of acute fat supplementation on sparing carbohydrate would depend on whether there was a concomitant increase in fat oxidation. As pointed out by Romijn and colleagues (26), fat supplementation would likely provide a benefit if plasma FFA availability was a limiting factor to fat oxidation as it appeared to be during 20 to 30 minutes of exercise at 85% $\dot{V}O_2max$. There was a 15% reduction in muscle glycogen degradation when the plasma FFA concentration was elevated above control. A reduced muscle glycogen degradation was found in other studies where plasma FFA concentration was elevated during exercise between 0.57 and 2.00 mM by Intralipid/heparin infusions during 15 to 60 minutes of moderate to high-intensity exercise (70% to 85% $\dot{V}O_2max$) (28–31) (Table 2–1). The controls in these studies had plasma FFA concentrations of approximately 0.34 mM. By contrast, Intralipid/heparin infusion did not

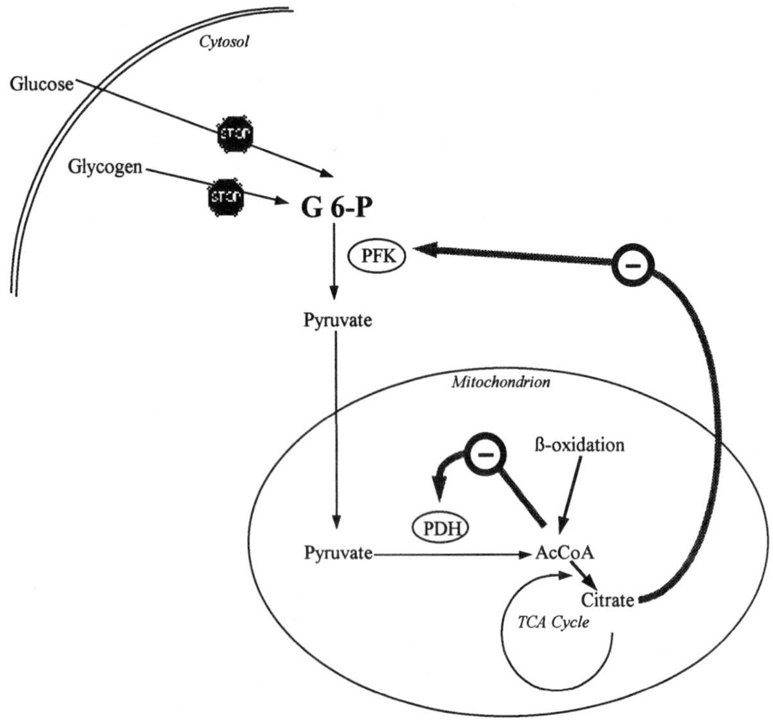

FIG. 2–2. The glucose-fatty acid cycle. *G6-P,* glucose-6-phosphate; *PFK,* phosphofructokinase; *PDH,* pyruvate dehydrogenase; *AcCoA,* acetyl-CoA; *TCA,* tricarboxylic acid.

TABLE 2–1. *Acute fat supplementation*

Reference	Subjects	Supplementation	Performance task	[FFA] during exercise (mM)	Glycogen sparing (%Δ from control)	Glucose sparing (%Δ from control)	Performance enhanced by fat supplementation?
Costill et al. (1977) (28)	T and UT	High-fat meal + heparin	30 min @ 70% V_{O_2}max	0.57–1.01	−40%	Not assessed	Not assessed
		5–6 h fast		~0.25			
Dyck et al. (1993) (30)	T and UT	Intralipid/heparin infusion	15 min @ 85% V_{O_2}max	1.27–1.42	−44%	Not assessed	Not assessed
		Saline infusion		~0.20			
Dyck et al. (1996) (29)	T and UT	Intralipid/heparin infusion	15 min @ 85% V_{O_2}max	1.00–1.12	−47%*	Not assessed	Not assessed
		Saline infusion		~0.36			
Hargreaves et al. (1991) (33)	T and UT	Intralipid/heparin infusion	1 h of one-legged exercise @ 80% max work load	0.91–1.40	No difference	−33%	Not assessed
		No infusion		0.48–0.65			
Okano et al. (1996) (34)	T	4 h preexercise fat meal	120 min @ 65% V_{O_2}max, then 85% V_{O_2}max to exhaustion	~0.80–1.30	Not assessed	Not assessed	No
		4 h preexercise CHO meal		~0.30–0.70			
Ravussin et al. (1986) (32)	UT	Intralipid/heparin infusion	150 min @ 44% V_{O_2}max	1.04–1.83	No difference	Not assessed	Not assessed
		Saline infusion		0.49–1.39			
Romijn et al. (1995) (26)	T	Intralipid/heparin infusion	20–30 min @ 85% V_{O_2}max	1.00–2.00	−15%	No difference	Not assessed
		No infusion		0.20–0.30			
Starling et al. (1997) (36)	T	12 h high-fat diet	Time trial	0.54–1.76	No difference	Not assessed	No
		12 h high-CHO diet		0.38–1.35			
Vukovich et al. (1993) (31)	UT	3 h preexercise fat meal or Intralipid/heparin infusion	60 min @ 70% V_{O_2}max	1.25–1.97	−28%	Not assessed	Not assessed
		3 h preexercise CHO meal		~0.33–0.75			

[FFA], concentration of plasma free fatty acid; mM, millimoles per liter; T, trained; UT, untrained; h, hour; CHO, carbohydrate; min, minutes; V_{O_2}max, maximal oxygen consumption; *7 of 11 subjects exhibited sparing.

significantly elevate fat oxidation or spare muscle glycogen at a low exercise intensity (44% $\dot{V}O_2max$) where plasma FFA availability was likely not limiting (32) or during one-legged knee extensions (32).

Little or no research supports an existence of the glucose–fatty acid cycle during exercise, however. Dyck and colleagues (30) observed no difference in citrate or acetyl-CoA concentrations or PDH activity between Intralipid/heparin–infused and control conditions during exercise. Romijn and associates (26) did not find a reduction in plasma glucose uptake with an elevated plasma FFA concentration, as would be predicted by the glucose–fatty acid cycle. An alternative mechanism for the sparing of carbohydrate with elevated plasma FFA concentration during exercise relates to the regulation of phosphorylase, the enzyme that catalyzes the degradation of glycogen (29). Intralipid/heparin infusion during high-intensity exercise attenuated the increase in free adenosine monophosphate (AMP), an activator of phosphorylase, resulting in the sparing of muscle glycogen in some subjects.

Although supplementing plasma FFA has been shown to spare muscle glycogen, the above studies have utilized infusion techniques that are not of practical use. More importantly, performance was not measured in these studies. Therefore, although these techniques may result in glycogen sparing, they have not been shown to alter endurance performance in humans.

Studies that have examined the effects of acute fat supplementation with high-fat meals on exercise performance have not found an effect on time to exhaustion or self-paced cycling performance (34–36). Starling and colleagues (36) fed endurance-trained athletes either a high-carbohydrate (83% carbohydrate) or high-fat (68% fat) diet for 12 hours following a 120-minute ride at 65% $\dot{V}O_2max$. The 12-hour feeding was followed by a 12-hour overnight fast and a self-paced cycling task. Although the high-fat diet increased IMTG concentration by 36%, it replaced only 13% of the muscle glycogen used during the 120-minute ride. The high-carbohydrate diet, on the other hand, did not significantly raise IMTG concentration, but it did replace 93% of muscle glycogen used. Following the high-fat diet, subjects had a lower respiratory exchange ratio (RER), indicating greater oxidation of fat, and a higher plasma FFA concentration during the self-paced cycling task compared to the high-carbohydrate diet. During the high-fat trial, subjects took significantly longer to perform the prescribed cycling task and exhibited a significant decrease in the percentage of $\dot{V}O_2max$ they were able to maintain by the end of the task. Although the high-fat diet increased the availability of plasma FFA and enhanced fat oxidation during exercise, self-paced cycling performance was decreased, likely as a result of inadequate muscle glycogen synthesis in the 24 hours preceding the task (33).

Okano and colleagues (34) fed endurance-trained athletes either a high-carbohydrate or high-fat meal 4 hours before a ride to exhaustion at 65% (0 to 120 minutes) and 85% $\dot{V}O_2max$ (120 minutes to exhaustion). The high-fat meal produced a lower RER, suggesting a greater reliance on fat and the possible sparing of carbohydrate. However, times to exhaustion were not significantly different between the conditions, and the possible sparing of muscle glycogen could not be assessed because muscle biopsies were not taken.

The rapid absorption and unregulated mitochondrial transport of MCFAs has led to the investigation of their efficacy as an ergogenic aid. Co-ingestion of medium-chain TG (MCT) and carbohydrate increased the amount of MCT oxidized during exercise (37). One study has shown improvements in endurance performance with MCT and carbohydrate co-ingestion (38). Others, however, have found that the amount of MCT that can be tolerated without gastrointestinal complaints contributes only 3% to 7% of total energy expenditure during prolonged exercise (37), even when muscle glycogen is reduced prior to exercise (39). In addition, MCT supplementation does not decrease muscle glycogen utilization during exercise (40).

Adaptations in Fat Metabolism with Endurance Training

Endurance training results in a greater reliance on fat oxidation during exercise at the same absolute intensity (41–43). This shift in substrate utilization is thought to be the result of the increase in the oxidative capacity of skeletal muscle.

Just as there is disagreement with respect to the source of carbohydrate sparing with training, there are two hypotheses regarding the source of increased fat utilization. Some investigators believe that training leads to an increased oxidation of plasma FFA (17,44,45). Support for this perspective comes from the findings that training increases the potential for rapid plasma FFA oxidation at the beginning of exercise (46), and that the expression of a fatty acid–binding protein thought to mediate skeletal muscle FFA uptake increases by 49% after 3 weeks of training (18). Many of the studies in this area have employed one-legged testing and training that results in much lower fluctuations in hormones that influence substrate utilization.

The other hypothesis proposes that the increased reliance on fat is due to increased IMTG oxidation (43,47–49). Hurley and colleagues (47) found that two-legged exercise at 64% of pretraining $\dot{V}O_2max$ after 12 weeks of training produced an increased oxidation of fat, a 41% decrease in muscle glycogen use, and a doubling of IMTG degradation during exercise. Martin (49) later reported reduced plasma FFA uptake and oxidation despite an increase in total fat oxidation after training.

The difference was thought to be accounted for by the increased oxidation of IMTG.

Chronic Fat Supplementation, Adaptation, and Endurance Performance

Starling and colleagues (36) demonstrated that acute high-fat feedings after prolonged exercise increased fat oxidation during exercise performed 24 hours later. Exercise performance was decreased and was likely the result of inadequate muscle glycogen repletion. Although acute fat supplementation may enhance fat oxidation during exercise, this may be counteracted by the low muscle glycogen stores that result from lower carbohydrate consumption. The next question is whether humans can adapt to chronic high-fat diets by improving their ability to oxidize fat during exercise, sparing carbohydrate stores, and thereby improving endurance training and possibly performance (Table 2–2).

Muoio and colleagues (50) fed trained runners a 7-day diet containing either 15%, 24%, or 38% of the energy intake from fat. Carbohydrate was 73%, 61%, and 50% of the total energy intake, respectively. Running time to exhaustion at 75% to 85% $\dot{V}O_2max$ were highest after the fat diet (38% fat) compared to the other two conditions. It was suggested that increased plasma FFA availability produced the improved performance and $\dot{V}O_2max$. However, RER values were equivalent between the conditions during the runs to exhaustion, suggesting that fat oxidation was the same despite differences in plasma FFA concentration. The results of this study must be viewed with caution because the order of the trials was not randomized and the percentage of fat provided to the subjects was not enough to be considered a high-fat diet.

Lambert and colleagues (51) fed trained cyclists either a high-carbohydrate (74% carbohydrate) or high-fat (67% fat) diet for 2 weeks. At the end of 2 weeks, subjects performed a Wingate test of maximal anaerobic power, a time to exhaustion test at 90% $\dot{V}O_2max$, and finally a time to exhaustion test at 60% $\dot{V}O_2max$ with rest periods between each test. There were no differences in maximal anaerobic power or time to exhaustion at 90% $\dot{V}O_2max$. The high-fat diet resulted in significantly longer time to exhaustion at 60% $\dot{V}O_2max$ despite lower muscle glycogen levels at the onset of exercise. It was suggested that the cyclists were able to adapt to the high-fat diet after 2 weeks and that this adaptation allowed them to spare endogenous carbohydrate during moderate-intensity exercise in a glycogen-depleted state.

Phinney and colleagues (52) found no difference in time to exhaustion at 64% $\dot{V}O_2max$ for trained cyclists before and after 4 weeks of consuming a high-fat diet despite a 47% decrease in resting muscle glycogen concentration. It was suggested that the subjects adapted to the high-fat diet and oxidized fat to a greater extent during exercise, and this spared carbohydrate. However, the extremely low carbohydrate intake (< 20 g carbohydrate$\cdot d^{-1}$) and ketogenic nature of this diet brings into question its applicability for athletes.

Helge and co-workers (53) performed the only study to examine the effects of a high-fat diet on the training-induced adaptations in fat metabolism of previously untrained subjects. Untrained subjects were fed either a high-carbohydrate (CHO) (65% carbohydrate, 20% fat, 6.8 g carbohydrate$\cdot kg^{-1}\cdot d^{-1}$) or high-fat diet (FAT) (62% fat, 22% carbohydrate, 2.4 g carbohydrate$\cdot kg^{-1}\cdot d^{-1}$) over an 8-week period during which both groups underwent identical endurance training. At the end of 7 weeks of training, both groups increased $\dot{V}O_2max$ by 11%. However, the CHO group increased time to exhaustion at 81% of pretraining $\dot{V}O_2max$ by nearly threefold while the FAT group only increased time to exhaustion by 1.8-fold.

The fact that the FAT group had a lower RER and

TABLE 2–2. *Chronic fat supplementation*

Reference	Subjects	% kcal Fat	% kcal CHO	Duration of diet (wk)	Training	Performance task	Glycogen sparing (%Δ from control)	Performance (min)
Helge et al. (1996) (53)	UT	62	20	7	3–4 d$\cdot$wk^{-1} 60–75 min 50–85% VO_2max	TTE @ 81% pretraining VO_2max	No difference	65*
		22	65	7				102
Lambert et al. (1994) (51)	T	67	7	2	Maintain habitual training	TTE @ 60% VO_2max	Not assessed	80*
		12	74	2				43
Muoio et al. (1994) (50)	T	38	50	1	Maintain habitual training	TTE @ 75–85% VO_2max	Not assessed	91*
		24	61	1				69
		15	73	1				76
Phinney et al. (1983) (52)	T	85	<2	4	Maintain habitual training	TTE @ 64% VO_2max	−79%	151
		29	57	1				147

kcal, kilocalories; CHO, carbohydrate; wk, weeks; min, minutes; T, trained; UT, untrained; d, day; VO_2max, maximal oxygen consumption; TTE, time to exhaustion; *significant difference between groups.

similar rates of glycogen degradation during exercise as the CHO group after 7 weeks of training suggested that plasma glucose uptake and oxidation was decreased in the FAT group. In addition to a lower RER during exercise, the FAT group also had plasma FFA concentrations similar to those of the CHO group despite greater glycerol levels. This implies that plasma FFA uptake and oxidation were greater in the FAT group, resulting in similar plasma FFA levels despite greater rates of lipolysis. Alternatively, this may suggest that there was a greater contribution of IMTG oxidation in the FAT group that increased plasma glycerol levels without increasing plasma FFA concentration. The exact pattern of fat utilization cannot be elucidated without the use of tracer techniques.

This study demonstrated that chronic fat supplementation while training resulted in the increased reliance on fat and sparing of carbohydrate during exercise. The source of the spared carbohydrate was likely liver glycogen and plasma glucose, however, as the rates of muscle glycogen degradation were not different between groups. While the sparing of plasma glucose for use as an alternate source of carbohydrate late in exercise is likely to improve endurance performance (54–57), the chronic high-fat diet may have given rise to a suboptimal adaptation in the ability of skeletal muscle to take up plasma glucose for oxidation. The FAT group may not have had the ability to oxidize plasma glucose late in exercise to the same degree as the CHO group, possibly explaining their attenuated improvement in endurance performance.

REFERENCES

1. Mayes PA. Lipid transport and storage. In: Murray RK, Granner DK, Mayes PA, Rodwell VW, eds. *Harper's biochemistry.* Norwalk, CT: Appleton and Lange, 1996:244–270.
2. Massicotte D, Peronnet F, Brisson GR, Hillaire-Marcel C. Oxidation of exogenous medium-chain free fatty acids during prolonged exercise: comparison with glucose. *J Appl Physiol* 1992;73:1334–1339.
3. Cahill GF, Aoki TT, Rossini AA. Metabolism in obesity and anorexia nervosa. *Nutr Brain* 1979;3:1–70.
4. Coyle EF. Fat metabolism during exercise. *Gatorade Sport Science Exchange* 1995;8.
5. Aarsland A, Chinkes D, Wolfe RR. Hepatic and whole-body fat synthesis in humans during carbohydrate overfeeding. *Am J Clin Nutr* 1997;65:1174–1182.
6. Kinsella JE. Lipids, membrane receptors, and enzymes: effects of dietary fatty acids. *J Parenter Enter Nutr* 1990;14:200S–217S.
7. Acheson KJ, Flatt J-P, Jequier E. Glycogen synthesis versus lipogenesis after a 500-g carbohydrate meal. *Metab Clin Exp* 1982;31:1234–1240.
8. Hellerstein MK, Christiansen M, Kaempfer S, et al. Measurement of de novo hepatic lipogenesis in humans using stable isotopes. *J Clin Invest* 1991;87:1841–1852.
9. Newsholme EA, Taylor K. Glycerol kinase activities in muscles from vertebrates and invertebrates. *Biochem J* 1969;112:465–474.
10. Romijn JA, Coyle EF, Sidossis LS, et al. Regulation of endogenous fat and carbohydrate metabolism in relation to exercise intensity and duration. *Am J Physiol* 1993;265:E380–E391.
11. Coppack SW, Jensen MD, Miles JM. In vivo regulation of lipolysis in humans. *J Lipid Res* 1994;35:177–193.
12. Arner P, Kriegholm E, Engfeldt P, Bolinder J. Adrenergic regulation of lipolysis in situ at rest and during exercise. *J Clin Invest* 1990;85:893–898.
13. Wolfe RR, Klein S, Carraro F, Weber JM. Role of triglyceride-fatty acid cycle in controlling fat metabolism in humans during and after exercise. *Am J Physiol* 1990;258:E382–E389.
14. Issekutz B, Bortz WM, Miller HI, Paul P. Turnover rate of plasma free fatty acids in humans and in dogs. *Metabolism* 1967;16:1001–1009.
15. Armstrong DT, Steele R, Altszuler N, Dunn A, Bishop JS, De-Bodo RC. Regulation of plasma free fatty acid turnover. *Am J Physiol* 1961;201:9–15.
16. Turcotte LP, Kiens B, Richter EA. Saturation kinetics of palmitate uptake in perfused skeletal muscle. *FEBS Lett* 1991;279:327–329.
17. Kiens B. Effect of endurance training on fatty acid metabolism: local adaptations. *Med Sci Sports Exerc* 1997;29:640–645.
18. Kiens B, Kristiansen S, Jensen P, Richter EA, Turcotte LP. Membrane associated fatty acid binding protein (FABPpm) in human skeletal muscle is increased by endurance training. *Biochem Biophys Res Commun* 1997;231:463–465.
19. van der Vusse GJ, Reneman RS. Lipid metabolism in muscle. In: Rowell LB, Shepherd RJ, eds. *Handbook of physiology, section 12: exercise: regulation and integration of multiple systems.* New York: Oxford University Press, 1996:952–994.
20. Coyle EF, Jeukendrup AE, Wagenmakers AJM, Saris WHM. Fatty acid oxidation is directly regulated by carbohydrate metabolism during exercise. *Am J Physiol* 1997;273:E268–E275.
21. Andres R, Cader G, Zierler KL. The quantitatively minor role of carbohydrate in oxidative metabolism by skeletal muscle in intact man in the basal state: measurements of oxygen and glucose uptake and carbon dioxide and lactate production in the forearm. *J Clin Invest* 1956;35:671–682.
22. Cahill GF, Herrara MG, Morgan AP, et al. Hormone-fuel interrelationships during fasting. *J Clin Invest* 1966;45:1751–1769.
23. Dohm GL, Beeker RT, Israel RG, Tapscott EB. Metabolic responses after fasting. *J Appl Physiol* 1986;61:1363–1368.
24. Keesey RE, Hirvonin MD. Body weight set-points: determination and adjustment. *J Nutr* 1997;127:1875S–1883S.
25. Turcotte LP, Hespel P, Richter EA. Circulating palmitate uptake and oxidation are not altered by glycogen depletion in contracting skeletal muscle. *J Appl Physiol* 1995;78:1266–1272.
26. Romijn JA, Coyle EF, Sidossis LS, Zhang X-J, Wolfe RR. Relationship between fatty acid delivery and fatty acid oxidation during strenuous exercise. *J Appl Physiol* 1995;79:1939–1945.
27. Randle PJ, Garland RB, Hales CN, Newsholme EA. The glucose-fatty acid cycle: its role in insulin sensitivity and the metabolic disturbances of diabetes mellitus. *Lancet* 1963;1:785–789.
28. Costill DL, Coyle E, Dalsky G, Evans W, Fink W, Hoopes D. Effect of elevated plasma FFA and insulin on glycogen usage during exercise. *J Appl Physiol* 1977;43:695–699.
29. Dyck DJ, Peters SJ, Wendling PS, Chelsey A, Hultman E, Spriet LL. Regulation of muscle glycogen phosphorylase activity during intense aerobic cycling with elevated FFA. *Am J Physiol* 1996;270:E116–E125.
30. Dyck DJ, Putman CT, Heigenhauser GJF, Hultman E, Spriet LL. Regulation of fat carbohydrate interaction in skeletal muscle during intense aerobic cycling. *Am J Physiol* 1993;265:E852–E859.
31. Vukovich MD, Costill DL, Hickey MS, Trappe SW, Cole KL, Fink WJ. Effect of fat emulsion infusion and fat feeding on muscle glycogen utilization during cycling exercise. *J Appl Physiol* 1993;75:1513–1518.
32. Ravussin E, Bogardus C, Schneidegger K, LaGrange B, Horton ED, Horton ES. Effect of elevated FFA on carbohydrate and lipid oxidation during prolonged exercise in humans. *J Appl Physiol* 1986;60:893–900.
33. Hargreaves M, Kiens B, Richter EA. Effect of increased plasma fatty acid concentrations on muscle metabolism in exercising men. *J Appl Physiol* 1991;70:194–201.
34. Okano G, Sato Y, Takumi Y, Sugawara M. Effect of 4 h preexercise high carbohydrate and high fat meal ingestion on endurance performance and metabolism. *Int J Sports Med* 1996;17:530–534.
35. Satabin P, Portero P, Defer G, Bricout J, Guezennec C-Y. Metabolic and hormonal responses to lipid and carbohydrate diets during exercise in man. *Med Sci Sports Exerc* 1987;19:218–223.

36. Starling RD, Trappe TA, Parcell AC, Kerr CD, Fink WJ, Costill DL. Effect of diet on muscle triglyceride and endurance performance. *J Appl Physiol* 1997;82:1185–1189.
37. Jeukendrup AE, Saris WHM, Schrauwen P, Brouns F, Wagenmakers AJM. Metabolic availability of oral medium chain triglycerides co-ingested with carbohydrates during prolonged exercise. *J Physiol* 1995;79:756–762.
38. van Zyl CG, Lambert EV, Hawley JA, Noakes TD, Dennis SC. Effects of medium-chain triglyceride ingestion on carbohydrate metabolism and cycling performance. *J Appl Physiol* 1996; 80:2217–2225.
39. Jeukendrup AE, Saris WHM, van Diesen R, Brouns F, Wagenmakers AJM. Effect of endogenous carbohydrate availability on oral medium-chain triglyceride oxidation during prolonged exercise. *J Appl Physiol* 1996;80:949–954.
40. Jeukendrup AE, Saris WHM, Brouns F, Halliday D, Wagenmakers AJM. Carbohydrate (CHO) metabolism after ingestion of CHO and medium chain triglycerides (MCT) during prolonged exercise. *Metabolism* 1996;45:915–921.
41. Christensen EH, Hansen O. Respiratorscher quotient und O_2-aufnahme. *Scand Arch Physiol* 1939;81:180–189.
42. Jansson E, Kaijser L. Substrate utilization and enzymes in skeletal muscle of extremely endurance-trained men. *J Appl Physiol* 1987;62:999–1005.
43. Phillips SM, Green HJ, Tarnopolsky MA, Heigenhauser GJF, Hill RE, Grant SM. Effects of training duration on substrate turnover and oxidation during exercise. *J Appl Physiol* 1996; 81:2182–2191.
44. Kiens B, Essen-Gustavsson B, Christiansen NJ, Saltin B. Skeletal muscle substrate utilization during submaximal exercise in man: effect of endurance training. *J Physiol (Lond)* 1993;469:459–478.
45. Turcotte LP, Richter EA, Kiens B. Increased plasma FFA uptake and oxidation during prolonged exercise in trained vs. untrained humans. *Am J Physiol* 1992;262:E791–E799.
46. Romijn JA, Klein S, Coyle EF, Sidossis LS, Wolfe RR. Strenuous endurance training increases lipolysis and triglyceride-fatty acid cycling at rest. *J Appl Physiol* 1993;75:108–113.
47. Hurley BF, Nemeth PM, Martin WH III, Hagberg JM, Dalsky GP, Holloszy JO. Muscle triglyceride utilization during exercise: effect of training. *J Appl Physiol* 1986;60:562–567.
48. Martin WH, Dalsky GP, Hurley BF. Effect of endurance training on plasma free fatty acid turnover and oxidation during exercise. *Am J Physiol* 1993;265:E708–E714.
49. Martin WH. Effect of endurance training on fatty acid metabolism during whole body exercise. *Med Sci Sports Exerc* 1997; 29:635–639.
50. Muoio DM, Leddy JL, Horvath PJ, Awad AB, Pendergast DR. Effect of dietary fat on metabolic adjustments to maximal $\dot{V}O_2$ and endurance in runners. *Med Sci Sports Exerc* 1994;26:81–88.
51. Lambert EV, Speechly DP, Dennis SC, Noakes TD. Enhanced endurance in trained cyclists during moderate intensity exercise following 2 weeks adaptation to a high fat diet. *Eur J Appl Physiol* 1994;69:287–293.
52. Phinney SD, Bistrian BR, Evans WJ, Gervino E, Blackburn GL. The human metabolic response to chronic ketosis without caloric restriction: preservation of submaximal exercise capability with reduced carbohydrate oxidation. *Metabolism* 1983;32:769–776.
53. Helge JW, Richter EA, Kiens B. Interaction of training and diet on metabolism and endurance during exercise in man. *J Physiol* 1996;492:293–306.
54. Coggan AR, Coyle EF. Effect of carbohydrate feedings during high-intensity exercise. *J Appl Physiol* 1988;65:1703–1709.
55. Coggan AR, Coyle EF. Reversal of fatigue during prolonged exercise by carbohydrate infusion or ingestion. *J Appl Physiol* 1987;63:2388–2395.
56. Coyle EF, Coggan AR, Hemmert MK, Ivy JL. Muscle glycogen utilization during prolonged strenuous exercise when fed carbohydrate. *J Appl Physiol* 1986;61:165–172.
57. Goodpaster BH, Costill DL, Fink WJ, et al. The effects of pre-exercise starch digestion on endurance performance. *Int J Sports Med* 1996;17:366–372.

Exercise and Sport Science,
edited by William E. Garrett, Jr., and Donald T. Kirkendall.
Lippincott Williams & Wilkins, Philadelphia © 2000.

CHAPTER 3

Protein Metabolism During Exercise

Peter W. R. Lemon

Beginning in the late 1960s, due to rapidly expanding interest in the area of muscle biochemistry, and specifically as a result of the increased availability of the needle biopsy technique reintroduced by the Scandinavians (1), knowledge about exercise metabolism (especially carbohydrate and fat metabolism) increased exponentially. Consequently, dietary recommendations for physically active individuals emphasizing the increased need for both energy and carbohydrate have become readily available. In contrast, protein metabolism received only sporadic attention during this time period; as recently as 1989, an expert panel of the National Academy of Sciences concluded that physical exercise had little effect on dietary protein need (2). Despite this opinion, athletes, especially those involved in strength training, have continued to believe that their dietary protein requirements are substantially higher than those of sedentary individuals. In fact, so entrenched is this belief that it is not unusual for strength athletes to consume at least twice and sometimes as high as six times the current protein recommendation of 0.8 $g \cdot kg^{-1} \cdot d^{-1}$ (2).

During the 1970s and early 1980s, a few published studies did suggest that exercise might actually cause significant changes in protein metabolism. Although largely unnoticed at the time, these studies created the stimulus for a renewed interest in the study of protein metabolism with exercise (3–8). Aided by the increased utilization of metabolic tracers, the result has been a considerable increase in the understanding of how exercise affects protein metabolism. For example, it is now known that significant acute decreases in protein synthetic rate and increases in degradation rate occur during and immediately following exercise (9–17). In addition, during exercise recovery (actual time course varies depending on a variety of factors including exercise type, frequency, duration, and intensity as well as type, quantity, and timing of nutrient intake) these responses flip-flop (Fig. 3–1). Consequently, assuming sufficient recovery between training sessions is available to avoid the net catabolic effects of overtraining, participation in regular exercise will lead to increased mitochondrial (endurance exercise) or contractile (strength exercise) protein. Moreover, there is accumulating evidence that the recommended protein intake for sedentary individuals is inadequate to support the increased muscle fuel needs of endurance athletes (18–23) and may even limit muscle development of individuals engaged in a strength training program (24–26).

Although poorly documented, it is also generally understood among athletes that exercise performance enhancements in a wide range of physical skills are possible if supplementary protein is consumed. Despite the renewed interest regarding the role of dietary protein for those regularly engaged in vigorous physical exercise, however, this area of study is still very controversial (5,7,8). For example, not only are the optimal protein needs for individuals involved in different types of exercise programs still unclear, but even the basic question of whether high protein intakes could result in adverse health effects is not yet resolved. Given the rather lucrative rewards available for successful performance in both human athletics and animal sporting events such as horse or dog racing, this seems very surprising. Although definitive answers to these protein metabolic questions are not yet possible based on current knowledge, there is a considerable amount of new information available. This chapter reviews the recent data collected on physically active individuals in an attempt to help clarify

P. W. R. Lemon: Department of Health Sciences, University of Western Ontario, London, Ontario, Canada.

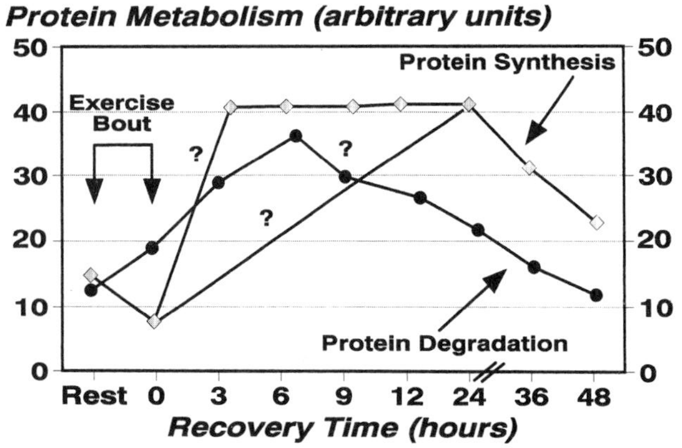

FIG. 3–1. Suspected effects of exercise on the time course of changes in muscle protein synthesis and degradation. Note that whether the net response is anabolic or catabolic could be influenced by the timing of the subsequent exercise session (e.g., catabolic, if exercise sessions are repeated before the anabolic phase can be realized fully), but specific recommendations relative to when sessions should occur to maximize the anabolic component are not yet possible because the point where the responses flip-flop is still unclear.

the ongoing debate about how regular exercise affects dietary protein needs.

THE PROTEIN REQUIREMENT DEBATE—WHAT'S THE CONTROVERSY?

Unfortunately, the controversy regarding how chronic exercise affects the protein requirement is complicated for a variety of reasons. First, there is a fair amount of contradictory information in the scientific literature likely due, at least in part, to the inability of investigators in some published studies to control and/or evaluate adequately the several confounding variables affecting either nutritional or exercise conditions. Second, the impact of the recent information has been reduced because the recommended dietary allowances in the United States, which incidentally do not recognize any increased protein need for chronic exercisers, were last revised in 1989 (2). Moreover, this information may be even more dated because the most recent citation on the protein requirement with exercise issue in this document is a 1977 paper. Third, although athletes frequently attribute impressive exercise performance results to the intake of diets high in protein, performance measures have been largely neglected in the scientific literature, so few scientific data support this opinion. Clearly, whether or how dietary protein needs are affected by regular physical activity is an area of study where much more work is needed.

PROTEIN METABOLISM SIMPLIFIED

To fully appreciate the protein requirement controversy it is necessary to have a working understanding of how the body metabolizes the component parts (amino acids) of dietary protein (Fig. 3–2). Central to this process is the body's amino acid supply, which exists in two locations—a small amount in a readily interchangeable pool located both in body tissues and the blood, and the vast majority bound as protein in body tissues. Although quantitatively small, the free pool is critical because before being utilized for any purpose all amino acids must pass through this pool. Excluding techniques used for experimental purposes (e.g., infusion of amino acid mixtures), there are only three ways amino acids can be made available to the free pool: (a) absorption of dietary protein (following meals), (b) degradation of tissue protein (an ongoing process), and (c) synthesis from a carbohydrate or fat source. This latter process requires a nitrogen source, can only produce some amino acids (the others must be consumed), and quantitatively contributes relatively small amounts of amino acids to the free pool, especially with an exercise treatment because carbohydrate and fat are used as muscle fuels preferentially. There are also three ways amino acids can leave this free pool: (a) oxidation (carbon excreted in breath, nitrogen in urine primarily but also in feces and sweat—the latter being quantitatively significant when sweat rates are high), (b) synthesis of tissue protein (carbon and nitrogen into tissue), and (c) incorporation into carbohydrate or fat for storage. As this latter process is energetically very demanding, it is thought to be quantitatively insignificant, especially with exercise.

Consequently, when considering an exercise treatment, there are basically two inputs and two outputs from the free pool for amino acids. If nonradioactively labeled (carbon [^{13}C] and/or nitrogen [^{15}N]) amino acids are infused directly into the bloodstream continuously (ingestion every few hours can also be used because absorption into the blood is continuous), it is possible

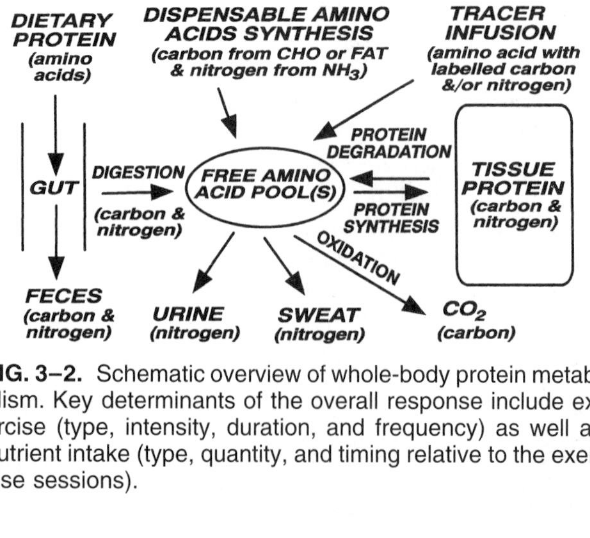

FIG. 3–2. Schematic overview of whole-body protein metabolism. Key determinants of the overall response include exercise (type, intensity, duration, and frequency) as well as nutrient intake (type, quantity, and timing relative to the exercise sessions).

to establish an isotopic steady state (where input and output are equal) and measure flux (turnover through the body) even during nonphysiologic steady states, such as with exercise (27). Then the various component parts of whole-body protein metabolism can be quantified as follows:

$$F = I + D = O \text{ (or } U) + S,$$

where F is the flux through the body, I is the dietary intake, D is the tissue protein degradation, O is the oxidation (when an amino acid carbon label is used), U is the urinary excretion (when an amino acid nitrogen label is used), and S is the protein synthesis. As dietary intake (food analysis) and oxidation (expired air analysis for carbon) or urine excretion (urinary analysis for nitrogen) can be easily quantified, calculations of whole-body protein degradation and/or synthesis rates can be completed without the need for invasive measures. Although the measured protein synthetic rate represents the whole-body average, this likely reflects changes in skeletal muscle metabolism in most situations because of the large contribution of this tissue to metabolism, especially with exercise. Finally, more direct measures of muscle synthetic or degradative rates are also possible if one obtains samples of skeletal muscle over a relevant time period. The latter requires only a small muscle sample and has become routine in many exercise laboratories using the needle biopsy technique (12–18).

These isotopic experiments, although more expensive, are clearly more informative than the classic nitrogen status (balance) experiments (where nitrogen intake and excretion data are collected and the net difference calculated) because they allow quantification of the component parts of protein metabolism rather than what is basically a black-box approach (that is, the internal workings are unknown; the overall process is understood, but not the details). Despite this fact, however, there is a substantial amount of nitrogen status data available, and it is still the method on which the current dietary recommendation for protein (0.8 $g \cdot kg^{-1} \cdot d^{-1}$) is based (2).

Most recently revised in 1989 (2), this recommended protein intake was obtained by adding a safety margin [+2 standard deviations (SD) for the sample studied, which is necessary to cover individual variability in the population] to the protein intake required to elicit nitrogen balance (i.e., nitrogen excretion = nitrogen intake) in a group of essentially sedentary individuals. This balance (status) technique has been criticized, not only because it is labor intensive for both subjects and investigators, but also because it has several inherent unexplained sources of error (25). Moreover, with an exercise treatment it is more questionable because even small changes in energy balance can invalidate the measure (28). The isotopic approach has also been used to assess protein/amino acid requirements, but this has not yet become widespread (29). Basically, this technique involves feeding varying intakes both above and below the expected requirement and measuring whole-body protein synthesis and/or oxidation. When these data are plotted as oxidation (or synthesis) versus protein intake, the requirement is thought to be the value where the rate of protein synthesis begins to plateau (Fig. 3–3), which should correspond to the point where oxidation begins to increase (Fig. 3–4), that is, where excess protein energy is irreversibly lost via oxidation. The latter response occurs because unlike carbohydrate and fat, there is no energy store for protein in the body; all protein is functional (enzymatic or structural). Data from these protein kinetic measurements do not necessarily agree with existing nitrogen status data, but this technique will likely become the method of choice to assess protein needs in the future as it is thought to be both more accurate and more reliable.

Unquestionably, some of the controversy regarding the effects exercise may have on dietary protein needs results from the use of these different assessment techniques. Moreover, although scientists focus on the effects of exercise on protein need as determined by nitrogen status or protein kinetic data, athletes/coaches concentrate on performance results. Clearly the best measure of success in athletics is performance itself. Consequently, the best way to determine if higher-protein diets are advantageous for athletes would likely be to examine exercise performance directly. In other words, regardless of the actual requirement, a performance benefit could result from some as yet unknown

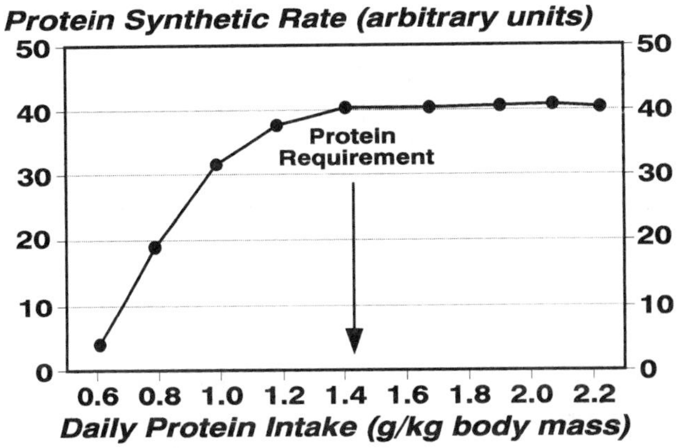

FIG. 3–3. Effects of exercise and protein intake on muscle protein synthesis. Note that protein synthesis increases linearly with increases in dietary protein until a point and then levels off. This maximum protein synthetic rate may be altered by several conditions such as strength training, inactivity, anabolic drugs, etc. The protein intake where the synthetic rate levels off represents the protein requirement. The dietary recommendation would be slightly higher because traditionally it includes a safety margin (+2 SD) to ensure that most (95%) of the population will not experience a deficiency.

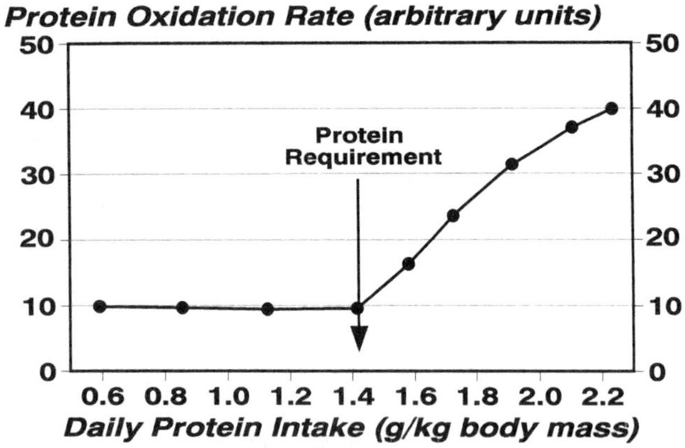

FIG. 3–4. Effects of exercise and protein intake on amino acid (protein) oxidation. Note that protein oxidation remains low and constant when protein intake is below the requirement as most of the available amino acids are used for protein synthesis; however, at some point oxidation begins to increase (nearly linearly) with increasing dietary protein. This point can also be changed by dietary or exercise interventions and is thought to represent the protein requirement. It should be at or near the protein intake where protein synthesis began to level off. The dietary recommendation would be this value +2 SD to ensure that 95% of the population will not experience a protein deficiency.

activating effect induced by diets high in protein. Countless possibilities could explain such a benefit, including, but not limited to, an effect on muscle development, on recovery/repair, or even on energetics. Perhaps the best place to start to resolve this protein controversy is to concentrate on well-controlled performance studies rather than on those investigating the requirement issue. Clearly, if performance in particular types of activities is consistently increased when dietary protein intakes are above the requirement determined using either nitrogen status or protein kinetic data, and assuming there are no adverse effects of such protein intakes, we would at least know that these type of diets are beneficial. The recent availability of good imaging techniques (e.g., magnetic resonance imaging) has dramatically improved our ability to assess changes in muscle size accurately, and these measures, although expensive, need to be utilized for these types of investigations. Once muscle size/performance enhancements are documented, the next step would be to focus on the underlying mechanism(s) responsible. Interestingly, there are some performance data that indicate that high-protein diets are beneficial, especially in strength power activities (24,30,31); however, there is a dearth of this type of data. Furthermore, most of it has been collected over a few weeks, which may have little or no relevance to an athlete who typically trains over several years. This time difference between the scientific studies and the athletes' experience could contribute to the different opinions about the value of diets high in protein.

SEMINAL DATA FROM THE 1970s AND EARLY 1980s

Although not widely recognized at the time, several studies published during a 10–15-year period in the 1970s and early 1980s provided evidence supporting the idea that dietary protein needs may be significantly increased with regular exercise. For example, exercise studies have demonstrated increases in the production of two amino acids in skeletal muscle (32,33), in urea accumulation (major metabolite of protein metabolism) in the blood beginning at about 70 to 80 minutes of endurance exercise (34), in urea accumulation/excretion during shorter time periods (<60 minutes) of aerobic exercise when carbohydrate availability was reduced prior to the exercise bout (35), in oxidation of several amino acids with endurance exercise (9,19–21,36–38), in the capacity for amino acid oxidation following endurance exercise training (39–41), and in decreases in nitrogen status (moving from positive to negative) when an exercise program was initiated while consuming 125% of the recommended protein intake (42).

RECENT STUDIES

Aerobic Exercise

With aerobic-type exercise, at least part of any increased protein need appears to be due to an exercise intensity–dependent increase in amino acid oxidation (38). The branched-chain amino acids (leucine, isoleucine, and valine) are likely the amino acids most utilized, and the mechanism of action is an exercise intensity–dependent activation of the limiting enzyme (branched-chain oxoacid dehydrogenase) in the oxidation pathway (43). This response may also account for the increased amino acid oxidation capacity in endurance-trained subjects (39–41) as both muscle and liver branched-chain oxoacid dehydrogenase activity increase with endurance training (41). Increased oxidation of these amino acids could also account for several of the other changes in protein metabolism observed previously, such as increased output of alanine and glutamine from active skeletal muscle, and increased ammonia and/or urea excretion (Fig. 3–5). In contrast, estimated urea production using tracer methods suggests that the increased amino acid oxidation with aerobic exercise is relatively small at least up to an intensity of 70% $\dot{V}O_2max$ (44). Moreover, some data indicate that moderate exercise increases nitrogen retention when dietary protein is at or near the sedentary requirement (45–47). These apparently conflicting data may have resulted from differences in the magnitude of the exercise stimulus, for example, intensity, frequency, and duration, and/or changes in metabolism at differing protein intakes. To fully assess the importance of these observations, however, more study of how other amino acids are affected by exercise is needed.

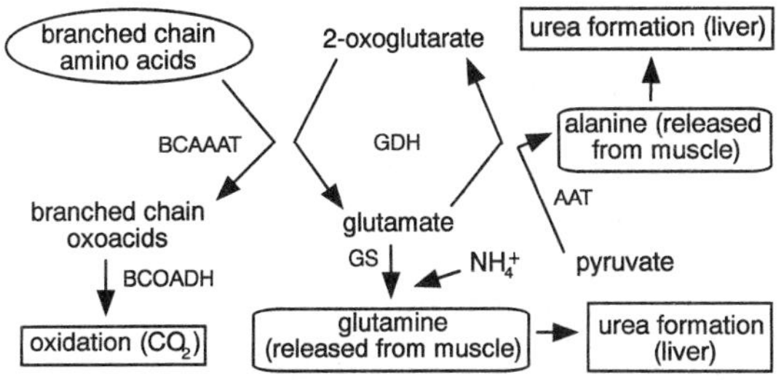

FIG. 3–5. Schematic overview of branched-chain amino acid oxidation showing production of the amino acids glutamine and alanine in skeletal muscle as well as the subsequent urea formation in the liver. *AAT,* alanine amino transferase; *BCAAAT,* branched-chain amino acid transferase; *BCOADH,* branched-chain oxoacid dehydrogenase; *CO_2,* carbon dioxide; *GDH,* glutamate dehydrogenase; *GS,* glutamine synthetase; *NH_4^+,* ammonium.

Exercise-induced amino acid deficiencies have not been documented in athletes; however, these exercise oxidation increases, if representative, could potentially lead to increased dietary requirements. Fortunately, the high energy intakes of most athletes should provide protein intakes above the current recommendation (4), but such may not always be the case for individuals who for whatever reason fail to increase their intake appropriately or who consume an unbalanced diet. Groups that are most vulnerable would include young athletes whose needs are already high because they are growing (children, adolescents), those who voluntarily restrict total energy or many types of food (dieters and vegetarians, especially young females due to the prevalence of disordered eating), or those with extremely high training energy expenditures.

Insufficient intake of the branched-chain amino acids could even limit endurance exercise performance by an indirect mechanism unrelated to fuel supply, for example, promoting increased production of the neurotransmitter serotonin in the brain leading to feelings of lethargy and what has been described as central fatigue (48). Specifically, serotonin is formed in the brain from the amino acid tryptophan, which competes with the branched-chain amino acids for the same blood–brain transporter (an increase in tryptophan and/or a decrease in the branched-chain amino acids should lead to a greater brain serotonin concentration). Consequently, a reduction in circulating branched-chain amino acids (caused by an increased exercise oxidation) in combination with a rising concentration of tryptophan with prolonged exercise (due to displacement of this amino acid from albumin by the increased mobilization of free fatty acids for energy) could result in increased central fatigue and therefore a reduction in performance. Some (49–51) but not all (52,53) data indicate that increasing circulating branched-chain amino acids via supplementation can enhance prolonged endurance performance. Although certainly these data are insufficient to indicate that exercise increases specific amino acid requirements or that individual amino acid supplements enhance performance, they are intriguing and suggest that more detailed investigation is warranted.

Based on data collected on individuals engaged in vigorous, regular aerobic exercise, several investigators (19–23,54) have recommended that a protein intake for aerobic-type athletes in the range of 1.1 to 1.4 $g \cdot kg^{-1} \cdot d^{-1}$ (about 38% to 75% above the current U.S. recommendation) is necessary to avoid a negative nitrogen status. Unfortunately, systematic aerobic performance studies of athletes consuming various protein intakes have not been conducted, so it is not possible to be certain that these or higher protein intakes can enhance performance in comparison to protein intakes near the recommended dietary allowance of 0.8 $g \cdot kg^{-1} \cdot d^{-1}$. These types of studies would be welcome, as they would provide the necessary objective information to determine whether supplemental protein and/or specific amino acids can in fact enhance aerobic performance.

Strength Exercise

With strength activities, there is good evidence that the current recommended protein will actually limit muscle growth (Fig. 3–6) (26). Optimal intakes appear to be in the range of 1.5 to 1.8 $g \cdot kg^{-1} \cdot d^{-1}$ (88% to 125% above the current protein recommended dietary allowance) (25,26); however, some data suggest that even greater intakes are beneficial (Fig. 3–7) (24,30,31,55). One explanation for this apparent contradictory information could involve the interacting effects of very high protein intakes and anabolic drugs (56,57). Although use of the

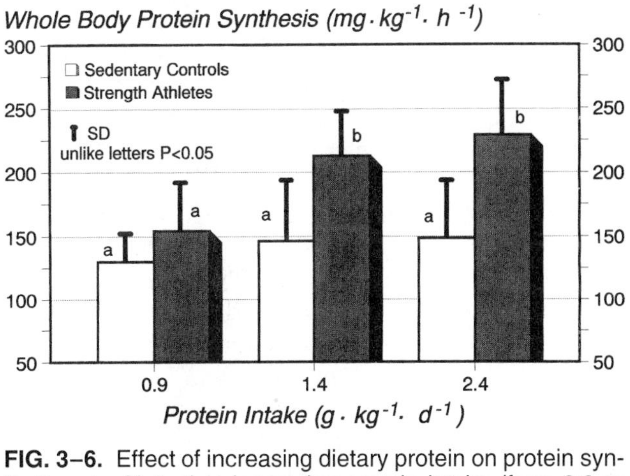

FIG. 3–6. Effect of increasing dietary protein on protein synthetic rate. Note that increasing protein intake (from 0.9 to 1.4 g/kg) increased protein synthesis in the strength athletes only and that further increases did not result when the protein intake was increased to 2.4 g/kg. (Adapted from ref. 26.)

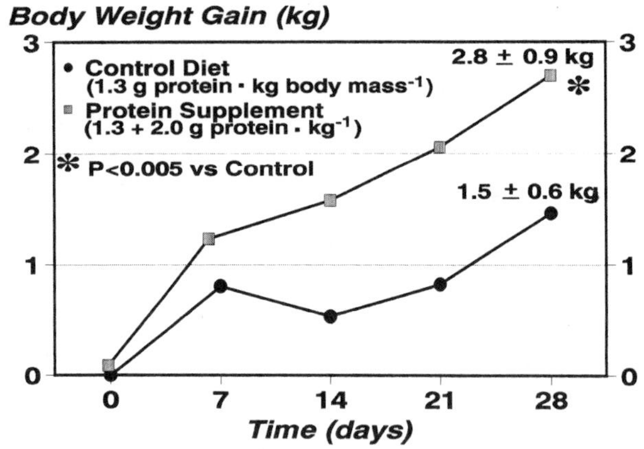

FIG. 3–7. Effect of very high protein intake and strength training on gains in body mass. Note the greater gains with the high (3.3 g/kg) protein intake. (Adapted from ref. 24.)

latter in sports since the 1970s is well documented, the influence of these anabolic agents on the data in many published studies of protein requirements is much less clear. For example, it could be that a ceiling effect relative to increased protein synthetic rates with strength exercise may occur at about 1.5 to 1.8 $g \cdot kg^{-1} \cdot d^{-1}$ in nondrug users (25,26) but at higher intakes when combined with other anabolic agents. If so, this could account for the conflicting opinions between scientists and strength athletes relative to how much dietary protein is optimal. More study is needed to determine if this is the main reason for the discrepancy or whether there are any other factors that contribute.

The timing of specific nutrient intake relative to the exercise stimulus may also be critical to overall muscle development. For example, it is often suggested that multiple small meals are better than a few large ones, presumably because they would make available a more constant supply of nutrients, that is, they would more adequately match supply to demand. Perhaps this suggestion can be refined to include specific nutrient supplementation a short time before (to provide fuel and/or to minimize the catabolic exercise stimulus) or after (to enhance further the subsequent anabolic stimulus induced by the exercise) strength training sessions. Although this topic is in its infancy, there is some evidence indicating that such practices are beneficial. For example, glycogen is a significant fuel during strength training (58), and it is clear that dietary manipulation can enhance muscle glycogen concentration (59). Moreover, due to exercise-induced increases in muscle sensitivity to both glucose and blood flow, nutrient intake in the immediate postexercise period is critical to fully replenish muscle glycogen (60). With strength exercise, the insulin response to dietary carbohydrate has been shown to enhance the already elevated protein synthetic rate in muscle following a strength training session (61). In addition, amino acid infusion following strength training also promotes muscle protein synthesis (62). Consequently, in an analogous manner to the known beneficial effects of appropriately timed carbohydrate intake to maximize aerobic exercise performance (59,60), it might be possible to maximize the muscle growth induced by strength training with specific recommendations about the timing and composition of nutrient intake both before and after strength training. If these kinds of results can be verified with subsequent experiments, the hot topic among strength athletes would likely expand from what combination of food supplements is best to include to what is the optimal time course of intake to maximize the anabolic stimulus of the training sessions. It is important to be careful with this kind of speculation before the data are available, however, because theoretical effects may not actually occur as anticipated. For example, many believe that the initial catabolic response in muscle with strength training is a critical stimulus for the subsequent muscle growth. If so, any specific nutrient intake recommendation that reduces this catabolic response may also minimize the resulting anabolic effect, leading to smaller gains in muscle size and strength.

The long-held belief by strength athletes that high-protein diets are important has resulted in very high meat intakes for these athletes. In fact, many believe that without large quantities of meat in the diet it is impossible to provide sufficient amino acids for the enhanced protein synthetic response induced by strength exercise. As mentioned, there is, in fact, some truth to this belief, at least for protein intakes up to perhaps 2.0 $g \cdot kg^{-1} \cdot d^{-1}$ (25,26), although these quantities of protein can also be reached with meat-free diets. However, recent data suggest that, in addition to the potential for enhanced muscle development, there may be additional benefits to meat intake for those active in strength training. For example, supplemental creatine (a nitrogen-containing compound found in meat and fish) intake appears to enhance short-term, intense exercise performance, especially if it is repeated (63–65). The mechanism is likely related to a more rapid regeneration of adenosine triphosphate from the increased muscle stores of phosphocreatine that result from supplementation (65). This ergogenic effect could also result in greater muscle development secondary to the ability to train harder, that is, a supertraining effect. Moreover, the increase in muscle creatine content may stimulate muscle protein synthesis indirectly via increasing muscle water content (66,67). If so, supplemental creatine intake could result in greater increases in muscle mass/strength than typically observed with strength training (68). Finally, there are other components in meat, for example, conjugated linoleic acid and carnosine, that may have ergogenic or anabolic effects.

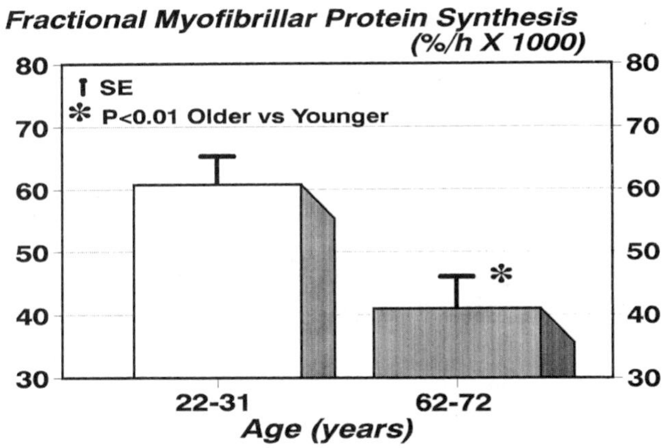

FIG. 3–8. Muscle protein synthetic rate in young versus older subjects. Note the reduced rate in the older subjects. (Adapted from ref. 73.)

Special Populations

Several specific populations have documented elevated dietary protein and/or energy needs relative to the average adult. Examples include children, adolescents, and pregnant women, because growth is occurring; nursing mothers, because protein synthetic rates are increased; and senior citizens, because protein synthetic rates are decreased (69–73) (Fig. 3–8). Although it is premature to conclude definitively, it may be that when individuals from any of these groups begin an exercise program of sufficient intensity, frequency, and duration, protein supplementation may be especially beneficial due to the possible potentiation of the exercise effect with their other condition. Moreover, as mentioned earlier, individuals who voluntarily restrict food intake (dieters) and/or reduce food variety for whatever reason are high-risk candidates. Unfortunately, very few studies have investigated protein needs in these populations.

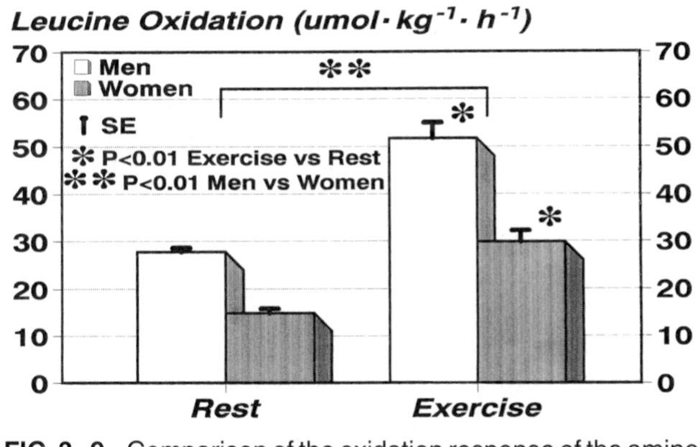

FIG. 3–9. Comparison of the oxidation response of the amino acid leucine at rest and during aerobic exercise in men versus women. Note that the rate is lower in women, both at rest and during exercise. (Adapted from ref. 23.)

Finally, some data indicate that the protein metabolic responses to exercise differ across the menstrual cycle (74), and that normally cycling women may rely less on carbohydrate and protein during exercise than men (23,75,76). These interesting data (Fig. 3–9), if substantiated with future study, could mean that dietary protein recommendations may need to differ between genders and perhaps even vary for women at various times during the menstrual cycle.

RECOMMENDATIONS

Clearly, it is difficult to make a conclusive protein intake recommendation for those active in vigorous regular exercise because of the complexity of the protein metabolic response to exercise. However, it also seems inappropriate to ignore the evidence that has been accumulating in recent years relative to the potential benefits of protein intakes exceeding the current recommendation. Moreover, based on the studies reviewed here and because there are no documented hazards to protein intakes up to at least 2.0 $g \cdot kg^{-1} \cdot d^{-1}$ (8), it appears that dietary protein intake recommendations in the range of 1.1 to 1.4 $g \cdot kg^{-1} \cdot d^{-1}$ for those active in aerobic exercise and 1.5 to 1.8 $g \cdot kg^{-1} \cdot d^{-1}$ for those participating in strength programs would be prudent. It is hoped that in the near future it will be possible to document further the benefits of these recommendations as well as whether adjustments need to be made for any of the populations with preexisting additional protein needs. Also, although exceptions exist, it is usually possible to obtain these protein intakes by small adjustments in one's present diet (4), as long as the diet contains both a wide variety of foods and sufficient energy to cover energy expenditure.

CONCLUSION

Dietary protein needs of physically active individuals have been debated for centuries. Until recently, scientists have disagreed with athletes, who generally believe that their protein needs are substantially greater than their less-active counterparts. Considerable, but not all, recent scientific data support the idea that beneficial effects may result if the diet has a protein content of 1.1 to 1.4 $g \cdot kg^{-1} \cdot d^{-1}$ (about 38% to 75% above the current recommendation) for aerobic athletes or 1.5 to 1.8 $g \cdot kg^{-1} \cdot d^{-1}$ (about 88% to 125% above the current recommendation) for strength athletes. The underlying mechanism responsible for the increased need appears to be related largely to increases in the muscle protein synthetic rate in strength athletes and to fuel use in aerobic athletes; however, there may be additional, more subtle responses or indirect beneficial effects of these moderately high protein diets (e.g., ergogenic effects of components of some high-protein foods and possible antifatiguing effects on brain metabolism). More study is necessary to assess the importance of these potential benefits as well as to determine whether more specific dietary protein recommendations are necessary for some special population groups whose dietary needs are already elevated for other reasons.

ACKNOWLEDGMENTS

Ongoing support of the author's laboratory by the Joe Weider Foundation is gratefully acknowledged.

REFERENCES

1. Bergstrom J. Muscle electrolytes in man. *Scand J Clin Lab Invest Suppl* 1962;14:1–110.
2. US Food & Nutrition Board. *Recommended dietary allowances.* Washington: National Academy Press, 1989.
3. Lemon PWR, Nagle FJ. Effects of exercise on protein and amino acid metabolism. *Med Sci Sports Exerc* 1981;13:141–149.
4. Lemon PWR. Protein and exercise: update 1987. *Med Sci Sports Exerc* 1987;19(suppl 5):S179–S190.
5. Butterfield GE. Amino acids and high protein diets. In: Williams M, Lamb D, eds. *Perspectives in exercise science and sports medicine, vol 4, ergogenics—the enhancement of exercise and sport performance.* Indianapolis: Benchmark Press, 1991:87–122.
6. Evans WJ. Exercise and protein metabolism. In: Simopoulos AP, Pavlou KN, eds. *Nutrition and fitness for athletes. World review of nutrition and dietetics.* Basel: Karger, 1993:21–33.
7. Rennie MJ, Bowtell JL, Millward DJ. Physical activity and protein metabolism. In: Bouchard C, Shephard RJ, Stephens T, eds. *Physical activity, fitness, and health.* Champaign, IL: Human Kinetics, 1994:432–450.
8. Lemon PWR. Dietary protein requirements in athletes. *Nutr Biochem* 1997;28:52–60.
9. Rennie MJ, Edwards RHT, Krywawych S, et al. Effect of exercise on protein turnover in man. *Clin Sci* 1981;61:627–639.
10. Booth FW, Watson PA. Control of adaptations in protein levels in response to exercise. *Fed Proc* 1985;44:2293–2300.
11. Devlin JT, Brodsky I, Scrimgeour A, Fuller S, Bier DM. Amino acid metabolism after intense exercise. *Am J Physiol* 1990; 258:E249–E255.
12. Carraro F, Stuart CA, Hartl WH, Rosenblatt J, Wolfe RR. Effect of exercise and recovery on muscle protein synthesis. *Am J Physiol* 1990;259:E470–E476.
13. MacDougall JD, Gibala MJ, Tarnopolsky MA, MacDonald JR, Interisano SA, Yarasheski KE. The time course of elevated muscle protein synthesis following heavy resistance exercise. *Can J Appl Physiol* 1995;20:480–486.
14. Phillips SM, Tipton KD, Aarsland A, Wolfe SE, Wolfe RR. Mixed muscle protein synthesis and breakdown after resistance exercise in humans. *Am J Physiol* 1997;273:E99–E107.
15. Yarasheski KE, Zachwieja JJ, Bier DM. Acute effect of resistance exercise on muscle protein synthesis rate in young and elderly men and women. *Am J Physiol* 1993;265:E210–E214.
16. Biolo G, Declan-Fleming RY, Wolfe RR. Physiologic hyperinsulinemia stimulates protein synthesis and enhances transport of selected amino acids in human skeletal muscle. *J Clin Invest* 1995;95:811–819.
17. Biolo G, Maggi SP, Williams BD, Tipton KD, Wolfe RR. Increased rates of muscle protein turnover and amino acid transport after resistance exercise in humans. *Am J Physiol* 1995;268:E514–E520.
18. Ferrando AA, Tipton KD, Bamman MM, Wolfe RR. Resistance exercise maintains skeletal muscle protein synthesis during bed rest. *J Appl Physiol* 1997;82:807–810.
19. Evans WJ, Fisher EC, Hoerr RA, Young VR. Protein metabolism and endurance exercise. *Phys Sports Med* 1983;11:63–72.
20. Tarnopolsky MA, MacDougall JD, Atkinson SA. Influence of protein intake and training status on nitrogen balance and lean body mass. *J Appl Physiol* 1988;64:187–193.
21. Meredith CN, Zackin MJ, Frontera WR, Evans WJ. Dietary protein requirements and protein metabolism in endurance-trained men. *J Appl Physiol* 1989;66:2850–2856.
22. Friedman JE, Lemon PWR. Effect of chronic endurance exercise on the retention of dietary protein. *Int J Sports Med* 1989; 10:118–123.
23. Phillips SM, Atkinson SA, Tarnopolsky MA, MacDougall JD. Gender differences in leucine kinetics and nitrogen balance in endurance athletes. *J Appl Physiol* 1993;75:2134–2141.
24. Fern EB, Bielinski RN, Schutz Y. Effects of exaggerated amino acid and protein supply in man. *Experientia* 1991;47:168–172.
25. Lemon PWR, Tarnopolsky MA, MacDougall JD, Atkinson SA. Protein requirements and muscle mass/strength changes during intensive training in novice bodybuilders. *J Appl Physiol* 1992; 73:767–775.
26. Tarnopolsky MA, Atkinson SA, MacDougall JD, Chesley A, Phillips S, Schwarcz H. Evaluation of protein requirements for trained strength athletes. *J Appl Physiol* 1992;73:1986–1995.
27. Wolfe RR. *Radioactive and stable isotope tracers in biomedicine: principles and practice of kinetic analysis.* New York: Wiley-Liss, 1992.
28. Munro HN. Carbohydrate and fat as factors in protein utilization and metabolism. *Physiol Rev* 1951;31:449–488.
29. Young VR, Bier DM, Pellet PL. A theoretical basis for increasing current estimates of the amino acid requirements in adult man with experimental support. *Am J Clin Nutr* 1989;50:80–92.
30. Vukovich MD, Sharp RL, King DS, Kershishnik K. The effect of protein supplementation on lactate accumulation during submaximal and maximal exercise. *Int J Sport Nutr* 1992;2:307–316.
31. Dragan GI, Vasiliu A, Georgescu E. Effect of increased supply of protein on elite weightlifters. In: Galesloot TE, Tinbergen BJ, eds. *Milk proteins '84.* Wageningen, the Netherlands: Pudoc, 1985:99–103.
32. Felig P, Wahren J. Amino acid metabolism in exercising man. *J Clin Invest* 1971;50:2703–2714.
33. Ruderman NB, Berger M. The formation of glutamine and alanine in skeletal muscle. *J Biol Chem* 1974;249:5500–5506.
34. Haralambie G, Berg A. Serum urea and amino nitrogen changes with exercise duration. *Eur J Appl Physiol* 1976;36:39–48.
35. Lemon PWR, Mullin JP. Effect of initial muscle glycogen levels on protein catabolism during exercise. *J Appl Physiol* 1980; 48:624–629.
36. Lemon PWR, Nagle FJ, Mullin JP, Benevenga NJ. In vivo leucine oxidation at rest and during two intensities of exercise. *J Appl Physiol* 1982;53:947–954.
37. Lemon PWR, Benevenga NJ, Mullin JP, Nagle FJ. Effect of daily exercise and food intake on leucine oxidation. *Biochem Med* 1985;33:67–76.
38. Babij P, Matthews SM, Rennie MJ. Changes in blood ammonia, lactate and amino acids in relation to workload during bicycle ergometer exercise in man. *Eur J Appl Physiol* 1983;50:405–411.
39. Dohm GL, Hecker AL, Brown WE, et al. Adaptation of protein metabolism to endurance training. *Biochem J* 1977;164:705–708.
40. Henderson SA, Black AL, Brooks GA. Leucine turnover in trained rats during exercise. *Am J Physiol* 1985;249:E137–E144.
41. Layman DK, Paul GL, Olken MH. Amino acid metabolism during exercise. In: Wolinsky I, Hickson JF, eds. *Nutrition in exercise and sport,* 2nd ed. Boca Raton: CRC Press, 1994.
42. Gontzea I, Sutzescu P, Dumitrache S. The influence of muscular activity on the nitrogen balance and on the need of man for proteins. *Nutr Rep Int* 1974;10:35–43.
43. Kasperek GJ, Snider RD. Effect of exercise intensity and starvation on the activation of branched-chain keto acid dehydrogenase by exercise. *Am J Physiol* 1987;252:E33–E37.
44. Carraro F, Kimbrough TD, Wolfe RR. Urea kinetics in humans at two levels of exercise intensity. *J Appl Physiol* 1993;75:1180–1185.
45. Garrel DR, Delmas PD, Welsh C, Arnaud MJ, Hamilton SE, Pugeat MM. Effects of moderate physical training on prednisone-induced protein wasting: a study of whole-body and bone protein metabolism. *Metabolism* 1988;37:257–262.
46. Todd KS, Butterfield GE, Calloway DH. Nitrogen balance in men

with adequate and deficient intake at three levels of work. *J Nutr* 1984;114:2107–2118.
47. Butterfield GE, Calloway DH. Physical activity improves protein utilization in young men. *Br J Nutr* 1984;51:171–184.
48. Newsholme EA, Parry-Billings M. Effects of exercise on the immune system. In: Bouchard C, Shephard RJ, Stephens T, eds. *Physical activity, fitness, and health.* Champaign, IL: Human Kinetics, 1994:451–455.
49. Blomstrand E, Hassmén P, Ekblom B, Newsholme E. Administration of branched-chain amino acids during sustained exercise: effects on performance and on plasma concentrations of some amino acids. *Eur J Appl Physiol* 1991;63:83–88.
50. Mittleman KD, Ricci MR, Baily SP. Branched-chain amino acids prolong exercise during heat stress in men and women. *Med Sci Sports Exerc* 1998;30:83–91.
51. Blomstrand E, Hassmén P, Ek S, Ekblom B, Newsholme EA. Influence of ingesting a solution of branched-chain amino acids on perceived exertion during exercise. *Acta Physiol Scand* 1997;159:41–49.
52. Madsen K, Maclean DA, Kiens B, Christensen D. Effects of glucose, glucose plus branched-chain amino acids or placebo on bike performance over 100 km. *J Appl Physiol* 1996;81:2544–2650.
53. Van Hall G, Raaymakers JSH, Saris WHM, Wagenmakers AJM. Ingestion of branched-chain amino acids and tryptophan during sustained exercise in man: failure to affect performance. *J Physiol* 1995;486:789–794.
54. Lemon PWR. Do athletes need more dietary protein and amino acids? *Int J Sport Nutr* 1995;5:S39–S61.
55. Laritcheva KA, Yalavaya NI, Shubin VI, Smornov PV. Study of energy expenditure and protein needs of top weightlifters. In: Parizkova J, Rogozkin VA, eds. *Nutrition, physical fitness and health.* Baltimore: University Park Press, 1978:155–163.
56. Griggs RC, Kingston W, Jozefowicz RF, Herr BE, Forbes G, Halliday D. Effect of testosterone on muscle mass and protein synthesis. *J Appl Physiol* 1989;66:498–503.
57. Bhasin S, Storer TW, Berman N, et al. The effects of supraphysiologic doses of testosterone on muscle size and strength in normal men. *N Engl J Med* 1996;335:1–7.
58. Tesch PA. Acute and longterm metabolic changes consequent to heavy-resistance exercise. In: Hebbelinck M, Shephard RJ, eds. *Medicine and sports science,* vol 26. Basel: Karger, 1987:67–89.
59. Sherman WM, Costill DL, Fink WJ, Miller JM. The effect of exercise and diet manipulation on muscle glycogen and its subsequent use during performance. *Int J Sports Med* 1981;2:114–118.
60. Ivy JL, Katz AL, Culter CL, Sherman WM, Coyle EF. Muscle glycogen synthesis after exercise: effect of time of carbohydrate ingestion. *J Appl Physiol* 1988;64:1480–1485.
61. Roy BD, Tarnopolsky MA, MacDougall JD, Fowles J, Yarasheski KE. Effect of glucose supplement timing on protein metabolism after resistance training. *J Appl Physiol* 1997;82:1882–1888.
62. Biolo G, Tipton KD, Klein S, Wolfe RR. An abundant supply of amino acids enhances the metabolic effect of exercise on muscle protein. *Am J Physiol* 1997;273:E122–E129.
63. Greenhaff PL, Casey A, Short AH, Harris R, Söderlund K. Influence of oral creatine supplementation of muscle torque during repeated bouts of maximum voluntary exercise in man. *Clin Sci* 1993;84:565–571.
64. Casey A, Constantin-Teodosiu D, Howell S, Hultman E, Greenhaff PL. Creatine ingestion favorably affects performance and muscle metabolism during maximal exercise in humans. *Am J Physiol* 1996;271:E31–E37.
65. Harris RC, Söderlund K, Hultman E. Evaluation of creatine in resting and exercising muscle of normal subjects by creatine supplementation. *Clin Sci* 1992;83:367–374.
66. Ingwall JS, Weiner CD, Morales MF, Davis E, Stockdale FE. Specificity of creatine in the control of muscle protein synthesis. *J Cell Biol* 1974;62:145–151.
67. Häussinger D, Roth E, Lang F, Gerok W. Cellular hydration state: an important determinant of protein catabolism in health and disease. *Lancet* 1993;341:1330–1332.
68. Krieder RB, Ferreira M, Wilson M, Grindstaff P, Plisk S. Effects of creatine supplementation on body composition, strength, and sprint performance. *Med Sci Sports Exerc* 1998;30:73–82.
69. Campbell WW, Crim MC, Dallal GE, Young VR, Evans WJ. Increased protein requirements in elderly people: new data and retrospective reassessments. *Am J Clin Nutr* 1994;60:501–509.
70. Campbell WW, Crim MC, Young VR, Joseph LJ, Evans WJ. Effects of resistance training and dietary protein intake on protein metabolism in older adults. *Am J Physiol* 1995;268: E1143–E1153.
71. Castaneda C, Charnley JM, Evans WJ, Crim MS. Elderly women accommodate to a low protein diet with losses in body cell mass, muscle function, and immune response. *Am J Clin Nutr* 1995; 62:30–39.
72. Castaneda C, Dolnikowski GG, Dallal GE, Evans WJ, Crim MC. Protein turnover and energy metabolism of elderly women fed a low protein diet. *Am J Clin Nutr* 1995;62:40–48.
73. Welle S, Thornton C, Statt M. Myofibrillar protein synthesis in young and old human subjects after three months of resistance training. *Am J Physiol* 1995;268:E422–E427.
74. Lamont LS, Lemon PWR, Bruot BC. Menstrual cycle and exercise effects on protein catabolism. *Med Sci Sports Exerc* 1987; 19:106–110.
75. Tarnopolsky LJ, MacDougall JD, Atkinson SA, Tarnopolsky MA, Sutton JR. Gender differences in substrate for endurance exercise. *J Appl Physiol* 1990;68:302–308.
76. Tipton KD, Ferrando AA Williams BD, Wolfe RR. Muscle protein metabolism in female swimmers after a combination of resistance and endurance exercise. *J Appl Physiol* 1996;81:2034–2038.

PART II

Physiology of Exercise

Exercise and Sport Science,
edited by William E. Garrett, Jr., and Donald T. Kirkendall.
Lippincott Williams & Wilkins, Philadelphia © 2000.

CHAPTER 4

Measurement of Work and Power in Sport

Jay T. Kearney, Kenneth W. Rundell, and Randall L. Wilber

WORK/POWER TESTS

One of the challenges confronting the sports scientist/sports medicine professional is to understand the factors contributing to successful performance. The ability to do work or generate power is a major determinant of performance in many sports. Consequently, it is important to be able to measure this capacity and incorporate the data in performance analysis and training feedback for athletes and coaches. The uses of work/power tests include:

1. Assessing current capacity and comparison with established norms.
2. Monitoring changes in physiologic capacity as a result of training.
3. Determining event characterization.
4. Establishing a goal for a rehabilitation program.
5. Identifying talent or providing guidance in event selection.
6. Serving as a motivational tool.

Although the objectives of testing, the instruments used, and the interpretation of results may be unique in each of these six applications, they are also interrelated.

Assessment of Current Status

The use of field or laboratory-based tests for measurement of work and/or power output capacity can provide an athlete and coach with information relative to the athlete's current physiologic capability and can allow them to compare that capacity to reference values for appropriate peer groups. The assessment of current status reveals strengths and limitations and serves as the basis for developing an optimal training program. It can also serve as the foundation for the development of a competitive strategy. For example, if athletes know they have very high power output capacity but limited endurance, their competition strategy should be designed to exploit this strength.

Consistent monitoring of work or power output capacity should be done at regular intervals throughout the year. A one-time assessment is only a snapshot and provides limited information. The relevance of a one-time assessment is to compare the athlete's current status with an appropriate reference group. Sports medicine/science professionals should design yearly programs so that athletes have the opportunity to be tested repeatedly at key times during the training cycle.

Efficacy of Training

One of the principal uses of field and/or laboratory-based work and power assessments is to monitor changes in physiologic capacity as a result of training. By using serial administration of appropriate test batteries, the coach can objectively track change that occurs as a result of training. The greater our ability to characterize training-induced changes, the more effective we can be in designing and modifying a training program. Responses to training are unique for each athlete; therefore, the training stimuli in a program need to be targeted as specifically as possible. For example, a coach training a group of sprint cyclists may be emphasizing strength training in October through December. Repetitive testing may reveal that only about half of the athletes are increasing their cycling sprint power. This information would allow the coach to reassess program design characteristics (days/week, number of sets, number of repetitions, specific exercises used, etc.) and traits of the nonresponding athletes in an attempt to improve the effectiveness of the training program. In this case, repeated application of appropriate tests is an invaluable aid.

J. T. Kearney and R. L. Wilber: Sport Science and Technology Division, United States Olympic Committee, Colorado Springs, Colorado 80909.

K. W. Rundell: Sport Science and Technology Division, United States Olympic Committee, 421 Old Military Road, Lake Placid, New York 12946.

Event Characterization

Field and laboratory-based assessments of work and power output capacity are a critical component of event characterization. Individuals who are successful in an event can be evaluated using work/power tests designed to determine the underlying physiologic capabilities, and thereby establish an event-specific profile. This profile of the successful athlete can be used in talent identification and event-selection programs, and can serve as a training goal for developing athletes. The sports medicine professional is cautioned that all performances are multifactorial, and thus strength or weakness on any single test will never guarantee or preclude success.

Rehabilitation

A well-designed rehabilitation program needs a reference point or goal. Work or power output capability assessments on an athlete, before an injury has occurred, or on the uninjured joint, can provide a target for the rehabilitation program. There are some individuals who believe that the goal of rehabilitation should actually be to elevate the performance capacity of the involved joint above the preinjury level. The theory behind this philosophy is that if the joint was unable to withstand the insult of the activity initially, it should be stronger or have a higher functional capacity in its rehabilitated state to prevent reinjury. Field and laboratory-based assessments can provide data to assist in development of rehabilitation goals.

Talent Identification or Event Selection

The work and power output requirements of different sports and events vary greatly. For example, if we consider the events in the continuum of track and field with times from 10 seconds to just over 2 hours, the power output or work capacity required of an athlete is obviously different. Similarly, the characteristics that allow an individual to be optimally successful in the shot put are very different from those that lead to successful performance as a pole vaulter. Field and laboratory-based testing provide an athlete and coach with information for the selection of an event in which the athlete may have the greatest likelihood of success. These physiologic capabilities should be combined with anthropometric, motoric, and psychologic characteristics. One of the factors that is critically important for individuals participating in sport is enjoyment. Most individuals enjoy achieving "success" in competitive sport. Therefore, it is important that we provide athletes with the capability of achieving success by directing their efforts toward events in which they have the greatest chance of success.

Motivation

The measurement of work or power output capacity has the potential to be a strong motivational aid. Initially, an athlete can use an appropriate norm or standard as a goal. The simple act of having an established nonperformance-specific goal can be motivational and less threatening than a performance-based goal or race. As athletes perform the work/power test over time, they can observe their improvement and have confidence that their training is effective. This motivational factor is strengthened if they can also observe a relationship between improvement on the test results and actual performance.

Terminology

The terms *force, work*, and *power* are often used to describe athletic activity. For example, a volleyball spike may be called "forceful," a 1500-m runner may be described as "working very hard to maintain the pace," or an Olympic weightlifter may be referred to as "a powerful athlete." From a scientific perspective, however, these terms have very precise meanings. It is critical to know the scientific definition of these terms to avoid confusion and inaccuracy. In addition, it is important to understand the interrelationships among force, work, and power as they apply in sports medicine and science.

Force

Force can be described as that which causes or tends to cause a change in an object's motion. More precisely, force (F) is defined as the product of mass (m) times acceleration (a). The SI unit of measure for force is a newton (N), which is equal to the force that accelerates a 1.0-kg mass at a rate of 1.0 m/s^2 (assuming the acceleration of gravity is 9.807 m/s^2). For example, a basketball player must apply a force of approximately 9.8 N to hold a basketball (mass ~1.0 kg) at waist height:

$$F = m \times a$$
$$F = 1.0\ \text{kg} \times 9.8\ \text{m/s}^2 \qquad [1]$$
$$F = 9.8\ \text{N}$$

Work

Work is defined as the product of the force (F) applied to an object and the linear distance (d) the object moves as a result of the applied force. The SI unit of measure for work is a joule (J), which is equal to the amount of work performed when an object is moved a linear distance of 1.0 m against an opposing force of 1.0 N. For example, when basketball players prepare to make an inbound pass, they raise the basketball (~1.0 kg) from below the waist to high above the head (~1.0 m). In doing so they perform 9.8 J of work as shown in Eq. 2:

$$Work = F \times d$$

$$Work = (1.0\ \text{kg} \times 9.8\ \text{m/s}^2) \times (1.0\ \text{m})$$

$$Work = (9.8\ \text{N}) \times (1.0\ \text{m}) \quad [2]$$

$$Work = 9.8\ \text{Nm}$$

[NOTE: 1 newton-meter (Nm) = 1 joule (J)]

$$Work = 9.8\ \text{J}$$

Power

Power is defined as the amount of work per unit of time (t):

$$P = Work/t \quad [3]$$

The SI unit of measure for power is a watt (W) (a work rate of 1.0 J/sec = 1 W). In the previous example, the basketball player performed 9.8 J of work in raising the basketball overhead in preparation for an inbound pass. If this movement is completed in approximately 1.5 sec, the basketball player produces 6.5 W of power as shown below:

$$P = Work/t$$

$$P = 9.8\ \text{J}/1.5\ \text{s}$$

$$P = 6.5\ \text{J/s}$$

$$P = 6.5\ \text{W}$$

Substituting Eq. 2 for work, Eq. 3 can be expressed as:

$$P = (F \times d)/t \quad [4]$$

$$P = [(1.0\ \text{kg} \times 9.8\ \text{m/s}^2) \times 1.0\ \text{m}]/1.5\ \text{s}$$

Equation 4 can be rewritten mathematically as:

$$P = F \times (d/t) \quad [5]$$

$$P = (1.0\ \text{kg} \times 9.8\ \text{m/s}^2) \times (1.0\ \text{m}/1.5\ \text{s})$$

Since velocity (v) is equal to linear displacement relative to the change in time (d/t), power can be expressed in final form as:

$$P = F \times v \quad [6]$$

Thus, power is precisely defined as the product of the force (F) exerted on an object directly against gravity, and the velocity (v) of the object in the direction in which the force is exerted. Using the basketball example and Eq. 6, power can be calculated as follows:

$$P = F \times v$$

$$P = (1.0\ \text{kg} \times 9.8\ \text{m/s}^2) \times (1.0\ \text{m}/1.5\ \text{s})$$

$$P = 9.8\ \text{N} \times (1.0\ \text{m}/1.5\text{s})$$

$$P = 9.8\ \text{Nm}/1.5\ \text{s}$$

$$P = 6.5\ \text{Nm/s}$$

$$P = 6.5\ \text{J/s}$$

$$P = 6.5\ \text{W}$$

Translational Versus Rotational Work

In the previous example, the basketball player raised a basketball from below the waist to high above the head in preparation for an inbound pass. This movement is defined as *linear* motion because it involves the linear movement of the basketball's center of mass from one point in space to another and directly against gravity. Movements that exhibit linear motion produce *translational* work. Translational work and power are defined by Eqs. 2 and 6, respectively.

In performing an arm curl, a weightlifter flexes/extends at the elbow while simultaneously keeping the shoulder and wrist joints in a "locked" position. The elbow joint serves as the pivot point with the biceps brachii and brachialis muscles involved in lifting and lowering the weight. In this exercise, the movement of the forearm can be defined as *rotary* motion because it involves the rotary or angular movement of an object around its axis of rotation, that is, the elbow joint. Movements that exhibit rotary motion produce *rotational* work. Rotational work is defined as the product of torque (T) and angular displacement (θ):

$$Work = T \times \theta \quad [7]$$

Torque ($F \times d\perp$) is defined as the product of a force (F) acting on an object or limb and the perpendicular distance ($d\perp$) from the line of action of the force to the axis of rotation. The SI unit of measure for torque is a newton-meter (Nm). Angular displacement (θ) is defined as the angle through which the object or limb rotates and is expressed in radians (1 radian = 57.30 degrees).

Similar to translational power, rotational power (P) can be defined as the amount of rotational work performed per unit of time (t):

$$P = Work/t \quad [8]$$

Substituting Eq. 7 for rotational work, Eq. 8 can be expressed as:

$$P = (T \times \theta)/t \quad [9]$$

Equation 9 can be rewritten mathematically as:

$$P = T \times (\theta/t) \quad [10]$$

Since angular velocity (ω) is equal to the change in angular position relative to the change in time (θ/t), rotational power can be expressed in final form as:

$$P = T \times \omega \quad [11]$$

Thus, rotational power is precisely defined as the product of the torque (T) exerted by an object or limb rotating about a fixed axis, and the angular velocity (ω) of the object or limb through the measured range of motion. Like translational power, the SI unit of measure for rotational power is a watt (W), but it is sometimes expressed in newton-meters per second [(Nm/s), 1 W = 1 Nm/s] or foot-pounds per second [(ft-lbs/s), 1 W = 0.7378 ft-lbs/s].

Although translational and rotational work can be individually defined and quantified, it is important to realize that many athletic movements and skills involve both. For example, when gymnasts perform a floor exercise, they usually include a somersault component, thereby combining both translational and rotational work. Gymnasts move linearly across the mat (translational work) while simultaneously performing a series of somersaults involving rotation around their center of gravity (rotational work).

Anaerobic Power and Capacity

The terms *anaerobic power* and *anaerobic capacity* are typically used in reference to the two anaerobic energy systems, adenosine triphosphate–creatine phosphate (ATP-CP) and anaerobic glycolysis. Traditionally, sport scientists have considered anaerobic power to be a measure of the ATP-CP system, and anaerobic capacity to be a measure of anaerobic glycolysis. In the 30-second Wingate test, for example, anaerobic power is defined as the maximum power (W, W/kg) generated, whereas anaerobic capacity is defined as the average power (W, W/kg) and/or total work (J, J/kg) calculated over the entire 30-second test. However, use of the terms *anaerobic power* and *anaerobic capacity* in reference to the ATP-CP and anaerobic glycolytic energy systems, respectively, may not be accurate. Recent research has suggested that anaerobic glycolysis makes a significant contribution (44%) to total energy produced during the first 10 seconds of a 30-second Wingate test (1). Similarly, the aerobic energy contribution during a 30-second Wingate test has been estimated to be between 18% and 28% of total energy production (1,2). Nevertheless, the "traditional" definitions of these terms are used in this chapter.

Test Characteristics

Desirable test characteristics are validity, reliability, and objectivity. For a test to provide useful information, all three characteristics must be present. A test is *valid* if it measures what it purports to measure. A valid field or laboratory-based test of work or power output capacity must therefore (a) be technically precise in recording the work or power being performed, and (b) measure a trait that is relevant to performance. For example, the 10-second version of the Wingate test requires that an athlete pedal a cycle ergometer, with a predetermined resistance, as rapidly as possible for 10 seconds. The technical validity of this power assessment relies on the calibration and accurate recording of the resistance applied by the ergometer and the distance that the flywheel travels during the time interval. An accurate assessment of an athlete's power output can then be made using the precisely measured resistance, distance, and time. The appropriateness of using a Wingate test for assessing or predicting performance capacity is the second necessary consideration in the evaluation of validity. For example, if we take three activities—the 100-m running sprint, the 200-m match sprint in cycling, and soccer—work and power output capacity are important determinants of performance in each. However, it is intuitive that the use of the Wingate test is most appropriate or valid for assessing 200-m match sprint capacity, intermediately related to 100-m running sprint ability, and probably only marginally related to soccer performance. There are also numerous research studies that document this conclusion (3).

The second necessary test characteristic is *reliability*, the ability to repeatedly obtain a similar score on the same subject over repeated administrations. Two groups of factors affect reliability: (a) biologic variability, and (b) experimental error. Biologic variability or consistency of performance on a test is impacted by factors such as circadian rhythms, residual impact of training or competition, subclinical illness, motivation, seasonal training effects, and habituation to the test. Factors associated with experimental error include standardized procedures, equipment calibration, and trained technicians. Some available methods (3a) attempt to establish the relative contribution of the technical and biologic elements to the reliability of assessment. A laboratory should have a reasonable estimate of the reliability of an assessment tool prior to its use on a client or athlete group. Denegar and Ball (4) present a treatise on the procedures that should be followed to establish reliability and precision of measurement. It is not unusual to have a variability of plus or minus 3% to 5% on repeated administration of the same test to the same individuals. This range of variability adds a challenge to interpretation of information for individuals at the high end of the performance spectrum. For example, if the variability of a test result, standard error of measurement, is as large as the expected rate of gain from training over the time period between repeated administrations of the test, the sports medicine professional cannot provide the athlete and coach with a definitive answer on the efficacy of training.

A third characteristic of assessment tools is *objectivity*. To be objective, a test must have the ability to obtain the same results when administered by different individuals and in different circumstances. One of the precautions that can be used to optimize objectivity is to very clearly describe the protocol, procedures, and conditions under which a test will be administered. The more specific these descriptions are, the more reliable and objective the results will be. As an example of objectivity, if athletes were tested at each of the three Olympic Training Centers, they would get comparable results.

Relationship Between Work, Power Output Capacity, and Competitive Success

In many sports endeavors, the relationship between an individual's work and power output capacity and performance ability is defined by an exponential relationship as illustrated in Fig. 4–1. As we progressively increase the velocity that an athlete wishes to achieve, the power output required to achieve each subsequent increment in velocity increases in exponential order. Interestingly, specific paces needed to achieve competitive success lie at the point on that curve where the power output requirement to gain an increase in velocity is very large. For example, in cycling, the increase in power output required to increase the velocity from 30 to 35 km/h is approximately 45 W. To increase from 40 to 45 km/h, approximately 75 W is required. The power output needed to increase from 50 to 55 km/h is significantly greater, and approaches 200 W. The consequence of this relationship is that within the range of competitive paces, the increase in work or power output capacity to make each small, incremental change in velocity becomes larger and larger. As such, it is important that the sports medicine professional and coach have the ability to make accurate assessments of the underlying power output capability of athletes in a particular sport event.

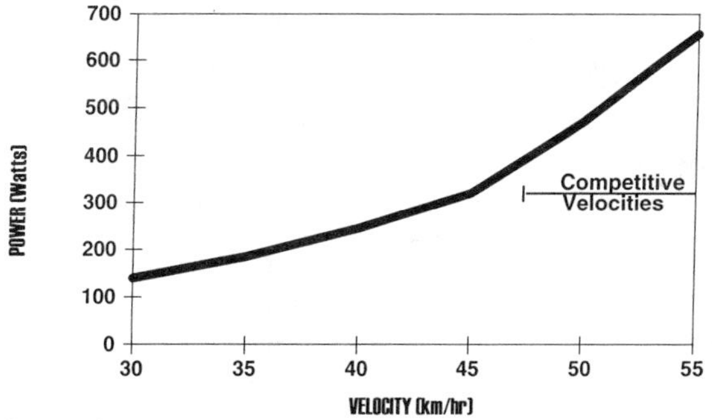

FIG. 4–1. Relationships among power output, velocity, and competitive performance.

SPORT-SPECIFIC TESTS

The testing philosophy employed at the Sport Science and Technology Division of the United States Olympic Committee (USOC) is based on the belief that work and/or power output capacity tests need to be sport-specific. With the exception of talent identification and event selection, each of the six applications of testing requires protocols selected or tailored to the requirements of the sport. In this section, we provide an overview of sport-specific tests, administration procedures, and information on interpretation of results for athletes and coaches.

Alpine Skiing

Alpine ski racing events range in duration from about 45 seconds to almost 3 minutes. Because of the aerodynamic "tuck" to reduce wind drag (at speeds that may exceed 140 km/h) and the high forces incurred during turns, exceptional leg strength and anaerobic power/capacity are characteristic of alpine racers. Muscle biopsy studies that have assessed the rate of glycogen utilization demonstrate that elite alpine skiers rely heavily on both slow- and fast-twitch muscle fibers. Post-race blood lactate levels typically reach 15 mmol/L (5). The high anaerobic energy contribution during alpine racing is thought to be in part a consequence of impaired blood flow to the quadriceps due to the required static component of the racing posture. In turn, this compromises aerobic energy metabolism by decreasing oxygen delivery to the working muscle. When compared to athletes of other sports, alpine skiers were found to have the highest enzyme activity of lactate dehydrogenase and creatine phosphokinase, enzymes important in anaerobic metabolism (6). Alpine skiers have traditionally been evaluated for anaerobic power and capacity by cycle ergometry and various field tests.

Wingate Test

The Wingate test has been successfully used to assess anaerobic power and capacity with durations of 30 and 90 seconds (7–11). The 30-second Wingate test is thought by some to be too short to exhaust anaerobic energy stores (12). Consequently, Simoneau and colleagues (13) suggested that a 90-second Wingate test be used to evaluate alpine skiers. This was supported by Stark and colleagues (10), who identified a crossover effect between slalom and downhill skiers at about 40 seconds. Slalom skiers demonstrated higher peak power with greater fatigue over 90 seconds, while downhill skiers were able to perform the test with less fatigue. More recent data support the use of the 90-second test (9). Significant correlations between Wingate test performance and racing ability have been found for both

TABLE 4–1. *Thirty-second Wingate power test results for international (Int), national (Nat), and regional (Reg) alpine skiers*

		Male			Female		
		Int $n = 12$	Nat $n = 8$	Reg $n = 11$	Int $n = 17$	Nat $n = 6$	Reg $n = 7$
Max. power (W/kg)	Mean	10.6	11.8	11.2	10.6	10.2	9.8
	SEM	0.30	0.36	0.28	0.21	0.37	0.30
Max. power (W)	Mean	836	859	772	669	650	572
	SEM	26	39	37	14	25	30

SEM, standard error of the mean. From White AT, Johnson SC. Physiological comparison of international, national, and regional alpine skiers. *Int J Sports Med* 1991;12:374–378.

30- and 90-second tests for females. Performance on the 90-second test is a superior predictor for males. Additionally, White and Johnson (11) reported significantly higher Wingate scores for international level skiers compared to regional level skiers. These data, summarized in Table 4–1, substantiate the critical importance of anaerobic power and endurance in alpine racing. The typical load used for alpine skiers (female and male) has been 7.5% of total body weight (kg) for both test durations. The U.S. Ski Team currently uses a 30-second Wingate test with a load of 7.5% of total body weight for both female and male athletes. The testing procedure is identical to that used for cyclists and is described in detail in the section devoted to cycling.

Field Tests

Various standardized field tests have been used to identify ski racing potential (7,8,11,14). The medals test used by the U.S. Ski Team includes 40- and 400-m sprints; a 1-mile run; a 90-second, 40-cm box jump; and a hexagonal obstacle test (11). The apparatus for the hexagonal obstacle test is a PVC pipe frame with outside barriers at heights between 20 and 30 cm. The test requires athletes to jump in and out of the frame until they have completed three revolutions both clockwise and counterclockwise. The Canadian Ski Federation uses a test battery that includes a 30-second Wingate test; a 20-m shuttle run; a double-leg jump test; a 90-second, 40-cm box jump; and a hexagonal obstacle jump. Of the seven field tests in the U.S. battery, only the hexagonal obstacle test and the box jump test have been shown to be related to racing performance (15). In a similar study, Anderson and colleagues (8) reported significant correlations between ski racing performance and the 90-second box jump (r = .80), double-leg jump (r = −0.86), and Hex test (r = 0.82). It is important to note, however, that the Hex test has been described as a measure of agility rather than specific anaerobic power (16). Performances for these levels of Canadian skiers are presented in Table 4–2.

Canoe/Kayak

There are two primary disciplines in Olympic canoe and kayak racing: sprint and slalom. In sprinting, men and women compete in single, double, and four-person kayaks, which are closed-hull boats paddled in a sitting position with a double-bladed paddle. Men also compete in single, double, and four-person canoes, which are open-hull boats paddled from a high kneeling position with a single-bladed paddle. Sprint races range in length from 200 m (35 to 40 seconds) to 1000 m (3 to 4 minutes), and are contested on a flat-water course similar to rowing.

Slalom racing involves single kayaks for men and women and single and double canoes for men. In competition, slalom boats are required to travel through desig-

TABLE 4–2. *Test battery results for the Canadian club, divisional and provincial alpine skiers*

		20-m shuttle run test (min)	60-s Wingate test: Peak power (W)	60-s Wingate test: Peak power (W/kg)	Hexagonal obstacle test (sec)	90-s high box jump test (jumps)	Double-leg jumping test (m)	Vertical jump test (cm)
Club	Mean	8.3	621.4	10.5	54.7	56.2	10.8	44.7
(n = 11)	SD	0.6	70.3	0.4	3.6	3.2	0.4	1.8
Divisional	Mean	10.6	836.3	12.2	36.4	85.3	13.1	53.4
(n = 14)	SD	0.3	27.3	0.5	1.1	3.3	0.2	1.8
Provincial	Mean	11.2	793.1	11.4	34.3	93.6	13.1	54.4
(n = 9)	SD	0.3	25.9	0.3	0.9	2.2	0.2	2.2

SD, standard deviation. From Andersen RE, Montgomery DL, Turcotte RA. An on-site test battery to evaluate giant slalom skiing performance. *J Sports Med Phys Fitness* 1990;30:276–282.

nated gates in rapidly flowing water. Racing requires a combination of sprinting, rapid turning, and paddling with and against the current. Typical races are 90 to 150 seconds in duration.

The laboratory and field tests described below are focused on the peak power and power endurance components of performance in both disciplines. Other protocols such as a paddling-specific oxygen uptake test would be included in a complete test battery.

Fifteen-Second Sprint

The objective of the 15-second sprint is to determine an athlete's anaerobic power, specifically peak power (W, W/kg), average power (W, W/kg) and time to peak power (s). The test is conducted on a commercially available paddling ergometer (K1, Roger Cargill, Garran, Australia) which is designed to simulate the kinematics of canoe and kayak paddling exercise, and can accurately measure power output via an optical sensor measuring device. An interface unit allows the optical sensor to relay data to a computer for calculation of power output. Prior to the test the athlete is required to warm up on the paddling ergometer. Upon completion of the warm-up, the test begins and the athlete performs the 15-second sprint at maximal effort. Verbal encouragement is provided throughout the test.

Two-Minute Race Simulation

The 2-minute simulated canoe/kayak race is also conducted on a K1 paddling ergometer and is typically administered in conjunction with the 15-second sprint. It is recommended that the 2-minute simulated race be performed approximately 60 minutes after the sprint to allow adequate recovery. The test consists of a 2-minute sustained effort during which time the athlete attempts to replicate the physiologic demands and power requirements of an actual race performance. After a thorough warm-up on the ergometer, the athlete begins the test and is periodically kept apprised of the time completed in order to allow him or her to use optimal pacing and sprint tactics. The recommended strategy during the test is to start strong, maintain a competitive pace during the first minute, build gradually during the second minute, and finish with a maximal sprint.

The primary objective of the 2-minute simulated race is to determine anaerobic capacity including average power (W, W/kg) and total work (J, J/kg). In addition, the percentage of 15-second sprint *peak* power (2-minute average power/15-second peak power) and the percentage of 15-second sprint *average* power (2-minute average power/15-second average power) are calculated for the purpose of determining a paddling athlete's ability to maintain maximal power output. These are important training parameters for canoe/kayak athletes since they compete in high-intensity, short-duration (35 seconds to 4 minutes) events requiring sustained and relatively high power output. Female sprint kayakers evaluated at the United States Olympic Training Centers (USOTC) were able to sustain 50% of the peak power (333 W) and 54% of the average power (306 W) generated during the 15-second sprint test. Male sprint canoeists and kayakers sustained 53% and 57%, respectively, of the peak power (canoe = 366 W, kayak = 571 W) and 66% and 67%, respectively, of the average power (canoe = 296 W, kayak = 491 W) produced in the 15-second sprint test.

Thirty-Second Upper Body Wingate Test

The 30-second upper body Wingate test is similar in format to the standard 30-second cycle ergometer Wingate test except that it is performed using the musculature of the upper body (arms, shoulders, chest, upper back) and therefore requires a more moderate test resistance. The objectives of the upper body Wingate test are to determine (a) anaerobic power [peak power (W, W/kg), time to peak power (s)], (b) anaerobic capacity [average power (W, W/kg), total work (J, J/kg)], and (c) fatigue rate (%). The test is conducted using a pan-loaded, mechanically braked arm crank ergometer used in conjunction with a commercially available optical sensor measuring system (SMI, St. Cloud, MN). A standard Monark 824E cycle ergometer (Monark, Stockholm, Sweden) can be easily adapted for this test by mounting it securely to a table or counter. The pedals are modified so that only the spindles (padded and taped) are used to crank the ergometer. It is recommended that athletes wear padded cycling gloves while performing the test.

The athlete is seated in front of the arm crank ergometer and positioned so that the glenohumeral joint is aligned with the center of the ergometer crank. A standardized warm-up on the ergometer precedes the test and consists of 5 minutes of moderate pedaling [1.0% total body weight (TBW) resistance for females and males] with a 5-second sprint (1.5% TBW resistance for females, 2.0% TBW resistance for males) done at the 2-, 3-, and 4-minute marks of the 5-minute warm-up. A 3-minute recovery period follows the warm-up. The test is initiated by having the athlete crank at a controlled cadence of 60 rpm. Upon completion of the final countdown, the athlete accelerates and the load is applied (3.0% TBW for females, 4.0% TBW for males). The athlete performs the 30-second maximal sprint and must stay seated during the test. Strong verbal encouragement is provided throughout the entire test. Values for female and male U.S. National Team slalom paddlers are provided in Table 4–3.

Ten × 10-Second K1 Sprint (Slalom)

The purpose of this test is to simulate the paddling effort experienced during a slalom race. The test is designed

TABLE 4–3. *U.S. National Team averages for 30-s and 5 × 30-s upper body (UB) Wingate tests*

	Resistance (% TBW)	Sprint number	Peak power (W)	Peak power (W/kg)	Avg. power (W)	Avg. power (W/kg)	Total work (J)	Total work (J/kg)
30-s UB Wingate								
Slalom kayak, female	3.0	1	335	5.4	308	4.9	9240	148
Slalom canoe/kayak, male	4.0	1	486	6.9	418	6.0	12,543	179
5 × 3 30-s UB Wingate								
Judo, female	2.5	1	225	3.8	199	3.3	5962	99
		2	185	3.1	167	2.7	4931	82
		3	180	3.0	158	2.6	4751	78
		4	166	2.7	146	2.4	4377	71
		5	173	2.8	149	2.4	4468	73
Judo, male	3.5	1	596	5.8	480	4.7	14,386	140
		2	386	3.8	300	2.9	8994	89
		3	333	3.4	253	2.5	7606	76
		4	267	2.9	212	2.1	6374	64
		5	308	3.0	239	2.4	7167	70
Wrestling, male	3.5	1	523	6.3	427	5.2	12,974	157
		2	390	4.7	319	3.9	9575	116
		3	305	3.8	254	3.2	7621	95
		4	276	3.5	232	2.9	6962	88
		5	278	3.5	226	2.8	6773	84

TBW, total body weight.

to examine peak power, 10-second average power, total work, and fatigue over a period of 200 seconds. The test is conducted on a commercially available paddling ergometer (K1, Roger Cargill, Garran, Australia) instrumented and computer-interfaced to measure and record 1-second power output values. Prior to the test, the athlete warms up on the K1 ergometer, interspersing short sprints during the warm-up. The test consists of ten 10-second sprints with a 10-second passive recovery interval between sprints. The athlete is instructed to perform each sprint maximally with no pacing during the test. Data are processed as 1-second peak power and 10-second mean power in W and W/kg for each 10-second bout. Total work (J, J/kg) for the 10 sprints is determined, and a fatigue factor is calculated as the difference between the first two and last two sprint averages divided by the first two sprint averages. Table 4–4 displays results obtained from top U.S. junior slalom paddlers, and Fig. 4–2 is a graphic representation of test results from an individual athlete.

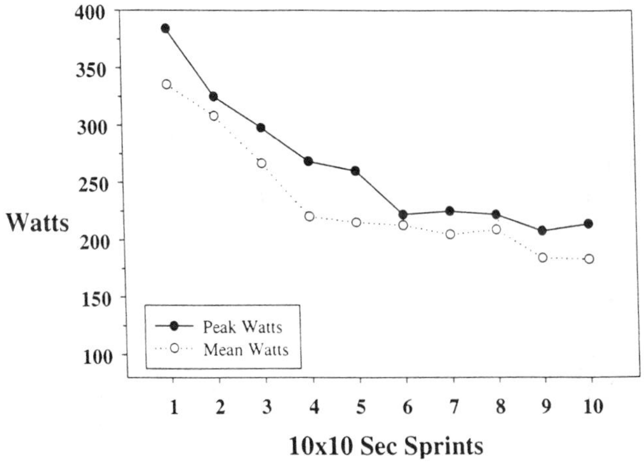

FIG. 4–2. Peak and mean power output (W) during ten × 10-second repeated sprints on K1 ergometer.

TABLE 4–4. *Values of absolute peak 1-s power, relative peak 1-s power, mean of absolute 10-s peak power, mean of relative 10-s peak power, peak % fatigue, mean % fatigue, total absolute work, and total relative work measured during 10-s sprints (10 trials) on a K1 ergometer*

	Peak 1-s (W)	Peak 1-s (W/kg)	Peak Mn 10-s (W)	Peak Mn 10-s (W/kg)	Peak % fatigue	Mean % fatigue	Total work (J)	Total work (J/kg)
Mean	274.7	4.2	240.0	3.7	42.2	40.7	17,530	266.3
SD	69.1	0.8	56.0	0.7	12.3	8.90	4129	47.5

Results are presented as the means and standard deviations (SD) (n = 9).

Combative Sports

Five × 30-Second Upper Body Wingate Test

The five × 30-second upper body Wingate test is used at the USOTC to measure the anaerobic power and capacity as well as the recovery capabilities of elite wrestlers and judo athletes. The test is designed to simulate the power demands of combative sports, which typically require several sequences of powerful, short-duration upper body maneuvers with minimal recovery. The test is conducted using a pan-loaded, mechanically braked arm crank ergometer in conjunction with a commercially available optical sensor measuring system (SMI, St. Cloud, MN). A standard Monark 824E cycle ergometer (Monark, Stockholm, Sweden) can be easily adapted for this test by mounting it securely to a table or counter. The pedals are modified as described in the 30-second upper body Wingate test (see the section on Canoe/Kayak, above) and athletes are encouraged to wear padded cycling gloves while performing the test.

The athlete is seated in front of the arm crank ergometer and positioned so that the glenohumeral joint is aligned with the center of the ergometer crank. A 5-minute warm-up is completed prior to the test at a resistance of 1.0% TBW for both females and males. Athletes are encouraged to perform a few sprints during the warm-up; however, no additional resistance is applied during the sprints. A 3-minute recovery follows the warm-up. The test is initiated by having the athlete pedal at a controlled cadence of 60 rpm. Upon completion of the final countdown, the athlete accelerates and the load is applied (2.5% TBW for females, 3.5% TBW for males). The athlete performs a 30-second maximal sprint and is verbally encouraged throughout the effort. Following a 30-second recovery (active or passive), the procedure is repeated until five 30-second sprints have been completed. The athlete must stay seated while performing each sprint.

The following parameters are measured for each 30-second sprint: (a) anaerobic power [peak power (W, W/kg), time to peak power (s)], (b) anaerobic capacity [average power (W, W/kg), total work (J, J/Kg)], and (c) fatigue rate (%). Values for female and male U.S. National Team athletes are provided in Table 4–3. For exceptionally well-trained wrestlers and judo athletes, the test is repeated twice [3 × (5 × 30-second sprint)] with a 60-minute recovery following each test. This protocol should be limited to well-trained elite athletes and is conducted for the purpose of simulating a competitive scenario in which the athlete is required to compete in several matches in 1 day.

Cycling

The work and/or power output tests used with cyclists must be carefully selected to match either the event requirements or training parameters targeted for evaluation. Cycling includes track events such as match sprints [200 m in 10 to 12 seconds, the kilo in 1:02 (minutes:seconds) to 1:15], individual and team pursuits (3:30 to 4:30) and longer races such as the points race. There is also a wide variety of formats and durations for road races. The tests described below can be used with athletes from a wide range of events depending on the objectives of the assessment.

Ten-Second Wingate Test

The 10-second Wingate test is conducted using a pan-loaded, mechanically braked cycle ergometer equipped with competition racing bars, saddle, pedals, and chain. The test bike is configured to match the exact dimensions (stem height, headset height, and saddle-to-headset distance) of the athlete's competition bicycle. Power output is measured using a commercially available optical sensor system (SMI). The objectives of the 10-second Wingate test are to determine (a) anaerobic power [peak power (W, W/kg), time to peak power (s)], and (b) fatigue rate (%).

A standardized warm-up on the ergometer precedes the test and consists of 5 minutes of moderate cycling (2.0% TBW resistance for females and males) with a 5-second sprint (5.0% TBW resistance for females, 6.6% TBW resistance for males) done at the 2-, 3-, and 4-minute marks of the 5-minute warm-up. A 3-minute recovery period follows the warm-up. The test is initiated by having the athlete pedal at a cadence of 135 rpm. Upon completion of the final countdown, the load is applied (10.0% TBW for females, 13.3% TBW for males) and the athlete performs the 10-second maximal sprint. These loads are significantly greater than the standard resistances recommended for Wingate tests with a normal population (3,17,18). Strong verbal encouragement is provided throughout the entire test. At the USOTC, the 10-second Wingate test is used to assess the anaerobic power of U.S. National Team track cyclists (sprint, 1000 m, 3000/4000 m individual pursuit, points race). Representative values for these athletes are provided in Table 4–5.

Thirty-Second Wingate Test

The 30-second Wingate test is used at the USOTC to evaluate track cyclists as well as endurance riders. The objectives of the 30-second Wingate test are to determine anaerobic power, similar to the 10-second Wingate test, and anaerobic capacity [average power (W, W/kg), total work (J, J/kg)]. The 30-second protocol varies depending on the athlete's event, however. When testing track cyclists (sprint, 1000 m, 3000/4000 m individual pursuit, points race), the 30-second Wingate protocol is identical to the 10-second protocol in terms of warm-

TABLE 4–5. *U.S. National Cycling Team averages for 10-s, 30-s, and 5 × 30-s Wingate tests*

	Resistance (% TBW)	Sprint number	Peak power (W)	Peak power (W/kg)	Avg power (W)	Avg power (W/kg)	Total work (J)	Total work (J/kg)
10-s Wingate								
Track, female	10.0	1	1104	18.7	1040	17.6	10,396	176
Track, male	13.3	1	1779	21.5	1504	18.2	15,044	182
30-s Wingate								
Track, female	10.0	1	—	—	—	—	—	—
Track, male	13.3	1	1730	19.4	1258	14.1	37,752	423
Endurance, female	7.5	1	667	10.9	546	8.9	16,371	268
Endurance, male	8.3	1	940	13.4	772	11.0	23,305	330
Off-road, female	7.5	1	649	11.2	466	8.0	13,975	242
Off-road, male	8.3	1	849	11.7	703	9.7	21,078	292
5 × 30-s Wingate								
Off-road, female	4.0	1	353	6.2	319	5.6	9559	168
		2	358	6.3	318	5.6	9526	167
		3	348	6.1	315	5.5	9464	166
		4	359	6.3	319	5.6	9560	168
		5	362	6.4	320	5.6	9613	169
Off-road, male	5.0	1	522	7.6	480	7.0	14,409	210
		2	519	7.6	482	7.0	14,461	211
		3	515	7.5	466	6.8	13,985	204
		4	519	7.6	462	6.7	13,866	202
		5	519	7.6	447	6.5	13,416	196

up, sprint, and test resistance. The only difference in procedure is that the initial pedaling cadence is 60 rpm in the 30-second Wingate test. When testing endurance cyclists (criterium: individual time trial and road), the warm-up, sprint, and test resistance are equivalent to 2.0%, 3.7%, and 7.5% TBW, respectively, for female athletes, and 2.9%, 4.1%, and 8.3% TBW, respectively, for male athletes. Similar to track cyclists, the test for endurance cyclists is initiated at a controlled cadence of 60 rpm. Values for the 30-second Wingate test for female and male U.S. National Team cyclists are provided in Table 4–5.

Five × 30-Second Wingate Test

At the USOTC, the five × 30-second Wingate test is used to measure the anaerobic power and capacity, as well as the recovery capabilities, of elite off-road endurance cyclists (mountain bikers). The test is designed to simulate those unique aspects of off-road cycling that require successive high-intensity efforts combined with minimal recovery, for example, a series of moderate to difficult hill climbs over technical terrain. The five × 30-second Wingate test is administered using the same equipment and measuring device as the 10-second and 30-second Wingate tests.

A 5-minute warm-up is completed at a resistance of 2.0% TBW for both females and males. Athletes are encouraged to perform a few sprints during the warm-up; however, no additional resistance is applied during the sprints. A 3-minute recovery follows the warm-up. Once the athlete is pedaling at a cadence of 60 rpm, a 5-second countdown is used to start the test. At the "go" signal the athlete accelerates and the load is applied (4.0% TBW for females, 5.0% TBW for males). The athlete performs a 30-second maximal sprint and is verbally encouraged throughout the effort. Following a 30-second recovery (active or passive), the procedure is repeated until five 30-second sprints have been completed. Representative values for female and male U.S. National Team mountain bikers are provided in Table 4–5.

Simulated Pursuit Ride

The purpose of the simulated pursuit test on the cycle ergometer is to replicate the physiologic demands and power output of a 3000-m (female) and 4000-m (male) individual pursuit race. The test is conducted on either a mechanically braked (interfaced with an optical sensor measuring device) or electrically braked cycle ergometer equipped with competition racing bars, saddle, and pedals; it is configured to match the exact dimensions of the athlete's competition bicycle.

The warm-up is done on the cycle ergometer and should simulate the precompetition warm-up in duration and intensity. A 5-minute recovery follows the warm-up. The athlete is instructed to maintain a pedaling cadence of 100 to 120 rpm. The test is initiated once the athlete has attained the appropriate cadence. Female and male athletes are required to ride to the completion of 90 and 120 kJ, respectively. Verbal encouragement is provided throughout the test. The athletes are periodically kept apprised of the work completed in order to allow them to use optimal pacing and sprint tactics. Total time (minutes:seconds) is recorded upon completion of the test. Typical times for U.S. National Team female and male pursuit riders tested at the USOTC are 235 to 250 sec (3:55–4:10) and 285 to 300 sec (4:45–5:00), respectively.

Aerobic/Anaerobic Capacity Test

The aerobic/anaerobic capacity test (AACT) is designed to (a) identify potential elite-level cyclists, (b) evaluate anaerobic and aerobic cycling capabilities, and (c) assess training responses (19). The test is conducted using a pan-loaded, mechanically braked cycle ergometer equipped with competition racing bars, saddle, pedals, and chain. The test bike is configured to match the exact dimensions of the athlete's competition bicycle. The AACT has also been modified for administration on a Computrainer (Computrainer, Seattle, WA) used in conjunction with the athlete's own bike. The AACT protocol involves a continuous series of 3-minute stages at progressively greater percentages (30%, 50%, 70%, 90%, 110%, and 130%) of the theoretically calculated power required to cycle at 35 km/h up a 1% grade. This calculation is based on drag components attributable to aerodynamics, rolling and frictional resistance, and climbing. The equation is as follows (20):

Power 100% =

$0.0119 \times FA \times V^3 +$	Aerodynamic
$0.022 \times M \times V$	Rolling and Friction
$2.715 \times \%\ \text{Grade} \times M \times V$	Climbing

where:

velocity (V) is in km/h,
mass (M) is in kg,
frontal area (FA) is calculated as $FA = 0.00179 \times M^{0.425} \times H^{0.725} \times$, where height ($H$) is in cm.

A sample of the work loads used for the test is presented in Table 4–6.

Performance on the test has been shown to effectively differentiate among athletes brought to the USOTC for talent screening. Results of 101 senior males initially used to develop the test also reveal that ride duration is independent of height ($r = 0.07$), weight ($r = -0.03$), and age ($r = -0.02$) (19). The data presented in Table 4–7 provide reference values for performance times on the AACT test for ages 10 years to senior level. It is important to note that the senior-level athletes were attending USA Cycling selection camps at the USOTC. Therefore, they were certainly better than average cyclists. All the data on younger subjects were collected as part of a broad-based talent identification program and represent a more heterogeneous group.

One-Hour Endurance Ride

Coyle and colleagues (20a) have developed a simulated time trial protocol that requires the athlete to ride at the highest power output possible for 60 minutes. Endurance performance is quantified as the average power

TABLE 4–6. *Example of work loads for aerobic/anaerobic capacity test: loads for an individual between 168 cm (5′6″) and 175 cm (5′9″)*

	Work loads at stages (% / Time)											
	30 0:00–3:00		50 3:01–6:00		70 6:01–9:00		90 9:01–12:00		110 12:01–15:00		130 15:01–18:00	
Weight (kg)	Kp	Watts	Kp	Watts	Kp	Watts	Kp	Watts	Kp	Watts	Kp	Watts
50–55	1.0	88.9	1.7	148.1	2.4	207.4	3.0	266.6	3.7	325.9	4.4	385.1
55–60	1.1	93.9	1.8	156.6	2.5	219.1	3.2	281.7	3.9	344.2	4.6	406.8
60–65	1.1	98.8	1.9	164.6	2.6	230.5	3.4	296.3	4.1	362.2	4.9	428.1
65–70	1.2	103.6	2.0	172.6	2.7	241.7	3.5	310.7	4.3	379.8	5.1	448.8
70–75	1.2	108.3	2.0	180.5	2.9	252.6	3.7	324.8	4.5	397.0	5.3	469.2
75–80	1.3	112.9	2.1	188.2	3.0	263.4	3.8	338.7	4.7	413.9	5.5	489.2
80–85	1.3	117.4	2.2	195.7	3.1	274.0	4.0	352.3	4.9	430.6	5.8	508.9
85–90	1.4	121.9	2.3	203.2	3.2	284.5	4.1	365.7	5.1	447.0	6.0	528.3
90–95	1.4	126.3	2.4	210.5	3.3	294.8	4.3	379.0	5.2	463.2	6.2	547.4
95–100	1.5	130.7	2.5	217.8	3.5	304.9	4.4	392.0	5.4	479.2	6.4	566.3
100–105	1.5	135.0	2.5	225.0	3.6	315.0	4.6	405.0	5.6	495.0	6.6	584.9
105–110	1.6	139.2	2.6	232.1	3.7	324.9	4.7	417.7	5.8	510.6	6.8	603.4

From Sjogaard C, Nielsen G, Mikkelsen F, Saltin B, Burke ER. Physiology of bicycling. Ithaca, NY: Mouvement Pub., Inc, 1984:9–16.

TABLE 4–7. *Performance norms for aerobic/anaerobic capacity test (AACT) by age and gender*

Female	Sample size	Mean score	25% score	Male	Sample size	Mean score	5th% score
Seniors	42	11:34	12:48	Seniors	101	14:34	17:04
17–18	14	9:36	10:41	17–18	81	12:18	15:25
15–16	27	8:29	10:06	15–16	117	10:28	15:02
13–14	22	5:27	6:38	13–14	88	7:08	10:47
11–12	51	4:18	4:42	11–12	79	5:42	8:26
10 & under	6	4:49	6:45	10 & under	22	5:14	7:14

output (W, W/kg) maintained on a cycle ergometer during the 1-hour test. The test is conducted on either a mechanically or electrically braked cycle ergometer equipped with competition racing bars, saddle, and pedals, and it is configured to match the exact dimensions of the athlete's competition bicycle.

Following a warm-up that includes 1- to 2-minute periods at the approximate performance work rate, the athlete is instructed to generate the highest power output possible throughout the 60-minute test. The athlete is required to complete the initial 8 minutes of the test at a power output estimated to be that which can be maintained for the entire 60-minute ride. This "predicted" power output is estimated from results of a lactate threshold test typically completed 1 to 2 days prior to the 1-hour endurance ride, and from the athlete's subjective perception during the test warm-up. After the initial 8 minutes, the athlete is free to increase or decrease the work load. During the test the athlete is verbally encouraged and provided with continuous visual feedback of the elapsed time, pedaling cadence, and power output. Average absolute power output ($\bar{X}$ = 346 W) measured during this 1-hour endurance test has been shown to be highly correlated with 40-km time trial performance ($r = -0.88$) in elite male cyclists (20). In addition, Bishop (21) has recently demonstrated that the 1-hour endurance performance test is a valid and reliable measure.

Ice Hockey

Ice hockey is a fast-paced "stop-and-start" sport in which exceptional leg power is a fundamental requirement. The game involves 30- to 40-second on-ice shifts that consist of repetitive sprint situations. The on-ice shift is interspersed with 2 to 3 minutes of recovery during which other players perform on-ice shifts. Although the players clearly approach $\dot{V}O_2$max during difficult shifts, the relatively modest $\dot{V}O_2$max values obtained on elite hockey players [typically 50 to 60 mL/kg^{-1}/min^{-1} for National Hockey League (NHL) players] suggest that high aerobic power is not critical to performance. In contrast, these players demonstrate relatively high peak power (22,23).

Wingate Test

Peak 5-second power data measured during a 30-second Wingate test demonstrate the high power characteristic of elite hockey players (1110 W, 12.7 W/kg; $n = 61$ top NHL draft picks). Other data on NHL players ($n = 31$) from a Wingate test (load = 9.0% TBW) indicates 5-second peak power values of 13.4 W/kg. The U.S. Women's National Team uses a 10-second Wingate test (load = 8.5% TBW) to evaluate 1-second peak power. Peak 1-second values average over 11 W/kg and correlate well with on-ice sprint times ($r = -0.79$). Protocols for administration of the 10-second and 30-second Wingate tests are described in the section devoted to cycling-specific tests.

On-Ice Testing

Several on-ice tests have been utilized to identify skating-specific skill, as well as the power strengths and weaknesses of hockey players. The tests involve a specific skating technique such as forward or backward crossovers, and short sprints (forward and backward) from a standing and/or flying start. The tests are done over standard distances and are timed with electronic timing eyes. The advantage of these tests over the laboratory tests is that they more closely simulate hockey-specific skills. Regrettably, most of these field tests have been team specific, and standardized protocols and norms are not available.

Nordic Sports

The Nordic sports of present-day Olympic competition include biathlon, cross-country skiing, ski jumping, and Nordic combined. Biathlon and cross-country have competitions for both genders, while ski jumping and Nordic combined hold competitions for males only. Each discipline has unique physiologic demands that are evaluated by both field testing and laboratory testing. Several tests overlap between disciplines, and the standard tests for aerobic fitness are covered in Chapter 18.

Biathlon

Biathlon combines cross-country skiing (skating technique) with rifle marksmanship. During competitions, the athletes are required to ski while carrying a rifle weighing a minimum of 3.5 kg. Competitions consist of skiing three to five relatively short (2.5–5 km) loops interspersed with two to four shooting stages, two for the sprint races (7.5 and 10 km for women and men, respectively), and four for the individual races (15 and 20 km for women and men, respectively). Although biathlon racing is primarily aerobic, the combination of rifle carriage and short race loops with relatively short, steep climbs necessitates relatively high strength and power. Current data (24,25) indicate that the upper body component during biathlon skiing is highly related to performance, with the best biathletes in the world demonstrating approximately 25% greater upper body power than U.S. biathletes. During uphill ski skating, the upper body can account for as much as 50% of the forward force impulse (26). The additional load of rifle carriage increases the upper body power component even more (27).

Current training/testing of U.S. biathletes reflects a strong focus on monitoring ski-specific upper body power/muscle endurance using a double-pole power test (25). Additionally, maximal double-poling aerobic power is evaluated during a roller ski double-pole ramp test on a motor-driven treadmill, where speed is increased at a constant 7% elevation until volitional exhaustion. The U.S. National Team standard for double-pole $\dot{V}O_2$ peak is to exceed 90% of running $\dot{V}O_2$ peak. As with many sports, the U.S. biathlon team also relies on a series of field tests to monitor athletes. Whole-body aerobic power and lactate threshold are evaluated during incremental treadmill running and treadmill roller skiing on a specially built treadmill.

Double-Pole Power Test

This test is performed on the Freestyle Arm Ergometer (Ergometrix, Minneapolis, MN) using a modified protocol from Rundell and Bacharach (25). After an initial warm-up, the athlete performs a progressive double-pole power test to determine absolute (W) and relative (W/kg) peak 10-second power. The initial work load is 50 W for women and 100 W for men. Thereafter, the work load is increased every 20 sec (20 W for women and 30 W for men). The test is terminated when the athlete can no longer maintain a flywheel velocity of 5 m/sec. Test times range from 4 to 6 minutes. The most recent results on the U.S. National Team were 316 ± 57 and 215 ± 25 W, or 4.2 ± 0.6 and 3.5 ± 0.4 W/kg, for the men and women, respectively.

Field Tests

The standard field tests used by the U.S. biathlon team are as follows:

Pull-ups: In this test the athlete uses a shoulder-width overhand grip on a pull-up bar. The movement must be controlled without bouncing. The test is scored as the maximum number of pull-ups the athlete can sequentially complete.

Sit-ups: The technique is a basic bent-knee sit-up with each hand resting on the opposite shoulder. During the movement, the buttocks should not leave the floor and the elbows must touch the top of the knee to complete the sit-up. The test is scored as the maximum number of sit-ups the athlete can complete in 60 seconds.

Box jump: One repetition begins with the athlete standing laterally to the box (51 × 60 cm) and jumping to the top of the box and ends with a jump to the ground on the other side of the box. The test is scored as the maximum number of jumps the athlete can complete in 60 seconds.

Dips: This test uses two benches for hand and feet suspension. Arms are flexed from straight to 90 degrees at the elbow and back up. Bouncing and pausing is not allowed, and the movement must remain continuous. The test is scored as the maximum number of dips the athlete can sequentially complete.

Ten hops: In this test the athlete leaps forward with either the right or left foot beginning and continues to bound with alternating feet. After the 10th bound the distance is measured and recorded. The U.S. National Team standards range from 19.8 m for junior women to 25.9 m for senior men. This test is a good indicator of explosive leg power.

Additional field tests: Additional tests used to evaluate U.S. National Team biathletes include the following: electronically timed 100-m sprint, 1.5-mile track run, 1-km double-pole uphill (5% grade) time trial (roller skis or on snow), and a 2.5-km trail run on a standard

TABLE 4–8. *Junior National Biathlon Team field test scores*

	Pull-ups (reps)	Sit-ups (reps/min)	Box jump (reps/min)	Dips (reps)	10 hops (feet)	1.5-mile run (min : s)	100-m dash (s)
Men (n = 8)	17	70	65	85	85	8:15	12.5
Women (n = 7)	8	55	55	50	70	9:45	14.5

TABLE 4–9. *National Cross-Country Ski Team field test scores*

	3000 m run (min:s)	40-yard dash (s)	Push-ups set 1	Push-ups set 2	Dips (dip bar) set 1	Dips (dip bar) set 2	Box jump	Vertical jump (inches)	Pull-ups set 1	Pull-ups set 2	Sit-ups set 1	Sit-ups set 2
Men	8:58	5.23	87	52	46	15	98	27.5	30	20	79	72
Women	10:49	5.75	48	18	20	11	79	17.0	10	5	69	64

loop at the Mount Van Hovenburg Biathlon range, Lake Placid, NY. Table 4–8 provides minimum test scores for the junior national team.

Cross Country

Cross-country skiing is the most aerobic of the Nordic disciplines, but, as with Biathlon, power plays an important role in the ability to ski fast (25,28). Maximal aerobic power is typically determined during a running protocol, unless treadmill roller skiing is available; then tests are performed using the classic and skating techniques. Upper-body evaluation is done as with the biathlon, that is, using the double-poling $\dot{V}O_2$ peak test and the double-poling power test previously described. In addition, the U.S. Ski Team uses nine field tests to assess cross-country athletes. Seven are general strength tests, one a flexibility measurement, and one a cardiovascular assessment. All are scored according to the specific test, and protocols are related to age. The field tests are similar to those used for biathlon, with the addition of a 3000-m run, 40-yard dash, vertical jump, and sit-and-reach flexibility test (data from the Cross-Country National Team are summarized in Table 4–9):

The 3000-m run: A timed test where the athlete runs 7.5 laps on a 400-m track.

Forty-yard dash: This test is a maximal sprint effort that measures explosive leg power. Ideally, an electronic timing system, start mat, and finish electronic eye are used for this test. If these are not available, the test can be administered on a standard track with hand-held timing.

Vertical jump: The Vertec vertical jump device (Questek Corp., Northridge, CA) is used to determine maximal jump height. The procedure involves a standing two-legged jump with no steps.

Flexibility: The sit-and-reach test is used to determine hamstring and low-back flexibility. Following a warm-up period, the athlete sits on the ground, with shoes off, and slowly reaches as far as possible along the top of a standard "sit-and-reach" box. The measurement is taken to the nearest 0.5 inch either past the toes (+ inches) or in front of the toes (− inches).

Ski Jumping

Ski jumping is the purest explosive power discipline of the Nordic sports. Strong relationships have been found for standing long jump distance, vertical jump height, and ski jumping performance. An explosive jump at the moment of takeoff effectively puts the jumper over the knoll and into flight position sooner. The U.S. Ski Jumping Team systematically evaluates jumping power by using a timing mat to determine jump height for a series of special jumps and applying the calculation:

$$h = 1/2a\,(t/2)^2$$

where:

$$a = 9.8\ \text{m/s}^2$$

$$t = \text{time in air}$$

The specialized jumps are described in detail below.

Ski Jump–Specific Vertical Jump Tests

In-run: This test measures a vertical jump height performed from the crouched, in-run position, with the trunk angle mimicking the in-run position.

Static: The athlete starts the jump from a static squat with the trunk in an upright position with hands at the waist.

Preloaded: This is a vertical jump performed with a countermovement to a squat position with hands at the shoulders, simulating a bar hold.

TABLE 4–10. *Comparison of vertical jump scores between top World Cup competitor and U.S. National Ski Jumping Team*

		In-run position (cm)	Static jump (cm)	Preload 0 kg (cm)	Preload 10 kg (cm)	Preload 30 kg (cm)	Preload 50 kg (cm)
Top World Cup competitor		—	61.8	67.1	55.9	40.5	30.7
U.S. National Team (*n* = 6)	Mean	48.7	43.7	45.3	38.3	29.2	24.1
	SD	6.0	5.6	7.5	6.5	5.8	2.8

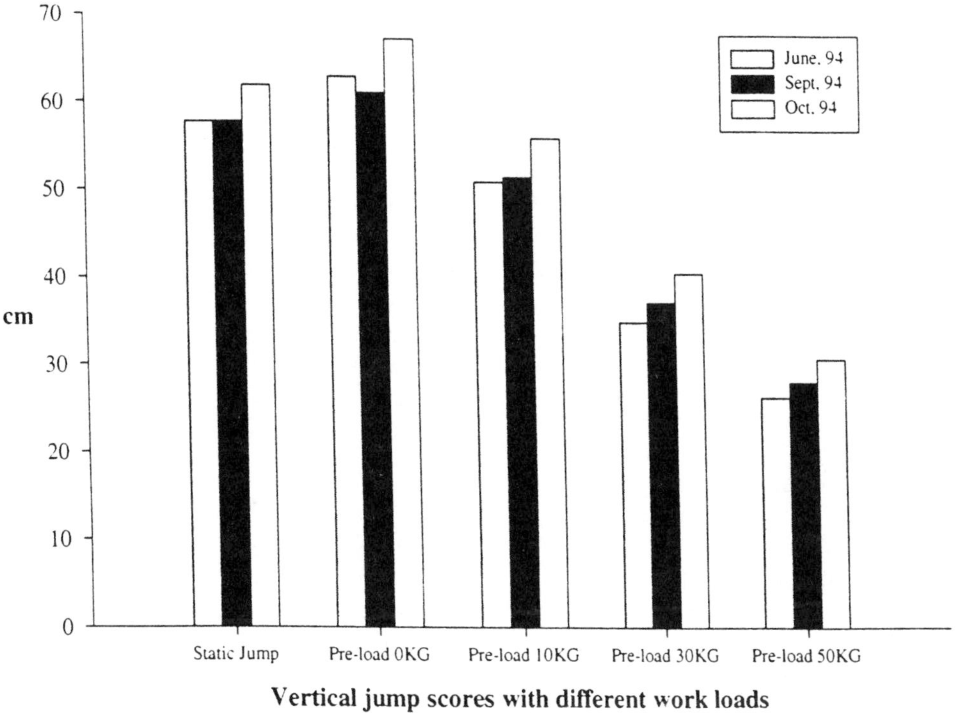

FIG. 4–3. Vertical jump scores of top World Cup competitor.

Preloaded 10 kg: Same as preloaded, but with a 10-kg bar placed on shoulders.

Preloaded 30 kg: Same as preloaded, but with a 30-kg bar placed on shoulders.

Preloaded 50 kg: Same as preloaded, but with a 50-kg bar placed on shoulders.

Data on the 1997–1998 U.S. National Team and one foreign World Cup competitor are presented in Table 4–10. The 1997–98 team was somewhat below the international standard in jumping, and these test data on a World Cup–level competitor highlight these differences. The use of sport-specific test procedures to monitor training is illustrated in Fig. 4–3, which tracks one athlete through a training session.

Nordic Combined

Nordic combined is a combination discipline that includes ski jumping and cross-country skiing. This unique combination requires that the athlete successfully compete in two events of conflicting physiologic requirements—explosive jumping and endurance-based cross-country skiing. Physical testing of these athletes includes those tests described for ski jumping and some of the laboratory tests described for biathlon and cross-country.

Rowing

Rowing is a traditional sport that lends itself to the assessment of work and/or power output capacity. For years, physiologists and coaches have used the ability to do external work on ergometers as an indication of oarsmen/oarswomen's potential on the water. In addition to helping to differentiate among athletes, the off-water tests have been used as indicators of training status and as off-season motivational tools. The development of valid and reliable ergometers has allowed rowers and their coaches to focus on rowing-specific power tests. The predominant ergometer used for testing today is the Concept II, Model C (Concept II, Morrisville, VT).

Two-Thousand-Meter Test

The classic test piece on a Concept II rowing ergometer was the time required to complete 2500 m. World-class Open men were able to complete this test in about 7:30. This translates to approximately 180 kJ of work. As competitive times have improved in recent years, the standard test duration has been shortened from 2500 m to 2000 m. For a world-class oarsman working at a power output of 500 W, this requires approximately 360 seconds or 6 minutes. Although this time is somewhat faster than the time required to complete a 2000-m competitive distance in a single, it is very comparable to the duration of competition in the larger boats. The advantage of a very sport-specific ergometer, such as the Concept II, is that it provides coaches and athletes with a reliable assessment of their performance capacity.

In a project completed at the 1994 World Championships in Indianapolis, Bouscaren and colleagues (29)

TABLE 4–11. *1998 U.S. National Team testing standards: 2000-meter time trial*

Classification	Women	Men
Elite open	6:55	6:04
Elite light	7:25	6:20
Elite junior	7:30	6:20
Developmental open	7:10	6:12
Developmental light	7:35	6:30
Developmental junior	7:40	6:30

surveyed the American crews in each of the major events. Their data indicated that the mean Concept II ergometer performance times of the crew members of the six medal-winning boats were all within 1.2% of the average of the eight best ergometer times recorded in the Crash-B Indoor World Championship rankings (described below). Additionally, only two boats compiled ergometer scores within this range and failed to win a medal. These data indicate that leading oarsmen also have the capacity to perform well on a rowing ergometer. It is important to note, however, that the inverse of this is not true. There are individuals who have demonstrated a significant capability for pulling excellent ergometer times who are not successful or competitive oarsmen/oarswomen. Clearly, the skill, balance, and finesse of applying the power that an athlete is capable of generating to the boat determines rowing performance. Therefore, when using a test such as the timed 2000-m ergometer piece, a sports medicine/sport science professional should be aware that the test assesses the work or power output capacity of the athlete, but it does not provide an evaluation of the event-specific skills necessary for successful on-water performance.

The 1998 U.S. National Team test standards for the 2000-m time trial are presented in Table 4–11.

A classic example of the use of a sport-specific test as a motivational tool is provided by the Crash-B Sprints, World Indoor Rowing Championships. This event held in Boston during February each year is the culmination of a series of regional and international qualifying regattas. It involves thousands of competitors and publishes a world ranking of ergometer times that can be submitted either in writing or achieved during one of the regional meets. These world rankings include competitors ranging in age from youth through Olympic athletes to men and women of 80 or more years of age. The rank list and percentile scores for all classes are available from Concept II.

Rowing Power Profile

Recently, the USOC Sport Science and Technology Division has evaluated the U.S. National Team using a profile of performance times on the Concept II in an attempt to assess each individual's relative strengths across a range of performance times (30). The times that have been selected for assessment are 15, 45, and 135 seconds, as well as the standard time required to complete 2000 m, or about 6 minutes. This battery of tests provides a profile of work capacities or power output across four time periods (Fig. 4–4). The time periods have been selected to provide an opportunity to assess an athlete's maximal non–oxygen-dependent power output capacity: two time periods (45 and 135 seconds) that involve assessment of anaerobic power and anaerobic capacity capabilities, and a 2000-m timed piece. The 2000-m time trial requires 6 to 7 minutes and is therefore heavily dependent on the ability to sustain a high oxidative capacity. In theory, comparing an athlete's performance across these four durations to a set of norms or other team members

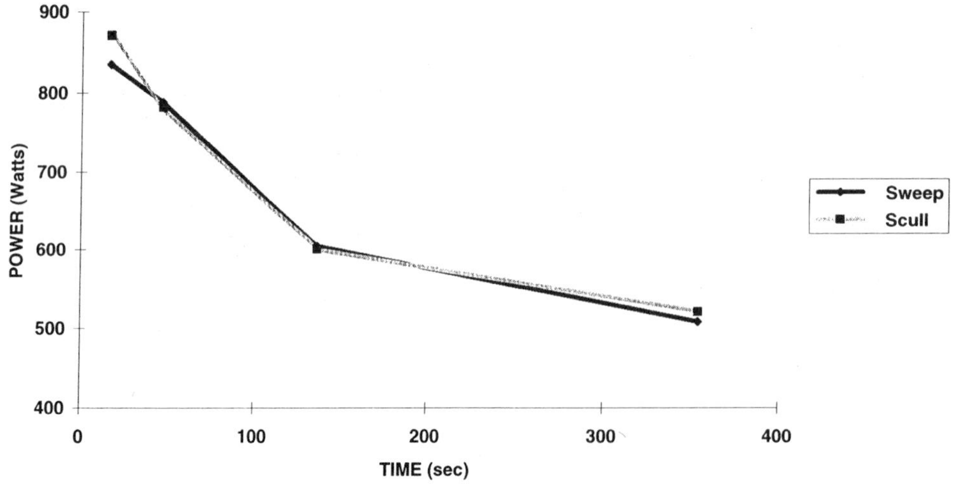

FIG. 4–4. Power output profiles: rowing.

should allow a coach or athlete to assess relative strengths and weaknesses. Knowledge of these characteristics facilitates individualized training in an attempt to maximize performance.

Running

Maximal Anaerobic Running Test

The maximal anaerobic running test (MART) was recently developed by Rusko and colleagues (31) for the purpose of providing a more accurate assessment of anaerobic capacity in sprinters and middle-distance runners. The test consists of a series of 20-second treadmill sprints performed at progressively faster velocities (calculated O_2 demand of 100% to 200% of $\dot{V}O_2$ max). A 5-second acceleration phase is allowed before each of the 20-second sprint intervals. Treadmill grade is maintained at 4 degrees throughout the entire test. Velocity for the initial 20-second sprint is calculated to allow the athlete to complete 8 to 12 sprints before exhausting. In general, the initial sprint should be performed at a velocity equivalent to the athlete's maximal aerobic power ($mL/kg^{-1}/min^{-1}$). This initial velocity can be estimated using standard formulas (32). Subsequent sprint velocities are increased by 1.37 km/h (~6 $mL/kg^{-1}/min^{-1}$) until volitional exhaustion. A 100-second recovery period follows each 20-second sprint. The test continues until the athlete is unable to complete an interval. After 40 seconds of recovery and at 2-, 5-, and 10-minutes postexhaustion, blood lactate is sampled. Upon completion of the MART, a blood lactate versus power curve is generated with power expressed as the oxygen demand ($mL/kg^{-1}/min^{-1}$) of running, and calculated according to the American College of Sports Medicine (ACSM) equation (32).

In the MART, power at exhaustion (P_{max}) and peak blood lactate (peak BLa) have been shown to be valid and reliable indices of anaerobic work capacity in sprinters (100 m, 400 m) and middle-distance runners (800 m, 1500 m) (32a,33), whereas power at 3, 5 and 10 mM blood lactate levels (P_{3mM}, P_{5mM}, and P_{10mM}) appear to be good indicators of anaerobic sprinting economy (32a,33). In addition, P_{max} can be used as a practical method for monitoring the effect of sprint training on anaerobic performance characteristics (34), while the running velocities at P_{3mM} and P_{10mM} have been shown to correspond to the velocities of *extensive* (100–600 m ≤79% of maximal velocity) and *intensive* interval training (60–600 m at 80% to 95% of maximal velocity), respectively, and therefore can be used to prescribe training for sprinters and middle-distance runners (34).

Sliding Sports: Bobsled and Luge

Bobsled and luge are the two Olympic sliding sports. Since the sleds must be maneuvered at extremely high speeds through tight corners down an approximately 1.6 km course, these sports are highly technical and skill dependent. The technical ability of the elite sliders is so finely tuned that the difference between first and fourth place is often measured in thousandths of a second. This homogeneity in technical ability among elite sliders has resulted in high emphasis being placed on the start. Time lost at the start could potentially be magnified threefold by the finish (35). Each sport relies on field testing and sport-specific start tests to evaluate the athletes.

Bobsled

Bobsled is a sport where two- and four-person teams slide down an approximately 1.6-km iced track. Speeds during competition may exceed 140 km/h. The bobsled start requires the athletes to accelerate the 200- to 250-kg bobsled in approximately 30 to 40 m while pushing on specially designed retractable bars attached to the sled. When the sled has reached optimum velocity during the push, athletes load for the ride to the bottom. A six-item field test is used to assess U.S. bobsled athletes (36). The six test events are explosive in nature and rely on both speed and strength. Additionally, the U.S. bobsled team evaluates athletes using a push-specific training/testing system. The system consists of a bobsled fitted with wheels that follows a metal railed track for 65 m, simulating the on-ice start section of a bobsled course. The track has a finish section that rises steeply to slow and eventually stop the sled.

Six-Item Field Test

The six-item test consists of a vertical jump, a two-arm underhand 7.3-kg shot toss, a five-hop test, and 30-, 60-, and 100-m sprints. Each item has a 150-point ceiling with a sliding point scale relative to event performance, giving a maximal total score of 900 points for the men. A minimal score of 625 points (arbitrarily selected by the U.S. Bobsled Federation) is required for brakemen and side pushers to compete on ice at the national level. The test follows the aforementioned order and is completed in 1 day. All events are scored as the best of three trials.

Vertical jump: The vertical jump is the difference between a standing reach and a standing, countermovement jump reach using the Vertec vertical jump apparatus. A maximal score of 150 points is assigned for a jump of 91.4 cm.

Underhand shot toss: The athlete assumes an upright position with feet shoulder width apart, braced against a rigid support and throws the shot (7.3 kg) underhand using both arms. A maximal score of 150 points is assigned for a toss of 17 m.

Five hops: The athlete performs five consecutive two-legged plyometric hops. Distance is measured in meters from a starting line to the athlete's heel at the completion of five hops. The athletes are encouraged to hop as quickly as possible. A maximal score of 150 points is assigned for a distance of 17 m.

The 30-, 60-, and 100-m sprints: Starting blocks and electric timing eyes are used for all running events. Timing is initiated when the athlete brakes a timing eye beam 1 m from the start line. Maximal scores of 150 points are assigned for times of 3.50 seconds, 6.65 seconds, and 10.80 seconds for the 30-, 60-, and 100-m sprints, respectively. Table 4–12 presents complete statistics on athletes selected and not selected for the world championship team in 1995.

Dry-Land Simulated Push

The National Bobsled Push Championships take place in August on the Lake Placid push track. The push procedure is similar to that conducted on ice. Briefly, for the brakemen, the athlete begins at the back of the sled with feet braced against a start block. On the start signal the athlete pushes the sled to top running speed and loads into the sled at approximately 40 m. Push time is recorded electronically for a 50-m section (with 5-m splits), measured between the 15- and 65-m timing eyes. Time for each athlete is given as an average from the best two of three trials. The side push is scored similarly, with the exception that the athlete pushes from the side position. Push time data are presented in Table 4–12.

The six-item test score correlates remarkably well ($r = -0.83$) to the dry-land push times, with multiple regression analysis demonstrating that the 30-m run and vertical jump are the best predictors of push performance (36). This observation is consistent with the high-speed/power requirement of performing the bobsled push start. Although the 7.3-kg underhand shot toss was not the best predictor of push time, the underlying purpose of including this event is to limit the bobsled athlete pool to include athletes who not only possess high speed and vertical jump height, but also are capable of rapidly accelerating a 200- to 250-kg bobsled from a standing start.

In 1995, the U.S. Bobsled Federation began a nationwide campaign to identify potential talent from a bobsled push contest using a two-man bobsled on a portable track. The contests are held throughout the country and are open to the general public. The contest involves pushing a 159-kg bobsled modified to run on wheels on a portable steel-railed track. A 20-m section of the track beginning 5 m after the start is electronically timed. A national team athlete attends these recruiting camps to set a standard push time to rank participants. If participants meet the criteria time standard, they are invited to the U.S. Bobsled Team Training Camp at Lake Placid for further testing and an opportunity to compete in the push championships. All but three of the 1998 U.S. Olympic bobsled team members were recruited through this program.

Luge

Luge is similar to bobsled in that the athletes slide down an approximately 1.6-km iced track where speeds may exceed 140 km/h. Maximum sled weight is 23 kg for a singles sled and 27 kg for a doubles sled. The athletes lie on their backs on the seat (pod) and steer by a combination of shoulder movement and runner control with the feet. The luge start begins with a pulling movement on start handles fixed on either side of the track. During the initial pull, the athlete is in a sitting position and typically does one or two countermovements, sliding the sled backward and forward and finishing with an explosive pull off the handles. The athlete then uses spiked gloves to perform three to four paddling movements to further accelerate the sled before settling into the prone position for the slide down the track. As in bobsled, the athlete must possess sufficient power to achieve the requisite fast start times. Unlike bobsled, the luge athlete relies almost exclusively on upper body power. USA Luge has developed a comprehensive strength/power training/testing program and requires athletes to achieve predetermined standards. Included in the battery of tests is the luge start, performed on a specially designed indoor start track.

Physical Tests

Eight events compose the luge physical tests. Test descriptions and order are as follows:

Standing long jump: The athlete performs a two-legged standing jump with arm swing countermovement allowed. The athletes are encouraged to extend their legs, land on their heels, and fall forward. Distance is measured in meters and the best of two trials is taken.

Push-ups: The athlete performs as many full strict push-ups as possible within 30 seconds.

Flexibility: This is the sit-and-reach test. The athlete sits with bare feet against a platform and flexes at the waist with outstretched arms while maintaining extended legs. Distance is measured in 0.5-inch increments from the edge of the foot platform. The best of three trials is taken.

Pull-ups: The athlete performs the maximum number of pull-ups possible in 15 seconds with a shoulder-width pronated grip. The chin must reach the top of the bar to be counted.

Sit-ups: This event is the maximum number of bent-knee sit-ups that can be performed in 60 seconds.

TABLE 4–12. *Push times and six-item test scores for 1995 U.S. Bobsled World Team athletes and those not selected for the team*

	Push time(s)		Six-item test	Vertical jump	Shot toss	5 hops	30-m run	60-m run	100-m run
	Brake	Side	(points)	(cm)	(m)	(m)	(s)	(s)	(s)
World Team (n = 11)									
Raw score	5.42* ± 0.07	5.48* ± 0.08	771* ± 54	82.3* ± 5.3	15.35* ± 1.00	15.53 ± 1.15	3.73* ± 0.08	6.75* ± 0.17	11.00* ± 0.42
Range	5.32–5.57	5.35–5.64	720–843	73.7–88.9	13.2–17.3	13.9–17.3	3.62–3.87	6.51–6.94	10.48–11.67
Non–World Team (n = 11)									
Raw score	5.64 ± 0.07	5.69 ± 0.06	633 ± 67	75.2 ± 6.6	13.52 ± 1.02	15.16 ± 0.72	3.90 ± 0.09	7.15 ± 0.22	11.70 ± 0.48
Range	5.55–5.78	5.58–5.85	490–740	64.8–83.8	11.3–14.9	14.3–15.9	3.76–4.07	6.87–7.63	11.16–12.74

Values are raw scores (mean ± SD).
*Selected athletes' scores are significantly better ($p < .05$).

Shot toss: This event is an over-the-back medicine-ball toss. Men use a 5.4-kg ball and women use a 3.6-kg ball. The ball is thrown with both hands over the head and behind the athlete. The scoring of the test is calculated by dividing the distance thrown by the body weight of the athlete (m/kg). The best of three throws is taken.

Thirty-meter sprint: This event is an electronically timed standing start sprint with timing eyes located at 1.25 and 31.25 m. The best of three sprints is taken for scoring.

Three-hundred-meter run: This event is an electronically timed standing start run with timing eyes located at 1.25 and 301.25 m. The best of two runs is taken for scoring.

Start Test

The Luge start test, done on the instrumented indoor track, is the most important item in the test battery. Although simple start time is the only data used as a selection criterion, impulse on the handles and a paddling index are monitored to assess athlete improvement. Physical and start test standards for luge are presented in Table 4–13.

Speed Skating

Ten-Second Wingate Test

The 10-second Wingate test is used with short-track speed skaters to evaluate anaerobic power. The ability to generate high peak power for quick speed changes and passing is an important component of short-track speed skating. Since short-track skaters often utilize the draft and typically do not make a move for the win until the last lap (an approximately 10-second maximal effort), the 10-second Wingate is an important test that relates well to a skater's ability to generate a fast lap. Additionally, the test is relevant to the critical need for a fast start in the short races (500 m). The test is conducted on a pan-loaded, mechanically braked cycle ergometer equipped with racing bars, saddle, and pedals. The cycle can be configured to fit individual athletes and is equipped with a computer-interfaced optical sensor (SMI, St. Cloud, MN). Peak power (W, W/kg), mean power (W, W/kg), and total work (J, J/kg) are recorded from the test. A 5-minute warm-up on the cycle at 2.0% TBW with three 5-second sprints (5.0% and 6.6% TBW for females and males, respectively) precedes the test. A 3-minute recovery period follows the warm-up. The test is initiated with a 5-second countdown at a pedaling cadence of 100 rpm. At the completion of the countdown, the test load (8.5% and 10.0% TBW for females and males, respectively) is applied and the athlete performs a 10-second maximal sprint. Top male and female U.S. National Team short-track speed skaters have achieved 1-second peak power values greater than 15 W/kg on this test.

Cycle Ergometer Time Trial

The purpose of the cycle ergometer time trial is to replicate the physiologic demands and power output of specific long-track speed skating events (3000 and 5000 m for women, 5000 m for men). The time trial format allows coaches and athletes to monitor training progress in a controlled, standardized off-ice setting. The test is conducted on either a mechanically braked (interfaced with an optical sensor measuring device) or electrically braked cycle ergometer equipped with competition racing bars, saddle, and pedals, and it is configured to match the exact dimensions of the athlete's training bicycle.

The warm-up is done on the cycle ergometer and should simulate the on-ice precompetition warm-up in duration and intensity. A 5-minute recovery follows the warm-up. If the test is conducted on a mechanically braked cycle ergometer, the athlete is instructed to maintain a pedaling cadence of 80 to 90 rpm. (A pedal-

TABLE 4–13. *Physical test standards for selection to the U.S. Luge Team*

	Senior men	Senior women	Junior men	Junior women
Standing long jump (m)	3.1	2.6	2.9	2.5
Pull-ups (15 s)	17	13	16	12
Sit and reach (inch)	11.0	12.0	9.5	10.5
Push-ups (30 s)	51	39	48	36
Sit-ups (60 s)	77	75	74	72
Shot toss (m/kg)	0.2	0.2	0.185	0.185
30-meter run (s)	3.73	4.30	3.85	4.45
300-meter run (s)	38.50	47.75	39.50	49.25
Singles start (s)	1.27	1.37	1.31	1.43
Doubles start (s)	1.27	—	1.33	—

Standards (distance or time) for maximum points (16) an athlete can earn in each test. Minimum number of points an athlete must score on nine tests is 90 combined points for senior team and 85 combined points for junior team (or 75 combined points on eight tests with no start test).

ing cadence greater than 90 rpm may result in premature exhaustion, i.e., "out too fast"). The test is started once the athlete has attained the appropriate cadence. Female and male long-track speed skaters are required to ride to the completion of 102 and 170 kJ, respectively. The comparable values for short-track skaters are 100 and 120 kJ. Verbal encouragement is provided throughout the test. The athletes are periodically kept apprised of the distance completed in order to allow them to use optimal pacing and sprint tactics. Total time (minute:second) is recorded upon completion of the time trial. Times for the 102 kJ time trial performed by U.S. National Team long-track female skaters have ranged from 4:33 to 5:00, whereas males have completed the 170 kJ test in times ranging from 6:37 to 7:10. Times for U.S. National Team short-track men on the 120 kJ test range from 4:33 to 5:20.

Water Ski

Progressive Five × 30-Second Wingate Test

The progressive Wingate test is used at the USOTC to measure the anaerobic power and capacity, as well as the recovery capabilities of elite water ski athletes. This seemingly unusual format of a test was designed to simulate the increasing physiologic demand of successive slalom runs—faster speeds or shorter rope. The test is conducted using a pan-loaded, mechanically braked cycle ergometer equipped with competition racing bars, saddle, pedals, and chain. Power output is measured using a commercially available optical sensor system (SMI). A 5-minute warm-up is completed prior to the test at a resistance of 1.0% TBW for both females and males. Athletes are encouraged to perform a few sprints during the warm-up; however, no additional resistance is applied during the sprints. A 3-minute recovery follows the warm-up.

The test is initiated by having the athlete pedal at a controlled cadence of 60 rpm. Upon completion of the final countdown, the athlete accelerates and the load is applied (3.0% TBW for females, 4.0% TBW for males). The athlete performs the first 30-second maximal sprint and is verbally encouraged throughout the effort. Following a 60-second recovery (active or passive), the procedure is repeated until four additional 30-second sprints have been completed at progressively greater work loads (4.0%, 5.0%, 6.0%, 7.0% TBW for females; 5.0%, 6.0%, 7.0%, 8.0% TBW for males). The following parameters are measured for each 30-second sprint: (a) anaerobic power [peak power (W, W/kg), time to peak power (s)], (b) anaerobic capacity [average power (W, W/kg), total work (J, J/kg)], and (c) fatigue rate (%).

CONCLUSION

This chapter has provided an overview of the terminology, units, and concepts used to discuss work and power tests accurately. Force, torque, work, and power with the relevant units of newtons, newton-meters, joules, and watts were discussed for translational and rotational situations. The interdependent terms of *anaerobic power* and *anaerobic capacity* as they relate to athletic performance were also reviewed. Sports medicine professionals were given access to information to allow them to effectively establish testing programs featuring the serial use of event or sports-specific tests that are valid, reliable, and objective. Data from these uses can assist with evaluation of current states of conditioning, monitoring of the efficacy of training, event or sport selection, and talent identification. The chapter presented sport-specific tests used for the evaluation of high-performance athletes at the U.S. Olympic Training Centers. For each of these tests we provided a rationale, administration procedures, and data on performance standards by our reference groups.

REFERENCES

1. Smith JC, Hill DW. Contribution of energy systems during a Wingate power test. *Br J Sports Med* 1991;25:196–199.
2. Seresse O, Lortie G, Bouchard C, et al. Estimation of the contribution of the various energy systems during maximal work of short duration. *Int J Sports Med* 1988;9:456–460.
3. Inbar O, Bar-Or O, Skinner JS. *The Wingate anaerobic test.* Champaign, IL: Human Kinetics, 1996.

3a. Pereira MA, Freedson PA. Intraindividual variation of running economy in highly trained and moderately trained males. *Int J Sports Med* 1997;18(2):118–124.

4. Denegar CR, Ball DW. Assessing reliability and precision of measurement: an introduction to interclass correlation and standard error of measurement. *J Sports Rehabil* 1993;2:35–42.
5. Tesch P, Larsson L, Eriksson A, Karlsson J. Muscle glycogen depletion and lactate concentration during downhill skiing. *Med Sci Sports* 1978;10:85–90.
6. Komi PV, Rusko H, Villka V. Anaerobic performance capacity in athletes. *Acta Physiol Scand* 1977;100:107–114.
7. Andersen RE, Montgomery DL. Physiological monitoring of divisional ski racers during the 1986–87 season. *Can J Sports Sci* 1987;12(3):3.
8. Andersen RE, Montgomery DL, Turcotte RA. An on-site test battery to evaluate giant slalom skiing performance. *J Sports Med Phys Fitness* 1990;30:276–282.
9. Bacharach DW, von Duvillard SP. Intermediate and long-term anaerobic performance of elite alpine skiers. *Med Sci Sports Exerc* 1995;27(3):305–309.
10. Stark RM, Reed AT, Wenger HJ. Power curve characteristics of elite slalom and downhill skiers performing a modified 90s wingate test. *Can J Sports Sci* 1987;12(3):24.
11. White AT, Johnson SC. Physiological comparison of international, national and regional alpine skiers. *Int J Sports Med* 1991; 12(4):374–378.
12. Vadewalle H, Peres G, Monod H. Standard anaerobic exercise tests. *Sports Med* 1987;4:268–289.
13. Simoneau JA, Lortie G, Boulay MR, Bouchard C. Tests of anaerobic alactic and lactic capacities: description and reliability. *Can J Sports Sci* 1983;8:266–270.
14. Brown SL, Wilkinson JG. Characteristics of national, divisional, and club male alpine ski racers. *Med Sci Sports Exerc* 1983; 15(6):491–495.
15. Shea JB. The alpine skiing assessment battery: the secret to picking the right people and training for the right things. *J US Ski Coaches Assoc* 1983;6:26–31.
16. Jasmin BJ, Montgomery DL, Hoshizaki TB. Applicability of the

hexagonal obstacle test as a measure of anaerobic endurance for alpine skiers. *Sports Training Med Rehab* 1989;1:155–163.
17. Bar-Or O. The Wingate anaerobic test—an update on methodology, reliability, and validity. *Sports Med* 1987;4:381–394.
18. Dotan R, Bar-Or O. Load optimization for the Wingate anaerobic test. *Eur J Appl Physiol* 1983;51:409–417.
19. Dengel D, Kearney JT. *Measurements of performance potential in cyclists.* Raleigh, NC: Olympic Festival Scientific Symposium, 1987.
20. Sjogaard C, Nielsen G, Mikkelsen F, Saltin B, Burke ER. Physiology of bicycling. Ithaca, NY: Mouvement Pub. Inc., 1984:9–16.
20a. Coyle EF, Feltner ME, Kautz SA, et al. Physiological and biomechanical factors associated with elite endurance cycling performance. *Med Sci Sports Exerc* 1991;23:93–107.
21. Bishop D. Reliability of a 1-h endurance performance test in trained female cyclists. *Med Sci Sports Exerc* 1997;29:554–559.
22. Cox MH, Miles DS, Verde TJ, Rhodes EC. Applied physiology of ice hockey. *Sports Med* 1995;19(3):184–201.
23. Twist P, Rhodes T. A physiological analysis of ice hockey positions. *Natl Strength Cond Assoc J* 1993;15(6):44–46.
24. Rundell KW. Treadmill roller ski test predicts biathlon roller ski race results of elite U.S. biathlon women. *Med Sci Sports Exerc* 1995;27(12):1677–1685.
25. Rundell KW, Bacharach DW. Physiological characteristics and performance of top U.S. biathletes. *Med Sci Sports Exerc* 1995;27(9):1302–1310.
26. Street GM. Technological advances in cross-country ski equipment. *Med Sci Sports Exerc* 1992;24:1048–1054.
27. Rundell KW, Szmedra L. Energy cost of rifle carriage in biathlon skiing. *Med Sci Sports Exerc* 1998;30:570-576.
28. Mygind E, Larsson B, Klausen T. Evaluation of a specific test in cross-country skiing. *J Sports Sci* 1991;9:249–257.
29. Bouscaren J, Auth T, Biglow J, Karlson K. Going fast at the world's: a study of U.S. team performance at the 1994 world rowing championships. Presented at U.S. Rowing Association Annual Convention, 1994.
30. Shannon MP, Kearney JT, Buono MJ. Physiological and power output capacity in elite U.S. oarsmen. In: *Congress Proceedings, Fourth IOC World Congress on Sports Science.* 1997:180.
31. Rusko H, Numella A, Mero M. A new method for the evaluation of anaerobic running power in athletes. *Eur J Appl Physiol* 1993;66:97–101.
32. American College of Sports Medicine. *Guidelines for graded exercise testing and exercise prescription,* 4th ed. Baltimore: Williams & Wilkins, 1995:269–287.
32a. Numella A, Alberts M, Rijntjes RP, et al. Reliability and validity of the maximal anaerobic running test. *Int J Sports Med* 1996;17(suppl 2):S97–S102.
33. Numella A, Mero M, Stray-Gundersen J, et al. Important determinants of anaerobic running performance in male athletes and nonathletes. *Int J Sports Med* 1996;17(suppl 2):S91–S96.
34. Numella A, Mero M, Rusko H. Effects of sprint training on anaerobic performance characteristics determined by the MART. *Int J Sports Med* 1996;17(suppl 2):S114–S119.
35. Leonardi LM, Komor A, Dal Monte A. *An interactive computer simulation of bobsled pushoff phase with a multimember crew. Biomechanics X-B.* Champaign, IL: Human Kinetics, 1987: 761–766.
36. Osbeck JS, Maiorca SN, Rundell KW. Validity of field testing to bobsled start performance. *J Strength Cond Res* 1996;10:239–245.

Exercise and Sport Science,
edited by William E. Garrett, Jr., and Donald T. Kirkendall.
Lippincott Williams & Wilkins, Philadelphia © 2000.

CHAPTER 5

Physiology of Intermittent Exercise

Jens Bangsbo

In many sports such as volleyball, basketball, badminton, road cycling, and soccer, athletes perform intermittent exercise (Fig. 5–1). In other sports, such as running, intermittent exercise is performed during training. Therefore, it is important to understand the physiology of intermittent exercise. Over the years this has been investigated systematically by changing one variable at a time. Such studies form the basis for understanding the physiology of intermittent exercise during sports performance. It has to be recognized, however, that in laboratory studies the variation in intensity and duration of the exercise is regular, whereas in many sports the changes in exercise intensity are irregular and often more frequent.

This chapter discusses energy production from aerobic and anaerobic sources, and substrate utilization and performance during intermittent exercise. When studying intermittent exercise, the intensity of the exercise should be considered. The intensity eliciting maximum oxygen uptake may be around 25% of peak maximum power; for example, an individual may obtain a peak power output of 1000 W during maximum cycling and reach $\dot{V}O_2max$ at an intensity of 250 W, with an individual range from 15% to 70%. The relative intensity corresponding to $\dot{V}O_2max$ will be even lower if it is expressed in relation to an individual's maximal power output, which may be several thousands of watts, as in a maximal jump. It is important to define the relative intensity when discussing the physiologic effects. For example, it is possible to perform 15-second exercise bouts interspersed by 15-second rest periods for a total duration of 60 minutes if the intensity is around the intensity eliciting $\dot{V}O_2max$, whereas the exercise can be performed for only a few minutes if the intensity is around 70% of maximum intensity. This chapter cites the intensity of the exercise periods when it is known.

J. Bangsbo: Institute of Exercise and Sport Sciences, Department of Human Physiology, University of Copenhagen, Copenhagen, Denmark.

AEROBIC ENERGY PRODUCTION DURING INTERMITTENT EXERCISE

At the start of exercise, the O_2 bound to myoglobin in muscle and hemoglobin in blood, and O_2 dissolved in the muscles, constitute direct O_2 sources that can be used. The total local oxygen store amounts to around 2 mmol O_2/kg dry weight (DW), corresponding to about 900 mL for an exercising individual who has about 20 kg of muscles. Nevertheless, the aerobic contribution is not sufficient to cover the energy demand, and energy will also be produced anaerobically. This insufficiency is referred to as the oxygen deficit, which will lead to an elevated oxygen uptake after exercise compared to rest (oxygen debt); it can last for several hours (1). This means that if the resting periods during intermittent exercise are not too long the oxygen uptake is elevated prior to the exercise bouts. Figure 5–2 demonstrates the pulmonary oxygen uptake during repeated 30-second high-intensity exercise (534 W) bouts separated by 4 minutes of recovery.

It has also been demonstrated that when intense exercise is repeated, the rise of the oxygen uptake by the contracting muscles in the initial phase of exercise is faster due to a more rapid increase in oxygen extraction (Fig. 5–3). The higher extraction has been associated with increased activity of pyruvate dehydrogenase (PDH), but it is unclear whether a more rapid decarboxylation of pyruvate is the cause of a more pronounced activation of the electron transport chain and greater extraction of oxygen when exercise is repeated.

The greater oxygen utilization when exercise is repeated will limit the oxygen deficit, but the oxygen uptake during exercise is still significantly lower than the

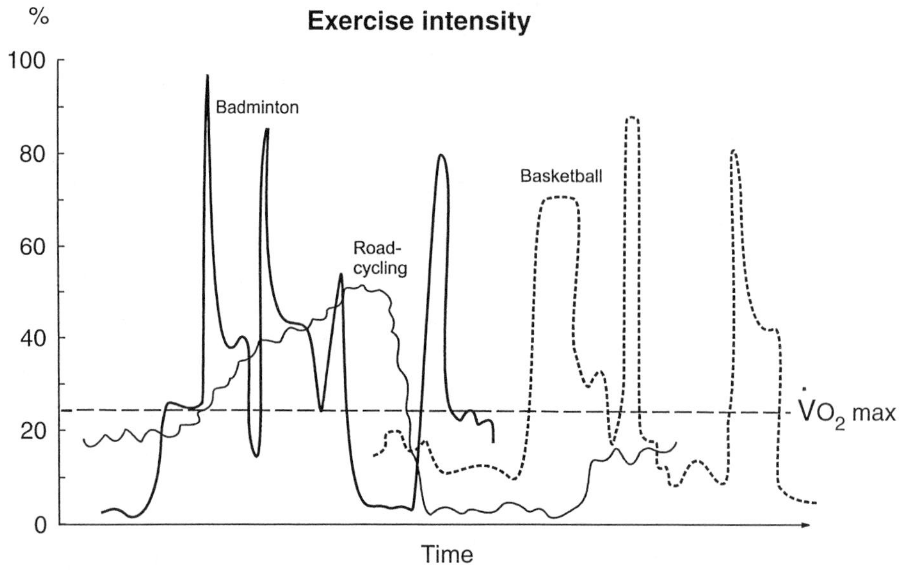

FIG. 5–1. Examples of pattern of exercise intensities in various sports. $\dot{V}O_2$max represents the intensity eliciting maximum oxygen uptake.

oxygen demand, leading to an oxygen deficit and greater oxygen utilization in the recovery periods than at rest. When the intensity during intermittent exercise is below the power output eliciting $\dot{V}O_2$max, the mean oxygen uptake appears to be the same whether the same work is performed continuously or intermittently (Figs. 5–4 and 5–5). This means that the oxygen deficit established in the initial phase of exercise is "paid back" in the recovery periods during intermittent exercise. In Fig. 5–4, the oxygen uptake during intermittent exercise alternating between 15 seconds at a running speed of 18 km/h and 10 seconds at 8 km/h is compared with the oxygen uptake during continuous exercise at the same speeds. The oxygen uptake at the low speed during intermittent exercise is higher than during continuous running, whereas the oxygen uptake for the high speed is lower during intermittent than during continuous running. If the exercise intensity is higher than that corresponding to $\dot{V}O_2$max, the mean oxygen uptake is higher during intermittent compared to continuous exercise (Fig. 5–5). The latter can be explained by findings that the oxygen debt after intense exercise is considerably higher than the oxygen deficit, which is related not only to greater oxygen uptake by the lungs and heart but also to elevated oxygen utilization of the exercised muscles. It has been observed that the muscle oxygen uptake in recovery from intense exercise to a significant extent exceeds resynthesis of phosphates such as adenosine triphosphate (ATP) and creatine phosphate (CP) as well as metabolism of lactate within the exercised muscle (2).

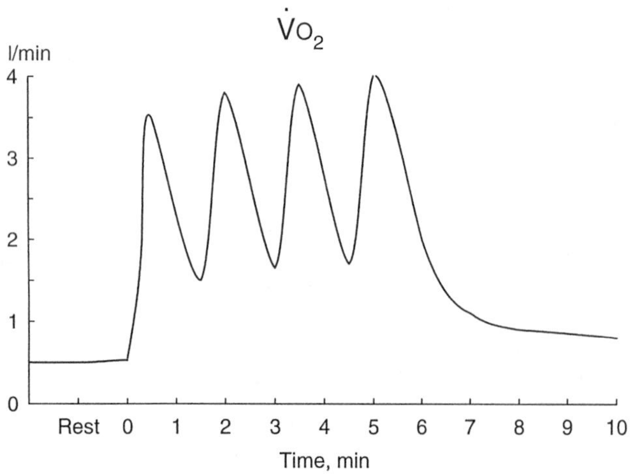

FIG. 5–2. Oxygen uptake measured breath by breath before and during intermittent cycling consisting of four 30-second-duration exercise periods (425 W) separated by 1-minute recovery periods.

Repeated maximal exercise even of short duration (a few seconds) also leads to a marked increase in oxygen uptake. For example, it was observed that the mean oxygen uptake was 2.85 L/min, corresponding to about 65% of $\dot{V}O_2$max, in the first 30 seconds of recovery after five repeated 5- to 6-second sprints separated by 30 seconds (3). The high demand on the aerobic system was also reflected in the finding of a mean heart rate of 173 beats/min during the first 30 seconds of recovery. The importance of aerobic energy production during repeated intense exercise can also be illustrated by findings in studies in which oxygen availability was changed. By increasing the hemoglobin (Hb) concentration through administration of erythropoietin, blood lactate and plasma hypoxanthine accumulation was lower after

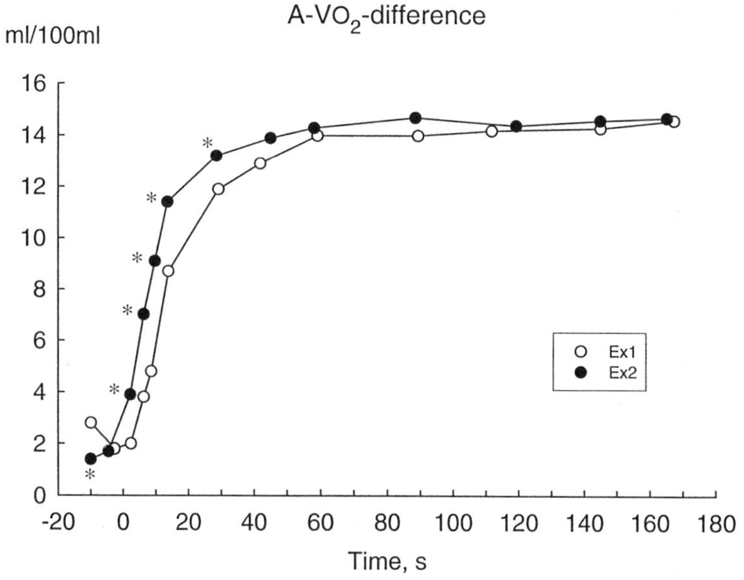

FIG. 5–3. Oxygen extraction of the exercising leg during repeated intense one-legged knee-extensor exercise (63 W). The two exercise periods were separated by a 6-minute rest period. Data presented as means. *, Significant difference between EX1 and EX2.

15 intense 6-second runs separated by 24-second recovery periods compared to a condition with normal Hb concentration (3). Furthermore, when subjects performed ten 6-second high-intensity bouts separated by 30-second rest periods under a hypoxic condition, performance was reduced and the accumulation of blood lactate was higher than in a normoxic condition (3).

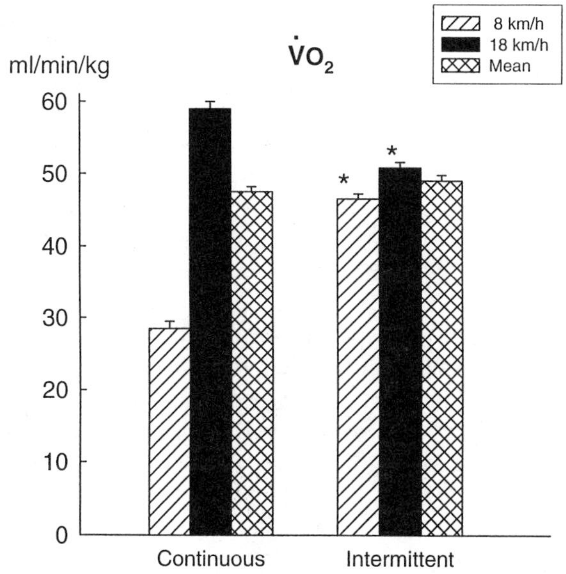

FIG. 5–4. Oxygen uptake ($\dot{V}O_2$) during continuous (*left*) and intermittent treadmill running alternating between 10 seconds at 8 km/h^{-1} and 15 seconds at 18 km/h^{-1} (*right*). Mean $\dot{V}O_2$ (*right-hatched bars*) is determined as [$\dot{V}O_2$ (at 8 km/h^{-1}; *left-hatched bars*) × 10 + $\dot{V}O_2$ (at 18 km/h^{-1}; *open bars*) × 15]/25. Data presented as means ± standard error of the mean (SEM). *, Significant difference between continuous and intermittent running.

ANAEROBIC ENERGY PRODUCTION DURING INTERMITTENT EXERCISE

Several studies have compared the anaerobic energy production during continuous and intermittent exercise at the same average work rate. At a mean exercise intensity corresponding to 50% of $\dot{V}O_2$max, it was observed that muscle lactate was lower during continuous compared to intermittent exercise consisting of 30-second running and 30-second rest periods (4). In a study by Essén and colleagues (5) the subjects performed continuous and intermittent cycle exercise for 1 hour at the same mean intensity. The intermittent exercise alternated between 15 seconds of rest and 15 seconds of exercise at a work rate that for continuous cycling demanded maximum oxygen uptake. No difference in muscle lactate was observed between continuous and intermittent exercise (Fig. 5–6), but a higher release of lactate was found during the intermittent exercise. Only small alterations occurred in ATP and CP during the continuous exercise, while in the intermittent exercise considerable fluctuations in these variables were observed (Fig. 5–7). After 5 minutes of the intermittent exercise, the CP concentration was 40% of the resting level after an exercise period, and it increased to about 70% of rest in the subsequent 15-second recovery period. Similar changes were found during the following 55 minutes of the intermittent exercise (Fig. 5–7). Figure 5–8 demonstrates a calculation of the contribution from aerobic and anaerobic sources during the exercise and recovery, based on the muscle metabolic data and the measured oxygen uptake (5).

The duration of the exercise bouts in an intermittent exercise program is important for the accumulation of

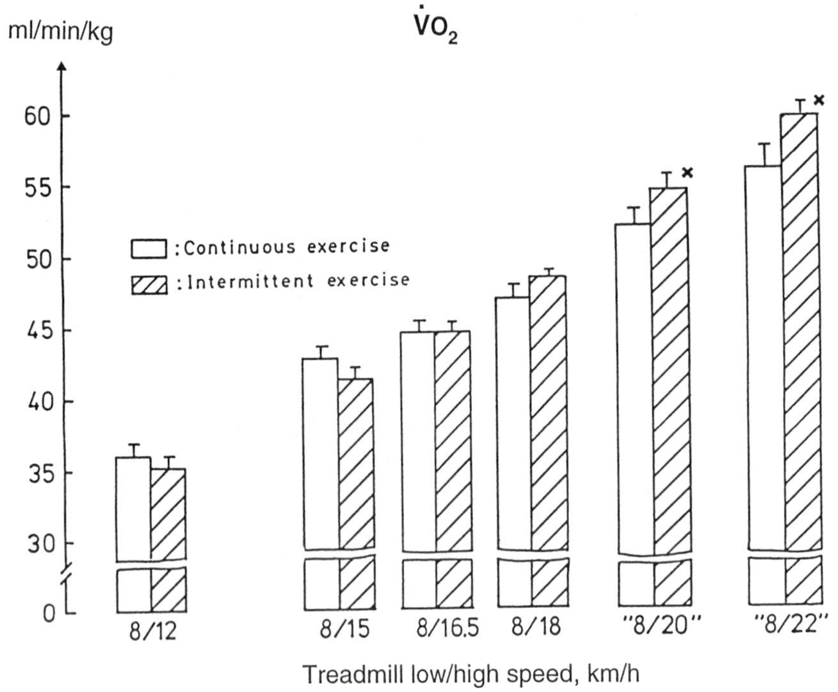

FIG. 5–5. Oxygen uptake ($\dot{V}O_2$) during continuous (*open bars*) and intermittent (alternating between 10 seconds at 8 km/h^{-1} and 15 seconds at a higher speed; *hatched bars*) treadmill running at the same mean speed. Oxygen uptake for the continuous exercise is estimated as [$\dot{V}O_2$ (at 8 km/h^{-1}) $\times$ 10 + $\dot{V}O_2$ (at the high speed) $\times$ 15]/25, except for "8/20" and "8/22," in which $\dot{V}O_2$ is determined during continuous running at the same speed as for the intermittent exercise (15.2 and 16.4 km/h^{-1}, respectively). Data presented as means $\pm$ SEM. *Significant difference between continuous and intermittent exercise.

lactate both in the blood and in the muscle. In a study by Saltin and Essén (6) the ratio between exercise and recovery was kept constant (1:2). The muscle and blood lactate concentrations were only slightly higher than at rest when the exercise time was 10 and 20 seconds, whereas the concentrations were considerably increased with exercise bouts of 30- and 60-second duration. Part of the difference can be explained by a higher aerobic contribution during the shorter exercise periods due to a greater total utilization of oxygen bound to myoglobin (Mb) and Hb in the muscles and blood.

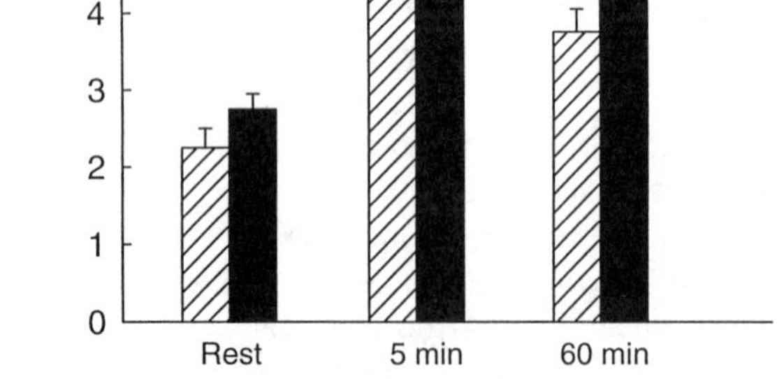

FIG. 5–6. Muscle lactate concentration at rest as well as after 5 and 60 minutes of continuous exercise at an intensity of 157 W (*open bar*) and of intermittent cycling alternating between 15-second exercise (299 W) and 15-second rest periods. Means $\pm$ SE are given. (Data adapted from ref. 5.)

Also, the intensity of the exercise affects to a great extent the metabolic response during intermittent exercise (Fig. 5–9). A subject performed 20-second running periods separated by 10-second rest periods at a speed of 22.0 km/h and on another occasion at 22.75 km/h. At the speed of 22.0 km/h the subject could exercise about an hour, whereas at the 22.75 km/h speed he became exhausted after about 25 minutes, and the rate of blood lactate accumulation was much higher than at the 22.0 km/h speed.

The metabolic response during intense intermittent exercise is also related to the duration of the rest periods in between the exercise bouts. In a study by Christensen and colleagues (7), one subject had lactate concentrations of 2.6 and 8.9 mmol/L when the 15-second exercise bouts were separated by 30 and 15 seconds of rest, respectively. Similarly, in a study by Margaria and colleagues (8), the subjects exercised repeatedly for 10 seconds at an intensity that led to exhaustion after 30 to 40 seconds, when performed continuously. Blood lactate increased progressively when the periods of exercise were separated by 10 seconds of rest, while it was only slightly elevated with 30 seconds of rest in between the exercise bouts.

Several studies have focused on intermittent exercise

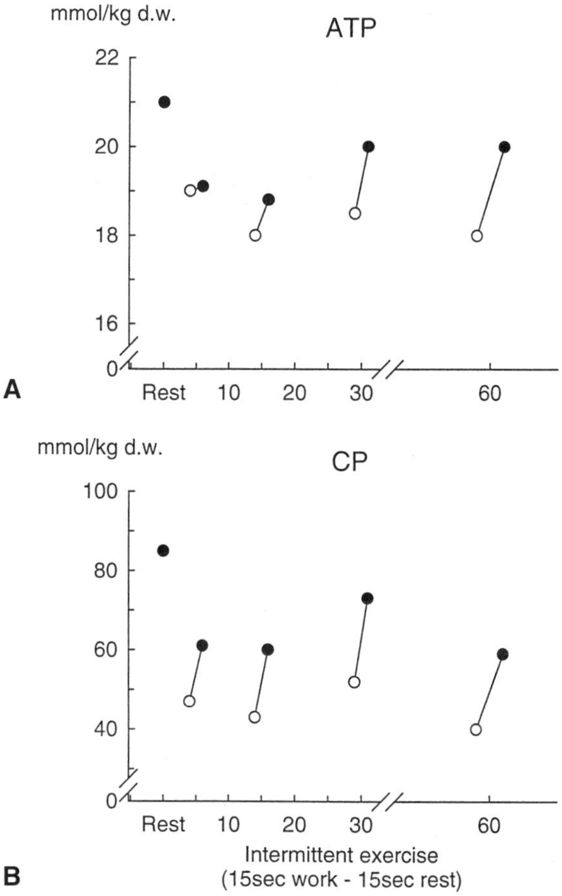

FIG. 5–7. Muscle adenosine triphosphate (ATP) (**A**) and creatine phosphate (CP) (**B**) concentration at rest and during intermittent cycling alternating between 15-second exercise and 15-second rest periods. *Open symbols* represent values immediately after exercise and *filled symbols* after 15 seconds of rest. (Data adapted from ref. 23.)

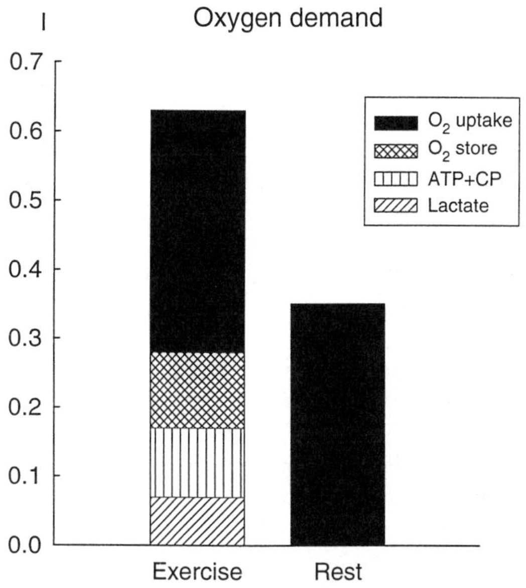

FIG. 5–8. Energy demand during the 15-second exercise periods (*left*) and oxygen uptake during the 15-second recovery periods (*right*) of intermittent cycling. The contribution to the oxygen deficit during the exercise periods from lactate accumulation, phosphagen depletion (ATP + CP) and oxygen stores, assuming a mass of active muscle of 11 kg, is indicated. Means ± SE are given. (Data adapted from ref. 5.)

in which the intensity was considerably higher than a power output eliciting $\dot{V}O_2max$ (supramaximal exercise). In one study supramaximal exercise was performed five times for 1 minute separated by 5-minute rest periods (9). The performance decreased progressively, and the muscle lactate concentration was the same at the end of the first, third, and fifth exercise bouts. Similar findings were obtained in other studies using repeated supramaximal exercise (10–15). In these studies, performance was gradually impaired, and muscle lactate accumulation decreased considerably as the intermittent exercise was continued. For example, when subjects repeated ten 6-second sprints on a cycle ergometer, Gaitanos and colleagues (13) found a 33% reduction in peak power and a 27% reduction in mean power output. The total anaerobic energy production during the 10th sprint was estimated to be about one-third of the production during the first sprint (Fig. 5–10). The glycogenolytic and glycolytic rates for the first sprint were 4.4 and 2.3 mmol/kg DW/s, respectively. By the 10th sprint the rate of both glycogenolysis and glycolysis (0.4 and 0.3 mmol/kg DW/s, respectively) was considerably lower. For the first exercise bout, net breakdown of ATP, CP, and energy release from glycolysis could account for 6%, 44%, and 50%, respectively, of the total anaerobic energy production, while the corresponding values for the 10th exercise bout were 4%, 80%, and 16% (Fig. 5–10).

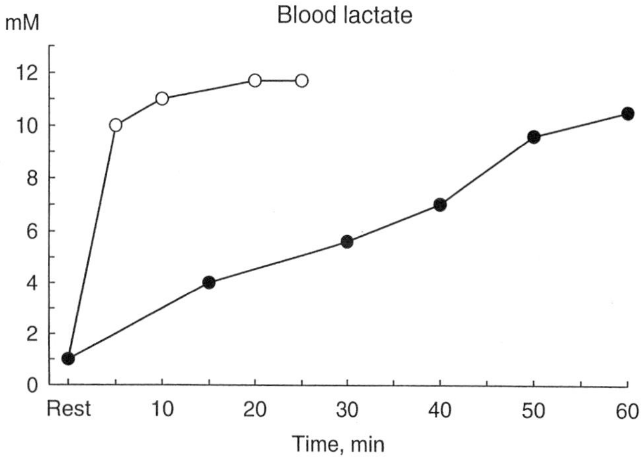

FIG. 5–9. Blood lactate concentration for a subject running to exhaustion at a speed of 22.75 km/h (*open circle*) and 22.00 km/h (*filled circle*). (Data adapted from ref. 6a.)

In line with these findings were observations in a nuclear magnetic resonance (NMR) study of repeated isometric contractions. The CP utilization was the same during each of four 30-second maximal voluntary contractions (MVCs) despite a lower work output during subsequent contractions (Fig. 5–11). These results indicate that muscle glycolysis was lower, which was supported by the finding of no change or a slight increase in muscle pH when the maximal contractions were repeated (Fig. 5–11).

The question to be raised is, What causes the lower rate of glycolysis when intense exercise is repeated? Only the most obvious possibilities will be discussed. A progressive decline in muscle glycogen concentration is an unlikely explanation, since it has been demonstrated in humans that glycogenolytic and glycolytic rates during short-term intense exercise are independent of initial muscle glycogen concentrations above about 50 mmol/kg wet weight (WW) (14). This value is lower than that observed in most of the studies showing a reduction in glycolysis.

A successive increase in the muscle H^+ concentration prior to the subsequent exercise bout may have impaired glycolysis, since it has been demonstrated that lower pH per se has an inhibitory effect on phosphorylase and phosphofructokinase (PFK), which are considered the key regulating enzymes of the glycogenolytic and glycolytic rate, respectively (16–18). However, the rate of lactate production was also significantly reduced when knee-extensor exercise was repeated after 1 hour of recovery, although muscle lactate and pH were at resting levels prior to the second exercise bout (14). Furthermore, it is questionable whether the reduction in pH during intense exercise is large enough to inhibit these enzymes *in vivo*. Studies on the allosteric regulation of PFK within the physiologic range have shown that the effect of pH is negligible if the pH is above 6.6 (19,20), which is lower than that observed in human studies showing a reduction in glycolysis (15). Thus, it appears that an elevated H^+ concentration is, at the least, not the only explanation for the reduction in the glycolytic rate during intermittent exercise.

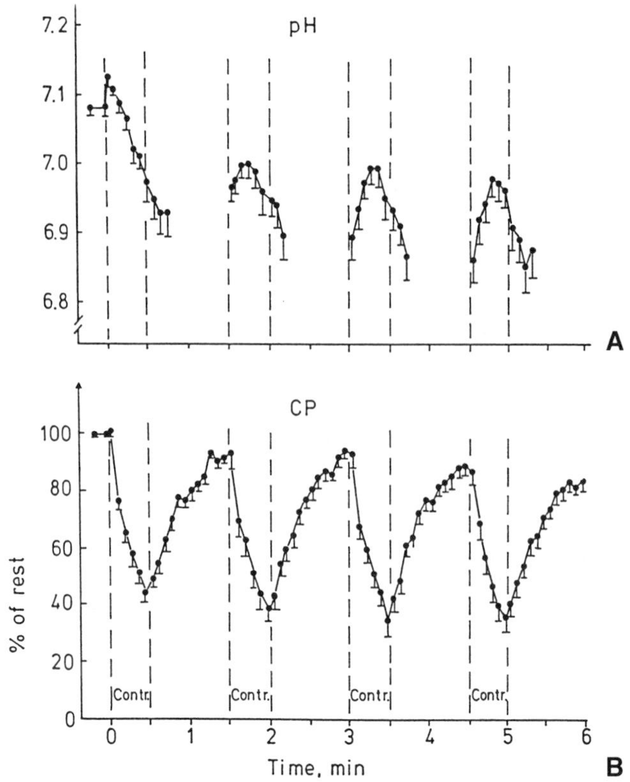

FIG. 5–11. Muscle CP concentration (**A**) and estimated muscle pH (**B**) determined by nuclear magnetic resonance (NMR) during repeated 30-second maximal isometric contractions. The CP concentration is expressed in relation to the concentration at rest. Means ± SEM are given. (Data adapted from ref. 25.)

Impairment of glycolysis when exercise is repeated could be due to accumulation of cytosolic citrate, as it has been demonstrated *in vitro* that citrate inhibits the

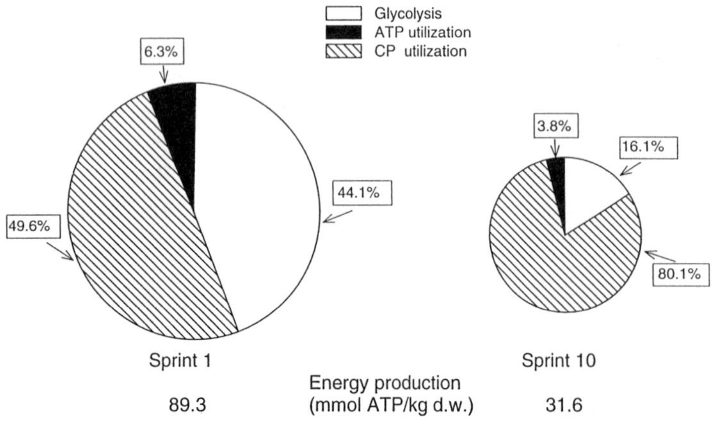

FIG. 5–10. Total muscle anaerobic energy production (not including energy production related to lactate release) and relative contribution of ATP and CP as well as glycolysis during the first and tenth 6-second sprints. The sprints were separated by 24 seconds of rest. (Data adapted from ref. 13.)

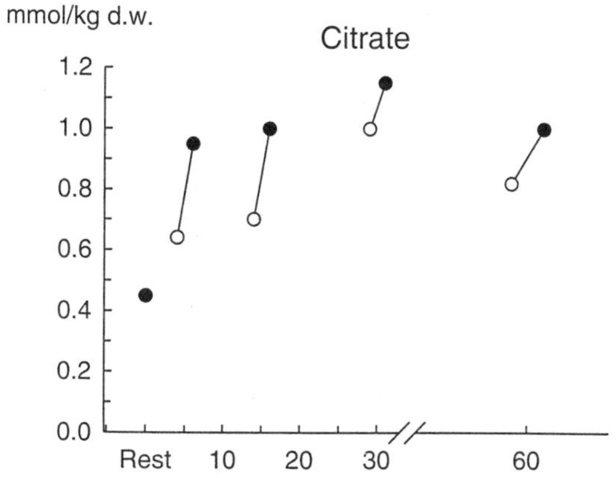

FIG. 5–12. Muscle citrate at rest and during intermittent cycling alternating between 15 seconds of exercise and 15 seconds of rest. *Open symbols* represent values immediately after exercise and *filled symbols* after 15 seconds of rest. (Data adapted from ref. 23.)

PFK activity by potentiating the inhibitory effect of ATP on PFK, and stimulates fructose-1,6-diphosphatase activity (17,21,22). It was observed by Essén (23) that the muscle citrate concentration was increased after 5, 10, and 30 minutes of intermittent cycling exercise consisting of 15 seconds of exercise, at a work rate eliciting $\dot{V}O_2$max, followed by 15 seconds of rest (Fig. 5–12). Furthermore, the muscle citrate concentration was higher at the end of the rest period than immediately after exercise. It was believed that this was caused by continuous acetylcoenzyme A (acetyl-CoA) production from β-oxidation together with decreased citric acid cycle activity during the rest periods. Essén (23) found that less glycogen was used, and lactate accumulation per unit of time was lower when intense exercise was performed intermittently as compared to continuously. It was suggested that the citrate accumulated during the intermittent exercise penetrated the mitochondrial membrane and retarded glycolysis, and that citrate was the primary cause of the metabolic changes.

It is possible that the citrate concentration at the onset of repeated supramaximal exercise is elevated and that this inhibits glycolysis, particularly at the initial phase of exercise. However, it is unlikely that the effect of citrate can account for all the impairment in glycolysis, since the effect of citrate within the physiologic range is small (24). Thus, it is unclear what causes the lower rate of glycolysis when intense exercise is repeated. (For an extended discussion of this topic, see ref. 25.)

SUBSTRATE UTILIZATION DURING INTERMITTENT EXERCISE

Essén (23) compared intermittent with continuous exercise performed at the same power output (corresponding to $\dot{V}O_2$max). The continuous exercise led to exhaustion within a few minutes, while the intermittent exercise could be sustained for 1 hour without reaching fatigue. The rate of glycogen utilization and accumulation of lactate during the continuous exercise at the high intensity was greater than during the intermittent exercise. Nevertheless, the intermittent exercise led to a progressive lowering of the muscle glycogen, which was similar to that observed during continuous exercise at the same mean intensity (Fig. 5–13). In general, carbohydrate oxidation was similar under the two conditions (Fig. 5–14). The rate of fat oxidation was considerably higher during the intermittent compared to the continuous exercise at the same intensity, and it resembled that occurring during continuous exercise at half the intensity (Fig. 5–14).

A marked difference in fiber type recruitment was also observed between the two types of exercise protocols. While it was mainly the slow-twitch (ST) fibers that were activated during the continuous exercise at half the intensity, both ST and fast-twitch (FT) fibers were involved in the intermittent exercise (Fig. 5–15) (23). The different pattern of fiber-type recruitment between continuous and intermittent exercise has important implications for training. By performing the training intermittently, it is possible to train some muscle fibers (FT fibers) that would have been recruited only after hours of submaximal continuous exercise. This is particularly relevant for sports in which high-intensity exercise frequently occurs. Intermittent exercise also allows prolonged high metabolic stress without fatiguing the fibers recruited.

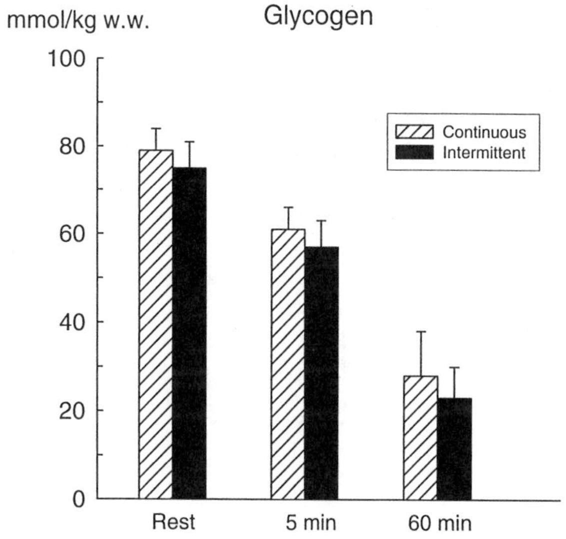

FIG. 5–13. Muscle glycogen concentration at rest as well as after 5 and 60 minutes of continuous exercise at an intensity of 157 W (*open bar*) and of intermittent cycling alternating between 15-second exercise (299 W) and 15-second rest periods. (*closed bar*). Means ± SE are given. (Data adapted from ref. 5.)

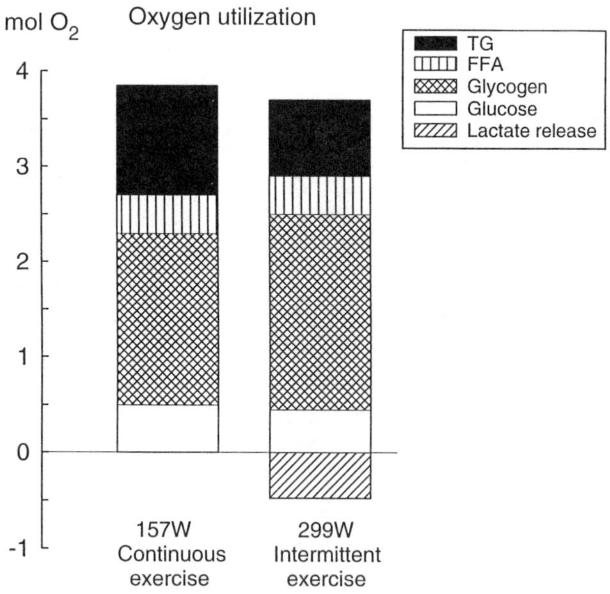

FIG. 5–14. Muscle substrate utilization during 60 minutes of continuous exercise at an intensity of 157 W (*open bar*) and of intermittent cycling alternating between 15-second exercise (299 W) and 15-second rest periods. The *total bar* shows the energy production based on measurements of leg oxygen uptake. The contribution from fat and carbohydrate oxidation is estimated from leg respiratory quotient (RQ) values. The uptake of FA and glucose from the blood and contribution to carbohydrate and fat oxidation, respectively, as well as lactate release, is also shown. The use of muscle glycogen is estimated as the difference between total oxidation of carbohydrates and glucose uptake, and the utilization of intramuscular/blood-borne triglycerides is determined as total fat oxidation subtracting oxidation related to fat uptake. (Data adapted from ref. 5.)

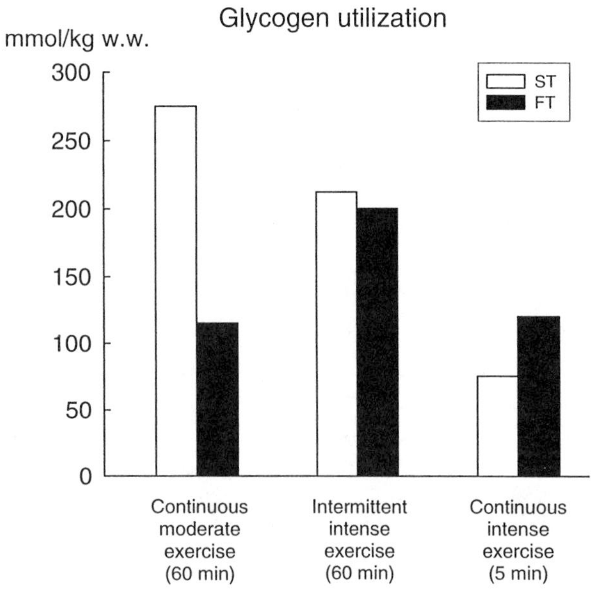

FIG. 5–15. Glycogen depletion in slow twitch (ST; *open bar*) and fast twitch (FT; *filled bar*) muscle fibers after 60 minutes of continuous exercise at an intensity of 157 W (*left*), of intermittent cycling alternating between 15-second exercise (299 W) and 15-second rest periods (*middle*) and continuous exhaustive exercise (299 W; 4–6 minutes, *right*). (Data adapted from ref. 23.)

During supramaximal exercise, primary energy sources are CP degradation and glycolysis, leading to pyruvate production for either oxidation or lactate formation. Creatine phosphate is in part resynthesized during the recovery periods, whereas muscle glycogen progressively decreases during intermittent exercise, since the rate of muscle glycogen synthesis during the recovery periods is low (2,14). Whereas muscle CP and glycogen are the main substrates during supramaximal exercise periods, in the recovery periods fat and glucose taken up from the blood are used more (2,11). The importance of fat oxidation during intense intermittent exercise is also illustrated by the finding of an elevated activity of the β-oxidative enzyme β-hydroxyacyl-CoA-dehydrogenase (HAD) after a period of anaerobic training (26).

PERFORMANCE DURING INTERMITTENT EXERCISE

Performance during intermittent exercise can be characterized by the ability to perform maximally, for example as determined by peak power during maximal cycling or by the ability to sustain a given power output after previous exercise. The time course of recovery from intense exercise may not be the same for these two types of muscle performance. Sahlin and Ren (27) reported that MVC force was restored 2 minutes after an intense muscle contraction, but the time to fatigue for an isometric contraction performed at 66% of MVC was reduced by 40%. Similarly, Bogdanis and colleagues (28) observed that peak power output during maximal cycling 3 minutes after a 30-second exercise bout had recovered to about 89% of peak power output during a single maximal exercise period, whereas Bangsbo and colleagues (14) found that the ability to maintain a given power output during one-legged knee-extensor exercise was lower by 10% even 1 hour after a 3-minute exhaustive exercise period. It appears that there is a long-lasting residual effect of intense exercise that does not influence maximal force development, but does affect the ability to sustain a high power output. This section discusses the cause of fatigue during intermittent exercise.

Fatigue during repeated intense exercise may be caused by a reduced neural activation of the muscle. It could be central (cortical), but it appears that in well-motivated subjects a substantial component of fatigue can be localized to the muscle (29). It is difficult to identify a single muscle factor responsible for the reduction in performance during intense intermittent exercise, but there are various suggestions for the cause of fatigue. This discussion is restricted to a few selected variables, such as ATP, lactate, protons, and potassium, which have been suggested to be involved in the development of fatigue during intense intermittent exercise in humans.

Availability of ATP and CP

Fatigue during intense repeated exercise does not appear to be related to a lack of energy, since muscle ATP rarely falls below 60% of preexercise levels during exhaustive voluntary exercise (15), and even in highly fatigued fibers the ATP concentration is over 100-fold higher than the micromolar amounts required for peak force (see ref. 30). In addition, it has been observed that when intense dynamic exercise was repeated, muscle ATP concentration was significantly lower at the end of the second exercise bout, indicating that lack of ATP was not the cause of fatigue during the first exercise period (15). In agreement with that suggestion, it has been observed that no fiber was totally depleted of ATP when single-fiber analysis was performed on muscle biopsies taken immediately after exercise, even after electrical stimulation that resulted in a large force decline (31,32). It cannot be excluded, however, that ATP is compartmentalized and that the ATP concentration can fall below a critical level in the vicinity of the ATP utilization sites, thereby causing a drop in contractile capacity.

Bogdanis and colleagues (28) observed an association between resynthesis of CP and recovery of peak power output after a maximal 30-second exercise bout. Furthermore, it has been observed that performance of high-intensity intermittent exercise was increased after a period of creatine intake, which in other studies has been shown to increase muscle creatine and CP, and it has been suggested that low CP levels are associated with fatigue (3,33). On the other hand, it has been observed that CP decreases rapidly in the initial phase of exercise, and that subjects are able to maintain the exercise intensity for several minutes even though the CP concentration remains low (34). Therefore, it is doubtful that low CP levels per se cause fatigue.

Accumulating Muscle Lactate and Protons

It is generally believed that lactic acid accumulation can cause fatigue during intense intermittent exercise. Lactate ions per se have been observed to inhibit rabbit sarcoplasmatic reticulum (SR) Ca^{2+} channel activity (35). Furthermore, increased lactate concentrations have been reported to impair tension development in intact dog muscle (36). However, lactate anions had no effect on maximal Ca^{2+} activated force in skinned fibers (37). Thus, it is questionable whether lactate causes fatigue. This notion is supported by findings in a study in which subjects repeated intense exhaustive knee-extensor exercise after a 60-minute recovery period (14). At the point of exhaustion the muscle lactate concentration in the second exercise bout was only 65% of the concentration at the end of the first exercise bout (Fig. 5–16).

A large production of lactate during intense exercise is associated with elevated acidity within the exercising muscles. Decreases in muscle pH from about 7.1 to 6.5–6.8 are often observed during intense exhaustive exercise (38–40); based on NMR studies, it has been suggested that pH in individual fibers can be even lower (41). This may affect the function of the muscle cells, as it is known from *in vitro* studies that low pH has an inhibitory effect on various functions within the muscle cell, such as the activity of phosphorylase and PFK, the excitation-contraction coupling, the affinity for Ca^{2+} to bind to troponin, and the coupling between the contractile elements and the reuptake of Ca^{2+} in the SR (37,42–46). However, pH may not be an exclusive determinant of fatigue. This was illustrated with observations in a human study (47). To examine the effect of muscle pH on development of fatigue during intensive exercise, seven subjects performed intense exhaustive leg exercise (3 to 5 minutes) on two occasions: with (leg-arm; LA) and without (leg; L) preceding intense intermittent arm exercise. The duration of the exercise was about 1 minute shorter in LA than in L. Before exercise, muscle pH was the same in L and LA, but at the end of exercise muscle pH was lower in LA (6.65) than in L (6.82). This finding suggests that there is no definitive muscle pH

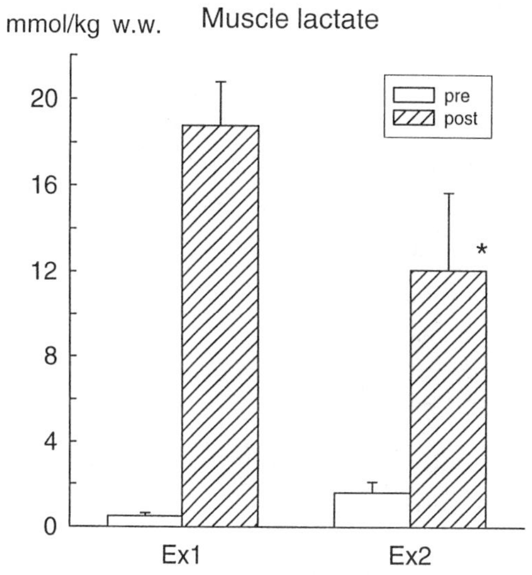

FIG. 5–16. Muscle lactate concentration prior to and at the end of two exhaustive knee-extensor exercise bouts separated by 1 hour of recovery. Note that the muscle lactate concentration at exhaustion was significantly lower at the end of exercise. (Data adapted from ref. 14.)

that leads to fatigue and that low pH is not the only factor causing fatigue during intense muscle contractions *in vivo*. This notion is supported in a study in which intense exercise was repeated after a 2.5-minute recovery period (15). Muscle pH tended to be higher at the point of fatigue, although muscle pH was significantly lower prior to the second exercise bout. Furthermore, muscle pH increased when intense static contractions were repeated, although force production was progressively reduced (see Fig. 5–11). Therefore, it is unlikely that low muscle pH per se causes fatigue. Along that line is the finding that the rapid phase of recovery of maximal force after intense exercise cannot be explained by the decline in H^+ accumulation, since muscle pH decreases after an intense muscle contraction (48, 49).

Accumulating Potassium in the Muscle Interstitium

It has been speculated that progressive accumulation of potassium in the interstitium during intense exercise may be implicated in the fatigue process (50). In the study mentioned above in which leg exercise was performed with and without prior arm exercise, the release of potassium during the exercise was greater in LA than in L (47). The greater release of potassium in LA led to the same arterial and venous potassium concentration at the point of exhaustion in LA and L, even though the exercise duration was about 1 minute shorter in LA. Furthermore, in both L and LA the potassium efflux to the blood was reduced at the end of exercise, suggesting that potassium in the interstitium accumulated progressively toward the end of exercise. Also, in studies using repeated intense knee-extensor exercise, it has been observed that the femoral arterial and venous potassium concentrations are the same at exhaustion, indicating that a given potassium concentration in the muscle interstitium leads to fatigue (14,15).

The mechanism behind the possible effect of potassium on the development of fatigue is unclear. It may be that the accumulating potassium stimulates sensory receptors of group III and IV nerve fibers, leading to inhibition at the spinal level (29,51). Another coupling between fatigue and potassium could be an inhibition of the propagation of the action potential due to ion disturbances over the sarcolemma and a possible block in its propagation into the t-tubules (50). The latter hypothesis is supported by the observation that rather small increments in extracellular potassium lead to a reduction in tension in subsequent contractions when isolated mouse muscles were stimulated (52). It is possible that a continuous efflux of potassium from the exercising muscle, together with a limited reuptake and a reduced release to venous blood, lead to a progressive accumulation of potassium in the interstitium, which may have been implicated in the fatigue process.

Other findings support the suggestion of a link between potassium and the fatigue processes during repeated intense exercise. The time course of change in muscle force and potassium, in recovery from exhaustive exercise, are similar and much faster than the changes in muscle pH (25). It is noteworthy that even though lowered pH does not cause fatigue, a decrease in pH may promote the development of fatigue during exercise by increasing the release of potassium from the muscle cell through potassium channels (47,53,54).

During intermittent exercise, it is likely that the exercising muscle releases potassium during the intense exercise periods and takes up potassium during rest or less-intense exercise periods. This is illustrated in a study in which subjects performed one-legged knee-extensor exercise at a rather high intensity (about 70% of peak $\dot{V}O_2$ for the exercising muscles) for 30 minutes. Twice during the exercise period, the work rate was increased further for 1 minute. It was found that the leg released potassium during the exercise, and a more pronounced efflux was observed during the periods when the intensity was elevated (Fig. 5–17). Immediately after the more intense bouts, a significant net uptake of potassium was noted, even though the subjects continued to exercise at the lower intensity. Thus, the intense exercise stimulated mechanisms such as Na^+/K^+ pumps sufficiently to counteract the release of potassium caused by the exercise. Apparently, the muscles have a high potential for reestablishing ion homeostatis, which probably occurs in recovery after the intense exercise periods in intermittent exercise. This means that fatigue related to accumulation of potassium is a transient phenomenon that can explain why performance can be temporally impaired in sports with intermittent exercise, for example in basketball after a fast break.

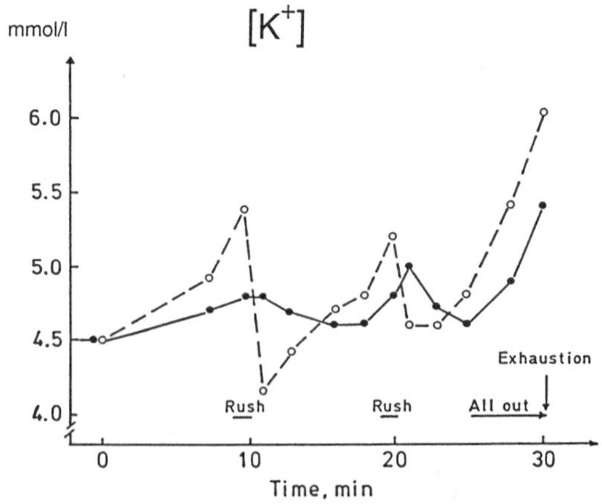

FIG. 5–17. Arterial (*filled circles*) and femoral venous (*open circles*) potassium (K^+) concentrations during knee-extensor exercise (60 W; kick frequency: 60 seconds) for one subject. Twice during exercise the kick frequency was elevated to 80 seconds for 1 minute (rush), and toward the end of the protocol the subject exercised to exhaustion (all-out). (Data adapted from ref. 25.)

The time needed to return to a normal level after intense exercise is dependent on a variety of factors such as the fitness level of the subject, the activity in the recovery period, and the intensity and duration of the preceding exercise. The latter is illustrated by the findings of Balsom and colleagues (3). They observed that running time (approximately 5.5 seconds) was progressively increased when a 40-m sprint was repeated 15 times, whereas performance was unaltered in 40 sprints of 15 m (approximately 2.5 seconds). In both cases the sprints were separated by a 30-second rest period. Thus, it appears that 30 seconds was sufficient to recover from approximately 3 seconds of maximal exercise, but not when the duration of the maximal exercise was about 6 seconds.

Muscle Glycogen and Fatigue During Prolonged Intermittent Exercise

Muscle glycogen does not appear to be linked to fatigue during a single bout of intense exercise unless muscle glycogen is low (<40 mmol/kg WW) (14,39). On the other hand, the type of fatigue that occurs during prolonged intermittent exercise may be related to a reduction in muscle glycogen.

Balsom and colleagues (55) examined the effect of different levels of muscle glycogen on performance during repeated intense exercise. The subjects were tested on two occasions: on one occasion the subjects consumed a diet containing a low amount of carbohydrate (LC) and on the other occasion a diet with a high-carbohydrate (HC) content was consumed in the days prior to the test, resulting in muscle glycogen levels of about 45 and 100 mmol/kg WW, respectively, prior to the test. At the test the subjects performed 15 6-second cycling bouts of an intensity of 958 W separated by 30 seconds on both occasions. The HC performance during the last four exercise bouts was significantly better than the LC, suggesting that the low muscle glycogen in LC inhibited performance (Fig. 5–18). On two separate days the subjects also performed repeated 6-second exercise bouts at intensities of about 700 to 800 W separated by a 30-second recovery period until exhaustion. The subjects could perform 111 and 294 bouts after having ingested a diet with low and high carbohydrate content, respectively, in the days before the test, leading to different muscle glycogen levels (45 vs. 135 mmol/kg WW, respectively). At the end of exercise the muscle glycogen concentration was around 14 and 45 mmol/kg WW. In agreement with these findings is the observation of an improved long-term intermittent exercise performance when subjects in the days prior to a test ingested a carbohydrate-rich diet that probably elevated the muscle glycogen concentrations (55a). It is also in accordance with the finding that the carbohydrate intake during prolonged intermittent exercise can increase performance (56).

The findings in the above-mentioned studies suggest that lower muscle glycogen is linked to fatigue during repeated prolonged intermittent exercise. It may be that the muscle fibers that are the most frequently recruited, and that have the lowest capacity to rebuild glycogen in the recovery periods, become depleted of glycogen (23). This probably reduces the number of fibers that can be recruited to compensate for a loss in muscle force, and the muscles may not be capable of generating sufficient tension during the high-intensity exercise periods.

It is unclear how a lower level of glycogen may cause fatigue during prolonged intermittent exercise. It has been suggested that attenuated glycogen concentrations result in a state of energetic deficiency, through an insuf-

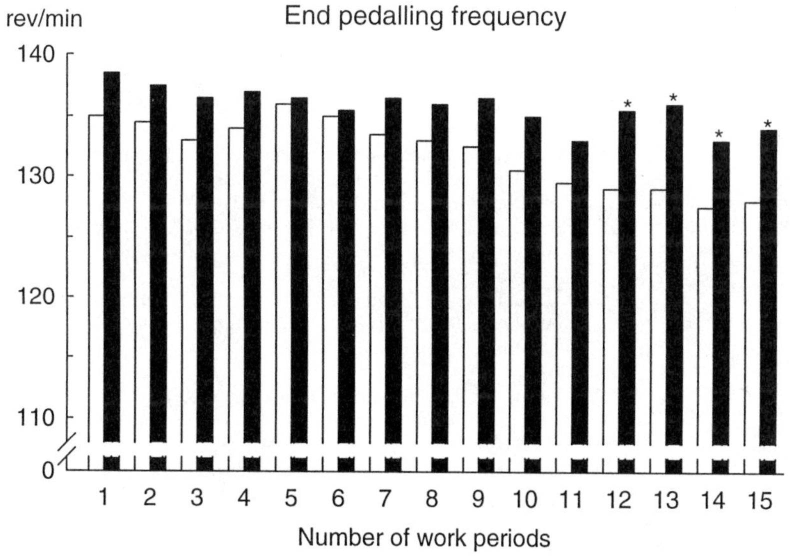

FIG. 5–18. Pedaling frequency during last 2 seconds of fifteen 6-second periods of intense cycling separated by 30-second rest periods with a diet low (*filled bars*) and high (*open bars*) in carbohydrates in the days before the test. The subjects were asked to maintain a pedaling frequency of 140 revolutions per minute. Note that after the high-carbohydrate diet the subjects' ability to keep a high pedaling frequency was better. (Data adapted from ref. 52a.) *Significant difference between high- and low-carbohydrate diet.

ficient rate of the tricarboxylic acid (TCA) cycle, which leads to impairment of the contractile processes (57,58). This theory is supported by the observation of a reduction in TCA intermediates as well as a drop in CP and a marked increase in inosine monophosphate (IMP) at the point of fatigue (58). However, the suggestion of an inadequate ATP regeneration as the cause of fatigue is not altogether clear, since the muscle ATP concentration is only moderately reduced at exhaustion of prolonged exercise (58,59).

It has to be recognized that fatigue during prolonged intermittent exercise may not always be related to muscle glycogen depletion. Also, other factors such as a reduction in the body water content may cause fatigue during such types of exercise (60).

CONCLUSION

The aerobic energy systems contribute significantly to the energy produced during intermittent exercise, during both the exercise and the recovery periods, whereas the anaerobic energy systems provide energy during the exercise bouts. Muscle glycogen is the primary substrate during the exercise periods. In the recovery periods fat oxidation is substantial, and glucose taken up from the blood is also a major substrate. When exercise at an intensity above that eliciting $\dot{V}O_2max$ is repeated, lactate production is reduced, which does not appear to be caused by a lowered muscle glycogen concentration or elevated concentrations of muscle lactate and H^+.

The issue of fatigue during intermittent exercise is complex, and it is difficult to identify a single factor in the muscle responsible for the reduction in performance during intense exercise. Based on measurements of ATP and CP in muscle biopsies obtained during and at the end of intense exhaustive exercise, it seems that muscle fatigue is not caused by lack of energy. Accumulation of lactate and a disturbance of the acid/base balance of skeletal muscle does not appear to be crucial for fatigue. Instead, fatigue during the intense exercise periods may be associated with an excitation-coupling failure and a reduced nervous drive due to reflex inhibition at the spinal level. In the latter hypothesis, accumulation of interstitial potassium in muscle may play a major role.

It is apparent that muscle glycogen depletion represents one important fatigue agent during prolonged intermittent activities, but other factors may also be involved in the fatigue processes.

REFERENCES

1. Bahr R. Excess postexercise oxygen consumption—magnitude, mechanisms and practical implications. *Acta Physiol Scand* 1992;144:3–70.
2. Bangsbo J, Gollnick PD, Graham TE, Saltin B. Substrates for muscle glycogen synthesis in recovery from intense exercise in humans. *J Physiol* 1991;434:423–440.
3. Balsom PD, Ekblom B, Söderlund K, Sjödin B, Hultman E. Creatine supplementation and dynamic high-intensity intermittent exercise. *Scand J Med Sci Sports* 1993;3:143–149.
4. Edwards RHT, Ekelund L-G, Harris C, et al. Cardiorespiratory and metabolic costs of continuous and intermittent exercise in man. *J Physiol* 1973;234:481–497.
5. Essén B, Hagenfeldt L, Kaijser L. Utilisation of blood-borne and intramuscular substrates during continuous and intermittent exercise in man. *J Physiol* 1977;265:489–506.
6. Saltin B, Essén B. Muscle glycogen, lactate, ATP and CP in intermittent exercise. In: Pernow B, Saltin B, eds. *Muscle metabolism during exercise: advances in experimental medicine and biology,* vol 2. New York: Plenum Press, 1971:419–424.

6a. Karlsson J, Hermansen L, Agnevite G, Saltin B. Energikraven vid löpning. *Idrottsfysiologi.* Stockholm, Sweden: Framtiden, 1967: Rapport 4.

7. Christensen EH, Hedman R, Saltin B. Intermittent and continuous running. A further contribution to the physiology of intermittent work. *Acta Physiol Scand* 1960;50:269–286.
8. Margaria R, Oliva RD, Di Prampero PE, Ceretelli P. Energy utilization in intermittent exercise of supramaximal intensity. *J Appl Physiol* 1969;26:752–756.
9. Karlsson J, Saltin B. Diet, muscle glycogen and endurance performance. *J Appl Physiol* 1971;31:203–206.
10. Wootton SA, Williams C. The influence of recovery duration on repeated maximal sprints. In: Knuttgen HG, Vogel JA, Poortmans J, eds. *Biochemistry of exercise.* International Series on Sports Sciences, vol 13. Champaign, IL: Human Kinetics, 1983:269–273.
11. McCartney N, Spriet LL, Heigenhauser JF, Kowalchuk JM, Sutton JR, Jones NL. Muscle power and metabolism in maximal intermittent exercise. *J Appl Physiol* 1986;60:1164–1169.
12. Spriet LL, Lindinger MI, McKelvie S, Heigenhauser GJF, Jones NL. Muscle glycogenolysis and H^+ concentration during maximal intermittent cycling. *J Appl Physiol* 1989;66:8–13.
13. Gaitanos GC, Williams C, Boobis LH, Brooks S. Human muscle metabolism during intermittent maximal exercise. *J Appl Physiol* 1993;75(2):712–719.
14. Bangsbo J, Graham TE, Kiens B, Saltin B. Elevated muscle glycogen and anaerobic energy production during exhaustive exercise in man. *J Physiol* 1992;451:205–222.
15. Bangsbo J, Graham T, Johansen L, Strange S, Christensen C, Saltin B. Elevated muscle acidity and energy production during exhaustive exercise in humans. *Am J Physiol* 1992: 263:R891–R899.
16. Danforth WH. Activation of glycolytic pathway in muscle. In: Chance B, Estrabrook BW, Williamson JR, eds. *Control of energy metabolism.* New York: Academic Press, 1965:287–297.
17. Bosca L, Aragon JJ, Sols A. Modulation of muscle phosphofructokinase at physiological concentration of enzyme. *J Biol Chem* 1995;260:2100–2107.
18. Amorena CF, Wilding TJ, Manchester JK, Roos A. Changes in intracellular pH caused by high K in normal and acidified frog muscle. *J Gen Physiol* 1990;96:959–972.
19. Spriet LL, Söderlund K, Bergström M, Hultman E. Skeletal muscle glycogenolysis, glycolysis and pH during electrical stimulation in men. *J Appl Physiol* 1987;62:616–621.
20. Dobson GP, Yamamoto E, Hochachka PW. Phosphofructokinase control in muscle: nature and reversal of pH-dependent ATP inhibition. *Am J Physiol* 1986;250:R71–R76.
21. Parmeggiani A, Bowman RH. Regulation of phosphofructokinase activity by citrate in normal and diabetic muscle. *Biochem Biophys Res Commun* 1963;12:268–273.
22. Wu TL, Davis EJ. Regulation of glycolytic flux in an energetically controlled cell-free system: The effects of adenine nucleotide ratios, inorganic phosphate, pH and citrate. *Arch Biochem Biophys* 1981;209:85–99.
23. Essén B. Studies on the regulation of metabolism in human skeletal muscle using intermittent exercise as an experimental model. *Acta Physiol Scand Suppl* 1978;454:1–32.
24. Peters SJ, Spriet LL. Skeletal muscle phosphofructokinase activity examined under physiological condition in vitro. *J Appl Physiol* 1995;78:1853–1858.

25. Bangsbo J. The physiology of soccer—with special reference to intense intermittent exercise. *Acta Physiol Scand* 1994; 151(suppl 610):1–157.
26. Pilegaard H, Domino K, Noland T, et al. Effect of high intensity exercise training on lactate/H^+ transport capacity in human skeletal muscle. *Am J Physiol* 1999;276:E255–E261.
27. Sahlin K, Ren JM. Relationship of contraction capacity changes during recovery from a fatiguing contraction. *J Appl Physiol* 1989;67:648–654.
28. Bogdanis G, Nevill ME, Lakomy HKA, Nevill AM. Recovery of power output and muscle metabolites following 30 s of maximal sprint cycling in man. *J Physiol* 1995;482:467–480.
29. Bigland-Ritchie B, Woods JJ. Changes in muscle contractile properties and neural control during human muscular fatigue. *Muscle Nerve* 1994;7:691–699.
30. Fitts RH. Cellular mechanisms of muscle fatigue. *Physiol Rev* 1994;74:49–94.
31. Jansson E, Dudley GA, Norman B, Tesch PA. ATP and IMP in single human muscle fibres after high intensity exercise. *Clin Physiol* 1987;7:337–345.
32. Söderlund K. *Energy metabolism in human skeletal muscle during intense contraction and recovery with reference to metabolic differences between type I and type II fibres* (thesis). Stockholm, Sweden: Huddings University Hospital, Karolinska Institute.
33. Greenhaff PL, Bodin K, Söderlund K, Hultman E. The effect of oral creatine supplementation on skeletal muscle phosphocreatine resynthesis. *Am J Physiol* 1994;266:E725–E730.
34. Karlsson J. Lactate and phosphagen concentrations in working muscle of man. *Acta Physiol Scand* 1971;suppl 358:7–72.
35. Favero TG, Zable AC, Colter D, Abramson JJ. Lactate inhibits Ca^{2+}-activated Ca^{2+}-channel activity from skeletal muscle sarcoplasmic reticulum. *J Appl Physiol* 1997;82:447–452.
36. Hogan MC, Gladden LB, Kurdak SS, Poole DC. Increased [lactate] in working dog muscle reduces tension development independent of pH. *Med Sci Sports Exerc* 1995;27:371–377.
37. Chase PB, Kushmerick MJ. Effects of pH on contraction of rabbit fast and slow skeletal muscle fibers. *Biophys J* 1988;53:935–946.
38. Sahlin K, Henriksson J. Buffer capacity and lactate accumulation in skeletal muscle of trained and untrained men. *Acta Physiol Scand* 1984;122:331–339.
39. Saltin B, Hermansen L. Glycogen stores and prolonged severe exercise. In: Blix G, ed. *Symposium of Swedish Nutrition Foundation.* Uppsala, Sweden: Almquist and Wiksell, 1967:32–46.
40. Bangsbo J, Graham TE, Johansen L, Saltin B. Lactate and H^+ fluxes from skeletal muscles in man. *J Physiol* 1993;462:115–133.
41. Wilson JR, McCully KK, Mancini DM, Boden B, Change B. Relationship of muscular fatigue to pH and diprotonated P_i in humans: a ^{31}P-NMR study. *J Appl Physiol* 1988;64:2333–2339.
42. Chasioltis D, Hultman E, Sahlin K. Acidotic depression of cyclic AMP accumulation and phosphorylase b to a transformation in skeletal muscle in man. *J Physiol* 1993;335:197–204.
43. Cooke R, Pate E. The inhibition of muscle contraction by the products of ATP hydrolysis. In: Sutton JR, Taylor AW, Gollnick PD, et al., eds. *Biochemistry of exercise,* vol 7. Champaign, IL: Human Kinetics, 1990:59–72.
44. Donaldson SBK. Fatigue of sarcoplasmic reticulum. Failure of excitation-contraction coupling in skeletal muscle. In: Taylor AW, Gollnick PD, Green HJ, et al., eds. *Biochemistry of exercise,* vol 7. Champaign, IL: Human Kinetics, 1990:49–57.
45. Edman KAP. The contractile performance of normal and fatigued skeletal muscle. In: Marconnet P, Komi PV, Saltin B, Sejersted OM, eds. *Muscle fatigue mechanisms in exercise and training. Med Sports Sci* Basel: Karger, 1992;34:20–42.
46. Lännergren J. Fatigue mechanisms in isolated intact muscle fibers from frog and mouse. In: Marconnet P, Komi PV, Saltin B, Sejersted OM, eds. *Muscle fatigue mechanisms in exercise and training. Med Sports Sci* Basel: Karger, 1992;34:43–53.
47. Bangsbo J, Madsen K, Kiens B, Richter EA. Effect of muscle acidity on muscle metabolism and fatigue during intense exercise in man. *J Physiol* 1996;495:587–596.
48. Metzer JM, Fitts RH. Role of intracellular pH in muscle fatigue. *J Appl Physiol* 1987:62;1392–1397.
49. Bangsbo J, Johansen L, Quistroff B, Saltin B. NMR and analytic biochemical evaluation of CrP and nucleotides in the human calf during muscle contraction. *J Appl Physiol* 1993;74:2034–2039.
50. Sjøgaard G. Exercise induced muscle fatigue: the significance of potassium. *Acta Physiol Scand Suppl* 1990;140(593):1–63.
51. Bigland-Ritchie B, Dawson NJ, Johansson RS, Leppold OCJ. Reflex origin for the slowing of motoneurone firing rates in fatigue of human voluntary contractions. *J Physiol (Lond)* 1986; 379:451–459.
52. Juel C. The effect of β_2-adrenoceptor activation on ion-shifts and fatigue in mouse soleus muscles stimulated in vitro. *Acta Physiol Scand* 1988;134:209–216.
52a. Balsom PD. *High intensity intermittent exercise* (thesis). Stockholm, Sweden: Karolinska Institute, 1995.
53. Fink R, Hase S, Lüttgau HC, Wettwer E. The effect of cellular energy reserves and internal calcium ions on the potassium conductance in skeletal muscle of the frog. *J Physiol* 1983; 336:211–228.
54. Davies NW. ATP-dependent K^+ channels and other K^+ channels of muscle: how exercise may modulate their activity. In: Marconnet P, Komi PV, Saltin B, Sejersted OM, eds. *Muscle fatigue mechanisms in exercise and training. Med Sports Sci* Basel: Karger, 1992;34:1–10.
55. Balsom PD. *High intensity intermittent exercise.* Doctoral thesis, Dept. of Physiology and Pharmacology, Physiology III, Karolinska Institute, Stockholm, Sweden 1995.
55a. Bangsbo J, Nörregaard L, Thorsoe EF. The effect of carbohydrate diet on intermittent exercise performance. *Int J Sports Med* 1992;13:152–157.
56. Nicolas CW, Williams C, Lakomy KHA, Phillips G, Nowitz A. Influence of ingesting a carbohydrate, electrolyte solution on endurance capacity during intermittent, high-intensity shuttle running. *J Sports Sci* 1995;13:283–290.
57. Wagenmakers AJM. Role of amino acids and ammonia in mechanisms of fatigue. In: Marconnet P, Komi PV, Saltin B, Sejersted OM, eds. *Muscle fatigue mechanisms in exercise and training. Med Sports Sci* 1992;34:69–86.
58. Spencer MK, Yan Z, Katz A. Effect of low glycogen on carbohydrate and energy metabolism in human muscle during exercise. *Am J Physiol* 1992;262:C975–C979.
59. Norman B, Sollevi A, Kaijser L. Jansson E. ATP breakdown products in human skeletal muscle during prolonged exercise to exhaustion. *Clin Physiol* 1987;7:503–509.
60. Maughan RE. The effects of dehydration on the body's performance. Proceedings from the symposium Metabolism and Nutrition in Sport, May 20–23, Barcelona, Spain, 1992.

Exercise and Sport Science,
edited by William E. Garrett, Jr., and Donald T. Kirkendall.
Lippincott Williams & Wilkins, Philadelphia © 2000.

CHAPTER 6

Nature of Training Effects

Atko Viru and Mehis Viru

BIOLOGIC ESSENCE OF EXERCISE TRAINING

Sports training consists of exercises performed systematically to improve physical abilities and to acquire skills connected with the technique of the performance of the sports event. Experience and, to a certain extent, the results of related studies suggest to the coach which exercises are necessary. The testing of physical abilities, visual evaluation of the performance technique, and competition results indicate the effectiveness of training. However, this usual understanding leaves a gap between exercise and the effects of its systematic repetition. In the guiding of training, an essential problem arises due to the fact that a couple of months is necessary before the training effects are demonstrated in physical abilities and physical working capacity to a measurable extent. Therefore, only delayed feedback information on training effects may be obtained by the tests of physical abilities and competition results. Moreover, the main shortcoming of this feedback information is that the concerned changes reflect an integral action of various exercises, training methods, and regimens.

Systematically performed physical exercises result in a great many changes in the organism. The changes take place on the levels of cellular structures, tissues, organs, and body build. The changes extend from cellular metabolic processes and their molecular mechanisms up to functional capacities of cellular structures as well as organs and their systems. Pronounced alterations have been found in the mechanisms of control of body functions and metabolic processes, including levels of cellular autoregulation, hormonal regulation, and neural regulation. Most of the training-induced changes express adaptation to the conditions of enhanced muscular activity.

A. Viru and M. Viru: Institute of Exercise Biology, University of Tartu, Tartu, Estonia.

Our general understanding of training will significantly improve if we consider that (a) all training effects are based on exercise-induced changes in the organism (Fig. 6–1), and (b) each change is specifically dependent on the exercise nature, intensity, and duration. Thus, each training exercise results in specific changes in the organism that are necessary to obtain a goal of the training. Collectively, the changes caused by various exercises warrant an increased level of sports performance.

In the practical organizing of training, the main advantages of this understanding are the following:

- Each exercise will be performed to achieve a concrete goal in the form of a certain change in the organism.
- The resulting changes make it possible to check the effectiveness of each exercise (or at least of a group of exercises).

In this way, "blind" exercising will be avoided and the training will become a well-controlled process. The changes in the organism will serve as means for the operative feedback control of the training effectiveness. This will be a specific feedback, allowing evaluation of the effect of the concrete exercise or group of exercises used.

The practical use of this approach requires knowing what changes are necessary to achieve the aim of training. The answer can be obtained by (a) an analysis of the factors limiting performance in the sport event, and (b) studies on top-level athletes to build a model of their organism.

The top-level performance depends on effective training as well as on genetic peculiarities. Therefore, the tasks of training and of sport selection have to be discriminated, but it must be emphasized that there are no genetically induced factors that directly determine the level of sports results in any event. The positive (or negative) significance of genetic factors becomes apparent in training. There exists a dual interrelationship:

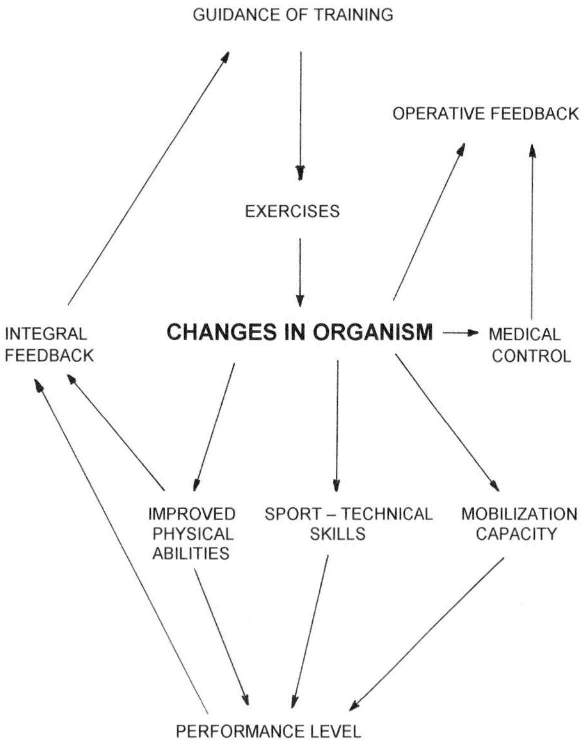

FIG. 6–1. Contemporary understanding of training.

Training makes possible the use of genetically induced manifestations (e.g., composition of muscle fibers of various types) in the improvement of sports performance. At the same time, the effectiveness of training in various directions depends on the susceptibility of the organism to the training action of various exercises. It is assumed that susceptibility to training actions is related to the genetic program (1). Besides the important role of the genotype in the corresponding sensitivity, the conditions of individual life and particularly previous muscular activity (maybe even at preschool age) may phenotypically induce corrections.

The task of training has to be distributed rationally across the 10 to 12 years it takes to make a prepubertal boy or girl an Olympic athlete. Training strategy has to determine how to distribute the tasks, taking into account the organism's development during adolescence. The most favorable periods have to be found to induce the necessary structural, metabolic, and functional changes. The training strategy also entails the distribution of various tasks within a year by training periods, and within training periods by mezo- and microcycles of training. Carrying out the induction of necessary changes is part of training tactics. Accordingly, the most rational way to organize training microcycles and training sessions has to be determined, and the necessary training methods and exercises have to be chosen.

MECHANISMS OF TRAINING EFFECTS

Adaptive Protein Synthesis

An intracellular mechanism interrelates the physiologic function and the genetic apparatus of cells. Through this mechanism the intensity of the functioning of cellular structures determines the activity of the genetic apparatus. Thereby protein synthesis is stimulated. It has been hypothesized that training exercises cause an accumulation of metabolites, which specifically induce the adaptive synthesis of structure and enzyme proteins related to the most active cellular structures and metabolic pathways. In addition, hormonal changes are induced by training sessions that amplify the inductor effect of metabolites. As a result, an effective renewal of protein structures, their enlargement, and an increase in the number of molecules of the most responsible enzymes will be created (Fig. 6–2).

The result of the activity of the cellular genetic apparatus is the production of specific messenger ribonucleic acids (mRNA), containing the information on the structure of the protein that has to be synthesized. Production of various species of mRNA and thereby transcription of the synthesis of the related protein has been found after training exercises (2) and during endurance training (3). The protein synthesis is controlled on three

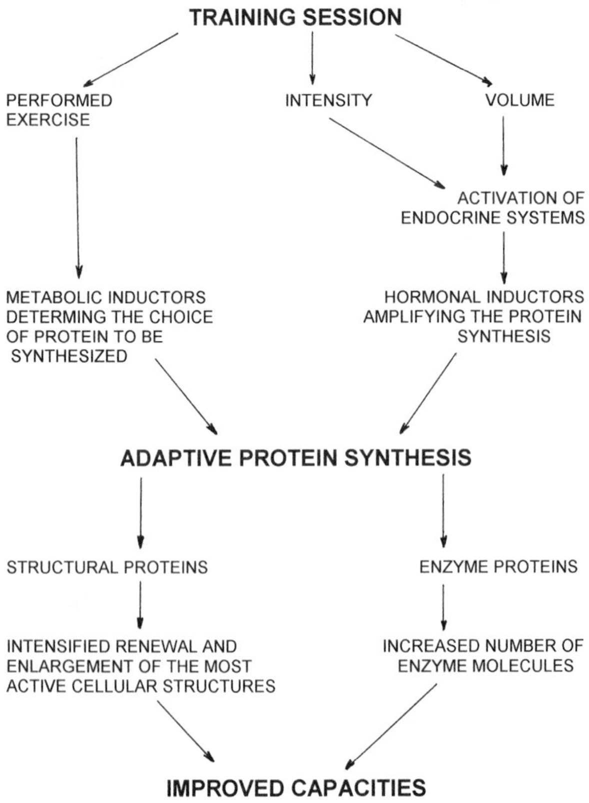

FIG. 6–2. Adaptive protein synthesis caused by a training session.

levels, however: transcription, translation (actualization of protein synthesis according to the information contained in the mRNA), and posttranslation levels (Fig. 6–3). The latter consists in regulation of the rate of degradation of concrete proteins in order to adjust the actual number of molecules of a protein to the actual need.

In muscular activity similar to endurance exercises, an increase in the production of mRNA for mitochondrial proteins has been found. Thus, the chronic adaptation to muscular activity of endurance type is based on the transcription control of the adaptive protein synthesis. Another situation appears in high-resistance training. After either concentric or eccentric exercise the synthesis rate of myofibrillar protein increases 50% to 60%. However, mRNAs for neither myofibrillar nor mitochondrial proteins changed after concentric exercises. While mitochondrial adaptation is not expected in heavy resistance training, the lack of change in mRNA for myofibrillar proteins suggests that myofibrillar protein synthesis might be stimulated through an increase in protein translation. (A milder resistance training program resulted in similar hypertrophy of the eccentric and concentric contracted muscle.) Nevertheless, the muscle hypertrophy was not found. Apparently, the increased protein synthesis rate, caused by translation control, was balanced by a comparable increase in protein degradation, resulting from posttranslation control. Eccentric exercises increased the formation of mRNA for a myofibrillar protein in combination with muscle hypertrophy. Therefore, the dominating mechanism was transcription control. Since the increase in myofibrillar proteins was lower than in the rate of synthesis of myofibrillar proteins, the posttranslation control participated as well (2).

It is possible to suggest that posttranslation control is essential to avoid muscular hypertrophy in endurance, speed, or power training.

The two main hormones participating in the induction of the adaptive protein synthesis in postexercise periods are male sex (testosterone) and thyroid (thyroxine/triiodothyronine) hormones (Fig. 6–4). Induction of myofibrillar proteins by testosterone makes it important in strength training-induced hypertrophy, as indicated by the prohibited using of androgen preparations of anabolic action (anabolic steroids) by athletes. However, the same action is provided by endogenous testosterone. Rat experiments have demonstrated that pharmacologic blockade of the cellular receptor for male sex hormones eliminates muscular hypertrophy during 2 weeks of electrical stimulation of gastrocnemius muscles (4). In this connection it is worth noting that, in training, skeletal muscle becomes more susceptible to the influence of testosterone: a rapid increase in the number of male sex hormone receptors has been found following electrical stimulation of rat muscles (5). The exercise-specific variability in hormonal control of the adaptive protein synthesis is emphasized by the fact that cellular hormonal receptors can be differently regulated in different fiber types in response to exercise of different types. Resis-

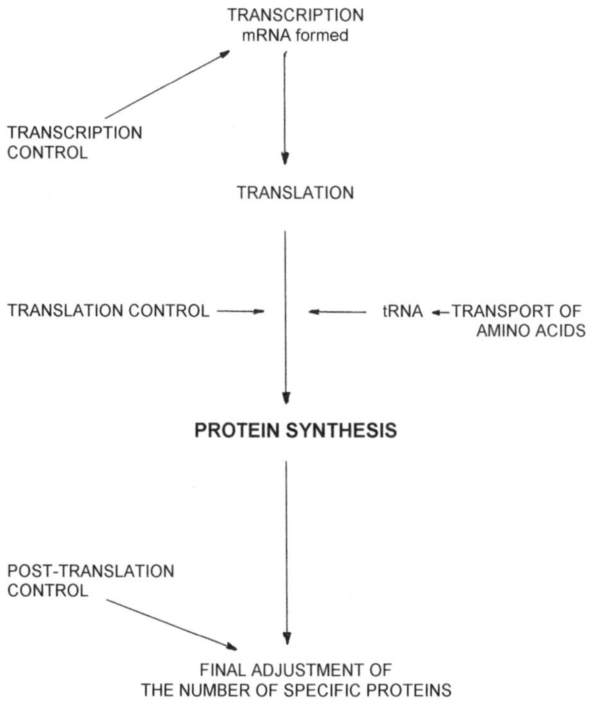

FIG. 6–3. The three levels of control in protein synthesis.

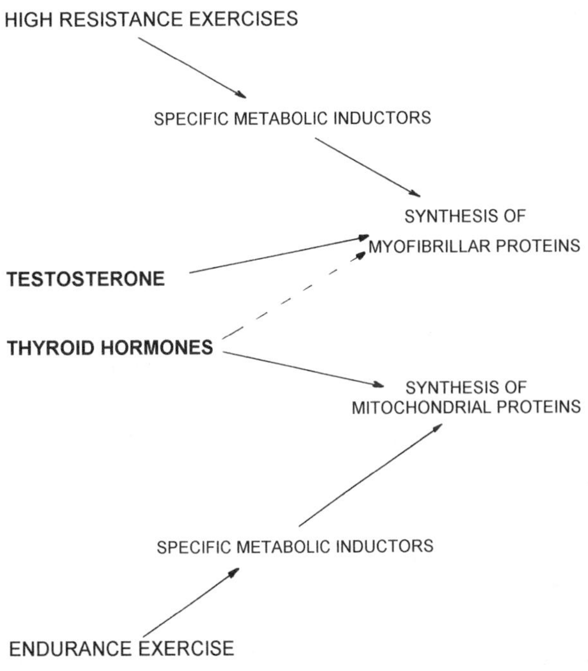

FIG. 6–4. Amplifying action of testosterone and thyroid hormones in exercise-induced adaptive protein synthesis.

tance exercise results in downregulation of androgen receptors in slow-twitch fibers and upregulation of these receptors in fast-twitch fibers (6). Consequently, the tissue susceptibility to the testosterone effect increases during resistance exercise selectively in fast-twitch muscle fibers.

By its antianabolic action, testosterone also participates in posttranslational control equilibrating the influence of endogenous catabolic agents. Administration of anabolic steroids diminished the decrease of myosin Mg^{2+}–adenosine triphosphatase (ATPase) activity in red muscle caused by forced training in rats (7).

Exogenous analogues of testosterone increase sarcotubular fraction (sarcoplasmic reticulum) in slow-twitch muscle fibers and enhance the activity of some mitochondrial enzymes in fast-twitch fibers. These effects were not potentiated by treadmill training (8).

Thyroid hormones are known to exert a stimulatory influence on the biosynthesis of mitochondria. The specific increase in the synthesis of mitochondrial protein in oxidative-glycolytic muscle fiber after an endurance exercise does not appear in hypothyroid rats (9). Accordingly, it has been demonstrated that treatment with triiodothyronine enhances the training-induced increase in activities of mitochondrial enzymes (10). Thyroid hormones are also capable of stimulating synthesis of myofibrillar proteins (11), altering the expression of myosin heavy-chain isozymes, modifying activity-induced changes in the expression of these isozymes, and influencing Ca^{2+}-pump function of sarcoplasmic reticulum (12).

The main hormonal regulators of the translation process are insulin and growth hormone; epinephrine and various metabolites also play a part. It has been suggested that growth hormone acts on the biochemical amplifying system for the cell's anabolic machinery. Thus, growth hormone determines the absolute change in muscle size that results from the influence of muscle activity (13). In adult humans with growth hormone deficiency, treatment with human growth hormone for 6 months increased the lean tissue, the total cross-sectional area of the thigh muscle, and the strength of the flexors and the limb girdle muscle, but not that of a number of other muscles (14). Increases were found also in $\dot{V}O_2max$, anaerobic ventilatory threshold and maximal power output (15). The stimulation of muscle protein synthesis by growth hormone has been evidenced in normal humans (16).

An increasing amount of evidence indicates the significance of insulin-like growth factors I and II in activity-induced muscle hypertrophy. The incidence of increased formation of insulin growth factors in hypertrophying rat muscle appears to be dependent on neither pituitary hormones, such as growth hormone (17), nor testosterone (18).

The meaning of the above results on hormone inductors of muscular hypertrophy has been underlined by results obtained in the training of athletes. In both male and female athletes heavy-resistance sessions resulted in significant increases in blood concentrations of growth hormone and insulin-like growth factor I. Males also demonstrated significant increases in blood serum testosterone value (19).

It has been thought that since the glucocorticoid hormones (cortisol and corticosterone) exert catabolic action, the increase in their level in blood blunts the effect of hormones stimulating protein synthesis. When the normal adrenocortical response during training exercises was blocked, training failed to increase endurance in rats (20). This fact may be related to the two regulatory effects of glucocorticoids. First, the glucocorticoid catabolic effect is necessary for mobilization of precursors (amino acids) for protein synthesis. Second, the same catabolic effects may be involved in intensive protein turnover and thereby an effective renewal of the most responsible protein structures.

In adrenalectomized rats, more pronounced cardiac hypertrophy than in normals was found after endurance training (21). This finding suggests that glucocorticoids may contribute to the determination of the optimal magnitude of structural changes of the myocardial cells, likely through the posttranslational control.

Adaptive Protein Synthesis in the Myocardium

No research suggests the existence of significant differences in the control of adaptive protein synthesis between skeletal and heart muscles. However, differences may exist in metabolic inductors and in conditions that are responsible for the production of necessary inductors. The main determinants of the cardiac hypertrophy are ventricular systolic stretch due to increased afterload and ventricular diastolic stretch due to increased preload. In the first case, a parallel sarcomere replication occurs that leads to an increased ventricular wall size. The result is a concentric hypertrophy. In the case of ventricular diastolic stretch series, sarcomere replication takes place, resulting in increased ventricular chambers—the eccentrical hypertrophy commonly observed in most athletes. However, eccentrical hypertrophy is also related to protein synthesis and protein degradation. The factors modulating these processes are the hormones catecholamines, somatotropin, thyroid hormones, insulin, and cortisol; the metabolites lactate, pyruvate, amino acids, and free fatty acids; as well as such factors as hemodynamic load and hypoxia.

Theory of Supercompensation

A supercompensation of energy stores after exercise has been established in animal experiments performed in the late 1940s and early 1950s. The postexercise repletion of energy stores does not cease after recovery of the initial store but continues further, resulting in a

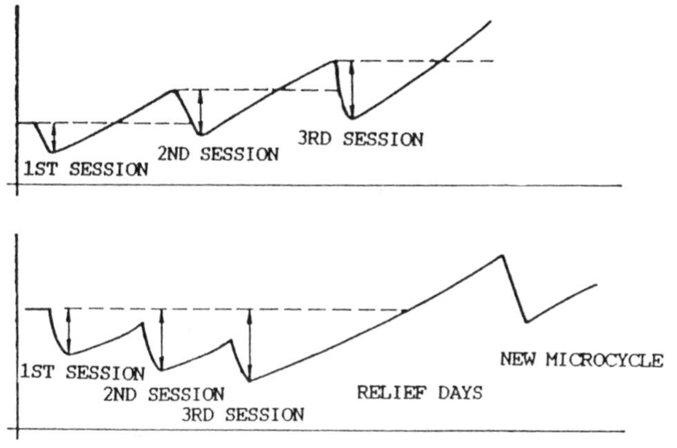

FIG. 6–5. Training-induced increase in the organism's energy reserve, based on the postexercise supercompensation.

transient increase of energy stores above the previous level. This phenomenon has been demonstrated in the content of glycogen in muscles and liver and the content of phosphocreatine in muscles.

Investigations on the postexercise supercompensation of energy stores led to an interesting finding. When the subsequent exercise set begins from the level of the supercompensated stores, the decrease in their levels of glycogen and phosphocreatine contents is greater than after the first exercise. The following supercompensation increases the energy stores to a higher level in comparison with supercompensation after the first exercise set (Fig. 6–5). Accordingly, in training the augmentation of energy stores is based on the performance of the subsequent exercise set from the level of supercompensation after the previous one (22).

Neural Adaptation

Training effects are related to the formation of new coordination mechanisms at various levels of the central nervous system (CNS), including formation of new systems of conditioned reflexes. This neural adaptation is related in part to the adaptive protein synthesis in nervous tissue (23). In exercised rats protein synthesis is intensified in neurons (24), including synthesis of mitochondrial proteins (25).

Most of the coordination mechanisms developed should have a specific dependence on the sports event and on the training exercises used. Regarding strength and power training, the significance of neural adaptation has been convincingly established (26,27). How muscle force is affected by different types of motor unit firing rates or frequencies is also an adaptive mechanism affected by heavy resistance training (28). Training adaptation entails developing the ability to recruit all motor units when needed to perform a strong contraction. The CNS structures are also capable of limiting force by engaging inhibitory mechanisms.

The neural adaptations are specifically related to the training goal; the athlete's performance can depend on the maximal forces applied, on the highest power output during a certain limited time interval, on the highest speed of movements, or on the most economical use of muscle forces.

An essential task in achieving high performance is the acquisition of specific sports skills in training. During competition the athlete's activity is programmed using previously acquired skills.

There are substantial differences between events in difficulties for forming the program of activity. Several groups of events may be distinguished: (a) programming and actualization of the program are simple during the competition (e.g., running events); (b) programs are formed in training, and in competition their actualization is exactly the same and there is no need to elaborate new programs; however, the actualization of the program is extremely complicated (e.g., gymnastics, figure skating, etc.); (c) during competition the programming of necessary activities is complicated due to the choice of the most suitable action and due to the time deficit resulting from the rapidly changing situation; the actualization of the program (e.g., sports, games, fencing) is also complicated. In chess, programming is extremely complicated but the actualization of the program is very simple.

ACTUALIZATION OF TRAINING EFFECTS

A single exercise is usually insufficient to evoke a training response. To obtain sufficient stimuli for training effects, a certain number of repetitions has to be performed during a training session. In other cases the training effect is based on the short (insufficient) rest intervals between exercise bouts, and thus the exercise sessions have a cumulative effect. In still other cases, a long period of continuous exercise is necessary to obtain the training effect. Accordingly, three principles of training can be discriminated:

1. the principle of repetition,
2. the principle of summation,
3. the principle of duration.

The benefits of adaptive protein synthesis, energy supercompensation, and improved neural coordination that arise from a single training session dissipate rapidly if subsequent exercise sessions are not held. Stable training benefits require a systematic exercise program with frequent training sessions of sufficient duration. At the same time, the demands of training must gradually increase, because the organism adapts to the same stimulus load after a certain number of repetitions.

Summary

The biologic foundation for improvement of the athlete's performance is the training-induced changes in the body. The molecular-cellular basis for these changes is the adaptive protein synthesis, which results in increases of the most active cellular structures and in the numbers of enzyme molecules catalyzing the most important metabolic pathways during training. The adaptive protein synthesis is controlled at levels of transcription, translation, and posttranslation. These controls are actualized by intracellular metabolites, bioactive substances produced during activity, and hormone secretion during and after training session. Testosterone plays an essential role in stimulating or amplifying the transcription, as it acts mainly on the synthesis of myofibrillar proteins. Thyroid hormones act mainly on the synthesis of mitochondria. Growth hormone and insulin contribute to the control of translation.

The effect of the adaptive protein synthesis is extended by neural adaptation and supercompensation of energy substrates (phosphocreatine and glycogen in muscular tissues and glycogen in hepatic tissues).

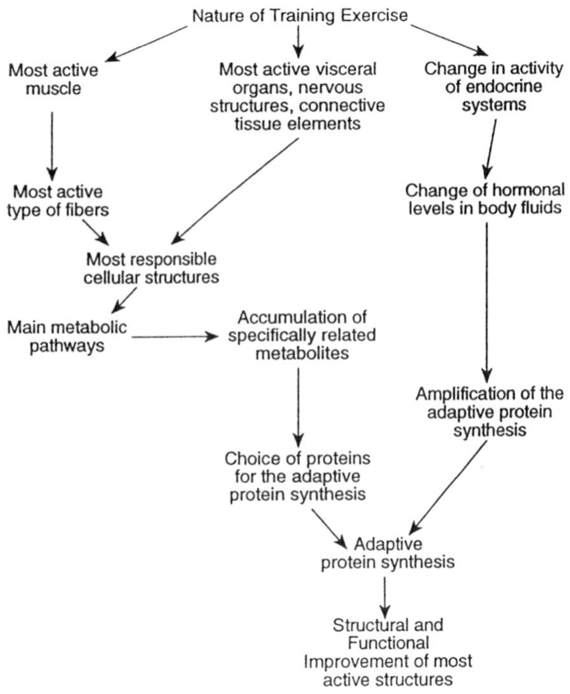

FIG. 6–6. Specific effects of training exercises.

SPECIFIC NATURE OF TRAINING ON SKELETAL MUSCLES

The principle of specific adaptation to various kinds of muscular activity was first formulated and argued by Yakovlev (29). Later, striking evidence of the specific nature of training effects was obtained from a great number of studies carried out in several laboratories.

Each exercise determines the degree of activity of various organs, different type of muscles, and motor units. Within each active cell the main metabolic pathways that permit the accomplishment of necessary functional tasks also depend on the nature of the training exercises. The activity of the metabolic control system at various levels as well as the activity of the system directly regulating bodily functions are also dependent on the nature of the training exercise. Correspondingly, the organism's adaptation bears the imprint of the type of exercise systematically used in training (Fig. 6–6).

Hypertrophy of Myofibrils

The most prominent result of training for improved strength is hypertrophy of skeletal muscles. A very pronounced muscle hypertrophy is displayed by athletes exposed to long-term vigorous strength training. Muscular hypertrophy is primarily the result of an increase in the size of the individual fiber (30,31), which, in turn, is based on the enlargement of myofibrils (32), due to the augmentation of myofibrillar proteins (33). Also, an increased number of myofibrils has been found, indicating some hyperplasia (22). It is assumed that the myogenic response to strength training involves mainly the synthesis of new contractile proteins.

The effect of training on strength differs from that of aerobic endurance training, which does not cause a substantial increase in the cross-sectional area of muscle fibers. However, a selective and moderate enlargement of slow-twitch oxidative (SO) fibers and in some cases also fast-oxidative glycolytic (FOG) fibers is possible in endurance training (34). In endurance training no enlargement of myofibrils was found. If an increase in the fiber diameter was found, it was due mainly to the elevated volume of sarcoplasm. The latter has been thought to be due to the glycogen content increase.

Endurance training induces an elevated rate of myosin heavy-chain and actin turnover in all fiber types. In sprint-trained rats, the increased turnover rate of the myosin heavy chain was found only in fast-glycolytic (FG) and FOG fibers in comparison with sedentary rats (35).

Sprint training increases the cross-sectional area of both slow-twitch and fast-twitch fibers, but less than high-resistance exercises. This effect is greatest for the fast-twitch fibers. The end result is that they occupy a slightly greater area in the sprint-trained athlete (36).

Running training induced greater areas of nerve terminals in the extensor digitorum longus muscle and the soleus muscle. The quantity of terminal branches as well as the cross-sectional area of motor nerve fibers increased as a result of speed or power training, but not as a result of endurance training. In cases of endurance training, a decrease of 15% in the cross-sectional area of motor nerve fibers was observed.

Hypertrophy Versus Hyperplasia

Results of a number of studies indicate the possibility of a longitudinal division of muscle fibers in training.

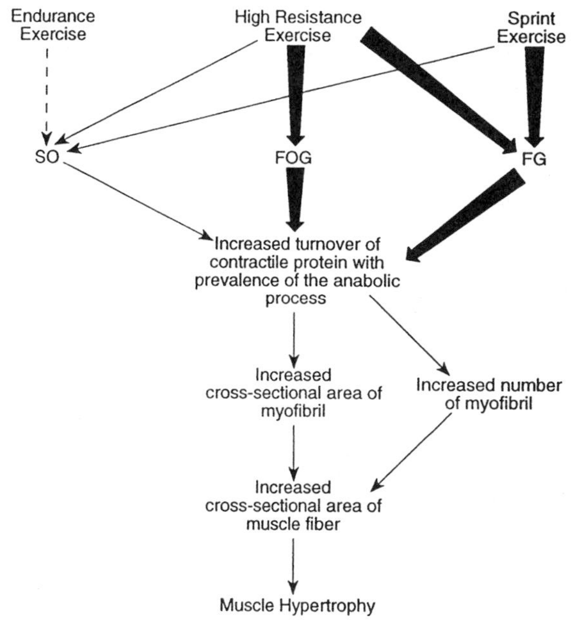

FIG. 6–7. Stimulation of the hypertrophy of muscle fibers by various exercises. The width of *arrows* shows the degree of influence.

The results suggest that motor nerve endings on newly formed muscle fibers develop from collateral branch endings springing from preterminal compartments of motor axons.

Calculations of total numbers of fibers were performed in the human biceps by measuring the total cross-sectional area of the muscle as determined by computed tomography. The area of the individual fibers was determined from biopsy samples. The obtained data demonstrate considerable variation in the numbers of fibers. However, there was no evidence of a systematic difference between sedentary and trained subjects. The greater total cross-sectional area in athletes was attributable to the larger cross-sectional area of individual fibers (37).

In conclusion, the stimulus for muscular hypertrophy depends on the resistance to muscle contraction as well as the total number of contractions performed against high resistance. Therefore, the main tool for muscle hypertrophy is high-resistance exercise (Fig. 6–7). The effect of power and sprint exercises is less pronounced. Endurance exercise is ineffective. Muscle hypertrophy appears mostly in FG fibers, to a lesser degree in FOG fibers, and inconsistently in SO fibers.

Sarcolemma

No data are available for evaluating the specific training effect on the excitation mechanism. It may only be speculated that there are individual differences in acetylcholine synthesis and release, cholinesterase activity, and maybe even ionic gradients. If this is the case, these differences may limit the transfer of high frequencies of nerve discharges to events initiating the contraction and determining the force or power output. Highly effective ionic pumps are necessary for avoiding decreases in the ionic gradient and thereby ensuring optimal conditions for excitation and excitation/coupling events. The plasma membrane of skeletal muscles has been frequently implicated in the process of fatigue (38). It was suggested that low-intensity fatigue may be the result of alterations in membrane structure in response to the activation of phospholipases and/or the production of free radicals. The latter can induce lipid peroxidation as well as direct modification of the transport systems. Training-induced adaptive response involves alterations in lipid peroxidation and scavenger enzyme activity (39).

A biopsy study showed that persons who for many years systematically exercised had increased concentrations of Na-K pumps in the vastus lateralis muscle. In comparison with age-matched untrained subjects, the swimming, running, and strength-trained subjects demonstrated increased density of Na-K pumps, indicated by a gain in concentrations of ^{3}H-ouabain–binding sites by 30%, 32%, and 40%, respectively (40). An intensive cycle-sprint training of 7 weeks resulted in an increase in ^{3}H-ouabain binding sites in the vastus lateralis muscle (41).

Sarcoplasmic Reticulum

The sarcoplasmic reticulum (SR) warrants sequestering Ca^{2+} for the contractile mechanism, and rebinding these ions again after the contraction. It has been established in rat experiments that the protein content of the SR increased in muscles as a result of swimming training when the exercise intensity was gradually increased, but not when the exercise intensity remained modest even if its duration was gradually prolonged (42). A comparison of effects of various training regimes in rats demonstrated increased rates of Ca^{2+} accumulation by the SR (calculated per milligram of protein) in the soleus muscle (containing slow-twitch oxidative fibers) after training in continuous aerobic running, sprint training, interval training, and strength training in fast clambering (Fig. 6–8). In the white portion of the quadriceps muscle (containing mainly fast-twitch glycolytic fibers) significantly increased rates were obtained after sprint, interval, or strength training, but not after continuous running. In both muscles the highest changes were caused by sprint and strength training. Training in continuous swimming decreased the Ca^{2+} accumulation in both muscles (43). Consequently, the training effect on the SR depends on the types of exercises used. As would be expected, adaptation to systematic use of highly intensive exercise stimulated an improvement in the function of the SR.

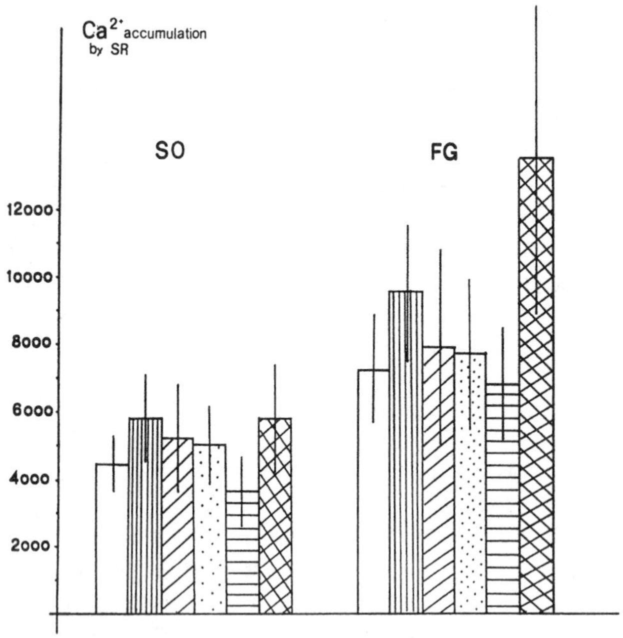

FIG. 6–8. Effect of various training programs on Ca^{2+} accumulation by sarcoplasmic reticulum (SR). Ca^{2+} accumulation was evaluated by cycles per minute (cpm) per milligram of protein (mean ± SEM).

Contractile Apparatus

Actomyosin ATPase Activity

Training experiments on rats showed that myofibrillar Ca^{2+}-ATPase activity was increased in the soleus muscle after sprint, interval, or strength training. In the white portion of the quadriceps the same changes have also been found after continuous running in addition to the effect obtained after sprint, interval, and strength training (Fig. 6–9). The greatest increase has been caused by strength training in glycolytic muscle. The effect of repeated short-term intensive running (sprint and interval training) was more pronounced than that of continuous running. Continuous swimming caused a decrease in the enzyme activity (43).

In humans the effect of strength training on the activity of myofibrillar ATPase is variable, showing both an increase and a decrease. Neither concentric nor combined eccentric and concentric resistance training regimes caused any strict changes in the Mg^{2+}-ATPase activity (44).

Thus, training may induce two different adaptations at the level of myofibrillar ATPase. One consists of an elevation of the enzyme activity, making possible a rapid liberation of energy for muscular contractions at a level of high-power output. This adaptation seems to be common for sprint and interval training as well as for strength training. The second adaptation takes place in continuous exercises of moderate intensity. The decreased myofibrillar ATPase may be considered essential for a more economical utilization of adenosine triphosphate (ATP) stores.

Characteristics of Contraction

Strength training induces changes in force-velocity curves of muscles (45). After heavy resistance training, the increase in the maximal voluntary force is most pronounced at slow velocities of contraction. After explosive types of strength (power) exercises, the improvement is greater in the high-velocity portion of the curve.

The time for producing a 30%, 60%, or 90% force level is shorter for wrestlers and bodybuilders than for power lifters (46). These differences can be explained by the various training exercises used. The training of bodybuilders and especially that of wrestlers involves more submaximal lifting at a higher speed, whereas the training of power lifters involves high-resistance, slow-contraction velocity exercises.

A program of sprint training shortened the time to peak tension of the rat soleus muscle, but it did not alter the contractile properties of the fast-twitch rectus femoris muscle (47). Treadmill endurance training resulted in a 14% decrease in the time to peak tension of the rat soleus muscle and increased the ability to maintain tetanic tension during a series of fatiguing contractions (48).

Mitochondria and Oxidative Enzymes

Typical for endurance training is an augmented number and volume of mitochondria observed and increased activity of oxidative enzymes. These changes are in association with increased working capacity and endurance.

Increased activity of enzymes of β-oxidation and a general enhancement of oxidative potential of muscle fibers make possible an elevated use of lipids during prolonged exercise, despite the high level of muscle lactate (49). A greater use of fat as a fuel after endurance training seems to be related to a more rapid translocation of the adenosine diphosphate (ADP) generated during contractions into the mitochondria. Consequently, there is tighter control over the glycolytic process, creating more favorable conditions for the entry of acetyl units derived from β-oxidation of fatty acids into the citric acid cycle (50).

When the endurance exercises are sufficiently intense, the increases in mitochondrial enzymes occur somewhat in parallel in all fiber types in the muscle (51). Consequently, glycolytic fibers become more oxidative, which is related to the peculiarity in motor units recruitment during prolonged exercise. Endurance exercises at approximately 60% $\dot{V}O_2max$ are initially performed through involvement of the activity of slow-twitch motor units. As the exercise continues, there is a progressive

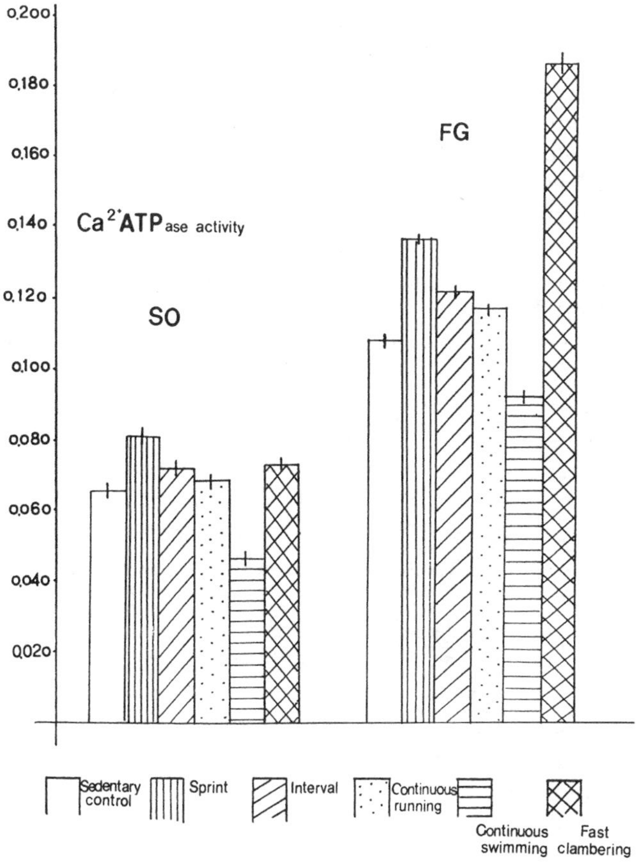

FIG. 6–9. Effect of various training programs on myofibrillar Ca^{2+}–adenosine triphosphatase (ATPase) activity [micromoles of released phosphate per milligram of protein in 1 minute; mean ± standard error of the mean (SEM)].

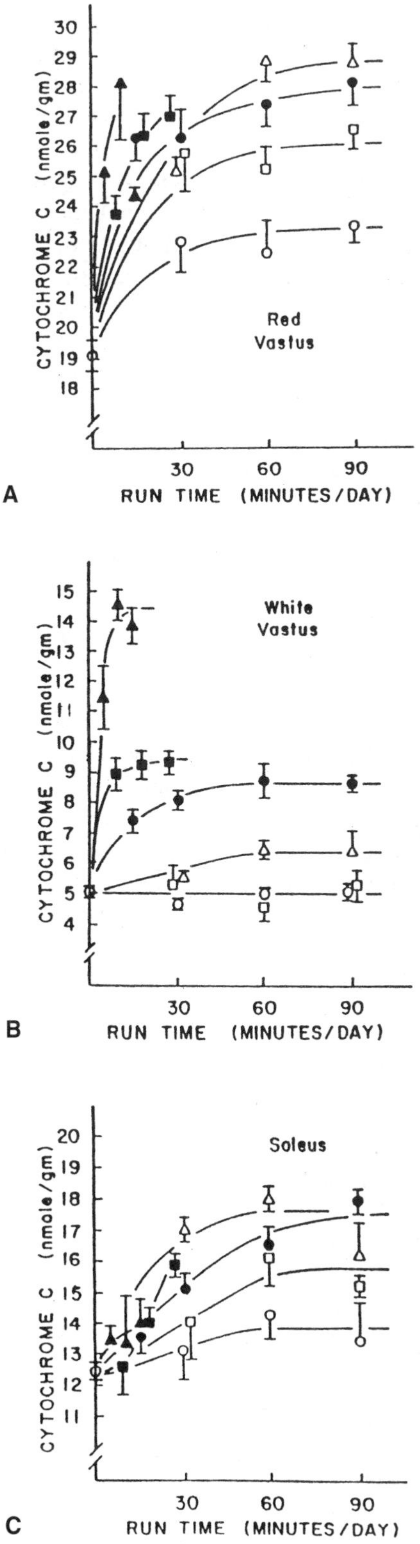

FIG. 6–10. Increase in cytochrome *c* concentration in fast-oxidative glycolytic (FOG) (**A**), fast-glycolytic (FG) (**B**), and slow-twitch oxidative (SO) (**C**) fibers as a function of duration of training exercises. The exercise intensity: (○) 10 m·min^{-1}, (□) 20 m·min^{-1}, (●) 30 m·min^{-1}, (△) 40 m·min^{-1}, (■) 50 m·min^{-1}, (▲) 60 m·min^{-1}. Adapted from Viru A. *Adaptation in sports training.* Boca Raton, FL: CRC Press, 1995, with permission.

recruitment of fast-twitch motor units. If exercise is carried out until exhaustion, all of the motor units in the muscle can be utilized (51). If the training exercise is moderate in intensity and duration, however, a difference may be found in the enzyme profile between various types of muscle fiber; for example, the β-hydroxybutyrate dehydrogenase activity increased 2.6-fold in SO and sixfold in FOG fibers, whereas no changes could be detected in FG fibers (52).

Training for improved strength usually does not cause a significant change in mitochondria number. After an intensive weight training program, a significant reduction has been found in mitochondrial volume density and mitochondrial to myofibrillar volume.

A linear increase is found in oxidative potential as the duration of training exercise increases (53). The results presented in Fig. 6–10 confirm that an increase in the duration of exercise brings about a greater adaptive response. When the running duration reached 60 minutes, however, a further prolongation of exercise did not further increase the cytochrome *c* concentration (54). When various running intensities were used in different training groups, the changes in markers of mitochondrial adaptation (increase in cytochrome *c* concentrations) depended on the fiber type studied. In FG fibers, the increase was found only when the running velocity was 30 $m \cdot min^{-1}$ or more (Fig. 6–11). In FOG fibers the training effect increased with running velocity up to 30 $m \cdot min^{-1}$. Then the effect leveled off at a steady-state level. In SO fibers the training effect was highest at a running velocity of 30 or 40 $m \cdot min^{-1}$. Lower and higher running velocities resulted in a less pronounced effect (54). Thus, an important point for rats was the running velocity of 30 $m \cdot min^{-1}$. This velocity results in an oxygen uptake of approximately 83% $\dot{V}O_2max$. This percent value seems to be close to the anaerobic threshold. If so, then from the anaerobic threshold onward the following occurs:

1. Training becomes effective in increasing oxidative potential in FG fibers.
2. The training effect levels off for the FOG fibers.
3. A further increase in exercise intensity reduces the training effect in SO fibers.

Although sprint training is usually ineffective in mitochondrial adaptation, a modest adaptation of mitochondrial enzymes is possible (55), perhaps related to the intermittent character of sprint exercises, in which a short period of activity with great power output is followed by a more prolonged recovery period for restoration of the levels of the muscle concentration of high-energy phosphate, furnished from oxidation energy. However, the effect of sprint training on mitochondrial enzymes is far from the effect of endurance training. When performed intermittently, isometric strength training also induces a modest increase in mitochondrial enzymes (56).

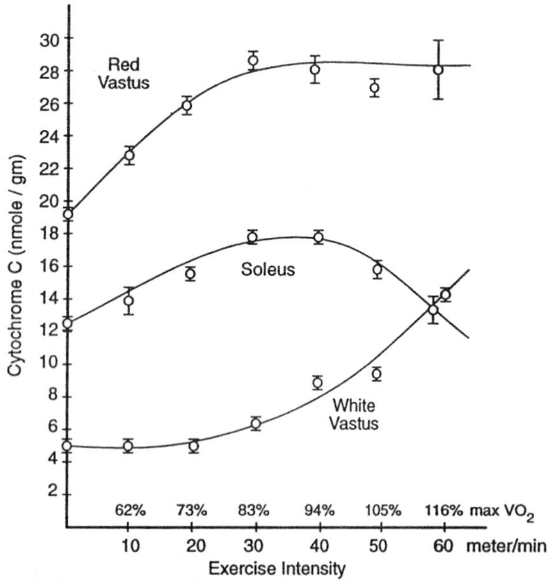

FIG. 6–11. Influence of exercise intensity on adaptive increase in oxidative capacity in working muscles of rat. On the abscissa the intensity of training exercises is shown as the running velocity and as the percentage of $\dot{V}O_2max$. Adapted from Viru A. *Adaptation in sports training.* Boca Raton, FL: CRC Press, 1995, with permission.

A study of muscle enzymes in track-and-field athletes demonstrated that the succinate dehydrogenase activity was highest in long- and middle-distance runners. A slight increase in activity was observed also in sprinters, but not in field athletes, compared to untrained subjects (57).

In rats, after 12 weeks of training, the succinate dehydrogenase activity was increased in the group continuously running (32 $m \cdot min^{-1}$, 85% $\dot{V}O_2max$, 120 minutes) in the soleus and vastus lateralis profundus, which contain SO and FOG fibers, respectively. A less-pronounced change occurred in the vastus lateralis superficialis (FG fibers). In a group undergoing sprint training (10-s dashes at 82 $m \cdot min^{-1}$, 160% $\dot{V}O_2max$) the enzyme activity increased only in the vastus lateralis superficialis (58).

While as a result of aerobic endurance training the activity of oxidative enzymes increases in combination with reduced activities of enzymes for anaerobic processes (59), anaerobic interval training increases the activities of enzymes catalyzing both processes (60). Greater mitochondrial changes were found following low-intensity compared with high-intensity interval training programs (55).

In conclusion, the adjustments on the mitochondrial level are common in training that entails a long exercise period of continuous or interrupted muscular activity (Fig. 6–12). The most effective seems to be continuous aerobic exercises close to the anaerobic threshold. Interrupted muscular activity becomes an effective tool for mitochondrial improvement when a high intensity of oxidation is required during the rest periods between the activity periods. This is the case with interval training. In sprint or strength training, prolonged rest periods are needed to produce optimal conditions for high force or

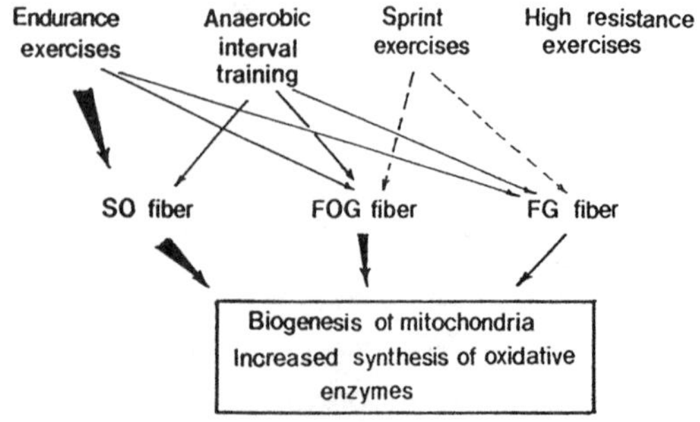

FIG. 6–12. Exercise-dependent specificity of effect on mitochondrial proliferation and activity on oxidative enzymes.

power output during the next repetition of exercise. Usually, only a part of these prolonged rest periods is necessary for recovery processes requiring a high oxidation rate. It is reasonable to suggest that the mitochondrial adjustments depend on (a) the total time of the persisting high level of oxidation in skeletal muscles, including the time for contractile activity, as well as the time for restitution based on high oxidation rate; and (b) the oxidation rate during these periods (the closer to the maximum oxidation rate, the more effective the training).

As a result of endurance training, active muscle starts to produce less lactate despite the same rate of glycogenolysis, which is partly related to the increased oxidation capacity. Additionally, one must recognize that endurance training influences lactate elimination from the blood rather than lactate production (61).

Anaerobic Enzymes

Creatine Kinase and Myokinase

The most rapid pathway of ATP resynthesis, the phosphocreatine mechanism, is related to the activity of creatine kinase. It should be expected that sprint training increases the activity of this enzyme. This possibility is supported by the fact that animals adapted to rapid dashes possess a high percentage of fast-twitch fibers and very high activities of creatine kinase, myokinase, and glycolytic enzymes in FG fibers (62). In the studies of Yakovlev (42) an increased activity of creatine kinase was found in rat skeletal muscles both after training with prolonged exercises of moderate intensity and after training with short-term intensive exercises. In rats 11 weeks of sprint training resulted in increased activity of creatine kinase in the soleus but not in the rectus femoris muscle (47).

In humans, sprint training's effect on the activity of muscle creatine kinase has not been confirmed (63). However, when fast maximal contractions were repeated five to eight times with brief rest intervals, creatine kinase and myokinase activities in muscle increased (59). Another program of strength training did not cause these changes (30).

Changes were found in creatine kinase isozymes in humans. In SO fibers of endurance-trained athletes, increased creatine kinase M and B subunit isozyme content was detected (64).

Glycolytic Enzymes

In exercises of submaximal power output lasting more than 30 seconds and less than 5 minutes, anaerobic glycogenolysis becomes critical for ATP resynthesis. Correspondingly, adaptive changes in enzymes of glycogenolysis are expected as the first order of training for improvement of sports performance in corresponding competitive exercises.

In the practice of sports training the main tool for improvement of anaerobic working capacity is interval training. Highly intensive exercises are repeated over rest intervals too short for elimination of accumulated lactate or for prevention of the summation from bout to bout of the consequences of anaerobic energy processes in the internal environment of the organism. The systematic use of interval training involves both aerobic and anaerobic enzymes, including the key enzyme of anaerobic glucogenolysis: phosphofructokinase activity (65).

Sprint training differs from interval training in that (a) it is a less-durable exercise (10- to 20-second dashes), (b) it has almost the highest exercise intensity, and (c) it has more prolonged rest intervals between repetitions. In humans, sprint training also resulted in an increase in phosphofructokinase activity (63). In rats, sprint training increased the phosphofructokinase activity in FOG and FG but not in SO fibers (58).

Endurance training with continuous exercises does not change the phosphofructokinase activity (58).

Strength training usually does not produce alterations in the activity of glycolytic enzymes. Shot-putters, weightlifters, and discus throwers have glycolytic enzyme activities well within the range of sedentary subjects, whereas sprinters, jumpers, and runners of 400 to 800 m usually have elevated levels of these enzymes (57).

Glycolytic enzymes have a short life span (between 1.5 hours and a few days). Therefore, what is essential is not an increase in number of enzyme molecules, but rather an enhanced sensitivity of rapidly renewing enzyme molecules to regulatory influences. Rat experiments used this version of adaptation in training. Phosphofructokinase activity decreased as a result of a 10-week period of anaerobic interval or continuous aerobic running both in SO and FG fibers. Sprint training caused this change in SO but not in FG fibers. Since 48 hours passed after the final training session before muscle samples were obtained, the time elapsed was enough to suggest that a rapid enzyme turnover eliminated the increased enzyme activity. However, an important result of this study was that 4 minutes of intensive running (at 60 m·min^{-1}) changed the muscle phosphofructokinase activity in a manner dependent on the training regimen used. In untrained control rats the test exercise induced a decrease in the enzyme activity in the oxidative muscle. In glycolytic muscle the activity did not change. Instead, a two- or threefold increase was found in muscles of rats trained by either interval or continuous running (Fig. 6–13). After test exercise, the enzyme activity was above the resting levels not only in these trained rats but also in sedentary control rats (43).

The effect of sprint training was different. The effect of the test exercise was to decrease muscle enzyme activ-

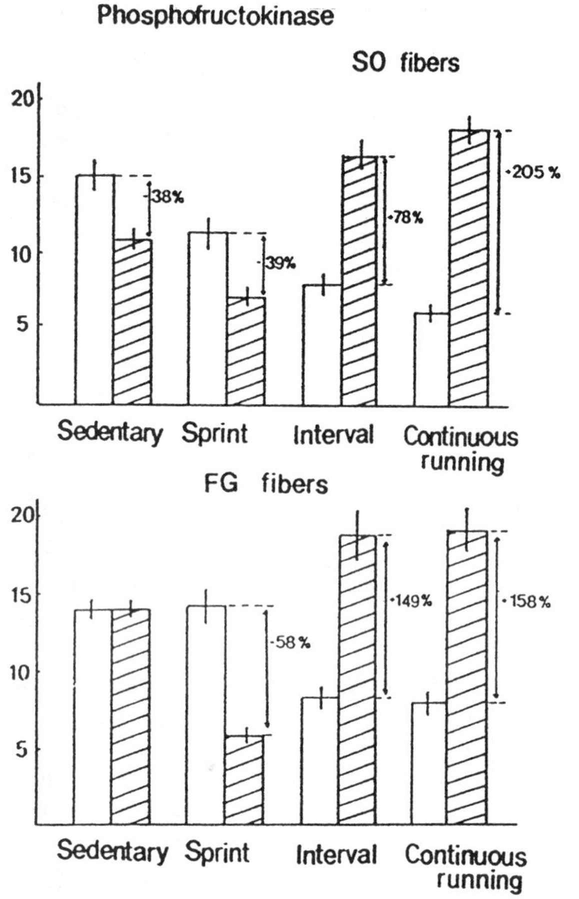

FIG. 6–13. Effects of sprint, interval, and continuous running on phosphofructokinase activity in the resting state (*open columns*) and after a 4-minute test running at 60 $m \cdot min^{-1}$ (*striated columns*) in rats. Phosphofructokinase activity is evaluated by the change in optical density during 30-s periods per 1 g protein (mean ± SEM).

ities in both types of fibers, but in SO fibers the change was greater than in the control group (43). The training-induced enhanced sensitivity of enzyme molecules was reflected in decreased enzyme activity due to dominating downregulation. During intense exercise the upregulation prevailed, and the combination of that together with enhanced sensitivity led to a pronounced increase in activity.

The specific adaptation to anaerobic exercises may affect the formation of isozymes less sensitive to a lowered pH value. However, this question has been investigated only in regard to hexokinase and in only one study (66).

Buffer Capacity

Since the possibilities of anaerobic glycolysis will be utilized during supramaximal exercises, training should increase the buffer capacity of skeletal muscles and the blood. This is a typical result of anaerobic interval training as well as sprint training (67). The buffer capacity is a contributing factor in enhanced anaerobic performance capacity.

Anaerobic Working Capacity

Anaerobic working capacity is the ability to perform highly intensive exercise using anaerobic processes for ATP resynthesis. Anaerobic working capacity implies (a) the highest possible power output during a specific time, and (b) the prevalence of anaerobic production of energy (resynthesis of ATP). The time factor discriminates the application of the anaerobic working capacity into three purposes: (a) energy that attains the maximal power output during exercises lasting up to 10 to 20 seconds, (b) energy that attains the submaximal power output during exercises lasting more than 20 to 30 seconds and less than 5 minutes, and (c) energy that attains great power output during exercises lasting from 5 to 30 minutes.

Accordingly, the first purpose of anaerobic working capacity concerns sprint exercises. In this case, anaerobic working capacity may be understood as the sprinter's capacity. ATP resynthesis has to be at the highest rate, which is provided by degradation of phosphocreatine. Due to the limited amount of phosphocreatine in muscles, the phosphocreatine mechanism of ATP resynthesis has to be complemented by anaerobic glycogenolysis. The phosphocreatine and the possibilities for its use in ATP resynthesis are important determinants in sprint performance. Highly significant also are the excitation-contraction mechanism, membrane functions including the Na-K pump, the function of the SR, the rate of cross-bridge formation, and the rate of ATP hydrolysis. The essential precondition for all of these is a high percentage of FG fibers.

The second and third purposes of anaerobic working capacity are anaerobic glycogenolysis and glycolysis. Frequently, the term *anaerobic working capacity* is used as it pertains to performance of exercise using anaerobic glycogenolysis and oxidative phosphorylation in ATP resynthesis. In exercises lasting from 30 seconds to 5 minutes, anaerobic glycolysis is prevalent; in exercises of 5 to 30 minutes oxidative phosphorylation is prevalent. In both groups of exercises, the contribution of anaerobic glycogenolysis is quantitatively related to the accumulation of lactate in the working muscles and blood. The increase in anaerobic working capacity as a result of exercise is summarized in Fig. 6–14.

Intramuscular Energy Stores and Myoglobin

Adenosine Triphosphate

There is no convincing evidence that training increases the ATP store in muscles. Only a minimal initial increase is possible at the beginning of training.

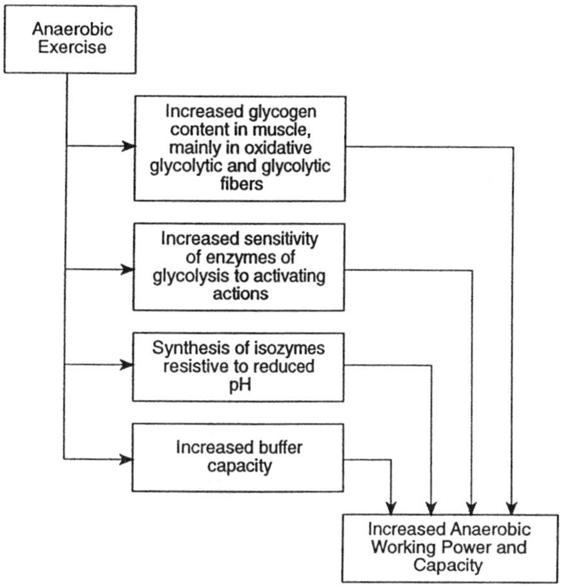

FIG. 6–14. Adaptation on anaerobic exercise.

Phosphocreatine

There is evidence that training elevates the phosphocreatine content in skeletal muscles. Rats trained by repeated short-term intensive exercise increased the phosphocreatine content in skeletal muscles, but the effect of continuous exercise was only modest (22). Some human biopsy studies confirm the increase in muscle phosphocreatine. However, an increased phosphocreatine store is not considered a common result of training.

Glycogen

The training effect on muscle glycogen store has been known since 1927. In rats, no difference was found between effects of training with continuous exercises and interval training, but the effect of high-power exercises was less pronounced (22). In humans, a higher level of muscle glycogen stores in trained than in sedentary individuals has been demonstrated repeatedly since the first biopsy studies (68). Both longitudinal and cross-sectional studies indicate that subjects undergoing strength, sprint, or endurance training programs possess a larger store of muscle glycogen than untrained persons or the same person before training. The augmentation of glycogen stores is clearly related to the increased glycogen synthetase activity in trained muscles (69).

Myoglobin

This protein increases the rate of O_2 diffusion in muscles, from the cytoplasm to the mitochondria. Endurance training increases the concentration of myoglobin in skeletal muscles of rats (70). Analogous results were obtained with speed and power training (22). In contrast, biopsy studies did not demonstrate an increased myoglobin content in endurance-trained humans.

Muscle Capillarization

An endurance training–induced increase in capillary densities was first detected in animal muscles six decades ago. Later it was confirmed that the human skeletal muscle also adapts to increased use by increasing the number of capillaries (71). This effect of endurance training becomes apparent with increases of capillaries per fiber, capillaries per square millimeter, and the number of capillaries found around a fiber. The increased muscle capillarity seems to be a specific phenomenon characteristic of endurance training.

Fiber-Type Transformation

Fast- and slow-twitch fibers can be distinguished by their specific myosin light chain patterns. Both fast and slow myosin were found in fast-twitch as well as in slow-twitch fibers, but in different ratios. Changes of these ratios are somewhat possible in training.

Under appropriate conditions muscle fibers are mutable. Perhaps the first of these situations occurs during maturation after birth. Studies demonstrate the change of slow-twitch to fast-twitch fibers during the early postnatal period. Fiber-type transformation is possible with cross-innervation and specific electrical stimulation. Chronically increased contractile activity by low-frequency stimulation induces a transformation of fast- into slow-twitch muscle fibers in the rabbit. Early changes in enzyme activities and isozymes of energy metabolism result in a "white to red" metabolic transformation. Simultaneously, cytosolic Ca^{2+} binding and Ca^{2+} sequestering are reduced. The fast to slow transformation is completed by an exchange of fast- with slow-type myosin isoforms (72). More recent studies have confirmed that endurance training can change the isomyosin pattern in fast- and slow-twitch muscles (73) and thereby alter the myosin fenotype of muscle fiber. In prolonged endurance training a transformation of type IIc fibers into type I fibers (74) and type IIb fibers into type IIa fibers (75) is possible. When the intensity of endurance exercises was above the anaerobic threshold, the training result was a decrease in type I fibers accommodated by an increase in type IIc fibers (76). According to the obtained results, it was suggested that in endurance training the following fiber type transformations may exist: IIa → IIc → I. Anaerobic interval training during a 15-week period also increased the percent of type I fibers (from 41% to 47%). Type IIb decreased from 17% to 12%, and the percent of type IIa did not change in the vastus lateralis muscle (77).

With sprint or strength training, changes in different

fiber types are restricted mainly to alterations in the myofibrillar to mitochondrial volume ratio. Nevertheless, one study demonstrated an increase in fast-twitch fibers, mainly type IIa fibers, as a result of sprint training (11,63).

Presently it seems correct to assume that, under certain appropriate conditions, an influence on the muscle cell genetic apparatus might be borne by training, resulting in switching of muscle fibers from one subgroup to another.

Summary

In skeletal muscles, the main manifestations of various forms and regimens of training are the following:

- myofibrillar hypertrophy,
- adaptation of myofibrillar ATPase,
- increased possibilities of the SR,
- improved function of Na-K pumps,
- increased activity of glycolytic enzymes or alterations of their susceptibility to activators and inhibitors,
- increased volume density of mitochondria and activity of oxidative enzymes,
- augmented capillarization,
- increased energy stores.

Resistance against muscle contraction is the main factor stimulating myofibrillar hypertrophy. Repeated strong contractions (heavy-resistance exercises) are necessary for actualization of this change. Continuous exercises of moderate intensity stimulate increases in the volume density of mitochondria, activity of oxidative enzymes, and capillarization. However, these alterations appear also in interrupted exercises of high intensity. Therefore, the most essential condition is a prolonged period of a high rate of oxidation, which may be warranted by prolonged continuous exercise, and by interrupted exercises if a high rate of oxidation persists during rest periods between exercise bouts. However, a question remains whether there is a limit for exercise intensity, bearing in mind the possibility that exaggerated accumulation of lactate and protons may suppress oxidation.

Adaptation of myofibrillar ATPase means, first of all, increased activity of the enzyme, which is a typical result of strength or speed training. In the case of endurance training, decreased enzyme activity is possible. While the increased myofibrillar ATPase activity is necessary for rapid and augmented transfer of chemical energy to mechanical energy, the decreased activity of myofibrillar ATPase enables economizing on the utilization of the produced energy.

Rapid sequestering and rapid reaccumulation of calcium ions are essential conditions in the performance of sprint or power exercises. The velocity of muscle contraction as well as the necessity to form a high number of cross-bridges in a short time are the factors stimulating the improvement of the function of the SR. Less effective are heavy-resistance exercises. Endurance exercises may exhibit an opposite effect. Again a question arises as to whether the latter is related to the sparing effect of endurance training.

Evidence has been obtained on the improved functions of the Na-K pump in trained muscles, but further detailed studies are necessary to specify the dependence of the improved Na-K pump functions on the exercises used.

The stimulus for adaptation at the level of glycolytic enzymes is provided by exercises based on a high rate of anaerobic glycogenolysis. The life span of glycolytic enzymes is rather short, however. Therefore, the increased activity of these enzymes, resulting from corresponding exercise, may persist for only a few hours or 1 to 2 days. Recently, it was found that anaerobic exercises may elevate the susceptibility of glycolytic enzymes to their activators and inhibitors, or they may induce a synthesis of isozymes resistive to low pH. These possibilities need further confirmation and specification.

The training effect on intramuscular energy stores is the most pronounced in regard to glycogen content. Endurance exercises seem to be more effective than sprint or strength exercises. Results are not unanimous in regard to increased phosphocreatine content. One may suggest that sprint exercises have to be the most effective in augmenting the phosphocreatine store, but this has not yet been convincingly evidenced. The increase of the ATP store is doubtful. Besides the function of energy donor, ATP possesses an essential role in the control of intracellular metabolism. The increased ATP content would mean decreased possibilities for mobilization of cellular resources during exercise performance.

All these training manifestations are dependent on the type of muscle fibers; some are favorable in FG, and others in SO fibers. This dependence is based on the differences in recruiting of various motor units and thereby fibers of various types. The increase in force application or intensity of performance makes it necessary to recruit more motor units. In heavy-resistance as well as highly intensive exercises, the recruiting of motor units is close to maximal. Therefore, the training effects of these exercises on muscle fibers of various types are less specific.

SPECIFIC NATURE OF TRAINING EFFECTS IN OTHER TISSUES AND ORGANS

Specificity of Training Effects on Aerobic Working Capacity

Anaerobic Threshold

Endurance training effects on the mitochondria facilitate the use of oxidative phosphorylation for ATP resynthesis during performance of more intensive exercises than before training. The so-called anaerobic threshold is likely a quantitative measure of the highest exercise intensity performed on the basis of oxidative phosphorylation without an extended use of anaerobic energy mechanisms. To put it more precisely, the anaerobic threshold expresses the highest exercise intensity during performance in which the pyruvate formation rate still does not exceed the maximal rate of oxidative phosphorylation. Accordingly, the formed lactate can be oxidized or used for gluconeogenesis by nonworking muscles, heart, and liver. Up to this qualitative point, an equilibrium exists between lactate formation and elimination (78).

Since the maximal oxygen uptake is obtained in exercise level, causing a pronounced lactate accumulation, exercise intensity at $\dot{V}O_2max$ does not indicate maximal performance on the basis of aerobic resynthesis of ATP. A study of elite road cyclists failed to show close coupling between the whole-body $\dot{V}O_2max$ and the oxidative capacity of a local muscle group during a competition season (79). A close relationship of these variables exists over the first 3 to 4 weeks of training. Thereafter, the increase in $\dot{V}O_2max$ levels off, but the activity of mitochondrial enzymes continues to rise (80). The $\dot{V}O_2$max of athletes may be twice that of untrained persons, whereas the activity of mitochondrial enzymes of their muscle is three- to fourfold higher than that of sedentary individuals. When training was discontinued, the activity of oxidative enzymes dropped to the initial level within 2 to 4 weeks, but $\dot{V}O_2max$ remained high for 6 weeks (80).

The anaerobic threshold is a variable that accurately predicts athletic endurance performance, particularly in running races of 10 to 42 km (Fig. 6–15), and in race walkers, rowers, and skiers. In 21 endurance-trained runners longitudinal changes in the anaerobic threshold and distance-running performance were in consistently high correlation over a 9-month training period (81).

For predicting the endurance performance level, exercise intensity at the anaerobic threshold is more important than the percent of $\dot{V}O_2max$ at this exercise intensity. A comparison of running velocity at 4 mmol·L^{-1} lactate in the best Swedish runners for 400 m to marathon distances showed that running velocity was the highest in 10,000-m or marathon runners (Fig. 6–16) (82).

In athletes the percent of slow-twitch oxidative fibers is significantly related to running velocity, corresponding to the blood lactate threshold, the average speed of the marathon race, and the average mechanical power output during running at the velocity corresponding to the blood lactate threshold (83).

An effective tool for improvement of the anaerobic threshold is aerobic endurance training. Aerobic training is most effective at intensities of exercises corresponding to the anaerobic threshold or at an intensity slightly higher than the anaerobic threshold. Training for 40 weeks at the anaerobic threshold (1 hour/day, 3 days/week) resulted in pronounced increases in the anaerobic threshold, maximal working capacity at 80% to 85% $\dot{V}O_2$max, and net efficiency of muscular work. However, there was no significant increase in $\dot{V}O_2max$ (84).

According to differences in anaerobic and aerobic training effects, the anaerobic threshold constituted 65.9% ± 0.3% of $\dot{V}O_2max$ in swimmers-sprinters, compared to 90.4% ± 0.1% in long-distance swimmers (85). In a case of a similar training protocol, running resulted in large improvements in the anaerobic threshold for both cycling and running, with a larger improvement in the running anaerobic threshold. Cycle training resulted in an improvement in the cycling anaerobic threshold with no change in the running anaerobic threshold (86). The difference between running and cycling training effect can be explained by the main influence on oxidative capacity of muscles most active during training exercises.

Exercise Economy

The increased oxidative capacity of working muscles makes it possible to use a smaller fraction of it for performance of exercises of moderate intensity. Accordingly, a successful long-distance run is dependent on the economical utilization of a highly developed aerobic capacity and the ability to employ a large fraction of that capacity with minimal accumulation of lactic acid. The endurance performance is related to this training effect (87).

Exercise economy and correspondingly the employed fractions of aerobic capacity are especially related to training exercises in two ways: (a) in the specific influence of exercises on the oxidative enzymes in most active muscles, and (b) in the specific improvement of muscle coordination that warrants the more accomplished biomechanical utilization of muscle forces, and thereby an increased mechanical efficiency.

Maximal Oxygen Uptake ($\dot{V}O_{2max}$)

An integral index of the aerobic capacity of the organism is maximal oxygen uptake. This index only partly depends on the oxidative capacity of muscles. $\dot{V}O_2max$ depends also on oxygen binding in erythrocytes. Moreover, fundamental studies have established that $\dot{V}O_2max$ is mainly set by cardiovascular determinants (88).

A great number of studies have demonstrated the relationship of individual $\dot{V}O_2max$ values to endurance performance. The high-performance capacity in sprint, power, strength, and skill events is not related to $\dot{V}O_2$max. The usual finding in endurance athletes is that the longer the main distance, the higher is the maximal

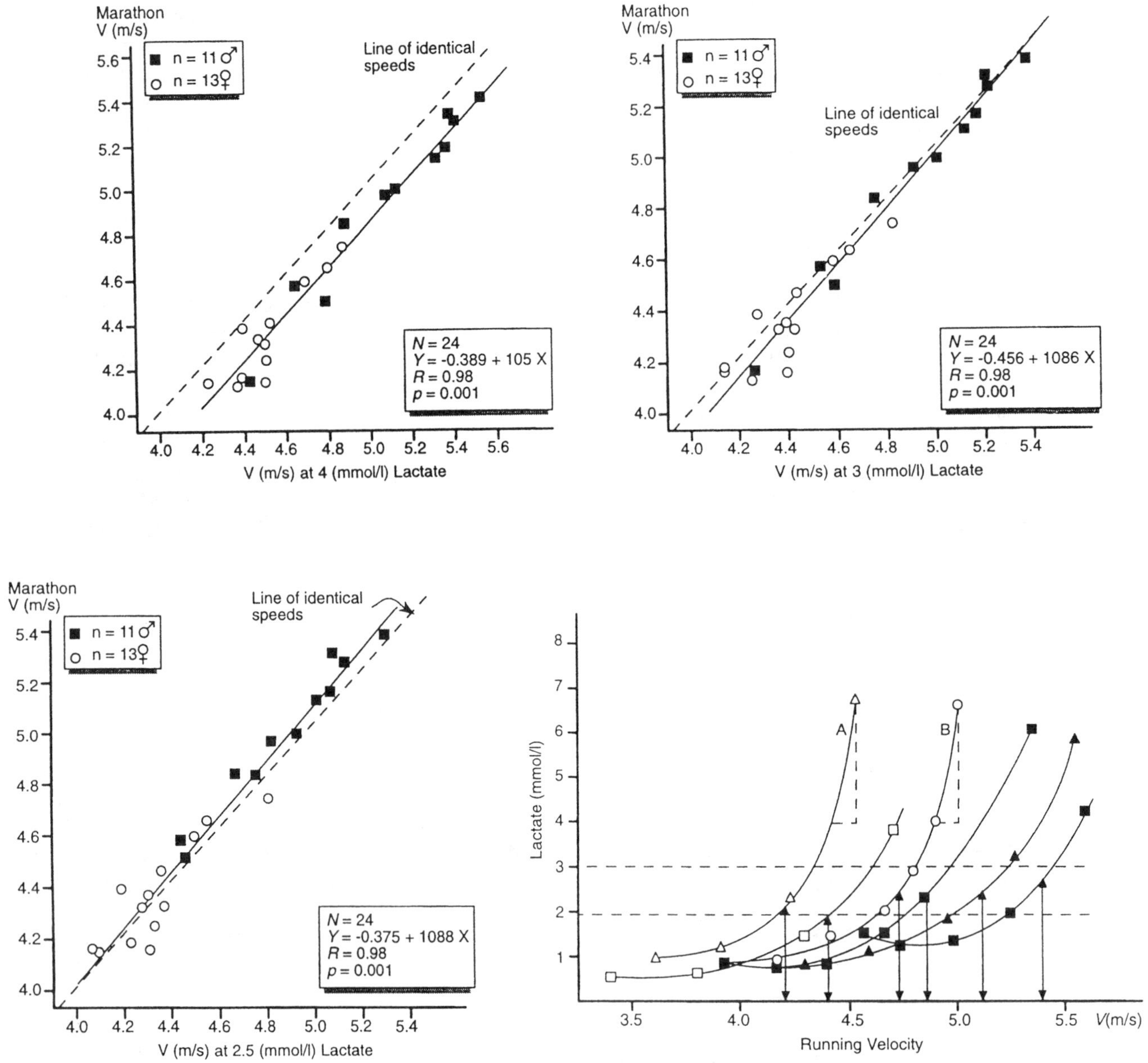

FIG. 6–15. Correlations of the marathon velocity with running velocities at lactate levels of 4 mmol·L^{-1}, 3 mmol·L^{-1}, 2.5 mmol·L^{-1}, determined in the incremental field test in female (*open symbols*) and male (*closed symbols*) runners, and individual lactate-running velocity relationship in female and male marathon runners. The average marathon velocity (*vertical arrows*) corresponds to the lactate-running velocity relationship determined in the incremental field test in the range 2 to 3 mmol·L^{-1} lactate. Adapted from Mader A. Evaluation of the endurance performance of marathon runners and theoretical analysis of test results. *J Sports Med Phys Fitness* 1991;31:1–19.

oxygen uptake, but changes in running performance with training may occur without equivalent changes in $\dot{V}O_2$max (89). $\dot{V}O_2$max was found to be a good predictor of endurance performance when a heterogeneous group of subjects with different athletic abilities was studied. However, it is a relatively poor predictor when athletes of similar ability are evaluated.

The specificity of training concept has been supported by researchers on training-induced changes in $\dot{V}O_2$max measured in various exercises. Significant differences were found when $\dot{V}O_2$max was compared in running versus swimming, running versus cycling, running versus rowing, and kayaking versus cycling. The specificity of training concept appears also to be present in regard to muscle groups utilized in training versus test exercises.

A specific effect of aerobic endurance training may be not only the improvement of maximal aerobic power, measured as $\dot{V}O_2$max, but also increased capacity to

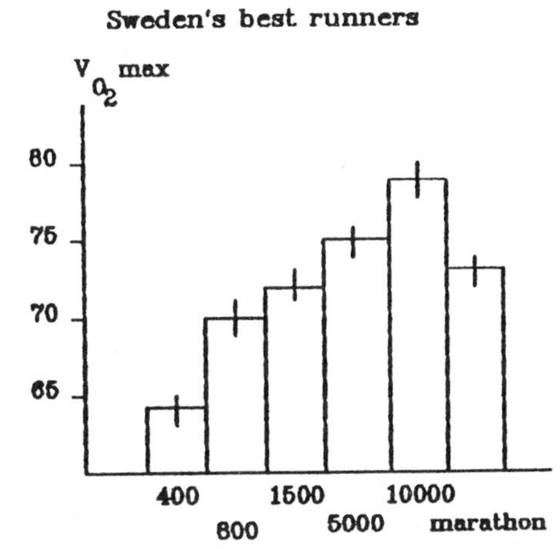

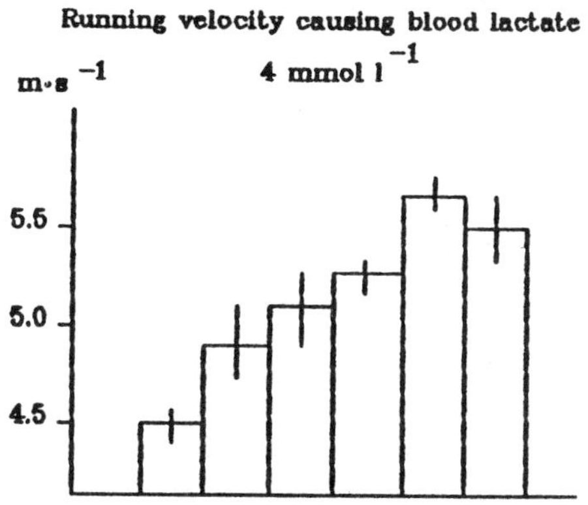

	n	The personal best mean	limits
400 m	2	46.96	45.63—48.33
800 m	6	1.46.41	1.47.64—1.50.42
800—1500 m	5	1.49.68	1.49.07—1.50.66
		3.41.86	3.38.51—3.46.43
1500—5000 m	6	3.44.7	3.41.9—3.48.1
		13.56.6	13.57.1—14.00.4
5000—10000	5	13.49.9	13.44.7—13.59.1
		26.57.9	28.36.6—29.21.0
1000-marathon	5	29.22.7	26.56.6—29.48.8
		2.16.18	2.12.07—2.21.04

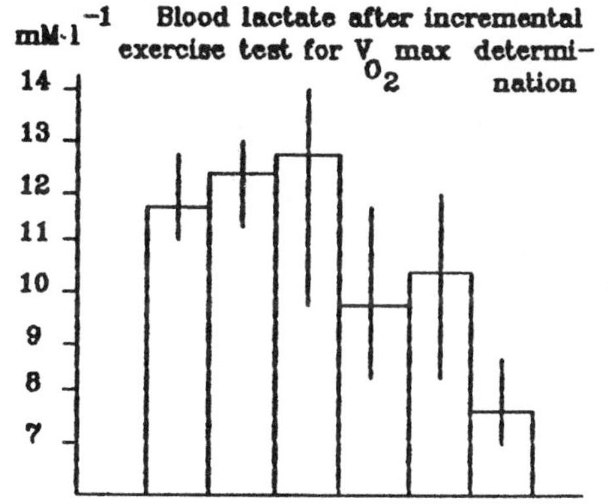

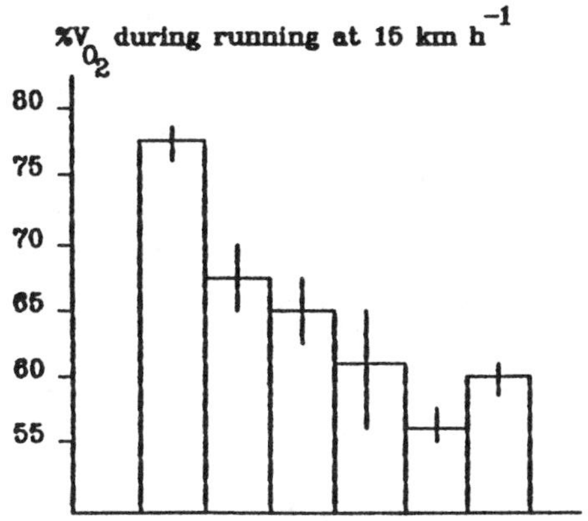

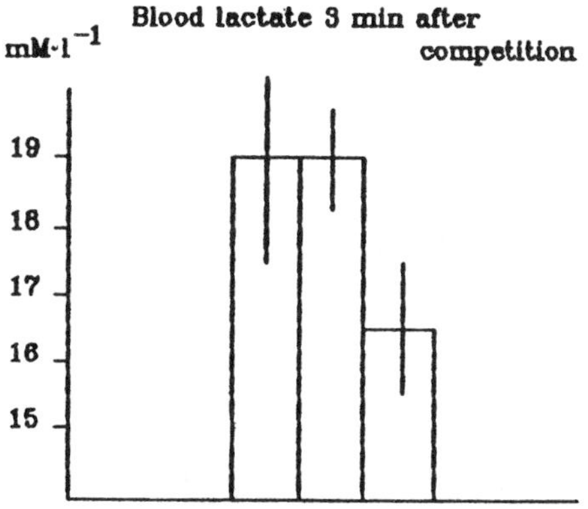

FIG. 6–16. $\dot{V}O_2$ and %$\dot{V}O_2$max during swimming at 15 km·h^{-1}, running velocity causing a blood lactate level of 4 mmol·L^{-1}, and blood lactate levels after incremental test exercise for $\dot{V}O_2$max determination and blood lactate levels at the finish of competition in the best Swedish runners. Adapted from Viru A. *Adaptation in sports training.* Boca Raton, FL: CRC Press, 1995, with permission.

perform prolonged aerobic exercise (maximal aerobic capacity). Aerobic training during a 20-week period enhanced the mean maximal aerobic power by 33% and maximal aerobic capacity by 51%. The latter was computed as the total work output accomplished during a 90-minute maximal ergocycle test (90).

$\dot{V}O_2$max increases as a result of continuous exercises performed at levels both above and below the anaerobic threshold. Effective are systematically performed continuous (35 to 45 minutes of duration) sets of aerobic dance or aerobic gymnastics. A number of studies as well as sports practice indicate the effectiveness of inter-

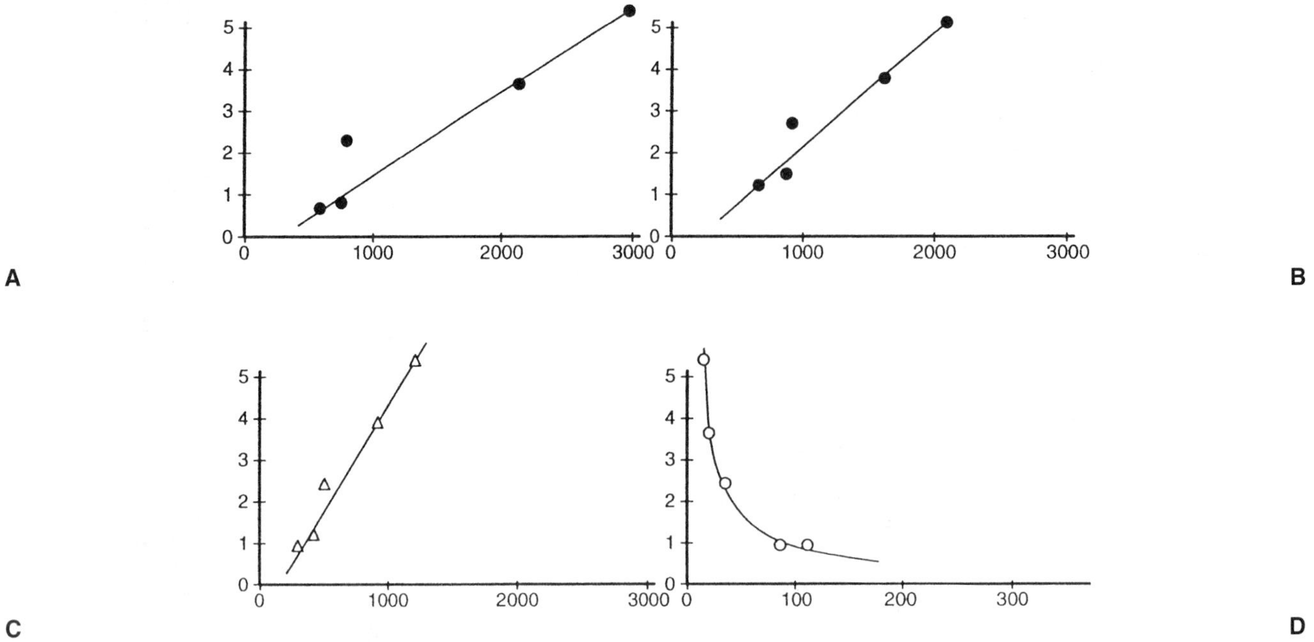

FIG. 6–17. Dependence of $\dot{V}O_2max$ improvement ($mL \cdot min^{-1} \cdot kg^{-1}$) on volume of various training exercises per year in kilometers. **A**: Total volume of running exercises. **B**: Volume of aerobic exercises. **C**: Volume of aerobic-anaerobic exercises. **D**: Volume of anaerobic exercises. Adapted from Viru A. *Adaptation in sports training.* Boca Raton, FL: CRC Press, 1995, with permission.

val training for improvement of $\dot{V}O_2max$. In contrast to aerobic and anaerobic endurance training, high-resistance strength training induces no increases in maximal oxygen uptake. Concurrent performance of endurance and resistance training does not affect the magnitude of increase in aerobic power induced by endurance training only. The situation may change in two cases: (a) when moderate resistance exercises are repeated over a prolonged period with short rest intervals between repetitions, and (b) when very intensive resistance exercises are used.

In runners the $\dot{V}O_2max$ improvement correlates with the total volume of running exercises, the volume of aerobic exercises, and the volume of anaerobic exercises during a training year (91). The relationship between $\dot{V}O_2max$ improvement and the volume of anaerobic exercises is inverted (Fig. 6–17).

Specificity of Training Effects on the Cardiovascular System

Cardiac Hypertrophy

Since the accurate chest percussion studies from the end of the nineteenth century, enlargement of the heart has been known as a typical result of endurance training. Subsequent x-ray studies confirmed this fact. The basis for heart enlargement in endurance athletes is both myocardial hypertrophy as well as enlargement of heart cavities. Three variants of heart dilation were discriminated: (a) myogenic dilation due to damage in the myocardium; (b) tonogenic dilation caused by loss in myocardial tone; and (c) regulative dilation, expressed by low myocardial tone in the resting state and by high contractility of myocardium in a strain situation caused by exercise or other factors (92). The latter variant is the usual result of endurance training. An expression of regulative dilations is the augmented residual blood volume in the heart during resting conditions and its almost maximal utilization for the increased stroke volume during exercise. In the resting state, endurance athletes showed a 3:1 ratio between residual and stroke volumes.

In sprinters, field athletes, gymnasts, and fencers, the heart volume, estimated from x-ray pictures, is close to values in untrained persons. Heart enlargement was found in weightlifters; however, in contrast with endurance athletes, the enlargement was mainly in the right ventricle. It has been assumed that the enlargement of the right heart ventricle is caused by exercise connected with short-term but intensive muscular effort and with respiration stop in the inspiration phase.

An enlarged heart in endurance athletes was confirmed by autopsy of athletes who had perished in accidents. Increased volume of heart cavities and increased heart weight were detected, but only in a single case did the weight of an athlete's heart exceed 500 g (92). This heart mass was considered critical. Larger human hearts were associated with cardiovascular efficiency. Accordingly, myocardial fiber thickness of more than 20 μm was considered critical.

The increased capillarity and capillary-to-fiber ratio in the myocardium of endurance-trained animals has been evidenced. Increased capillary diffusion capacity, precapillary vascularity and total size of the coronary tree, development of extra coronary collaterals, and increased coronary artery lumina have been found (93,94).

A further specification of training effects on the human heart became possible with the use of echocardiography. Cross-sectional echocardiographic studies demonstrated larger right and left ventricular diameters and calculated left ventricular masses in endurance athletes as compared to sedentary persons (95). Different patterns of left ventricular hypertrophy exist among different types of athletes. In athletes trained primarily with combined dynamic and static exercises (wrestlers), the main changes were increased wall thickness and increased volume. In dynamically trained athletes (runners), increased heart volume was found (96). In contrast with a previous theory, the echocardiographic studies showed that resistance training increases absolute left ventricular wall thickness and left ventricular mass (97).

In adolescent boys $\dot{V}O_2max$ increased significantly together with a slight enlargement of calculated left ventricular mass as a result of endurance training. In a group that underwent sprint training, these changes were insignificant. In a strength-trained group a less-pronounced increase was found in the left ventricular mass in combination with a pronounced rise in muscular strength (98). Endurance-trained female athletes also exhibit trends toward higher left ventricular end-diastolic dimensions and volumes, stroke volume, left ventricular mass, and left atrial dimensions when data were standardized for body surface area (99).

Morganroth and colleagues (100) considered concentric hypertrophy the training effect on the heart in power athletes as opposed to pure dilation (eccentric hypertrophy) in endurance athletes. They took into consideration the increased pressure work during static or power exercises and the predominant volume work during dynamic exercises, respectively. However, Rost (101) did not confirm concentric hypertrophy in power athletes. He found only some examples of such hypertrophy in power athletes, but for an unknown reason this could also be found in endurance athletes. He assumed that cardiac hypertrophy takes place in a uniform way as eccentric hypertrophy. The differences between the hearts of athletes of various events are only quantitative, according to his data. A common result of many years of training is the increased volume of the left ventricle at the end of diastole during exercise.

Cardiac Performance

The major adaptation to endurance training is the generation of a greater stroke volume at any given level of exercise intensity as well as a greater maximal stroke volume. This training effect is related to increased blood volume, enlarged heart cavities, and enhanced contractility of myocardium. The latter is related to decreased end-systolic volume.

The endurance-training effects on the myocardium contractility have been proved in various kinds of animal experiments, including experiments on isolated preparations of myocardium and on isolated perfused heart. Two versions of heart adaptation to training have been suggested. One is connected with myocardial hypertrophy, which in rats appears mainly as a result of swimming training. The other is connected with adjustments that do not necessarily include heart muscle hypertrophy, increased amounts of contractile protein, and elevated activity of ATPase in myofibrils. This version of adaptation is revealed mainly as a result of running training and seems to be related to adjustments in the level of intracellular Ca^{2+} metabolism (102).

Neither endurance nor other kinds of training increase the amount of cardiac mitochondrial proteins per gram of tissue or the activity of mitochondrial enzymes. In the untrained organism the oxidative capacity of heart already exceeds that of the slow-twitch oxidative fibers of skeletal muscles by approximately threefold. With training, the skeletal muscle can approximately double its oxidative capacity (see above), while that of the heart remains unaffected under intense training regimes. The myocardial mitochondria is chronically maintained in a maximal upregulated state. This property permits the heart to maintain a positive energy balance in the face of a constantly changing availability of substrates. Hence, the endurance training effect on skeletal muscle mitochondria implies the reduction of differences between skeletal and heart muscles' oxidative capacities. In regard to the heart muscle, it was assumed that training induced a proportional increase in myofibrillar and mitochondrial protein (103). At the same time endurance training suppresses the free radical oxidation of lipids in myocardiums.

Coronary vasodilation during exercise can produce a three- to fivefold increase in coronary flow. Even in strenuous exercise the myocardial oxygen delivery appears to be adequate and the existing flow reserve seems capable of handling the increased oxygen demand (104). There is a difference between the effect of endurance and high-resistance training on myocardial vascularity. Endurance-trained rats exhibited a higher left and total coronary cast weight when compared to either sedentary control or resistance-trained rats. In resistance-trained rats, a higher right coronary cast weight was observed in comparison with their sedentary counterparts. It has been concluded that exercises that substantially increase the cardiac output and coronary blood flow stimulate a neovascular response at least at the capillary level (105).

Endurance training increases the glycogen store in the myocardium, but no changes were found in the contents of phosphocreatine, ATP, ADP, and adenosine monophosphate (AMP). Myocardial triglycerides, phospholipids, and cholesterol are not altered with training.

Stimulus for Cardiac Adaptation

As cited above, it had been suggested that the stimulus for myocardial adaptation arises from either ventricular diastolic stretch or work against the increased aortic pressure. During most exercises, both aortic pressure and venous return have been raised to high levels. Therefore, the dependence of myocardial adaptation on training exercise cannot be very specific. The relation between cardiac preload due to venous inflow and cardiac afterload due to the pressure work is altered in cases of short-term respiration stop during strong muscle effort. In this way a different adaptation to endurance and high-resistance exercises can be caused.

The difference between chronic effects of continuous aerobic endurance exercises and intensive anaerobic interval training is negligible. The stimulus for myocardial adaptation depends on duration of cardiac activity on high levels but not on the duration of an exercise or on the total duration of short-term exercise bouts. Certainly, high heart activity is necessary not only during the exercise but also during the first part of the recovery period to ensure elevated oxidative metabolism for restitution processes. In the 1960s, Reindell and co-workers (92) suggested that the stimulus for cardiac adaptation is determined by the duration of heart activity with maximal stroke volume. Since their study showed that during exercise the stroke volume is maximal when heart rate is above 130 beats per minute (106), they assumed that the duration of heart activity above this level is required for a trainable effect. Accordingly, the effect of anaerobic interval training is related to the total time of the session, including both exercise bouts and short-term recovery intervals between them. However, in this way a stimulus arises mainly for adaptation on the level of cardiac myofibrils. On the level of cardiac mitochondria, adaptive changes have not been demonstrated, and a different situation seems to exist on the level of the sarcoplasmic reticulum. Thus, it is suggested that the function of myocardial sarcoplasmic reticulum (both the calcium sequestering and its binding again by the sarcoplasmic reticulum) improves depending on the total time of heart rate at higher levels than 130 beats per minutes during a training session. Perhaps heart rate levels of 160 to 180 beats per minutes are necessary.

Long duration of the necessary level of heart activity seems to be essential both for improvement of cardiac myofibrils and for sarcoplasmic reticulum. Therefore, it is understandable that short-term exercise bouts (high-resistance, power, or speed exercise) that are interchanged by relatively prolonged rest intervals are not effective for induction of adaptive changes in the heart.

Additional Adaptive Changes in the Oxygen Transport System

The adaptation to endurance exercises is connected with an increased capillarization of the lung alveolus, as well as changes in the respiratory muscles. In the diaphragm, activity of oxidation enzymes increases. Increased glycogen content was found in type I and type IIb fibers of the diaphragm but not in type IIa. No changes in the oxidation enzymes were found in the intercostal muscles.

Endurance training stimulates erythropoietic processes in the bone marrow, resulting in an increase in total hemoglobin content of blood. This effect may be measured by the sports anemia related to plasma expansion, intensified hemolysis, or iron deficiency.

Specificity of Training Effects on Neural Control

Neural adaptation takes place at the level of spinal motoneurons as well as at higher levels of the CNS. The existence of neural adaptation explains why (a) the changes in cross-sectional area of muscle fibers are much smaller than the changes in maximal force production; (b) training-induced increases in voluntary strength may occur without increases in twitch and tetanic tension evoked by electrical stimulation; (c) training of one limb causes increases in strength of both the ipsilateral and contralateral limbs; and (d) increases in voluntary strength are specific to the movement pattern, joint position, contraction type, and movement velocity used in training.

Neural adaptation is related to improved coordination or training, increased activation of prime mover muscles, and changes in the recruitment pattern of motor units. One of the expressions is a better synchronization of the activity of motor units. Correlations were found between the increases in voluntary strength and the increases in integrated electromyogram (Fig. 6–18), indicating that strength-trained subjects can more fully activate prime-mover muscles for maximal voluntary contractions (107).

As discussed above, in each sport event the muscular activity is based on specific motor programming that takes place in the premotor cortex, the supplementary motor areas, and other association areas of the brain cortex. Inputs from these areas, from the cerebellum, and, to some extent, from the basal ganglia converge

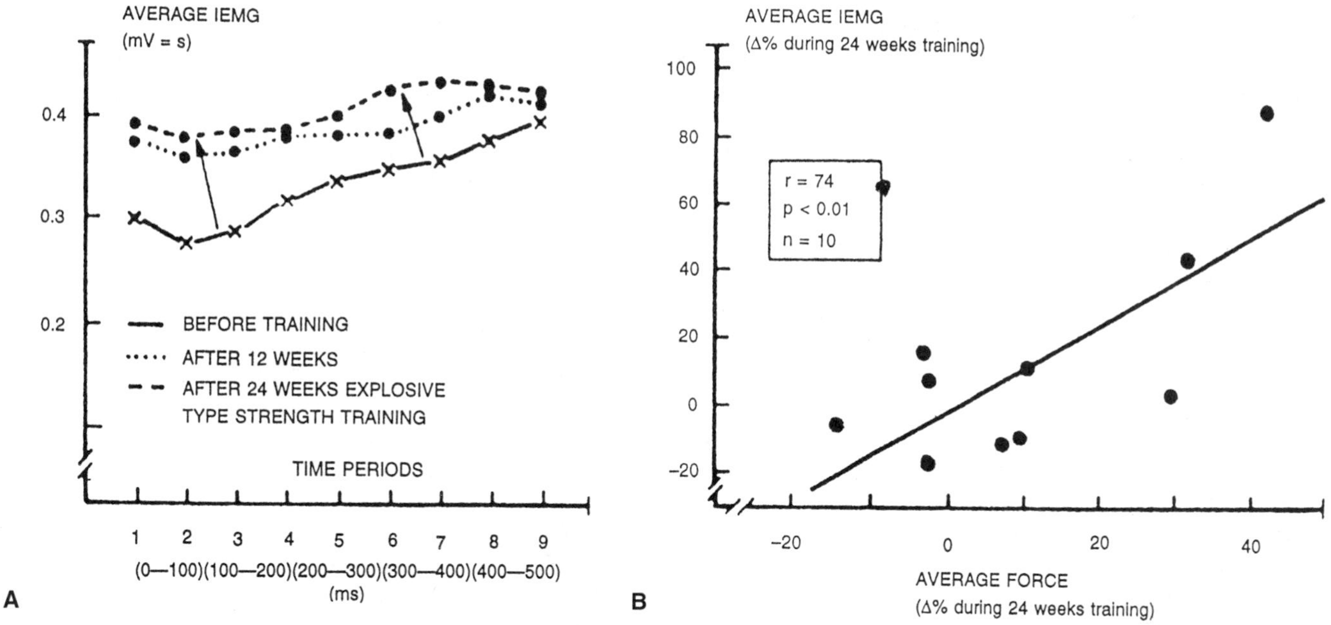

FIG. 6–18. Average integrated electromyogram (IEMG) time curves calculated from averaged IEMGs of the vastus lateralis, vastus medialis, and rectus femoris muscles produced during the early 500 ms in rapid maximal isometric bilateral leg extension in the subjects accustomed to strength training before and after the 12- and 24-week explosive-type strength training (**A**) and the relationship between the relative changes in average early IEMG and the relative changes in average early force (**B**) after the corresponding 24-week training. Adapted from Viru A. *Adaptation in sports training.* Boca Raton, FL: CRC Press, 1995, with permission.

on the primary motor cortex and finally excite or inhibit the corticobulbar and corticospinal neurons of the motor cortex. These output neurons of the motor cortex have a powerful influence on interneurons and motoneurons of the brainstem and of the spinal cord. Accordingly, the primary motor cortex can influence spinal motoneurons directly via the pyramidal tract and indirectly by modulating the activity of the descending brainstem system (the vestibulospinal and reticulospinal tracts). The final point is the spinal α-motoneuron. The net membrane current of the motoneuron determines the firing pattern of the motor unit and, thus, the muscular activity (108).

Possible mechanisms of neural adaptation in training are the following (27):

1. increased activation of agonists
2. selective recruitment of motor units within agonists
3. selective activation of agonists within a muscle group
4. co-contraction of antagonists.

In addition, the training effects on motoneuron excitability and lability have to be considered. Strength training with weightlifting or isometric exercises causes an increase in the reflex potentiation of electromyogram (EMG) response (28). Enhanced reflex potentiation has been found also in elite sprinters (109).

Isometric strength training resulted in an elevated ability of subjects to discharge motor units at regular firing intervals, whereas high-repetition dynamic training resulted in a trend toward reduced ability to maintain regular firing intervals (110). In a 60-day training period with the aid of maximal isokinetic knee extensions, hypertrophy accounted for 40% of the increase in force while the remaining 60% was attributable to an increased neural drive and possibly to changes in muscle architecture (111).

A training program that included various types of jumping exercises resulted in an earlier preactivation of leg extensor muscles before impact in the performance of test exercises. This was associated with a more powerful eccentric working phase. Higher preactivation of muscle, higher flexion of knee, and increased dorsiflection of ankle joints at the beginning of contact caused an increased tendomuscular stiffness, possibly through the more powerful reflex activation (112).

The main difference between exercise applied in heavy resistance and that applied in power training is time of development of peak force during movements. In heavy-resistance exercise the aim is to apply the highest possible force or one close to it. The time for force development is not the main condition of these exercises. In power exercises the aim is to achieve the highest possible power output by the movement. Therefore, the time of force development becomes a main determinant.

Correspondingly, there are substantial differences in the results of the systematic use of heavy-resistance or power exercises. These differences have to be related to adaptive changes on the muscular level (hypertrophy versus improvement of the excitation-coupling system, sarcoplasmic reticulum function, and cross-bridge formation rate) or on the level of CNS control. Usually, both groups of adaptive changes occur together. Only the ratio between them is different depending on the training exercises. There also seems to be a certain time sequence in the development of various adaptive changes in training for improved strength. Early changes in voluntary strength can usually be accounted for largely by neural factors, with a gradually increasing contribution of hypertrophy factors as the training proceeds (27). During prolonged heavy-resistance training the capacity of the neuromuscular system for fast force production may even decrease after the initial slight improvement.

The neural adaptation includes training effects on spinal motoneuron size (113) and their oxidative potential (114). These adaptations are specific to motor unit types and cannot be generalized beyond motor unit population. The neural adaptation is related also to training-induced changes in neuromuscular junctions, for example, increased presynaptic nerve terminal area (115) and density of both acetylcholine vesicles and receptors in the synapse (116). The noted changes in neuromuscular junctions are related to running intensity in training.

In conclusion, neural adaptations make possible an increased activation of prime movers in a specific movement and appropriate changes in the activation of synergists and antagonists. These manifestations are essential not only for improved muscular strength and power, but also for improved speed of movement and endurance.

Specifics of Training Effects on Endocrine Function

Capacities of Endocrine Systems

A great body of data has been published indicating that the activation of the adrenal cortex and medulla, of pancreatic α-cells, and of growth hormone production is reduced during moderate exercise due to training (mainly endurance training). The decrease in the blood insulin level becomes less pronounced. These alterations are related to changes in the individual threshold intensity for inducing endocrine responses to exercise. Therefore, exercise that before the training exceeded the threshold appeared to be under the threshold after training. A more intense exercise, exceeding the new threshold level, induced a pronounced hormonal response after training. Such responses to high-intensity exercises have usually been observed in highly fit athletes. Consequently, when a high output of endocrine systems is required, the hormonal responses of athletes are not reduced but magnified. Training increases the functional capacity of endocrine systems, which enables very pronounced changes in extreme exercises. In supramaximal exercises, blood levels of catecholamines, corticotropin, cortisol, β-endorphin, and growth hormone rise in trained athletes more (in some cases several times more) than in less-trained subjects. Increased functional capacity of endocrine systems may be related to maintaining high hormone levels in blood during prolonged exercise.

The hypertrophy of most active endocrine glands (in most cases of both adrenal medulla and cortex) and adaptive changes in cell structures offer a plausible explanation for the increased functional capacity of endocrine systems. Adrenal hypertrophy induced by endurance training is associated with increased numbers of mitochondria, their vesicular cristae, elements of endoplasmic reticulum and of polysomes in cells of zona fasciculata, as well as with an elevated content of cytochrome a to a_3 in the adrenal cortex (117). Mitochondria and endoplasmic reticulum are the main sites of biosynthesis of glucocorticoids. Consequently, the training-induced morphofunctional improvement has to be reflected in an augmented potential for hormone biosynthesis. The elevated capacity of the adrenal medulla for hormone secretion is reflected by augmented stores of epinephrine and norepinephrine as well as by enzymatic adaptations in medullar cells.

Three specific variants of training effects on endocrine functions may be discriminated. When training is directed to the improvement of sports performance in sprint or highly intensive anaerobic exercises, the development of an opportunity for rapid and intensive adrenaline output is expected. The potential for enhanced epinephrine secretion in training has been demonstrated (118). After a sprint training period, running at maximum speed for 30 seconds caused a higher rise in blood norepinephrine level than before the training (119).

The second variant is common for endurance training. In a number of studies, endurance-training effects on the functional stability of the sympathoadrenal and pituitary-adrenocortical systems have been shown, along with a corresponding relationship with endurance capacity. However, since these findings resulted from maintaining a stable high level of hormone excretion with urine, they have to be reexamined with more methodologic precision.

A morphometric analysis, together with the other data, showed four sets of alterations in the adrenal medulla and cortex of rats, depending on the training regime: (a) an adrenal hypertrophy, due to enlargement of the medulla and the glomerular zone, was characteristic of adaptation to short-term sprint exercises during the first week of training; (b) a pronounced adrenal hypertrophy due to enlargement of the fascicular and reticular zones and the medulla, without any pronounced changes in the adrenal corticosterone content, was characteristic of adaptation to prolonged continuous exercise; (c) a slight adrenal hypertrophy due to enlargement of the fascicular and reticular zones, accompanied by an augmented adrenal corticosterone content, was connected with adaptation to anaerobic exercises; (d) a slight adrenal hypertrophy accompanied by a decrease in the adrenal corticosterone content was specific for prolonged adaptation to short-term sprint exercises (117).

The third variant of the specificity of training effects on the endocrine function may be the strength-training influence on the potential to produce testosterone, stimulating muscular hypertrophy. Almost nothing is known about whether training alters the capacity for testosterone secretion and whether such an effect is specifically related to training for improved strength. However, data were obtained suggesting that resistance training stimulates testosterone production. A two-year study showed that even in elite athletes a prolonged intensive strength training leads to increased serum levels of testosterone. The correlation of change in maximal force with changes both in testosterone/cortisol ratio and in free testosterone level suggests that the increase in testosterone production creates optimal conditions for strength improvement (120).

Basal Level of Hormones in Blood

Several changes related to training have been found in basal hormone levels. Endurance training increases the level of epinephrine and reduces levels of insulin, testosterone, and cortisol in the blood. The reduction in blood testosterone has been particularly well demonstrated (121). A diminished blood cortisol level is in accordance with findings in endurance-trained males of higher levels of $\dot{V}O_2$max associated with lower levels of blood cortisol, compared with untrained subjects (122). However, cortisol level tends to increase during periods of high volume and/or intensity training in endurance athletes but not in strength athletes. Therefore, in endurance athletes the decline in blood cortisol level induced by endurance training may be counteracted by the opposite influence of hard training.

In sprinters the basal testosterone level was found to be higher than in cross-country skiers or soccer players (123).

Cellular Reception of Hormones

The effect of strength exercise on the density of the cellular receptor for testosterone in skeletal muscles was discussed above. However, endurance training did not increase the binding of androgens by cytoplasmic proteins of various muscles in rats (124). Variable results have been obtained on the influence of training on adrenoreceptors in various tissues. In brain tissue endurance training caused a preliminary downregulation of β-adrenoreceptor with normalization after 2 weeks of training. In liver cells β-receptor number did not change initially. After 2 weeks of training, a significantly increased density of β-receptor was found (125). The myocardium density of β-receptors decreases with endurance training (126). Studies on endurance athletes showed lower density of β-receptor in blood granulocytes and lymphocytes compared with untrained subjects, weightlifters, and wrestlers (127). In blood platelets the density of α-adrenoreceptors was decreased in endurance and increased in strength-trained athletes (128).

A common result is an increased lipolytic effect of epinephrine, but not of norepinephrine, in adipocytes isolated from subcutaneous fat of endurance-trained athletes. However, the total number of β-adrenoreceptors was unaffected by training in rats, although the increased lipolytic effect of adrenaline was found also in adipose cells of this species (129). Training increases the lipolytic capacity of adipocytes at a metabolic step distal to adrenoreceptors.

Endurance training also increases the sensitivity to insulin. In adipose cells the rates of glucose uptake and oxidation, as well as the lipogenetic effect of insulin, are increased in the trained organism. In comparison with active athletes, former endurance athletes (4 to 8 years after finishing their participation in high-level competitions) showed an increased basal rate of lipolysis and reduced sensitivity to lipogenic action of insulin (130). These changes may have significance for avoiding an augmentation of the adipose tissue after a drop in energy expenditure due to decreased physical activity.

Human experiments with insulin euglycemic clamp techniques demonstrated that insulin action on glucose metabolism is significantly higher in long-distance runners and weightlifters in comparison with control subjects. The results obtained by using various insulin doses suggested that the enhancement of insulin action by training is due to the increase in insulin sensitivity rather than insulin responsiveness. Endurance training appeared to be more effective than strength training for the improvement of insulin sensitivity (131).

Increased insulin sensitivity is associated with changes at the cellular receptors for insulin. Endurance training increases the specific binding of labeled insulin in the blood monocytes together with a gain in $\dot{V}O_2$max (132). Another result of endurance training is the elevated number of insulin receptors in skeletal muscles (133).

Intensive exercises for 10 days reduced the number of glucocorticoid receptors in myocardial cells (134). After a more prolonged training period, no changes in cardiac glucocorticoid or androgen receptors were observed. In contrast, when training caused a dramatic cardiac enlargement (30%), the specific binding of glucocorticoids increased without a change in the binding of androgens (124).

Training Effects on the Connective Tissue

Tendons and Ligaments

Animal studies demonstrate that endurance training increases the maximum strength of tendons and ligaments. Accordingly, the breaking load of ligaments and tendons increases. These changes were accompanied by an increased mass of tendons and ligaments. Listed changes were found in young but not in old animals. In male animals the changes were more pronounced than in female animals.

The main types of connective tissue (ligaments, tendons, collagenous structures within muscles, bone, and cartilage) contain collagen, which is extracellularly located and constitutes 25% to 30% of the total body protein. Collagens can be measured by determining the hydroxyproline content. A training-induced rise in breaking strength of tendons and ligaments parallels the increase of hydroxyproline concentration and accelerated rate of collagen turnover.

Sprint training enhances ligament weight and the weight/length ratio (135), as does high-resistance training. The maximum voluntary contraction represents approximately 30% of the maximum tensile strength of tendons. This leaves a great safety margin.

Exercise for improved flexibility involves stretching ligaments and tendons. Stretching of a tendon to 108% of its original length alters the tendon's qualities. The tendon remains at 104% of its original length when unloaded. In the second trial the tendon will be stretched more. Nevertheless, there are no changes observed in the maximal load at breaking.

Bone and Cartilage Tissue

Systematic physical activity also increases bone density and mass. The bone mass of the main active limbs increases. The major factors for changes in the bone tissue are training intensity and load bearing (136). However, there are differences in stimulation of bone density and bone length. Low-intensity training may stimulate bone growth (in length and girth) in growing animals. Relatively high-intensity training inhibits these processes, but results in increased bone density. Lower-intensity training does not change the density.

Increased bone density with high-intensity training or increased load bearing is based on increases in calcium and hydroxyproline concentration in bones. Bone enlargement together with increased bone density, collagen concentration, and mineral content increase the breaking strength (137).

The thickness of cartilage in all joints is greater in trained than in nontrained animals.

Endomyseal Connective Tissue

Compensatory hypertrophy of insulin after ablating the synergist group of muscles or severing their tendons is accompanied by increased collagen content. In young men, strength training stimulates endomyseal connective tissue growth. In bodybuilders the collagen amount was increased in the biceps muscle, but the proportion of collagen in the total amount of noncontractile proteins was similar in untrained persons and elite and novice bodybuilders (138).

Endurance exercises do not increase the collagen of the endomyseal connective tissue, but lifelong endurance training maintains a higher level of biosynthesis collagen in the soleus muscle (139). Endurance training increases myocardial collagen content depending on age: an increase was found in 4-month-old rats, but not in 8-month-old rats (140).

General Comments on the Training Responses

Training-induced changes in the body are founded on morphofunctional improvements at the level of cellular structures. On the one hand, there are enlargements of most active cellular structures. On the other hand, the increased number of enzyme molecules and more perfected regulation of enzyme activity raise the potential for the actualization of cellular activities, which is supported by augmented intracellular energy reserves. The morphofunctional changes at the cellular level are due to morphologic and functional perfection of organs and their systems, reflected in increased functional capacities of organ systems and of the whole body.

Changes from the level of cellular structures up to the level of organs and their systems take place in organs involved directly in the tasks of muscular activity (skeletal muscles), in organs attaining the function of muscles (cardiovascular and respiratory systems, liver), in tissues supporting muscle function (skeletal and other connective tissue elements), and in organs coordinating the functions of muscles and integrating the metabolic processes and functional manifestations (central and peripheral nervous structures, endocrine glands).

On the integrative level of the whole-body activities, the following general training responses may be distinguished:

1. Hypertrophy of organs: skeletal muscles (based on the myofibrillar hypertrophy), myocardium, adrenals, and bones (to which the muscles are attached, performing strong contractions).
2. Increased functional capacities of organ systems: Several approaches have been used to assess the functional capacities of organ systems:

   a. incremental exercise tests (stepwise increase in exercise intensity), to obtain the highest possible parameters of the function;
   b. assessment of the exercise intensity (mechanical power output, speed of movement) at a specific level of functional activity of an organ or organ system (e.g., the physical working capacity test called PWC_{170} test, estimating the exercise intensity at heart rate 170 beats per min);
   c. evaluation of the recovery time or summarized functional activity during a specific period of postexercise recovery, for example, total number of heart beats, excess oxygen consumption (oxygen dept), planimetry of the postexercise function (parameter) above the resting baseline after an exercise demanding utilization of close to the maximum capacity of a functional system (e.g., Harvard step test);
   d. assessment of a critical level of exercise intensity or duration above which functional disturbances appear (e.g., decrease of stroke volume or blood pressure, negative changes in electrocardiogram, chest pain in cardiac patients);
   e. comparison of the functional activity during maximal effort in performance of the competition exercise and in laboratory tests to assess the maximal functional parameters.
3. Functional stability: the capacity to maintain the necessary functional activity during prolonged exercise despite developing fatigue.
4. Functional reserve: the difference between resting basal level and the highest possible level of a function or functional parameter.
5. Energy reserves of the body: using needle biopsy, glycogen and phosphocreatine content of skeletal muscles can be determined. Evaluation of liver glycogen reserve is possible only indirectly.
6. Efficiency of functioning and energy processes: using the most effective pathway for increasing the function in a concrete exercise (e.g., relation between heart rate and stroke volume, breathing rate and tidal volume). An important parameter for energy metabolism is mechanical efficiency of muscle work. The efficiency of energy processes may be assessed by determining the oxygen uptake at a specific exercise level and expressing the result either in absolute units of oxygen uptake or in percent of $\dot{V}O_2max$. The functional and energy efficiencies together are expressed by changes of functions (e.g., heart rate during submaximal exercises). The training-induced bradycardia as well as several other similar parameters, estimated in the resting state, express the efficiency of basal activities of the body.
7. Perfected coordination, regulation, and control of body functions and metabolic processes: evaluation requires a specific approach depending on the aim of the investigation (the processes or functions and the exercises or conditions).
8. Motor abilities:
   a. maximal voluntary isometric, dynamic or functional strength;
   b. strength deficit (difference between maximal voluntary strength and strength of muscle contraction evoked by supramaximal electric stimulation);
   c. speed of reaction, speed or frequency of simple movements, velocity in performance of certain exercises or locomotor acts;
   d. power output for a single movement (e.g., jump or throw), also called explosive strength;
   e. power output in performance of a certain short-term exercise (e.g., 200- or 400-m runs, Wingate test, Bosco jumping test);
   f. speed endurance (possibility of maintaining the highest speed for a specific distance);
   g. strength or power endurance (possibility of maintaining a specific level of strength or power output during prolonged exercise; may be estimated by duration of exercise performed without change in application of muscle force or in power output, or by the assessment of muscle strength that can be maintained for a specific number of repeated contractions [e.g., 1 repetition maximum (RM), 3 RM, 8 RM, etc.];
   h. anaerobic endurance (performance of exercise demanding utilization of a great fraction of anaerobic working capacity);
   i. aerobic endurance (performance of prolonged exercises at an intensity that enables use solely of the aerobic energy metabolism);
   j. flexibility;
   k. general and specific skills.
9. Power, capacity, and efficiency of energy mechanisms. These criteria express the potential for ATP resynthesis on the account of energy released either in breakdown of phosphocreatine or glycogen (glucose), or in oxidative phosphorylation. The problem is that the corresponding parameters of related biochemical processes have to be evaluated based on data obtained in the whole organism; Table 6–1 lists various approaches.

Some of the listed training responses can be recorded in the resting state. Those are morphologic changes and parameters related to increased functional efficiency and reduced basal metabolic rate. An example is the training bradycardia, which is considered to express the increased parasympathetic tone. However, the bradycardia is impossible to use if the heart rate does not ensure the necessary rate of blood circulation (e.g., in cardiac patients). Most of the training responses need exercise tests for their evaluation. Most frequently, max-

TABLE 6–1. *Opportunities for assessment of power, capacity, and efficiency of three pathways of ATP resynthesis in skeletal muscles*

	Power	Capacity	Efficiency
Phosphocreatine mechanism (ATP resynthesis at the expense of phosphocreatine breakdown)	Maximal power output in exercises of the highest possible rate (duration 3 to 7 s); maximal rate of phosphocreatine breakdown in exercises of the highest possible rate (by results of analysis of muscle biopsy samples)	Time of all-out exercise at the highest possible level of power output; phosphocreatine content in skeletal muscles (by results of muscle biopsy)	Relationship between maximal rate of phosphocreatine breakdown and actual power output
Anaerobic glycolysis (ATP resynthesis at expense of glycogen or glucose breakdown up to formation of lactate)	Highest power output in "pure" anaerobic exercises (duration 30–60 s); maximal rate of lactate production (by analysis of blood or muscle biopsy samples)	Maximal O_2 dept; maximal amount of lactate accumulation and the highest pH shift in blood or muscles	Mechanical equivalent of lactate formation
Oxidative phosphorylation in "pure" aerobic exercises	The power output (velocity, work rate) at the anaerobic threshold	The highest amounts of exercise performed at the level of the anaerobic threshold	Mechanical efficiency; ratio between oxidation of carbohydrates and lipids; mechanical efficiency
In aerobic-anaerobic exercises	Maximal oxygen uptake	The highest amount of exercise performed at the level of $\dot{V}O_2max$	

ATP, adenosine triphosphate.

imal efforts are necessary. However, evaluation of functional and mechanical efficiencies requires results obtained mainly in submaximal exercise tests. In these cases the training response is expressed by reduced functional changes. In maximal exercise tests, however, the improved functional capacities are expressed by far more pronounced changes than in less-trained persons (Fig. 6–19).

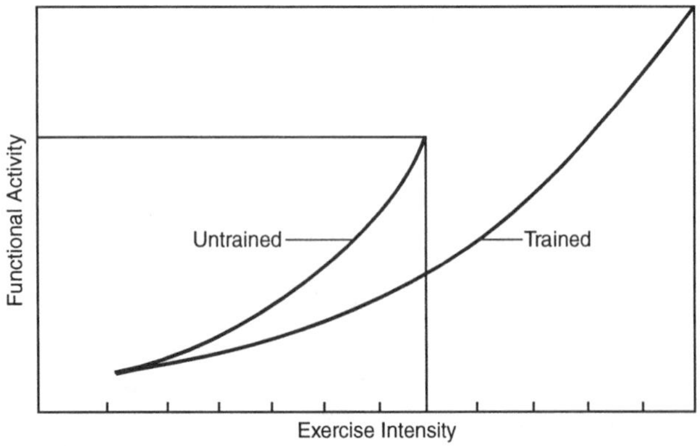

FIG. 6–19. Differences in changes of functional parameters between trained and untrained persons in dependence on exercise intensity.

REFERENCES

1. Bouchard C, Boulay MR, Simoneau JA, Lortie G, Pérusse L. Heredity and trainability of aerobic and anaerobic performance. An update. *Sports Med* 1988;5:69–73.
2. Booth FW, Thomason DB. Molecular and cellular adaptation of muscle in response to exercise: perspectives of various models. *Physiol Rev* 1991;71:541–585.
3. Marone JR, Falduto MT, Essig DA, Hickson RC. Effects of glucocorticoids and endurance training on cytochrome oxidase expression in skeletal muscle. *J Appl Physiol* 1994;77:1685–1690.
4. Inoue K, Yamasaki S, Fushiki T, Okada Y, Sugimoto E. Androgen receptor antagonist suppresses exercise-induced hypertrophy of skeletal muscle. *Eur J Appl Physiol* 1994;69:88–91.
5. Inoue K, Yamasaki S, Fushiki T, et al. Rapid increase in the number of androgen receptors following electrical stimulation of the rat muscle. *Eur J Appl Physiol* 1993;66:134–140.
6. Deschenes M, Kraemer WJ, Maresh CM, Crivello JF. Endurance and resistance exercise induce muscle fiber type specific responses in androgen binding capacity. *J Steroid Biochem Mol Biol* 1994;50:175–179.
7. Viru A, Kõrge P. Role of anabolic steroids in the hormonal regulation of skeletal muscle adaptation. *J Steroid Biochem* 1979;11:931–932.
8. Saborido A, Vila J, Molano F, Megios A. Effect of anabolic steroids on mitochondria and sarcotubular system of skeletal muscle. *J Appl Physiol* 1991;70:1038–1043.
9. Konovalova G, Masso R, Ööpik V, Viru A. Significance of thyroid hormones in post-exercise incorporation of amino acids into muscle fibers in rats: an autoradiographic study. *Endocrin Metab* 1997;4:25–31.
10. Kraus H, Kinne R. Regulation der bei longandauerdem körperlichen Adaptation und Leistungssteingerung durch Thyroid-hormone. *Pflugers Arch Ges Physiol* 1970;331:332–345.

11. Ianuzzo D, Patel P, Chen V, O'Brian P, Williams C. Thyroidal trophic influence on skeletal muscle myosin. *Nature* 1977;270:74–76.
12. Caiozzo VJ, Haddad F. Thyroid hormone modulation of muscle structure, function and adaptive responses to mechanical loading. *Exerc Sport Sci Rev* 1996;24:321–361.
13. Goldberg AK, Goodman HM. Relationship between growth hormone and muscular work in determining muscle size. *J Physiol* 1969;200:655–665.
14. Cuneo RC, Salomon F, Wills CM, Sönksen PH. Growth hormone treatment in growth hormone-deficient adults. I. Effects on muscle mass and strength. *J Appl Physiol* 1991;70:688–694.
15. Cuneo RC, Salomon F, Wills CM, Hesp R, Sönksen PH. Growth hormone treatment in growth hormone-deficient adults. II. Effects on exercise performance. *J Appl Physiol* 1991;70:695–700.
16. Fryburg DA, Gelfand RA, Barnett EJ. Growth hormone acutely stimulates forearm muscle protein synthesis in normal humans. *Am J Physiol* 1991;26:E499–E504.
17. Devol DL, Rotwein P, Sadow JL, Novanofski J, Bechtel PJ. Activation of insulin-like growth factor gene expression during work-induced skeletal muscle growth. *Am J Physiol* 1990;259: E89–E95.
18. Urban RJ, Bodenburg YH, Gilkison C, et al. Testosterone administration to elderly man increases skeletal muscle strength and protein synthesis. *Am J Physiol* 1995;269:E820–E826.
19. Kraemer WJ, Gordon SE, Fleck SJ, et al. Endogenous anabolic hormonal and growth factor responses to heavy resistance exercise in males and females. *Int J Sports Med* 1991;12:167–256.
20. Viru A. The role of adrenocortical response to exercise in the increase of body working capacity. *Byull Eksp Biol Med (Moscow)* 1976;82:774–776.
21. Viru A, Seene T. Peculiarities of adaptation to systematic muscular activity in adrenalectomized rats. *Endocrinologie* 1982;80: 235–237.
22. Jakowlew NN. *Sportbiochimie.* Leipzig: Borth, 1977.
23. Dunn AJ, Rees HD. Brain RNA and protein synthesis during training: the interpretation of changes of precursor incorporation. In: McGough JL, Drucker-Colin RK, eds. *Neurobiology of sleep and memory.* New York: 1977:33–54.
24. Altman J. Differences in the utilization of tritiated leucine by single neurones in normal and exercised rats: an autoradiographic investigation with microdensitometry. *Nature* 1963;199: 777–780.
25. Hamberger A, Gregson N, Lehninger AL. The effect of acute exercise on amino acid incorporation in to mitochondria of rabbit tissue. *Biochim Biophys Acta* 1969;186:373–383.
26. Enoka R. Muscle strength and its development: new perspectives. *Sports Med* 1988;6:146–168.
27. Sale DG. Neural adaptation to strength training. In: Komi P, ed. *Strength and power in sports.* Oxford: Blackwell, 1992:249–265.
28. Sale DG, MacDougall JD, Upton ARM, McComas AJ. Effect of strength training upon motoneuron excitability in man. *Med Sci Sports Exerc* 1983;15:57–68.
29. Jakovlev NN. Biochemical foundations of muscle training (in Russian). *Usp Sovrem Biol (Moscow)* 1949;27:257–271.
30. Thorstenson A, Hultrén B, von Döbeln W, Karlsson J. Effect of strength training on enzyme activities and fibre characteristics in human skeletal muscle. *Acta Physiol Scand* 1976;96:392–398.
31. MacDougall JD, Elder GCB, Sale DG, Moroz JR, Sutton JR. Effects of strength training and immobilization on human muscle fibers. *Eur J Appl Physiol* 1980;43:25–34.
32. Lüthi JM, Howald H, Claasen H, Rösler K, Vock P, Hoppler H. Structural changes in skeletal muscle tissue with heavy-resistance exercise. *Int J Sports Med* 1986;7:123–127.
33. McDonagh MJM, Davies CTM. Adaptive response of mammalian muscle to exercise with high loads. *Eur J Appl Physiol* 1984;52:139–159.
34. Howald H, Hoppeler H, Claassen H, Mathieu O, Straub R. Influence of endurance training on the ultrastructural composition of the different muscle fiber types in humans. *Pflugers Arch Ges Physiol* 1985;403:369–376.
35. Seene T, Alev K. Effect of muscular activity on the turnover rate of action and myosin heavy and light chains in different types of skeletal muscle. *Int J Sports Med* 1991;12:204–207.
36. Saltin B, Nazar K, Costill DL, et al. The nature of the training response, peripheral and central adaptations to one-legged exercise. *Acta Physiol Scand* 1976;96:289–305.
37. Nygaard E. Number of fibers in skeletal muscle of man. *Muscle Nerve* 1980;3:268–276.
38. Tibbits GF. Role of the sarcolemma in muscle fatigue. In: Taylor AW, et al., eds. *Biochemistry of exercises,* vol 7. Champaign, IL: Human Kinetics, 1990:37–47.
39. Alession HM, Goldfarb AH. Lipid peroxidation and scavenger enzymes during exercise: adaptive response to training. *J Appl Physiol* 1988;64:1333–1336.
40. Klitgaard H, Clausen T. Increased total concentration of Na,K-pump in vastus lateralis muscle of old trained human subjects. *J Appl Physiol* 1989;67:2491–2494.
41. McKenna MJ, Schmidt TA, Hargreaves H, Cameron L, Skinner SL, Kjeldsen K. Sprint training increases human skeletal muscle Na^+-K^+-ATPase concentration and improves K^+ regulation. *J Appl Physiol* 1993;75:173–180.
42. Jakovlev NN. Biochemische and morphologische veränderungen der muskelfasern in abhängigkeit von der art des training. *Med Sport (Berlin)* 1978;18:161–164.
43. Viru M. Differences in effects of various training regimes on metabolism of skeletal muscles. *J Sports Med Phys Fitness* 1994;34:217–227.
44. Tesch PA, Thorsson A, Colleander EB. Effects of eccentric and concentric resistance training on skeletal muscle substrates, enzyme activities and capillary supply. *Acta Physiol Scand* 1990;140:575–580.
45. Häkkinen K. Neuromuscular and hormonal adaptations during strength and power training. *J Sports Med Phys Fitness* 1989;29:9–26.
46. MacDougall JD, Ward D, Sale G, Sutton JR. Biochemical adaptation of human skeletal muscle to heavy resistance training and immobilization. *J Appl Physiol* 1977;43:700–703.
47. Staude HW, Exner GU, Pette D. Effects of short-term, high intensity (sprint) training on some contractile and metabolic characteristics of fast and slow muscle of the rat. *Pflugers Arch Ges Physiol* 1973;344:159–168.
48. Fitts RH, Holloszy JO. Contractile properties of rat soleus muscle effects of training and fatigue. *Am J Physiol* 1977;233:86–91.
49. Holloszy JO. Biochemical adaptations to exercise: aerobic metabolism. *Exerc Sport Sci Rev* 1973;1:45–71.
50. Gollnick PD, Riedy M, Quintiskie JJ, Bertocci LA. Differences in metabolic potential of skeletal muscle fibers and their significance for metabolic control. *J Exp Biol* 1985;115:191–199.
51. Terjung RL. Muscle fiber involvement during training of different intensities and durations. *Am J Physiol* 1976;230:946–950.
52. Winder WW, Baldwin KM, Holloszy JO. Enzymes involved in ketone utilization in different types of muscles: adaptation to exercise. *Eur J Biochem* 1974;47:461.
53. Fitts RH, Booth FW, Winder WW, Holloszy JO. Skeletal muscle respiratory capacity, endurance and glycogen utilization. *Am J Physiol* 1975;228:1029.
54. Dudley GA, Abraham WM, Terjung RL. Influence of exercise intensity and duration on biochemical adaptations in skeletal muscle. *J Appl Physiol* 1982;53:844–850.
55. Hickson RC, Heusner WW, VanHuss WD. Skeletal muscle enzyme alteration after sprint and endurance training. *J Appl Physiol* 1975;40:868–872.
56. Thorstensson A, Sjödin B, Karlsson J. Enzyme activities and muscle strength after sprint training in man. *Acta Physiol Scand* 1975;94:313–318.
57. Costill DL, Daniels J, Evans W, Fink W, Krahusbuhl G, Saltin B. Skeletal muscle enzymes and fiber composition in male and female track athletes. *J Appl Physiol* 1976;40:149–154.
58. Gillespie AC, Fox LE, Merola AJ. Enzyme adaptations in rat skeletal muscle after two intensities of treadmill training. *Med Sci Sports Exerc* 1982;14:461–466.
59. Green HJ, Thomson JA, Daub WD, Houston ME, Ranney DA. Fiber composition, fiber size and enzyme activities in vastus lateralis of elite athletes involved in high intensity exercise. *Eur J Appl Physiol* 1979;41:109–117.
60. Pfister M, Moesch H, Howald H. Beeinflussung glykolytischer and oxidativer skelettmuskelenenzyme des mensschen durch an-

aerobes training oder anabols steroide. *Schweiz Zeitsch Sportmed* 1981;29:45–52.
61. Donovan CM, Brooks GA. Endurance training affects lactate clearance, not lactate production. *Am J Physiol* 1983;244:E83–E92.
62. Hochacka PW, Somero GN. *Biochemical adaptation.* Princeton, NJ: Princeton University Press, 1984.
63. Jacobs I, Esbjörsson M, Sylven C, Holm I, Jansson E. Sprint training effects on muscle myoglobin, enzymes, fiber types and blood lactate. *Med Sci Sports Exerc* 1987;19:368–374.
64. Jansson E, Sylvén C. Creatine kinase MB and citrate synthetase in type I and type II muscle fibers in trained and untrained men. *Eur J Appl Physiol* 1985;54:207–209.
65. Roberts AD, Balleter R, Howald H. Anaerobic muscle enzyme changes after interval training. *Int J Sports Med* 1982;3:18–21.
66. Goldberg ND. Changes of activity and isozyme spectra of hexokinase of skeletal muscles and brain in adaptation to intensive physical exercise (in Russian). *Ukr Biokhim Zh* 1985;52(2):46–51.
67. Parkhause WS, McKenzie DC. Possible contributions of skeletal muscle buffers to enhanced anaerobic performance: a brief review. *Med Sci Sports Exerc* 1983;16:328–338.
68. Hultman E. Studies on muscle metabolism of glycogen and active phosphate in man with special references to exercise and diet. *Scand J Clin Lab Invest* 1967;19(suppl 94):1–63.
69. Taylor AW, Thayer R, Rao S. Human skeletal muscle glycogen synthetase activities with exercise and training. *Can J Physiol Pharmacol* 1972;50:411–415.
70. Lowrie RA. Effect of enforced exercise on myoglobin concentration in muscle. *Nature* 1983;171:1069–1070.
71. Andersen P, Henriksson J. Capillary supply of the quadriceps femoris muscle of man: adaptive response to exercise. *J Physiol* 1977;270:677–690.
72. Pette D, Remirez BA, Müller W, Simon R, Exner GU, Hildebrand R. Influence of intermittent long-term stimulation of contractile, histochemical and metabolic properties of fiber population in fast and slow rabbit muscles. *Pflugers Arch Ges Physiol* 1975;361:1–7.
73. Fitsimons DP, Diffee GM, Herrick RE, Baldwin KM. Effect of endurance exercise on isomyosin pattern in fast- and slow-twitch skeletal muscles. *J Appl Physiol* 1990;68:1950–1955.
74. Jansson E, Sjödin B, Thorntensson A, Hultèn B, Frith K. Changes in muscle fibre type distribution in man after physical exercise. A sign of fibre type transformation? *Acta Physiol Scand* 1978;104:235–237.
75. Andersen P, Hendriksson J. Training induced changes in subgroups of human type II skeletal muscle fibers. *Acta Physiol Scand* 1977;123–125.
76. Jansson E, Esbjörnsson M, Holm I, Jacobs I. Increase in the proportion of fast-twitch muscle fibers by sprint in males. *Acta Physiol Scand* 1990;140:359–363.
77. Simoneau J-A, Lortie G, Boulay MR, Marcotte M, Thibault M-C, Bouchard C. Human skeletal muscle fiber alteration with high-intensity intermittent training. *Eur J Appl Physiol* 1985;54:250–253.
78. Brooks GA. Anaerobic threshold: review of the concept and direction for further research. *Med Sci Sports Exerc* 1985;17:22–31.
79. Sjogaard G. Muscle morphology and metabolic potential in elite road cyclists during a season. *Int J Sports Med* 1984;5:250–254.
80. Hendriksson J, Reitman JS. Time course of changes in human skeletal muscle succinate dehydrogenase and cytochrome oxidase and maximal oxygen uptake with physical activity and inactivity. *Acta Physiol Scand* 1977;99:91–97.
81. Farrell PA, Wilmore JH, Coyle EF, Billing JE, Costill DL. Plasma lactate accumulation and distance running performance. *Med Sci Sports Exerc* 1979;11:338–344.
82. Svedenhag J, Sjödin B. Maximal and submaximal oxygen uptakes and blood lactate levels in elite male middle and long-distance runners. *Int J Sports Med* 1984;5:255–261.
83. Komi PA, Ito A, Sjödin B, Wallensstein R, Karlsson J. Muscle metabolism, lactate breaking point, and biomechanical features of endurance running. *Int J Sports Med* 1981;2:148–153.
84. Denis C, Fouquet R, Poty P, Geyssant A, Lacour JR. Effect of 40 weeks of endurance training on the anaerobic threshold. *Int J Sports Med* 1982;3:208–214.
85. Smith BW, McMurray RG, Symanski JD. A comparison of the anaerobic threshold of sprint and endurance trained swimmers. *J Sports Med Phys Fitness* 1984;24:94–99.
86. Pierce EF, Weltman A, Seip RL, Snead D. Effects of training specificity on the lactate threshold and $\dot{V}O_2$max. *Int J Sports Med* 1990;11:267–272.
87. Conley DL, Kranhenbuhl GS. Running economy and distance running performance. *Med Sci Sports Exerc* 1980;12:357–360.
88. Saltin B, Strange S. Maximal oxygen uptake: old and new arguments for a cardiovascular limitation. *Med Sci Sports Exerc* 1992;24:30–37.
89. Daniels JT, Yarbrough RA, Foster C. Changes in $\dot{V}O_2$max and running performance with training. *Eur J Appl Physiol* 1978;39:249–254.
90. Lortie G, Simoneau JA, Hamal P, Borday MR, Landry F, Bouchard C. Responses of maximal aerobic power and capacity to aerobic training. *Int J Sports Med* 1984;5:232–236.
91. Volkov NI. *Human bioenergetics in strenuous muscular activity and pathways for improved performance in sportsmen.* Moscow: Anokhin Research Institute of Normal Physiology, 1990.
92. Reindell H, Klepzig H, Steim H, Musshoff K, Rosskamm H, Schildge F. *Herz- und Kreislaufkrankheiten und Sport.* München: J.A. Barth, 1960.
93. Koerner JE, Terjung RL. Effect of physical training on coronary collateral circulation of the rat. *J Appl Physiol* 1982;52:376–387.
94. Laughlin MH, Tomanek RJ. Myocardial capillarity and maximal capillary diffusion in exercise-trained dogs. *J Appl Physiol* 1987;63:1481–1486.
95. Gilbert CA, Nutter DO, Felner JM, Perkins JV, Heysfield SB, Schlant RC. Echocardiographic study of cardiac, dimensions and functions in the endurance-trained athletes. *Am J Cardiol* 1977;40:528–533.
96. Cohen JL, Segal KR. Left ventricular hypertrophy in athletes: an exercise-echocardiographic study. *Med Sci Sports Exerc* 1985;17:695–700.
97. Dickhuth HH, Simon G, Kindermann W, Wildberg A, Keed J. Echocardiographic studies on athletes of various sport-type and non-athletic persons. *Zeitsch Kardiol* 1979;68:449–453.
98. Ricci G, Lajoie D, Petitclerc R, et al. Left ventricular size following endurance, sprint, and strength training. *Med Sci Sports Exerc* 1982;14:344–347.
99. Rubal BJ, Al-Muhailani A-R, Rosentswieg J. Effects of physical conditioning on the heart size and wall thickness of college women. *Med Sci Sports Exerc* 1987;19:423–429.
100. Morganroth J, Maron BJ, Henry WL, Epstein SE. Comparative left ventricular dimensions in trained athletes. *Ann Intern Med* 1975;82:521–524.
101. Rost R. The frontiers between physiology and pathology in the athlete's heart: to what limits can it be enlarged and beat slowly? In: Lubich T, Venerando A, Zeppelini P, eds. Bologna: Aulo Gaggi, 1989:187–198.
102. Tibbits G, Koziol BJ, Roberts NK, Baldwin KM, Barnard RJ. Adaptation of the rat myocardium to endurance training. *J Appl Physiol* 1978;44:85–89.
103. Oscai LB, Molé PA, Holloszy JO. Effects of exercise on cardiac weights and mitochondria in male and female rats. *Am J Physiol* 1971;220:1944–1948.
104. Bove AA. Effects of strenuous exercise on myocardial blood flow. *Med Sci Sports Exerc* 1985;17:517–521.
105. Scheuer J. Effect of physical training on myocardial vascularity and perfusion. *Circulation* 1982;66:491–495.
106. Musshoff K, Reindell H, Klepzig H. Stroke volume, arteriovenous difference, cardiac output and physical working capacity and their relationship to heart volume. *Acta Cardiol* 1959;14:427–452.
107. Häkkinen K, Komi PV. Electromyographic changes during strength training and detraining. *Med Sci Sports Exerc* 1983;15:455–460.
108. Noth J. Cortical and peripheral control. In: Komi PV, ed. *Strength and power in sport.* Oxford: Blackwell Scientific, 1992:9–20.
109. Upton ARM, Radford PF. Motoneuron excitability in elite

sprinters. In: Komi PV, ed. *Biomechanics Va.* Baltimore: University Park Press, 1975:82–87.

110. Cracraft JD, Petajan JH. Effect of muscle training on the pattern of firing of single motor units. *Am J Phys Med* 1977;56:183–194.
111. Narici MV, Roi GS, Landoni L, Minetti AE, Ceretelli P. Changes in force, cross-sectional area and neural activation during strength training and detraining of the human quadriceps. *Eur J Appl Physiol* 1989;59:310–319.
112. Kyröläinen H, Komi PV, Kim DH. Effect of power training on neuromuscular performance and mechanical efficiency. *Scand J Med Sci Sports* 1991;1:78–87.
113. Gilliam TB, Roy RR, Taylor JF, Heusner WW, VanHuss WD. Ventral motor neuron alteration in rat spinal cord after chronic exercise. *Experientia* 1977;15:665.
114. Gerchman LB, Edgerton VR, Carrow RE. Effect of physical training on the histochemistry and morphology of central motor neurons. *Exp Neurol* 1975;49:790.
115. Andonian MJ, Fahins MA. Effects of endurance exercise on the morphology of mouse neuromuscular junctions during aging. *J Neurocytol* 1987;16:589–599.
116. Deschenes MR, Maresh CM, Crivello JF, Armstrong LE, Kraemer WJ, Covault J. The effects of exercise training of different intensities on neuromuscular morphology. *J Neurocytol* 1993;22:603–615.
117. Viru A, Seene T. Peculiarities of adjustments in the adrenal cortex to various training regimes. *Biol Sports* 1985;2:91–99.
118. Kjaer M. Epinephrine and some other hormonal responses to exercise in man. With special reference to physical training. *Int J Sports Med* 1989;10:1–15.
119. Nevill ME, Boabis LH, Brooks S, William C. Effect of training on muscle metabolism during treadmill sprinting. *J Appl Physiol* 1989;67:2376–2382.
120. Häkkinen K, Pakarinen A, Alén M, Kauhanen H, Komi PV. Neuromuscular and hormonal adaptations in athletes to strength training in two years. *J Appl Physiol* 1988;65:2406–2412.
121. Hackney AC. The male reproductive system and endurance exercise. *Med Sci Sports Exerc* 1996;28:180–189.
122. Viru A, Smirnova T. Independence of physical working capacity from increased glucocorticoid level during short-term exercise. *Int J Sports Med* 1982;3:80–83.
123. Bosco C, Viru A. Testosterone and cortisol levels in blood of male sprinters, soccer players and cross-country skiers. *Biol Sport* 1998;15:3–8.
124. Hickson RC, Kurowski TT, Capaccio JA, Chatterton RT. Androgen cytosol binding in exercise-induced sparing of muscle atrophy. *Am J Physiol* 1984;247:E597–E603.
125. Nakamura T, Kitayama I, Nomura J. Effect of force-running stress on β-adrenergic receptors in rat brain and liver. *Neurosci Res* 1989;(suppl 9):151.
126. Werle EO, Strobel G, Weicker H. Decrease in rat cardiac beta$_1$ and beta$_2$-adrenoceptors by training and endurance exercise. *Life Sci* 1990;46:9–17.
127. Jost J, Weiß M, Weicker H. Comparison of sympatho-adrenergic regulation at rest and of the adrenoceptors system in swimmers, long-distance runners, weight-lifters, wrestlers and untrained men. *Eur J Appl Physiol* 1989;58:596–604.
128. Lehmann M, Hasler K, Bergdolt E, Keul J. Alpha 2-adrenoreceptor density on intact platelets and adrenaline-induced platelet aggregation in endurance and nonendurance trained subjects. *Int J Sports Med* 1986;7:172–176.
129. Bukowiecki L, Lupien J, Follea N, Paradis A, Richard D, LeBlanc J. Mechanism of enhanced lipolysis in adipose tissue of exercise-trained rats. *Am J Physiol* 1980;239:E422–E429.
130. Viru A, Toode K, Eller A. Adipocyte responses to adrenaline and insulin in active and former sportmen. *Eur J Appl Physiol* 1992;64:345–349.
131. Sato J, Osawa I, Oshida Y, et al. Effects of different types of physical training on insulin action in human peripheral tissues-use of the euglycemic clamp technique. 8th International Biochemistry of Exercise Conference, Nagoya,1991:133.
132. Soman VR, Koivisto VA, Deibert D, Felig P, DeFronzo RA. Increased insulin sensitivity and insulin binding to monocytes after physical training. *N Engl J Med* 1979;301:1200–1204.
133. Dohm GL, Sinha MK, Caro JF. Insulin receptor binding and protein kinase activity in muscles of trained rats. *Am J Physiol* 1987;252:E170–E175.
134. Eller A, Nyskas C, Szabo G, Endröczi B. Corticosterone binding in myocardial tissue of rats after chronic stress and adrenalectomy. *Acta Physiol Acad Sci Hung* 1981;53:205–211.
135. Tipton CM, Matthes RD, Maynard JA, Carey RA. The influence of physical activity on ligaments and tendons. *Med Sci Sports Exerc* 1975;7:165–175.
136. Stone MH. Implications for connective tissue and bone alterations resulting from resistance exercise training. *Med Sci Sports Exerc* 1988;20(suppl):S162–S168.
137. Kiiskinen A, Heikkinen E. Effect of prolonged physical training on the development of connective tissues in growing mice. In: Howald H, Poortmans JR, eds. *Metabolic adaptation to prolonged physical exercise.* Basel: Birkhäuser Verlag, 1975:253–261.
138. MacDougall JD, Sale DG, Alway SE, Sutton JR. Muscle fiber number in biceps brachii in body builders and control subjects. *J Appl Physiol* 1984;57:1399–1403.
139. Kovanen V, Suominen H. Age- and training-related changes in collagen metabolism of rat skeletal muscle. *Eur J Appl Physiol* 1989;58:765–771.
140. Bartosová D, Chavapil M, Karecky B, et al. The growth of the muscular and collagenous parts of the rat heart in various forms of cardiomegaly. *J Physiol* 1969;200:285–295.

SELECTED READINGS

Åstrand P-O, Rodahl K. *Textbook of work physiology,* 2nd ed. New York: McGraw-Hill, 1986.

Booth FW, Gould EW. Effects of training and disuse on connective tissue. *Exerc Sport Sci Rev* 1975;3:83–112.

Brooks GA, Fahey TD, White TP. *Exercise physiology. Human bioenergetics and its application,* 2nd ed. Mountain View, CA: Mayfield, 1996.

Carson JA. The regulation of gene expression in hypertrophying skeletal muscle. *Exerc Sport Sci Rev* 1997;25:301–320.

Essig DA. Contractile activity-induced mitochondrial biogenesis in skeletal muscle. *Exerc Sport Sci Rev* 1996;24:289–319.

Kraemer WJ, Fleck SJ, Evans WJ. Strength and power training: physiological mechanisms of adaptation. *Exerc Sport Sci Rev* 1996; 24:363–397.

Mader A. Evaluation of the endurance performance of marathon runners and theoretical analysis of test results. *J Sports Med Phys Fitness* 1991;31:1–19.

Saltin B, Gollnick PD. Skeletal muscle adaptability: significance for metabolism and performance. In: Peachy LD, Adrian RH, Geiger SR, eds. *Handbook of physiology. Section 10: skeletal muscle.* Baltimore: Williams & Wilkins, 1983;555–631.

Viru A. *Adaptation in sports training.* Boca Raton, FL: CRC Press, 1995.

Wilmore JH, Costill DL. *Physiology of sport and exercise.* Champaign, IL: Human Kinetics, 1994.

Exercise and Sport Science,
edited by William E. Garrett, Jr., and Donald T. Kirkendall.
Lippincott Williams & Wilkins, Philadelphia © 2000.

CHAPTER 7

Fatigue from Voluntary Motor Activity

Donald T. Kirkendall

The factors that contribute to fatigue from voluntary activity are numerous and interact in a complex multifactorial phenomenon. Virtually every step in the chain of events that leads to muscular contraction has been studied under a variety of circumstances. As a result, many theories of fatigue have been discussed. The lack of a singular factor inducing fatigue across the gamut of sporting activities points to the multitude of mechanisms that protect muscle from a relentless progression toward irreversible rigor. Because there are so many different factors that contribute to fatigue, physical training designed to delay fatigue is a complex matter.

An underlying tenet in the exercise sciences is the concept of *specificity.* A specific type of exercise results in a specific type of physiologic response that, if performed repeatedly, will lead to a specific adaptation. The concept of specificity must also be extended to include fatigue; specific exercise also leads to a specific mechanism of fatigue. And while the intensity-duration relationship forms a foundation for nearly every discussion in exercise science, fatigue is often omitted when it rightly should be in the forefront, as all training is designed to delay the onset of fatigue.

Historically, investigators have focused on two basic conceptual locations for fatigue. Central fatigue involves mechanisms within the brain and spinal cord, whereas peripheral fatigue includes the motor neuron and the muscle fiber. The bulk of studies have addressed peripheral fatigue, including neuromuscular junction transmission, impulse propagation, excitation-contraction coupling, calcium regulation by the sarcoplasmic reticulum, metabolites, and cross-bridge interaction. Central mechanisms have been implied when there was a decline in performance in the absence of peripheral changes, and they were often attributed to psychologic factors because of the lack of objective measures to study. These psychologic factors were frequently thought to be due to lack of motivation or lack of familiarity with the experimental procedure.

This chapter discusses the evidence for both central and peripheral fatigue. The operational definition of fatigue is the failure to maintain an expected power output. The various mechanisms of fatigue that have been discussed in relation to voluntary activity are summarized in Fig. 7–1.

CENTRAL FATIGUE

Evidence of Central Nervous System Involvement in Fatigue

Determining the presence of a central nervous system (CNS) component in a voluntary motor activity can be problematic. One of the first methods used was the twitch interpolation technique. Investigators would look at the force during a maximal voluntary contraction (MVC), then see if the force would increase in response to controlled electrical stimulation (1). Usually, force during MVC or enhanced by twitch interpolation would decline in parallel during fatiguing contractions (2–4), leading one to conclude that CNS drive was not a factor in fatigue. However, it is quite difficult to hold an MVC under these circumstances if the subject is not well practiced and highly motivated to activate all available motor units, which is difficult in concentric contractions (5,6) or at a high altitude (7).

Frequently, evidence of a CNS role in fatigue is set aside as psychologic factors, such as inadequate motivation, lack of attention, effort perception, and pain. Indeed, force generation and the electromyogram (EMG) are enhanced with verbal encouragement (8,9). Furthermore, force output is enhanced in subjects who concentrate on the task, in contrast with subjects who are dis-

D. T. Kirkendall: Department of Orthopaedics, University of North Carolina, Chapel Hill, North Carolina 27549-7055.

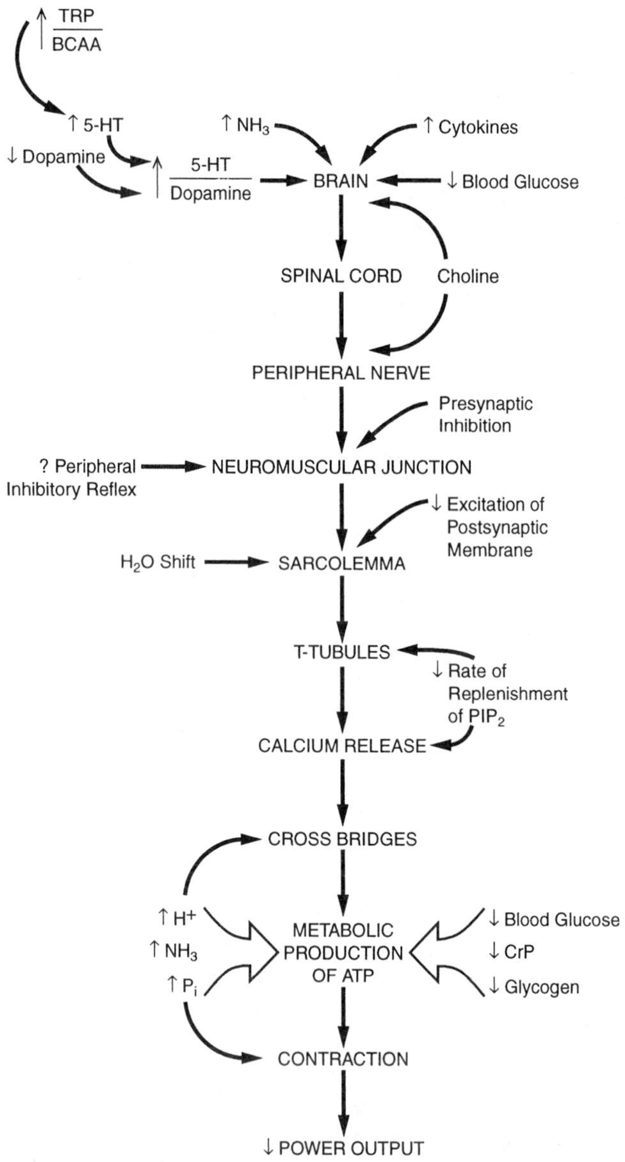

FIG. 7–1. Summary of neuromuscular pathway leading to contraction and probable mechanisms of fatigue.

tracted (9,10). It has long been known that the sum of the force output of each leg exceeds the force output of both legs (8). Specificity of training comes into play when subjects trained either one leg or both legs. Subjects fatigued more rapidly during the task for which they did not train (8), further indicating that CNS drive differed in one-legged versus two-legged training and that part of the training adaptation involved the CNS.

The first clue that muscle will fail to maintain the desired power output is the increased perception of effort, not the reduction in force output. Therefore, neuropsychologic mechanisms must be considered. Reduction in the activation of the motoneuron can be due to either fewer descending impulses arriving at the motoneuron or some inhibition of the motoneuron. Evidence for the latter hypothesis comes from Bigland-Ritchie and colleagues (3), who suggested that the motoneuron could be inhibited by feedback from local mechanoreceptors or free nerve endings that are sensitive to metabolic by-products building up during fatigue. The CNS would then alter its activation pattern based on this feedback to maintain overall force output.

Were this to be true, then in fatiguing contractions there should be a change in the overall pattern of activation all the way back to the motor cortex. Evidence for this sensory feedback hypothesis (4) can be seen in monkeys performing isometric elbow flexion where neuron discharge rates from the motor cortex decline during repetitive fatiguing contractions (11). CNS activation of the motoneuron in humans can be studied using transcranial magnetic stimulation (12), in which motor responses were briefly decreased in response to fatiguing exercise, leading to the conclusion of an alteration of neurotransmitters in the CNS prior to the level of the corticospinal neurons.

A central role in fatigue can be examined by studying patients with chronic fatigue syndrome (CFS). The CFS patient has a normal cardiovascular response to graded exercise but higher perceptions of effort, and they cease voluntary exercise prior to reaching their physiologic limit (13–15). When appropriately motivated, most CFS patients do not have problems generating force, and the mechanisms generally associated with peripheral fatigue (16) are similar to those of normal subjects, but the patients routinely rate the perception of effort higher (17). While it is premature to assign a central site for the fatigue, it appears that CFS patients have the necessary ability to perform work but are unable or unwilling to work to their maximum.

The Role of Neurotransmitters in Central Fatigue

Until the late 1980s, there was little proposed as an objective, verifiable hypothesis on central fatigue. In 1987, Newsholme and colleagues (18) proposed a role for serotonin (5-hydroxytryptamine, 5-HT) because of its established links to arousal, mood, sleepiness, and lethargy, which could modify the perception of muscular effort.

5-HT in the brain increases in response to an added delivery of its precursor, tryptophan (TRP). While most TRP circulates loosely bound to albumin, the free tryptophan (fTRP) can cross the blood–brain barrier through a mechanism of transport that is shared with other amino acids (19), especially the branched-chain amino acids (BCAAs) of leucine, isoleucine, and valine. An increase in 5-HT in the brain occurs when the ratio of fTRP to the plasma concentration of BCAAs increases. During sustained exercise, this increase could occur because BCAAs can be taken up by skeletal muscle and oxidized as fuel. This ratio could also be increased when there is an increase in circulating free fatty acids because free fatty acids can displace TRP from its binding sites on albumin, leading to an increase in fTRP.

Chaouloff and colleagues (20–23) and Blomstrand and colleagues (24) ran rats for 1 to 2 hours on a treadmill and showed increases in fTRP and brain concentrations of TRP, 5-HT, and the primary metabolite of 5-HT, 5-hydroxyindoleacetic acid (5-HIAA). Similar increases in TRP and 5-HIAA were found in the cerebrospinal fluid before returning to normal 1 hour after exercise. While these studies did not address fatigue directly, they did provide evidence that increasing fTRP and an increase in the fTRP/BCAA ratio lead to an increase in brain 5-HT from sustained exercise.

Bailey and colleagues (25) extended the study of regional brain amino acids and their metabolites to fatigue in the rat. They focused on 5-HT and dopamine (DA, a neurotransmitter for arousal, motivation, and motor control). Rats ran on a treadmill at approximately 60% to 65% of $\dot{V}O_2$max and were sacrificed at 1 hour or at fatigue (about 3 hours). Sections of the brain (midbrain, striatum, hippocampus, and hypothalamus) were analyzed for 5-HT and DA as well as the primary metabolite of each, 5-HIAA and dihydrophenylacetic acid, respectively. In most regions, 5-HT was increased after 1 hour of exercise and at fatigue, whereas DA was increased after 1 hour of exercise but decreased at fatigue. In addition to the continuing increase in 5-HT, the decrease in DA at fatigue may reflect reduced motivation, arousal, and muscular coordination.

To see whether changes in 5-HT could influence time to fatigue, Bailey and colleagues (25–27) administered drugs that were agonistic or antagonistic to 5-HT and demonstrated a dose-related relationship. 5-HT agonists reduced time to exhaustion, while the administration of a 5-HT antagonist increased time to exhaustion. When a 5-HT agonist (paroxetine) was given acutely to humans, running time to exhaustion at 70% of $\dot{V}O_2$max was reduced (28). Thus, a low ratio of 5-HT to DA favors performance, while a higher ratio decreases performance (29).

A Role for Nutrition on Markers of Central Nervous System Fatigue

The difficulty in obtaining tissue samples of CNS markers requires either animal experimentation or sampling peripheral markers of TRP availability to the brain. Blomstrand and colleagues (30) documented elevations in fTRP and reductions in BCAA after marathon running, cross-country skiing, and soccer, which are consistent with elevated TRP availability for the brain. This should lead to elevated 5-HT and the opportunity for central fatigue. As such, nutritional strategies to decrease the fTRP/BCAA ratio would reduce 5-HT synthesis. Either administration of BCAA or carbohydrate supplementation should decrease this ratio and delay the central component of fatigue.

In a field setting, the subjects of Blomstrand and colleagues (31,32) showed improved marathon, cross-country skiing, and mental performance after the administration of BCAA. Delaying fatigue in the lab has not met with as much success (33–35), and Blomstrand and colleagues (36) have failed to improve human performance in a controlled laboratory setting. To make a physiologically important change in the fTRP/BCAA ratio requires large doses of BCAAs, but large doses can lead to a transient buildup of ammonia; this can have effects on both the brain and the contracting muscle's ability to produce energy.

The other option is to increase carbohydrate intake. This would suppress the release of free fatty acids that compete for binding sites on albumin with fTRP. With few free fatty acids in circulation, more fTRP combines with albumin, and the subsequent fTRP/BCAA ratio declines. Ingestion of moderate and high concentrations of a carbohydrate-electrolyte solution reduced fTRP indirectly, and carbohydrate concentration and cycle ergometer rides to exhaustion were increased (35). Peripheral fatigue did not appear to play a role in this model.

Other Variables in Central Nervous System Fatigue

Choline/Acetylcholine

The most common neurotransmitter in the body is acetylcholine, and in the CNS it is associated with temperature regulation, memory, and awareness. As with all transmitters, its synthesis is based on the availability of its main precursor, in this case choline. Depletion of choline could be a factor in CNS fatigue. Restricting choline intake can slow impulse transmission speed in skeletal muscle (37), and plasma choline levels are markedly reduced following a marathon run (38). However, a study on choline supplementation failed to determine the time to exhaustion during prolonged or intense cycle ergometer exercise (39).

Brain Dopamine

Dopamine (DA) was probably the first transmitter studied, possibly in response to the use of amphetamines by athletes as an ergogenic aid. Dopaminergic activity seems necessary for endurance performance, as destruction of these neurons impairs performance (40), and amphetamine use improves performance (41,42). How DA affects performance is not fully understood. It is possible that fatigue is delayed because of the ability of DA to inhibit the synthesis and metabolism of 5-HT. In addition, reductions of DA lead to lower efficiency through a loss of coordination and motivation (29).

Cytokines

Fatigue from viral infections and CFS may be due to substances released from immune cells that directly affect the CNS (43). For example, α-interferon can lead to a host of neuropsychiatric symptoms and fatigue (44,45). Cytokines may also be implicated in the depressed exercise response in patients with bacterial or other viral infections (46,47).

Ammonia

Ammonia is toxic to the brain (48) and can alter membrane permeability to the precursors of numerous neurotransmitters, but any elevation is brief and reversible. Ammonia is elevated from increased myokinase activity, particularly in the fast-twitch type muscle fibers (49) and from the catabolism of BCAA (50,51). Regardless of the mechanism, ammonia accumulations in the brain can impair coordination and motor control (centrally) as well as local oxidative metabolism (48).

PERIPHERAL FATIGUE

Beyond the brain and spinal cord, there are numerous locations that potentially can be a focal point for fatigue. The motor nerve, neuromuscular junction, sarcolemma, transverse tubules, excitation-contraction coupling, cross-bridge formation, and the contractile process have all been studied and in selected circumstances may be the primary mechanism of fatigue.

Neuromuscular Junction

Naess and Storm-Mathisen (52) first proposed the junction as a potential site of fatigue. There are studies that favor (53,54) and dispute (55,56) the role of the junction as a factor in fatigue. But there are numerous potential mechanisms at the junction that must be considered. For example, there may be some inhibition of the presynaptic endings or inadequate transmitter substance, or the postsynaptic membrane may be unable to be excited (57). Perhaps a decrease in the motoneuron firing rate is due to a peripheral reflex that inhibits the firing of the motoneuron, which would lead to a reduction in the firing of the muscle fiber in the absence of junctional dysfunction (58). An interesting finding is an increase in junctional cholinesterase following endurance training in the rat (59).

Sarcolemma

A change in the excitability of the muscle fiber membrane would most certainly affect the excitability of the cell. Changes in the concentration balance of sodium and potassium as a result of water shifts would alter the membrane potential of the fiber. Shifts in fluid and electrolytes as a result of exercise could make it more difficult to excite the membrane, leading to a reduction in the overall tension production by the muscle, which is fatigue.

Excitable cells will cease propagating an impulse in response to a constant depolarizing stimulus of 20 to 30 millivolts (mV) (60). Fatiguing contractions can lead to a substantial efflux of potassium (61), which can change the resting membrane potential by that 20 mV (62). So there is real evidence to warrant further investigation into the sarcolemma's being a key factor in fatigue of the muscle cell.

Models of local muscle fatigue involving reciprocal knee extensions, cycle ergometry, and swimming were developed. Arterial-venous blood sampling and muscle biopsies were used to study the role of the membrane in fatigue (63–68).

Sjogaard (66) had subjects exercise for 2 hours at 60% of $\dot{V}O_2$max. While there was substantial, but not complete, depletion of muscle glycogen, and lactate levels were similar to levels seen at rest, the calculations showed a continual loss of potassium from the vastus lateralis. The author calculated a change in the membrane potential from 88 to 80 mV. He concluded that this 10% change may have influenced the muscle's ability to produce tension. A similar study on swimming failed to show the same results due to the minimal involvement of the vastus lateralis in swimming (63).

An increase in intensity and reduction in duration led to greater changes in the membrane potential. Sjogaard and colleagues (68) exhausted their subjects by having them perform 10 minutes of knee extensions at 55% of $\dot{V}O_2$max followed by 6 to 7 minutes at 100%. There was some glycogen breakdown, lactate production, and a fall in pH, as expected. Muscle cell potassium fell and water increased. The calculated membrane potential changed from 89 to 75 mV.

Cellular potassium was taken up by other cells and tissues, and rapidly returned to the fatigued cells upon relaxation. We are familiar with the performance of high-intensity fatiguing exercise that, with a brief period of recovery, can be reinitiated for a short time. Perhaps fatigue of the membrane is the mechanism of fatigue in such activities.

Excitation-Contraction Coupling

This process couples the excitation of the membrane with the actual contraction of the cross-bridges. If the membrane can be a factor in fatigue, then so too could the coupling process. Donaldson (69) suggests that the trigger to calcium release by the sarcoplasmic reticulum is a transverse tubule membrane, polyphosphoinositide (PIP_2). When hydrolyzed, inositol trisphosphate (IP_3) diffuses to the sarcoplasmic reticulum, triggering the release of calcium. Should the rate of hydrolysis of PIP_2 exceed replenishment, then the subsequent fall in IP_3 would result in less calcium released from the sarcoplasmic reticulum, and we know that calcium is a requirement for muscle contraction.

Metabolic Considerations in Fatigue

Once inside the muscle cell, metabolic factors come into play in fatigue. The gain or loss of selected variables can ultimately affect cross-bridge interaction. These factors are important, and these changes prevent the muscle from depleting adenosine triphosphate (ATP) and progressing toward irreversible rigor. Two hypotheses have been broadly discussed: exhaustion and accumulation.

Exhaustion Hypothesis

Upon the initiation of submaximal exercise, energy is obtained from stored phosphagens and glycolysis. Continuation of the work leads to aerobic metabolism as the primary source of energy. With adequate blood and oxygen, the Krebs cycle is able to compete for pyruvic acid, which can lead to a slowing of the rate of glycogen depletion because energy from fatty acids increases. This increases the total work output relative to the stores of glycogen. If the exercise continues to the point of glycogen depletion, then the power output will have to decrease to a level that can be supported solely by fats, around 50% of $\dot{V}O_2max$ (70).

A reduction in blood glucose has long been considered a main factor in fatigue, but mostly from its role as the primary energy fuel for the brain and its resultant role in mood and motivation. The discussion about central fatigue illustrates how complex the interaction of metabolites can be. However, maintenance of blood glucose during endurance exercise has been shown to offer an alternative fuel source for the exercising muscle, increasing the time to exhaustion (71).

Fatigue from short-term anaerobic work is not generally due to whole-muscle glycogen depletion, yet there is some selective depletion of glycogen from the high-tension output IIb fibers that can lead to a reduction in power output (72,73). ATP depletion at the cross-bridge head is a possibility, but magnetic resonance spectroscopy shows minimal changes in ATP, adenosine diphosphate (ADP), or adenosine monophosphate (AMP). Creatine phosphate reduction tends to parallel reduction in force production under conditions in which glycolysis is poisoned (74,75). Eventually, continued contraction would lead to rigor. However, if glycolysis was not poisoned, force production did not parallel creatine phosphate decline, but rather was inversely related to lactate production. While creatine phosphate levels had declined to 25% of prefatigue levels, tension output was still 85% of control. Thus, glycolysis served to protect the cell from progressing to rigor.

It is well known that during long-term low-intensity exercise and during some games, glycogen depletion is a primary component in fatigue. When glycogen levels become depleted, the power output must be supplied by energy solely from fat metabolism, and the rate of exercise that can be supported by fats is around 50% of $\dot{V}O_2max$ (70). Nutritional strategies that augment stored muscle glycogen and delay fatigue are commonplace in endurance sports.

Accumulation Hypothesis

The accumulation of selected metabolites can interfere with tension production. The primary metabolites are hydrogen ions, inorganic phosphate, and ammonia.

Hydrogen Ions

High-intensity exercise leads to an increase in hydrogen ions from glycolytic energy production, mostly in the type II muscle fibers. Ions build up because nearly all the lactic acid produced is ionized at physiologic pH. Most of these ions are buffered, yet the changes in pH are due to the nearly 0.001% of ions that go unbuffered (74,76).

The accumulation of hydrogen ions and the resultant fall in pH can affect a variety of factors in tension production. Action potentials, calcium flux, and muscle enzymes are all sensitive to pH. For example, as the pH of the extracellular environment decreases, so does the excitability of the membrane (77). Falling pH has two effects on calcium: more calcium is required for similar tension levels (78,79), and release of calcium for the sarcoplasmic reticulum is reduced (57).

Muscle enzymes are particularly sensitive to changes in pH. The conversion of the inactive form of phosphorylase to its active form is reduced by a falling pH (76). The often-considered rate-limiting enzyme of glycolysis, phosphofructokinase (PFK), is thought to be inactive at a pH of 6.5 (80–82). Slowing the activity of PFK backs up glycolytic intermediates (e.g., glucose-6-phosphate), which inhibit both hexokinase and phosphorylase, while physiologic concentrations of lactic acid inhibit lactate dehydrogenase and adenosine triphosphatase (ATPase) (70). Declining pH also favors the creatine kinase reaction (76,83) and limits free fatty acid release by adipose tissue (57).

Because fatigue is related to a declining pH and training effectively delays fatigue, then training must have some effect on the buffering capacity of skeletal muscle. Cross-sectionally, game sport participants (ice hockey, soccer) have a higher buffer capacity than nonathletes (84). In a study of sprint cycle training, lactic acid production and total work output increased along with buffer capacity (85). The buffer capacity of endurance-trained athletes is not appreciably different from that of untrained subjects (84).

Inorganic Phosphate

An isolated skinned muscle preparation has shown that inorganic phosphate may bind myosin, thereby limiting force production (57). Add to this the acid form of phosphate (H_2PO_4), and the potential for a reduction in force output is possible (86).

Ammonia

Very intense exercise can require the fast type II fibers to generate energy through the myokinase reaction. Myokinase converts two ADP molecules to one ATP and one AMP. In the presence of water, the AMP is converted to NH_3 and inosine monophosphate (IMP). Ammonia can influence a variety of factors such as membrane function (87), PFK activity (70,88), the Krebs cycle (70,89–91), gluconeogenesis (57), or oxidation by the mitochondria (63,70). Any of the above would lead to increased lactic acid production and glycogen depletion (92). For high-intensity exercise, there are some who think that pH decline might be secondary to the production of ammonia (57,92).

The characterizations of fatigue commonly include the word *failure* in their definition. Perhaps it is wiser to view fatigue as a method to protect the muscle from progressing toward irreversible damage. From the view of the athlete, much of training is designed to delay the onset of fatigue. The type of training should be specific to the mechanism(s) of fatigue for any given activity. It appears that the interaction of intensity and duration plays a role in peripheral fatigue. Historically, the overriding mechanisms of fatigue have been located in the periphery, but current investigations into a role for the CNS indicate that the CNS may indeed be a concern that needs to be addressed in the design and implementation of training programs (Fig. 7–1). The multitude of possibilities and interactions make the study of fatigue and training to delay fatigue a most complex undertaking.

REFERENCES

1. Hales JP, Gandevia SC. Assessment of maximal voluntary contraction with twitch interpolation: an instrument to measure twitch responses. *J Neurosci Methods* 1988;25:97–102.
2. Bigland-Ritchie B, Cafarelli E, Vollestad NK. Fatigue of submaximal static contractions. *Acta Physiol Scand* 1986;128(suppl 556):137–148.
3. Bigland-Ritchie B, Thomas B, Rice CK, Howarth JV, Woods JJ. Muscle temperature, contractile speed and motoneuron firing rates during human voluntary contractions. *J Appl Physiol* 1992;73:2457–2461.
4. Enoka RM, Stuart DG. Neurobiology of muscle fatigue. *J Appl Physiol* 1992;72:1631–1648.
5. Tesch PA, Dudley GA, Duvoisin MR, Hatcher BM, Harris RT. Force and EMG signal patterns during repeated bouts of concentric and eccentric muscle actions. *Acta Physiol Scand* 1990;138:263–271.
6. Westing SH, Cresswell AG, Thorstensson A. Muscle activation during maximal voluntary eccentric and concentric knee extension. *Eur J Appl Physiol* 1991;62:104–108.
7. Garner SH, Sutton JR, Burse RL, McComas AJ, Cymerman A, Houston CS. Operation Everest II: neuromuscular performance under conditions of extreme simulated altitude. *J Appl Physiol* 1990;68:1167–1172.
8. Rube N, Secher NH. Paradoxical influence of encouragement on muscle fatigue. *Eur J Appl Physiol* 1981;46:1–7.
9. Secher NH. Motor unit recruitment: a pharmacological approach. *Med Sports Sci* 1987;26:152–162.
10. Asmussen E, Mazin B. Recuperation after muscular fatigue by "diverting activities." *Eur J Appl Physiol* 1978;38:1–8.
11. Maton B. Central nervous changes in fatigue induced by local work. In: Atlan G, Beliveau L, Bouissou P, eds. *Muscle fatigue: biochemical and physiological aspects.* Paris: Masson, 1991:207–221.
12. Brasil-Neto JP, Pascual-Leone A, Valls-Sole J, Cammarota A, Cohen LG, Hallett M. Postexercise depression of motor evoked potentials: a measure of central nervous system fatigue. *Exp Brain Res* 1993;93:181–184.
13. Gibson H, Carroll JE, Clague E, Edwards RHT. Exercise performance and fatigability in patients with chronic fatigue syndrome. *J Neurol Neurosurg Psychiatry* 1993;56:993–998m.
14. Riley MS, O'Brien CJ, McClusky DR, Bell NP, Nicholls DP. Aerobic work capacity in patients with chronic fatigue syndrome. *Br Med J* 1990;301:953–956.
15. Stokes MJ, Cooper RG, Edwards RHT. Normal muscle strength and fatigability in patients with effort syndromes. *Br Med J* 1988;297:1014–1017.
16. Kent-Braun JA, Sharma KR, Weiner MW, Massie B, Miller RG. Central basis of muscle fatigue in chronic fatigue syndrome. *Neurology* 1993;43:125–131.
17. Lloyd AR, Gandevia SC, Hales JP. Muscle performance, voluntary activation, twitch properties and perceived effort in normal subjects and patients with chronic fatigue syndrome. *Brain* 1991;114:85–98.
18. Newsholme EA, Acworth IN, Blomstrand E. Amino acids, brain neurotransmitters and a functional link between muscle and brain that is important in sustained exercise. In: Benzi G, ed. *Advances in myochemistry.* London: John Libbey Eurotext, 1987:127–133.
19. Chaouloff F, Elghozi JL, Guezennec Y, Laude D. Effects of conditioned running on plasma, liver and brain trytophan and on brain 5-hydrotryptamine metabolism of the rat. *Br J Pharmacol* 1985;86:33–41.
20. Chaouloff F, Kennett GA, Serrerier B, Merina D, Cutson G. Amino acid analysis demonstrates that increased plasma free trytophan causes the increase in brain trytophan during exercise in the rat. *J Neurochem* 1986;46:1647–1650.
21. Chaouloff F, Laude D, Guezennec Y, Elghozi JL. Motor activity increases trytophan, 5-hydroxyindoleacetic acid and homovanillic acid in ventricular cerebrospinal fluid of the conscious rat. *J Neurochem* 1986;46:1313–1316.
22. Chaouloff F, Laude D, Merino D, Serrurier B, Guezennec Y, Elghozi JL. Amphetamine and alpha-*p*-tyrosine affect the exercise induced imbalance between the availability of trytophan and synthesis of serotonin in the brain of the rat. *Neuropharmacology* 1987;26:1099–1106.
23. Chaouloff F, Laude D, Elghozi JL. Physical exercise: evidence for differential consequences of trytophan on 5-HT synthesis and metabolism in central serotonergic cell bodies and terminals. *J Neural Transm* 1989;78:121–130.
24. Blomstrand E, Perrett D, Parry-Billings M, Newsholme EA. Effect of sustained exercise on plasma amino acid concentrations and on 5-hydroxytryptamine metabolism in six different brain regions in the rat. *Acta Physiol Scand* 1989;136:473–481.
25. Bailey SP, Davis JM, Ahlborn EN. Neuroendocrine and substrate responses to altered brain 5-HT activity during prolonged exercise to fatigue. *J Appl Physiol* 1993;74:3006–3012.
26. Bailey SP, Davis JM, Ahlborn EN. Brain serotonergic activity

affects endurance performance in the rat. *Int J Sports Med* 1993;6:330–333.

27. Bailey SP, Davis JM, Ahlborn EN. Effect of increased brain serotonergic (5-HT_{1c}) activity on endurance performance in the rat. *Acta Physiol Scand* 1992;145:75–76.
28. Wilson WM, Maughan RJ. Evidence for a possible role of 5-hydrotryptamine in the genesis of fatigue in man: administration of paroxetine, a 5-HT re-uptake inhibitor, reduces the capacity to perform prolonged exercise. *Exp Physiol* 1992;77:921–924.
29. Davis JM, Bailey SP. Possible mechanisms of central nervous system fatigue during exercise. *Med Sci Sports Exerc* 1997;29:45–57.
30. Blomstrand E, Celsing F, Newsholme EA. Changes in plasma concentrations of aromatic and branched-chain amino acids during sustained exercise in man and their possible role in fatigue. *Acta Physiol Scand* 1988;133:115–121.
31. Blomstrand E, Hassmen P, Newsholme EA. Effect of branched-chain amino acid supplementation on mental performance. *Acta Physiol Scand* 1991;136:473–481.
32. Blomstrand E, Hassmen P, Ekblom B, Newsholme EA. Administration of branched-chain amino acids during sustained exercise: effects on performance and on plasma concentration of some amino acids. *Eur J Appl Physiol* 1991;63:83–88.
33. Varnier M, Sarto P, Martines D. Effect of infusing branched-chain amino acids during incremental exercise with reduced muscle glycogen content. *Eur J Appl Physiol* 1994;69:26–31.
34. Verger PH, Aymard P, Cynobert L, Anton G, Luigi R. Effects of administration of branched-chain amino acids vs. glucose during acute exercise in the rat. *Physiol Behav* 1994;55:523–526.
35. Davis J, Bailey SP, Woods JA, Galiano FJ, Hamilton M, Bartoli WP. Effects of carbohydrate feedings on plasma free trytophan and branched-chain amino acids during prolonged cycling. *Eur J Appl Physiol* 1992;65:513–519.
36. Blomstrand E, Andersson S, Hassmen P, Ekblom B, Newsholme EA. Effect of branched-chain amino acid and carbohydrate supplementation on the exercise-induced change in plasma and muscle concentration of amino acids in human subjects. *Acta Physiol Scand* 1995;153:87–96.
37. Xia N. *Effects of dietary choline levels on human muscle function.* MS thesis, Boston University College of Engineering, 1991.
38. Conlay LA, Sabounjian AL, Wurtman RJ. Exercise and neuromodulators: choline and acetylcholine in marathon runners. *Int J Sports Med* 1992;13(suppl 1):S141–142.
39. Spector SA, Jackman MA, Sabounjian LA, Sakkas C, Landers DM, Willis WT. Effects of choline supplementation on fatigue in trained cyclists. *Med Sci Sports Exerc* 1995;27:668–673.
40. Heyes MP, Garnett ES, Coates G. Nigrostriatal dopaminergic activity is increased during exhaustive exercise stress in rats. *Life Sci* 1988;42:1537–1542.
41. Bhagat B, Wheeler N. Effect of amphetamine on the swimming endurance of rats. *Neuropharmacol* 1973;12:711–713.
42. Gerald MC. Effect of (+)-amphetamine on the treadmill endurance performance of rats. *Neuropharmacology* 1978;17:703–704.
43. Hart BL. Biological basis of the behavior of sick animals. *Neurosci Biobehav Rev* 1988;12:123–137.
44. Mannering GJ, Deloria LB. The pharmacology and toxicology of the interferons: an overview. *Annu Rev Pharmacol Toxicol* 1986;26:455–515.
45. Wills RJ, Denis S, Spiedel HE, Gibson DM, Nadler PI. Interferon kinetics and adverse reactions after intravenous, intramuscular and subcutaneous injection. *Clin Pharmacol Ther* 1984;35:722–727.
46. Lloyd AR, Hales JP, Gandevia SC. Muscle strength, endurance and recovery in the post-infection fatigue syndrome. *J Neurol Neurosurg Psychiatry* 1988;51:1316–1322.
47. Lloyd AR, Wakefield RD, Broughton C, Dwyer J. Immunological abnormalities in the chronic fatigue syndrome. *Med J Aust* 1989;151:122–124.
48. Banister EW, Cameron BJC. Exercise-induced hyperammonemia: peripheral and central effects. *Int J Sports Med* 1990;11(suppl 2):S129–S142.
49. Meyer RA, Dudley GA, Terjung RL. Ammonia and IMP in different skeletal muscle fibers after exercise in rats. *J Appl Physiol* 1980;49:1037–1041.
50. Wagenmakers AJ, Bechers EJ, Brouns F. Carbohydrate supplementation, glycogen depletion, and amino acid metabolism during exercise. *Am J Physiol* 1991;260:E883–E890.
51. Wagenmakers AJM, Coakley JH, Edwards RHT. Metabolism of branched-chain amino acids and ammonia during exercise: clues from McArdle's disease. *Int J Sports Med* 1990;11:S101–S113.
52. Naess K, Storm-Mathisen A. Fatigue and sustained tetanic contractions. *Acta Physiol Scand* 1955;34:351–366.
53. Marsden CD, Meadows JC, Merton PA. "Muscular wisdom" that minimized fatigue during prolonged effort in man: peak rates of motoneuron discharge and slowing of discharge during fatigue. In: Desmedt JE, ed. *Motor control mechanisms in health and disease.* New York: Raven Press, 1983:169–211.
54. Stephans JA, Taylor A. Fatigue of maintained voluntary muscle contraction in man. *J Physiol* 1972;220:1–19.
55. Bigland-Ritchie B, Kakula CB, Lippold LJ, Woods JJ. The absence of neuromuscular junction failure in sustained maximal voluntary contractions. *J Physiol (Lond)* 1982;330:265–278.
56. Merton PA. Voluntary strength and fatigue. *J Physiol (Lond)* 1954;123:553–564.
57. MacLaren DPM, Gibson B, Parry-Billings M, Edwards RHT. A review of metabolic factors in fatigue. *Exerc Sports Sci Rev* 1989;17:29–68.
58. Woods JJ, Furbish F, Bigland-Ritchie BR. Evidence for fatigue-induced reflex inhibition of motoneuron firing rates. *J Neurophysiol* 1987;58:125–137.
59. Crockett JL, Edgerton VR, Max SR, Barnard RJ. The neuromuscular junction in response to endurance training. *Exp Neurol* 1976;51:207–215.
60. Hodgkin AL, Huxley AF. The dual effect of membrane potential on sodium conductance in the giant axon of loligo. *J Physiol (Lond)* 1952;116:487–506.
61. Mainwood GW, Lucher GE. Fatigue and recovery in isolated frog sartorius muscles: effects of bicarbonate concentration and associated potassium loss. *Can J Physiol Pharmacol* 1972;50:132–142.
62. Locke S, Soloman HC. Relation of resting potential in rat gastrocnemius and soleus muscle to innervation activation and the Na-K pump. *J Exp Zool* 1967;166:377–386.
63. Nielsen B, Sjogaard G, Bonde-Petersen F. Cardiovascular, hormonal and body fluid changes during prolonged exercise. *Eur J Appl Physiol* 1984;53:63–70.
64. Sjogaard G. Electrolytes in slow and fast muscle fibers at rest and with dynamic exercise. *Am J Physiol* 1983;245:R25–R31.
65. Sinkeler SPT, Daaren HAM, Wevers RA, Oel L, Joosten EMG, Binkhorst RA. Relation between blood lactate and ammonia in ischemic handgrip exercise. *Muscle Nerve* 1985;8:523–527.
66. Sjogaard G. Water and electrolyte shifts during exercise and their relation to muscular fatigue. *Acta Physiol Scand* 1986;128(suppl 556):129–136.
67. Sjogaard G, Saltin B. Extra and intracellular water spaces in muscles of man at rest and with dynamic exercise. *Am J Physiol* 1982;243:R271–R280.
68. Sjogaard G, Adams RP, Saltin B. Water and ion shift in skeletal muscles of humans with intense knee extensions. *Am J Physiol* 1985;245:R190–R196.
69. Donaldson SK. Mammalian muscle fiber types: comparison of excitation-contraction coupling mechanisms. *Acta Physiol Scand* 1986;128(suppl 556):157–166.
70. Newsholme EA, Leech AR. *Biochemistry for the medical sciences.* New York: Wiley, 1983.
71. Coyle EF, Hagberg JM, Hurley BF. Carbohydrate feeding during prolonged strenuous exercise can delay fatigue. *J Appl Physiol Respir Environ Exerc Physiol* 1983;55:230–235.
72. Edgerton VR, Saltin B, Essen B, Simpson DR. Glycogen depletion in specific types of human skeletal muscle fibers in intermittent continuous exercises. In: Howald H, Poortmans JR, eds. *Metabolic adaptation to prolonged exercise.* Basel: Birkhauser Verlag, 1975:402–415.
73. Gollnick PD, Karlsson J, Piehl K, Saltin B. Selective glycogen depletion in skeletal muscle fibers in man following sustained contractions. *J Physiol* 1974;241:59–67.
74. Sahlin K. Effects of acidosis on energy metabolism and force generation in skeletal muscle. In: Knuttgen HG, Vogel H, eds.

Biochemistry of exercise. Champaign, IL: Human Kinetics, 1983:151–160.

75. Sahlin K. Muscle fatigue and lactic acid production accumulation. *Acta Physiol Scand* 1986;128(suppl 556):83–91.
76. Sahlin K, Harris RC, Hultman E. Creatine kinase equilibrium and lactate content compared with muscle pH in tissue samples obtained after isometric contraction. *Biochem J* 1975;152:173–180.
77. Orchardson P. The generation of nerve impulses in mammalian axons by changing the concentrations of the normal constituents of extracellular fluid. *J Physiol* 1978;275:177–189.
78. Fabiato A, Fabiato F. Effects of pH on the myofilaments and the sarcoplasmic reticulum of skinned cells from cardiac and skeletal muscles. *J Physiol (Lond)* 1978;276:233–255.
79. Robertson S, Kerrick W. The effects of pH on submaximal calcium ion activated tension I skinned frog skeletal fibers. *Biophys J* 1976;16:37A.
80. Danforth WH. Activation of the glycolytic pathway in muscle. In: Chance B, Estabrook RW, eds. *Control of energy metabolism.* New York: Academic Press, 1965:287–298.
81. Trivedi B, Danforth WH. Effects of pH on the kinetics of frog muscle phosphofructokinase. *J Biol Chem* 1966;241:4110–4114.
82. Ui M. A role of phosphofructokinase in pH dependent regulation of glycolysis. *Biochim Biophys Acta* 1966;124:310–322.
83. Sahlin K, Harris RC, Hultman E. Resynthesis of creatine phosphate in human muscle after exercise in relation to intramuscular pH and availability of oxygen. *Scand J Lab Invest* 1979;39:551–557.
84. Sahlin K, Henriksson J. Buffer capacity and lactate accumulation in skeletal muscle of trained and untrained men. *Acta Physiol Scand* 1984;122:331–339.
85. Sharp RL, Costill DL, Fink WJ, King DS. Effects of eight weeks of bicycle ergometer sprint training on buffer capacity. *Int J Sports Med* 1983;7:13–17.
86. Wilkie DR. Muscular fatigue: effects of hydrogen ions and inorganic phosphate. *Fed Proc* 1986;45:2921–2933.
87. Heald DE. Influence of ammonium ions of mechanical and electrophysiological responses of skeletal muscle. *Am J Physiol* 1975;229:1174–1179.
88. Lowenstein JM. Ammonia production in muscle and other tissues: the purine nucleotide cycle. *Physiol Rev* 1972;52:382–414.
89. Aragon JJ, Tornheim K, Goodman MN, Lowenstein JM. Replenishment of citric acid cycle intermediates by the purine nucleotide cycle in rat skeletal muscle. *Curr Top Cell Regul* 1981;18:131–149.
90. Katanuma N, Arada M, Nishii Y. Regulation of the urea cycle and TCA cycle by ammonia. In: Weaver G, ed. *Advances in enzyme regulation,* vol 4. New York: Pergamon Press, 1966:317–339.
91. Worcel A, Erechinska M. Mechanism of inhibitory action of ammonia on the respiration of rat-liver mitochondria. *Biochim Biophys Acta* 1964;67:27–33.
92. Mutch BA, Banister EW. Ammonia metabolism in exercise and fatigue. *Med Sci Sports Exerc* 1983;14:41–50.

PART III

Systemic Exercise

Exercise and Sport Science,
edited by William E. Garrett, Jr., and Donald T. Kirkendall.
Lippincott Williams & Wilkins, Philadelphia © 2000.

CHAPTER 8

Cardiovascular Responses to Exercise and Training

Barry A. Franklin

The cardiac profile of individuals who participate regularly in vigorous, isotonic exercise is characterized by left ventricular volume overload with increased left ventricular internal dimension, end-diastolic volume, stroke volume, and myocardial mass (1). These changes are associated with enhanced left ventricular performance and peripheral adaptations (e.g., increases in the size and number of skeletal muscle mitochondria, myoglobin content, oxidative enzymes, and capillary density) that facilitate a significantly higher aerobic capacity compared with similarly aged control subjects.

This chapter reviews the physiologic effects of exercise on cardiovascular function, with specific reference to energy production, submaximal and maximal oxygen consumption ($\dot{V}O_2max$), acute cardiorespiratory responses to exercise, measurement of the $\dot{V}O_2max$, physiologic variations in the $\dot{V}O_2max$, cardiovascular and metabolic adaptations to training, and dynamic versus static exercise.

ENERGY SYSTEMS FOR EXERCISE

The energy required for muscle contraction or other forms of biologic work is produced by anaerobic and aerobic pathways. Adenosine triphosphate (ATP; Fig. 8–1) breaks down inside muscle cells and becomes a source of energy. Although not all ATP is formed aerobically, the amount of ATP yielded by anaerobic glycolysis is extremely small (Table 8–1). Nevertheless, anaerobic mechanisms provide a rapid source of ATP, which is particularly important at the beginning of exercise and during high-intensity activity that can be sustained only for brief periods.

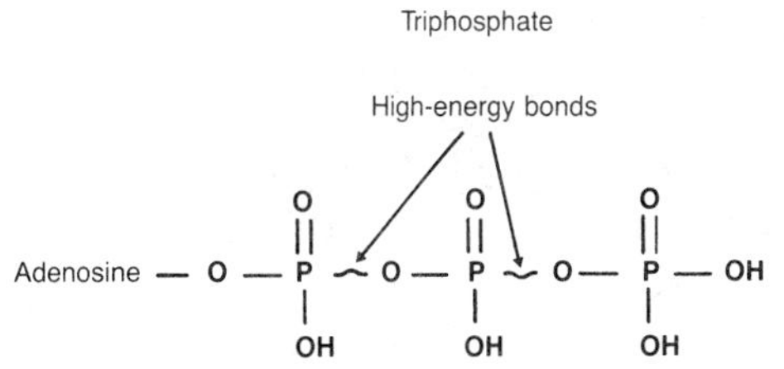

FIG. 8–1. Simplified structure of an adenosine triphosphate (ATP) molecule. The symbol ~ represents the high energy bonds.

The aerobic system, which uses glycogen, fats, and proteins as energy substrates, provides large amounts of ATP for muscular energy (2). However, oxygen delivery to the cell is critical; hence, the capacity to provide oxygen to the tissues usually determines the intensity of physical activity that an individual can perform.

OXYGEN CONSUMPTION

The most widely recognized measure of cardiopulmonary fitness is the aerobic capacity or maximal oxygen consumption ($\dot{V}O_2max$). This variable is defined physiologically as the highest rate of oxygen transport and use that can be achieved at peak physical exertion.

Somatic oxygen consumption ($\dot{V}O_2$) may be expressed mathematically by a rearrangement of the Fick equation:

$$\dot{V}O_2 = HR \times SV \times (CaO_2 - C\bar{v}O_2)$$

where $\dot{V}O_2$ is oxygen consumption in milliliters per min-

B. A. Franklin: Department of Physiology, School of Medicine, Wayne State University, Detroit, Michigan 48201; Cardiac Rehabilitation and Exercise Laboratories, Cardiology Department, William Beaumont Hospital, Royal Oak, Michigan 48073; and Beaumont Rehabilitation and Health Center, Cardiac Rehabilitation Department, Birmingham, Michigan, 48009.

TABLE 8–1. *Characteristics of the two mechanisms by which adenosine triphosphate (ATP) is formed*

Mechanism	Food or chemical fuel	Oxygen required?	Relative ATP yield
Anaerobic			
Phosphocreatine	Phosphocreatine	No	Extremely limited
Glycolysis	Glycogen (glucose)	No	Extremely limited
Aerobic			
Krebs cycle and electron transport system	Glycogen, fats, proteins	Yes	Large

Adapted from ref. 2.

ute; HR is heart rate in beats per minute; and $CaO_2 - C\bar{v}O_2$ is the arteriovenous oxygen difference in milliliters of oxygen per deciliter of blood. Thus, it is apparent that both central and peripheral regulatory mechanisms affect the magnitude of body oxygen consumption.

In physiologic terms, a maximal test exercises an individual to a work load beyond which further work increases will not be accompanied by increased oxygen consumption (i.e., there is a leveling off or plateauing in $\dot{V}O_2$). At this point, the individual has attained his or her maximal oxygen uptake—the true state of cardiovascular fitness (3).

Rest Versus Exercise

Typical circulatory data at rest and during maximal exercise in a healthy, sedentary 30-year-old man and a world-class endurance athlete of similar age are shown in Table 8–2. By dividing the absolute resting oxygen consumption (0.25 L/min) by body weight in kilograms (70 kg), one derives the energy requirement for basal homeostasis, termed one metabolic equivalent (MET), approximating 3.5 milliliters of oxygen per kilogram of body weight per minute (3.5 mL/kg/min) (4). This expression of resting oxygen consumption is extremely important in exercise physiology, being relatively constant for all persons, regardless of age, body weight, or fitness level. Furthermore, multiples of this value are often used to quantify relative levels of energy expenditure and aerobic fitness (5). For example, an activity that requires 14 mL/kg/min corresponds to 4 METs (14/3.5 = 4) or four times the resting energy expenditure.

The 10-fold increase in oxygen transport and utilization in the sedentary individual is contrasted by a 23-fold increase in the endurance athlete, corresponding to $\dot{V}O_2$max values of 35 and 80 mL/kg/min, respectively. The increased aerobic capacity in the athlete appears to be primarily the result of increased maximal cardiac output, due to a greater increment in heart rate and, to a lesser extent, stroke volume, rather than an increased peripheral extraction of oxygen (6). Because there is little variation in maximal heart rate and maximal systemic arteriovenous oxygen difference with training, $\dot{V}O_2$max virtually defines the pumping capacity of the heart. Therefore, it is of major importance in the cardiovascular evaluation of the athlete.

$\dot{V}O_2$max values in elite and national-class athletes vary from a high of 94 mL/kg/min, reported in a cross-country skier, to values in the low- to mid-40s for athletes participating in anaerobic-type sports (Fig. 8–2). Most world-class endurance athletes have a $\dot{V}O_2$max greater than 70 mL/kg/min, whereas many other championship athletes demonstrate values between 60 and 70 mL/kg/min. In contrast, the reported $\dot{V}O_2$max of national-class body-

TABLE 8–2. *Hypothetical circulatory data at rest and during maximal exercise for a 30-year-old sedentary man versus a world-class endurance athlete*

Condition	Oxygen consumption (L/min)	(mL/kg/min)	(METs)	Cardiac output (L/min)	Heart rate (beats/min)	Stroke volume (mL/beat)	Arteriovenous oxygen difference (mL/dL blood)
Sedentary man (70 kg)							
Rest	0.25	3.5[a]	1	6.1	70	87	4.0
Maximal exercise	2.50	35.0	10	17.7	190	93	14.0
World-class endurance athlete (70 kg)							
Rest	0.25	3.5[a]	1	6.1	45	136	4.0
Maximal exercise	5.60	80.0	23	35.0	190	184	16.0

[a] 3.5 mL/kg/min = 1 metabolic equivalent (MET); average resting metabolic rate expressed per unit body weight.

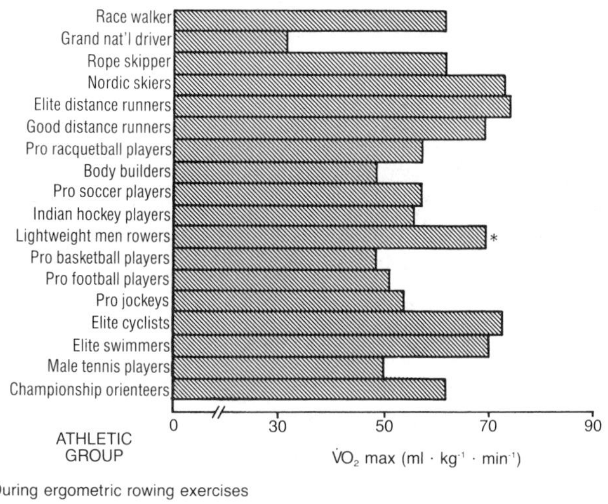

FIG. 8–2. Average $\dot{V}O_2$max (mL/kg/min) values for various athletic groups.

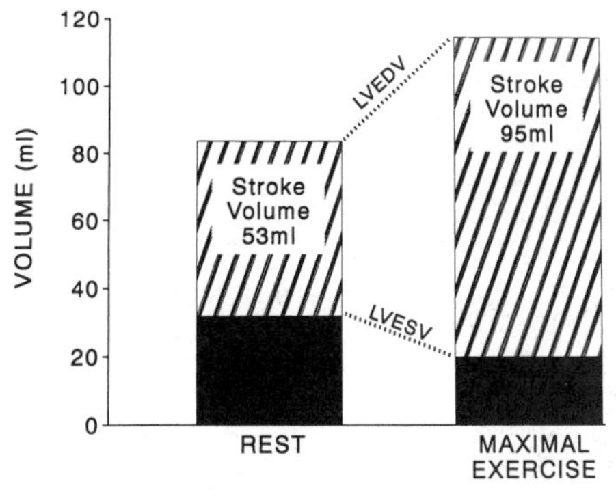

FIG. 8–3. Changes in stroke volume from rest to maximal upright exercise are shown in young, healthy men. *LVEDV*, left ventricular end-diastolic volume; *LVESV*, left ventricular end-systolic volume. (Adapted from ref. 8.)

builders and of professional football, tennis, and basketball players is between 40 and 50 mL/kg/min. Although intense physical training may increase the $\dot{V}O_2$max by 25% or more, it has become increasingly apparent that natural endowment (i.e., "selecting the right parents"), rather than training per se, plays a major role in producing world-class endurance athletes (6).

ACUTE CARDIORESPIRATORY RESPONSES

Many cardiorespiratory mechanisms function collectively to support the increased metabolic demands on active muscle. The overall effect of these changes in heart rate, stroke volume, cardiac output, arteriovenous oxygen difference, blood flow, blood pressure, and pulmonary ventilation is to deliver blood to the active tissues and provide oxygenation of that blood.

Heart Rate

Heart rate generally increases progressively as a function of exercise intensity; there is a roughly linear relationship between heart rate and work load or power output (7). Although heart rate will generally level off within 2 to 3 minutes at a given submaximal work load, at higher work loads it takes progressively longer to plateau or attain a steady-state rate. At even higher work loads a definable maximum heart rate is attained, which decreases with age. The equation 220 − age provides an approximation of the maximal heart rate in normal healthy men and women, but the variance for any given age is considerable (standard deviation $\pm \sim 10$ beats/min).

Stroke Volume

The stroke volume response to exercise is highly dependent on hydrostatic pressure effects. Stroke volume at rest in the erect position generally varies between 60 and 100 mL/beat among healthy adults, while maximum stroke volume approximates 100 to 120 mL/beat. When exercising in the erect position, stroke volume increases curvilinearly with the work load until it reaches a near-maximum value at approximately 50% of the individual's maximal aerobic capacity (3), increasing only slightly thereafter. Although it has been suggested that stroke volume may actually decrease at higher heart rates due to the disproportionate shortening in diastolic filling time, this issue remains unsettled.

Within physiologic limits, enhanced venous return increases the heart's end-diastolic volume, stretching cardiac muscle fibers and increasing their force of contraction. During exercise there is an increase in stroke volume resulting from both the Frank-Starling mechanism and a decreased end-systolic volume (Fig. 8–3) (8). The latter is due to increased ventricular contractility, secondary to catecholamine-mediated sympathetic stimulation.

Cardiac Output

Cardiac output in healthy adults generally increases linearly with increases in work load, from a resting value of approximately 5 L/min to a maximum of about 20 L/min during upright exercise, corresponding to a fourfold increase. Maximum values of cardiac output are dependent on many factors, however, including body size and the level of physical conditioning. At exercise levels of up to 50% of a person's $\dot{V}O_2$max, the increase in cardiac output is accomplished through increases in both heart rate and stroke volume (3). At higher exercise intensities, the increase results almost solely from the continued rise in heart rate.

Arteriovenous Oxygen Difference

As the exercise intensity progresses from moderate to heavy loads, an increased extraction of oxygen from the arterial blood supply occurs at the muscle. The arterial and mixed venous oxygen content at rest are approximately 20 and 15 mL of oxygen per 100 mL (dL) of blood, respectively. As the work load approaches the point of exhaustion, however, the mixed venous oxygen content typically decreases to 5 mL/dL blood or lower, thus widening the arteriovenous oxygen difference from 5 to 15 mL/dL blood, corresponding to a threefold increase (3).

Blood Flow

At rest, only 15% to 20% of the cardiac output is distributed to the muscles; 80% to 85% goes to the visceral organs (stomach, liver, spleen, kidneys), the heart, and the brain (9). However, during exercise there is a shunting of blood so that the working muscles receive as much as 85% to 90% of the cardiac output through vasodilation, while blood flow to the visceral organs is simultaneously decreased by vasoconstriction. Blood flow to the myocardium is increased in proportion to the increased metabolic activity of the heart, whereas that to the brain is maintained via autoregulation at resting levels (10).

During exercise, cutaneous blood flow is also greatly increased to facilitate heat dissipation. When maximal exertion is approached, however, the body sacrifices cutaneous circulation in order to meet the increasing metabolic requirements of working muscles, and consequently core temperature may quickly rise (11).

Blood Pressure

There is a linear increase in the systolic blood pressure with increasing levels of exercise, with maximal values typically reaching 170 to 220 mm Hg. Diastolic blood pressure generally remains unchanged or decreases slightly from rest to maximum exercise in the normal, healthy adult.

Pulmonary Ventilation

Pulmonary or minute ventilation ($\dot{V}_E$), the volume of air inspired or expired per minute, increases from approximately 6 L/min at rest to more than 100 L/min in the average sedentary adult male when exercising. This substantial increase in ventilation is accomplished through three- and fivefold increases in respiratory rate and tidal volume, respectively. For the most part, the increase in pulmonary ventilation is directly proportional to the increase in somatic oxygen consumed ($\dot{V}O_2$) and carbon dioxide produced ($\dot{V}CO_2$). At moderate to high levels of exercise, however, $\dot{V}_E$ increases disproportionately relative to $\dot{V}O_2$, but not to $\dot{V}CO_2$.

Anaerobic or Ventilatory Threshold

The abrupt increase in minute ventilation (also known as the gas exchange anaerobic threshold) presumably signifies the peak level of submaximal exercise at which energy demands exceed the circulation's ability to sustain aerobic metabolism (12). The physiology underlying the inflection in $\dot{V}_E$ may be attributed, at least in part, to the buffering of lactic acid by sodium bicarbonate in the blood, according to the following reaction:

$$\underset{\text{(lactic acid)}}{HLa} + \underset{\text{(sodium bicarbonate)}}{NaHCO_3} \rightarrow \underset{\text{(sodium lactate)}}{NaLa} + \underset{\text{(carbonic acid)}}{H_2CO_3}$$

$$\rightarrow H_2O + CO_2$$

As a result, CO_2 is released in excess of that produced by muscle metabolism, presumably providing an additional stimulus for minute ventilation. Accordingly, values for $\dot{V}_E$ and CO_2 production increase out of proportion to the intensity of exercise performed, suggesting an abrupt increase in serum lactate (13). Although there is controversy surrounding the mechanisms responsible for the anaerobic or ventilatory threshold (14), several studies now suggest that this variable represents an important predictor of performance in endurance events (15–17).

MEASUREMENT OF $\dot{V}O_2$max

Submaximal and maximal oxygen consumption can be assessed noninvasively by measuring the volume and analyzing the oxygen content of expired air, corrected to standard temperature and pressure dry, using the following equation:

$$\dot{V}O_2 = \dot{V}_E\,(F_{IO_2} - F_{EO_2})$$

where: $\dot{V}_E$ is the expired measured volume per minute;

F_{IO_2} is the concentration of oxygen in the inspired air; normal room air is 0.2093; and

F_{EO_2} is the directly measured concentration of oxygen in the expired air.

Traditionally, $\dot{V}O_2$max has been measured during the final minutes of exercise using an open circuit or Douglas bag technique. However, several automated systems are now available.

Maximal oxygen consumption may be expressed on an absolute basis in liters per minute, reflecting total body energy output and caloric expenditure, where each liter of oxygen is equivalent to approximately 5 kilocalories (kcal). However, since large persons usually have a large absolute oxygen consumption simply by virtue of their large muscle mass, physiologists generally divide this value by body weight in kilograms (kg) to allow a more equitable comparison between individuals of different size. This variable, when expressed in millili-

TABLE 8–3. *Average $\dot{V}O_2max$ values (mL/kg/min) of healthy active and sedentary men and women per decade*[a]

Age (years)	Men: Active 69.7 − 0.612 years	Men: Sedentary[b] 57.8 − 0.445 years	Women: Active 42.9 − 0.312 years	Women: Sedentary[b] 42.3 − 0.356 years
20	57.5	48.9	36.7	35.2
30	51.3	44.5	33.5	31.6
40	45.2	40.0	30.4	28.1
50	39.1	35.6	27.3	24.5
60	33.0	31.1	24.2	20.9
70	26.9	26.7	21.1	17.4

[a] $\dot{V}O_2max$ for any age can be predicted using the above-referenced regression equations (from ref. 19).
[b] Defined as subjects who do not exert themselves sufficiently to develop sweating at least once a week.

ters of oxygen per kilogram per minute (mL/kg/min), is considered the best single index of physical work capacity or cardiorespiratory fitness (18).

Average values of $\dot{V}O_2max$, expressed as mL/kg/min, expected in healthy men and women can be predicted from the regression equations shown in Table 8–3 (19).

Estimation of $\dot{V}O_2max$

Because it is inconvenient to measure oxygen consumption directly, as it requires sophisticated equipment, technical expertise, and frequent calibration, physiologists have increasingly sought to predict or estimate $\dot{V}O_2max$ from the treadmill speed and percentage grade (Fig. 8–4), or the cycle ergometer work load, expressed as kilogram meters per minute. The conventional Bruce treadmill protocol (Fig. 8–5) is perhaps the most familiar and widely used because it offers a rapid and safe exercise progression for which normative values for heart

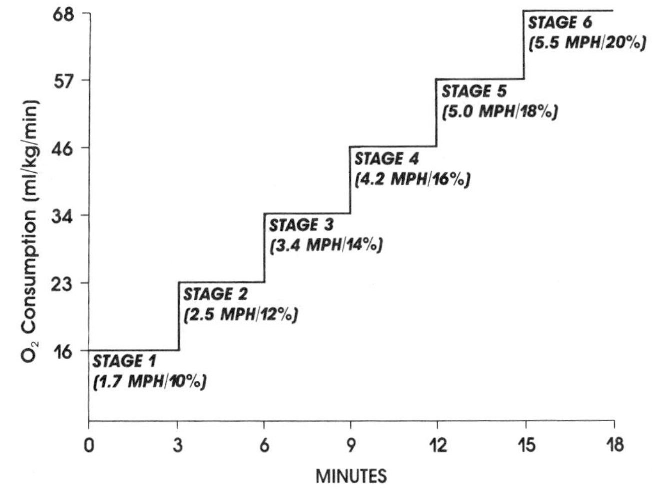

FIG. 8–5. The standard Bruce treadmill protocol showing progressive stages (speed, percentage grade) and the corresponding aerobic requirement, expressed as mL/kg/min.

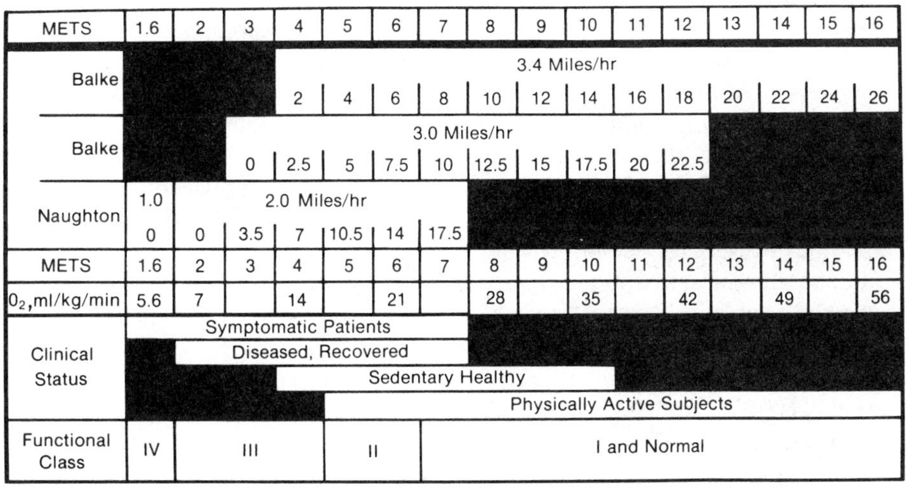

METS 1.6 2 3 4 5 6 7 8 9 10 11 12 13 14 15 16
Balke
3.4 Miles/hr
2 4 6 8 10 12 14 16 18 20 22 24 26
Balke
3.0 Miles/hr
0 2.5 5 7.5 10 12.5 15 17.5 20 22.5
Naughton
1.0
2.0 Miles/hr
0 0 3.5 7 10.5 14 17.5
METS 1.6 2 3 4 5 6 7 8 9 10 11 12 13 14 15 16
O2,ml/kg/min 5.6 7 14 21 28 35 42 49 56
Clinical Status
Symptomatic Patients
Diseased, Recovered
Sedentary Healthy
Physically Active Subjects
Functional Class
IV
III
II
I and Normal

FIG. 8–4. Metabolic cost of selected treadmill test protocols. Numbers refer to treadmill speed (miles/hour) and percentage grade. Oxygen consumption is expressed as mL/kg/min and as metabolic equivalents (METs).

rate, blood pressure, and oxygen uptake have been established (19).

The variability of O_2 consumption (expressed as liters per minute) on the cycle ergometer is small because of the constant external work load or power output (expressed in kilogram meters per minute [kgm/min]) and comparable efficiency among subjects. Because cycle ergometer testing is independent of body weight, there is a marked variability in O_2 consumption expressed on a relative basis as milliliters per kilogram per minute. With treadmill exercise, where the body weight is supported by the legs at a given speed and percentage grade, one sees a similar $\dot{V}O_2$ for all individuals when expressed as milliliters per kilogram per minute, and a larger variation when it is reported as liters per minute.

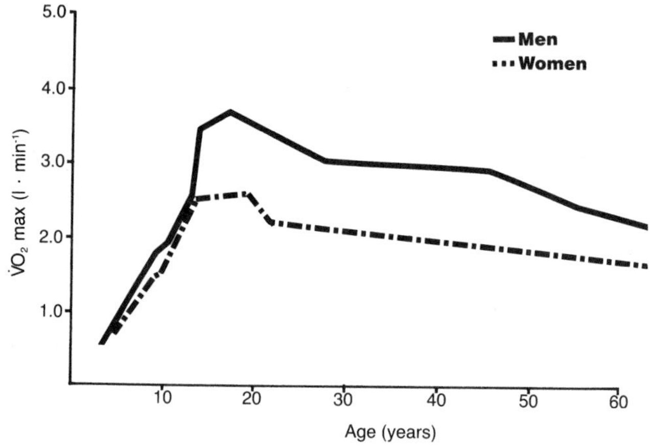

FIG. 8–6. Influence of age on maximal oxygen consumption ($\dot{V}O_2$max) in males and females. Before the age of 12, the values for boys and girls are comparable. A peak in $\dot{V}O_2$max occurs between 15 and 20 years of age followed by a gradual decline with advancing age. (Adapted from ref. 22.)

PHYSIOLOGIC VARIATIONS IN MAXIMAL OXYGEN CONSUMPTION

The functional reserve capacity of the cardiovascular and respiratory systems, largely reflected by the $\dot{V}O_2$max, is adversely affected by age, disuse, and disease. Differences in body size, muscle mass, extremities involved (arms versus legs), age, gender, habitual level of activity, physical conditioning, and athletic training also account for much of the physiologic variation in $\dot{V}O_2$max.

Numerous studies have examined the relationships among $\dot{V}O_2$max, body size, and muscle mass (18,20). Collectively, these findings suggest that the $\dot{V}O_2$max, expressed as L/min, is highly dependent on the amount of lean tissue in the body. Because large persons usually have a large absolute $\dot{V}O_2$max simply by virtue of their greater muscle mass, this cardiorespiratory variable is frequently expressed relative to body weight, that is, in mL/kg/min, to provide a more equitable comparison between persons of different size.

Maximal oxygen consumption ($\dot{V}O_2$max) during arm exercise generally approximates 70% ± 10% of the leg $\dot{V}O_2$max (21). Consequently, an individual with a leg $\dot{V}O_2$max of 35 mL/kg/min (10 METs) would have an estimated arm $\dot{V}O_2$max of 24.5 mL/kg/min or 7 ± 1 METs. Because leg and arm exercise testing generally offers only a poor to fair predictor of arm and leg aerobic capacity, respectively, arm exercise testing appears to be the functional evaluation of choice for persons whose recreational and/or athletic training activities are dominated by upper extremity efforts.

The influence of age and gender on maximal oxygen consumption is shown in Fig. 8–6. Although there is little difference in $\dot{V}O_2$max (L/min) among prepubertal boys and girls, considerable differences are apparent between the sexes following the onset of the teen years (22). $\dot{V}O_2$max values for adult women average approximately 20% ± 5% lower than for men. These differences may be related to changes in the habitual level of physical activity as well as physiologic variations, including more body fat, less metabolically active muscle mass, and lower hemoglobin concentrations in women than men.

Cross-sectional and longitudinal studies have shown that after the age of 20, $\dot{V}O_2$max typically declines by about 1% per year (23). Part of this decline is the inevitable result of biologic aging, with associated decreases in pulmonary and tissue gas exchange, maximum breathing capacity, maximum heart rate, stroke volume, and muscle mass, but part is probably also a consequence of increased sedentary living.

A classic study in the late 1960s showed that the effect of prolonged bed rest on aerobic fitness is exactly opposite of that of exercise (24). After 3 weeks of bed rest, healthy subjects had a 27% lower $\dot{V}O_2$max. The reduction in aerobic capacity was primarily attributed to a 29% decrease in maximal stroke volume, since maximal arteriovenous oxygen difference and heart rate remained essentially unchanged. Fortunately, the baseline (i.e., pre–bed rest) aerobic fitness of these subjects returned within weeks of resuming physical activity. The higher the initial level of fitness of the subject, the longer the period of training that was required to restore the pre–bed rest aerobic capacity.

Endurance-type exercise training generally augments the $\dot{V}O_2$max by ~15%; however, even greater relative improvements are observed in unfit or deconditioned persons. Among previously sedentary middle-aged and older men and women, this may be extrapolated to a 15-year functional rejuvenation (i.e., aerobic capacity approximates that of an untrained individual who is 15 years younger). Improvement in aerobic capacity with exercise training generally shows an inverse relationship with age, habitual physical activity, and initial $\dot{V}O_2$max, and a positive correlation with the conditioning frequency, intensity, and duration.

CARDIOVASCULAR AND METABOLIC ADAPTATIONS TO TRAINING

Exercise physiologists have traditionally regarded oxygen transport, particularly increased maximal cardiac output, as the primary mechanism of improvement in $\dot{V}O_2$max after training. Cardiovascular morphologic characteristics such as central blood volume and total hemoglobin appear to increase with regular exercise (25). Enlargement in cardiac dimension (e.g., left ventricular end-diastolic volume) and improved pump function (increased cardiac output and stroke volume) are also consistent findings in athletes and other healthy persons after physical conditioning (1).

Advances in our understanding of the adaptations to physical training have highlighted the importance of peripheral mechanisms as well in enhancing the $\dot{V}O_2$max. Specifically, studies involving the biopsy removal of human muscle tissue have shown an improvement in the metabolic preparedness of the muscle cells as a result of structural and enzymatic adaptations.

Endurance exercise training has been shown to increase the oxidative capacity of skeletal muscle through increases in the size and/or number of skeletal muscle mitochondria, as well as increases in oxidative enzymes (26). Increases in skeletal muscle capillary density also occur with regular training. The result appears to be a decreased cardiac output and muscle blood flow at any given submaximal work load or oxygen uptake; that is, the muscle needs and receives a smaller blood flow than before training. Thus, there is better utilization of available blood flow, resulting in economy and reserve capacity with respect to cardiac work.

The hemodynamic advantage of a more efficient distribution of cardiac output and increased oxidative capacity of skeletal muscle is reflected by a decreased lactate release and a lowered respiratory exchange ratio at any given level of exercise, with increases in arteriovenous oxygen difference at submaximal and maximal exercise. It is interesting that peripheral adaptations occur in both athletes and young, healthy individuals who show an increased arteriovenous oxygen difference at maximal exercise, whereas with middle-aged and older individuals the increases in $\dot{V}O_2$max are predominantly due to increases in stroke volume and cardiac output (27). Thus, improvement in $\dot{V}O_2$max may be achieved by the central and/or peripheral adaptations listed in Table 8–4.

TABLE 8–4. *Mechanisms responsible for ↑ $\dot{V}O_2$max with physical conditioning*

Central
1. ↑ cardiac output and stroke volume at maximal exercise (predominantly normals)
2. ↑ central blood volume and total hemoglobin
Peripheral
1. ↑ size and number of skeletal muscle mitochondria
2. ↑ myoglobin (↑ O_2 storage)
3. ↑ oxidative enzymes (e.g., succinate dehydrogenase, cytochrome oxidase)
4. ↑ skeletal muscle capillary density
5. ↓ cardiac output (↓ muscle blood flow) at a given submaximal work load
6. ↑ arteriovenous oxygen difference at submaximal and maximal work loads

↑, increase; ↓, decrease. The brackets signify that, collectively, variables 1–4 lead to the adaptations shown in 5 and 6.

Training Specificity

Numerous studies have investigated the cardiorespiratory and metabolic adaptations of trained versus untrained muscles to physical conditioning. Results have generally shown that arm and leg training cause only minor improvements in submaximal and maximal leg and arm exercise responses, respectively. After endurance training of one limb or set of limbs, several investigators have reported increases in $\dot{V}O_2$max and anaerobic (ventilatory) threshold or decreases in heart rate (Fig. 8–7) (28), blood lactate (29), pulmonary ventilation (30), ventilatory equivalent (Fig. 8–8), blood pressure, and perceived exertion during submaximal exercise with trained but not untrained limbs. These limb-specific training effects imply that a substantial portion of the conditioning response is attributed to peripheral factors, for example, alterations in blood flow and cellular and enzymatic adaptations in the trained limbs alone (26).

DYNAMIC VERSUS ISOMETRIC EXERCISE

Isometric exertion involves sustained muscle contraction against an immovable load or resistance with no change in length of the involved muscle group or joint motion. Stroke volume remains largely unchanged except at high levels of tension, where it may decrease (31). The result is a moderate increase in cardiac output, which is nevertheless high for the increase in metabolism. Despite the increased cardiac output, blood flow to the noncontracting muscle does not significantly increase, probably because of reflex vasoconstriction. The combination of vasoconstriction and increased cardiac output causes a disproportionate rise in systolic, diastolic, and mean blood pressure. Thus, a significant pres-

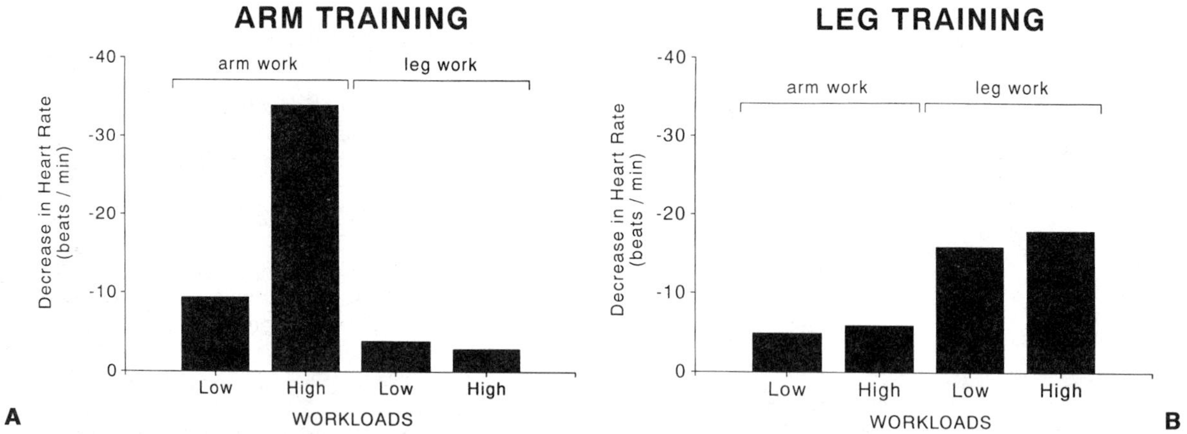

FIG. 8–7. **A**: Arm training using a cycle ergometer markedly decreased the heart rate responses during arm exercise at low and high work loads, whereas the heart rate reduction during leg work was small. **B**: Similarly, leg training markedly decreased the heart rate during leg work, whereas the heart rate reduction during arm work was minimal. (Adapted from ref. 28.)

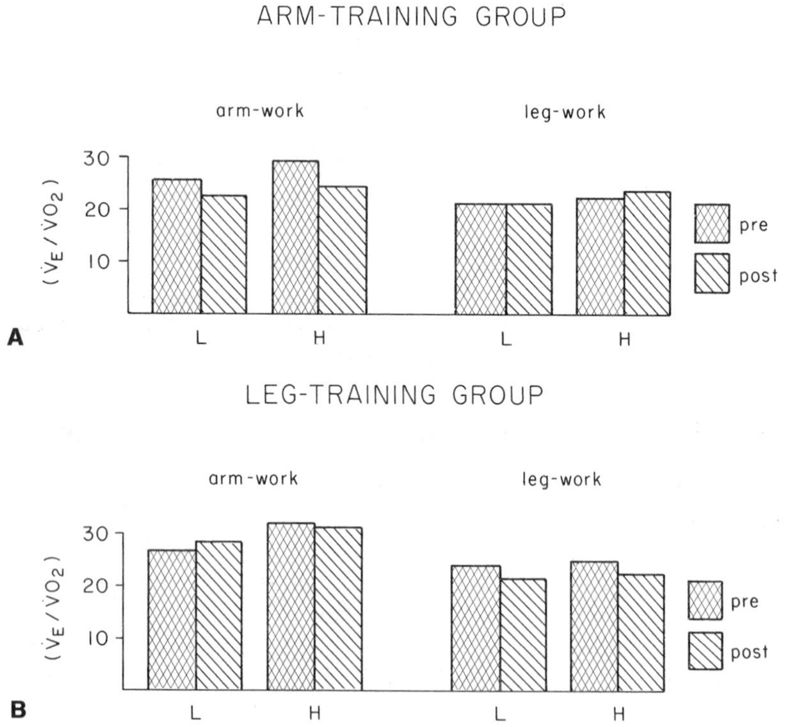

FIG. 8–8. Ventilatory equivalents ($\dot{V}_E/\dot{V}O_2$) during light (*L*) and heavy (*H*) submaximal arm and leg work before and after (**A**) arm training and (**B**) leg training. (Adapted from ref. 30.)

TABLE 8–5. *Comparison of the relative hemodynamic responses to dynamic and static exertion*

	Dynamic (isotonic)	Static (isometric)
Cardiac output	++++	+
Heart rate	++	+
Stroke volume	++	0 → −
Peripheral resistance	−	+++
Systolic blood pressure	+++	++++
Diastolic blood pressure	0 → −	++++
Mean arterial pressure	0 → +	++++
Left ventricular work	Volume load	Pressure load

+, increase; −, decrease; 0, unchanged.

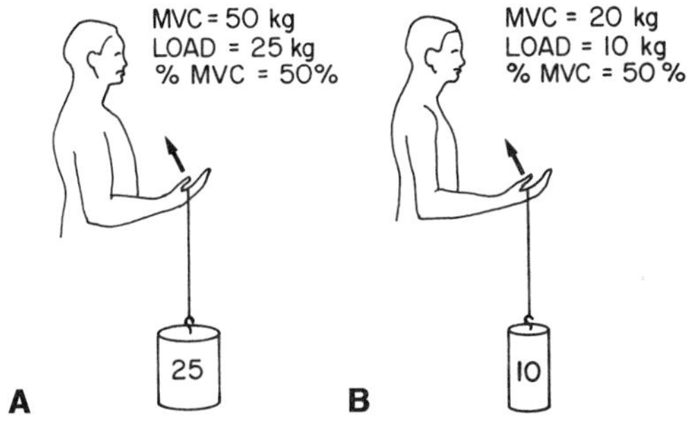

FIG. 8–9. The hemodynamic response to isometric exertion is proportional, in part, to the percentage of maximal voluntary contraction (% MVC) of the muscle group involved. The heart rate and blood pressure response depend on the tension exerted relative to the greatest tension possible in the muscle group. A high degree of tension exerted by a stronger person (**A**) will produce approximately the same heart rate and blood pressure response as a low tension representing an equivalent relative tension (% MVC) developed by a weaker person (**B**), if all other factors are equal.

sure load is imposed on the heart, presumably to increase perfusion to the active (contracting) skeletal muscle. A comparison of the relative hemodynamic responses to dynamic and isometric exercise is shown in Table 8–5.

Sustained isometric exertion is characterized by a pressor response that is proportionate to the relative intensity [percentage of maximal voluntary contraction (Fig. 8–9)] (31), duration, and muscle mass involved (32). Consequently, increased muscular strength should result in attenuated heart rate and blood pressure responses to any given load (33), since the load now represents a lower percentage of the maximal voluntary contraction.

REFERENCES

1. Kaimal KP, Franklin BA, Moir TW, et al. Cardiac profiles of national-class race walkers. *Chest* 1993;104:935–938.
2. Mathews DK, Fox EL. *The physiological basis of physical education and athletics,* 2nd ed. Philadelphia: WB Saunders, 1997:14.
3. Mitchell JH, Blomqvist G. Maximal oxygen uptake. *N Engl J Med* 1971;284:1018–1022.
4. Balke B. Experimental studies on the functional capacities of middle-aged and aging persons. *J Okla State Med Assoc* 1961;54:120–123.
5. Wilson PK, Bell CW, Norton AC. *Rehabilitation of the heart and lungs.* Fullerton, CA: Beckman Instruments, 1980:68.
6. Franklin BA, Fletcher GF, Gordon NF, et al. Cardiovascular evaluation of the athlete. *Sports Med* 1997;24(2):97–119.
7. Wilmore JH, Norton AC. *The heart and lungs at work: a primer of exercise physiology.* Schiller Park, IL: Beckman Instruments, 1975:2.
8. Poliner LR, Dehmer GJ, Lewis SE. Left ventricular performance in normal subjects: a comparison of the responses to exercise in the upright and supine position. *Circulation* 1980;62:528–534.
9. Rowell LB. Circulation. *Med Sci Sports* 1969;1:15–22.
10. Zobl EG, Talmers FN, Christensen RC, et al. Effect of exercise on the cerebral circulation and metabolism. *J Appl Physiol* 1965;20:1289–1293.
11. Rowell LB, Murray JA, Brengelmann GL, et al. Human cardiovascular adjustments to rapid changes in skin temperature during exercise. *Circ Res* 1969;24:711–724.
12. Wasserman K, Whipp BJ, Koyal SN, et al. Anaerobic threshold and respiratory gas exchange during exercise. *J Appl Physiol* 1973;35:236–243.
13. Davis JA, Vodak P, Wilmore JH, et al. Anaerobic threshold and maximal aerobic power for three modes of exercise. *J Appl Physiol* 1976;41:544–550.
14. Jones N, Ehrsam R. The anaerobic threshold. *Exerc Sport Sci Rev* 1982;10:49–83.
15. Costill DL. Physiology of marathon running. *JAMA* 1972;221:1024–1029.
16. Costill DL, Fox EL. Energetics of marathon running. *Med Sci Sports* 1969;1:81–86.
17. Costill DL, Thomason H, Roberts E. Fractional utilization of the aerobic capacity during distance running. *Med Sci Sports* 1973;5:248–252.
18. Buskirk E, Taylor HL. Maximal oxygen intake and its relation to body composition, with specific reference to chronic physical activity and obesity. *J Appl Physiol* 1957;2:72–78.
19. Bruce RA, Kusumi F, Hosmer D. Maximal oxygen intake and nomographic assessment of functional aerobic impairment in cardiovascular disease. *Am Heart J* 1973;85:546–562.
20. Von Dobeln W. Human standard and maximal metabolic rate in relation to fat-free body mass. *Acta Physiol Scand* 1956;37(suppl 126).
21. Franklin BA. Exercise testing, training and arm ergometry. *Sports Med* 1985;2:100–119.
22. Åstrand PO. *Health and fitness.* Stockholm: Universaltryck, 1973:12.
23. Dehn MM, Bruce RA. Longitudinal variations in maximal oxygen intake with age and activity. *J Appl Physiol* 1972;33:805–807.
24. Saltin B, Blomqvist G, Mitchell JH, et al. Response to exercise after bed rest and after training. *Circulation* 1968;38(suppl 7): 1–78.
25. Grande F, Taylor H. Adaptive changes in the heart, vessels, and patterns of control under chronically high loads. In: Hamilton WF, ed. *Handbook of physiology—Circulation,* vol 3. Washington, DC: American Physiological Society, 1965:2615–2677.
26. Henriksson J, Reitman JS. Time course of changes in human skeletal muscle succinate dehydrogenase and cytochrome oxidase activities and maximal oxygen uptake with physical activity and inactivity. *Acta Physiol Scand* 1977;99:91–97.
27. Hartley LH, Grimby G, Kilbom A, et al. Physical training in sedentary middle-aged and older men: III. Cardiac output and gas exchange at submaximal and maximal exercise. *Scand J Clin Lab Invest* 1969;24:335–344.
28. Clausen JP, Trap-Jensen J, Lassen NA. The effects of training on the heart rate during arm and leg exercise. *Scand J Clin Lab Invest* 1970;26:295–301.
29. Klausen K, Rasmussen B, Clausen JP, et al. Blood lactate from

exercising extremities before and after arm or leg training. *Am J Physiol* 1974;227:67–72.
30. Rasmussen B, Klausen K, Clausen JP, et al. Pulmonary ventilation, blood gases and blood pH after training of the arms or the legs. *J Appl Physiol* 1975;38:250–256.
31. Lind AR, McNichol GW. Muscular factors which determine the cardiovascular responses to sustained and rhythmic exercise. *Can Med Assoc J* 1967;96:706–715.
32. Mitchell JH, Payne FC, Saltin B, et al. The role of muscle mass in the cardiovascular response to static contractions. *J Physiol* 1980;309:45–54.
33. McCartney N, McKelvie RS, Martin J, et al. Weight-training-induced attenuation of the circulatory response of older males to weightlifting. *J Appl Physiol* 1993;74:1056–1060.

Exercise and Sport Science,
edited by William E. Garrett, Jr., and Donald T. Kirkendall.
Lippincott Williams & Wilkins, Philadelphia © 2000.

CHAPTER 9

Pulmonary Responses to Exercise and Training

Dale D. Brown

The primary role of the respiratory system is that of a support system for the maintenance of cellular function. As depicted in Fig. 9–1, the respiratory system is one of several bodily systems that function with an integrated approach aimed at optimizing cellular activity. Although each system on its own is important, all systems are interdependent for the functions of each system to be achieved. This integrated approach can be represented by the Fick equation, which describes bodily function with respect to oxygen consumption:

$$\underset{\text{Oxygen consumption}}{\dot{V}O_2\,(\text{L/min})} = \underset{\text{Cardiac output}}{Q\,(\text{L/min})} \times \underset{\text{Arteriovenous oxygen difference}}{a - vO_2\,(\text{mL/L})} \quad [1]$$

Although the equation appears simple in form, numerous systems and factors affect the functionality of the Fick equation. Whereas total body oxygen consumption (i.e., cellular function) is obviously dependent on blood flow produced by the cardiovascular system, the ability to produce adequate cardiac output is a complex component affected by many different variables. Factors such as stroke volume, heart rate, diastolic filling time, contractility, venous return, blood viscosity, neural and endocrine cardiac-control mechanisms, vascular resistance, intrathoracic pressure, and others are all contributors to overall cardiovascular function. Additionally, the arteriovenous oxygen difference, although obvious in its presence in the Fick equation and simple in definition, is affected by and dependent on numerous physiological factors. Determinants of arteriovenous oxygen difference can be divided into those factors that affect the components of arterial oxygenation versus the mixed venous oxygen component. Although the respiratory system anatomy and physiology mainly affect arterial oxygenation, venous oxygenation is dependent on cellular activity. Arterial oxygenation is obviously dependent on adequate airflow and gas exchange produced by the respiratory system, but the ability to produce adequate arterial oxygenation is affected by numerous variables. Factors such as tidal volume, respiratory rate, distribution of ventilatory volume (i.e., alveolar and dead-space ventilation), chest-wall mechanics, altitude, inspired and alveolar oxygen pressures, red blood cell volume, pulmonary blood flow distribution, pulmonary capillary transit time, lung disease, and others are all contributors to overall effective arterial oxygenation. Venous oxygenation is no less complex, with factors such as cellular oxygen extraction, redistribution of blood flow, the dynamic nature of the oxygen–hemoglobin dissociation curve, cellular metabolic demand, cellular fuel supply, and other factors affecting venous oxygenation. The Fick equation therefore represents an integrated approach to understand bodily function rather a simple way of describing or calculating oxygen consumption.

Equally impressive as the complexity of the Fick equation are the adaptations in the components of the equation that occur from the resting state to one of physical exercise (Table 9–1). Whereas the changes in cardiovascular responses during the transition from rest to exercise are substantial (five- to sevenfold increases in cardiac output and two- to threefold increases in both heart rate and stroke volume), the acute adaptations to exercise for the respiratory system are even more remarkable. Respiratory rate has a four- to fivefold increase during exercise in comparison to resting conditions, tidal volume increases five- to sevenfold, and minute ventilation can increase 20 to 30 times over resting airflow values. The effect of respiratory system alterations is the maintenance of arterial oxygenation at or near preexercise levels, even in very heavy exercise.

D. D. Brown: Department of Health, Physical Education, and Recreation, Illinois State University, Normal, Illinois 61790-5120.

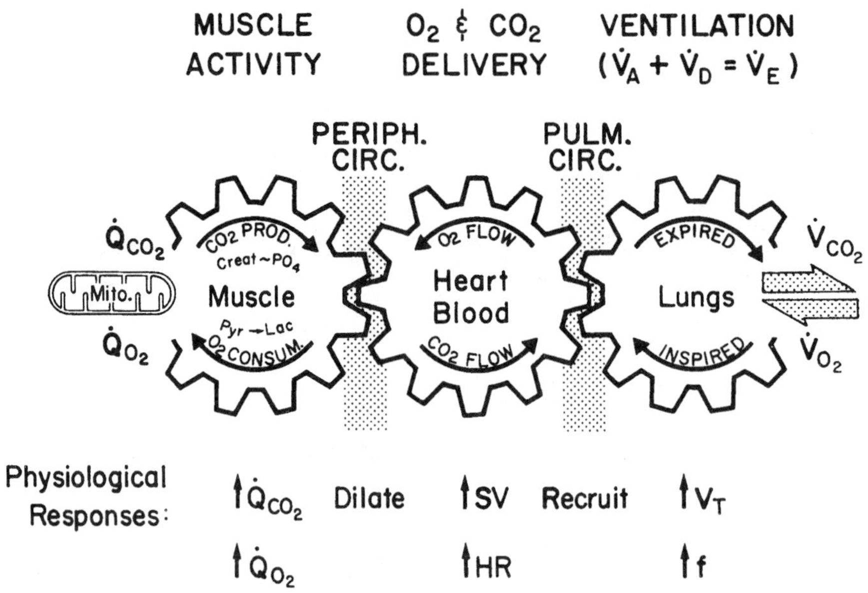

FIG. 9–1. A scheme illustrating the gas-transport mechanisms for coupling cellular (internal) to pulmonary (external) respiration. The gears represent the functional interdependence of the physiological components of the system. The large increase in O_2 use by the muscles (Qo_2) is achieved by increased extraction of O_2 from the blood perfusing the muscles, the dilatation of selected peripheral vascular beds, an increase in cardiac output (stroke volume and heart rate), an increase in pulmonary blood flow by recruitment and vasodilatation of pulmonary blood vessels, and finally, an increase in ventilation. O_2 is taken up (Vo_2) from the alveoli in proportion to the pulmonary blood flow and degree of O_2 desaturation of hemoglobin in the pulmonary blood. In the steady state, $Vo_2 = Qo_2$. Ventilation [tidal volume (*VT*) and breathing frequency (*f*)] increase in relation to the newly produced CO_2 (Qco_2) arriving at the lungs and the drive to achieve arterial CO_2 and hydrogen ion homeostasis. These variables are related in the following way:

$$Vco_2 = VA \times P_aco_2/PB$$

where Vco_2 is the minute CO_2 production, VA is the minute alveolar ventilation, P_aco_2 is the arterial CO_2 tension, and PB is the barometric pressure. The representation of gears as uniformly sized is not intended to imply equal changes in each of the components of the coupling. For instance, the increase in cardiac output is proportionally smaller than the increase in metabolic rate. This results in an increased extraction of O_2 from, and CO_2 loading into, the blood by the muscle. In contrast, at moderate work intensities, minute ventilation increases in approximate proportion to the new CO_2 brought to the lungs by the venous return. The development of metabolic acidosis, at heavy and very heavy work intensities, results in an increased ventilation to provide respiratory compensation for the metabolic acidosis. From ref. 41, with permission.

TABLE 9–1. *Alterations in the Fick equation variables from rest to maximal exercise*

	Vo_2 (mL/min)	=	HR (beats/min)	×	SV (L/beat) (EDV − ESV)	×	(ao_2 − vo_2) (mL/L)		(mL/L)
Untrained subject at rest	280	=	80	×	0.070 (0.120 − 0.050)	×	200	−	150
Untrained subject during exercise	3080	=	200	×	0.110 (0.155 − 0.045)	×	200	−	60
Trained subject during exercise	3458	=	190	×	0.130 (0.165 − 0.035)	×	200	−	60
Endurance-trained subject during exercise	5595	=	190	×	0.190 (0.220 − 0.030)	×	200	−	45

TABLE 9–2. *Nonrespiratory functions of the respiratory system*

Nonrespiratory function	Specific example
Elimination of volatile substances: chemicals that can be transformed and eliminated from the body through respiratory system function	Alcohol, garlic, acetone, dimethyl sulfoxide (DMSO), etc.
Detoxification of the blood: degradation of blood-borne chemicals occurs as a result of the respiratory system activity	Hormone degradation (e.g., prostaglandins, norepinephrine)
Biosynthesis of molecules: production of various chemicals is the result of respiratory system activity	Mucus, lipid (surfactant), proteins (anti-trypsin)
Endocrine functions: in addition to detoxification of various hormones, the respiratory system produces hormones	Hormone synthesis (e.g., angiotensin, heparin, histamine, serotonin)
Immunologic function: as the system of contact between the body and the external environment, the respiratory system contains defense mechanisms	A variety of immunologic functions occur as the first line of defense against infection for the body
Phonation	Formation of speech sounds

With arterial oxygenation maintained, the threefold increase in the arteriovenous oxygen difference is therefore accomplished as the venous oxygenation decreases because of greater cellular extraction of arterial oxygen. The net effect of these and other physiological adaptations to exercise is a 20- to 25-fold increase in oxygen consumption over resting values. This is truly a remarkable feat.

ROLE OF THE RESPIRATORY SYSTEM

With that preface in mind, this chapter focuses specifically on the respiratory system anatomy and physiology and their contributions to human body function. In general the respiratory system has two main functions: ventilation and gas exchange. Although cellular oxygen consumption is commonly cited as a third function of the respiratory system, oxygen consumption more accurately reflects cellular activity rather than any particular changes associated with the respiratory system, other than being the location where it is conveniently measured. In addition to the respiratory functions, the respiratory system provides several, less-often-mentioned vital nonrespiratory functions (Table 9–2). These homeostatic functions are not only required for optimal function of the respiratory system but are also vital in the regulation and coordination of the human body (1). Although these nonrespiratory functions are important, the remaining discussion examines the respiratory system anatomy and physiology pertinent to accomplishing the respiratory functions of ventilation and gas exchange.

RESPIRATORY SYSTEM ANATOMY

Anatomically the respiratory system can be divided into three general structural areas: the respiratory pump, the respiratory passageways, and the air that is ventilated. The ability to produce the respiratory functions of the respiratory system is dependent on the interaction and interrelation of these three accompanying anatomic structures. The anatomic structures associated with each of these respiratory components are identified in Table 9–3.

TABLE 9–3. *Respiratory system anatomy*

Respiratory pump (thorax)	Respiratory passageways (airways)	Room air (gases)
Bones	Conducting division	Oxygen, 20.93%
Sternum	Nasal cavity	Carbon dioxide, 0.03%
Ribs	Oral cavity	Nitrogen, 79.04%
Vertebrae	Pharynx	
Muscles	Larynx	
Inspiratory	Trachea	
Diaphragm	R & L primary bronchi	
External intercostals	Secondary bronchioles	
Scalenus	Segmental bronchioles	
Sternocleidomastoid	Terminal bronchioles	
Pectoralis minor	Respiratory division	
Expiratory	Respiratory bronchioles	
Internal intercostals	Alveolar duct	
Abdominals	Alveolar sacs (alveoli)	
Pleura and pleural cavity	(type I & II alveolar cells)	
Parietal pleura		
Visceral pleura		
Pleural fluid		

Respiratory System Pump

The respiratory pump or thorax is made up of skeletal and soft-tissue structures (skeletal muscles and pleural membranes). Although the rigid nature of the skeletal components of the thorax provides structural support, protection, and an attachment for skeletal muscles, it remains flexible and dynamic, thereby facilitating the alternating inspiratory and expiratory movements of the respiratory system. Contraction and relaxation of the inspiratory and expiratory muscles result in changes in thoracic cavity volume, which alters intrapulmonary pressure, allowing inspiration and expiration (i.e., pulmonary ventilation). The inspiratory phase of pulmonary ventilation is an active, energy-requiring process involving contraction of inspiratory muscles. During inspiratory muscle contraction, the thorax and thoracic cavity volume increase, producing a reduction in intrapulmonary pressure, causing pulmonary inspiration (1–4). Depending on the ventilatory needs, two different types of inspiration can occur. Normal quiet inspiration (such as that during resting situations) relies on the activity of the primary inspiratory muscles (diaphragm and external intercostals), which alter the thoracic cavity volume vertically and anteroposteriorly (Fig. 9–2). During the forced deep inspiration that accompanies heavy breathing (coughing, exercise, disease conditions), the secondary or accessory muscles augment the activity of the primary inspiratory muscles (3,4). Contraction of the scalenes, pectoralis minor, and sternocleidomastoid muscles increases the thorax vertically and anteroposteriorly, further increasing thoracic cavity volume and decreasing intrathoracic pressure to a larger extent than normal quiet inspiration (1,3–6). The anteroposterior movements produced by inspiratory muscle activity result in a 20% anteroposterior thickening of the thorax from maximal inspiration to expiration (5).

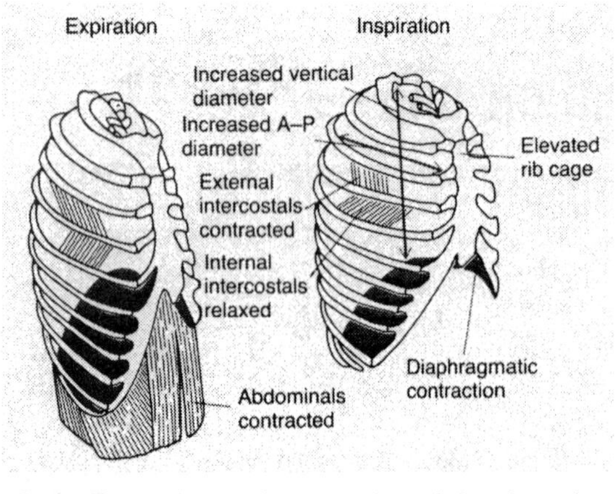

FIG. 9–2. Expansion and contraction of the thoracic cage during expiration and inspiration, illustrating especially diaphragmatic contraction, elevation of the rib cage, and function of the intercostals. From ref. 5, with permission.

The expiratory phase of pulmonary ventilation can be both an active, energy-requiring and a passive process. Whereas normal quiet expiration is a passive process produced by the recoil or relaxation of inspiratory muscles, forced expiration (e.g., coughing, sneezing, and heavy breathing) is an active process requiring contraction of expiratory muscles (1,5,7). During normal quiet expiration, the thoracic cavity volume is decreased due to the passive recoil of the inspiratory muscles. The result is an increased intrapulmonary pressure, causing pulmonary expiration to occur. When pulmonary ventilation demands increase during heavy or labored breathing, expiratory muscle contraction is needed to compress the thoracic cavity rapidly and forcefully. Expiratory muscle contraction of the thorax produces a decrease in thoracic cavity volume, increasing intrapulmonary pressure, resulting in pulmonary expiration. Contraction of the abdominal muscles (external and internal obliques, transverse abdominal, and rectus abdominis groups) occurs when the elastic recoil of the inspiratory muscles cannot provide adequate expiratory flow. Their contraction increases the intraabdominal pressure, forcing the diaphragm upward, decreasing the size of the thorax, and reducing thoracic cavity volume vertically and anteroposteriorly (1,5,7). The resulting effect is an increase in intrapulmonary pressure, causing expiration to occur. The activity of inspiratory and expiratory muscles is dependent on the metabolic demands placed on the body. As those demands are altered, respiratory muscle activity is altered to accommodate those demands. Progressive increases in ventilation or the need for ventilation requires the recruitment of additional inspiratory and expiratory muscles, with significant increases in ventilation (>100 L/min, requiring the recruitment of all inspiratory muscles) (Table 9–4) (1).

Respiratory System Airways

Alternating inspiratory and expiratory thoracic pump activity and the accompanying pressure fluctuations effectively produce pulmonary ventilation through respiratory passageways. The respiratory passageways that transport air from the external environment to the gas-exchange areas deep within the lungs are subdivided into conducting and respiratory division structures (Fig. 9–3). Branching of the respiratory passageways results in the development of numerous smaller-diameter airways. The tracheal branching into the right and left primary bronchi starts the formation of the bronchial tree, in which each airway branch (i.e., z-generation) divides into additional smaller branches, resulting in the formation of thousands of airways leading into the respiratory division of the respiratory system (Fig. 9–3*A*) (8,9). Continued branching of the airways in the respiratory zone yields millions of alveoli within the right and left lungs, thereby producing the location of

TABLE 9–4. *Summary of respiratory muscle action*

Level	Inspiration	Expiration
Quiet ventilation	Diaphragm in all subjects Intercostals in most subjects Scalenes in some subjects	Some persistence of inspiratory muscle contraction in expiration
Modest increase in ventilation (<50 L/min)	Diaphragm in all subjects Intercostals in most subjects Scalenes in some subjects	Some persistence of inspiratory muscle contraction in expiration
Moderate increase in ventilation (50–100 L/min)	Diaphragm in all subjects Intercostals in most subjects Scalenes in most subjects Sternocleidomastoid action toward end inspiration	Some persistence of inspiratory muscle contraction Abdominal and intercostals at end expiration
Significant increase in ventilation (>100 L/min)	All inspiratory accessories active	Abdominals active throughout inspiration

Reprinted with permission from Scanlon CL. *Egan's fundamentals of respiratory care.* 6th ed. St. Louis: Mosby, 1995.

greatest surface area within the respiratory system (Fig. 9–3*B*). Histologic characteristics associated with the z-generations dictates each structure's function. Whereas the respiratory division (z-generations 17 to 23) is composed of small-diameter, thin-walled structures, the conducting division (z-generations 1 to 16) anatomy is larger-diameter, thicker-walled components. The airways transform from cartilaginous, mucus-secreting, ciliated airways on the tracheal end of the conducting division to noncartilaginous, nonciliated, muscular airways in the bronchial end of the conducting division (Fig. 9–3*C*) (1,5,8,9). The changes of a reduction in hyaline cartilage and increasing percentage distribution of smooth muscle across the conducting division results in the smaller-sized bronchioles being the point of greatest resistance to airflow (1,5,9). This becomes most notable in the asthmatic individual, in whom bronchial constriction drastically alters normal airflow patterns as the airway becomes obstructed (10–12). Given the histologic characteristics and the wall thickness created by the tissues of the conducting division, these structures are incapable of allowing gas exchange to occur (Fig. 9–3*C*). The air ventilated into these areas then is considered to be occupying dead space; hence the term *anatomic dead-space ventilation* or *dead-space volume.* Although the conducting-division structures are not directly involved in gas exchange, they provide a large surface area for humidification, filtering, and warming of the ventilated inspiratory air (1,5,8,9).

Eventually the airways develop into single-celled air sacs at the point of the alveolus within the respiratory division of the respiratory system. In contrast to the conducting division, the respiratory-division airway structures are thin-walled structures made of a single cell layer, specifically the type I and type II alveolar cells (1,5,8,9). The air ventilated into these areas is considered to be occupying alveolar space; hence the term *alveolar volume* or *ventilation.* The walls of the respiratory-division structures are made up predominantly of squamous epithelial cells, called type I alveolar cells. The abundance of type I alveolar cells and their thinness yields a large surface area for gas exchange between the alveolar air and the pulmonary capillary blood (Fig. 9–4). The type II alveolar cells compose a much smaller proportion of the alveolar area and are more compact and not so effective as a gas-exchange structure. The type II alveolar cells produce and secrete surfactant that, when released, reduces the surface tension of alveolar fluids, discouraging alveolar collapse (1,5,8,9,13). The type I and II alveolar cells compose one side of the respiratory membrane; the other portion is made up of the endothelial cell layer of the pulmonary capillary bed. These cells are also squamous epithelial cells, which provide an effective area of the capillary for gas exchange to continue through the respiratory membrane. The two cell layers, alveolar epithelium and capillary epithelium, are separated by the interstitial fluid–filled interstitial space. Collectively these structures compose the respiratory membrane (see Fig. 9–4) (5). Although the respiratory membrane is relatively simple by design, several factors can affect gas exchange across this membrane, thereby affecting the rate of oxygen and carbon dioxide diffusion. Those factors are (a) thickness of the respiratory membrane, (b) surface area, (c) permeability of the respiratory membrane, (d) pressure gradient across the membrane for the O_2 and CO_2, (e) red blood cell and hemoglobin concentrations, and (f) capillary transit time.

Whereas the total volume of air ventilated in the respiratory system can vary from breath to breath, the maximal lung volume (i.e., total lung capacity) is relatively fixed, based on the anatomic constraints of the individual, although it varies among individuals (14,15). Total lung capacity can be subdivided into four primary lung volumes: (a) tidal volume, (b) inspiratory reserve volume, (c) expiratory reserve volume, and (d) residual

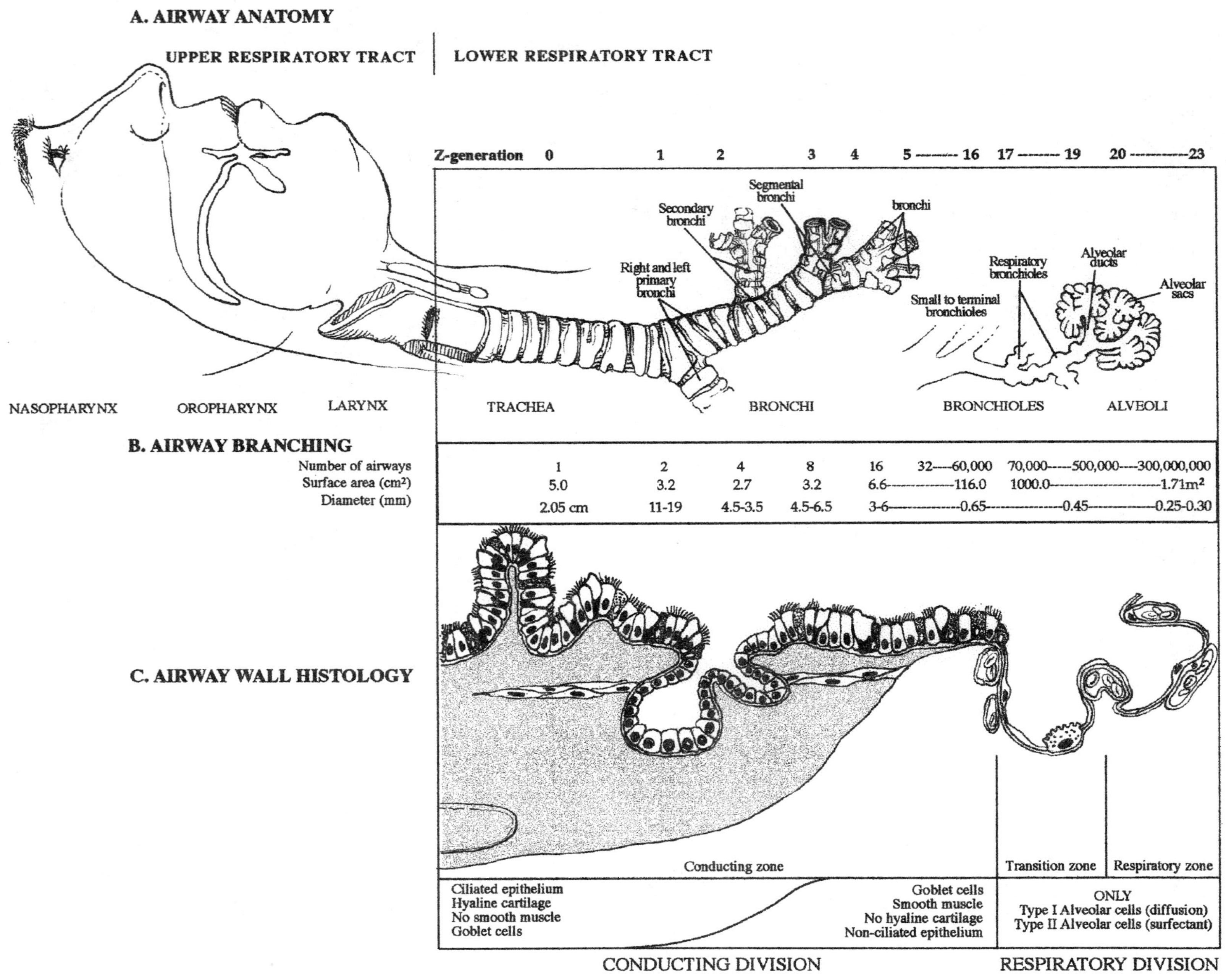

A. AIRWAY ANATOMY
UPPER RESPIRATORY TRACT
LOWER RESPIRATORY TRACT
Z-generation 0 1 2 3 4 5 ------- 16 17 ------- 19 20 ----------23
Secondary bronchi
Segmental bronchi
bronchi
Right and left primary bronchi
Respiratory bronchioles
Alveolar ducts
Alveolar sacs
Small to terminal bronchioles
NASOPHARYNX
OROPHARYNX
LARYNX
TRACHEA
BRONCHI
BRONCHIOLES
ALVEOLI
B. AIRWAY BRANCHING
Number of airways 1 2 4 8 16 32----60,000 70,000-----500,000----300,000,000
Surface area (cm²) 5.0 3.2 2.7 3.2 6.6--------------116.0 1000.0----------------------1.71m²
Diameter (mm) 2.05 cm 11-19 4.5-3.5 4.5-6.5 3-6--------------0.65---------------0.45-------------0.25-0.30
C. AIRWAY WALL HISTOLOGY
Conducting zone
Transition zone
Respiratory zone
Ciliated epithelium
Hyaline cartilage
No smooth muscle
Goblet cells
Goblet cells
Smooth muscle
No hyaline cartilage
Non-ciliated epithelium
ONLY
Type I Alveolar cells (diffusion)
Type II Alveolar cells (surfactant)
CONDUCTING DIVISION
RESPIRATORY DIVISION

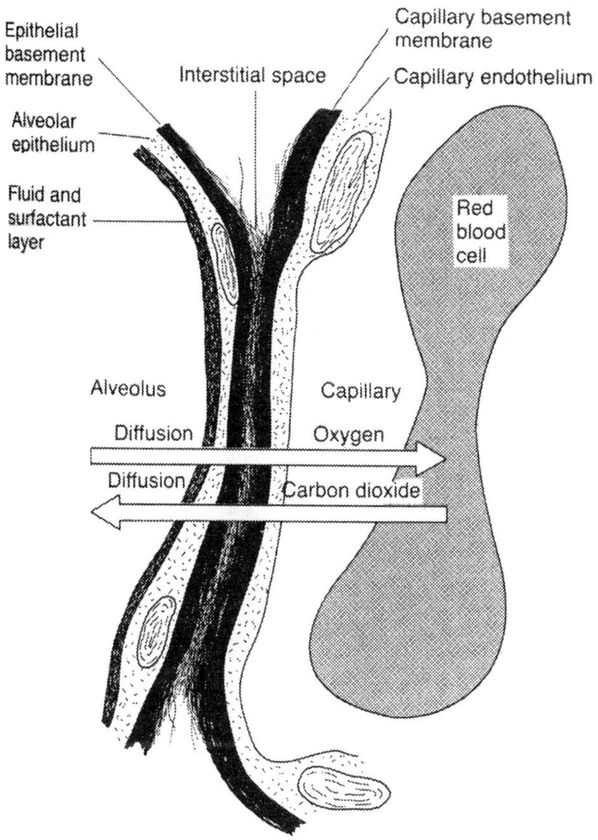

FIG. 9–4. Ultrastructure of the respiratory membrane as shown in cross section. From ref. 5, with permission.

volume (Fig. 9–5) (16). Tidal volume represents the amount of air ventilated per breath (either inspiration or expiration), but inspiratory and expiratory reserve volumes represent the amount of "unused" lung volume. Tidal volume and both inspiratory and expiratory reserve volumes exist in an inverse relation, such that as tidal volume increases, inspiratory and expiratory lung volumes decrease, and vice versa (see Fig. 9–5) (17–20). Whereas both reserve capacities are decreased with increases in tidal volume, the reductions are not equal, with a slightly greater reduction in inspiratory reserve volume as compared with expiratory reserve volume (21–24). From a functional standpoint, the potential volume of air that could be ventilated to accommodate airflow demand could equal the sum of the reserve volumes and tidal volume (i.e., vital capacity) (see Fig. 9–5). As the metabolic demand continues to increase, tidal volume would appear to be able to increase to the volume equaling vital capacity; however, the maximal tidal volume usually peaks at about 60% of an individual's vital capacity (17–19).

Residual volume reflects the air that remains in the respiratory passageways after a maximal forced expiration (Fig. 9–5) and typically averages 0.8 to 1.4 L, depending on gender, age, and body size (15). Although the respiratory system's response to the increased metabolic demand during exercise obviously necessitates the need for greater air flow (i.e., tidal volume increases), increases in residual volume also have been observed associated with exercise. Postexercise residual volume has been shown to increase by 10% to 20% immediately after exercise, and eventually it returns to preexercise levels, usually within 24 hours (25–33). It has been speculated that the reason for this change may be associated with the closure of small airways and an accumulation of pulmonary extravascular fluid accompanying exercise; however, the exact underlying mechanism explaining this change is not known (14).

PULMONARY RESPONSE TO ACUTE EXERCISE

Ventilation is the process of providing sufficient airflow through the respiratory passageways filling the gas-exchange areas in an attempt to accommodate the cellular needs of oxygen delivery and carbon dioxide removal. Whereas the resting ventilatory responses typically range from a respiratory rate of 10 to 12 breaths per minute, a tidal volume of approximately 0.5 L per breath and an airflow rate (i.e., minute ventilation) response of 5 to 6 L per minute, the exercise ventilation responses vary, depending on the intensity of the exercise. Changes in ventilatory dynamics during exercise alter these variables, producing acute adaptations to exercise for the respiratory system that are profoundly remarkable. Respiratory rate can increase five- to sixfold during maximal exercise with respiratory rates of 50 to 60 breaths per minute frequently reported. Accordingly, tidal volume is substantially altered from rest, with fivefold to sevenfold increases during maximal exercise and tidal volumes of greater than 3 L commonly observed. The net effect on minute ventilation is an astonishing 30- to 40-fold increase over resting airflow values with airflow rates approaching and exceeding 200

←

FIG. 9–3. Anatomy of the respiratory airways. **A**: Airway anatomy with corresponding z-generations for branches of the airways. **B**: Number of structures, surface area, and diameter of structures corresponding to the different z-generations. **C:** Respiratory airway histologic changes across the z-generations.

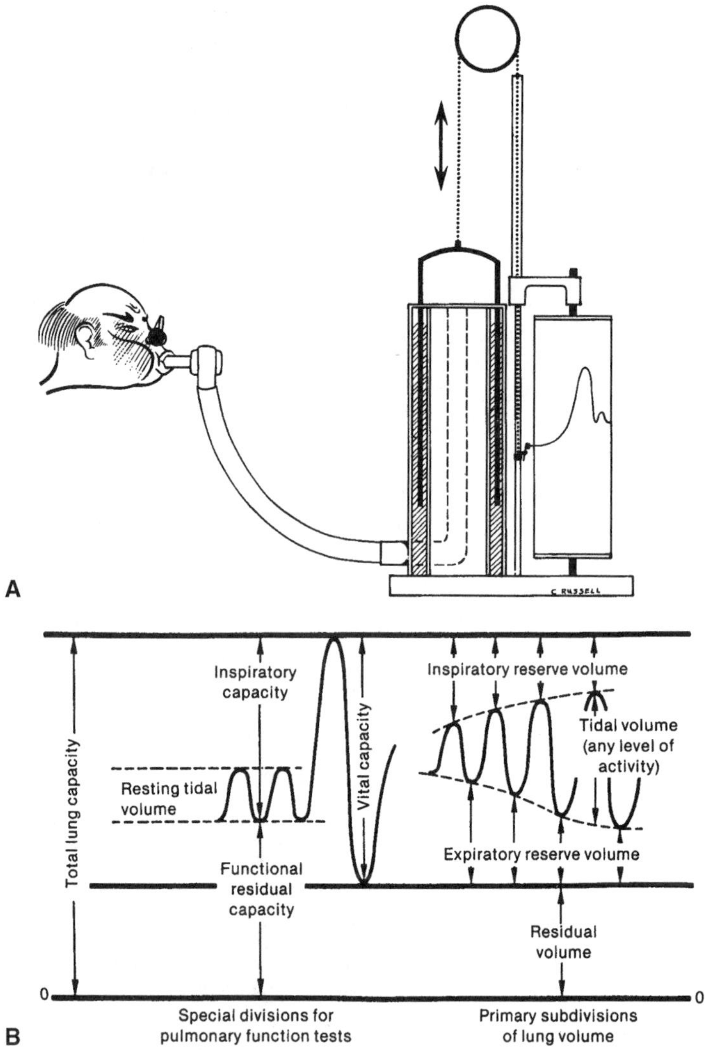

FIG. 9–5. A: A type of spirometer. Spirometers measure the volume of gas that the lungs inhale and exhale, usually as a function of time. They are used to measure the volume changes and flow rates of spontaneous breathing and various breathing maneuvers. **B**: Subdivisions of lung volumes. From ref. 16, with permission.

L per minute during maximal exercise in the highly trained male athlete. Although not as remarkable as the highly trained athlete, the untrained individual can produce some rather impressive changes in ventilatory dynamics during exercise. The extent to which these differences are related to physical training, anatomic limitations, or gender differences is not known, although it is logical to assume that the individual who is physically trained has better strength and endurance of the respiratory muscles.

The respiratory system's adaptation to the cellular demands during exercise is immediate, with an initial increase in ventilatory response occurring before exercise actually begins (34–38). These changes in pulmonary minute ventilation from rest to exercise can be summarized in three different phases of the ventilatory response (Fig. 9–6). Although the overall main regulatory force behind the exercise pulmonary ventilation response is associated with the chemical state of the blood, other factors contribute to the ventilatory response (39–41). The initial phase (anticipatory increase and rapid increase) is relatively short in duration and occurs immediately before the onset of exercise through the first 10 to 20 seconds of exercise. During this phase, pulmonary minute ventilation increases abruptly, and it is believed that the primary force behind this increase is produced by neurogenic and mechanoreceptor stimulation from the cerebral cortex (central command) as an individual "prepares" for exercise (Table 9–5). The next phase (leveling off) yields a steady progressive increase in ventilation, with changes occurring more slowly than the initial ventilatory response. Whereas the control mechanisms from initial phase continue to be the driving force for ventilation, inputs from central and peripheral chemoreceptors provide an additional regulatory input, helping to control and "fine tune" the ventilation response. Pulmonary ventilation may slowly continue to increase until a "leveling off" or steady-

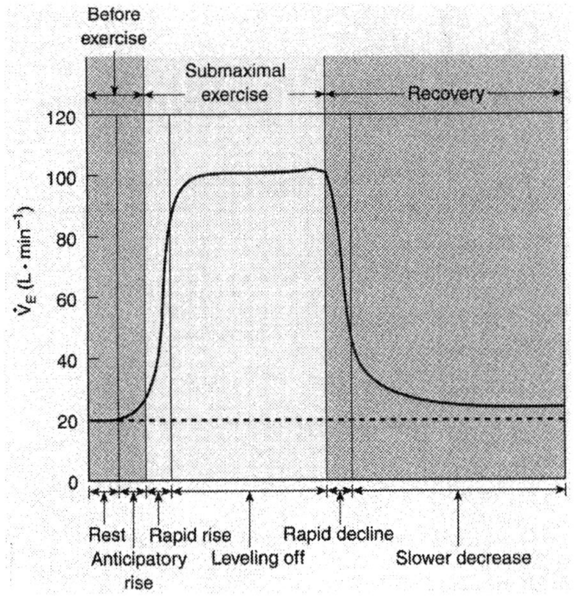

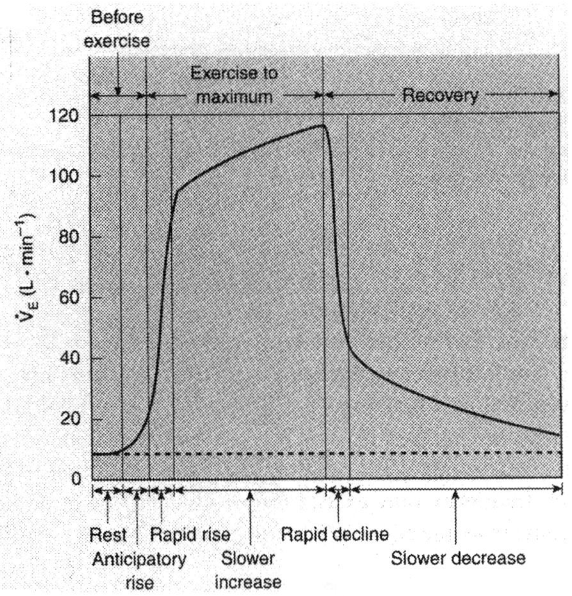

FIG. 9–6. Minute ventilation (V_E) increases even before exercise begins. Immediately after exercise starts, ventilation increases rapidly, and then levels off (submaximal exercise as shown in **A**) or continues to increase (maximal exercise as shown in **B**). During recovery, ventilation decreases more rapidly at first, and then gradually moves toward resting values. From ref. 34, with permission.

state ventilation is attained, with this response typically evident in submaximal-intensity exercise (Fig. 9–6*A*). As exercise intensity progresses to maximal effort, ventilation progressively and continuously increases as the need for airflow/oxygen delivery increases. Unlike submaximal-intensity exercise in which ventilation tends to level off, maximal-intensity exercise yields a continuous increase in ventilation (Fig. 9–6*B*). Ventilatory control factors during the later phase are produced primarily through central and peripheral chemoreceptor feedback as blood homeostasis of oxygen, carbon dioxide, hydrogen ion concentration, and temperature attempts to be maintained (Table 9–5) (39–42). On the cessation of exercise, the rapid decline in recovery minute ventilation is reflective of the reduction in regulatory inputs from "central command" and mechanoreceptors, whereas the slower decrease appears to be related more to the matching of pulmonary ventilation with blood chemical stimuli as the resting state is restored (40–42).

TABLE 9–5. *Ventilatory changes before, during, and after exercise*

Phase	Change	Controlling mechanism
1. Rest	—	Central and peripheral chemoreceptors influencing intrinsic pattern established by the medulla
2. Before exercise	Moderate increase	↑ Central command (cerebral cortex)
3. During exercise		
a. Immediate	Rapid increase	↑ Central command and possibly ↑ neural stimuli to medulla caused by activation of muscle/joint receptors
b. Mid	Steady-state or slower increase	Central or peripheral chemoreceptors reacting to ↑ P_{CO_2} and ↓ pH in blood or cerebrospinal fluid
c. End	Continued or rapid (hyperventilation) increase	Same as above, with possible additional input from ↑ blood potassium, ↑ blood catecholamines, ↑ body temperature, and ↑ central command
4. Recovery		
a. Immediate	Rapid decrease	↓ Central command
b. Later	Slower decrease toward rest	↓ Input from central and peripheral chemoreceptors as P_{CO_2} and pH normalize

Reprinted with permission from Fox ML, Keteyian SJ. *Fox's physiological basis for exercise and sport.* 6th ed. Boston: WCB McGraw-Hill, 1998.

Ventilation through the respiratory passageways can be initially achieved with inspiration through the nasal passageways with sufficient airflow accomplished through the nose. As ventilatory demands increase (e.g., exercise, heavy breathing), the nasal cavity becomes the flow-limiting segment of the respiratory passageway in its ability to deliver sufficient airflow. The relatively small diameter of the external nares of the nose increases nasal airway resistance as airflow demand increases and accounts for approximately 50% to 60% of the total respiratory resistance (43–45). As an individual switches to more oronasal breathing, the nasal passageways still can contribute 40% to 60% of the total airflow (46). The result is a greater involvement of the oral cavity in the ventilation process. In highly trained athletes, in whom small changes in normal function can be of tremendous benefit in enhancing athletic performance, attempts have been made to reduce nasal airway resistance with the hope that greater nasal airflow rates could be achieved. Devices such as external nasal dilators, when applied to the bridge of the nose, flare the nostrils and reduce nasal airway resistance. Although the reduction in nasal resistance is impressive, subsequent improvements in exercise performance have not accompanied these changes. Research has found no significant improvements for ventilation, respiratory rate, tidal volume, power output, oxygen consumption, and other physiological variables during both aerobic and anaerobic exercise or during recovery when wearing these devices (47–53). Aside from the possible psychological benefits of wearing such devices, ventilatory responses at rest and during exercise are more than capable of providing and maintaining normal ventilatory function.

Once air is ventilated into the respiratory passageways, it is distributed throughout the conducting and respiratory divisions of the respiratory system. Dead-space ventilation (V_D) and alveolar ventilation (V_A) define the distribution of the ventilatory tidal volume into the conducting and respiratory divisions of the respiratory system, respectively. The distribution of tidal volume is described by the V_D/V_T ratio, which normally ranges between 25% and 35% at rest or a 150 mL V_D from an average resting V_T of 500 mL (17,41). This ratio not only reflects the distribution of ventilation within the anatomic dead space but also indicates alveolar ventilation and physiological dead-space ventilation. When the V_D/V_T ratio is low, distribution of ventilatory tidal volume within the alveolar spaces is high, indicating a high degree of matching of pulmonary alveolar ventilation and pulmonary capillary blood flow (17,19,41). To accommodate the energy demands during exercise, the distribution of tidal volume changes with the V_D/V_T ratio, decreasing to ranges of 5% to 20% and thereby increasing external gas-exchange potential (17,19,41). Although dead-space volume increases during exercise (54,55), these increases are relatively small and are overshadowed by the substantial increases in tidal volume, which affect the decrease in the V_D/V_T ratio to a larger extent than do changes in V_D (Fig. 9–7) (17,19,41,55,56). Additionally, changes in tidal volume are the major contributor to increases in pulmonary minute ventilation in light- to moderate-intensity exercise, whereas at higher exercise intensities, tidal volume tends to plateau once approximately 60% of vital capacity is reached (14,17,41). At the point of tidal volume plateau, further increases in pulmonary minute ventilation can be attributed to continued increases in breathing rate (Fig. 9–8) (17,37,41,55,56).

The increase in airflow is typically linearly related to the metabolic demand of increased oxygen consumption and carbon dioxide elimination accompanying light- to moderate-intensity exercise. As exercise intensity continues to increase, eventually reaching or exceeding 55% to 65% of maximal aerobic capacity, the increased ventilation is more related to the physiologic need of carbon dioxide elimination rather than oxygen consumption (Fig. 9–9) (14,17,34,41). This "break point" at which a disproportionate increase in ventilation and carbon dioxide production occurs, in contrast to the linear changes observed in oxygen consumption, has received much attention and debate as to the physiological reasoning for its occurrence. Although numerous names describe this break point (e.g., "anaerobic threshold," "ventilatory threshold," "lactate inflection point"), its occurrence is related to higher exercise intensities at which the ability to sustain energy production through aerobic energy systems becomes strained (41,57–63). As the metabolic energy-production pathways shift to a greater reliance on anaerobic glycolysis, the by-products (specifically lactic acid) from that catabolic process accumulate at a rate greater than that at which those substrates can be eliminated (59–62). With the rate of lactic acid production exceeding the lactic acid removal rate, buffering of lactic acid in the blood becomes imperative to maintain homeostasis (14,17,18,41). The buffering of lactic acid through the bicarbonate system yields nonmetabolically produced carbon dioxide, as indicated in the following chemical reaction:

$$La^- + H^+ + NaHCO_3 \rightarrow NaLa + H_2CO_3 \qquad [2]$$

Lactic acid + sodium bicarbonate yields sodium lactate + carbonic acid.

$$H_2CO_3 \rightarrow H_2O + CO_2 \qquad [3]$$

Carbonic acid rapidly dissociates, yielding water + carbon dioxide.

The resulting effect is a much more rapid production of carbon dioxide in the cardiovascular system, as carbon dioxide is produced both metabolically and nonmetabolically through lactic acid buffering (60–63). As a result, the production of metabolic and nonmetabolic

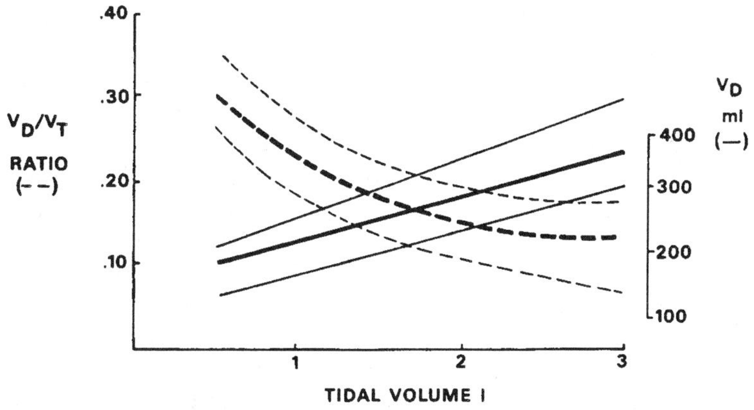

FIG. 9–7. Physiologic dead space (V_D) and the V_D/V_T ratio, mean values for male subjects (*thick lines*) and range (*thin lines*). From ref. 17, with permission.

sources of carbon dioxide during heavy exercise create a rapid increase in blood carbon dioxide load. This is in contrast to the smaller carbon dioxide load produced during light- to moderate-intensity exercise, in which the predominant source of carbon dioxide originates directly from metabolic activity of the Krebs cycle in the catabolism of acetyl-coenzyme A (CoA). Regardless of the source for carbon dioxide production, the respiratory centers of the central nervous system respond to the regulatory feedback by stimulating an increase in pulmonary minute ventilation (i.e., excess ventilation) that mirrors the changes in carbon dioxide production (Figs. 9–9 and 9–10).

The changes in ventilatory dynamics are more than sufficient to maintain adequate pulmonary airflow throughout the respiratory passageways during exercise. With these tremendous adaptations in airflow rates during physical exertion, one might think that gas-exchange efficiency would be compromised. Whereas the total time for pulmonary capillary blood flow at rest equals 0.75 seconds, external gas exchange of oxygen and car-

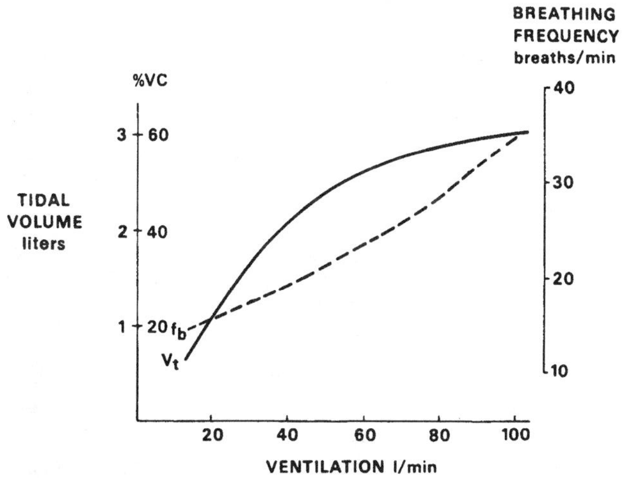

FIG. 9–8. Tidal volume and breathing frequency in normal male subjects. From ref. 17, with permission.

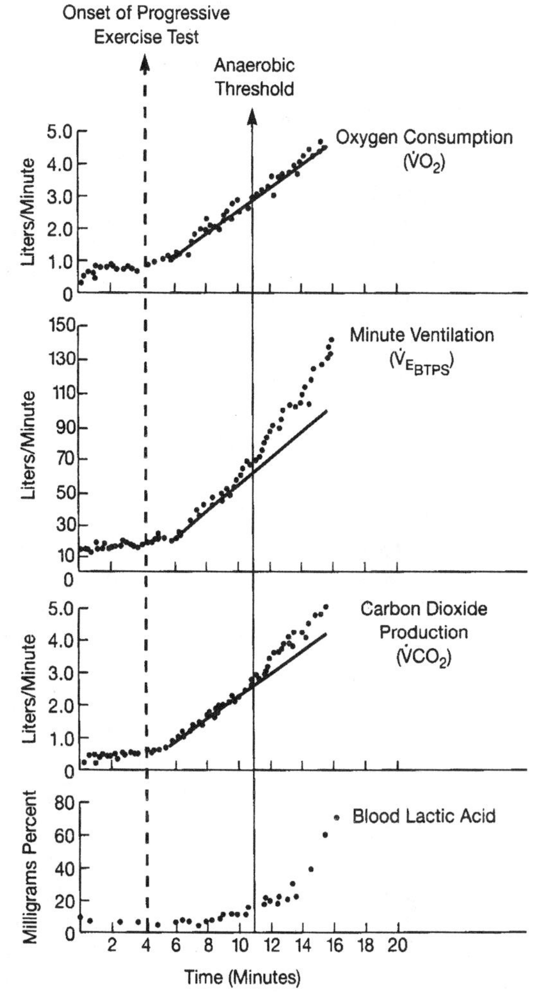

FIG. 9–9. Relation of minute ventilation to the anaerobic threshold. Minute ventilation (V_{EBTPS}) and carbon dioxide production (V_{CO_2}) start to increase sharply at the anaerobic threshold (*thin vertical line*), coinciding with the steep increase in blood lactic acid. The dashed vertical lines denote the start of the progressive exercise test. From ref. 34, with permission.

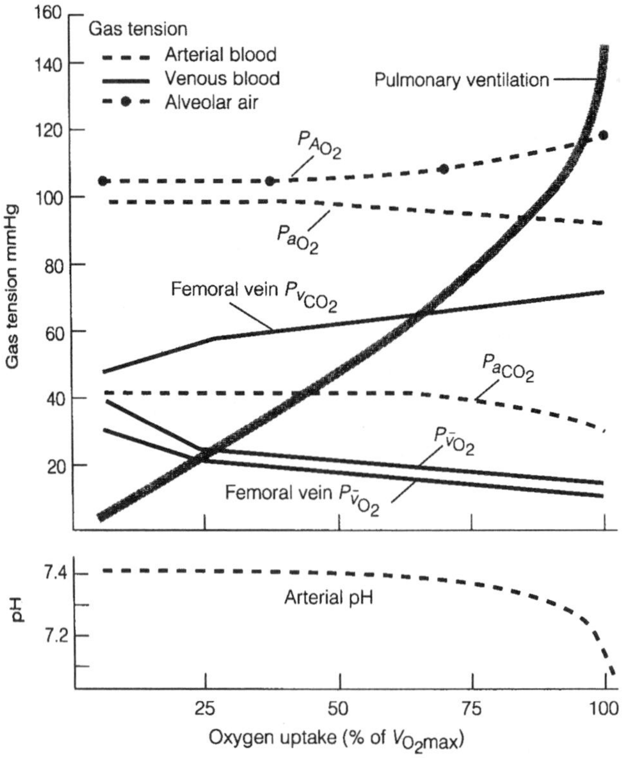

FIG. 9–10. Oxygen and carbon dioxide partial pressures in alveolar air (*PA*), arterial blood (*Pv*) during rest and graded exercise. Note that as relative effort increases, the partial pressure of O_2 in arterial blood (P_aO_2) remains constant or decreases only slightly. Because of the shape of the hemoglobin dissociation curve, arterial O_2 content remains close to resting levels of approximately 95% to 98% saturation. From ref. 61, with permission.

bon dioxide with the arterial blood requires only about 50% of that time (Fig. 9–11). To accommodate the physiological adaptations at the respiratory membrane during exercise, pulmonary capillary blood volume expands to 3 times its resting value, and its increase is linearly related to the changes in pulmonary blood flow (19,64). Exercise pulmonary capillary transit time decreases to approximately 0.4 seconds; however, this does not significantly affect the exchange of oxygen and carbon dioxide in the pulmonary capillary bed (19,64). As indicated in Fig. 9–10, with progressive increases in pulmonary minute ventilation accompanying continuous changes in exercise intensity, arterial oxygen and carbon dioxide pressure are maintained at near-resting levels. It is not until exercise intensity reaches near-maximal levels, with pulmonary minute ventilation responses increasing at a much greater rate, that the arterial oxygen and carbon dioxide pressure show slight alterations from resting levels. Although these changes could represent a potential limitation in gas-exchange efficiency, the fact is, as noted by Dempsey (64), that in normal healthy individuals exercising at sea level (a) alveolar capillary-diffusion distances are maintained; (b) the average capillary transit time of red blood cells through the pulmonary capillaries is maintained within about one-half the resting time; (c) ventilation-to-perfusion ratios of the lungs are high and fairly uniformly distributed; and (d) arterial oxygen pressure is maintained at resting values. The resulting effect of the respiratory system performance is the maintenance of arterial oxygen and carbon dioxide concentrations at or near normal resting values throughout a wide range of exercise intensities. As summarized in Table 9–6, the respiratory system responses to a variety of exercise situations are relatively consistent, with the most notable and significant changes occurring after the transition into more anaerobic, heavy-intensity-type exercise situations.

PULMONARY RESPONSE TO CHRONIC EXERCISE

The responses and adaptations of the respiratory system to prolonged training are considerably less remarkable than those observed in other body systems. Whereas other systems show significant improvements with long-term training, the respiratory system responses remain relatively similar between trained and untrained individuals (Table 9–7). This lack of adaptation to prolonged activity in the respiratory system is not necessarily all that surprising when one considers the tremendous reserves that accompany the respiratory system, even without physical training. No other bodily system has the ability to expand its response to a wider range, regardless of the level of physical training, than does the respiratory system. With the capacity of ventilation to increase 20- to 40-fold and of respiratory rate and tidal volume to increase 4- to 6-fold that of resting values, the respiratory system is designed for maximal function without the requirement of adaptations through prolonged physical training. Research by Dempsey (64), addressing the question "is the lung built for exercise?," showed that the respiratory system is not considered the "weak link" or the limiting factor to exercise performance in the majority of untrained and trained individuals. It has been postulated that two physiologic extremes can limit maximal exercise performance (Fig. 9–12). In most individuals (untrained and trained), exercise performance becomes limited because of the "weak link" of the oxygen-transport system and oxidative capacity of the muscular system (64). This notion is supported by research that has shown no significant relationship among level of physical training, method of physical training, and the adaptations in lung capacity and volumes. In fact, studies that have examined wrestlers, football players, distance runners, and other types of athletes revealed no significant differences in pulmonary-function responses to prolonged exercise when compared with controls matched for body weight,

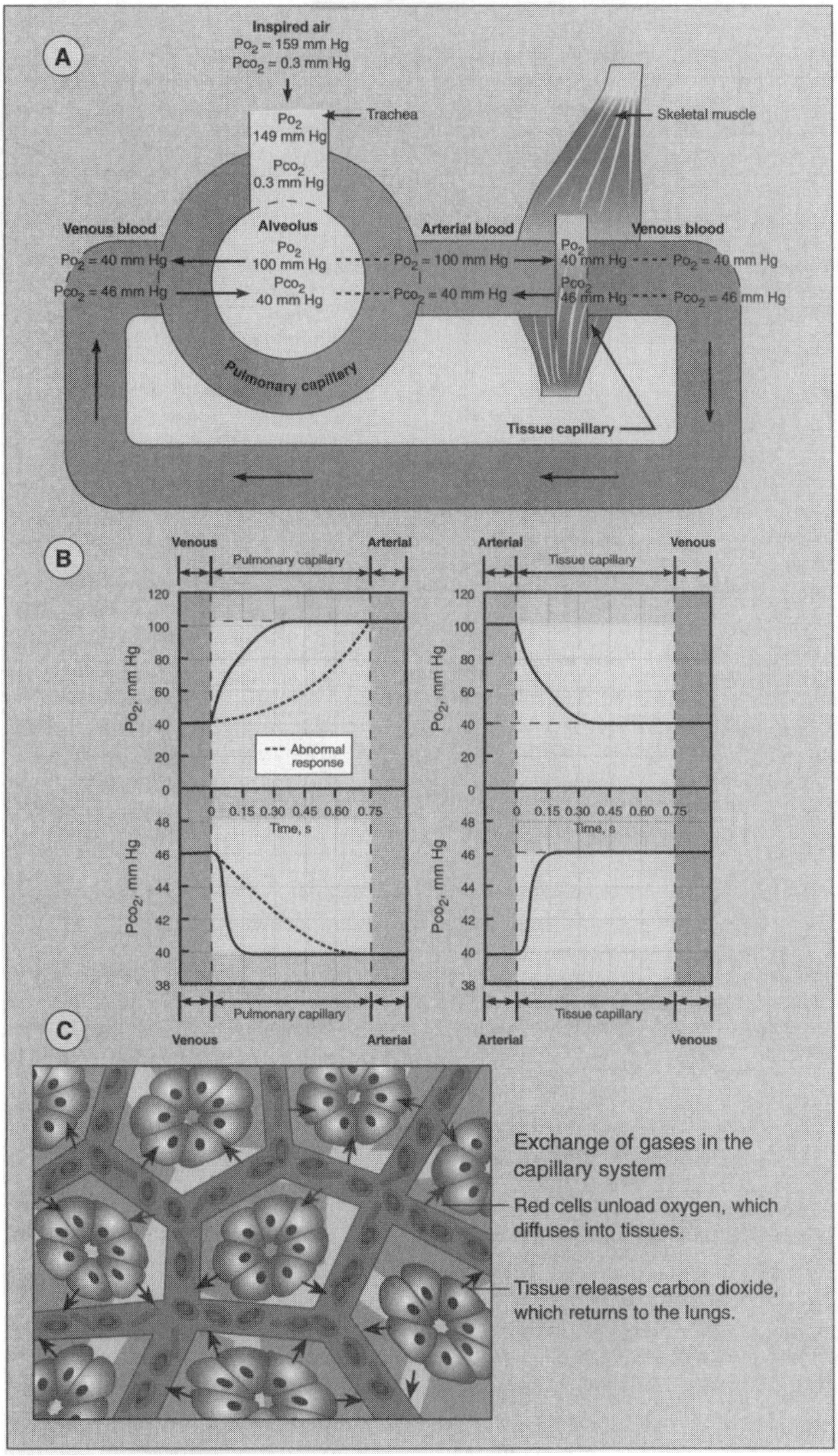

FIG. 9–11. Pressure gradients for gas transfer in the body at rest. **A**: The Po_2 and Pco_2 of ambient, tracheal, and alveolar air are shown, along with these gas pressures in venous and arterial blood and muscle tissue. Movement of gas at the alveolar–capillary and tissue–capillary membranes is always from an area of higher partial pressure to one of lower partial pressure. **B**: The time required for gas exchange. At rest, blood remains in the pulmonary and tissue capillaries for about 0.75 seconds. In pulmonary disease (*dashed line*), the rate of gas transfer across the alveolar–capillary membrane is impaired, thus prolonging the time for equilibrium of gases. During maximal exercise, the transit time is reduced to about 0.4 seconds, but this is usually still adequate in the healthy lung for complete aeration of the blood. **C**: The exchange of gases in the capillary system. From ref. 14, with permission.

TABLE 9–6. *Respiratory responses to exercise*

	Light- to moderate-intensity, short-term submaximal exercise[a]	Heavy, long-duration submaximal exercise	Incremental-to-maximum exercise	Static exercise
Pulmonary ventilation				
$\dot{V}_E$	Increases rapidly; levels off	Increases rapidly; levels off; drifts upward	Shows initial rectilinear increase; has two breakpoints	All responses the same as for light- to moderate-intensity, short-term submaximal exercise
V_D	Decreases	Decreases	Decreases	
V_T	Increases rapidly; levels off	Increases rapidly; levels off	Has truncated, inverted U-shaped curve; increases greatly; has incomplete reversal	
f	Slowly increases; levels off	Increases slowly; levels off; drifts upward	Has exponential curvilinear increase	
V_D/V_T	Decreases initially; levels off	Decreases rapidly initially; levels off	Decreases rapidly initially; levels off at 60% of maximum and is maintained	
External respiration				
$\dot{V}_A$	Increases rapidly; levels off	Increases rapidly; levels off; drifts upward	Shows initial rectilinear increase; has two breakpoints	
P_AO_2	Shows no change	Shows no change	Shows no change until approximately 75% of maximum; then has exponential increase	
P_aO_2	Shows no change	Has small U-shaped curve	Shows no change until approximately 75% of maximum; then increases slightly	
$(A\text{-}a)PO_2$ diff	Decreases slightly or shows no change (light); increases slightly (moderate)	Has truncated, inverted U-shaped curve; increases rapidly initially; has incomplete reversal	Shows no change until approximately 75% of maximum; then has exponential increase[b]	
$SaO_2\%$	Decreases 1%; has U-shaped curve	—	—	
Internal respiration				
P_aCO_2	Is level; then decreases slightly	Is level; then decreases slightly	Is level; then decreases	
P_vCO_2	Shows slight linear increase	Shows linear increase; levels off	Has sharp increase; levels slightly	
P_vO_2	Decreases rapidly; levels off	Decreases rapidly; levels off	Decreases sharply; levels off	
$S_vO_2\%$	Decreases initially; levels off	Decreases initially; levels off	Decreases sharply; never reaches 0	↓
$a\text{-}vO_2$ diff	Increases rapidly; levels off	Increases rapidly; levels off	Shows rectilinear increase to highest possible value that is maintained to maximum	Shows no change or decreases slightly

Resting values are taken as baseline.
[a] The difference between leveling during the light to moderate short-term and heavy long-duration submaximal exercise responses is one of magnitude; that is, leveling occurs at a higher value with higher intensities.
[b] Hypoxemia may occur at higher altitudes.
Reprinted with permission from Plowman SA, Smith DL. *Exercise physiology for health, fitness, and performance.* Boston: Allyn & Bacon, 1997.

gender, and age (Table 9–7) (15,65–71). The exception to this appears to be with athletes who participate in water-based sports (swimming and diving), in which pulmonary adaptations occur, resulting in greater lung volumes and capacities as compared with the matched land-based trained and untrained controls (Table 9–7) (67,72–75).

In contrast, on the other end of the physiologic continuum, in the elite, highly trained individual, with significant improvements from long-term training to their cardiovascular and musculoskeletal systems and minimal pulmonary adaptations, the respiratory system may become the rate-limiting step in the oxygen-consumption equation. In the healthy untrained and trained individual, alveolar-to-arterial gas exchange appears to be maintained at or near normal levels, but the highly trained, elite individual exhibits a somewhat different response. In the elite athlete, the rate-limiting step may

TABLE 9–7. *Respiratory training adaptations*

	Rest	Submaximal exercise	Maximal exercise
Lung volumes and capacities	Show no changes from land-based activities; swimming and diving show increases, especially in total lung capacity and vital capacity	—	—
Pulmonary ventilation			
$\dot{V}_E$	Shows no change	Decreases	Increases
V_T	Increases	Increases	Increases
f	Decreases	Decreases	Increases
External respiration, $(A\text{-}a)Po_2$ diff	Shows no change	Decreases	Shows no change
Internal respiration			
P_VCO_2		Decreases	—
Oxygen-dissociation curve	—	Curve shifts to the right	Curve shifts to the right
$a\text{-}vO_2$ diff	Shows no change in children; increases in young adults	Shows no change in children; inconsistent changes in adults	Shows no change in children; increases in young adults

Reprinted with permission from Plowman SA, Smith DL. *Exercise physiology for health, fitness, and performance.* Boston: Allyn & Bacon, 1997.

become the anatomic and physiologic constraints of the respiratory system, resulting in widening of the alveolar and arterial oxygen pressure, producing an exercise-induced hypoxemia (EIH; arterial oxygen–hemoglobin saturation of 91% or less) (64,76,77). Although the exact mechanism and prevalence of the exercise-induced hypoxemia in elite, highly trained athletes remains unknown, some studies suggested an incidence of 50% of the athletes examined (78). Although numerous investigations reported arterial oxygen–hemoglobin desaturation in highly trained individuals during maximal exercise (79–83), the validity of those findings remains in question. The initial studies regarding EIH in elite, highly trained athletes determined HbO_2 saturation by using invasive blood gas measurements, but many subsequent studies relied on noninvasive ear-oximetry technology. This technology has proven to be very effective and beneficial in resting situations, but its ability to be valid and reliable during exercise situations can be questioned. Research has shown that the incidence of EIH in highly trained athletes may be overestimated when HbO_2 saturations are determined noninvasively as compared with invasive arterial blood sampling (84). The prevalence and extent to which highly trained athletes exhibit limitations in the respiratory system at meeting the demands of maximal exercise is still unknown, although it does appear to occur.

One the few consistent adaptations that appear to occur with prolonged training, regardless of the mode of activity, is the change in pulmonary ventilatory dynamics. With repeated bouts of regular physical exercise, pulmonary minute ventilation is increased during

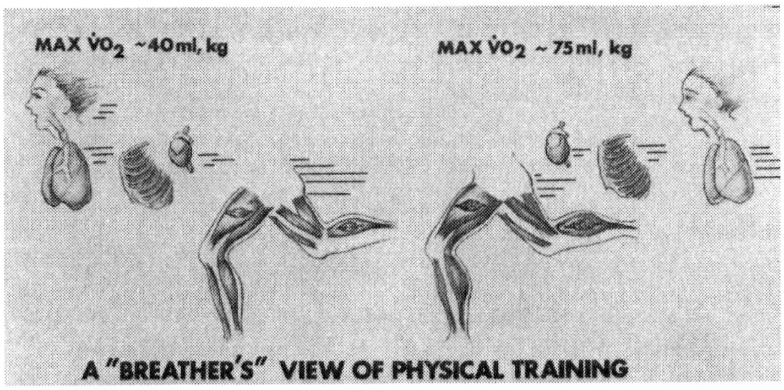

FIG. 9–12. Hypothesis: In the untrained, the capacity for O_2 transport by the pulmonary system (lungs and chest wall) far exceeds that of the cardiovascular system and the oxidative capacity of the limb locomotor muscles. Physical training primarily causes adaptation in the skeletal muscles and in the systemic cardiovascular system, with little change in the pulmonary system. Thus eventually the capacity of the pulmonary system for O_2 transport cannot meet the superior demands imposed by the limbs and cardiovascular system; arterial blood gas and acid–base homeostasis fail, and the lungs become a significant limitation to performance capacity. From ref. 64, with permission.

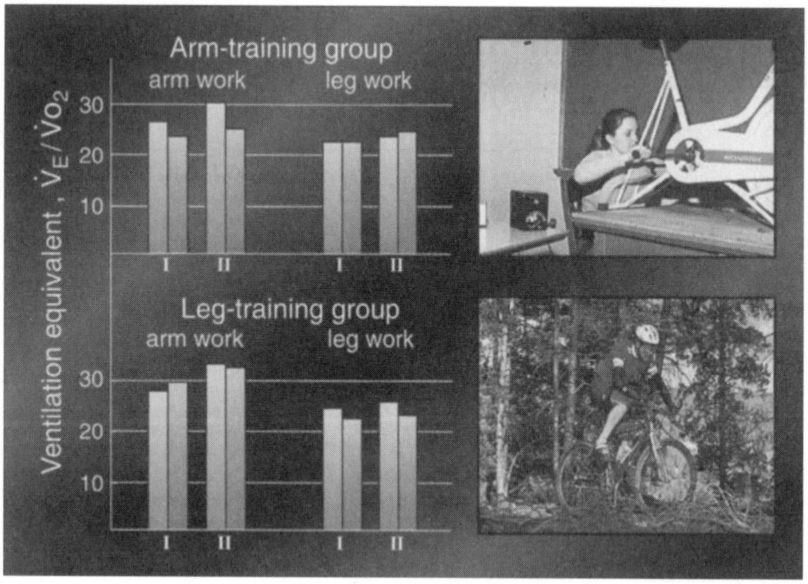

FIG. 9–13. Ventilation equivalents during light (*I*) and heavy (*II*) submaximal arm and leg exercise before and after arm training (*top*) and leg training (*bottom*). Bars on the left indicate pretraining values, whereas bars on the right indicate posttraining values. From ref. 14, with permission.

maximal-exercise and decreased during submaximal-exercise intensities. These changes are accompanied by adaptations in the ventilatory dynamics of tidal volume and respiratory rate. Regular physical training increases tidal volume both at rest and during submaximal and maximal exercise (Table 9–7). In contrast, after prolonged exercise, respiratory rate is reduced both at rest and during submaximal exercise and increased during maximal exercise when compared with matched controls. Physiologically this would make sense, because a greater depth and slower rate of breathing during submaximal exercise would ensure adequate alveolar ventilation and greater time for external gas exchange to occur. During maximal exercise, the demand for airflow is extremely high and can best be met through an increase in both respiratory rate and tidal volume, yielding the tremendously large airflow rates observed in highly trained athletes (17,36,41,85–87). Additional adaptations in the respiratory muscles to prolonged physical activity are evident in improvements in respiratory muscle strength and endurance (88,89). Ventilatory equivalents for oxygen decrease with physical training, indicating an improvement in respiratory muscle function in terms of both strength and endurance (17,36,41, 90–93). These adaptations, in which a smaller amount of air is ventilated to provide the same amount of oxygen, are specific to the method of training, but consistent across the intensity of exercise (Fig. 9–13) (14). The finding of a training-specific response to prolonged exercise training would indicate that not only are there improvements in respiratory muscle function, both in terms of strength and endurance, but there probably are also local adaptations in the specific muscle groups being trained (76,90,92).

CONCLUSION

The maintenance of cellular activity is dependent on the interaction of numerous body systems that provide an integrated approach to oxygen supply, delivery, uptake, and use. Each body system makes tremendous adaptations to short- and long-term physical activity, but the unified efforts between body systems at maintaining cell function continue to be achieved. The respiratory system anatomy and physiology allow a continued maintenance of ventilation and gas exchange, even during situations in which airflow responses are increased 30 to 40 times those of the resting values. Although the acute response of the respiratory system to physical activity can actually occur before exercise begins, the long-term adaptations are much less impressive. With the reserve capacities that are inherent in the respiratory system, it is evident that it is geared to maintenance of cellular function in a wide variety of situations.

REFERENCES

1. Scanlon CL. *Egan's fundamentals of respiratory care.* 6th ed. St. Louis: Mosby, 1995.
2. Leech JA, Ghezzo H, Stevens D, Becklake MR. Respiratory pressures and function in young adults. *Am Rev Respir Dis* 1983;128:17.
3. Farkas GA, Decramer M, Rochester DF, De Troyer A. Contractile properties of intercostal muscles and their functional significance. *J Appl Physiol* 1985;59:528–535.
4. Celli BR. Clinical and physiologic evaluation of respiratory muscle function. *Clin Chest Med* 1989;10:199.
5. Guyton AC, Hall JE. *Human physiology and mechanisms of disease.* 6th ed. Philadelphia: WB Saunders, 1997.
6. Martin BJ, Sparks KE, Zwillich CW, Weil JV. Low exercise ventilation in endurance athletes. *Med Sci Sports Exerc* 1979;11:181–185.
7. Sharp JT, Goldberg NB, Druz WS, Danon J. Relative contribu-

tions of rib cage and abdomen to breathing in normal subjects. *J Appl Physiol* 1975;39:601.
8. Beachey W. *Respiratory care anatomy and physiology.* St. Louis: Mosby, 1998.
9. Des Jardins T. *Cardiopulmonary anatomy and physiology: essentials for respiratory care.* 2nd ed. Albany, NY: Delmar, 1993.
10. Mahler D. Exercise-induced asthma. *Med Sci Sports Exerc* 1993;25:554.
11. McFadden ER, Gilbert IA. Current concepts in exercise-induced asthma. *N Engl J Med* 1994;330:1362.
12. Hough DO, Dec KL. Exercise-induced asthma and anaphylaxis. *Sports Med* 1994;18:162.
13. Clements JA, et al. Pulmonary surface tension and alveolar stability. *J Appl Physiol* 1972;16:144.
14. McArdle WD, Katch FI, Katch VL. *Exercise physiology: energy, nutrition, and human performance.* 4th ed. Baltimore: Williams & Wilkins, 1996.
15. Wilmore JH, Haskell WL. Body composition and endurance capacity of professional football players. *J Appl Physiol* 1972;33:564.
16. Irwin S, Tecklin JS. *Cardiopulmonary physical therapy.* 3rd ed. St. Louis: Mosby, 1995.
17. Jones NL, Campbell EJM. *Clinical exercise testing.* 4th ed. Philadelphia: WB Saunders, 1997.
18. Wasserman K. Breathing during exercise. *N Engl J Med* 1978;298:780–785.
19. Dempsey JA, Bidruk EH, Mastenbrook SM. Pulmonary control systems in exercise. *Fed Proc* 1980;39:1498–1505.
20. Johnson BD, Aaron EA, Babcock MA, Dempsey JA. Respiratory muscle fatigue during exercise: implications for performance. *Med Sci Sports Exerc* 1996;28:1129–1137.
21. Koyal SN, Whipp BJ, Huntsman D, Bray GA, Wasserman K. Ventilatory responses to the metabolic acidosis of treadmill and cycle ergometry. *J Appl Physiol* 1976;40:864–867.
22. Pearce DH, Milhorn HT. Dynamic and steady-state respiratory responses to bicycle exercise. *J Appl Physiol* 1977;42:959–967.
23. Turner JM, Mead J, Wohl ME. Elasticity of human lungs in relation to age. *J Appl Physiol* 1968;25:664–671.
24. Younes M, Kivinen G. Respiratory mechanics and breathing pattern during and following maximal exercise. *J Appl Physiol* 1984;57:1773–1782.
25. Buono MJ, Constable SH, Morton AR, Rotkis TC, Stanforth PR, Wilmore JH. The effects of an acute bout of exercise on selected pulmonary function measurements. *Med Sci Sports Exerc* 1981;5:290–293.
26. Cordain L, Rode EJ, Gotshall RW, Tucker A. Residual lung volume and ventilator muscle strength changes following maximal and submaximal exercise. *Int J Sports Med* 1994;15:158–161.
27. Farrell PA, Maron MB, Hamilton LH, Maksud MG, Foster C. Time course of the lung volume changes during prolonged treadmill exercise. *Med Sci Sports Exerc* 1983;4:319–324.
28. Katch FI. Pre and post-test changes in the factors that influence computed body density changes. *Res Q* 1971;3:280–285.
29. Maron MB, Hamilton LH, Maksud MG. Alterations in pulmonary function consequent to competitive marathon running. *Med Sci Sports Exerc* 1979;3:244–249.
30. Miles DS, Cox MH, Bomze JP, Gotshall RW. Acute recovery profile of lung volumes and function after running 5 miles. *J Sports Med* 1991;2:243–248.
31. Miles DS, Durbin RJ. Alterations in pulmonary function consequent to a 5-mile run. *J Sports Med* 1985;25:90–97.
32. Stubbing DG, Pengelly LD, Morse JL, Jones NL. Pulmonary mechanics during exercise in normal males. *J Appl Physiol* 1980;3:506–510.
33. Quindry JQ, Brown DD, Thomas DQ, McCaw ST. Implications of residual lung volume responses to exercise on the estimation of body composition. *Med Sci Sports Exerc* 1997;29:S330.
34. Fox ML, Keteyian SJ. *Fox's physiological basis for exercise and sport.* 6th ed. Boston: WCB McGraw-Hill, 1998.
35. Pardy RL, Hussain SNA, Macklein PT. The ventilatory pump in exercise. *Clin Chest Med* 1984;5:35–49.
36. Whipp BJ. The hyperpnea of dynamic muscular exercise. In: Hutton RS, ed. *Exercise sport science review.* Vol 5. Santa Barbara, CA: Journal Publishing Affiliates, 1977:295–311.
37. Whipp BJ, Ward SA. Ventilatory control dynamics during muscular exercise in men. *Int J Sports Med* 1980;1:146–159.
38. Whipp BJ, Ward SA, Lamarra N, Davis JA, Wasserman K. Parameters of ventilatory and gas exchange dynamics during exercise. *J Appl Physiol* 1982;52:1506–1513.
39. Eldridge FL. Central integration of mechanisms in exercise hyperpnea. *Med Sci Sports Exerc* 1994;26:319–327.
40. Jones NL. Dyspnea in exercise. *Med Sci Sports Exerc* 1984;16:14–19.
41. Wasserman K, Hansen JE, Sue DY, Whipp BJ, Casaburi R. *Principles of exercise testing and interpretation.* 2nd ed. Philadelphia: Lea & Febiger, 1994.
42. Whipp BJ. Peripheral chemoreceptor control of exercise hyperpnea in humans. *Med Sci Sports Exerc* 1994;26:337–347.
43. Saketkhoo K, Kaplan I, Sackner M. Effect of exercise on nasal mucus velocity and nasal airflow resistance in normal subjects. *J Appl Physiol* 1979;46:369–371.
44. Schreck S, Sullivan KJ, Chang HK. Correlations between flow resistance and geometry in a model of the human nose. *J Appl Physiol* 1993;75:1767–1775.
45. Daubenspeck JA. Influence of small mechanical loads on variability of breathing patterns. *J Appl Physiol* 1981;50:229–306.
46. Niinimaa V, Cole P, Mintz S. Oronasal distribution of respiratory airflow. *Respir Physiol* 1981;43:69–75.
47. Brown DD, Rodgers J, Steurer RA. The effect of external nasal dilators on submaximal exercise responses. *Med Sci Sports Exerc* 1997;29:S1670.
48. Huffman MS, Huffman MT, Brown DD, Quindry JC, Thomas DQ. Exercise responses using the Breathe Right external nasal dilator. *Med Sci Sports Exerc* 1996;28:S418.
49. Clapp AJ, Bishop PA. Effect of the Breathe Right external nasal dilator during light to moderate exercise. *Med Sci Sports Exerc* 1996;28:S88.
50. Papanek PE, Brown JA, Young CC. The effects of an external nasal dilator on respiratory flow volume. *Med Sci Sports Exerc* 1997;29:S285.
51. Thomas DQ, Bowdoin BA, Brown DD, McCaw ST. Nasal strips and mouthpieces do not affect power output during anaerobic exercise. *Res Q Exerc Sport* 1998;69:201–204.
52. Trocchio M, Wimer JW, Parkman AW, Fisher J. Oxygenation and exercise performance-enhancing effects attributed to the Breathe Right nasal dilator. *J Athlet Train* 1995;30:211–214.
53. Young L, Sowash J, Lever D, Wygand J, Otto RM. The effect of Breatherite aids on acute anaerobic performance and recovery. *Med Sci Sports Exerc* 1996;28:S17.
54. Asmussen E, Nielsen M. Physiological dead-space and alveolar gas pressures at rest and during muscular exercise. *Acta Physiol Scand* 1956;38:1.
55. Grimby G. Respiration in exercise. *Med Sci Sports Exerc* 1969;1:9–14.
56. Wasserman K, Van Kessel AL, Burton GG. Interaction of physiological mechanisms during exercise. *J Appl Physiol* 1967;22:71–85.
57. Loat CER, Rhodes EC. Relationship between the lactate and ventilatory thresholds during prolonged exercise. *Sports Med* 1993;15:104–115.
58. Skinner JS, McLellan TH. The transition from aerobic to anaerobic metabolism. *Res Q Exerc Sport* 1980;51:234–298.
59. Brooks GA. Anaerobic threshold: review of the concepts and directions for the future. *Med Sci Sports Exerc* 1985;17:91–98.
60. Davis JA. Anaerobic threshold: review of the concepts and directions for the future. *Med Sci Sports Exerc* 1985;17:6–18.
61. Brooks GA, Fahey TD, White TP. *Exercise physiology: human bioenergetics and its application.* 2nd ed. Mountain View, CA: Mayfield Publishing, 1996.
62. Wasserman K, McIlroy MB. Detecting the threshold of anaerobic metabolism. *Am J Cardiol* 1964;14:844–852.
63. Wasserman K, Whipp BJ, Koyal SN, Beaver WL. Anaerobic threshold and respiratory gas exchange. *J Appl Physiol* 1973;35:236–243.
64. Dempsey JA. Is the lung built for exercise? *Med Sci Sports Exerc* 1986;18:143–155.
65. Astrand PO, Rodahl K. *Textbook of work physiology.* New York: McGraw-Hill, 1986.
66. Bachman JC, Horvath SM. Pulmonary function changes which

accompany athletic conditioning programs. *Res Q Exerc Sport* 1968;39:235–239.
67. Cordain L, Tucker A, Moon D, Stager JM. Lung volumes and maximal respiratory pressures in collegiate swimmers and runners. *Res Q Exerc Sport* 1990;61:70–74.
68. Dempsey JA, Fregosi RF. Adaptability of the pulmonary system of changing metabolic requirements. *Am J Cardiol* 1985;55:59D–67D.
69. Kaufmann DA, Swenson EW, Fencl J, Lucas A. Pulmonary function of marathon runners. *Med Sci Sports Exerc* 1974;6:114–117.
70. Niinimaa V, Shepard RJ. Training and oxygen conductance in the elderly: I. The respiratory system. *J Gerontol* 1978;33:354–361.
71. Reuschlein PS, Reddan WG, Burpee J, Gee JBL, Rankin J. Effect of physical training on the pulmonary diffusing capacity during submaximal work. *J Appl Physiol* 1968;24:152–158.
72. Leith DG, Bradley M. Ventilatory muscle strength and endurance training. *J Appl Physiol* 1976;41:508–516.
73. Andrew GM, Becklake MR, Guleria JS, Bates DV. Heart and lung functions in swimmers and nonathletes during growth. *J Appl Physiol* 1972;32:245–251.
74. Clanton TL, Dixon GF, Drake J, Gadek JE. Effects of swim training on lung and inspiratory muscle conditioning. *J Appl Physiol* 1987;62:39–46.
75. Mahler DA, Shuhart CR, Brew E, Stukel TA. Ventilatory responses and entrainment of breathing during rowing. *Med Sci Sports Exerc* 1991;23:186–192.
76. Dempsey JA, Johnson BD, Saupe KW. Adaptations and limitations in the pulmonary system during exercise. *Chest* 1990;97:81S–87S.
77. Dempsey JA, Hanson PG, Henderson KS. Exercise-induced arterial hypoxaemia in healthy human subjects at sea level. *J Physiol (Lond)* 1984;355:161–175.
78. Powers SK, Dodd S, Lawler J, et al. Incidence of exercise induced hypoxemia in elite endurance athletes at sea level. *Eur J Appl Physiol* 1988;58:298–302.
79. Hopkins SR, McKenzie DC. Hypoxic ventilatory response and arterial desaturation during heavy work. *J Appl Physiol* 1989;67:1119–1124.
80. Powers SK, Dodd S, Freeman J, Ayers GD, Samson H, McKnight T. Accuracy of pulse oximetry to estimate HbO_2 fraction of total Hb during exercise. *J Appl Physiol* 1989;67:300–304.
81. Powers SK, Lawler J, Dempsey JA, Dodd S, Landry G. Effects of incomplete pulmonary gas exchange on $V_{O_2}max$. *J Appl Physiol* 1989;66:2491–2495.
82. Powers SK, Williams J. Exercise-induced hypoxemia in highly trained athletes. *Sports Med* 1987;4:46–53.
83. Smyth RJ, D'Urzo AD, Slutsky AS, Galko BM, Rebuck AS. Ear oximetry during combined hypoxia and exercise. *J Appl Physiol* 1986;60:716–719.
84. Brown DD, Knowlton RG, Szurgot BT, Sanjabi PB. Re-examination of the incidence of exercise induced hypoxaemia in highly trained subjects. *Br J Sports Med* 1993;27:167–170.
85. Rasmussen B, Klausen K, Clausen JP, TrapJensen J. Pulmonary ventilation, blood gases, and blood pH after training of the arms or the legs. *J Appl Physiol* 1975;38:250–256.
86. Wilmore JH, Royce J, Girandola RN, Katch FI, Katch VL. Physiological alterations resulting from a 10 week program of jogging. *Med Sci Sports Exerc* 1970;2:7–14.
87. Coast JR, Clifford PS, Henrich TW, Stray-Gundersen J, Johnson RL. Maximal inspiratory pressure following maximal exercise in trained and untrained subjects. *Med Sci Sports Exerc* 1990;22:811–815.
88. Byrne-Quinn E, Weil JV, Sodal IE, Filley GF, Grover RF. Ventilatory control in the athlete. *J Appl Physiol* 1971;30:91–98.
89. Miyamura M, Yamashina T, Honda Y. Ventilatory responses to CO_2 rebreathing at rest and during exercise in untrained subjects and athletes. *Jpn J Physiol* 1976;26:245–254.
90. Chevrolet JC, Tschopp JM, Blanc Y, Rochat T, Junod A. Alterations in inspiratory and leg muscle force and recovery pattern after a marathon. *Med Sci Sports Exerc* 1993;25:501–507.
91. Johnson BD. Exercise induced diaphragmatic fatigue in healthy humans. *J Physiol (Lond)* 1993;460:385.
92. Cassaburi R. Effect of endurance training on possible determinants of V_{O_2} during heavy exercise. *J Appl Physiol* 1987;62:199.
93. Martin BJ, Weil JV, Sparks KE, McCullough RE, Grover RF. Exercise ventilation correlates positively with ventilatory chemoresponsiveness. *J Appl Physiol* 1978;45:557–564.

Exercise and Sport Science,
edited by William E. Garrett, Jr., and Donald T. Kirkendall.
Lippincott Williams & Wilkins, Philadelphia © 2000.

CHAPTER 10

Endocrine Responses to Exercise and Training

Robert G. McMurray and Anthony C. Hackney

The nature of the human body is such that it cannot survive without some method of internal communications. Humans have evolved two such internal-communication systems: the nervous system, which responds quickly by using specific neural pathways to receive and send information throughout the body; and the endocrine system, a loosely affiliated group of glands, which regulates physiologic processes at a much slower rate than does the nervous system (Table 10–1). The endocrine glands use the circulatory system to carry highly specialized chemical substances, hormones, to target tissues. Through the interaction of these two communication systems, the body maintains homeostasis, as well as responding and adapting to stress. This chapter focuses on the endocrine system and how the stress of exercise causes this system to respond and adapt.

Different types of activities (walking, running, jumping, lifting, throwing, etc.) can be classified as exercise. Each of these activities has varying degrees of muscular movement patterns (i.e., contractile characteristics that are unique to the activities). For example, an activity can involve "dynamic" muscular contractions (isotonic contractions), or "static" muscular contractions (isometric contractions), or some combination of the two. Even this can be further subdivided, as isotonic contractions can be concentric and eccentric in nature. Furthermore, an activity can be of "short" or "prolonged" duration relative to the amount of time in which it is performed. Unfortunately, in the literature, the actual time duration denoting short versus prolonged is not well defined. For the purposes of this chapter, however, short duration is less than 30 minutes, whereas prolonged is more than 30 minutes. Finally, when considering these factors, it becomes necessary to view these effects as in response to more frequent, repetitive exercise bouts (prolonged exposure; e.g., training effects).

The topic presented in this chapter could warrant a book in and of itself; however, space and time limitations prevent such a lengthy undertaking. Therefore, we limit our discussion to certain topics in an attempt to be concise and focus attention on key, selected aspects of endocrinology as related to exercise. One final comment on this last point. It has become apparent that many tissues and organs in the human body have some degree of endocrine-like function and capacity (e.g., adipose releases leptin and prostaglandins), but space limitations prevent full discussions of these new and exciting additions to the endocrine world. The primary foci are the hormones from the pituitary gland, thyroid gland, pancreas, adrenal gland, and the female and male gonads. In addition, because not all exercise results in the same stress, we examine our state of knowledge of the endocrine responses that occur during four types of exercise: (a) short-term aerobic exercise, (b) prolonged aerobic exercise, (c) short-term high-intensity anaerobic exercise, and (d) resistance or strength training. A short summary of the effects of exercise training on the hormonal system also is included. The chapter is organized by endocrine gland rather than by metabolic process. The end of the chapter contains a short summary that attempts to consolidate the hormones by metabolic function.

Methodologically, human endocrine evaluations are typically limited to the measurement of hormonal concentrations in the blood. Such measurements are a "snapshot" of what is occurring within a constantly changing and ever-dynamic system. That is, hormonal concentrations are the product of glandular secretion versus metabolic clearance, and during exercise these two factors may be constantly changing. Thus scientists are limited in what can be interpreted from such snap-

R. G. McMurray and A. C. Hackney: Department of Physical Education, Exercise and Sport Science, University of North Carolina, Chapel Hill, North Carolina 27599-8700.

TABLE 10–1. *Metabolic half-life ($T_{1/2}$) of the exercise-related hormones*

Hormone	$T_{1/2}$
Adrenocorticotropin	20–25 min
Antidiuretic	15–20 min
Aldosterone	~20 min
Catecholamines	2–2.5 min
Cortisol	60–70 min
Estradiol	60 min
Follicle stimulating hormone	180 min
Glucagon	5 min
Growth hormone	20–25 min
Insulin	10 min
Luteinizing	30 min
Parathyroid hormone	4–6 min
Testosterone	70 min
Thyroid stimulating hormone	50 min
Thyroxine (T_4)	6.5 days
Triiodothyronine (T_3)	1 day

shots. Nonetheless, this limitation must be lived with and always kept in mind when evaluating hormonal responses.

OVERVIEW OF THE ENDOCRINE SYSTEM

The endocrine system consists of a loosely associated group of nine glands and some specific tissues found throughout the body. These glands secrete hormones into the blood, which then cause some perturbation within a target tissue. The release of hormone is usually controlled by a feedback mechanism. The glands sense the need for the hormone, usually from the blood. The hormone is released, travels to the target tissue, and corrects the disturbance. Once corrected, signals are sent back to the gland, once again usually by the blood, to reduce release of the hormone. For example, elevated blood glucose levels cause the pancreas to release insulin, resulting in an increased cellular uptake of glucose. The increased cellular uptake reduces blood glucose toward normal levels, which is then sensed by the pancreas, causing a reduction in the output of insulin. The example presents a very simple feedback mechanism; however, some of the feedback mechanisms are very complex and involve multiple organs and glands. Regardless of the feedback mechanism, the purpose of the endocrine response still remains the same: maintain the existence of the human organism.

There are two chemical classifications of hormones: those based on amino acids and those based on steroids (1). Steroid hormones are synthesized from cholesterol in the gonads and adrenal cortex. These hormones are lipid soluble and can therefore diffuse directly into the cell. Once inside the cell, these hormones combine with an intracellular receptor, which in turn translocates to the DNA-associated receptor protein, initiating gene activity. The majority of hormones are amino acid based. These range in size from simple amino acid complexes to large molecules. Some amino acid–based hormones enter the cell through exocytosis to bring about a response, but most do not typically enter directly into the cell. They usually combine at a receptor site on the cell membrane, which activates another compound in the cytoplasm, a "second messenger," to bring about the response within the cell.

There appear to be three second messengers for amino acid–based hormones: cyclic adenosine monophosphate (cAMP), cyclic guanosine monophosphate (cGMP), and inositol triphosphate (1,2). The most studied second messenger is cAMP. It was first noted in the study of epinephrine, but it is now believed that at least eight hormones use cAMP as their second messenger. The influence of cAMP appears to be related to the target tissue and cells. In general, cAMP can (a) activate protein kinase, which causes protein catabolism in the liver or thyroxin production in the thyroid; (b) cause glycogen to be converted to glucose-6-phosphate (G-6-P) in muscle cells; (c) activate phosphofructokinase, which enhances glycolysis; (d) activate lipase in the adipocytes to increase free fatty acids (FFAs) in circulation; (e) enhance skeletal and cardiac muscle contractility; (f) increase steroid hormone synthesis; and (g) enhance water retention in the kidney. Thus the effects of cAMP are quite diverse. Of the hormones that are influenced by exercise, adrenocorticotropin hormone (ACTH), thyroid-stimulating hormone (TSH), antidiuretic hormone (ADH), glucagon, and epinephrine work through cAMP. Other exercise-responding hormones such as insulin and norepinephrine work through other second messengers, cGMP or inositol triphosphate.

PITUITARY

Pars Nervosa

The posterior lobe of the pituitary gland secretes ADH, sometimes called *vasopressin*. ADH, an amino acid–based hormone, causes water conservation in the kidneys. The release of ADH is controlled by two mechanisms (Fig. 10–1). Osmoreceptors in the hypothalamus monitor the solute concentration in the blood. Blood normally has an osmolality of 280 to 300 mOsm/L. The exact neurostimulus is unknown, although research has indicated that the ADH is not regulated by endogenous opioids but may in some way be affected by γ-aminobutyric acid (GABA)ergic pathways (3). Regardless of the specific neuromechanism, an increase in osmolality to more than 290 mOsm/L causes the osmoreceptors to signal hypothalamic neurons to synthesize ADH. The ADH travels down the axon (axoplasmic flow) and is released into the blood system in the posterior lobe of the pituitary (4). Once released, ADH travels to the collecting duct of the nephron in the kidney and causes

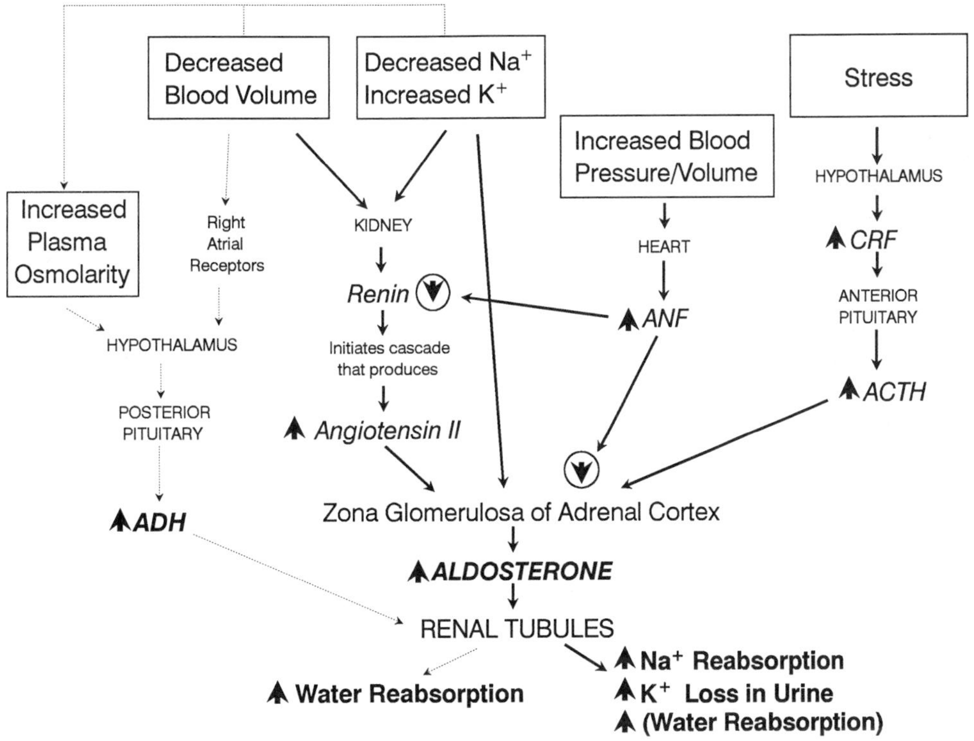

FIG. 10–1. Schematic representation of the hormonal involvement with water and sodium/potassium balance. The *arrows pointing upward* indicate increase, and the *arrows pointing downward* indicate decreased effect.

water retention. This effect is mediated by the second messenger, cAMP. Conversely, a reduction in plasma osmolality to less than 275 to 285 mOsm/L causes ADH to be suppressed, ultimately resulting in diuresis—increased urine output (4,5).

The other mechanism of release of ADH involves the right atrial receptors. These stretch receptors sense the filling pressure in the right atrium of the heart (6). A loss of pressure causes signals to be sent to the hypothalamus to increase ADH synthesis and release. A gain in pressure causes a suppression of ADH. The pressure gain is most obvious during immersion in water, which results in enhanced venous return and right atrial engorgement; there is a concomitant suppression of ADH, causing diuresis (7).

ADH also was shown to have a pressor or vasoconstriction effect at high levels of secretion. The pressor effect appears to be limited to the visceral blood vessels; however, it can result in an increase in systemic blood pressure. In theory then, ADH would help maintain blood pressure during dehydration; however, not all data support this theory (8).

Exercise Responses

Research has indicated that a maximal exercise test that uses a ramp-type protocol lasting 15 minutes or less may (9) or may not (10) increase ADH. The reasons for these equivocal results are unclear. However, exercise sessions of 20 to 60 minutes appear to cause small increases (less than 50%) in circulating ADH concentrations, when the intensity is 50% of maximal capacity or greater (11–14). This effect appears to be intensity related, in that high-intensity exercise causes a greater increase of ADH than does moderate-intensity exercise (13,15). Because total body water during short-term exercise is redistributed rather than lost from the body, the importance of this response is not well understood. The cause of the increase in ADH is still equivocal, but it is probably related to the hemoconcentration or osmolality changes that occur during exercise (11,16). It also is possible that the increased catecholamine response that occurs with high-intensity exercise causes the ADH to be released (17); however, this mechanism is controversial (18). The response also may be related to production or clearance rates. In a hydrated exerciser participating in 30 minutes of exercise, plasma volume is reconstituted in approximately 1 hour. Interestingly, ADH also returns to normal within an hour of the short-term exercise. Thus the ADH response may simply be a result of decreased clearance during this type of exercise and not increased production (14).

The effect of exercise intensity on ADH is magnified by the state of dehydration; the more dehydrated the person, the greater the effect (13,14). Exercising for 20 minutes at 65% of maximal capacity results in a 25% increase in ADH. However, the same exercise with a dehydration of 3% of body weight results in a 75% to 100% increase in ADH, whereas a dehydration of 5% during the exercise results in a 200% increase in ADH (13). During prolonged exercise, considerable sweating occurs, and body water and plasma volume are lost. Water conservation becomes critical for the exercise to continue and, in some cases, for the exerciser to survive. As expected, prolonged exercise seems to cause the greatest ADH response (19,20).

There appears to be no effect of training on ADH. Because endurance training has been shown to increase plasma volume, a modification of the ADH response would be expected. However, no effect has been seen (21). The lack of an effect suggests that there may be some resetting of the volume receptors to allow retention of the greater fluid volume. This is purely speculation at this time.

ADH also can have an effect during rehydration after exercise. If the rehydration solution is very hypotonic and the volume of water ingested is quite large (more than 1000 mL), the solution will result in a very sudden and large increase in plasma water, which can suppress ADH, even though rehydration is not complete (22,23). The suppression of ADH can lead to diuresis—increases of urinary water loss—at a time when water retention is critical, compromising rehydration. These results suggest that care should be taken with regard to the volume and tonicity of the fluid given to rehydrate.

Pars Distalis

Six hormones are secreted by the anterior pituitary; *adrenocorticotropin* (ACTH), *growth hormone* (hGH), *thyroid-stimulating hormone* (TSH), *follicle-stimulating hormone* (FSH), *luteinizing hormone* (LH), and *prolactin*. ACTH regulates glucocorticoid and mineralocorticoid production in the adrenal cortex. Growth hormone regulates postneonatal growth and protein synthesis. TSH regulates thyroid secretions. FSH, LH, and prolactin are related to reproductive functions. There is an intimate relationship between ACTH and adrenal mineralocorticoids; therefore ACTH is discussed in detail in the section on the adrenal cortex. Similarly, an intimate relationship exists between TSH and thyroid function; thus this hormone pairing is discussed in the section on the thyroid gland.

Growth Hormone

Growth hormone, or somatotropin, is an amino acid–based hormone that stimulates protein synthesis and the use of lipids for energy production. It is essential for bone, connective tissue, and muscle growth. The release of hGH is controlled by two hypothalamic-releasing factors or hormones: growth hormone–releasing factor (GHRF), also called somatocrinin, and growth hormone–inhibiting factor (GHIF), also referred to as somatostatin. GHRF is triggered by low hGH levels and a number of the secondary factors including hypoglycemia, low circulating FFAs, norepinephrine, certain amino acids, and generalized stress. GHRF then travels to the cells of the anterior pituitary to cause the release of hGH. Conversely, GHIF inhibits the output of hGH when circulating hGH levels are high. GHIF also is triggered during hyperglycemia, hyperlipidemia, and obesity. In a nonstressful state, the releases of hGH occur in pulses, with greatest pulsations occurring about 2 hours after the onset of sleep (24).

As with all amino acid–based hormones, hGH appears to exert its effects within the cell through a second messenger. The messenger mechanism is still not completely defined, but the present state of knowledge indicates that *insulin-like growth factors* (IGF-I and IGF-II) are involved (1). These IGFs also are called *somatomedins*; however, we refer to them as IGFs. IGF-I is known to increase cellular uptake of amino acids and glycogen synthesis, and can stimulate cell mitosis. The role of IGF-II is not well understood; however, it may have many effects similar to IGF-I (25). IGF-I appears to be more sensitive to growth hormone than is IGF-II.

Growth hormone targets the bone by promoting proliferation of epiphyseal cartilage. This normally occurs before puberty; thus, under normal circumstances, this purpose may not be significant in adulthood. Growth hormone causes proliferation of the connective tissues by stimulating both amino acid and sulfur uptake. In muscle tissue, hGH increases amino acid uptake by the cells and protein synthesis. In adipose tissue, hGH stimulates lipolysis. While in the liver, hGH causes increased fat oxidation and glycogenolysis to produce more glucose and therefore increases liver glucose output. Thus it appears that hGH influences not only protein metabolism but also fat and carbohydrate metabolism (26).

Exercise Responses

Exercise of as little as 8 to 9 minutes in duration has the potential to cause a significant elevation of hGH levels (27–29). The elevation appears to be influenced by the intensity of exercise, duration of exercise, age and gender of the exerciser, and the fitness level of the exerciser. VanHelder and associates (29,30) showed that hGH response to exercise is linearly related to the oxygen demand or exercise intensity, whether the exercise be weightlifting, continuous aerobic cycling, or intermittent anaerobic cycling. High-intensity sprinting for 30 to 60 seconds can even elevate hGH levels more than occurs during submaximal exercise (31,32). The hGH response to the very-short-term exercise may be delayed, however (31,32). Other studies have also shown that anaerobic exercise results in a four- to eightfold increase in hGH, whereas 20 to 30 minutes of moderate-intensity aerobic exercise results in only a one- to three-fold increase (27–30,33,34), and mild exercise appears to exert no effect (35). Thus sufficient data exist to support an effect of intensity of exercise-induced hGH response; however, not all studies are in total agreement (35,36). The purpose of the elevated hGH level during short-term high-intensity exercise is not well understood. However, the cause of the release may be related to norepinephrine, which is known to have exercise intensity–dependent release and concomitantly cause a release of hGH (37–40).

The influence of duration of exercise on hGH is not clear. Karagiorgos and colleagues (41) noted that 30 minutes of exercise at 50% of maximal capacity results in a twofold increase in hGH, whereas 60 minutes of exercise at the same intensity results in a 10-fold increase. Other studies have also noted a progressive increase during 40 to 60 minutes of exercise (42,43), but hGH levels appear to level off at about 60 minutes and, in some cases, may actually decline at exhaustion (35,44). This potential effect at exhaustion appears not to occur in all individuals, as research has noted that marathon runners have elevated hGH levels at the end of their prolonged runs (45,46). Because little anabolic activity occurs during exercise, the need for the elevation of hGH levels may simply be related to attempts to increase lipid metabolism and conserve glucose.

Several studies have reported that intermittent exercise, like interval training, causes a greater hGH response than continuous exercise (30,32,41). This generalization can be somewhat misleading, because all of these studies used higher-intensity exercise for their intermittent protocols. For example, Karagiorgos and co-workers (41) used 45% of maximal intensity for their continuous exercise and 80% of maximal intensity for their intermittent exercise. Similarly, Van Helder and colleagues (30) used almost triple (285 W vs. 100 W) the work load for the intermittent cycling exercise compared with their continuous exercise. From what was stated earlier, it appears that the intensity of the intermittent exercise may have been the cause of the elevated hGH levels rather than the intermittent nature of the exercise. This is an area in need of further study.

Resistance exercise (strength training) has been shown to elevate hGH levels. McMurray and co-workers (24) showed that a high-intensity resistance exercise program elevates hGH levels by about 500%. Kraemer and colleagues (47) showed a three- to fivefold elevation of hGH levels during resistance exercise. As with other forms of high-intensity exercise, the reason for the increase is not clear. If the purpose was to increase protein synthesis for repair or muscle building, then a prolonged elevation of hGH levels would be expected. Most studies have shown, however, that hGH returned to normal levels within an hour after exercise (24,47,48). In addition, one study evaluated overnight hormonal responses to resistance training and found no differences in hGH between a control night and the night after a heavy resistance-training session (24). Furthermore, resistance training does not appear to have a consistent effect on IGF-I (47), suggesting that whatever the purpose of the elevated hGH levels, it may not be mediated by, or through, IGF-I. Thus, although resistance exercise enhances hGH output, the specific purpose is not understood.

Growth hormone can have a direct effect on muscle or can indirectly stimulate IGF-I to cause protein synthesis and cell mitosis. IGF-I appears to be more closely associated with hGH, whereas IGF-II appears to be less dependent on hGH (49). Because the actions of hGH can be mediated through IGFs, it is important to determine the effects of exercise on these growth factors. This process is complicated by the fact that IGFs have a very slow response, taking 3 to 6 hours to respond to a growth-hormone infusion and peaking 16 to 28 hours after infusion (50). Thus studies that focus on IGF response to exercise must monitor responses during the next 24 hours. A 24-hour evaluation is complicated by nutrition, as an inadequate caloric balance reduces IGFs (51). Thus caloric balance must be maintained.

The acute effects of exercise on IGF-I are controversial. Cappon and colleagues (52) found that IGF-I levels were elevated after 10 minutes of exercise and remained elevated for an additional 20 minutes after exercise. However, this elevation followed the same pattern as changes in plasma volume and may not have been directly related to exercise. Cappon and co-workers did monitor the IGF levels over the next 24 hours and found no significant increase, even though hGH increased during the exercise session. Schwarz and co-workers (53) found that 10 minutes of either low- or high-intensity exercise caused a significant increase in IGF-I. Once again, when the exercise-induced loss of plasma volume was taken into account, the increase in IGF was not evident. Furthermore, the increase in IGF-I reported by Schwarz and colleagues came at a time when hGH had not reached its peak response. This response suggests an independence of IGF and hGH during exercise. Henriksen (54) reported that IGF-I levels in rats were slightly elevated after an exhaustive swim. The increase was associated with increased cellular uptake of glucose independent of insulin. Thus prolonged exercise may have an effect. Human studies on prolonged exercise (more than 2 hours) showed that IGF-I is not affected even though hGH increases significantly (45,55,56). However, some of the binding proteins for IGF may be increased for up to 24 hours (56). At present the relevance of the binding-protein changes is not known.

Because resistance training develops muscle mass, it is reasonable to expect that such exercise should increase

IGF-I, but the data do not support this contention. A single weightlifting session appears to result in no acute change in IGF-I, even though hGH increases. In addition, there seems to be no delayed effect of the resistance training on IGF-I (47). Other studies found no consistent effect of resistance training on IGF-I (57,58). Thus it appears that exercise does not exert a strong influence on IGF, and in fact the growth-hormone response to exercise may not mediate an IGF-I response.

It is possible that exercise does not result in an increase in IGF-I but does cause an increased receptor-binding capacity. This response has been demonstrated in mice (59). Such an increase in binding capacity would allow a greater effect of IGF-I without a noticeable increase in IGF-I. Such an effect could account for the insulin-independent increased glucose uptake, as shown by Henriksen (54), and the increased protein synthesis that occurs after exercise.

Endurance training modifies the hGH response to exercise. Studies have shown that resting hGH levels may be elevated in trained individuals (60–62). The elevated resting hGH levels may be related to a lower resting cortisol level that occurs with training, as hGH release has been noted to be negatively related to cortisol (63,64). However, not all studies agree (44,47,65). The reason for these differing results may be related to the intensity of training. Weltman and colleagues (34) noted that when exercise training occurs below the lactate threshold, no effect on resting hGH pulse amplitude is seen. Conversely, when training occurs above the lactate threshold, resting hGH pulse amplitudes were increased compared with controls. An elevated resting hGH level may be necessary to maintain or develop muscle, bone, and connective tissues. This is purely speculation, but the hypothesis appears logical when one considers that training also elevates resting IGF-I levels (66), which are known to mediate protein synthesis.

Several studies have noted that the hGH response to a given submaximal exercise intensity is greater in the untrained individual compared with a trained individual. Chang and co-workers (60) noted a 25% to 30% lower hGH response during 30 minutes of moderate-intensity submaximal exercise. Similarly, Galbo (67) found that the hGH response was lower for trained individuals than for untrained individuals, when exercising at equivalent work loads. In contrast, it appears that the hGH response to high-intensity exercise is greater in the trained individual. Several studies have shown that when exercise intensity exceeds 80% of maximal capacity, the hGH response is 25% to 45% greater in the trained person (44,60,62,68–70). The increased response could be related to the greater lipid oxidation occurring in the trained person. This is only speculation, and the specific purpose is unknown.

Other factors influence hGH. Women have higher resting hGH levels than do men (44,47), but the hGH responses of women during submaximal and maximal exercise may either be similar to those of men (44) or greater than those of men (46,47). Obese individuals appear to have a blunted exercise response (67). High-carbohydrate diets may increase resting hGH (27,71). The influence of dietary composition on hGH exercise response is controversial, however, as one study found that high-fat diets increase the hGH response more than high-carbohydrate diets (71), whereas another study found just the opposite (52). Low caloric intake can elevate resting hGH levels and decrease IGF-I (27). Finally, aging is associated with a reduction in resting hGH levels (48,72) and a blunted exercise-induced hGH response (48,73). The low resting hGH and IGF-I levels and the lack of an exercise-induced hGH effect in older individuals could contribute to the decline in muscle mass associated with aging.

Prolactin

Prolactin is a protein-based hormone also released by the anterior pituitary. Its production is inhibited by dopamine [referred to in reference to prolactin as prolactostatin (PIH)] and is stimulated by thyroliberin (or TRH), although on this last point opinions differ as to whether an additional specific prolactin-releasing hormone actually exists (74). In women prolactin specifically induces breast development and lactogenesis during pregnancy. In both males and females, prolactin release also is associated with a stress response (emotional or physical). For this reason, it has been used as a marker of stress-reactivity in people. In addition, both sexes can develop reproductive problems and disorders from excessive prolactin release. In women, oligomenorrhea and amenorrhea have been reported, whereas in men, oligospermia and testicular atrophy are associated with high levels of prolactin (see references 74 and 75 for more details). The physiologic roles for these observed changes in prolactin during exercise are not understood, but the cause of the response may be related to the overall physical and emotional stress of exercise.

Exercise Responses

Prolactin concentrations in the blood increase during exercise, with the magnitude of the increase somewhat proportional to the intensity of the activity (67). Whether there is a minimal threshold of intensity necessary to induce a response is unclear, but evidence suggests that work above the anaerobic threshold is necessary to elicit substantial changes (67). Provided that intensity is adequate, the increase in blood levels occurs quite rapidly. With short-term exercise, however, the increase in prolactin may peak after the exercise bout if a steady state has not been achieved (76). In some situations, excessive emotional stress can cause an increase before the exercise event even commences [i.e., psychologically induced anticipatory increase (77)].

As for prolonged exercise, as noted earlier, the prolactin response seems proportional to the exercise intensity (64,67). However, extending the duration of the exercise bout can augment the magnitude of the prolactin response (77). Furthermore, as is the case with the hGH response, the prolactin response to prolonged exercise is enhanced when a diet rich in fat is consumed, if an extended fast has occurred first, by conditions in which there is an increase in body temperatures, and after administration of β-adrenergic blockage (67). However, prolactin release is conversely inhibited by α-adrenergic blockade (67). Additionally, during the night, after prolonged endurance exercise during the daytime, prolactin levels are 2 to 3 times greater than when no daytime exercise was performed (77).

Research has shown that the peak prolactin response to repetitive, high-intensity anaerobic exercise (110% $\dot{V}O_2max$) exceeds that found during prolonged submaximal aerobic exercise (78). It is important to note, however, that if the intensity of the exercise is sufficient and the duration is short, the peak prolactin levels in the blood may not occur until the recovery from the exercise bout. Additionally, as noted earlier, the psychological stress of high-intensity work can result in an increase before an exercise bout begins (44).

Repetitive or prolonged maximal isometric muscular contractions are associated with increased prolactin levels, typically during the recovery period (79). Whether similar responses are seen during dynamic resistance exercise is unclear, but preliminary evidence suggests that responses are proportional to the intensity and volume of resistance work completed (Hackney, unpublished results). Although we can demonstrate significant elevations of prolactin levels during a number of different exercise events, the purpose of the response remains an enigma.

The data are contradictory with regard to the effect of exercise training on basal prolactin levels. Some studies have found increases, and others have found decreases (77,80–82). The contradictions are most likely related to the differences in training protocols (intensity, volume duration). In men, Hackney and colleagues (77) showed that the prolactin response to submaximal exercise became attenuated, whereas the response to maximal exercise is augmented as an individual becomes more exercise trained (67). Relative to women, the data are equally contradictory, most likely because of the lack of controls for menstrual status or menstrual-phase considerations.

Gonadotropins: FSH and LH

The gonadotropins are *luteinizing hormone* (LH) and *follicle-stimulating hormone* (FSH), which are released from the anterior pituitary in males and females. The glycoprotein-based gonadotropins are released in responses to a gonadotropin-releasing hormone (GnRH) stimulus from the hypothalamus. GnRH is released in bursts or pulses through the activity of the pulse-generator tissue. The pulsatility of GnRH results in LH and FSH concentrations that also are pulsatile. However, the pulse amplitude and frequency of concentration changes are different for LH and FSH and vary between the genders (see refs. 1 and 83 for more detail). The gonadotropins target the gonads (female ovaries, male testes) and stimulate sex steroid hormone production as well as some aspects of the reproductive processes [i.e., menstruation and spermatogenesis (74)]. The regulation of the gonadotropin concentrations in the blood is under the control of the hypothalamic–pituitary–gonadal axis, which is a complicated feedback-loop mechanism. These two hormones do not directly relate to exercise metabolism; however, prolonged strenuous exercise may modulate these hormones, resulting in an alteration in pubescence in youth, menstrual cycle in women, and possibly spermatogenesis in men.

Exercise Responses

Research indicates that concentrations in the blood of the gonadal hormones may increase during short-term exercise, the increase being more pronounced the higher the work load (43,81,84). These changes are probably due to decreased hepatic blood flow and clearance of the hormones. However, some investigators have reported significant decreases or no changes at all in the gonadotropins in response to exercise (78,82). The reason for the contradictions in the literature appears to be related to methodologic problems in studies. In many cases researchers used infrequent blood-sampling techniques to assess the gonadotropins, which are released in a highly pulsatile fashion.

The prolonged exercise-induced responses of LH and FSH in the blood vary considerably for both men and women (64). Evidence of significant increases, decreases, and no changes at all has been reported (44,64,67). As noted, the reasons for these discrepancies in the findings may relate primarily to methodologic differences between studies. Gender differences in the responsiveness of the gonadotropins may exist, as evidence suggests that the hypothalamic–pituitary–gonadal axis in women is a more sensitive regulatory system than that in men (85).

The research examining short-term supramaximal exercise is limited. Available evidence suggests that LH concentrations are either unaffected or increased slightly in response to this type of exercise (64). More research exists on the responses in relation to maximal exercise. Nonetheless, the findings for maximal exercise are contradictory (44,64), but the majority of the evidence indicates that small, transient increases would occur in the gonadotropins (44,64,67,81). However, the outcomes of these studies, and thus the interpretations, are subject to the same methodologic limitations as noted earlier.

Resistance exercise has been shown to cause an increase in the gonadotropins in women (86). Similar findings are reported for men; however, the amount of research available for this type of exercise is limited in both sexes (87). Further work in needed to determine more clearly the effects of this type of exercise on the gonadotropins.

The major effect of exercise training on the gonadotropins is on the resting, basal concentrations. Several studies report resting LH levels to be elevated after training, whereas others report slight decreases or no change at all (80,82,88–90). The resting pulsatile characteristics of LH seem more consistently affected than the overall concentration levels. Evidence suggests that the pulse amplitude and frequency are compromised after training in both men and women (82,86). The findings for FSH relative to these issues are inconsistent at best (85,91). Whether the responses of the gonadotropins to an acute bout of exercise are consistently affected after training is unclear (64). Work by Duclos and colleagues (89) suggests that submaximal exercise responses (only LH measured) are very similar in the trained and untrained states. Likewise, Hackney and co-workers (81) reported no effect of training in the response of LH or FSH to maximal exercise. Clearly more research is needed regarding the influence of exercise and training on the gonadotropins.

THYROID PHYSIOLOGY

The thyroid gland secretes two amino acid (tyrosine)–based hormones: *thyroxine* (T_4) and *triiodothyronine* (T_3). These two hormones are essential for normal body functioning by modulating metabolic rate and affecting glucose, fat, and protein metabolism. All tissues of the human body except the brain, anterior pituitary gland, spleen, testis, uterus, and thyroid gland appear to be influenced by thyroid hormones. Thyroid hormones increase oxidative metabolism in the mitochondria. These hormones increase tissue responsiveness to the catecholamines (1), which also are known to influence metabolic rate and have a cardiogenic effect (increase heart rate and contractility). Thyroid hormones also increase all aspects of lipid metabolism. High levels of thyroid hormones also cause liver glycogenolysis and protein degradation. Conversely, low levels of these hormones cause protein synthesis and the conversion of glucose to glycogen. Thus thyroid hormones also aid in tissue growth and development.

The thyroid hormones are under the control of *thyroid-stimulating hormone* (TSH), a glycoprotein-based hormone released from the anterior pituitary gland. The anterior pituitary releases TSH in response to thyroid-releasing factor (TRF) from the hypothalamus. Thus control of the release involves a negative feedback loop that includes TRF, TSH, and the thyroid hormones. This regulatory loop is refered to as the hypothalamic–pituitary–thyroid axis. TSH uses cAMP as its second messenger to signal the thyroid gland to release T_4 and T_3. Both T_3 and T_4 exist in bound (primary carrier protein is thyroglobulin, or sometimes called thyroid-binding globulin) and in the free, unbound forms. The free form is the biologically active form. Both T_4 and T_3 act directly in the cell to stimulate metabolism and are essential for muscular contraction (see ref. 92 for a detailed discussion). In the blood, the concentration of T_4 exceeds that of T_3, but T_3 is the biologically more viable of the hormones. The turnover rate of the thyroid hormones is very small, relative to the large extracellular hormone pool that exists. This makes it difficult to detect changes, even large ones, in thyroid function.

Exercise Responses

During short-term exercise, plasma TSH concentrations increase progressively with increasing work loads, with a critical intensity threshold of approximately 50% $\dot{V}O_2max$ being necessary to induce significant changes (84). Although TSH appears to increase, most of the literature on short-term exercise indicates that the concentrations of total and free T_4 and T_3, as well as rT_3 (3,3′,5′-triiodothyronine, peripherally produced), and the clearances of these hormones are essentially unchanged (84,93). Some studies indicate significant increases for total levels of the hormones; however, these findings are most likely brought about by the exercise-induced hemoconcentration (44). An increase in TSH levels might be expected to stimulate the thyroid gland, but a delay is inherent in the stimulus–secretion events at the thyroid gland (92). Thus it is not surprising that a number of studies report the blood concentrations of thyroid hormones (T_4, T_3, and rT_3) as essentially unchanged during a single bout of exercise (64,84). The situation is compounded by the fact that in previous research the influence of environmental factors, food ingestion, and diurnal changes were not always separated from the influence of exercise. Nor has the issue been resolved as to whether exercise-induced changes in thyroid hormone concentrations in the blood may be entirely due to changes in the concentrations of binding proteins.

The influence of prolonged exercise on thyroid function, despite extensive research, is still controversial. Several investigations, which used different exercise protocols, found no effect on the concentration of TSH in the blood (94,95). In contrast, other studies found TSH concentration to increase progressively with higher work load and to reach an elevated steady-state level after approximately 40 minutes of prolonged exercise (96,97). As previously mentioned, an increase in TSH might be expected to cause in increase in T_4 or T_3, but physiologically the issue is much more complicated with the thyroid hormones.

Berchtold and colleagues (97) reported that, during prolonged submaximal exercise (about 3 hours), total T_4 remained constant but then declined during recovery. In the same study, the levels of T_3 were found to decline continuously during exercise. Others have reported total T_3 to remain unchanged, but total T_4 to be increased by 60 minutes of submaximal exercise (98). Galbo (67) suggested that strenuous, prolonged exercise will result only in an increase in the concentration of free T_4 levels. Obviously, more work is necessary in this area to delineate these contradictory results and to determine the physiologic consequences of these responses.

Acute bouts of anaerobic exercise may influence the thyroid hormones. Hackney and Gulledge (98) reported that high-intensity (about 110% $\dot{V}O_2max$) intermittent exercise increases total T_4 levels for several hours into recovery. However, whether these were hemoconcentration-induced changes or due to metabolic clearance rate (MCR) decreases was not determined. Galbo and co-workers (96) showed small, transient increases in the thyroid hormones in response to a maximal graded exercise test ($\dot{V}O_2max$ test). Again, the physiological significance of these findings remains to be determined.

Research on the effect of resistance exercise on thyroid hormones is lacking and is a credible area for future research study. The studies that have been conducted were limited by some of the factors noted earlier and thus had equally contradictory findings. McMurray and colleagues (24) performed a well-controlled study that produced interesting results. These investigators examined total T_4 and T_3 responses immediately after an intensive resistance-training session, as well as for approximately 12 hours into recovery, throughout the night. Transient elevations in T_4 and T_3 were seen immediately after the exercise and were related to hemoconcentration. However, significant nocturnal elevations in T_3 levels were observed as compared with a control night before which no daytime exercise occurred. Physiologically, the elevations of T_3 levels are logical because the resistance exercise would require increased metabolism to repair tissue and increase protein synthesis, both exacerbated by thyroid hormones (1).

The effects of training or chronic exercise exposure on TSH and thyroid function are equivocal (99). Basal and TRF-stimulated blood TSH concentrations were shown to be similar in trained and in weight-matched animals (93) and humans (100). Generally it appears that TSH is not influenced by training, but some human studies showed the rate of T_4 secretion to be higher in trained individuals than that in untrained individuals (101,102). Conversely, Galbo (67) reported that short-term, intensive training periods (1 to 2 weeks) resulted in significant reductions in thyroid hormones. Still other studies did not confirm either of these results, and found that the T_4 secretion rate was similar in trained and in weight-matched control subjects (93,96). The discrepancy in these findings may be related to the fact that these studies failed to account for nutrient balance or thyroid-turnover rate. That is, a negative energy balance has been shown to reduce thyroid hormones (1). Furthermore, work by Irvine (103) suggested that the turnover rate of thyroid hormones may be increased in trained athletes. Obviously, more research is necessary to define the relation between exercise training and thyroid function.

ADRENAL GLAND

Cortex

The adrenal cortex is responsible for the production and release of three major types of steroid-based hormones: glucocorticoids, mineralocorticoids, and gonadocorticoids. The essential function of the *glucocorticoids* is to influence carbohydrate, lipid, and protein metabolism of cells and to assist in providing resistance to stressors. These hormones are essential to sustain life (1,2). Although three forms of glucocorticoids exist in the human, cortisol is the most prevalent. The purpose of the *mineralocorticoids* is to regulate electrolyte concentrations, mainly sodium and potassium, in the extracellular fluid. Although there are several mineralocorticoids, aldosterone makes up about 95% of the total production. The *gonadocorticoids* are male (androgens) and female (estrogens) sex hormones and, as such, are responsible for the development of male or female characteristics. The adrenal cortex provides the only source of androgen in the female and, under normal circumstances, the importance of these gonadocorticoids appears minimal (1). Once these steroid hormones are produced, they easily diffuse into circulation, where the major portion of the hormone is bound to a protein, albumin or corticosteroid-binding globulin (CBG), for transport. Once bound, these hormones are biologically inactive. Thus the minor portion, or free hormone, becomes important, as this portion is the biologically active form of the hormone.

Glucocorticoids

Glucocorticoids are steroid-based hormones essential for life. Their most significant role is to maintain blood glucose levels, and they appear to have an important role in stress adaptation. The most active of the glucocorticoids is *cortisol*, but cortisone, corticosterone, and deoxycorticosterone are other glucocorticoids. These hormones have a direct effect on the liver, where they stimulate gluconeogenesis, which, in turn, elevates blood glucose levels. In the adipose tissue, glucocorticoids, in combination with epinephrine, stimulate lipolysis. Glucocorticoids also have a catabolic effect on liver and muscle protein stores, in some cases creating a negative nitrogen balance. These hormones also appear to have a minor effect on the kidneys, where they facilitate water loss, and on immune function; in large doses, they are immunosuppressive and reduce the inflammatory response. Stress, either physiological or psychological, causes the release of glucocorticoids. The effect of stress is mediated through the central nervous system, probably residing in the sympathetic nervous system, also including the hypothalamus and anterior pituitary gland.

Glucocorticoids are under the control of ACTH, an amino acid–based hormone, the which is secreted from the anterior pituitary. The release of ACTH is controlled by a negative-feedback loop that originates in the hypothalamus and involves both the anterior pituitary and adrenal cortex: the hypothalamic–pituitary–adrenal axis. Corticotropin-releasing factor (CRF) is released from the hypothalamus in response to stress (emotional and physical) and to decreasing blood glucose levels (104). CRF causes the anterior pituitary to release ACTH, which in turn stimulates the release of cortisol. The increasing levels of cortisol feedback modulate the release of CRF, and thus ACTH. The cortisol ultimately enters the cell and targets the nucleus to stimulate muscle proteolysis, adipose lipolysis, and hepatic gluconeogenesis (74).

Both blood ACTH and cortisol levels follow daily patterns that are affected by circadian rhythms, eating, and exercise patterns (1). ACTH and cortisol levels are typically high during the early morning but decrease after the morning meal. As the day progresses, the levels of each hormone will increase again after the midday and evening meals, but in general the overall levels later in the day are lower than those in the morning.

Exercise Responses

The secretion of ACTH during short-term submaximal exercise has mostly been inferred from estimates of cortisol production. However, direct measurements of ACTH concentrations in the blood have been made by a few researchers. There appears to be a delay of 10 to 15 minutes before changes in blood levels are noted (67,84,105–107). Furthermore, exercise of low intensity does not appear to cause a response (67). However, Kjaer and colleagues (108) showed that two-legged knee-extensor static contractions at only 21% maximal voluntary contraction, maintained for approximately 10 minutes, resulted in an ACTH increase. Barwich and co-workers (109) reported that 20 minutes of cycle exercise at 70% of $\dot{V}O_2max$ caused a significant increase in ACTH. Galbo (67) found that ACTH concentration increases with the duration of dynamic exercise, as long as the exercise intensity is higher than 25% of $\dot{V}O_2max$. Similarly, Farrell and colleagues (105) noted that ACTH levels increase about 10% to 15% during moderate-intensity exercise, compared with a 100% increase during high-intensity exercise and a 400% to 500% increase during maximal-intensity exhaustive exercise. Thus the exercise response appears to be related to intensity. The reason for the elevation of ACTH levels is not well understood. Short-term submaximal exercise does not result in decreasing blood glucose levels, nor does it present significant stress, unless the intensity is greater than 50% to 60%. Research has suggested that there is considerable neural interaction with CRF release (110). Because there is a direct proportional relationship between stress and sympathetic activity, it is possible that the neural response to the stress is the cause of the release.

Because cortisol release is under the influence of ACTH, when exercise starts, there tends to be a short lag time (several minutes) for the cortisol response to occur, but the levels increase at a rate proportional to the exercise intensity. This is provided that the intensity is above a critical threshold of approximately 50% to 60% $\dot{V}O_2max$ (111). The final maximal cortisol levels reached are dependent on the total duration of the exercise bout (112). Obviously then, short-duration exercise (especially at very high intensity) may not allow enough time for peak cortisol response to occur during exercise. Furthermore, at work loads less than 50% of $\dot{V}O_2max$, the cortisol concentration in the blood usually decreases because the rate of removal of cortisol from the blood is higher during such low-intensity exercise than at rest, and the secretion rate appears to be lower than at rest (67,84).

During intense prolonged exercise, ACTH concentrations increase dramatically, resulting in significant release of cortisol (67,104). The magnitudes of the responses are modulated by both the relative intensity and duration of the exercise; the greater the intensity and the longer the duration, the greater the release. With prolonged exercise, however, additional factors have time to develop and can result in a further augmentation of the ACTH and cortisol responses. There is evidence that the responses are exaggerated in hypoglycemic and hypoinsulinemic states (64,84). Furthermore, increases in body temperatures may promote exaggerated responses to exercise and psychological stresses, which can influence secretion during exercise (44,46, 64,67). Research has also shown that the responses can be greater during hypoxic exercise than under normoxic conditions (84). Thus prolonged exercise has the potential to stimulate the pituitary–adrenal axis maximally. Although prolonged exercise may elevate ACTH and cortisol levels, it should be noted that several research studies have reported no increase or even a decrease in cortisol level with prolonged exercise (113–115). In some cases, however, the duration of the exercise in these studies appeared insufficient, diurnal circadian patterns were controlled for, or the intensity of the work was below the anaerobic threshold (64).

The magnitude of ACTH–cortisol responses to acute anaerobic exercise is modulated by several of the factors noted earlier, principally relative intensity and exercise duration (64). Anaerobic exercise (more than 100% $\dot{V}O_2max$) is at an intensity great enough to elicit ACTH–cortisol responses, but the duration of activities is typically so short that the increased concentrations in the blood for these hormones may not occur until during the recovery from exercise (44). For example, Buono and co-workers (116) reported a significant increase in ACTH and cortisol levels after 1-minute exercise at 120% $\dot{V}O_2max$. The ACTH increase occurred immediately after the exercise, whereas the cortisol increases were evident at 5 and 15 minutes into the recovery period after the exercise. Viru (64) reported that the exercise-induced increase in ACTH is not only very rapid, but is also very intensive and seems to be the primary mechanism for inducing cortisol increase, because dexamethasone administration abolishes the exercise-induced increase in cortisol (107). Alternatively, a sympathetic–adrenal connection should not be discounted entirely (84,108). Finally, anticipation of the stressful nature of such activities may, however, result in a psychologically induced increase in these hormones before any activity begins (46,64).

Increased ACTH–cortisol concentrations have typically been observed after single acute bouts of hard resistance (weightlifting) exercise (87,117–119). Changes have been observed for varieties of different types of resistance-exercise routines: strength, body building, powerlifting, and Olympic weightlifting (24,86,87). Some studies have reported no changes at all (28,117,118). In this latter situation, methodologic concerns and limitations have compromised the validity of the results. As with many types of activities, there seems to be an intensity-threshold effect necessary to elicit a cortisol response to resistance exercise. It appears that the greater the intensity of the resistance exercise, the larger the magnitude of the cortisol response.

Resting, basal levels of ACTH–cortisol do not seem to show consistent changes in response to exercise training, and most research suggests that no differences exist (80,99). This issue is complicated by the length of time individuals have been involved with their training and whether they are displaying overt symptoms of being overtrained (85). Although resting levels may be unaffected, the exercise response may be modulated. When compared at the same submaximal work loads, trained persons in some research studies have been found to have a smaller increase in blood ACTH and cortisol levels than do untrained persons (46,120). The magnitude of metabolic responses to a given absolute exercise work load declines after a period of endurance training and could account for the lessened hormonal response (101,102,121). However, there also may be a higher rate of disappearance of the hormones from the blood in trained subjects (67). These findings are not universal, as others have reported no differences in cortisol responses to submaximal exercise after exercise training (89) or an increased response (64,122). Relative to maximal exercise, after exercise training, subjects typically have a hormonal response that is greater than or identical to the responses of untrained subjects (121). This phenomenon is due to the trained person's reaching a greater absolute work load; therefore a greater stress is placed on the hypothalamic–pituitary–adrenal axis (46,85).

Mineralocorticoids

Aldosterone is produced in the outer layer (zona glomerulosa) of the adrenal cortex. Its primary function is to control sodium balance. Although produced in the adrenals, its target organs are the nephrons of the kidneys, salivary glands, and sweat glands. At all three sites, aldosterone causes sodium ion reabsorption from the secreted solution of the gland (urine, saliva, sweat) and enhances elimination of potassium and hydrogen ions from the extracellular fluid (blood and interstitial fluid). In addition, aldosterone assists with water balance. Because water appears to move passively with sodium, any reabsorption of sodium would also result in water reabsorption. The combined effect of sodium and water retention influences blood volume and blood pressure.

Aldosterone is regulated by three mechanisms, presented schematically in Fig. 10–1: (a) plasma concentrations of sodium and potassium, (b) ACTH from the anterior pituitary, and (c) the renin–angiotensin system. A decrease in plasma sodium content or an increase in plasma potassium content is directly sensed by the cells of the zone glomerulosa, which causes the release of aldosterone. Conversely, an increase in sodium or a decrease in potassium inhibits the release of aldosterone. A loss of sodium and/or potassium is a common result of dehydration. ACTH becomes important only during very stressful events. During such events, a large amount of ACTH may be released, which appears to cause a modest release of aldosterone.

The major regulator of aldosterone is the renin–angiotensin system. Specialized cells in the juxtaglomerular apparatus of the kidneys respond when (a) renal blood pressure or blood flow declines, (b) there is a decrease in sodium or an increase in potassium in the cell medium, and (c) they are stimulated by the sympathetics or catecholamines (123). These cells release renin into the circulation. The renin initiates a series of reactions that causes angiotensinogen, a protein already present in the blood, to form angiotensin II. Angiotensin II circulates to the adrenal cortex, where it is a potent stimulator of aldosterone release. Angiotensin also is a vasoconstrictor, which causes an increase in blood pressure.

A loss of blood volume or dehydration reduces plasma volume. This causes a reduction in renal blood pressure or flow and modifies sodium and potassium concentrations. Concomitantly, the loss of volume increases catecholamines or causes a sympathetic-induced renal constriction that limits blood flow through the renal arterioles (124–126). All of these initial responses ultimately cause a release of aldosterone. Each of these mechanisms can become important during different types of exercise.

The renin–angiotensin system can be modified by a hormone secreted by the heart, *atrial natriuretic peptide* (ANP). An increase in blood pressure or blood volume in the atria of the heart causes ANP to be released (1,2). The ANP blocks renin, thus reducing aldosterone release. Therefore the overall effect of ANP is to allow more sodium (and water) to be eliminated by the kidneys, thus reducing blood pressure. The response appears to be independent of sympathetic or catecholamine influences (123).

Exercise Responses

The release of aldosterone (and renin) during exercise appears to be partially dependent on intensity (13,124). One investigation reported that 20 minutes of mild exercise caused aldosterone to increase by about 12%. Moderate exercise of the same duration results in about a 50% increase in aldosterone, whereas higher-intensity exercise results in about 75% to 80% increase (13). A high-intensity run at 80% maximal capacity until exhaustion caused a 10-fold increase in aldosterone (15). The mechanism appeared to be related to the sympathetic nervous system and the catecholamines. Exercise enhances sympathetic–catecholamine activity in proportion to the intensity. This in turn would activate the β-adenoreceptors in the renal arterioles, which would reduce renal blood perfusion, causing renin to increase, ultimately increasing aldosterone. This hypothesis also is supported by research on graded exercise testing (20 to 30 minutes), in which increased plasma catecholamines, renin, and aldosterone were found to be related to the catecholamine responses (127).

However, the intensity-dependent relation is not always apparent. One study found that exercise for 20 minutes at 40% to 50% maximal capacity results in an approximately 100% increase in plasma renin and a similar increase in aldosterone (128). Another study found that 30 minutes of exercise at 60% maximal capacity caused plasma renin to increase about 80%, while aldosterone increased only 30% to 70% (129). In contrast to these studies, short-term (less than 10 minutes) peak exercise was shown to elevate angiotensin more than aldosterone levels, probably because of reduced renal degradation or a delayed response on the part of aldosterone (130). Although these reports appear inconsistent, they indicate that the aldosterone response to exercise appears to take approximately 20 minutes to become evident and, furthermore, even mild- to moderate-intensity exercise is sufficient to cause the response.

Although the mechanism for the aldosterone response to short-term exercise is probably related to changes in renal blood flow and sympathetic activity, the purpose remains unclear. There are no significant amounts of sodium or water loss. In addition, movements of potassium into the plasma and sodium out of the plasma are transient and return to normal within an hour. Thus no physiological purpose for the increased aldosterone is readily evident.

The elevation of aldosterone levels in response to more severe, prolonged exercise seems logical. Prolonged exercise, in which considerable sweating occurs, reduces blood volume. There is a concomitant vasoconstriction (including the kidneys) that redistributes blood away from the kidneys to maintain muscle blood flow. This response causes increased renin and aldosterone. In addition, to enhance heat loss, more blood would be distributed to the periphery, which would reduce central blood volume; this would reduce renal blood flow, and once again, cause renin to be released. Dehydration also is associated with an increased sodium loss, which directly stimulates aldosterone release. Dehydration is clearly a factor influencing the release of aldosterone, as a 5% body-weight dehydration can cause a threefold increase in aldosterone compared with similar exercise in a hydrated state (13). Ninety minutes of exercise at 60% maximal capacity results in a 200% to 300% increase in aldosterone (131). Marathon runs cause 5- to 10-fold increases in aldosterone, which may remain elevated 22 hours after exercise. Thus the research is clear that all prolonged exercise to exhaustion results in large increases in aldosterone.

There appears to be little effect of training on the aldosterone response to exercise or dehydration (12,15, 21,132). Because training attenuates sympathetic/catecholamine responses at a given absolute work load, an effect would be expected. This suggests that aldosterone may not be as tightly coupled to the sympathetic nervous system as indicated earlier. Although there appears to be little training effect, there is evidence of an important role for aldosterone during training. Endurance training induces an expansion of plasma volume, which may be partially accounted for by an effect of aldosterone. Luetkemeier and colleagues (133) trained men for 2 hours per day at 65% maximal capacity for 3 days. They then blocked aldosterone with spironolactone and found a smaller increase in plasma volume and reduced aldosterone activity compared with controlled training without the aldosterone block. They estimated that approximately 40% of the training-induced plasma volume expansion could be accounted for by aldosterone activity. Thus aldosterone may be important during training to assist with plasma volume expansion. The increased plasma volume may be an effect of the aldosterone causing sodium retention, which would passively result in water retention. Endurance training also causes partial heat acclimation. Heat acclimation results in plasma volume expansion. Previous research suggests that heat acclimation results in higher circulating aldosterone, which may be the cause of the increased blood volume (134). The information on training and heat acclimation, taken together, suggests that any effect of training may be a result of the increased core temperatures that occur during the exercise training and may not be related to any change in the sympathetic nervous system activity. Such a response may be the reason that no training effects were evident when the exercise-training session lasted less than an hour. This duration of training may not have been sufficient to produce a significant heat load.

The effect of exercise on ANP has been documented. Short-term high-intensity exercise increases ANP (135,136). Similarly, ANP has been shown to increase 100% with a 15-minute graded exercise test (9). Although the specific physiologic role is unknown, the increased ANP may reduce vascular resistance and thus improve blood flow (135). Prolonged exercise of 150 minutes at 70% has been shown to increase ANP 200% to 300% (135). Theoretically this response would not be expected because elevated ANP would adversely affect blood volume through its diuretic effects. However, the sympathetic-induced decrease in renal blood flow may attenuate this effect. The importance during exercise may not be related to fluid volume control but may be related to ANP ability to cause vasodilatation, which could (a) subdue the vasoconstrictive effects of angiotensin, (b) improve muscle perfusion, and (c) enhance heat dissipation through the skin (135).

Adrenal Medulla

The inner portion of the adrenal gland is the adrenal medulla. It is actually part of the autonomic nervous system, deriving its tissues from the same source. The secretions of this tissue are intimately involved with the "fight-or-flight" mechanism, mobilizing the individual's capacity to meet the needs of a crisis. The active substances released by the medulla are the *catecholamines*: epinephrine, norepinephrine, and dopamine. Because of the significant interaction of the catecholamines and the sympathetic nervous system, the far-reaching effects of the catecholamines, and the lack of a specific target tissue (Table 10–2), the catecholamines are not considered true hormones by some endocrinologists (1). Because of their importance during exercise, however, they are incorporated in this chapter.

The adrenal medulla is activated by the sympathetic nervous system; the greater the sympathetic activity, the greater the catecholamine responses. The medullary secretions consist of approximately 75% to 80% epinephrine, 20% to 25% norepinephrine, and small amounts of dopamine. For comparison purposes, the sympathetic nervous system releases predominantly (75% to 80%) norepinephrine and small amounts (20% to 25%) of epinephrine. Therefore under resting conditions, the plasma levels of norepinephrine are 5- to 10-fold greater than those of epinephrine (1). However, in severe stress when the adrenal medulla is stimulated, as in high-intensity or prolonged exercise, epinephrine levels can increase 10- to 20-fold.

Neither norepinephrine or epinephrine can enter the cell; thus the specific cell functions are mediated through

TABLE 10–2. *Effects of catecholamines on the various tissues directly involved with exercise*

Receptor	Target tissue/organ	Response
β_1	Heart	Increased rate, contractility
β_2	Arterioles	Vasodilatation of muscle and coronary arteries
α	Vascular system	Vasoconstriction
β_2	Respiratory system	Bronchial dilation
β_2	Pancreas	Increased insulin secretion
α_2	Pancreas	Decreased insulin & increased glucagon secretion
β_2	Skeletal muscle	Activated phosphorylase & phosphofructokinase
β_2	Adipose tissue	Increased lipolysis
β_2	Liver	Increased glycogenolysis, gluconeogenesis, & lipolysis
β_2	GI system	Decreased contractility
α	GI system	Vasoconstriction
α	Skin	Increased sweat production
β_1	Kidneys	Increased renin secretion

Adapted from ref. 1, with permission.

a second messenger. Epinephrine generally works through the adenyl cyclase–cAMP system, whereas norepinephrine may work though PIP as the second messenger (1). However, the hormone/second-messenger match for the catecholamines is not always that clear. The actions of epinephrine and norepinephrine are mediated through separate types of adrenergic receptors, classified as α and β receptors (Table 10–2). There also are subclassifications of each of these receptors: α_1, α_2, β_1, and β_2. The distribution of these receptors is unique throughout the body. Although both catecholamines can stimulate α and β receptors, the catecholamines appear to have different affinities for each type of receptor. Norepinephrine has a greater affinity than epinephrine for α receptors, particularly α_2. These α_2 receptors are located in greater numbers in the periphery, pancreas, and organs of the urogenital system. During exercise, stimulation of these receptors causes generalized vasoconstriction, decreased insulin output, and increased sweat rate. The β receptors are found in higher concentrations in adipose tissue, heart muscle, skeletal muscle, the gastrointestinal (GI) system, and the urogenital system. Epinephrine seems to have a greater affinity for β receptors. During exercise, epinephrine stimulates the β receptors, particularly β_2, which enhances metabolism. The β_1 receptor, which is responsible for the increased heart rate during exercise, seems to be equally stimulated by epinephrine and norepinephrine. The issue is further confused in that stimulation of some receptors causes an excitatory effect at some target tissues but an inhibitory effect at others. For example, stimulation of the β_2 receptor causes increased metabolism in the muscle cells and also relaxation of the bronchial muscles.

Epinephrine is a potent stimulator of metabolism. It can increase phosphorylase activity, which causes glycogen to be converted back to G-6-P (137). It activates phosphofructokinase (PFK), which increases the rate of glycolysis and can increase lactate formation (137). In addition, epinephrine can increase lipolysis, which presents metabolically active cells with more FFA as a source of energy production (137). The increased phosphorylase activity affects glycogenolysis both in the liver and in the muscle cells. Thus epinephrine helps to maintain blood glucose levels. The increased PFK activity appears to occur in the muscle cells, whereas the increased lipolysis occurs mostly in the adipose tissue. Epinephrine also has an inhibitory effect on insulin release and an excitatory effect on glucagon release (137). Thus the effects of epinephrine support blood glucose levels.

In the cardiovascular system, both epinephrine and norepinephrine stimulate heart rate during exercise. However, the cardiac effect is not evident until the heart rate increases about 25 beats/min above rest (138). Norepinephrine causes a generalized vasoconstriction, whereas epinephrine causes dilation of the skeletal and coronary blood vessels (1). These responses work synergistically to increase cardiac output and active muscle blood flow.

The catecholamine responses and effects on other physiologic systems also are important to exercise. Epinephrine also causes dilation of the bronchial smooth muscle to reduce resistance to airflow, and through the central nervous system, effects can increase rate and depth of respiration. The catecholamines also reduce renal blood flow, constrict bladder sphincter muscles, reduce digestion, and increase renin secretion. Such responses would support the demands of high-intensity exercise.

Exercise Responses

The response of the catecholamines to exercise is dependent on the intensity and duration of the exercise. Several studies have shown that norepinephrine increases with the intensity of exercise (40,138,139). Small increases are evident even during low-intensity exercise. The low-intensity response is related to the sympathetic nervous system more than to the adrenals (138). Disproportionate increases are evident during high-intensity exercise (140). The augmented output during high-intensity exercise is related to both sympathetic nervous and adrenal output. Unlike norepinephrine, it appears that epinephrine does not increase during light-intensity exercise and becomes evident only during moderate-intensity exercise (138). Studies have reported small increases in epinephrine at 40% maximal capacity (40,140) and significant increases thereafter (40,139). Thus the intensity-related response of epinephrine may be somewhat delayed. The increases in catecholamine during submaximal exertion are quite notable in comparison to other hormones. Twenty minutes of exercise at 60% maximal capacity can double the circulating levels of norepinephrine and triple the levels of epinephrine (40,141). The same duration of exercise, but at 80% maximal capacity, results in a 350% increase in norepinephrine and a 500% increase in epinephrine (40,141). By comparison, maximal- and supramaximal-intensity exercise was shown to cause a 10-fold to 15-fold increase (1000% to 1500%) in both epinephrine and norepinephrine (140,142) levels. The reasons for the increased catecholamines during high-intensity exercise are to support the greater need for cellular glucose uptake, glycolysis, increased heart functioning, vasoconstriction to redistribute blood volume to exercising muscle, and increased ventilatory needs.

As the duration of exercise increases (at a given intensity), the catecholamine output also increases. One study showed that a 50-minute run at 60% to 70% maximal intensity resulted in a 300% to 400% increase in epinephrine and a 600% to 900% increase in norepinephrine (142). Ninety minutes of exercise caused an 11-fold increase in epinephrine and a 10-fold increase in norepinephrine (102). Finally, moderate exercise (about 50% maximal capacity) to exhaustion resulted in a 28-fold increase in norepinephrine and a similar increase in epinephrine (67). The increased catecholamines during prolonged exercise support the increased muscle cell need for glucose by enhancing liver glycogenolysis, increasing glucagon output from the pancreas, and increasing lipolysis in the adipose tissue. The catecholamines also help with heat dissipation by increasing sweating and redistributing blood flow from the nonactive tissues (splanchnic area) to the skin for better heat convection. Finally, the increased catecholamines also help with water conservation by decreasing renal blood flow and increasing renin output, affecting aldosterone.

Endurance training reduces the catecholamine response during submaximal exercise. The reduced medullary output is evident both at a given absolute metabolic rate (liters O_2/min or milliliters O_2/kg/min) and also at a given percentage of maximal metabolic rate (102,121,143,144). To counter the lower catecholamine output, it appears that there is an increased receptor sensitivity, and not increased receptor number (145), which results in a greater response for a given amount of catecholamines. Although the submaximal response is attenuated in the trained individual, the maximal response is increased (143,146). This enables the trained individual to sequester more glucose and glycogen to sustain the high metabolic requirements. The training response occurs in less than 3 weeks (102).

PANCREAS

The endocrine portion of the pancreas is involved with blood glucose regulation. Minute cell clusters are dispersed throughout the gland, known as the islets of Langerhans. These islets contain predominantly two types of cells, the alpha and beta cells. The alpha cells secrete the hormone *glucagon*, which functions to elevate blood glucose levels, whereas the beta cells secrete *insulin*, which reduces blood glucose levels. Although these hormones have opposing effects, it does not necessarily follow that when one is elevated, the other is suppressed. Their control appears to be independent to some degree.

Normal blood glucose concentrations are 70 to 110 mg/dL (3.9 to 6.1 mmol/L). Levels less than 70 mg/dL (3.9 mmol/L) are considered hypoglycemia and result in an elevation of glucagon levels. Conversely, glucose levels above approximately 120 mg/dL (6.7 mmol/L) are considered hyperglycemic and result in an elevation of insulin levels (147). These appear to be the typical responses for insulin and glucagon in a normal, healthy individual. However, these responses are modified by the disease diabetes mellitus and exercise. Diabetes mellitus can be a result of a hyposecretion of insulin or a hypoactivity of insulin, which results in an elevation of blood glucose levels due to a reduction in cellular uptake. The cause can be a lack of production of insulin by the beta cells (type I) or a resistance of cells to insulin's effects (type II). A complete discussion of diabetes mellitus is beyond the scope of this chapter.

Insulin

Insulin is a small protein-based hormone that causes blood glucose levels to decrease by increasing cellular uptake of glucose, particularly in the muscle cells. Insulin activates tyrosine kinase, which allows the insulin to be internalized into the cell (148). Once inside the cell, insulin causes a translocation of glucose transporters from the cytoplasm to the plasma membrane, which allows more glucose to be delivered into the cell. Insulin appears to have little effect on the liver, kidneys, and brain, but has its major effect on striated muscle cells. In these muscle cells, the GLUT4 transporter molecule is the most abundant. The GLUT4 transporter assumes a very prominent role during exercise.

The effect of insulin is not limited to just cellular uptake of glucose. Once glucose is inside the cell, insulin encourages glucose to form glycogen. If glycogen stores are full, insulin can cause the conversion of glucose to fat, particularly in the adipose tissue (1,2). In addition to these effects, insulin attenuates the use of fats for energy, glycogenolysis, and gluconeogenesis. Insulin also attenuates protein degradation and enhances cellular uptake of amino acid, thereby promoting protein anabolism. Thus insulin affects the metabolism of all three major nutrients.

Exercise Responses

Most forms of exercise cause a reduction in insulin levels, as long as an increase in blood glucose does not occur (149). The cause of the exercise-induced reduction in insulin is not completely understood, but it has been shown that the beta cells have α-adrenergic receptors, which, when stimulated, decrease insulin secretion. Exercise elevates sympathetic activity, which would stimulate these α-adrenergic receptors, reducing insulin. The effect was found to occur during short-term (10- to 30-minute) submaximal exercise at an intensity of 40% or more maximal exercise capacity (64,102,150), prolonged submaximal exercise of 60 to 180 minutes (151–153), maximal-intensity exercise (154), and even during resistance or strength exercises (155). The effect does not appear to be intensity dependent at greater than 40% maximal capacity (64,156) but is directly related to duration of exercise (149). In addition, this effect can last from just a few hours (157,158) up to 48 hours (159).

Insulin normally declines during exercise, yet cellular

uptake of glucose can increase up to 20-fold (160). A decrease in insulin theoretically should result in a decrease in cellular uptake of glucose; however, noninsulin mechanisms are used to cause the muscular uptake. First, exercise increases blood flow, which presents the cells with more glucose. Second, catecholamines in some way stimulate cellular uptake of glucose. Third, the exercise directly stimulates translocation of GLUT4 transporters to the sarcolemma to enhance glucose uptake. The exact mechanism of stimulation is not completely known; however, it is known that nitrous oxide–dependent (161) and calcium-dependent (162) mechanisms exist. Therefore the increased blood flow, increased catecholamines, and GLUT4 translocation all work synergistically to enhance muscle cell glucose uptake. Thus the reduction in insulin is appropriate, or the combined effect of exercise and elevated insulin levels would cause too fast a rate of cellular uptake of glucose, resulting in hypoglycemia. The low levels of insulin also permit mobilization of glucose from liver stores, fat use for energy, and gluconeogenesis (1), all necessary responses during prolonged exercise.

Some exercisers ingest glucose or sugars (solids or liquids) 30 to 60 minutes before exercise. They believe that these sugars will serve as a source of energy during the exercise. Some research has shown that this practice causes an increase of insulin that is maintained during the initial 30 minutes of exercise. The combined effect of the insulin and exercise has been shown to cause transient hypoglycemia (163). In addition, the elevated insulin level also suppresses energy production by beta-oxidation. If this effect occurs during prolonged exercise, there may be a loss in performance and possibly early fatigue due to premature use of glycogen stores (164). In contrast, if the ingestion of high-sugar drinks occurs during exercise, the exercise effect on insulin is suppressed, thus insulin stays low, and detrimental effects are not evident (165).

Endurance training results in a lower resting insulin; however, the response to exercise does not appear to be changed (102). Research has shown increases in insulin sensitivity (159,166) and GLUT4 transporter content of the muscle in as little as 7 days (167–169). The improved sensitivity and transporter changes appear to be complete in 2 weeks; however, they last only 3 to 6 days after the cessation of training (159,169).

Glucagon

Glucagon is a polypeptide hormone released from the alpha cells of the islets in response to hypoglycemia. Thus its major effects appears to oppose those of insulin. Glucagon is a very potent hormone in that very small amounts of glucagon will cause large increases in plasma glucose. The elevation of blood glucose levels is accomplished at the liver by causing the release of any glucose contents, causing stores of glycogen to be converted to glucose (glycogenolysis), causing the synthesis of glucose from lactic acid, and causing the liver to produce glucose from fatty acids and amino acids (gluconeogenesis). In adipose tissue, glucagon promotes lipolysis; thus more fatty acids are available for energy production. Glucagon uses cAMP as its second messenger inside the cell. The cAMP activates protein kinase, which through a series of events activates the enzymes necessary to bring about the necessary responses at the target tissue.

Exercise Responses

Our knowledge of glucagon responses to exercise is quite elementary compared with what is known about insulin. There appears to be no response during the first 10 minutes of submaximal exercise (64); however, short-term maximal exercise, as in a stress test, which may last 13 to 15 minutes, does result in a small (about 30%) increase in glucagon (170). Once the delayed response begins, there is a slow, steady increase. The increase in glucagon continues slowly for approximately the first 30 minuts of exercise; thereafter it may level off or continue to increase at a slower rate (149,150). The overall effect of exercise on plasma glucagon is small compared with the effect on other hormones. Most human studies have found increases of less than 100%. For example, mild exercise at 40% maximal capacity for durations of 40 to 120 minutes results in only about a 20% increase in glucagon (153,160). Moderate-intensity exercise (55% to 65% maximal capacity) for 90 minutes results in a 40% to 50% increase (102). It appears that the longer the exercise duration, the greater the glucagon response (102,149). This is particularly evident in untrained subjects (102).

Several factors have been found to influence the glucagon response to exercise. The most obvious is the reduction of blood glucose levels. Bottger and colleagues (171) found that hypoglycemic-induced release of glucagon can account for about 48% of the hepatic glucose production. This finding suggests that more than 50% of the stimulus for liver glucose production is not directly tied to glucagon. Exercise must be prolonged for this response to occur, however, and it is known that glucagon is increased fairly quickly in exercise. The alpha cells of the pancreas have β-adrenergic receptors that respond to increasing epinephrine (172). Exercise increases epinephrine, which could serve as the initial stimulus for glucagon release. Studies have shown that when epinephrine levels are manipulated during exercise, glucagon release follows a similar pattern (172,173). Researchers have also hypothesized that increased use of fats for energy during exercise may serve as a stimulus for glucagon (64,149,173). Insulin must decline for fat oxidation to be increased, and it is known that a decrease in insulin sensitizes liver cells to glucagon (149). Thus several factors appear to control glucagon during exercise.

Endurance training has been shown to blunt the glucagon response during submaximal exercise lasting less than 120 minutes (102,171). The reason for this effect appears to be twofold. First, trained individuals conserve glucose and glycogen stores. They have increased muscular glycogen stores; thus liver stores are not required until late in exercise. In addition, they have increased capacities to use fats for energy, which delays use of the liver glycogen further into exercise. Second, training reduces the epinephrine response to submaximal exercise (102); thus there would be less adrenergic stimulus for glucagon release.

Figure 10–2 illustrates the relation between insulin and glucagon during exercise. Exercise causes an increase in catecholamines. The norepinephrine has a suppressive effect on insulin, which accounts for the reduction of insulin during exercise. The epinephrine has a stimulatory effect on glucagon, which can account for the early increase. For cells to maintain or increase glucose uptake with declining insulin, the exercise stimulates a translocation of the glucose receptors. Thus more receptors on the membrane provide more sites for facilitated transport and therefore greater glucose uptake. As the exercise continues, the use of fats for energy may provide feedback to stimulate glucagon release; this further mobilizes FFAs from adipose stores, thus providing more fats for energy, which would conserve glycogen and glucose stores. During exercise, the body attempts to match glucose production with cellular uptake. Glucagon stimulates the liver to release its glucose stores, convert glycogen stores to glucose, or convert fats and amino acids to glucose. These mechanisms work in synchronization to attempt to maintain blood glucose and muscular glucose uptake during exercise.

TESTIS

Testosterone is the major male sex hormone. In men testosterone production is signaled by hormones from the hypothalamus and anterior pituitary. Specifically, low circulating testosterone feeds back to cause the release of gonadotropin-releasing factor (GnRF) from the hypothalamus. The GnRF stimulates the release of FSH and LH from the anterior pituitary, in a pulsatile fashion. The LH in turn stimulates the cells of Leydig in the testis to produce and release testosterone. In men, this interaction of hormones and glands is refered to as the hypothalamic–pituitary–gonadal axis (85). For women, testosterone is released primarily from the adrenal cortex through a mechanism that also implements the release of the glucocorticoids and/or mineralocorticoids (i.e., the hypothalamic–pituitary–adrenal axis). For both sexes, circulating testosterone exists in free

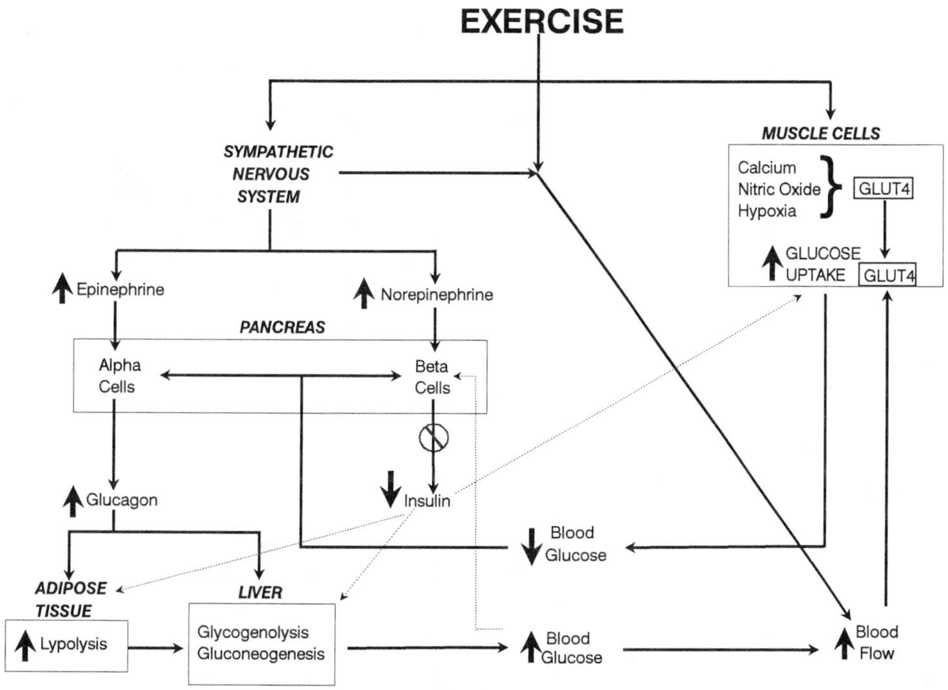

FIG. 10–2. Schematic representation of the control mechanism for the release of insulin and glucagon in the pancreas. *Arrows pointing downward* indicate a reduced effect, whereas *arrows pointing upward* indicate an increased effect. The *dotted lines* indicate pathways that are evident at rest but are suppressed during exercise.

and bound forms. Approximately 3% or less of the total testosterone is in the free form; the remainder is bound. The primary binding protein for testosterone is sex hormone–binding globulin (SHBG), sometimes referred to as sex steroid–binding globulin (74,92). Physiologically, testosterone, a steroid-based hormone, has both anabolic and androgenic roles in each sex and is considered essential for proper growth, development, sex differentiation, and reproductive function. With respect to exercise, the anabolic functions are more significant than the androgenic functions. These functions include increased protein synthesis, long-bone growth, enzyme activation, and increased erythrocyte formation. Testosterone is under regulation by the hypothalamus and anterior pituitary gland.

Exercise Responses

Numerous studies indicate that during short-term exercise, the total and free testosterone levels increase, and this increase is proportional to the relative intensity of the work load being performed (64,67,90,174,175). Whether an exact critical threshold intensity of exercise is necessary to elicit a response is debatable. Evidence indicates that the increases are due to a combination of factors: (a) a decrease in metabolic clearance rate (MCR), (b) an increase in secretion production (mediated possibly by circulating catecholamines, sympathetic activity), and/or (c) exercise-induced hemoconcentration (85).

During prolonged exercise, the testosterone responses appear quite variable (64). There are findings suggesting that testosterone concentrations are either increased or decreased with prolonged exercise (64, 176). The reason for these contrasting results seems to be related to the intensity and duration of the exercise bout. As noted earlier, testosterone responses are proportional to the intensity of the exercise; as higher intensities are performed, testosterone levels increase. However, if the duration of an exercise bout is long enough, 60 to 90 minutes or longer, hormonal levels start to decline, because of either an increased MCR or a slightly decreased testicular secretion production. If the exercise duration is substantial, then the testosterone levels can decline below preexercise concentrations and the reduction can persist for up to several days (96,177).

In response to maximal exercise, testosterone levels are significantly increased (96,175). The reasons for this increase seem to be hemoconcentration, decreased MCR, and catecholamine-stimulated gonadal secretion production (91,96,175). Supramaximal exercise also results in increased testosterone concentrations, most likely for the reasons just noted (78,177). As with many hormones, the duration of anaerobic exercise is typically so short that the increase observed in testosterone may not occur until the recovery period. Regardless, all changes brought about by acute bouts of anaerobic exercise seem very transient and short lived in nature.

Studies indicate that testosterone is increased after resistance-based exercise (24,87,119). However, this finding is not completely universal (178,179). The magnitude of the testosterone increase appears dependent on several variables, including the intensity of exercise (i.e., percentage of one repetition maximum), the volume of the exercise (i.e., mass lifted × repetition number × number of sets), the amount of muscle tissue used in the exercise protocol, and the age of the subject (87,180). Research also suggests that there is a threshold intensity, volume, and muscle-mass involvement necessary to produce increases in testosterone concentrations (87). The extent to which these variables interact with one another results in individual-based thresholds and does not allow generalizations as to the exact point where the threshold occurs. Furthermore, other factors may affect the response, such as rest-period length or combining session lifting formats (low resistance, high volume vs. high resistance, low volume), but the degree of the effect remains to be determined. The responses of testosterone (or androgens) seem somewhat consistent in both men and women. Nonetheless, the magnitude of the increase after exercise may be less in women (this may be related to the lower basal levels of the hormone found in women) and may also be influenced by the phase of the menstrual cycle (178). On this issue, however, there are fewer studies with women as subjects, and the data are more contradictory than those found in men.

Training causes adaptations in the acute responses of testosterone to exercise. In the case of dynamic activity such as treadmill running, there seems to be an attenuation of the normal increase in the concentrations in response to submaximal exercise (64). The increase is still proportional to the intensity of the exercise, but the absolute and relative changes appear to be smaller (181). Research on the maximal exercise responses after training point to equivocal results (90). One of the most notable changes in this hormone with training is in the basal concentrations (81,82). Research has shown that the longer a man is involved with exercise training (i.e., running), the lower the basal testosterone concentrations. The magnitude of these reductions in basal testosterone levels can be on the order of 25% to 75% of the pretraining levels (85). The research to determine whether these changes at rest are reversible or occur in other forms of training (e.g., swimming) is inconclusive. Evidence indicates that there may be a relationship between these reduced testosterone concentrations and the development of male infertility (182). However, much further research is necessary to substantiate this potential relation. The lower testosterone levels may be related to training-related changes in LH such as altered pituitary release and pulse characteristics (90). However, the details of this mechanism are still equivocal.

Research suggests that resting testosterone concentrations remain unaltered by resistance training (87, 179). However, Stone and colleagues (180) reported increased resting levels during the course of a 12-week resistance program in middle-aged men. Conversely, Arce and co-workers (183) reported that men involved with resistance training had lower resting testosterone levels than age-matched men who were nonexercisers. Thus the responses of testosterone to resistance training are in need of further research examination. The acute testosterone response to a bout of resistance exercise after training appears variable. Some studies have shown increases in the testosterone response, whereas others have shown no change after training (87,179). Some of the reasons for the equivocal results may relate to issues of subject age, as young subjects may show a greater tendency to have increases after training. The duration of the exposure to resistance-training programs, gender, and the subjects' experience with resistance training are other factors that should be considered.

OVARIAN HORMONES

The ovaries secrete two types of hormones: *estrogens*, which include estradiol, esterone, and estriol, and *progesterone*. As with testosterone, the majority of these hormones circulate throughout the body attached to SHBG. Only 1% to 2% are actually free form, and it is this 1% to 2% that are biologically active. These steroid-based hormones are intimately involved with reproduction and the development of the female secondary-sex characteristics. Estrogen has some other characteristics that might have some implications for exercise. Estrogen may cause glycogen conservation or sparing during submaximal exercise due to an increased metabolism of lipids (184,185). Estrogens also may have a role in water retention and maintaining plasma volume (186). During heat exposure, estrogens have been implicated as promoters of heat loss independent of sweating (186). Estrogens have a role in epiphyseal closure at the end of pubescence in girls. Thus ovarian hormones are of minimal importance during exercise.

Exercise Responses

Limited research has focused on the acute responses of ovarian hormones to exercise. Most of the research has focused on the effect of exercise training. The research on acute responses has shown that 30 minutes of exercise results in an increase in both estrogens and progesterone. For example, Bonen and colleagues (187) noted that in general, 30 minutes of exercise at 70% maximal intensity causes an estimated 38% increase in progesterone and about a 14% increase in estradiol, with no changes in FSH or LH. Furthermore, the increases appear to be somewhat related to the intensity of the exercise, as the study also found that as exercise intensity increased from 62% to 78% maximal capacity, both hormones increased. Jurkowski and co-workers (188) also reported an intensity-related increase in progesterone; however, the results were not as consistent with respect to estrogen, as significant increases occurred only during exhaustive exercise. The same study also noted that the exercise must be greater than 33% maximal intensity to cause a significant increase in progesterone. Other studies have also found increases in ovarian hormones during short-term and prolonged submaximal exercise (189,190). The elevation of estrogen and progesterone levels during submaximal exercise appears to be related to changes in hepatic clearance; Keizer and co-workers (191) found that during the follicular phase, 40 minutes of exercise resulted in a 50% reduction in MCR.

The response to exercise is dependent on the phase of the menstrual cycle. Bonen (187) noted that during the luteal phase, progesterone increases 40%, and estradiol increases about 21%. The increase in progesterone during menses was similar in the luteal phase, but estradiol actually decreased about 17%. These differences in response have the potential to influence glycogen metabolism during exercise. Research has shown that high-intensity exercise during the luteal phase results in a greater use of fats for energy (glycogen sparing) than occurs during the follicular phase (188). Furthermore, the glycogen-sparing effect that occurs during the luteal phase has the potential to improve exercise times to exhaustion by as much as 40% (184). Thus the phase of the menstrual cycle complicates the study of the ovarian hormonal responses to exercise.

The response of the ovarian hormones to chronic exercise or exercise training has been the focus of several investigations. The majority have reported that these forms of exercise cause a decrease in resting levels of estrogens and progesterone (189,192,193). The low levels have been related to lower FSH and LH in some studies (192,193). Low levels of both gonadotropins and ovarian hormones have resulted in menstrual irregularities in some athletes and even in some moderate exercisers (194). The more prolonged and intense the exercise, however, the greater the risk of menstrual irregularities and amenorrhea or loss of menstrual cycle (194). There are several theories as to why the irregularities occur. We know that exercise causes an increase in β-endorphin. Grossman and co-workers (195) showed that opioids, including β-endorphin, have the ability to block the release of GnRF from the hypothalamus. Thus reduced GnRF suppresses LH and FSH, resulting in low estrogens and progesterone. We also know that exercise increases prolactin and hypothalamic CRF (192). Both of these hormones inhibit GnRF, which would result in the same cascade of events, leading to the irregularities. Chronic exposure to exercise that keeps prolactin, CRF, or opioids elevated could therefore result in a loss of menstrual cycle. Another potential confounder is loss of body fat, as Elias and Wilson (194) found that as athletes lose body fat, the number of menstrual irregularities increases. The exact mechanism is still speculative and in need of further research.

OTHER HORMONES AND NONCLASSIC HORMONES

β-Endorphin

Besides the numerous releasing factors or releasing hormones already discussed, the hypothalamus also is responsible for secreting *β-endorphin* (β-END). β-END, a neuropeptide, is a natural opiate that reduces perceptions of pain and modulates the output of some hormones. β-END is found throughout the brain and in measurable levels in the circulation. Research has suggested that there is a relation between brain and blood levels (196). At the anterior pituitary, proopiomelanocortin (POMC) is a precursor polypeptide for ACTH. The ACTH formed in this way can be further processed to melanocyte-stimulating hormone, y-lipotropin, and β-END (74). The physiological significance of β-END is still a question of some debate, but it has been associated with mood-state alteration (i.e., improved positive affect), insulin and glucose metabolism (197), and possibly cardiovascular regulatory function and regulation of glucose (74,196,198).

Exercise Responses

As both intensity and duration of dynamic exercise reach a critical level, there is an increase in β-END (40,199,200). A minimal relative work load of approximately 55% $\dot{V}O_2max$ is probably needed to induce significant increases in β-END concentration (201). However, there is considerable variability in the magnitude of the increase in β-END concentration during short-term exercise (64,202).

As noted earlier, there does appear to be a critical threshold for exercise intensity to elicit an increase in β-END concentrations. Thus, provided that an intensity of 55% to 60% $\dot{V}O_2max$ is obtained, β-END levels will increase during prolonged exercise (40,196,200,201). The same intensity of exercise also is necessary to elicit a cortisol response, and cortisol is regulated by ACTH, which can be processed to form β-END. There can be a delay in the onset of the increase from the initiation of submaximal exercise (5 to 10 minutes). Once above the threshold intensity, the magnitude of the β-END increase is proportional to exercise intensity and approaches 2 to 5 times resting levels (64,201). Data from Pestell and colleagues (203) have suggested that if the intensity of exercise is below the threshold level, regardless of the duration, β-END will not increase. Potential causes of the release are lactate and pH changes, as both of these have been positively correlated to changes in β-END (194), but not in all studies (204). In addition, some studies have shown a loose relation between catecholamines and β-END (40). However, there is need for much further study to obtain a clear understanding of the causes of elevations of β-END levels during exercise.

At very high exercise intensities (i.e., more than 100% $\dot{V}O_2max$), the short duration of the exercise bout results in β-END levels reaching a peak after the stopping of exercise (64,205). However, at very high work loads that can be maintained for at least 3 minutes (about 100 $\dot{V}O_2max$), reports have shown an increase in β-END levels at the very end of the exercise (206).

The data on prolonged exercise are fairly clear, in that runs ranging from 2 to 26 miles resulted in 25% to 350% increases in circulating β-END (204). Furthermore, the elevation of β-END levels was associated with an improved General Affect Scale score (204). Thus there appears to be a mood-enhancement role for β-END during prolonged exercise. It also is possible that the elevated β-END level is stimulated by hypoglycemia (207) or that β-END stimulates insulin release after exercise, which would hasten the rate of glycogen replenishment from circulating glucose (197). The specific role of β-END during exercise is still the subject of debate.

Resistance exercise is typically associated with increases in β-END levels. However, the studies are somewhat contradictory. Melchionda and co-workers (208) reported no change in β-END levels, whereas Walberg-Rankin and colleagues (209) showed significant elevations. Still others reported β-END increases only after cessation of such activity, during recovery (108). The lack of agreement in the findings may be related to the type of muscular contraction involved with the resistance exercise (static isometric vs. dynamic isotonic or isokinetic) as well as the degree of intensity and the volume of resistance work performed by subjects (87).

The literature regarding the influence of training on β-END is controversial. Goldfarb and associates (201) compared the β-END responses of trained and untrained men at various submaximal exercise intensities (60%, 70%, and 80% $\dot{V}O_2max$). Results from this study indicated that training status had no significant effect on the magnitude of the β-END response at any intensity, although the results showed that there was a tendency for the untrained subjects to have a slightly greater response. In contrast, several other studies showed that, after exercise training, a decrease in resting β-END levels occurs (207,210), and a decreased response to submaximal exercise also is evident (211,212). During maximal exercise, trained subjects have the ability to exercise to higher absolute work loads when reaching

$\dot{V}O_2max$. Thus the hormonal responses to maximal exercise tend to be higher (or at least identical) to those observed before training (81,84,108).

Disturbances in basal β-END levels brought about by exercise training have been postulated as a mechanism for the development of menstrual problems in female athletes (193,196,208,213,214). To date, no direct linking has been drawn to β-END and the development of oligo- or amenorrhea in female athletes. However, much further work is necessary on this issue, and the question has yet to be resolved.

Calcium-Balance Hormones

Two hormones are involved with calcium balance: *parathyroid hormone* (PTH) from the parathyroid gland and *calcitonin* from the thyroid gland. These two hormones work in opposition to each other, responding to changing levels of calcium in the blood by affecting calcium levels of bone, renal absorption or excretion rates, and intestinal absorption rate. *Calcitonin* functions to reduce blood calcium levels. It does so by decreasing bone resorption, which allows better calcium uptake. Calcitonin also may increase urinary calcium output and limit GI uptake. Conversely, PTH functions to increase blood calcium levels. PTH causes calcium efflux from the bone, stimulates calcium reabsorption in the kidneys, and may increase intestinal absorption of calcium (1).

Exercise Responses

Little is known about the influence of exercise on the calcium-balance hormones. A search revealed only a single study focusing on calcitonin and only a few articles on PTH. The research produced differing results with regard to PTH. Some studies (215–217) found no increase in PTH during exercise. In addition, research using short-term submaximal or intense exercise failed to find any change in PTH (218,219). Furthermore, some studies reported a decrease in serum PTH after either 45 minutes of submaximal cycle ergometry (220) or intermittent anaerobic exercise (221). However, other studies indicated that PTH increases during exercise (222,223). The increases seen were on the order of about 25% to 30% during prolonged submaximal exercise (222,224) and about 60% increase after a 50-minute incremental run to exhaustion (223). In these studies, the increase in PTH was independent of any change in blood calcium levels. The differing results could be related to techniques for the measurement of PTH, as newer techniques are better at detecting the intact molecule. Also, because PTH has a half-life in plasma of 4 to 6 minutes, the time of sampling after exercise could be a factor. Most studies report no significant change in blood calcium, so the cause of the response is obscure. Speculation suggests that the increase may be caused by the catecholamines, as previous research indicated that epinephrine can stimulate PTH release (225). In addition, a statistical relation exists between lactate and PTH; however, this may not indicate a true cause–effect relation. The increase in PTH may allow bone to disperse the calcium stores to those areas of greater stress for remodeling. Thus PTH may have both a catabolic and an anabolic effect on skeletal bone (223).

Two studies attempted to evaluate a training response of PTH. One study noted a decrease in serum PTH with training in adolescent girls (226). The other (223), completed in male subjects, found that trained runners had serum PTH levels approximately 50% greater than fire fighters. Clearly, more research is necessary to solve this conundrum.

Erythropoietin

Erythropoietin (EPO) is an amino acid–based hormone produced primarily in the kidneys. EPO stimulates red cell formation and development. The major factor influencing EPO is tissue oxygenation, as it has been shown that exposure to high altitudes (16,000 ft or 4900 m) increases EPO within 12 hours of arrival (227). However, both androgens and hGH also can stimulate EPO (1).

Exercise Responses

Exercise up to 60 minutes at high intensities appears to have little immediate effect on EPO (228–230), particularly when diurnal variations are taken into consideration (231). Although Klausen and colleagues (229) reported a 19% increase after 60 minutes at 85% to 95% maximal capacity, the increase was found to be related to exercise-induced hemoconcentration. However, one study reported that 31 hours after prolonged exercise, EPO level was significantly elevated (232). This suggests a delayed response of EPO. Perhaps studies should evaluate EPO 24 to 48 hours after exercise rather than immediately after exercise.

Athletes in general have increased red cell mass. Additionally, athletes may have elevated resting hGH. Thus EPO would be expected to be elevated in trained athletes. One study inferred this response from detraining. Klausan and co-workers (229) detrained marathon runners for 3 weeks and found about a 20% decrease in resting EPO. They then trained these same runners for 2 weeks and found an increase over the untrained state, suggestive of a training effect. However, the same primary author also reported no significant differences in 24-hour EPO diurnal responses when comparing trained and untrained healthy young men (231). Similar results also were reported in studies by Weight (230) and Schmidt and colleagues (233). Thus, at present, the responses of EPO during exercise, as well as the occurrence of a training effect, are in need of further research.

CONCLUSION

As evidenced in the discussion above, knowledge of the hormonal responses and their effects during exercise is limited, and there is need for further study. However, our present state of knowledge can be summarized in Table 10–3. In anticipation of exercise, the catecholamines, ACTH, and cortisol may increase. The increase is directly related to the perception of the difficulty of the exercise. During submaximal short-term exercise, most hormone levels are elevated, with the exception of insulin, which declines, and the thyroid hormones, which do not respond. The increase may be related to the sympathetic nervous system or catecholamines, but it may also serve the body by attempting to maintain optimal cellular glucose uptake. However, the specific purpose of some of the hormonal responses is not known and may be related to nothing more than a stress-reactivity within the endocrine system.

Most studies have shown that higher-intensity exercise results in greater increase in the stress-responding hormones: ACTH, cortisol, catecholamines, and prolactin. The increase of these hormones influences not only metabolism but also the cardiovascular, respiratory, digestive, and renal systems. Other hormones also are increased such as hGH, ADH, and aldosterone, theoretically to improve energy sources, water retention, and sodium balance. However, the real need for these hormones is not completely understood. The gonadotropin and gonadal hormones also increase, but present knowledge suggests that the increase is related to a reduced MCR rather than an increased production. Resistance or strength exercises are usually considered very high intensity. Therefore those hormones that respond to high-intensity exercise also respond similarly to resistance exercises.

Prolonged exercise causes an elevation of those hormones that support substrate availability and metabolism. These include hGH, cortisol, glucagon, and catecholamines. At the same time, insulin declines. Because prolonged exercise is accompanied by sweat loss, hormones related to water and electrolyte balance also are increased: ADH and aldosterone.

Training appears to have a profound effect on the hormonal system, particularly with regard to the stress hormones and the metabolic hormones. Most studies have shown that resting levels of ACTH, cortisol, catecholamines, insulin, and glucagon are lower in trained individuals. This may be related to the greater energy stores in the body of a trained individual. The response also may be related to some reduced perceptions of life stresses. In addition, the gonadotropin and gonadal hormones also appear to decline because of some disruption of the feedback mechanisms.

The information presented in this chapter emphasizes the importance of the endocrine system in modulating exercise physiology. Future studies on the physiology of exercise cannot overlook the importance of the endocrine system. The physiology of many of these hormones is not well understood, nor is the significance of many exercise responses. The development of new molecular and histochemical techniques, however, should allow future exercise endocrinologists to complete our knowledge of the causes and reasons for many of the hormonal responses to exercise.

TABLE 10–3. *Summary of the known hormonal responses to different types of exercise*

Hormone	Anticipation	Short-term submaximal	High intensity	Prolonged exercise	Resistance exercise	Aerobic training
Antidiuretic	0	+ (>50%)	++	++	?	0
Growth	0	+	++	++	++	+
ACTH	+	+	++	++	++	−
TSH	0	+	+ or 0	+ or 0	?	0
Prolactin	0	+	++	+	+	+ or −
FSH	0	+	+ or 0	+, 0, −	++	−
LH	0	+	+ or 0	+, 0, −	++	−
T_3 & T_4	0	0	0	+ or −	0	0 or −
Parathyroid	?	+	+	+	?	?
Insulin	0	−	−	−	−	−
Glucagon	0	+	+	++	?	−
Cortisol	+	+ (>60%)	++	++	++	−
Catecholamines	+	+	++	++	++	−
Aldosterone	0	+	++	++	+	0
Testosterone	0	+	+	+ or −	+	0 or −
Estrogens	0	+	+	?	?	− or 0
Progesterone	0	+	+	?	?	− or 0

+, increase; ++, strong increase; 0, no change; −, decrease; ?, unknown.

REFERENCES

1. Hedges GA, Colby HD, Goodman RL. *Clinical endocrine physiology.* Philadelphia: WB Saunders, 1987.
2. Marieb EN, *Human anatomy and physiology* 4th ed. Redwood City, CA: Benjamin/Cummings Publishing Co., 1997.
3. Chiodera P, Volpi R, Maffei ML, et al. Role of GABA and opioids in the regulation of vasopressin response to physical exercise in normal men. *Regul Pept* 1993;49:57–63.
4. Hammer M, Ladefoged J, Olgaard K. Relationship between plasma osmolality and plasma vasopressin in human subjects. *Am J Physiol* 1979;238:E313–E317.
5. Moses AM. Osmotic thresholds for AVP release with the use of plasma and urine AVP and free water clearance. *Am J Physiol* 1989;256:R892–R897.
6. Wang BC, Sundet WD, Hakumaki MOK, et al. Cardiac receptors influences on the plasma osmolality-plasma vasopressin relationship. *Am J Physiol* 1984;246:H360–H368.
7. Epstein M, Pins DS, Miller M. Suppression of ADH during water immersion in normal man. *J Appl Physiol* 1975;38:1038–1044.
8. Fejes-Toth G, Naray-Fejes-Toth A, Ratge D. Evidence against role of antidiuretic hormone in support of blood pressure during dehydration. *Am J Physiol* 1985;249:H42–H48.
9. Perrault H, Melin B, Jimenez C, et al. Fluid-regulating and sympathoadrenal hormonal responses to peak exercise following transplantation. *J Appl Physiol* 1994;76:230–235.
10. Ueda K, Takahashi M, Yamada T, et al. Evaluation of changes in hepatic energy metabolism during exercise by ketone body ratio in humans. *J Cardiol* 1997;29:95–102.
11. Convertino VA, Keil LC, Greenleaf JE. Plasma volume, renin, and vasopressin responses to graded exercise after training. *J Appl Physiol* 1983;54:508–514.
12. Geyssant A, Geelen G, Denis CH, et al. Plasma vasopressin, renin activity, and aldosterone: effect of exercise and training. *Eur J Appl Physiol* 1981;46:21–30.
13. Mountain SJ, Laird JE, Latzka WA, Sawaka MN. Aldosterone and vasopressin responses in the heat: hydration level and exercise intensity effects. *Med Sci Sports Exerc* 1997;29:661–668.
14. Wade CE, Claybaugh JR. Plasma renin activity, vasopressin concentration, and urinary excretory responses to exercise in men. *J Appl Physiol* 1980;49:930–936.
15. Melin B, Echache JP, Geelen G, et al. Plasma AVP, neurophysin, renin activity, and aldosterone during submaximal exercise performed until exhaustion in trained and untrained men. *Eur J Appl Physiol* 1980;44:141–151.
16. Grant SM, Green HJ, Phillips SM, et al. Fluid and electrolyte hormonal responses to exercise and acute plasma volume expansion. *J Appl Physiol* 1996;81:2386–2392.
17. Brunner DB, Burnier M, Brunner HR. Plasma vasopressin in rats: effect of sodium, angiotensin, and catecholamines. *Am J Physiol* 1983;244:H259–H265.
18. Kimura T, Shoji M, Itake K, et al. The role of central β_1 and β_2 adrenoceptors in the regulation of vasopressin release and the cardiovascular system. *Endocrinol* 1984;114:1426–1432.
19. Ghaemmaghami F, Gauquelin G, Gharib C, et al. Effects of treadmill running and swimming on plasma and brain vasopressin levels in rats. *Eur J Appl Physiol* 1987;56:1–6.
20. Greenleaf JE, Brock PJ, Keil LC, Morse JT. Drinking and water balance during exercise and heat acclimation. *J Appl Physiol* 1983;54:414–419.
21. Carroll JF, Convertino VA, Wood CE, et al. Effects of training on blood volume and plasma hormone concentrations in the elderly. *Med Sci Sports Exerc* 1995;27:79–84.
22. Glace BW, Gleim GW, Zabetakis PM, Nicholas JA. Systemic effects of ingesting varying amounts of a commercial carbohydrate beverage postexercise. *J Am Coll Nutr* 1994;13:268–276.
23. Maughan RJ, Owen JH, Shirreffs SM, Leiper JB. Post-exercise rehydration in man: effects of electrolyte addition to ingested fluids. *Eur J Appl Physiol* 1994;69:209–215.
24. McMurray RG, Eubank TK, Hackney AC. Nocturnal hormonal responses to resistance exercise. *Eur J Appl Physiol* 1995; 72:121–126.
25. Zapf J, Froesch ER. Insulin-like growth factors/somatomedins: structure, secretion, biological actions and physiological role. *Horm Res* 1986:24:121–130.
26. Davidson MB. Effect of growth hormone on carbohydrate and lipid metabolism. *Endocrinol Rev* 1987;8:115–131.
27. McMurray RG, Proctor CR, Wilson WL. Effect of caloric deficit and dietary manipulation on aerobic and anaerobic exercise. *Int J Sports Med* 1991;12:167–172.
28. Nazar K, Jezova D, Kyealik-Borowka E. Plasma vasopressin, growth hormone and ACTH responses to static hand grip in healthy subjects. *Eur J Appl Physiol* 1989;58:400–404.
29. VanHelder WP, Casey K, Radomski WM. Regulation of growth hormone during exercise by oxygen demand and availability. *Eur J Appl Physiol* 1987;56:628–632.
30. VanHelder WP, Goode RC, Radomski MW. Effect of anaerobic and aerobic exercise of equal duration and work expenditure on plasma growth hormone levels. *Eur J Appl Physiol* 1984;52: 255–257.
31. Gordon SE, Kraemer WJ, Vos NH, Lynch JM, Knuttgen HG. Effect of acid-base balance on the growth hormone response to acute high-intensity cycle exercise. *J Appl Physiol* 1994;76: 821–829.
32. Nevill ME, Holmyard DJ, Hall GM, et al. Growth hormone responses to treadmill sprinting in sprint- and endurance-trained athletes. *Eur J Appl Physiol* 1996;72:460–467.
33. Sutton JR, Jones NL, Toews CJ. Growth hormone secretion in acid-base alterations at rest and during exercise. *Clin Sci Mol Med* 1976;50:241–247.
34. Weltman A, Weltman JY, Womack CJ, et al. Exercise training decreases the growth hormone (GH) response to acute constant-load exercise. *Med Sci Sports Exerc* 1997;29:669–767.
35. Hartley LH. Growth hormone and catecholamine response to exercise in relation to physical training. *Med Sci Sports Exerc* 1975;7:34–36.
36. Tater P, Kozlowski S, Vigas M, et al. Endocrine response to physical efforts with equivalent total work loads but different intensities in man. *Endocrinol Exp* 1984;18:233–239.
37. Chwalbinski-Moneta J, Krkysztofiak H, Ziemba A, et al. Threshold increases in plasma growth hormone in relation to plasma catecholamine and blood lactate concentrations during progressive exercise in endurance-trained athletes. *Eur J Appl Physiol* 1996:73:117–120.
38. Kjaer M, Secher NH, Bach FW, et al. Hormonal and metabolic responses to dynamic exercise in man: effect of sensory nervous blockade. *Am J Physiol* 1989;257:E95–E101.
39. Kozlowski S, Chwalbinski-Moneta J, Vigas M, et al. Greater serum GH response to arm than to leg exercise performed at equivalent oxygen intake. *Eur J Appl Physiol* 1983;52:132–135.
40. McMurray RG, Forsythe WA, Mar MH, Hardy CJ. Exercise intensity-related responses of β-endorphin and catecholamines. *Med Sci Sports Exerc* 1987;19:570–574.
41. Karagiorgos A, Garcia JF, Brooks GA. Growth hormone response to continuous and intermittent exercise. *Med Sci Sports Exerc* 1979;11:302–307.
42. Lassare C, Girard F, Durand J, Raynaud J. Kinetics of human growth hormone during submaximal exercise. *J Appl Physiol* 1974;37:826–830.
43. Raynaud J, Caperou A, Martineau JP, et al. Intersubject variability in growth hormone time course during different types of work. *J Appl Physiol* 1983;55:1682–1687.
44. Bunt JC, Boileau RA, Bahr JM, Nelson RA. Sex and training differences in human growth hormone levels during prolonged exercise. *J Appl Physiol* 1986;61:1796–1801.
45. Banfi G, Merinelli M, Roi GS, et al. Growth hormone and insulin-like growth factor I in athletes performing a marathon at 4000 m of altitude. *Growth Regul* 1994;4:82–86.
46. Shephard RJ, Sidney KH. Effects of physical exercise on plasma growth hormone and cortisol levels in human subjects. In: Wilmore J, Keogh E, eds. *Exercise and sports science review.* New York: Academic Press, 1975:1–30.
47. Kraemer RR, Kilgore JL, Kraemer GR, Castracane VD. Growth hormone, IGF-I and testosterone responses to resistive exercise. *Med Sci Sports Exerc* 1992;24:1346–1352.
48. Hakkinen K, Pakarinen A. Acute hormonal responses to heavy

resistance exercise in men and women at different ages. *Int J Sports Med* 1995;16:507–513.
49. Nissley SP, Rechler MM. Insulin-like growth factors: biosynthesis, receptors and IGF-carrier proteins. In: Li CH, ed. *Hormonal proteins and peptides*. New York: Academic Press, 1985:127–203.
50. Copeland KC, Underwood LE, Van Wyk JJ. Induction of immunoreactive somatomedin-C in human serum by growth hormone: dose response relationship and effect on chromatographic profiles. *J Clin Endocrinol Metab* 1980;50:690–697.
51. Isley WL, Underwood LE, Clemmons DR. Dietary components that regulate serum somatomedin-C concentrations in humans. *J Clin Invest* 1983;71:175–182.
52. Cappon J, Brasel JA, Mohan S, Cooper DM. Effect of brief exercise on circulating insulin-like growth factor I. *J Appl Physiol* 1994;76:2490–2496.
53. Schwarz AJ, Brasel JA, Hintz RL, et al. Acute effect of low- and high-intensity exercise on circulating insulin-like growth factor (IGF) I, II, and IGF binding protein-3 and its proteolysis in young healthy men. *J Clin Endocrinol Metab* 1996;81:3492–3497.
54. Henriksen EJ, Louters LL, Stump CS, Tipton CM. Effects of prior exercise on the action of insulin-like growth factor I in skeletal muscle. *Am J Physiol* 1992;263:E340–E344.
55. Hopkins NJ, Jakeman PM, Hughes SC, Holly JMP. Changes in circulating insulin-like growth factor-binding protein-I (IGFBP-I) during prolonged exercise: effect of carbohydrate feeding. *J Clin Endocrinol Metab* 1994;79:1887–1890.
56. Koistinen H, Koistinen R, Selenius L, et al. Effect of marathon run on serum IGF-I and IGF-binding protein 1 and 3 levels. *J Appl Physiol* 1996;80:760–764.
57. Kraemer WJ, Gordon SE, Fleck SJ, et al. Endogenous anabolic hormonal and growth factor responses to heavy resistance exercise in males and females. *Int J Sports Med* 1991;12:228–235.
58. Kraemer WJ, Marchitelli L, McCurry D, et al. Hormonal and growth factor responses to heavy resistance exercise protocols. *J Appl Physiol* 1990:69:1442–1450.
59. Willis PE, Chadan S, Baracos V, Parkhouse WS. Acute exercise attenuates age-associated resistance to insulin-like growth factor I. *Am J Physiol* 1997;272:E397–E404.
60. Chang FE, Dodds WG, Sullivan M, et al. The acute effects of exercise on prolactin and growth hormone secretion: comparison between sedentary women and women runners with normal and abnormal menstrual cycles. *J Clin Endocrinol Metab* 1986; 62:551–556.
61. Walsh BT, Buig-Antich J, Goetz R, et al. Sleep and growth hormone secretion in women athletes. *Electroencephalogr Clin Neurophysiol* 1984;57:528–531.
62. Weltman A, Weltman JY, Schurrer R, et al. Endurance training amplifies the pusatile release of growth hormone: effects of training intensity. *J Appl Physiol* 1992;72:2188–2196.
63. Dinan TG, Thakor J, O'Keane V. Lowering cortisol enhances growth hormone response to growth releasing hormone in healthy subjects. *Acta Physiol Scand* 1994;151:413–416.
64. Viru A. Plasma hormones and physical exercise. *Int J Sports Med* 1992;13:201–209.
65. Hackney AC, Ness RJ, Schrieber A. Effects of endurance exercise on nocturnal hormone concentrations in males. *Chronobiol Int* 1989;6:341–346.
66. Poehlman ET, Rosen CJ, Copeland KC. The influence of endurance training on insulin-like growth factor-I in older individuals. *Metabolism* 1994;43:1401–1405.
67. Galbo H. *Hormonal and metabolic adaptations to exercise*. New York: Georg Thieme Verlag, 1983:1–116.
68. Barreca T, Reggiani E, Franceschini F, et al. Serum prolactin, growth hormone and cortisol in athletes and sedentary subjects after submaximal and exhaustive exercises. *J Sports Med* 1988;28:89–92.
69. Kraemer RR, Blair MS, McCaferty R, Castracane VD. Running-induced alterations in growth hormone, prolactin, triiodothyronine, and thyroxine concentrations in trained and untrained men and women. *Res Q Exerc Sport* 1993;64:69–74.
70. Snegovaskaya V, Viru A. Elevation of cortisol and growth hormone levels in the course of further improvement of performance capacity in trained rowers. *Int J Sports Med* 1993;14:202–206.
71. Quirion A, Brisson G, De Carufel D, et al. Influence of exercise and dietary modifications on plasma human growth hormone, insulin and FFA. *J Sports Med Phys Fitness* 1988;28:352–353.
72. Vollotton MB. Endocrine functions and aging: a summary. *Horm Res* 1995;43:5–7.
73. Pyka G, Wiswell RA, Marcus R. Age-dependent effect of resistance exercise on growth hormone secretion in people. *J Clin Endocrinol Metab* 1992;75:404–407.
74. Despopoulos J, Silbernagi S. *Color atlas of physiology*. Stuttgart: Georg Thieme Verlag, 1991:232–271.
75. Dale E, Gerlach DG, Whilhite AL. Menstrual dysfunction in distance runners. *Obstet Gynecol* 1979;54:47–53.
76. Gawel MJ, Alaghband-Zadeh J, Park DM, Rose FC. Exercise and hormonal secretion. *Postgrad Med J* 1979;55:373–376.
77. Hackney AC, Sharp RL, Runyon W, et al. Effects of intensive training on the prolactin response to submaximal exercise in males. *J Iowa Acad Sci* 1989;96:52–53.
78. Hackney AC, Premo MC, McMurray RG. Influence of aerobic vs. anaerobic exercise on the relationship between reproductive hormones in men. *J Sport Sci* 1995;13:305–311.
79. Noel GL, Suh HK, Stone JG, Frantz AG. Human prolactin and growth hormone release during surgery and other conditions of stress. *J Clin Endocrinol Metab* 1972;35:840–851.
80. Hackney AC, Sinning WE, Bruot BC. Comparison of resting reproductive hormonal profiles in endurance trained and untrained men. *Med Sci Sports Exerc* 1988;20:60–65.
81. Hackney AC, Fahrner CL, Stupnicki R. Reproductive hormonal responses to maximal exercise in endurance trained men with low testosterone levels. *Clin Exp Endocrinol Diabetes* 1997;105: 291–295.
82. Wheeler GD, Singh M, Pierce WD, et al. Endurance training decreases serum testosterone levels in men without changing luteinizing hormone pulsatile release. *J Clin Endocrinol Metab* 1991;72:422–425.
83. Griffin JE. Odjeda SR, eds. *Textbook of endocrine physiology*. 3rd ed. New York: Oxford University Press, 1996.
84. Galbo H, Kjaer M, Mikines KJ. Neurohormonal system. In: Skinner J, Corbin CB, Landers DM, et al., eds. *Future directions in exercise and sport science research*. Champaign, IL: Human Kinetics Publishers, 1989:339–345.
85. Hackney AC. The male reproductive system and endurance exercise. *Med Sci Sports Exerc* 1996;28:180–189.
86. Cumming DC, Wall SR, Galbraith MA, Belcastro A. Reproductive hormonal responses to resistance exercise. *Med Sci Sports Exerc* 1987;19:234–238.
87. Kraemer WJ. Endocrine response to resistance exercise. *Med Sci Sports Exerc* 1988;20:S152–S157.
88. Bonen A, Belcastro AN, Ling WY, Simpson AA. Profiles of selected hormones during menstrual cycles of teenage athletes. *J Appl Physiol* 1981;50:545–551.
89. Duclos M, Corcuff JB, Rashedi M, Fougere V. Does functional alteration of the gonadotropic axis occur in endurance trained athletes during or after exercise? A preliminary study. *Eur J Appl Physiol* 1996;73:427–433.
90. Hackney AC, Sinning WE, Bruot BC. Hypothalamic-pituitary-testicular axis function in endurance trained males. *Int J Sports Med* 1990;11:298–303.
91. Hackney AC. Endurance training and testosterone levels. *Sports Med* 1989;8:117–127.
92. Griffin JE. The thyroid. In: Griffin JE, Odjeda SR, eds. *Textbook of endocrine physiology* 3rd ed. New York: Oxford University Press, 1996:260–283.
93. Wirth A, Holm G, Lindstedt G, et al. Thyroid hormones and lipolysis in physically trained rats. *Metabolism* 1981;30:237–241.
94. Brisson G, Nolle MA, Desharnaris D, Tanka M. A possible submaximal exercise-induced hypothalamo-hypophyseal stress. *Horm Metab Res* 1980;12:201–205.
95. Terjung RL, Tipton CM. Plasma thyroxine and TSH levels during submaximal exercise in humans. *Am J Physiol* 1971;220:1840–1845.
96. Galbo H, Hummer L, Peterson IB, et al. Thyroid and testicular hormonal responses to graded and prolonged exercise in men. *Eur J Appl Physiol* 1977;36:101–106.
97. Berchtold P, Berger M, Cuppers HJ, et al. Non-glucoregulatory hormones (T_4, T_3, rT_3, TSH and testosterone) during physical

exercise in juvenile type diabetics. *Horm Metab Res* 1978;10: 269–273.
98. Hackney AC, Gulledge TP. Thyroid responses during an 8 hour period following aerobic and anaerobic exercise. *Physiol Res* 1994;43:1–5.
99. DeSouza MJ, Arce JC, Pescatello LS, et al. Gonadal hormones and semen quality in male runners: a volume threshold effect of endurance training. *Int J Sports Med* 1994;15:383–391.
100. Hohtari H, Pakarinen A, Kauppila A. Serum concentrations of thyrotropin, thyroxine, triiodothyronine and thyroxine binding globulin in female endurance runners and joggers. *Acta Endocrinol* 1987;114:41–46.
101. Winder WW, Hagberg JM, Hickson RC, et al. Time course of sympathoadrenergic adaptation to endurance exercise training in man. *J Appl Physiol* 1978;45:370–374.
102. Winder WW, Hickson RC, Hagberg JM, et al. Training-induced changes in hormonal and metabolic responses to submaximal exercise. *J Appl Physiol* 1979;46:766–771.
103. Irvine CHG. Effect of exercise on thryoxine degradation in athletes and non-athletes. *J Clin Endocrinol* 1968;28:942–948.
104. Brooks GA, Fahey TD, White TP. *Exercise physiology: human bioenergetics and its application.* Mountain View, CA: Mayfield Publishing, 1996:144–172.
105. Farrell PA, Garthwaite TL, Gustafson AB. Plasma adrenocorticotropin and cortisol responses to submaximal and exhaustive exercise. *J Appl Physiol* 1983;55:1441–1444.
106. Nazar K, Jezova D, Kowalik-Borowka E. Plasma vasopressin, growth hormone and ACTH responses to static handgrip in healthy subjects. *Eur J Appl Physiol* 1989;58:400–404.
107. Viru A, Smirnova T. Independence of physical working capacity from increased glucocorticoid level during short term exercise. *Int J Sports Med* 1982;3:80–83.
108. Kjaer M, Secher NH, Bach FW, et al. Hormonal, metabolic and cardiovascular responses to static exercise in man: influence of epidural anesthesia. *Am J Physiol* 1991;261:E214–E220.
109. Barwich D, Klett G, Eckert W, Weicker H. Exercise-induced lipolysis in patients with central Cushing's disease. *Int J Sports Med* 1980;1:120–126.
110. Gann DS, Bereiter DA, Carlson DE, Thrivikraman KV. Neural interaction in control of adrenocorticotropin. *Fed Proc* 1985;44: 162–167.
111. Davis CTM, Few JD. Effects of exercise on adrenocortical function. *J Appl Physiol* 1973;35:887–891.
112. Brandenberger G, Follenius M. Influence of timing and intensity of muscle exercise on temporal patterns of plasma cortisol levels. *J Clin Endocrinol Metab* 1975;40:845–849.
113. Cuneo RC, Espiner EA, Nichalls MG, Yemdle TG. Exercise induced increase in plasma natriuretic peptide and effect of sodium loading in normal man. *Horm Metab Res* 1988;20:115–117.
114. Kuoppasalmi K, Naveri H, Kosunen K, et al. Plasma steroid levels in muscular exercise. In: Poortmans J, Niset G, eds. *Biochemistry of exercise* IV. Baltimore: University Park Press, 1981:149–160.
115. Staehlin D, Labhart A, Froesch R, Kagi HR. The effect of muscular exercise and hypoglycemia on the plasma levels of 17-hydroxysteroids in normal adults and in patients with andrenogenital syndrome. *Acta Endocrinol* 1955;18:521–529.
116. Buono MJ, Yeager JE, Hodgdon J. Plasma adrenocorticotropin and cortisol responses to brief high-intensity exercise in humans. *J Appl Physiol* 1986;61:1337–1339.
117. Guezennec Y, Leger F, Hostr FL, et al. Hormonal and metabolic responses to weightlifting training sessions. *Int J Sports Med* 1986;7:100–105.
118. Lukaszewska J, Biczoswa B, Hobilewicz D, et al. Effect of physical exercise on plasma cortisol and growth hormone levels in young weightlifters. *Endokrynol Pol* 1976;2:149–158.
119. Passelegue P, Robert A, Lac G. Salivary cortisol and testosterone variations during an official and simulated weight-lifting competition. *Int J Sports Med* 1995;16:298–303.
120. Buono MJ, Yeager JE, Sucec AA. Effect of aerobic training on the plasma ACTH response to exercise. *J Appl Physiol* 1987;63:2499–2501.
121. Bloom SR, Johnson RH, Park DM, et al. Differences in the metabolic and hormonal response to exercise between racing cyclists and untrained individuals. *J Physiol (Lond)* 1976;258: 1–18.
122. Fellmann N, Coudert J, Jarrige J, et al. Effects of endurance training on the androgenic response to exercise in man. *Int J Sports Med* 1985;6:215–219.
123. Kantola I, Tarssanen L, Scheinin M, et al. Beta-blockade, atrial natriuretic peptide and exercise. *Int J Clin Pharmacol Ther* 1996;34:12–16.
124. Fallo F. Renin-angiotensin-aldosterone system and physical exercise. *J Sports Med Phys Fitness* 1993;33:306–312.
125. Fray JCS, Lush DJ, Vanentine ND. Cellular mechanism of renin secretion. *Fed Proc* 1983;42:3150–3154.
126. Saitoh M, Yanagawa T, Kondoh T, et al. Neurohumoral factor responses to mental (arithmetic) stress and dynamic exercise in normal subjects. *Intern Med* 1995;34:618–622.
127. Guezennec CY, Defer G, Cazorla G, et al. Plasma renin activity, aldosterone and catecholamine levels when swimming and running. *Eur J Appl Physiol* 1986;54:632–637.
128. Wolf JP, Nguyen NU, Dumoulin G, Berthelay S. Plasma renin and aldosterone changes during twenty minutes' moderate exercise. *Eur J Appl Physiol* 1986;54:602–607.
129. Stephenson LA, Kolka MA, Francesconi R, Gonzalez RR. Circadian variations in plasma renin activity, catecholamines and aldosterone during exercise in women. *Eur J Appl Physiol* 1989;58: 756–764.
130. Suzuki M, Sudoh M, Matsubara S, et al. Changes in renal blood flow measured by radionuclide angiography following exhaustive exercise in humans. *Eur J Appl Physiol* 1996;74:1–7.
131. Zappe DH, Helyar RG, Green HJ. The interaction between short-term exercise training and a diuretic-induced hypovolemic stimulus. *Eur J Appl Physiol* 1996;72:335–340.
132. Lehmann M, Knizia K, Gastmann U, et al. Influence of 6-week, 6 days per week, training on pituitary function in recreational athletes. *Br J Sports Med* 1993;27:186–192.
133. Luetkemeier MJ, Flowers KM, Lamb DR. Spironolactone administration and training-induced hypervolemia. *Int J Sports Med* 1994;15:295–300.
134. Nielsen B, Hales JR, Strange S, et al. Human circulatory and thermoregulatory adaptations with heat acclimation and exercise in a hot, dry environment. *J Physiol (Lond)* 1993;460:467–485.
135. Goodman JM, Logan AG, McLaughlin PR, et al. Atrial natriuretic peptide during acute and prolonged exercise in well-trained men. *Int J Sports Med* 1993;14:185–190.
136. Opstad PK, Haugen AH, Sejersted AM, Bahr R, Skrede KK. Atrial natriuretic peptide in plasma after prolonged physical strain, energy deficiency and sleep deprivation. *Eur J Appl Physiol* 1994;68:122–126.
137. Richter EA, Sonne B, Christensen NJ, Galbo H. Role of epinephrine for muscular glycogenolysis and pancreatic hormonal secretion in running rats. *Am J Physiol* 1981;240:E526–E532.
138. Christensen NJ, Galbo H, Hansen JF, Hesse B, Richter EA, Trap-Jensen J. Catecholamines and exercise. *Diabetes* 1979; 28:58–62.
139. Kotchen TA, Hartley LH, Rice TW, Mougey EH, Jones LG, Mason JW. Renin, norepinephrine, and epinephrine responses to graded exercise. *J Appl Physiol* 1971;31:178–184.
140. Keul VJ, Lehmann M, Wybitul K. Zur siung von burnotrolol auf hertzfrequenz, metabolishe grossen bei korperarbeit and leistungsverhalten. *Arzneimittelforshung* 1981;31:1–16.
141. Favier R, Pequignot JM, Desplanches D, et al. Catecholamines and metabolic responses to submaximal exercise in untrained men and women. *Eur J Appl Physiol* 1983;50:393–404.
142. Kinderman W, Schnabel A, Schmitt WM, et al. Catecholamines, growth hormone, cortisol, insulin, and sex hormones in anaerobic and aerobic exercise. *Eur J Appl Physiol* 1982;49:389–399.
143. Hull EM, Young SH, Ziegler MG. Aerobic fitness affects cardiovascular and catecholamine responses to stressors. *Psychophysiology* 1984;21:353–360.
144. Svedenhag J, Martinsson A, Ekblom B, Hjemdahl P. Altered cardiovascular responsiveness to adrenaline in endurance-trained subjects. *Acta Physiol Scand* 1986;126:539–550.
145. Takeda N, Dominiak P, Turck D, et al. The influence of endurance training on mechanical catecholamine responsiveness,

β-adrenoceptor density and myosin isoenzyme pattern of rat ventricular myocardium. *Basic Res Cardiol* 1985;80:88–99.
146. Kjaer M, Galbo H. Effect of physical training on the capacity to secrete epinephrine. *J Appl Physiol* 1988;64:11–16.
147. Kaplan LA, Pesce AJ. *Clinical chemistry: theory, analysis and correlations.* St. Louis: CV Mosby, 1989.
148. Jacobs S, Cuatrecasas P. Insulin receptor: structure and function. *Endocrinol Rev* 1981;2:251–263.
149. Wasserman DH, O'Dherty RM, Zinker BA. Role of the endocrine pancreas in control of fuel metabolism by the liver during exercise. *Int J Obesity* 1995;19(suppl 4):S22–S30.
150. Gyntelberg F, Rennie MJ, Hickson RC, Holloszy JO. Effect of training on the response of plasma glucagon to exercise. *J Appl Physiol* 1977;43:302–305.
151. Araujo-Vilar D, Osifo E, Kirk M, et al. Influence of moderate physical exercise on insulin-mediated and non-insulin-mediated glucose uptake in healthy subjects. *Metabolism* 1997;46:203–209.
152. Koivisto VA, Yki-Jarvinen H. Effect of exercise on insulin binding and glucose transport in adipocytes of normal humans. *J Appl Physiol* 1987;63:1319–1323.
153. Lavoie C, Ducros F, Bourque J, et al. Glucose metabolism during exercise in man: the role of insulin and glucagon in the regulation of hepatic glucose production and gluconeogenesis. *Can J Physiol Pharmacol* 1997;75:26–35.
154. Hartley LH, Mason JW, Hogan RP, et al. Multiple hormonal responses to graded exercise in relation to physical training. *J Appl Physiol* 1972;33:602–606.
155. Miller WJ, Sherman WM, Ivy JL. Effect of strength training on glucose tolerance and post glucose insulin response. *Med Sci Sports Exerc* 1984;16:539–543.
156. Ben-Ezra V, Jankowski C, Kendrick K, Nichols D. Effect of intensity and energy expenditure of postexercise insulin responses in women. *J Appl Physiol* 1995;79:2029–2034.
157. Brambrink JK, Fluckey JD, Hickey MS, Craig BW. Influence of muscle mass and work on post-exercise glucose and insulin responses in young untrained subjects. *Acta Physiol Scand* 1997;161:371–377.
158. Treadway JL, James DE, Burcel E, Ruderman B. Effect of exercise on insulin receptor binding and kinase activity in skeletal muscle. *Am J Physiol* 1989;256:E138–E144.
159. Mikines KJ, Sonne B, Farrell PA, Tronier B, Galbo H. Effect of physical exercise on sensitivity and responsiveness to insulin in humans. *Am J Physiol* 1988;254:E248–E259.
160. Felig P, Wahren J. Fuel homeostasis in exercise. *N Engl J Med* 1975;293:1078–1084.
161. Roberts CK, Barnard RJ, Scheck SH, Balon TW. Exercise-stimulated glucose transport in skeletal muscle is nitric oxide dependent. *Am J Physiol* 1997;273:E220–E225.
162. Holloszy JO, Narahara HT. Enhanced permeability of sugar associated with muscle contraction: studies of the role of Ca^{++}. *J Gen Physiol* 1967;50:551–562.
163. Horowitz JF, Coyle EF. Metabolic responses to preexercise meals containing various carbohydrates and fats. *Am J Clin Nutr* 1993;58:235–241.
164. Hargreaves M, Costill DL, Fink WJ, et al. Effects of pre-exercise carbohydrate feeding on endurance cycling performance. *Med Sci Sports Exerc* 1987;19:33–36.
165. Neufer PD, Costill DL, Flynn MG, et al. Improvements in exercise performance: effects of carbohydrate feeding and diet. *J Appl Physiol* 1987:62:683–688.
166. James DE, Kraegen EW, Chisholm DJ. Effect of exercise training on whole-body insulin sensitivity and responsiveness. *J Appl Physiol* 1984;56:1217–1222.
167. Etgen GJ Jr, Jensen J, Wilson CM, et al. Exercise training reverses insulin resistance in muscle by enhanced recruitment of GLUT-4 to the cell surfaces. *Am J Physiol* 1997;272:E864–E869.
168. Gulve EA, Spina RJ. Effect of 7-10 days of cycle ergometer exercise on skeletal muscle GLUT-4 protein content. *J Appl Physiol* 1995;79:1562–1566.
169. Vukovich MD, Arciero PJ, Kohrt WM, Racette SB, Hansen PA, Holloszy JO. Changes in insulin action and GLUT-4 with 6 days of inactivity in endurance runners. *J Appl Physiol* 1996;80: 240–244.
170. Menshikov VV, Gitel EP, Bolshakova TD, et al. Endocrine function of the pancreas during exercise. In: Knuttgen HG, Vogel JA, Poortmans J, eds. *Biochemistry of exercise.* Champaign, IL: Humans Kinetics Publishers, 1983:688–693.
171. Bottger I, Schlein EM, Faloona GR, et al. The effect of exercise on glucagon secretion. *J Clin Endocrinol Metab* 1972;35:117–125.
172. Luyckx AS, Lefebvre PJ. Mechanisms involved in the exercise-induced increase in glucagon secretion in rats. *Diabetes* 1974;23: 81–93.
173. Jimenez C, Melin B, Koulmann N, et al. Effects of various beverages on the hormones involved in energy metabolism during exercise in the heat in previously dehydrated subjects. *Eur J Appl Physiol* 1997;76:504–509.
174. Wilkerson JE, Horvath SM. Plasma testosterone during treadmill running. *J Appl Physiol* 1980;49:249–253.
175. Sutton JR, Coleman MJ, Casey J. Androgen responses to physical exercise. *Br Med J* 1973;1:520–522.
176. Kindermann W, Schmitt W. Verhalten von testosteron im blutserum bei körperarbeit unterschiedlicher dauer und intensität. *Dtsch Z Sportmed* 1985;36:99–104.
177. Kuoppasalmi K, Naveri H, Harkonen M, Adlercreutz H. Plasma cortisol, androstenedione, testosterone and LH in running exercise of different intensities. *Scand J Clin Lab Invest* 1980;40: 403–409.
178. Kraemer RR, Heleniak RJ, Tryniecki JL, et al. Follicular and luteal phase hormonal responses to low-volume resistive exercise. *Med Sci Sports Exerc* 1995;27:809–817.
179. Nicklas BJ, Ryan AJ, Treuth MM, et al. Testosterone, growth hormone, and IGF-I responses to acute and chronic resistive exercise in men aged 55-70 yr. *Int J Sports Med* 1995;16:445–450.
180. Stone MH, Byrd R, Johnson C. Observations on serum androgen responses to short term resistance exercise in middle-aged sedentary males. *Natl Cond Assoc J* 1984;5:40–65.
181. Viru A, Karelson K, Smirnova T. Stability and variability in hormonal response to prolonged exercise. *Int J Sports Med* 1992;13:230–235.
182. Arce JC, DeSouza MJ. Exercise and male factor infertility. *Sports Med* 1993;15:146–169.
183. Arce JC, DeSouza MJ, Pescatello S, Luciano AA. Subclinical alterations in hormone and semen profiles in athletes. *Fertil Steril* 1993;59:398–404.
184. Kendrick ZV, Steffen CA, Rumsey WL, Goldberg DI. Effect of estradiol on tissue glycogen metabolism in exercised oophorectomized rats. *J Appl Physiol* 1987;63:492–496.
185. Wenz M, Berend JZ, Lynch NA, et al. Substrate oxidation at rest and during exercise: effects of menstrual cycle phase and diet composition. *J Physiol Pharmacol* 1997;48:851–860.
186. Tankersley CG, Nicholas WC, Deaver DR, et al. Estrogen replacement in middle-aged women: themoregulatory responses to exercise in the heat. *J Appl Physiol* 1992;73:1238–1245.
187. Bonen A, Ling WY, MacIntyre KP, et al. Effects of exercise on the serum concentrations of FSH, LH, progesterone, and estradiol. *Eur J Appl Physiol* 1979;42:15–23.
188. Jurkowski JE, Jones NL, Walker WC, et al. Ovarian hormonal responses to exercise. *J Appl Physiol* 1978;44:109–114.
189. Bullen BA, Skrinar GS, Beitins IZ, et al. Endurance training effects on plasma hormonal responsiveness and sex hormone excretion. *J Appl Physiol* 1984;56:1453–1463.
190. Keizer HA, Kuipers H, De Haan J, et al. Multiple hormonal responses to physical exercise in eumenorrheic trained and untrained women. *Int J Sports Med* 1987;8:139–150.
191. Keizer HA, Poortmans J, Bunnik GSJ. Influence of physical exercise on sex-hormone metabolism. *J Appl Physiol* 1980;48: 765–769.
192. Keizer HA, Rogol AD. Physical exercise and menstrual cycle alterations: what are the mechanisms? *Sports Med* 1990;10: 218–235.
193. Bonen A, Belcastro AN, Ling WY, Simpson AA. Profiles of selected hormones during menstrual cycles of teenage athletes. *J Appl Physiol* 1981;50:545–551.
194. Elias AN, Wilson AF. Exercise and gonadal function. *Hum Reprod* 1993;8:1747–1761.
195. Grossman A, Moult PJA, Gaillard RC, et al. The opioid control of LH and FSH release: effects of a met-enkephalin analogue and naloxone. *Clin Endocrinol* 1981;14:41–47.

196. Storzo GA. Opioids and exercise, an update. *Sports Med* 1988;7:109–184.
197. Farrell PA, Sonne B, Mikines K, Galbo H. Stimulatory role for endogenous opioid peptides on postexercise insulin secretion in rats. *J Appl Physiol* 1988;65:744–749.
198. Stassen J, Fiocchi R, Bouillon R, et al. The nature of opioid involvement in the hemodynamic respiratory and humoral responses to exercise. *Circ* 1985;72:982–990.
199. Rahkila P, Hakala E, Alen M, et al. Beta-endorphin and corticotropin release is dependent on a threshold intensity of running exercise in male endurance athletes. *Life Sci* 1988;43:551–557.
200. Schwarz L, Kindermann W. Beta-endorphin, catecholamines and cortisol during exhaustive endurance exercise. *Int J Sports Med* 1989;10:324–328.
201. Goldfarb A, Hatfield BD, Potts J, Armstrong D. Beta-endorphin time course of response to intensity of exercise: effect of training status. *Int J Sports Med* 1991;12:264–268.
202. Farrell PA. Exercise and endorphins: male responses. *Med Sci Sports Exerc* 1985;17:89–93.
203. Pestell RG, Hurley DM, Vandongen R. Biochemical and hormonal changes during a 100 km ultra-marathon. *Clin Exp Pharmacol Physiol* 1989;16:353–361.
204. McMurray RG, Berry MJ, Vann RT, et al. The effect of running in an outdoor environment on plasma beta endorphins. *Ann Sports Med* 1988;3:230–233.
205. Farrell PA, Kjaer M, Bach FW, Galbo H. Beta-endorphin and adrenocorticotropin response to supra-maximal treadmill exercise in trained and untrained males. *Acta Physiol Scand* 1987; 130:619–625.
206. Kraemer WJ, Patton JF, Knuttgen HG, et al. Hypothalamic-pituitary-adrenal responses to short-duration high-intensity cycle exercise. *J Appl Physiol* 1989;66:161–166.
207. Mikines KJ, Kjaer M, Hagen C, et al. The effect of training on responses of β-endorphin and other pituitary hormones to insulin-induced hypoglycemia. *Eur J Appl Physiol* 1985;54: 476–479.
208. Melchionda A, Clarkson P, Denko C, et al. The effect of local isometric exercise on serum levels of beta-endorphin/beta-lipotropin. *Phys Sports Med* 1984;12:102–109.
209. Walberg-Rankin J, Frank WD, Gwazdauskas FC. Response of beta-endorphin and estradiol to resistance exercise in females during energy balance and energy restriction. *Int J Sports Med* 1992;13:542–547.
210. Lobstein DD, Ismail AH. Decreases in resting plasma endorphin/-lipotropin after endurance training. *Med Sci Sports Exerc* 1989;21:161–166.
211. Appenzeller O, Appenzeller J, Standefer J, Skipper B, Atkinson R. Opioids and endurance training; longitudinal study. *Ann Sports Med* 1984;2:22–25.
212. Howlett TA, Tomlin S, Ngahfoong L, et al. Release of β-endorphin and met-enkephalin during exercise in normal women: response to training. *Br Med J* 1984;288:1950–1952.
213. Dale E, Gerlach DG, Whilhite AL. Menstrual dysfunction in distance runners. *Obstet Gynecol* 1979;54:47–53.
214. Shangold M, Freeman R, Thyson B, Gatz M. The relationship between long-distance running, blood progesterone and luteal phase length. *Fertil Steril* 1979;31:130–133.
215. Aloia JF, Rasulo P, Deftos IJ, et al. Exercise-induced hypercalcemia and the calciotropic-hormones. *J Lab Clin Invest* 1985;106: 229–232.
216. O'Neill ME, Wilkerson M, Robinson BG, et al. The effect of exercise on circulating immunoreactive calcitonin in men. *Horm Metab Res* 1990;22:546–550.
217. Vora NM, Kukreja SC, York PAJ, et al. Effect of exercise on serum calcium and parathyroid hormone. *J Clin Endocrinol Metab* 1983;57:1067–1069.
218. Ljunghall S, Joborn H, Benson L, et al. Effects of physical exercise on serum calcium and parathyroid hormone. *Eur J Clin Invest* 1984;14:469–473.
219. Ljunghall S, Joborn H, Lundin L, et al. Regional and systemic effects of short-term intense muscular work on plasma concentrations and content of total and ionized calcium. *Eur J Clin Invest* 1985:15:248–252.
220. Grimston SK, Tanguay KE, Gundberg CM, Hanley DA. The calciotropic hormone response to changes in serum calcium during exercise in female long distance runners. *J Clin Endocrinol Metab* 1993;76:867–872.
221. Takada H, Washino K, Nagashima M, Iwata H. Response of parathyroid hormone to anaerobic exercise in adolescent female athletes. *Acta Paediatr Jpn* 1998;40:73–77.
222. Ljunghall S, Joborn H, Roxin LE, et al. Increase in serum parathyroid hormone levels after prolonged physical exercise. *Med Sci Sports Exerc* 1988:20:122–125.
223. Salvesen H, Johansson AG, Foxdal P, et al. Intact serum parathyroid hormone levels increase during running exercise in well-trained men. *Calcif Tissue Int* 1994;54:256–261.
224. Ljunghall S, Joborn H, Roxin LE, et al. Prolonged low-intensity exercise raises the serum parathyroid hormone levels. *Clin Endocrinol* 1986;25:535–542.
225. Brown EM, Hurwitz S, Aurbach GD. Beta adrenergic stimulation of cyclic AMP content and parathyroid hormone release from isolated bovine parathyroid cells. *Endocrinology* 1977;100: 1609–1612.
226. Takada H, Washino K, Hanai T, Iwata H. Response of parathyroid hormone to exercise and bone mineral density in adolescent female athletes. *Environ Health Prevent Med* 1999;2:161–166.
227. Siri WE, Van Dyke DC, Winchell HS, et al. Early erythropoietin, blood, and physiological responses to severe hypoxia in man. *J Appl Physiol* 1966;21:73–80.
228. Gareau R, Caron C, Brisson GR. Exercise duration and serum erythropoietin level. *Horm Metab Res* 1991;23:355.
229. Klausen T, Breum L, Fogh-Andersen N, et al. The effect of short and long duration exercise on serum erythropoietin concentrations. *Eur J Appl Physiol* 1993;67:213–217.
230. Weight LM, Alexander D, Elliot T, Jacobs P. Erythropoietic adaptations to endurance training. *Eur J Appl Physiol* 1992;64: 444–448.
231. Klausen T, Dela F, Hippe E, Galbo H. Diurnal variations of serum erythropoietin in trained and untrained subjects. *Eur J Appl Physiol* 1993;67:545–548.
232. Schwandt HJ, Heyduck B, Gunga HC, Rocker L. Influence of prolonged physical exercise on the erythropoietin concentration in blood. *Eur J Appl Physiol* 1991;63:463–466.
233. Schmidt W, Eckardt KU, Hilgendorf A, et al. Effect of maximal and submaximal exercise under normoxic and hypoxic conditions on serum erythropoietin level. *Int J Sports Med* 1991;12:457–461.

Exercise and Sport Science,
edited by William E. Garrett, Jr., and Donald T. Kirkendall.
Lippincott Williams & Wilkins, Philadelphia © 2000.

CHAPTER 11

Muscular Responses to Exercise and Training

Robert S. Staron and Robert S. Hikida

ANATOMY

Muscle Structure

Skeletal muscle has unique properties that are highly susceptible to adaptive changes. This plasticity is manifested by its changes induced by exercise or altered activity. Some of the important factors to be considered in examining skeletal muscle adaptations are (a) the nuclei are postmitotic; (b) the cells are multinucleated, consisting of several hundred to several thousand nuclei per centimeter length of a fiber; (c) different isoforms of structural proteins and enzymes are manifested; and (d) space constraints within a fiber limit the noncontractile components (mitochondria, lipids, and other sarcoplasmic contents), so muscle fibers must maximize the use of the space available to them.

Nuclei

The two characteristics of muscle-fiber nuclei (multinucleation and postmitotic condition) create unique problems for the fiber. Because of its multinucleated condition, the muscle fiber is divided into a mosaic of overlapping regions, or domains (1,2), each controlled by a nucleus. The nucleus generally controls the structural proteins within its domain. As muscle growth occurs during postnatal development, more nuclei must be added to accommodate the increased fiber size. If this incorporation of additional nuclei is inhibited, then growth does not occur (3).

A comparison of myonuclear density produces a wide range of values, depending on the animal, age, sample size, and technique for measurement. Many studies have compared the number of myonuclei per length of fiber, although this does not take into account the differences in cross-sectional area. When nuclear distribution is measured in this way, slow type I fibers usually contain more nuclei than the fast type II fibers. However, a more meaningful measurement is obtained by measuring number of myonuclei per volume of muscle fiber. This can be done by considering the section of tissue as infinitely thin or by calculating the cross-sectional area and multiplying by its length. The former yields nuclei per square micrometer, and the latter, nuclei per cubic micrometer.

Table 11–1 gives a summary of several studies quantifying nuclear numbers in control animal muscles (4–11; Hikida, unpublished data). Some values have been estimated from the data in the articles. What becomes apparent from this table is that the volume per nucleus between type I (slow) and II (fast) fibers varies considerably between studies, and in most studies the volume per nucleus is higher in fast than in slow fibers. Furthermore, the range of nuclei counted in different studies varies widely (45 to 145 nuclei/mm for fast fibers, 47 to 168 nuclei/mm for slow fibers). In most cases, the methods for measuring these nuclei involved analysis of single teased fibers. This necessitated very small sample sizes (fewer than 10 fibers) in many of the studies. Because of the small sample sizes for most of the studies and the variability, it is difficult to generalize about the nuclear domains between fiber types at this time. Our recent studies (9,12) used a different method to determine these parameters, and this method analyzed several hundred fibers per muscle. The results of using these different methods are similar to the results of the other studies, suggesting that this method may be a valid and more valuable way to establish the nucleocytoplasmic relations than using single fibers. In spite of the question of accuracy of domain size, the molecular studies showed this to be an important aspect of muscle biology.

R. S. Staron and R. S. Hikida: Department of Biomedical Sciences, College of Osteopathic Medicine, Ohio University, Athens, Ohio 45701.

TABLE 11–1. *Myonuclear numbers*

	Fast type II fibers			Slow type I fibers		
Species/ref	XSA	No./mm	μm³/n	XSA	No./mm	μm³/n
Cat plant/4	1729	70	26,000	1176	88	14,000
sol/4	1950			2529	126	20,650
Rat sol/5	1950	137	14,500	2100	168	13,000
Rat plant/6	4066	44	112,000	1373	47	34,000
Rat sol/6	1731	54	40,000	3135	116	30,000
J.rat tib/7	1150	57	22,000			
J-gast/7	900	50	18,000			
Rat plant/8	4423	76	65,000	2967	98	30,000
Rat sol/8	4270	145	29,000	4671	154	33,000
Rat sol/9	2037	43	47,400	2360	57	41,000
J-rat sol/10					76	
J-rat tib/10		44				
Rat semit/11		100				
Rabbit add/11		118				
Human vl[a]	4786	139	34,000	4046	105	39,000

XSA, Cross-sectional area in μm²; No./mm, number of myonuclei per mm of muscle-fiber length; μm³/n, volume of sarcoplasm per nucleus; Species/ref, animal used, muscle, reference; j, juvenile animals; plant, plantaris; sol, soleus; tib, tibialis anterior; gast, gastrocnemius; semit, semitendinosus; add, adductor magnus; vl, vastus lateralis.
[a] Hikida, unpublished data.

The incorporation of nuclei into the muscle fiber is done by satellite cells, which are undifferentiated myogenic cells that lie dormant beside the muscle fiber and enclosed within the muscle fiber's basal lamina. A satellite cell is thought to undergo mitosis, and one of the daughter nuclei becomes incorporated into the fiber as a new myonucleus (13). It is this division of satellite cells that can be inhibited to stop muscle growth.

This relation between nuclear domains and nuclear incorporation by satellite cell activation has become of interest recently in terms of muscular atrophy and hypertrophy. The hypothesis tested by various studies is to determine whether the nuclear domain size is tightly controlled in adult muscle fibers. This question has been examined in fibers that have atrophied because of the reduced gravity of space flight (5,7,9), and, conversely, in muscle fibers induced to undergo hypertrophy because of resistance training (12, and Hikida, unpublished data).

Surprisingly, two of three studies (5,9) showed, by using different techniques, that rat muscles atrophied by space flight had fewer nuclei than those of their ground-based littermates. This occurred after only 6 to 14 days in space and indicated a loss of myonuclei as the muscle fibers atrophied. In contrast, little information is available about hypertrophy and nuclear increase. Myonuclei do not increase in hypertrophied elderly human muscle (12). Preliminary results suggest that muscle fibers from young and elderly human subjects respond differently to resistance training (Hikida, unpublished data). These results suggest that the satellite cells may have less capability to be activated in the elderly, and this may be due to satellite cells undergoing senescence, as was indicated in early studies of rat muscles (14).

Mitochondria

The major noncontractile components of muscle fibers are mitochondria. These mitochondria occur in two populations: subsarcolemmal and intermyofibrillar. The subsarcolemmal population accumulates within oxidative (type I and IIA) fibers, and a high population is often adjacent to a capillary in oxidative fibers. The mitochondrial distribution has been studied in red, white, and intermediate (presumably I, IIB, and IIA) fibers of human muscles by an elegant scanning electron microscopic study (15). This study showed that the type I and IIA fibers had similar distributions of mitochondria, with short, thick branches oriented perpendicular to the myofibril at the I-band, and extensions running across the sarcomere at the A-band (to produce the intermyofibrillar portion). Although type I and IIA fibers had similar distributions of mitochondria, the intermediate fibers had thinner and longer mitochondria. The white type IIB fibers had thin mitochondria that extended perpendicular to the myofibrils at the I-band levels. No subsarcolemmal population occurred in the white (IIB) fibers.

The volume occupied by mitochondria can change quickly in response to altered activity levels. This again reflects the adaptability of the fiber to maximize its use of space in response to the activity.

Myofibrils

The muscle fiber consists of myofibrils, with mitochondria and a sarcotubular membrane system occurring between them (Fig. 11–1). Oxidative fibers also contain lipid (triglyceride) droplets, usually associated with the

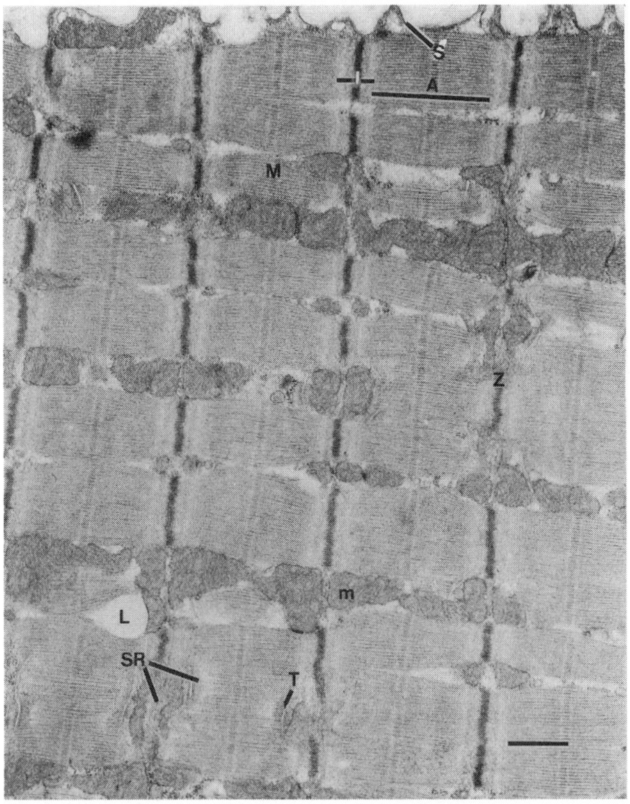

FIG. 11–1. Normal ultrastructure of a muscle fiber showing the fiber surface with its sarcolemma (*S*). The sarcomere components are indicated as the A-band (*A*), I-band (*I*), Z-line (*Z*), and M-line (*M*). The myofibrils are incompletely separated by mitochondria (*m*), sometimes associated with lipid droplets (*L*). The sarcotubular system is represented here by the transverse tubules (*T*) and sarcoplasmic reticulum (*SR*). Scale bar is 1 μm.

mitochondria. Another organelle, which increases with aging, is the lipofuscin granule, thought to be related to lysosomal residual bodies.

Myofibrils are made up of interdigitated thick (myosin) and thin (actin) filaments, this interdigitation forming the striation pattern (see Fig. 11–1). Several isoforms of myosin molecules exist, and these isoforms are associated with different muscle fiber types. Because the myosin molecule is an adenosine triphosphatase (ATPase) enzyme, fibers that contain different myosin isoforms have different myofibrillar ATPase activities, as described below.

Although myosin isoforms differ in the thick filaments, the sarcomere pattern is relatively homogeneous in human skeletal muscle fiber types, except for two features: the Z-line and the M-line. These two structures differ in the different muscle fiber types. A clear distinction in fiber types is seen in the lower mammals (16), but the human fiber type differences are more subtle. The widths of the Z-lines are known to differ between fiber types, as first shown by Payne and colleagues (17), and subsequently confirmed by Prince and co-workers (18). The type I slow fibers have the thickest Z-widths and are progressively thinner in the IIA and IIB fibers. In addition, Payne and colleagues (17) quantified the M-line thickness, indicating that the thickest were in the type I, and they became progressively thinner in the IIA and IIB fibers.

Shortly after the studies measuring M-line and Z-line widths, studies by Sjostrom's group (19) demonstrated that the fiber types had specific ultrastructural differences in the M-line. Type I fibers had five strong M-line bridges, IIB fibers had three strong bridges, and IIA fibers had three strong bridges flanked on either side by a single weak bridge (19) (Fig. 11–2). These were correlated with the Z-line widths, which showed the variation in thickness according to the fiber types, as shown previously. This study pointed out that different observers produced consistently different ranges of measurements of Z-line widths, although obtaining a bimodal (type I vs. type II) distribution. Therefore the Z-line width varies depending on the interpretation of its structural limits. This inconsistency of interpretation and the significant overlap of values between fiber types

A
B
C

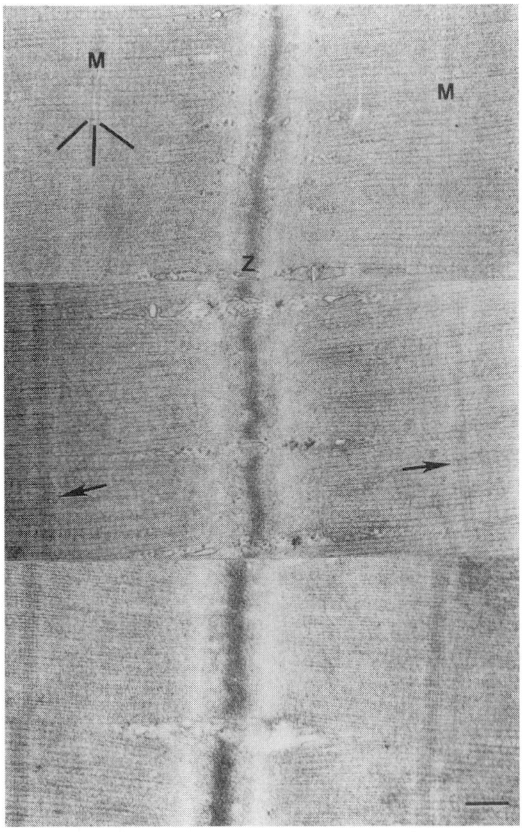

FIG. 11–2. The Z-lines and M-lines of the three primary muscle fiber types are shown here at high magnification. The type IIB (**A**) fiber has three bands making up the M-line, the IIA fiber (**B**) has three heavy bands flanked by an indistinct band on either side, and the type I fiber (**C**) has five distinct bands. Scale bar is 100 nm.

suggest that Z-line width is not so good a discriminator of fiber types as is M-line structure (19).

Sarcotubular System

The sarcotubular system [sarcoplasmic reticulum and transverse tubular (T-system)] is highly developed and organized in the muscles of vertebrates other than humans (20–23). The complexity and elaboration appear to be related to the speed of the muscle contraction and relaxation. Human muscles, however, have a relatively rudimentary sarcoplasmic reticular system. The A-band reticulum is least developed, and the I-band reticulum is relatively extensive (15). The striking feature of human sarcotubular interactions is that the terminal cisternae of the sarcoplasmic reticulum do not attach almost continuously to the T-tubule as they do in other fast vertebrate muscles.

Cytoskeleton and Fiber Integrity

A cytoskeletal network holds the myofibrils together. This network consists of the intermediate filament, desmin, and the cytoskeletal actin (or microfilament). These filaments interconnect the myofibrils to hold the fibrils in register and also connect the fibrils to the sarcolemma. The attachment to the sarcolemma occurs by means of an anchoring protein, dystrophin, that connects the actin to the dystrophin-associated glycoproteins at the sarcolemma (24,25). The dystrophin itself is connected to the connective tissue of the extracellular space by means of dystrophin-associated glycoproteins (26). In this way, the movement of the sarcomeres is transmitted by the cytoskeleton to the sarcolemma and then to the surrounding connective tissue (25).

The cytoskeleton of a skeletal muscle fiber is any structure primarily involved in connecting protein filaments to each other or to anchoring sites (27). Because the cytoskeletal network maintains the myofibrils in register, any damage to the muscle, as described below, will cause myofibrillar disruption; this is most likely caused by disruption of the cytoskeleton. When components of this complex are lacking, muscular dystrophy and other muscle disorders result in humans (25).

mATPase-Based Fiber Types

Human skeletal muscle is composed of a variety of fiber types that can be delineated on the basis of differences in histochemical, immunohistochemical, biochemical, morphologic, and physiological properties (28). For example, fibers can be separated based on contractile speed (slow and fast twitch) or on the basis of differences in myoglobin and capillary content (red and white). Attention must be given to the method used to delineate fiber types, as not all methods are compatible (e.g., not all red fibers are slow twitch). One of the most popular methods for delineating fiber types uses differences in the pH sensitivity of myofibrillar ATPase (mATPase). This enzyme hydrolyzes ATP to release energy for contraction and is associated with the thick filament.

In 1962 Engel (29) described the delineation of two groups of fibers (which he termed type I and type II) by using an assay for mATPase activity. Under the alkaline conditions of the assay, the type I fibers (which were later found to be slow twitch) exhibited low ATPase activity, and the type II fibers (found to be fast twitch) had high activity. Subsequently it was determined that the type I fibers were not only alkali labile (low activity), but also that they were acid stable (high activity), and the type II fibers were the reverse: alkali stable and acid labile (30). This histochemical method allowed an easy identification of two major fiber types differing in their mATPase stability. Careful investigation of the pH sensitivity of mATPase revealed the existence of additional fiber types and led to the currently used nomenclature of I, IIA, IIB, and IIC (31). This mATPase-based classification scheme was more recently expanded to include a few additional "hybrid" fiber types: IIAB, IIAC, and IC (for review, see ref. 28). Therefore the entire range of mATPase-based fiber types in human limb and trunk muscles consists of I, IC, IIC, IIAC, IIA, IIAB, and IIB (Figs. 11–3 and 11–4).

The histochemical staining of these fiber types is such that the type I fibers have mATPase activity that is stable in the acid ranges (pH 4.3 and 4.6) but labile at an alkaline pH of 10.4, whereas type IIA fibers display the reverse pattern (Figs. 11–3 and 11–4). All fibers stable at pH 4.6 and 10.4 but labile at pH 4.3 are classified as either type IIB or IIAB, depending on their staining intensity after preincubation at pH 4.6. After being exposed to this pH, the type IIAB fibers will have a staining intensity that is between the dark type IIB

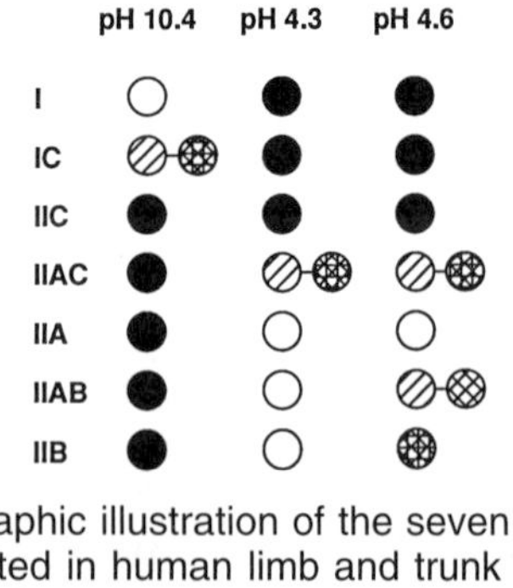

FIG. 11–3. Graphic illustration of the seven fiber types that can be delineated in human limb and trunk musculature by using mATPase histochemistry after preincubation at the various pH values. Muscle fibers cut in cross section (*circles*), and the various levels of shading correspond to the actual staining intensities. Possible gradations of staining intensity between the two given extremes are shown (*connected circles*). Compare with micrograph of actual staining in Fig. 11–2. From ref. 32, with permission.

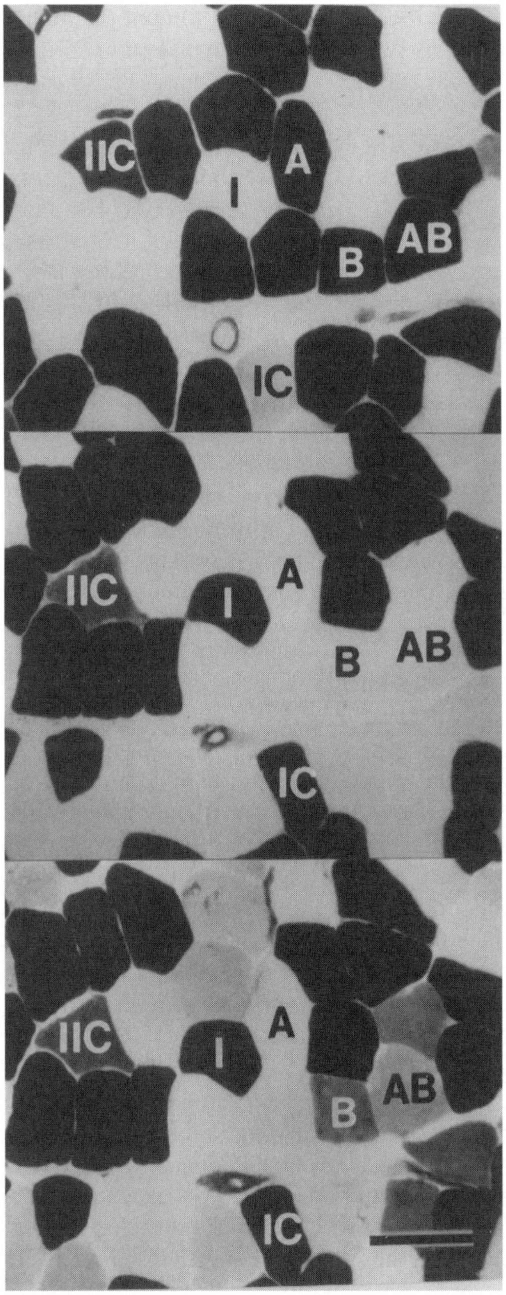

A

B

C

FIG. 11–4. Serial cross sections assayed for myofibrillar ATPase activity after preincubation at pH values of 10.4 (**A**), 4.3 (**B**), and 4.6 (**C**). Six muscle fiber types have been delineated corresponding to the format given in Fig. 11–1. *I*, type I; *IC*, type IC; *IIC*, type IIC; *A*, type IIA; *AB*, type IIAB; *B*, type IIB. Scale bar is 100 μm. From Staron RS, Malicky ES, Leonardi MJ, Falkel JE, Hagerman FC, Dudley GA. Muscle hypertrophy and fast fiber type conversions in heavy resistance-trained women. *Eur J Appl Physiol* 1990;60:71–79, with permission.

fibers and the light type IIA fibers (see Fig. 11–4). Fibers classified as C (types IC, IIC, IIAC) remain stable, to varying degrees, throughout the entire pH range of 4.3 to 10.4 (see Fig. 11–4). Those fibers that are histochemically more similar to type I (indistinguishable from the type I fibers after either of the acid preincubations but intermediate staining after the alkaline preincubation) are termed type IC. Those fibers more similar to the type II fibers (indistinguishable from the fast fibers after the alkaline preincubation but intermediate staining after the acid preincubation of pH 4.3) are type IIAC. Some fibers remain darkly stained throughout the entire pH range and are classified as type IIC. Although the C fibers normally make up a minor portion of most adult human muscles (0 to 5%), significant numbers (greater than 15%) have been found in limb muscles of untrained and trained individuals (e.g., 32).

It is important to understand that under physiologic conditions, all fibers retain their mATPase activity. The mATPase activity is stable well outside the narrow range of possible *in vivo* pH fluctuations (range of approximately pH 6.2 to 7.0). Indeed, histochemical methods showed that mATPase activity is retained *in vitro* throughout a range of approximately 4.7 to 10.0 (33). It should also be noted that mATPase histochemistry is not a measure of the amount of ATPase activity but is merely a qualitative method used to separate fibers into groups.

Although some studies have delineated human fast-fiber subtypes by using a metabolic enzyme-based classification scheme (e.g., 34–36), the assumption that metabolic properties correlate with mATPase characteristics is not justified. Although it is true that, as a group, the type I fibers in human muscle are the most oxidative and the IIB the least, there is a wide range of metabolic enzyme activity levels within each specific mATPase-based fiber type (37,38). Microphotometric analysis of succinate dehydrogenase activity levels revealed a complete overlap between the type IIA and IIB fibers in human muscle (39). Even the type I fibers represent a metabolically heterogeneous population within a muscle (40). In addition, metabolic enzyme activity levels of the various fibers depend on the training state of the muscle (41). Alterations in oxidative capacity could, therefore, take place without accompanying changes in other components of the cell (e.g., myosin heavy chain). As such, similar to the contractile-based versus color-based systems mentioned earlier, the metabolic enzyme–based and the mATPase-based classification schemes are not compatible. This is especially true when considering the subgrouping of the fibers in human muscle. Subgrouping (creating groups in addition to the two major groups) appears to be more reliably accomplished by using differences in mATPase sensitivity as compared with using histochemical reactions for oxidative and/or glycolytic enzymes (42).

Myosin Heavy Chain–Based Fiber Types

The major component of the thick filament is the myosin molecule. Myosin is a hexameric protein consisting of two heavy portions of approximately 200 kDa each (myosin heavy chains) and four lighter portions of approximately 20 kDa each (myosin light chains). The myosin heavy chains (MHCs) contain the mATPase activity (which is located on the cross-bridges) (43). Fibers separated on the basis of differences in the pH sensitivity of their mATPase activity also differ in their MHC content and thus differ with regard to specific contractile properties (44,45). As such, the three major fiber types in human skeletal muscle (I, IIA, and IIB) have been found to correspond to the expression of three MHCs, termed MHCI, MHCIIa, and MHCIIb, respectively.

More recently a method was devised to analyze electrophoretically single fiber fragments from freeze-dried cross sections cut in series to sections used for mATPase histochemistry (46). Applying this method to human muscle has increased our understanding of the correlation between the mATPase-based and MHC-based fiber types (32,47) (Fig. 11–5). The seven mATPase-based fiber types correspond to a specific MHC profile. Each of the histochemically identified fiber types (I, IIA, and IIB) contains one type of MHC (MHCI, MHCIIa, and MHCIIb, respectively), whereas the "hybrid" fiber types (types IIAB, IC, IIC, and IIAC) are made up of fibers that contain two MHCs. Type IIAB fibers coexpress MHCIIa and MHCIIb, and the C fibers (IC, IIC, and IIAC) coexpress MHCI and MHCIIa (32,47).

Although the human genome contains at least 10 genes for MHC (48,49), only seven have thus far been identified in mature human extrafusal fibers. Most muscles in the human appear to express three MHC isoforms: a slow MHCI, which is similar to MHCβcard (50), and two fast MHCs (MHCIIa and MHCIIb). In the limb and trunk musculature of small mammals, a third fast MHC (termed MHCIId or MHCIIx) has been identified (51–53). Recently it was shown that the type IIB fibers in human muscle contain MHC transcripts similar to those found in the IIX (also termed IID) fibers of the rat (54,55). Thus some of the recent studies on human muscle have been renaming fibers formerly classified as type IIB as either IIX or IID.

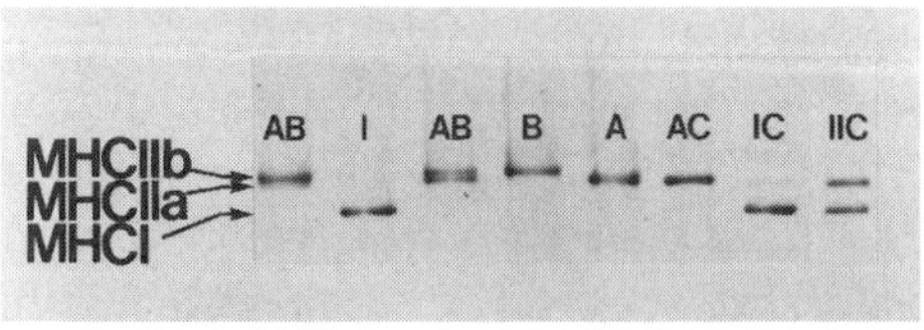

FIG. 11–5. Electrophoretic separation of single-fiber fragments of human vastus lateralis muscle demonstrating the myosin heavy chain (MHC) content of specific histochemically identified fiber types. *I*, type I; *IC*, type IC; *IIC*, type IIC; *AC*, type IIAC; *A*, type IIA; *AB*, type IIAB; *B*, type IIB. Note the varying proportions of MHCIIa and MHCIIb in the two type IIAB fibers and the varying proportions of MHCI and MHCIIa in the three C fibers. Modified from refs. 28, 32, and 47, with permission.

SHORT-TERM RESPONSES TO EXERCISE AND TRAINING

Sarcolemmal Damage

Damage to skeletal muscle causes leakage of muscle-specific components into the bloodstream through membrane disruptions. The most commonly assayed component is creatine kinase (CK), although myoglobin, lactate dehydrogenase, and muscle structural proteins also have been used as indicators of muscle damage. Although CK is commonly used, the specific mechanism by which this enzyme is released is unclear, mainly because of the time course of its presence in the blood. In most studies, the peak levels of CK usually occur between 2 and 4 days after the damaging exercise. Many studies have examined the time course of changes, and the variability is puzzling. Downhill walking results in a maximal serum CK level at 24 hours, whereas biceps curls produced a maximum at 3 or 4 days in the same study of inactive men (56). Men doing leg resistance exercises attained a maximal CK value at 4 or 5 days after exercise (57). Clarkson and colleagues have done many studies by using CK as an assay for muscle damage. Among these, they showed that eccentric exercise of the forearm flexors in young versus elderly women produced CK levels that were still increasing at 5 days (58,59). They also compared women exercising with both arms versus one arm, such that one group did twice as many eccentric actions (60). Peak CK was measured either 3 or 4 days after the exercise, and no significant difference in CK levels occurred between groups, even though twice as much muscle damage presumably occurred in one group as in the other. Based on this study, then, the amount of serum CK does not reflect the amount of damage done to the muscle.

Although these studies show that maximal serum CK levels occur several days after the exercise, Apple and co-workers (61) demonstrated that the CK levels can increase significantly as early as 2 hours after eccentric biceps activity in young untrained men. Although total CK did not increase significantly even after 6 hours, various isoforms of CK, assayed by isoelectric focusing, increased significantly after 2 hours.

It was mentioned earlier that damage to both arms produced no higher CK levels than that to a single arm (60). Our group, however, showed that damage to as few as 2000 muscle fibers in the vastus lateralis muscle of men increases the total serum CK levels at between 3 and 8 hours after the damage (62). The damage was induced by taking muscle biopsies involving an average of 1800 fibers and measuring CK levels at intervals thereafter. Although an increase in CK was observed, the CK increase with damage to 1800 muscle fibers was insignificant compared with most exercise-induced damage or injuries.

A review by Noakes (63) suggested that men had higher serum CK levels than women after similar activities (such as running a marathon). This gender difference may be related to hormonal levels, as there is some indication that estrogen inhibits enzyme release (64), as demonstrated by ovariectomy. The estrogen effect is long lasting, however, because ovariectomy of mature female rats produced less CK release after running than it did in rats having ovariectomies when sexually immature. According to Noakes (63), serum CK peaks at 24 to 48 hours after the prolonged exercise, and athletes running races at 15 km and 21.1 km had no serum CK increases. Serum CK levels increased significantly with marathon length (42.2 km) races, but subjects running 56-km and 90-km races had twice the CK levels of those running a marathon (42 km). The peaks of all these occurred at 24 hours after the race.

It is clear that the serum CK not only signifies damage to the muscle fiber membrane, but it is also associated with breakdown of the myofibrillar apparatus. This is shown by an identical time course of increase in serum levels of CK, myoglobin, MHC fragments, and troponin 1 (65) after eccentric exercise inducing immediate muscle damage.

Significance of the Time Course of Creatine Kinase Changes

Most studies have indicated a period of 1 to 5 days between the damaging exercise and the maximal CK measured in the bloodstream, and there are often at least 2 days before a significant increase is detectable. Because direct muscle damage (initiated by a muscle biopsy) results in the CK levels increasing after 3 hours and before 6 hours (62), it must take at least 4 hours for the muscle enzymes to appear in sufficient quantities to be detectable in the bloodstream. This further suggests that those studies that show a 5-day lag time must have membrane leakage occurring as a factor secondary to the changes initiated by the damaging activity. It is reasonable to assume that maximal CK at 5 days after exercise is due to a factor such as destruction by inflammatory cells occurring after the exercise, which probably did not initially disrupt the membrane. In this scenario, the activity itself does not produce immediate membrane disruption. Instead, some damage secondarily signals an inflammatory reaction, which in turn causes a delayed breakdown of muscle fibers. Correspondingly, those activities resulting in significant CK release within 24 hours should be a result of the activity directly injuring the muscle fiber membranes.

The changes proposed here might be related to structural changes, such as Z-line streaming, being the initiator of the inflammatory reaction by perhaps disrupting the cytoskeletal elements that connect the myofibrillar apparatus to the extracellular matrix.

Structural Changes with Exercise

Skeletal muscle responds to unaccustomed or strenuous exercise with several types of morphologic alterations. The initial response shows Z-line streaming (Fig. 11–6), which may be accompanied by intracellular edema. This is evident in the muscle immediately after the activity and remains for approximately 3 days (Hikida, unpublished observations). This was observed in vastus lateralis muscles of untrained subjects who had been tested for maximal leg strength [1 repetition maximum (RM)]. Biopsies were taken either before or up to 5 days after this, and Z-line streaming was observed only 1 to 3 days after the 1-RM measurement. This Z-line streaming may be the universal response of skeletal muscle to altered activity. It has been seen after various types of activities: muscles of amino acid–supplemented swimming rats (66), eccentric contractions (67,68), and after a marathon (69). Surprisingly, it also was observed after prolonged bedrest (70).

Although Z-line streaming is a common and initial response to unaccustomed eccentric muscular activity, this type of activity is not necessarily required to induce streaming. In fact, activity may not be required at all. Hindlimb unweighting by suspension of rats, spaceflight, and bedrest studies have all shown that muscle biopsies

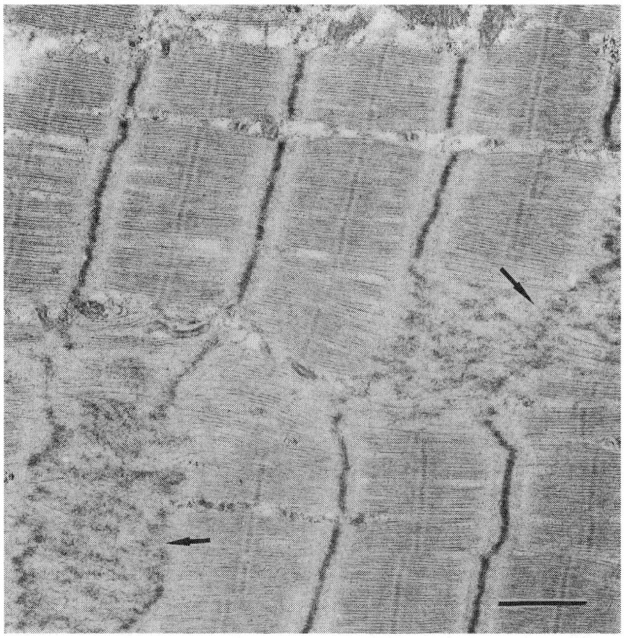

FIG. 11–6. Exercise-induced muscle damage, reflected by Z-line streaming and myofibril disruption (*arrows*). Scale bar is 1 μm.

taken after these procedures show myofibrillar disruption and Z-line streaming (70–74). In most of these studies, the muscle samples were taken after return to normal gravity or release from suspension, and one could not determine whether the structural damage was due to unweighting or reloading. Krippendorf and Riley (75) compared hindlimb suspended rats not exposed to reloading with those returned to normal activity for various periods after the suspension. They found evidence for myofibrillar disruption in both, based on light microscopy, but could not quantify the results. A later study (73) compared muscles removed from rats *in space* after 13 days of spaceflight versus muscles from rats 2 to 7 hours after landing. The muscles from in-space rats showed no damage, whereas those returning to gravity had the Z-line streaming, indicating that damage was induced by reloading to normal gravity.

In spite of the studies describing a return to normal weighting as inducing the myofibrillar alterations, several studies have shown that altered activity is not required for the sarcomere lesions to occur. Hikida and colleagues (70) found extensive lesions in soleus muscles of subjects exposed to 30 days of bedrest, before the subjects returned to ambulation. Similarly, Lancha and co-workers (66) compared muscles from swimming rats that had amino acid supplementation with those with no supplementation and found Z-line streaming in the supplemented rats. These studies showed that the lesions can occur with reduced activity or in the absence of eccentric load. Therefore the Z-line streaming, perhaps induced by cytoskeletal changes, reflects the initial response to altered activity patterns of muscle, and not only to strong eccentric activity.

Cytoskeletal Changes and Myofibril Disruption

Many studies have shown that cytoskeletal elements are abnormal or lacking in neuromuscular disorders and myopathies (76–80). Although many structural alterations are observed in these muscle disorders, it is possible that cytoskeletal disruptions are a common cause for the myofibrillar disorganization. The cytoskeletal intermediate filament composed of desmin interconnects myofibrils by a skelemin attachment, and the desmin intermediate filaments are correspondingly connected to the muscle fiber sarcolemma by means of attachment proteins such as vinculin, spectrin, ankyrin, or talin (27,81,82).

The exosarcomeric cytoskeleton, with desmin as its major component, was proposed to be disrupted when exercise-induced Z-line streaming occurred (83,84). Lieber and associates (85) showed that desmin disruption occurs almost immediately after eccentric exercise-induced damage, and this is consistent with the time course of Z-line streaming (Hikida, unpublished data). To investigate this interaction between the intermediate filaments and exercise-induced damage, Lieber's group (85) induced eccentric damage to rabbit muscles and examined the early changes in cytoskeletal proteins with immunohistochemistry. Desmin disappeared within 15 minutes of the damaging exercise, affecting 25% of the fibers of the extensor digitorum longus muscle after 1 day. Significantly, all affected fibers were type II low-oxidative (IIB) fibers. This study is important for at least two reasons. First, the results suggest that myofibrillar organization is disrupted because the organizational cytoskeletal network is removed or reduced. This further reinforces the role and importance of the cytoskeleton in maintaining the integrity of the fiber organization. The second significant finding is that loss of desmin occurred only in glycolytic fibers. This revisits the proposal that exercise-induced damage may be fiber-type specific or at least may occur preferentially in IIB fibers (69,86).

In spite of Z-line streaming and desmin loss occurring simultaneously in supporting the hypothesis that intermediate filaments are involved in the Z-line streaming process, Vater and colleagues (87) have results that do not agree. Snake venom toxin was used to induce degeneration and regeneration in rat soleus muscles, and myofibrillar disruption occurred in regions where desmin occurred, as determined by immunocytochemistry (88). This discrepancy may be due to desmin being present, but depolymerized and not present as intact filaments, or if intact, desmin filaments may not be anchored to the myofibrils. Desmin was present and well organized in early myotubes, indicating its importance in myofibril alignment. Further work must be done to clarify these relations.

In a related study, these authors examined dystrophin changes in the degeneration and regeneration process (88). At 3 hours, even though necrosis was occurring, dystrophin distribution was normal. By 6 hours, the dystrophin was present only in sporadic patches and had disappeared completely by 12 hours. The dystrophin returned several days after regeneration had begun, indicating that myotubes of these regenerating muscles do not need dystrophin. The time course of these changes is interesting, showing that in this model necrosis precedes membrane disruption.

Another possible cause of Z-line streaming might be alterations in titin. Lieber and colleagues (85) demonstrated increased titin staining with eccentric damage. Because there is evidence that titin attaches not only to Z-lines, but also to the actin near the Z-lines (89), it is possible that part of the Z-line streaming may be the result of titin accumulating in these regions.

A question that arises from these studies is why desmin composition increases in diseased and regenerating muscle while becoming reduced in exercise-damaged fibers. Many studies demonstrated increased desmin staining in patients with muscular disorders

(76,77,79,90). A further problem arises when considering the results of a study by Vater and colleagues (87). This group studied changes in desmin and titin correlated with ultrastructural changes of the rat soleus muscle during degeneration and regeneration induced by a myotoxic snake venom. The early degeneration (1 hour after injection) showed hypercontraction or stretching of fibers; after 3 hours there was phagocytic infiltration and edema. Desmin had not changed until 3 hours, when some fibers had lost their desmin. The fibers without desmin had no Z-lines. After 2 days, the muscle fibers began regenerating. This regeneration was associated with enhanced desmin staining, which was not localized (at the Z-line) as in control muscle fibers. By day 7, when the muscle fibers appeared mostly mature, the desmin composition and localization were similar to those of the controls. This study shows that the early degenerative response is to lose the desmin, whereas the regenerative response is associated with increased desmin composition. This suggests that the increased desmin content in muscle diseases may be an attempt by the muscle to regenerate, because desmin content is high during muscle-fiber development and regeneration (78).

A second question related to the concept of desmin and muscle damage is how a muscle can be protected from soreness and additional damage after the first damaging activity. It is well known that the initial induction of muscle soreness protects the muscle from soreness and damage for several weeks after the first event. Does the change in desmin distribution have any relation to this? It seems likely that after the initial loss of desmin, the expression of desmin is enhanced shortly thereafter to levels much higher than in the normal muscle fiber. This sequence of events would be similar to that demonstrated by the experimental studies of Vater and coworkers (87,88). This regenerative response, which most likely occurs after the initial damage, produces a cytoskeletal network that is much more extensive than in the normal adult muscle fiber. It is possible that this enhanced cytoskeletal network protects the muscle fibers from additional damage during the regenerative phase of the injury process.

Later Structural Alterations

Severe exercise often results in changes that have a longer time course than Z-line streaming, and these changes are associated with inflammation, membrane disruption, enzyme leakage, and necrosis. These delayed-onset, more serious muscular changes have been attributed to a number of causes such as oxygen-reactive radicals, calpain, and ubiquitin. In spite of the many potential causes, it appears that most of these are associated with damage to the membrane (91) and subsequent inflammatory changes (reviewed in refs. 92 and 93). These inflammatory changes result in reactions that attract macrophages to clean up debris from damaged muscle fibers and to initial muscle regeneration. Many of these inflammatory changes were described in a series of changes after marathon running (69).

Because the time course of delayed-onset muscle soreness closely matches the time course of inflammatory changes, it was proposed that the soreness was related to the inflammation (94), and that this might be related to intracellular edema induced by the exercise (95).

LONG-TERM RESPONSES TO EXERCISE AND TRAINING

Although one fiber type may predominate, all human muscles contain a mixture of fiber types; these vary greatly between muscles and among individuals. This heterogeneity affords human skeletal muscle with a wide range of functional capabilities and thus plays an important role in athletic performance (96,97). It must, however, be remembered that muscle fibers are not static structures but are continually adjusting to altered functional demands, hormonal signals, and neural input (98–100).

Comparative studies have shown that athletes competing in strength/power versus endurance events possess muscles with very different percentages of fast and slow fibers (28). The muscles of elite strength/power athletes (weightlifters, sprinters, shot putters, discus throwers, etc.) usually contain a predominance of fast fibers, whereas elite endurance athletes (marathoners, rowers, long-distance swimmers, cyclists, etc.) have a predominance of slow fibers. There is currently much debate over whether individuals can alter the overall percentage of fast and slow fibers in a muscle with training. Most of the data accumulated from training studies on human muscle indicate that genetic factors appear to play a large role in determining the fast and slow fiber composition of a muscle. In support of this, it is not uncommon to find untrained individuals with a predominance of either fast or slow fibers in their muscles.

It is not that the muscle is not capable of fast-to-slow transformations. Indeed, such transitions can be artificially induced by long-term low-frequency stimulation in small mammals (101). This, however, requires extremely long periods of stimulation. For example, it took 60 days of continuous stimulation (24 h/day) of the rabbit tibialis anterior muscle to cause a complete shift from fast to slow (102). Thus it is perhaps easy to understand that training does not appear to represent enough of a stimulus to cause a change from fast to slow.

Although it appears that little or no transition will take place between the fast and slow groups with training, the muscle can still adapt to altered functional demands. Indeed, fiber-type composition is but one factor responsible for athletic performance. Other factors (e.g., cardiovascular fitness, biomechanics, neural adaptations, motivation, technique, equipment, body type, nutrition) also play important roles in determining performance. In addition, lack of a transition between fast and slow does not mean that a muscle cannot increase its endurance or force output. Changes within the muscle such as increasing or decreasing the size of specific fibers can be an extremely beneficial adaptation. For example, a strength athlete with a predominance of slow fibers (e.g, 40% fast) may have caused dramatic hypertrophy of the fast fibers through training, so that they now make up 60% to 70% of the area.

Although the overall percentage of the major fiber types (fast and slow) appears to be fixed shortly after birth, the percentage of the fast fiber types IIA and IIB can be altered with training or detraining (Fig. 11–7). Thus if the type IIB fibers are recruited often enough and for a long enough period during training, the type IIB fibers will be transformed into type IIA. This being the case, regardless of the overall percentage of fast and slow fibers in a muscle, if the muscle is highly trained the fast fiber population will be either all or almost all type IIA. With detraining, the reverse transformation (IIA to IIB) will take place (103,104). Research appears to indicate that the "hybrid" fibers (especially the type IIAB) represent transitional states (Fig. 11–7). For example, fibers transforming from type IIB to IIA at some point are type IIAB. Although most research indicates that a complete transformation from type I to IIA (or vice versa) either does not occur or does not occur to any great extent in exercise-trained human muscle, the C fibers represent the pathway for such a transition.

Endurance training promotes the improvement of oxygen delivery and use. At the muscle, this implies alterations to improve the ability to perform repeated contractions at a submaximal level. As such, changes within the muscle include increases in capillaries, mitochondrial content, aerobic oxidative enzyme activity levels, and so on (41,96). In addition, endurance training tends to decrease the size of the muscle. This makes sense because the concern is not maximizing force output but maximizing the ability to contract repeatedly. Thus a hypotrophic (decreased cross-sectional area) response will decrease the diffusion distances for the oxygen/carbon dioxide exchange and thus improve aerobic capacity. Endurance training also causes changes within the fast-fiber population such that type IIB fibers become type IIA. Such a change is not entirely understood. As a group, however, the type IIA are more oxidative compared with the type IIB. Indeed, the ability to extract and use oxygen maximally correlates inversely with the amount of type IIB fibers present (105). Thus as all

TRAINING

I ⇆ IC ?/? IIC ⇆ IIA ⇆ IIB

SEDENTARY

FIG. 11–7. Schematic representation of possible fiber-type conversions with training and detraining (sedentary). From ref. 28, with permission.

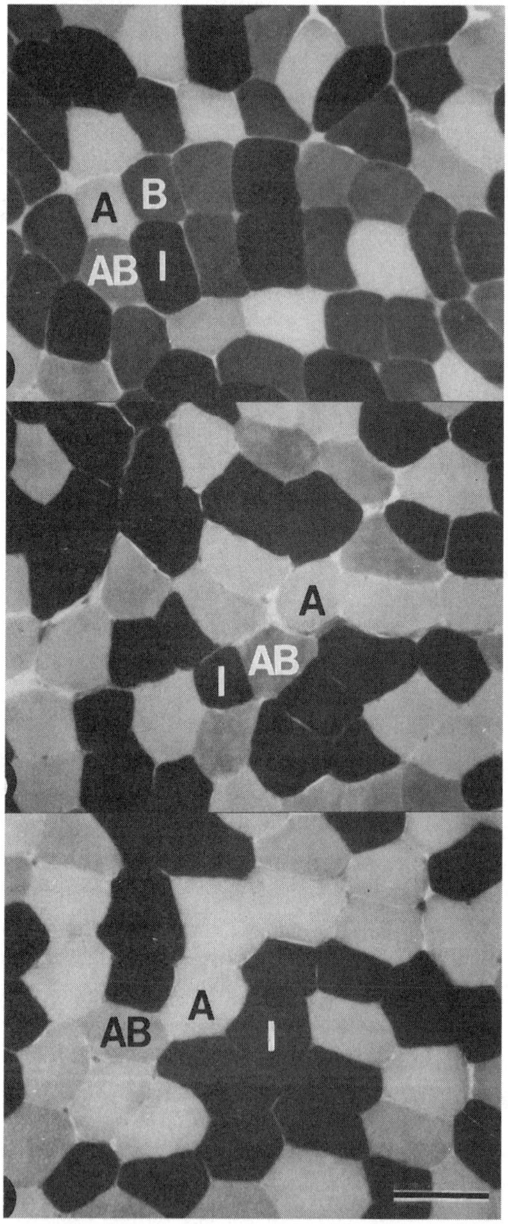

A B C

FIG. 11–8. Cross sections of vastus lateralis muscle samples taken from one subject and assayed simultaneously for myofibrillar adenosine triphosphatase (ATPase) activity (preincubation pH 4.6) before (**A**), and after 6 (**B**) and 13 (**C**) weeks of resistance training. Note the disappearance of fibers classified as type IIB and the increase in the cross-sectional area of the fibers. *I*, type I; *A*, type IIA; *AB*, type IIAB; *B*, type IIB. Bar = 100 μm. From ref. 103, with permission.

fibers are increasing their oxidative capacity in response to endurance training, some are transforming from type IIB to IIA, and some perhaps from type IIA to IIAC (see Fig. 11–7).

With resistance training, the adaptations within the muscle primarily concern maximizing force output. Because the cross-sectional area of a muscle (and muscle fiber) correlates with force output, increases in strength relate, in large part, to increases in size. Although the hypertrophic (increased cross-sectional area) response affects all fiber types, the fast fibers appear to be the most affected. The increase in size appears to be the result of an increase in protein synthesis. It has been shown that a single bout of heavy resistance exercise can increase muscle protein synthesis for up to 24 hours after exercise (106). The increased rates of protein synthesis contribute to an increase in the amount of contractile material, which ultimately leads to a significant increase in cross-sectional area. This addition of thick and thin filaments is obviously a gradual process, taking approximately 6 to 8 weeks to become detectable (107).

Although significant changes in the cross-sectional area appear to take at least 2 months, the exchange of fast MHCs and thus fast fiber types occurs earlier. It was demonstrated that as little as 2 weeks (approximately five workouts) can cause a significant decrease in the percentage of type IIB fibers in a muscle (107) (Fig. 11–8). Continued training appears to cause a complete disappearance of fibers classified as type IIB fibers, with only a few type IIAB fibers, and a concomitant increase in the number of fibers classified as type IIA (Fig. 11–9). Although resistance training stresses the muscle very differently compared with endurance training, both types of training cause a similar fiber-type shift (IIB to IIA). Whereas the body's ability to extract and use oxygen has not changed as a result of resistance training, the transformation of fibers from IIB to IIA may improve local muscular endurance. In support of this concept, Staron (104) found a significantly higher volume percentage of mitochondria in the muscles of weightlifters compared with untrained controls. In addition, various studies have demonstrated an improvement in cycle endurance performance after strength training (108,109). Therefore the transformation of IIB to IIA may be one of the factors responsible for increasing the number of possible repetitions and/or sets.

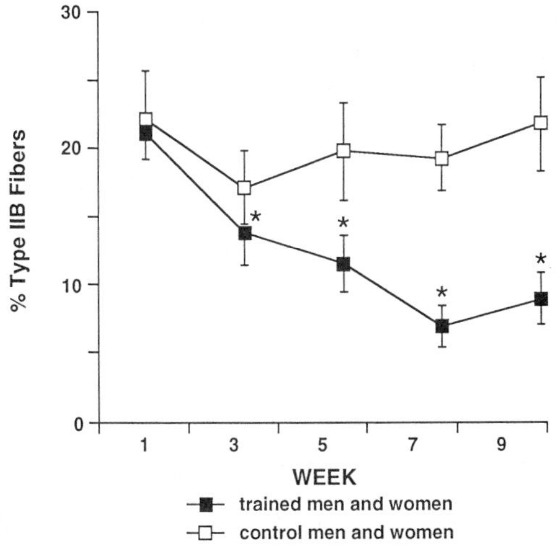

FIG. 11–9. Effect of resistance training on mATPase-based fiber-type distribution in the vastus lateralis muscle over time. Biopsies are taken every 2 weeks from men and women undergoing an 8-week heavy-resistance training program (*solid squares*) and from control subjects (*open squares*). Note the significant decrease over time in the trained subjects. Values expressed as mean ± SD. *Significantly different ($p \leq .05$) from week 1 values. Plotted from the data of ref. 107, with permission.

CONCLUSION

Skeletal muscle is a highly adaptable tissue. Components of the muscle fiber that play important roles in this plasticity are the myonuclei, mitochondria, myofibrils (particularly the myosin molecules), sarcotubular system, and cytoskeleton. One of the distinguishing features of skeletal muscle is its heterogeneity. Indeed, a total of seven fiber types can be identified in human limb and trunk musculature based on the pH stability/lability of mATPase. For most human muscles, mATPase-based fiber types correlate with the MHC content. Thus each histochemically identified fiber type has a specific MHC profile.

Unaccustomed exercise (especially using eccentric contractions) can cause sarcolemmal damage, which releases muscle-specific components into the bloodstream. Creatine kinase is an excellent marker for exercise-induced skeletal muscle damage. A novel bout of exercise or strenuous training also can lead to various morphologic alterations within a muscle including Z-line streaming, cytoskeletal changes, and myofibrillar disruption, which if severe enough can cause necrosis. Favorable adaptations take place with long-term exercise and training. Endurance training causes alterations within and around the muscle, increasing its ability to contract repeatedly, whereas strength training causes increases in force output. Although the major populations of fast and slow fibers are, for the most part, established shortly after birth, alterations take place within the fast-fiber population. Interestingly, both strength and endurance training cause a similar shift within the fast fibers, consisting of type IIB to IIA.

REFERENCES

1. Hall ZW, Ralston E. Nuclear domains in muscle cells. *Cell* 1989;59:771–772.
2. Pavlath GK, Rich K, Webster SG, Blau HM. Localization of

muscle gene products in nuclear domains. *Nature* 1989; 337:570–573.
3. Rosenblatt JD, Yong D, Parry DJ. Satellite cell activity is required for hypertrophy of overloaded adult rat muscle. *Muscle Nerve* 1994;17:608–613.
4. Allen DL, Monke SR, Talmadge RJ, Roy RR, Edgerton VR. Plasticity of myonuclear number in hypertrophied and atrophied mammalian skeletal muscle fibers. *J Appl Physiol* 1995;78:1969–1976.
5. Allen DL, Yasui W, Tanaka T, et al. Myonuclear number and myosin heavy chain expression in rat soleus single muscle fibers after spaceflight. *J Appl Physiol* 1996;81:145–151.
6. Tseng BS, Kasper CE, Edgerton VR. Cytoplasm-to-myonucleus ratios and succinate dehydrogenase activities in adult rat slow and fast muscle fibers. *Cell Tissue Res* 1994;275:39–49.
7. Kasper CE, Xun L. Cytoplasm-to-myonucleus ratios following microgravity. *J Muscle Res Cell Motil* 1996;17:595–602.
8. Kasper CE, Xun L. Cytoplasm-to-myonucleus ratios in plantaris and soleus muscle fibres following hindlimb suspension. *J Muscle Res Cell Motil* 1996;17:603–610.
9. Hikida RS, Van Nostran S, Murray JD, Staron RS, Gordon SE, Kraemer WJ. Myonuclear loss in atrophied soleus muscle fibers. *Anat Rec* 1997;247:350–354.
10. Schmalbruch H, Hellhammer U. The number of nuclei in adult rat muscles with special reference to satellite cells. *Anat Rec* 1977;189:169–176.
11. Burleigh IG. Observations on the number of nuclei within the fibres of some red and white muscles. *J Cell Sci* 1977;23:269–284.
12. Hikida RS, Hagerman FC, Staron RS, Kaiser E, Shell S, Hervey S. Satellite cells and myonuclei in young and elderly muscles: effect of training. *Med Sci Sports Exerc* 1997;29:S290.
13. Bischoff R. The satellite cell and muscle regeneration. In: Engel AE, Franzini-Armstrong C, eds. *Myology I.* 2nd ed. New York: McGraw Hill, 1994:97–118.
14. Schultz E, Lipton BH. Skeletal muscle satellite cells: changes in proliferation potential as a function of age. *Mech Ageing Dev* 1982;20:377–383.
15. Ogata T, Yamasaki Y. Ultra-high resolution scanning electron microscopy of mitochondria and sarcoplasmic reticulum arrangement in human red, white, and intermediate muscle fibers. *Anat Rec* 1997;248:214–223.
16. Gauthier GF. On the relationship of ultrastructural and cytochemical features to color in mammalian skeletal muscle. *Z Zellforsch Mikrosc Anat* 1969;95:462–482.
17. Payne CM, Stern LZ, Curless RG, Hannapel LK. Ultrastructural fiber typing in normal and diseased human muscle. *J Neurol Sci* 1975;25:99–108.
18. Prince FP, Hikida RS, Hagerman FC, Staron RS, Allen WH. A morphometric analysis of human muscle fibers with relation to fiber types and adaptations to exercise. *J Neurol Sci* 1981; 49:165–179.
19. Sjostrom M, Kidman SIW, Henriksson-Larsen K, Angquist K-A. Z- and M-band appearance in different histochemically defined types of human skeletal muscle fibers. *J Histochem Cytochem* 1982;30:1–11.
20. Peachey LD. The sarcoplasmic reticulum and transverse tubules of the frog's sartorius. *J Cell Biol* 1965;25:209–231.
21. Hikida RS. The structure of the sarcotubular system in avian muscle. *Am J Anat* 1972;134:481–496.
22. Schmalbruch H. *Skeletal muscle.* Berlin: Springer-Verlag, 1985.
23. Ogata T, Yamasaki Y. Ultra-high resolution scanning electron microscopic studies on the sarcoplasmic reticulum and mitochondria in various muscles: a review. *Scan Microsc* 1993;7:145–156.
24. Brown RH. Dystrophin-associated proteins and the muscular dystrophies. *Annu Rev Med* 1997;48:457–466.
25. Henry MD, Campbell KP. Dystroglycan: an extracellular matrix receptor linked to the cytoskeleton. *Curr Opin Cell Biol* 1996; 8:625–631.
26. Ohlendieck K. Towards an understanding of the dystrophin-glycoprotein complex: linkage between the extracellular matrix and the membrane cytoskeleton in muscle fibers. *Eur J Cell Biol* 1996;69:1–10.
27. Stromer MH. Immunocytochemistry of the muscle cell cytoskeleton. *Microsc Res Techn* 1995;31:95–105.
28. Staron RS, Johnson P. Myosin polymorphism and differential expression in adult human skeletal muscle. *Comp Biochem Physiol* 1993;106B:463–475.
29. Engel WK. The essentiality of histo- and cytochemical studies of skeletal muscle in the investigation of neuromuscular disease. *Neurology* 1962;12:778–784.
30. Guth L, Samaha FJ. Qualitative differences between actomyosin ATPase of slow and fast mammalian muscle. *Exp Neurol* 1969; 25:138–152.
31. Brooke MH, Kaiser KK. Three "myosin ATPase" systems: the nature of their pH lability and sulfhydryl dependence. *J Histochem Cytochem* 1970;18:670–672.
32. Staron RS, Hikida RS. Histochemical, biochemical, and ultrastructural analyses of single human muscle fibers with special reference to the C fiber population. *J Histochem Cytochem* 1992;40:563–568.
33. Staron RS, Hikida RS, Hagerman FC. Myofibrillar ATPase activity in human muscle fast-twitch subtypes. *Histochemistry* 1983; 78:405–408.
34. Edgerton VR, Smith JL, Simpson DR. Muscle fibre type populations of human leg muscles. *Histochem J* 1975;7:259–266.
35. Prince FP, Hikida RS, Hagerman FC. Muscle fiber types in women athletes and non-athletes. *Pflugers Arch* 1977; 371:161–165.
36. Staron RS, Hagerman FC, Hikida RS. The effects of detraining on an elite power lifter: a case study. *J Neurol Sci* 1981; 51:247–257.
37. Essén B, Jansson E, Henriksson J, Taylor AW, Saltin B. Metabolic characteristics of fibre types in human skeletal muscle. *Acta Physiol Scand* 1975;95:153–165.
38. Hintz CS, Coyle EF, Kaiser KK, Chi MM-Y, Lowry OH. Comparison of muscle fiber typing by quantitative enzyme assays and by myosin ATPase staining. *J Histochem Cytochem* 1984; 32:655–660.
39. Reichmann H, Pette D. A comparative microphotometric study of succinate dehydrogenase activity levels in type I, IIA and IIB fibres of mammalian and human muscles. *Histochemistry* 1982; 74:27–41.
40. Askanas V, Engel WK. Distinct subtypes of type I fibers of human skeletal muscle. *Neurology* 1975;25:879–887.
41. Saltin B, Gollnick PD. Skeletal muscle adaptability: significance for metabolism and performance. In: Peachey LD, Adrian RH, Geiger SR, eds. *Handbook of physiology*. Baltimore: Williams & Wilkins, 1983:555–631.
42. Sjogaard G, Houston ME, Nygaard E, Saltin B. Subgrouping of fast twitch fibres in skeletal muscle of man. *Histochemistry* 1978;58:79–87.
43. Wagner PD, Giniger E. Hydrolysis of ATP and reversible binding of F-actin b myosin heavy chains free of all light chains. *Nature* 1981;292:560–562.
44. Larsson L, Moss RL. Maximum velocity of shortening in relation to myosin isoform composition in single fibres from human skeletal muscles. *J Physiol (Lond)* 1993;472:595–614.
45. Harridge SDR, Bottinelli R, Canepari M, et al. Whole-muscle and single-fibre contractile properties and myosin heavy chain isoforms in humans. *Pflugers Arch* 1996;432:913–920.
46. Staron RS, Pette D. Correlation between myofibrillar ATPase activity and myosin heavy chain composition in single rabbit muscle fibers. *Histochemistry* 1986;86:19–23.
47. Staron RS. Correlation between myofibrillar ATPase activity and myosin heavy chain composition in single human muscle fibers. *Histochemistry* 1991;96:21–24.
48. Appelhans H, Vosberg H-P. Characterization of a human genomic DNA fragment coding for a myosin heavy chain. *Hum Genet* 1983;65:198–203.
49. Saez L, Leinwand LA. Characterization of diverse forms of myosin heavy chain expressed in adult human skeletal muscle. *Nucleic Acids Res* 1986;14:2951–2970.
50. Jandreski MA, Sole MJ, Liew C-C. Two different forms of beta myosin heavy chain are expressed in human striated muscle. *Hum Genet* 1987;77:127–131.
51. Schiaffino S, Saggin L, Viel A, Gorza L. Differentiation of fibre types in rat skeletal muscle visualized with monoclonal antimyosin antibodies. *J Muscle Res Cell Motil* 1985;6:60–61.

52. Schiaffino S, Gorza L, Sartore S, et al. Three myosin heavy chain isoforms in type 2 skeletal muscle fibres. *J Muscle Res Cell Motil* 1989;10:197–205.
53. Bär A, Pette D. Three fast myosin heavy chains in adult rat skeletal muscle. *FEBS Lett* 1988;235:153–155.
54. Smerdu V, Karsch-Mizrachi I, Campione M, Leinwand L, Schiaffino S. Type IIx myosin heavy chain transcripts are expressed in type IIb fibers of human skeletal muscle. *Am J Physiol* 1994;36:C1723–C1728.
55. Ennion S, Pereira JS, Sargeant AJ, Young A, Goldspink G. Characterization of human skeletal muscle fibres according to the myosin heavy chains they express. *J Muscle Res Cell Motil* 1995;16:35–43.
56. Thompson HS, Hyatt J-P, De Souza MJ, Clarkson PM. The effects of oral contraceptives on delayed onset muscle soreness following exercise. *Contraception* 1997;56:59–65.
57. Vincent HK, Vincent KR. The effect of training status on the serum creatine kinase response, soreness, and muscle function following resistance exercise. *Int J Sports Med* 1997;18:431–437.
58. Clarkson PM, Dedrick ME. Exercise-induced muscle damage, repair, and adaptation in old and young subjects. *J Gerontol* 1988;43:M91–M96.
59. Ebbeling CB, Clarkson PM. Muscle adaptation prior to recovery following eccentric exercise. *Eur J Appl Physiol* 1990;60:26–31.
60. Nosaka K, Clarkson PM. Relationship between post-exercise plasma CK elevation and muscle mass involved in the exercise. *Int J Sports Med* 1992;13:471–475.
61. Apple FS, Hellsten Y, Clarkson PM. Early detection of skeletal muscle injury by assay of creatine kinase MM isoforms in serum after acute exercise. *Clin Chem* 1988;34:1102–1104.
62. Hikida RS, Staron RS, Hagerman FC, et al. Serum creatine kinase activity and its changes after a muscle biopsy. *Clin Physiol* 1991;11:51–59.
63. Noakes TD. Effect of exercise on serum enzyme activities in humans. *Sports Med* 1987;4:245–267.
64. Amelink GJ, Bar PR. Exercise-induced muscle protein leakage in the rat: effects of hormonal manipulation. *J Neurol Sci* 1986; 76:61–68.
65. Sorichter S, Mair J, Koller A, et al. Skeletal troponin I as a marker of exercise-induced muscle damage. *J Appl Physiol* 1997;83:1076–1082.
66. Lancha AH, Santos MF, Palanch AC, Curi R. Supplementation of aspartate, asparagine and carnitine in the diet causes marked changes in the ultrastructure of soleus muscle. *J Submicrosc Cytol Pathol* 1997;29:405–408.
67. Jones C, Allen T, Talbot J, Morgan DL, Proske U. Changes in the mechanical properties of human and amphibian muscle after eccentric exercise. *Eur J Appl Physiol* 1997;76:21–31.
68. Friden J, Sjostrom M, Ekblom B. Myofibrillar damage following intense eccentric exercise in man. *Int J Sports Med* 1983; 4:170–176.
69. Hikida RS, Staron RS, Hagerman FC, Sherman WM, Costill DL. Muscle fiber necrosis associated with human marathon runners. *J Neurol Sci* 1983;59:185–203.
70. Hikida RS, Gollnick PD, Dudley GA, Convertino VA, Buchanan P. Structural and metabolic characteristics of human skeletal muscle following 30 days of simulated microgravity. *Aviat Space Environ Med* 1989;60:664–670.
71. Riley DA, Slocum GR, Bain JLW, Sedlak FR, Sowa TE, Mellender JW. Rat hindlimb unloading: soleus histochemistry, ultrastructure, and electromyography. *J Appl Physiol* 1990;69:58–66.
72. Riley DA, Ellis S, Geometti G, et al. Muscle sarcomere lesions and thrombosis after spaceflight and suspension unloading. *J Appl Physiol* 1992;73(suppl):33S–43S.
73. Riley DA, Ellis S, Slocum GR, et al. In-flight and postflight changes in skeletal muscles of SLS-1 and SLS-2 spaceflown rats. *J Appl Physiol* 1996;81:133–144.
74. D'Amelio F, Daunton NG. Effects of spaceflight in the adductor longus muscle of rats flown in the Soviet Biosatellite COSMOS 2044: a study employing neural cell adhesion molecule (N-CAM) immunocytochemistry and conventional morphological techniques (light and electron microscopy). *J Neuropathol Exp Neurol* 1992;51:415–431.
75. Krippendorf BB, Riley DA. Distinguishing unloading- versus reloading-induced changes in rat soleus muscle. *Muscle Nerve* 1993;16:99–108.
76. Bornemann A, Schmalbruch H. Anti-vimentin staining in muscle pathology. *Neuropathol Appl Neurobiol* 1993;19:414–419.
77. Vita G, Migliorato A, Baradello A, et al. Expression of cytoskeleton proteins in central core disease. *J Neurol Sci* 1994;124:71–76.
78. Gallanti A, Prelle A, Moggio M, et al. Vimentin as markers of regeneration in muscle diseases. *Acta Neuropathol* 1992; 85:88–92.
79. Sarnat HB. Vimentin and desmin in maturing skeletal muscle and developmental myopathies. *Neurology* 1992;42:1616–1624.
80. Goebel HH. Desmin-related neuromuscular disorders. *Muscle Nerve* 1995;18:1306–1320.
81. Price MG, Gomer RH. Skelemin, a cytoskeletal M-disc periphery protein, contains motifs of adhesion/recognition and intermediate filament proteins. *J Biol Chem* 1993;268:21800–21810.
82. Thornell LE, Price MG. The cytoskeleton in muscle cells in relation to function. *Biochem Soc Trans* 1991;19:1116–1120.
83. Friden J, Kjörell U, Thornell LE. Delayed muscle soreness and cytoskeletal alterations: an immunocytological study in man. *Int J Sports Med* 1984;5:15–18.
84. Waterman-Storer CM. The cytoskeleton of skeletal muscle: is it affected by exercise? A brief review. *Med Sci Sports Exerc* 1991;23:1240–1249.
85. Lieber RL, Thornell LE, Friden J. Muscle cytoskeletal disruption occurs within the first 15 min of cyclic eccentric contraction. *J Appl Physiol* 1996;80:278–284.
86. Lieber RL, Friden J. Selective damage of fast glycolytic muscle fibres with eccentric contraction of the rabbit tibialis anterior. *Acta Physiol Scand* 1988;133:587–588.
87. Vater R, Cullen MJ, Harris JB. The fate of desmin and titin during the degeneration and regeneration of the soleus muscle of the rat. *Acta Neuropathol* 1992;84:278–288.
88. Vater R, Cullen MJ, Nicholson LVB, Harris JB. The fate of dystrophin during the degeneration and regeneration of the soleus muscle of the rat. *Acta Neuropathol* 1992;83:140–148.
89. Trombitas K, Granzier H. Actin removal from cardiac myocytes shows that near Z-line titin attaches to actin while under tension. *Am J Physiol* 1997;273:C662–C670.
90. Thornell LE, Edstrom L, Eriksson A, Henriksson KG, Angqvist K-A. The distribution of intermediate filament protein (skeletin) in normal and diseased human skeletal muscle. *J Neurol Sci* 1980;47:153–170.
91. Armstrong RB. Initial events in exercise-induced muscular injury. *Med Sci Sports Exerc* 1990;22:429–435.
92. Camus G, Deby-Dupont G, Deby C, Juchmes-Ferir A, Pincemail J, Lamy M. Inflammatory response to strenuous muscular exercise in man. *Mediators Inflamm* 1993;2:335–342.
93. Tidball JG. Inflammatory cell response to acute muscle injury. *Med Sci Sports Exerc* 1995;27:1022–1032.
94. Hagerman FC, Hikida RS, Staron RS, Sherman WM, Costill DL. Muscle damage in marathon runners. *Physician Sports Med* 1984;12:39–48.
95. Howell JN, Chila AJ, Ford G, David D, Gates T. An electromyographic study of elbow motion during postexercise muscle soreness. *J Appl Physiol* 1985;58:1713–1718.
96. Saltin B, Henriksson J, Nygaard E, Andersen P, Jansson E. Fiber types and metabolic potentials of skeletal muscles in sedentary man and endurance runners. *Ann NY Acad Sci* 1977;301:3–29.
97. Gollnick PD, Matoba H. The muscle fiber composition of skeletal muscle as a predictor of athletic success: an overview. *Am J Sports Med* 1984;12:212–217.
98. Pette D, Staron RS. Cellular and molecular diversities of mammalian skeletal muscle fibers. *Rev Physiol Biochem Pharmacol* 1990;116:1–76.
99. Pette D, Staron RS. The molecular diversity of mammalian muscle fibers. *NIPS* 1993;8:153–157.
100. Pette D, Staron RS. Mammalian skeletal muscle fiber type transitions. *Int Rev Cytol* 1997;170:143–223.
101. Pette D, Vrbová G. Adaptation of mammalian skeletal muscle fibers to chronic electrical stimulation. *Rev Physiol Biochem Pharmacol* 1992;120:116–202.
102. Staron RS, Pette D. Myosin polymorphism in single fibers of

chronically stimulated rabbit fast-twitch muscle. *Pflugers Arch* 1987;408:444–450.
103. Staron RS, Leonardi MJ, Karapondo DL, et al. Strength and skeletal muscle adaptations in heavy-resistance-trained women after detraining and retraining. *J Appl Physiol* 1991;70:631–640.
104. Staron RS. Human skeletal muscle fiber types: delineation, development, and distribution. *Can J Appl Physiol* 1997;22:307–327.
105. Staron RS, Hikida RS, Hagerman FC, Dudley GA, Murray TF. Human skeletal muscle fiber type adaptability to various workloads. *J Histochem Cytochem* 1984;32:146–152.
106. Chesley A, MacDougall JD, Tarnopolsky MA, Atkinson SA, Smith K. Changes in human muscle protein synthesis after resistance exercise. *J Appl Physiol* 1992;73:1383–1388.
107. Staron RS, Karapondo DL, Kraemer WJ, et al. Skeletal muscle adaptations during early phase of heavy-resistance training in men and women. *J Appl Physiol* 1994;76:1247–1255.
108. Hickson RC, Rosenkoetter MA, Brown MM. Strength training effects on aerobic power and short-term endurance. *Med Sci Sports Exerc* 1980;12:336–339.
109. Marcinik EJ, Potts J, Schlabach G, Will S, Dawson P, Hurley B. Effects of strength training on lactate threshold and endurance performance. *Med Sci Sports Exerc* 1991;23:739–743.

Exercise and Sport Science,
edited by William E. Garrett, Jr., and Donald T. Kirkendall.
Lippincott Williams & Wilkins, Philadelphia © 2000.

CHAPTER 12

Exercise, the Immune System, and Infectious Disease

David C. Nieman

Athletes are at risk for several types of infectious diseases, including hepatitis, human immunodeficiency virus (HIV) infection, various skin infections, upper respiratory tract infections (URTI), and other miscellaneous infections (1,2). The most common infectious agents are viruses, but a variety of fungi and bacteria also have been reported among athletes and military recruits (3–11).

Participation in competitive sports has been identified periodically with infectious disease outbreaks, and these have been related to person-to-person, common-source, and airborne routes (3). Risk of infection can be potentially high among athletes because of several factors:

- Athletes often perform in an environment in which certain pathogenic microorganisms are particularly widespread;
- Depending on the type of sport, abrasions or other tissue injury may be more likely, allowing the transfer of microbial agents (12);
- Athletes are liable to cross-infection from others with whom they are in close contact (e.g., sharing of contaminated drinking utensils);
- They are exposed to alien environmental pathogens during foreign travel, and lack of specific immunity (13);
- There is a potential for immunosuppression from both psychosocial and physiological stress that can arise during periods of heavy training and competition (14,15).

In this chapter, emphasis will be placed on four types of infections: viral hepatitis B, HIV infection, skin infections, and URTI. The chronic and acute immune response to both heavy and moderate exercise are reviewed, with guidelines provided for prevention and management of URTI in athletes.

VIRAL HEPATITIS B

Viral hepatitis B occurs worldwide, with particularly high rates of infection occurring in Africa and Asia (16). Approximately 5% of the adult U. S. population has serologic evidence of previous infection, with 0.2% to 0.9% being chronic carriers of the hepatitis B virus (HBV). Severity ranges from inapparent cases detectable only by liver-function tests to fulminating, fatal cases of acute hepatic necrosis.

HBV has been found in virtually all body secretions and excretions; however, only blood, saliva, semen, and vaginal fluids have been shown to be infectious. Transmission occurs by percutaneous and permucosal exposure to infective body fluids, as may occur in sexual and perinatal exposure, contamination of skin lesions, or by exposure of mucous membranes to infective blood.

Detecting the asymptomatic carrier has proven to be virtually impossible. Protection of open wounds and avoidance of unsafe sexual contact are essential. HBV vaccination is recommended for various high-risk groups such as people living or working with HBV patients or carriers, or travelers staying more than 6 months in high-level HBV areas.

The United States Olympic Committee (USOC) has emphasized that because HBV is more easily transmitted than HIV, overall risk of HBV infection in athletic settings is substantially higher (17). During 1957 through 1966, for example, more than 600 cases of hepatitis were reported among orienteers in Sweden (9,18). In nearly all cases, HBV appeared to have been transmitted

D. C. Nieman: Department of Health, Leisure, and Exercise Science, Appalachian State University, Boone, North Carolina 28608.

through scratches and wounds inflicted from thorns and bushes during the competitions.

The USOC recommends that prophylactic hepatitis B vaccine be considered for athletes in high-risk sports such as boxing, tae kwon do, and wrestling, and in moderate-risk sports such as basketball, field hockey, ice hockey, judo, soccer, and team handball (17). The USOC also recommends that

- Voluntary testing for HBV and educational information be made available to all athletes in high- and moderate-risk sports;
- Gloves be worn when contact with blood or other body fluids is anticipated, and skin surfaces washed and cleaned with soap and a diluted solution of household bleach (1:10 dilution) immediately if contaminated;
- Athletes in the high-risk sports be required to wear mouthpieces;
- Matches be interrupted when an athlete has a wound in which a large amount of exposed blood is present to allow the blood flow to be stopped and the area and athletes cleaned;
- Open wounds be covered with dressings to prevent contamination; and
- Athletes and officials in the high-risk sports wear protective eyewear to reduce the possibility of bloody body fluids entering the eyes.

There are several reports of food- and water-borne hepatitis A outbreaks among athletes and military recruits (6,11). Hepatitis A is spread through fecal–oral routes, and improved sanitation and aggressive use of postexposure prophylaxis are recommended.

Does exercise before or during hepatitis infection alter the course of the disease? In general, most researchers have reported that strenuous exercise does not appear to have any adverse effect (19–21). In one report of five patients with severe cases of fulminating hepatitis, all had undertaken vigorous exercise during the early stages of the illness (22). The authors of the report suggested that strenuous exertion should be avoided when hepatitis is first suspected.

HIV INFECTION

Acquired immunodeficiency syndrome (AIDS) is a major public health problem, first recognized as a distinct syndrome in 1981 (16). Within several weeks to several months after infection with HIV, many individuals develop an acute self-limited mononucleosis-like illness lasting for a week or two. Most persons infected with HIV develop detectable antibodies within 1 to 3 months, although occasionally there may be a more prolonged interval.

HIV-infected persons may be free of clinical signs or symptoms for many months to years before onset of clinical illness, which starts with a constellation of nonspecific symptoms (AIDS-related complex or ARC) before proceeding to AIDS. Fully developed AIDS infection also includes more than a dozen additional opportunistic infections and several cancers. Although the vast majority of HIV-infected persons is projected to develop AIDS within 15 to 20 years, with modern therapy the incubation period is expected to be considerably longer. Without specific therapy, the case fatality rate of AIDS has been very high, with 80% to 90% of patients dying within 3 to 5 years after diagnosis.

The primary target of this virus is the T-helper/inducer cell because it binds directly to the CD4 surface membrane receptor and kills the cell as replication proceeds. As a result, AIDS patients have a marked reduction in the number of CD4 cells. When CD4 cell counts decrease to less than 50 cells/mm^3, patients develop the most serious of the opportunistic infections associated with AIDS. According to the Centers for Disease Control and Prevention (CDC), when CD4 cell counts decrease to less than 200 cells/mm^3, this is one criterion among others indicating that AIDS should be diagnosed in HIV-infected patients.

Pertinent questions have been raised regarding HIV transmission during sports that require close physical contact. Most patients diagnosed with active AIDS are acutely and chronically ill and are not likely to participate in athletic endeavors. For each patient with clinically apparent AIDS, however, many more are infected with HIV, are free of clinical manifestations, and may be capable of normal participation in sports (23).

Routine social or community contact with an HIV-infected person carries no risk of transmission; only sexual exposure and exposure to blood or tissues carries a risk. Whereas HIV has been found in saliva, tears, urine, and bronchial secretions, there is no evidence that the virus can be transmitted after contact with these secretions (16).

There are several situations, however, in which the transmission of HIV is of concern in athletic settings. In sports in which athletes can be cut, such as boxing or wrestling, or in other contact sports such as football, basketball, and baseball, risk of HIV transmission exists when the mucous membranes of a healthy athlete are exposed to the blood of an infected athlete. At present, the feeling is that testing all athletes before sports participation is impractical, unethical, and unrealistic (23–25). Therefore the team physician and athletic trainer are urged to provide information about the transmission of HIV, recommended behavior to reduce risks, and referral for care or diagnosis.

These concerns and concepts have been summarized by several consensus reports from the World Health Organization and International Federation of Sports Medicine (26), USOC (17), American Academy of Pediatrics (27), and National Football League (28). These organizations have made recommendations concerning HIV infection in the athletic setting, and these are summarized in the next several paragraphs.

- No evidence exists for a risk of transmission of HIV when infected persons, without bleeding wounds or skin lesions, engage in sports. Thus athletes infected with HIV should be allowed to participate in all competitive sports.
- There is no medical or public-health justification for testing or screening for HIV infection before participation in sports activities. HIV testing should remain voluntary.
- There is a very low risk of HIV transmission during combative sports when an infected athlete with a bleeding wound or a skin lesion with exudate comes in contact with another athlete who has a skin lesion or an exposed mucous membrane. Olympic sports with the greatest risk include boxing, tae kwon do, and wrestling; basketball, field and ice hockey, judo, soccer, and team handball pose only moderate risk, however.
- It should be the responsibility of any athlete participating in a combative sport who has a wound or other skin lesion to report it immediately to a responsible official and to seek medical attention. Athletes who know they are infected with HIV should seek medical counseling about further participation in sports, especially in sports such as wrestling or boxing that involve a high theoretic risk of contagion to other athletes.
- Each coach and athletic trainer should receive training in how to clean skin and athletic equipment surfaces exposed to blood or other body fluids. These procedures are the same as outlined previously in this chapter for HBV.

Can exercise training be used as a method to delay the progression from HIV infection to AIDS? Few investigators have published results in this area (29–33). One descriptive study of long-surviving persons with AIDS found that nearly all engaged in physical fitness or exercise programs (34). However, many other factors may explain this association.

Rigsby and colleagues (30) studied the effects of an exercise program (three 1-hour sessions per week of strength training and aerobic exercise) on 37 HIV-infected subjects who spanned the range of HIV disease progression from asymptomatic to a diagnosis of AIDS (CD4 cell counts ranged from 9 to 804 cells/mm^3). Subjects were randomly assigned to either a 12-week exercise-training or a counseling control group. Although exercise training had the expected effect in improving both strength and cardiorespiratory fitness in exercise subjects, no significant change in CD4 cell counts or the CD4/CD8 ratio was found for either condition. These results are similar to those of LaPerriere and co-workers (29).

The increase in strength with weight training, which also was reported by Spence and colleagues (31) in AIDS subjects, is noteworthy in that muscle atrophy and nervous system disorders are common among ARC and AIDS patients. Weight training may provide one means of retarding the wasting syndrome that accompanies AIDS and of improving the quality of life for these individuals.

One tentative conclusion that can be made from these studies is that appropriately supervised exercise training does not appear to affect HIV-infected individuals adversely. Several potential benefits of both aerobic and strength training by HIV-infected individuals, especially when initiated early in the disease state, include improvement in psychological coping, maintenance of health and physical function for a longer period, and attenuation of negative immune system changes. Improved quality of life is perhaps the chief benefit of regular exercise by HIV-infected patients (23–25). It is recommended that exercise prescriptions for all HIV-infected individuals be made on an individual basis, with appropriate initial screening. The exercise prescription should emphasize both cardiorespiratory and musculoskeletal training components.

SKIN INFECTIONS

Athletic clothing and footwear provide a warm, moist environment for several types of bacteria and viruses (35). During athletic participation, frictional trauma can damage the skin, increasing adherence and penetration of these microorganisms (12). Skin infections that can be acquired by person-to-person contact in such sports as wrestling and rugby (especially in the scrum) include streptococcal impetigo, folliculitis, erysipelas, herpes simplex, and tinea barbae. These infections have been appropriately termed "scrumpox." Abrasions and the wearing of facial stubble facilitate the inoculation of the infecting agent during grinding physical contact.

Prevention of the spread of such infections is best achieved by the combined efforts of the athletes and medical personnel. Newly acquired cuts and abrasions should be treated with soap, water, and topical antiseptics. Oral and topical antibiotics are effective against mild infections. Open wounds should be covered, and athlete-to-athlete skin contact should be discontinued until healing has occurred (36).

Herpes simplex is a viral infection characterized by a localized primary lesion, latency, and a tendency to localized recurrence (16). Cutaneous and ocular infection with herpes simplex virus type I (HSV-1) was initially recognized as a health risk for wrestlers and rugby players in the 1960s and was labeled "herpes gladiatorum" (37). Herpes is highly infectious, spreading rapidly from person to person by droplet spread or where skin surfaces are directly opposed, as in contact sports, or indirectly by the sharing of eating utensils, infected towels, clothing, and equipment (38).

Several major outbreaks of herpes gladiatorum have been reported among high-school wrestlers attending intensive-training camps (37). Lesions were found on all parts of the body where skin-to-skin contact was effected. Constitutional symptoms, including fever, chills, sore throat, and headache, were common. Control efforts should emphasize the early identification of skin lesions and prompt exclusion of potentially infected wrestlers. Routine skin examinations by coaches or trainers may be helpful because some athletes are reluctant to report skin lesions that would bar them from competition.

Infections also can be acquired from the environment of changing facilities, with the most frequent being the superficial dermatophyte infections of skin, tinea pedis ("athlete's foot") and tinea cruris ("jock itch") (13). Several species of fungi survive well in the moist environment of dressing and shower rooms, and fungal infections are more prevalent in hot, humid climates and during warm seasons (39). Definitive diagnosis can be made with a potassium hydroxide preparation, a test quickly and easily performed in most physicians' offices. Treatment is usually simple and consists of antifungal medication and alteration of the warm, moist environment of the affected area. For prevention, athletes are encouraged to keep the skin area as cool and dry as possible; to wear loose, absorbent clothing rather than tight garments or those made of synthetic fabrics; and to not share towels, soaps, or sports equipment with other athletes.

UPPER RESPIRATORY TRACT INFECTION

Among elite athletes and their coaches, a common perception is that heavy exertion lowers resistance and is a predisposing factor to URTI (40). Many elite athletes including Sebastian Coe, Uta Pippig, Liz McColgan, Michelle Akers-Stahl, Alberto Salazar, and Steve Spence have reported significant bouts with infections that have interfered with their ability to compete and train (40). During the Winter and Summer Olympic Games, it has been regularly reported by clinicians that "upper respiratory infections abound" (41) and that "the most irksome troubles with the athletes were infections" (42).

On the other hand, there is also a common belief among many individuals that regular exercise confers resistance against infection. For example, a 1989 *Runner's World* subscriber survey revealed that 61% of 700 runners reported fewer colds since beginning to run, whereas only 4% thought that they had experienced more (43). In a survey of 170 nonelite marathon runners (personal best time, average of 3 hours 25 minutes) who had been training for and participating in marathons for an average of 12 years, 90% reported that they definitely or mostly agreed with the statement that they "rarely get sick" (unpublished personal observations). A survey of 750 masters athletes (ranging in age from 40 to 81 years) showed that 76% perceived themselves as less vulnerable to viral illnesses than their sedentary peers (46).

The CDC has estimated that more than 425 million URTIs occur annually in the United States, resulting in $2.5 billion in lost school and work days and in medical costs (44). The National Center for Health Statistics reports that acute respiratory conditions (primarily the common cold and influenza) have an annual incidence rate of 90 per 100 persons (45). Understanding the relationship between exercise and infection has potential implications for public health; for the athlete, it may mean the difference between being able to compete and performing at a subpar level or missing the event altogether because of illness.

It has been proposed that the relationship between exercise and URTI may be modeled in the form of a "J" curve (40) (Fig. 12–1). This model suggests that although the risk of URTI may decrease below that of a sedentary individual when one engages in moderate exercise training, risk may increase to above average during periods of excessive amounts of high-intensity exercise.

At present, there is more evidence, primarily epidemiologic, exploring the relation between heavy exertion and infection, and these data are reviewed first, followed by a brief section on moderate exercise training and infection. Much more research with larger subject pools and improved research designs is necessary before this model can be wholly accepted or rejected.

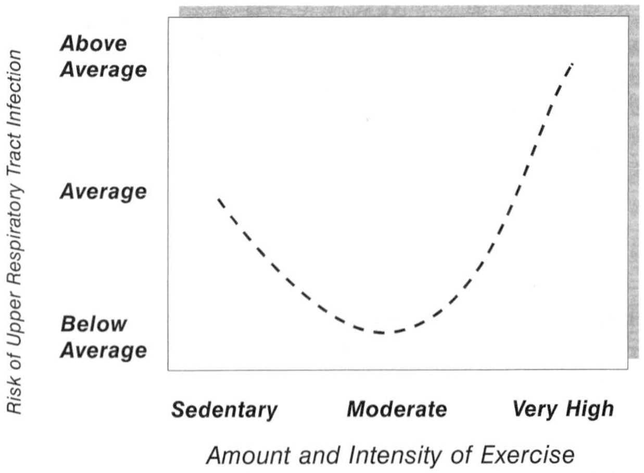

FIG. 12–1. "J"-shaped model of relation between varying amounts of exercise and risk of upper respiratory tract infections (URTI). This model suggests that moderate exercise may reduce risk of URTI, whereas excessive amounts may increase the risk.

TABLE 12–1. *Epidemiologic and clinical research on the relationship between exercise and upper respiratory tract infections (URTI)*

Investigators	Subjects	Method of determining URTI	Major finding
Peters & Bateman (49) (1982)	141 South African marathon runners vs. 124 live-in controls	2-wk recall of URTI incidence and duration after 56-km race	URTI incidence twice as high in runners after 56-km race vs. controls (33.3% vs. 15.3%)
Linde (48) (1987)	44 Danish elite orienteers vs. 44 matched nonathletes	URTI symptoms self-recorded in daily log for 1 yr	Orienteers vs. controls had 2.5 vs. 1.7 URTIs during year
Nieman, Johanssen, & Lee (47) (1989)	294 California runners training for race	2-mo recall of URTI incidence; 1 wk recall after March 5-, 10-, 21-km races	Training 42 vs. 12 km/wk associated with lower URTI; no effect of race participation on URTI
Peters (51) (1990)	108 South African marathon runners vs. 108 live-in controls	2-wk recall of URTI incidence and duration after 56-km race	URTI incidence 28.7% in runners vs. 12.9% in controls after 56-km race
Nieman et al. (47) (1990)	2311 Los Angeles marathon runners	2-mo recall of URTI incidence during training for marathon; 1-wk recall after March race	Runners training ≥97 vs. <32 km/wk at higher URTI risk; odds ratio 5.9 for participants vs. nonparticipants 1 wk after 42.2-km race
Nieman et al. (52) (1990)	36 mildly obese, inactive women, California	Daily logs using self-reported, precoded, URTI symptoms	Walking group reported fewer days with URTI symptoms than controls (5.1 vs. 10.8)
Heath et al. (53) (1991)	530 runners, South Carolina	1-yr daily log using self-reported, precoded, symptoms	Increase in running distance positively related to increased URTI risk
Peters et al. (50) (1993)	84 South African marathon runners vs. 73 nonrunner controls	2-wk recall of URTI incidence and duration after 90-km race	URTI incidence 68% in runners vs. 45% in controls after 56-km race; 33% in runners using vitamin C vs. 53% of controls
Nieman et al. (55) (1993)	42 elderly women (30 inactive, 12 athletes), North Carolina	Daily logs using self-reported, precoded URTI symptoms	Incidence of URTI 8% in athletes; inactives randomized to 12 wk walking vs. controls, 21% in walkers, 50% in sedentary controls

Heavy Exertion and URTI: Epidemiologic Evidence

Several epidemiologic reports suggest that athletes engaging in marathon-type events and/or very heavy training are at increased risk of URTI (Table 12–1). Nieman and co-workers (47) researched the incidence of URTI in a group of 2311 marathon runners who varied widely in running ability and training habits. Runners retrospectively self-reported demographic, training, and URTI episode and symptom data for the 2-month period (January, February) before and the 1-week period immediately after the 1987 Los Angeles Marathon race. During the week after the race, 12.9% of the marathoners reported a URTI compared with only 2.2% of control runners who did not participate (odds ratio, 5.9; Fig. 12–2). Forty percent of the runners reported at least one URTI episode during the 2-month winter period before the marathon race. Controlling for various confounders, it was determined that runners training more than 96 km/week doubled their odds for sickness compared with those training less than 32 km/week.

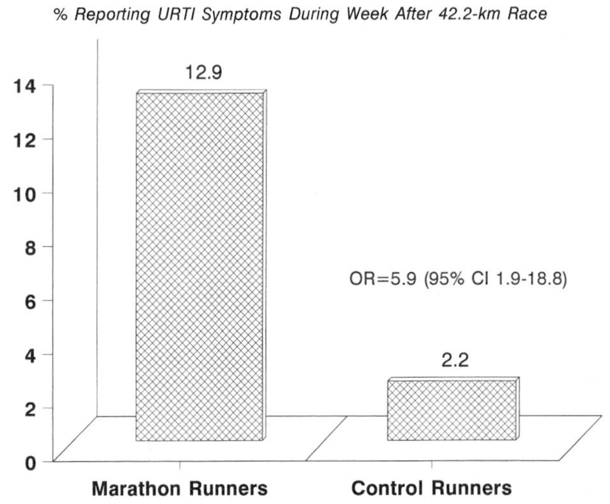

FIG. 12–2. Self-reported upper respiratory tract infections (URTI) in 2300 Los Angeles marathon runners during the week after the 1987 Los Angeles Marathon. From ref. 47, with permission.

Other epidemiologic data support these findings. Linde (48) studied URTI in a group of 44 elite orienteers and 44 nonathletes of the same age, sex, and occupational distribution during a 1-year period. The orienteers experienced significantly more URTI episodes during the year in comparison to the control group (2.5 vs. 1.7 episodes, respectively).

Peters and Bateman (49) studied the incidence of URTI in 150 randomly selected runners who took part in a 56-km Cape Town race in comparison to matched controls who did not run. Symptoms of URTI occurred in 33.3% of runners compared with 15.3% of controls during the 2-week period after the race and were most common in those who achieved the faster race times.

Two subsequent studies from this group of researchers confirmed this finding (50,51). During the 2-week period after the 56-km Milo Korkie Ultramarathon in Pretoria, South Africa, 28.7% of the 108 subjects who completed the race reported non–allergy-derived URTI symptoms as compared with 12.9% of controls (53). In the most recent report from Peters and co-workers (50), 68% of runners reported the development of symptoms of URTI within 2 weeks after the 90-km Comrades Ultramarathon. By using a double-blind placebo research design, it was determined that only 33% of runners taking a 600-mg vitamin C supplement daily for 3 weeks before the race developed URTI symptoms. The authors suggested that because heavy exertion enhances the production of free oxygen radicals, vitamin C, which has antioxidant properties, may be required in increased quantities.

URTI risk after a race event may depend on the distance, with an increased incidence conspicuous only after marathon or ultramarathon events. For example, Nieman and co-workers (52) were unable to establish any increase in prevalence of URTI in 273 runners during the week after 5-km, 10-km, and 21.1-km events as compared with the week before. URTI incidence also was measured during the 2-winter-month period before the three races, and in this group of recreational runners, 25% of those running 25 or more km/week (average of 42 km/week) reported at least one URTI episode, as opposed to 34% training less than 25 km/week (average of 12 km/week; $p = .09$). These findings suggest that, in recreational running, an average weekly distance of 42 km versus 12 km is associated with either no change in or even a slight reduction in URTI incidence. Furthermore, they suggest that racing 5 km to 21.1 km is not related to an increased risk of sickness during the ensuing week.

Together these epidemiologic studies imply that intense and prolonged acute or chronic exercise is associated with an increased risk for URTI (40,53). The risk appears to be especially high during the 1- or 2-week period after marathon-type race events. Among runners varying widely in training habits, the risk for URTI is slightly increased for the longest-distance runners, but only when several confounding factors are controlled.

Moderate Exertion and Upper Respiratory Tract Infections

What about the common belief that moderate physical activity is beneficial in decreasing URTI risk? Very few studies have been carried out in this area, and more research is certainly warranted to investigate this interesting question.

No published epidemiologic reports have retrospectively or prospectively compared incidence of URTI in large groups of moderately active and sedentary individuals. Two randomized experimental trials with small numbers of subjects have provided important preliminary data in support of the viewpoint that moderate physical activity may reduce URTI symptoms (see Table 12–1). In one randomized, controlled study of 36 women (mean age, 35 years), exercise subjects walked briskly for 45 minutes, 5 days a week, and experienced half the days with URTI symptoms during the 15-week period compared with those of the sedentary control group (5.1 ± 1.2 days vs. 10.8 ± 2.3 days; $p = .039$; Fig. 12–3) (54).

In a study of elderly women, the incidence of the common cold during a 12-week period in the fall was measured to be lowest in highly conditioned, lean subjects who exercised moderately each day for about 1.5 hours (8%). Elderly subjects who walked 40 minutes, 5 times a week had an incidence of 21%, as compared with 50% for the sedentary control group ($\psi^2 = 6.36$; $p = .042$) (55). These data suggest that elderly women not engaging in cardiorespiratory exercise are more likely than those who do exercise regularly to experience a URTI during the fall season.

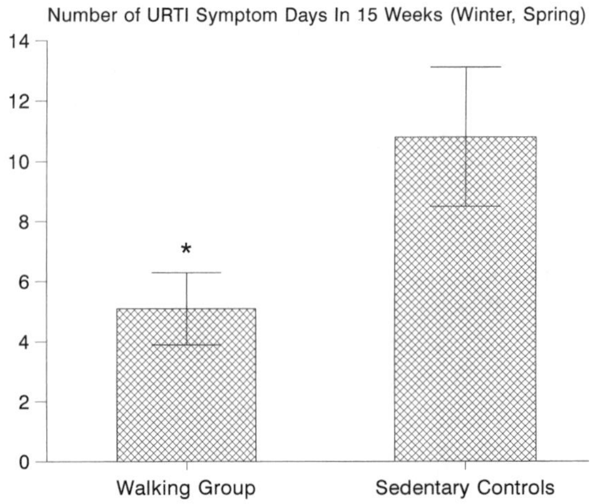

FIG. 12–3. Moderate exercise training effects on the number of symptom days from upper respiratory tract infections (URTI) during a 15-week period in 18 walkers versus 18 sedentary controls. *$p < .05$. From ref. 54, with permission.

EFFECTS OF EXERCISE ON THE IMMUNE SYSTEM

It naturally follows that if heavy and fatiguing exertion lead to an increased risk of URTI, various measures of immune function should be negatively affected. And conversely, if moderate exercise decreases URTI risk, there should be some aspect of immune function that is chronically or at least transiently improved.

Resting Immunity in Endurance Athletes Versus Nonathletes

In this section, data currently available on cross-sectional comparisons of human endurance athletes and nonathletes for natural killer cell activity (NKCA) (56–60), neutrophil function (phagocytosis and oxidative burst) (61–70), and lymphocyte proliferative response (T-cell function) (55,57,58,60,61,71–73) are reviewed.

Natural Killer Cell Activity

Natural killer (NK) cells are large granular lymphocytes that can mediate non–major histocompatibility complex (MHC)–restricted cytolytic reactions against a variety of neoplastic and viral- or bacteria-infected cells (74). NK cells also exhibit key noncytolytic functions and can inhibit microbial colonization and growth of certain viruses, bacteria, fungi, and parasites.

The majority of cross-sectional studies have supported the finding of enhanced NKCA in athletes when compared with nonathletes, in both younger and older groups (56–60). Figure 12–4 summarizes NKCA data comparing 22 experienced marathon runners and 18 sedentary controls (58). NKCA was 57% higher in the marathon runners (373 ± 38 vs. 237 ± 41 total lytic units; $p = .02$). The data of Tvede and colleagues (60) supported a higher NKCA in elite cyclists during the summer months (intensive-training period) when compared with the winter (low-training period).

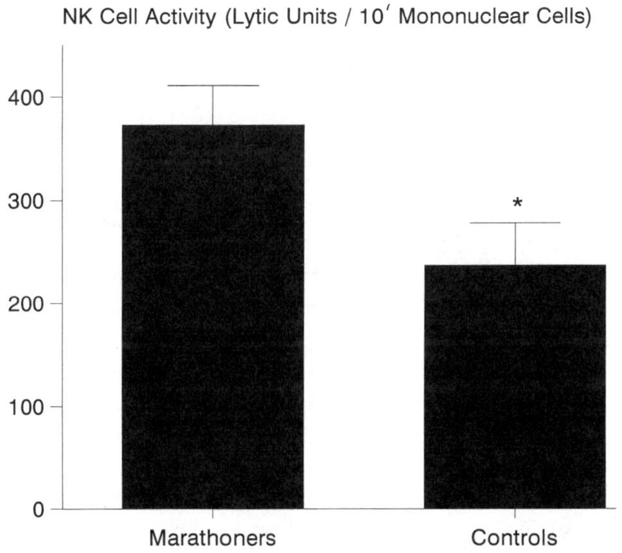

FIG. 12–4. Natural killer cell cytotoxic activity was 57% higher in the marathon runners versus sedentary controls when expressed in lytic units per 107 mononuclear cells. *$p < .05$.

Several prospective studies that used moderate endurance-training regimens over a period of 8 to 15 weeks have reported no significant elevation in NKCA relative to sedentary controls (55,75,76). Together these data imply that endurance exercise may have to be intensive and prolonged (i.e., at athletic levels) before NKCA is chronically elevated.

Neutrophil Function

Neutrophils are important components of the innate immune system, aiding in the phagocytosis of many bacterial and viral pathogens and the release of immunomodulatory cytokines (66).

The neutrophil function cross-sectional data are in contrast to those for NKCA (another component of the innate immune system). No researcher has reported an increase in neutrophil function (both phagocytic and oxidative burst) among endurance athletes when compared with nonathletes (61–70). Instead, during periods of high-intensity training, neutrophil function was reported to be suppressed in athletes. This is especially apparent in the studies by Hack and co-workers (64) and Baj and co-workers (61), in which neutrophil function in athletes was similar to that in controls during periods of low-training work loads, but it was significantly suppressed during the summer months of intensive training. Pyne and colleagues (68) reported that elite swimmers undertaking intensive training have a significantly lower neutrophil oxidative activity at rest than do age- and sex-matched sedentary individuals, and that function is further suppressed during periods of strenuous training before national-level competition.

In that neutrophils are considered the body's best phagocyte, suppression of neutrophil function during periods of heavy training is probably a significant factor explaining the increased URTI risk among athletes. Muns (70) reported that neutrophils in the upper-airway passages of athletes have a decreased phagocytic capacity when compared with those of nonathletes, and that after heavy exertion, a further suppression is experienced for 1 to 3 days. Repeated cycles of heavy exertion may thus put the athletes at increased risk of URTI.

Lymphocyte Proliferative Response

Determination of the proliferative response of human lymphocytes to stimulation with various mitogens *in vitro* is a well-established test to evaluate the functional capacity of T and B lymphocytes. Mitogen stimulation of lymphocytes *in vitro*, by using optimal and suboptimal doses, is believed to mimic events that occur after antigen stimulation of lymphocytes *in vivo*.

Data on the lymphocyte proliferative response to athletic endeavor are less clear than those for NK cells and neutrophils, but generally support no significant difference between athletes and nonathletes (55,57, 58,60,61,71–73). Baj and co-workers (61) reported no difference between elite cyclists and nonathletes during low-training periods (March); there were, however, increased levels in the athletes for phytohemagglutinin (PHA) and anti-CD3 monoclonal antibody (mAb), but not concanavalin A (Con A) or pokeweed mitogen (PWM), during intensive training. Interleukin-2 generation, however, was suppressed in the athletes versus controls during intensive training. These data contrast with those of Tvede and colleagues (60), who found no difference between athletes and nonathletes during both low- and high-training periods.

Among highly conditioned elderly women, PHA-induced lymphocyte proliferative response was reported to be 56% higher than among sedentary controls (55). Data from Japan also support enhanced T-cell function among trained elderly men versus untrained controls (73). These data are interesting because T-cell function tends to diminish with age. Moderate exercise training for 12 weeks failed to alter T-cell function in elderly women, however, indicating that an unusual commitment to vigorous exercise may be necessary before an effect on T-cell function can be measured in the elderly population (55).

Other Measures of Immunity

Other components of immunity have been less well studied among human athletes and nonathletes. Tomasi and co-workers (77) reported that resting salivary immunoglobulin A (IgA) levels were lower in elite cross-country skiers than in age-matched controls, but this was not confirmed in a follow-up study of elite cyclists (78). As reviewed by Mackinnon and Hooper (79), the secretory immune system of the mucosal tissues of the upper respiratory tract is considered the first barrier to colonization by pathogens, with IgA the major effector of host defense. Secretory IgA inhibits attachment and replication of pathogens, preventing their entry into the body. Although several studies have shown that salivary IgA concentration decreases after a single bout of intense endurance exercise, further research is needed to determine the overall long-term effect (79,80).

Complement but not serum immunoglobulins (especially when adjusted for the higher plasma volumes of athletes) was reported to be lower in marathon runners versus sedentary controls (81,82). Most studies have failed to demonstrate any important effects of regular exercise training on concentrations of circulating total leukocytes or lymphocytes or their various subpopulations (55,57,58,62).

Together these data support the concept that the innate immune system responds differentially to the prolonged stress of intensive exercise, with NKCA tending to be enhanced while neutrophil function is suppressed. The adaptive immune system in general seems to be largely unaffected, although the research data at present are mixed. Further research is needed with larger groups of athletes and nonathletes to allow a more definitive comparison.

The Acute Immune Response to Aerobic Exercise

As reviewed earlier, epidemiologic studies have suggested that marathon and ultramarathon race events are associated with a significant increase in risk of URTI during the 1- to 2-week recovery period. In light of the mixed results regarding the effect of chronic, intensive training on resting immune function, several authors have posited that prolonged cardiorespiratory endurance exercise (defined in this chapter as 2 hours or more) leads to transient but significant perturbations in immunity and host defense, providing a physiological rationale for the epidemiologic data (40,79,83).

For example, NKCA (84–91) (Fig. 12–5), mitogen-induced lymphocyte proliferation (88,92–97) (Fig. 12–6), upper-airway neutrophil phagocytosis and blood neutrophil oxidative burst (70,98,99), and salivary IgA concentration (77–80,100) have all been reported to be suppressed for at least several hours during recovery from prolonged, intense endurance exercise. During this "window of decreased host protection," viruses and bacteria may gain a foothold, increasing the risk of subclinical and clinical infection. This may be especially apparent when the athlete goes through repeated cycles of heavy exertion.

Natural Killer Cell Activity

The acute response of NKCA to prolonged endurance exercise by 50 marathon runners is depicted in Fig. 12–5. These data, based on several studies conducted in my laboratory, show that NKCA is decreased 45% to 62% for at least 6 hours after 2.5 to 3 hours of high-intensity running (84,86). Although some have reasoned that the decrease in NKCA can be ascribed to numeric shifts in NK cells (41,87,90,91), others have reported that prostaglandins from activated monocytes and neutrophils (83,89,101) or elevated stress hormone levels (84) suppressed the ability of NK cells to function appropriately. Preincubation of blood mononuclear cells *in vitro* with indomethacin (an inhibitor of prostaglandin) did not

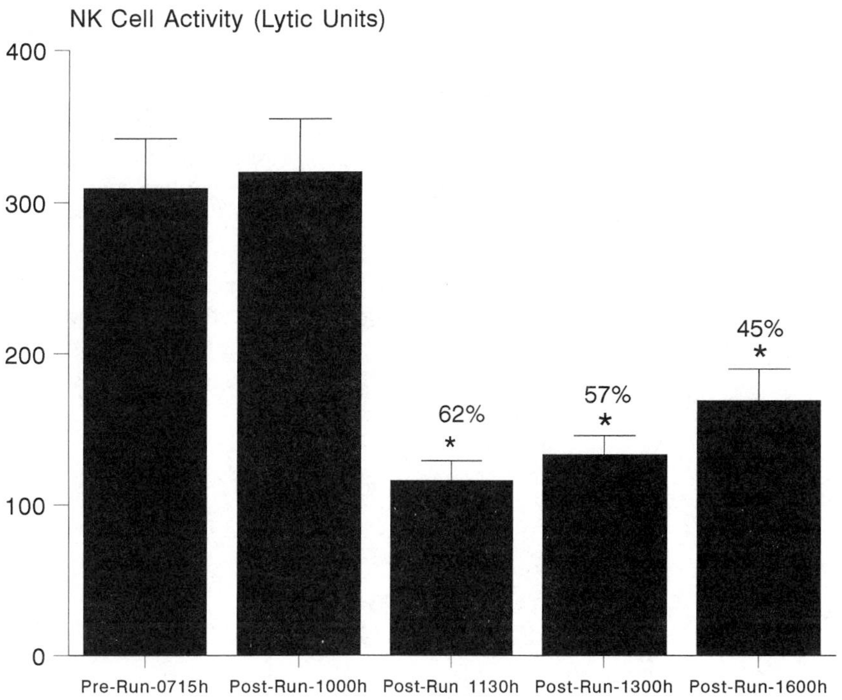

FIG. 12–5. The pattern of change in natural killer cell activity over time in 50 marathon runners who ran 2.5 to 3 hours at 75.9% ± 0.9% $\dot{V}O_2max$. From ref. 86 and unpublished data from the laboratory at Appalachian State University. $^*p < .001$, comparison with before exercise.

attenuate the postexercise reduction in the marathoners depicted in Fig. 12–5 (86). When NKCA was adjusted on a per–NK cell basis, however, the postexercise decline in NKCA was eliminated. NKCA data from this study and others suggest that even though the per–NK cell function is not impaired after exercise, the loss of NK cells from the circulation means that the blood compartment as a whole has a transient decrease in NKCA capacity. Whether this is important for total body host protection is unknown.

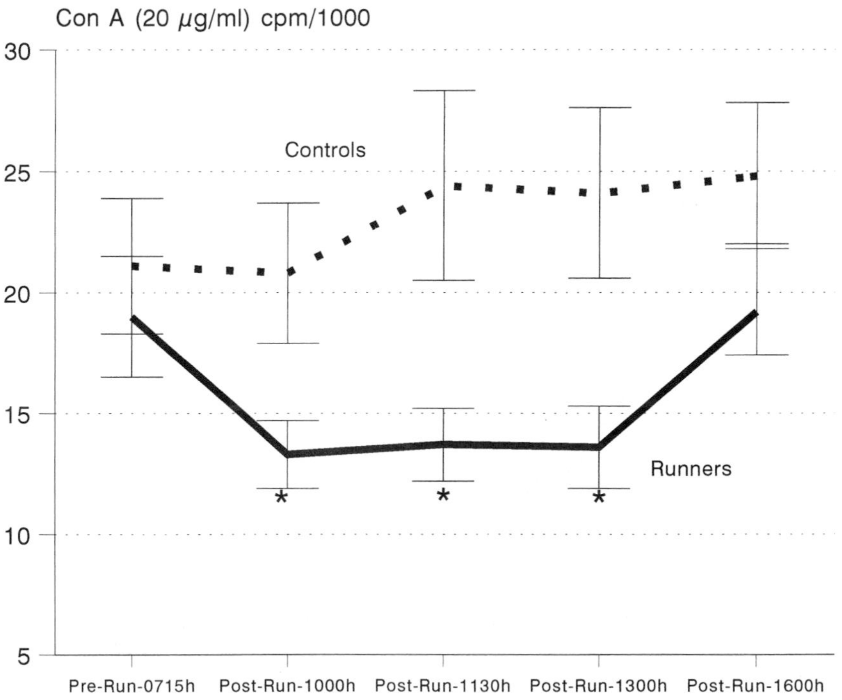

FIG. 12–6. Whole blood, concanavalin A (Con A)–induced lymphocyte proliferative response to 2.5 hours of running at about 75% $\dot{V}O_2max$ in marathon runners compared with values obtained from resting, sedentary control subjects. The pattern of change was significantly different between groups [$F(4, 116) = 2.51$, $p = .045$]. $^*p < .0125$, between groups at a given time. From ref. 95, with permission.

Lymphocyte Proliferative Response

Figure 12–6 shows that the mitogen-induced lymphocyte proliferative response (T-cell function) after 2.5 hours of running at high intensity is suppressed for several hours relative to control levels (95). Eskola and coworkers (92), Gmünder and colleagues (93), and Shinkai and associates (88) also reported significant decreases in T-cell function after prolonged, intense aerobic exercise. There is evidence that elevation of both serum cortisol and plasma epinephrine levels inhibits mitogen-induced lymphocyte proliferation (94–96). Various monocyte functions are inhibited in the presence of cortisol; because monocytes are important as accessory cells in many T- and B-lymphocyte responses, cortisol-induced inhibition of monocyte function indirectly contributes to the decrement in the ability of T cells to proliferate in response to Con A (102).

After 2.5 hours of running at high intensity, serum cortisol concentrations are significantly increased above control levels for several hours (86) (Fig. 12–7). Cortisol has been related to many of the immunosuppressive changes experienced during recovery (102,103). Glucocorticoids administered *in vivo* have been reported to cause neutrophilia, eosinopenia, lymphocytopenia, and a suppression of both NK- and T-cell function, all of which occur during recovery from prolonged, high-intensity cardiorespiratory exercise. A significant correlation exists between the change in serum cortisol and the change in the neutrophil/lymphocyte ratio after 2.5 to 3 hours of running (95). The neutrophil/lymphocyte ratio, which increases strongly after heavy, prolonged exertion, has been proposed as an excellent index of the physiologic stress on the immune system (95).

Taken together, these data suggest that the immune system is suppressed and stressed after prolonged endurance exercise, decreasing host protection against viruses and bacteria. There are few convincing data at this time, however, that exercise-induced changes in immune function explain the increased risk of URTI suggested by epidemiologic data (104,105). In a small study of elite squash and hockey athletes, Mackinnon and colleagues (104) demonstrated that low salivary IgA concentrations precede URTI. However, exercise training–induced changes in T-cell or neutrophil function have not been significantly associated with URTI (68,97).

MANAGEMENT OF THE ATHLETE DURING INFECTION

Endurance athletes are often uncertain of whether they should exercise or rest during an infectious episode. Few data are available in humans to provide definitive answers. Most clinical authorities in this area recommend that if the athlete has symptoms of a common cold with no constitutional involvement, then regular training may be safely resumed a few days after the resolution of symptoms (38,106–108). Mild exercise during sickness with a common cold does not appear to be contraindicated, but there is insufficient evidence at

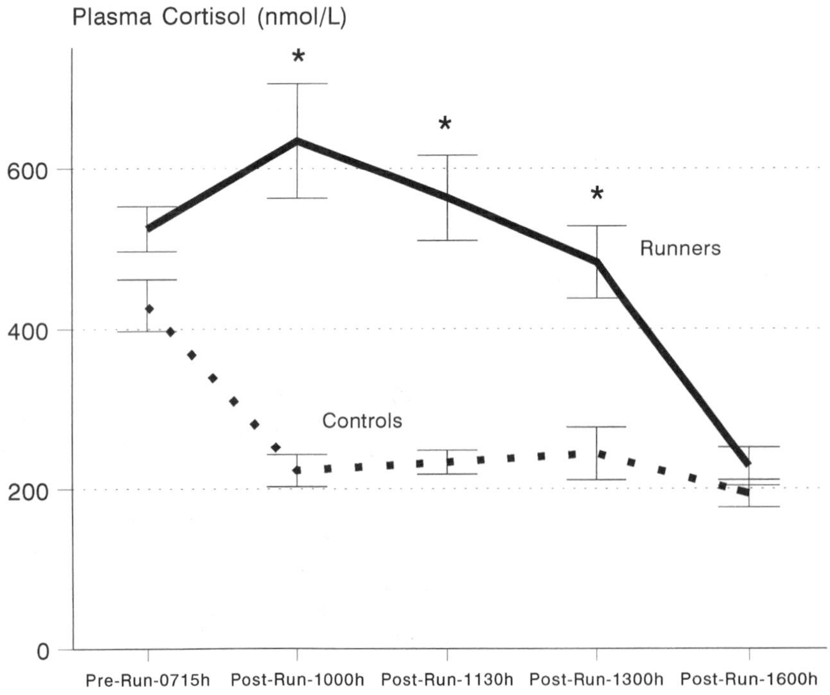

FIG. 12–7. Serum cortisol response to 2.5 hours of running at about 75% $\dot{V}O_2max$ in marathon runners compared with values obtained from resting, sedentary controls. The pattern of change was significantly different between groups [$F(4, 27) = 9.39$, $p < .001$]. $^*p < .0125$, between groups at a given time. From ref. 95, with permission.

present to say one way or the other. If, however, there are symptoms or signs of systemic involvement (fever, extreme tiredness, muscle aches, swollen lymph glands, etc.), then 2 to 4 weeks should probably be allowed before resumption of intensive training.

These recommendations are speculative, however, and are primarily based on animal studies and on some case reports of humans who died after bouts of vigorous exercise during an acute viral illness (40). Depending on the pathogen (with some more affected by exercise than others), animal studies generally support the finding that one or two periods of exhaustive exercise after inoculation of the animal lead to a more frequent appearance of infection and a higher fatality rate (109).

It is well established that various measures of physical-performance capability are reduced during a systemic infectious episode (but not during the common cold) (107,110–115). Although causes are debated, muscle protein catabolism, circulatory deregulation, and mitochondrial abnormalities have been reported (112, 116,117). Several case histories have been published demonstrating that sudden and unexplained deterioration in athletic performance can in some individuals be traced to either recent URTI or subclinical viral infections that run a protracted course (38,107,108). In some athletes, a viral infection may lead to a severely debilitating state known as post–viral fatigue syndrome (PVFS) (116,117). The symptoms can persist for several months and include lethargy, atypical depression, excessive sleep, night sweats, easy fatigability (made worse by exercise), and myalgia.

For elite athletes who may be undergoing heavy-exercise stress in preparation for competition, several precautions may help them reduce their risk of URTI. Considerable evidence indicates that two other environmental factors, improper nutrition (118) and psychological stress (119), can compound the negative influence that heavy exertion has on the immune system. Based on current understanding, the athlete is urged to eat a well-balanced diet, keep other life stresses to a minimum, avoid overtraining and chronic fatigue, obtain adequate sleep, and space vigorous workouts and race events as far apart as possible (40). Immune system function appears to be suppressed during periods of low caloric intake and weight reduction (120), so when necessary the athlete is advised to lose weight slowly during noncompetitive training phases. Cold viruses are spread both by personal contact and by breathing the air near sick people (121–123). Therefore, if at all possible, athletes should avoid being around sick people before and after important events. If the athlete is competing during the winter months, a flu shot is recommended.

Some preliminary data indicate that various immunomodulator drugs or nutrient supplements may afford athletes some protection against infection during competitive cycles (124–132). Much more research is needed before any of these can be recommended.

CONCLUSION

In this chapter, emphasis is placed on four types of infections: viral hepatitis B, HIV infection, skin infections, and URTI. For viral hepatitis B and HIV infection, an emphasis on the "universal precautions" is made. At this time, various professional organizations do not recommend prohibiting HIV-infected athletes from competing in athletic endeavors, nor do they see the necessity of widespread screening.

The chronic and acute immune response to both heavy and moderate exercise is reviewed, with guidelines provided for prevention and management of URTI in athletes. The epidemiologic data suggest that endurance athletes are at increased risk for URTI during periods of heavy training and the 1- to 2-week period after marathon-type race events. At present, there is no clear indication that either acute or chronic alterations in immune function explain the increased risk. For example, although several researchers have reported a diminished neutrophil function in athletes during periods of intense and heavy training, others have shown an enhanced NKCA. After acute bouts of prolonged heavy endurance exercise, several components of the immune system demonstrate suppressed function for several hours. This has led to the concept of the "open window" theory, described as the 3- to 12-hour period after prolonged endurance exercise when host defense is decreased and risk of URTI is increased (128). Further research is needed to provide a better understanding of underlying mechanisms before definitive clinical conclusions can be drawn. Nonetheless, there is sufficient evidence to caution athletes to practice various hygienic measures to reduce their risk of URTI and to avoid heavy exertion during systemic illness.

REFERENCES

1. Nieman DC. Physical activity, fitness and infection. In: Bouchard C, Shephard RJ, Stephens T, eds. *Exercise, fitness, and health.* Champaign, IL: Human Kinetics Publishers, 1994:796–813.
2. Nieman DC. Exercise immunology: practical applications. *Int J Sports Med* 1997;18(suppl 1):S91–S100.
3. Goodman RA, Thacker SB, Solomon SL, Osterholm MT, Hughes JM. Infectious diseases in competitive sports. *JAMA* 1994;271:862–867.
4. Alexander JP, Chapman LE, Pallansch MA, et al. Coxsackievirus B2 infection and aseptic meningitis: a focal outbreak among members of a high school football team. *J Infect Dis* 1993; 167:1201–1205.
5. Ikeda RM, Kondracki SF, Drabkin PD, Birkhead GS, Morse DL. Pleurodynia among football players at a high school: an outbreak associated with coxsackievirus B1. *JAMA* 1993; 270:2205–2206.
6. Rubertone MV, DeFraites RF, Krauss MR, Brandt CA. An outbreak of hepatitis A during a military field training exercise. *Mil Med* 1993;158:37–41.
7. Lee DJ, Meehan RT, Robinson C, Mabry TR, Smith ML. Im-

mune responsiveness and risk of illness in U.S. Air Force Academy cadets during basic cadet training. *Aviat Space Environ Med* 1992;63:517–523.
8. Bailey DM, Davies B, Budgett R, Gandy G. Recovery from infectious mononucleosis after altitude training in an elite middle distance runner. *Br J Sports Med* 1997;31:153–154.
9. Berg R, Ringertz O, Espmark A. Australia antigen in hepatitis among Swedish trackfinders. *Acta Pathol Microbiol Scand* 1971; B79:423–427.
10. Glezen WP, DeWalt JL, Lindsay RL, Dillon HC. Epidemic pyoderma caused by nephritogenic streptococci in college athletes. *Lancet* 1972:1:301–304.
11. Morse LJ, Bryan JA, Hurley JP, Murphy JF, O'Brien TF, Wacker WEC. The Holy Cross College football team hepatitis outbreak. *JAMA* 1972;219:706–708.
12. Conklin RJ. Common cutaneous disorders in athletes. *Sports Med* 1990;9:100–119.
13. Girdwood RWA. Infections associated with sport. *Br J Sports Med* 1988;22:117.
14. Nieman DC, Nehlsen-Cannarella SL. The effects of acute and chronic exercise on immunoglobulins. *Sports Med* 1991; 11:183–201.
15. Nieman DC. Immune response to heavy exertion. *J Appl Physiol* 1997;82:1385–1394.
16. Benenson AS. *Control of communicable diseases in man.* Washington, DC: American Public Health Association, 1990.
17. United States Olympic Committee, Sports Medicine and Science Committee. Transmission of potentially lethal infectious agents during athletic competition. Unpublished internal memorandum, 1991.
18. Ringertz O, Zetterberg B. Serum hepatitis among Swedish track finders: an epidemiologic study. *N Engl J Med* 1967;276:540–546.
19. Nelson RS, Sprinz H, Colbert JW, Cantrell FP, Havens WP, Knowlton M. Effect of physical activity on recovery from hepatitis. *Am J Med* 1954;16:780–789.
20. Repsher LH, Freebern RK. Effects of early and vigorous exercise on recovery from infectious hepatitis. *N Engl J Med* 1969; 281:1393–1396.
21. Edlund A. The effect of defined physical exercise in the early convalescence of viral hepatitis. *Scand J Infect Dis* 1971; 3:189–196.
22. Krikler DN, Zilberg B. Activity and hepatitis. *Lancet* 1966; 2:1046–1047.
23. Calabrese LH, LaPerriere A. Human immunodeficiency virus infection, exercise and athletics. *Sports Med* 1993;15:6–13.
24. Lawless D, Jackson CGR, Greenleaf JE. Exercise and human immunodeficiency virus (HIV-1) infection. *Sports Med* 1995; 19:235–239.
25. Eichner ER, Calabrese LH. Immunology and exercise: physiology, pathophysiology, and implications for HIV infection. *Med Clin North Am* 1994;78:377–388.
26. Goldsmith MF. World Health Organization Consensus Statement. Consultation on AIDS and sports. *JAMA* 1992;267:1312–1314.
27. American Academy of Pediatrics: Committee on Sports Medicine and Fitness. Human immunodeficiency virus [acquired immunodeficiency syndrome (AIDS) virus] in the athletic setting. *Pediatrics* 1991;88:640–641.
28. Brown LS, Phillips RY, Brown CL, Knowlan D, Castle L, Moyer J. HIV/AIDS policies and sports: the National Football League. *Med Sci Sports Exerc* 1994;26:403–407.
29. LaPerriere AR, Fletcher MA, Antoni MH, et al. Aerobic exercise training in an AIDS risk group. *Int J Sports Med* 1991; 12(suppl 1):S53–S57.
30. Rigsby LW, Dishman RK, Jackson AW, Maclean GS, Raven PB. Effects of exercise training on men seropositive for the human immunodeficiency virus-1. *Med Sci Sports Exerc* 1992; 24:6–12.
31. Spence DW, Galantino MLA, Mossberg KA, Zimmerman SO. Progressive resistance exercise: effect on muscle function and anthropometry of a select AIDS population. *Arch Phys Med Rehabil* 1990;71:644–648.
32. Birk TJ, MacArthur RD. Chronic exercise training maintains previously attained cardiopulmonary fitness in patients seropositive for human immunodeficiency virus type 1. *Sports Med Train Rehabil* 1994;5:1–6.
33. MacArthur RD, Levine SD, Birk TJ. Supervised exercise training improves cardiopulmonary fitness in HIV-infected persons. *Med Sci Sports Exerc* 1993;25:684–688.
34. Solomon GF. Psychosocial factors, exercise, and immunity: athletes, elderly persons, and AIDS patients. *Int J Sports Med* 1991;12(suppl 1):S50–S52.
35. Scheinberg RS. Stopping skin assailants: fungi, yeasts, and viruses. *Phys Sports Med* 1994;22:33–39.
36. Beller M, Gessner BD. An outbreak of tinea corporis gladiatorum on a high school wrestling team. *J Am Acad Dermatol* 1994;31:197–201.
37. Belongia EA, Goodman JL, Holland EJ, et al. An outbreak of herpes gladiatorum at a high-school wrestling camp. *N Engl J Med* 1991;325:906–910.
38. Sharp JCM. Viruses and the athlete. *Br J Sports Med* 1989; 23:47–48.
39. Ramsey ML. How I manage jock itch. *Phys Sports Med* 1990; 18:63–72.
40. Nieman DC. Exercise, infection, and immunity. *Int J Sports Med* 1994;15:S131–S141.
41. Hanley DF. Medical care of the US Olympic team. *JAMA* 1976;12:147–148.
42. Jokl E. The immunological status of athletes. *J Sports Med* 1974;14:165–167.
43. Anonymous. Up with people. *Runner's World*, April 1990:77.
44. The Office of Disease Prevention and Health Promotion, U.S. Public Health Service, U.S. Department of Health and Human Services. *Disease prevention/health promotion: the facts.* Palo Alto: Bull Publishing Company, 1988.
45. Adams PF, Benson V. Current estimates from the National Health Interview Survey: National Center for Health Statistics. *Vital Health Stat* 1991;10:1–232.
46. Shephard RJ, Kavanagh T, Mertens DJ, Qureshi S, Clark M. Personal health benefits of Masters athletics competition. *Br J Sports Med* 1995;29:35–40.
47. Nieman DC, Johanssen LM, Lee JW, et al. Infectious episodes in runners before and after the Los Angeles Marathon. *J Sports Med Phys Fitness* 1990;30:316–328.
48. Linde F. Running and upper respiratory tract infections. *Scand J Sport Sci* 1987;9:21–23.
49. Peters EM, Bateman ED. Respiratory tract infections: an epidemiological survey. *S Afr Med J* 1983;64:582–584.
50. Peters EM, Goetzsche JM, Grobbelaar B, et al. Vitamin C supplementation reduces the incidence of postrace symptoms of upper-respiratory-tract infection in ultramarathon runners. *Am J Clin Nutr* 1993;57:170–174.
51. Peters EM. Altitude fails to increase susceptibility of ultramarathon runners to post-race upper respiratory tract infections. *S Afr J Sports Med* 1990;5:4–8.
52. Nieman DC, Johanssen LM, Lee JW. Infectious episodes in runners before and after a roadrace. *J Sports Med Phys Fitness* 1989;29:289–296.
53. Heath GW, Ford ES, Craven TE, et al. Exercise and the incidence of upper respiratory tract infections. *Med Sci Sports Exerc* 1991;23:152–157.
54. Nieman DC, Nehlsen-Cannarella SL, Markoff PA, et al. The effects of moderate exercise training on natural killer cells and acute upper respiratory tract infections. *Int J Sports Med* 1990;11:467–473.
55. Nieman DC, Henson DA, Gusewitch G, et al. Physical activity and immune function in elderly women. *Med Sci Sports Exerc* 1993;25:823–831.
56. Brahmi Z, Thomas JE, Park M, et al. The effect of acute exercise on natural killer-cell activity of trained and sedentary human subjects. *J Clin Immunol* 1985;5:321–328.
57. Nieman DC, Brendle D, Henson DA, et al. Immune function in athletes versus nonathletes. *Int J Sports Med* 1995;16:329–333.
58. Nieman DC, Buckley KS, Henson DA, et al. Immune function in marathon runners versus sedentary controls. *Med Sci Sports Exerc* 1995;27:986–992.
59. Pedersen BK, Tvede N, Christensen LD, et al. Natural killer

cell activity in peripheral blood of highly trained and untrained persons. *Int J Sports Med* 1989;10:129–131.
60. Tvede N, Steensberg J, Baslund B, et al. Cellular immunity in highly-trained elite racing cyclists and controls during periods of training with high and low intensity. *Scand J Sports Med* 1991;1:163–166.
61. Baj Z, Kantorski J, Majewska E, et al. Immunological status of competitive cyclists before and after the training season. *Int J Sports Med* 1994;15:319–324.
62. Green RL, Kaplan SS, Rabin BS, et al. Immune function in marathon runners. *Ann Allergy* 1981;47:73–75.
63. Hack V, Strobel G, Rau J-P, et al. The effect of maximal exercise on the activity of neutrophil granulocytes in highly trained athletes in a moderate training period. *Eur J Appl Physiol* 1992; 65:520–524.
64. Hack V, Strobel G, Weiss M, et al. PMN cell counts and phagocytic activity of highly trained athletes depend on training period. *J Appl Physiol* 1994;77:1731–1735.
65. Lewicki R, Tchórzewski H, Denys A, et al. Effect of physical exercise on some parameters of immunity in conditioned sportsmen. *Int J Sports Med* 1987;8:309–314.
66. Pyne DB. Regulation of neutrophil function during exercise. *Sports Med* 1994;17:245–258.
67. Smith JA, Telford RD, Mason IB, et al. Exercise, training and neutrophil microbicidal activity. *Int J Sports Med* 1990; 11:179–187.
68. Pyne DB, Baker MS, Fricker PA, et al. Effects of an intensive 12-wk training program by elite swimmers on neutrophil oxidative activity. *Med Sci Sports Exerc* 1995;27:536–542.
69. Petrova IV, Kuzmin SN, Kurshakova TS, et al. Phagocytic activity of neutrophils and humoral factors of systemic and local immunity during intensive physical loads. *Zh Mikrobiol Epidemiol Immunobiol* 1983;12:53–57.
70. Muns G. Effect of long-distance running on polymorphonuclear neutrophil phagocytic function of the upper airways. *Int J Sports Med* 1993;15:96–99.
71. Oshida Y, Yamanouchi K, Hayamizu S, et al. Effect of acute physical exercise on lymphocyte subpopulations in trained and untrained subjects. *Int J Sports Med* 1988;9:137–140.
72. Papa S, Vitale M, Mazzotti G, et al. Impaired lymphocyte stimulation induced by long-term training. *Immunol Lett* 1989; 22:29–33.
73. Shinkai S, Kohno H, Kimura K, et al. Physical activity and immune senescence in men. *Med Sci Sports Exerc* 1995;27:1516–1526.
74. Lewis CE, McGee JOD, eds. *The natural killer cell.* New York: Oxford University Press, 1992:175–203.
75. Nieman DC, Cook VD, Henson DA, et al. Moderate exercise training and natural killer cell cytotoxic activity in breast cancer patients. *Int J Sports Med* 1995;16:334–337.
76. Baslund B, Lyngberg K, Andersen V, et al. Effect of 8 wk of bicycle training on the immune system of patients with rheumatoid arthritis. *J Appl Physiol* 1993;75:1691–1695.
77. Tomasi TB, Trudeau FB, Czerwinski D, et al. Immune parameters in athletes before and after strenuous exercise. *J Clin Immunol* 1982;2:173–178.
78. Mackinnon LT, Chick TW, Van As A, et al. The effect of exercise on secretory and natural immunity. *Adv Exp Med Biol* 1987; 216A:869–876.
79. Mackinnon LT, Hooper S. Mucosal (secretory) immune system responses to exercise of varying intensity and during overtraining. *Int J Sports Med* 1994;15:S179–S183.
80. Mackinnon LT, Jenkins DG. Decreased salivary immunoglobulins after intense interval exercise before and after training. *Med Sci Sports Exerc* 1993;25:678–683.
81. Nieman DC, Nehlsen-Cannarella SL. The effects of acute and chronic exercise on immunoglobulins. *Sports Med* 1991; 11:183–201.
82. Nieman DC, Tan SA, Lee JW, et al. Complement and immunoglobulin levels in athletes and sedentary controls. *Int J Sports Med* 1989;10:124–128.
83. Pedersen BK, Ullum H. NK cell response to physical activity: possible mechanisms of action. *Med Sci Sports Exerc* 1994; 26:140–146.
84. Berk LS, Nieman DC, Youngberg WS, et al. The effect of long endurance running on natural killer cells in marathoners. *Med Sci Sports Exerc* 1990;22:207–212.
85. Mackinnon LT, Chick TW, Van As A, et al. Effects of prolonged intense exercise on natural killer cell number and function. *Exerc Physiol* 1988;3:77–89.
86. Nieman DC, Ahle JC, Henson DA, et al. Indomethacin does not alter natural killer cell response to 2.5 hours of running. *J Appl Physiol* 1995;79:748–755.
87. Nieman DC, Nehlsen-Cannarella SL. Effects of endurance exercise on immune response. In: Shephard RJ, Ästrand PO, eds. *Endurance in sport.* Oxford: Blackwell Scientific Publications, 1992:487–504.
88. Shinkai S, Kurokawa Y, Hino S, et al. Triathlon competition induced a transient immunosuppressive change in the peripheral blood of athletes. *J Sports Med Phys Fitness* 1993;33:70–78.
89. Pedersen BK, Tvede N, Klarlund K, et al. Indomethacin in vitro and in vivo abolishes post-exercise suppression of natural killer cell activity in peripheral blood. *Int J Sports Med* 1990;11: 127–131.
90. Shinkai S, Shore S, Shek PN, et al. Acute exercise and immune function: relationship between lymphocyte activity and changes in subset counts. *Int J Sports Med* 1992;13:452–461.
91. Nieman DC, Miller AR, Henson DA, et al. The effects of high-versus moderate-intensity exercise on natural killer cell cytotoxic activity. *Med Sci Sports Exerc* 1993;25:1126–1134.
92. Eskola J, Ruuskanen O, Soppi E, et al. Effect of sport stress on lymphocyte transformation and antibody formation. *Clin Exp Immunol* 1978;32:339–345.
93. Gmünder FK, Lorenzi G, Bechler B, et al. Effect of long-term physical exercise on lymphocyte reactivity: similarity to space-flight reactions. *Aviat Space Environ Med* 1988;59:146–151.
94. Nieman DC, Miller AR, Henson DA, et al. Effects of high-versus moderate-intensity exercise on circulating lymphocyte subpopulations and proliferative response. *Int J Sports Med* 1994;15:199–206.
95. Nieman DC, Simandle S, Henson DA, et al. Lymphocyte proliferation response to 2.5 hours of running. *Int J Sports Med* 1995;16:404–408.
96. Crary B, Borysenko M, Sutherland DC, et al. Decrease in mitogen responsiveness of mononuclear cells from peripheral blood after epinephrine administration in humans. *J Immunol* 1983; 130:694–699.
97. Oshida Y, Yamanouchi K, Hayamizu S, Sato Y. Effect of acute physical exercise on lymphocyte subpopulations in trained and untrained subjects. *Int J Sports Med* 1988;9:137–140.
98. Fukatsu A, Sato N, Shimizu H. 50-mile walking race suppresses neutrophil bactericidal function by inducing increases in cortisol and ketone bodies. *Life Sci* 1996;58:2337–2343.
99. Gabriel H, Kindermann W. The acute immune response to exercise: what does it mean? *Int J Sports Med* 1997;18(suppl 1): S28–S45.
100. Müns AL, Liesen H, Riedel H, Bergmann KC. Einfluss von langstreckenlauf auf den IgA-gehalf in nasensekret und speichel. *Dtsch Z Sportmed* 1989;40:63–65.
101. Tvede N, Kappel M, Halkjaer-Kristensen J, et al. The effect of light, moderate, and severe bicycle exercise on lymphocyte subsets, natural and lymphokine activated killer cells, lymphocyte proliferative response and interleukin 2 production. *Int J Sports Med* 1993;14:275–282.
102. Cupps TR, Fauci AS. Corticosteroid-mediated immunoregulation in man. *Immunol Rev* 1982;65:133–155.
103. Munck A, Guyre PM, Holbrook NJ. Physiological functions of glucocorticoids in stress and their relation to pharmacological actions. *Endocr Rev* 1984;5:25–44.
104. Mackinnon LT, Ginn EM, Seymour GJ. Temporal relationship between decreased salivary IgA and upper respiratory tract infection in elite athletes. *Aust J Sci Med Sport* 1993;25:94–99.
105. Lee DJ, Meehan RT, Robinson C, Mabry TR, Smith ML. Immune responsiveness and risk of illness in U.S. Air Force Academy cadets during basic cadet training. *Aviat Space Environ Med* 1992;63:517–523.
106. Burch GE. Viral diseases of the heart. *Acta Cardiol* 1979;34:5–9.

107. Roberts JA. Loss of form in young athletes due to viral infection. *Br J Med* 1985;290:357–358.
108. Roberts JA. Viral illnesses and sports performance. *Sports Med* 1986;3:296–303.
109. Chao CC, Strgar F, Tsang M, et al. Effects of swimming exercise on the pathogenesis of acute murine *Toxoplasma gondii* Me49 infection. *Clin Immunol Immunopathol* 1992;62:220–226.
110. Daniels WL, Sharp DS, Wright JE, et al. Effects of virus infection on physical performance in man. *Mil Med* 1985;150:8–14.
111. Friman G, Ilbäck NG, Crawford DJ, et al. Metabolic responses to swimming exercise in *Streptococcus pneumoniae* infected rats. *Med Sci Sports Exerc* 1991;23:415–421.
112. Friman G, Wesslen L, Karjalainen J, Rolf C. Infectious and lymphocytic myocarditis: epidemiology and factors relevant to sports medicine. *Scand J Med Sci Sports* 1995;5:269–278.
113. Ilbäck NG, Friman G, Crawford DJ, et al. Effects of training on metabolic responses and performance capacity in *Streptococcus pneumoniae* infected rats. *Med Sci Sports Exerc* 1991;23:422–427.
114. Weidner TG, Anderson BN, Kaminsky LA, Dick EC, Schurr T. Effect of a rhinovirus-caused upper respiratory illness on pulmonary function test and exercise responses. *Med Sci Sports Exerc* 1997;29:604–609.
115. Parker S, Brukner P, Rosier M. Chronic fatigue syndrome and the athlete. *Sports Med Train Rehabil* 1996;6:269–278.
116. Maffulli N, Testa V, Capasso G. Post-viral fatigue syndrome. a longitudinal assessment in varsity athletes. *J Sports Med Phys Fitness* 1993;33:392–399.
117. Behan PO, Behan WM, Gow JW, Cavanagh H, Gillespie S. Enteroviruses and postviral fatigue syndrome. *Ciba Found Symp* 1993;173:146–159.
118. Chandra RK. 1990 McCollum award lecture: Nutrition and immunity: lessons from the past and new insights into the future. *Am J Clin Nutr* 1991;53:1087–1101.
119. Cohen S, Tyrrell DA, Smith AP. Psychological stress and susceptibility to the common cold. *N Engl J Med* 1991;325:606–612.
120. Boyum A, Wiik P, Gustavsson E, et al. The effect of strenuous exercise, calorie deficiency and sleep deprivation on white blood cells, plasma immunoglobulins and cytokines. *Scand J Immunol* 1996;43:228–235.
121. Ansari SA, Springthorpe VS, Sattar SA, et al. Potential role of hands in the spread of respiratory viral infections: studies with human parainfluenza virus 3 and rhinovirus 14. *J Clin Microbiol* 1991;29:2115–2119.
122. Jackson GG, Dowling HG, Anderson TO, et al. Susceptibility and immunity to common upper respiratory viral infections: the common cold. *Ann Intern Med* 1960;53:719–738.
123. Jennings LC, Dick EC. Transmission and control of rhinovirus colds. *Eur J Epidemiol* 1987;3:327–335.
124. Ghighineishvili GR, Nicolaeva VV, Belousov AJ, et al. Correction by physiotherapy of immune disorders in high-grade athletes. *Clin Ter* 1992;140:545–550.
125. Weib M. Infect prophylaxis with polyvalent immunoglobulins in top athletes: a discussion on the occasion of the application in the German Boxing Team before the Olympic Games of 1992. *Dtsch Z Sportmed* 1993;44:466–471.
126. Lindberg K, Berglund B. Effect of treatment with nasal IgA on the incidence of infectious disease in world-class canoeists. *Int J Sports Med* 1995;17:235–238.
127. Garagiola U, Buzzetti M, Cardella E, et al. Immunological patterns during regular intensive training in athletes: quantification and evaluation of a preventive pharmacological approach. *J Int Med Res* 1995;23:85–95.
128. Pedersen BK, Bruunsgaard H. How physical exercise influences the establishment of infections. *Sports Med* 1995;19:393–400.
129. Nehlsen-Cannarella SL, Fagoaga OR, Nieman DC, et al. Carbohydrate and the cytokine response to 2.5 h of running. *J Appl Physiol* 1997;82:1662–1667.
130. Nieman DC, Fagoaga OR, Butterworth DE, et al. Carbohydrate supplementation affects blood granulocyte and monocyte trafficking but not function after 2.5 h of running. *Am J Clin Nutr* 1997;66:153–159.
131. Peters EM. Vitamin C, neutrophil function, and upper respiratory tract infection risk in distance runners: the missing link. *Exerc Immunol Rev* 1997;3:32–52.
132. Mackinnon LT, Hooper SL. Plasma glutamine and upper respiratory tract infection during intensified training in swimmers. *Med Sci Sports Exerc* 1996;28:285–290.

Exercise and Sport Science,
edited by William E. Garrett, Jr., and Donald T. Kirkendall.
Lippincott Williams & Wilkins, Philadelphia © 2000.

CHAPTER 13

Exercise and Gastrointestinal Function

Michiel A. van Nieuwenhoven, Fred Brouns, and Robert-Jan M. Brummer

This chapter is divided into two halves. First we consider the anatomy of the gastrointestinal tract, and in the second half we discuss the effect of physical exercise on the various parts of the gastrointestinal system.

ANATOMY

Introduction

The gastrointestinal (GI) tract can be considered a luminal, muscular tube, beginning at the mouth and ending at the anus. The diameter of this tube is not the same over its entire length; wider and narrower places can be discriminated. This makes it possible to divide the GI tract into compartments such as esophagus, stomach, small bowel, and large bowel (Fig. 13–1). Some of these compartments are separated from each other by sphincter muscles, which can open and close at certain times, which allows regulation of the quantity of the ingested meal from one compartment to another and prevents the ingested meal from moving in the wrong direction. The wall structure of the GI tract is basically the same throughout. From the lumen, the following layers can be distinguished (Fig. 13–2):

- The mucosa, which serves as the barrier between the internal and external environments. It consists of an epithelial layer and a thin muscular layer, the muscularis mucosae. The mucosa contains mucus cells.
- The submucosa, a connective tissue layer that consists mainly of collagen and elastic fibers. A network of nerve fibers, the submucosal plexus, is located here.
- The muscularis, which consists of two muscular layers; the inner part is a circular muscle layer, and the outer part is a longitudinal smooth-muscle layer. A second nerve plexus, the myenteric plexus, is located between these layers. This plexus plays an important role in GI motility. The submucosal and myenteric plexus together form the enteral nerve system (ENS). This ENS consists of a number of networks, which contain

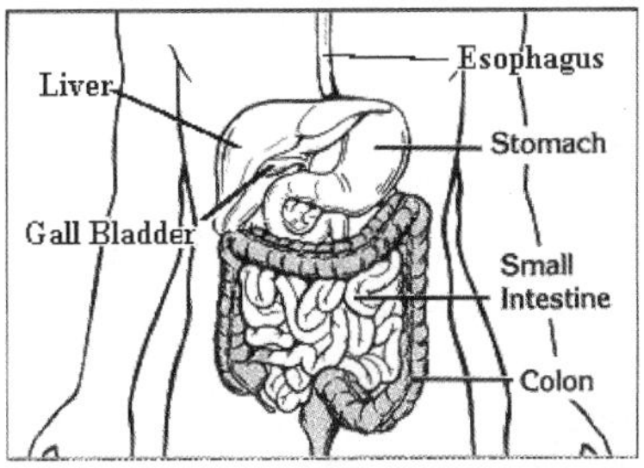

FIG. 13–1. Overview of the digestive tract.

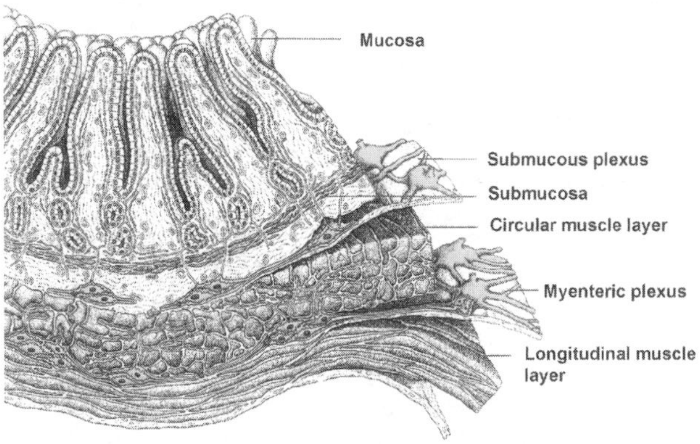

FIG. 13–2. Overview of the wall structure of the gastrointestinal tract. (Courtesy of Janssen Pharmaceutica Ltd.)

M. A. van Nieuwenhoven: Department of Human Biology and Gastroenterology, Maastricht University, Maastricht, The Netherlands.
F. Brouns: Sandoz Nutrition, Maastricht, The Netherlands.
R-J. M. Brummer: Nutrition and Toxicology Research Institute, Maastricht University; Department of Gastroenterology and Hepatology, University Hospital Maastricht, Maastricht, The Netherlands.

ganglia. These ganglia are connected to each other via a network of nerve fibers, the primary plexus. The ENS contains more than 10 million nerve cells.

- The outer layer of the GI tract, which consists mainly of connective tissue and elastic fibers. In the abdominal part of the GI tract, this is the serosa, which contains blood vessels and nerve fibers. In the esophagus, the outer layer is nonserosal.

Esophagus/Lower Esophageal Sphincter

Anatomy and Innervation

The esophagus is a tube with a length of approximately 20 cm. It is composed of skeletal (striated) and smooth muscle. The proximal 5% of the esophagus is striated; the middle 40% is mixed. The proportion of smooth muscle increases distally. The distal 50% to 60% consists entirely of smooth muscle. The proximal end of the esophagus is connected to the pharynx with the upper esophageal sphincter (UES). This consists of the musculus cricopharyngeus, which is connected to the cricoid. Both the circular and the longitudinal muscle layer of the esophagus are attached to the UES. The distal end is connected to the stomach via the lower esophageal sphincter (LES), which angles obliquely upward from the lesser to the greater curvature of the stomach and is contiguous with the circular muscle of the esophagus. The maximal thickness of the LES occurs at the greater curvature of the stomach. Toward the stomach, the LES is split into two segments: one forms short transverse muscle clasps around the esophagus, and the other forms long oblique loops in the stomach. The LES is characterized anatomically and manometrically as a zone of approximately 3 cm of specialized muscle that maintains a tonic activity. It is situated within the esophageal hiatus of the diaphragm, which usually is formed by the fibers of the right diaphragmatic crus. It is assumed that extrinsic compression of the LES by the diaphragmatic crus represents a component of the intraluminal LES pressure.

In the smooth-muscle part of the esophagus, the myenteric plexus contains relay neurons between the vagus and the smooth muscle. The function of these neurons in the striated muscle part is obscure. The submucosal plexus contains only sparse neurons. The extrinsic innervation of the esophagus occurs via the vagal fibers. The striated muscle of the esophagus is innervated by axons of lower motor neurons, with their cell bodies in the nucleus ambiguus. The smooth muscle of the esophagus is innervated by the dorsal motor nucleus of the vagus. The extrinsic innervation of the LES occurs via fibers of the nervus hypoglossus, the vagus, and fibers with their neurons located in the cervical superior ganglion.

Function/Physiology

The function of the esophagus is to transport food from the mouth to the stomach. As soon as food enters the hypopharynx, a swallow reflex occurs. This is a coordinated process of contraction of the hypopharynx and relaxation of the UES. Subsequently a peristaltic contraction occurs in the esophagus, which transmits distally. Before the peristaltic contraction enters the distal esophagus, relaxation of the LES occurs via inhibitory nitric oxide neurons. This allows the food to enter the stomach. This swallow-induced peristalsis is called primary peristalsis. When gastric content enters the esophagus (reflux), it causes distention of the esophagus wall, which induces a peristaltic movement as well; this is secondary peristalsis, which also leads to LES relaxation. Other motility events in the esophagus occur as well; they include nontransmitted, simultaneous, and retrograde contractions. Inappropriate or transient LES relaxations occur spontaneously. These relaxations are not associated with swallowing, and especially occur when the fundus is distended, thus allowing the release of ingested air. Spontaneous reflux episodes in healthy persons are almost entirely caused by inappropriate LES relaxations (1).

Measurement of Esophagus and Lower Esophageal Sphincter

The most important technique for investigating esophageal motility is manometry. This can be both stationary, which is the clinical gold standard, and ambulatory. For stationary manometry, a transnasal catheter is used. The catheter contains several lumens, which are connected with a pressure transducer. The lumens are continuously perfused with water, at a constant flow of 0.2 to 0.3 mL/min. The pressure transducer transforms a pressure event in the esophagus into an electrical signal, which can be recorded outside the body. The LES pressure can be determined by introducing the catheter into the fundus of the stomach and by subsequently pulling the catheter slowly back through the LES, while the pressure is continuously recorded. The most recent method of studying esophageal motility is with a catheter containing solid-state pressure sensors (2). This method does not require perfusion and therefore allows long-term manometric measurements in an ambulatory subject. Manometry of the LES by using the conventional technique often leads to an inadequate measurement, because a small movement of the sensor can result in a shift in proximal or distal direction. Therefore the gold standard for a long-term LES manometry is the Dent sleeve (3). This is a sensor that contains a membrane of a few centimeters length, which is continuously perfused. This sensor is positioned in the LES and allows the registration of the highest pressure in the whole LES section. Solid-state sphinctometers have been developed that allow ambulatory measurement of LES motility, because no perfusion is required (4).

Measurement of Gastroesophageal Reflux

The pH in the esophagus and/or in the stomach can be monitored by using a small-caliber transnasal electrode. pH-Isfet and glass–antimony electrodes are commonly used. Reflux can be assessed by the standard position of the pH electrode 5 cm above the LES (5). The electrode catheter is connected to a portable data logger, which allows long-term ambulatory pH measurement.

Recently advanced thin-caliber catheters were developed, which offer the opportunity of measuring esophageal motility, LES motility, gastric pH, and gastroesophageal reflux simultaneously (Fig. 13–3). These catheters contain solid-state pressure and pH sensors and are connected with a portable data logger, which allows ambulatory measurements as well (6).

Stomach

Anatomy and Innervation

The stomach is an expanded section of the digestive tube between the esophagus and small intestine. Structurally, the stomach is a pouch. It can be divided into the proximal and the distal stomach. The proximal stomach consists of the fundus and the proximal corpus, and it has a tonic activity. The distal part consists of the distal corpus and the antrum, and it has phasic activity. The antrum is separated from the duodenum by the pyloric sphincter.

The right side of the stomach contains the greater curvature. Gastric pacemaker cells are located in this area and are responsible for a basal gastroelectrical activity of 3 cycles/min (cpm). The left side of the stomach contains the lesser curvature. The wall of the stomach is structurally similar to other parts of the digestive tube, with the exception that the stomach has an extra, oblique layer of smooth muscle inside the circular layer, which aids in the performance of complex grinding motions. In the empty state, the stomach is contracted, and its

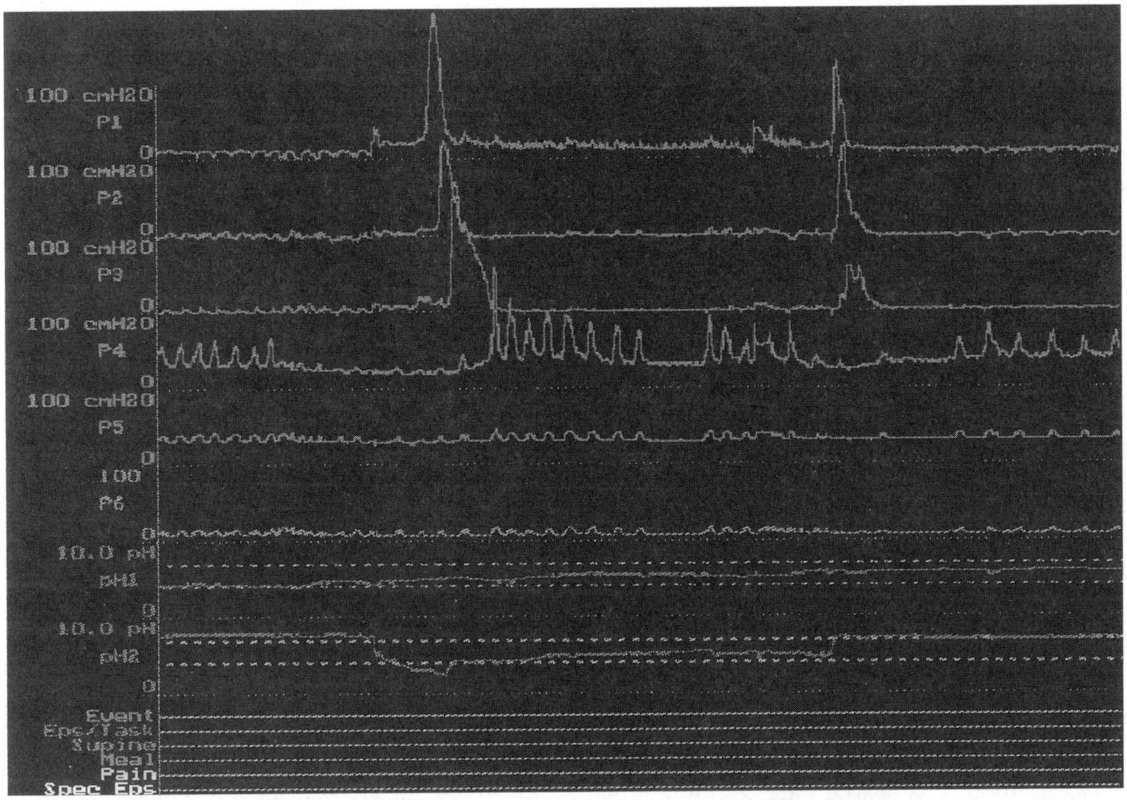

FIG. 13–3. A transient lower esophageal sphincter (LES) relaxation (*P4*) followed by a reflux episode (*pH 2*). Channels *P1* to *P3* represent the esophageal pressure in the distal direction, respectively. The pressure sensors are separated from each other by 5 cm. Channel *P4* represents the LES pressure, and channels *P5* and *P6* represent the fundic pressure. Channels *pH 1* and *pH 2* represent the pH in the stomach and in the esophagus, respectively.

mucosa and submucosa are thrown up into distinct folds called rugae; when the stomach is distended with food, the rugae will flatten and disappear.

Within the stomach there is an abrupt transition from stratified squamous epithelium extending from the esophagus to a columnar epithelium dedicated to secretion. This transition is very close to the esophageal orifice. The inner lining of the stomach is a thick mucous membrane that has many small openings, located at the end of the gastric glands, which are called gastric pits. Within these gastric glands lie multiple secretory cells: mucous cells, chief cells, parietal cells, and G cells. Mucous cells can be found in the necks of the glands near the openings of the gastric pits, but both chief cells and parietal cells are located in deeper parts of the glands. Each of these cells secretes a substance that has a role in the digestive process. The chief cells secrete the proenzyme pepsinogen. The parietal cells release hydrochloric acid. When pepsinogen interacts with the hydrochloric acid produced by parietal cells, it is converted into the active proteolytic enzyme pepsin. Mucous cells secrete large amounts of mucus, which acts as a protective coating against pepsin. When combined, these substances form the gastric juice. The G cells produce the gastric hormone gastrin. Gastrin increases the secretory activity of the gastric glands and has a trophic effect throughout the GI system.

Branches of the vagus nerve regulate the extrinsic parasympathetic innervation of the stomach. These branches contain both efferent fibers, which play a stimulating role in gastric motility, and afferent (sensory) fibers, which inform the brain about the condition of the stomach. Branches from the thoracolumbal part of the spinal cord regulate the sympathetic innervation. Branches originating from this part of the spinal cord arrive in the sympathetic ganglia (ganglion coeliacum). Here the fibers synapse with postganglionic nerve cells, which end in the intramural plexus. Noradrenalin is the most important neurotransmitter. The result of sympathetic stimulation is inhibition of GI motility. The intrinsic innervation of the stomach is regulated by the ENS and plays a role in GI motility. The myenteric plexus of the fundus contains a relatively small number of ganglion cells. The antrum, however, contains relatively many and large ganglion cells and a well-developed primary plexus. The submucosal plexus contains relatively few ganglion cells.

Function/Physiology

The functions of the stomach are (a) storing ingested food, (b) mixing food with gastric juice and initiating the digestion of proteins, and (c) emptying the contents of the stomach into the small intestine.

The function of the proximal stomach is mainly storage of consumed food. This part of the stomach exhibits tonic activity. The pressure in the proximal stomach is regulated by receptive relaxation. This relaxation occurs directly after swallowing, which induces a relaxation of the fundus for about 20 seconds. Hence, the pressure decreases, and the fundus is able to receive the swallowed bolus. Adaptive relaxation of the stomach occurs as well; if food accumulates in the stomach, the pressure would normally increase in equal proportion. Stretch-sensitive receptors in the stomach are stimulated by distention of the stomach, and relaxation of the proximal stomach occurs via a vago–vagal reflex. The result is maintenance of gastric pressure at a constant level. At a certain level, no further relaxation will take place.

Directly after the onset of meal consumption, the basal rhythmic activity of 3 cpm leads to peristaltic contractions of the distal stomach (postprandial pattern). These contractions always run from corpus to antrum and are initiated by stimulation of stretch-sensitive receptors.

The function of these contractions is crushing of food particles and mixing with gastric juice, thus stimulating the process of digestion, especially the protein degradation by pepsin. The result of this peristalsis is transport of chymus toward the pyloric sphincter. This sphincter is usually contracted in such a way that a small opening is present. This allows liquids and very small food particles to enter the duodenum if a pressure difference between the two compartments exists. If a peristaltic wave approaches the pyloric sphincter, it will close, and the majority of the chymus will be squirted back in the oral direction. Only a small quantity of the chymus will leave the stomach before the pyloric sphincter closes.

When all the food particles (except larger indigestible particles) have left the stomach, the movements of the distal stomach and the intestine fade away. This is called phase I from the interdigestive pattern generated by the ENS, and it lasts usually for about 40 minutes. Subsequently peristaltic movements will appear gradually. This is called phase II, and lasts for about 40 minutes as well. Only a small number of depolarizations of the smooth muscle result in a peristaltic movement. This number, however, increases suddenly to a regular frequency of three contractions per minute: phase III. This lasts approximately 10 minutes. Subsequently the contractions will fade away, and the stomach returns to phase I. This rhythmic pattern of gastric movement is repeated every 90 minutes and is called the interdigestive migrating motor complex (MMC). During phase III of the MMC, the gastric contractions have sufficient power, and the pylorus is opened wide enough to allow larger indigestible food particles to enter the duodenum. The MMC migrates from the stomach toward the terminal ileum, in conjunction with an increased production of gastric juice, pancreatic juice, and bile. The MMC is thought to serve a "housekeeping" role, as it sweeps residual undigested material through the digestive tube. This results in cleaning the stomach and the small bowel and preventing bacterial overgrowth in the small bowel (7).

The parameter that describes gastric emptying is the time after which the stomach has emptied half of its contents: the gastric-emptying half-time ($T_{1/2}$). The rate of gastric emptying is strongly influenced by both volume and composition of the consumed meal. Liquids empty quickly from the stomach. The stomach becomes distended, but there are no solids to grind and liquefy; after the liquid reaches the small intestine, not much processing is required before absorption. Therefore the rate of gastric emptying of liquids is fast and is dependent only on the type/composition of the liquid. The gastric-emptying rate (GER) is lower with liquids with a high caloric content (8,9), to prevent caloric overload of the intestine. A temperature that deviates considerably from the normal gastric temperature delays the GER (10). An increase in volume leads to more gastric distention, which accelerates the GER (11). The GER of liquids as a function of time can be described as an exponential relation, which, with a concomitant increase in caloric content of the liquid, shifts toward a linear relation.

The gastric-emptying pattern of solids is different from that of liquids. The stomach needs to process the ingested meal before it can empty into the duodenum. Therefore a lag-phase occurs, because the process of emptying is delayed. The duration of this lag-phase depends on the composition of the meal. The emptying pattern of the solid meal displays a linear relation in time, which is also dependent on the caloric content of the meal.

Therefore the rate of gastric emptying of any meal can be predicted rather accurately by knowing its nutrient density. Nutrient density is sensed predominantly in the small intestine by osmoreceptors and chemoreceptors and is relayed to the stomach as inhibitory neural and hormonal messages that delay emptying by altering the patterns of gastric motility. The hormones involved in this inhibiting process are cholecystokinin (CCK) (12), polypeptide YY (PYY) (13), and glucagon-like peptide-1 (GLP-1) (14). Both PYY and GLP-1 are associated with inhibition of gastric secretion (15,16). Their release is triggered by the presence of nutrients in the ileum and colon. The presence of fat in the small intestine is a very potent inhibitor of gastric emptying (17,18), which induces relaxation of the proximal stomach and diminished contractions of the distal stomach. When the fat has been absorbed, the inhibitory stimulus is removed, and productive gastric motility resumes.

Measurement of Gastroelectric Activity

Measurement of the surface electrogastrography (EGG) is a technique to record myoelectrical activity of the stomach noninvasively, by using electrodes on the abdominal surface. The human EGG signal is a 3-cycles/min (cpm) sinusoid, which is difficult to distinguish from background noise. Because of the poor signal-to-noise ratio, the electrode type, electrode position, leads, filter settings, and proper skin preparation (abrasion) are very important. Application of Fourier transformation to the raw EGG signal in the time domain results in a frequency spectrum. The amplitude of each frequency in the spectrum indicates the extent of contribution to the raw signal. The power of a frequency component is the squared amplitude of that component. This means that a Fourier-transformed EGG signal has two major characteristics: the frequency of the dominant component, and its power (Fig. 13–4). Interpretation of an EGG signal is difficult, and its clinical significance is not yet fully established. One parameter that can be derived from EGG analysis is the postprandial power change. This is the ratio of the power of the mean spectrum of the postprandial state to that of the fasting state. This ratio is referred to as the power ratio (PR). Normally the postprandial-to-fasting PR is 2. The postprandial power increase is probably caused by a change in waveform of the intracellular source signal, induced by postprandial antral contractions, combined with distention of the stomach. Another parameter that can be derived from EGG analysis is the dominant frequency. The normal dominant frequency is 2.4 to 3.6 cpm. After a meal, a short downward frequency shift of approximately 20% can be seen for about 10 minutes. After this shift, a frequency overshoot is usually seen. Tachygastria is defined as a frequency of 3.6 to 10.8 cpm, not of respiratory origin, and lasting at least 2 minutes. Bradygastria is defined as a frequency of 2.6 cpm, in absence of a normal 3 cpm frequency. Nausea, vomiting, and gastric motility disorders are often associated with gastric dysrhythmias (19).

Measurement of Gastric Emptying

Scintigraphy

The gold standard for the measurement of gastric emptying is scintigraphy (20,21). This technique provides an excellent means of measuring gastric emptying of solids and liquids simultaneously. In this method, a radionuclide marker is incorporated into the test meal, and its radioactivity in the stomach is measured by using an externally positioned gamma-scintillation camera. ^{99m}Technetium and ^{113}indium diethylenetriamine pentaacetic acid (DPTA) are the most commonly used radionuclide markers for the solid phase and the liquid phase. Solid and liquid phase can be tracked independently and simultaneously. The test is physiologic, because ordinary meals can be used; it is noninvasive and quantitative. Disadvantages are, however, the costs of

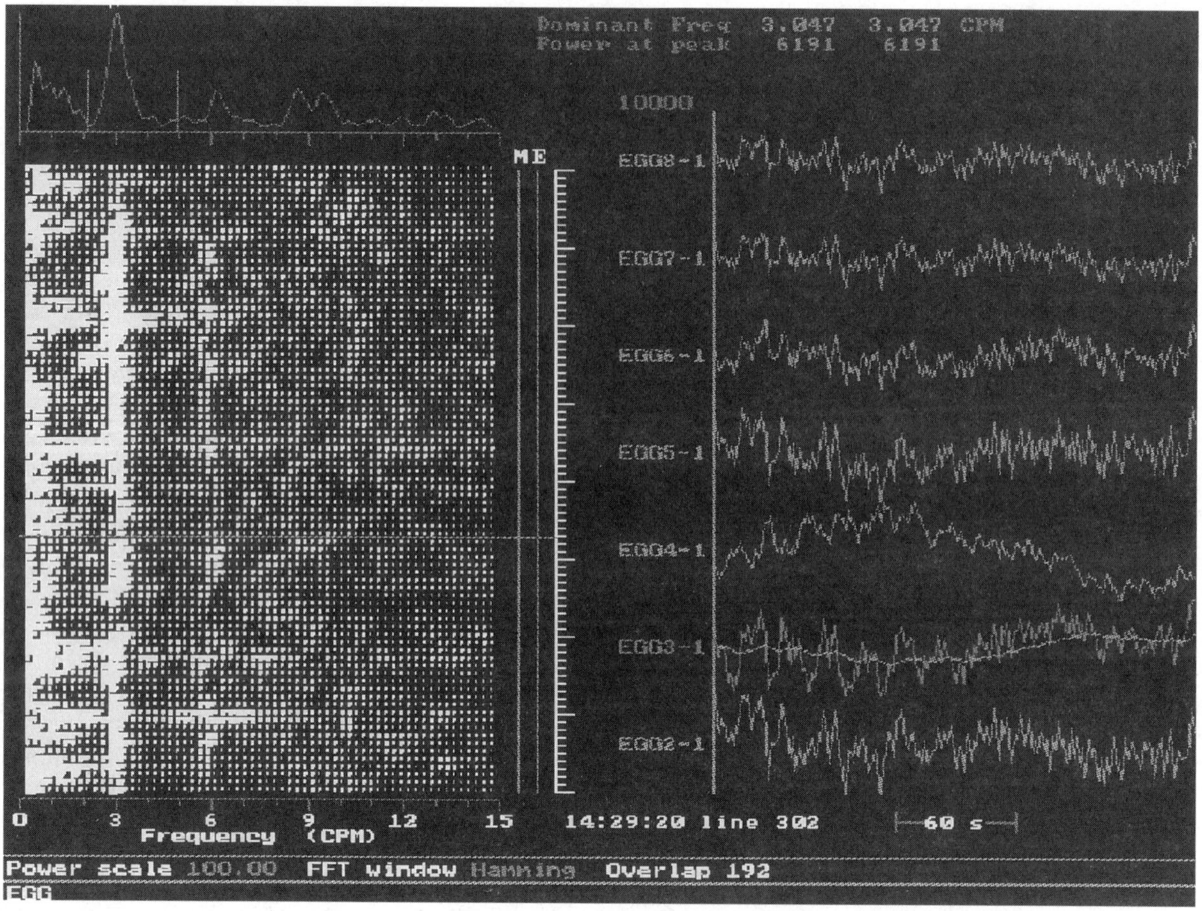

FIG. 13–4. An overview of an electrogastrographic registration. **Right:** A representation of bipolar signals of electrogastric activity in the time domain. **Left:** A gray-scale plot representing the Fourier-transformed frequency domain. A dominant frequency of approximately 3 cpm is visible as a vertical white band.

the tests and the equipment; the test must be standardized within each nuclear medicine laboratory and the small radiation load to the subject. Moreover, test results vary between laboratories because there is a lack of uniformity in size, composition, and caloric content of the administered test meal, as well as a number of technical factors such as the availability of a tissue-attenuation correction.

Double-Sampling Aspiration Technique

The double-sampling technique is a cheap and relatively simple method that allows the measurement of gastric emptying of liquids (22,23). The test can be carried out in an ambulatory setting, which makes it suitable for gastric-emptying measurements during physical exercise. The method depends on the determination of dye concentration (phenol red) in gastric samples obtained before and after the addition of a known amount of dye to the stomach contents. Disadvantages of this method include nasogastric intubation, which is uncomfortable and may influence the process of gastric emptying itself in sensitive subjects, as well as the fact that only emptying of liquids can be studied.

The Stable Isotope Breath Technique

Methods for the measurement of gastric emptying by using stable nonradioactive isotope methods have been proposed (24). The principle of this test is based on the oxidation of a ^{13}C-labeled tracer to $^{13}CO_2$ after emptying of the tracer together with the test meal from the stomach and after absorption in the duodenum. The $^{13}CO_2$ enrichment in the breath then reflects the process of gastric emptying. The method is based on the observation that the ^{13}C-labeled tracer is not absorbed in the stomach. It is furthermore assumed that the substrate is immediately absorbed in the intestine after gastric emptying, and that the delay between intestinal absorption, intracellular oxidation, and appearance of $^{13}CO_2$ is minimal. A half-emptying time can then be calculated, assuming that the time needed for absorption and oxidation of the [^{13}C]acetate is constant. If all these assumptions are valid, then it is axiomatic that the time needed for the appearance of $^{13}CO_2$ in the breath would be directly proportional to the GER of the substrate. [^{13}C]Octanoic acid has been described as a useful label to determine the gastric emptying of solids, whereas [^{13}C]acetate has been described as a label to determine the GER of liquids and semisolids under resting conditions (25). The advantages of the stable isotope breath technique include their simplicity, the safety because stable isotopes are used, and the possibility for widespread clinical applications. It also is possible to perform gastric-emptying studies in children, pregnant women, or immobilized patients. The technique also can be used in the field or during physical exercise because breath samples can be obtained and transported to a mass spectroscopy or infrared spectroscopy facility for analysis. The disadvantage of this technique, however, is that, apart from the need of mass spectroscopy availability, the breath enrichment reflects not only gastric emptying but also the processes of intraduodenal absorption, oxidation, and exhalation via the body bicarbonate pool. It is not certain that a calculated $T_{1/2}$, which assumes a constant rate of absorption, oxidation, and exhalation, is valid under all circumstances (26), for instance, during physical exercise. Therefore determination of the time of peak breath enrichment (^{13}C-TTP) may provide a reliable but relative parameter of gastric emptying, because good correlations have been observed between scintigraphic $T_{1/2}$ and ^{13}C-TTP for solids (24), for liquids and semisolids (25), and for liquids at rest and during physical exercise (Fig. 13–5) (27).

The Paracetamol and Sulfamethizole Absorption Tests

The paracetamol (28) and sulfamethizole absorption tests (29) have been described as useful techniques to measure relative gastric emptying of liquids. The technique is based on measurement of plasma paracetamol or sulfamethizole concentration after ingestion of a liquid meal labeled with these substances. The advantage of the technique is that it is cheap. However, the method is indirect, it requires blood sampling, and it assumes that the increase in plasma concentration depends only on the GER and that the renal clearance and hepatic metabolism of the drugs are constant processes.

Applied Potential Tomography

Gastric emptying can be measured noninvasively by using applied potential tomography (APT), also known as electrical impedance tomography (30). It is a convenient and simple technique that generates tomographic images of changes in resistivity to a small electrical current at 50 to 100 kHz frequency. The principle of APT is similar to that of computed tomography (CT), which requires x-ray, but instead of radiation an electrical method is used. To perform the investigation, electrodes are placed around the upper abdomen, and a small current is passed between two adjacent electrodes; the potential differences are measured at the remaining electrode pairs. When each of the electrodes has acted as a drive electrode, one cycle has been performed. To form a data set, 150 cycles are added together. By introducing food into the stomach, the resistivity of the stomach area is changed. When the stomach empties, there is a further change in resistivity; these changes are measured and analyzed by the APT analysis program. The advantage of this method is its noninvasive character; it is a direct measurement, it is nonradioactive and cheap, and the analysis can be done rapidly. The disadvantages include the need for sophisticated equipment and the limitation that only liquids can be measured. Moreover, the subjects are required to lie on a bed, which makes the method unsuitable for ambulatory measurement.

Small Bowel

Anatomy and Innervation

The adult small bowel is an elongated mobile tube 3.5 to 6.5 m long and predominantly located intraperitoneally. Only the proximal 30 cm, which is denoted the duodenum, is retroperitoneal and hence immobile. The duodenum is anatomically related to the pancreas, liver, and gallbladder. Bile and pancreatic juice drain into the vertical (second) part of the duodenum through an orifice called papilla of Vater (papilla major). The accessory papilla (papilla minor) is located some centimeters proximal of the papilla major and drains the dorsal part of the duct of Santorini of the pancreas, but this orifice is often not patent, and all pancreatic juice drains via the duct of Wirsung (ventral part of the pancreas) into the duodenum. The second and third parts of the small bowel are denoted the jejunum and ileum, respectively, and are suspended from a mesentery that allows optimal mobility in combination with guaranteed blood and nerve supply. No specific anatomic mark separates the jejunum from the ileum, and arbitrarily the jejunum is defined as the proximal two fifths and is predominantly located in the upper and left abdomen. The distal three fifths of the small bowel (except the duodenum) is considered the ileum and is located primarily in the lower and left abdomen. The ileocecal junction is usually fixed to the posterior abdominal wall. Normally, the diameter and wall thickness of the small bowel gradually decrease toward the distal ileum (Fig. 13–6).

Unlike that in the proximal duodenum, the mucosa in the remaining small bowel has a villous structure, which amplifies the digestive and absorptive areas enormously. The intraluminal content, comprising nutrients

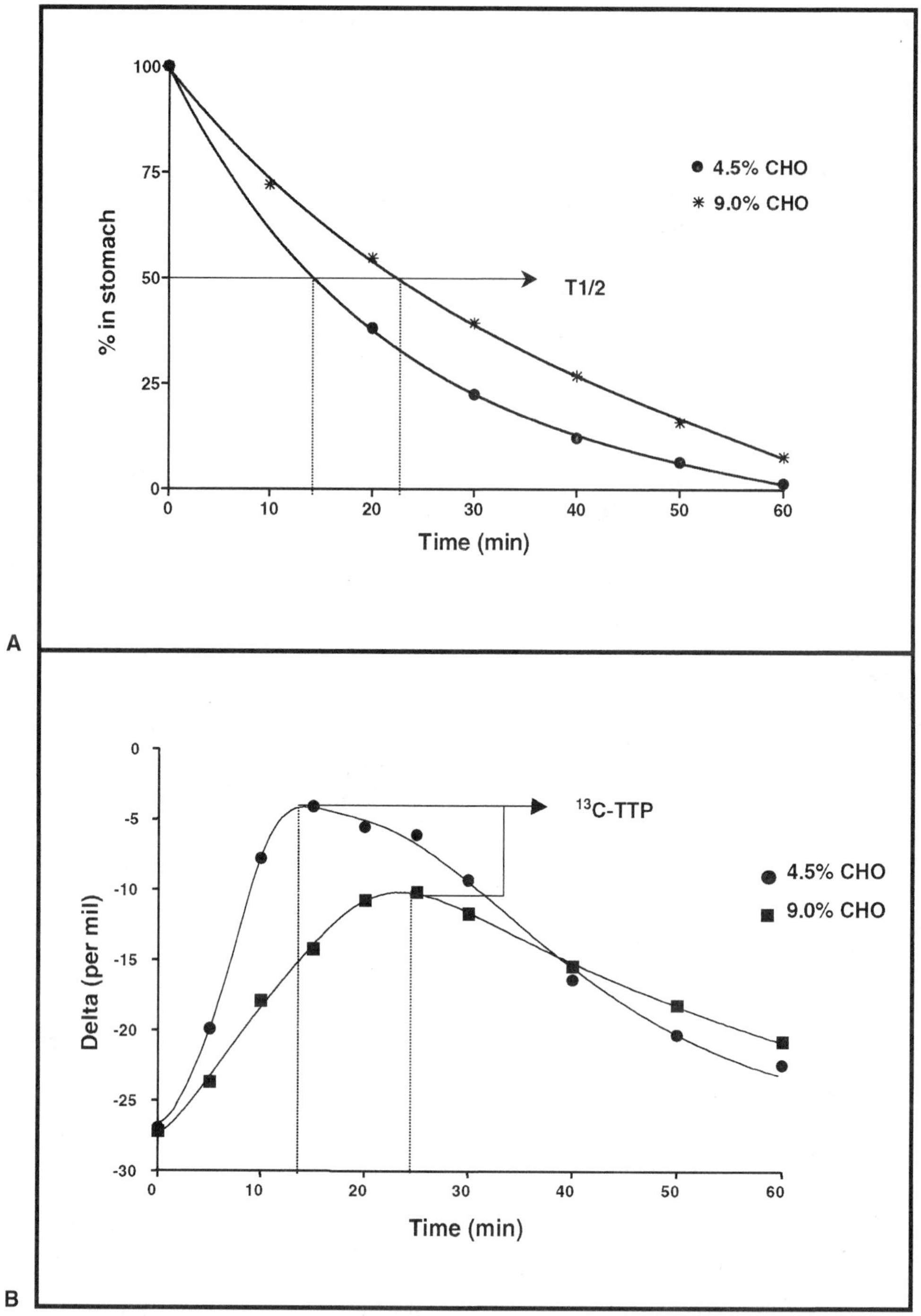

FIG. 13–5. A: The gastric-emptying curves of a 4.5% and a 9% carbohydrate solution, obtained via the double-sampling technique. **B**: The breath-enrichment curves of these two solutions. There is a good correlation between the gastric-emptying half-time ($T_{1/2}$), obtained via the double-sampling technique, and the time of peak breath enrichment (^{13}C-TTP), obtained via the [^{13}C]acetate breath test.

and some bacteria, is important for the integrity of the villi and the mucosa. The epithelial cells are connected to each other by cytoskeleton-associated tight junctions, which serve as intestinal barriers for microorganisms and bacterial endotoxins. They allow, however, for some paracellular permeation of smaller molecules (e.g., sugars). Under pathologic conditions, as in ischemia, this tightness decreases, and hence permeability may increase.

The superior mesenteric artery supplies the entire small bowel except for the first and second parts of the duodenum, which are supplied by the gastroduodenal

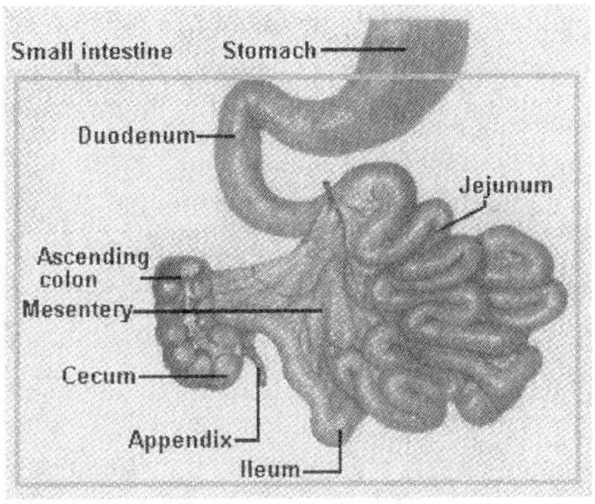

FIG. 13–6. An overview of small-bowel anatomy.

artery, a branch of the celiac trunk. The latter also supplies the stomach, pancreas, and usually the liver as well.

The parasympathetic innervation of the small bowel occurs by a branch of the vagal nerve. The vagal nerve is a mixed nerve with 80% afferent sensoric fibers. Sympathetic fibers reach the intramural plexus via paravertebral sympathetic ganglia. The myenteric plexus of the small bowel resembles that of the antrum with a high number of ganglia and a dense neural network. The submucosal plexus is well developed, and two interconnected networks can be distinguished. The serosal layer of the small bowel also contains some small nerve networks.

Peptide hormones, secreted by endocrine cells in the small bowel, act on the GI tract itself and the pancreas and sometimes even have a substantial systemic effect, as, for example, on the central nervous system. These hormones are responsible for a number of effects such as the modulation of gut motility, mucosal growth and development; Table 13–1 shows a number of GI hormones and their action sites (31). CCK not only is responsible for gallbladder emptying but also retards intestinal transit. Motilin is thought to play a role in the induction of phase III of the interdigestive motor pattern (see "Function and Physiology," below), which explains the effect of motilin agonists such as erythromycin (32). Recently PYY, secreted in the terminal ileum and the colon, attracted increased attention because of its regulatory role in splanchnic blood flow, intestinal secretion, and motility. Especially the so-called ileal-brake phenomenon, responsible for the delay in gastric emptying and the transport of intraluminal contents from the distal ileum via the ileocecal valve toward the colon, is dedicated to the action of PYY (33,34).

Function and Physiology

The small bowel is the main site of fluid and electrolyte absorption as well as of food digestion and nutrient absorption. Although the daily fluid intake normally does not exceed 2 L, the total fluid load to the small intestine is about 7 to 9 L daily because of the salivary, gastric, pancreatic, and biliary secretions. Furthermore, there is fluid secretion by the intestine. Normally, the small intestine is able to absorb up to 80% of the fluid load, which results in a daily ileocecal flow of approximately 1.5 L. Sodium, chloride, and potassium are absorbed, whereas bicarbonate is excreted. The fluid absorbed in the small intestine is isotonic, and the sodium absorption is limited. It is well known that, because of the related process of water and glucose absorption, intraluminal glucose facilitates water absorption.

The initial step of digestion of food partitioned by chewing and antral motility starts in the duodenal and

TABLE 13–1. *Functions regulated (at least partly) by GI hormones*

Function	Action	Hormone
Pancreatic secretion of fluid and bicarbonate	Stimulation	Secretin
Pancreatic secretion of enzymes	Stimulation	Pancreozymin
Pancreatic secretion of fluid, bicarbonate, and enzymes	Inhibition	Pancreotone
Pancreatic secretion of hormones	Inhibition or stimulation	Enteroinsular axis; for insulin, incretin
Gallbladder emptying	Stimulation	Cholecystokinin
Choleresis	Stimulation	Secretin
Gastric secretion	Stimulation	Gastrin, entero-oxyntin
	Inhibition	Enterogastrone, antral chalone, bulbogastrone
Villous motility	Stimulation	Villikinin
Lower esophageal sphincter motility		
Gastric motility	Inhibition	Enterogastrone
Trophic effects on GI tract		
Intestinal motility	Stimulation	Motilin
Intestinal secretion and absorption	Stimulation	Enterocrinin, duocrinin

The left-hand column lists the regulatory functions; the center column indicates whether regulation is stimulatory or inhibitory or both; and the right-hand column lists designations of the (often hypothetical) responsible humoral agent.

jejunal lumen under the influence of pancreatic enzymes and bile. The final step of digestion takes place in the intestinal brush border, after which the process of transport (absorption) takes place. Triglycerides are split into fatty acids and monoglycerides by pancreatic lipase, which, under the influence of bile salts, build together with phospholipids and cholesterol an intraluminal soluble complex, denoted the micelle. The fat-soluble vitamins (A, D, E, and K) are also included in the micelle. Before lipid absorption in the mucosal epithelial cell can take place, three diffusion barriers should be passed: the unstirred water layer (UWL), the mucous coat layer covering the brush border, and the lipid bilayer membrane. By disaggregation of the micelle at the intestinal surface, bile salts remain to facilitate the formation of new micelles in the small bowel and will eventually be absorbed in the distal ileum; after that transport via the portal system to the liver takes place, before the next turn of secretion in the bile (enterohepatic cycle). Normally, only approximately 5% of the luminal bile salts escape from absorption in the distal ileum.

The main carbohydrate sources in the human diet are starch, sucrose, and lactose. In the duodenum, starch is rapidly digested by intraluminal pancreatic amylase (the contribution of salivary amylase is rather small) to maltotriose, maltose, and α-limit dextrins. These products, together with the dietary disaccharides sucrose and lactose, must be hydrolyzed to the final monosaccharide constituent in the brush border by dedicated enzymes. The final transport/absorption by the intestinal cell takes place via at least two different processes. Glucose and galactose are actively cotransported with sodium via the Na^+/K^+/adenosine triphosphatase (ATPase), but permitting transport against a gradient. Fructose is passively transported by facilitated diffusion.

Protein digestion starts with pepsin in the stomach, but the contribution of the stomach is small and not essential. The pancreas secretes precursor proteases, which are activated by the duodenal mucosal surface enzyme enterokinase and by activated trypsin. This results in the formation of the endopeptidases (trypsin, chymotrypsin, and elastase), which produce peptides that sequentially can be digested by the exopeptidases (carboxypeptidases). The final products are dipeptides and oligopeptides (up to six amino acids). At the level of the brush border, oligopeptidases continue the process of peptide hydrolization. It is evident that, apart from transport of free amino acids in the intestinal cell, an intact transport exists for certain dipeptides and tripeptides.

The smooth muscle cells of the small bowel have a basal rhythmic electrical activity with a frequency of 12 depolarizations per minute proximally, decreasing to 8 per minute in the ileum. If depolarization is followed by an action potential, a contraction (motor activity) occurs. As in the stomach, the peristalsis of the small bowel should be divided into a fasting and a postprandial motility pattern. During fasting, three phases can be distinguished. Phase I of the interdigestive motility patterns is characterized by motor quiescence. This is followed by a gradual increase of motor activity during phase II. This accumulates to a sudden formation of regular high-amplitude contractions with a frequency of approximately 12 per minute in the duodenum, with a duration of about 10 minutes. This phase III, or MMC, moves slowly along the small bowel with a velocity of 5 to 10 cm/min, during which the amplitude of the contractions gradually decreases and the duration of the MMC increases (Fig. 13–7). In optimal antroduodenal coordination, the MMC starts in the stomach. Not all MMCs reach the terminal ileum. During phase II and especially phase III, the delivery of bile and pancreatic juice to the duodenum is increased. The most important function of the MMC is to keep the small bowel clean from bacterial and undigested particles, and hence it deserves its nickname "the intestinal housekeeper" (7).

During the postprandial phase, rather irregular phasic motor activity occurs with propulsion along a short distance. The frequency and amplitude of the contractions is dependent on the composition of the food delivered from the stomach. The meal consistency has, in contrast with the stomach, a rather limited effect on postprandial motor activity. Normally after approximately 2 hours, the interdigestive motor pattern has reoccurred.

To facilitate optimal gastric emptying, to prevent the stomach from an excessive exposition of bile acids, and to protect the duodenum from too much gastric acid, it is of utmost importance that the antrum, pylorus, and duodenum act in harmony. This phenomenon is called "antroduodenal coordination."

Measurement of Small Bowel Function

Measurement of the electrical activity of the small bowel can be performed only by using intramucosal electrodes, which is rather unfeasible in humans. Small bowel motor activity is normally investigated by using a manometry system connected to an intraluminal tube, positioned under radiographic guidance with or without the help of a guide wire and an endoscopic device. This allows recordings reaching far beyond the Treitz ligament in the jejunum. Originally, water-perfused multilumen tubes with side holes at regular distances were connected to stationary pressure transducers, and the analog signals were recorded on a multichannel paper polygraph. A/D converters now allow recording of the signals on a personal computer system with the advantage of easier data storage and evaluation and the possibility of automatic data analysis. Manometric catheters with solid-state transducers facilitate the ambulatory measurement of the motility pattern by using a portable

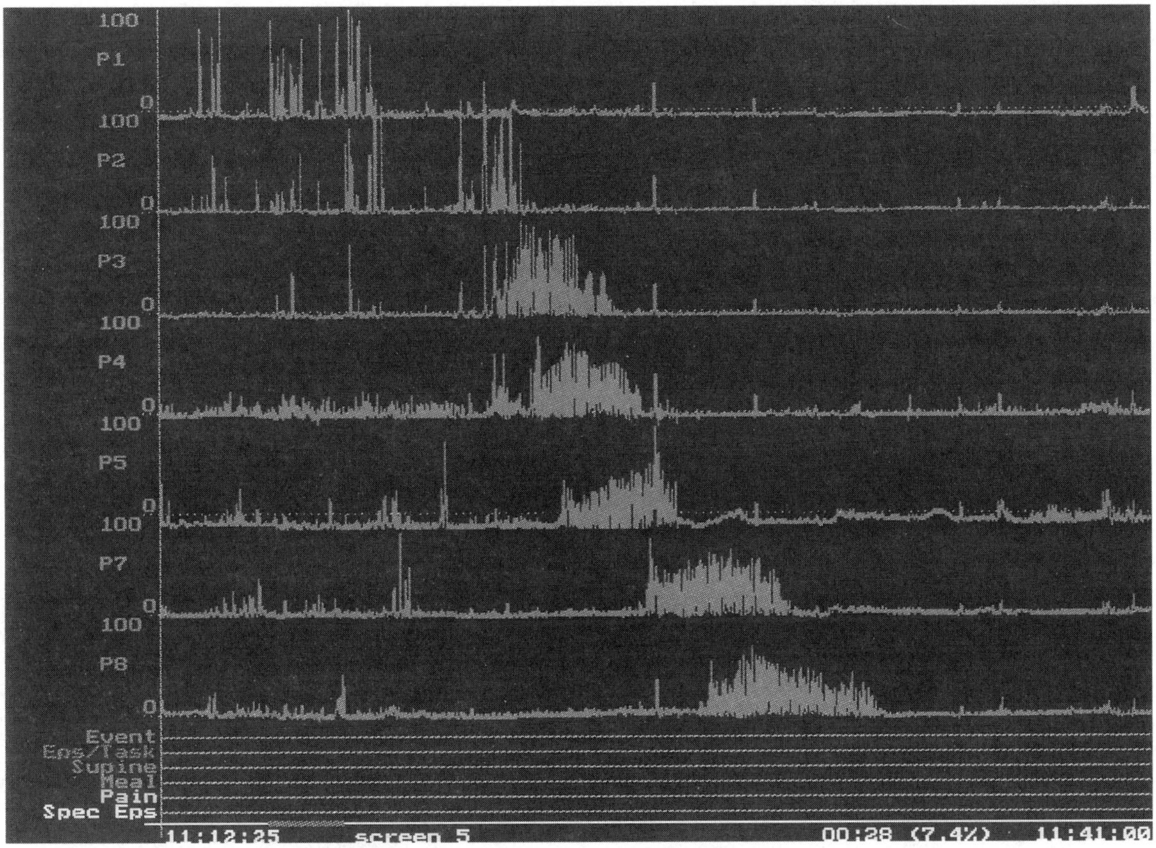

FIG. 13–7. A migrating motor complex (MMC) in the small bowel. Channels *P1-8* represents pressure events on different locations in the small bowel, in a distal direction.

data logger. These systems are, however, much more expensive and less reliable than the water-perfused systems. In antroduodenal manometry, the side holes/transducers at the level of the antrum, near the pylorus, are spaced 1 to 2 cm apart, whereas the intestinal side holes/transducers are spaced 10 to 20 cm apart. During the recording, some catheter dislocation is caused by the patient and intestinal movements, as well as change of stomach configuration after food ingestion. The measurement of transpyloric potential difference allows the identification of the pylorus, which facilitates data analysis, especially in ambulatory recordings. Ambulatory recordings during exercise are possible, although strong body movements may cause recording artifacts induced by catheter dislocation, as occurs during running.

Based on the principle that fermentation of indigestible carbohydrates will be delayed until they arrive in the colon (because of the near absence of bacterial flora in the small bowel) and that this fermentation leads to production of hydrogen, which will rapidly be absorbed from the intestinal lumen and will subsequently be expired, the orocecal transit time (OCTT) can be assessed by the oral administration of a small amount of lactulose and the repeated measurement of end-expiratory H_2 concentration (35). However, lactulose itself may induce an accelerated small bowel transit because of its osmotic effect. By using a sophisticated breath analyzer and with a number of precautions (36), a lactulose dose as low as 5 g is sufficient to perform a reliable OCTT. It is obvious that the lactulose H_2-breath test is unable to distinguish between gastric emptying and small bowel transit.

With the use of a radioisotope-labeled meal and dedicated scintigraphic hardware and software, it is possible to evaluate small bowel transit (37,38). A standard ^{99m}Tc-labeled meal, for the scintigraphic determination of gastric emptying, is appropriate. Small bowel transit is calculated by subtracting the elapsed time for a certain amount of the marker (10% or 50%) to empty from the stomach from the elapsed time for the same amount of radioisotope to arrive in the colon. Deconvolution analysis may be applied to enhance the validity of the test. The scintigraphic analysis of small bowel transit is superior to a radiologic study with barium, because the administration of barium is nonphysiologic, and it passes the small bowel more rapidly than does normal food. Furthermore, with the use of an isotope-labeled meal, the radiation exposure does not increase as more scans are obtained by the gamma camera.

In contrast to the lactulose H_2-breath test, the scinti-

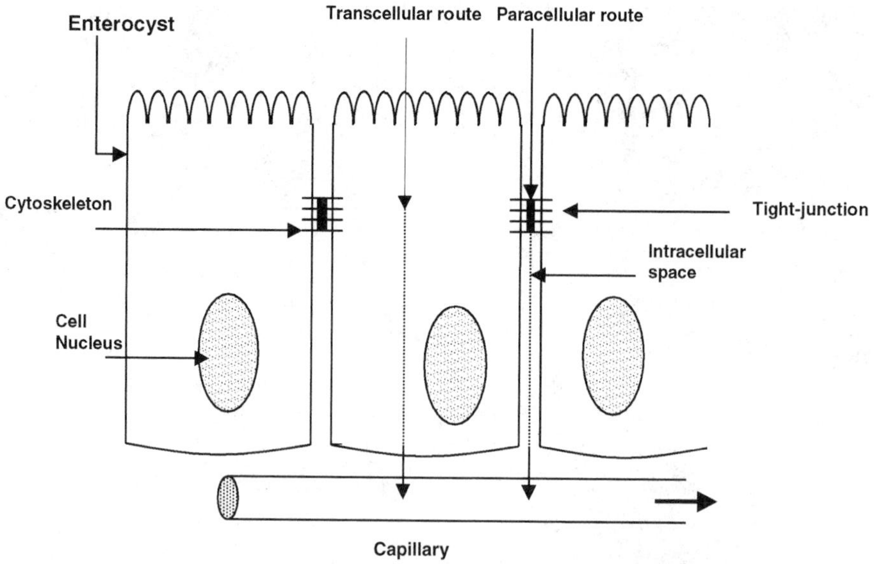

FIG. 13–8. Different permeation routes of the intestinal mucosa. Larger molecules can pass the mucosa via the paracellular route, whereas smaller molecules can pass transcellularly as well.

graphic analysis of small bowel transit cannot be used during exercise, as a steady position in front of the gamma camera must be obtained/guaranteed.

Intestinal Permeability

The intestinal permeability can be evaluated by measuring urinary excretion of orally administered water-soluble, nondegradable test probes. This barrier-function test is based on the comparison of intestinal permeation of a larger molecule with that of a smaller molecule by measuring the ratio of urinary excretion. These two probes follow different routes of intestinal permeation; the larger molecules are assumed to permeate paracellularly, and the smaller molecules are assumed to permeate transcellularly (Fig. 13–8). Preabsorption factors such as gastric emptying and dilution by secretion and intestinal transit rate, and postabsorption factors such as systemic distribution and renal clearance are assumed to affect both molecules equally. Therefore the urinary-excretion ratio is considered to be a parameter for intestinal permeability (Fig. 13–9) (39–41). Knowledge about the intestinal-barrier function has implications for the etiology and the pathogenesis of various intestinal and systemic disorders, such as celiac disease, inflammatory bowel disease, immunodeficiency syndromes, ankylosing spondylitis, cystic fibrosis, iron deficiency, atopic eczema, cardiopulmonary bypass, kwashiorkor, ileostomy, viral hepatitis, viral gastroenteritis, diabetes mellitus, and food allergies. Some drugs such as nonsteroidal antiinflammatory drugs (NSAIDs), cytostatics, and choleretics have been reported to increase intestinal permeability. Other factors that can increase intestinal permeability include alcohol abuse, enteral feeding, prolonged parenteral nutrition, and

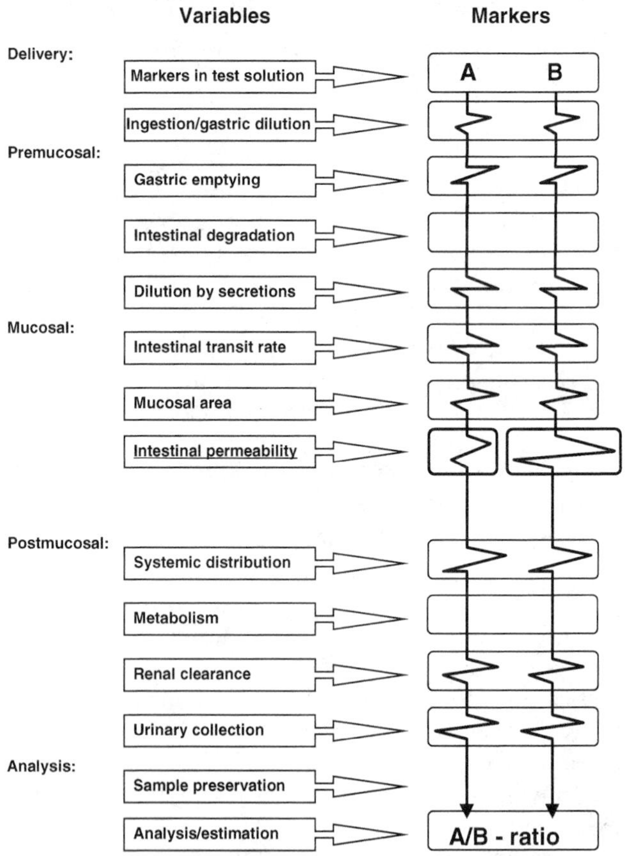

FIG. 13–9. The concept of the intestinal-permeability measurement. Both markers (*A* and *B*) are equally affected by pre- and postmucosal factors. The only difference is the intestinal-permeation route. This difference is reflected in the urinary-excretion ratio.

strenuous exercise (39). Several probes for the determination of intestinal permeability have been described. The larger probes are usually disaccharides, such as lactulose or cellobiose. Other probes such as ^{51}Cr-EDTA, ^{99m}Tc-DPTA, polyethylene glycols (PEGs), and Dextran also have been used. The smaller probes are usually the monosaccharides rhamnose and mannitol (39–41). A detailed examination of the various publications revealed that different probes were used in varying dosages. The reason for these differences may be the local availability of analysis techniques, which makes comparisons between the various studies very difficult.

Small-Bowel Absorption/Secretion

Over the last few decades, several methods involving intestinal intubation and perfusion have been used for the investigation of intestinal absorption and secretion *in vivo.* The first method described was the double-lumen perfusion technique, introduced by Fordtran and colleagues in 1961 (42). With this technique, two tubes are introduced into the part of the intestine under investigation. The solution to be investigated is perfused via one tube into the intestine at a constant rate. Subsequently, samples are drawn from the contents of the intestine at a measured distance distal from the perfusion site. If a nonabsorbable marker, such as PEG, is added to the test solution, the water flux in the part of the intestine under investigation can be calculated from the difference in concentration of this marker in the test solution and the intestinal sample. Because this method does not take into account the endogenous secretion of the intestine, the technique has been improved. The triple-lumen perfusion technique (TLPT) was presented as a reliable method to measure absorption or secretion of water and water-soluble substances (minerals, carbohydrates, amino acids, drugs) in the intestine (43,44). In this technique, three tubes, which are cemented together, are used. The different tubes have openings at specific distances. One tube is used to perfuse the original test solution into the intestine. The other two tubes have an opening at 15 and 45 cm farther down the intestine. The 15 cm between the perfusion site and the first or proximal opening is called the mixing segment, and the 30 cm between the proximal and distal opening is called the test segment. Samples from the intestinal lumen are drawn via these two openings. By measuring the concentration difference between these two samples, it is possible to calculate net absorption or secretion. A steady-state condition is essential for accurate absorption measurements.

Colon

Anatomy and Innervation

The length of the colon in adults is approximately 1 to 1.5 m; from proximal to distal, the following segments can be distinguished: cecum, ascending colon, transverse colon, descending colon, sigmoid colon, and rectum. The two sharp angulations, the hepatic and splenic flexures, mark the transition between ascending colon and transverse colon, and between the transverse colon and descending colon, respectively. Only the transverse colon and the descending colon have a mesentery, which allows some mobility. The diameter of the colon diminishes from the cecum aborally (Fig. 13–10). The outer longitudinal muscle layer of the colon forms three separate bands, the taeniae coli. The circular folds due to contraction of the inner muscular layer give rise to the haustrae, which form the characteristic picture of the colon. Distally, this inner circular muscle layer transforms to the internal anal sphincter. The external sphincter comprises striated muscle.

The absorptive surface of the colonic epithelium is rather flat, and villi are absent, in contrast to the small bowel. Some area enhancement occurs because of tubular crypts. The mucosa contains a large number of mucus-producing goblet cells.

The superior mesenteric artery supplies the cecum, ascending colon, and proximal transverse colon via three major branches—the ileocolic, right colic, and middle colic arteries—which together form arcades and connect to the arcades originating from the inferior mesenteric artery, forming the marginal artery. These arcades supply the colon via end-arteries, which have few if any anastomotic connections. Relative distal vascular occlusion may give rise to segmental infarctions. The inferior mesenteric artery supplies the distal transverse colon, descending colon, sigmoid colon, and proximal rectum. Sometimes an anastomosis exists between the middle colic artery and the left colic artery. This is a branch of the inferior mesenteric artery, which is de-

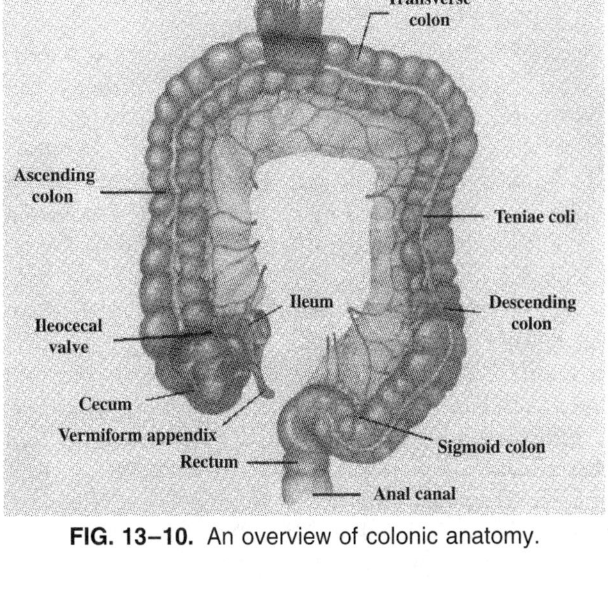

FIG. 13–10. An overview of colonic anatomy.

noted the meandering mesenteric artery or "the arc of Riolan" and serves as a collateral supply in the event of occlusion of one of the larger arteries. The arterial blood flow of the distal rectum is supplied by branches of the internal iliac arteries.

The celiac branches of the vagal nerve are responsible for the parasympathetic innervation of the cecum, the ascending colon, and the proximal transverse colon. The remaining colon, the rectum, and the internal anal sphincter receive parasympathetic innervation along the nervi erigentes, which have their origin at the level of the sacral segments 2, 3, and 4. These nerves join the hypogastric nerves to form the pelvic plexuses, which also contain sympathetic and afferent fibers and many autonomic ganglia. The external anal sphincter is innervated by the nonautonomic pudendal nerve. The sympathetic innervation occurs from thoracolumbal segments of the spine. These nerves synapse with the vertebral and prevertebral ganglia. Nerves with their cell bodies in the superior and inferior mesenteric ganglion innervate the right and left side of the colon, respectively. The pelvic ganglion innervates the rectum. The autonomic nerves connect to the myenteric and submucosal plexuses of the ENS. The density of ganglia in the myenteric plexus diminishes aborally, and the two-layer submucosal plexus is less dense than that of the small bowel.

The hormonal regulation of the colon is still unclear, but PYY, involved in the ileal-brake phenomenon, probably inhibits colonic motility.

Function and Physiology

The main function of the colon in humans is to reabsorb water and electrolytes from the approximately 1.5 L of semiliquid ileal effluent. About 90% of the water and electrolytes in the ileal effluent are absorbed by the colon. In contrast to the small bowel, the colon is characterized by a relatively high passive diffusion, the absence of glucose-enhanced water and electrolyte transport, the absence of active nutrient absorption, and the fact that mineralocorticoids secreted by the adrenal gland influence electrolyte transport. Intestinal electrolyte transport is stimulated by aldosterone, glucocorticoids, somatostatin, and certain catecholamines. The GI hormone vasoactive intestinal polypeptide (VIP) is known to stimulate fluid secretion. The presence of several endotoxins also induces fluid and electrolyte excretion.

Unabsorbed carbohydrates delivered to the colon are fermented by colonic bacteria into short-chain fatty acids (propionate, acetate, and butyrate), which are partly absorbed in the colon. Butyrate is an essential nutrient for the colonic mucosa and is known to facilitate water absorption in the right colon (45).

The motility pattern of the colon is less clear than that of the small bowel. The movements of the right colon contribute primarily to the mixing of the feces, whereas in the left colon a more propulsive movement can be observed. The electrical activity of the colon is irregular most of the time. Besides the difficulty of detecting slow waves, three types of rapid electrical activity can be observed: the frequently occurring nonpropagated short spike bursts, the stationary or propagating (over a short segment) long spike bursts, and the migrating long spike bursts. Generally, two types of contractility patterns can be distinguished. The phasic contractions usually hold for more than 10 seconds and give rise to the typical appearance of the colon. The location of these contractions moves continuously along the colon. The episodic "mass movements" have a much more intense propulsive effect. These movements rapidly propel (about 1 cm/second) the colonic contents aborally a few times per day. If these contractions occur in the sigmoid colon, an urge to defecate may follow. The combination of fecal contact to the mucosa of the upper anal canal and rectal distention are perceived as the need to defecate. The motility process of defecation is very complex and is characterized by straightening of the recto–anal angle due to relaxation of the puborectalis muscle, rectal contractions, inhibition of the tonic contractions of the internal anal sphincter, and voluntary relaxation of the external anal sphincter.

Colonic motility increases shortly after meal ingestion, the "gastro–colic response," which proceeds for about 30 to 60 minutes and is mediated by gastrin and cholecystokinin.

Measurement of Colonic Function

With the help of colonoscopy, a manometric catheter can be introduced into the right colon to obtain a colonic-motility recording. However, the large variation of wall-movement patterns and the rather unpredictable propulsive action induced by these movements limit the scientific and clinical benefit of this investigation. Furthermore, a prepared colon is necessary to introduce the colonoscope into the cecum, which is an unphysiologic situation. Without preparation of the colon, a manometric catheter cannot be positioned farther than in the distal left colon.

A conventional radiographic study of the colon by using a barium enema may yield some useful information concerning wall movements of the colon and can reveal atony, spasms, stenosis, or a dilatation.

Measurement of colonic transit time can be obtained either by the use of radiopaque markers, which can be detected by a series of conventional radiographs, or by radionuclide markers and scintigraphy. Furthermore, the measurement of total colonic transit time should be distinguished from the more sophisticated determination of segmental colonic transit.

The ingestion of a number of radiopaque markers followed by serial radiographic examinations of the abdomen or the stool is the most common method of determining colonic transit time. Total oral–anal transit time can be calculated by counting the number of markers excreted in the stool (46). This method is often inadequate with diarrhea, however. Several modified methods exist to calculate segmental colonic transit time, often after administration of the markers during several consecutive days (47–49). These methods necessitate several abdominal roentgenograms, which increase the radiation exposure considerably. Without orocecal intubation, all these methods have in common the fact that orocecal transit time is determined rather than colonic transit time *per se.*

The invention of delayed-release capsules, in which the pH-sensitive coating dissolves at a pH of about 7, and taking advantage of the pH gradient of the small bowel, allow the delivery of a bolus of isotope-labeled pellets from the distal ileum into the cecum (37,38,50). By defining regions of interest according to the segments of the colon on the serial scans, and applying simple mathematics, an accurate and reproducible determination of segmental colonic transit can be obtained with low radiation exposure of the investigated subject.

A variety of techniques exist to investigate anorectal motility, of which anal manometry, electromyography, and defecography/evacuation proctography are the most important (51–53).

THE EFFECT OF PHYSICAL EXERCISE ON GASTROINTESTINAL FUNCTION

Introduction

Participation in endurance events has become very popular. Many people participate in races, some of which last more than 15 hours. Participants frequently have abdominal pains, abnormal defecation, heartburn, nausea, and vomiting, which suggests that exercise can influence GI function. Although some people seem to have such problems in almost every endurance race, it seems very difficult to find a specific cause because many factors may play roles in the etiology of a specific GI disturbance. The chance that there is a race participant with a GI disease that is not related to exercise increases with the number of participants. Such a person may experience GI symptoms during exercise, although exercise itself is not the causative factor (54) (Fig. 13–11).

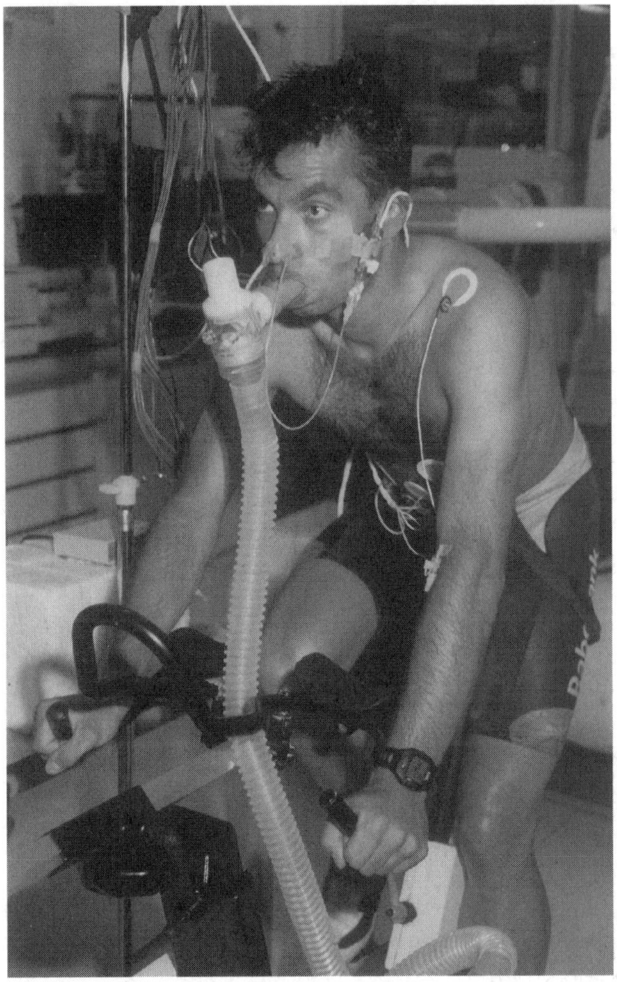

FIG. 13–11. An example of gastrointestinal measurements during exercise. An advanced transnasal solid-state pressure and pH catheter, connected to an ambulatory data logger, allows esophageal and lower esophageal sphincter motility and gastroesophageal reflux measurements. A thin catheter with a latex balloon placed in the pharynx allows recording of swallows. Breath sampling allows the determination of both gastric emptying (by using the [^{13}C]acetate breath test) and orocecal transit time (by using the H_2 breath test).

Epidemiology, Types, and Frequencies of Gastrointestinal Disturbances

Exercise-induced GI symptoms have gained scientific attention only recently. A number of studies have been performed in which questionnaires have been given to participants in endurance events. Keeffe and colleagues (55) surveyed 1700 participants in a marathon race. Lower GI symptoms, such as diarrhea, abdominal cramps, urge to defecate, flatulence, and GI bleeding, were found to be more common than upper GI symptoms, such as nausea, vomiting, heartburn, bloating, and side ache. The most common symptom experienced was urge to defecate (36% to 39% of the participants), both during and immediately after running. Bowel movements (35%) and diarrhea (19%) were reported relatively frequently, immediately after running. During the race, some runners had to stop for a bowel movement (16% to 18%), and some runners had to stop because of diarrhea (8% to 10%). Bloody bowel movements were reported by 1% to 2% of the participants. Lower GI symptoms were more common in women than in men, and some symptoms were more frequently reported by younger than by older participants. Comparable results were obtained by Riddoch and Trinick (56). They also reported lower GI symptoms as the most common; they observed more symptoms in women than in men and more symptoms in younger than in older people. Worobetz and co-workers (57) compared the effects of swimming, cycling, and running on the prevalence of GI symptoms. They demonstrated that the frequency of GI symptoms was low during cycling and swimming. Running, however, was associated with a high frequency of gastroesophageal and colonic symptoms. This was probably caused by mechanical stress due to the up-and-down movements of the abdominal organs during running. The need to defecate was the most common reason for interrupting exercise. This indicates that the type of exercise can affect the etiology of GI symptoms. It also appeared that both upper and lower GI symptoms were affected by exercise intensity, recency of meals, and intake of specific foods during exercise, such as fiber-rich food, coffee, and orange juice. Anxiety seemed to influence the occurrence of lower GI symptoms. Women were more likely to experience abdominal cramps during menstruation. Rehrer and colleagues (58) made an attempt to correlate dietary intake (including food and fluid intake) during triathlon competition and the occurrence of GI symptoms. It was observed that, in general, triathletes who consumed hypertonic carbohydrate solutions during exercise and those who consumed food products high in dietary fiber, fat, or protein before competition had more GI symptoms. The last three factors were especially related to vomiting and gastroesophageal reflux. In addition, the time of the last meal played a role; triathletes who consumed a solid meal shortly before exercise had more vomiting. Peters and colleagues (59) investigated the relation between GI symptoms and the type of consumed meal during exercise. They studied three different types of meals: a semisolid carbohydrate meal, a liquid carbohydrate meal, and a water placebo. They observed only a small difference in duration of nausea between the water placebo and the semisolid carbohydrate meal; nausea lasted longer after ingestion of the water placebo.

Other factors can initiate exercise-induced GI symptoms. Sandell and co-workers (60) reported that inadequate training, no carbohydrate-rich meal consumption beforehand, hypoglycemia, no breakfast on the race day, prerace illness, and hypothermia can play roles in exercise-induced GI symptoms.

Etiology

The underlying etiology of GI symptoms associated with exercise, especially running, has been little studied and remains speculative. Nevertheless it appears that gastric emptying, intestinal transit and intestinal absorption, and secretion may be involved. These functions are largely regulated by nervous and hormonal processes, which in turn are influenced by the immediate physiologic activity level (i.e., metabolic demand and blood supply). The question then arises whether exercise alters these functions by influencing the regulating factors. At the onset of exercise, many physiologic and biochemical processes adapt to the increased degree of physical activity. The most important alterations are immediate local changes in tissue biochemistry, such as changes in oxygen saturation, concentration of energy-rich phosphates, and accumulation of metabolites, as well as changes in sympathetic and parasympathetic output and circulating hormones (54,61). The muscular blood flow is increased, and the GI tract receives less blood during exercise (62,63). Rowell and co-workers (64) demonstrated a 60% to 70% reduction in splanchnic blood flow in subjects exercising at an intensity of 70% $\dot{V}O_2max$. Clausen (65) reported that blood flow may be reduced to 20% of the resting level during maximal exercise, in both trained and untrained people. Sympathetic output plays a major role in redistributing blood flow during exercise. Blood flow may be decreased to critical levels during maximal sympathetic stimulation, and maximal hormonal changes, which take place when hyperthermia, dehydration, hypoglycemia, hypoxia, or a combination of these factors may cause fatigue and exhaustion. The plasma noradrenalin concentration has been shown to vary inversely with the oxygen saturation of mixed venous blood. Hyperthermia and hypoglycemia lead to highly increased sympathetic stimulation and plasma catecholamine levels and may therefore influence blood flow significantly (64,66). Continuing dehydration (more than 3% body weight) leads to tissue dehydration and decreased capillary blood supply in peripheral tissues such as muscle and skin, and may reduce intestinal blood flow to practically zero. In addition, blood viscosity is known to be affected by exercise-induced hyperthermia. Plasma viscosity is temperature dependent and shows a 10% increase at 40°C. Whole-blood viscosity, which may further affect intestinal capillary blood flow, is influenced by hydration status (67). Dehydration, reduced splanchnic blood flow, and tissue hypoxia strongly influence the occurrence of GI symptoms associated with the lower GI tract especially. A lack of oxygen may induce acute energy deficits, which may influence active, energy-dependent absorption of nutrients, such as glucose or amino acids, and may also interfere with Na^+/K^+-ATPase activity. As a result, GI motility, intestinal absorption, and mucosal integrity may be disturbed.

Effect of Exercise on Esophageal Motility and Gastroesophageal Reflux

Athletes frequently have exercise-induced GI symptoms (61,68). As stated above, these symptoms can be divided into lower- and upper-GI symptoms. Upper-GI symptoms include nausea, vomiting, belching, and heartburn (70). GI symptoms ascribed to the esophagus include heartburn and chest pain. These symptoms indicate disturbances in esophageal motility and an increased incidence of gastroesophageal reflux, and therefore the general belief that exercise-induced chest pain suggests a cardiac rather than a GI origin is not true in exercise-induced esophageal complaints. The primary pathophysiologic event of noncardiac chest pain is an abnormal exposure of the esophagus to gastric juice. Two main factors can play roles in the pathogenesis: an increased rate of reflux episodes, and/or a decreased rate of esophageal clearance via primary and secondary peristalsis. The composition of the refluxate, especially the acidity and the quantity of pepsin, and the sensitivity of the esophageal mucosa for the refluxate can play roles in the perception of heartburn as well.

Because the ambulatory measurement of reflux, LES, and esophageal motility are relatively recent techniques, only a small number of studies on the effect of exercise on gastroesophageal reflux have been carried out (Fig. 13–12).

In 1989 Clark and co-workers (71) studied exercise-induced gastroesophageal reflux in 12 healthy volunteers. The subjects were studied on two different occasions: fasted and after a meal. They underwent a rest–exercise protocol, and esophageal pH was measured. The exercise consisted of 15 minutes of cycling, 15 minutes of a weight routine, and 15 minutes of running on a treadmill. Five minutes of rest followed each exercise bout, and the exercise was conducted at near-maximal effort. The results indicated that strenuous exercise could induce gastroesophageal reflux in normal volunteers. It also was observed that running caused the most reflux, and cycling produced less reflux. In the weight-routine bout, gastroesophageal reflux was induced in some subjects, but no particular exercise was associated with more reflux. Postprandial exercise showed a pattern of gastroesophageal reflux similar to reflux during exercise under the fasted condition, but it was quantitatively larger. This finding is consistent with the known postprandial increase of gastroesophageal reflux in healthy sedentary subjects. The exercise-induced increase in gastroesophageal reflux was not associated with an increase in upper-GI symptoms. Kraus and colleagues (72) studied gastroesophageal reflux in runners in a rest–exercise protocol comprising a 1 hour baseline

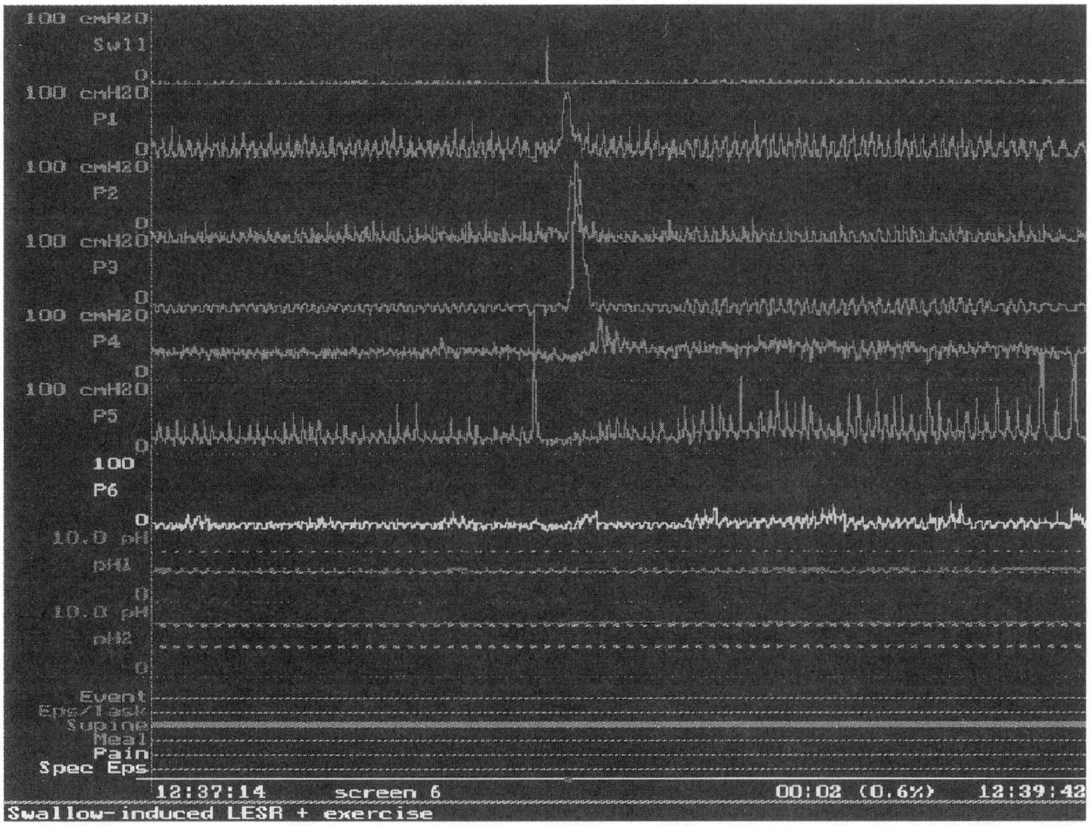

FIG. 13–12. An example of swallow, esophageal motility, lower esophageal sphincter (LES) pressure, and gastroesophageal reflux measurements during physical exercise. The registration shows a swallow-induced LES relaxation (*P4*). Channel 1 (*Swll*) represents swallows, recorded in the pharynx. Channels *P1–P3* represent esophageal pressure in a distal direction, respectively. The pressure sensors are separated from each other by 5 cm. Channel *P4* represents the LES pressure, and channels *P5* and *P6* represent the fundic pressure. Channels *pH 1* and *pH 2* represent the pH in the stomach and in the esophagus, respectively.

recording and 1 hour of near-maximal running on a treadmill. The effect of ranitidine versus a placebo was studied as well. They observed that gastroesophageal reflux was prevalent in many subjects, and that symptoms, primarily belching, were more frequent during running than at rest. These symptoms were associated with reflux episodes. Ranitidine reduced the acidity of the refluxate and the duration of reflux episodes as well.

Soffer and colleagues (73,74) carried out two studies in which they investigated the effect of exercise intensity on esophageal motility and gastroesophageal reflux in both trained and untrained subjects. The untrained subjects underwent a rest–exercise protocol, and the exercise consisted of four periods of cycling at 40%, 60%, 75%, and 90% of their maximal oxygen uptake ($\dot{V}O_2$max). They were encouraged to exercise for as long as they could in each session, with a resting period between each cycling session. At the highest intensity, the load could not be maintained longer than 2 to 3 minutes. The trained subjects underwent a protocol consisting of 60 minutes at 60% $\dot{V}O_2$max, 45 minutes at 75% $\dot{V}O_2$max, and 10 minutes at 90% $\dot{V}O_2$max. A 30-minute rest followed each cycling session. Similar results were obtained in both groups; the duration, amplitude, and frequency of esophageal contractions declined with increasing exercise intensity, and the differences reached significance for all three parameters at 90% $\dot{V}O_2$max.

The number and duration of reflux episodes were increased during the highest intensity, but not at lower intensities. The underlying mechanism for this increase in gastroesophageal reflux may be an exercise-induced decrease of the LES pressure. Van Nieuwenhoven and colleagues (6) observed no increase in gastroesophageal reflux in 10 well-trained subjects who cycled for 90 minutes at 70% of their maximal work capacity. This does not rule out the possibility that gastroesophageal reflux is increased at higher, near-maximal intensities, or during running-type exercises. Peters and co-workers (75) studied the LES pressure in healthy volunteers before and immediately after 30 minutes of cycling at an increasing intensity. They observed that the LES pressure decreased with severe exercise. Schoeman and associates (76) studied reflux and LES pressure in ambulatory subjects. During the 24-hour registration, the subjects performed a standardized exercise program consisting of three 10-minute periods of exercise with vigorous cycling on an exercise bicycle, walking at steady-state pace on a treadmill, and walking as fast as possible on a treadmill. The intensities were not standardized. They observed, during exercise, an increase in gastroesophageal reflux and a decrease in basal LES pressure, which was, however, unrelated to the occurrence of reflux. The majority of the reflux episodes were associated with transient LES relaxations (TLESR). The number of TLESRs was not increased during exercise.

However, it is unclear how exercise affects the characteristics of LES motility. The relation between the rate of gastric emptying and reflux at high-intensity exercise, and the possible long-term effects of exercise-induced reflux, are areas to be clarified in the future.

Effect of Exercise on Gastric Emptying

For the last 2 decades, substantial attention has been given to the effects of dehydration and rehydration in the exercising athlete. This has been reviewed in a number of articles (8,11,77–80). Although low-intensity exercise increases solid-meal GERs (81), during exercise predominantly liquids are consumed. Generally, after swallowing a liquid down to the stomach, gastric emptying is considered the first limiting step in making fluid available to the circulation. The stomach functions as a reservoir from which no significant absorption takes place and from which fluid has to be emptied into the intestine before absorption.

In relation to exercise, the GER depends on

- Exercise intensity,
- Volume of the drink,
- Energy density of the drink,
- Temperature of the drink,
- Osmolality of the drink,
- Body temperature/dehydration level,
- Type of exercise,
- Psychological stress level.

These factors are discussed below.

Exercise Intensity

From studies done at rest and during exercise, it appears that up to exercise-intensity levels of 70% to 80% $\dot{V}O_2$max, there is no difference in the regulation of the GER between the conditions. At higher intensities, the GER has been found to be reduced. The significance of this finding for the exercising athlete is low, however, because exercise at intensities of more than 80% $\dot{V}O_2$max generally cannot be performed long enough to cause a limitation in fluid availability. Even if this happened, the exercise-induced hyperventilation would be so intense that drinking would cause a direct disturbance of breathing patterns, and with it the ability to perform well (e.g., a 10,000-m run in the heat would not allow drinking). It appears that factors related to the quantity of the fluid consumed and to its chemical composition are of prime importance in making fluid available for absorption.

Volume of the Drink

When a meal or fluid bolus enters the stomach, it allows for volume adjustment (i.e., the gastric wall distends). The result of this adaptation is that the volume increases without an increase in pressure. The latter will occur only after the capacity to distend has been maximized. Once contractions of the corpus are initiated, the quantity emptied from the stomach is larger if the gastric content is large. This effect can be observed in most GER studies and is presented by a more or less exponential GE response after the ingestion of fluids. First, there is a rapid emptying phase followed by a phase of reduced emptying once the volume of the stomach has been reduced to about 30% of its initial content.

Energy Density of the Drink

This volume effect can be overruled by the chemical composition of a drink. For example, drinks with a high nutrient content (thus also a high caloric value/energy density) do not exert an exponential response but empty almost linearly from the stomach. Two important conclusions can be drawn from these findings: (a) for substantial fluid replacement, drinks should have a relatively low nutrient content; and (b) volume drinking may have advantages over frequent "small-body drinking" (11).

Because athletes deal with two major limiting factors to perform endurance exercise in the heat [i.e., fluid and carbohydrate (CHO) availability], it is important to determine how high the CHO content of a drink should be, without limiting fluid availability. Many studies have been done in this respect. Generally, these show that the addition of CHO in quantities up to 4% (40 g/L) does not inhibit the GER. Higher quantities progressively reduce GER (9,82,83). Yet there is some degree of freedom to use slightly higher CHO contents during exercise (i.e., 6% to 8%). Observations on the quantity of fluid usually consumed during endurance exercise highlight the fact that runners seldom ingest more than 500 mL/h (84), whereas cyclists can ingest more (i.e., 500 to 800 mL/h). Both quantities are substantially less than the maximal GER. Therefore, the fact that drinks containing 40 to 80 g CHO/L are more slowly emptied from the stomach may not necessarily be of physiologic significance when relatively small to moderate fluid volumes are consumed. As a general rule, drinks for the endurance athlete exercising in the heat may contain 40 to 80 g CHO/L, whereas drinks with a higher CHO content may be more beneficial to support CHO availability and oxidation in conditions in which sweat loss is small. Maximal oral CHO oxidation has been observed to approximate 0.5 to 1.0 g/min, requiring 600 to 750 mL of an 8% solution (85).

Osmolality

A high content of simple CHO causes a drink to have a high osmotic pressure. In the early 1970s, it was believed that osmolality is one of the most important factors in the control of the GER. However, osmolality and content of simple or short-chain CHO are related, and increasing the CHO content will increase osmolality. For that reason we recently performed a study to compare the effect of six drinks with osmolalities ranging from 240 to 390 mOsm/L, but all with a CHO content of 60 g/L. It was observed that all drinks emptied at the same rate (82). Thus although osmolalities may reduce GER (83), this does not seem to be an important factor in relation to most sports drinks consumed (range, 200 to 400 mOsm/L).

Temperature

When considering the effect of temperature on the total time to empty liquids from the stomach, the effect can be considered physiologically unimportant. Athletes are advised to adjust drink temperature to personal preference and tolerance during exercise, and cooled drinks may offer some benefit in taking up heat from the body. In contrast, with exercise in cold conditions, warm drinks may offer a psychological benefit.

Stress Level

Psychological and severe physical stress are known to affect GI motility and to reduce the GER. Changes in plasma stress hormones and GI hormones related to stress and exercise are discussed below. The only remedy to reduce such effects is adequate training and mental preparation. Stress due to dehydration in the heat (i.e., hyperthermia) is known to coincide with heat exhaustion and intestinal upset. Studies on the effect of exercise dehydration–induced hyperthermia showed that the GER slows (8) and that GI upset may occur (86). This is most probably caused by stress-related hormonal changes and a significant decrease in GI blood flow (54).

Type of Exercise

Running exercise leads to a much higher incidence of GI problems compared with gliding types of exercise such as cycling, cross-country skiing, swimming, and skating (54,77). Consequently, fluid intakes during running events are small and range from 150 to maximally 600 mL/h (84), and the incidence of dehydration and related GI upset is larger (86). This may have a direct effect on GI motility and the GER. When different types of exercise are compared in controlled laboratory circumstances, however, GI problems generally do not occur, and differences in the GER are not observed (86).

Women are observed to have a slower GER compared with men, but during ovulation this is reversed (87). Women also have lower sweat-production rates than men. If women and men drink equal volumes during endurance exercise, this causes more gastric complaints of distention in women compared with men (23). Thus both men and women should monitor body-weight loss as a result of endurance exercise to calculate the required fluid replacement.

Keys for Practice

- Drinks remaining in the stomach are not available to the body;
- Drinks with a high energy content reduce the fluid delivery to the gut;
- Temperature, osmolality, and training status are not considered to be of great importance to the GER;
- Optimally, rehydration drinks to be ingested during exercise in the heat should contain fewer than 80 g CHO/L;
- Drinks to be ingested in conditions in which fluid loss is not performance limiting (i.e., during winter) may contain more CHO and may also be warm; and
- Athletes should find out their personal preferences and tolerances for both drink volume and drink temperature in training sessions.

The Effect of Exercise on Small Bowel Motility

Intense exercise can cause GI symptoms, reduced intestinal blood flow (54), and elevated plasma concentrations of catecholamines, endorphins (88), and all types of GI hormones (89), each of which can affect intestinal motility. The few reports concerning the effect of exercise on intestinal motor function are conflicting, however. Studies of intestinal motility during exercise are obstructed by the technical problems associated with recording during physical exercise. Cammack and colleagues (90) carried out one of the first studies on small intestinal transit during a low-intensity 60 km cycle ride, by using the breath-hydrogen technique. No effect was observed. Keeling and co-workers (91,92), however, reported an acceleration in OCTT in both men and women during walking at 5.6 km/h. They also used the breath-hydrogen technique. It must be noted that quite a large quantity of the nondigestible carbohydrate lactulose was used: 20 g. In contrast, Meshkinpour (93) reported a delay in OCTT during walking. Lactulose (10 g) was administered in this study. Soffer and co-workers (94) measured the effect of cycling at different intensities on duodenojejunal motor activity and OCTT in eight well-trained cyclists. It was observed that exercise at higher intensities can affect intestinal postprandial motor activity. In a number of subjects, interruptions of the fed pattern by a burst of rhythmic activity resembling an activity front that propagated from the duodenum to the jejunum were observed. This effect was exercise-intensity dependent, but not related to GI symptoms. The OCTT was measured as well, and it appeared to be unchanged by short, intense exercise. Peters (95) studied the effect of prolonged physical exercise and fluid supplementation (water vs. carbohydrate solution) in triathletes on antroduodenal motility. He observed an early reappearance of phase III during exercise, especially with carbohydrate, which was unexpected because no phase IIIs were present before exercise and energy intake in the morning before the exercise. Koffler and associates (96) studied OCTT in untrained middle-aged and elderly men, after a 13-week total body strength training period. They also were unable to observe an effect of physical exercise on OCTT. These results were confirmed by Liu and Toda (97) in a study in which nine physically active elderly men were studied after a period of 2 weeks of inactivity. Intestinal markers to study intestinal transit also have been used. Harrison and co-workers (98) used oral radiopaque markers in recreational runners and observed no differences in intestinal transit between active and inactive periods. Evans and colleagues (99) used jejunal pressure-sensitive radiotelemetry capsules, attached to a wire, to study 20 fasted male subjects at rest and during exercise. They observed a decreased occurrence of MMC, which indicates a delayed intestinal transit. In another study, the intestinal transit of capsules was reported to be delayed (100). Ollerenshaw and associates (101) used radioactive-labeled raisin beans to study the effect of three different intensity levels on mean intestinal transit time. No differences in transit time could be observed.

Summarizing, it can be concluded that the effect of exercise, or exercise intensity, on intestinal transit remains unclear. Studies carried out so far show conflicting results. Various methods to measure intestinal transit, different types of subjects, and different quantities of lactulose to determine OCTT have been used, which makes it difficult to compare the studies. More standardized research is needed to elucidate the role of exercise on intestinal motility. Its relation to gastric emptying, intestinal absorption, and exercise-induced GI symptoms are areas to be elucidated in the future as well.

The Effect of Exercise on Small Bowel Absorption

Impaired intestinal fluid and electrolyte absorption cause an osmotic load, which may result in GI distress and diarrhea. Most studies on small intestinal absorption in exercise have applied the triple-lumen perfusion technique (61). In one of the first studies with this technique (102), no effect of 1 hour of treadmill running at an exercise intensity of 70% $\dot{V}O_2$max was found on water glucose and electrolyte absorption in five athletes. Barclay and Turnberg (103), however, observed that exercise of moderate intensity (45% to 50% of $\dot{V}O_2$max) significantly reduced jejunal absorption of water, sodium, chloride, and potassium. It has been suggested that a reduction of mesenteric blood flow by more than 50% causes a linear decrease in the rate of glucose absorption (104). By using deuterium oxide as a tracer for water absorption, Maughan and colleagues (105) observed impaired water absorption when exercise was performed at 80% $\dot{V}O_2$max compared with 42% or 61% $\dot{V}O_2$max.

It was suggested that the intraluminal concentration of carbohydrates and sodium affects fluid absorption, because carbohydrate and sodium share a coupled active transport system in the intestinal wall (106). Sodium may not necessarily be of physiologic significance for the rate of glucose absorption, however (107). Rehrer and co-workers (108) observed, by using deuterium oxide–enriched beverages, that net jejunal water absorption occurred if a beverage was consumed containing either water, 4.5% glucose, or 17% maltodextrin, whereas net secretion took place if 17% glucose was consumed, during 80 minutes at 70% $\dot{V}O_2$max. By using the triple-lumen technique, it was shown that differences in osmolality of the beverages were eliminated within the proximal duodenum and that 6% carbohydrate solutions with osmolalities ranging from 186 to 403 mOsm/kg did not produce significant differences in fluid homeostasis (plasma volume) at the end of an 80-minute test period (109). Generally, fluid absorption in small intestinal segments after water perfusion is smaller (about 1 ml/cm/h) compared with well-composed carbohydrate solutions with an absorption rate of about 3 to 4 ml/cm/h (110). The rate of water absorption may even be enhanced by using a relatively low carbohydrate content (3% to 4%) and a low osmolality (240 to 270 mOsm/L) (111,112). However, such a low carbohydrate administration limits the effects on exercise performance. Drinks with a very high absorption rate have not been shown to result in better water retention, probably because a rapid increase in plasma volume stimulates urine production by pressure receptors.

The Effect of Exercise on Intestinal Permeability

The role of the physiologic barrier function of the small bowel and its possible role in health and disease have attracted much attention during the 1990s. The intact intestinal mucosa serves as a barrier between the nonsterile lumen and the sterile interior of the body. Microorganisms or endotoxins such as toxic lipopolysaccharides may sometimes penetrate this barrier. This process is named *translocation*. In a normal healthy subject, translocation causes only a limited bacteremic/endotoxemic challenge, which can be cleared by the defense systems (mesenteric lymph nodes and the hepatic reticuloendothelial system) of the body (113). Under conditions of an ischemic intestinal mucosa, the leakage of bacteria and/or endotoxins through the more permeable intestinal mucosa may be increased, resulting in a condition that may give rise to GI symptoms. It has been shown in an animal study that reduction of the small intestinal blood supply of more than 50% induces detectable tissue injury (114).

Exercise may lead to a substantial decrease in GI blood flow of more than 50% (62,63). Rowell and co-workers (64) demonstrated a 60% to 70% reduction in splanchnic blood flow in subjects exercising at an intensity of 70% $\dot{V}O_2$max, and Clausen (65) reported a reduction in splanchnic blood flow of 80% of the resting level during maximal exercise. It also may lead to an alteration in intestinal motility. Mechanical trauma due to running, for instance, may occur as well. These factors may lead to an injury of the intestinal mucosa, and as a consequence, an increase in intestinal permeability. Recently there has been increasing evidence that, in addition to the mucosal injury taking place under ischemic conditions, intestinal injury also takes place at reperfusion (115). The underlying mechanism of reperfusion damage is generally believed to be an increased production of oxygen-derived free radicals. There are few data available concerning the effect of exercise on intestinal permeability. Øktedalen and associates (116) studied two groups of long-distance runners for the effect of marathon running on the GI mucosa. They observed gastric erosions in five of nine subjects, and a substantial increase in the 24 hour urinary excretion of ^{51}Cr-labeled EDTA after oral intake of this probe. This indicates an increased intestinal permeability, caused by damage of the intercellular junctions of adjacent enterocytes. However, they did not use a control probe besides the ^{51}Cr-EDTA; therefore it cannot be excluded that factors other than changes in intestinal permeability caused the increase in urinary excretion. Moreover, ^{51}Cr-EDTA is nondecomposable by bacteria, and therefore reflects colonic permeation as well (41). None of the subjects experienced GI symptoms during the marathon. Moses and colleagues (117) reported an increased permeability within 6 hours to oral PEG-400 combined with 6% glucose solution in asymptomatic subjects who underwent a protocol of 90 minutes of alternating high-intensity (15 minutes of 60% to 85% $\dot{V}O_2$max) treadmill running with 30 second sprints to exhaustion. PEG-400 consists of polymers with molecular masses ranging from 190 to 500 Da. Therefore they may follow variable routes of intestinal permeation. PEG-400 also exhibits variable urinary excretion (26% to 69%) after intravenous administration. For these reasons, interpretation of the results is difficult. Van Nieuwenhoven and co-workers (118) reported no changes in intestinal lactulose/rhamnose permeability in both symptomatic and asymptomatic subjects who ran on a treadmill for 90 minutes at a velocity of 70% of their maximal speed. No differences were found between the two groups, and between the preexercise, the exercise, and the 24 hour postexercise periods. This was confirmed by a study of Ryan and colleagues (119). They evaluated the effect of exercise and aspirin intake on intestinal permeability by using a hyperosmotic lactulose/mannitol test solution. The exercise was composed of 60 minutes of treadmill running at 65% $\dot{V}O_2max$. An increase in intestinal permeability was observed because of aspirin ingestion but not because of exercise. Running was not associated with GI symptoms. To summarize, it can be concluded that the influence of physical exercise on intestinal permeability is not yet clear. It cannot be excluded that changes in intestinal permeability may occur during more severe or prolonged exercise, eventually in combination with hyperthermia and/or dehydration. The use of antiinflammatory drugs, during exercise, to reduce pain may lead to adverse GI effects and should thus not be recommended.

Effect of Exercise on Colonic Function

There is a general belief that inactivity is a risk factor for constipation, and that increasing the level of physical exercise is effective against chronic constipation (97,120). The substantial evidence that physical activity reduces the risk for colon cancer may be associated with the change in GI transit (121). Other circumstantial evidence for the effect of exercise on colonic motility is the fact that many long-distance runners often experience diarrhea and the urge to defecate (56,122). Furthermore, the amount of exercise was reported to correlate with the prevalence of diarrhea. Colonic transit normally lasts for about 20 to 60 hours, with a wide interindividual and intraindividual variation. Hence, gut transit is mainly a colonic event, and exercise-induced diarrhea is often considered the result of a colonic function disorder. Now the specific transit of a segment of the gut can be determined with sophisticated transit measurements. The different compartments of the GI tract should not be regarded as independent organs, however. The gastrocolonic response is a typical illustration of the functional cohesion of the GI system. According to this phenomenon, the acceleration of colonic transit due to mass movements originates at the level of the stomach.

Only a few studies have investigated the effect of exercise on colonic motility, and the results are rather conflicting. Cordain and co-workers (123) found transit to be accelerated by an aerobic training program, whereas Bingham and Cummings (124) did not find an effect of exercise. Moderate aerobic exercise in healthy men with a sedentary lifestyle did not significantly change total and segmental colonic transit (125,126), although a trend toward accelerated right colonic transit was observed. In contrast to these findings, a comparative study between soccer players and age-matched sedentary controls showed that right colonic transit was considerably slower in the soccer players, whereas left colonic and rectal transit were slightly accelerated (127). By using a sophisticated manometric device, the acute colonic response to moderate aerobic exercise was studied (128). During exercise, a shift toward increased frequency and intensity of the contractions was observed.

It is well known that several factors may influence the results of studies on the effect of exercise on colonic motility, such as duration and intensity of exercise, mode of exercise, training status, hydration state, diet, and gender.

Periods of intensive long-lasting exercise induce changes in the dietary intake of several nutrients. Generally, dietary fiber increases fecal mass, which reduces colonic transit, and the metabolism of minerals, nitrogen, and bile acids is affected (129,130).

In athletes, both dietary fiber and secretion changes will affect intestinal transit in periods of intensive exercise. This is most pronounced in athletes who consume vegetarian diets (131). Rehrer and associates (132) observed that triathletes who ingested pregame meals relatively rich in dietary fiber had more GI symptoms during exercise.

The etiology of the experience of an urge to defecate during exercise, especially running, is still a matter of debate. Early work of DeYoung (133) in dogs, by using intracolonic balloons, showed a rapid increase in colonic pressure shortly after the start of exercise, followed by relative relaxation and decreased sphincter pressure. This combination of events was assumed to cause defecation. Cordain and co-workers (123) hypothesized that sympathetic stimulation causes a relaxation of the GI tract. This relaxation could facilitate the passage of intraluminal contents from the colon into the rectum during the up-and-down bouncing motion associated with running. This would be followed by the urge to defecate.

Many other explanations of diarrhea and urge to defecate during exercise could be proposed. Direct exercise-induced irritation by a hypertrophied psoas muscle on the rectosigmoid colon has been shown (134), but its significance has never been proven. Several GI hormones may affect internal anal sphincter pressure (135).

It should be emphasized that GI complaints due to (often latent) preexisting GI disorders, such as irritable bowel syndrome, lactose malabsorption, celiac disease, and giardiasis infection, may be aggravated during intense exercise. Furthermore, the frequently administered NSAIDs to alleviate muscle and joint complaints have a detrimental effect on GI mucosal integrity, causing gastritis, duodenitis, and often (unobserved) GI blood loss. The administration of NSAID-containing suppositories does not prevent these complications, as these drugs exert their effects systemically through the inhibition of prostaglandin synthesis. The suppositories may in fact also induce a proctitis and hence rectal symptoms such as urge to defecate.

The Effect of Exercise on Gastrointestinal Hormones

Gastrointestinal function is partially under hormonal control. Therefore exercise-induced changes in GI hormones and peptides may play a role in the etiology of exercise-induced GI symptoms. Many hormones associated with GI function can be influenced by physical activity. These hormones and peptides consist of catecholamines (which were discussed earlier), VIP, secretin, pancreatic polypeptide, somatostatin, gastrin, motilin, glucagon, PYY, cholecystokinin (CCK), GLP-1, endorphins, and prostaglandins. Several of these hormones have a metabolic function as well, which makes exercise-induced alterations in plasma levels very difficult to interpret. The possible effect of exercise on circulating GI hormones was studied by Hilsted and associates (136). They observed significant increases in VIP, pancreatic polypeptide, somatostatin, glucagon, and secretin in subjects during 3 hours of low-intensity cycling. These observations were confirmed by Sullivan and coworkers (137), who studied runners during a 30-km run. They also found an increase in plasma gastrin and motilin. Øktedalen and colleagues (138) also found increases in secretin and VIP during a 90-km ski race. Riddoch and Trinick (56,139) found an increase in VIP, motilin, gastrin, pancreatic polypeptide, and secretin, besides elevations in some neuropeptides, such as peptide, histidine, methionine, and neurotensin, after a marathon. Although these observations suggest a relation between the plasma elevation of several hormone levels and the occurrence of GI symptoms, it is unclear whether these hormonal elevations were caused by GI dysfunction, or whether the hormonal elevations were the underlying reason for GI dysfunction. The increase in GI hormones may have had more of a metabolic origin, in the response to energy demands, rather than being specifically related to alterations in GI function. In a study by MacLaren and colleagues (140), gastrin and VIP were elevated after 90 minutes of treadmill running, and VIP was more increased if no fluid was ingested, compared with ingestion of an 8% maltodextrin solution. This suggests that carbohydrate drinks can counteract possible adverse effects of accumulating VIP levels on GI function. Philipp and colleagues (141) studied the influence of long-distance running on the secretion of CCK and gastrin. Several stress hormones were measured as well. The hormones were measured before and after a competitive marathon run, and a few weeks later as a control measurement. CCK and the stress hormones were elevated under prerun conditions compared with control conditions. It is suggested that CCK may induce the type of endocrine response normally associated with the action of a stressful stimulus. The endocrine effect of CCK in relation to stress could be explained by a direct action at the pituitary level, where it may stimulate adrenocorticotropic (ACTH) release. Therefore this study suggests that CCK, which delays gastric emptying, inhibits gastric acid secretion, reduces the LES pressure, enhances small-bowel motility, and stimulates gallbladder contraction (142), may be an important regulatory factor in response to anticipatory stress. Therefore it may play a role in the occurrence of GI symptoms during stressful competitive events. O'Connor and colleagues (89) studied GI hormones in relation to GI symptoms in subjects immediately after finishing a marathon run and then 30 minutes after finishing. They measured VIP, gastrin, secretin, pancreatic polypeptide, neurokinin A, pancreastatin, insulin, and GLP-1. All these hormones, except insulin, were increased after the race. It would appear that some hormones are secreted in quantities that may be linked to a variety of GI symptoms. Elevated levels of VIP can induce watery diarrhea by reducing absorption of water and electrolytes and enhancing water, chloride, and bicarbonate secretion. The VIP levels after the marathon exceed the VIP levels seen in patients with watery diarrhea hydrochloracidemia (WDHA syndrome). No relation between VIP levels and exercise-induced diarrhea could be observed, however. Gastroesophageal reflux, nausea, and vomiting were suggested to be caused by an increased gastric acid production, which, in turn, may be caused by an elevated gastrin level. Banfi and colleagues (143) studied plasma gastrin and cortisol combined with plasma pepsinogen in mountain marathon runners before and immediately after the race, with the aim to establish their interrelation with exercise-induced GI symptoms. They concluded that, after endurance exercise, correlations between GI symptoms and a change in plasma levels of GI hormones do not exist. Therefore it can be concluded that exercise-induced GI symptoms do not necessarily correlate with plasma levels of GI hormones. This is surprising if the magnitude of the hormonal changes is taken into account. Other factors may contribute, including duration of elevation of GI hormone levels, sensitivity to the GI hormones, intestinal contents, and adaptation. Further intervention studies are required to elucidate the mechanisms of release and action of GI hormones during exercise and possibly under other physiologic conditions.

REFERENCES

1. Dent J, Dodds WJ, Friedman RH, et al. Mechanism of gastroesophageal reflux in recumbent asymptomatic human subjects. *J Clin Invest* 1980;65:256–267.
2. Barham CP, Gotley DC, Mills A, Alderson D. A new 24-hour pH and motility recording system. *Gut* 1993;34:444–449.
3. Dent J, Chir B. A new technique for continuous sphincter pressure measurement. *Gastroenterology* 1976;71:263–267.
4. Gotley DC, Barham CP, Miller R, Arnold R, Alderson D. The sphinctometer: a new device for measurement of lower oesophageal spincter function. *Br J Surg* 1991;78:933–935.
5. Johnson FL. Methods of testing esophageal clearance. In: Dubois A, Castrell DO, eds. *Esophageal and gastric emptying.* Boca Raton: CRC Press, 1984.

6. van Nieuwenhoven MA, Brouns F, Brummer R-JM. Ambulatory measurement of esophageal motility, LES pressure and gastro-esophageal reflux during exercise [Abstract]. *Gastroenterology* 1996;110:A704.
7. Code CF, Schlegel JF. The gastrointestinal housekeeper: motor correlates of the interdigestive myoelectric complex of the dog. In: *Proceedings of the 4th International Symposium on Gastrointestinal Motility.* Vancouver: Mitchell Press, 1974:631–634.
8. Rehrer NJ, Brouns F, Beckers EJ, Saris WHM. The influence of beverage composition and gastrointestinal function on fluid and nutrient availability during exercise. *Scand J Med Sci Sports* 1994;4:159–172.
9. Vist GE, Maughan RJ. Gastric emptying of ingested solutions in man: effect of beverage glucose concentration. *Med Sci Sports Exerc* 1994;26:1269–1273.
10. McArthur KE, Feldman M. Gastric acid secretion, gastrin release, and gastric emptying in humans as affected by liquid meal temperature. *Am J Clin Nutr* 1989;49:51–54.
11. Noakes TD, Rehrer NJ, Maughan RJ. The importance of volume in regulating gastric emptying. *Med Sci Sports Exerc* 1991; 23:307–313.
12. Beglinger C. Effect of cholecystokinin on gastric motility in humans. *Ann N Y Acad Sci* 1994;713:219–225.
13. Sheikh SP. Neuropeptide Y and peptide YY: major modulators of gastrointestinal blood flow and function. *Am J Physiol* 1991;261:G701–G715.
14. Holst JJ. Glucagonlike peptide 1: a newly discovered gastrointestinal hormone. *Gastroenterology* 1994;107:1848–1855.
15. Gomez G, Padilla L, Udupi V, et al. Regulation of peptide YY by gastric acid and gastrin. *Endocrinology* 1996;137:1365–1369.
16. Layer P, Holst JJ, Grandt D, Goebell H. Ileal release of glucagon-like peptide-1 (GLP-1): association with inhibition of gastric acid secretion in humans. *Dig Dis Sci* 1995;40:1074–1082.
17. Hunt JN. Control of gastric emptying. *Am J Dig Dis* 1968; 13:372–375.
18. Welch I, Cunningham KM, Read NW. Regulation of gastric emptying by ileal nutrients in humans. *Gastroenterology* 1988; 94:401–404.
19. Chen JZ, McCallum RW. *Electrogastrography: principles and applications.* New York: Raven Press, 1984.
20. Heading RC, Tothill P, McLoughlin GP, Shearman DJC. Gastric emptying rate measurement in man: a double isotope scanning technique for simultaneous study of liquid and solid components of a meal. *Gastroenterology* 1976;71:45–50.
21. Collins PJ, Horowitz M, Cook DJ, Harding PE, Shearman DJC. Gastric emptying in normal subjects: a reproducible technique using a single scintillation camera and computer system. *Gut* 1983;24:1117–1125.
22. George JD. New clinical method for measuring the rate of gastric emptying: the double sampling technique. *Gut* 1968;9:237–242.
23. Beckers EJ, Rehrer NJ, Brouns F, Ten Hoor F, Saris WHM. Determination of total gastric volume, gastric secretion and residual meal using the double sampling technique of George. *Gut* 1988;29:1725–1729.
24. Ghoos YF, Maes BD, Geypens BJ, et al. Measurement of gastric emptying rate of solids by means of a carbon-labeled octanoic acid breath test. *Gastroenterology* 1993;104:1640–1647.
25. Braden B, Adams S, Duan L-P, et al. The [^{13}C]-acetate breath test accurately reflects gastric emptying of liquids in both liquid and semisolid test meals. *Gastroenterology* 1995;108:1048–1055.
26. Choi M-G, Camilleri M, Burton DB, Zinsmeister AR, Forstrom LA, Spreekumaran Nair K. [^{13}C]Octanoic acid breath test for gastric emptying of solids: accuracy, reproducibility, and comparison with scintigraphy. *Gastroenterology* 1997;112:1155–1162.
27. van Nieuwenhoven MA, Wagenmakers AJM, Senden JMG, Brouns F, Brummer R-JM. The assessment of gastric emptying of liquids during exercise using a [^{13}C]-acetate breath test. *Gastroenterology* 1997;112:A843.
28. Heading RC, Nimmo J, Prescott LF, Tothill P. The dependence of paracetamol absorption on the rate of gastric emptying. *Br J Pharmacol* 1973;47:415–421.
29. Hirakawa K, Iida M, Fuchigami T, Murata S, Matsumoto T, Fujishama M. Sulfamethizole absorption test for the assessment of gastric emptying. *Scand J Gastroenterol* 1995;30:133–138.
30. Avill R, Mangnall YF, Bird NC, et al. Applied potential tomography new non-invasive technique for measuring gastric emptying. *Gastroenterology* 1987;92:1019–1026.
31. Holst JJ, Schmidt P. Gut hormones and intestinal function. *Baillieres Clin Endocrinol Metab* 1994;8:137–164.
32. Peeters TL, Matthijs G, Depoortere I, Cachet T, Hoogmartens J, Vantrappen G. Erythromycin is a motilin receptor agonist. *Am J Physiol* 1989;257:G469–G474.
33. Pironi L, Stanghellini V, Miglioli M, et al. Fat-induced ileal brake in humans: a dose-dependent phenomenon correlated to the plasma levels of peptide YY. *Gastroenterology* 1993;105:733–739.
34. Lin HC, Zhao X-T, Wang L, Wong H. Fat-induced ileal brake in the dog depends on peptide YY. *Gastroenterology* 1996; 110:1491–1495.
35. Brummer R-M, Armbrecht U, Bosaeus I, Dotevall G, Stockbrügger RW. The hydrogen (H_2) breath test: sampling methods and the influence of dietary fibre on fasting levels. *Scand J Gastroenterol* 1985;20:1007–1013.
36. Armbrecht U, Jensen J, Edén S, Stockbrügger RW. Assessment of orocoecal transit time by means of a hydrogen (H_2) breath test as compared with aradiologic control method. *Scand J Gastroenterol* 1986;21:669–677.
37. Von der Ohe MR, Camilleri M. Measurement of small bowel and colonic transit: indications and methods. *Mayo Clin Proc* 1992;67:1169–1179.
38. Kamm MA. The small intestine and colon: scintigraphic quantitation of motility in health and disease. *Eur J Nucl Med* 1992; 19:902–912.
39. Bjarnason I, MacPherson A, Hollander D. Intestinal permeability: an overview. *Gastroenterology* 1995;108:1566–1581.
40. Hollander D. The intestinal permeability barrier: a hypothesis as to its regulation and involvement in Crohn's disease. *Scand J Gastroenterol* 1992;27:721–726.
41. Travis S, Menzies I. Intestinal permeability: functional assessment and significance. *Clin Sci* 1992;82:471–488.
42. Fordtran JS, Levitan R, Bikerman V, Burrows BA. The kinetics of water absorption in the human intestine. *Trans Assoc Am Physician* 1961;42:195–205.
43. Cooper H, Levitan R, Fordtran JS, Ingelfinger FJ. A method for studying absorption of water and solute from the human small intestine. *Gastroenterology* 1966;50:17.
44. Whalen GE, Harris JA, Geenen JE, Soergel KH. Sodium and water absorption from the human small intestine: the accuracy of the perfusion method. *Gastroenterology* 1966;51:975–984.
45. Cummings JH, Englyst HN. Gastrointestinal effects of food carbohydrates. *Am J Clin Nutr* 1995;61(suppl):938S–945S.
46. Hinton JM, Lennard-Jones JE, Young AC. A new method for studying gut transit times using radioopaque markers. *Gut* 1969;10:842–847.
47. Cummings JH, Wiggins HS. Transit through the gut measured by analysis of a single stool. *Gut* 1976;17:219–223.
48. Arhan P, Devroede G, Jehannin B, et al. Segmental colonic transit itime. *Dis Colon Rectum* 1981;24:625–629.
49. Metcalf AM, Philips SF, Zinsmeister AR, MacCarty RL, Beart RW, Wolff BG. Simplified assessment of segmental colonic transit. *Gastroenterology* 1987;92:40–47.
50. Krevsky B, Malmud LS, D'Ercole F, Maurer AH, Fisher RS. Colonic transit scintigraphy: a physiologic approach to the quantitative measurement of colonic transit in humans. *Gastroenterology* 1986;91:1102–1112.
51. Kamm MA, Lennard-Jones JE, eds. *Constipation.* Petersfield, UK: Wrighton Biomedical Publishing, 1994.
52. Kuijpers JHC. Transit time measurement. In: Buchman P, Bruhlman W, eds. *Investigations of anorectal function disorders.* Berlin: Springer Verlag, 1993:115–118.
53. Goei R. Anorectal function in patients with defecation disorders and asymptomatic subjects: evaluation with defecography. *Radiology* 1990;174:121–123.
54. Brouns F. Etiology of gastrointestinal disturbances during endurance events. *Scand J Med Sci Sports* 1991;1:66–77.
55. Keeffe EB, Lowe DK, Gross JR, Wayne R. Gastrointestinal symptoms of marathon runners. *West J Med* 1984;141:481–484.
56. Riddoch C, Trinick TR. Gastrointestinal disturbances in marathon runners. *Br J Sports Med* 1988;22:71–74.

57. Worobetz LJ, Gerrard DF. Gastrointestinal symptoms during exercise and endurance athletes: prevalence and speculations of the etiology. *N Z Med J* 1985;98:644–646.
58. Rehrer NJ, Beckers EJ, Brouns F, Ten Hoor F. Effects of dehydration on gastric emptying and gastrointestinal distress while running. *Med Sci Sports Exerc* 1990;22:790–795.
59. Peters HPF, van Schelven FW, Verstappen PA, et al. Gastrointestinal problems as a function of carbohydrate supplements and mode of exercise. *Med Sci Sports Exerc* 1993;25:1211–1225.
60. Sandell RC, Pascoe MD, Noakes TD. Factors associated with collapse during and after ultramarathon foot races: a preliminary study. *Physician Sports Med* 1988;16:86–94.
61. Brouns F, Beckers EJ. Is the gut an athletic organ? Digestion, absorption and exercise. *Sports Med* 1993;15:242–257.
62. Konturek S, Falser J, Obtulowicz W. Effect of exercise on gastrointestinal secretions. *J Appl Physiol* 1973;34:324–328.
63. Wade OL, Combes B, Chilos AW, et al. The effect of exercise on the splanchnic blood flow and splanchnic blood volume in normal men. *Clin Sci* 1956;15:457–463.
64. Rowell LR, Blackmon JR, Bruce RA. Indocyanin green clearance and estimated blood flow during mild to maximal exercise in upright man. *J Clin Invest* 1964;43:1677–1690.
65. Clausen JP. Effect of physical training on cardiovascular adjustments to exercise in man. *Physiol Rev* 1977;57:779–815.
66. Galbo H. Gastroenteropancreatic hormones. In: Galbo H, ed. *Hormonal and metabolic adaptation to exercise.* New York: Thieme, 1983:59–61.
67. Vandewalle HC, Lacombe JC, Lereivre A, Poirot C. Blood viscosity after 1 hr submaximal exercise with and without drinking. *Int J Sports Med* 1988;9:104–107.
68. Moses FM. The effect of exercise on the gastrointestinal tract. *Sports Med* 1990;9:159–172.
69. Reference deleted in proofs.
70. Shawdon A. Gastro-oesophageal reflux and exercise: important pathology to consider in the athletic population. *Sports Med* 1995;20:109–116.
71. Clark CS, Kraus BB, Sinclair J, Castell DO. Gastroesophageal reflux induced by exercise in healthy volunteers. *JAMA* 1989;261:3599–3601.
72. Kraus BB, Sinclair JW, Castell DO. Gastroesophageal reflux in runners: characteristics and treatment. *Ann Intern Med* 1990; 112:429–433.
73. Soffer EE, Merchant RK, Duethman G, Launspach J, Gisolfi C, Adrian TE. Effect of graded exercise on esophageal motility and gastroesophageal reflux in trained athletes. *Dig Dis Sci* 1993; 38:220–224.
74. Soffer EE, Wilson J, Duethman RK, Launspach J, Adrian TE. Effect of graded exercise on esophageal motility and gastroesophageal reflux in nontrained subjects. *Dig Dis Sci* 1994; 39:193–198.
75. Peters O, Peters P, Clarys JP, De Meirleir K, Devis G. Esophageal motility and exercise. *Gastroenterology* 1988;94:A351.
76. Schoeman MN, Tippett MD, Akkermans LMA, Dent J, Holloway RH. Mechanisms of gastroesophageal reflux in ambulant healthy human subjects. *Gastroenterology* 1995;108:83–91.
77. Brouns F, Saris WHM, Rehrer NJ. Abdominal complaints and gastrointestinal function during long-lasting exercise. *Int J Sports Med* 1987;8:175–189.
78. Sherman WM, Lamb DR. Nutrition and prolonged exercise. In: Lamb DR, Murray RM, eds. *Perspectives in exercise science and sports medicine. Volume 1: Prolonged medicine.* Indianapolis: Benchmark Press, 1988:261–264.
79. Maughan RJ. Fluid and electrolyte loss and replacement in exercise. *J Sports Sci* 1991;7:117—142.
80. Murray R. The effects of consuming carbohydrate-electrolyte beverages on gastric emptying and fluid absorption during and following exercise. *Sports Med* 1987;4:22–51.
81. Moore JG, Datzl FL, Christian PE. Exercise increases solid meal gastric emptying rates in men. *Dig Dis Sci* 1990;35:28–32.
82. Brouns F, Senden J, Beckers EJ, Saris WHM. Osmolarity does not affect the gastric emptying rate of oral rehydration solutions. *J Parenter Enter Nutr* 1995;19:403–406.
83. Vist GE, Maughan RJ. The effect of osmolality and carbohydrate content on the rate of gastric emptying of liquids in man. *J Physiol* 1995;486:523–531.
84. Noakes TD, Adams BA, Myburgh KH, Greeff C, Lotz T, Nathan M. The danger of an inadequate water intake during prolonged exercise. *Eur J Appl Physiol* 1988;57:210–219.
85. Hawley JA, Dennis SC, Noakes TD. Oxidation of carbohydrate ingested during prolonged endurance exercise. *Sports Med* 1992;14:27–42.
86. Rehrer NJ, Brouns F, Beckers EJ, Ten Hoor F, Saris WHM. Gastric emptying with repeated drinking during running and bicycling. *Int J Sports Med* 1990;11:238–243.
87. Notivol R, Carrio I, Cano L, Estorch M, Vilardell F. Gastric emptying of solid and liquid meals in healthy young subjects. *Scand J Gastroenterol* 1984;19:1107–1113.
88. McMurray RG, Forsythe WA, Mar MH, Hardy CJ. Exercise intensity-related responses of beta-endorphin and catecholamines. *Med Sci Sports Exerc* 1987;19:570–574.
89. O'Connor AM, Johnston CF, Buchanan KD, Boreham C, Trinick TR, Riddoch CJ. Circulating gastrointestinal hormone changes in marathon running. *Int J Sports Med* 1995;16:283–287.
90. Cammack JN, Read W, Cann A, et al. Effect of prolonged exercise on the passage of a solid meal through the stomach and the small intestine. *Gut* 1982;23:957–962.
91. Keeling WF, Martin BJ. Gastrointestinal transit during mild exercise. *J Appl Physiol* 1987;63:978–981.
92. Keeling WF, Harris A, Martin BJ. Orocecal transit during mild exercise in women. *J Appl Physiol* 1990;68:1350–1353.
93. Meshkinpour H, Kemp C, Fairshter R. Effect of aerobic exercise on mouth-to-cecum transit time. *Gastroenterology* 1989;96: 938–941.
94. Soffer EE, Summers RW, Gisolfi C. Effect of exercise on intestinal motility and transit time in athletes. *Am J Physiol* 1991; 260:G698–G702.
95. Peters HPF. Gastrointestinal symptoms and dysfunction during prolonged exercise. Thesis, Utrecht University, 1995.
96. Koffler KH, Menkes A, Redmon RA, et al. Strength training accelerates gastrointestinal transit in middle-aged and older man. *Med Sci Sports Exerc* 1992;24:415–419.
97. Liu F, Toda Y. Brief physical inactivity prolongs colonic transit time in elderly men. *Int J Sports Med* 1993;14:465–467.
98. Harrison RJ, Leeds AR, Bolster NR. Exercise and wheat bran: effect on whole gut transit. *Proc Nutr Soc* 1980;32:22A.
99. Evans DF, Foster GE, Hardcastle DJ. Does exercise affect the migrating motor complex in man? In Roman C, ed. *Gastrointestinal motility*. Boston: MTP Press, 1984:277–284.
100. Evans DF, Foster GE, Hardcastle DJ. Does exercise affect small bowel motility in man? *Gut* 1989;24:A1012.
101. Ollerenshaw KJ, Norman S, Wilson CG, Hardy JG. Exercise and small intestinal transit. *Nucl Med Commun* 1987;8:105–110.
102. Fordtran JS, Saltin B. Gastric emptying and intestinal absorption during prolonged severe exercise. *J Appl Physiol* 1967;23: 331–335.
103. Barclay GR, Turnberg LA. Effect of moderate exercise on salt and water transport in the human jejunum. *Gut* 1988;29:816–820.
104. Winne D. Models of the relationship between drug absorption and the intestinal blood flow. In: Shepherd AP, Granger DN, eds. *Physiology of intestinal circulation.* New York: Raven Press, 1984:289.
105. Maughan RJ, Leiper JB, McGaw A. Effects of exercise intensity on absorption of ingested fluids in man. *Exp Physiol* 1990; 75:419–421.
106. Sladen GEG. *Methods of studying intestinal absorption in man: intestinal absorption in man.* London: Academic Press, 1975.
107. Heargraves M, Costill D, Burke L, et al. Influence of sodium on glucose bioavailability during exercise. *Med Sci Sports Exerc* 1994;26:365–368.
108. Rehrer NJ, Wagenmakers AJM, Beckers EJ, et al. Gastric emptying, absorption and carbohydrate oxidation during prolonged exercise. *J Appl Physiol* 1992;72:468–475.
109. Shi X, Summers RW, Schedl HP, Chang RT, Lambert GP, Gisolfi CV. Effects of solution osmolality on absorption of select fluid replacement solutions in human duodenojejunum. *J Appl Physiol* 1994;77:1178–1184.
110. Gisolfi CV, Duchman SM. Guidelines for optimal replacement

beverages for different athletic events. *Med Sci Sports Exerc* 1992;24:679–687.
111. Hunt JB, Elliot EJ, Faiclough PD, et al. Water and solute absorption from hypotonic glucose-electrolyte solutions in the human jejunum. *Gut* 1992;33:479–483.
112. Leiper JB, Maughan RJ. Comparison of absorption rates from two hypotonic and two isotonic rehydration solutions in the intact human jejunum. *Clin Sci* 1988;75:22P.
113. Haglund U. Gut ischemia. *Gut* 1994;35:S73–S76.
114. Bulkley GB, Kvietys PR, Parks DA, et al. Relationship of blood flow and oxygen consumption to ischemic injury in the canine small intestine. *Gastroenterology* 1985;89:852–857.
115. Schoenberg MH, Fredholm B, Haglund U, et al. Studies on the oxygen radical mechanism involved in the small intestinal reperfusion damage. *Acta Physiol Scand* 1985;124:581–589.
116. Øktedalen O, Lunde OC, Opstad PK, Aabakken L, Kvernebo K. Changes in the gastrointestinal mucosa after long-distance running. *Scand J Gastroenterol* 1992;27:270–274.
117. Moses F, Singh A, Smoak B, et al. Alterations in intestinal permeability during prolonged high-intensity running. *Gastroenterology* 1991;100:A472.
118. van Nieuwenhoven MA, Geerling BJ, Deutz NEP, Brouns F, Brummer R-JM. Gut permeability test in subjects with and without exercise-induced gastrointestinal symptoms. *Gut* 1996; 39(suppl 3):A247.
119. Ryan AJ, Chang R-T, Gisolfi CV. Gastrointestinal permeability following aspirin intake and prolonged running. *Med Sci Sports Exerc* 1996;28:698–705.
120. Donald IP, Smith RG, Cruickahank JG, Elton RA, Stoddart ME. A study of constipation in the elderly living at home. *Gerontology* 1985;31:112–118.
121. Colditz GA, Cannuscio CC, Frazier AL. Physical activity and reduced risk of colon cancer: implications for prevention. *Cancer Causes Control* 1997;8:649–667.
122. Sullivan SN. The gastrointestinal symptoms of running. *N Engl J Med* 1981;304:915.
123. Cordain L, Latin RW, Behnke JJ. The effects of an aerobic running program on bowel transit time. *J Sports Med* 1986; 26:101–104.
124. Bingham SA, Cummings JH. Effect of exercise and physical fitness on large intestine function. *Gastroenterology* 1989;97: 1389–1399.
125. Robertson G, Meshkinpour H, Vandenberg K, James N, Cohen A, Wilson A. Effects of exercise on total and segmental colon transit. *J Clin Gastroenterol* 1993;16:300–303.
126. Robertson G, Meshkinpour H, Vandenberg K, James N, Cohen A, Wilson A. Effects of exercise on total and segmental colon transit. *Gastroenterology* 1990;98:A385.
127. Sesboue B, Arhan P, Devroede G, et al. Colonic transit in soccer players. *J Clin Gastroenterol* 1995;20:211–214.
128. Cheskin LJ, Crowell MD, Kamal N, Rosen B, Schuster MM, Whitehead WE. The effects of acute exercise on colonic motility. *J Gastrointest Motil* 1992;4:173–177.
129. Cummings JH. Diet and transit through the gut. *J Plant Foods* 1978;3:83–95.
130. Stephan AM, Cummings JH. Mechanism of action of dietary fibre in the human colon. *Nature* 1980;284:283–284.
131. Niemann DC. Vegetarian dietary practices and endurance performance. *Am J Clin Nutr* 1988;48:754–761.
132. Rehrer NJ, van Kemenade MC, Meester TA, Brouns F, Saris WHM. Gastrointestinal complaints in relation to dietary intakes in triathletes. *Int J Sports Nutr* 1992;2:48–59.
133. DeYoung VR, Rice HA, Steinhaus AH. Studies in the physiology of exercise. VII. The modification of colonic motility induced by exercise and some indications for a nervous mechanism. *Am J Physiol* 1931;99:52–63.
134. Dawson DJ, Khan AN, Shreeve DR. Psoas muscle hypertrophy: mechanical cause for "jogger's trots?" *Br Med J* 1985;291: 787–788.
135. Nurko S, Dunn BM, Rattan S. Peptide histidine isoleicine and vasoactive intestinal polypeptide cause relaxation of opposum internal anal sphincter via two distinct receptors. *Gastroenterology* 1989;96:403–413.
136. Hilsted J, Galbo M, Sonne B, et al. Gastroenteropancreatic hormonal changes during exerise. *Am J Physiol* 1980;239:G136–G140.
137. Sullivan SN, Champion MC, Christofides ND, Adrian TE, Blom SR. Gastrointestinal regulatory peptides responses in long distance runners. *Physician Sports Med* 1984;12:77–82.
138. Øktedalen O, Opstad P, Schaffalitzky de Muckadel OB. The plasma concentrations of secretin and vasoactive intestinal polypeptide (VIP) after long-term, strenuous exercise. *Eur J Appl Physiol* 1983;52:5–8.
139. Riddoch CJ. Exercise-induced gastrointestinal symptoms, hormonal involvement. Thesis. Queens University, 1990, Belfast, Ireland.
140. MacLaren DP, Raine NM, O'Connor AM, Buchanan KD. Human gastrin and vasoactive intestinal polypeptide responses to endurance running in relation to training status and fluid ingested. *Clin Sci* 1995;89:137–143.
141. Philipp E, Wilckens T, Friess E, Platte P, Pirke K-M. Cholecystokinin, gastrin and stress hormone responses in marathon runners. *Peptides* 1992;13:125–128.
142. Grider JR. Role of cholecystokinin in the regulation of gastrointestinal motility. *J Nutr* 1994;124:1334S–1339S.
143. Banfi G, Marinelli M, Bonini P, Gritti I, Roi GS. Pepsinogens and gastrointestinal symptoms in mountain marathon runners. *Int J Sports Med* 1996;17:554–558.

Exercise and Sport Science,
edited by William E. Garrett, Jr., and Donald T. Kirkendall.
Lippincott Williams & Wilkins, Philadelphia © 2000.

CHAPTER 14

Renal Responses to Exercise and Training

Gilbert W. Gleim

Classic exercise physiology pays little attention to the kidneys and their function in exercising animals. Unlike other important organs during exercise, blood flow and oxygen consumption are apt to decline in the kidneys. By doing so, the kidneys play the starring role in helping to maintain vascular volume, which is of paramount importance in the preservation of cardiac output. Reestablishing the balance of electrolytes and water following exercise is another important aspect of renal function, as is the clearance of nitrogenous waste products, which are in greater supply following exercise and meals. The kidneys also have important endocrine functions that are necessary for both acute exercise and adaptations to chronic exercise, especially at altitude and in hot environments. Even though the kidneys do not seem to exhibit any major conditioning effects from exercise training, without functioning kidneys maximal training effects are impossible to attain.

ANATOMY AND PHYSIOLOGY OF THE KIDNEYS

At rest, the kidneys receive about 20% of total cardiac output so that the entire blood volume circulates through the kidneys approximately 288 times per day. About 10% of the blood volume (around 125 mL/min) that enters into the kidneys is filtered into the urinary space. Consequently, if it were not for the miraculous ability to reabsorb fluids, electrolytes, and other substances small enough to be filtered, the kidneys would dispose of the entire fluid volume of the body in less than 45 minutes. This remarkable function is made possible by a filtration and reabsorption system based on an anatomic structure that takes advantage of fundamental physical principles, diffusion, and countercurrent exchange, as well as active transport processes. While the body is naturally endowed with a pair of kidneys, the loss of one kidney is without effect on normal homeostasis.

G. W. Gleim: Research Institute, Mission St. Joseph's Hospital, Asheville, North Carolina 28801; Department of Physiology, New York Medical College, Valhalla, New York 10458.

RENAL BLOOD FLOW

The aorta gives rise to bilateral renal arteries, which upon entering the kidneys branch into interlobar arteries. Interlobar arteries in turn give rise to arcuate arteries. The extensive branching of the arcuate arteries into afferent arterioles marks the beginning of the functional unit of the kidneys, the nephron. Upon entering the glomerulus the afferent arterioles give rise to the glomerular capillaries, which terminate in another arteriole, the efferent arteriole. This unique arrangement provides vascular smooth muscle on either side of the capillary bed in the glomerulus, thus allowing for hydrostatic pressure regulation within the glomerular capillaries either upstream or downstream (Fig. 14–1). Increasing smooth muscle tone in the afferent arterioles results in decreased glomerular hydrostatic pressure, while increased efferent arteriolar tone results in increased glomerular hydrostatic pressure. It is important to understand this concept since it forms the basis of blood flow regulation and glomerular filtration by the kidneys.

The efferent arteriole gives rise to the peritubular capillary network in the renal cortex. It also gives rise to the vasa recta, another capillary network that plunges deep into the renal medulla and surrounds the loop of Henle. By running in the opposite direction of the filtrate, it takes advantage of the countercurrent exchange principle. The important characteristic of blood within these capillary networks is that it has already passed through the glomerulus and is thus filtered of many of the normal constituents of blood. These capillaries

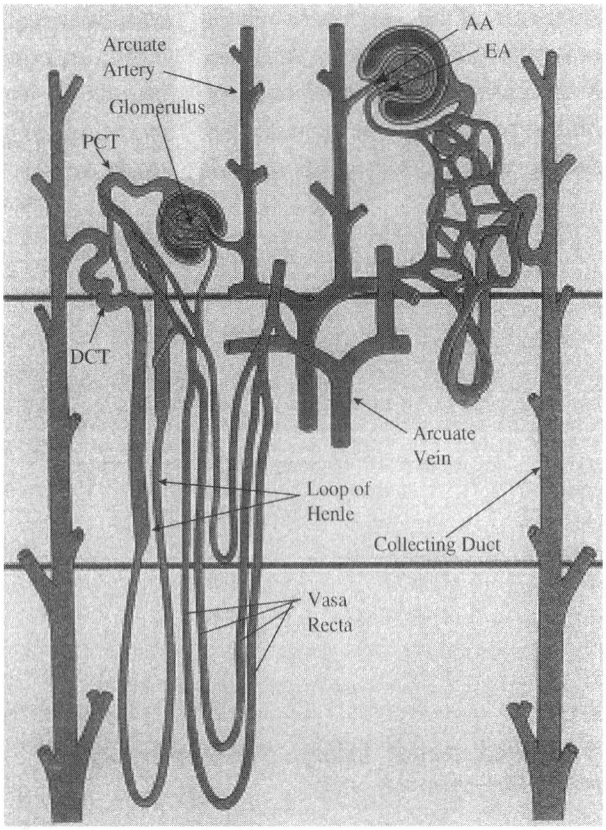

FIG. 14–1. Two adjacent nephrons with the left being juxtamedullary and the right being juxtacortical. *Top horizontal line* represents demarcation between renal cortex (*above*) and renal medulla (*below*). Second *vertical line* represents demarcation between superficial and deep medulla. Common collecting ducts accept many nephrons. *AA*, afferent arteriole; *EA*, efferent arteriole; *DCT*, distal convoluted tubule; *PCT*, proximal convoluted tubule.

coalesce into the arcuate veins, which in turn drain into the interlobar veins.

THE URINARY SPACE

Bowman's capsule contains the glomerular capillaries as well as the beginning of the urinary space of the kidneys. The cells that surround the glomerular capillary cells consist of endothelial cells, which are perforated by numerous small holes called fenestrae. A basement membrane of collagen and proteoglycans is on the other side, and finally epithelial cells line the outer surface of the glomerulus. This discontinuous layer of cells contains numerous slit pores for passage of water and other molecules.

The glomerular space leads next to the proximal tubule. The proximal tubule continues to the loop of Henle, which, depending on the location of that particular nephron (cortical or juxtamedullary), plunges down and up through the medulla. The loop of Henle terminates in the distal tubule, which in turn drains into the cortical collecting ducts (see Fig. 14–1). Cortical collecting ducts drain into collecting ducts and into the renal pelvis. Urine exits the kidneys through the ureter.

Nephrons that are located near the outer surface of the kidneys are called juxtacortical nephrons and are characterized by a shorter loop of Henle. Deeper nephrons that plunge down deeply into the medulla are called juxtamedullary nephrons and are characterized by longer loops of Henle. Because they penetrate into renal parenchyma, which has a higher osmolality, they are better at creating a concentrated urine. It is possible that filtration characteristics of juxtamedullary and juxtacortical glomeruli differ, and that renal blood flow (RBF) changes perfusion of these nephrons during exercise so that the deeper nephrons are used. In discussing nephron characteristics, we tend to treat all nephrons as if they were the same. This simplification is necessary since it is nearly impossible to study function of deeper nephrons that do not allow for micropuncture characterization. As a result, the heterogeneity of nephron function remains a relatively unexplored area of renal physiology.

GLOMERULAR FILTRATION

Movement of fluid, solutes, and larger-molecular-weight substances across the glomerulus is a function of hydrostatic pressure, colloid osmotic pressure, and the size, and, to some extent, the ionic charge of the glomerular pores.

By the time blood has passed to the end of the afferent arteriole, its hydrostatic pressure has dropped to around 60 mm Hg, and by the end of the glomerular capillary bed it has dropped further to about 15 mm Hg. Pressures this high are atypical for most capillary beds and provide for a high force favoring filtration from the blood into the urinary space. Because the hydrostatic pressure drops some 45 mm Hg across the glomerular capillaries, forces favoring filtration from the blood are stronger at the beginning of the glomerular capillary bed (Fig. 14–2).

Colloid osmotic pressure is primarily a function of the protein content of the blood. Because proteins (primarily albumin by amount in the blood) are large-molecular weight substances, they do not pass readily through the glomerular membrane. Colloid osmotic pressures at the beginning of the glomerulus are about 28 mm Hg and have increased to about 36 mm Hg by the end of the glomerulus because of loss of fluid (about 20%) into the urinary space. The combined effects of hydrostatic pressure and colloid osmotic pressure favor filtration at the beginning of the glomerulus (by about 60 − 28 mm Hg or 32 mm Hg) and reabsorption at the end of the glomerulus (by about 15 − 36 mm Hg or −21 mm Hg).

Physical characteristics of the glomerular membrane

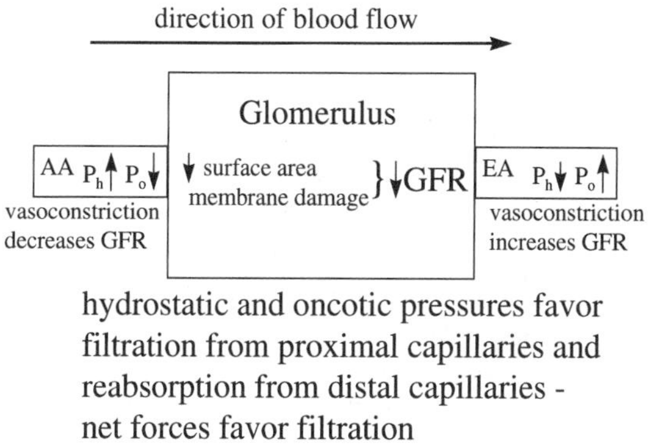

FIG. 14–2. Schematic diagram depicting factors that influence glomerular filtration rate (GFR). *AA*, afferent arteriole; *EA*, efferent arteriole; *Ph*, hydrostatic pressure; *Po*, osmotic pressure.

also have a large influence upon what is filtered. The size of the pores in the membrane is about 8 nanometers (nm), which allows for the passage of all electrolytes and substances having molecular weights up to 10,000. Albumin, the primary protein of the blood, has a molecular weight of 69,000 and a molecular diameter of about 6 nm. Theoretically, its size should allow it to pass through the glomerular membrane with relative ease as well, but the proteoglycan basement membrane has a net negative charge as does the albumin molecule. The similar charge causes the albumin to be repelled by the basement membrane, with the net effect being that very little albumin normally passes into the urinary space (perhaps 0.5%). Notably, all types of blood cells are much too large to pass through the glomerular membrane under normal circumstances.

Mathematically, it is possible to express the glomerular filtration rate (GFR) as an equation reflecting the above-mentioned factors:

$$\text{GFR} = (P_{\text{hydrostatic}} - P_{\text{oncotic}}) \times K_f$$

K_f is referred to as the ultrafiltration coefficient and is a reflection of the physical factors that affect the filtration membrane. In addition to the above-mentioned characteristics, glomerular surface area will have an effect on the K_f, and factors that decrease the surface area will decrease K_f. $P_{\text{hydrostatic}}$ refers to the hydrostatic pressures and P_{oncotic} refers to the colloid osmotic pressures. In humans, the normal GFR is 125 mL/min.

Often it is convenient to express the GFR as a percentage of renal plasma flow (RPF), and when multiplied by 100 this term is called the filtration fraction [FF = (GFR/RPF) × 100].

The composition of the glomerular filtrate is markedly similar to the blood, less the proteins and cellular constituents. In fact, the filtrate has the same concentrations as the blood for the following substances: sodium, potassium, calcium (ionized), magnesium, chloride, bicarbonate, phosphate ions, sulfate, glucose, urea, uric acid, and creatinine. Concentrations of major proteins (globulins and albumin) are detectable but negligible. The urine that is ultimately formed has significantly lower concentrations of sodium, bicarbonate, and glucose (which should be undetectable in the urine). Alternatively, the urine has significantly increased concentrations of potassium, magnesium, chloride, phosphate, sulfate, urea, uric acid, and creatinine.

Because concentrations of substances change as they pass through the kidney tubules, we know that some are reabsorbed and others are actively secreted. Therefore, any substance that is used to measure GFR must satisfy the following criteria: it must be freely filtered at the glomerulus and it must not be reabsorbed or secreted by the tubules. Inulin, a sugar, is such a substance that is not made by the body; when it is infused into the blood to establish a constant concentration and its excretion is measured in the urine, one has the most precise determination of GFR. Creatinine, the principal breakdown product of creatine, is a surrogate marker for GFR, but it is actually secreted to some extent by the proximal tubules. Further, creatinine generation is constant only when metabolic rate is constant and when no exogenous creatine from the diet is introduced. *Since creatinine generation is not constant during or following exercise, its use as a measure of GFR during and following exercise is flawed.* Nevertheless, much of what we assume to be true about glomerular function during exercise in humans is based on the measurement of creatinine.

TUBULAR FUNCTION

An important aspect of the blood leaving the glomerulus is that it has a higher colloid osmotic pressure than the filtrate, thus favoring fluid reabsorption, and it has a similar concentration of many freely filterable substances, as mentioned above. Additionally, the hydrostatic pressures in the blood vessels that have left the glomerulus and ultimately surround the tubules are below 15 mm Hg and thus favor reabsorption as well.

By far the greatest proportion of the glomerular filtrate is reabsorbed by the proximal tubule, so that by the time the filtrate reaches the loop of Henle only 35% remains. The highly active cells in the proximal tubule have numerous ways of reabsorbing sodium and water, and the composition of the filtrate by the end of the proximal tubule is isosmotic with the plasma. Importantly, under normal circumstances, none of the filtered glucose reaches the loops of Henle unless the amount filtered, such as might occur in poorly controlled diabetics or with an epinephrine surge at the end of exercise, exceeds the tubular maximum of the proximal tubules. Glucose passing through the proximal tubule will appear in the final urine because no other cells distal to this point have the ability to cotransport glucose back into the bloodstream. Similarly, many amino acids are cotransported back. Finally, the vast majority of filtered proteins are reabsorbed by the process of pinocytosis so that normally only trace amounts are excreted daily.

The rest of the kidneys are directed at reabsorbing more water and certain solutes by virtue of the concentration gradients that develop in the kidneys as the tubules migrate deeper into the medulla and because different segments of the kidneys are selectively impermeable to some ions as well as water. The net result with respect to water reabsorption is that only 0.7% of what is filtered remains in the urine, with the greatest changes made possible in the collecting duct under the control of vasopressin.

Two major waste products that are concentrated in the urine are urea and creatinine. Urea is produced at a rate of 25 to 30 g per day and will be higher in individuals consuming a high-protein diet. Generally speaking, about 60% of the urea that is filtered by the glomerulus appears in the urine, but this amount will decrease if GFR falls and urea remains in the tubules for prolonged periods of time. The urea that is reabsorbed is an important component of the increased osmolality of the renal medulla, an important physical force promoting water reabsorption in the collecting duct. It is beyond the scope of this chapter to detail the myriad mechanisms responsible for the composition of the final urine, and the reader is urged to consult one of the renal physiology texts referenced at the end of the chapter.

HORMONE INFLUENCES ON THE COMPOSITION OF THE URINE

Two important hormones that increase in concentration during exercise are aldosterone and vasopressin (antidiuretic hormone, ADH). A third important hormone, which is made by the kidneys, is renin, and this hormone results ultimately in the formation of angiotensin II.

Aldosterone, a mineralocorticoid, is secreted by the adrenal medulla in response to a number of factors. Angiotensin II and high potassium levels are the primary stimuli to aldosterone release. It is possible that aldosterone release is nonselectively stimulated by adrenocorticotropic hormone (ACTH) as well. All of these factors are evident during exercise and all are likely to promote the aldosterone release that is evident even at low levels of exercise. Aldosterone has its most specific action on the distal tubule of the nephron and promotes the exchange of sodium for potassium, reabsorbing sodium and secreting potassium. Since sodium is the primary osmole of the extracellular fluid, its retention by the kidneys helps to maintain water volume in the vascular space.

Vasopressin is produced by the posterior pituitary gland in response to increased osmolality of the blood and decreased blood volume. The decrease in urine volume produced by vasopressin is rapid, and it exerts its effect by increasing the permeability to water of the cells of the collecting duct. Without vasopressin, these cells are normally impermeable to water, but in its presence they allow water to follow its osmotic pressure gradient into the renal medulla. The net effect is that a more concentrated urine is produced when blood volume is reduced or its osmotic concentration is increased.

Angiotensin II is one of the most powerful vasoconstrictors produced by the body. In addition to its effects on vascular smooth muscle, it causes contraction of certain cells (mesangial cells) composing the glomerulus. Because the GFR is influenced by the surface area of the filtration membrane, the reduction caused by angiotensin II will result in a decrease in GFR and a reduction in urine formation. Angiotensin II also increases resistance to blood flow in the kidneys, and this will also decrease GFR.

HORMONE PRODUCTION BY THE KIDNEYS

Renin

As mentioned above, the kidneys produce a hormone called renin. Granules containing renin are located in specialized cells of the afferent and efferent arterioles called juxtaglomerular cells. These cells are innervated by nerves of the sympathetic nervous system. At this point in the nepron the distal convoluted tubule contacts the juxtaglomerular (JG) cells as well. Both the neural innervation and the contact with the distal convoluted tubule influence release of renin by the JG cells.

Increased sympathetic nervous stimulation to the kidneys results in renin release, as do increased levels of epinephrine. The increased sympathetic stimulation will decrease blood flow past the JG cells; because the cells sense this, by perhaps decreased contact with the distal convoluted tubule, renin is released. Renin will also be released by direct stimulation of beta receptors on the JG cells as well. Finally, if the volume of filtrate in the distal tubule is small, this too is sensed by the JG cells and causes them to release renin. It is noteworthy that there are redundant mechanisms available for the release of renin because this protein is responsible for the powerful mechanisms available to the body for maintaining vascular volume and retaining sodium.

Renin causes the cleaving of an α_2-globulin circulating in the blood to form angiotensin I. Angiotensin I has minimal biologic activity until it is converted to angiotensin II by an enzyme found in great supply in the pulmonary circulation—converting enzyme. Angiotensin II is the active component of the renin cascade. Converting enzyme inhibitors are a popular choice for antihypertensive medication because they are associated with minimal side effects, and they have never been shown to impact exercise performance.

Erythropoietin

The other major hormone produced by the kidneys is erythropoietin (EPO). It is a glycoprotein weighing between 39,000 and 70,000 atomic mass units (u) and is produced in minute amounts when the kidneys are subjected to hypoxia. It is believed that in reality the kidneys do not directly produce EPO but rather an erythropoietic factor that acts on a globulin within the blood to split away the EPO molecule. EPO acts on the bone marrow to stimulate red blood cell production.

Any form of chronic hypoxia will increase the production of EPO by the kidneys. Typically, athletes travel to high altitudes (>5000 feet) to stimulate its production, but the increase in red blood cell mass that results takes at least 5 days. Living at high altitude is much more important than training at altitude because short exposures to hypoxia are not as useful in promoting EPO production. Any pathologic condition, such as heart failure, lung failure, or anemia, that creates hypoxia in the kidneys will also promote increased EPO production. In addition, end-stage renal disease results in a near-total lack of EPO, and until recombinant EPO was manufactured the resulting anemia was profound. Today, patients with end-stage renal disease are routinely given EPO to maintain a hematocrit in the range of 32%. Higher levels are associated with an increased likelihood of strokes. This is a useful point about which to remind the athlete who is trying to increase red blood cell mass with this banned substance.

ACUTE RESPONSES TO EXERCISE

Blood Flow and Glomerular Filtration Rate

Normal blood flow to the kidneys is about 4 mL/min/g tissue, compared to only 0.04 mL/min/g muscle at rest. The situation changes dramatically with exercise, and with high intensities RBF may decrease by 30% to 40% based on the clearance of para-amino hippuric acid (1). By comparison, active muscle blood flow may be as high as 5 to 8 mL/min/g (2). The decline in RBF is especially striking in light of the 300% to 400% increase in cardiac output. Declines in blood flow are intensity dependent.

Decreased RBF results from increased renal vascular resistance, due primarily to both afferent and efferent arteriolar constriction. Increased sympathetic stimulation to the kidneys is the primary determinant of the increased vascular tone (3). Angiotensin II levels are also increased from increased plasma renin activity, and this may be a response to the increased sympathetic activity to the JG cells as well as a result of decreased renal blood, GFR, and sodium in the tubular filtrate. The net effect is that two powerful vasoconstricting agents (norepinephrine and angiotensin) are maintaining the increase in renal vascular resistance (Fig. 14–3).

Both norepinephrine and angiotensin promote the formation of vasodilating prostaglandins within the kidney medulla. It is felt that these autocoids are of paramount importance in helping to maintain blood flow to the deep nephrons, providing oxygen for the active metabolic processes of concentrating the urine. Inhibition of prostaglandin synthesis with nonsteroidal antiinflammatory drugs (NSAIDs) has been associated with acute renal failure in athletes, such as marathon runners, who have experienced prolonged and potentially dehydrating exercise. While these are rare occurrences, athletes who habitually use NSAIDs are at an increased risk for acute renal failure following prolonged dehydrating exercise.

Despite the pronounced decline in RBF with exercise of increasing intensity, GFR is protected in its decline until higher-intensity exercise is encountered. This phenomenon is a function of autoregulation of GFR. In essence the percentage of RBF that is filtered by the glomerulus (filtration fraction) is increased. Remembering the factors that determine GFR, filtration fraction can be increased by increasing the efferent arteriolar resistance more than the afferent arteriolar resistance, which would increase intraglomerular hydrostatic pressures. An alternative explanation is that K_f is increased.

With exercise of sufficient intensity, GFR will eventually decline. A decline in the amount of filtered substrate will result in a decrease in fluid and electrolyte excretion as well. It should be remembered, however, that protein catabolism is increased during exercise and nitrogenous waste (urea) and creatinine formation are increased as a result. That being the case, it is likely that GFR must be increased following exercise either transiently or for some period of time, but this is a little known aspect of renal function. If this were not the case, individuals who habitually exercise vigorously would eventually accumulate high levels of nitrogenous waste products, and this is certainly not evident in that population.

Paradoxically, low levels of exercise have been associated with increases in urine flow and sodium excretion (4). Furthermore, it has been shown that urine flow rate correlates highly to GFR during dynamic exercise ($r = 0.91$) and that increases in urine flow rates at low intensities of exercise (25%) are associated with modest increase in GFR (5). These same authors demonstrated that atrial natriuretic hormone was modestly increased at this work rate and that vasopressin was mildly decreased. Either change could explain the increase in urine flow, although atrial natriuretic hormone levels continue to increase during exercise. At sufficiently high levels of exercise (80%), GFR declined dramatically but urine osmolality actually decreased, suggesting that urine concentrating ability may be compromised at sufficiently high intensities of exercise. Figure 14–4 demon-

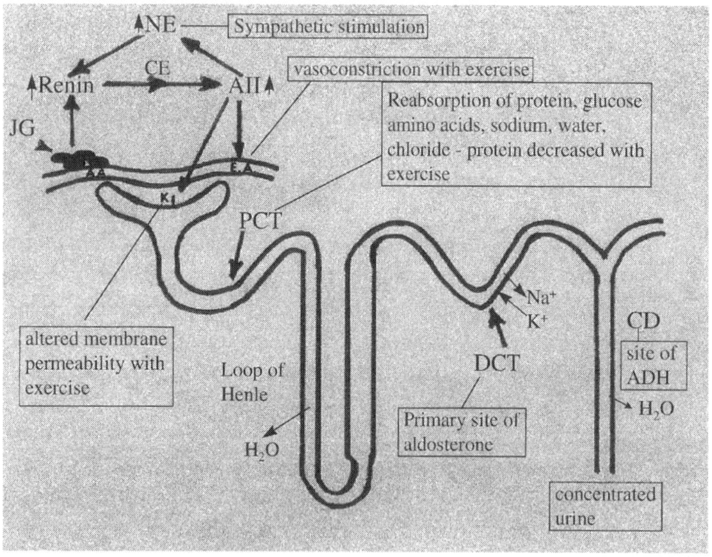

FIG. 14–3. A summary of changes occurring in the kidneys during exercise. *AA,* afferent arteriole; *ADH,* antidiuretic hormone; *AII,* angiotensin II; *CD,* collecting duct; *CE,* converting enzyme; *DCT,* distal convoluted tubule; *EA,* efferent arteriole; *JG,* juxtaglomerular cells; K_f, ultrafiltration coefficient; *NE,* norepinephrine; *PCT,* proximal convoluted tubule. (See text for details.)

strates changes in RBF, GFR, and urine flow during exercise of increasing intensity.

People with compromised renal function may experience falls in GFR even at low levels of exercise. Normal subjects who exercised at a heart rate barely exceeding 100 beats per minute (BPM) experienced some decline in RBF with no change in GFR, while patients with moderate renal impairment experienced about a 33% decline in GFR (6). This would mean that such patients have compromised autoregulation of GFR.

Plasma renin activity (PRA) is increased significantly only when high-enough levels of exercise are encountered. We have demonstrated that PRA can be shown to be related to the lactate threshold (7). Consequently, this represents a point during exercise when the kidneys are experiencing profound decreases in blood flow or augmented sympathetic stimulation. Inhibition of angiotensin II formation by converting enzyme inhibitors was without effect on urinary parameters in nine subjects exercising at 60% of maximum oxygen consumption for 45 minutes, although this degree of blockade did produce a decline in mean arterial blood pressure preceding, during, and following exercise (8). Aldosterone levels do not seem to be related to any threshold phenomena and demonstrate significant increases even with mild levels of exercise (9). Aldosterone release during exercise may be responding to increases in serum potassium levels that occur even with mild exercise.

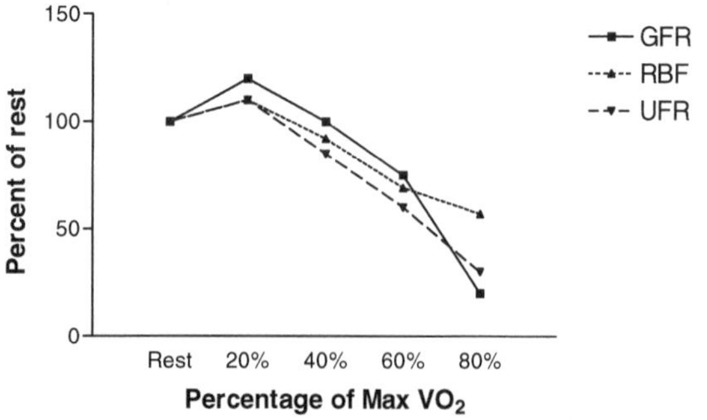

FIG. 14–4. Graph depicting relative changes in renal function following about 15 to 20 minutes of exercise at the indicated percentages of maximum oxygen consumption ($\dot{V}O_2max$). *GFR,* glomerular filtration rate; *RBF,* renal blood flow; *UFR,* urine flow rate. Note that with low levels of exercise intensity, there are likely to be actual increases in GFR, RBF, and UFR.

Changes in Urine Composition

Osmolality of the urine is markedly influenced by the baseline hydration status of the individual. Normal osmolality of the blood is about 300 mOsm/L. With massive fluid ingestion, the kidneys can produce large amounts of free water clearance so that the osmolality is as low as 65 mOsm/L. Under maximal states of dehydration, urine osmolality can attain levels as high as 1200 mOsm/L or perhaps slightly higher. Short-term acute exercise of moderate intensity is associated with an increase in urine osmolality of about 40 mOsm/L. Higher-intensity exercise is associated with declines in tubular function as noted above, and urine osmolality can actually decrease as a result (5). Notably, the volume of urine production is typically depressed at high levels of exercise because of the pronounced declines in GFR and the antidiuretic and antinatriuretic hormone milieu evident with high levels of exertion.

Normally cells of the collecting duct are impermeable to water, and this serves to prevent further concentration of the urine as the collecting duct passes through the deep levels of the renal medulla where osmolality is high (up to 1200 to 1400 mOsm). During exercise of sufficient intensity, vasopressin levels are increased. Cells of the collecting duct respond to this increase by allowing water to follow the concentration gradient from the urine to the peritubular space. Hence, the increased levels of vasopressin further serve to cause an increase in the osmolality of the urine and decrease the amount of urine produced. The extent to which vasopressin levels are elevated depends to a large degree on the hydration status of the exercising individual as well as the ambient temperature and rate of fluid loss.

The responses of vasopressin to water exercise are complicated by the known effects of immersion on increases in central blood volume and the subsequent suppression of vasopressin. Typically, water immersion is associated with a diuresis, natriuresis, and kaliuresis. Subjects who are exercised in water respond with a decreased natriuresis and diuresis. Consequently, the exercise stimulus is sufficient to prevent the suppression of vasopressin release and may be associated with an increased release (10). Nevertheless, comparable levels of exercise in water vis-à-vis on land are likely to be associated with a less-pronounced decline in urine flow rate.

A known consequence of intense exercise is proteinuria, which under other conditions could indicate underlying renal pathology. Young individuals without any evidence of renal disease increased albumin excretion from a resting level of 6.5 μg/min to more than 24 μg/min following 25 minutes of exercise at a heart rate of 155 BPM (11). Increases in protein excretion have been noted as high as 100-fold following intense exercise (12).

Changes in glomerular permeability are likely to be a part of the reason that protein excretion is increased during intense exercise. Remembering that filtration fraction is increased (by up to 50%) it is possible that even though renal blood is dramatically reduced, hydrostatic pressures may be increased in the glomerulus with relatively greater efferent arteriolar vasoconstriction than afferent arteriolar vasoconstriction. Increased glomerular permeability may also be due to changes in the charges associated with the pores in the glomerulus, and this has been implicated in some diseases. It is also thought that there is a partial inhibition of tubular reabsorption of the plasma proteins that normally pass through the glomerulus (13), and this too will result in increased levels of protein in the urine. Changes in plasma volume and the extent of dehydration do not seem to be related to the rate at which protein levels in the urine return to normal, and increased albumin excretion can be evident even when normal levels of creatinine excretion have been reestablished 2 hours following exercise (14). Individuals who already have indications of proteinuria at rest will have even greater evidence of proteinuria following exercise.

Because proteinuria is not uncommon following exercise, especially intense exercise, it is useful to question athletes about the last time they exercised when obtaining a urine sample for routine medical tests. If elevations in protein levels are found in the urine within 48 hours of athletic activity, the assessment should be repeated after the athlete has been instructed to rest for 24 to 48 hours. Generally speaking, proteinuria from exercise has never been associated with any long-term sequelae (15).

Microscopic hematuria is another abnormality that may appear in an athlete or military recruit following intense exercise of longer duration. Originally designated as "march" hematuria following prolonged treks by military personnel, it has been more recently named sports hematuria, and there may be a number of causes. Initially, it was thought that disruption of red blood cells in the feet caused by mechanical pounding released hemoglobin into the blood and subsequently some of this appeared in the urine. Now, following documentation by cystoscopy of bleeding in the urinary bladder, the most likely source of red blood cells in the urine is mechanical trauma to the posterior bladder wall on the trigone. It has been proposed that keeping some urine in the bladder may help to prevent this occurrence (16). Hypoxic damage to the kidneys from intense exercise represents a possible, albeit remote, etiology for sports hematuria. Finally, direct trauma to the kidneys from physical contact may represent a potentially fatal circumstance, and it is usually associated with gross hematuria and physical symptoms such as flank pain and hypotension. Contusions to the kidneys that result in frank hematuria require immediate medical management.

The iron-containing pigments hemoglobin and myoglobin are toxic to the renal tubules. Intense exercise, whether associated with dehydration or not, can result in rhabdomyolysis and massive release of myoglobin into the bloodstream. Even though the ingestion of large quantities of water may not be the most rapid way of replacing intracellular stores of water, the production of high urine flow rates following exercise serves to maintain a dilute urine and will mitigate the toxic effects of myoglobin or hemoglobin that is filtered into the urinary space. Acute tubular necrosis resulting from these pigments may not be evident until 24 hours or longer following exercise or physical exertion. Individuals who are unaccustomed to exercise are at the greatest risk of acute renal failure following exercise (17).

RESPONSES TO CHRONIC EXERCISE

Blood Flow and Glomerular Filtration Rate

Despite the pronounced changes that occur in RBF and GFR with higher-intensity exercise, no one has documented any adaptive long-term changes in renal function. Since GFR can decline substantially during exercise and remain suppressed for at least some period following exercise, it is surprising that no one has documented renal function for a long-enough period of time following exercise to observe any increase in GFR to compensate for the lower GFR during exercise. Since exercise represents a catabolic state for protein, production of urea and uric acid must be increased. Increased urea excretion, over and above what would be expected in a resting state, has never been documented following exercise.

A single study in mice documented an increase in kidney weight/body weight ratio in older trained mice as well as an increase in mesangial damage and capillary lumen obliteration that was not evident in younger trained mice or older controls (18). No study has been able to corroborate these results in humans, and there exists no epidemiologic evidence to suggest that chronic, lifelong exercise is associated with decrements in renal function. Older individuals have been shown to have lower resting RBF and to experience less of a decline in flow when exercising at similar intensity (50% max $\dot{V}O_2$max) as younger individuals. Additionally, RBF remained depressed during recovery for a longer period of time in the older group (19). GFR was not measured in that study.

The blood pressure–lowering effects of exercise can theoretically be related to changes in renal function since the kidneys play a primary role in the long-term maintenance of blood pressure. In this regard, exercise training sufficient to lower blood pressure and to increase $\dot{V}O_2$max by 12% in habitually sedentary, healthy men has been shown to lower sympathetic activity to the kidneys without an apparent effect on cardiac sympathetic activity, even though resting heart rate was decreased (presumably by increased vagal tone). The increase in total body vascular conductance was explained in part by an increase in renal vascular conductance (20). It is possible that the decrease in sympathetic stimulation to the kidneys represents a long-term conditioning effect enabling the body to more readily dissipate salt and volume overloads. This is speculative at this time.

EXERCISE TRAINING IN CHRONIC RENAL FAILURE AND END STAGE RENAL DISEASE

Despite the falls in GFR that occur with higher levels of exercise and the increased protein excretion associated with higher levels of exercise, one is hard pressed to find any evidence in the literature that exercise contributes to renal disease or to a more rapid decline in renal function in those with chronic renal failure. Alternatively, exercise training has never been associated with an amelioration of chronic renal failure or to a decreased incidence of renal disease, contrary to the effects of physical activity on cardiovascular disease. The incidence of renal diseases is much lower than that of cardiovascular disease, and this may make any epidemiologic association difficult to discern.

In the early 1980s a number of facilities were interested in the effects of exercise on hemodialysis patients, since this is a population that suffers from significant cardiovascular morbidity. Before the time when routine recombinant EPO therapy was available, we found that dialysis patients had an average maximum oxygen consumption of around 5 metabolic equivalents (METs) and that a walking and jogging program could improve this value some 20% (21). A number of other investigators have also documented similar numbers (22). Thus, the disability of chronic renal failure coupled with life-maintaining renal replacement therapy is profound. EPO therapy has improved the functional status of these patients somewhat, but even the ability of these patients to return to work is low and is unlikely to exceed 20%.

REFERENCES

1. Castenfors J. Renal clearances and urinary sodium and potassium excretion during supine exercise in normal subjects. *Acta Physiol Scand* 1967;70:207–214.
2. Guyton AC. *Textbook of medical physiology*, 6th ed. Philadelphia: WB Saunders, 1981:344.
3. Tidgen B, Hjemdahl P, Theodorsson E, Nussberger J. Renal neurohormonal and vascular responses to dynamic exercise in humans. *J Appl Physiol* 1991;70:2279–2286.
4. Kachadorian WA, Johnson RE. Renal responses to various rates of exercise. *J Appl Physiol* 1970;28:748–752.
5. Freund BJ, Shizuru EM, Hashiro GM, Claybaugh JR. Hormonal, electrolyte, and renal responses to exercise are intensity dependent. *J Appl Physiol* 1991;70:900–906.
6. Taverner D, Craig K, Mackay I, Watson ML. Effects of exercise on renal function in patients with moderate impairment of renal function compared to normal men. *Nephron* 1991;57:288–292.
7. Gleim GW, Zabetakis PM, Depasquale EE, Michelis MF, Nicholas JA. Plasma osmolality, volume and renin activity at the "anaerobic threshold." *J Appl Physiol* 1984;56:57–63.
8. Mittleman KD. Influence of angiotensin II blockade during exercise in the heat. *Eur J Appl Physiol* 1996;72:542–547.
9. Gleim GW, Zabetakis PM, Coplan NL, Michelis MF, Nicholas JA. Hyperkalemia during progressive dynamic exercise. *J Cardiopulmon Rehab* 1988;8:33–37.
10. Rim H, Yun YM, Lee KM, et al. Effect of physical exercise on renal response to head-out water immersion. *Appl Human Sci* 1997;16:35–43.
11. Torffvit O, Castenfors J, Agardh CD. A study of exercise-induced microalbuminuria in type I (insulin-dependent) diabetes mellitus. *Scand J Urol Nephrol* 1991;25:39–43.
12. Poortmans JR. Post exercise proteinuria in humans—facts and mechanisms. *JAMA* 1985;253:236–240.
13. Poortmans JR. Renal response to exercise in healthy and diseased patients. *Nephrologie* 1995;16:317–324.
14. Poortmans JR, Rampaer L, Wolfs J-C. Renal protein excretion after exercise in man. *Eur J Appl Physiol* 1989;58:476–480.
15. Cianflocco AJ. Renal complications of exercise. *Clin Sports Med* 1992;11:437–451.
16. Eichner ER. Hematuria: a diagnostic challenge. *Phys Sports Med* 1990;18:53–63.

17. Knochel JP. Rhabdomyolysis and myoglobinuria. *Semin Nephrol* 1981;1:75.
18. Lichtig C, Levy J, Gershon D, Reznick AZ. Effect of aging and exercise on the kidney. *Gerontology* 1987;33:40–48.
19. Kenny WL, Zappe DH. Effect of age on renal blood flow during exercise. *Aging Clin Exp Res* 1994;6:293–302.
20. Meredith IT, Friberg P, Jennings GL, et al. Exercise training lowers resting renal but not cardiac sympathetic activity in humans. *Hypertension* 1991;18:575–582.
21. Zabetakis PM, Gleim GW, Pasternak FL, Saraniti A, Nicholas JA, Michelis MF. Long-duration submaximal exercise conditioning in hemodialysis patients. *Clin Nephrol* 1982;18:17–22.
22. Painter PL. Exercise in end-stage renal disease. In: Pandolf KB, ed. *Exercise and sports science reviews,* vol 16. New York: Macmillan, 1988:305–339.

SUGGESTED READINGS (General Renal Physiology)

Brenner BM, Rector FL Jr. *The Kidney,* vol 1, 2nd ed. Philadelphia: WB Saunders, 1981.

Guyton AC. *Textbook of medical physiology,* 6th ed. Philadelphia: WB Saunders, 1981:403–445.

Schrier RK, Gottschalk CW. *Diseases of the kidney,* vol 1, 5th ed. Boston: Little, Brown, 1993.

Exercise and Sport Science,
edited by William E. Garrett, Jr., and Donald T. Kirkendall.
Lippincott Williams & Wilkins, Philadelphia © 2000.

CHAPTER 15

Skeletal Responses to Exercise and Training

Diane M. Cullen, Urszula T. Iwaniec, and M. Janet Barger-Lux

The skeleton is a living, dynamic system that adapts to the mechanical loads of exercise. Mechanical forces regulate bone size and structure in combination with genetics, nutrition, and biochemistry (1–4). Compared to other systems, such as the cardiovascular and muscular systems, bone adaptation to exercise is slower and the increments in size and strength are smaller. As a result, bone adaptation is more difficult to measure. Wolff first discussed the relationship between daily forces and bone structure in 1870, and a full century elapsed before human exercise intervention studies for bone were published (5–7).

The exercise benefits for bone are now so widely accepted that exercise is recommended for the prevention of osteoporosis (8). Despite the widespread acceptance of exercise, limited information is available on effective exercise prescription for bone health. Most of our knowledge on exercise prescription comes from animal studies in which exercise and lifestyle variables are controlled and invasive techniques permit accurate quantification of the stimulus and response. The most effective human exercise programs use knowledge from these studies while maximizing diet and hormonal variables (9–11). This chapter presents a conceptual framework for mechanical regulation of bone and summarizes the results from effective exercise programs.

MECHANICAL REGULATION OF BONE MASS AND SIZE

Bone activation with mechanical loading begins with tissue distortion and continues until the size and shape of the bone have been altered to prevent further distortion and fracture.

Strain as a Stimulus for Bone Adaptation

One function of bones in our body is to serve as stiff levers and beams for support and movement. Forces from muscle contraction and impact loading create compression, tension, torsion, and shear stresses within bone that result in minuscule shape distortions, bending, or deformation. The degree of deformation is measured by gauges attached directly to the bone surface and recorded as strain (ε), or the change in length relative to original length. Forces that create $-1000\ \mu\varepsilon$ compress or shorten bone by 0.1%. The degree of distortion or strain magnitude during loading is directly proportional to the applied forces and inversely proportional to the size and distribution of the bone (Fig. 15–1). Moment of inertia (MI) measures the distribution of bone tissue relative to a neutral axis and reflects the resistance of bone to bending. The greater the bone mass and the farther the mass is located from the neutral axis, the greater the MI and the lower the strain for any given force. The bone adapts to repeated high strains by increasing MI and creating resistance to continued distortion.

Strain as a measure of bone adaptation is analogous to heart rate as a measure of cardiovascular adaptation. With training, the heart muscle strength increases in terms of maximal stroke volume, while bone strength increases in terms of maximal breaking strength. The larger and more efficient the heart, the lower the heart rate at a given metabolic level during training. Similarly with bone, the larger, stiffer, and stronger the bone, the lower the strain during loading at a given force (see Fig. 15–1). As a marker of intensity during exercise, target heart rates for training and maximal heart rates are fairly similar among individuals. In parallel, target bone strains for hypertrophy and maximal strain before failure are also fairly stable. Both heart rate and strain are relative markers for intensity of stimulation and fitness.

Although exercise stimulates systemic cardiovascular and hormonal responses, exercise interventions act di-

D. M. Cullen, U. T. Iwaniec, and M. J. Barger-Lux: Creighton University, Osteoporosis Research Center, Omaha, Nebraska 68131.

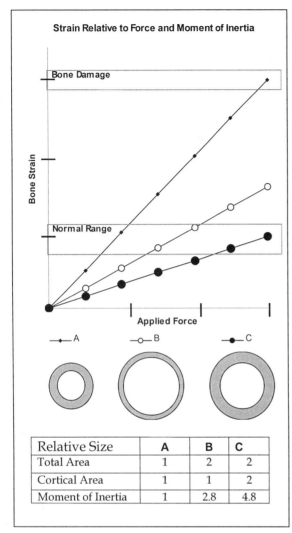

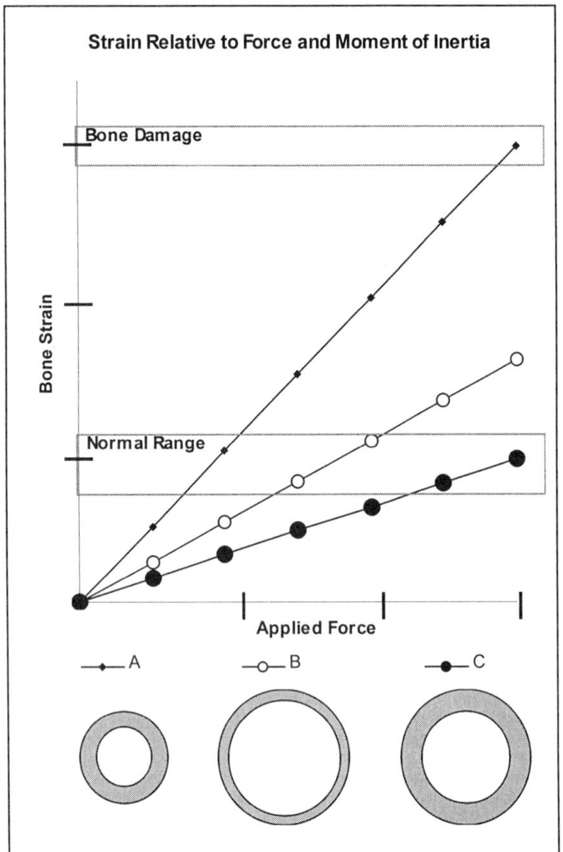

Relative Size	A	B	C
Total Area	1	2	2
Cortical Area	1	1	2
Moment of Inertia	1	2.8	4.8

FIG. 15–1. The graph and drawing represent three bone sizes: (*A*) small, dense; (*B*) large, low density; and (*C*) large, dense. Bone size and structure are reported relative to the smallest bone. During loading, strain increases in proportion to the applied force, but is inversely proportional to moment of inertia. Bone adapts to maintain an acceptable or normal range of peak strains. These bones have adapted to different ranges of forces. Low forces in *A* (sedentary) create normal daily peak strains, moderate forces in *B* (mild activity), and high forces in *C* (athletic). As a result, bone damage will occur at lower forces for bone *A* than *B* or *C*.

rectly on the loaded bones, causing localized adaptations to prevent failure or fracture. Activities that create strains stimulate formation in loaded or targeted bones, but not in nonloaded bones (12–15). Strain or bending of the bones is the mechanical signal that triggers a biochemical response. Physical deformation of bone tissue creates local fluid flow in canaliculi and matrix, cell cytoskeletal distortion, and streaming potentials within the tissue. These stimulate bone cell production of autocrine and paracrine factors for cell proliferation, differentiation, and bone formation (16). This local release of growth factors is an efficient mechanism to increase mass and strength selectively at the loaded bone sites.

The primary stimulus for bone activation is strain magnitude or the degree of shape distortion (17). Other important factors include strain rate, number and frequency of load repetitions, and angle of load application (18–20). With large strains, relatively few repetitions are needed to initiate formation, but as strain magnitude decreases, the number of repetitions needed increases exponentially (21). Activities such as gymnastics and ballet that create high impact, require rapid acceleration and deceleration, and involve strong muscle contractions most effectively increase bone mass (22,23).

The Mechanical Set-Point for Bone Size and Shape

In healthy young individuals, daily loading patterns and strains regulate bone formation and resorption to establish sufficient bone mass and appropriate structure to prevent excessive strain and fracture. Bone shape and size are maintained so that there is a wide safety margin between peak strains during movement and strains that will create bone damage. Peak strains are the highest strains measured during loading. In most animal species, the peak bone strains during such varied activities as running, flying, and chewing range from 2100 to 3200 $\mu\varepsilon$ (Table 15–1) (24). Shear strains in humans range from 800 $\mu\varepsilon$ in walking to 2000 $\mu\varepsilon$ in vigorous cross-country running (25). A single load that produces strains threefold greater than these peaks will result in bone damage, while strains fivefold greater will result in fracture (24). Figure 15–1 depicts the relationship between bone stiffness and force in terms of normal and bone-damaging strains. Bone A, which has adapted to lower forces than bones B and C, will experience bone-damaging strains at lower forces than the stiffer bones (B and C).

Strain as the controlling variable for mechanical regulation of bone is described by Frost's (26) mechanostat theory. This paradigm suggests that bone mass is regulated around a mechanical set-point so that normal daily peak strains are within an acceptable range. Daily peak strains might be viewed as loading intensity, representing a composite of strain magnitude, number, and rate

TABLE 15–1. *Strain in activity and fracture (24)*

Bone activity	Strain ($\mu\varepsilon$)
Peak strain measured in animal	2100–3200
Bone damage (yield load)	6800
Bone fracture (ultimate load)	15,700
Threshold for formation (theoretical) (108)	1500

of repetitions. Adaptation begins when training creates an overload and cells detect strains above the normal strain range. Adaptation ceases when the exercise is no longer an overload and strains return to the normal range. The bone formation response is a transient period of increased formation that results in greater resistance to bending. As the bone adapts to the new training or loading level, formation returns to normal baseline levels. The minimum effective strain (MES) required to stimulate significant bone formation in healthy young adults is postulated to be 1500 $\mu\varepsilon$ (27). This is consistent with animal artificial loading models where strains greater than 1000 $\mu\varepsilon$ are sufficient to initiate formation (17,28). Based on *in vivo* human tibia strain measurements, 1500 $\mu\varepsilon$ can be achieved in well-trained subjects by vigorous activity (25).

The mechanostat theory suggests that systemic variables such as hormones and pharmaceutical agents can alter the mechanical set-point, either increasing or decreasing sensitivity and response to strain. With aging and menopause, sensitivity is decreased and the safety margin between normal strains and bone damage decreases until fractures occur during routine activities.

Bone Adaptation to Altered Mechanical Loads

Four mechanical usage windows or levels are disuse, adapted, mild overload, and pathologic overload (26). The adapted window represents normal daily strains and activities that maintain, but do not stimulate, new bone formation. This normal strain range could be achieved with running and jumping by an athlete, or walking by a sedentary person. Bone mass and shape remain stable, but bone turnover occurs through remodeling to replace damaged bone or maintain homeostasis. Remodeling is a tightly coupled process of osteoclast bone resorption immediately followed by osteoblast bone formation at the same site. The resorption phase lasts 4 to 6 weeks and the entire process of resorption and formation lasts 4 to 6 months. Ideally, by the end of the remodeling period bone mass is unchanged (26). With aging, menopause, and calcium deficiency, remodeling often results in bone loss.

Disuse is the removal of normal high strains, and it results in bone loss. It is seen most dramatically with bed rest, immobilization, or space flight, but it also occurs to a smaller extent with lifestyle changes that eliminate intense activities and increase sedentary activities. Bone loss occurs as osteoclast activity increases without an equal increase in osteoblast activity, and the net result is incomplete filling of the remodeling site.

Bone Response to Mild Overloads

Bone adapts to increased loading by increasing its resistance to bending through modeling. Modeling is the process of bone growth in which bone-forming cells (osteoblasts) and bone-resorbing cells (osteoclasts) work on different bone surfaces to model or shape bone. It normally results in a net increase in bone mass. This process predominates in growing children, increasing the outer diameter and the marrow cavity, and tapering the long bones at the metaphysis to form the diaphysis (26). It was believed that modeling occurred only in adults with fracture healing, but exercise has been shown to initiate modeling in adult bone (12,29). In exercise-induced modeling in adults, osteoblasts initiate bone formation on new surfaces and osteoclasts are suppressed (29–31). This differential effect on osteoblasts and osteoclasts is unique to mechanical loading. The cellular responses are usually greater on the surfaces with the greatest change in strain, such as the outer periosteal surface. The net effect is a dose-response increase in bone mineral content and bone area (17,28).

Bone Response to Pathologic Overloads

Excessive activities that apply high loads or high repetitions of loads over a period of a couple of weeks are pathologic and can lead to stress fractures (32). Although the normal strains during physical activity are only one-third of that required for fracture with one repetition, lower loads can result in fracture if repeated often enough (33). The number of repetitions to fracture increases exponentially as force decreases. Bones are predicted to fracture after one repetition at 15,000 $\mu\varepsilon$ and after 1 million repetitions at 2000 $\mu\varepsilon$. These fractures are first evident as microdamage or cracks in bone. The internal damage weakens the structure and decreases the bone stiffness, making it more susceptible to fracture with continued loading. Remodeling is subsequently stimulated to remove and replace the damaged tissue. As the damaged tissue is resorbed, porosity increases, causing a transient bone loss. The already weakened bone is most susceptible to fracture during this phase. As the overload continues or increases, further damage and resorption sites are initiated, compounding the risks of fracture. In military basic training, fractures are most common in the first 4 to 6 weeks when fatigue damage resorption is predicted to be greatest (34). If loading is decreased when injury is diagnosed and the bone has time to complete the remodeling and repair process, then bone mass and strength should be restored. As in military recruits, stress fractures are common in athletes, especially those with negative calcium balance due to poor diet or amenorrhea (35).

The Calcium and Bone Relationship

The relationship between calcium and bone is unique among nutrients. The skeleton is a mineral storehouse as well as an engineering structure; to meet immediate metabolic needs, the structural function will be sacrificed to meet the metabolic needs. Calcium can be withdrawn from the skeleton only by tearing down bone. A chronic shortage of calcium (secondary to low intake, poor absorption, excessive loss, or any combination of these) prevents "borrowed" bone from being fully replaced. Thus, excessive withdrawals of skeletal calcium inevitably reduce bone mass and strength. This process eventually produces permanent damage by destroying portions of the trabecular plates and struts that cannot be replaced. Without a sufficient nutrient supply of calcium, mechanical loading cannot maintain or increase bone strength.

The body of an adult woman includes roughly 900 to 1100 g of calcium, 99% in the skeleton (bone is 20% to 25% calcium by weight), 7 to 8 g in cells, and 1 g in fluids and blood. As the concentration of ionized calcium in the extracellular fluid (ECF, which includes the fluid fraction of blood) falls (e.g., as calcium is withdrawn to mineralize new bone), the amount of parathyroid hormone (PTH) released into the circulation increases. PTH acts in several ways. It stimulates new osteoclast formation and indirectly enhances bone resorption, thereby increasing input of calcium from bone into the ECF. PTH also increases renal tubular calcium reabsorption, thereby reducing urinary calcium loss. This effect, like the level of a dam at the downstream end of a pond, is the principal determinant of ECF calcium level. PTH also promotes the kidney conversion of 25-hydroxyvitamin D into a more active hormone, calcitriol (1,25-dihydroxyvitamin D). Calcitriol enhances calcium entry into the ECF by increasing the efficiency of intestinal calcium absorption and osteoclastic bone resorption.

Both direct and indirect evidence supports the hypothesis that early humans had high calcium intakes. Archaeologic evidence reveals that the hunter-gatherers who lived before the dawn of agriculture had heavy skeletons and were comparable in stature to present-day groups. A careful examination of the foods available to those early hunter-gatherers indicates that daily calcium intakes in excess of 1800 mg were likely (36,37). Given adequate skeletal reserves and dietary calcium, it is not surprising that humans did not develop an appetite and a taste for calcium-rich foods analogous to the drive to consume salt, a scarce component in the diets of early hunter-gatherers. Calcium intake must be consciously maintained if adequate amounts are to be available for mechanical regulation of bone.

Indirect evidence that the customary diets of our distant ancestors were calcium rich and sodium poor persists in the physiology of present-day humans. Calcium is absorbed and conserved quite inefficiently. Healthy, nonpregnant adults typically absorb only about 15% to 35% of ingested calcium. Digestive juices carry about 150 mg of calcium into the gut lumen each day, with only a similar fraction reabsorbed. The daily loss of calcium in urine is ordinarily about 110 mg, and 24-hour losses in excess of 200 mg are not unusual. The loss of calcium in sweat is apparently uncontrolled, and the limited evidence that is available suggests that athletes may lose large quantities of calcium in this way (38). In contrast, the gut absorbs sodium completely. If sodium intake is restricted, urine sodium and sweat sodium can be reduced virtually to zero.

The Basics of Calcium Nutrition

The recommendations of the 1994 Consensus Panel on Optimal Calcium Intake, convened by the National Institutes of Health, are listed in Table 15–2 (39). Roughly two-thirds of the calcium in the United States food supply is in dairy products, and a daily diet without calcium-rich foods provides only about 200 to 300 mg of calcium. Because low-calcium diets are usually also deficient in many other nutrients, simply taking a calcium supplement cannot repair the nutritional error of avoiding calcium-rich foods (40). The most recent national data show that median calcium intake among U.S. women and girls peaks at age 8 and hovers at only about 600 mg throughout adult life. Relatively few adult women in the United States ingest calcium in recommended quantities (41). Findings for males are only slightly less discouraging.

Intakes of protein and salt affect the individual requirement for calcium. Persons who ingest diets that are very low in both protein and salt may be able to maintain calcium balance and avoid diet-related bone

TABLE 15–2. *Recommendations for calcium intake (optimal 1998)*

Category	Ages (years)	Calcium intake (mg/day)
Children and yound adults	11 to 24	1200 to 1500
Premenopausal women	25 to 50	1000
Pregnant women		Age-specific value + 400
Postmenopausal women taking estrogen	Less than 65	1000
Postmenopausal women not taking estrogen	Less than 65	1500
Men	Less than 65	1000
Men and women	65 and over	1500

loss while ingesting as little as 400 mg of calcium a day. Conversely, calcium intakes of more than 2000 mg a day may be required to avoid diet-related bone loss when intakes of protein and salt are high. For every gram of protein ingested, urine calcium increases by about 1 mg; protein in the form of meat shifts part of this loss to the gut, but the loss occurs nonetheless (42). The 1989 estimates for typical daily salt (sodium chloride) consumption by U.S. adults was 10 to 14.5 g, with roughly one-third intrinsic to the foods, one-third added during processing, and one-third added at the table (43). The Salt Institute, the U.S. industry group that represents producers and marketers, estimates typical daily salt intake, worldwide, at 6 to 10 grams. On average, for every gram of salt ingested, urine calcium increases by about 9 mg (44). However, salt intake has been largely ignored as a factor in calcium nutrition. The effects of rigorous athletic training on individual requirements for calcium, protein, and salt have not been clearly defined.

The net effect of moderate caffeine consumption on calcium nutrition is small (45). It is presently unclear whether soft drinks have a deleterious effect on calcium balance. Different acids are used to produce acid tartness in citrus-type and cola-type soft drinks. Though the effect has not been demonstrated clinically, it is physiologically plausible to suspect that the phosphoric acid of colas may have a negative effect on calcium balance, an effect that the citric acid of citrus-type soft drinks is unlikely to evoke. However the principal threat of coffee, tea, and soft drinks to calcium nutrition probably occurs when they consistently replace milk as a dietary choice. A recent review by Heaney (46) provides further details of calcium nutrition.

Vitamin D is essential to human health and is required for optimal calcium absorption. Its natural source is sun exposure. The ultraviolet radiation that produces the precursor of vitamin D in skin (a process that plateaus after only about 15 minutes of sun exposure) is ineffective at temperate latitudes during winter. The process is also blocked by glass, sunscreen, and clothing, and is diminished in persons with dark skin and older adults. In the United States, milk (but not other dairy products) is regularly fortified with vitamin D. Other food sources of vitamin D (liver, butter, fatty fish, and egg yolks) are currently out of favor (as is sun exposure), and multivitamins are variably effective sources of vitamin D (47).

Normal ranges for 25-hydroxyvitamin D often extend down to 20 to 40 nmol/L (8 to 16 ng/mL), because, in the mistaken notion that what is abnormal is also rare, it has been customary to derive reference values from the prevailing values of ostensibly healthy adults. It is the emerging consensus among researchers, however, that vitamin D status is probably suboptimal if circulating 25-hydroxyvitamin D falls below about 80 nmol/L (32 ng/mL) (48,49). To ensure a positive calcium balance for bone accretion, both calcium intake and vitamin D levels need to be optimal.

THE EXERCISE RESPONSE IN BONE

Although the magnitude of the bone response to mechanical forces depends on the forces and strains created during exercise, hormonal milieu, and dietary intake, additional contributing factors include genetic potential and age.

Genetic Potential and Exercise

In studies that show bone gain with exercise, the variation in response to exercise intervention studies ranges from +4% to −2% in college-age women and from +15% to −7% in postmenopausal women (10,50). Undoubtedly some of the variation is due to measurement error, but some may be associated with individual potential for either exercise or bone gain. Genetic factors have been associated with 60% to 80% of the variance in bone mass (51). Genes associated with high and low bone mass or hormonal effects on bone are currently under investigation (52).

The potential for bone mass accretion with exercise may be genetically regulated, just as the potential for muscle hypertrophy varies with body type (mesomorph, endomorph, and ectomorph). In mice, there are breed differences in bone density and the bone formation response to mechanical loading (53,54). Cross-sectional studies have shown moderate correlations between bone mineral content (BMC) or bone mineral density (BMD) and body weight, height, and body composition that could potentially reflect the genetic regulation of musculoskeletal adaptation, simultaneous stimulation during exercise, or inherited body type and size. These relationships cannot be differentiated in cross-sectional studies because activity level is self-selected and self-reported. The persistence of individuals in strenuous exercise could result directly from genetic endowment and adaptive potential.

Physical Activity and Bone Across the Life Span

The potential effectiveness of exercise to alter bone mass varies with age and development. In the growing child, bone modeling is rapid, with formation increasing bone size and resorption shaping the bone. Peak bone mass is achieved by the end of the third decade (55). In adults, the skeleton is continuously remodeling or turning over, but bone mass remains stable with little or no modeling. With aging, a remodeling imbalance between resorption and formation results in 5% bone loss per decade (56). With the loss of estrogen at menopause, this imbalance can result in 10% to 15% bone loss within 10 years (56). Exercise has been shown to modulate each of these developmental phases.

Growth and Peak Bone Mass

Early in life, genetic and early developmental factors determine skeletal size. Body weight at 1 year and height at 5 years are the best predictors of total body BMC in college-age adults (57). The body weight to BMC ratio remains fairly constant with growth. In cross-sectional studies, exercise is sometimes a predictor of BMD (58–60), and calcium intake is sometimes associated with low BMD (60). However, weight and Tanner stage are stronger and more consistent predictors of bone mass during growth (58–65). These data suggest that lifestyle factors only act to modify achieved peak bone mass relative to genetic potential either by maximizing or diminishing the potential bone mass.

The exercises with the greatest association with bone size in childhood are high-impact, weight-bearing activities. Cross-sectional studies show a positive relationship between BMD and current weight-bearing activity (66). In competitive weightlifters and gymnasts, but not swimmers, bone mass is greater than in nonexercisers (67–69).

Prospective studies with prepubescent girls show that aerobic weight-bearing exercise increases BMD 2% to 10% higher than normal growth in nonexercisers (70). Similarly, 1-year elite gymnasts showed 32% to 85% greater gain in BMD than controls (71). Compared to controls, however, the gymnasts' bones tended to be shorter and thicker. These data are consistent with strenuous exercise in growing animals where bone length and width are smaller, but mass and density are greater than in controls (72). Strenuous weight-bearing exercise during growth appears to be positively associated with increase in bone mass, but it may suppress longitudinal growth.

Retrospective studies show that general physical activity before puberty and through college may have the greatest potential for increasing bone mass (59,73,74). Prepubertal training in tennis, gymnastics, and ballet has been associated with greater adult BMC. Adult female tennis players average 2% to 23% greater BMC in their dominant than their nondominant arm. The difference is two- to fourfold greater in women who began training before rather than after puberty (75). Former gymnasts, 25 years old and retired for 8 years, have higher bone mass than average, apparently retaining training benefits for years after training has ceased (71). In adult retired ballet dancers the differences from controls in proximal femur BMD were positively correlated with hours of training at ages 10 to 12 (76). Middle-aged former elite tennis players have greater lumbar and femoral neck BMD than controls and greater dominant than nondominant forearm BMD (77). These retrospective data conflict with the traditional cliché "use it or lose it" and suggest that prepubertal skeletal gains due to mechanical loading may have long-term positive effects on peak bone mass.

Peak bone mass is achieved by the late 20s, and physical activity during this period can still have a positive impact on bone mass (55). The goal during this development stage is to optimize peak bone mass and then maintain it through adulthood. From cross-sectional data, physical activity was the best lifestyle factor for predicting bone mass at the femoral neck and lumbar spine in college women (57). Longitudinal studies show that college gymnasts increase lumbar bone density during the training season (22,23). Running and weightlifting interventions during this period can increase lumbar bone density but are less effective at the hip (50).

Exercise with Amenorrhea or Oligomenorrhea

Metabolic state has a direct effect on bone cell activity and balance. Calcium balance, as discussed above, and gonadal hormones cause the most significant problems or conflicts with bone accretion from exercise. Circulating estrogen suppresses osteoclast resorption, and estrogen deficiency increases bone remodeling by activating osteoclasts. Amenorrheic and oligomenorrheic athletes are good examples of the conflict between systemic signals for bone loss and local stimuli for bone gain. In addition to overtraining, poor nutrition is often a contributing factor for amenorrhea, and calcium deficiency can compound the effects of estrogen deficiency on bone. In athletic amenorrhea, exercise can reduce this effect in loaded bones, but it has no effects in nonloaded skeletal regions. Bone density appears directly related to menstrual history; the more years and the greater the menstrual irregularity, the lower the bone density (78).

Although exercise should be a stimulus for increased bone mass, the bone density in the lower limbs and spine for amenorrheic athletes can be up to 19% less than in eumenorrheic athletes (79,80). Stress fractures in the loaded bones are more common in amenorrheic than eumenorrheic athletes. Both groups are applying similar forces, but the osteopenic bones in amenorrheic athletes have compromised strength. The nonloaded bone of amenorrheic and oligomenorrheic women is below normal and are susceptible even to low trauma fracture (35,78).

Primary amenorrhea in athletes before the attainment of peak bone mass may have lifelong consequences. Evidence suggests that bone gains attained during growth may persist into adulthood. Negative factors that slow or inhibit bone acquisition will minimize genetic potential and may permanently limit peak bone mass. These individuals will enter adulthood and menopause with lower bone mass and a higher risk of fracture than predicted by their genetic profiles.

Low bone density with intense training is not unique to women, as highly competitive male athletes also show lower than predicted bone mass (81). Although within normal ranges, triathletes and runners tend to have lower testosterone levels and bone density than controls in cross-sectional studies (82,83). In these studies bone density correlates with measures of training intensity, but not with serum testosterone. Although there is no direct evidence, a possibility exists that male gonadal hormone suppression with intense training may limit bone response to loading as it does in female athletes. Another potential possibility is that sweat calcium loss in these heavily trained men may exacerbate nutritional calcium deficiency and lead to bone loss (38).

Menopause Reduces Peak Bone Mass

In healthy women, peak bone mass is first threatened at menopause. The permanent loss of estrogen, either through menopause or surgical removal of the ovaries, stimulates resorption, with an imbalance between resorption and formation resulting in net bone loss. Although exercise does not take the role of estrogen in bone, its bone-forming stimulus can temper loss in loaded bones (84). The exercise effect may be similar for pre- and postmenopausal women (85). When the metabolic conditions for bone retention are maximized through estrogen replacement therapy, the exercise training can result in even greater bone density (11,86).

Two meta-analyses of exercise studies in postmenopausal women found that the exercise effect was significant, but that exercise did not increase lumbar bone density (87,88). Nonexercisers averaged 2.83% greater bone loss than aerobic exercise participants (87). Meta-analyses for the arm and hip found no significant exercise effects (88). This is not surprising since most of the aerobic and resistive programs were not designed to increase forearm bone mass, and the hip has proven difficult to affect with exercise. Several intervention studies that have used resistance training for the forearms have found significant bone gains (15,89). The success or failure of exercise programs to maintain bone after menopause can be explained in most cases by the type of stimulation in terms of movement pattern or strain intensity, measurement site relative to loaded regions, duration of training period, or metabolic conditions.

Fracture Prevention in the Elderly

Pharmaceutical treatments designed to prevent bone loss with aging and even to increase bone mass (e.g., bisphosphonates) are now available for the elderly. These treatments are systemic and alter total body bone balance. However, exercise intervention studies for older adults can also reduce bone loss and increase bone mass (7,90). One advantage of exercise-related bone gain is that the gains are localized to mechanically stimulated bone regions and should act to strengthen weak sites at greatest risk of fracture.

Exercise for bone in the elderly is difficult in the presence of other diseases. The level and intensity of activity required for bone gains may not be reasonable if joint disability, cardiovascular disease, or systemic problems related to other diseases or drugs limit mobility or aerobic capacity. In sedentary individuals for whom intense athletic activity is not appropriate, bone gains may be achieved with a lower level of exercise. Exercise with known positive effects include walking and seated exercises. Walking performed vigorously (1.7 m/s) several hours a week (2.6 hrs/wk) has been shown to increase calcaneal bone properties in sedentary women (91). Seated activities that require arm strength such as throwing medicine balls, squeezing tennis balls, or performing dynamic resistive exercises can be an effective way to maintain or increase arm bone density (89,92,93).

The effectiveness of exercise to prevent hip fracture probably depends more on the ability to increase mobility than the ability to strengthen the femoral neck. Based on work by Hayes and colleagues (94), most hip fractures occur when the body weight force upon landing from a sideward fall is concentrated directly on the greater trochanter. In women, these forces can range from 5000 to 6500 N and far exceed the fracture threshold for the femoral neck. For women with a femoral neck BMD value of 0.6 g/cm^2, the fracture threshold is predicted to be 3400 to 4200 N. A BMD of 1 g/cm^2 has a predicted fracture threshold of 7000 N. The primary benefits for exercise for the elderly may include increased flexibility, strength, endurance, and balance, which can all contribute to decreased risk of falls (95).

Bone Adaptation to Mechanical Load Reduction

Detraining

Whereas bone adapts to mechanical loading by increasing bone mass, the mechanostat theory predicts that the opposite occurs with unloading or disuse. In one study with postmenopausal women, a 5.2% gain in lumbar BMD after 9 months of training was reduced to baseline levels after 13 months of detraining (10). A similar but nonsignificant trend was observed in the lower limbs of young women after 1 year of training followed by 3 months of detraining (96).

Cross-sectional data from retired athletes suggests that high bone mass associated with early athletic training may be retained in adulthood, despite decreased activity (71,75,76). In a prospective study, bone gains in premenopausal women after 18 months of high-impact training were generally maintained (97). These finding are not inconsistent with Frost's mechanostat theory. Although the threshold for the mild overload window that will initiate bone formation is predicted to be relatively high (1500 $\mu\varepsilon$), the threshold for the disuse window may be very low (50 $\mu\varepsilon$). Removing all mechanical loads and reducing strains to near zero results in rapid bone loss. However, decreasing activity so that strains remain in the adapted window should not trigger a remodeling response that results in bone loss. Retired athletes and high-impact exercisers may have worked hard enough and long enough for the bones to fully adapt. When they ceased the strenuous activity of the moderate overuse window but maintained a physically active lifestyle, most of the bone gains were retained.

Inactivity and Weightlessness

Even if temporary, immobilization or removal of all mechanical loads is detrimental for bone health. Severe localized disuse osteopenia is clearly documented in the lower limbs of paraplegic individuals (98–100). Immediately after spinal cord injury, bone loss is rapid and averages 1% to 2% per month for the femur and twice that for the tibia. Temporary immobilization including bed rest results in bone loss averaging 1% per week (101–103). The lower limb bones demonstrate the greatest BMC losses, while the upper limbs show minimal loss even after prolonged bed rest. In the calcaneus, bone loss can be as high as 1.8% per week and ranges from 0.13% to 0.27% per week in the tibia, femur, and spine. The difference in bone loss rates with bed rest between lower and upper limbs can be accounted for by the greater relative unloading in the weight-bearing bones when going from normal mobility to bed rest. Bone recovery after disuse takes at least twice as long as the initial bone loss (101). Studies have shown that, even after 6 months, young men do not regain initial bone mass (103). Bone loss of the hip and lumbar spine with bed rest may be more detrimental for older, sedentary individuals with osteoporotic vertebral fractures than for young, healthy individuals. The recommendation for bed rest to relieve back pain after fracture may induce additional bone loss and muscle atrophy and can lead to increased risk of subsequent fracture. In addition, older individuals may never recover bone mass due to diminished exercise capacity after prolonged bed rest.

Space flight removes normal gravitational loads from bone and creates more extreme disuse than bed rest. This weightless environment results in a marked decline in bone mass (104,105). As with bed rest, greater bone loss occurs in the lower than in the upper limb bones. Bone mineral loss averages 1% per month, even when combined with a strenuous exercise program (104). A challenge to the research community is to devise methods for simulating normal skeletal loads in microgravity to prevent irreversible bone losses during space flight.

Appropriate Exercises

Low-intensity (load $\times$ repetitions) interventions that create very little bone strain are not effective for increasing bone in most subjects (15,106–108). The biggest gains or differences in bone mass are seen in elite athletes training in high-impact sports such as gymnastics. These exercises have the greatest effect on bone because they generate high and varied forces at multiple angles and frequencies to create maximal strains in bone. Many cross-sectional studies show the advantages in lumbar and femoral bone mass for athletes in racket sports, volleyball, basketball, dance, and weightlifting in comparison to either controls or swimmers. The advantage of competitive sports training is that athletes are encouraged for years to continually increase exercise intensity. By pushing their physical limits, they maintain a training overload to stimulate incremental gains. In contrast, the typical recreational exercise regime starts with massive overloads but eventually tapers to a comfortable routine that does not create daily overloads. Without continued overload, bone mass will no longer increase and will be maintained until metabolic factors such as menopause, calcium balance, or disease disrupt bone balance.

The best and most effective recommendations for maximizing bone mass and maintaining it might be the following:

1. Optimize metabolic conditions, such as calcium balance, by proper nutrition.
2. For maximal bone gain, exercise must stress the targeted bones with adequate force, repetitions, and varied movements.
3. For a healthy skeleton, start moving and playing young, keep it up throughout life, and adjust activities for maximum fun, fitness, and safety.
4. For sedentary people, it is never too late to start or restart an exercise program as long as the exercises are appropriate for metabolic and musculoskeletal ability.

REFERENCES

1. Carter DR. Mechanical loading history and skeletal biology. *J Biomech* 1987;20:1095–1109.
2. Cowin SC, Moss-Salentyn L, Moss ML. Candidates for the mechanosensory system in bone. *J Biomech Eng* 1991;113:191–197.
3. Frost HM. Skeletal structural adaptations to mechanical usage (SATMU): 1. Redefining Wolff's law: the bone modeling problem. *Anat Rec* 1990;226:403–413.
4. Lanyon LE. The success and failure of the adaptive response to functional load-bearing in averting bone fracture. *Bone* 1992; 13:S17–S21.
5. Roesler H. The history of some fundamental concepts in bone biomechanics. *J Biomech* 1987;11/12:1025–1034.
6. Aloia JF, Cohn SH, Babu T, Abesamis C, Kalici N, Ellis K. Skeletal mass and body composition in marathon runners. *Metabolism* 1978;2778:1793–1796.
7. Smith EL, Reddan W, Smith PE. Physical activity and calcium modalities for bone mineral increase in aged women. *Med Sci Sports Exerc* 1981;13:60–64.

8. U.S. Department of Health and Human Services. *A report of the Surgeon General, 1996.* Atlanta, GA: US Department of Health and Human Services, Centers for Disease Control and Prevention, National Center for Chronic Disease Prevention and Health Promotion.
9. Friedlander AL, Genant HK, Sadowsky S, Byl NN, Gluer CC. A two-year program of aerobics and weight training enhances bone mineral density of young women. *J Bone Miner Res* 1995; 10:574–585.
10. Dalsky GP, Stocke KS, Ehsani AA, Slatopolsky E, Lee WC, Birge SJ. Weight-bearing exercise training and lumbar bone mineral content in postmenopausal women. *Ann Intern Med* 1988; 108:824–828.
11. Kohrt WM, Snead DB, Slatopolsky E, Birge SJ. Additive effects of weight-bearing exercise and estrogen on bone mineral density in older women. *J Bone Miner Res* 1995;10:1303–1311.
12. Raab DM, Crenshaw TD, Kimmel DB, Smith EL. A histomorphometric study of cortical bone activity during increased weight-bearing exercise. *J Bone Miner Res* 1991;7:741–749.
13. Tommerup LJ, Raab DM, Crenshaw TD, Smith EL. Does weight bearing exercise affect non-weight bearing bone? *J Bone Miner Res* 1993;8:1053–1058.
14. Raab-Cullen DM, Akhter MP, Kimmel DB, Recker RR. Periosteal bone formation stimulated by externally induced bending strains. *J Bone Miner Res* 1994;9:1143–1152.
15. Kerr D, Morton A, Dick I, Prince R. Exercise effects on bone mass in postmenopausal women are site-specific and load-dependent. *J Bone Miner Res* 1996;11:218–224.
16. Brighton CT, Fisher JRS, Levine SE, et al. The biochemical pathway mediating the proliferative response of bone cells to a mechanical stimulus. *J Bone Joint Surg* 1996;78A:1337–1347.
17. Rubin CT, Lanyon LE. Regulation of bone mass by mechanical strain magnitude. *Calcif Tissue Int* 1985;37:411–417.
18. Rubin CT, Lanyon LE. Regulation of bone formation by applied dynamic loads. *J Bone Joint Surg* 1984;66A:397–402.
19. O'Connor JA, Lanyon LE, MacFie H. The influence of strain rate on adaptive bone remodelling. *J Biomech* 1982;15:767–781.
20. Lanyon LE. Using functional loading to influence bone mass and architecture: objectives, mechanisms, and relationship with estrogen of the mechanically adaptive process in bone. *Bone* 1996;18:37s–43s.
21. Whalen RT, Carter DR, Steele CR. Influence of physical activity on the regulation of bone density. *J Biochem* 1988;21:825–837.
22. Nichol DL, Sanborn CF, Bonnick SL, Gench B, DiMarco NM. The effect of gymnastics training on bone mineral density. *Med Sci Sports Exerc* 1994;26:1220–1225.
23. Taaffe DR, Robinson TL, Snow CM, Marcus R. High-impact exercise promotes bone gain in well-trained female athletes. *J Bone Miner Res* 1997;12:255–260.
24. Rubin CT, Lanyon LE. Limb mechanics as a function of speed and gait: a study of functional strains in the radius and tibia of horse and dog. *J Exp Biol* 1982;101:187–211.
25. Burr DB, Milgrom C, Fyhrie D, et al. In vivo measurement of human tibial strains during vigorous activity. *Bone* 1996; 18:405–410.
26. Frost HM. Perspectives: bone's mechanical usage windows. *Bone Miner* 1992;19:257–271.
27. Frost HM. Bone mass and the mechanostat: a proposal. *Anat Rec* 1987;219:1–9.
28. Turner CH, Forwood MR, Rho JY, Yoshikawa T. Mechanical thresholds for lamellar and woven bone formation. *J Bone Miner Res* 1994;9:878–897.
29. Pead MJ, Skerry TM, Lanyon LE. Direct transformation from quiescence to bone formation in the adult periosteum following a single brief period of bone loading. *J Bone Miner Res* 1988; 3:647–655.
30. Hillam RA, Skerry TM. Inhibition of bone resorption and stimulation of formation by mechanical loading of the modeling rat ulna in vivo. *J Bone Miner Res* 1995;10:683–689.
31. Boppart MD, Cullen DM, Yee JA, Kimmel DB. Time course for osteoblast appearance after in vivo loading. *J Bone Miner Res* 1996;11:S266(abst).
32. Burr DB, Forwood MR, Fyhrie DP, Martin RB, Schaffler MB, Turner CH. Bone microdamage and skeletal fragility in osteoporotic and stress fractures. *J Bone Miner Res* 1997;12:6–9.
33. Carter DR, Caler WE, Spengler DM, Frankel VH. Fatigue behavior of adult cortical bone: the influence of mean strain and strain range. *Acta Orthop Scand* 1981;52:481–490.
34. Margulies JY, Simkin A, Leichter I, et al. Effect of intense physical activity on the bone-mineral content in the lower limbs of young adults. *J Bone Joint Surg* 1986;68A:1090–1093.
35. Myburg KH, Hutchins J, Fataar AB, Hough SF, Noakes TD. Low bone density is an etiologic factor for stress fractures in athletes. *Ann Intern Med* 1990;113:754–759.
36. Eaton SB, Konner M. Paleolithic nutrition. *N Engl J Med* 1985; 312:283–289.
37. Eaton SB, Nelson DA. Calcium in evolutionary perspective. *Am J Clin Nutr* 1991;54:281S–287S.
38. Klesges RC, Ward KD, Shelton ML, et al. Changes in bone mineral content in male athletes—mechanisms of action and intervention effects. *JAMA* 1996;276:226–230.
39. NIH Consensus Conference. Optimal calcium intake. NIH Consensus Development Panel on Optimal Calcim Intake. *JAMA* 1994;272:1942-1948.
40. Barger-Lux MJ, Heaney RP, Packard PT, Lappe JM, Recker RR. Nutritional correlates of low calcium intake. *Clin Appl Nutr* 1992;2:39–44.
41. Alaimo K, McDowell MA, Briefel RR, et al. Dietary intake of vitamins, minerals, and fiber in persons ages 2 months and over in the United States: Third National Health and Nutrition Examination Survey, Phase 1, 1988–1991. Advance data from vital and health statistics, no. 258, 1994.
42. Heaney RP. Protein intake and the calcium economy. *J Am Dietetic Assoc* 1993;93:1259–1260.
43. National Research Council. *Diet and health: implications for reducing chronic disease risk.* Washington, DC: National Academy Press, 1989:72–73.
44. Nordin BEC, Need AG, Morris HA, Horowitz M. Sodium, calcium and osteoporosis. In: Burckhardt P, Heaney RP, eds. *Nutritional aspects of osteoporosis. Serono symposia.* New York: Raven Press, 1991:85,279–295.
45. Barger-Lux MJ, Heaney RP, Lanspa SJ, Healy JC, DeLuca HF. An investigation of sources of variation in calcium absorption efficiency. *J Clin Endocrinol Metab* 1995;80:406–411.
46. Heaney RP. Calcium. In: Bilekikian JP, Raisz LG, Rodan GA, eds. *Principles of bone biology.* San Diego: American Press, 1996:1007–1018.
47. Utiger RD. The need for more vitamin D. *N Engl J Med* 1998;338:828–829.
48. Heaney RP. Interpreting trials of bone-active agents. *Am J Med* 1995;98:329–330.
49. McKenna MJ, Freaney R. Defining hypovitaminosis D in the elderly. In: Burckhardt P, Dawson-Hughes B, Heaney RP, eds. *Nutritional aspects of osteoporosis.* New York: Springer-Verlag, 1998: 268–277.
50. Snow-Harter C, Bouxsein ML, Lewis BT, Carter DR, Marcus R. Effects of resistance and endurance exercise on bone mineral status of young women: a randomized exercise intervention trial. *J Bone Miner Res* 1992;7:761–769.
51. Johnston CC Jr, Slemenda CW. Determinants of peak bone mass. *Osteoporosis Int* 1993;3(suppl 1):S54–55.
52. Johnson ML, Gong G, Kimberling W, Recker S, Kimmel DB, Recker RR. Linkage of a gene causing high bone mass to human chromosome 11 (11q12-13). *Am J Hum Genet* 1997;60:1326–1332.
53. Beamer WG, Donahue LR, Rosen CJ, Baylink DJ. Genetic variability in adult bone density among inbred strains of mice. *Bone* 1996;18:397–403.
54. Akhter MP, Cullen DM, Kimmel DB, Recker RR. Bone response to in vivo mechanical loading in C3H/HeJ mice. *Calcif Tissue Int* 1999;65:41–46.
55. Recker RR, Davies KM, Hinders SM, Heaney RP, Stegman MR, Kimmel DB. Bone gain in young adult women. *JAMA* 1992;268:2403–2408.
56. Heaney RP. Estrogen-calcium interactions in the postmenopause: a quantitative description. *Bone Miner* 1990;11:67–84.
57. Cooper C, Cawley M, Bhalla A, et al. Childhood growth, physical

activity, and peak bone mass in women. *J Bone Miner Res* 1995;10:940–947.
58. Boot AM, De Ridder MAJ, Pols HAP, Krenning EP, De Muinck Keizer-Schrama SMPF. Bone mineral density in children and adolescents: relation to puberty, calcium intake, and physical activity. *J Clin Endocrinol Metab* 1997;82:57–62.
59. Welten DC, Kemper HCG, Post GB, et al. Weight-bearing activity during youth is a more important factor for peak bone mass than calcium intake. *J Bone Miner Res* 1994;9:1089–1096.
60. Ruiz JC, Mandel C, Garabedian M. Influence of spontaneous calcium intake and physical exercise on the vertebral and femoral bone mineral density of children and adolescents. *J Bone Miner Res* 1995;10:675–682.
61. Katzman DK, Bachrach LK, Carter DR, Marcus R. Clinical and anthropometric correlates of bone mineral acquisition in healthy adolescent girls. *J Clin Endocrinol Metab* 1991;73:1332–1339.
62. Lappe JM, Recker RR, Malleck MK, Stegman MR, Packard PP, Heaney RP. Patellar ultrasound transmission velocity in healthy children and adolescents. *Bone* 1995;16:251S–256S.
63. Grimston SK, Morrison K, Harder JA, Hanley DA. Bone mineral density during puberty in Western Canadian children. *Bone Miner* 1992;19:85–96.
64. Nordstrom P, Thorsen K, Nordstrom G, Bergstrom E, Lorentzon R. Bone mass, muscle strength, and different body constitutional parameters in adolescent boys with a low or moderate exercise level. *Bone* 1995;17:351–356.
65. Nordstrom P, Thorsen K, Bergstrom E, Lorentzon R. High bone mass and altered relationships between bone mass, muscle strength, and body constitution in adolescent boys on a high level of physical activity. *Bone* 1996;19:189–195.
66. Slemenda CW, Miller JZ, Hui SL, Reister TK, Johnston C. Role of physical activity in the development of skeletal mass in children. *J Bone Miner Res* 1991;6:1227–1233.
67. Conroy BP, Raab DM, Kimmel DB, Recker RR. Interaction of parathyroid hormone (PTH) treatment and in vivo mechanical loading. *J Bone Miner Res* 1993;8:S280(abst).
68. Daly RM, Rich PA, Klein R. Influence of high impact loading on ultrasound bone measurements in children: a cross-sectional report. *Calcif Tissue Int* 1997;60:401–404.
69. Courteix D, Lespessailles E, Peres L, Obert P, Germain P, Benhamou CL. Effect of physical training on bone mineral density in prepubertal girls: a comparative study between impact-loading and on-impact-loading sports. *Osteoporosis* 1998;8:152–158.
70. Morris FL, Naughton GA, Gibbs JL, Carlson JS, Wark JD. Prospective ten-month exercise intervention in premenarcheal girls: positive effects on bone and lean mass. *J Bone Miner Res* 1997;12:1453–1462.
71. Bass S, Pearce G, Bradney M, et al. Exercise before puberty may confer residual benefits in bone density in adulthood: studies in active prepubertal and retired female gymnasts. *J Bone Miner Res* 1993;13:500–507.
72. Forwood MR, Parker AW. Effect of exercise on bone growth: mechanical and physical properties studied in the rat. *Clin Biomech* 1987;2:185–190.
73. Tsuji S, Katsukawa F, Onishi S, Yamazaki H. Period of adolescence during which exercise maximizes bone mass in young women. *J Bone Miner Metab* 1996;14:89–93.
74. Tylavsky FA, Anderson JJB, Talmage RV, Taft TN. Are calcium intakes and physical activity patterns during adolescence related to radial bone mass of white college-age females? *Osteoporosis Int* 1992;2:232–240.
75. Kannus P, Haapasalo H, Sankelo M, et al. Effect of starting age of physical activity on bone mass in the dominant arm of tennis and squash players. *Ann Intern Med* 1995;123:27–31.
76. Khan KM, Bennell KL, Hopper JL, et al. Self-reported ballet classes undertaken at age 10–12 years and hip bone mineral density in later life. *Osteoporosis* 1998;8:165–173.
77. Etherington J, Harris PA, Nandra D, et al. The effect of weight-bearing exercise on bone mineral density: a study of female ex-elite athletes and the general population. *J Bone Miner Res* 1996;11:1333–1338.
78. Pearce G, Bass S, Young N, Formica C, Seeman E. Does weight-bearing exercise protect against the effects of exercise-induced oligomenorrhea on bone density? *Osteoporosis Int* 1996;6: 448–452.
79. Rencken ML, Chesnut CH, Drinkwater B. Bone density at multiple skeletal sites in amenorrheic athletes. *JAMA* 1996; 276:238–240.
80. Myburg KH, Bachrach LK, Lewis B, Kent K, Marcus R. Low bone mineral density at axial and appendicular sites in amenorrheic athletes. *Med Sci Sports Exerc* 1993;25:1197–1202.
81. Bennell KL, Brukner PD, Malcolm SA. Effect of altered reproductive function and lowered testosterone levels on bone density in male endurance athletes. *Br J Sports Med* 1996;30:205–208.
82. Smith R, Rutherford OM. Spine and total body bone mineral density and serum testosterone levels in male athletes. *Eur J Appl Physiol* 1993;67:330–334.
83. Hetland ML, Haarbo J, Christiansen C. Low bone mass and high bone turnover in male long distance runners. *J Clin Endocrinol Metab* 1993;77:770–775.
84. Krolner B, Toft B, Nielsen SP, Tondevold E. Physical exercise as prophylaxis against involutional vertebral bone loss: a controlled trial. *Clin Sci* 1983;64:541–546.
85. Smith EL, Gilligan C, McAdam M, Ensign CP, Smith PE. Deterring bone loss by exercise intervention in premenopausal women and postmenopausal women. *Calcif Tissue Int* 1989;44:312–321.
86. Notelovitz M, Martin D, Tesar R, et al. Estrogen therapy and variable-resistance weight training increase bone mineral in surgically menopausal women. *J Bone Miner Res* 1991;6:583–590.
87. Kelley G. Aerobic exercise and lumbar spine bone mineral density in postmenopausal women: a meta-analysis. *J Am Geriatr Soc* 1998;46:143–152.
88. Berard A, Bravo G, Gauthier P. Meta-analysis of the effectiveness of physical activity for the prevention of bone loss in postmenopausal women. *Osteoporosis Int* 1997;7:331–337.
89. Simkin A, Ayalon J, Leichter I. Increased trabecular bone density due to bone-loading exercises in postmenopausal osteoporotic women. *Calcif Tissue Int* 1987;40:59–63.
90. Rundgren A, Aniansssom A, Ljungberg P, Wetterqvist H. Effects of a training programme for elderly people on mineral content of the heel bone. *Arch Gerontol Geriatr* 1984;3:243–248.
91. Jones PRM, Hardman AE, Hudson A, Norgan NG. Influence of brisk walking on the broadband ultrasonic attenuation of the calcaneus in previously sedentary women aged 30–61 years. *Calcif Tissue Int* 1991;49:112–115.
92. Smith EL, Smith PE, Ensign CJ, Shea MM. Bone involution decrease in exercising middle-aged women. *Calcif Tissue Int* 1984;36:s129–s138.
93. Beverly MC, Rider TA, Evans MJ, Smith R. Local bone mineral response to brief exercise that stresses the skeleton. *Br Med J* 1989;299:233–235.
94. Hayes WC, Myers ER, Robinovitch SN, Van Den Kroonenberg A, Courtney AC, McMahon TA. Etiology and prevention of age-related hip fractures. *Bone* 1996;18:77s–86s.
95. Grabiner MD, Enoka RM. Changes in movement capabilities with aging. In: Holloszy JO, ed. *Exercise and sport sciences reviews*. Philadelphia: Williams & Wilkins, 1995:65–104.
96. Vuori I, Heinonen A, Sievanen H, Kannus P, Pasanen M, Oja P. Effects of unilateral strength training and detraining on bone mineral density and content in young women: a study of mechanical loading and deloading on human bones. *Calcif Tissue Int* 1994;55:59–67.
97. Heinonen A, Oja P, Sievanen H, et al. Maintenance of increased bone mineral density after an effective 18-months exercise intervention. *Med Sci Sports Exerc* 1997;29:S5(abst).
98. Hancock DA, Reed GW, Atkinson PJ, Cook JB, Smith PH. Bone and soft tissue changes in paraplegic patients. *Paraplegia* 1980;17:267–271.
99. Kiratli BJ. *Skeletal adaptation to disuse: longitudinal and cross-sectional study of the response of the femur and spine to immobilization (paralysis)*. Madison: University of Wisconsin, 1989.
100. Biering-Sorensen F, Bohr H, Schaadt O. Longitudinal study of bone mineral content in the lumbar spine, the forearm and the lower extremities after spinal cord injury. *Eur J Clin Invest* 1990;20:330–335.

101. Donaldson CL, Hulley SB, Vogel JM, Hattner RS, Bayers JH, McMillan DE. Effect of prolonged bed rest on bone mineral. *Metabolism* 1970;19:1071–1084.
102. Hulley SB, Vogel JM, Donaldson CL, Bayers JH, Friedman RJ, Rosen SN. The effect of supplemental oral phosphate on the bone mineral changes during prolonged bed rest. *J Clin Invest* 1971;50:2506–2518.
103. LeBlanc AD, Schneider VS, Evans HJ, Engelbretson DA, Krebs JM. Bone mineral loss and recovery after 17 weeks of bed rest. *J Bone Miner Res* 1990;5:843–850.
104. Leblanc A, Schneider V, Shackelford L, et al. Bone mineral and lean tissue loss after long duration spaceflight. *J Bone* 1996;11:S323(abst).
105. Collet P, Uebelhart D, Vico L, Hartmann G, Roth M, Alexandre C. Effects of 1- and 6-month spaceflight on bone mass and biochemistry in two humans. *Bone* 1997;20:547–551.
106. Sinaki M, Wahner HW, Bergstralh EJ, et al. Three-year controlled, randomized trial of the effect of dose-specified loading and strengthening exercises on bone mineral density of spine and femur in nonathletic, physically active women. *Bone* 1996; 19:233–244.
107. Cavanaugh DJ, Cann CE. Brisk walking does not stop bone loss in postmenopausal women. *Bone* 1988;9:201–204.
108. Frost HM. The role of changes in mechanical usage set points in the pathogenesis of osteoporosis. *J Bone Miner Res* 1992; 7:253–261.

Exercise and Sport Science,
edited by William E. Garrett, Jr., and Donald T. Kirkendall.
Published by Lippincott Williams & Wilkins, Philadelphia, 2000.

CHAPTER 16

Skin Responses to Exercise and Training

Dean L. Kellogg, Jr., and Pablo Pérgola

The primary role of the skin during periods of systemic exercise is to facilitate thermal homeostasis through increases in skin blood flow (SkBF) and sweating. The processes of contraction, shortening, and relaxation of skeletal muscle are thermogenic, inherently leading to an increase in body temperature. Thermoregulatory reflexes are then activated to reduce body heat and maintain thermal homeostasis to protect the central nervous system. Thermoregulatory reflexes evoke significant increases in cutaneous blood flow; however, the primary role of the cardiovascular system during periods of systemic exercise is the delivery of sufficient amounts of oxygen and nutrients to active muscle. Thus, thermoregulatory reflexes induced by thermogenic exercise often conflict with nonthermoregulatory cardiovascular reflex adaptations to exercise. For example, during strenuous dynamic exercise, or during exercise in a warm environment, competing demands for high blood flow to active skeletal muscle and skin are placed on the human cardiovascular system. These demands center around providing adequate blood flow to meet the metabolic needs of active skeletal muscle, to maintain systemic arterial pressure, and to prevent internal temperature from reaching deleterious levels through increasing SkBF and sweating (1). The first two demands often conflict with the third. In the first conflict, demand for blood flow by active muscle to maintain exercise and demand for blood flow to skin to maintain thermal homeostasis compete for cardiac output. In the second conflict, increased SkBF to maintain thermal homeostasis reduces the ability of the baroreflex to maintain systemic blood pressure.

In general, these competing demands are resolved by increasing cardiac output; however, dynamic exercise at moderate work loads, especially when combined with heat stress, can exceed the ability to increase cardiac output. This inadequacy is generally compensated for by increased vasoconstriction in inactive regional circulations. Approximately two-thirds of the demand for increased SkBF is met by increasing cardiac output, and the remainder is met through redistribution of flow from other vascular beds including the splanchnic and renal circulations (2–6). However, these compensatory mechanisms may be inadequate to resolve deficits resulting from combined strenuous exercise and heat stress, leading to cardiovascular collapse.

MECHANISMS OF HEAT TRANSFER

To maintain thermal homeostasis, humans must balance heat production with heat loss according to the following equation:

$$\Delta S = M - E \pm R \pm C \pm K - W$$

Where ΔS = change in heat storage

M = metabolic energy production

E = evaporative heat loss

R = radiant heat gain or loss

C = convective heat gain or loss

K = conductive heat gain or loss

W = useful work done on an external system

If ΔS is greater than zero, the body is gaining heat and body temperature rises. If ΔS is less than zero, the body is losing heat and body temperature falls.

Metabolic energy production (M) is the rate of transformation of chemical energy into heat and mechanical work and can be expressed as $M = H + W$, where H is metabolic heat production and W is useful work. Evaporation (E) is the sum of heat loss by evaporation

D. L. Kellogg, Jr., and P. Pérgola: Division of Geriatrics and Gerontology, Department of Medicine, University of Texas Health Science Center at San Antonio; Department of Geriatrics and Extended Care, Audie L. Murphy Memorial Veterans Administration Hospital, San Antonio, Texas 78284.

of water primarily from sweat on the skin's surface with a minor component from water evaporation from the respiratory tract. E is therefore highly dependent on the rate of sweat production, the surface area available for evaporation, and water vapor pressure in the air. Convective heat transfer (C) is heat exchange due to the forced movement of a fluid. C is responsible for transfer of heat to the body surface by SkBF and for some of the heat transfer between the body surface and environment by air flow. C is dependent on body surface area, the difference of skin temperature and ambient temperature, and the rate of blood flow and/or airflow. Conductive heat transfer (K) represents the flow of heat down a temperature gradient as between tissues and the blood, between the blood and the skin, and between the skin and the environment. Radiant heat transfer (R) represents heat transfer by emission and absorption of electromagnetic (infrared) energy. This accounts for 50% to 60% of heat loss in normothermia, but it can convert to a net heat gain in direct sunlight.

During heat stress at rest, factors R, C, and K can become positive so that heat is transferred from the environment to the body, resulting in a positive ΔS. This elicits a purely thermoregulatory reflex response. During dynamic exercise, factor M becomes positive, thus leading to a positive ΔS. During exercise in a hot environment, factors M, E, R, C, K, and W become positive, leading to a greatly positive ΔS. In these two cases, thermoregulatory reflexes are activated by the positive ΔS and are integrated with the nonthermoregulatory reflex adaptations to exercise.

ANATOMY OF THE SKIN

The skin makes up approximately 5% of total body weight in humans (7). In adults the skin covers about 1.8 m^2 and averages 1 to 2 mm in thickness. Its primary function is to provide a protective, waterproof covering for the body's surface. In humans, the skin has a unique role in thermoregulation because its blood flow can be varied and because of its ability to produce sweat.

The skin consists of two layers: a superficial layer, the epidermis, and a deep layer, the dermis. The epidermis is made up of keratinized squamous epithelial cells and is waterproof. The dermis has a more complex histology and contains blood vessels, afferent and efferent nerves, sweat glands, sebaceous glands, and hair follicles.

Blood vessels in human skin are arranged in several plexuses that are arranged in deep and superficial layers that parallel the skin surface. Most vessels are found in the superficial or papillary plexus, which is made up of high-resistance terminal arterioles, papillary loops, and postcapillary venules. Papillary loops are true capillaries and are often referred to as "nutritional vessels." Across these papillary loops, which are located close to the dermal-epidermal junction, the temperature gradient from blood to epidermal tissue is the greatest because epidermal temperature is closest to that of the environment. In addition, the surface area of the papillary loops is quite high, thus favoring heat exchange. Thus, an important function of blood flow through the papillary loops is to deliver heat from the blood to the skin's surface, where a highly efficient heat exchange occurs. This arrangement thus facilitates thermal homeostasis.

All areas of skin contain papillary loops; however, in acral skin (i.e., the skin of the fingers, lips, ears, palms, and plantar aspects of the feet) arteriovenous anastomoses (AVAs) are also found. AVAs are coiled vessels with thick muscular walls and dense innervation. AVAs lie deep to the papillary plexus and superficial to sweat gland coils. AVAs directly connect arterioles and venules, bypassing the high-resistance arterioles and capillaries of the papillary plexus. AVAs are involved in local vasodilation during exposure to extremely cold environmental temperatures. This vasodilation brings warm blood into the tissue to maintain tissue temperature, and thus preserve tissue viability. AVAs also dilate in response to hyperthermia, thus providing for a second mechanism for heat loss to the environment (8). However, because AVAs are deeper in the dermis and have a lower surface area, the AVA system is not as efficient as papillary loops in heat transfer.

In addition to the cutaneous vasculature, eccrine sweat glands play a major role in thermoregulation. Their principal function is to enhance heat loss during exposure to a hot environment or during exercise by evaporation of sweat. Eccrine sweat glands are found over almost the entire body surface. The density of the glands varies from 64 glands/cm^2 on the back to 700 glands/cm^2 in palmar and plantar skin (9). Each gland consists of a secretory coil deep in the dermis. A duct extends from the coil through the dermis and epidermis and empties onto the skin's surface. Sweat is secreted as a nearly isotonic fluid by the coils and conducted to the surface via the ducts. Partial reabsorption of NaCl occurs within the ducts so that the sweat delivered to the skin surface is hypotonic (10).

THERMOREGULATION AND THE SKIN

More is known about SkBF and its control in humans than in any other species. Under resting circumstances, flow in the forearm skin averages approximately 30 to 40 mL/min/100 g of skin; however, the absolute amount of blood in the skin can vary from nearly zero during periods of maximal vasoconstriction to as much as 8 L/min distributed to all skin during maximal vasodilation.

The cutaneous circulation is a major effector of human thermoregulatory reflex responses. During heat stress, elevated internal temperature (T_{int}) and skin temperature (T_{sk}) lead to a reflex cutaneous vasodilation. Conversely, during cold stress, reduced temperatures lead to cutaneous vasoconstriction. In apical regions (palms, plantar aspect of feet, nose, and ears), cutaneous arterioles are innervated solely by noradrenergic sympathetic vasoconstrictor nerves (11–14). All thermoregulatory reflexes in apical skin regions are therefore mediated by changes in vasoconstrictor tone (12–14). In nonapical areas of skin (limbs, head, and trunk), reflex changes in SkBF are mediated by two branches of the sympathetic nervous system: noradrenergic vasoconstrictor nerves, which elicit cutaneous vasoconstriction, and active vasodilator nerves, which elicit a cutaneous vasodilation (14) (Fig. 16–1).

Dual-vasomotor neural systems were first suggested in 1931 by Lewis and Pickering (15); however, the first definitive evidence came from work by Grant and Holling (16). They measured blood flow in the human forearm and found large increases in SkBF in response to heat stress that could be abolished by sympathectomy or nerve blockade. They noted that while sympathectomy or nerve blockade caused only a slight cutaneous vasodilation during normothermia, heat stress elicited a much greater increase in SkBF. In addition, nerve blockade during established hyperthermia and vasodilation abolished the increase in SkBF. These results suggested that nonapical cutaneous vessels received sympathetic active vasodilator as well as vasoconstrictor innervation. If the nonapical cutaneous circulation was controlled solely by vasoconstrictor nerves, sympathectomy should have caused a near maximal vasodilation instead of the small response they observed. In addition, heat stress would have had no additional effect after sympathectomy. Their findings were later confirmed by Edholm and colleagues (17), who found that blockade of cutaneous sympathetic nerves during heat stress produced significant reductions in SkBF. They concluded that an active neural process caused cutaneous vasodilation. Similar conclusions were drawn by Roddie and colleagues (18), who measured oxygen saturation from veins selectively draining either superficial (cutaneous) or deep (muscle) forearm structures in combination with either superficial (cutaneous) or deep (muscle) nerve blockade. They found that blockade of cutaneous nerves during heat stress produced a decrease in oxygen saturation in veins draining skin. This suggested an active vasodilator system in the skin. More recently it was shown that bretylium tosylate (a prejunctional noradrenergic neuronal blocking agent) abolishes the cutaneous vasoconstriction induced by cold stress but does not alter the vasodilator responses induced by heat stress (19). This confirmed that dual efferent systems control the cutaneous arterioles.

Cutaneous vasoconstrictor nerves are noradrenergic and act through postjunctional alpha-1 and alpha-2 receptors (13,20). This system is activated during periods of cold stress to reduce SkBF and conserve body heat (1,12–14,20–22). The specific neurotransmitter of the vasodilator nerves is not known, although an indirect relationship to cholinergic sudomotor nerve activity has been postulated (11,23,24). Sweat glands are innervated by postganglionic sympathetic cholinergic and adrenergic fibers (25). These nerves appear to contain a variety of neuropeptides as well (26). Classically, sweat glands are activated by cholinergic nerves in response to elevated T_{int}. Sweating works in conjunction with the papillary loops to facilitate thermal homeostasis during hyperthermia through evaporative cooling.

Drawing on work done with salivary glands, Fox and Hilton (27) proposed that cholinergic activation of sweat glands elicited a glandular production of kininogenase, which ultimately resulted in bradykinin production via

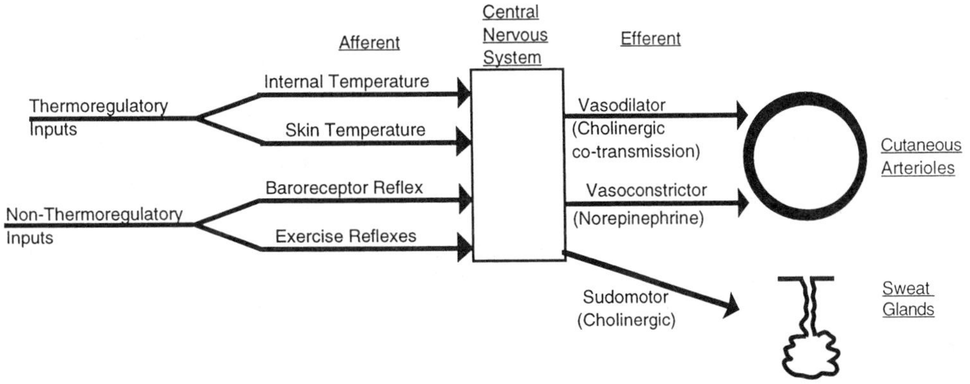

FIG. 16–1. Summary of reflex control of skin blood flow (SkBF). Thermoregulatory reflexes arise from changes in internal temperature and skin temperature. Nonthermoregulatory reflexes include baroreceptor reflexes and reflexes associated with exercise. Efferent control of SkBF is mediated by noradrenergic active vasoconstrictor nerves and by cholinergic active vasodilator nerves through a cotransmitter system. Cholinergic sudomotor nerves innervate sweat glands, but whether the sudomotor and vasodilator nerves are one and the same remains unclear.

an enzymatic cascade. Bradykinin was proposed as the effector of vasodilation (27). Their proposal was based on observations that atropine completely blocked sweat production but only slightly delayed active vasodilation during heat stress. They also detected a bradykinin-forming enzyme in human sweat (27). Subsequent work has not confirmed this proposal. Frewin and colleagues (24) were unable to find any kinins or kininogenases in human sweat.

An alternative to the foregoing hypothesis was proposed by Hökfelt and colleagues (28) with supporting evidence derived from studies in the cat. According to this scheme, a single set of neurons could control both active vasodilation of cutaneous arterioles and sweating by releasing both acetylcholine (Ach) and the cotransmitter vasoactive intestinal peptide (VIP). Ach would control sweating and VIP would effect active vasodilation (28). This colocalization mechanism could explain why atropine blocks sweating but inconsistently affects active vasodilation (18,29).

Current evidence supports a cotransmitter mechanism in human cutaneous active vasodilation (29). Cutaneous active vasodilation is completely abolished by intradermal botulinum toxin, which prevents release of Ach and all other neurotransmitters from cholinergic nerves (29). Muscarinic receptor blockade with atropine slightly reduces and delays vasodilator responses to hyperthermia although it completely abolishes the vasodilation induced by exogenous Ach (18,29). These observations strongly suggest that active vasodilation is effected by a cholinergic cotransmitter system in humans. The failure of atropine to block cutaneous vasodilation has generally been taken as evidence against a role for Ach as the neurotransmitter involved. However, the fact that there was some effect of atropine on the process, albeit incomplete, suggests a role for Ach (30).

The suggestion that Ach may play a role in active vasodilation likewise suggests a mechanistic role for nitric oxide (NO) in the process. Ach effects vasodilation through increasing NO levels. Work in humans has shown that NO donors can increase SkBF (31) and that NO contributes to a basal dilator tone in forearm and finger skin (32). Recently, we found that blockade of NO synthase with either N^G-nitro-L-arginine-methyl ester (L-NAME) or N^G-monomethyl-L-arginine (L-NMMA) attenuates, but does not abolish, thermoregulatory reflex-mediated cutaneous active vasodilation in humans. Thus, NO generation is involved in the mechanism of cutaneous active vasodilation in humans.

Overall, the active vasodilator system is responsible

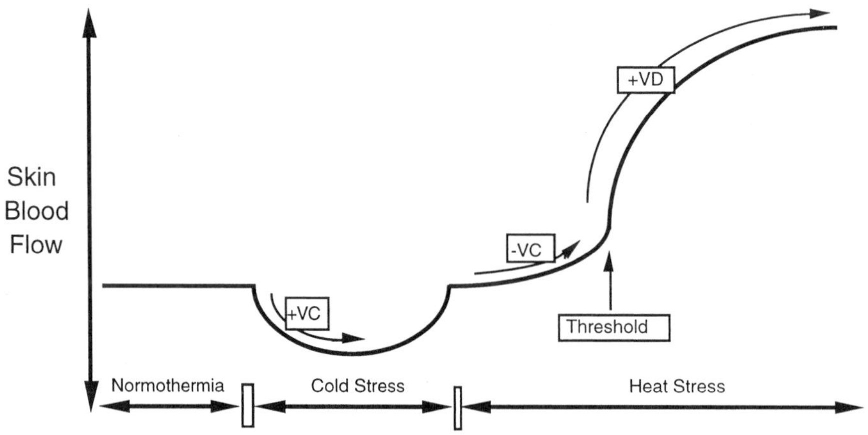

FIG. 16–2. Mechanisms of thermoregulatory reflexes. This diagram summarizes the efferent neural mechanisms that control the cutaneous circulation in three thermoregulatory conditions: normothermia, cold stress, and heat stress. In normothermia, cutaneous arterioles receive little neural stimulation; hence, the smooth muscle cells of the cutaneous arterioles are at basal tone. With cold stress, falling skin and internal temperatures initiate a thermoregulatory reflex to conserve body heat. This reflex is mediated by increased noradrenergic vasoconstrictor tone directed to the cutaneous arterioles. This increased tone leads to an arteriolar vasoconstriction and a decrease in SkBF. Conversely, with heat stress, rising skin and internal temperatures initiate a thermoregulatory reflex to facilitate body cooling. The initial response is the abolition of any extant vasoconstrictor tone. As internal temperature continues to rise, it reaches a threshold value at which cutaneous vasodilation begins. Sweating also begins at approximately the same internal temperature. At this threshold, active vasodilator tone to the cutaneous arterioles is enhanced. Vasodilator tone increases with further increases in internal temperature. This increase in neural activity mediates a decrease in smooth muscle tone, an arteriolar vasodilation, and hence an increase in SkBF. High SkBF delivers heat to the body surface, where it is dissipated to the environment in conjunction with the evaporation of sweat. *+VC*, increased active vasoconstrictor nerve activity; *−VC*, decreased active vasoconstrictive nerve activity; *+VD*, increased active vasodilator activity; *Threshold:* internal temperature at which cutaneous vasodilation and sweating begin.

for 80% to 95% of the elevation in SkBF accompanying heat stress (1). Since whole-body SkBF can achieve levels approaching 8 L per minute, or 60% of cardiac output during heat stress (1), it is clear that this vasodilator system is important both to thermoregulatory responses and to systemic hemodynamics.

As illustrated in Fig. 16–1, thermoregulatory reflexes are affected by the afferent neural inputs of T_{int} and T_{sk}. During cold stress, as T_{sk} falls, there is a progressive increase in efferent noradrenergic vasoconstrictor nerve activity. This reduces SkBF and conserves body heat. If this vasoconstriction is insufficient to preserve thermal homeostasis and T_{int} and T_{sk} continue to fall, metabolic production of heat is increased through shivering.

During body heating, there is initially an abolition of any extant vasoconstrictor activity, causing a small increase in SkBF. As heat exposure continues, internal and skin temperatures rise. When T_{int} reaches a threshold of approximately 37°C, efferent active vasodilator and sudomotor nerves are activated. Increased vasodilator nerve activity acts to increase SkBF and facilitate heat dissipation by increased delivery from deep body tissues to the body surface, where it can be transferred to the environment. Increased sudomotor activity enhances sweat production, leading to increased heat transfer to the environment by evaporative cooling (1,11–13) (Fig. 16–2).

INITIATION OF DYNAMIC EXERCISE

Reflex adaptations to dynamic exercise involve reductions in blood flow to inactive regional circulations (14). These reductions in vascular conductance provide additional blood flow to meet the increased metabolic demands of active skeletal muscle. The cutaneous circulation participates in this redistribution of blood flow with dynamic exercise, especially in the early phases of exercise.

In normothermic humans, the initiation of exercise causes a reduction in SkBF to supply additional blood flow to working muscle (12,14). Such reflex cutaneous vasoconstriction has been documented in the hands, feet, trunk, and forearm (33–39). The cutaneous vasoconstriction due to exercise initiation also appears to be graded with work loads over 125 W (40,41). Johnson and Park (42) found that the degree of vasoconstriction due to exercise initiation is partially dependent on the preexercise level of SkBF; specifically, the cutaneous vasoconstriction is greater during hyperthermia than under normothermic conditions (12,42). This demonstrates how the cutaneous vascular responses to nonthermoregulatory reflexes could be modified by simultaneously occurring thermoregulatory reflexes. The net result of these competing reflexes is an integrated cutaneous vascular response.

By what efferent mechanisms does the cutaneous vasculature respond to competing thermoregulatory and nonthermoregulatory reflexes? The answer, as far as is known, varies between body regions. In apical regions (hands, feet, nose, and ears), cutaneous arterioles are innervated solely by noradrenergic sympathetic vasoconstrictor nerves (11–14). All thermoregulatory and nonthermoregulatory reflexes in apical skin regions are therefore mediated by alterations in active vasoconstrictor tone (12–14).

In nonapical regions (head, limbs, and trunk), the dual-efferent innervation adds complexity. If the effects of one system could be removed, analysis would be much simplified. Such an approach was used by Blair and colleagues (43,44) by employing intraarterial injection of bretylium tosylate to abolish norepinephrine release from sympathetic nerves. They found that bretylium abolished the fall in forearm blood flow elicited by the initiation of dynamic leg exercise. The authors concluded that this fall was due to vasoconstriction in nonexercising forearm muscle only, and that the cutaneous vessels were not affected. However, other studies have clearly demonstrated that the initiation of exercise does induce a cutaneous vasoconstriction under normothermic conditions (33–35,40–42). In light of these other studies, the vasoconstriction observed by Blair and colleagues (43) was likely due to a decrease in skin rather than muscle blood flow.

During hyperthermia, the neural mechanisms responsible for exercise-induced falls in SkBF were unclear due to the dual-vasomotor innervation of the cutaneous arterioles. Reductions in SkBF could be caused by (a) increased vasoconstrictor tone, (b) reduced vasodilator tone, or (c) a combination of increased vasoconstrictor and reduced vasodilator tones. This problem was overcome using a combination of laser-Doppler flowmetry (LDF) with the local iontophoresis of bretylium tosylate (19), a technique that has proved invaluable in defining efferent neural control mechanisms in the skin. LDF monitors SkBF from small volumes of skin (approximately 1 mm^3). The measurement is specific to skin, being uninfluenced by blood flow from deeper tissues (45). Bretylium tosylate is an antiadrenergic neuronal agent that can be applied to small areas of skin by local iontophoresis (19). It is taken up by prejunctional noradrenergic neurons and selectively abolishes active vasoconstrictor influences on cutaneous arterioles without significantly altering active vasodilator control. By monitoring SkBF at the bretylium-treated site with no functional vasoconstrictor control, and at an adjacent untreated site with both vasoconstrictor and vasodilator control, the roles of the separate neural systems were studied.

The combination of bretylium iontophoresis and LDF was used to investigate the efferent vasomotor mechanism that causes the cutaneous vasoconstriction induced by exercise initiation (46). Under normothermic condi-

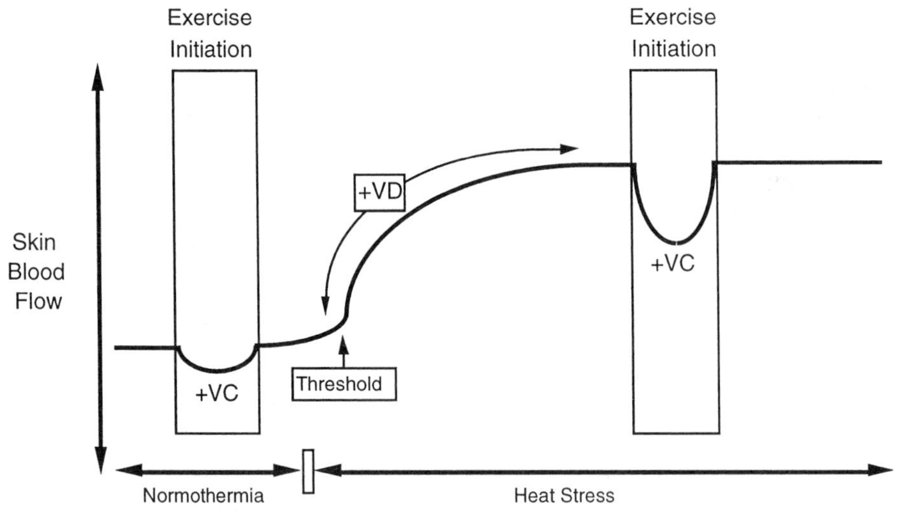

FIG. 16–3. Mechanisms of integration of thermoregulatory and exercise initiation reflexes. This diagram summarizes the efferent neural mechanisms that control the cutaneous circulation during dynamic exercise initiation in two conditions—normothermia and heat stress—as revealed by bretylium blockade of the active vasoconstrictor system. In normothermia, exercise initiation elicits a cutaneous vasoconstriction mediated by an increase in active vasoconstrictor tone directed at the cutaneous arterioles. During heat stress at rest, thermoregulatory reflexes are activated. SkBF is increased through enhanced vasodilator and reduced vasoconstrictor nerve activity. Under such conditions, exercise initiation reflexes are integrated with thermoregulatory reflexes by enhanced active vasoconstrictor nerve activity superimposed on tonically high vasodilator activity. These competing neural tones are summated at the level of the cutaneous arterioles, producing a net vasoconstriction. *+VC,* increased active vasoconstrictor nerve activity; *+VD,* increased active vasodilator activity; *Threshold,* internal temperature at which cutaneous vasodilation begins.

tions with no vasodilator tone, bretylium treatment abolished the vasoconstriction due to the initiation of exercise; this verifies that when exercise starts in normothermia, vasoconstrictor tone to the cutaneous arterioles is enhanced, reducing SkBF (46). When the thermoregulatory reflex responses to heat stress were fully developed with high active vasodilator tone, exercise initiation significantly reduced the SkBF at untreated sites while SkBF was unchanged at bretylium-treated sites. Since bretylium blockade of norepinephrine release (and hence blockade of vasoconstrictor function) abolished the response, the vasoconstriction induced by exercise initiation in hyperthermia must have been due solely to an increase in active vasoconstrictor tone. The initiation of exercise did not directly affect the active vasodilator system. At untreated sites, hyperthermia had activated the vasodilator system. Subsequent exercise initiation activated the vasoconstrictor system. Cutaneous arterioles thus received simultaneous and competing inputs from both systems. The net outcome of this competition was an integrated response of the nonthermoregulatory, exercise-induced increase in active vasoconstrictor activity and the thermoregulatory reflex-mediated high vasodilator activity. This implies that the site of integration between these competing reflexes must have been at the level of the cutaneous arterioles. That is, the cutaneous arterioles summated competing high vasoconstrictor activity (due to exercise) and high vasodilator activity (due to heat stress). The net outcome of the summation was an arteriolar smooth muscle contraction and hence an arteriolar vasoconstriction (Fig. 16–3).

In contrast to the cutaneous vasomotor responses to exercise initiation, van Beaumont and Bullard (47) found that sweat rate increased dramatically within 1.5 to 2 seconds after the initiation of dynamic leg exercise. Their results indicate that sudomotor nerve activity is enhanced at the onset of exercise, independent of effects of internal temperature. A combination of increased sudomotor activity and the lack of any change in active vasodilator activity would imply that the sudomotor and vasodilator systems are mediated by different sets of nerves.

INTERMEDIATE-DURATION DYNAMIC EXERCISE

Another reflex adaptation to dynamic exercise derives from the thermogenic nature of muscle activity. Dynamic exercise, with its attendant metabolic heat production, increases T_{int}. If exercise is performed long enough, T_{int} reaches a threshold at which thermoregulatory reflexes for heat dissipation are evoked (12,14,48). Above this threshold, thermoregulatory demands begin to exert control over SkBF and effect an active cutaneous vasodilation to facilitate heat loss (14,38,49).

When compared to the temperature threshold at which cutaneous vasodilation begins at rest (approximately 37.0°C), the threshold during dynamic exercise is higher (approximately 37.2°C) (40,49). Taylor and colleagues (40) found that this threshold shift was greater as work loads increased above 125 W. Pérgola and colleagues (50) also found the threshold shift to be greater when exercise was performed at low T_{sk}. Under such conditions T_{int} thresholds for vasodilation approach 38°C. This threshold elevation, or shift, can be viewed as an integrated reflex response, with partial sacrifice of thermoregulatory stability and a consequently higher T_{int} in order to provide additional blood flow to exercising muscle. The combination of bretylium iontophoresis and LDF was used to study the efferent mechanisms responsible for this integrated response. Dynamic exercise induced similar threshold shifts at both bretylium-treated and -untreated sites. Since SkBF at bretylium-treated sites was controlled exclusively by the vasodilator system, the threshold shift must have been due to an exercise-induced delay in activation of the vasodilator system. That is, exercise increases the internal temperature level for activation of vasodilation (Fig. 16–4). This contrasts with exercise initiation, which alters SkBF through changes in vasoconstrictor tone.

Activation of the sudomotor system during thermogenic dynamic exercise has also been examined. Johnson and Park (49) measured the T_{int} threshold for activation of sweating during dynamic exercise as induced by two-leg dynamic exercise at moderate work loads. They found that the internal temperature threshold for the onset of sweating was not altered by exercise, although the threshold for vasodilation was increased. Their results indicate that dynamic exercise does not alter the internal temperature threshold for enhancement of sudomotor activity. Similar results were reported by Kellogg and colleagues (51). They measured sweat rate and cutaneous vasodilator threshold shifts induced by two-leg dynamic exercise at moderate work loads. Blood flow measurements were made with LDF combined with blockade of noradrenergic vasoconstrictor function with bretylium. As in the work by Johnson and Park (49), they found that the internal temperature threshold for the onset of sweating was not altered by exercise, but

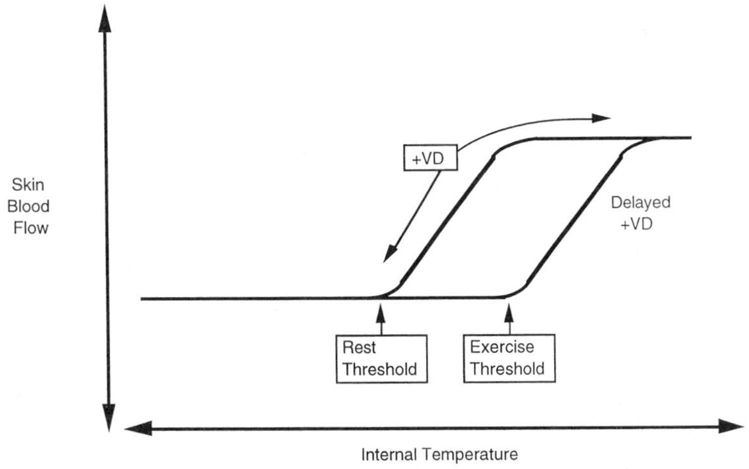

FIG. 16–4. Mechanisms of integration of thermoregulatory and exercise reflexes. This diagram summarizes the efferent neural mechanisms involved in internal temperature threshold shifts during dynamic exercise. Exercise results in heat production from active skeletal muscle. As exercise continues, this heat production leads to a rise in internal temperature. Elevated temperature causes an increased thermoregulatory drive and, eventually, cutaneous vasodilation when internal temperature reaches a threshold value of about 37.0°C at rest and 37.2°C during moderate work-load exercise. The resultant increase in skin blood flow thus occurs at a higher internal temperature during exercise than during heat stress at rest. Relative to resting conditions, exercise increases the internal temperature threshold for cutaneous vasodilation by delaying increases in vasodilator tone until a higher internal temperature is reached. This implies that dynamic exercise reflexes directly control the internal temperature threshold at which cutaneous active vasodilation begins. Furthermore, this observation implies some integration of thermoregulatory reflexes, and the reflex adaptations to dynamic exercise occur within the nervous system. The threshold during exercise in a cool environment (with a low skin temperature) is increased above threshold during exercise in a warm environment (with a warm skin temperature). This is due to an additional delay in activation of the vasodilator system by the lower skin temperature. *+VD*, increased active vasodilator activity; *Rest Threshold*, internal temperature at which cutaneous vasodilation begins at rest; *Exercise Threshold*, internal temperature at which cutaneous vasodilation begins during dynamic exercise.

that the vasomotor threshold was increased. Thus, the vasomotor threshold shift was due to a shift in activation of the active vasodilator system. The divergence of the sudomotor and vasodilator responses suggests that the vasodilator and sudomotor systems are independently controlled, and it questions their mechanistic relationship.

The finding that exercise reflexes directly control the vasodilator system implies that integration of exercise and the thermoregulatory reflexes with respect to the vasodilator threshold occurs within either the central nervous system or the peripheral nervous system. If any aspects of integration occurred at the cutaneous arteriolar level, the thresholds of treated and untreated sites would have differed; they did not. Thus, integration must have occurred proximal to the cutaneous arterioles, within the nervous system.

Whether the neural site of integration between simultaneous thermoregulatory and nonthermoregulatory reflexes occurs within the central nervous system or peripheral nervous system is not clear. It is likely that integration occurs at the hypothalamic level. For example, the threshold shift for vasodilation may represent an increase in a hypothalamic "set-point" for activation of thermoregulatory reflexes (52). Several studies have suggested that dynamic exercise increases the hypothalamic set-point temperature (53,54); however, other studies have suggested that dynamic exercise decreases (55) or does not change (49) this set-point. It is not possible to base a firm conclusion regarding this issue on the peripheral measurements of SkBF. One can say that exercise elevates the threshold internal temperature at which the cutaneous active vasodilator system is engaged and that this probably happens within central nervous system interaction. However, it is not clear that the threshold shift represents an increase in the set-point per se. A more likely scenario is that a single central set-point for body temperature has thermoregulatory control over both vasomotor and sudomotor functions. Nonthermoregulatory reflexes associated with exercise may not change the set-point but instead may modify vasomotor and sudomotor functions, inhibiting active vasodilator outflow relative to that for sudomotor control. Such a scheme would permit increases of the vasomotor threshold without changing that for sweating (49). This mechanism for central integration would also allow a reduced central set-point (47,55). Regardless of any reduction in central set-point due to exercise, the cutaneous vasoconstriction induced by the vasoconstrictor system and the higher threshold internal temperature for activation of the cutaneous vasodilator system would each contribute to retarding heat loss and, hence, to the higher internal temperature of exercise. This would be beneficial by providing some additional blood flow to exercising muscle by forgoing some degree of thermal homeostasis.

PROLONGED DYNAMIC EXERCISE (Fig. 16–5)

As exercise duration increases, rising internal temperature causes further cutaneous vasodilation (48,56). This vasodilation is initially rapid as the T_{int} threshold is exceeded and is followed by a slow, steady increase to an average value of about 15 mL/100 mL forearm/min (48). This SkBF plateau is approximately 40% to 60% of maximal SkBF at rest and represents a modification of thermoregulatory reflexes by prolonged exercise. Thus, in addition to causing an initial cutaneous vasoconstriction and altering the vasodilator threshold, dynamic exercise places a limit on the capacity of the skin to vasodilate; that is, prolonged dynamic exercise functionally limits maximal cutaneous vasodilation.

During dynamic exercise in the upright position in a warm environment, SkBF increases linearly with temperature beyond a T_{int} threshold of about 37.2°C (12,57–61). As T_{int} approaches 38°C the increase in SkBF with respect to T_{int} is attenuated (12,57–60,62,63). This reduction in the slope of the SkBF-T_{int} relationship results in little further increase in SkBF as T_{int} exceeds 38°C. Even at such a high T_{int} during exercise, SkBF is not maximal as would have been the case at rest.

The plateau of SkBF during prolonged exercise has been found to be a consequence of limitation of active vasodilation activity. Kenney and colleagues (63) found that systemic α_1-adrenoreceptor blockade with prazosin had no effect on the plateau of SkBF during prolonged exercise in the heat. However, cutaneous arterioles also have α_2-adrenoreceptors and thus norepinephrine may have caused the plateau of SkBF by activating these receptors. To clarify this issue, Kellogg and colleagues (51) used prejunctional blockade of noradrenergic vasoconstrictor nerves by local iontophoresis of bretylium. They showed that the attenuation or plateau phase of the SkBF-T_{int} relationship was due to a limitation of active vasodilator activity rather than to enhanced vasoconstrictor tone (51). This was evidenced by the failure of bretylium to alter the plateau phase of the relationship, which would have been higher had enhanced vasoconstrictor tone been responsible for the plateau. Furthermore, the presence of a functioning vasoconstrictor system was associated with a less marked plateau phase, suggesting that vasoconstrictor tone was being slowly withdrawn during the later stage of prolonged dynamic exercise.

Given the hypothesized mechanistic link between the active vasodilator system and sweat gland activity, one might expect that sweat rate would show a similar attenuated rate of rise with SkBF-T_{int}. This was found to be the case; however, the degree of attenuation of the SkBF-T_{int} relationship is significantly greater than for the sweat rate–T_{int} relationship (51).

The baroreflex is known to control the active vasodilator system at rest (64). Baroreceptor unloading has been

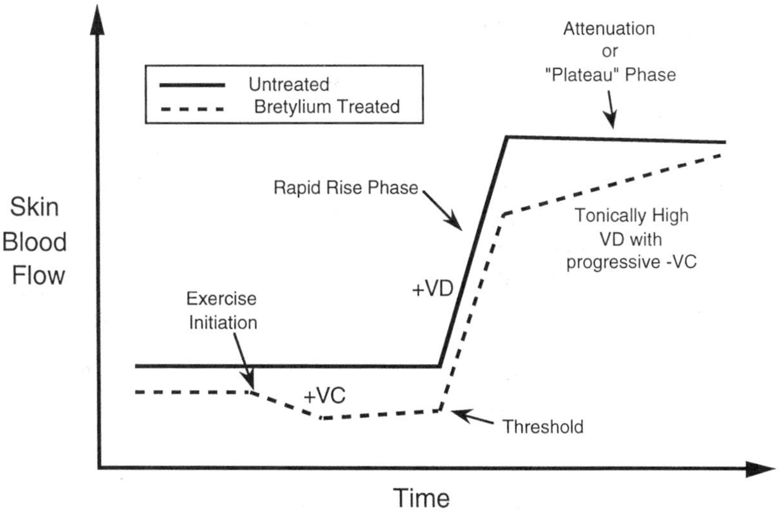

FIG. 16–5. Summary of the cutaneous vascular responses to prolonged dynamic exercise. During exercise, internal temperature rises. At a threshold internal temperature, a rapid rise in SkBF (rapid rise phase) occurs. Since this phase is not significantly altered by prejunctional blockade of noradrenergic active vasoconstrictor nerves by bretylium, the rapid rise in blood flow is due to increased active vasodilator tone. As internal temperature continues to rise in the later phase of exercise, an internal temperature is reached, above which further increases in SkBF are attenuated (plateau or attenuation phase). Interestingly, the attenuation is less pronounced after prejunctional blockade of noradrenergic active vasoconstrictor nerves. Thus, the plateau phase is characterized by an attenuation of further increases in active vasodilator tone despite further increases in internal temperature. These results also imply that the increase in vasoconstrictor tone effected by exercise initiation is withdrawn during this phase of exercise. *+VC*, increased active vasoconstrictor nerve activity; *+VD*, increased active vasodilator activity; *−VC*, decreased active vasoconstrictor activity; *Threshold*, internal temperature at which cutaneous vasodilation begins.

suggested to limit vasodilator activity during the plateau phase of exercise. Nielsen and colleagues (62) found that performance of exercise during water immersion to the xiphoid, which prevented baroreceptor unloading, was not accompanied by a plateau phase of the SkBF-T_{int} relationship. Similarly, Nose and colleagues (60) found that saline infusion during dynamic exercise in the heat also abolished the plateau phase. Finally, reduction of blood volume further restricts the level of SkBF during dynamic exercise in the heat, providing additional support for this role of the baroreflex (58,61).

LOCAL SKIN TEMPERATURE AND DYNAMIC EXERCISE

Local temperature of the skin participates in the control of SkBF: local warming effects a vasodilation through a NO-dependent mechanism (65) while local cooling causes vasoconstriction. Local cooling exerts its effects partially by altering noradrenergic function. Prejunctionally, local cooling enhances norepinephrine release (66,67), enhances α_2-adrenoreceptor affinity for norepinephrine (68–70), and enhances a nonadrenergic vasoconstrictor mechanism (67). These effects of local cooling or warming on the cutaneous circulation are unaltered by nerve blockade, suggesting a mechanism independent of central control (67). Pérgola and colleagues (50) investigated the individual roles of local skin temperature and general skin temperature in the cutaneous reflex responses to dynamic exercise at moderate work loads (100–125 W). As mentioned previously, they found that a cool skin temperature (28°C) increased the T_{int} threshold for active vasodilation and that bretylium blockade of noradrenergic vasoconstriction did not affect this shift. The rate of increase of SkBF with T_{int} was reduced by local cooling of the skin, an effect abolished by bretylium. This demonstrated that exercise in a cool environment results in a reflex inhibition of the onset of active vasodilation and a reduced rate of rise of SkBF with T_{int}. This reduced rate is partially due to norepinephrine release stimulated by a low local skin temperature. Thus, the effect of a cool skin temperature on the cutaneous vascular responses to dynamic exercise is to suppress increases in SkBF through delayed onset of active vasodilation and enhanced norepinephrine release from vasoconstrictor nerves.

ISOMETRIC EXERCISE AND THE SKIN

Isometric exercise differs from dynamic exercise in that there is little or no increase in heat production. Studies of the vasomotor response to handgrip exercise find that SkBF increases in direct proportion to blood pressure in nonacral skin. These studies indicate that isometric exercise appears to elicit only passive, rather than active (neural), cutaneous responses (71).

Studies of cutaneous efferent nerves suggest that there can be a simultaneous activation of multiple fiber types by isometric exercise, although results have not been consistent. For example, Bini and colleagues (72, 73) found that isometric exercise reduced cutaneous vasoconstriction tone, but Vissing and colleagues (74) reported increased vasoconstrictor tone. In contrast to the vasomotor nerves, studies of sweat gland activity indicate that sudomotor nerve activity increases during isometric exercise (74,75).

Crandall and colleagues (76) used bretylium iontophoresis to block vasoconstrictor nerves to elucidate whether SkBF was altered by isometric handgrip exercise during normothermia and heat stress. Sweat rate responses were also examined. Under normothermic conditions, isometric handgrip exercise did not affect SkBF or sweat rate; however, during hyperthermia SkBF was reduced regardless of vasoconstrictor nerve blockade with bretylium (Fig. 16–6). Furthermore, sweat rate increased during handgrip exercise in hyperthermia. Thus, under normothermic conditions, no evidence was found for enhanced vasoconstrictor, vasodilator, or sudomotor nerve activity. During heat stress, however, these results showed that vasodilator activity was reduced while sudomotor activity increased. These results suggest that the vasodilator and sudomotor systems can be independently controlled, and they further question their mechanistic relationship.

ACCLIMATION TO ENVIRONMENTAL CONDITIONS AND TRAINING EFFECTS

Repeated exercise in a warm environment produces an acclimatization of responses such that T_{int} is lower at a given level of exercise. The major adaptation responsible for this acclimatization is an increase in sweating at a given T_{int} (77–81). Increased sweating is accomplished by lowering the T_{int} threshold for initiation of sweating and perhaps by an increase in the sweat rate per degree increase in T_{int}. The threshold for vasodilation is also shifted to a lower T_{int}; however, the rate of increase of SkBF per degree increase in T_{int} is not altered (77,80).

Acclimation appears to be accomplished by both training effects and adaptation to a warm environment (80). Roberts and colleagues (80) found that training in a normothermic environment reduced the T_{int} threshold for vasodilation by 0.2°C. Additional training by bouts of

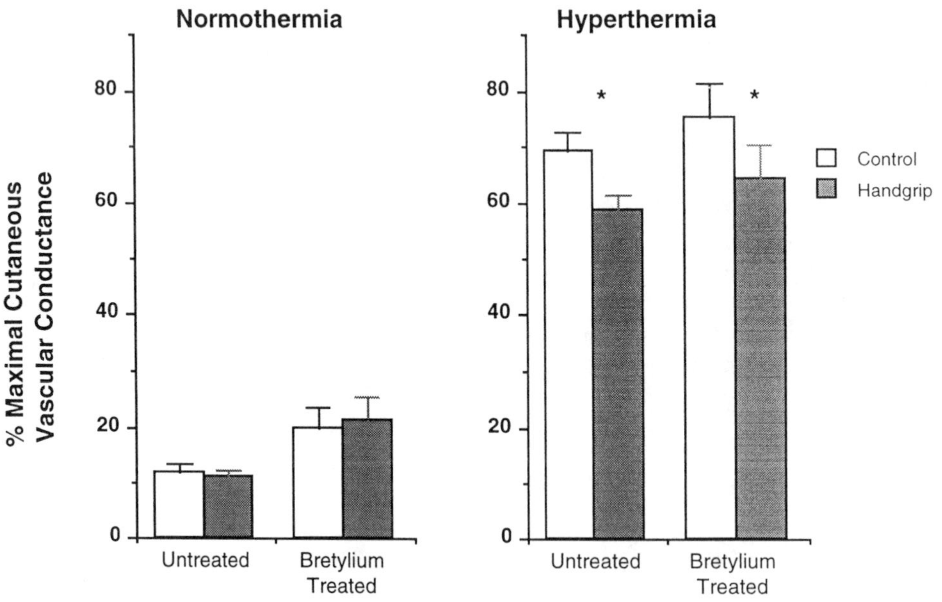

FIG. 16–6. Responses of cutaneous vascular conductance to 3 minutes of isometric handgrip exercise at 30% maximal voluntary contraction under normothermia and hyperthermia. Responses from untreated sites and sites pretreated with bretylium to abolish vasoconstrictor function are shown. Under normothermic conditions, isometric handgrip exercise had no effect; however, during heat stress, isometric handgrip exercise reduced cutaneous vascular conductance significantly ($p < .05$) at both the untreated and bretylium-treated sites. Since the response in hyperthermia was not altered by bretylium blockade of the vasoconstrictor system, the reduction in cutaneous vascular conductance during isometric handgrip exercise is mediated by withdrawal of vasodilator tone, rather than increases in vasoconstrictor tone. (Modified from ref. 76.)

exercise in a warm environment reduced the threshold further (0.26°C). Similar effects were found for sweating (80). Such shifts allow heat elimination to balance heat production at lower temperatures. It is unclear how these chronic changes in the control of the cutaneous responses to exercise are accomplished. It is possible that neural, endocrinologic, or even structural changes play roles in acclimation and training effects.

CONCLUSION

The cutaneous vasculature and sweat glands participate in the reflex adaptations to dynamic exercise. Cutaneous vessels are controlled by efferent neural systems of two types: a noradrenergic active vasoconstriction system and a cholinergic cotransmitter active vasodilator system. Sweat glands are controlled by cholinergic nerves.

The skin participates in reflex adaptations to both dynamic and isometric exercise. When dynamic exercise is initiated, SkBF is reduced by increased active vasoconstrictor tone. The thermogenic aspect of muscle activity increases T_{int} to a threshold level at which the active vasodilator system is activated, effecting a rapid increase in SkBF. Sudomotor nerve activity increases, initiating sweat production. After rising rapidly, SkBF levels off despite further increases in T_{int}. This limitation of SkBF is due to a limitation of active vasodilator activity. During the later stages of prolonged exercise, any remaining vasoconstrictor tone is withdrawn, further increasing SkBF.

Cutaneous vascular responses to isometric exercise have been difficult to demonstrate in normothermia. During hyperthermia, cutaneous vessels appear to vasoconstrict during isometric exercise due to withdrawal of active vasodilator tone.

REFERENCES

1. Rowell LB. *Human circulation: regulation during physical stress.* New York: Oxford University Press, 1986.
2. Hales JRS, Rowell LB, King RB. Regional distribution of blood flow in awake heat-stressed baboons. *Am J Physiol* 1979; 237(Heart Circ. Physiol. 6):H705–H712.
3. Eisman MM, Rowell LB. Renal vascular response to heat stress in baboons—role of renin-angiotensin. *J Appl Physiol* 1977; 43:739–746.
4. Proppe DW. Effect of sodium depletion on peripheral vascular responses to heat stress in baboons. *J Appl Physiol* 1987;62:1538–1543.
5. Rowell LB. Human cardiovascular adjustments to exercise and thermal stress. *Physiol Rev* 1974;54:75–159.
6. Rowell LB. Cardiovascular adjustments to thermal stress. In: Shepherd JT, Abboud FM, eds. *Handbook of physiology: the cardiovascular system,* vol sec. 2, vol. 3, pt. 2. Bethesda, MD: American Physiological Society, 1983:967–1024.
7. Leider M. On the weight of the skin. *J Invest Dermatol* 1949; 12:187–191.
8. Johnson JM, Proppe DW. Cardiovascular adjustments to heat stress. In: Fregly M, Blatteis C, eds. *Handbook of physiology—environmental physiology,* vol 1. New York: Oxford University Press, 1996:215–243.
9. Sato K. The physiology, pharmacology, and biochemistry of the eccrine sweat gland. *Rev Physiol Biochem Pharmacol* 1977;79: 51–131.
10. Sato K, Sato F. Nonisotonicity of simian eccrine primary sweat induced in vivo. *Am J Physiol* 1987;252:R1099–1105.
11. Fox RH, Edholm OG. Nervous control of the cutaneous circulation. *Br Med Bull* 1963;19:110–114.
12. Johnson JM. Nonthermoregulatory control of human skin blood flow. *J Appl Physiol* 1986;61:1613–1622.
13. Johnson JM, Brengelmann GL, Hales JRS, Vanhoutte PM, Wenger CB. Regulation of the cutaneous circulation. *Fed Proc* 1986; 45:2841–2850.
14. Rowell LB. Reflex control of the cutaneous vasculature. *J Invest Dermatol* 1977;69:154–166.
15. Lewis T, Pickering GW. Vasodilation in the limbs in response to warming the body; with evidence for sympathetic vasodilator nerves in man. *Heart* 1931;16:33–51.
16. Grant RT, Holling HE. Further observations on the vascular responses of the human limb to body warming; evidence for sympathetic vasodilator nerves in the normal subject. *Clin Sci* 1938; 3:273–285.
17. Edholm OG, Fox RH, MacPherson RK. Vasomotor control of the cutaneous blood vessels in the human forearm. *J Physiol (Lond)* 1957;139:455–465.
18. Roddie IC, Shepherd JT, Whelan RF. The contribution of constrictor and dilator nerves to the skin vasodilation during body heating. *J Physiol (Lond)* 1957;136:489–497.
19. Kellogg DL Jr, Johnson JM, Kosiba WA. Selective abolition of adrenergic vasoconstrictor responses in skin by local iontophoresis of bretylium. *Am J Physiol* 1989;257(*Heart and Circ Physiol* 26): H1599–1606.
20. Lindblad LR, Ekenvall L. Alpha-adrenoreceptors in the vessels of human finger skin. *Acta Physiol Scand* 1986;128:219–222.
21. Ekenvall L, Lindblad LE. Is vibration white finger a primary sympathetic nerve injury? *Br J Ind Med* 1986;43:702–706.
22. Ekenvall L, Lindblad LE, Norbeck O, Etzell B. Sympathetic alpha-adrenoreceptors and cold-induced vasoconstriction in human finger skin. In: Ekenvall L, ed. *Vibration syndrome: clinical and pathogenic aspects.* Stockholm: Karolinska Institute, 1987.
23. Brengelmann GL, Freund PR, Rowell LB, Olerud JE, Kraning KK. Absence of active vasodilation associated with congenital absence of sweat glands in humans. *Am J Physiol* 1981;240(Heart and Circ. Physiol 9):H571–H575.
24. Frewin DB, McConnell DJ, Downey JA. Is a kininogenase necessary for human sweating? *Lancet* 1973;2:744.
25. Uno H. Sympathetic innervation of the sweat glands and piloerector muscle of macaques and humans. *J Invest Dermatol* 1977; 69:112–130.
26. Sato K, Kang H, Saga K, Sato KT. Biology of sweat glands and their disorders. I. Normal sweat gland function. *J Am Acad Dermatol* 1989;20:537–563.
27. Fox RH, Hilton SM. Bradykinin formation in human skin as a factor in heat vasodilation. *J Physiol (Lond)* 1958;142:219–232.
28. Hökfelt TM, Johansson O, Ljungdahl A, Lundberg JM, Schultzberg M. Peptidergic neurones. *Nature* 1980;284:515–521.
29. Kellogg DL Jr, Pérgola PE, Kosiba WA, Grossmann M, Johnson JM. Cutaneous active vasodilation in humans is mediated by cholinergic nerve co-transmission. *Circ Res* 1995;77:1222–1228.
30. Kellogg DL Jr, Crandall CG, Liu Y, Charkoudian N, Johnson JM. Nitric oxide and cutaneous active vasodilation during heat stress in humans. *J Appl Physiol* 1998;85:824–829.
31. Toda N, Okamura T. Role of nitric oxide in neurally induced cerebroarterial relaxation. *J Pharmacol Exp Ther* 1991;258:1027–1032.
32. Coffman JD. Effects of endothelium-derived nitric oxide on skin and digital blood flow in humans. *Am J Physiol* 1994;267(*Heart and Circ Physiol* 36):H2087–H2090.
33. Bevegärd BS, Shepherd JT. Reaction in man of resistance and capacity vessels in forearm and hand to leg exercise. *J Appl Physiol* 1966;21:123–132.
34. Bishop JW, Donald KW, Taylor SH, Wormald PN. The blood flow in the human arm during leg exercise. *Circ Res* 1961;9:264–274.
35. Christensen EH, Nielsen M, Hannisdahl B. Investigations of the circulation in the skin at the beginning of muscular work. *Acta Physiol Scand* 1942;4:162–170.

36. Hirata K, Nagasaka T, Hirai A, Harashita M, Takahata T. Peripheral vascular tone during heat load is modified by exercise intensity. *Eur J Appl Physiol* 1983;51:7–15.
37. Johnson JM, Park MK. Reflex control of skin blood flow by skin temperature: role of core temperature. *J Appl Physiol* 1979; 47:1188–1193.
38. Johnson JM, Rowell LB, Brengelmann GL. Modification of the skin blood flow-body temperature relationship by upright exercise. *J Appl Physiol* 1974;37:880–886.
39. Taylor WF, Johnson JM, O'Leary D, Park MK. Modification of the cutaneous vascular response to exercise by local skin temperature. *J Appl Physiol* 1984;57(6):1878–1884.
40. Taylor WF, Johnson JM, Kosiba WA, Kwan CM. Graded cutaneous vascular responses to dynamic leg exercise. *J Appl Physiol* 1988;64:1803–1809.
41. Zelis R, Mason DT, Braunwald E. Partition of blood flow to the cutaneous and muscular beds of the forearm at rest and during leg exercise in normal subjects and in patients with heart failure. *Circ Res* 1969;24:799–806.
42. Johnson JM, Park MK. Effect of heat stress on cutaneous vascular responses to the initiation of exercise. *J Appl Physiol* 1982; 53:744–749.
43. Blair DA, Glover WE, Roddie IC. Vasomotor responses in the human arm during leg exercise. *Circ Res* 1960;9:264–274.
44. Blair DA, Glover WE, Kidd BSL, Roddie IC. Peripheral vascular effects of bretylium tosylate in man. *Br J Pharmacol* 1960; 15:466–475.
45. Saumet JL, Kellogg DL Jr, Taylor WF, Johnson JM. Cutaneous laser-Doppler flowmetry: influence of underlying muscle blood flow. *J Appl Physiol* 1988;65:478–481.
46. Kellogg DL Jr, Johnson JM, Kosiba WA. Competition between the cutaneous active vasoconstrictor and vasodilator systems during exercise in man. *Am J Physiol* 1991;261(Heart and Circ. Physiol 30):H1184–H1189.
47. van Beaumont W, Bullard RW. Sweating exercise stimulation during circulatory arrest. *Science* 1966;152:1521–1523.
48. Johnson JM, Rowell LB. Forearm skin and muscle vascular responses to prolonged leg exercise in man. *J Appl Physiol* 1975;39:916–924.
49. Johnson JM, Park MK. Effect of upright exercise on threshold for cutaneous vasodilation and sweating. *J Appl Physiol* 1981;50:814–818.
50. Pérgola PE, Johnson JM, Kellogg DL Jr, Kosiba WA. Control of skin blood flow by whole body and local skin cooling in exercising humans. *Am J Physiol* 1996;270(Heart. Circ Physiol 39):H208–H215.
51. Kellogg DL Jr, Johnson JM, Kenney WL, Pérgola PE, Kosiba WA. Mechanisms of control of skin blood flow during prolonged exercise in humans. *Am J Physiol* 1993;265:H562–H568.
52. Hammel HT, Jackson DC, Stolwijk JAJ, Hardy JD, Stremme SB. Temperature regulation by hypothalamic proportional control with adjustable set point. *J Appl Physiol* 1963;18:1146–1154.
53. Nielsen M. Die regulation der körpertemperatur bei muskelarbeit. *Skand Arch Physiol* 1938;79:193–230.
54. Nielsen B, Davies CTM. Temperature regulation during exercise in water and air. *Acta Physiol Scand* 1976;98:500–508.
55. Tam H-S, Darling RC, Cheh H-Y, Downey JA. Sweating response: a means of evaluating the set-point theory during exercise. *J Appl Physiol* 1978;45:451–458.
56. Kamon E, Belding HS. Dermal blood flow in the resting arm during leg exercise. *J Appl Physiol* 1969;26:317–320.
57. Brengelmann GL, Johnson JM, Hermansen L, Rowell LB. Altered control of skin blood flow during exercise at high internal temperatures. *J Appl Physiol* 1977;43:790–794.
58. Fortney SM, Nadel ER, Wenger CB, Bove JR. Effect of acute alterations of blood volume on circulatory performance in humans. *J Appl Physiol* 1981;50:292–298.
59. Nadel ER, Cafarelli E, Roberts MF, Wenger CB. Circulatory regulation during exercise in different ambient temperatures. *J Appl Physiol* 1979;46:430–437.
60. Nose H, Mack GW, Shi X, Morimoto K, Nadel ER. Effect of saline infusion during exercise on thermal and circulatory regulation. *J Appl Physiol* 1990;69:609–616.
61. Nishiyasu T, Shi X, Mack GW, Nadel ER. Effect of hypovolemia on forearm vascular resistance control during exercise in the heat. *J Appl Physiol* 1991;71:1382–1386.
62. Nielsen B, Rowell LB, Bonde-Petersen F. Cardiovascular responses to heat stress and blood volume displacement during exercise in man. *Eur J Appl Physiol* 1984;52:370–374.
63. Kenney WL, Tankersley CG, Newswanger DL, Puhl SM. α_1-Adrenergic blockade does not alter control of skin blood flow during exercise. *Am J Physiol* 1991;260(*Heart Circ Physiol* 29):H855–H861.
64. Kellogg DL Jr, Johnson JM, Kosiba WA. Baroreflex control of the cutaneous active vasodilator system in humans. *Circ Res* 1990;66:1420–1426.
65. Kellogg DL Jr, Liu Y, Kosiba IF, et al. Nitric oxide mediates increases in skin blood flow during local warming in humans. *FASEB J* 1997;11:A43.
66. Lindblad LE, Ekenvall L, Klingstedt C. Neural regulation of vascular tone and cold induced vasoconstriction in human finger skin. *J Auton Nerv Sys* 1990;30:169–174.
67. Pérgola PE, Kellogg DL Jr, Johnson JM, Kosiba WA. Role of sympathetic nerves in the vascular effects of local temperature in human forearm skin. *Am J Physiol* 1993;265(*Heart Circ Physiol* 34):H785–H792.
68. Bodelsson M, Arneklo-Nobin B, Nobin A, Owman C, Sollerman C, Tornebrandt K. Cooling enhances alpha 2-adrenoreceptor-mediated vasoconstriction in human hand veins. *Acta Physiol Scand* 1990;138:283–291.
69. Faber JE. Effect of local tissue cooling on microvascular smooth muscle and post-junctional α_2-adrenoreceptors. *Am J Physiol* 1988;255(Heart Circ. Physiol. 24):H121–H130.
70. Flavahan NA. The role of vascular alpha-2-adrenoreceptors as cutaneous thermosensors. *News Physiol Sci* 1991;6:251–255.
71. Taylor WF, Johnson JM, Kosiba WA. Roles of absolute and relative load in skin vasoconstrictor responses to exercise. *J Appl Physiol* 1990;69(3):1131–1136.
72. Bini G, Hagbarth K-E, Hynninen P, Wallin BG. Thermoregulatory and rhythm-generating mechanisms governing the sudomotor and vasoconstrictor outflow in human cutaneous nerves. *J Physiol (Lond)* 1980;306:537–552.
73. Bini G, Hagbarth KE, Wallin BG. Cardiac rhythmicity of skin sympathetic activity recorded from peripheral nerves in man. *J Auton Nerv Syst* 1981;4:17–24.
74. Vissing SF, Scherrer U, Victor RG. Stimulation of skin sympathetic nerve discharge by central command. *Circ Res* 1991; 69:228–238.
75. Saito M, Maito M, Mano T. Different responses in skin and muscle sympathetic nerve activity to static muscle contraction. *J Appl Physiol* 1990;69:2085–2090.
76. Crandall CG, Musick J, Hatch JP, Kellogg DL Jr, Johnson JM. Cutaneous vascular and sudomotor responses to isometric exercise in humans. *J Appl Physiol* 1995;79(6):1946–1950.
77. Fox RH, Goldsmith R, Kidd DJ, Lewis HE. Acclimatization to heat in man by controlled elevation of body temperature. *J Physiol (Lond)* 1963;166:530–547.
78. Fox RH, Goldsmith R, Kidd DJ, Lewis HE. Blood flow and other thermoregulatory changes with acclimatization to heat. *J Physiol (Lond)* 1963;166:548–562.
79. Gonzalez RR, Pandolf KB, Gagge AP. Heat acclimation and decline in sweating during humidity transients. *J Appl Physiol* 1974;36:419–425.
80. Roberts MF, Wenger CB, Stolwijk JAJ, Nadel ER. Skin blood flow and sweating changes following exercise training and heat acclimation. *J Appl Physiol* 1977;43:133–137.
81. Rowell LB, Kraning KK II, Kennedy JW, Evans TO. Central circulatory responses to work in dry heat before and after acclimatization. *J Appl Physiol* 1967;22:509–518.

Exercise and Sport Science,
edited by William E. Garrett, Jr., and Donald T. Kirkendall.
Lippincott Williams & Wilkins, Philadelphia © 2000.

CHAPTER 17

Molecular Biology of Exercise

James A. Carson and Frank W. Booth

The molecular biology of exercise is a broadly applied subject, as the definitions given below indicate. Molecular biology can be considered as just another tool that can be employed to improve human performance. This chapter discusses muscle hypertrophy and the increase of mitochondrial density through enhanced aerobic exercise, with an emphasis on molecular biologic information. The chapter also considers the molecular biologic information that complements epidemiologic studies on how daily physical activity decreases the risk of many chronic diseases.

DEFINITIONS

Definition of Exercise Physiology

Exercise physiology is a multidisciplinary discipline including the fields of aging, cell biology, developmental biology, epidemiology, genomics, immunology, molecular biology (biochemistry, genetics, and biophysics), clinical medicine, neurosciences, pediatrics, pharmacology, physiology, preventive medicine, and public health. The ultimate model of exercise is the unanesthetized human being during maximal physical exertion. Those who investigate responses to exercise must be broadly trained and knowledgeable in most biologic disciplines. Molecular biology is merely one of many powerful tools that can be employed by exercise physiologists to explain how human beings are able to exercise at maximal exertion and how they are able to adapt at the molecular, organelle, cellular, tissue/organ, and systemic levels to increase their capacity for exercise, whether it is extending their limits for intensity or duration.

J. A. Carson: Department of Exercise Science, South Carolina University, Columbia, South Carolina 29208.
F. W. Booth: Department of Integrative Biology, Pharmacology and Physiology, University of Texas Medical School, Houston, Texas 77030.

Definition of Molecular Biology

Molecular biology is intimidating to many unfamiliar with its terminology. However, molecular biology can be thought of merely as a new set of biologic tools to answer questions in exercise sciences. The *Oxford Medical Companion* (1) defines molecular biology as the study of the chemical structures and processes underlying biologic events, in particular the formation, organization, and activity of the macromolecules essential to life such as nucleic acids and proteins, and the detailed structure and function of chromosomes and subcellular organelles. Kendrew (2) reports that the boundaries between biochemistry, genetics, molecular biology, and biophysics have become less and less well defined. Thus, molecular biology can be thought of as a tool to answer the integrative questions posed by exercise physiologists.

OVERVIEW OF MUSCLE HYPERTROPHY

Skeletal muscle provides the force that allows the body to undergo locomotion and perform work. Properties intrinsic to skeletal muscle can affect the rate and duration of our body's locomotion, as well as its ability to produce force. Some of these intrinsic properties include the muscle's phenotype, oxidative capacity, and cross-sectional area (3). Determining the limits of human performance has been an interest of humankind since the time of the ancient Greeks. Physical competitions have traditionally been used to determine these performance limits, including how fast or long a person can perform a task, as well as how much power or force the person can produce. The work capacity of the recruited muscle can alter these performance parameters. The worldwide attention the Olympic Games receive every 4 years clearly demonstrates that defining the limits of human performance continues to be a major interest of humankind.

Skeletal muscle is a dynamic tissue, and its intrinsic properties change throughout a human's life span. Skeletal muscle grows with the body's frame until maturity. Several maturation-induced alterations in skeletal muscle occur during aging and include a gradual decrease in muscle mass, a shift in the muscle phenotype, and a decreased ability to recover from injury (4). Skeletal muscle's dynamic properties are also demonstrated by the specific adaptations muscle exhibits to different stimuli. Overload is an example of a powerful stimulus that can induce skeletal muscle adaptation.

Healthy skeletal muscle can respond to increased external loading by increasing mass. The primary adaptation for muscle mass enlargement by intermittent resistance exercise in humans is increased muscle fiber cross-sectional area (5). The radial enlargement of existing muscle fibers increases the muscle's force-generating capacity. It is a well-documented phenomenon that heavy physical labor and sports such as gymnastics, swimming, wrestling, and weightlifting produce muscular enlargement. The mechanisms producing the muscle hypertrophy have not been clearly defined, however. Understanding the regulation of muscle hypertrophy at the molecular level should provide definitive evidence for the cellular processes contributing to overload-induced enlargement. This knowledge will impact the way athletes as well as older individuals train to maintain or gain muscle mass.

Inducing Skeletal Muscle Hypertrophy

A multitude of exercise routines have been devised to produce human skeletal muscle hypertrophy; however, the major theme of the vast majority of these routines is intermittent resistance exercise using concentric and eccentric contractions against a resistance. Strength training is usually progressive, with either the resistance or the repetitions being increased as the muscle's work capacity improves.

Resistance exercise in previously untrained individuals produces extremely rapid strength, and this adaptation has a significant neural component involving a more efficient recruitment of the contracting muscles (6). Resistance exercise–induced increases in muscle mass occur at a slower rate and plateau after a period of training (6). Thus, not only is the growth rate of resistance-trained muscle slow, but the growth capacity appears limited. The difficulty in producing extreme muscle hypertrophy has caused many athletes and recreational weightlifters to turn to the expanding market of legal and illegal ergogenic aids to produce increased muscle mass.

In contrast to human resistance exercise, animal studies employing chronic stretch or compensatory overload produce a rapid and extremely large growth to the loaded muscles. These hypertrophy models have a large chronic loading component where the muscle is under a constant stretch or load. During human resistance exercise the working muscle undergoes intermittent active contractions against a resistance. Chronic loading appears to be important for the large increases in skeletal muscle mass. Animal models that either employ intermittent loading or mimic human resistance exercise produce less muscle mass increases than chronic loading models (7–9). Thus, the nature of the loading stimulus provided to the muscle appears to regulate the extent of overload-induced muscle hypertrophy. Determining the molecular pathways activated by chronic loading and comparing those to the events occurring in intermittent-loaded muscle will help delineate the rate-limiting mechanisms when inducing skeletal muscle hypertrophy in humans.

MOLECULAR ADAPTATION IN HYPERTROPHIED SKELETAL MUSCLE

Determinants of Protein Expression

Protein abundance within a muscle fiber is a consequence of both protein synthesis and degradation rates. Both protein synthesis and degradation are upregulated during hypertrophy (10,11). Protein degradation may demonstrate specificity for certain proteins, such as myosin isoforms, during overload-induced muscle growth (10). However, at this time there is not a good understanding of protein degradation regulation during overload-induced hypertrophy, when compared to the body of literature regarding protein synthesis regulation. Translational mechanisms are involved in messenger ribonucleic acids (mRNAs) being translated into protein. Alterations in the capacity and/or efficiency of the muscle's translation machinery are mechanisms for this type of regulation. Increasing the abundance of ribosomes and translational cofactors affecting 5′-cap–mediated ribosomal binding to the mRNA contributes to an increased translational capacity in the fiber. The family of eukaryotic initiation factors (eIFs) comprises cofactors that alter translation efficiency by altering cap-dependent ribosome binding. The activity of eIFs can be altered by posttranslational modifications such as phosphorylation (12). These modifications can alter the efficiency of the translation process (Fig. 17–1).

Pretranslational events also influence protein synthesis by altering the abundance of specific mRNAs available for translation. mRNA abundance is regulated at the levels of synthesis, processing, and stability, and mRNA synthesis is controlled at the level of gene transcription. Specific deoxyribonucleic acid (DNA) regulatory sequences found that both 5′ and 3′ in the coding region of the gene, as well as within the coding sequence, can regulate the gene's transcription rate. The promoter region of a gene contains regulatory sequences at 5′

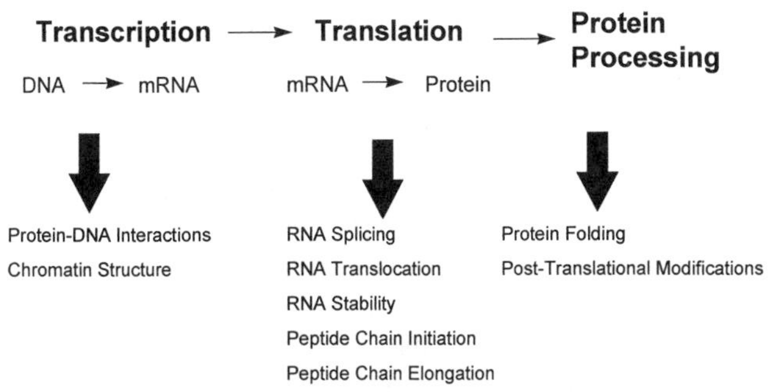

FIG. 17–1. The basic sequence of cellular gene expression.

of the gene's transcription start site. DNA regulatory elements located within the promoter region influence transcription by binding specific proteins and/or protein complexes. A DNA-binding protein's activity can be modified by dimerization with other proteins and by posttranslational modifications of the proteins (i.e., phosphorylation).

Protein synthesis rates increase in both human and animal skeletal muscle after hypertrophy-producing resistance exercise (13,14). Indirect and direct evidence point to both pretranslational and translational control mechanisms in hypertrophying skeletal muscle, and multiple factors appear to influence molecular regulation during overload-induced growth. Protein function must be considered when examining expression patterns. An example of this important distinction of function is whether a given gene can be classified as an immediate early gene, where synthesis of other proteins is not required for expression. Immediate early gene expression, such as c-*fos,* is tightly regulated, undergoing massive shifts in protein and RNA abundance. This can be in stark contrast to the regulation of muscle structural proteins, such as skeletal α-actin, where gene expression is already at a high level. Structural proteins are expressed at constitutive levels. Protein isoform shifts are another factor that can affect gene regulation during skeletal muscle hypertrophy. Skeletal muscle protein isoforms can have their expression levels dramatically increased or decreased during overload-induced hypertrophy (3). The expression of myosin heavy chain isoforms during hypertrophy is an excellent example of this regulation. Other factors involved in the molecular regulation of gene expression during skeletal muscle hypertrophy include the muscle's growth rate and the time point analyzed during the time course of hypertrophy (i.e., rapid vs. slowed growth phases) (15). The above-mentioned factors must be considered to give the context of a specific gene's regulation during hypertrophy.

In muscle atrophy produced by unloading, a sequence of events occurs in the slow-twitch soleus muscle: protein synthesis decreases within hours of unloading, protein degradation increases after 3 days, and then the rise in protein degradation decreases after the 14th day of unloading until it falls to less than control values, so that both protein synthesis and degradation are similar to, but less than, control values at the 21st day of unloading (16).

Translational Control in Overloaded Skeletal Muscle

Skeletal muscle protein synthesis increases after a bout of isotonic resistance training in both humans and rodents (13,14). Skeletal muscle protein synthesis rates also increase during hypertrophy induced by chronic loading (10,11,17). Considerable evidence points to translational and/or posttranslational regulation being important for increased muscle protein synthesis after either a single bout of resistance exercise or at the onset of chronic loading. Much of this evidence is indirect, however, since direct measures of translational regulation during overload-induced hypertrophy have not been performed at this time (Fig. 17–2).

The quantification of the muscle's total RNA pool

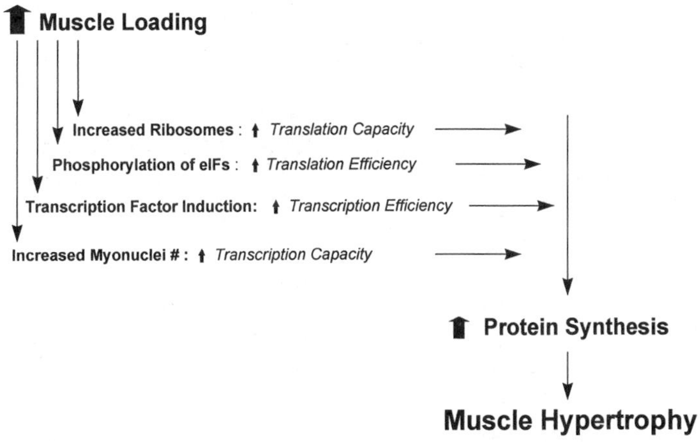

FIG. 17–2. Potential stages of molecular regulation during overload-induced hypertrophy.

and RNA activity can be used to estimate translational regulation changes in the hypertrophying muscle (10,11,13). The majority of the total RNA pool in skeletal muscle is 18S and 28S ribosomal RNAs. Thus, an increase in total RNA serves to increase the ribosomal capacity of the muscle and enlarge its translational capacity. RNA activity represents the quantity of protein synthesized per day for a given quantity of RNA. Increased RNA activity implies that an increase in the muscle's translational capacity and/or translational efficiency is important for increased protein synthesis during hypertrophy. No change in RNA activity implies that increased RNA abundance is important for increasing protein synthesis. Total RNA and RNA activity have been quantified to provide insight into the mechanisms regulating gene expression during overload-induced hypertrophy.

The rat gastrocnemius and plantaris muscles hypertrophy after isotonic resistance exercise training, and translational control has been shown to be important for increased protein synthesis after a bout of resistance exercise (13). This resistance exercise regime induced an increase in myofibril protein synthesis 17 hours postexercise; the increase was maintained for at least 41 hours postexercise. Protein synthesis increases after resistance exercise and appears not to be driven by increased mRNA abundance, since the mRNA levels for skeletal α-actin were not changed postexercise. Both the total RNA pool and RNA activity were increased in the exercised muscle, however. Although translational control appears important after a single bout of resistance exercise, a 10-week isotonic resistance training program increased skeletal α-actin mRNA abundance (9). This implies that in order to support the growth of the hypertrophying muscle, mRNA abundance is increased over time to drive protein for continued muscle enlargement.

Translational mechanisms also appear important for increases in muscle protein synthesis at the onset of chronic overload (10,11). Stretch overloading the chicken anterior latissimus dorsi (ALD) increases muscle protein synthesis, and this increased protein synthesis is accompanied by increased total RNA and RNA activity (11). Additionally, at the onset of stretch overload in the ALD muscle actin protein synthesis rates increase (10), while the skeletal α-actin mRNA concentration is significantly reduced (18). RNA activity also increases, at the onset of chronic stretch, the rat extensor digitorum longus (EDL) muscle (19). Chronic stretch of the rabbit EDL muscle dramatically increases the muscle's total RNA pool (20). These studies provide more evidence for the importance of translational regulation at the onset of stretch-induced hypertrophy (Fig. 17–3).

The hypertrophying chicken ALD muscle appears to shift from translational mechanisms toward transcriptional mechanisms to support protein synthesis for muscle growth. RNA activity in the stretch overloaded ALD muscle, after an initial increase, returns to control levels after 3 days of stretch overload (11). mRNA abundance appears to become more critical for maintaining increased protein synthesis rates as muscle growth continues. A decreased reliance on translational mechanisms is also supported by the fact that skeletal α-actin mRNA concentration in the stretch overload in the ALD is increasing between the third and sixth days of stretch overload (18). Increased mRNA abundance may be necessary for maintaining the rapid and large hypertrophy induced by chronic stretch.

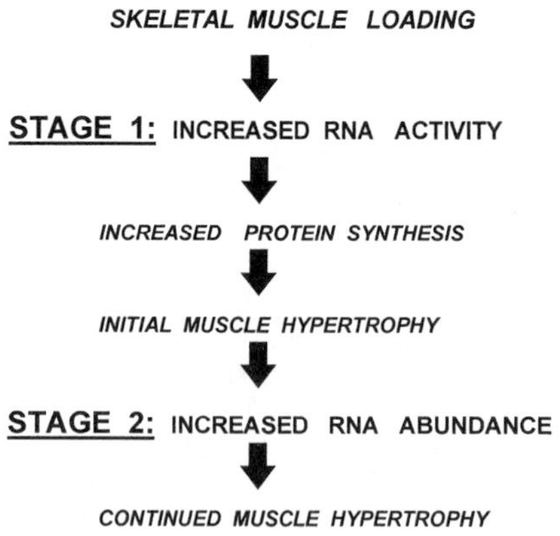

FIG. 17–3. A multistage model for gene expression regulation during skeletal muscle hypertrophy.

These observations from animal models have accurately predicted the responses of human skeletal muscle to weightlifting. MacDougall's group (14,21) has shown that muscle protein synthesis rate was significantly elevated in the biceps brachii muscle of male subjects for 24 hours postexercise and had returned to control levels by 36 hours. Moreover, while RNA activity increased (implying increased translational efficiency), RNA capacity remained unchanged (21). These observations suggest that animal models are appropriate for some aspects of human resistance training.

Although there is growing interest in the regulation of translation, very little is known about translational regulation in hypertrophying skeletal muscle. In atrophying skeletal muscle, however, decreased protein synthesis is associated with a decreased elongation rate of nascent polypeptide chains (22). Translational initiation factors serve to regulate translation by binding to and forming a complex at the mRNA 5′-cap (m^7GpppN) (23). The eIFs can mediate 5′-cap–regulated binding of ribosomes, increasing translational efficiency, and their activity can be altered by phosphorylation events (23). eIF-4e phosphorylation is correlated with increased protein synthesis rates in the pressure-overloaded canine left ventricle (24). There is also evidence for a decreased association of 70-kd heat shock protein (HSP-70) with the polysome (25). A better understanding of translational regulation in overloaded skeletal muscle should dramatically increase our understanding of the stimulus involved in inducing the process. Delineating the signaling cascades responsible for altering the phosphorylation of eIFs and the regulation of HSP-70 may be some of the first important steps in this direction.

Control of Transcription in Overloaded Skeletal Muscle

Transcriptional regulation serves to increase or decrease mRNA template synthesis in muscle, but measuring mRNA abundance in the muscle does not serve as an indicator of that transcriptional regulation. mRNA abundance is a function of its turnover rate, which involves both synthesis and degradation. The nuclear run-on assay, which measures the transcription rate of a specific mRNA, is the standard for providing direct evidence of transcriptional regulation. At this time there are no studies providing direct evidence of either increased or decreased transcriptional control during skeletal muscle hypertrophy. There is strong indirect evidence, however, for transcriptional control during overload-induced skeletal muscle hypertrophy.

Indirect evidence of transcriptional control in hypertrophied skeletal muscle involves the analysis of muscle promoter regions directing the expression reporter genes. Promoter regulation analysis during hypertrophy has been performed in animal models using transgenic or plasmid injection technologies (18,26,27). Transgenic mice have a transgene inserted into the mouse's genome. The transgene contains the promoter regulatory region of a specific gene and directs the expression of a reporter gene. The reporter gene encodes a protein that is not normally expressed in skeletal muscle. Measurement of the reporter protein's activity gives the activity of a specific promoter. Plasmid DNA injected into a muscle contains promoter and reporter gene regulation as transgenic technology; however, plasmid injection is a transient assay since the plasmid DNA remains episomal and is not integrated into the genome. Promoter regulation studies along with the corresponding mRNA measurements support the fact that transcriptional control is an important control point in hypertrophying skeletal muscle.

Both positive and negative gene regulation appear to be invoked during skeletal muscle hypertrophy. The type of regulation is dependent on the function of the protein encoded by the gene and the phenotype of the hypertrophying muscle. Muscle creatine kinase (MCK) serves to maintain adenosine triphosphate (ATP) levels in the muscle during periods of intense contraction, and it is more predominant in fast-twitch muscles (28). Compensatory overload studies using transgenic mice have demonstrated that MCK mRNA levels and a −3300–base pair (bp) length of the MCK promoter directing reporter gene expression decrease in the hypertrophying rat PLAN muscle (26). Deletions of the MCK promoter have demonstrated that a 2146-bp region between −3300 and −1256 bp is critical for the repression of transcription (26). Unlike the MCK regulation, β-myosin heavy chain (MHC) mRNA and promoter-directed reporter gene activity increase in the hypertrophying PLAN muscle (29). A region between −293 and +120 bp of the transcription start site appears sufficient for this response (30). Both MCK and β-MHC appear to be regulated at the level of the gene during compensatory overload in the PLAN muscle. MCK and β-MHC expression patterns mirror the fast to slow phenotype switch occurring in the hypertrophying PLAN muscle. Further work may provide important insight into the question of whether the two different genes use similar DNA regulatory elements to both activate and repress transcription during muscle phenotype transitions. Furthermore, even if the DNA regulatory elements are not similar between the two genes during the overload-induced phenotype switch, it will be interesting to discover if the signaling cascade regulating repression of one gene and activation of another gene are shared. This will provide important insight into the molecular signaling involved in muscle phenotype transitions during exercise or loading.

Transcriptional regulation also appears important for regulation of skeletal α-actin regulation during chronic stretch overload (27). The stretch overloaded ALD muscle appears to follow a sequence of regulation during the first week of chronic stretch overload. Although skeletal α-actin mRNA concentration is initially decreased at the onset of stretch overload, it returns to control levels by day 6 of overload (18). Actin promoter–directed reporter gene expression is also increased at the sixth day of stretch. The first 100 bp of the skeletal α-actin promoter are sufficient for increased promoter activity. Interaction between two DNA regulatory elements, serum response element-1 (SRE1, CArG box) and transcription enhancer factor-1 (TEF-1, MCAT) binding sites, located within the 100-bp region, appears necessary for stretch overload activation (18). Studies analyzing cardiac myocytes' hypertrophy in culture have found that the first 100 bp of the skeletal α-actin promoter can confer its transactivation by transforming growth factor-β (31) and α-adrenergic induction (32). Considerable knowledge will be gained regarding the regulation of skeletal muscle hypertrophy by understanding the protein-protein interactions and kinase cascades involved at the SRE1 and TEF-1 binding sites during chronic stretch overload.

The importance of protein-protein interactions and possibly intracellular kinase cascades for the induction of gene expression during hypertrophy can be demonstrated with the skeletal α-actin gene. SRE1 and TEF-1 DNA regulatory elements bind nuclear transcription factor proteins to influence skeletal α-actin gene transcription (33,34). The TEF-1 binding site binds TEF-1 protein, and SRE1 has affinity for two proteins: serum response factor (SRF) and yin yang-1 (YY1). SRF binds to SRE1 as a homodimer and is an important activator of the skeletal α-actin promoter (34). YY1 functions as a repressor of skeletal α-actin promoter activity by competing for the SRE1 binding site with SRF. Additionally, SRF binding to the SRE in the c-*fos* promoter is necessary for serum induction of the promoter in culture (35). DNA binding assays with ALD nuclear extracts have demonstrated that the SRF-SRE1 complex has a faster migration complex during native gel electrophoresis (18). There is the possibility that a post-translational modification of the SRF protein, such as phosphorylation, may be responsible for this altered mobility.

Delineating the signaling mechanisms that translate a loading stimulus into altered gene regulation in the nucleus of the myofiber will have an enormous impact on our understanding of overload-induced hypertrophy. There are several interesting candidates for the mechanism(s) involved in the regulation of overload-induced growth. These mechanisms include growth factor signaling, anabolic and catabolic steroid action, and integrin-mediated signaling pathways. The extracellular domain of the integrin-receptor complex interacts with the extracellular matrix (ECM), while propagation of integrin signaling to the nucleus occurs via cytoplasmic domain of the receptor initiating signaling cascades (36). These signaling cascades allow integrin signaling to alter myofiber gene expression. Components of integrin-mediated signaling, including Rho, a Ras-related guanosine triphosphate (GTP)-binding protein, and focal adhesion kinase (FAK), are good candidates for the signaling cascades' mediating of overload- or stretch-induced skeletal muscle growth. Further work is needed to link components of mechanical signaling to specific changes in gene expression during hypertrophy.

The regulation of gene expression in skeletal muscle appears complex. During skeletal muscle hypertrophy, certain genes are induced while other genes are repressed. Several mechanisms are available to the myofiber to alter protein synthesis, and transcriptional regulation is one of these regulatory options. During the time course of skeletal muscle hypertrophy, there appears to be a sequential hierarchy of these regulatory mechanisms (15). Further research will provide answers pointing to the molecular mechanisms signaling transcriptional regulation in hypertrophying skeletal muscle; however, a more significant question involves understanding the cellular signaling that creates a demand for transcriptional control during skeletal muscle hypertrophy. These insights will provide a much clearer picture of the regulation of overload-induced muscle growth.

MOLECULAR SIGNALS IN SKELETAL MUSCLE HYPERTROPHY

Insulin-Like Growth Factors

Insulin-like growth factor-I and -II (IGF-I and -II) are polypeptides that can regulate functions in many cell types (37). The IGFs stimulate myoblast proliferation and differentiation in cell culture, and growth hormone's actions on skeletal muscle are also thought to be mediated through the IGF system (38). IGFs can exert effects on skeletal muscle by binding to their respective IGF-I or -II receptor on the sarcolemma of the muscle fiber. Receptor binding propagates signaling into the myofiber by the activation of tyrosine residues located on the cytosolic domain of the receptor. The phosphorylated receptor can then initiate signaling cascades in the myofiber, which can alter gene expression in the nucleus or cellular regulation in the cytosol. IGFs can regulate skeletal muscle in either an autocrine or paracrine manner. IGF-I and -II can be synthesized endogenously and secreted by muscle fibers; however, they are also synthesized by most tissues in the body and found in the circulation (37). The muscle's extracellular matrix is also a rich source of growth factors, including the IGFs (38). The interaction of IGF-binding proteins with circulating IGFs is a point of regulation for the growth factor's biologic activity (38).

Animal and cell culture studies have provided much of the evidence for IGFs biologic function on skeletal muscle. IGFs appear able to induce skeletal muscle hypertrophy, and endogenously produced IGFs appear important for this response. Cultured myotubes administered IGF-I exhibit hypertrophy (39). Additionally, transgenic mice that overexpress IGF-I only in skeletal muscle exhibit myofiber hypertrophy (40). Mechanical stimuli that induce skeletal muscle hypertrophy also increase the loaded muscle's endogenous IGF gene expression. IGF-I protein secretion increases in cultured myotubes during intermittent stretch-induced hypertrophy (41). Additionally, during overload-induced hypertrophy IGF-I mRNA concentration increases in the rat soleus (42), rat plantaris (42), rabbit EDL (20), and chicken patagialis muscles (43). Interestingly, IGF-I mRNA is induced to a greater degree when passive stretch is combined with electrical stimulation, when compared to passive stretch of the rabbit EDL alone (12-fold vs. 40-fold) (20). IGF-II mRNA also increases during hypertrophy in the rat hind-limb muscles (42). The endogenous synthesis of IGF-I and IGF-II mRNAs appears to increase in enlarging skeletal muscle. Endogenously produced IGFs could use an autocrine mechanism to signal skeletal muscle growth. The molecular targets of IGF signaling in hypertrophying muscle remain to be determined.

The IGF response in humans undergoing resistance exercise has also been examined. Protein synthesis is increased post–resistance exercise (14). Circulating IGF-I levels are not increased after a bout of heavy resistance exercise, however, even though growth hormone levels are dramatically elevated (44). Circulating levels of IGFs may not be a good indicator of changes in function. The biologic activity of circulating IGFs can also be regulated by their association with IGF-binding proteins. Further work will be needed to determine if IGFs could be working in an autocrine manner after resistance exercise in humans. IGF-I mRNA levels are increased in the skeletal muscle of elderly men receiving testosterone administration (45). Endogenous increases of skeletal muscle IGF-I mRNA seem to correlate with muscle growth. Further work will help define the targets activated by IGF signaling and will define signaling cascades that alter IGF expression in hypertrophying muscle. In short, determining at what level(s) the IGF system signals overload-induced enlargement of skeletal muscle will greatly increase our understanding of, and ability to manipulate, skeletal muscle hypertrophy.

Testosterone

Pharmaceutical derivatives of testosterone, an anabolic-androgenic steroid, have been widely used for decades by recreational, amateur, and professional athletes trying to increase muscle mass (46). It has been known for some time that testosterone administration has an anabolic effect on skeletal muscle in castrated animals (47). It has been demonstrated that testosterone administration increases fat-free mass, muscle size, and muscle strength in hypogonadal men (48). Testosterone administration increases muscle strength and protein synthesis in nonexercising elderly men (45). Although initial scientific studies using testosterone administration in normal exercising humans did not demonstrate a consistent effect on muscle mass, anabolic steroid use remained high among strength and power athletes, their general perception being that anabolic steroid usage did indeed enhance resistance training–induced increases in muscle mass.

Bhasin and colleagues (49), controlling many of the variables ignored in previous studies and giving supraphysiologic doses of testosterone, demonstrated that anabolic steroids could enhance overload-induced hypertrophy in human skeletal muscle. Additionally, the area of the triceps and quadriceps muscles increased in the testosterone treatment group without exercise. The mechanism by which supraphysiologic doses of testosterone increase muscle mass appears not to be dependent on loading; however, there appeared to be synergism between resistance exercise and supraphysiologic doses of testosterone on the increase in quadriceps muscle mass (49).

The molecular targets of testosterone-mediated signaling during overload-induced hypertrophy have not been identified. General cellular regulation by steroids works through their binding to specific receptors in the cytoplasm, being transported into the nucleus, and forming complexes in the nucleus that alter gene transcription (50). It will be interesting to determine the mechanisms and point of regulation involved in augmented testosterone-induced muscle growth. Supraphysiologic doses of testosterone may either override and/or act synergistically with regulatory events occurring in resistance-trained muscle. Steroid-induced activation of histone acetyltransferases allows restructuring of chromatin to expose the DNA regulatory site, which serves to form a stable preinitiation complex and increase gene transcription (50). It is possible that steroid signaling during overload-induced hypertrophy could involve alterations in chromatin structure that allow previously inaccessible DNA regulatory elements to have DNA-protein interactions and alter gene transcription. Determining the target genes, the cofactors involved, and specific regulatory elements involved in testosterone-induced increases in muscle mass will lead to a better ability to manipulate muscle mass in older individuals, as well as in disease states causing skeletal muscle wasting. Additionally, insight may also be provided into maximizing resistance-training-program efficiency for producing muscle hypertrophy by constructing training regimes that could activate similar signaling mechanisms as anabolic steroids.

The authors of the study showing that supraphysiologic doses of testosterone increased muscle mass cautioned that their results should in no way justify the use of anabolic-androgenic steroids in sports (49). They state that with extended use these drugs have potentially serious adverse side effects on the cardiovascular system, prostate, lipid metabolism, and insulin sensitivity. However, Bhasin and colleagues (49) suggest that the short-term administration of androgens could have beneficial effects in immobilized patients, during space travel, and in patients with cancer-related cachexia, disease caused by human immunodeficiency virus, or other chronic wasting conditions.

Satellite Cells

Skeletal muscle fibers are multinucleated, and a fiber's myonuclear population is not fixed but rather is dynamic. A muscle fiber adds additional nuclei during growth due to either maturation or overload (51–53). The number of myonuclei in a myofiber also decreases during disuse atrophy (53). The addition of myonuclei to growing fibers is thought to be a function of a myonucleus having a finite cytoplasmic domain (54). The concept of a limited nuclei/cytoplasm ratio in skeletal muscle is based on the idea that a given myonucleus can support transcription only for a given volume of fiber. The nuclear domain hypothesis would support the idea that the ability for skeletal muscle nuclei to increase transcription efficiency (transcription per nucleus) is limited, and an important point of regulation is to increase the enlarging muscles' transcriptional capacity (number of nuclei).

The source of additional myonuclei for enlarging myofibers is the muscle's satellite cell population (51). The satellite cell is a quiescent myogenic stem cell that can be induced to proliferate by a variety of stimuli. Activators of quiescent satellite cells include IGFs, fibroblast growth factor, testosterone, and skeletal muscle injury (55,56). Mitotically active satellite cells have several fates including continued proliferation, internalization by an existing fiber, or fusion with other satellite cells to form myotubes that can develop into newly synthesized fibers (55). Satellite cells have been shown to become mitotically active in hypertrophying muscle due to stretch or compensatory overload (52,57). The functions of mitotically active satellite cells in hypertrophying skeletal muscle include the repairing of muscle damage induced by the loading stimulus and de novo fiber formation in the stretch-overloaded chicken ALD muscle (58) and after eccentric contractions in human resistance training (21). Satellite cell proliferation is important for normal maturation-induced growth of turkey pectoralis muscle (59) and compensatory overload-induced hypertrophy of the rat EDL muscle (60). If satellite cell proliferation is prevented, muscle hypertrophy does not occur (60). Although satellite cell activation appears important for skeletal muscle growth, a reduced capacity for stretch overload–induced muscle growth in the quail ALD with aging is not accompanied by a change in satellite cell activation (61). Thus, satellite cell activation appears necessary for overload-induced hypertrophy in the rodent hind limb; however, mechanisms controlling satellite cell differentiation may also play a critical role during hypertrophy.

Many factors have been identified that can induce satellite cells into a proliferative state (55,56). However, very little information is available regarding the molecular signals involved in recruiting satellite cells into existing myofibers to support growth. The nuclear domain hypothesis suggests that additional myonuclei are necessary to sustain growth. Important questions in overload-induced hypertrophy are the following: Why are additional myonuclei needed? How does the myofiber sense the need for an increased transcription capacity? Could the regulation of both sensing the demand and recruiting additional myonuclei be rate limiting when trying to produce overload-induced hypertrophy? Understanding the need for increased transcriptional capacity in hypertrophying skeletal muscle will allow a better ability to understand, as well as manipulate, overload-induced muscle growth.

Rehabilitative Growth of Skeletal Muscle

Skeletal muscle atrophies during repair of joint and bone injuries. The restoration of function of the atrophied muscle is vital. Recent studies report that skeletal muscle from both adult and elderly rats has an inability to completely recover mass after damage by the myotoxin bupivacaine (62). The mechanism for this failure to restore muscle strength and function is not known. Future molecular studies should determine this cause so that better rehabilitation can occur in individuals 30 years of age or older.

MITOCHONDRIAL ADAPTATIONS

Endurance-Trained Skeletal Muscle Has Increased Oxidative Capacity

Oxidative capacity is defined as the maximal utilization of oxygen possible by a muscle fiber. If oxygen were to become near limiting, or limiting, to a muscle fiber, the appropriate adaptive response would be for all muscle proteins involved in delivery of oxygen to increase. Indeed, this is essentially the adaptive response of skeletal muscle to endurance training.

Adaptive Changes in Oxygen and Substrate Extractability by Endurance-Trained Skeletal Muscle

Most (11 to 12 of the 14 proteins/structures listed in the center column of Table 17–1) of the changes in protein composition in endurance-trained skeletal muscle function to improve the transfer of oxygen/substrates into ATP in the muscle. The two that do not increase are submaximal blood flow per unit of muscle mass and glycolytic enzyme levels. If the peripheral vasculature were to be entirely vasodilated, the volume of blood needed to perfuse it would exceed the maximal cardiac output (63). Glycolytic capacity decreases in endurance-trained skeletal muscle, which contributes to glycogen sparing and a greater utilization of fatty acids for oxidation to ATP at the same absolute work load after training.

Several studies have found that endurance types of exercise increase mitochondrial density in skeletal muscle. In 1967, Holloszy (64) showed that white muscles in rats would become redder if rats were endurance trained. Holloszy presented the rationale that the differences in color between inactive (white) and active (red) muscles might be due to not only genetic differences but also an adaptive process. A doubling in the capacity

TABLE 17–1. *Most processes involved in transfer of oxygen and substrates increase in response to endurance types of training*

Item transferred	Protein/structure involved in transfer	Directional change to endurance types of training
Blood	Capillary density	↑
	Mean capillary transit time (at a given Q)	↑
	Blood flow through muscle	
	Same submaximal work intensity	→
	Maximal work	↑
Oxygen	Arterial-venous O_2 difference	
	Small mass of exercising muscle	→
	Large mass of exercising muscle	↑
	Myoglobin	
	Animals	↑
	Human beings	→
	Krebs cycle enzyme activities	↑
	Electron transport chain activities	↑
Glucose	GLUT-4	↑
	Glycolytic enzyme activities	
	1–2 hours exercise/day	↓ type IIa ↑ type I
	8–24 hours continuous stimulation/day	↓
Fatty acids	Lipoprotein lipase	↑
	Albumin	↑
	Fatty acid binding protein	↑
	Carnitine palmitoyltransferase	↑
	Capacity to oxidize fatty acids	↑

From ref. 3, with permission (contains the references for this table).

of (a) mitochondria to oxidize pyruvate, (b) activities and concentrations of Krebs cycle and electron transport enzymes, and (c) the capacity to produce ATP in the gastrocnemius muscle of rats occurred after rats ran 2 hours per day on a motor-driven treadmill (64). Consequently, it was shown that increases in capillary density and myoglobin occurred in endurance-trained muscles of the rat. While endurance-trained humans were then shown to have an increased mitochondrial concentration and capillary density in their skeletal muscles, myoglobin did not increase. Thus, it was established that endurance training increases the redness of skeletal muscle due to increases in heme proteins, which have a reddish-brown color (hemoglobin in capillaries, myoglobin in the sarcoplasm, and cytochromes in the electron transport chain).

The reddening of skeletal muscle by endurance training can be further appreciated by a comparison of muscle colors in the chicken. The whiteness of the breast muscle of a chicken is due to the low amount of heme-containing protein in a muscle with low capillaries, myoglobin, and mitochondria. Chickens do not flap their wings much and breast muscles are presumably white in color because they are not endurance trained. On the other hand, the leg muscles of chickens, which are used for standing, or the breast muscles of pigeons who fly, are reddish-brown in appearance because of a high density of capillaries, myoglobin, and mitochondria.

Functional Significance of Increased Mitochondrial Density

Many functions seem to be elicited from the increase in capillaries, myoglobin, and mitochondria in skeletal muscle. If the density of mitochondria is twice as much in one skeletal muscle compared to another, then each mitochondrial unit has to produce half as much ATP at the same absolute work intensity in the muscle with more mitochondria (64). Thus, at the same contractile activity, a smaller decrease in ATP and creatine phosphate (CP) concentrations; smaller increases in inorganic phosphate (P_i), creatine, and adenosine diphosphate (ADP) concentrations; slower glycogen depletion; lower lactate production; and a greater reliance on fatty acid oxidation for energy occur in the muscle with the higher mitochondria (64). Since training increases mitochondrial density in skeletal muscle, the trained individual will show smaller changes in the aforementioned factors than the untrained individual working at the same absolute work load (64). These smaller disruptions in the cellular homeostasis serve to lengthen exercise time to exhaustion at a given absolute submaximal work load after endurance training.

MECHANISM OF INCREASED MITOCHONDRIAL DENSITY IN TRAINED MUSCLE

The mechanism as to how aerobic-type activities, but not resistance training, increase mitochondrial density has been the subject of numerous investigations. Essig (65) has synthesized existing data into a model that classifies mitochondrial biogenesis into three stages during endurance types of exercise.

Early Response Phase

Genes for mitochondrial biogenesis responding early (stage 1) are 5′-aminolevulinate synthase (ALAS), HSP-70, and the RNA subunit of mitochondrial RNA-processing enzyme (MRP RNAse). ALAS is the first and rate-limiting enzyme in heme biosynthesis. Heme is a prosthetic group of cytochromes and is the oxygen-binding portion of cytochrome a_3, the final protein at the end of the electron transport chain in mitochondria. The increase in ALAS occurs after a single bout of endurance exercise and precedes any observable increase in cytochrome *c*. Cytoplasmic HSP-70 functions in the unfolding of newly synthesized proteins. Without the unfolding, these proteins would not be imported into the mitochondria. The increase in HSP-70 occurs after a single bout of exercise. MRP RNAse increased threefold above control values 24 hours after initiation of 10-Hz nerve stimulation. Williams's group (66) suggests that this early increase could be preparing the mitochondrial DNA to switch from a transcriptional to replicative mode since mitochondrial DNA copy increases with chronic stimulation of skeletal muscle.

Middle Response Phase

The middle phase of mitochondrial biogenesis, as coined by Essig (65), entails increases in proteins involved in metabolic pathways. These include the enzymes of Krebs cycle, β-oxidation, and electron transport, and are termed oxidative enzymes here because of their role in aerobic metabolism. It takes 3 and 8 days to observe increases in these oxidative enzymes in endurance and chronic stimulation studies, respectively. Most of these enzymes increase in parallel and by similar percentages during increases in contractile activity (67). There is a dose-response relationship between the increases in oxidative enzymes and the intensity and duration of the exercise up to a maximal value. For example, the longer the daily duration of training, the greater is the percentage increase in oxidative enzymes of mitochondria (68). Furthermore, if the intensity of endurance training is increased, a greater percentage increase in oxidative enzymes for a given daily duration of training occurs (68), likely because the greater intensity recruits a higher percentage of motor units (muscle fibers).

Late Response Phase

The major event associated with this phase is the apparent replication of mitochondrial DNA. The presumed functional consequence is an increase in the coding capacity and restoration of homeostasis to transcription from the mitochondrial genome (65). In the soleus muscle of endurance-trained rats, it took longer than 6 weeks of training to increase mitochondrial DNA (69). In chronic stimulation, mitochondrial DNA was unchanged during the first 5 days (70).

EXERCISE MOLECULAR MEDICINE*

Incidence of Chronic Disease in the United States and the Potential Role of Physical Activity in Prevention

Current estimates report that 45% of Americans have one or more chronic diseases (a medical condition lasting for a period of years), and in 1987 these conditions accounted for 75% of U.S. health care expenditures. In 1990, chronic conditions cost $659 billion in the United States. The Centers for Disease Control and Prevention, the American College of Sports Medicine (71), the Surgeon General of the United States (72), and ourselves (73) have cited the references that support the contention that appropriately performed physical activities or exercise reduces the risk of breast and female reproductive cancers, claudication, coronary artery disease, depression, diseases arising from chronic bed rest, hypertension, non–insulin-dependent diabetes mellitus, obesity, postmenopausal osteoporosis, sleep apnea associated with obesity, stroke, back pain, colon cancer, congestive heart failure, and loss of independence of living. Based on a knowledge of when disease processes start, Table 17–2 speculates on the age ranges during which individuals should perform endurance types of activities/exercise in order to decrease the risk of certain of these chronic diseases.

Application of emerging new tools in molecular biology and genetics will enable determinations of answers to two sets of questions in the next 20 years regarding how exercise decreases the risk of disease. The first question is, What is the exercise duration and intensity required to reduce the risk of a chronic disease listed in Table 17–2? An answer to this question will be obtained, in part, from the new field of genomics. Chronic

* Written with the assistance of Brian S. Tseng.

TABLE 17–2. *Speculated age ranges for endurance exercises*

Disease (see refs. 76–80)	Exercise decreases risks of	Exercise treats disease	Ages during which exercise decreases disease risk (years)			
			0–20	20–40	40–60	60–100
Breast and female reproductive cancers	X		—	—	→	
Claudication	X	X	—	—	—	→
Coronary artery disease	X	X	—	—	—	→
Depression	X		—	—	—	→
Diseases arising from chronic bed rest	X	X	—	—	—	→
Hypertension	X	X	—	—	—	→
Type I diabetes mellitus (insulin dependent)		X	—	—	→	
Type II diabetes mellitus (non–insulin dependent)	X	X	—	—	→	
Obesity	X	X	—	—	—	→
Osteoporosis (postmenopausal)	X	X	—	—	—	→
Severe acute pancreatitis	X	X	—	—	—	→
Sleep apnea associated with obesity	X	X	—	—	—	→
Stroke	X		—	—	—	→
Back pain	X	X		—	—	→
Colon cancer	X			—	→	
Congestive heart failure	X			—	→	
Loss of independence with aging	X	X		—	—	→
Severe gastrointestinal hemorrhage	X					→
Rheumatoid arthritis		X				→

From ref. 73, with permission.

diseases are polygenic, and a fraction of these genes will be susceptible to changes in their expression by physical exercise. Exercise may decrease the protein made from a gene that predisposes to a disease, or it may increase the expression of a gene that lowers the risk of a disease. The second question that can be answered in future years is, What is the variability of this response? It is well known that there are responders and nonresponders to environmental perturbations. About one-fourth of genes have polymorphisms. It is likely that some of these polymorphisms account for responders and nonresponders. Finally, the mechanistic determination of how increased physical activity decreases the risk of certain chronic diseases will clearly fortify the rationales for health care professionals to prescribe exercise as a necessary part of their patients' lives.

Potential Role of Exercise on Disease-Associated Genes

It is likely that most, if not all, diseases have a genetic basis. However, the absolute number of human diseases purely heritable from a single gene is relatively uncommon as compared to the frequency of multifactorial human diseases, for example, diabetes, coronary artery disease, and cancer. The recent increase in chronic diseases, such as the sixfold increase of non–insulin-dependent diabetes mellitus from 1958 to 1993 in the United States, is due not to mutations in human DNA but to dramatic changes in lifestyle (activity and diet). Multifactorial diseases, including all chronic diseases, are caused by environmental and temporal factor(s) impinging on genes. With the gigantic effort that will completely define the DNA sequence for the entire human genome by the year 2002, the identification of all genes and variant sequence(s) of specific genes that may correlate with susceptibility, severity, and lethality of many human diseases will be possible. We expect that each multifactorial disease will involve multiple genes—some "good" and some "bad." All humans have essentially the same genetic template, yet DNA sequence variations (polymorphisms) within individual genes can also modulate predisposition to certain diseases. We define the term *disease-associated gene* as a gene that increases or decreases the susceptibility for a disease. Such a disease-associated gene will not be the sole cause of disease, but its expression clearly lowers or raises (predisposes) the likelihood threshold for a person to develop a disease. Exercise will be shown in future years to play a role as important as pharmaceutical medicines in the prevention and therapeutic management of chronic disease by activating or suppressing critical disease-associated genes. Many chronic diseases begin early in childhood. Thus, pediatric sports medicine professionals should consider preventive medicine of chronic disease as important as the healing of sports injuries. In the future, sports medicine personnel will have the tools to diagnose in their recreational and athletic patients the occurrence of disease-associated genes whose expression predisposes to chronic diseases. They will be able to practice preventive medicine.

Clinical Utility of Exercise with Molecular Biology

A carcinogen in tobacco smoke has been shown to mutate a critical cell cycle gene in lung cells called p53, whose protein product may cause or at least facilitate the development of some lung cancers (74). This molecular-science inquiry has added strong evidence supporting the causal relationship between tobacco smoke and the development of some lung cancers. Certainly other genetic and nongenetic factors are also involved. This example provides a template for how exercise might modulate disease-associated genes. The association of certain lifestyle types on the progression of various chronic diseases has been implied by seminal epidemiologic human data, but at this time it lacks the additional credibility that defined molecular mechanisms can provide in understanding pathophysiology and ultimately orient clinical endeavors such as prevention and therapy.

To address causal relationships of sedentary lifestyle type with chronic disease, we postulate that diet and activity levels interplay profoundly with genetic backgrounds of each individual to determine the threshold for clinical expression, type, progression, and severity of specific disease(s). This paradigm provides a fruitful opportunity for exercise researchers to apply their skills to study the interaction of physical activity and low-fat diets as environmental influences on the expression of specific disease-associated genes. Animal models of disease-associated genes should be developed, and exercise studies performed on these animals might determine the mechanisms of how physical activity suppresses the expression of some "bad" genes or stimulates other "good" genes for modulating disease progression. This will be a significant new area of research in exercise. It will integrate molecular biology and clinical exercise physiology. A delineation of how lifestyle (activity and diet) influences the expression of both disease-susceptible and disease-resistant genes with molecular biologic tools will provide a better scientific basis for the prescription of exercise and diet to decrease the risk of chronic diseases. If more individuals increased their daily physical activity to appropriate levels, then more chronic diseases would be prevented, quality of life would improve, health care costs would decrease, worker productivity would increase, and fewer people would suffer loss of independent living.

FUTURE RESEARCH

Outstanding Questions in Exercise Physiology

A number of major questions remain unanswered in sports medicine and exercise physiology. A short list of these questions demonstrates the importance of a multidisciplinary approach: How does exercise strengthen connective tissues (ligaments, bones, and tendons) so that joint injuries are prevented? How does exercise compensate for osteoporosis with aging? How does resistance exercise produce muscle hypertrophy? How does resistance exercise compensate for age-induced muscle loss? What is the mechanism for muscle atrophy when skeletal muscles are unloaded? How does aerobic training increase the number of muscle mitochondria? What are the molecular changes that lead to the changes that allow trained muscles to fatigue less at the same absolute work load after training? How does aerobic exercise increase the expression of genes beneficial for health, such as lipoprotein lipase, which lowers blood triglycerides and contributes to an increase in blood high-density lipoprotein (HDL)? How does exercise prevent cardiovascular disease? How does aerobic exercise prevent obesity and non–insulin-dependent diabetes mellitus? What is the signal that converts myosin isoforms from rapid velocity of contraction to a slower velocity during endurance training? How does moderate exercise improve immune function, and how does overtraining depress immune function? What is the mechanism for the good feeling experienced after exercise? How does exercise training compensate for the 10% loss in maximal oxygen consumption with aging? What is the mechanism for improved insulin sensitivity of skeletal muscle after training? What is the molecular mechanism for muscle soreness? Is muscle injury obligatory for muscle hypertrophy? How does endurance training compensate for aging effects on the heart? Answering these and other major questions will require an interdisciplinary approach, including molecular biology tools. Space limitations prevent us from addressing the current status of answers to all the above questions.

CONCLUSION

Improvements in human performance are usually based on science. As new techniques in science are found, it is a challenge to exercise scientists to determine whether and how new techniques can be applied to outstanding unanswered questions, such as those cited above. This chapter cited examples of the application of molecular biologic techniques to answer these questions. At this time the application of molecular biology is in its infancy. The future delineation of the entire sequence of the human genome will open unparalleled opportunities to improve both human performance and health.

ACKNOWLEDGMENTS

We thank the National Institutes of Health (NIH) for support in the research for this chapter. The chapter was written with support from U.S. Public Health Service NIH grants R01 AR19393 and R01 AR44208 (F.W.B.), F32 AR 8328 (J.A.C.), and National Shriner's Hospital for Crippled Children Research Project #5953 (Brian Tseng), and the M.D.-Ph.D. program at the University of Texas Medical School (Brian Tseng).

REFERENCES

1. Wilkinson JL. Molecular biology in medicine. In: Walton J, ed. *Oxford medical companion.* Oxford: Oxford University Press, 1994.
2. Kendrew JC. Molecular biology. In: *The encyclopedia of molecular biology.* Oxford: Blackwell Scientific and Oxford University Press, 1994:664.
3. Booth FW, Baldwin KM. Muscle plasticity: energy demand/supply processes. In: Rowell LB, Shepherd JT, eds. *Handbook of physiology: section 12: integration of motor, circulatory, respiratory, and metabolic control during exercise.* New York: Oxford University Press, 1996:1075–1123.
4. White TP. Skeletal muscle structure and function in older mammals. In: Lamb DR, Gisolfi CV, Nadel E, eds. *Perspectives in exercise science and sports medicine: exercise in older adults*, vol 5. Carmel, IN: Cooper, 1995:115–174.
5. Abernathy PJ, Jurimae J, Logan PA, Taylor AW, Thayer RE. Acute and chronic response of skeletal muscle to resistance exercise. *Sports Med* 1994;17(1):22–38.
6. Sale DG. Neural adaptations to strength training. In: Komi PV, ed. *Strength and power in sport.* Oxford, England: Blackwell Scientific, 1992:249–265.
7. Antonio J, Gonyea WJ. The role of muscle fiber hypertrophy and hyperplasia in intermittently stretched avian muscle. *J Appl Physiol* 1993;74:1893–1898.
8. Gonyea WJ, Ericson GC. An experimental model for the study of exercise-induced muscle hypertrophy. *J Appl Physiol* 1976; 40:630–633.
9. Wong TS, Booth FW. Skeletal muscle enlargement with weight-lifting exercise by rats. *J Appl Physiol* 1988;65:950–954.
10. Gregory P, Gagnon J, Essig DA, Reid SK, Prior G, Zak R. Differential regulation of actin and myosin isoenzyme synthesis in functionally overloaded skeletal muscle. *Biochem J* 1990;265:525–532.
11. Laurent GJ, Sparrow MP, Millward DJ. Turnover of muscle protein in the fowl. Changes in rates of protein synthesis and breakdown during hypertrophy of the anterior and posterior latissimus dorsi muscles. *Biochem J* 1978;176:407–417.
12. Morris DR. Growth control of translation in mammalian cells. In: Owens IS, Ritter JK, eds. *Progress in nucleic acids research and molecular biology*, vol 51. New York: Academic Press, 1996:339–363.
13. Wong TS, Booth FW. Protein metabolism in rat gastrocnemius muscle after stimulated chronic concentric exercise. *J Appl Physiol* 1990;69:1709–1717.
14. MacDougall JD, Gibala MJ, Tarnopolsky MA, MacDonald JR, Interisano SA, Yarasheski KE. The time course for elevated muscle protein synthesis following heavy resistance exercise. *Can J Appl Physiol* 1995;20:480–486.
15. Carson JA. Molecular regulation in overloads skeletal muscle. In: Holloszy JO, ed. *Exercise and sports science reviews.* Baltimore: Williams & Wilkins, 1997:301–320.
16. Thomason DB, Booth FW. Atrophy of the soleus muscle by hindlimb unweighting. *J Appl Physiol* 1990;68:1–12.
17. Goldspink DF. Exercise related changes in protein turnover in mammalian striated muscle. *J Exp Biol* 1991;160:127–148.
18. Carson JA, Schwartz RJ, Booth FW. SRF and TEF-1 control of chicken skeletal α-actin gene during slow-muscle hypertrophy. *Am J Physiol* 1996;270:C1624–C1633.
19. Goldspink DF. The influence of immobilization and stretch on protein turnover in mammalian striated muscle. *J Physiol* 1977; 264:267–282.
20. Goldspink DF, Cox VM, Smith SK, et al. Muscle growth in response to mechanical stimuli. *Am J Physiol* 1995;268:E288–E297.
21. Chesley A, MacDougall JD, Tarnopolsky MA, Atkinson SA, Smith K. Changes in human muscle protein synthesis after resistance exercise. *J Appl Physiol* 1992;73:1383–1388.
22. Ku Z, Thomason DB. Soleus muscle nascent polypeptide chain elongation slows protein synthesis rate during non-weight bearing activity. *Am J Physiol* 1994;267:C115–C126.
23. Sonenberg N. Translational control. In: Hershey JWB, Mathews MB, Sonenberg N, eds. *Translational control.* Cold Spring Harbor, NY; Cold Spring Harbor Laboratory Press, 1996:245–270.
24. Wada H, Ivester CT, Carabello BA, Cooper G, McDermott PJ. Translational initiation factor eIF-4e, a link between cardiac load and protein synthesis. *J Biol Chem* 1996;271:8359–8364.
25. Ku Z, Yang J, Menon V, Thomason DB. Decreased polysomal HSP-70 may slow polypeptide elongation during skeletal muscle atrophy. *Am J Physiol* 1995;268:C1369–C1374.
26. Tsika RW, Hauschka SD, Gao L. M-creatine kinase gene expression in mechanically overloaded skeletal muscle of transgenic mice. *Am J Physiol* 1995;269:C665–C674.
27. Carson JA, Yan Z, Booth FW, Coleman ME, Schwartz RJ, Stump CS. Regulation of skeletal α-actin promoter in young chickens during hypertrophy caused by stretch overload. *Am J Physiol* 1995;268:C918–C924.
28. Yamashita K, Yoshioka T. Profiles of creatine kinase isoenzyme compositions in single muscle fibers of different types. *J Muscle Res Cell Motil* 1991;12:37–44.
29. Wiedenman JL, Rivera-Rivera I, Vyas D, et al. β-MHC and SMLC1 transgene induction in overloaded skeletal muscle of transgenic mice. *Am J Physiol* 1996;270:C1111–C1121.
30. Wiedenman JL, Tsika GL, Gao L, et al. Muscle-specific and inducible expression of 293-base pair β-myosin heavy chain promoter in transgenic mice. *Am J Physiol* 1996;271:R688–R695.
31. Maclellan WR, Lee TC, Schwartz RJ, Schneider MD. Transforming growth factor-β response elements of skeletal α-actin gene. *J Biol Chem* 1994;269:16754–16760.
32. Karns LR, Kariya K, Simpson PC. M-CAT, CArG, and SP1 elements are required for α_1-adrenergic induction of the skeletal α-actin promoter during cardiac myocyte hypertrophy. *J Biol Chem* 1995;270:410–417.
33. Chow KL, Schwartz RJ. A combination of closely associated positive and negative cis-acting promoter elements regulates transcription of the skeletal α-actin gene. *Mol Cell Biol* 1990;10:528–538.
34. Lee TC, Chow K-L, Fang P, Schwartz RJ. Activation of skeletal α-actin gene transcription: the cooperative formation of serum response factor-binding complexes over positive cis-acting promoter serum response elements displaces a negative-acting nuclear factor enriched in replicating myoblasts and nonmyogenic cells. *Mol Cell Biol* 1991;11:5090–5100.
35. Treisman R. The SRE: a growth factor responsive transcription regulator. *Semin Cancer Biol* 1990;1:47–58.
36. Schwartz MA, Schaller MD, Ginsberg MH. Integrins: emerging paradigms of signal transduction. *Annu Rev Cell Dev Biol* 1995; 11:549–599.
37. Cohick WS, Clemmons DR. The insulin-like growth factors. *Annu Rev Physiol* 1993;55:131–153.
38. Florini JR, Ewton DZ, Coolican SA. Growth hormone and the insulin-like growth factor system in myogenesis. *Endocr Rev* 1996;17:481–517.
39. Vandenburgh HH, Karlisch P, Shansky J, Feldstein R. Insulin and IGF-I induce pronounced hypertrophy of skeletal myofibers in tissue culture. *Am J Physiol* 1991;260:C475–C484.
40. Coleman ME, DeMayo F, Yin KC, et al. Myogenic vector expression of insulin-like growth factor I stimulates muscle cell differentiation and myofiber hypertrophy in transgenic mice. *J Biol Chem* 1995;270:12109–12116.
41. Perrone CE, Fenwick-Smith D, Vandenburgh HH. Collagen and stretch modulate autocrine secretion of insulin-like growth factor-I and insulin-like growth factor binding proteins from differentiated skeletal muscle cells. *J Biol Chem* 1995;270:2099–2106.
42. Devol DL, Rotwein P, Sadow JL, Novakofski J, Bechtel PJ. Activation of insulin-like growth factor gene expression during work-induced skeletal muscle growth. *Am J Physiol* 1990;259:E89–E95.
43. Czerwinski SM, Martin JM, Bechtel PJ. Modulation of IGF mRNA abundance during stretch-induced skeletal muscle hypertrophy and regression. *J Appl Physiol* 1994;76:2026–2030.
44. Kraemer WJ, Aguilera BA, Terada M, et al. Responses of IGF-1

to endogenous increases in growth hormone after heavy resistance exercise. *J Appl Physiol* 1995;79:1301–1315.
45. Urban RJ, Bodenburg YH, Gilkison C, et al. Testosterone administration to elderly men increases skeletal muscle strength and protein synthesis. *Am J Physiol* 1995;269:E820–E826.
46. Wilson JD. Androgen abuse by athletes. *Endocr Rev* 1988; 9:181–199.
47. Mooradian AD, Morley JE, Korenman SG. Biological actions of androgens. *Endocr Rev* 1987;8:1–20.
48. Bhasin S, Storer TW, Berman N, et al. Testosterone replacement increases fat-free mass and muscle size in hypogonadal men. *J Clin Endocrinol Metab* 1997;82:407–413.
49. Bhasin S, Storer TW, Berman N, et al. The effects of supraphysiologic doses of testosterone on muscle size and strength in normal men. *N Engl J Med* 1996;335:1–7.
50. Spencer TE, Jenster G, Burcin MM, et al. Steroid receptor coactivator-1 is a histone acetyltransferase. *Nature* 1997;389:194–198.
51. Moss FP, Leblond CP. Satellite cells as the source of nuclei in muscles of growing rats. *Anat Rec* 1971;170:421–436.
52. Winchester PK, Gonyea WJ. A quantitative study of satellite cells and myonuclei in stretched avian slow tonic muscle. *Anat Rec* 1992;232:369–377.
53. Allen DL, Monke SR, Talmadge RJ, Roy RR, Edgerton VR. Plasticity of myonuclear number in hypertrophied and atrophied mammalian skeletal muscle fibers. *J Appl Physiol* 1995; 78:969–976.
54. Cheek DB, Holt AB, Hill DE, Talbert JL. Skeletal muscle mass and growth: the concept of the deoxyribonucleic acid unit. *Pediatr Res* 1971;5:312–328.
55. Schultz E, McCormick KM. Skeletal muscle satellite cells. *Rev Physiol Biochem Pharmacol* 1994;123:213–257.
56. Bischoff R. The satellite cell and muscle regeneration. In: Engel AG, Franzini-Armstrong C, eds. *Myology,* vol 1. New York: McGraw-Hill, 1995:97– 118.
57. Schiaffino S, Bormioli SP, Aloisi M. The fate of newly formed satellite cells during compensatory muscle hypertrophy. *Virchows Arch [B]* 1976;21:113–118.
58. McCormick KM, Schultz E. Mechanisms of nascent fiber formation during avian skeletal muscle hypertrophy. *Dev Biol* 1992; 150:319–334.
59. Mozdziak PE, Schultz E, Cassens RG. Myonuclear accretion is a major determinant of avian skeletal muscle growth. *Am J Physiol* 1997;272:C565–C571.
60. Rosenblatt JD, Parry DJ. Gamma irradiation prevents compensatory hypertrophy of overloaded mouse extensor digitorum longus muscle. *J Appl Physiol* 1992;73:2538–2543.
61. Carson JA, SE Alway. Stretch overload-induced satellite cell activation in slow tonic muscle from adult and aged Japanese quail. *Am J Physiol* 1996;270:C578–C584.
62. Marsh DR, Criswell DS, Hamilton MT, Booth FW. Association of insulin-like growth factor mRNAs are expression with muscle regeneration in young, adult, and old rats. *Am J Physiol* 1997; 273:R353–R358.
63. Rowell LB. Muscle blood flow in humans: how high can it go? *Med Sci Sports Exerc* 1988;20(5 suppl):S97–S103.
64. Holloszy JO. Biochemical adaptations in muscle. *J Biol Chem* 1967;242:2278– 2282.
65. Essig DA. Contractile activity-induced mitochondrial biogenesis in skeletal muscle. *Exerc Sports Sci Rev* 1996;24:289–319.
66. Ordway GA, Li K, Hand GA, Williams RS. RNA subunit of mitochondrial-processing enzyme is induced by contractile activity in striated muscle. *Am J Physiol* 1993;265:C1511–C1516.
67. Pette D, Vrbova G. Adaptation of mammalian skeletal muscle fibers to chronic stimulation. *Rev Physiol Biochem Pharmacol* 1992;120:115–202.
68. Dudley GA, Abraham WM, Terjung RL. Influence of exercise intensity and duration on biochemical adaptations in skeletal muscle. *J Appl Physiol* 1982;53:844–850.
69. Murakami Y, Shimomura Y, Fujisuka N, et al. Enzymatic and genetic adaption of soleus muscle to physical training in rats. *Am J Physiol* 1994;267:E388–E395.
70. Williams RS, Salmons S, Newsholme EA, Kaufman RE, Mellor J. Regulation of nuclear and mitochondrial gene expression by contractile activity in skeletal muscle. *J Biol Chem* 1986; 261:376–380.
71. Pate RR, Pratt M, Blair SN, et al. Physical activity and public health. A recommendation from the Centers for Disease Control and Prevention and the American College of Sports Medicine. *JAMA* 1995;273:402–407.
72. U.S. Department of Health and Human Services. *Physical activity and health: a report of the surgeon general.* Atlanta, GA: U.S. Department of Health and Human Services, Centers for Disease Control and Prevention, National Center for Chronic Disease Prevention and Health Promotion, 1996.
73. Booth FW, Tseng BS. America needs to exercise for health. *Med Sci Sports Exerc* 1995;27:462–465.
74. Denissenko MF, Pao A, Tang M, Pfeifer GP. Preferential formation of benzo[a]pyrene adducts at lung cancer mutational hotspots in p53. *Science* 1996;274:430–432.

PART IV

Applied Topics

Exercise and Sport Science,
edited by William E. Garrett, Jr., and Donald T. Kirkendall.
Lippincott Williams & Wilkins, Philadelphia © 2000.

CHAPTER 18

Individual Assessment of the Aerobic-Anaerobic Transition by Measurements of Blood Lactate

Axel Urhausen, Bernd Coen, and Wilfried Kindermann

MAXIMAL PERFORMANCE PARAMETERS

The traditional principle for performance testing in a laboratory is represented by spiroergometry, which usually includes the determination of maximal performance as well as maximal oxygen uptake ($\dot{V}O_2max$) and is usually based on a stepwise increasing exercise test either on a cycle ergometer or on a treadmill. Additional determinations of the heart volume demonstrate adaptations of cardiac dimensions, such as an athlete's heart induced by long-term and intensive endurance training. However, a considerable discrepancy between specific performance development and the so-called performance parameters clearly appears when looking at the changes over several decades in $\dot{V}O_2max$ and heart volume in sports with easily measurable performance, such as long-distance running. The values of $\dot{V}O_2max$ and heart volume measured in the 1960s and 1970s are similar to those measured during later decades. $\dot{V}O_2max$ values of 80 $ml{\cdot}min^{-1}{\cdot}kg^{-1}$ or above as well as enlarged heart volumes were already reported 30 years ago (1). An interesting study compares Caucasian and African-American long-distance runners with identical $\dot{V}O_2max$ (3). During identical submaximal running velocities, African-American long-distance runners both produce less lactic acid and are able to compete with a higher percentage of their $\dot{V}O_2max$ than Caucasian long-distance runners. There has been no difference concerning the running economy. The presented examples indicate that a performance diagnostic that only considers maximal indicators is insufficient and inappropriate for performance diagnosis and monitoring of training.

A. Urhausen, B. Coen, and W. Kindermann: Institute of Sports and Preventive Medicine, University of Saarland, Saarbrücken, Germany.

SUBMAXIMAL PERFORMANCE PARAMETERS: THE ANAEROBIC THRESHOLD CONCEPT

The measurement of maximal performance parameters was gradually complemented by concepts based on submaximal values. In this context, the registration of changes in the metabolism of the skeletal muscles by means of both respiratory dimensions and concentrations of blood lactate are of fundamental importance (4). At the beginning of the 20th century, Fletcher and Hopkins (5) recognized the increase of blood lactate during physical exercise, which they attributed to an inadequate oxygen supply of the working muscles. In the early 1920s, Hill and Lupton described this phenomenon as O_2 deficit (6). In 1959, Hollmann (7) identified the so-called point of optimal efficiency of ventilation by means of incremental graded exercise. The coincidence of the beginning of the curvilinear increase of the minute ventilation with the increase of the blood lactic acid could be shown. The "O_2-Dauerleistungsgrenze" (limit of O_2 endurance performance) was defined as a work-load level that, if remaining underneath this level, leads to a constant amount of O_2 deficit independent of the exercise duration (8). In the 1960s and 1970s, Wasserman and McIlroy (9) developed the concept of the anaerobic threshold, which precisely indicates the exercise intensity that provokes the ventilatory parameters to be less linear and to disproportionately increase in relation to the oxygen uptake. Based on the findings of Hollmann and colleagues, Wasserman and McIlroy found an exercise intensity that leads to the initial increase in concentration of lactic acid, if compared to rest values, by measuring only respiratory parameters. This increase was interpreted as the beginning of the anaerobic metabolism and was designated the *anaerobic threshold.* Now this overproportional increase of ventilation is called the *ventilatory threshold* (10). During the 1980s and

1990s, numerous investigations dealt with threshold concepts based on the easier-to-determine parameter of lactic acid to evaluate physiologic performance capacity.

By means of an empirical investigation with differently trained subjects, Mader and colleagues (11) determined the aerobic-anaerobic threshold at a fixed concentration of 4 mmol·L^{-1} of lactic acid (11). The onset of blood lactate accumulation (OBLA) was also described at a fixed concentration of 4 mmol·L^{-1} of lactic acid (12). To avoid the developing confusion concerning different terms referring to the anaerobic threshold, Kindermann and colleagues (13) suggested the term *aerobic-anaerobic transition*. This transition starts with the aerobic threshold, which marks the first increase of lactic acid and is generally identical to the anaerobic threshold named by Wasserman and thus to the ventilatory threshold. Its intensity ranges between 50% and 65% of $\dot{V}O_2max$, depending on the type of exercise, and the concentration of lactic acid is between 1.5 and 2 mmol·L^{-1}. In English-language references this aerobic threshold is occasionally called the lactate break point (14). The aerobic-anaerobic transition ends with the anaerobic threshold (13). By definition, this anaerobic threshold represents the maximal blood lactate steady state. Even slightly higher intensities lead to a gradual increase of lactic acid during exercises with constant work loads. In general, the anaerobic threshold refers to about 70% to 80% of $\dot{V}O_2max$. According to the usual biologic processes, this threshold is exceeded gradually, not abruptly. Heck (15) confirmed the essentials of Mader and colleagues' (11) report through endurance exercises over a period of 30 minutes. The average values for the maximal lactate steady state in this study were 4.02 ± 0.7 mmol·L^{-1} (treadmill) and 4.30 ± 1.1 mmol·L^{-1} (cycle ergometer). The individual values were between 2.3 and 6.8 mmol·L^{-1}. During stepwise increasing exercises with step duration less than 4 minutes, the threshold of Mader and colleagues has to be modified to a 3.5 mmol·L^{-1} lactate threshold (16).

Fixed points of the lactate performance curve, and thus an identical concentration of blood lactate in different subjects, do not necessarily imply an identical metabolic situation and therefore may have a different meaning in different athletes. Highly trained endurance athletes are usually overstrained during longer-lasting endurance exercises conducted with an intensity of 4 mmol·L^{-1} of lactic acid. Therefore, those athletes usually practice with lower exercise intensities. It has been shown that both the ventilatory threshold and the lactate break point do not occur at a fixed lactate concentration of 2 and 4 mmol·L^{-1}, respectively (14). Therefore, the development of different individual threshold concepts began in the early 1980s (17–21). By investigating 60 lactate performance curves Keul and colleagues (19) found a mean tangent angle of 51°34′ at 4 mmol·L^{-1} during stepwise increasing exercise. Thus, the developed individual anaerobic threshold did not occur at a fixed lactate concentration but at a fixed incline of the lactate performance curve. By applying the identical method to different subjects, Simon (20) found a tangent angle of 45 degrees. Simon evaluated this point of the lactate performance curve as a signal for a break in the metabolism that occurs at an identical increase of lactic acid but at different lactate values. Bunc and colleagues (17) defined their individual anaerobic threshold as that point of the lactate performance curve where the incline of the curve maximally changes. Tangents were fitted to the lactate performance curve both at the point of lowest work load and at a lactate concentration of 15 mmol·L^{-1}. The bisector of the angle at the point of intersection of both tangents crosses the lactate performance curve at the point of the individual anaerobic threshold. A further method to determine the individual anaerobic threshold was introduced by Hagberg and Coyle (18) for stepwise increasing race walking, by Simon (20) for swimming, and by Dickhuth and colleagues (22) for running tests. The addition of 1 or 1.5 mmol·L^{-1} lactate to the baseline lactate concentration determined the threshold, which can be described as a "quasi-individual" threshold.

The measurement of lactic acid during physiologic tests under both laboratory and field conditions does not occur inside the muscle but by taking blood samples—either from the arterialized capillary blood of the earlobe or, rarely, from the fingertip or (less precise) from venous blood samples. For that reason many factors have to be taken into consideration when interpreting lactate values. The blood lactate concentration depends not only on the production of lactic acid within the working muscles but also on the diffusion of lactate from the muscle to the blood as well as on the elimination in the heart, liver, kidneys, and in resting as well as moderately working muscles (23). At the range of low work loads during stepwise increasing exercise with resulting low diffusion rates, an increasing elimination of lactate and a simultaneously increased velocity of its diffusion can be assumed. The lactate concentration in the capillary blood at the end of low exercise steps remains unchanged or increases only minimally in spite of increasing exercise intensity. With further increasing intensity, the diffusion velocity also increases. The steeper part of the lactate performance curve can be explained by a lower elimination rate if compared to the diffusion rate.

The kinetic model to determine the individual anaerobic threshold (IAT) was developed in 1981 by Stegmann and colleagues (21). It indicates the highest work load that still results in a balance of both lactate diffusion and lactate elimination velocity, corresponding to the maximal lactate steady state. It is the only concept that determines the anaerobic threshold by taking into consideration the change of lactate concentration during

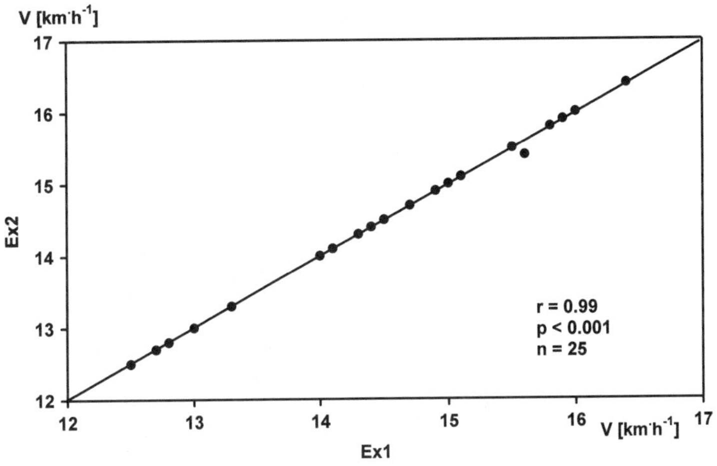

FIG. 18–1. Linear regression between the results of two experienced examiners (Ex1 and Ex2) concerning the graphic determination of the individual anaerobic threshold (IAT).

the recovery after exercise. Besides a diminished lactate production in working muscles (24), training induces a faster rate of lactate diffusion as well as a faster lactate clearance (25–27). So it is appropriate that the model of IAT calculation takes into account the changes of blood lactate not only during exercise but also during the early (approximately 10-minute) recovery phase. Because of the findings of lower lactate concentrations during practice in better-trained endurance athletes, the mean lactate concentrations accompanying the IAT are actually lower in those sports that entail a greater aerobic energy supply (28).

In recent years our institution conducted a series of investigations both on a treadmill and on an indoor track with 176 subjects (specifically trained in running) to evaluate the scientific quality and possible methodologic factors that are relevant to the determination of the IAT.

REPRODUCIBILITY AND RELIABILITY OF THE IAT

The examiner's influence on the results was investigated by using several examiners with different levels of experience in the method of IAT determination. The interobserver variability is very low in experienced examiners (Fig. 18–1). There are also only slight variations in the results of moderately experienced examiners (r = 0.98). We found two (out of 25) individual differences that were relevant—differences in recommendations of running velocity of about 10 seconds for 1000 m during intensive endurance training.

The reliability assessed during test-retest comparisons is very high (29). In 25 athletes the correlation coefficient between both tests was 0.98 for the running velocity at the IAT and 0.82 for the heart rate velocity at the IAT (both significant at $p <.001$). The findings confirm the results of other working groups that demonstrated high reliability and reproducibility of the IAT during cycle ergometry (30). A low, though statistically significant, shift to the right of the lactate performance curve during the retests, probably resulting from adaptation effects, does not affect the running velocity or performance on the IAT. Consequently, training recommendations resulting from the IAT are not affected. The mean running velocity at fixed lactate concentrations was increased by 0.4 km·h^{-1} on average.

VALIDITY OF THE IAT—A PHYSIOLOGIC THRESHOLD?

The IAT can be assumed to describe a valid measure for the maximal lactate steady state (Fig. 18–2). During endurance exercises lasting at least 30 to 45 minutes, each performed with different constant work loads and different percentages of the intensity at the IAT, a lactate steady state can be found at different levels of

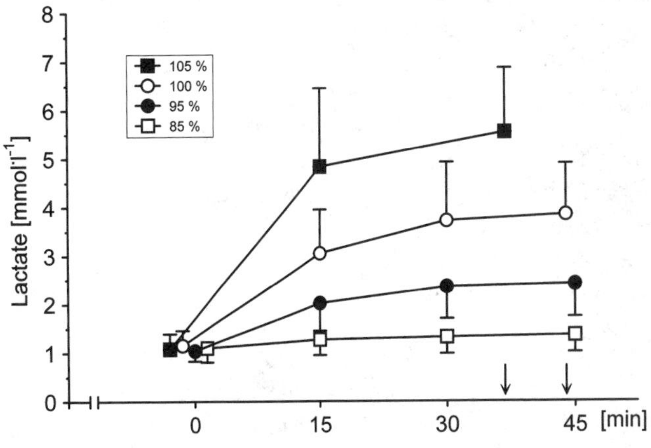

FIG. 18–2. Lactate values during endurance running exercises with different intensities (85% to 105% IAT). (From ref. 31, with permission.)

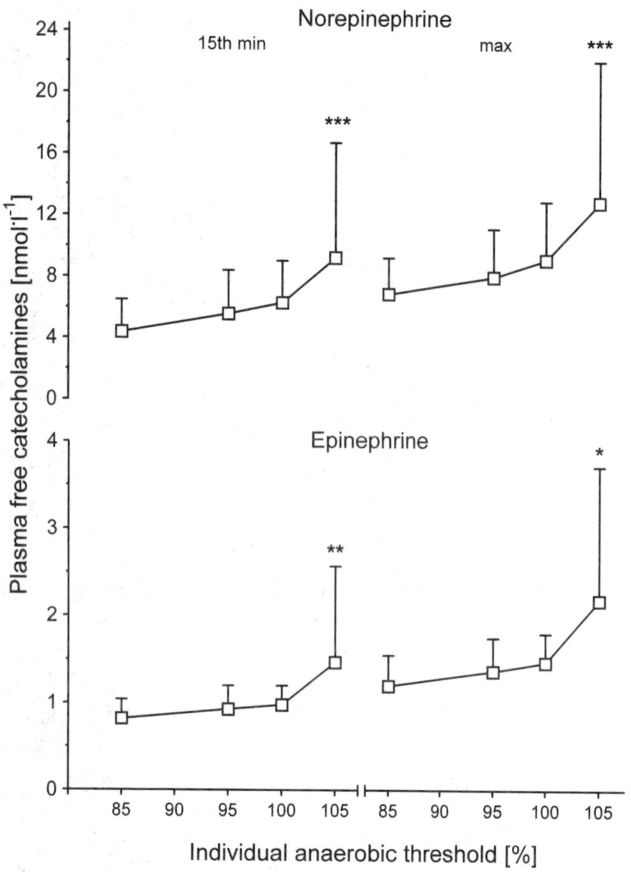

FIG. 18–3. Free plasma epinephrine and norepinephrine during endurance running exercises with different percentages of the IAT. (From refs. 38 and 51, with permission.)

lactate as long as the intensity is below or identical to the IAT (28,31). Individual analysis shows that endurance exercises with an intensity of up to 95% IAT always result in a lactate steady state. A lactate steady state was found in 93% of our subjects during endurance exercises with exactly the intensity of the IAT, performed either on a cycle ergometer by 35 rowers or cyclists, or on a treadmill by 26 runners or physically active students (28,32,33). These results were confirmed by McLellan and Cheung (34) on a cycle ergometer. A small increase of the intensity of the IAT by 5% leads to continuously increasing lactate concentrations or premature abandonment of exercise (see Fig. 18–2). An exercise intensity of 10% above the IAT exceeds the maximal lactate steady state in all cases. Comparable investigations of high methodologic expenditure [increase by 50 W or 0.5 km·h^{-1} (15)] also found the IAT at the maximal lactate steady state.

Additional measurements of the free plasma catecholamines epinephrine and norepinephrine were made in order to draw conclusions about the sympathetic activity. These determinations include indications about the psychic stress during exercise conditions (35) that cannot be determined only by looking at the changes in lactic acid. Epinephrine and norepinephrine correlate with the exponential increase in lactic acid (36). During longer-lasting aerobic exercises, however, epinephrine and norepinephrine increase with the increasing exercise duration. This increase is lower than during shorter, highly intensive, anaerobic lactic exercises that also lead to a higher epinephrine/norepinephrine ratio (37). During longer-lasting exercises performed up to an intensity of 100% IAT, the free catecholamines show few differences within this range of intensities. When increasing the intensity by only 5% above the IAT, an overproportional increase of the catecholamines as an indicator of a higher sympathetic activation can be recognized (38) (Fig. 18–3). These findings correspond to the results of other authors who measured a time-dependent increase of concentrations of epinephrine and norepinephrine during exercise intensities lower than the aerobic-anaerobic transition (about 70% of $\dot{V}O_2$max), whereas exercise intensities with increased anaerobic energy supply were time and intensity dependent (36). The changes in the catecholamines together with the findings concerning the maximal lactate steady state lead to the conclusion that the IAT describes a real physiologic break point.

METHODOLOGIC EFFECTS

In a daily routine, increased lactate values at the onset of a stepwise increasing exercise test cannot always be avoided because of exercises performed prior to the test, such as an intensified warm-up period or other exercise tests. In our investigation initial lactate values of around 4 mmol·L^{-1} had no significant effect on the performance at the IAT. This confirms earlier findings (15). The corresponding heart rates are increased by three to six beats per minute, however. This finding has to be taken into consideration when formulating the intensity recommendations for endurance training mainly according to heart rates (15,29).

The management of the immediate recovery has been reported not to affect the IAT determination (39), although an active recovery phase accelerates the elimination of blood lactate if compared to a passive recovery phase (40). Nevertheless, we recommend a standard passive recovery phase. Only the first minute after (exhaustive) cycle ergometer tests should be active in order to avoid circulatory complications (collapse).

The effect of both longer duration and lower increment of each exercise step is also of interest, because of different physiologic test systems (29). An extension of the step duration from 3 to 5 minutes leads to a steeper incline of the lactate performance curve above the threshold. The IAT itself is only slightly but not significantly lower, whereas the fixed 4 mmol·L^{-1} lactate threshold is clearly lower if compared to shorter step durations (Fig. 18–4). A change in the increment, however, has a significant effect on the IAT parameters. A reduction of the increment from 2 to 1 km·h^{-1} results

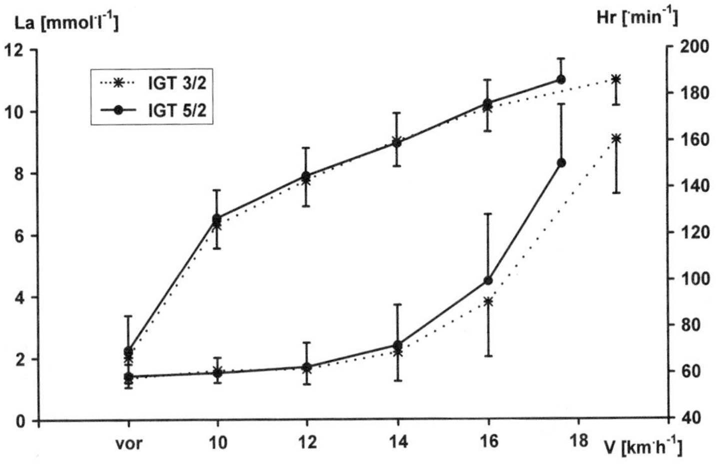

FIG. 18–4. Lactate (*La*) and heart rate (*Hr*) performance curves for stepwise incremental graded exercise tests (*IGT*) with different step duration (3 min vs. 5 min; increments of 2 km·h^{-1}, respectively).

in a relevant average increase of the velocity at the IAT of 0.9 km·h^{-1} (6%) with simultaneously increased heart rates and lactate concentrations by an average of 5 beats·min^{-1} and 0.6 mmol·L^{-1}, respectively. Heck (15) found similar results during investigations on a cycle ergometer.

A lower exhaustion level at the end of stepwise increasing exercise may lead to a slight underestimation of the endurance capacity if assessed on the basis of the IAT. A difference in running velocity of 0.2 to 0.3 km·h^{-1} on average, however, has no relevant effect on the results of performance diagnostics or the velocities recommended for endurance training. On the other hand, individual variations may reach 1.0 km·h^{-1} and thus have significant effect on the test results. Above a maximal lactate concentration of 7 to 8 mmol·L^{-1} there exists no relevant difference (29). The main problem of the submaximal tests is the slight overhang during the early recovery period (only a small difference between the blood lactate concentration at the end of exercise and the highest lactate value in the early recovery phase), with the resulting difficulty in applying the method of IAT determination.

The lactate performance curve as well as anaerobic threshold calculations that use fixed lactate concentrations may be affected by the state of the muscular glycogen stores (42). A decreased glycogen filling caused by either previous exercise or an insufficient supply of carbohydrates lowers the level of the lactate performance curve and therefore results in a higher performance at the 4 mmol·L^{-1} lactate threshold. In contrast, extremely loaded glycogen stores in the muscles lift the level of the lactate performance curve, which reaches the 4 mmol·L^{-1} lactate level at a lower exercise intensity. It was proved that the exercise intensity at the IAT remains unchanged (43), however, probably because of its taking into consideration the lactate kinetics during as well as after exercise. The concentration of lactate is shifted downward (lower values in cases of lower glycogen storage), while the performance at the IAT, however, does not change. Therefore, determining the endurance capacity on the basis of the IAT and the resulting recommendations for the intensity of endurance exercise do not depend on the level of the glycogen deposits during the step test.

SPORTS-SPECIFIC APPLICATIONS

The concept of IAT is valid not only for testing procedures under laboratory conditions but also for sports-specific field tests with gradually increasing exercise intensities. Besides the running test on an indoor or outdoor track (e.g., increasing every 3 minutes by 2 km·h^{-1} per step), a 5 × 800 m test, which is comfortable in a daily routine, provides comparative results (B. Coen, unpublished data). Sports with significant demands on the aerobic energy supply and simultaneously involving more complex motions or technical skills require more specific methods of testing. The practicality and validity of these procedures under field conditions was demonstrated for swimming, cycling (unpublished data), racquet sports such as tennis (44) and badminton (45), rowing (46,47), and ice speed skating (41). These tests, however, are partly dependent on external (e.g., weather) conditions and difficulties in standardization, which may affect the reliability and validity of the results.

The assessment of competition results or race times by using calculations of the IAT derived from sports-specific running tests is possible to some extent in longer-lasting events. The IAT itself accounts for approximately 30% to 65% of the variance in competitive performance from 1500 m races up to marathon races in specifically trained athletes (12). A marathon is usually performed with a running speed of 95% IAT to slightly above the IAT (48). In shorter endurance events (e.g., 800 and 1500 m), maximal aerobic ($\dot{V}O_2max$) and anaerobic performance capacities (e.g., maximal performance) also have to be taken into account. Very similar results (49) were found for the concept of the individual anaerobic threshold by Simon (20) and Dickhuth and colleagues (22).

THE IAT AND MONITORING OF TRAINING

Endurance training is performed at different intensities. These intensities may be monitored by means of the lactate performance curve. A randomized study under field conditions was performed in order to confirm a concept for the monitoring of running endurance training by means of the IAT. The subjects ran 10 km with a randomly assigned intensity of 70%, 80%, 90%, 95%, and 100% of the velocity at the IAT with an accompanying control of lactate and heart rate (50).

Within the regenerative or low extensive range of endurance (70% to 80% IAT, corresponding to 55% to 63% $\dot{V}O_2max$), the energy supply is guaranteed by aerobic processes and the level of lactic acid does not increase. Within the extensive range of endurance (80% to 90% IAT, corresponding to 63% to 71% $\dot{V}O_2max$), the lactate values are slightly increased if compared to rest conditions, and endurance-trained runners usually do not exceed 2 to 2.5 mmol·L^{-1}. Within the intensive range of endurance (90% to 95% IAT), the energy supply can be guaranteed only by including anaerobic processes with a corresponding increase in the level of lactate concentration. So-called threshold runs with an intensity of 100% IAT (around 80% $\dot{V}O_2max$) result in (stable) lactate values above the lactate concentration at the IAT assessed during stepwise increasing exercises. Even exceeding this critical intensity of 100% IAT by a small amount would clearly increase the sympathetic stress response and, if repeated too often, may induce an overtraining syndrome in the long term (51,52).

In the control of exercise intensity in endurance training, it is important to consider the different selectivity of heart rate and lactate values (Fig. 18–5). Small changes of intensity up to 80% IAT may be better assessed by controlling the heart rate; lactate remains unchanged or even decreases at these low intensities. At intensities above 85% to 90% IAT, the selectivity of lactate is improved because of the steep increase of lactate if compared to the heart rate, even when considering only small increases of the intensity. Therefore, the general rules for the training heart rates resulting from our data (Table 18–1) are less accurate with increasing intensity (50).

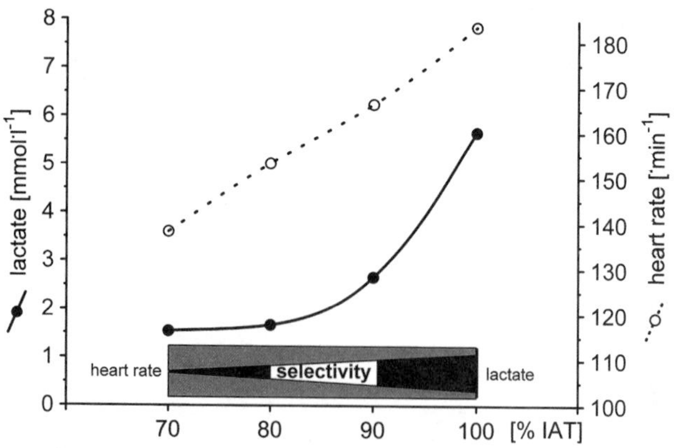

FIG. 18–5. Changes of lactate and heart rate during endurance runs with different intensities (70% to 100% IAT) and corresponding intensity-dependent selectivity of the parameters. (From ref. 50, with permission.)

INTERVAL TRAINING

Interval training above the IAT can also be monitored on the basis of IAT data (53). Figure 18–6 shows the example of a 5 × 1000 m program with rests of 4.5 minutes after each run. Different lactate values can be targeted by means of the regression line between percent IAT and the lactate concentration. The close correlation between lactate and percentage of threshold intensity is remarkable. Similar interval programs are suitable training sessions not only for runners but also for players of such sports as soccer and handball. Series of somewhat shorter and faster runs are more accepted by those athletes than endurance runs. For these exten-

TABLE 18–1. *Means of lactate (La) and heart rate (Hr), and rough rates for Hr during endurance runs*

% IAT	% $\dot{V}O_2$max	La [mmol · l^{-1}]	% La IAT	Hr [· min^{-1}]	% Hr IAT	% Hr max	Rough formula [· min^{-1}]
70	55	1.54	45	138	80	72	165 − age
80	63	1.67	50	154	89	80	180 − age
90	71	2.67	80	166	96	86	195 − age
95	75	3.53	105	175	101	91	203 − age
100	79	5.67	165	183	106	95	210 − age

Lactate and heart rates are either absolute values or percentages of the corresponding threshold and maximal values. Endurance runs are of intensities varying from 70% to 100% of individual anaerobic thresholds (IATs), corresponding to 55% to 79% of $\dot{V}O_2$max. From ref. 50, with permission.

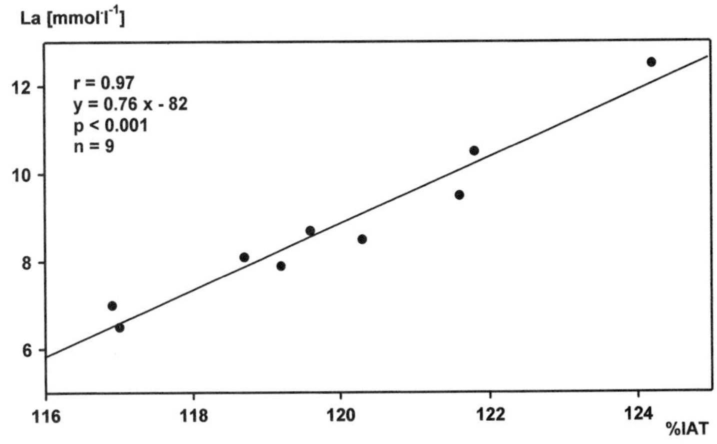

FIG. 18–6. Linear regression between lactate (*La*) and percent IAT during 5 × 1000-m interval running programs. (From ref. 53, with permission.)

sive interval sessions, intensities between 110% and 115% IAT corresponding to lactate concentrations of 4 to 6 mmol·L^{-1} seem to be appropriate for these players. In high performance athletes, however, training recommendations on the basis of data resulting from performance diagnostics have to be verified under field conditions because of individual variations and unquantifiable effects.

OVERTRAINING

In the state of overtraining the (individual) anaerobic threshold usually remains unchanged or is even slightly increased because of the somewhat lower submaximal lactate concentrations (52). This is a false higher endurance performance because it cannot be realized during training or competition. The diagnosis of an overtraining syndrome is not possible by using submaximal lactate performance curves; it requires the assessment of maximal performance parameters (e.g., lactate) (51,52).

EXERCISE IN CARDIAC REHABILITATION

The IAT can also be used to recommend the work loads of aerobic exercise (by means of heart rate guidelines) during ambulant rehabilitation for coronary patients (54). The concentration of lactic acid at the IAT usually can be expected to be around 3 mmol·L^{-1}. But this recommendation is valid only as long as no clinical complaints occur within the given range of intensity. Patients with limited myocardial function often have to abandon the exercise at an intensity that is lower than the anaerobic threshold. In these cases the heart rate recommendations have to be based on the onset of cardiac complaints instead of on the IAT.

CONCLUSION

Performance diagnostics and monitoring of training on the basis of anaerobic thresholds are controversial, because of the multitude of existing thresholds and the resulting confusion and because of the insufficient descriptions of the corresponding physiologic and biochemical factors. Changes of energy supply occur gradually, not abruptly. It is appropriate to determine thresholds, however, because of the pronounced changes in the course of both respiratory parameters and lactate concentrations, which frequently can be visually recognized as break points. Thresholds allow the quantification of defined areas or transition and the demarcation of exercise intensities by determining the aerobic energy supply and the anaerobic energy supply. Several threshold concepts are suitable for performance diagnostics and monitoring of training, but threshold models on the basis of both lactate and respiratory parameters should be scientifically evaluated under laboratory and field test conditions before being used in sports. Furthermore, the interpretation of performance diagnostic data by using threshold calculations must not overlook the observations of the lactate performance curve at other ranges of intensities. Further valid characteristic points or areas of the lactate performance curve, for example the incline of the lactate performance curve, should be investigated in the near future in order to improve the analysis of performance data.

Lactate performance curves determined under either laboratory or field conditions represent expressive and practical procedures for performance diagnostics and monitoring of training in sports with endurance components. The test procedures, however, have to be validated and their appropriate application has to be critically assessed. Training recommendations on the basis of lactate measurements must be verified under specific field conditions. Effective and efficient performance diagnostics on the basis of lactate measurements may represent an important step in optimizing performance.

REFERENCES

1. Saltin B, Astrand PO. Maximal oxygen uptake in athletes. *J Appl Physiol* 1967;23:353–358.
2. Reference deleted in proofs.
3. Coetzer P, Noakes TD, Sanders B, et al. Superior fatigue resistance of elite black South African distance runners. *J Appl Physiol* 1993;75:1822–1827.
4. Anderson GS, Rhodes EC. A review of blood lactate and ventilatory methods of detecting transition thresholds. *Sports Med* 1989;8:43–55.
5. Fletcher WM, Hopkins FG. Lactic acid in amphibian muscle. *J Physiol (Lond)* 1907;35:247–309.
6. Hill AV, Lupton H. Muscular exercise, lactic acid and the supply and utilization of oxygen. *Q J Med* 1923;16:135–171.
7. Hollmann W. The relationship between pH, lactic acid, potassium in the arterial and venous blood, the ventilation (PoW) and pulse frequency during increasing spirometric work in endurance-trained and untrained persons. Pan American Congress for Sports Medicine, Chicago, 1959.
8. Hollmann W. Die ärztliche beurteilung der körperlichen höchstund dauerleistungsfähigkeit. *Umschau Wissenschaft Technik* 1961;22:689–692.
9. Wasserman K, McIlroy MB. Detecting the threshold of anaerobic metabolism in cardiac patients. *Am J Cardiol* 1964;14:844–852.
10. Brooks GA. Anaerobic threshold: review of the concept and directions for future research. *Med Sci Sports Exerc* 1985;17:22–34.
11. Mader A, Liesen H, Heck H, et al. Zur beurteilung der sportartspezifischen ausdauerleistungsfähigkeit im labor. *Sportarzt Sportmed* 1976;27:80–88,109–112.
12. Sjödin B, Jacobs I, Karlsson J. Onset of blood lactate accumulation and enzyme activities in m. vastus lateralis in man. *Int J Sports Med* 1981;2:166–170.
13. Kindermann W, Simon G, Keul J. The significance of the aerobic-anaerobic transition for the determination of work load intensities during endurance training. *Eur J Appl Physiol* 1979;42:25–34.
14. Davis JA, Caiozzo VJ, Lamarra N, et al. Does the gas exchange anaerobic threshold occur at a fixed blood lactate concentration of 2 or 4 mM? *Int J Sports Med* 1983;4:89–93.
15. Heck H. *Laktat in der leistungsdiagnostik.* Schorndorf, Germany: Hofmann, 1991.
16. Heck H, Mader A, Hess G, Mucke S, Muller R, Hollmann W. Justification of the 4-mmol/l lactate threshold. *Int J Sports Med* 1985;6:117–130.
17. Bunc V, Heller J, Novack J, Leso J. Determination of the individual anaerobic threshold. *Acta Universitatis Carolinae Gymnica* 1985;27:73–81.
18. Hagberg JM, Coyle EF. Physiological determinants of endurance performance as studied in competitive racewalkers. *Med Sci Sports Exerc* 1983;15:287–289.
19. Keul J, Simon G, Berg A, Dickhuth H-H, Goertler I, Kübel R. Bestimmung der individuellen anaeroben schwelle zur leistungsbewertung und trainingsgestaltung. *Dtsch Z Sportmed* 1979; 30:212–218.
20. Simon G. Trainingssteuerung im schwimmsport. *Dtsch Z Sportmed* 1986;37:376–379.
21. Stegmann H, Kindermann W, Schnabel A. Lactate kinetics and individual anaerobic threshold. *Int J Sports Med* 1981;2:160–165.
22. Dickhuth H-H, Wohlfahrth B, Hildebrand D, Rokitzki L, Huonker M, Keul J. Jahreszeitliche schwankungen der ausdauerleistungsfähigkeit von hochtrainierten mittelstreckenläufern. *Dtsch Z Sportmed* 1988;39:346–353.
23. Weicker H. Interaktion zwischen aerober und anaerober energieproduktion, laktatproduktion, release und elimination. In: Clasing D, Weicker H, Böning D, eds. *Stellenwert der Laktatbestimmung in der leistungsdiagnostik.* Stuttgart: Gustav Fischer, 1994:11–25.
24. Favier RJ, Constable SH, Chen M, Holloszy JO. Endurance exercise training reduces lactate production. *J Appl Physiol* 1986; 61:885–889.
25. Freund H, Zouloumian P. Lactate after exercise in man: I. Evolution kinetics in arterial blood. *Eur J Appl Physiol* 1981;46:121–133.
26. MacRae HS, Dennis SC, Bosch AN, Noakes TD. Effects of training on lactate production and removal during progressive exercise in humans [see comments]. *J Appl Physiol* 1992;72:1649–1656.
27. Messonnier L, Freund H, Bourdin M, Belli A, Lacour JR. Lactate exchange and removal abilities in rowing performance. *Med Sci Sports Exerc* 1997;29:396–401.
28. Urhausen A, Coen B, Weiler B, Kindermann W. Individuelle anaerobe schwelle und laktat steady state bei ausdauerbelastungen. In: Clasing D, Weicker H, Böning D, eds. *Stellenwert der laktatbestimmung in der leistungsdiagnostik.* Stuttgart: Gustav Fischer, 1994:37–46.
29. Coen B, Urhausen A, Kindermann W. Influence of the exercise protocol on the individual anaerobic threshold determined during an increasing exercise test. *Int J Sports Med* 1996;17(suppl 1):S18.
30. McLellan TM, Jacobs I. Reliability, reproducibility and validity of the individual anaerobic threshold. *Eur J Appl Physiol* 1993; 67:125–131.
31. Urhausen A, Coen B, Weiler B, Kindermann W. Individual anaerobic threshold and maximum lactate steady state. *Int J Sports Med* 1993;14:134–139.
32. Schnabel A, Kindermann W, Schmitt WM, Biro G, Stegmann H. Hormonal and metabolic consequences of prolonged running at the individual anaerobic threshold. *Int J Sports Med* 1982; 3:163–168.
33. Stegmann H, Kindermann W. Comparison of prolonged exercise tests at the individual anaerobic threshold and the fixed anaerobic threshold of 4 mmol·l(-1) lactate. *Int J Sports Med* 1982;3:105–110.
34. McLellan TM, Cheung KS. A comparative evaluation of the individual anaerobic threshold and the critical power. *Med Sci Sports Exerc* 1992;24:543–550.
35. Frankenhaeuser M. Behavior and circulating catecholamines. *Brain Res* 1971;31:241–262.
36. Lehmann M, Kapp R, Himmelsbach M, Keul J. Time and intensity dependent catecholamine responses during graduated exercise as an indicator of fatigue and exhaustion. In: Knuttgen HG, Vogel JA, Poortmans J, eds. *Biochemistry of exercise.* Champaign, IL: Human Kinetics, 1983:738–748.
37. Kindermann W, Schnabel A, Schmitt WM, Biro G, Cassens J, Weber F. Catecholamines, growth hormone, cortisol, insulin, and sex hormones in anaerobic and aerobic exercise. *Eur J Appl Physiol* 1982;49:389–399.
38. Urhausen A, Weiler B, Coen B, Kindermann W. Plasma catecholamines during endurance exercise of different intensities as related to the individual anaerobic threshold. *Eur J Appl Physiol* 1994; 69:16–20.
39. McLellan TM, Cheung KS, Jacobs I. Incremental test protocol, recovery mode and the individual anaerobic threshold. *Int J Sports Med* 1991;12:190–195.
40. McLellan TM, Skinner JS. Blood lactate removal during active recovery related to the aerobic threshold. *Int J Sports Med* 1982; 3:224–229.
41. Reference deleted in proofs.
42. Yoshida T. Effect of dietary modifications on lactate threshold and onset of blood lactate accumulation during incremental exercise. *Eur J Appl Physiol* 1984;53:200–205.
43. Fröhlich J, Urhausen A, Seul U, Kindermann W. Beeinflussung der individuellen anaeroben schwelle durch kohlenhydratarme und reiche ernährung. *Leistungssport* 1989;19:18–20.
44. Urhausen A, Kullmer T, Schillo C, Kindermann W. Performance diagnosis in tennis: the influence of basic aerobic endurance (field step test) and tennis-specific skills (ball machine test) on the performance in playing tennis. *Dtsch Z Sportmed* 1988;39:340–346.
45. Coen B, Urhausen A, Weiler B, Huber G, Wiberg F, Kindermann W. Specific performance diagnostic in badminton. *Int J Sports Med* 1998;19(suppl):22.
46. Coen B, Schell W, Urhausen A, Weiler B, Kindermann W. The 4 × 6 min increasing exercise water test in rowing. *Int J Sports Med* 1996:17(suppl 1):S25.

47. Urhausen A, Weiler B, Kindermann W. Heart rate, blood lactate, and catecholamines during ergometer and on water rowing. *Int J Sports Med* 1993;14(suppl 1):S20–S23.
48. Rieder T, Kullmer T, Kindermann W. Aerobic and anaerobic treadmill tests: their validity for the competitive performance capacity in middle and long distance running. *Dtsch Z Sportmed* 1987;38:318–322.
49. Röcker K, Schotte O, Niess A, Heitkamp HC, Dickhuth H-H. Treadmill testing and the prediction of race results in distance running. *Dtsch Z Sportmed* 1997;48:315–323.
50. Coen B, Urhausen A, Herrmann S, Weiler B, Kindermann W. Belastungsdosierung von dauerläufen unterschiedlicher intensität anhand der parameter herzfrequenz, laktat und katecholamine. *Sportorthopädie-Sporttraumatologie* 1996;12:96–101.
51. Urhausen A, Gabriel H, Kindermann W. Blood hormones as markers of training stress and overtraining. *Sports Med* 1995; 20:251–276.
52. Urhausen A, Gabriel H, Weiler B, Kindermann W. Ergometric and psychological findings in overtraining. A prospective long-term follow-up study in endurance athletes. *Int J Sports Med* 1998;19:114–120.
53. Coen B, Schwarz L, Urhausen A, Kindermann W. Control of training in middle- and long-distance running by means of the individual anaerobic threshold. *Int J Sports Med* 1991;12:519–524.
54. Kindermann W. Laktatdiagnostik II. In: Reindell H, Bubenheimer P, Dickhuth H-H, Görnandt L, eds. *Funktionsdiagnostik des gesunden und kranken herzens.* Stuttgart: Thieme 1988: 221–228.

Exercise and Sport Science,
edited by William E. Garrett, Jr., and Donald T. Kirkendall.
Lippincott Williams & Wilkins, Philadelphia © 2000.

CHAPTER 19

Exercise for Successful Aging

William J. Evans

Advancing age is associated with a remarkable number of changes in body composition. Reductions in lean body mass have been well characterized. This decreased lean body mass occurs primarily as a result of losses in skeletal muscle mass (1,2). This age-related loss in muscle mass has been termed *sarcopenia* (3). Loss in muscle mass accounts for the age-associated decreases in basal metabolic rate, muscle strength, and activity levels, which, in turn cause the decreased energy requirements of the elderly. In sedentary individuals, the main determinant of energy expenditure is fat-free mass, which declines by about 15% between the third and eighth decades of life. It also appears that declining caloric needs are not matched by an appropriate decline in caloric intake, with the ultimate result being an increased body fat content with advancing age. Increased body fat along with increased abdominal obesity are thought to be directly linked to the greatly increased incidence of type II diabetes among the elderly. This chapter discusses the extent to which regularly performed exercise can affect nutritional needs (with particular emphasis on protein needs) and functional capacity in the elderly.

Sarcopenia is a direct cause of the age-related decrease in muscle strength. Our laboratory examined muscle strength and mass in 200 healthy 45- to 78-year-old men and women and concluded that muscle mass (not function) is the major determinant of the age- and sex-related differences in strength (1). This relationship is independent of muscle location (upper vs. lower extremities) and function (extension vs. flexion). Reduced muscle strength in the elderly is a major cause of their increased disability. With advancing age and very low activity levels seen in the very old, muscle strength and power are critical components of walking ability (4). The high prevalence of falls among the institutionalized elderly may be a consequence of their lower muscle strength.

The question that we have been addressing is: To what extent are these changes inevitable consequences of aging? Data examining young and middle-aged endurance-trained men demonstrate that body fat stores and maximal aerobic capacity were not related to age but rather to the total number of hours of exercise per week (5). Even among sedentary individuals, energy spent in daily activities explains more than 75% of the variability in body fatness among young and older men (6). These data and the results of other investigators indicate that levels of physical activity are important in determining energy expenditure and ultimately body fat accumulation. However, cross-sectional data of Klitgaard and colleagues (7,8) found that older endurance athletes (runners and swimmers) display fat-free mass and muscle strength similar to those seen in sedentary aged-matched controls, an indication that endurance exercise alone may not prevent sarcopenia.

AEROBIC EXERCISE

Maximal aerobic capacity ($\dot{V}O_2max$) declines with advancing age (9). This age-associated decrease in $\dot{V}O_2max$ has been shown to be approximately 1% per year between the ages of 20 and 70. This decline is likely due to a number of factors, including decreased levels of physical activity, changing cardiac function (including decreased maximal cardiac output), and reduced muscle mass. Flegg and Lakatta (10) determined that skeletal muscle mass accounted for most of the variability in $\dot{V}O_2max$ in men and women above the age of 60. Recently, Rosen and colleagues (11) examined predictors of this age-associated decline in $\dot{V}O_2max$. They found that $\dot{V}O_2max$ declines at the same rate in athletic and

W. J. Evans: Nutrition, Metabolism, and Exercise Laboratory, Veterans Affairs Medical Center, North Little Rock, Arkansas 72114.

sedentary men and that 35% of this decline is due to sarcopenia.

Aerobic exercise has long been an important recommendation for the prevention and treatment of many of the chronic diseases typically associated with old age. These include non–insulin-dependent diabetes mellitus (NIDDM) (and those with impaired glucose tolerance), hypertension, heart disease, and osteoporosis. Regularly performed aerobic exercise increases insulin action. The responses of initially sedentary young (age 20 to 30) and older (age 60 to 70) men and women to 3 months of aerobic conditioning (70% of maximal heart rate, 45 minutes per day, 3 days per week) were examined by Meredith and colleagues (12). They found that the absolute gains in aerobic capacity were similar between the two age groups. The mechanism for adaptation to regular submaximal exercise appears to be different between old and young people, however. Muscle biopsies taken before and after training showed a more than twofold increase in oxidative capacity of the muscles of the older subjects, while those of the young subjects showed smaller improvements. In addition, skeletal muscle glycogen stores in the older subjects, significantly lower than those of the young men and women initially, increased significantly. The degree to which the elderly demonstrate increases in maximal cardiac output in response to endurance training is still largely unanswered. Seals and co-workers (13) found no increases after 1 year of endurance training, while Spina and colleagues (14) observed that older men increased maximal cardiac output and healthy older women demonstrated no change in response to endurance exercise. If these gender-related differences in cardiovascular response are real, they may explain the lack of response in maximal cardiac output when older men and women are included in the same study population.

EXERCISE AND CARBOHYDRATE METABOLISM

The 2-hour plasma glucose level during an oral glucose tolerance test (OGTT) increases by an average of 5.3 mg/dL per decade, and fasting plasma glucose increases by an average of 1 mg/dL per decade (15). The National Health and Nutrition Examination Survey (NHANES II) demonstrated a progressive increase of about 0.4 mM/decade of life in mean plasma glucose value 2 hours after a 75-g OGTT (n = 1678 men and 1892 women) (16). Shimokata and co-workers (17) examined glucose tolerance in community-dwelling men and women ranging in age from 17 to 92. By assessing level of obesity, pattern of body fat distribution, activity, and fitness levels, they examined the independent effect of age on glucose tolerance. They found no significant differences between the young and middle-aged groups; however, the old groups had significantly higher glucose and insulin values (following a glucose challenge) than young or middle-aged groups. They concluded: "The major finding of this study is that the decline in glucose tolerance from the early-adult to the middle-age years is entirely explained by secondary influences (fatness and fitness), whereas the decline from mid-life to old age still is also influenced by chronologic age. This finding is unique. It is also unexplained." It must be pointed out, however, that anthropometric determination of body fatness becomes increasingly less accurate with advancing age and does not reflect the intraabdominal and intramuscular accumulation of fat that occurs with aging (18). The results of this study may be due more to an underestimation of true body fat levels than age per se. These age-associated changes in glucose tolerance can result in NIDDM and the broad array of associated abnormalities. It has been estimated that 13% of men and women between the ages of 60 and 74 had impaired glucose tolerance, and an additional 17% had NIDDM (18a). In a large population study of elderly men and women (≥55 years), serum glucose and fructosamine levels were seen to be higher in subjects with retinopathy compared with those without, and in the groups with retinopathy, serum glucose was significantly associated with the number of hemorrhages (19). These relationships were independent of body composition, abdominal obesity, or the presence of NIDDM.

The relationships among aging, body composition, activity, and glucose tolerance were also examined in 270 female and 462 male factory workers aged 22 to 73 years, none of whom were retired (20). Plasma glucose levels, both fasting and after a glucose load, increased with age, but the correlation between age and total integrated glucose response following a glucose load was weak; in women only 3% of the variance could be attributed to age. When activity levels and drug use were factored in, age accounted for only 1% of the variance in women and 6.25% in men.

The fact that aerobic exercise has significant effects on skeletal muscle may help explain its importance in the treatment of glucose intolerance and NIDDM. Seals and co-workers (21) found that a high-intensity training program showed greater improvements in the insulin response to an oral glucose load compared to lower-intensity aerobic exercise. However, their subjects began the study with normal glucose tolerance. Kirwan and co-workers (22) found that 9 months of endurance training at 80% of the maximal heart rate (4 days per week) resulted in reduced glucose-stimulated insulin levels; however, no comparison was made to a lower-intensity exercise group. Hughes and co-workers (23) demonstrated that regularly performed aerobic exercise without weight loss resulted in improved glucose tolerance, rate of insulin-stimulated glucose disposal, and increased skeletal muscle GLUT-4 (the glucose transporter protein in skeletal muscle) levels in older glucose-intolerant subjects. In this investigation, a moderate-intensity aerobic exercise program was compared to a higher-intensity program (50% vs. 75% of maximal heart rate reserve, 55 minutes per day, 4 days per week for 12 weeks). No differences were seen between the moderate- and higher-intensity aerobic exercise on glucose tolerance, insulin sensitivity, or muscle GLUT-4 levels, indicating perhaps that a prescription of moderate aerobic exercise should be recommended for older men and women with NIDDM or a high risk for NIDDM to help ensure compliance with the program.

Endurance training and dietary modifications are generally recommended as the primary treatment in the NIDDM patient. Cross-sectional analysis of dietary intake supports the hypothesis that a low-carbohydrate/high-fat diet is associated with the onset of NIDDM (24). This evidence, however, is not supported by prospective studies in which dietary habits have not been related to the development of NIDDM (25,26). The effects of a high-carbohydrate diet on glucose tolerance have been equivocal (27,28). Hughes and colleagues (29) compared the effects of a high-carbohydrate (CHO) (60% CHO and 20% fat)/high-fiber (25 g dietary fiber/1000 kcal) diet with and without 3 months of high-intensity (75% maximum heart rate reserve, 50 minutes per day, 4 days per week) endurance exercise in older, glucose-intolerant men and women. Subjects were fed all of their food on a metabolic ward during the 3-month study and were not allowed to lose weight. These investigators observed no improvement in glucose tolerance or insulin-stimulated glucose uptake in either the diet or the diet-plus-exercise group. The exercise–plus–high-carbohydrate diet group demonstrated a significant and substantial increase in skeletal muscle glycogen content, and at the end of the training the muscle glycogen stores would be considered saturated. Since the primary site of glucose disposal is skeletal muscle glycogen stores, the extremely high muscle glycogen content associated with exercise and a high-carbohydrate diet likely limited the rate of glucose disposal. Thus, when combined with exercise and a weight-maintenance diet, a high-carbohydrate diet had a counterregulatory effect. It is likely that a high-carbohydrate/high-fiber diet in the treatment of excess body fat may be an important cause of the impaired glucose tolerance. Schaefer and co-workers (30) demonstrated that older subjects consuming an ad libitum high-carbohydrate diet lost weight.

There appears to be no attenuation of the response of elderly men and women to regularly performed aerobic exercise when compared to that seen in young subjects. Increased fitness levels are associated with reduced mortality and increased life expectancy. They have also been shown to prevent the occurrence of NIDDM in those who are at the greatest risk for developing this disease (31). Thus, regularly performed aerobic exercise is an important way for older people to improve their glucose tolerance.

Aerobic exercise is generally prescribed as an important adjunct to a weight-loss program. Aerobic exercise combined with weight loss has been demonstrated to increase insulin action to a greater extent than weight loss through diet restriction alone. In a study by Bogardus and colleagues (32), diet therapy alone improved glucose tolerance, mainly by reducing basal endogenous glucose production and improving hepatic sensitivity to insulin. Aerobic exercise training, on the other hand, increased carbohydrate storage rates; therefore, "diet therapy plus physical training produced a more significant approach toward normal." However, aerobic exercise (as opposed to resistance training) combined with a hypocaloric diet has been demonstrated to result in a greater reduction in resting metabolic rate (RMR) than diet alone (33). Heymsfield and co-workers (34) found that aerobic exercise combined with caloric restriction did not preserve fat-free mass (FFM) and did not further accelerate weight loss when compared with diet alone. This lack of an effect of aerobic exercise may have been due to a greater decrease in RMR in the exercising group. In perhaps the most comprehensive study of its kind, Goran and Poehlman (35) examined components of energy metabolism in older men and women engaged in regular endurance training. They found that endurance training did not increase total daily energy expenditure due to a compensatory decline in physical activity during the remainder of the day. In other words, when elderly subjects participated in a regular walking program, they rested more, so that activities outside of walking decreased and thus 24-hour calorie expenditure was unchanged. However, older individuals who had been participating in endurance exercise for most of their lives have been shown to have a greater RMR and total daily energy expenditure than did age-matched sedentary controls (36). Ballor and colleagues (37) compared the effects of resistance training to those of diet restriction alone in obese women. They found that resistance exercise training results in increased strength and gains in muscle size as well as a preservation of FFM during weight loss. These data are similar to the results of Pavlou and colleagues (38), who used both aerobic and resistance training as adjuncts to a weight-loss program in obese men.

STRENGTH TRAINING

While endurance exercise has been the more traditional means of increasing cardiovascular fitness, strength or resistance training is currently recommended by the American College of Sports Medicine as an important component of an overall fitness program. This is particularly important in the elderly, in whom loss of muscle mass and weakness are prominent deficits.

Strength conditioning or progressive resistance training is generally defined as training in which the resistance against which a muscle generates force is progressively increased over time. Progressive resistance training involves few contractions against a heavy load. The metabolic and morphologic adaptations resulting from resistance and endurance exercise are quite different. Muscle strength has been shown to increase in response to training between 60% and 100% of the one repetition maximum (1 RM), which is the maximum amount of weight that can be lifted with one contraction. Strength conditioning will result in an increase in muscle size, and this increase in size is largely the result of increased contractile proteins. The mechanisms by which the mechanical events stimulate an increase in ribonucleic acid (RNA) synthesis and subsequent protein synthesis are not well understood. Lifting weight requires that a muscle shorten as it produces force. This is called a concentric contraction. Lowering the weight, on the other hand, forces the muscle to lengthen as it produces force. This is an eccentric muscle contraction. These lengthening muscle contractions have been shown to produce ultrastructural damage that may stimulate increased muscle protein turnover (39).

Our laboratory examined the effects of high-intensity resistance training of the knee extensors and flexors (80% of 1 RM, 3 days per week) in older men (age 60 to 72). The average increases in knee flexor and extensor strength were 227% and 107%, respectively. Computed tomography (CT) scans and muscle biopsies were used to determine muscle size. Total muscle area by CT analysis increased by 11.4%, while the muscle biopsies showed an increase of 33.5% in type I fiber area and 27.5% increase in type II fiber area. In addition, lower body $\dot{V}O_2max$ increased significantly, while upper body $\dot{V}O_2max$ did not, indicating that increased muscle mass can increase maximal aerobic power. It appears that the age-related loss in muscle mass may be an important determinant in the reduced maximal aerobic capacity seen in elderly men and women (10). Improving muscle strength can enhance the capacity of many older men and women to perform many activities such as climbing stairs, carrying packages, and even walking.

We have applied this same training program to a group of frail, institutionalized elderly men and women (mean age 90 ± 3 years, range 87 to 96) (40). After 8 weeks of training, the 10 subjects in this study increased muscle strength by almost 180% and muscle size by 11%. A similar intervention with frail nursing home residents demonstrated not only increases in muscle strength and size but also increased gait speed, stair climbing power, and balance (41). In addition, spontaneous activity levels increased significantly, while the activity of a nonexercised control group was unchanged. In this study the effects of a protein/calorie supplement [240-mL liquid supplying 360 kcal in the form of carbohydrate (60%), fat (23%), and soy-based protein (17%), which was designed to augment caloric intake by about 20%, and provide one-third of the recommended dietary allowance (RDA) for vitamins and minerals] combined with exercise were also examined. While no interaction was seen with muscle strength, functional capacity, or muscle size (no differences in improvements between the supplemented group and a nonsupplemented control group), the men and women who consumed the supplement and exercised gained weight compared to the three other groups examined (exercise/control, non–exercise supplemented, and nonexercise control). The nonexercising subjects who received the supplement reduced their habitual dietary energy intake so that total energy intake was unchanged. It should be pointed out that this was a very old, very frail population with diagnoses of multiple chronic diseases. The increase in overall levels of physical activity has been a common observation in our studies (41–43). Since muscle weakness is a primary deficit in many older individuals, increased strength may stimulate more aerobic activities like walking and cycling.

Strength training may increase balance through the improvement in strength of the muscles involved in walking. Indeed, ankle weakness has been demonstrated to be associated with increased risk of falling in nursing home patients (44). However, balance training, which may demonstrate very little improvement in muscle strength, size, or cardiovascular changes, has also been demonstrated to decrease the risk of falls in older people (45). Tai chi, a form of dynamic balance training that requires no new technology or equipment, has been demonstrated to reduce the risk of falling in older people by almost 50% (46). As a component of the National Institute on Aging FICSIT trials (Frailty and Injuries: Cooperative Studies of Intervention Techniques), individuals aged 70+ were randomized to Tai chi (TC), individualized balance training (BT), and exercise control education (ED) groups for 15 weeks (47). In a follow-up assessment 4 months postintervention, 130 subjects responded to exit interview questions about perceived benefits of participation. Both TC and BT subjects reported increased confidence in balance and movement, but only TC subjects reported that their daily activities and their overall life had been affected; many of these subjects had changed their normal physical activity to incorporate ongoing TC practice. The data suggest that when mental as well as physical control is perceived to be enhanced, with a generalized sense of improvement in overall well-being, older persons' motivation to continue exercising also increases.

Province and colleagues (48) examined the overall effect of many different exercise interventions in the FICSIT trials on reducing falls. While each these separate interventions was too underpowered to draw conclusions about their effects on the incidence of falls in an elderly population, they did draw the following conclusion:

> All training domains, taken together under the heading of "general exercise" showed an effect on falls. This probably demonstrates the "rising tide raises all boats" principle, in which training that targets one domain may improve performance somewhat in other domains as a consequence. If this is so, then the differences seen on fall risk due to the exact nature of the training may not be as critical compared with the differences in not training at all.

The use of a community-based exercise program for frail older people has been examined (49). Participants were predominantly sedentary women over age 70 with multiple chronic conditions. The program was conducted with peer leaders to facilitate its continuation after the research demonstration phase. In addition to positive health outcomes related to functional mobility, blood pressure maintenance, and overall well-being, this intervention was successful in sustaining active participation in regular physical activity through the use of peer leaders selected by the program participants.

In addition to its effect on increasing muscle mass and function, resistance training can also have an important effect on energy balance of elderly men and women (50). Men and women participating in a resistance training program of the upper and lower body muscles required approximately 15% more calories to maintain body weight after 12 weeks of training when compared to their pretraining energy requirements. This increase in energy needs came about as a result of an increased resting metabolic rate, the small energy cost of the exercise, and what was presumed to be an increase in activity levels. While endurance training has been demonstrated to be an important adjunct to weight-loss programs in young men and women by increasing their daily energy expenditure, its utility in treating obesity in the elderly may not be great. This is because many sedentary older men and women do not spend many calories when they perform endurance exercise, due to their low fitness levels. Thirty to 40 minutes of exercise may increase energy expenditure by only 100 to 200 kcal with very little residual effect on calorie expenditure. Aerobic exercise training will not preserve lean body mass to any great extent during weight loss. Because resistance training can preserve or even increase muscle mass during weight loss, this type of exercise for those older men and women who must lose weight may be of genuine benefit.

BONE HEALTH

The increased calorie need resulting from strength training may be a way for the elderly to improve their overall nutritional intake when the calories are derived from nutrient-dense foods. In particular, calcium is an important nutrient to increase since calcium intake was found to be one of the few limiting nutrients in the diet of free-living elderly men and women in the Boston nutritional status survey, which assessed free-living and institutionalized elderly men and women (51). Careful nutritional planning is needed to reach the recommended calcium levels of 1500 mg/d for postmenopausal women with osteoporosis or using hormone replacement therapy, and 1000 mg/d for postmenopausal women taking estrogen. An increased calorie intake from calcium-containing food is one method to help achieve this goal.

In one of the very few studies to examine the interaction of dietary calcium and exercise, we studied 41 postmenopausal women consuming either high-calcium (1462 mg/d) or moderate-calcium (761 mg/d) diets. Half of these women participated in a year-long walking program (45 minutes per day, 4 days per week, 75% of heart rate reserve). Independent effects of the exercise and dietary calcium were seen. Compared with the moderate-calcium group, the women consuming a high-calcium diet displayed reduced bone loss from the femoral neck, independent of whether the women exercised. The walking prevented the loss of trabecular bone mineral density seen in the nonexercising women after 1 year. Thus, it appears that calcium intake and aerobic exercise are each independently beneficial to bone mineral density at different sites. The effects of 52 weeks of high-intensity resistance exercise training were examined in a group of 39 postmenopausal women (42). Twenty were randomly assigned to the strength training group (2 days per week, 80% of 1 RM for upper and lower body muscle groups). At the end of the year significant differences were seen in lumbar spine and femoral bone density between the strength-trained and sedentary women. Unlike other pharmacologic and nutritional strategies for preventing bone loss and osteoporosis, however, resistance exercise affects more than just bone density. The women who strength trained improved their muscle mass, strength, balance, and overall levels of physical activity. Thus, resistance training can be an important way to decrease the risk for an osteoporotic bone fracture in postmenopausal women.

PROTEIN NEEDS AND AGING

Previous estimates of dietary protein needs of the elderly using nitrogen balance have ranged from 0.59 to 0.8 $g \cdot kg^{-1} \cdot d^{-1}$(52–54). However, the low value was reported by Zanni and colleagues (54), who preceded their 10-day dietary protein feeding with a 17-day protein-free diet, which was likely to improve nitrogen retention during the 10-day balance period. Our group (55) reassessed the nitrogen balance studies mentioned above using the currently accepted, 1985 World Health Organization (WHO) (56) nitrogen-balance formula. These newly recalculated data were combined with nitrogen balance data collected on 12 healthy older men and women (age range 56 to 80 years, 8 men and 4 women) consuming the current RDA for protein or double this amount (0.8 $g \cdot kg^{-1} \cdot d^{-1}$ and 1.6 $g \cdot kg^{-1} \cdot d^{-1}$, respectively) in our laboratory. Our subjects consumed the diet for 11 consecutive days, and nitrogen (N) balance ($mg \cdot kg^{-1} \cdot d^{-1}$ N) was measured during days 6 to 11. The estimated mean protein requirements from the three retrospectively assessed studies and the current study can be combined by weighted averaging to produce an overall protein requirement estimate of 0.91 ± 0.043 $g \cdot kg^{-1} \cdot d^{-1}$. The combined estimate excluding the data from our 12 subjects is 0.894 ± 0.048 $g \cdot kg^{-1} \cdot d^{-1}$ protein.

The current RDA in the United States of 0.8 $g \cdot kg^{-1} \cdot d^{-1}$ is based on data collected, for the most part, on young subjects. The RDA includes an upward adjustment based on the coefficient of variability of the average requirement established in these studies (0.6 $g \cdot kg^{-1} \cdot d^{-1}$). Based on the coefficient of variability (CV) previously established for nitrogen balance studies, an adequate dietary protein level for 97.5% of the elderly population would be provided by an intake of 25% [twice the standard deviation (SD)] above the mean protein requirement. Our data suggest that the safe protein intake for elderly adults is 1.25 $g \cdot kg^{-1} \cdot d^{-1}$. On the basis of the current and recalculated short-term N-balance results, a safe recommended protein intake for older men and women should be set at 1.0 to 1.25 $g \cdot kg^{-1} \cdot d^{-1}$ high-quality protein. It has been reported that approximately 50% of 946 healthy, free-living men and women above the age of 60 living in the Boston, Massachusetts, area consume less than this amount of protein, and 25% of the elderly men and women in this survey consume, respectively, <0.86 and <0.81 $g \cdot kg^{-1} \cdot d^{-1}$ protein (51). A large percentage of homebound elderly people consuming their habitual dietary protein intake (0.67 $g \cdot kg^{-1} \cdot d^{-1}$ mixed protein) have been shown to be in negative N balance (57).

We examined the effects of marginal dietary protein intake in 12 sedentary healthy women, aged 66 to 79. They were admitted into a 9-week metabolic study and consumed a meat-free diet containing 0.45 or 0.93 $g \cdot kg^{-1} \cdot d^{-1}$ protein. The nonprotein energy in the diet was provided by carbohydrates (65%) and fat (35%). Six-day nitrogen-balance periods were measured during study days 16 to 21 (week 3), and 56 to 61 (week 9). In addition to N balance, body composition [total body potassium, body density (underwater weighing), and dual-energy x-ray absorptiometry], whole-body leucine kinetics ([1-^{13}C]leucine infusion), muscle fiber area, immune function (delayed hypersensitivity), urinary creatinine and 3-methylhistidine, muscle strength, and plasma insulin-like growth factor-I (IGF-I) were measured while the women consumed 1.2 $g \cdot kg^{-1} \cdot d^{-1}$ protein at baseline and after adaptation to the two different dietary protein levels (week 9). This study demonstrated that long-term adaptation to 0.45 $g \cdot kg^{-1} \cdot d^{-1}$ protein resulted in an accommodation resulting in reductions in ^{40}K (active cell mass), skeletal muscle mass, muscle strength, and immune function. Leucine oxidation rates were a more sensitive index of the adequacy of protein intake than synthesis, flux, or metabolic rate. N balance was negative in the low-protein group. The greatest losses in body nitrogen occurred during the first balance period; however, the women on the low-protein intake remained in negative N balance throughout the trial. The change in IGF-I levels was significantly associated with the change in nitrogen balance, body cell mass, muscle fiber size, skeletal muscle, and immune function. Inadequate dietary protein intake may be an important cause of sarcopenia. These data demonstrate that the compensatory response to long-term decreases in dietary protein intake is a loss in lean body mass.

We recently examined adequacy of the current RDA for protein for healthy elderly men and women by examing the effects of long-term (15 weeks) consumption of a eucaloric diet providing 0.8 $g \cdot kg^{-1} \cdot d^{-1}$ protein. CT scans of the thigh muscle show that the subjects who consumed the RDA for protein and did not exercise lost a significant amount of skeletal muscle, confirming our hypothesis that the RDA for protein is inadequate for older individuals. Muscle biopsies taken from the m. vastus lateralis confirm the CT scan data by demonstrating a significant reduction in muscle-fiber-area of type II muscle cells in the sedentary group of subjects.

High-intensity resistance training appears to have profoundly anabolic effects in the elderly. Data from our laboratory demonstrate a 10% to 15% decrease in N excretion at the initiation of training that persists for 12 weeks. That is, progressive resistance training improved N balance; thus, older subjects performing resistance training have a lower mean protein requirement than do sedentary subjects. These results are somewhat at variance with our previous research (58), which demonstrated that regularly performed aerobic exercise causes an increase in the mean protein requirement of middle-aged and young endurance athletes. This difference likely results from increased oxidation of amino acids during aerobic exercise that may not be present during resistance training.

We recently examined the effects of resistance training on nitrogen balance in subjects with mild to moderate chronic renal failure (CRF). Five women (age 62 ± 10 years, body mass index = 30.3 ± 4 kg/m^2, creatinine clearance = 56 ± 22 mL/min) were studied before and after a 4-week resistance training protocol (two upper body and three lower body exercises, three sets of eight repetitions, at 80% of the 1 RM, 3 days per week). All of the women consumed a diet providing 0.6 $g \cdot kg^{-1} \cdot d^{-1}$ protein for 3 weeks before and during the training period. Body weight was maintained at ±0.5 kg of baseline weight. At week 3 of baseline and week 4 of resistance training, 24-hour urine collections and food homogenates were collected during 4 consecutive days, and analyzed for total nitrogen by the Kjeldahl method. With resistance training, strength increased 11% ± 6% for upper body (p <.05) and 17% ± 6% (p <.01) for the lower body. Glomerular filtration rate estimated by insulin clearance (57 ± 26 mL/min), renal plasma flow estimated by *p*-aminohippurate clearance (277 ± 146 mL/min), and percent body fat (42.3% ± 6.2%) and fat-free mass estimated by underwater weighing (44.8 ± 4.2 kg) did not change during the intervention. Urinary nitrogen excretion decreased 10.7% ± 7.9% (0.56 ± 0.4 g N/day, p <.05) and estimated nitrogen balance increased from −0.34 ± 0.58 to 0.08 ± 0.41 g N/day, p <.05). These results demonstrate that resistance training in CRF patients is safe, increases nitrogen retention, and reduces renal handling of nitrogen. Strength training, therefore, may be an important clinical tool in the treatment of CRF, especially to prevent muscle wasting.

MUSCLE STRENGTH TRAINING IN THE ELDERLY

Muscle strength training can be accomplished by virtually anyone. Many health care professionals have directed their patients away from strength training in the mistaken belief that it can cause undesirable elevations in blood pressure. With proper technique, the systolic pressure elevation during aerobic exercise is far greater than that seen during resistance training. Muscle strengthening exercises are rapidly becoming a critical component to cardiac rehabilitation programs as clinicians realize the need for strength as well as endurance for many activities of daily living.

CONCLUSION

There is no other group in our society that can benefit more from regularly performed exercise than the elderly. While balance, aerobic, and strength conditioning are highly recommended, only strength training can stop or reverse sarcopenia. Increased muscle strength and mass in the elderly can be the first step toward a lifetime of increased physical activity and a realistic strategy for maintaining functional status and independence.

REFERENCES

1. Frontera WR, Hughes VA, Evans WJ. A cross-sectional study of upper and lower extremity muscle strength in 45–78 year old men and women. *J Appl Physiol* 1991;71:644–650.
2. Tzankoff SP, Norris AH. Longitudinal changes in basal metabolic rate in man. *J Appl Physiol* 1978;33:536–539.
3. Evans W. What is sarcopenia? *J Gerontol* 1995;50A(special issue):5–8.
4. Bassey EJ, Fiatarone MA, O'Neill EF, Kelly M, Evans WJ, Lipsitz LA. Leg extensor power and functional performance in very old men and women. *Clin Sci* 1992;82:321–327.
5. Meredith CN, Zackin MJ, Frontera WR, Evans WJ. Body composition and aerobic capacity in young and middle-aged endurance-trained men. *Med Sci Sports Exerc* 1987;19:557–563.
6. Roberts SB, Young VR, Fuss P, et al. What are the dietary energy needs of adults? *Int J Obes* 1992;16:969–976.
7. Klitgaard H, Mantoni M, Schiaffino S, et al. Function, morphology and protein expression of ageing skeletal muscle: a cross-sectional study of elderly men with different training backgrounds. *Acta Physiol Scand* 1990;140:41–54.
8. Klitgaard H, Zhou M, Schiaffino S, Betto R, Salviati G, Saltin B. Ageing alters the myosin heavy chain composition of single fibres from human skeletal muscle. *Acta Physiol Scand* 1990;140:55–62.
9. Buskirk ER, Hodgson JL. Age and aerobic power: the rate of change in men and women. *Fed Proc* 1987;46:1824–1829.
10. Fleg JL, Lakatta EG. Role of muscle loss in the age-associated reduction in $\dot{V}O_2$max. *J Appl Physiol* 1988;65:1147–1151.
11. Rosen MJ, Sorkin JD, Goldberg AP, Hagberg JM, Katzel LI. Predictors of age-associated decline in maximal aerobic capacity: a comparison of four statistical models. *J Appl Physiol* 1998; 84:2163–2170.
12. Meredith CN, Frontera WR, Fisher EC, et al. Peripheral effects of endurance training in young and old subjects. *J Appl Physiol* 1989;66:2844–2849.
13. Seals DR, Hagberg JM, Hurley BF, Ehsani AA, Holloszy JO. Endurance training in older men and women: cardiovascular responses to exercise. *J Appl Physiol: Respirat Environ Exercise Physiol* 1984;57:1024–1029.
14. Spina RJ, Ogawa T, Kohrt WM, Martin WH III, Holloszy JO, Ehsani AA. Differences in cardiovascular adaptation to endurance exercise training between older men and women. *J Appl Physiol* 1993;75:849–855.
15. Davidson MB. The effect of aging on carbohydrate metabolism. A review of the English literature and a practical approach to the diagnosis of diabetes mellitus in the elderly. *Metabolism* 1979;28:688–705.
16. Hadden WC, Harris MI. *Prevalence of diagnosed diabetes, undiagnosed diabetes, and impaired glucose tolerance in adults 20–74 years of age: United States, 1976–1980.* DHHS PHS publ. no. 87-1687. Washington, DC: U.S. Govt. Printing Office, 1987.
17. Shimokata H, Muller DC, Fleg JL, Sorkin J, Ziemba AW, Andes R. Age as independent determinant of glucose tolerance. *Diabetes* 1991;40:44–51.
18. Borkan GA, Hultz DE, Gerzoff AF. Age changes in body composition revealed by computed tomography. *J Gerontol* 1983; 38:673–677.

18a. Harris MI, Hadden WC, Knowles WC, Bennett PH. Prevalence of diabetes and impaired glucose tolerance and plasma glucose levels in U.S. population aged 20–47 yr. *Diabetes* 1987;36:523–534.

19. Stolk RP, Vingerling JR, de Jong PTVM, et al. Retinopathy, glucose and insulin in an elderly population: the Rotterdam study. *Diabetes* 1995;44:11–15.
20. Zavaroni I, Dall'Aglio E, Bruschi F, et al. Effect of age and environmental factors on glucose tolerance and insulin secretion in a worker population. *J Am Geriatr Soc* 1986;34:271–275.
21. Seals DR, Hagberg JM, Hurley BF, Ehsani AA, Holloszy JO. Effects of endurance training on glucose tolerance and plasma lipid levels in older men and women. *JAMA* 1984;252:645–649.
22. Kirwan JP, Kohrt WM, Wojta DM, Bourey RE, Holloszy JO. Endurance exercise training reduces glucose-stimulated insulin levels in 60- to 70-year-old men and women. *J Gerontol* 1993; 48:M84–M90.
23. Hughes VA, Fiatarone MA, Fielding RA, et al. Exercise increases muscle GLUT 4 levels and insulin action in subjects with impaired glucose tolerance. *Am J Physiol* 1993;264:E855–E862.
24. Marshall JA, Hamman RF, Baxter J. High-fat, low-carbohydrate diet and the etiology of non-insulin-dependent diabetes mellitus: the San Luis Valley Diabetes Study. *Am J Epidemiol* 1991; 134:590–603.
25. Feskens EJM, Kromhout D. Cardiovascular risk factors and the 25-year incidence of diabetes mellitus in middle-aged men. *Am J Epidemiol* 1989;130:1101–1108.
26. Lundgren J, Benstsson C, Blohme G, et al. Dietary habits and

incidence of noninsulin-dependent diabetes mellitus in a population study of women in Gothenburg, Sweden. *Am J Clin Nutr* 1989;52:708–712.
27. Garg A, Grundy SM, Unger RH. Comparison of effects of high and low carbohydrate diets on plasma lipoprotein and insulin sensitivity in patients with mild NIDDM. *Diabetes* 1992;41:1278–1285.
28. Borkman M, Campbell LV, Chisholm DJ, Storlien LH. Comparison of the effects on insulin sensitivity of high carbohydrate and high fat diets in normal subjects. *J Clin Endocrinol* 1991; 72:432–437.
29. Hughes VA, Fiatarone MA, Fielding RA, Ferrara CM, Elahi D, Evans WJ. Long term effects of a high carbohydrate diet and exercise on insulin action in older subjects with impaired glucose tolerance. *Am J Clin Nutr* 1995;62:426–433.
30. Schaefer EJ, Lichtenstein AH, Lamon-Fava S, et al. Body weight and low-density lipoprotein cholesterol changes after consumption of a low-fat ad libitium diet. *JAMA* 1995;274:1450–1455.
31. Helmrich SP, Ragland DR, Leung RW, Paffenbarger RS Jr. Physical activity and reduced occurrence of non-insulin-dependent diabetes mellitus. *N Engl J Med* 1991;325:147–152.
32. Bogardus C, Ravussin E, Robbins DC, Wolfe RR, Horton ES, Sims EAH. Effects of physical training and diet therapy on carbohydrate metabolism in patients with glucose intolerance and non-insulin-dependent diabetes mellitus. *Diabetes* 1984;33:311–318.
33. Phinney SD, LaGrange BM, O'Connell M, Danforth E Jr. Effects of aerobic exercise on energy expenditure and nitrogen balance during very low calorie dieting. *Metabolism* 1988;37:758–765.
34. Heymsfield SB, Casper K, Hearn J, Guy D. Rate of weight loss during underfeeding: relation to level of physical activity. *Metabolism* 1989;38:215–223.
35. Goran MI, Poehlman ET. Endurance training does not enhance total energy expenditure in healthy elderly persons. *Am J Physiol* 1992;263:E950–E957.
36. Withers RT, Smith DA, Tucker RC, Brinkman M, Clark DG. Energy metabolism in sedentary and active 49- to 70-year-old women. *J Appl Physiol* 1998;84:1333–1340.
37. Ballor DL, Katch VL, Becque MD, Marks CR. Resistance weight training during caloric restriction enhances lean body weight maintenance. *Am J Clin Nutr* 1988;47:19–25.
38. Pavlou KN, Steffee WP, Lerman RH, Burrows BA. Effects of dieting and exercise on lean body mass, oxygen uptake, and strength. *Med Sci Sports Exerc* 1985;17:466–471.
39. Evans WJ, Cannon JG. The metabolic effects of exercise-induced muscle damage. In: Holloszy JO, ed. *Exercise and sport sciences reviews.* Baltimore: Williams & Wilkins, 1991:99–126.
40. Fiatarone MA, Marks EC, Ryan ND, Meredith CN, Lipsitz LA, Evans WJ. High-intensity strength training in nonagenarians. Effects on skeletal muscle. *JAMA* 1990;263:3029–3034.
41. Fiatarone MA, O'Neill EF, Ryan ND, et al. Exercise training and nutritional supplementation for physical frailty in very elderly people. *N Engl J Med* 1994;330:1769–1775.
42. Nelson ME, Fiatarone MA, Morganti CM, Trice I, Greenberg RA, Evans WJ. Effects of high-intensity strength training on multiple risk factors for osteoporotic fractures. *JAMA* 1994;272:1909–1914.
43. Frontera WR, Meredith CN, O'Reilly KP, Evans WJ. Strength training and determinants of $\dot{V}O_2$ max in older men. *J Appl Physiol* 1990;68:329–333.
44. Whipple RH, Wolfson LI, Amerman PM. The relationship of knee and ankle weakness to falls in nursing home residents. *J Am Geriatr Soc* 1987;35:13–20.
45. Wolfson L, Whipple R, Judge J, Amerman P, Derby C, King M. Training balance and strength in the elderly to improve function. *J Am Geriatr Soc* 1993;41:341–343.
46. Wolf SL, Barnhart HX, Kutner NG, McNeely E, Coogler C, Xu T. Reducing frailty and falls in older persons: an investigation of Tai Chi and computerized balance training. Atlanta FICSIT Group. Frailty and Injuries: Cooperative Studies of Intervention Techniques [see comments]. *J Am Geriatr Soc* 1996;44:489–497.
47. Kutner NG, Barnhart H, Wolf SL, McNeely E, Xu T. Self-report benefits of Tai Chi practice by older adults. *J Gerontol B Psychol Sci Soc Sci* 1997;52:P242–246.
48. Province MA, Hadley EC, Hornbrook MC, et al. The effects of exercise on falls in elderly patients: a preplanned meta-analysis of the FICSIT trials. *JAMA* 1995;273:1341–1347.
49. Hickey T, Sharpe PA, Wolf FM, Robins LS, Wagner MB, Harik W. Exercise participation in a frail elderly population. *J Health Care Poor Underserved* 1996;7:219–231.
50. Campbell WW, Crim MC, Young VR, Evans WJ. Increased energy requirements and body composition changes with resistance training in older adults. *Am J Clin Nutr* 1994;60:167–175.
51. Sahyoun N. Nutrient intake by the NSS elderly population. In: Hartz SC, Russell RM, Rosenberg IH, eds. *Nutrition in the elderly: The Boston nutritional status survey.* London: Smith-Gordon, 1992:31–44.
52. Gersovitz M, Munro H, Scrimshaw N, Young V. Human protein requirements: assessment of the adequacy of the current recommended dietary allowance for dietary protein in elderly men and women. *Am J Clin Nutr* 1982;35:6–14.
53. Uauy R, Scrimshaw N, Young V. Human protein requirements: nitrogen balance response to graded levels of egg protein in elderly men and women. *Am J Clin Nutr* 1978;31:779–785.
54. Zanni E, Calloway D, Zezulka A. Protein requirements of elderly men. *J Nutr* 1979;109:513–524.
55. Campbell WW, Crim MC, Dallal GE, Young VR, Evans WJ. Increased protein requirements in the elderly: new data and retrospective reassessments. *Am J Clin Nutr* 1994;60:167–175.
56. WHO/FAO/UNU. *Energy and protein requirements.* WHO Technical Report Series. Geneva: World Health Organization, 1985:724.
57. Bunker V, Lawson M, Stansfield M, Clayton B. Nitrogen balance studies in apparently healthy elderly people and those who are housebound. *Br J Nutr* 1987;57:211–221.
58. Meredith CN, Zackin MJ, Frontera WR, Evans WJ. Dietary protein requirements and body protein metabolism in endurance-trained men. *J Appl Physiol* 1989;66:2850–2856.

Exercise and Sport Science,
edited by William E. Garrett, Jr., and Donald T. Kirkendall.
Published by Lippincott Williams & Wilkins, Philadelphia, 2000.

CHAPTER 20

Effects of Air Pollutants on Exercise

Lawrence J. Folinsbee

Air pollution is not a new problem and, in one form or another, has likely been encountered by humans since prehistoric times. Our lungs are continuously being exposed to trace amounts of various air contaminants, and the extent and type of this exposure is dictated largely by where we live, work, and exercise. Since the late 1950s, considerable progress has been made in improving air quality both in the ambient atmosphere and in the workplace. Air pollution can have both acute and chronic health impacts on the lungs and other organs. In some cases, exposure to air pollutants can also impact exercise performance (1). Concern has also been expressed that training in the urban air atmosphere may increase the risk of some chronic health effects from air pollutants.

Despite control measures, urban air pollution continues to be a problem in many densely populated areas. Air pollutants come from both mobile (e.g., cars, trucks) and stationary sources (e.g., refineries, power plants, other industrial processes). The air pollutants that we are most concerned about in the vicinity of many North American cities include ozone, sulfur dioxide, carbon monoxide, lead, and particulate matter or aerosols. Air pollutants such as ozone (O_3) and fine respirable particulate matter (including acidic aerosols) are regional pollutants since their concentrations are more uniform across a broad geographic area. These pollutants are formed as a result of secondary chemical reactions of primary pollutants, such as NO_2, CO, and SO_2 in the atmosphere. Ozone is produced by a complex series of reactions involving NO_2, hydrocarbons, oxygen, and sunlight. In addition to daily variation, ambient pollution concentrations vary seasonally but are often at their worst during certain atmospheric conditions such as air stagnation and inversions. For example, ozone and acid aerosols are more prevalent in the summer months and may be transported over large distances.

Table 20–1 lists air quality standards for the United States and guidelines of the World Health Organization, along with some of the world's cities in which comparatively high levels of these pollutants may occur.

Human physiologic responses to air pollutants are influenced by the amount of pollutant inhaled and subsequently delivered to the lungs and other organs. The major factors that determine the exposure dose are the concentration of the pollutant, the duration of the exposure, and the volume of air inhaled (i.e., the ventilatory volume). Because inhaled volume and inspiratory flow rate increase proportionately with the intensity of exercise, the responses to air pollutants are increased in individuals engaged in activity. Some fraction of the particulate air pollutants that are inhaled is deposited in the airways and alveoli. Although almost all the particles are cleared within 24 hours, some particles, especially insoluble ones, may not be cleared for many months. The deposition of particles depends not only on the factors above, which determine the inhaled quantity (i.e., exposure duration, concentration, and ventilation), but also on the size of the particles. Other factors such as chemical reactions (modifying or neutralizing the air pollutant) or production of secondary products within the body may also modify the "dose."

In addition to a discussion of the effects of various air pollutants on health, this chapter focuses on the effects of air pollutants on exercise or work performance (2). There are a number of potential mechanisms for air pollutants to impact work performance. Many air pollutants are irritating to the respiratory mucosal surfaces and lead to symptoms such as cough or breathing discomfort. Other pollutants may cause changes in oxygen delivery by reducing blood oxygen transport. In some cases, worsening of existing respiratory (e.g.,

L. J. Folinsbee: Department of Medicine, University of North Carolina, Chapel Hill; Environmental Media Assessment Branch, National Center for Environmental Assessment, U.S. Environmental Protection Agency, Research Triangle Park, North Carolina 27711.

TABLE 20–1. *Present National Ambient Air Quality Standards (USA), guideline concentrations established by the World Health Organization (WHO), and some world cities that have problematic levels of these pollutants*

Pollutant	USA primary standard[a]	WHO guidelines	Example cities with high levels
Ozone	0.08 ppm, 8 h average[b]	0.06 ppm, 8 h average*	Los Angeles, São Paulo, Mexico City, Houston
Sulfur dioxide	0.03 ppm annual mean; 0.14 ppm max 24 h average	0.017 ppm annual mean; 0.044 ppm max 24 h average	Pittsburgh, Seoul, Prague, Beijing, Mexico City
Particulate matter PM_{10}	150 $\mu g/m^3$ 24 h[c]; 50 $\mu g/m^3$ annual mean	70 $\mu g/m^3$ 24 h*	Beijing, Shanghai, Bangkok, Bombay
Particulate matter $PM_{2.5}$	65 $\mu g/m^3$ 24 h[d]; 15 $\mu g/m^3$ annual mean		
Nitrogen dioxide	100 $\mu g/m^3$ annual average	40 $\mu g/m^3$ annual average *	Los Angeles, Athens, Mexico City, Moscow
Carbon monoxide	9 ppm, 8 h average; 35 ppm, 1 h average	10 mg/m^3, 8 h average	Mexico City

[a] Standard to be exceeded not more than once per year on average.
[b] 4th highest daily maximum.
[c] 99th percentile of 24 h means.
[d] 98th percentile of 24 h means.
* Revisions under consideration or pending approval.
Source: World Health Organization. *Urban air pollution in megacities of the world.* Oxford: Blackwell, 1992.

asthma) or cardiovascular disease may be induced by air pollutants.

EXPOSURE TO AIR POLLUTANTS

Athletes and others who spend a great deal of time outdoors constitute a group at increased risk from exposure to air pollutants. The potential effects of air pollutants on exercise performance are associated with pollutant concentrations and the intensity and duration of exercise. Pulmonary health effects that occur after exposure to low ambient levels of pollutants are typically associated with moderate or heavy exercise during the exposure. There are at least three important factors to consider in assessing the health risks posed by air pollution exposure. These include the likelihood of being exposed to one or more pollutants, the amount of pollutant delivered to the target tissues in the lungs or other organs, and the individual susceptibility of the person being exposed.

In the temperate zones of the industrialized world, a large portion of the day is spent indoors. In fact, the typical adult spends no more than an hour or two outdoors, on a daily basis (3). In warmer regions or during the warmer parts of the year, children may spend, on average, as much as 3 hours per day outdoors. The amount of air pollution present indoors depends on whether there is an indoor source (e.g., NO_2 from gas stoves), how reactive the air pollutant is (for example, ozone reacts quickly with surfaces), and whether or not the air pollutant penetrates from the outdoor to the indoor environment. Proximity to the source of primary air pollutants is an obvious determinant of exposure (e.g., SO_2 from industrial boilers burning coal or oil, CO from street level automobile exhaust). Many people within a geographic region may be exposed to similar levels of secondary pollutants (e.g., ozone) whose concentrations are more evenly distributed and who are also subject to long-range transport. Depending on the geographic region, the problem pollutants may differ considerably. For example, high concentrations of ozone are well known for the Los Angeles and Mexico City air basins. On the other hand, eastern North America and many industrial areas of Europe and Asia have higher levels of SO_2 and particulate matter, including acidic aerosols. Remote rural areas typically have minimal air pollutant levels.

The amount of pollutant that reaches pulmonary tissues depends on numerous factors. Beyond the amount that enters the respiratory tract (i.e., concentration · time · minute ventilation), other factors that influence deposition of gases include the mode of breathing [i.e., either nasal (through the nose) or oronasal (through the mouth and nose)], the solubility of the gas in the surface liquids of the upper and lower airways (e.g., SO_2 is highly soluble in water), and chemical reactions that may occur in the air or on the airway surface. For example, under resting breathing conditions, very little inhaled SO_2 gets beyond the mouth and nose because of its high solubility (4,5). Low concentrations of inhaled acidic gases or aerosols are partially or completely neutralized by ammonia present at high concentrations in the mouth (from bacterial action) and at much lower concentrations in the lungs (6).

Humans are primarily nasal breathers. During periods of increased ventilation, especially during exercise, we breathe through both mouth and nose (i.e., oronasal). The transition from nasal to oronasal breathing depends in part on the ventilation rate. A typical ventilation for the switch-over is about 35 L/min (7). Other factors—such as the duration of exercise, nasal resistance [which is dramatically reduced during exercise (8,9)], and the size of the individual—may also influence the transition from nasal to oronasal breathing.

Deposition of airborne particles or aerosols is highly dependent on their size. Larger particles (>10 μm), such as road or trail dust, will tend to be deposited either in the upper airways or in the larger pulmonary airways. Smaller (<2 μm) particles are more likely to penetrate to the alveoli. The amount of particles smaller than about 5 to 6 mm that will be deposited in the alveoli will be increased if mouth breathing is increased. Most of the clearance of particles from the lungs is accomplished by the mucociliary clearance mechanism. Particles deposited on the mucus layer are transported toward the oropharynx by the action of cilia that move the mucus layer. Once mucus from either the trachea or the nasal passages is transported to the oropharynx, it is usually swallowed. Particles that are deposited in the alveoli are cleared by alveolar macrophages that engulf the particles. A few particles may persist in the lungs for long periods (many months), although a very large percentage of deposited particles are cleared within 24 hours.

With air pollutants as well as with many other stimuli, there is a range of response to a given stimulus, some of which is due to random variability and some to specific differences in responsiveness. Some of the individual characteristics that render certain individuals more susceptible to some air pollutants are easily identified; others are not well understood. For example, asthmatics, because of preexisting airway hyperresponsiveness, are typically about 10 times more responsive to SO_2 than nonasthmatics (10). Patients with coronary artery disease are more susceptible to the decreased oxygen-carrying capacity caused by CO exposure (11). Asthmatics are typically more responsive to ozone, nitrogen dioxide, and acidic aerosols. People who exercise outdoors are more likely to be exposed to air pollution, and thus their increased responses are primarily due to the increased amount of air pollution that they inhale as a result of increased ventilation during exercise.

Many air pollutants induce responses in the airways and the lungs, although effects can occur in other organs. Methods of measuring these responses include lung function measurements such as spirometry, airway resistance, pulmonary diffusion, and changes in the breathing pattern. To determine if air pollution may have caused the airways to become hyperresponsive, an airway challenge with bronchoconstricting agents, such as exercise, cold air, histamine, or methacholine, can be used. A more invasive technique, bronchoalveolar lavage, can be used to sample airway fluids and tissues in order to study the responses of airway cells and inflammatory mediators. For pollutants such as CO, which have cardiovascular effects, electrocardiography and measures of cardiac output or $\dot{V}O_2max$ can be used to evaluate changes in cardiac function. A more detailed discussion of response measures and experimental exposure techniques can be found elsewhere (12).

CHRONIC EFFECTS OF EXPOSURE TO AIR POLLUTION

With increasing age, the chest wall becomes less compliant (i.e., stiffer) and the lungs show decreased elastic recoil (13). Among the consequences of these changes is that vital capacity is decreased and residual volume is increased. Chronic exposure to air pollution may also accelerate this age-related decline in lung function. Pulmonary function is also worsened by habitual cigarette smoking, an addiction that involves about 25% of American adults. In patients with chronic respiratory diseases, who already have compromised lung function, long-term exposure to polluted ambient air may have an even greater effect. Changes in the thickness of airway epithelial cells, deposition of collagen, and a persistent airway inflammation in response to air pollutants may all contribute to "aging" of the lungs.

For residents of communities with high levels of air pollution, the decline in lung function may be accelerated in adults, or lung growth and development may be impaired in children. Thus, athletes who train in polluted air on a routine basis should be concerned about the potential long-term effects of the air environment on their lungs. Unfortunately, there have been no systematic studies of the effects of air pollution on people who engage in regular outdoor activity or athletic training. As an appropriate preventive measure, whenever possible training should be conducted during the early morning or late evening hours, especially during the summer months when ozone levels are at their highest. Of course, these are the same hours that are appropriate for the avoidance of excessive heat exposure. Because minor pulmonary damage does not necessarily cause symptoms, the absence of chronic lung responses cannot be assumed just because the ventilatory response to exercise is normal and symptoms are absent.

INDOOR AIR

Although we are justifiably concerned with the quality of our outdoor environment, Americans, in general, spend much more time indoors. It is quite possible that exposure to air contaminants in the indoor environment may have greater consequences for long-term health effects than outdoor exposures. There continue to be more and more energy-efficient homes that have reduced air turnover, which increases the potential for increased concentrations of indoor air pollutants. The presence of radon is known to increase lung cancer risk. Environmental tobacco smoke (ETS) can influence lung function, including lung growth and development, and respiratory illness in children. Other carcinogenic compounds possibly present in the home, in addition to ETS and radon, include volatile organic compounds and wood smoke. Although wood smoke (and smoke from other types of fires) is less of a risk in the modern North American home, the high levels of wood smoke in primitive dwellings of some Third World countries may be associated with chronic lung diseases, including cancer (14). Formaldehyde is often present in many newly manufactured household furnishings and can cause symptoms such as headache, eye irritation, and irritation of mucous membranes.

Swimmers spend a great deal of time training indoors during the cooler months. Because they exercise at high intensities at the surface of the water, they are exposed to higher concentrations of the chemicals that are used to treat the water. The concentrations of chlorine and chlorination by-products, such as chloramines and chloroform, are generally higher at the water surface than in the pool enclosure. Chloroform levels in the blood of indoor swimmers have been shown to be higher than in outdoor swimmers (15). The levels of such compounds in the air of enclosed swimming pools are affected by the air turnover rate in the building as well as by the amount of activity in the water (16,17). Problems can arise when pool chemistry is not properly attended to, the air turnover rate is too low because of malfunctioning equipment, or there is a misguided attempt to conserve energy by reducing air turnover. Chronic exposure of young swimmers to the air in swimming pool enclosures has been associated with an increased incidence of airway hyperreactivity (18). This can be a factor in the longer-term exacerbation of asthma, although swimming is less likely than other forms of exercise to induce asthma (i.e., exercise-induced asthma). Other effects of swimming pool water exposure include conjunctivitis and staining or damage to teeth (19). With proper pool maintenance and adequate building ventilation, many of these problems can be avoided.

OZONE

Ozone is a secondary regional air pollutant produced by photochemical oxidation of products of combustion, especially internal combustion engines. Ozone is a potent airway irritant and can cause marked effects on respiratory symptoms and lung function, which can lead to impairment of exercise performance, even at levels that exist in the ambient air of some major metropolitan areas. Symptoms that are typical of ozone exposure include cough, pain in the throat or larynx, pain beneath the sternum after taking a deep breath, and a feeling of chest tightness.

Ozone air pollution is typically associated with cities with large populations and large numbers of motor vehicles. The first evidence that ozone could impair exercise performance came from a study published in 1967 that indicated that high school cross-country runners racing in Los Angeles experienced poorer performance on days when the prerace ozone concentrations were elevated (20). Experimental controlled exposure studies of the effects of ozone on exercise performance showed that ozone causes both peak oxygen consumption and endurance time to be reduced (21–23) (Fig. 20–1). In addition there were several cases in which individuals were unable to complete the planned exercise regime (24,25). Respiratory discomfort, including cough, chest pain on deep inspiration, and a rapid shallow breathing pattern, accompanied the decline in exercise performance. Impaired exercise performance may be seen in trained athletes with exposure to as little as 0.18 ppm ozone, levels that are often exceeded in cities such as Los Angeles and Mexico City. At ozone levels higher than 0.18 ppm, many more people would experience symptoms, and the effects on exercise performance and lung function would be greater. Figure 20–2 illustrates the decline in forced expiratory volume in 1 second (FEV_1) associated with a 1-hour exposure to ozone in exercising subjects.

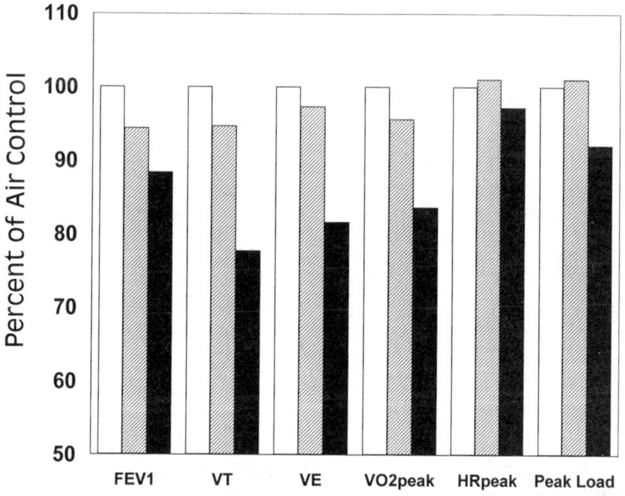

FIG. 20–1. Decreased maximum exercise performance in cyclists exposed to 0.12 and 0.20 ppm ozone for 1 hour while exercising at approximately 70% of maximal oxygen consumption. *Clear bars* represent end-exposure maximum exercise tests while breathing air, *hatched bars* represent 0.12 ppm exposures, and *black bars* indicate 0.20 ppm exposures. *FEV*$_1$, forced expiratory volume in 1 second; *VT*, tidal volume at peak V; *VE*, highest ventilation attained at maximum exercise; *VO2 peak*, highest oxygen uptake attained; *HR peak*, heart rate at maximum exercise; *peak load*, highest ergometer load setting. (Date from ref. 23.)

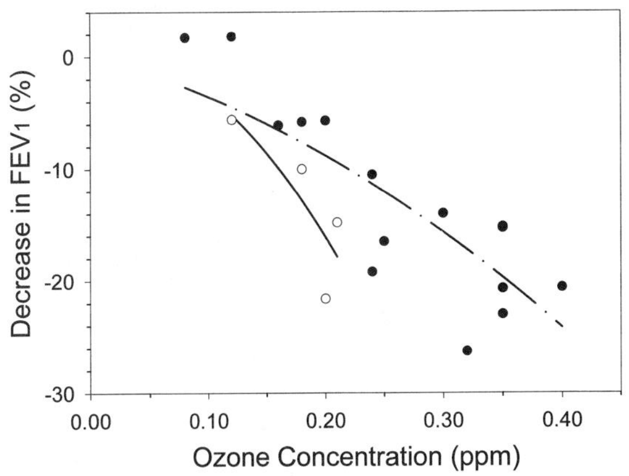

FIG. 20–2. Percentage decline in FEV_1 following a 1-hour exposure to ozone while exercising continuously. The *dashed line* (*closed circles*) represents responses for trained persons performing exercise requiring a ventilation of 55 to 80 L/min, and the *solid line* (*open circles*) represents persons performing heavy exercise requiring a ventilation of 80 to 100 L/min (very heavy training). (Modified from ref. 2.)

Respiratory system factors that can limit exercise performance include large increases in resistive or elastic work of breathing (26). Ozone only increases airway resistance slightly and does not change lung elasticity (27). These observations suggest that ozone does not influence exercise performance by causing an increase in the work of breathing. Also, ozone does not appear to cause changes in cardiac output or maximal heart rate (21,28). At much higher concentrations than occur in ambient air, ozone inhalation can cause pulmonary edema (27). Somewhat lower concentrations of ozone that cause lung cell damage and airway inflammation (29) could potentially lead to mild interstitial edema that could impair diffusion of oxygen across the alveolar-capillary membrane. At environmentally realistic levels, however, highly trained runners breathing 0.18 ppm ozone for 1 hour while performing a simulated training run (about 70% $\dot{V}O_2max$) had no alterations in arterial oxygen saturation associated with ozone exposure (30). Thus, it appears that breathing ozone at ambient levels does not compromise the major physiologic systems responsible for oxygen delivery during exercise.

In addition to the cross-country runners cited above, there are anecdotal reports of athletes who felt that their performance was or would be compromised by exposure to air pollution (31,32). Performance of maximum exercise after ozone exposure is difficult for both athletes and nonathletes. One of the responses to the irritation produced by ozone exposure is that tidal volume is reduced and breathing frequency is increased during exercise. This is a reflex response probably caused by stimulation of irritant receptors or bronchial C-fiber receptors in the airways (33). People who have been exposed to ozone repeatedly, either in the laboratory or in the ambient air, appear to have changed their breathing patterns intentionally in order to avoid the discomfort that occurs when they take a deep breath. The rapid, shallow breathing pattern allows them to achieve the necessary ventilation with minimal discomfort. This response is most evident during moderate to heavy exercise. Cyclists and runners who have been exposed to ozone during competition have reported that air pollution, especially in locales with high oxidant levels (i.e., ozone), had previously led to breathing discomfort and may have compromised their performance. In addition, some well-trained competitive athletes who have participated in controlled ozone exposure studies indicated that, under competitive conditions, if they had experienced the symptoms that resulted from the controlled ozone exposure, they probably would have been unable to perform optimally. After an hour or more of training, with ventilation in the range of 70 to 100 L/min, symptoms may be sufficiently annoying to cause a limitation of exercise performance at ozone concentrations in the range of 0.16 to 0.20 ppm. Some individuals may be much more severely affected by breathing ozone than others, and their performance is more likely to be affected.

Decrements in common measures of lung function such as spirometry are sensitive noninvasive indicators of the acute effects of ozone on the lungs. Ozone induces a reflex inhibition of inspiration, probably also caused by stimulating bronchial C-fiber or airway irritant receptors. Although ozone causes some bronchoconstriction, the inability to take a deep breath appears to be primarily responsible for the decrease in spirometry (Fig. 20–3). The spirometric response can be rapidly reversed (either partially or completely) by local anesthesia of the airways (e.g., with lidocaine) or by administration of analgesics that block the pain sensation arising from airway receptors (34,35) (see also Fig. 20–7).

With as little as 2 hours of exposure to ozone concentrations of about 0.12 ppm, significant decrements will occur, in some individuals, in tests such as forced vital capacity or FEV_1. As discussed above, the response is dependent on the dose or amount of pollutant inhaled, and therefore the magnitude of these responses depends on the duration of the exposure, the exercise intensity, and the ozone concentration. People who are routinely outdoors, possibly because of their occupation or exercise habits, could be expected to respond to even lower concentrations of ozone. It has been shown that exposure to levels as low as 0.08 ppm, which are not uncommon during the summer, can result in small decrements in lung function if the exposure is prolonged (i.e. 6 to 8 hours) (36). However, it is likely that only the most sensitive individuals would experience an effect on exercise performance at these lower ozone levels, and even then only if they were exercising at a fairly intense pace.

In addition to changes in lung function, ozone also

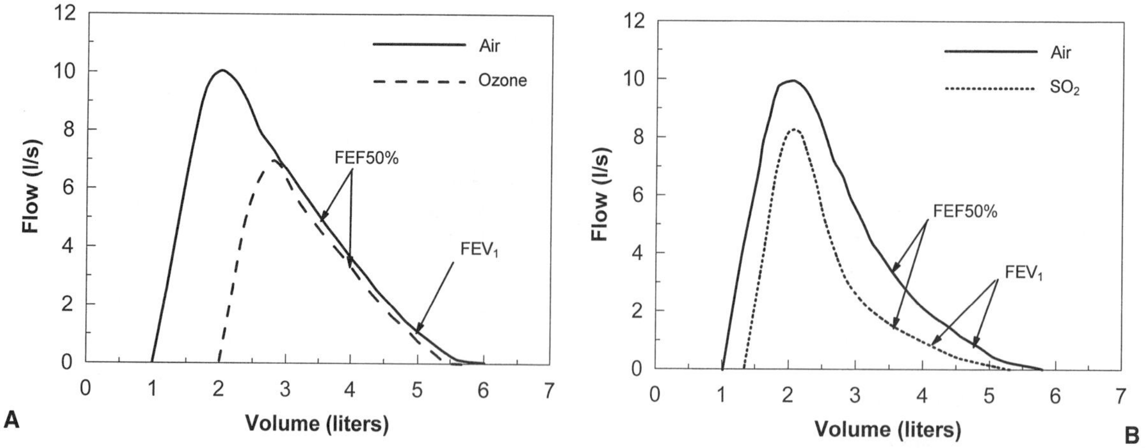

FIG. 20–3. Schematic expiratory flow-volume curves showing the effect of ozone on healthy adults and the effect of SO_2 on mild asthmatics. The ordinate is flow in liters/second, and the abscissa is volume in liters. **A**: Ozone reduces the maximum inspiratory position (*left*) and may slightly reduce the maximum expiratory position (*right*). Reduction in maximum inspiration reduces the forced vital capacity (FVC) and FEV_1. This causes a reduction in expiratory flow measurements [e.g., forced expiratory flow at 50% of FVC expired (FEF50%)]. Since ozone causes only a small change in resistance, the relationship between flow and volume is not changed to a large extent. **B**: SO_2 causes an increase in airway resistance in asthmatics and hence reduced expiratory flow at a given lung volume, also leading to decreased FEV_1 and FEF50%.

induces hyperresponsiveness to bronchoconstrictive drugs such as methacholine or histamine (these chemicals are routinely used in an inhalation challenge to test airway hyperresponsiveness in asthmatics). Ozone causes damage to the airway epithelium, leading to increased epithelial permeability and inflammation of the airways (Fig. 20–4) (29). It has recently been demonstrated that ozone exposure can also cause increased responses to inhaled allergens such as grass pollen or dust mite antigens in asthmatics who are allergic to these materials (37). Thus, allergic asthmatics who are exposed to ozone while exercising not only may be at risk because they are more acutely responsive to ozone but also could experience exacerbation of the allergic component of their asthma.

Asthmatics, especially those who routinely use medication to control their asthma symptoms, often have larger decreases in FEV_1 and airway resistance than nonasthmatics exposed to ozone. Asthmatics also experience greater airway inflammatory responses than healthy individuals exposed to ozone. Such responses include increased levels of inflammatory mediators (interleukin-8) and increased inflammatory cells (neutrophils, eosinophils) (38). The use of a typical β-adrenergic agonist inhaler (e.g., albuterol) partially reverses the lung function responses in asthmatics (39) but is ineffective in nonasthmatics (27).

Although exercise enhances the response of asthmatics to ozone, moderate exposure to ozone does not appear to exacerbate exercise-induced bronchoconstriction (EIB), which is typically induced by relatively heavy

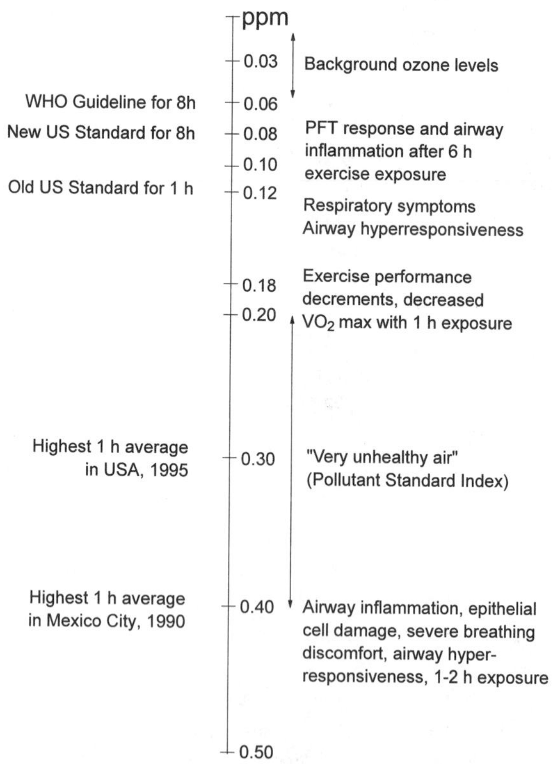

FIG. 20–4. Ozone concentration line indicating the levels of various standards and guidelines as well as levels at which effects may be expected in heavily exercising subjects. *WHO*, World Health Organization; *PFT*, pulmonary function test. U.S. standard is the concentration level of the National Ambient Air Quality Standard.

exercise (40). It has been shown that preexposure to ozone did not cause exercise-induced asthma in mild asthmatics who do not typically experience EIB, nor did it enhance the EIB in asthmatics who typically had a 20% or greater decline in FEV_1 in response to heavy submaximal exercise. The two studies that have examined the effects of ozone on EIB have used relatively mild exposure conditions (40,41). Thus, it is possible that with a greater ozone exposure and more pronounced changes in lung function and airway responsiveness, EIB may be increased.

Symptoms and lung function responses may take some time to be noticed during exposure to ozone. After this initial lag period, symptoms intensify; if the exposure lasts long enough and is not too severe, the responses may reach a plateau where they do not get any worse even with continued exposure. After exposure ends or is reduced, the decrements in lung function and the respiratory symptom responses begin to resolve. Usually within a few hours, symptomatic and spirometric responses are reversed, although some minimal dysfunction may last for up to 24 hours or even longer with severe responses. Inflammation of the airways has been observed at least 18 hours after exposure and probably persists for at least 24 hours, if not longer. Damage to pulmonary cells is repaired over a longer period of several days as the damaged cells are replaced by new cells that are typically more resistant to ozone exposure. If people are exposed to high concentrations (0.25 to 0.50 ppm) of ozone on 2 or more consecutive days, the effect on pulmonary function and respiratory symptoms is sometimes greater on the second day, but with subsequent exposures the individual's response to ozone becomes attenuated. Thus, a person who continues to be exposed to ozone will often not have symptoms nor experience lung function changes. However, it is now clear that ozone continues to damage epithelial cells in the lungs with repeated exposures (42).

Recurrent exposures to ozone, as would occur from regular training in a polluted city, result in decreased responsiveness to ozone. Residents of urban areas who experience frequent exposure to high summer ozone concentrations typically experience fewer ozone-induced respiratory symptoms and lung function effects in the fall than they do from similar levels in the spring, suggesting that repeated intermittent ozone exposure may induce a short-lasting acclimatization to ozone (43). Athletes training in the cities that have higher levels of oxidant air pollution (e.g., Los Angeles) generally report more breathing discomfort with exercise during the spring, when the smog season begins. Even though symptoms are minimal after initial exposures, this does not eliminate the possibility that continued regular exposures could induce effects in the lungs that might lead to chronic respiratory problems. For example, studies of communities with frequent ozone exposure have suggested that the decline in lung function with age may be more rapid in areas with high levels of air pollution. In addition, children who grow up in areas with high oxidant pollution tend to have slightly poorer lung function than when they become adults (44).

Medications, such as ibuprofen and indomethacin, that inhibit the cyclooxygenase pathway of arachidonic acid metabolism (responsible for the formation of mediators like prostaglandin E_2 or thromboxane B_2) can at least partially block the effects of ozone on spirometry and respiratory symptoms. These medications do not prevent ozone-induced epithelial cell damage or prevent inflammatory cells from entering the lungs, however (45). There is some evidence, especially from laboratory animal studies, that antioxidants such as vitamin C or E may reduce the responses to ozone (46). However, the extent to which supplementation with these vitamins can inhibit the effects of ozone in humans is undergoing further study.

CARBON MONOXIDE

Carbon monoxide (CO) is emitted from combustion sources including motor vehicle engines and fires. Ambient CO exposure occurs in areas with high concentrations of automobile or diesel exhaust, such as close to roadways and in parking garages and traffic tunnels. In the indoor environment, CO exposure can be caused by exposure to wood smoke or tobacco smoke (especially active smoking). Carbon monoxide exposure is well known as a cause of death and has been the cause of many accidental deaths dating back thousands of years. Small amounts of CO in the blood can also cause impairment of exercise performance by reducing the blood's oxygen-carrying capacity.

Carbon monoxide binds reversibly with hemoglobin to form carboxyhemoglobin (COHb). Hemoglobin has an affinity for CO about 250 times that of oxygen (47). This high affinity is important in clearing endogenously produced CO (which comes from the metabolic degradation of hemoglobin and other heme proteins) from the tissues. When occupied by CO, binding sites on the hemoglobin molecule are no longer available to transport oxygen to the tissues. Thus, an exposure to CO resulting in a blood level of 5% COHb means that the oxygen-carrying capacity of the blood is reduced by 5%. COHb levels in healthy nonsmokers are normally less than 1%, indicating that the clearance of endogenously produced CO is accomplished effectively. This normal process of CO excretion via the lungs is reversed by low inspired levels of CO (25 to 50 ppm), however, and COHb levels will increase rapidly. The presence of increased COHb levels also causes a leftward shift in the hemoglobin-oxygen dissociation curve that makes it more difficult to unload oxygen at the tissue level, which in turn leads to a lower partial pressure of oxygen (PO_2) in the tissues. Both the reduced O_2-carrying capacity and decreased tissue unloading can impair exercise performance (48,49) by reducing maximal oxygen uptake (Fig. 20–5).

Because of its high affinity for hemoglobin, the clearance of CO from the blood is relatively slow, requiring between 2 to 4 hours to eliminate half the accumulated CO (50). CO can build up in the blood as a result of prolonged exposure to low near-ambient concentrations (10 to 30 ppm) or brief exposure to higher concentrations (>100 ppm). After an hour of heavy exercise near heavily traveled roadways where average levels of CO might reach 7 to 10 ppm and peak exposures could exceed 100 ppm, COHb levels may increase to about 3% to 4% of the oxygen-carrying capacity of hemoglobin. In smokers, for comparison, the COHb levels are chronically about 5%. COHb levels in this range (3% to 7%) may also be seen in fire fighters working in close proximity to fires for a prolonged period (e.g., forest fires) (51). Once CO combines with hemoglobin, continued exposure to relatively low levels (~10 ppm) can slow the rate at which CO is cleared from the blood. Continued exposure reduces the partial pressure difference across the alveolar-capillary membrane necessary for elimination of CO by diffusion.

In nonsmokers at sea level, maximal oxygen uptake is decreased by about 10% as a result of increasing the COHb level to about 10%. The relationship between the decrease in $\dot{V}O_2max$ and COHb levels is linear (see Fig. 20–5), but statistically significant effects on maximal exercise performance have not been seen with COHb levels less than about 4% to 5%. Carbon monoxide reduces peak $\dot{V}O_2$ primarily by reducing the oxygen-carrying capacity of the blood; maximal cardiac output is not decreased. Despite these reductions in peak $\dot{V}O_2$, moderate submaximal exercise performance (30% to 60% maximum) is not affected in healthy individuals. With submaximal exercise, tissue oxygen delivery is maintained by an increase in cardiac output to compensate for the reduced oxygen-carrying capacity (52). Cardiac compensation is effective for COHb levels below about 15%. At the exercise levels reached by highly trained athletes (75% to 90% maximum), an increase in cardiac output is unable to increase blood flow sufficiently, and at these high levels of effort even the submaximal oxygen uptake must be reduced. In addition to reduction of peak $\dot{V}O_2$, increased COHb leads to a reduction of the lactic acidosis threshold (LAT). This leads to increased ventilation at work rates that exceed the LAT in order to compensate for the acidosis (53). For patients with cardiovascular disease in whom the ability to increase cardiac output in response to exercise is limited, a decrease in oxygen-carrying capacity caused by elevated COHb levels will increase hypoxic stress on the heart.

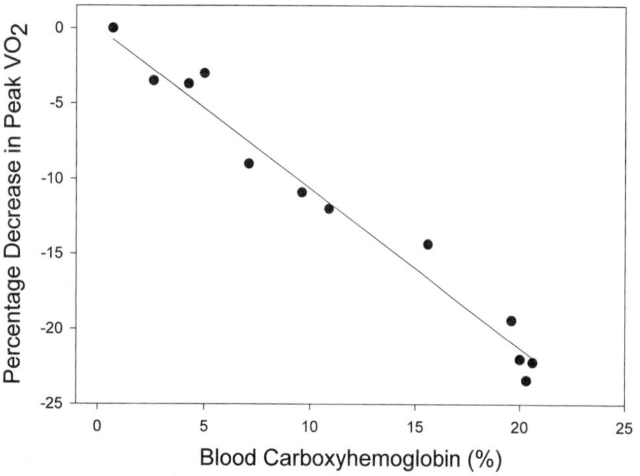

FIG. 20–5. Decrease (%) in peak oxygen uptake (peak $\dot{V}O_2$) associated with an increase in blood carboxyhemoglobin (COHb) concentration (%). The *line* represents the linear regression. (Modified from ref. 77 and includes new data.)

Because CO inhalation contributes to tissue hypoxia, it follows that the combined stress of CO and other factors that affect tissue oxygen delivery such as anemia and altitude hypoxia could potentially lead to greater hypoxic stress and hence even greater effects on exercise performance. Because of the lower barometric pressure at altitude, however, the partial pressure of a given concentration of CO is less and consequently the rise in COHb is also less at altitude (54). On a practical note, it is not uncommon for mountaineers to use gas stoves to cook inside their tents or for less hardy campers to use space heaters inside tents or trailers. This practice can lead to elevated CO levels, especially if the tent is poorly ventilated (55). In some cases the COHb could be increased to as much as 10%, a level that can cause a significant reduction in peak $\dot{V}O_2$. An increase in COHb of this magnitude is approximately equivalent to a gain of 1000 m in altitude.

Cardiac patients who experience angina or silent ischemia will be at greater risk of myocardial ischemia if they are exposed to CO. In patients with coronary artery disease who breathe CO-containing air, exercise-induced angina (or chest pain) occurs at lower exercise intensities than without CO exposure. Such individuals also show more electrocardiographic evidence of myocardial ischemia. In one major study, the duration of exercise prior to ischemic responses was shorter when the patients had elevated levels of COHb (56). When the COHb level was increased to 4% from the normal background level of about 1%, the exercise time required to induce ischemic changes in the electrocardiogram (ECG) was decreased about 12%. Time to the onset of chest pain (angina) was reduced by only 7%, however. This relatively low level of COHb (i.e., 4%)

may be experienced by many people from time to time, including freeway commuters, police officers, auto tunnel workers, garage attendants, or people exercising in proximity to dense traffic. At only slightly higher levels of COHb (6%), performance of the left ventricle may be affected (as shown by a reduction in the left ventricular ejection fraction) (57).

Electrical instability of the myocardium can also result from hypoxia due to CO. This in turn may lead to arrhythmia, which can increase the risk of sudden death, especially in elderly patients with cardiopulmonary disease. Increased exercise-related arrhythmias, such as premature ventricular depolarizations, have been seen in cardiac patients with COHb levels greater than 5% (58). At lower COHb levels (59,60), a significant increase in ventricular ectopic beats was not seen. Patients with heart or lung disease should avoid exposure to CO. Because of the slow clearance of CO from the body, exposure that may have occurred as much as 2 hours earlier could still have a significant effect on COHb levels and hence on tissue hypoxia. There is evidence that traffic tunnel workers have greater mortality from arteriosclerotic heart disease (61). In addition to high concentrations of motor vehicle exhaust, they are routinely exposed to 40 to 50 ppm CO, with even higher levels during daily rush hours.

Carbon monoxide can clearly impair exercise performance in healthy athletes. The reduced oxygen-carrying capacity caused by CO exposure is especially harmful for patients with cardiopulmonary disease who already have compromised oxygen delivery to the heart and other organs.

SULFUR DIOXIDE

SO_2 is emitted primarily as a result of combustion of fossil fuels (e.g., coal or oil fired power plants) but also from refineries, cement plants, and pulp and paper mills, collectively referred to as point sources. SO_2 is the primary pollutant involved in the secondary formation of acid aerosols and acid rain. From a health standpoint, considering SO_2 levels that are typical of outdoor exposure in the United States, even heavily exercising healthy individuals will not experience respiratory symptoms or lung function or exercise performance effects. People with asthma are nearly 10 times more sensitive to SO_2 than nonasthmatics (10), however, and they experience airway narrowing or bronchoconstriction following even brief (2- to 5-minute) exposures (Fig. 20–6) to SO_2 (62). Even so, most asthmatics respond to SO_2 only when they are exercising during the exposure. For asthmatics who exercise regularly, the greatest concern would be exposure to high concentrations of SO_2 near a point source. Approximately 5% to 6% of the population has asthma and the disease is somewhat more prevalent among young men (63). The proportion

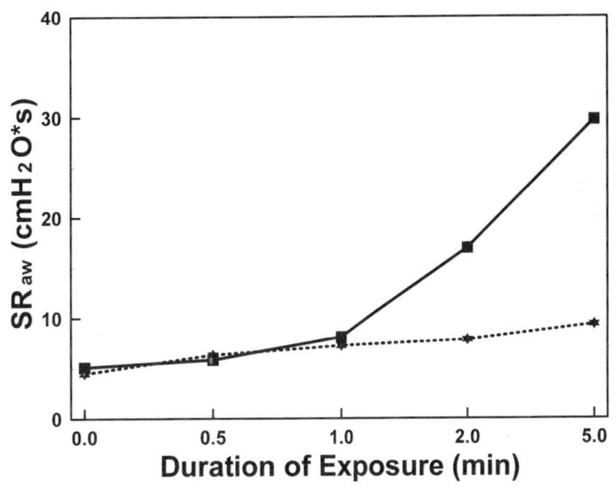

FIG. 20–6. Increase in airway resistance in asthmatic subjects following exposure to 1.0 ppm SO_2 (*solid line*) lasting from 0 to 5 minutes. The *dotted line* represents clean air exposures. (Data from ref. 62.)

of athletes who have asthma symptoms may run as high as 10% (64).

SO_2 causes airway narrowing by initiating a reflex leading to cholinergically mediated stimulation of airway smooth muscle. Effects of SO_2 may be mediated through histamine release from mast cells (65,66). Histamine is a potent stimulus for airway narrowing and is often used clinically to evaluate airway responsiveness in asthmatics. One asthma medication, cromolyn sodium, can partially or completely block the effects of SO_2 by preventing degranulation (i.e., histamine release) of mast cells. Other common asthma medications such as β-adrenergic agonists can reverse or prevent the airway narrowing caused by SO_2. Both cromolyn sodium and β_2-agonists (e.g., albuterol) are medications that are on the approved list of the International Olympic Committee. SO_2-induced bronchoconstriction during exercise can be avoided by using either of the above medications, which are often used by asthmatics to avoid EIB. However, some asthma medications are not effective in blocking the effects of SO_2. These include theophylline (a direct smooth muscle relaxant), some anticholinergics (ipratropium bromide), and inhaled steroids (e.g., beclomethasone). Figure 20–7 illustrates some potential pathways for the effects of SO_2 and ozone on the respiratory tract that could lead to reductions in expiratory airflow.

The risk of exposure of asthmatics to SO_2 levels of 0.40 ppm or higher, a level sufficient to induce bronchoconstriction, is quite small. Levels of SO_2 are highest in an air plume coming directly from an SO_2 source. In addition, the effects are usually experienced only in conjunction with increased levels of ventilation such as during exercise. Nevertheless, only 2 to 5 minutes of exposure to such levels are necessary to cause bronchoconstriction, wheezing, or chest tightness that is severe

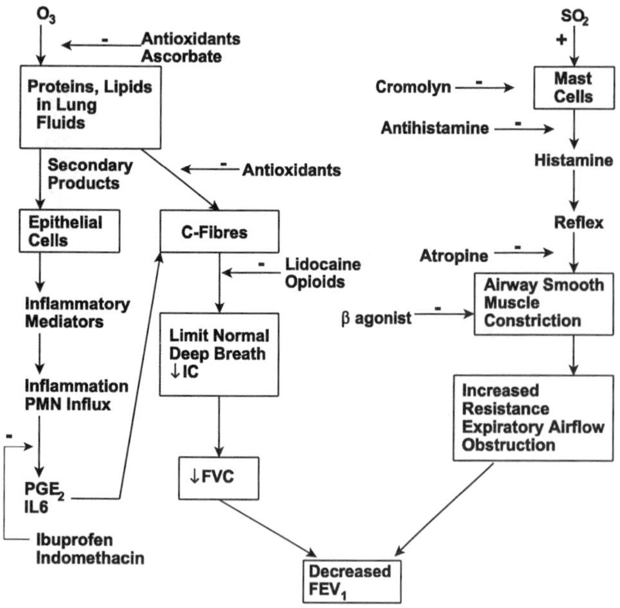

FIG. 20–7. Comparison of the response mechanisms leading to a decrease in FEV_1 in asthmatics exposed to SO_2 and nonasthmatics exposed to ozone. Ozone interacts with surface fluids and associated compounds to produce secondary reaction products, which then initiate a cascade of events resulting in the limitation of taking a deep breath (see also Fig. 20–3*A*). SO_2 probably causes release of histamine from mast cells and may also act directly to cause a cholinergically mediated reflex stimulation of airway smooth muscle resulting in airway narrowing, increased airway resistance, and obstruction of expired air flow. Although both gases cause a reduction in expired flow, SO_2 does so through airway narrowing and ozone does so through inhibition of taking of a deep breath.

enough, in the most sensitive asthmatics, to require the use of medication. The response quickly reaches a maximum level and does not get much worse after 5 to 10 minutes of exposure.

A large amount of inhaled SO_2 is removed in either the oral or nasal passages because SO_2 is highly soluble in the moist surface of the airways, especially the nose (4,5). Typically, a very small percentage of inhaled SO_2 (about 1% to 2%) actually reaches the trachea in resting people breathing through their nose. During exercise, the inspired flow rate is increased, reducing the time for gas absorption, and there is more mouth breathing, where SO_2 absorption is less efficient; thus, more SO_2 is delivered to the lower airway. This leads to increased bronchoconstriction. If an individual has increased nasal resistance, possibly due to congestive allergic rhinitis, as many asthmatics do, this may result in more mouth breathing and thus increased SO_2 exposure.

It is well known that breathing cold, dry air during exercise increases EIB (67). Clinical tests of EIB often use dry, subfreezing air to help elicit it. Cold, dry air tends to dry the surfaces of the upper airways, leaving less fluid available for the absorption of SO_2. Therefore, during exercise under these conditions, an increased amount of SO_2 would be delivered to the airways. It has been shown that the combination of cold dry air and SO_2 is worse for an asthmatic because the two stimuli are additive (68). Thus, exercise during cold, dry winter conditions combined with SO_2 exposure would be more likely to lead to breathing difficulties for an asthmatic athlete.

The effect of exercise on SO_2 responses cannot be estimated simply by the product of SO_2 concentration and ventilation (i.e., estimating the amount SO_2 inhaled) because the rate of absorption of SO_2 in the upper airway decreases as the inspiratory flow rate increases. In addition, the amount of EIB in asthmatics varies with the intensity of exercise, the temperature and dryness of the air, and current severity of the disease. The maximal decrease in FEV_1 or increase in airway resistance that occurs as a result of SO_2 exposure is similar to the maximal response to other nonimmunologic stimuli such as exercise or voluntary eucapnic hyperpnea with cold, dry air. Exercise and SO_2 appear to cause similar types of effects on the airway and may cause bronchoconstriction by a similar efferent pathway. SO_2 exposure will add to the effect of mild EIB but, if a near-maximal level of EIB is induced following a period of heavy submaximal exercise in cold air, the additional amount of bronchoconstriction added by SO_2 would be minimal, if any (69). The specific effect of SO_2 on maximal or heavy submaximal exercise performance in asthmatics has not been examined.

Bronchoconstriction caused by SO_2 is typically short lasting. In people with mild asthma, spontaneous recovery usually occurs in less than an hour. If SO_2 exposure occurs again in the next 3 hours or so, however, the response is usually much less than it was on the first exposure. This is not an adaptation but a state of refractoriness (i.e., reduced responsiveness) to SO_2 and is similar to the refractory period that follows EIB and lasts for about the same period of time.

PARTICULATE MATTER

Another important constituent of air pollution, both indoors and out, is particulate matter (PM). PM that can be inhaled is generally composed of particles less than 15 μm in diameter. PM exists in many shapes and has a diverse chemical composition coming from a variety of sources including dusts from the earth's crust; biologic material such as bacteria, pollen, and fungal spores; and smaller particles formed by gaseous pollutants reacting and aggregating in the atmosphere to form particles. Exposure to high concentrations of PM is known to have caused numerous premature deaths during past air pollution disasters (e.g., the London fog of 1952). Epidemiologic studies have demonstrated that increased exposure to PM increases the risk of cardiorespiratory mortality, especially in elderly patients with chronic respiratory disease (70,71). A comprehensive review of the health effects of and exposures to PM is available elsewhere (72).

Respirable PM consists of a coarse fraction (PM >2 to 3 μm, mainly crustal and biologic material) and a fine fraction (PM <1 to 2 μm, including acidic aerosols, metals, and combustion products). Coarse PM may be associated with respiratory symptoms in asthmatics since increased asthma attacks have been associated with increased levels of coarse PM (73). The spores or pollen contained in this fraction can also exacerbate allergic asthma. Exposure to high levels of coarse PM is more likely to occur in areas with an abundance of dust, such as rural areas with unpaved roads. Athletes may encounter high coarse PM levels while exercising on unpaved roadways (running or cycling) and hiking or mountain biking in dry, mountainous areas. Such exposures could lead to respiratory symptoms, such as cough, in nonasthmatics and could increase the risk of an asthma attack in asthmatics. During heavy exercise more air and hence more particles will pass through the mouth than through the nose, where they would be more efficiently removed. The likelihood of large particles reaching the lungs is thus increased with mouth breathing. Because of increased airflow rates, however, a larger fraction of the particles is deposited in the airways. The use of a mask in dusty areas can dramatically reduce the amount of PM that is inhaled.

Higher concentrations of fine PM are often found in urban areas. In the atmosphere, sulfur oxides and nitrogen oxides can be converted to aerosol sulfate and nitrate, which are important constituents of fine PM. Acidic aerosols (e.g., sulfuric acid) can cause slowing of particle clearance from the lungs and can also cause lung function changes in asthmatics, but these responses are usually seen only at concentrations that are higher than in the ambient air (74). Thus there is little reason to expect that acid aerosols, sulfates, or nitrates would impact exercise performance. Smoke from fires also contains many fine particles; prolonged exposure to smoke, as in forest fire fighting, can cause decreases in lung function that may be persistent (51).

NITROGEN OXIDES

Nitrogen monoxide (NO) is one of the primary exhaust emissions and, together with nitrogen dioxide (NO_2), is involved in the formation of ozone. Even at the highest levels that have been seen in ambient air, NO_2 causes no known acute effects in normal healthy adults, and NO appears to have few effects at low ambient concentrations. At much higher concentrations (e.g., in silos), NO_2 can cause severe pneumonitis and lung damage. At the highest levels that occur in ambient air (<0.5 ppm), however, the main effects of NO_2 may be to increase airway responsiveness in asthmatics, the main consequence of which would be increased responses to inhaled allergens (75). Exposure to NO_2 followed by exposure to other pollutants, such as ozone, or to antigens could result in a greater response to the other pollutant. Indoor exposure to NO_2 (from gas appliances) has also been associated with increased respiratory illness in children (76). There are no known effects of NO_2 on exercise performance.

CONCLUSION

Air quality can have important effects on breathing discomfort, lung function, and exercise performance. The major pollutants affecting exercise performance are ozone, which causes respiratory symptoms and lung function decrements, and carbon monoxide, which interferes with the ability of hemoglobin to transport oxygen. For asthmatics, other pollutants, especially sulfur dioxide, may cause exercise performance impairment. Air pollutants are also implicated in general respiratory health (77,78), as they are associated with respiratory morbidity (asthma attacks, hospitalization for respiratory disease, etc.) and mortality from cardiopulmonary causes.

DISCLAIMER

This chapter has been reviewed in accordance with U.S. Environmental Protection Agency policy and approved for publication. It does not necessarily reflect the views of the agency and no official endorsement should be inferred. Mention of trade names or commercial products does not constitute endorsement or recommendation for use.

REFERENCES

1. Adams WC. Effects of ozone exposure at ambient air pollution episode levels on exercise performance. *Sports Med* 1987;4: 395–424.
2. Folinsbee LJ. Ambient air pollution and endurance performance. In: Shephard RJ, Åstrand P-O, eds. *Endurance in sport (the encyclopedia of sports medicine,* vol 2). Oxford: Blackwell Scientific, Human Kinetics, 1992:479–486.
3. Johnson TR, McCoy M, Capel J, Wijnberg L, Ollison W. A comparison of ten time/activity databases: effects of geographical location, temperature, demographic group, and diary recall method. In: Vostal JJ, ed. *Tropospheric ozone: nonattainment and design value issues.* Proceedings of the 1992 International Conference on Tropospheric Ozone. Pittsburgh: Air & Waste Management Assoc, 1993:255–276.
4. Speizer FE, Frank NR. A comparison of changes in pulmonary flow resistance in healthy volunteers acutely exposed to SO_2 by mouth and by nose. *Br J Ind Med* 1966;23:75–79.
5. Bethel RA, Erle DJ, Epstein J, Sheppard D, Nadel JA, Boushey HA. Effect of exercise rate and route of inhalation on sulfur-dioxide-induced bronchoconstriction in asthmatic subjects. *Am Rev Respir Dis* 1983;128:592–596.
6. U.S. Environmental Protection Agency (Environmental Criteria

and Assessment Office). *An acid aerosols issue paper, health effects and aerometrics.* Publ. no. EPA/600/8-88/005F. Research Triangle Park, NC: EPA, 1989.
7. Niinimaa V, Cole P, Mintz S, Shephard RJ. The switching point from nasal to oronasal breathing. *Respir Physiol* 1980;42:61–67.
8. Forsyth RD, Cole P, Shephard RJ. Exercise and nasal patency. *J Appl Physiol* 1983;55:860–865.
9. Olson LG, Strohl KP. The response of the nasal airway to exercise. *Am Rev Respir Dis* 1987;135:356–359.
10. Folinsbee LJ. Sulfur oxides: controlled human exposure studies. In: Lee SD, Schneider T, eds. *Comparative risk analysis and priority setting for air pollution issues.* Proceedings of the 4th U.S.-Dutch International Symposium, June 1993, Keystone, CO. Pittsburgh: Air & Waste Management Assoc, 1995:326–334.
11. Allred EN, Bleecker ER, Chaitman BR, et al. Short term effects of carbon monoxide exposure on the exercise performance of subjects with coronary artery disease. *N Engl J Med* 1989;321: 1426–1432.
12. Folinsbee LJ, Kim CS, Kehrl HR, Devlin RB, Prah J. Methods in human inhalation toxicology. In: Massoro EJ, ed. *Handbook of human toxicology.* Boca Raton, FL: CRC Press, 1997:607–670.
13. Agostoni A, Hyatt RE. Static behavior of the respiratory system. In: Macklem PT, Mead J, eds. *Handbook of physiology, the respiratory system,* vol 3. Bethesda, MD: American Physiological Society, 1986:113–130.
14. Mumford JL, He XZ, Chapman RS, et al. Lung cancer and indoor air pollution in Xuan Wei, China. *Science* 1987;235:217–220.
15. Aiking H, van Acker MB, Scholten RJPM, Feenstra JF, Valkenburg HA. Swimming pool chlorination: a health hazard? *Toxicol Lett* 1994;72:375–380.
16. Drobnic F, Freixa A, Casan P, Sanchis J, Guardino X. Assessment of chlorine exposure in swimmers during training. *Med Sci Sports Exerc* 1996;28:271–274.
17. Potts J. Factors associated with respiratory problems in swimmers. *Sports Med* 1996;21:256–261.
18. Zwick H, Popp W, Budik G, Wanke T, Rauscher H. Increased sensitization to aeroallergens in competitive swimmers. *Lung* 1990;168:111–115.
19. Rose KJ, Carey CM. Intensive swimming: can it affect your patients smiles? *J Am Dent Assoc* 1995;126:1402–1406.
20. Wayne WS, Wehrle PF, Carroll RE. Oxidant air pollution and athletic performance. *JAMA* 1967;199:151–154.
21. Folinsbee LJ, Silverman FS, Shephard RJ. Decrease of maximum work performance following exposure to ozone. *J Appl Physiol* 1977;42:531–536.
22. Foxcroft WJ, Adams WC. Effects of ozone exposure on four consecutive days on work performance and VO_2max. *J Appl Physiol* 1986;61:960–966.
23. Gong H, Bradley PW, Simmons MS, Tashkin DP. Impaired exercise performance and pulmonary function in elite cyclists during low-level ozone exposure in a hot environment. *Am Rev Respir Dis* 1986;134:726–733.
24. Avol EL, Linn WS, Venet TG, Shamoo DA, Hackney JD. Comparative respiratory effects of ozone and ambient oxidant pollution exposure during heavy exercise. *JAPCA* 1984;34:804–809.
25. Schelegle ES, Adams WC. Reduced exercise time in competitive simulations consequent to low level ozone exposure. *Med Sci Sports Exerc* 1986;18:408–414.
26. Deno NS, Kamon E, Kiser DM. Physiological responses to resistance breathing during short and prolonged exercise. *Am Ind Hyg Assoc J* 1981;42:616–623.
27. U.S. Environmental Protection Agency, National Center for Environmental Assessment. *Air quality criteria for ozone and other photochemical oxidants.* Publ. no. EPA/600/p-93/004aF-cF. Research Triangle Park, NC: EPA, 1996.
28. Superko RH, Adams WC, Daly PW. Effects of ozone inhalation during exercise in selected patients with heart disease. *Am J Med* 1984;77:463–470.
29. Koren HS, Devlin RB, Graham DE, et al. Ozone-induced inflammation in the lower airways of human subjects. *Am Rev Respir Dis* 1989;139:407–415.
30. Folinsbee LJ, Horstman DH, Vorona RD, Prince JM. Determinants of endurance performance during ozone inhalation (#P217.04). *Proc Int Union Physiol Sci* 1986;16:176.
31. Adams WC, Schelegle ES. Ozone and high ventilation effects on pulmonary function and endurance performance. *J Appl Physiol* 1983;55:805–812.
32. Folinsbee LJ, Bedi JF, Horvath SM. Pulmonary function changes after 1 h continuous heavy exercise in 0.21 ppm ozone. *J Appl Physiol* 1984;57:984–988.
33. Coleridge JCG, Coleridge HM, Schelegle ES, Green JF. Acute inhalation of ozone stimulates bronchial C-fibers and rapidly adapting receptors in dogs. *J Appl Physiol* 1993;74:2345–2352.
34. Hazucha MJ, Bates DV, Bromberg PA. Mechanism of action of ozone on the human lung. *J Appl Physiol* 1989;67:1535–1541.
35. Passannante A, Hazucha MJ, Bromberg PA, Seal E, Folinsbee L, Koch G. Nociceptive mechanisms modulate ozone-induced human lung function decrements. *J Appl Physiol* 1998;85:1863–1870.
36. Horstman DH, Folinsbee LJ, Ives PJ, Abdul-Salaam S, McDonnell WF. Ozone concentration-pulmonary response relationships for 6.6 hour exposures with five hours of moderate exercise to 0.08, 0.10, and 0.12 ppm. *Am Rev Respir Dis* 1990;142:1158–1163.
37. Jörres R, Nowak D, Magnussen H. Effects of ozone exposure on allergen responsiveness in subjects with asthma or rhinitis. *Am J Respir Crit Care Med* 1995;153:56–64.
38. Scannell CH, Chen LL, Aris R, et al. Greater ozone-induced inflammatory responses in subjects with asthma. *Am J Respir Crit Care Med* 1996;154:24–29.
39. Horstman DH, Ball BA, Brown J, Gerrity TR, Folinsbee LJ. Comparison of pulmonary responses of asthmatic and nonasthmatic subjects performing light exercise while exposed to a low level of ozone. *Toxicol Ind Health* 1995;11:369–385.
40. Weymer AR, Gong H, Lyness A, Linn WS. Pre-exposure to ozone does not enhance or produce exercise-induced asthma. *Am J Respir Crit Care Med* 1994;149:1413.
41. Fernandes AL, Molfino NA, McLean PA, et al. The effect of pre-exposure to 0.12 ppm ozone on exercise-induced asthma. *Chest* 1994;106:1077–1082.
42. Devlin RB, Folinsbee LJ, Biscardi FH, et al. Inflammation and cell damage induced by repeated exposure of humans to ozone. *Inhal Toxicol* 1997;9:211–235.
43. Linn WS, Avol EL, Shamoo DA, et al. Repeated laboratory ozone exposures of volunteer Los Angeles residents: an apparent seasonal variation in response. *Toxicol Ind Health* 1988;4:505–520.
44. Kunzli N, Lurmann F, Segal M, Ngo L, Balmes J, Tager IB. Association between lifetime ambient ozone exposure and pulmonary function in college freshmen—results of a pilot study. *Environ Res* 1997;72:8–23.
45. Hazucha MJ, Madden MC, Pape C, et al. Effects of cyclooxygenase inhibition on ozone-induced respiratory inflammation and lung function changes. *Eur J Appl Physiol Occup Med* 1996; 73:17–27.
46. Chatham MD, Eppler JH, Sauder LR, Green D, Kulle TJ. Evaluation of the effects of vitamin C on ozone-induced bronchoconstriction in normal subjects. *Ann NY Acad Sci* 1987;498:269–279.
47. Roughton FJW, Darling RC. The effect of carbon monoxide on the oxyhemoglobin dissociation curve. *Am J Physiol* 1944;141: 17–31.
48. Pirnay F, DuJardin J, DeRoanne R, Petit JM. Muscular exercise during intoxication by carbon monoxide. *J Appl Physiol* 1971; 31:573–575.
49. Horvath SM, Raven PB, Dahms TE, Gray DJ. Maximal aerobic capacity at different levels of carboxyhemoglobin. *J Appl Physiol* 1975;38:300–303.
50. Landaw SA. The effects of cigarette smoking on total body burden and excretion rates of carbon monoxide. *J Occup Med* 1973; 15:231–235.
51. Materna BL, Jones JR, Sutton PM, Rothman N, Harrison RJ. Occupational exposures in California wildland fire fighting. *Am Ind Hyg Assoc J* 1992;53:69–76.
52. Vogel JA, Gleser MA. Effect of carbon monoxide on oxygen transport during exercise. *J Appl Physiol* 1972;32:234–239.
53. Koike A, Wasserman K, Armon Y, Weiler-Ravell D. The work-rate–dependent effect of carbon monoxide on ventilatory control during exercise. *Respir Physiol* 1991;85:169–183.
54. Horvath SM, Agnew JW, Wagner JA, Bedi JF. *Maximal aerobic capacity at several ambient concentrations of carbon monoxide at*

several altitudes. Health Effects Institute research report no. 21. Cambridge, MA: Health Effects Institute, 1988.
55. Pugh LGCE. Carbon monoxide hazard in Antarctica. *Br Med J* 1959;1:192–196.
56. Allred EN, Bleecker ER, Chaitman BR, et al. Short term effects of carbon monoxide exposure on the exercise performance of subjects with coronary artery disease. *N Engl J Med* 1989;321: 1426–1432.
57. Adams KF, Koch G, Chaterjee B, et al. Acute elevation of blood carboxyhemoglobin to 6% impairs exercise performance and aggravates symptoms in patients with ischemic heart disease. *J Am Coll Cardiol* 1988;12:900–909.
58. Sheps DS, Herbst MC, Hinderliter AL, et al. Production of arrhythmias by elevated carboxyhemoglobin in patients with coronary artery disease. *Ann Intern Med* 1990;113:343–351.
59. Hinderliter AL, Adams KF, Price CJ, Herbst MC, Koch G, Sheps DS. Effects of low-level carbon monoxide exposure on resting and exercise-induced ventricular arrhythmias in patients with coronary artery disease and no baseline ectopy. *Arch Environ Health* 1989;44:89–93.
60. Dahms TE, Younis LT, Wiens RD, Zarnegar S, Byers SL, Chaitman BR. Effects of carbon monoxide exposure in patients with documented cardiac arrhythmias. *J Am Coll Cardiol* 1993;21: 442–450.
61. Stern FB, Halperin WE, Hornung RW, Ringenburg VL, McCammon CS. Heart disease mortality among bridge and tunnel officers exposed to carbon monoxide. *Am J Epidemiol* 1988;128:1276–1288.
62. Horstman DH, Seal E, Folinsbee LJ, Ives PJ, Roger LJ. The relationship between exposure duration and sulfur dioxide-induced bronchoconstriction in asthmatic subjects. *Am Ind Hyg Assoc J* 1988;49(1):38–47.
63. National Institutes of Health, National Asthma Education and Prevention Program. *Guidelines for the diagnosis and management of asthma.* Expert panel report 2. NIH publication #97-4051. Bethesda, MD: NIH, 1997.
64. Voy RO. The U.S. Olympic Committee experience with exercise-induced bronchospasm, 1984. *Med Sci Sports Exerc* 1986;18: 328–330.
65. Sheppard D, Nadel JA, Boushey HA. Inhibition of sulfur dioxide-induced bronchoconstriction by disodium cromoglycate in asthmatic subjects. *Am Rev Respir Dis* 1981;124:257–259.
66. Sheppard D, Wong WS, Uehara CF, Nadel JA, Boushey HA. Lower threshold and greater bronchomotor responsiveness of asthmatic subjects to sulfur dioxide. *Am Rev Respir Dis* 1980; 122:873–878.
67. McFadden ER. Respiratory heat and water exchange: physiological and clinical implications. *J Appl Physiol* 1983;54:331–336.
68. Sheppard D, Eschenbacher WL, Boushey HA, Bethel RA. Magnitude of the interaction between the bronchomotor effects of sulfur dioxide and those of dry (cold) air. *Am Rev Respir Dis* 1984; 130:52–55.
69. Bethel RA, Sheppard D, Geffroy B, Tam E, Nadel JA, Boushey HA. Effect of 0.25 ppm sulfur dioxide on airway resistance in freely breathing, heavily exercising, asthmatic subjects. *Am Rev Respir Dis* 1985;131:659–661.
70. Schwartz J, Marcus A. Mortality and air pollution in London: a time series analysis. *Am J Epidemiol* 1990;131:185–194.
71. Schwartz J, Dockery DW. Increased mortality in Philadelphia associated with daily air pollution concentrations. *Am Rev Respir Dis* 1992;145:600–604.
72. U.S. Environmental Protection Agency, National Center for Environmental Assessment. *Air quality criteria for particulate matter.* Publ. no. EPA/600/AP-95/001aF-cF. Research Triangle Park, NC: EPA, 1996.
73. Gordian ME, Ozkaynak H, Xue J, Morris SS, Spengler JD. Particulate air pollution and respiratory disease in Anchorage Alaska. *Environ Health Perspect* 1996;104:209–217.
74. Koenig JQ, Pierson WE, Horike M. The effects of inhaled sulfuric acid on pulmonary function in adolescent asthmatics. *Am Rev Respir Dis* 1983;128:221–225.
75. Tunnicliffe WS, Burge PS, Ayres JG. Effect of domestic concentrations of nitrogen dioxide on airway responses in inhaled allergen in asthmatic patients. *Lancet* 1994;344:1733–1736.
76. U.S. Environmental Protection Agency, Environmental Criteria and Assessment Office. *Air quality criteria for oxides of nitrogen,* Document no. EPA-600/8-91-049F. Research Triangle Park, NC: EPA, 1991.
77. Folinsbee LJ. Heat and air pollution. In: Pollock MJ, Schmidt DH, eds. *Heart disease and rehabilitation.* Champaign IL: Human Kinetics, 1995:327–342.
78. Folinsbee LJ. Human health effects of air pollution. *Environ Health Perspect* 1993;100:45–56.

Exercise and Sport Science,
edited by William E. Garrett, Jr., and Donald T. Kirkendall.
Lippincott Williams & Wilkins, Philadelphia © 2000.

CHAPTER 21

Free Radicals and Antioxidants in Exercise and Sports

Li Li Ji

Research over the past 2 decades has shown that oxygen free radical generation is a major cause for cell and tissue injury associated with rigorous physical exertion (1–3). Reactive oxygen species (ROS) resulting from either increased oxygen consumption or specific pathways activated during or after exercise can elicit a series of biochemical modifications to the various cellular components, causing a more oxidized environment within the cell, generally termed "oxidative stress." To counteract the detrimental effects of ROS, higher organisms have developed effective antioxidant systems during the course of evolution (4–6). Antioxidant systems consist of antioxidant enzymes, several vitamins or their precursors (ascorbic acid, α-tocopherol and β-carotene), glutathione (GSH), and other low-molecular-weight antioxidants. Each of these antioxidants plays a unique role in the cell, and they complement each other geographically and functionally (4). Furthermore, certain antioxidants such as GSH may be transported between organs (7). In general, the cell has adequate antioxidant reserve to cope with mild oxidative stress so that serious and long-term damage does not occur. The protective margin of most antioxidants is relatively small, however. Therefore, when ROS production is excessive, or when antioxidant defense is compromised because of inactivation or nutritional deficiency, extensive cell and tissue damage may occur, leading to various pathogenic disorders (5). The resulting oxidative damage can induce further ROS production, thus forming a vicious cycle. There is increasing evidence that unaccustomed and strenuous exercise may inflict an imbalance between ROS and antioxidant defenses in favor of the former (8,9). This disturbance of antioxidant homeostasis is implied in numerous physiological disorders occurring during and after exercise, such as fatigue, muscle soreness, myofibril disruption, and impairment of immune function (3,10,11).

The purpose of this chapter is to provide up-to-date knowledge about (a) the major theories proposing possible mechanisms by which exercise may lead to cellular oxidative stress and damage, and (b) the short- and long-term strategies that cells use to protect against ROS-inflicted oxidative stress.

FREE RADICAL GENERATION DURING EXERCISE

Except for strict anaerobes, most organisms use oxygen as the terminal electron acceptor to oxidize the various metabolic fuels so that stored energy is released for various biologic activities (5). During this process, which occurs primarily in the mitochondria of eukaryotic cells, most oxygen molecules are reduced to water. However, molecular oxygen cannot accept four electrons required for its complete reduction at once because of the spin-restriction rule; instead, it has to take one electron at a time. This process gives rise to several univalently reduced oxygen intermediates and their protonated derivatives. The main species are superoxide ($O_2^{\cdot-}$), hydrogen peroxide (H_2O_2), and hydroxyl radical ($^{\cdot}OH$), representing one-, two-, and three-electron reductants of oxygen, respectively (5). All three ROS have a strong tendency to extract electrons to reach a chemically more stable state and therefore are capable of eliciting serious damage to the cellular components, but their chemical properties and detrimental potential are different (4). $^{\cdot}OH$ is the most reactive ROS and attacks all biologic materials at a diffusion-limited rate. H_2O_2, although not

L. L. Ji: Departments of Kinesiology and Nutritional Science, University of Wisconsin–Madison, Madison, Wisconsin 53706.

a free radical by definition, has considerable stability and diffusibility, making it accessible to many targets distant from its generation sites. In addition to the mitochondrial respiratory chain, cells generate ROS to assist in the elimination of xenobiotics through phagocytosis that involves a respiratory burst (11). Although this process is generally considered desirable, it can indiscriminately subject the cell to potential oxidative damage (3). In addition, oxygen serves as an electron acceptor for several other metabolic pathways in the cell such as purine nucleotide degradation, D-amino acid oxidation, cytochrome P_{450}, and catecholamine autooxidation. It is estimated that a normal cell produces 2×10^{10} $O_2^{\cdot-}$ and H_2O_2 per day, which amounts to 3.3×10^{-14} moles (12). The constant contact and reaction of the cellular constituents (including genetic materials) with ROS have been proposed to be a main mechanism for organism aging (13).

The first implication in the literature that ROS may play an important role in exercise-induced tissue damage occurred in the late 1970s and early 1980s (14–16). It is now widely accepted that many of the disorders at the cell, tissue, or organ levels observed either immediately after heavy exercise or during post-exercise recovery may be attributed to ROS generation (1–3,8,9). By using electron paramagnetic resonance (EPR) spectroscopy as a tool, several authors have provided direct data showing that exercised muscle and heart tissues produce higher levels of free radicals than do those in rested controls (15,17–19). By using a synthetic intracellular probe dichlorofluorescin (DCFH), Reid and colleagues (20) have demonstrated that contracting diaphragm muscle generates $O_2^{\cdot-}$, which is released from muscle cell. My laboratory recently found that both muscle and heart homogenates from acutely exercised rats exhibit a higher rate of DCFH oxidation than do those from their rested counterparts (21,22). The biochemical mechanism(s) by which ROS production is enhanced during exercise is still largely hypothetical, however. Several biochemical pathways, which may be activated under different physiological conditions and in different organs, tissues, and cellular locations, have been either identified or postulated.

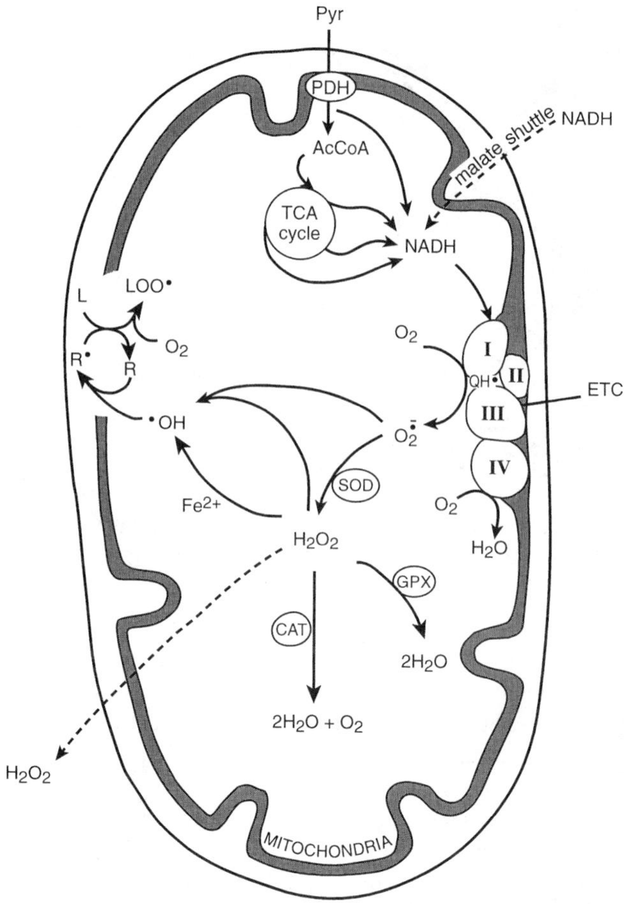

FIG. 21–1. Generation of reactive oxygen species in the mitochondria. *CAT*, catalase; *ETC*, electron transport chain; *GPx*, glutathione peroxidase; *LOO·*, lipid peroxy radical; *PDH*, pyruvate dehydrogenase complex; *QH·, semiquinone; R·*, alkyl radical; *SOD*, superoxide dismutase. Reactions are not balanced stoichiometrically.

Mitochondrial Electron-Transport Chain

The majority of oxygen consumed by the eukaryotes is reduced in the mitochondria through the electron-transport chain (ETC). Both NADH-ubiquinone reductase and ubiquinone-cytochrome *c* reductase generate $O_2^{\cdot-}$ and H_2O_2 (4). Because transition from two-electron carrier (NADH and $FADH_2$) to one-electron carrier (ubiquinone) involves the formation of semiubiquinone (QH·), this segment of the ETC becomes a primary site for $O_2^{\cdot-}$ production (4,15) (Fig. 21–1). $O_2^{\cdot-}$ is readily reduced to H_2O_2 by mitochondrial superoxide dismutase (SOD; Mn containing). A metal-catalyzed Fenton reaction or Haber–Weiss reaction may give rise to ·OH (5). It is estimated that liver mitochondria produce 24 nmol $O_2^{\cdot-}$/min per gram of tissue, reaching a steady-state $O_2^{\cdot-}$ concentration of 8×10^{-8} mol/L in the presence of Mn SOD (4). Heart mitochondria generate 0.3 to 0.6 H_2O_2 nmol/min/mg protein, representing 2% of the tissue's total oxygen consumption. Mitochondrial H_2O_2 production can be increased with increased O_2 tension, making it a viable source of ROS when metabolic rate and oxygen consumption are increased (23).

The premise that exercise increases mitochondrial ROS production is based on the well-known fact that tissue and whole-body oxygen consumption are increased proportionally with increased workload during aerobic exercise. During maximal exercise, whole-body oxygen consumption ($\dot{V}O_2$max) can increase up to 20-fold, while VO_2 at the muscle fiber level is estimated to be elevated by as much as 100-fold above the resting levels (3). Assuming that the percentage of O_2 to be converted to $O_2^{\bar{\cdot}}$ remains the same (i.e., ETC efficiency maintains the same), ROS production will increase roughly proportionally. It may be argued that $O_2^{\bar{\cdot}}$ production has been found to be lower in state 3 (ADP-stimulated) than state 4 (basal) respiration in isolated mitochondria (4). It is doubtful that a more efficient oxidative phosphorylation can completely compensate for the electron leakage, however, due to a much greater O_2 flux during heavy exercise. Furthermore, there is evidence that heavy exercise may induce mitochondrial uncoupling due to inner membrane damage and hyperthermia (15,24). However, the actual rate of ROS production from mitochondrial source during exercise is unknown.

The hypothesis that mitochondria comprise a primary site of ROS generation during exercise has been implicated in numerous studies. By using the EPR method, Davies and colleagues (15) were able to show that free radical signals recorded in muscle and liver homogenate from exercised rats were significantly greater than those from the rested controls. Because tissues were taken immediately from exhaustively exercised rats and the free radicals were identified as semiquinone ($g = 2.004$), it was reasonable to assume that mitochondria were the origins of the free radicals detected in the study. By using isolated mitochondrial preparations, several authors showed that state 4 respiration is increased in muscle and liver mitochondria (15) and heart mitochondria (25) after exhaustive exercise, suggesting a possible inner-membrane leakage inflicted by ROS. Respiratory control index in these studies was decreased as a result of the augmented state 4 respiration, with no change or a proportionally smaller increase in state 3 respiration. These changes coincided with the observation that mitochondria from exercised rats exhibited enhanced lipid peroxidation, loss of membrane integrity (15), decreased protein thiol content, and inactivation of oxidative enzymes (26). As supporting evidence, both muscle and heart mitochondria from animals involved in high-intensity chronic exercise demonstrated compromised respiratory control and disturbance of GSH redox status (27,28). The mitochondrial hypothesis of ROS production also is consistent with training adaptation of mitochondrial antioxidant enzymes. Higuchi and co-workers (29) showed that mitochondrial (Mn) SOD activity was increased after endurance training, whereas cytosolic (CuZn) SOD was unaffected. Muscle mitochondrial GPX was found to have a greater training adaptation than cytosolic GPX in rat (30). These data provided strong evidence that mitochondria are probably a major source of ROS production, because ROS generated in other cellular locations are unlikely to migrate to mitochondria to elicit the observed effects.

The observations that the extent of tissue oxidative damage is proportional to the workload of aerobic exercise may be viewed as indirect evidence to support the mitochondrial hypothesis of ROS generation. Alessio and Goldfarb (31) showed that lipid peroxidation measured by thiobarbituric acid reactive substance (TBARS) correlated with treadmill workload in rats. Kanter and colleagues (32) reported a proportionally increased pentane production in expired air of human subjects with increased workload. Ji and colleagues (33) showed that the oxidation of GSH to glutathione disulfide (GSSG) in skeletal muscle increased as a function of treadmill speed and incline in rats. Despite these findings, two lines of direct evidence supporting the mitochondrial hypothesis of ROS production are still missing: (a) the ROS detected in the various studies are indeed generated in the mitochondria from exercised animals; and (b) mitochondrial production of ROS is quantitatively related to O_2 consumption and workload.

Xanthine/Xanthine Oxidase Pathway

Xanthine oxidase (XO)–catalyzed reactions have been well established as one of the major sources of free radical generation in the ischemic-reperfused (I-R) heart (34). During ischemia, adenosine triphosphate (ATP) is degraded to adenosine diphosphate (ADP) and adenosine monophosphate (AMP) because of the energy demand of contracting myocardium. Without sufficient oxygen to replenish ATP by oxidative phosphorylation, AMP is continuously degraded, leading to accumulation of hypoxanthine, which is converted to xanthine and uric acid by XO, coupled with the one-electron reduction of O_2 and generation of $O_2^{\bar{\cdot}}$ and H_2O_2 (35) (Fig. 21–2). To activate this pathway, several conditions must be met. First, sufficient amounts of hypoxanthine and xanthine must be present in the tissue as the substrates. Second, XO must be present in oxidized form, because the reduced form of XO (xanthine dehydrogenase) uses NAD^+ rather than O_2 as the electron acceptor and does not produce $O_2^{\bar{\cdot}}$ (36). Third, O_2 must be available as the electron acceptor. I-R tissues apparently provide all these prerequisites.

There is some evidence that high-intensity exercise simulates the situation of heart I-R and may activate the XO pathway (37,38). Hypoxanthine was reportedly accumulated after intense muscular contraction as a result of adenine nucleotide degradation (39), and uric acid concentration was shown to increase in both contracting arm muscle and in the plasma (40). These findings suggest that XO was active, because contribution of the other pathways to uric acid production is negligible. Sahlin and associates (41) showed that blood hypoxanthine and xanthine concentrations increased dramatically in human subjects after intense exercise. Skeletal muscle was thought to be the source of these purine metabolites resulting from AMP breakdown. Radak

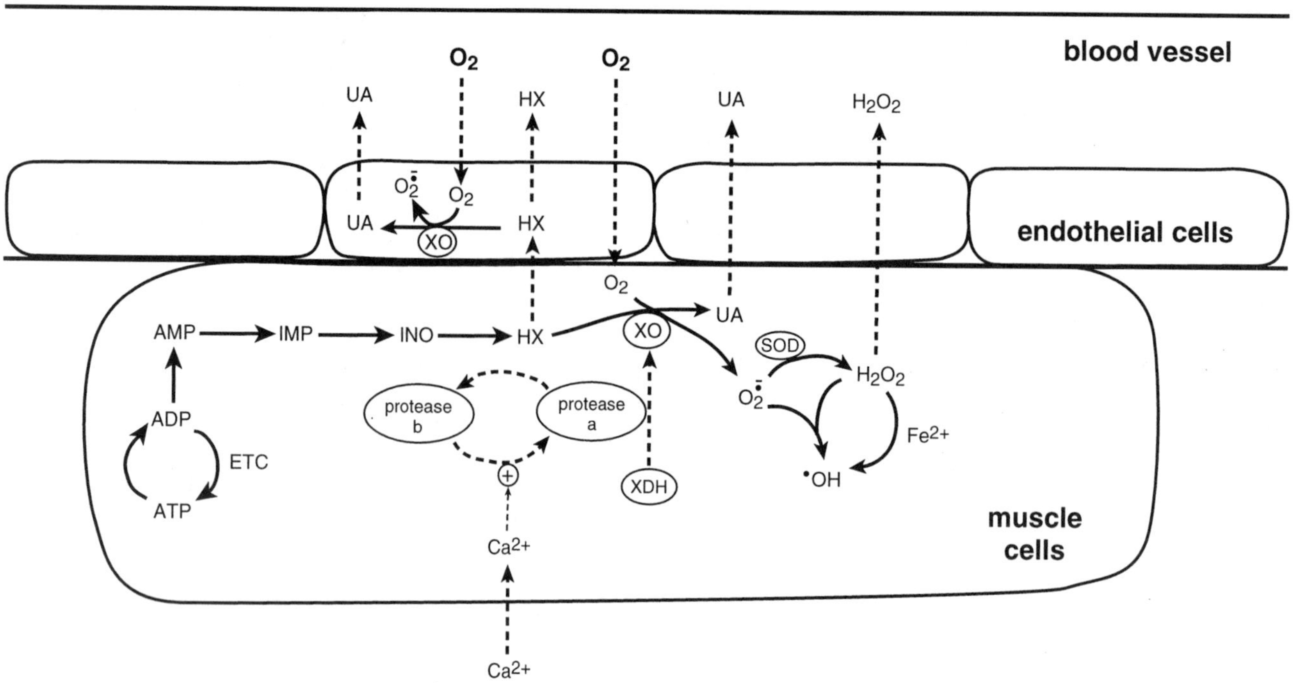

FIG. 21–2. The role of xanthine oxidase (*XO*) in free radical generation in the muscle and endothelial cells. *ETC*, electron transport chain; *HX*, hypoxanthine; *UA*, uric acid; *XDH*, xanthine dehydrogenase. Reactions are not balanced stoichiometrically.

and colleagues (42,43) showed that XO activity was increased 10-fold in the plasma and liver of rats after repeated high-intensity running to exhaustion, and plasma XO activity correlated to lactate concentration. The authors proposed that the origin of the enzyme was from the endothelial cells of the muscle, where xanthine dehydrogenase was converted to XO via a Ca^{2+}-activated protease. A recent study by Rasanen and co-workers (44) showed that strenuous exercise in horses increased peroxyl radical production and XO activity in the plasma. Furthermore, uric acid concentration increased exponentially in relation to workload, indicating a rapid degradation of purine products.

Several potential problems argue against the xanthine–XO hypothesis of free radical production during exercise. First, hypoxanthine and xanthine tend to accumulate during intense muscle contraction only during ischemic exercise or relative ischemic exercise, such as arm exercise, when blood flow and oxygen supply to the muscle are low. Dynamic exercise involving a large muscle mass does not result in an appreciable accumulation of purine nucleotide degradation products (41). Second, the increased uric acid levels observed in the blood could have been formed through xanthine dehydrogenase rather than XO (41). Third, XO activity is low in skeletal muscle, and data of muscle XO activity in response to exercise are currently not available. Whether the XO activity detected in the plasma after strenuous exercise comes from skeletal muscle remains to be verified. However, Hellsten and co-workers (45) were able to show an increase in XO-immunoreactive cells, presumably capillary endothelial and leukocyte cells, in human subjects after 7 days of intense exercise training. Thus it is reasonable to conclude that the XO hypothesis has merit at least under the conditions that skeletal muscle encounters an adenine nucleotide deficit and/or hypoxia followed by reoxygenation. This may occur during isometric contraction such as weightlifting and sprinting exercise.

Respiratory Burst and Neutrophils

Although there has been increasing research with respect to exercise and immune function, it became clear only recently that ROS may be involved in tissue inflammatory response to injury and that polymorphoneutrophils (PMNs) play a key role in this process (3,11,46). PMNs are part of the white blood cell family that are especially important in defending tissues from viral and bacterial infection during the acute-phase response. In response to blood-borne signals released from the injured tissues (such as interleukins), PMNs migrate to the injury site and release two primary factors for phagocytosis, lysozymes and $O_2^{\cdot-}$ (46). Lysozymes facilitate the breakdown of damaged proteins, whereas $O_2^{\cdot-}$ is produced by NADPH oxidase (47). If the initial injury

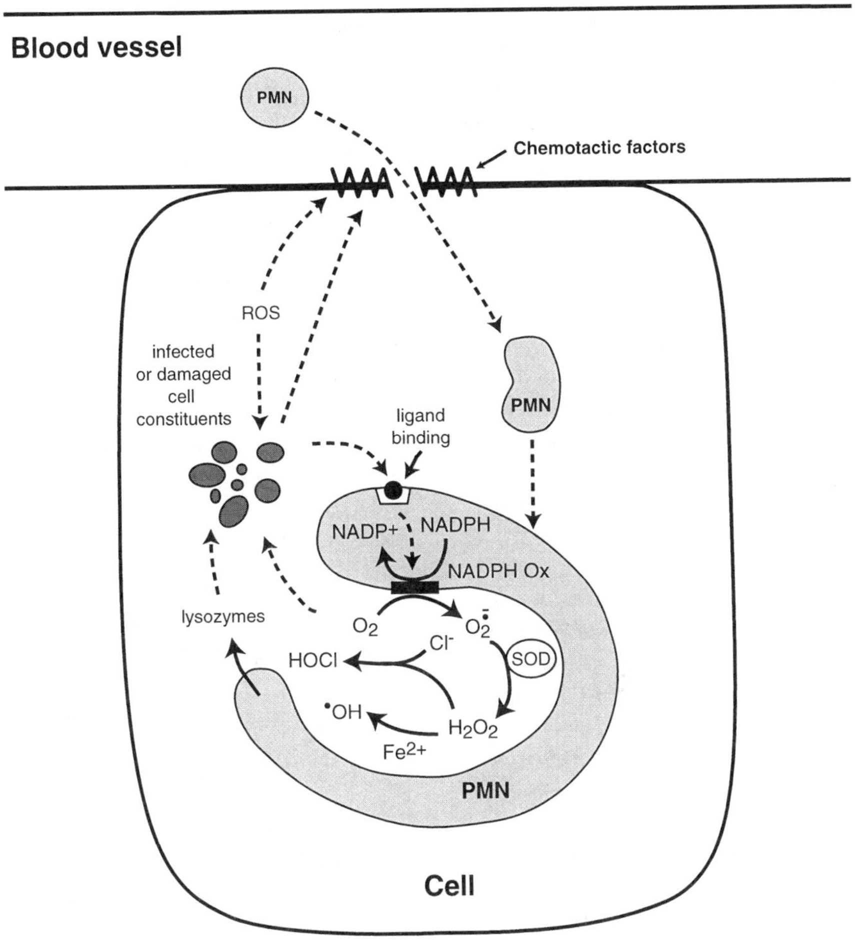

FIG. 21–3. The process of polymorphoneutrophil (*PMN*) infiltration and activation in the cell. *NADPH Ox*, NADPH oxidase; *ROS*, reactive oxygen species; *SOD*, superoxide dismutase. Reactions are not balanced stoichiometrically.

is caused by oxidative damage, ROS can activate chemotactic factors that attract neutrophils (44). This process resembles that of sepsis, wherein they share a common mediator, ROS (48). Figure 21–3 shows the process of neutrophil activation and ROS production during an acute-phase response in the cell.

Unaccustomed strenuous exercise has long been recognized to cause muscle injury accompanied by an inflammatory response, which is characterized by increased protease and lysozymal enzyme activities in working muscle (16). The response can last from several hours to several days after the cessation of exercise, depending on the intensity and duration of exercise. Furthermore, it was discovered that the biomarkers of the inflammatory responses often coincide with increase of antioxidant enzyme activities such as glutathione peroxidase (GPx) and catalase (16). These findings prompted some investigators to hypothesize that ROS might be produced in postexercise tissues, possibly caused by inflammation and neutrophil invasion (49). Although this inflammatory response is considered critical in removing damaged proteins and preventing bacterial and viral infection, ROS released from neutrophils also can cause secondary damage (3). Hack and associates (50) showed that an acute bout of exhaustive exercise in humans significantly increased cell counts of leukocytes, lymphocytes, and neutrophils. Phagocytosis assays revealed that ingestion capacity was increased immediately after exercise up to 24 hours after exercise, whereas significant increase in $O_2^{\cdot-}$ production was noticed only at 24 hours after exercise. Meydani and colleagues (49) showed that after an acute bout of eccentric exercise in sedentary men, circulating cytokine (interleukin-1; IL-1) levels were significantly elevated. Because eccentric exercise is known to cause muscle tissue injury and IL-1 can be induced by $O_2^{\cdot-}$ *in vitro* (11), this study suggests that interleukins may be involved in mobilizing PMNs during or after muscle injury. Furthermore, vitamin E administration attenuated urinary markers of lipid peroxidation found during the postexercise period, indicative of the oxidative nature of the injury (49). Smith and colleagues (51) have reported that H_2O_2 generation in neutrophils collected 1 hour after an acute bout of moderate exercise was increased threefold under *in vitro* challenge, accompanied by an enhanced receptor expression. Although available data provided some strong evidence that an interaction between neutrophil activation and ROS production occurs in injured tissues, it is obvious that ROS generated by PMNs are not the primary etiologic cause for the damage. Given the time required for neutrophil infiltration, this pathway probably is not a major source of free radical production during short-term exercise. However, it may serve as an important secondary mechanism for oxidative stress in muscle during prolonged exercise or during recovery from heavy eccentric exercise or exhaustive exercise.

Other ROS-Generating Pathways

Peroxisomes are organelles in the cell involved in nonmitochondrial oxidation of fatty acids and D-amino acids. Under physiologic conditions, peroxisomes contribute to the steady-state production of H_2O_2 but not $O_2^{\bar{\cdot}}$ (4). At rest, liver is the primary organ where peroxisomal contribution to H_2O_2 production is important. Prolonged starvation has been shown to increase H_2O_2 generation mainly because of the increased fatty acid oxidation in this organelle. Starvation for 48 hours in rats has been shown to decrease the hepatic GSH:GSSG ratio, accompanied by an increased malonaldehyde (MDA) content in liver and skeletal muscle (52). During prolonged exercise, fatty acids are the primary energy substrate for the myocardium and skeletal muscle; therefore peroxisomes are potential sites for ROS production. The findings that catalase activity is increased after an acute bout of exercise in muscle seem to support this hypothesis (31,33).

Under physiologic conditions, liver microsomes generate oxygen free radicals primarily through the cytochrome P-450 system (4,6). Mixed-function oxygenase is the key enzyme to catalyze NADPH oxidation, producing $O_2^{\bar{\cdot}}$, which is then dismuted to H_2O_2. The rate of H_2O_2 production also is known to increase when oxygen consumption in the microsome is increased (5). However, whether this pathway contributes to overall ROS production during exercise is unclear. There is some indication that exercise may alter ROS production in the liver microsomal system. Kim and associates (53) have reported that ROS production is increased in liver microsomes from old versus young rats, and that chronically active animals produce less ROSs than do their sedentary counterparts. Another situation wherein exercise is expected to alter ROS production by this pathway is when large doses of prooxidant drugs, such as acetaminophen, are administered before exercise. Hepatic blood flow is decreased during exercise, which could cause changes in the pharmacokinetics and pharmacodynamics of drug metabolism and thus microsomal exposure to these oxidants (54).

The heart releases norepinephrine from sympathetic nerve endings under various stressful conditions, including heavy exercise. Circulating catecholamines released from adrenal medulla also are increased during prolonged exercise. Catecholamines enhance myocardial and skeletal muscle oxidative metabolism via activation of β-adrenergic receptors, thereby increasing ROS production through a mitochondrial pathway. β-Blockade has been shown to reduce oxidative-stress markers in plasma of human subjects working at high intensity (55). Furthermore, autooxidation of adrenaline to adrenochrome is associated with $O_2^{\bar{\cdot}}$ formation, which is considered a source of ROS production during heart I-R (56). However, the quantitative importance of catecholamine as a source of ROS production during exercise has not been investigated and remains unclear.

ANTIOXIDANT DEFENSE SYSTEMS

Cellular antioxidant defenses are conventionally classified into two groups, enzymatic and nonenzymatic. Primary antioxidant enzyme SOD, catalase (CAT), and GPx catalyze the one-electron reduction of $O_2^{\bar{\cdot}}$ or H_2O_2 (4). A number of enzymes are involved in the supply of substrates and reducing power (NADPH) for primary antioxidant enzymes, such as glutathione reductase (GR) and glucose-6-phosphate dehydrogenase (G6PDH), but they do not directly remove ROS. Antioxidant vitamins directly scavenge $O_2^{\bar{\cdot}}$ and $^{\cdot}OH$ as well as singlet oxygen (6). GSH and other low-molecular-weight antioxidants play an important role in maintaining the substrate levels for GPx and keeping vitamins E and C in the reduced state (57). From a nutritional point of view, it may also be useful to divide antioxidants into two categories. The first category of antioxidants can be synthesized within the body and are inducible under oxidative stress. This includes most antioxidant enzymes and GSH (Table 21–1). The second category of antioxidants cannot be synthesized or

TABLE 21–1. *Inducible and noninducible antioxidants*

Inducible antioxidants	Noninducible antioxidants
Superoxide dismutase	α-Tocopherol (vitamine E)
Glutathione peroxidase	Ascorbic acid (vitamin C)
Catalase	β-Carotene (vitamin A precursor)
Glutathione reductase	Dihydrolipoate(?[a])
Glutathione-*S*-transferase	
Glutathione	
Ubiquinone	

[a] α-Lipoic acid was classified as a vitamin after it was isolated, but it was later found to be synthesized by animals and humans. See ref. 149 for details.

TABLE 21–2. *Antioxidant enzyme activity in various tissues*

	SOD			GPX			CAT	GR	GST	G6PDH
Tissues	Cu/Zn (unit/mg)	Mn	Total (unit/g ww)	Cyto (unit/mg)	Mito	Total (unit/g ww)	(unit/g ww)			
Liver	500	50	14,400	550	430	85	670	40	940	8.0
Heart	65	21	2610	150	70	17	84	1.3	2.5	10.9
Soleus	n.d.	n.d.	1300	n.d.	n.d.	13	61	0.8	1.1	n.d.
DVL	21	8	1360	23	17	2	18	0.4	0.5	0.6
SVL	n.d.	n.d.	887	n.d.	n.d.	0.9	15	0.3	0.2	n.d.
Erythrocytes	n.a.	n.a.	8.8	n.a.	n.a.	25	10	35	1.0	2.3

Units of enzyme activity in rat tissues: Cu/Zn & Mn SOD, unit/mg protein; SOD total, unit/g wet wt; cytosolic & mitochondrial GPX, nmol/min/mg protein; GPX total, nmol/min/g wet wt; catalase, K × 10^{-2}/g wet wt; activity for other enzymes, μmol/min/g wet wt; activity in human erythrocytes: units per g Hb; n.a., not applicable; n.d., not determined.

induced, and they must be taken from the diet. This includes vitamin E, vitamin C, and β-carotene. However, even the inducible antioxidants are influenced by dietary intake of trace elements and micronutrients (58). Thus nutrition has a significant impact on cellular antioxidant systems.

Antioxidant Enzymes

Functions, Properties, and Regulation

Superoxide Dismutase

The first line of defense against ROS in the cell is provided by SOD, which catalyzes the following reaction.

$$2\ O_2^{\cdot-} + 2\ H^+ \rightarrow H_2O_2 + O_2$$

Three types of SOD isozymes depend on the metal ion bound to its active site (5). CuZn SOD is a highly stable enzyme found primarily in the cytosolic compartment of the eukaryotic cells such as yeast, plants, and animals, but not generally in the prokaryotes such as bacteria and algae (5). CuZn SOD is a dimer (MW, 32,000) and sensitive to cyanide and H_2O_2 inhibition (59). It is interesting that although Cu and Zn are both required for the synthesis of the enzyme, the copper ion plays the primary function of dismutation with alternative oxidation and reduction, whereas the Zn appears to have no catalytic role except stabilizing the enzyme (5). Mn SOD is a tetramer with a much larger MW of 88,000. Mn SOD is present in the mitochondrial matrix of eukaryotes and is insensitive to cyanide and H_2O_2. It is not as stable as CuZn SOD, however, and it can be inhibited by SDS and chloroform/ethanol treatments (60). This distinction of cyanide sensitivity has been used to measure the activity of the two SODs in tissue extracts without isolating mitochondria and cytosol (29). In addition to CuZn and Mn SOD, bacteria contain a third type of SOD that requires Fe as a prosthetic group. In mammals, the highest SOD activity is found in the liver, followed by kidney, brain, adrenal gland, and heart (5). In the skeletal muscle, SOD activity is similar to that in the heart, and there are relatively small differences between muscle-fiber types (Table 21–2).

Unlike most enzymes, SOD lacks a Michaelis constant (K_m). The enzyme is partially occupied by its substrate ($O_2^{\cdot-}$), and its catalytic activity increases with increasing $O_2^{\cdot-}$ concentration within a wide range (4). High levels of H_2O_2 have been shown to inhibit SOD *in vitro* (61). Because of the previously mentioned kinetic properties, assays of SOD are usually based on indirect methods involving the inhibition of a reaction in which $O_2^{\cdot-}$ is generated by using a variety of electron donors (62). Therefore it is difficult to compare maximal activity between studies by using different assay methods.

The two types of SOD have quite different characteristics in terms of protein turnover. Recombinant human SOD (r-h SOD) studies reveal that CuZn SOD has a half-life ($t_{1/2}$) of 6 to 10 minutes, whereas Mn SOD has a much longer $t_{1/2}$ of 5 to 6 hours (63). This information has provided us with an important clue as to how SOD gene regulation is controlled. The relative abundance of CuZn SOD messenger RNA (mRNA) displays clear tissue-specific differences, with the liver possessing the highest levels, followed by kidneys, heart, lung, and then the skeletal muscle (Fig. 21–4). Among different muscle fibers, CuZn SOD mRNA levels are the highest in type 1 muscle (soleus), followed by mixed muscle-fiber type (plantaris), and then type 2 muscle (vastus lateralis and gastrocnemius). Consistent with the mRNA levels, type 1 muscle also has a higher level of CuZn SOD protein content than type 2 muscle (60). These findings suggest that, at rest, CuZn SOD gene expression is regulated at the pretranslational level.

In general, Mn SOD activity, content, and mRNA abundance follows the same order across tissues as that displayed by CuZn SOD. Mn SOD in the eukaryotic cells is encoded by a nuclear gene. A large precursor enzyme form is made in the cytosol and transported into the mitochondria by an energy-dependent process (64). Mn SOD has been shown to be inducible under

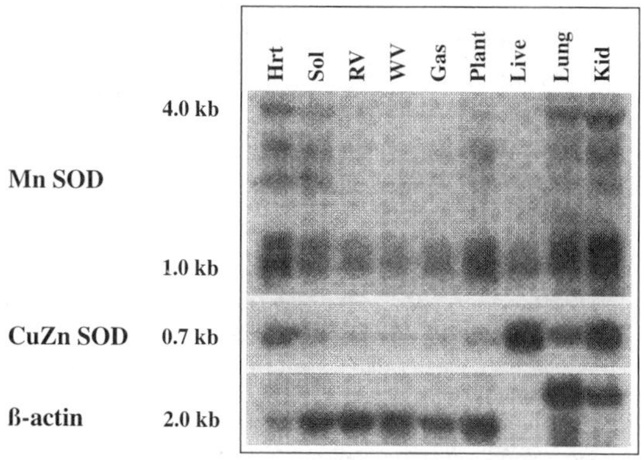

FIG. 21–4. Northern blots of messenger RNA for Cu-Zn SOD and Mn SOD in the various rat tissues. *Hrt*, heart; *Sol*, soleus; *RV*, red vastus lateralis; *WV*, white vastus lateralis; *Gas*, gastrocnemius; *Plant*, plantaris; *Kid*, kidney. β-Actin was used as a housekeeping gene. The cDNA probes for CuZn SOD and Mn SOD were kind gifts of Dr. Ye-Shih Ho, Wayne State University, Detroit, Michigan.

oxidative stress, and the upregulation of Mn SOD gene expression is mediated at least partially by a transcriptional mechanism (65). A number of potential inducers of Mn SOD have been identified, including tumor necrosis factor–α (TNF-α), IL-1, and lipopolysaccharide (66). The Mn SOD promoter contains both nuclear factor (NF)κB and AP-1 binding sites, and the effects of TNF-α and IL-1 on Mn SOD gene expression were mediated in part by a thio-redox modulation of NF-κB activation (67). Furthermore, intracellular oxygen tension seems to play a major role in regulating Mn SOD gene expression (68).

Catalase

The primary function of CAT is to decompose H_2O_2 to H_2O (4). It shares this function with GPx, although substrate specificity and affinity as well as the cellular location of the two antioxidant enzymes are different (see below).

$$2\,H_2O_2 \rightarrow 2\,H_2O + O_2$$

CAT is a tetramer with a relatively large MW of ~240,000. Fe^{3+} is a required ligand to be bound to the enzyme's active site for its catalytic function. CAT resembles SOD in many kinetic properties such as the lack of an apparent K_m and V_{max}. Its activity increases enormously with an increase in H_2O_2 concentration (4). In the presence of H_2O_2, CAT is also capable of reducing a limited number of hydroperoxides (peroxidatic function), but not *t*-butyl hydroperoxide, to their respective aldehydes (4). Azide and cyanide are both inhibitors of CAT. This inhibition is often used to partition CAT activity from GPx activity in enzyme assays by using crude tissue extracts (69). CAT is widely distributed within the cell with a high concentration found in the peroxisomes. Mitochondria and other intracellular organelles also contain considerable CAT activity, however (70). As shown in Table 21–2, the activities of CAT among mammalian tissues follow the order of SOD, with liver the highest and skeletal muscle the lowest. Interfiber difference of muscle CAT activity, however, is much greater for CAT than for SOD.

Murine CAT gene regulation has been studied extensively. A single gene (Cs) located on chromosome 2 is responsible for coding the primary structure of the enzyme (71). Once synthesized, the polypeptide may be modified epigenetically in terms of sulfhydryl groups and carbohydrate or protein moieties. The normal (N) and epigenetically modified (E) polypeptidal subunits can produce five tetrameric isozymes, similar to the isozyme patterns of lactate dehydrogenase (72).

As a peroxisomal enzyme, CAT is more sensitive to oxidative stress in the liver and lung. For example, administration of ciprofibrate, a peroxisome proliferator, increased hepatic CAT activity possibly due to enhanced β-oxidation and generation of H_2O_2 (73). In the lung of prenatal guinea pigs, there is a coordinated elevation of mRNA levels for Mn SOD, CAT, and GPx, which correlate with activities of these enzymes, suggesting a pretranslational control mechanism (74). In contrast, liver mRNA levels for SOD and CAT are significantly increased only after birth. Relatively little is known about the gene regulation of CAT in skeletal muscle.

Glutathione Peroxidase

GPx catalyzes the reduction of H_2O_2 and organic hydroperoxide to H_2O and alcohol, respectively, by using GSH as the electron donor (75).

$$2\,GSH + H_2O_2 \rightarrow GS\text{-}SG + 2\,H_2O$$

or

$$2\,GSH + ROOH \rightarrow GS\text{-}SG + ROH$$

GPx refers only to the Se-dependent enzyme (EC 1.11.1.9). The so-called Se-independent GPx is actually a fraction of the GST (EC 2.5.1.18) activity, which also removes ROOH (76). The primary function of GST, however, is to catalyze the conjugation of GSH with a variety of xenobiotic substances as the initial step for their metabolism. GPx is highly specific for its hydrogen donor GSH but has low specificity for hydroperoxide, ranging from H_2O_2 to complex organic hydroperoxide including long-chain fatty acid hydroperoxide and nucleotide-derived hydroperoxides (75). This kinetic characteristic of GPx makes it a versatile hydroperoxide remover in the cell and thus serves an important role in inhibiting lipid peroxidation and preventing damage to DNA and RNA. It also is important to recognize that although GPx and CAT have an overlap of substrate H_2O_2, GPx (at least in mammals) has a much greater affinity for H_2O_2 at low concentrations (K_m = 1 μ/L) than CAT (K_m = 1 m × mol/L) (6). GPx is susceptible to $O_2^{\cdot-}$ and hydroperoxide *in vitro* because of the oxidation of the selenocysteine residue at the enzyme's active site (61). Both SOD and GSH prevent the inactivation of GPx by removing $O_2^{\cdot-}$ and reducing the sulfhydryls of the enzyme, respectively. GPx is located in both the cytosol and mitochondrial matrix of the cell, with a distribution ratio of about 2:1 (4). This allows it to reach a number of cellular sources of hydroperoxide generation. The activity of GPx is high in the liver and erythrocytes, moderate in the brain, kidney, and heart, and low in the skeletal muscle (see Table 21–2). However, the oxidative type 1 muscle (soleus) possesses a GPx activity close to the level in the heart (77).

GPx is a homotetramer with each 22-kDa subunit bound by a selenium atom existing as a selenocysteine. The expression of the GPx gene, *hgpx1*, occurs in a wide range of tissues controlled by different mechanisms in mammalian tissues (78). First, GPx expression is influenced by oxygen tension. Thus lung and erythrocytes have a higher GPx activity compared with other tissues. Second, metabolic rate seems to play a significant role in GPx expression, as liver, kidney, and pancreas have higher GPx activities than other tissues (75). Third, GPx appears to be developmentally regulated. GPx activity in the lung of prenatal rats increased dramatically several days before birth in anticipation of high oxygen tensions (78). Finally, toxins and xenobiotics can induce GPx, especially in the liver (5).

Glutathione Reductase

Regeneration of GSH from glutathione disulfide (GSSG) is accomplished by the flavin-containing enzyme GR. NADPH is used as the reducing power of this reaction, which is coupled with G6PDH in erythrocytes and some other tissues (75). When H_2O_2 concentration is increased in the red cells, there is a tendency toward an elevated GSSG, which appears to affect the regulation of the hexose monophosphate shunt in the following manner. First, GSSG activates G6PDH directly; second, regeneration of GSH decreases NADPH level, which is normally inhibitory to G6PDH; and third, consumption of NADPH elevates $NADP^+$, which is a substrate and allosteric activator of G6PDH (75). In skeletal muscle, isocitrate dehydrogenase may play a more important role in supplying NADPH for GR than does G6PDH (79). Thus although not classified as an antioxidant enzyme, GR has a subcellular distribution similar to that of GPx and is essential for normal antioxidant function.

Other Enzymes Offering Antioxidant Protection

In addition to the primary antioxidant enzymes mentioned, the cell has a number of enzyme systems that function either to reduce the production of ROS or to facilitate the removal of ROS and their by-products. Cytochrome *c* oxidase is the terminal enzyme in the mitochondrial respiratory chain, catalyzing the electron transfer from cytochrome a_3 to O_2. Chance and colleagues (4) emphasized the importance of this enzyme in preventing the release of $O_2^{\cdot-}$ and H_2O_2 outside the respiratory chain by binding these ROS tightly with the enzyme. Yu (6) expanded the concept of antioxidant defenses to those enzymes participating in the degradation, removal, and repair of the damaged cell constituents. For example, phospholipase A_2 plays an important role in the removal of oxidized lipids, thus preventing extensive lipid peroxidation (6). Degradation of oxidized protein is another important function performed by certain proteases that are activated to degrade oxidized protein preferentially (80).

Protection During Acute Exercise

Because of the specific kinetic properties discussed, antioxidant enzymes are capable of increasing their activities in response to increased substrate levels (4). Within the physiologic range, this is probably accomplished by activating the existing enzyme molecules via allosteric and/or covalent modification rather than by synthesizing new enzyme proteins (8). Because an acute bout of exercise has been shown to increase free radical production in several tissues including liver, heart, and skeletal muscle (15,18), certain antioxidant enzyme activities in these tissues are expected to increase in response to exercise. Because of the wide range of endogenous enzyme activity and levels of ROS production in the various tissues, antioxidant enzymes have demonstrated different exercise responses.

SOD activity has been shown to increase after an acute bout of exercise in liver (26,30,31,81), skeletal muscle (81–84), heart (25,83), and blood (85–88). With a few exceptions (83), most of the studies also indicated that exercise increases CuZn SOD rather than Mn SOD activity. This activation of SOD has been proposed to be caused by increased $O_2^{\cdot-}$ production during exercise according to *in vitro* SOD kinetics (89). Because we now know that CuZn SOD has a relatively fast turnover rate and a short $t_{1/2}$ in the range of minutes (see the previous section), *de novo* synthesis of new enzyme protein cannot be ruled out in explaining the observed CuZn SOD response to acute exercise. Radak and coworkers (42) have shown that CuZn and Mn SOD activities and immunoreactive enzyme contents in rat soleus and tibialis muscles were significantly increased after a single bout of exhaustive running. CuZn SOD activity and content gradually returned to resting levels after 1 to 3 days, whereas Mn SOD activity and protein content continued to increase during the postexercise period. These findings suggest that the stimulating effects of exercise on CuZn SOD and Mn SOD gene expression may be different in terms of the threshold and time course of induction.

Similar to SOD, GPx activity has demonstrated variable responses to an acute bout of exercise in the various types of skeletal muscle. Some studies showed no exercise effect on muscle GPx activity (81,90–92), whereas others reported a significant elevation (33,42,93–96). Liver GPx seems to be unaffected in all studies reported (8). A few studies showed an increase in GPx activity in the heart (96) and platelets (88).

Most of the previous studies revealed no significant alteration in CAT activity with acute exercise (3,8). However, there were exceptions when CAT activity was found to increase significantly after an acute bout of exercise to exhaustion in the deep portion of vastus lateralis (DVL) muscle in rats (33,93). Although CAT is located primarily in the peroxisomes, muscle mitochondria have been reported to contain a significant fraction of CAT activity (70). Thus it is possible that the observed increase in muscle CAT activity reflected an activation of mitochondrial CAT due to the increased H_2O_2 production.

Recently there has been increased effort to examine the effect of acute exercise on gene regulation of antioxidant enzymes. Oh-Ishi and colleagues (95) reported a significant downregulation of mRNA levels for both CuZn and Mn SOD isozymes in soleus muscle of untrained rats after an acute bout of exercise, but in the trained rats no exercise downregulation was observed. We recently investigated the effects of a prolonged exercise bout on mRNA abundance of muscle antioxidant enzymes and NF-κB binding patterns in rats (97). Relative abundance of CuZn SOD, Mn SOD, and CAT mRNA were not altered by exercise, but exercise decreased GPx mRNA levels by 21.6% and 60.8% ($p < .05$) in DVL and the superficial vastus lateralis (SVL), respectively. NF-κB binding was significantly decreased in DVL with exercise but showed no change in SVL. We suspect that an acute bout of exhaustive exercise may alter either the transcription or the mRNA stability of GPx, Mn SOD, and CuZn SOD in certain muscle fibers because of the changes in cellular metabolic and redox status. The altered binding of the redox-sensitive transcriptional regulator NF-κB implies an involvement of transcriptional control in antioxidant enzyme regulation during exercise.

In summary, antioxidant enzymes may be selectively activated during an acute bout of strenuous exercise. This activation may depend on the oxidative stress imposed on the specific tissue as well as the intrinsic antioxidant enzyme property. Skeletal muscles are subjected to a greater oxidative stress than are liver and heart because of increased oxygen consumption during exercise; therefore the muscles need greater antioxidant protection against potential oxidative damage. Understanding the mechanism for the observed rapid increases in antioxidant enzyme activity during acute exercise remains a challenge.

Adaptation to Chronic Exercise

Tissues involved in strenuous exercise training are under great oxidative challenge. Increased energy demand accomplished by increased oxidative metabolism means a large oxygen flux through the mitochondria, rendering the tissue to a high level of ROS exposure. If exercise intensity is heavy enough to cause a net deficit of adenine nucleotides and/or muscle injury, xanthine oxidase, and neutrophil pathways may be activated to produce additional ROS in the tissue (see previous sections). Furthermore, training may deplete nonenzymatic antioxidant reserves such as vitamin E and glutathione if dietary intakes are not increased to match the demand (see below). Thus as a long-term strategy cells may activate *de novo* antioxidant enzyme synthesis to cope with the enhanced oxidative stress.

SOD activity in skeletal muscle has been reported to increase significantly after training in rats (29,77,95,98–101). Many studies failed to detect SOD training adaptation, however, even though similar training protocols were used (31,89,102). Furthermore, a recent study by Tiidus and associates (103) failed to detect a training effect on SOD activity in human leg muscle after 8 weeks of bicycle exercise. The discrepancies between studies may be explained by a relatively small training adaptation of Mn SOD, which could be masked when total SOD activity was measured. To identify which SOD isozyme is induced by training, Higuchi and colleagues (29) demonstrated that Mn SOD is primarily responsible for the increased SOD activity. Ji and associates (26), although showing no difference in muscle Mn SOD activity expressed as per milligram of mitochondrial protein between trained and untrained rats, clearly demonstrated that trained rats had a greater mitochondrial protein content. Therefore muscle Mn SOD activity per gram of muscle weight apparently was increased with training. Oh-Ishi and co-workers (95) showed that CuZn SOD activity was significantly increased with training, but the enzyme protein content and mRNA level were not altered. In contrast, Mn SOD showed both an increased activity and protein content, without affecting mRNA levels. Hollander and co-workers (104) reported that training induction of Mn SOD is muscle fiber specific. Significant increases in both Mn SOD activity (+70%) and enzyme protein content (+26%) were found in rat DVL muscle after 10 weeks of treadmill running, with only marginal changes occurring in soleus muscle. Consistent with the findings of Oh-Ishi and colleagues (95), resting mRNA levels for both Mn and CuZn SOD were lowered with training. These data suggest that training induction of both SODs is caused by posttranscriptional mechanisms and that Mn SOD training adaptation may be more important because of mitochondrial ROS production during exercise.

CAT activity has been shown to increase after training in skeletal muscle by some authors (95,96,98), but most studies have reported no change in muscle CAT with training (cf. 1,3,8). A few studies even reported a decrease (99,102). There are more consistent reports on GPx adaptation to training, with a majority of studies showing an increase in GPx activity (26,30,77,82, 95,99,100–102). GPx adaptation also demonstrates a muscle fiber–specific pattern, with type 2a muscle the most adaptive to training. Powers and associates (100) showed a 45% increase in GPx activity in red gastrocnemius muscle after endurance training in rats, and the level of increment appeared to be dependent on running time rather than on speed during training sessions. Soleus and white gastrocnemius muscles revealed no training effect of GPx regardless of training intensity and duration. Leeuwenburgh and co-workers (77) reported a 62% increase in GPx activity in DVL (type 2a) muscle in response to treadmill training with 2 h/day at moderate intensity (25 m/min, 10%), whereas soleus and myocardium showed no training effect. Because GPx has a wider range of substrate specificity and a lower K_m with respect to peroxides than does CAT, an increased GPx activity would facilitate the removal of both H_2O_2 and lipid peroxides generated in the mitochondrial inner membrane (105).

Why do different antioxidant enzymes display different characteristics of training adaptation? The answer may be multifaceted, depending on the specific pattern of gene expression for each enzyme, the threshold of ROS required for induction, and their interactions. *De novo* synthesis of an enzyme is energy demanding and relatively slow, and it is probably reserved as the last resort to cope with oxidative stress. SOD activities appear sufficiently high and relatively uniform across tissues and various muscle types (see Table 21–1), suggesting that the removal of superoxide anion may not be a rate-limiting step. In comparison, GPx destroys the end products of the ROS generation pathway (i.e., hydrogen peroxide and organic peroxide, including lipid peroxide), and its activity is relatively low. This may explain why GPx usually displays a greater training adaptation than SOD and CAT. After studying the kinetics of SOD, CAT, and GPx in vitro, Remacle and associates (106) proposed that GPx is the most important antioxidant enzyme for cell survival because of its higher sensitivity to intracellular ROS levels and its greater adaptability to oxidative stress.

Glutathione and Thiols

Biochemical Property and Cellular Distribution

GSH is a thio-containing tripeptide found in high concentrations in virtually all animal and plant cells and in some bacteria. GSH serves multiple roles in the cellular antioxidant defense (7,57). The most important antioxidant function of GSH is to serve as a substrate for GPx to remove hydrogen and organic peroxides. Another critical role of GSH is to keep other antioxidants such as vitamin E (α-tocopherol), vitamin C (ascorbic acid), and dihydrolipoate in the reduced state (107). GSH also is capable of scavenging $^{\cdot}$OH and other free radicals (5).

GSH concentration in the cell is in the millimolar range, but there is a great variability in GSH content in different organs depending on their function and oxidative capacity. Eye lens has the highest concentration of GSH in the body (10 m*M*) because of the constant exposure to light (5). Liver contains 5 to 7 m*M* GSH, the second highest GSH content in the body, and plays a central role for GSH homeostasis and detoxification (see below). Other important organs such as the lung, kidney, and heart contain 2 to 3 m*M* GSH. In the blood, erythrocytes and plasma maintain two separate GSH pools with a much higher GSH concentration in the former (~2 m*M*) than the latter (<0.05 m*M*). Skeletal muscle GSH concentration varies widely depending on muscle-fiber type and animal species (108). In rats, type 1 fibers (e.g., soleus) have sixfold higher GSH content (~3 m*M*) than type 2b fibers (e.g., SVL). Despite the differences in content, the GSH/GSSG ratio is remarkably consistent across various fiber types (8).

Intracellular GSH levels are determined by both GSH use and GSH synthesis, but most organs and tissues do not synthesize GSH *de novo*. Instead, GSH is translocated from extracellular sources into the cell in a complicated process known as the γ-glutamyl cycle (7). The membrane-borne γ-glutamyltranspeptidase (GGT) first cleaves plasma GSH, and the ingredient amino acids glutamate, cysteine, and glycine are transported across the cell membrane into the cell. γ-Glutamylcysteine synthetase (GCS) and GSH synthetase (GS) catalyze the formation of the tripeptide in a series of ATP-dependent steps. GCS is considered the rate-limiting enzyme for GSH synthesis.

The majority of *de novo* GSH synthesis occurs in the liver, supplying approximately 90% of the circulating GSH under physiologic conditions (57). Hepatic GSH synthesis is controlled by both substrate (amino acids) availability and hormonal regulation. Insulin and glucocorticoids stimulate hepatic GSH synthesis through induction of GCS (109). In contrast, glucagon and several other cyclic adenosine monophosphate (cAMP)–stimulating agents downregulate hepatic GSH synthesis by phosphorylating and inhibiting GCS (110). GSH release from the liver is promoted by catecholamines, glucagon, and vasopressin (111,112).

GSH turnover is rapid in most mammalian tissues. The turnover rate for the liver, kidneys, and skeletal muscle is estimated to be 4.5, 2.7, and 1.6 μmol/hour, respectively (113). At rest, the kidneys are the most

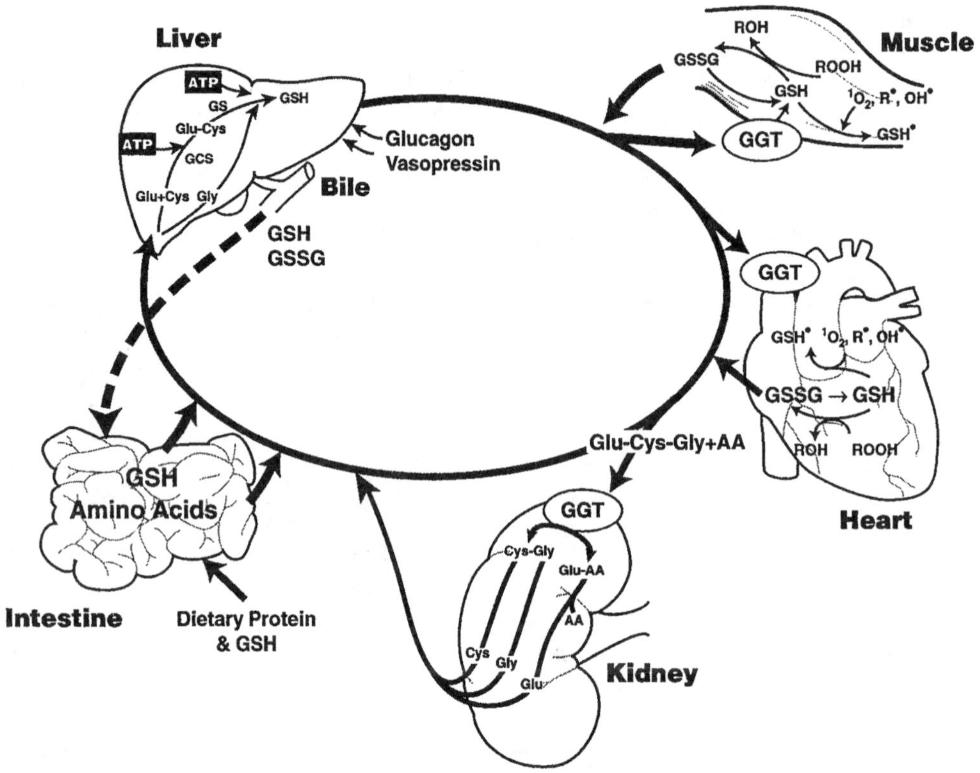

FIG. 21–5. Postulated outline of interorgan transport of glutathione. *GSH,* glutathione; *GSSG*, glutathione disulfide; *GS*$^-$, glutathione thiyl radical; *ROOH, hydrogen peroxide; ROH*, alcohol; *GGT*, γ-glutamyltranspeptidase.

important organ for GSH turnover, wherein GSH is broken down to glutamate, cysteine, and glycine; these are subsequently released to the blood circulation. GSH turnover is relatively slow in the noncontracting skeletal muscle. However, muscle constitutes a large GSH pool due to its mass (~40% of the body weight), and it may exert an important influence on plasma GSH levels and whole-body GSH homeostasis under certain physiologic and pathologic conditions (113,114). Figure 21–5 illustrates the interorgan GSH transport and regulation in mammals.

After donating a pair of hydrogen ions to neutralize peroxide, GSH is oxidized to GSSG. Reduction of GSSG is catalyzed by GR, a flavin-containing enzyme, wherein NADPH is used as the reducing power. This reaction couples the reaction catalyzed by GPx, thus providing a redox cycle for the regeneration of GSH (75). GSSG levels in most tissues are kept very low, whereas the intracellular ratio of GSH to GSSG is kept very high (probably greater than 100) (115,116). When oxidation of GSH to GSSG exceeds the reducing capacity of GR, skeletal muscle fibers, cardiac myocytes, and liver cells are all capable of exporting GSSG to maintain the GSH/GSSG ratio (57). This is an important protection for the cell because high levels of GSSG disturb intracellular redox status, which can inactivate certain enzymes regulated by thio-disulfide exchange mechanism and causes protein cross-linkage (5).

GSH Homeostasis During Exercise

Muscle GSH status is influenced by both enzyme activities and substrate levels in the γ-glutamyl cycle. During heavy aerobic exercise, ROS production is increased in skeletal muscle, which requires more NADPH to regenerate GSH and maintain the GSH/GSSG ratio. However, NADPH production via hexose monophosphate shunt (pentose shunt) and isocitrate dehydrogenase reaction may be limited, in part because of the competition for glucose-6-phosphate from glycolysis. Intracellular resynthesis of GSH from amino acids also requires ATP, which may decline because of an increased demand by muscular contraction. All of these factors contribute to a decreased GSH and an accumulation of GSSG in the cell. Indeed, an acute bout of exhaustive exercise has been shown to increase GSSG content significantly in rat skeletal muscle (33,93,117). GSSG increment appears to depend on exercise intensity and muscle-fiber type (33). Accumulation of GSSG in exercising muscle is associated with an activation of GPx and GR, suggesting an increased hydroperoxide production. In contrast to heavy exercise, prolonged exercise at moderate intensity results in no accumulation of GSSG in skeletal muscle of mice (91) and rats (94), indicating a relatively stable GSH homeostasis.

The ratio of GSH to GSSG, an indicator of intracellular redox status, was reported to be dramatically decreased in human skeletal muscle biopsy after marathon running (118). In rodent studies, however, most authors have found only moderate decrease or no change in the GSH to GSSG ratio after acute exercise, although the reported GSH/GSSG values varied greatly from study to study (from 10 to several hundred) (33,91,93,117).

It is now clear that some body tissues are capable of adapting to chronic exercise training by increasing their GSH content. However, training effect on GSH content seems to vary greatly between animal species and tissues. High levels of endurance training have been shown to increase GSH content in the hindlimb muscles of dogs (81,101,114) and rats (77,99,101). Increased GSH content in the trained muscle groups may be explained by an enhanced ability to take up GSH from extramural sources, reflected by a training adaptation of GGT, GCS, and GS (81,101).

A closer look reveals that training adaptation of GSH is muscle fiber specific. Activities of the γ-glutamyl cycle enzymes seem to play an important role. For example, DVL muscle, which has the highest GGT activity among various muscle types, demonstrated a prominent training adaptation of GSH, whereas soleus and SVL showed no training effect (77). No significant difference in GCS activity was noticed between various types of skeletal muscle, suggesting that the translocation of amino acids rather than intracellular assembly of GSH may be the rate-limiting step. In contrast to skeletal muscle, hepatic GSH status does not seem to be affected by training.

Physically trained human subjects and animals generally demonstrate a greater tolerance of exercise-induced disturbance of blood GSH status (86,119–121). Kretzschmar and colleagues (120) found that both young and old trained individuals had higher resting plasma GSH concentrations than did their sedentary counterparts. Furthermore, erythrocyte GSH content has been shown to increase significantly after 20 weeks of physical training in previously sedentary men (122). Blood GSH concentration has been reported to be higher in trained runners compared with sedentary subjects, and it appears to be elevated with increased running distance (121).

GSH Deficiency and Supplementation

The physiologic role of GSH is best illustrated when tissues deprived of GSH are subjected to an oxidative challenge. Several chemical agents known to deplete tissue GSH were shown to disturb GSH homeostasis during exercise. Kramer and associates (123) found that rats injected with diethylmaleate, a GSH conjugater, 2 hours before exercise showed a significant impairment of swimming performance. Diethylmaleate treatment in the diaphragm muscle was shown to be associated with a significant reduction of maximal tetanic tension and twitch tension (124).

A more established procedure to deplete tissue GSH is through the administration of L-buthionine SR-sulfoximine (BSO), an irreversible inhibitor of GCS (125,126). Rats receiving BSO by i.p. injections and exercising until exhaustion decreased total glutathione contents in the liver, lung, blood, and plasma by ~50%, and in skeletal muscle and heart by 80% to 90% (91). Exhaustive exercise increased the GSSG/GSH ratio in the skeletal muscle, especially in the GSH-depleted animals (127). Furthermore, a 50% decrease of endurance time was observed in the GSH-depleted rats, suggesting that GSH plays an essential role in maintaining exercise performance during high-intensity treadmill running (127). GSH depletion also was shown to be associated with a significant increase in lipid peroxidation in the heart, skeletal muscles, and plasma of rats. Liver MDA content was found to correlate inversely with GSH concentration in both the GSH-adequate and depleted mice (91). GSH depletion was not found to affect endurance performance during the moderate swim exercise, however.

Supplementation of GSH and GSH analogues has been used for therapeutic purposes such as drug-induced oxidative stress and radiation therapy (126). However, access of the target tissues to exogenously supplemented GSH is limited by GGT activity, which in most tissues, except for the kidneys, is quite low (57). Furthermore, GCS, the rate-limiting enzyme of GSH synthesis, is strongly feedback inhibited by GSH. To overcome these limitations, cysteine analogues such as L-2-oxothiazolidine-4-carboxylate or *N*-acetylcysteine (NAC) have been used to promote GSH synthesis. GSH monoester also was used to transport GSH directly into the cell (126). Human subjects receiving 400 mg NAC/day for 2 days with an additional 800 mg before exercise showed an attenuated blood GSSG response during a maximal treadmill test (128). However, the sparing effect of NAC on the exercise-induced blood GSH oxidation in humans was not so pronounced as that in rats. Running performance of the animals was not different between the NAC-supplemented and control groups. Oral supplementation of NAC and GSH was found to be effective in preventing the increase in GSSG levels during exercise in rats (129). NAC supplementation by intravenous bolus attenuated the rate of diaphragmatic fatigue during repetitive isometric contraction (130). None of the mentioned studies demonstrated an increase in tissue or blood GSH with NAC administration, however. Recently Reid and colleagues (131) showed that NAC administration improved muscle contractile functions and reduced low-frequency fatigue in humans.

Supplementation of free GSH generated limited

promise in increasing tissue GSH contents. Although repeated injection of GSH increased plasma and kidney GSH significantly, it did not lead to a desirable increase in GSH content in skeletal muscle, heart, liver, or lung (127,132). Exercise endurance was reported to be unchanged with GSH supplementation (127). Novelli and co-workers (133), however, showed that acute GSH injection doubled swimming endurance time in mice. Total swimming time in that study was only 2 to 3 minutes, and tissue GSH levels were not measured; therefore it is difficult to evaluate the contribution of GSH to endurance performance. Leeuwenburgh and Ji (132) also reported a benefit of acute GSH supplementation on exercise performance in mice. Intraperitoneal injection of GSH and GSH ethyl ester (6 mmol/kg) increased swimming endurance from 4 to 6 hours, albeit with no change in tissue GSH levels observed. Oral administration of GSH was found effective in preventing an exercise-induced oxidation of GSH to GSSG (129). Thus supplementing GSH during exercise appears to hold some promise, but the mechanisms of action and desirable protocols remain to be examined in future studies.

Antioxidant Vitamins

Vitamins E, C, and β-carotene play a critical role in protecting the cells from ROS-induced oxidative stress (5,6,107). Because humans cannot synthesize these vital antioxidants, they are dependent exclusively on dietary intake. Recent research suggests that several other low-molecular-weight compounds, such as ubiquinone, uric acid, and α-lipoic acid, also serve important antioxidant functions (6). There is an abundance of evidence that tissue content of certain antioxidant vitamins (e.g., vitamin E) are decreased as a result of acute and chronic exercise, narrowing their protective margin against ROS. Ironically, exercise tends to alter the dietary habits of an individual, thus affecting antioxidant intake. So far, there are no clear guidelines regarding optimal dietary intake of antioxidants for physically active individuals beyond the Recommended Dietary Allowance (RDA).

Vitamin E

α-Tocopherol is the most well-known lipid-soluble free radical scavenger. Its unique location in the cell membrane enhances its efficiency to quench free radicals originating from the mitochondrial inner membrane and other biomembranes (107). The importance of vitamin E during exercise is best illustrated in studies in which animals are depleted of tissue vitamin E by feeding a vitamin E–deficient diet beginning at an early stage of life. Davies and colleagues (15) found that vitamin E deficiency exacerbated muscle and liver free radical production and enhanced lipid peroxidation and mitochondrial dysfunction in exhaustively exercised rats. Endurance performance also was reported to decrease in rats fed a vitamin E–deficient diet (15,133a). Vitamin E deficiency has been shown to enhance lipid peroxidation, disturb GSH/GSSG redox status, and cause early fatigue in the diaphragm muscle during resistance breathing in rats (124).

Skeletal muscle contains approximately 30 to 50 nmol of vitamin E per gram of wet weight, with considerable differences between muscle-fiber types, whereas the concentration of vitamin E in the heart and liver amounts to 60 to 70 nmol/g (134,135). Although an acute bout of exercise does not seem to affect vitamin E content in tissues significantly, its concentration has been shown to decrease in a number of tissues, such as skeletal muscle, liver, and heart, in rats after endurance training (135–137). More dramatic changes were observed when tissue vitamin E levels were expressed per unit of mitochondrial ubiquinone content (134). The reduction of mitochondrial vitamin E after training probably reflects the increased free radicals production at the ETC on the mitochondrial inner membrane.

Dietary supplementation of vitamin E may increase tissue resistance to exercise-induced lipid peroxidation. Kanter and co-workers (32) showed that daily supplementation of a vitamin mixture containing 600 mg α-tocopherol for 6 weeks significantly decreased levels of serum MDA and expired pentane both at rest and after 30 minutes of treadmill exercise at 60% and 90% $\dot{V}O_2$max. Goldfarb and colleagues (138) reported that rats supplemented with 250 IU vitamin E/kg diet for 5 weeks had lower TBARS and lipid peroxide levels in plasma and leg muscles than did controls after 1 hour treadmill exercise. Sumida and co-workers (139) also demonstrated a protective effect of vitamin E supplementation (300 mg/day) in reducing serum MDA concentration and enzyme markers of tissue damage during exercise. Kumar and associates (18) showed that dietary supplementation of vitamin E for 60 days abolished exercise-induced free radical production and lipid peroxidation in rat myocardium. These findings support the recommendation by Packer (107) that humans living an active lifestyle consider increasing daily dietary vitamin E intake. Despite the aforementioned beneficial effects, however, no study demonstrated improved physical performance as a result of vitamin E supplementation (8,140).

Vitamin C

Ascorbic acid is a water-soluble antioxidant existing in the cytosol and extracellular fluid. Its chemical properties allow it to interact directly with $O_2^{\cdot-}$ and $\cdot OH$, thus functioning as an antioxidant (141). It also can reduce oxidized vitamin E, wherein ascorbate is oxidized to dihydroascorbate (DHA). DHA may be reduced by a GSH and/or dihydrolipoic acid redox cycle (5,142). Vitamin C is especially efficient in scavenging free radicals formed in the aqueous phase, such as plasma, thus preventing damage to erythrocyte membrane (141). The importance of vitamin C in protecting against exercise-induced oxidative stress is not well established, partly because most mammalian species synthesize vitamin C, making a deficiency study rather difficult. Vitamin C also performs numerous functions not related to that of an antioxidant (143). By reducing dietary vitamin C content to 10% of the normal values (0.2 g/kg), Packer and colleagues (144) demonstrated that myocardial capacity to oxidize pyruvate, 2-oxoglutarate, and succinate was significantly reduced in guinea pigs (which cannot synthesize vitamin C). As a result, running time to exhaustion was significantly shortened in vitamin C–deficient animals.

It is well known that given at high doses, vitamin C can behave as a prooxidant (6). This is because ascorbate reacts with transition metal irons to form ROS, including $^{\cdot}OH$ (5,6). Thus it is interesting to note that in the aforementioned study, a group of guinea pigs supplemented with twice the normal amount of vitamin C in the diet also exhibited similar metabolic defects in the heart and early fatigue during prolonged exercise, possibly due to oxidative stress caused by excessive vitamin C. Because one of the primary antioxidant functions of vitamin C is to recycle vitamin E, Gohil and coworkers (133) investigated the effect of dietary vitamin C supplementation on vitamin E–deficient rats during training. Vitamin C could not prevent a decrease of endurance time and mitochondrial dysfunction caused by vitamin E deficiency.

The effect of dietary supplementation of vitamin C has not been well studied in human subjects involved in physical exercise. Although some authors claimed that large doses of vitamin C intake reduced fatigue and muscle damage, no specific oxidative stress markers were measured; therefore it is difficult to determine whether the observed benefits were related to the antioxidant functions of vitamin C (140).

Ubiquinone (Q10)

As an electron carrier, ubiquinone is rich in the mitochondrial inner membrane. An early study by Gohil and associates (134) showed that training could significantly increase Q_{10} content in skeletal muscle and adipose tissues. Reduced Q_{10} acts as an antioxidant *in vitro,* and its role as an antioxidant *in vivo* has been proposed (145). Tissue slices from rats fed a high-Q_{10} diet demonstrated more resistance to hydroperoxide-induced lipid peroxidation than those from rats fed a control diet (146). These antioxidant properties prompted several studies using dietary supplementation of Q_{10} to evaluate its protective function during exercise. For example, Shimomura and associates (147) reported that Q_{10} administration attenuated muscle creatine kinase and lactate dehydrogenase release in rats caused by downhill running. These studies did not clearly establish the role of Q_{10} as an antioxidant *in vivo*, however. Furthermore, few data are available regarding the interaction of Q_{10} with other antioxidants during exercise.

Uric Acid

Uric acid is the end product of purine metabolism, appearing in high concentrations in the circulation after heavy muscular contraction and in the effluent of ischemia–reperfused organs (37). This results from an insufficient intramuscular ATP supply, causing excessive adenine nucleotide degradation and accumulation of hypoxanthine and xanthine (38–41). These purine metabolites are released from the muscle into the blood, and a portion of these compounds presumably is converted to uric acid by XO located in the endothelial cells of the blood vessels. Uric acid's function as a potential antioxidant has been emphasized (6). Besides being an excellent scavenger of $^{\cdot}OH$, uric acid may preserve plasma ascorbic acid under oxidative stress (148). Because an acute bout of exercise has been shown to increase blood uric acid concentrations in human subjects (41,42), it is not unreasonable to speculate that the increased uric acid may serve as one of the protectants again blood-borne sources of ROS, thus reducing oxidative stress to erythrocytes and other tissues. However, there currently are no data to substantiate the antioxidant function of ubiquinone in exercise.

α-Lipoic Acid

α-Lipoic acid is a well-known cofactor for the oxidative decarboxylation catalyzed by ketoacid dehydrogenases. Recently a great deal of attention has been given to the antioxidant potential of its reduced form, dihydrolipoic acid (DHLA). Both α-lipoic acid and DHLA exhibited specific scavenging capacity for a variety of free radicals such as $O_2^{\cdot-}$, $^{\cdot}OH$, $^1O_2$, peroxyl radical, and hypochlorous radical (149). They are chelators of transition metal ions, thereby preventing damaging free radical chain reactions. DHLA is capable of regenerating other antioxidants such as vitamin E and vitamin C from their radical forms, either directly or indirectly via the GSH-GSSG redox cycle. Thus DHLA prevents vitamins E and C deficiencies, possibly through increasing intracellular GSH levels (149). Perhaps the most intriguing and complex biologic function of DHLA is its proposed effect on gene expression of antioxidant enzymes via the regulation of nuclear factor NF-κB. DHLA was shown to influence both the dissociation of the inhibitory subunit IκB from NF-κB complex and the binding of the activated NF-κB (p50 and p65) to DNA. The overall effect could be either stimulatory or inhibitory, depending on the redox state of the cell and the relative concentrations of α-lipoic acid and DHLA (9,149).

β-Carotene

β-Carotene, a major carotenoid precursor of vitamin A, has recently received broad attention as an antioxidant (5,6). Although its best-defined antioxidant function is to quench singlet oxygen, it may also be involved in other free radical reactions (150). β-Carotene has an inhibitory effect on lipid peroxidation initiated by oxygen- or carbon-centered free radicals (6). There is little information about its efficacy in protecting against exercise-induced lipid peroxidation or other forms of oxidative tissue damage, however (140).

CONCLUSION

Production of ROS is a normal process in aerobic life. Both direct and indirect evidence suggests that heavy physical exercise can enhance free radical production in skeletal muscle and other tissues that increase their metabolic rate. Although increased oxygen flux through the mitochondrial ETC is considered the main source of ROS, other pathways of ROS generation such as xanthine oxidase and polymorphoneutrophil also may be activated during or after exercise. Furthermore, these sources may be additive, escalating ROS generation.

Cellular antioxidant systems play a vital role in protecting the tissues from ROS-induced oxidative damage. Acute and chronic exercise may perturb antioxidant homeostasis, however. The impact of exercise on antioxidant systems depends on the biochemical properties and the intrinsic levels of each antioxidant. SOD, GPX, and GSH have demonstrated considerable adaptability to exercise-induced oxidative stress, whereas vitamin E appears to narrow its protective margin because of increased interaction with free radicals. These different responses to acute and chronic exercise may have important implications in considering pharmacologic intervention with and/or dietary supplementation of antioxidants.

ACKNOWLEDGMENT

I wish to thank the American Heart Association National Center and Wisconsin Affiliate, the University of Wisconsin Alumni Foundation, and the Vilas Trust Fund for their financial support for the work presented in the chapter.

REFERENCES

1. Jenkins RR. Free radical chemistry: relationship to exercise. *Sport Med* 1988;5:156–170.
2. Jenkins RR. Exercise, oxidative stress and antioxidant: a review. *Int J Sports Nutr* 1993;3:356–375.
3. Meydani M, Evans WJ. Free radicals, exercise, and aging. In: Yu BP, ed. *Free radicals in aging.* Boca Raton: CRC Press, 1993:183–204.
4. Chance B, Sies CH, Boveris A. Hydroperoxide metabolism in mammalian organs. *Physiol Rev* 1979;59:527–605.
5. Halliwell B, Gutteridge JMC. *Free radicals in biology and medicine.* 2nd ed. Oxford: Clarendon Press, 1989.
6. Yu BP. Cellular defenses against damage from reactive oxygen species. *Physiol Rev* 1994;74:139–162.
7. Deneke SM, Fanburg BL. Regulation of cellular glutathione. *Am J Physiol* 1989;257:L163–L173.
8. Ji LL. Exercise and oxidative stress: role of the cellular antioxidant systems In: Holloszy JO, ed. *Exercise sport science reviews.* Baltimore: Williams & Wilkins, 1995:135–166.
9. Sen CK. Oxidants and antioxidants in exercise. *J Appl Physiol* 1995;79:675–686.
10. Reid MB, Haack KE, Franchek KM, Valberg PA, Kobzik L, West MS. Reactive oxygen in skeletal muscle I: intracellular kinetics and fatigue in vitro. *J Appl Physiol* 1992;73:1797–1804.
11. Cannon JG, Blumberg JB. Acute phase immune responses in exercise. In: Sen CK, Packer L, Hanninen O, eds. *Exercise and oxygen toxicity.* New York: Elsevier Science, 1994:447–479.
12. Ames BN, Shigenaga MK, Hagen TM. Mitochondrial decay in aging. *Biochim Biophys Acta* 1995;1271:165–170.
13. Harman D. Aging: a theory based on free radical and radiation chemistry. *J Gerontol* 1956;11:298–300.
14. Dillard CJ, Litov RE, Savin WM, Dumclin EE, Tapple AL. Effect of exercise, vitamin E, and ozone on pulmonary function and lipid peroxidation. *J Appl Physiol* 1978;45:927–932.
15. Davies KJA, Quintanilha TA, Brooks GA, Packer L. Free radical and tissue damage produced by exercise. *Res Biochem Biophys Commun* 1982;107:1198–1205.
16. Salminen A, Vihko V. Endurance training reduces the susceptibility of mouse skeletal muscle to lipid peroxidation in vitro. *Acta Physiol Scand* 1983;117:109–113.
17. Jackson MJ, Edwards RHT, Symons MCR. Electron spin resonance studies of intact mammalian skeletal muscle. *Biochim Biophys Acta* 1985;847:185–190.
18. Kumar CT, Reddy VK, Prasad M, Thyagaraju K, Reddanna P. Dietary supplementation of vitamin E protects heart tissue from exercise-induced oxidative stress. *Mol Cell Biochem* 1992; 111:109–115.
19. Somani SM, Arroyo CM. Exercise training generates ascorbate free radical in rat heart. *Ind J Physiol Pharmacol* 1995; 39:323–329.
20. Reid MB, Stokic DS, Koch SM, Khawli FA, Lois AA. *N*-acetylcysteine inhibits muscle fatigue in humans. *J Clin Invest* 1994;94:2468–2474.
21. Bejma J, Ji LL. Aging and acute exercise enhance free radical generation in rat skeletal muscle. *J Appl Physiol* 1999;87: 465–470.
22. Ji LL, Bejma J, Ramires P, Donahue C. Free radical generation and oxidative stress in the heart are intensified during aging and exhaustive exercise. *Med Sci Sports Exerc* 1998;30:S322.
23. Boveris A, Chance B. The mitochondrial generation of hydrogen peroxide: general properties and effect of hyperbaric oxygen. *Biochem J* 1973;134:707–716.
24. Salo DC, Donovan CM, Davies KJA. HSP70 and other possible heat shock or oxidative stress proteins are induced in skeletal muscle, heart, and liver during exercise. *Free Radic Biol Med* 1991;11:239–246.
25. Ji LL, Mitchell EW. Effects of Adriamycin on heart mitochondrial function in rested and exercised rats. *Biochem Pharmacol* 1994;47:877–885.
26. Ji LL, Stratman FW, Lardy HA. Enzymatic down regulation with exercise in rat skeletal muscle. *Arch Biochem Biophys* 1988;263:137–149.
27. Chandwaney R, Leichtweis S, Leeuwenburgh C, Ji LL. Oxidative stress and mitochondrial function in skeletal muscle: Effects of aging and exercise training. *Age* 1998;21:109–117.
28. Leichtweis S, Leeuwenburgh C, Fiebig R, Parmelee D, Yu XX,

Ji LL. Rigorous swim training impairs mitochondrial function in post-ischemic rat heart. *Acta Physiol Scand* 1997;160:139–148.
29. Higuchi M, Cartier LJ, Chen M, Holloszy JO. Superoxide dismutase and catalase in skeletal muscle: adaptive response to exercise. *J Gerontol* 1985;40:281–286.
30. Ji LL, Stratman FW, Lardy HA. Antioxidant enzyme systems in rat liver, and skeletal muscle: influences of selenium deficiency, chronic training and acute exercise. *Arch Biochem Biophys* 1988;263:150–160.
31. Alessio HM, Goldfarb AH. MDA content increases in fast- and slow-twitch skeletal muscle with intensity of exercise in a rat. *Am J Physiol* 1988;255:C874–877.
32. Kanter MM, Nolte LA, Holloszy, JO. Effect of an antioxidant vitamin mixture on lipid peroxidation at rest and postexercise. *J Appl Physiol* 1993;74:965–969.
33. Ji LL, Fu RG, Mitchell E. Glutathione and antioxidant enzyme in skeletal muscle: effect of fiber type and exercise intensity. *J Appl Physiol* 1992;73:1854–1899.
34. Downey JM. Free radicals and their involvement during long-term myocardial ischemia-reperfusion. *Annu Rev Physiol* 1990; 52:487–504.
35. Kuppasamy P, Zweier JL. Characterization of free radical generation by xanthine oxidase: evidence for hydroxyl radical generation. *J Biol Chem* 1989;264:9880–9884.
36. Hearse DJ, Manning AS, Downey JM, Yellon DM. Xanthine oxidase: a critical mediator of myocardial injury during ischemia and reperfusion? *Acta Physiol Scand* 1986;548:65–78.
37. Sjodin B. Westing H, Apple S. Biochemical mechanisms for oxygen free radical formation during exercise. *Sports Med* 1990;10:236–254.
38. Hellsten Y. Xanthine dehydrogenase and purine metabolism in man: with special reference to exercise. *Acta Physiol Scand* 1994;621:1–73.
39. Norman B, Sovelli A, Kaijser L, Jansson E. ATP breakdown products in human muscle during prolonged exercise to exhaustion. *Clin Physiol* 1987;7:503–510.
40. Hellsten-Westing Y, Balsom PD, Norman B, Sjodin B. The effect of high-intensity training on purine metabolism in man. *Acta Physiol Scand* 1993;149:405–412.
41. Sahlin K, Ekberg K, Cizinsky S. Changes in plasma hypoxanthine and free radical markers during exercise in man. *Acta Physiol Scand* 1991;142:273–281.
42. Radak Z, Asano K, Inoue M, et al. Superoxide dismutase derivative reduces oxidative damage in skeletal muscle of rats during exhaustive exercise. *J Appl Physiol* 1995;79:129–135.
43. Radak Z, Asano K, Inoue M, et al. Superoxide dismutase derivative prevents oxidative damage in liver and kidney of rats induced by exhausting exercise. *Eur J Appl Physiol Occup Physiol* 1996;72:189–194.
44. Rasanen LA, Wiitanen PAS, Lilius EM, Hyyppa S, Poso AR. Accumulation of uric acid in plasma after repeated bouts of exercise in the horse. *Comp Biochem Physiol* 1996;114B: 139–144.
45. Hellsten Y, Hansson HA, Johnson L, Frandsen U, Sjodin B. Increased expression of xanthine oxidase acid insulinlike growth factor (IGF-1) immunoreactivity in skeletal muscle after strenuous exercise in humans. *Acta Physiol Scand* 1996;157:191–197.
46. Pyne DB. Regulation of neutrophil function during exercise. *Sports Med* 1994;17:245–258.
47. Petrone WF, English DK, Wong K, McCord JM. Free radicals and inflammation: superoxide-dependent activation of a neutrophil chemotactic factor in plasma. *Proc Natl Acad Sci USA* 1980;77:1159–1163.
48. Camus G, Deby-Dupont G, Duchateau J, Deby C, Pincemail J, Lamy M. Are similar inflammatory factors involved in strenuous exercise and sepsis? *Intens Care Med* 1994;20:602–610.
49. Meydani M, Evans W, Andelman G, et al. Antioxidant response to exercise-induced oxidative stress and protection by vitamin E. *Ann N Y Acad Sci* 1992;669:363–364.
50. Hack V, Strobel G, Rau JP, Weicker H. The effect of maximal exercise on the activity of neutrophil granulocytes in highly trained athletes in a moderate training period. *Eur J Appl Physiol Occ Physiol* 1992;65:520–524.
51. Smith JA, Gray AB, Pyne DB, Baker MS, Telford RD, Weidemann MJ. Moderate exercise triggers both priming and activation of neutrophil subpopulations. *Am J Physiol* 1996;39:R838–R845.
52. Godin DV, Wohaieb SA. Nutritional deficiency, starvation, and tissue antioxidant status. *Free Radic Biol Med* 1988;5:165–176.
53. Kim JD, McCarter RJM, Yu BP. Influence of age, exercise, and dietary restriction on oxidative stress in rats. *Aging Clin Exp Res* 1996;8:123–129.
54. Somani S, Kamimori GH. The effects of exercise on absorption, distribution, metabolism, excretion, and pharmacokinetics of drugs, In: Somani S, ed. *Pharmacology in exercise and sports.* New York: CRC Press, 1996:1–38.
55. Pincemail J, Camus G, Roesgen A, et al. Exercise induces pentane production and neutrophil activation in humans: effect of propranolol. *Eur J Appl Physiol Occ Physiol* 1990;61:319–322.
56. Simpson PJ, Lucchesi BR. Free radicals and myocardial ischemia and reperfusion injury. *J Lab Clin Med* 1987;19:1195–1206.
57. Meister A, Anderson ME. Glutathione. *Annu Rev Biochem* 1983;52:711–760.
58. Harris ED. Regulation of antioxidant enzymes. *FASEB J* 1992;6:2675–2683.
59. Fridovich I. Superoxide radical and superoxide dismutases. *Annu Rev Biochem* 1995;64:97–112.
60. Ohno H, Suzuki K, Fujii J, et al. Superoxide dismutases in exercise and disease. In: Sen CK, Packer L, Hanninen O, eds. *Exercise and oxygen toxicity.* New York: Elsevier Science, 1994:127–161.
61. Blum J, Fridovich, I. Inactivation of glutathione peroxidase by superoxide radical. *Arch Biochem Biophys* 1985;240:500–508.
62. Fridovich I. Quantitation of superoxide dismutase. In: Greenwald RA, ed. *Handbook of methods for oxygen free radical research.* Boca Raton: CRC Press, 1985:211–215.
63. Gorecki M, Beck Y, Hartman JR, et al. Recombinant human superoxide dismutases: production and potential therapeutical uses. *Free Radic Res Commun* 1991;12,13:401–410.
64. Zhang N. Characterization of the 5′-flanking region of the human Mn SOD gene. *Biochem Biophys Res Commun* 1996;220: 171–180.
65. Whitsett JA, Clark JC, Wispe JR, Pryhuber GS. Effects of TNF-α and phorbol ester on human surfactant protein and Mn SOD gene transcription *in vitro. Am J Physiol* 1992;262:688–693.
66. Visner GA, Dougall WC, Wilson JM, Burr IM, Nick HS. Regulation of manganese superoxide dismutase by lipopolysaccharide, interleukin-1, and tumor necrosis factor. *J Biol Chem* 1990; 265:2856–2864.
67. Das KC, Lewis-Molock Y, White CW. Thiol modulation of TNF and IL-1 induced Mn SOD gene expression and activation of NF-κB. *Mol Cell Biochem* 1995;148:45–57.
68. Cowan DB, Weisel RD, Williams, WG, Mickle DAG. The regulation of glutathione peroxidase gene expression by oxygen tension in cultured human cardiomyocytes. *J Cell Cardiol* 1992;24:423–433.
69. Aebi H. 1984. Catalase. *Methods Enzymol* 1984;105:121–126,
70. Luhtala TA, Roecker EB, Pugh T, Feuers RJ, Weindruch R. Dietary restriction attenuates age-related increases in rat skeletal muscle antioxidant enzyme activities. *J Gerontol* 1994;49:B321–B328.
71. Holmes RS, Duley JA. Biochemical and genetic studies of peroxisomal multiple enzyme systems: alpha-hydroxyacid oxidase and catalase. In: Markert DL, ed. *Isozymes I. Molecular structure.* New York: Academic Press, 1975:191–211.
72. Holmes RS, Master CJ. Epigenetic interconversions of the multiple forms of mouse liver catalase. *FEBS Lett* 1970;11:45–48.
73. Dhaunsi G, Singh I, Orak JK, Kingh AK. Antioxidant enzymes in ciprofibrate-induced oxidative stress. *Carcinogen* 1994;15: 1923–1930.
74. Yuan HT, Bingle CD, Kelly FJ. Differential patterns of antioxidant enzyme mRHA expression in guinea pig lung and liver during development. *Biochim Biophys Acta* 1996;1305:163–171.
75. Flohe L. Glutathione peroxidase brought into focus. In: Pryor W, ed. *Free radical in biology and medicine.* Vol 5. New York: Academic Press, 1982:223–253.
76. Habig WH, Pabst JB, Jakoby WB. Glutathione *S*-transferases. *J Biol Chem* 1984;249:7130–7139.
77. Leeuwenburgh C, Hollander J, Leichtweis S, Fiebig R, Gore M, Ji LL. Adaptations of glutathione antioxidant system to endurance

training are tissue and muscle fiber specific. *Am J Physiol* 1997;272:R363–R369.
78. Moscow JA, Morrow CS, He R, Mullenbach GT, Cowan KH. Structure and function of the 5′-flanking sequence of the human cytosolic selenium-dependent glutathione peroxidase gene (*hgpx1*). *J Biol Chem* 1992;267:5949–5958.
79. Reed D. Regulation of reductive processes by glutathione. *Biochem Pharmacol* 1986;35:7–13.
80. Oliver CN, Ahn B, Moerman EJ, Goldstein S, Stadtman ER. Age-related changes in oxidized proteins. *J Biol Chem* 1987;262:5488–5491.
81. Marin E, Kretzschmar M, Arokoski J, Hanninen O, Klinger W. Enzymes of glutathione synthesis in dog skeletal muscle and their response to training. *Acta Physiol Scand* 1993;147:369–373.
82. Lawler JM, Powers SK, Visser T, Van Dijk H, Korthuis MJ, Ji LL. Acute exercise and skeletal muscle antioxidant and metabolic enzymes: effect of fiber type and age. *Am J Physiol* 1993; 265:R1344–R1350.
83. Quintanilha AT, Packer L. Biology of vitamin E. In: Porter R, Whelan J, eds. *Ciba Foundation Symposium 101*. London: Pitman, 1983:56–59.
84. Quintanilha AT, Packer L, Davies JMS, Racanelli T, Davies JKA. Membrane effects of vitamin E deficiency: bioenergetics and surface charge density studies of skeletal muscle and liver mitochondria. *Ann N Y Acad Sci* 1982;399:32–47.
85. Lukaski H, Hoverson BS, Gallagher SK, Bolonchuck WW. Physical training and copper, iron, and zinc status of swimmers. *Am J Clin Nutr* 1990;51:1093–1099.
86. Mena P, Maynar M, Gutierrez JM, Maynar J, Timon JJ, Campillo JE. Erythrocyte free radical scavenger enzymes in bicycle professional racers: adaptation to training. *Int J Sports Med* 1991;12:563–566.
87. Ohno H, Sato Y, Yamashita K, et al. The effect of brief physical exercise on free radical scavenging enzyme systems in human red blood cells. *Can J Physiol Pharmacol* 1986;64:1263–1265.
88. Buczynski A, Kedziora J, Tkaczewski W, Wachowicz B. Effect of submaximal physical exercise on antioxidative protection of human blood platelets. *Int J Sports Med* 1991;12:52–54.
89. Ji LL. Antioxidant enzyme response to exercise and aging. *Med Sci Sports Exerc* 1993;25:225–231.
90. Brady PS, Brady LJ, Ullrey DE. Selenium, vitamin E and the response to swimming stress in rats. *J Nutr* 1979;109:1103–1109.
91. Leeuwenburgh C, Ji LL. Glutathione depletion in rested and exercised mice: biochemical consequence and adaptation. *Arch Biochem Biophys* 1995;316:941–949.
92. Vihko V, Salminen A, Rantamaki J. Oxidative lysosomal capacity in skeletal muscle of mice after endurance training. *Acta Physiol Scand* 1978;104:74–79.
93. Ji LL, Fu RG. Responses of glutathione system and antioxidant enzymes to exhaustive exercise and hydroperoxide. *J Appl Physiol* 1992;72:549–554.
94. Leeuwenburgh C, Ji LL. Glutathione regulation during exercise in unfed and refed rats. *J Nutr* 1996;126:1833–1843.
95. Oh-Ishi S, Kizaki T, Nagasawa I, et al. Effects of endurance training on superoxide dismutase activity, content, and mRNA expression in rat muscle. *Clin Exp Pharmacol Physiol* 1997; 24:326–332.
96. Quintanilha AT. The effect of physical exercise and/or vitamin E on tissue oxidative metabolism. *Biochem Soc Trans* 1984; 12:403–404.
97. Gore M, Fiebig R, Hollander J, Ji LL. Acute exercise alters mRNA abundance of antioxidant enzyme and nuclear factor B activation in skeletal muscle, heart and liver. *Med Sci Sports Exerc* 1997;29:229.
98. Jenkins RR. The role of superoxide dismutase and catalase in muscle fatigue. In: Knuttgen HG, Vogel JA, Poortmans J, eds. *Biochemistry of exercise.* Vol 13. Champaign: Human Kinetics Publishers, 1983:467–471.
99. Leeuwenburgh C, Fiebig R, Chandwaney R, Ji LL. Aging and exercise training in skeletal muscle: response of glutathione and antioxidant enzyme systems. *Am J Physiol* 1994;267:R439–R495.
100. Powers SK, Criswell D, Lawler J, et al. Influence of exercise intensity and duration on antioxidant enzyme activity in skeletal muscle differing in fiber type. *Am J Physiol* 1994;266:R375–R380.
101. Sen CK, Marin E, Kretzschmar M, Hanninen O. Skeletal muscle and liver glutathione homeostasis in response to training, exercise and immobilization. *J Appl Physiol* 1992;73:1265–1272.
102. Laughlin MH, Simpson T, Sexton WL, Brown OR, Smith JK, Korthuis RJ. Skeletal muscle oxidative capacity, antioxidant enzymes, and exercise training. *J Appl Physiol* 1990;68:2337–2343.
103. Tiidus PM, Pushkarenko J, Houston ME. Lack of antioxidant adaptation to short-term aerobic training in human muscle. *Am J Physiol* 1996;271:R832–R836.
104. Hollander J, Gore M, Fiebig R, Bejma J, Ookawara T, Ohno H, Ji LL. Superoxide dismutase gene expression in skeletal muscle-fiber-specific adaptation to endurance training. *Am J Physiol* 1999 (*in press*).
105. Nanji AA, Griniuviene B, Sadrzadeh SMH, Levitsky S, McCully JD. Effect of type of dietary fat and ethanol on antioxidant enzyme mRNA induction in rat liver. *J Lipid Res* 1995;36: 736–744.
106. Remacle J, Lambert D, Raes M, Pigeolet E, Michiels C, Toussaint O. Importance of various antioxidant enzymes for cell stability: Confrontation between theoretical and experimental data. *Biochem J.* 1992;286:41–46.
107. Packer L. Protective role of vitamin E in biological systems. *Am J Clin Nutr* 1991;53:1050S–1055S.
108. Ji LL, Leeuwenburgh C. Glutathione and exercise In: Somani S, ed. *Pharmacology in exercise and sports.* New York: CRC Press, 1996:97–123.
109. Lu SC, Ge JL, Kulenkamp J, Kaplowitz N. Insulin and glucocorticoid dependence of hepatic-glutamylcysteine synthetase and glutathione synthesis in the rat. *J Clin Invest* 1992;90:260.
110. Lu SC, Kulenkamp J, Garcia-Ruiz C, Kaplowitz N. Hormone-mediated down-regulation of hepatic glutathione synthesis in the rat, *J Clin Invest* 1991;88:260.
111. Lu SC, Garcia-Ruiz C, Kuhlenkamp J, Ookhtens M, Salas-Prato M, Kaplowitz N. Hormonal regulation of glutathione efflux. *J Biol Chem* 1990;265:16088–16095.
112. Sies H, Graf P. Hepatic thiol and glutathione efflux under the influence of vasopressin, phenylephrine and adrenaline. *Biochem J* 1985;226:545–549.
113. Griffiths OW, Meister A. Glutathione: interorgan translocation, turnover, and metabolism. *Proc Natl Acad Sci USA* 1979;76: 5606–5610.
114. Kretzschmar M, Muller D. Aging, training and exercise: a review of effects of plasma glutathione and lipid peroxidation. *Sports Med* 1993;15:196–209.
115. Asuncion JGD, Millan A, Pla R, et al. Mitochondrial glutathione oxidation correlates with age-associated oxidative damage to mitochondrial DNA. *FASEB J* 1996;10:333–338.
116. Vina J, Sastre J, Asensi M, Packer L. Assay of blood glutathione oxidation during physical exercise. *Methods Enzymol* 1995;251: 237–243.
117. Lew H, Pyke S, Quintanilha A. Change in the glutathione status of plasma, liver and muscle following exhaustive exercise in rats. *FEBS Lett* 1985;185:262–266.
118. Corbucci GG, Montaanari G, Cooper MB, Jones DA, Edards RHT. The effect of exertion of mitochondrial oxidative capacity and on some antioxidant mechanisms in muscle from marathon runners. *Int J Sports Med* 1984;5:135S.
119. Ji LL, Katz A, Fu RG, Parchert M, Spencer M. Alteration of blood glutathione status during exercise: the effect of carbohydrate supplementation. *J Appl Physiol* 1993:74:788–792.
120. Kretzschmar M, Pfeifer U, Machnik G, Klinger W. Influence of age, training and acute physical exercise on plasma glutathione and lipid peroxidation in man. *Int J Sports Med* 1991;12:218–222.
121. Robertson JD, Maughan RJ, Duthie GG, Morrice PC. Increased blood antioxidant systems of runners in response to training. *Clin Sci* 1991;80:611–618.
122. Evelo CTA, Palmen NG, Artur Y, Janssen GME. Changes in blood glutathione concentrations, and in erythrocyte glutathione reductase and glutathione *S*-transferase activity after running training and after participation in contests. *Eur J Appl Physiol* 1992;64:354–358.
123. Kramer K, Dijkstra H, Bast A. Control of physical exercise of rats in a swimming basin. *Physiol Behav* 1993;53:271.

124. Anzueto A, Andrade FH, Maxwell LC, et al. Diaphragmatic function after resistive breathing in vitamin E-deficient rats. *J Appl Physiol* 1993;74:267–271.
125. Martensson J, Meister A. Mitochondrial damage in muscle occurs after marked depletion of glutathione and is prevented by giving glutathione monoester. *Proc Natl Acad Sci USA* 1989;86: 471–475.
126. Meister A. Glutathione deficiency produced by inhibition of its synthesis, and its reversal: application in research and therapy. *Pharmacol Ther* 1991;51:155–194.
127. Sen CK, Atalay M, Hanninen O. Exercise-induced oxidative stress: glutathione supplementation and deficiency. *J Appl Physiol* 1994;77:2177–2187.
128. Sen CK, Rankinen T, Vaisanen S, Rauramaa R. Oxidative stress following human exercise: effect of *N*-acetylcysteine supplementation. *J Appl Physiol* 1994;76:2570–2577.
129. Sastre J, Asensi M, Gasco E, et al. Exhaustive physical exercise causes oxidation of glutathione status in blood: prevention by antioxidant administration. *Am J Physiol* 1992;263:R992–R995.
130. Shindoh C, DiMarco A, Thomas P, et al. Effect of *N*-acetylcysteine on diaphragm fatigue. *J Appl Physiol* 1990;68:2107.
131. Reid MB, Stokic DS, Koch SM, Khawli FA, Lois AA. *N*-acetylcysteine inhibits muscle fatigue in humans. *J Clin Invest* 1994;94:2468–2474.
132. Leeuwenburgh C, Ji LL. Glutathione and glutathione ethyl ester supplementation of mice alter glutathione homeostasis during exercise. *J Nutr* 1998;128:2420–2426.
133. Novelli GP, Falsini S, Bracciotti G. Exogenous glutathione increases endurance to muscle effort in mice. *Pharmacol Res* 1991;23:149–155.
133a. Gohil K, Packer L, deLumen B, Brooks GA, Terblanche SE. Vitamin E deficiency and vitamin C supplementation: exercise and mitochondrial oxidation. *J Appl Physiol* 1986;60:1986–1991.
134. Gohil K, Rothfuss L, Lang J, Packer L. Effect of exercise training on tissue vitamin E and biquinone content. *J Appl Physiol* 1987;63:1638–1641.
135. Tiidus PM, Houston ME. Vitamin E status does not affect the responses to exercise training and acute exercise in female rats. *J Nutr* 1993;123:834–840.
136. Aikawa KM, Quintanilha AT, deLumen BO, Brooks GA, Packer L. Exercise endurance training alters vitamin E tissue levels and red blood cell hemolysis in rodents. *Biosci Rep* 1984;4:253–257.
137. Packer L, Almada AL, Rothfuss LM, Wilson DS. Modulation of tissue vitamin E levels by physical exercise. *Ann N Y Acad Sci* 1989;570:311–321.
138. Goldfarb AH, McIntosh MK, Boyer BT, Fatouros J. Vitamin E effects on indexes of lipid peroxidation in muscle from DHEA-treated and exercised rats. *J Appl Physiol* 1994;76:1630–1635.
139. Sumida S, Tanaka K, Kitao H. Nakadomo F. Exercise-induced lipid peroxidation and leakage of enzymes before and after vitamin E supplementation. *Int J Biochem* 1989;21:835–838.
140. Kanter MM. Free radicals and exercise: effects of nutritional antioxidant supplementation. In: Holloszy JO, ed. *Exercise and sport science reviews.* Baltimore: Williams & Wilkins, 1995: 375–398.
141. Beyer RE. The role of ascorbate in antioxidant protection of biomembranes: interaction with vitamin E and coenzyme Q. *J Bioenerg Biomembr* 1994;26:349–358.
142. Niki E, Kawakami A, Saito M, Yamamoto Y, Tsuchiya J, Kamiya Y. Effect of phytyl side chain of vitamin E on its antioxidant activity. *J Biol Chem* 1985;260:2191–2196.
143. Bendich A, Langseth L. The health effects of vitamin C supplementation: a review. *J Am Coll Nutr* 1995;14:124–136.
144. Packer L, Gohil K, DeLumen B, Terblanche SE. A comparative study on the effects of ascorbic acid deficiency and supplementation on endurance and mitochondrial oxidative capacities in various tissues of the guinea pig. *Comp Biochem Physiol* 1986;83B:235–240.
145. Beyer RE. The relative essentiality of the antioxidant function of coenzyme Q: the interactive role of DT-diaphorase. *Mol Aspects Med* 1994;15:S117–129.
146. Leibovitz B, Hu ML, Tappel AL. Dietary supplements of vitamin E, beta-carotene, coenzyme Q10 and selenium protect tissues against lipid peroxidation in rat tissue slices. *J Nutr* 1990;120: 97–104.
147. Shimomura Y, Suzuki M, Sugiyama S, Hanaki Y, Ozawa T. Protective effect of coenzyme Q10 on exercise-induced muscular injury. *Biochem Biophys Res Comm* 1991;176:349–355.
148. Sevanian A, Davies KJA, Hochstein P. Conservation of vitamin C by uric acid in the blood. *J Free Radic Biol Med* 1985;1:117–124.
149. Packer L, Witt EH, Tritschler HJ. α-Lipoic acid as a biological antioxidant. *Free Radic Biol Med* 1995;19:227–250.
150. Mascio PD, Murphy ME, Sies H. Antioxidant defense systems: the role of carotenoids, tocopherols, and thiols. *Am J Clin Nutr* 1991;53:194S–200S.

Exercise and Sport Science,
edited by William E. Garrett, Jr., and Donald T. Kirkendall.
Lippincott Williams & Wilkins, Philadelphia © 2000.

CHAPTER 22

Body Composition in Sports: Measurement and Applications for Weight Loss and Gain

Richard A. Boileau and Craig A. Horswill

A long-standing interest in the variability of the physiques of elite athletes is documented in several seminal reviews of the somatotype and anthropometry of Olympic and champion athletes (1–3). The body composition of athletes also has been of interest since the early 1940s, when Welhem and Behnke (4) first measured the body composition of All-American collegiate football players and demonstrated that these athletes were overweight by normal height and weight standards but were not obese.

The wide range of body size and composition characteristics among elite athletes demonstrates the potential importance of physique for high-level performance in many sports. Although it is recognized that the determinants of sports performance are complex, involving an array of biochemical, physiologic, psychological, and morphologic factors, body size and composition must clearly be considered as either enhancing or limiting both metabolic and mechanical aspects of performance. For example, a tall stature is typically needed for success in basketball, whereas a smaller stature is advantageous in gymnastics. Similarly, a large body mass is important for sumo wrestling, but a relatively low body weight is required for distance running. In addition to body-size considerations, the constitutional makeup of the body in terms of body-composition components also may be important. Excess body fat is detrimental to performance in most sports, but fat-free body mass (FFB) is normally associated with enhancing performance. Because of these generally well-documented associations, exercise and dietary regimens to reduce fat to a minimum and develop FFB mass to an optimum have become commonplace in most sports-training programs. The quest for an optimal body-composition performance profile has at times been overemphasized and inappropriate, however, compromising the health of athletes. This problem may particularly be exacerbated in sports in which appearance and weight-classification systems are considerations.

Perhaps in part due to the importance of the influence of body composition on performance, but also because of the potential health consequences of altering body composition, interest in the assessment and management of body composition among coaches, athletic trainers, and sports physicians has intensified. This chapter focuses on the influence of body size and composition on athletic performance, use of body-composition measurements to assess and monitor the body weight of athletes, and issues concerning rapid and long-term weight change in athletes.

INFLUENCE OF BODY COMPOSITION ON PHYSICAL PERFORMANCE

High-level performance appears to be enhanced by specific physique characteristics in terms of body size, composition, and structure, as seen in the profiles of athletes in various sports. Later in this chapter we will provide a compilation of sport-specific data on elite male and female athletes and we will discuss how to use such data to estimate an ideal weight. In this section, however, the focus is on the potential influences of body size and composition on performance in a generic sense, perhaps the better to understand sport-specific profiles of top performers in various sports. Body composition can be functionally divided into two components: FFB, includ-

R. A. Boileau: Departments of Kinesiology and Nutritional Sciences & Internal Medicine, University of Illinois, Urbana, Illinois 61801.

C. A. Horswill: Department of Research and Development, Gatorade Exercise Physiology Laboratory, The Quaker Oats Company, Barrington, Illinois 60010.

ing those tissues and components that are functionally involved in the production and conduction of force; and body fat. The influence of FFB and fat components is complex, having both negative and positive effects, depending on the type of physical tasks to be performed. For example, in running performance, fat represents dead weight that must be moved, whereas the FFB component includes the force-producing and conducting tissues (e.g., muscle). In swimming, in contrast to running, a certain amount of fat may have a positive influence on buoyancy; however, a very high relative FFB may have a negative influence, including decreased buoyancy, which may increase energy requirements to move the body in water.

In general, body fatness negatively influences performance both mechanically and metabolically in most physical tasks that require translocation of body weight. Mechanically, excess fatness is detrimental to performance in which acceleration of the body either horizontally or vertically is required, because it adds non–force-producing mass to total body weight. Because acceleration is proportional to the force but inversely proportional to the mass, excess body fatness at a given level of force application impedes change in velocity, an important component in many sports. However, a certain level of body fat appropriately positioned may be useful in sports in which absorbing force is important and when momentum is important, as in contact sports. Metabolically, however, excess fatness increases the metabolic cost of performing work in activities requiring movement of the total body mass. One would expect, then, that in most types of performance involving translocation of the body mass, a low relative fatness (%Fat) is advantageous from both mechanical and metabolic perspectives. This concept is demonstrated in the body-composition profiles of elite athletes in most sports.

Fat-free weight, on the other hand, tends to have a positive relation with physical performance. An excess of FFB mass may be a negative factor in selected sports, however. Certainly in activities in which force must be applied against external objects, a large FFB mass is often required, because force is generated in the skeletal muscle, which comprises 40% to 50% of the FFB mass. A large FFB mass may have a negative influence on performances requiring translocation of the body mass, because it, like fat, adds to the mass of the body, as in running, jumping, and agility events. Excess FFB mass also may be detrimental in certain types of activities in which the energy cost of the activity is important.

Several studies have documented these theoretical relations in both young and adult athletes. Cureton and colleagues (5) studied the association of several physical-performance items (e.g., pull-ups, sit-ups, shuttle run, standing broad jump, 50-yard dash, softball throw, and 600-yard run) with body-composition components in 49 prepubescent boys. A lower fat content, estimated by densitometry, was significantly associated with good performances in the pull-up, standing broad jump, 50-yard dash, and 600-yard run, and FFB was significantly correlated with power activities including the standing broad jump and softball throw. Teeple and co-workers (6), by using multiple regression analysis, demonstrated that physical performance can be more precisely predicted in children when fat and FFB are considered in addition to their age, height, and weight. Cureton and associates (7), by using a path-analysis model to study running performance in 196 boys and girls, found %Fat to have a negative and significant influence on distance-running performance as reflected in the 600-yard and 1-mile run times. McLeod and colleagues (8) reported on the association of body fatness and physical performance in 2342 male and 832 female high school athletes. Their data also demonstrated the negative influence of body fat on performance in an array of physical-performance tests. Data from our laboratory (9) on 374 boys and 121 girls found the FFB to be positively related to performance on the standing broad-jump test ($r = 0.65$) and grip strength ($r = 0.87$), but %Fat was negatively correlated with performances on the standing broad jump ($r = -0.33$) and 600-yard run time ($r = -0.38$). Although the significance of body composition is undeniable to performance in the young athlete, it is important that interventions not be imposed that would interrupt the normal course of growth and development simply to enhance performance.

In general, the relation of body composition to physical performance also is observed in adults (10), although most studies on adults have focused primarily on the influence of body fat on running performance. Studies showed that %Fat is significantly associated with poorer performances at distances ranging from 800 to 10,000 m (r values = 0.49 to 0.69) in trained runners (11,12). Another study conducted on trained male runners reported a correlation of 0.78 (13) between %Fat and time in the 2-mile run. In a novel experiment in part to assess the significance of the difference in body-fatness levels between trained male and female subjects, Cureton and Sparling (14) noted that when male subjects were externally weight loaded to off-set the difference in fat weight carried by their female counterparts, the difference between the female and male performance times was significantly reduced.

In summary, body size and composition are important factors determining one's performance ability. In general, body fat negatively influences athletic performances involving agility, speed, endurance, running, and jumping. On the other hand, the FFB is positively associated with and may be required for athletic activities in which force must be applied such as lifting, pushing, throwing, and blocking.

BODY-COMPOSITION ASSESSMENT

Body-composition assessment is an important aspect in the evaluation of health, physical fitness, and nutritional status. The conceptualization and measurement of human body composition received a major impetus in the 1940s and 1950s with pioneering work on whole-body chemical cadaver analysis (15–17) and the development of *in vivo* densitometric and hydrometric methods (18–21). This early work formed the basis of the classic two-component model, fat and FFB, as well as other conceptualizations of body composition (22) used with present methods.

Criterion Methods for Assessing Body Composition

Many *in vivo* body-composition methods have been used, including densitometry, hydrometry, body potassium, neutron-activation analysis, creatinine excretion and other muscle metabolites, basal metabolic rate, and anthropometry (23,24). In addition to the earlier established methods, new and emerging technologies have been developed such as bioelectric impedance (25) and total-body conductivity (26), dual x-ray absorptiometry (27), infra-red interactance (28), magnetic resonance imaging, and computed axial tomography (CAT) scanning (29). A recently published book, *Human Body Composition* (30), provides a comprehensive review of most of these methods. Because much of the past and present information on body composition of athletes is based on densitometry, however, and because most of the field/clinical techniques are validated and calibrated by densitometry, discussion will focus primarily on this method and a few other methods that can be applied outside of the research laboratory.

Densitometry

Body density (D_B) is the ratio of body weight to body volume. Total body volume is normally measured by hydrostatic weighing (31) with correction for pulmonary residual volume (32). A more recent technique for measuring body volume by air displacement is being evaluated (33). Body density measured as grams per cubic centimeter (g/cc) must be transformed into the components of fat and FFB to be effectively used.

Conceptually, total body density is a function of the additive densities of four components including fat, and those of the FFB consisting of water, mineral, and residual components. The residual component consists mostly of protein, and thus it is referred to as protein hereafter. Therefore, D_B can be represented by the proportions and densities of its parts as follows:

$$D_B = 1/(f/d_f + w/d_w + m/d_m + p/d_p) \quad [1]$$

The whole body mass is assumed to be equal to unity (one); thus the sum of the parts can be represented as fractions of the whole, accordingly: $1 = f + w + m + p$. The lower-case letters (f, w, m, p) represent the fractions of fat, water, mineral, and protein, respectively, and lower-case letter d with its subscripts indicates the densities of the individual components. This formulation is the basis of several densitometric models.

Among the densitometric body-composition paradigms, the two-component model, consisting of fat and FFB, is the most commonly used. Several equations have been developed based on both theoretic and empiric assumptions associated with the two-component model. To estimate %Fat from densitometry by using the two-component model, assumptions are made about the densities of both components based on adult cadaver data. Because fat is a solitary component, it is reasonable to assume that the density of fat, 0.900 g/cc, is somewhat constant. However, the assumption that the FFB, which consists of several components, is constant with regard to proportions of its respective components is less tenable, particularly during growth and aging. Moreover, there appears to be variability in the FFB component among racial groups, which is of considerable importance in the athletic population. Most of the body-composition literature on athletes is based on the Siri (21) equation, which was derived through the two-component model by assuming the constants for the density of fat (D_f) of 0.900 g/cc and the density of FFB (D_{FFB}) of 1.100 g/cc by using the following general equation:

$$\%Fat = 1/D_B[(D_f \times D_{FFB})/(D_{FFB} - D_f)] - [D_f/(D_{FFB} - D_f)] \times 100 \quad [2]$$

By using these constants for D_f and D_{FFB} in Eq. 2, the Siri equation (21) can be formulated as follows:

$$\%Fat = (4.95/D_B - 4.50) \times 100 \quad [3]$$

Fat-free body is calculated as:

$$FFB = \text{Body weight (BW)} - (\%Fat/100) \times BW \quad [4]$$

To use the most appropriate equation for estimating %Fat from D_B, the D_{FFB} representative of the group being assessed must be known to compute accurate body-composition estimates. Unfortunately, information on the D_{FFB} for age and racial groups is extremely sparse, and as yet no studies have defined the variability in D_{FFB} among athletic groups. Recent work in this regard has focused on measuring the D_{FFB} during various stages of growth and development. There appears to be consensus that the D_{FFB} changes at various stages of the growth process, and that specific equations are needed to adjust for changes in the D_{FFB} more accurately to estimate fat and FFB of children and adolescents. Several review articles have summarized the available data pertaining to variability in D_{FFB} during growth and development (34,35). The following equations have been proposed to account for the apparent growth-related changes in the D_{FFB} and are recommended for the adolescent athlete to estimate %Fat from body density (34):

$$\text{Boys aged 13 to 15 years: \%Fat} = (5.075/D_B - 4.639) \times 100 \quad [5]$$

$$\text{Girls aged 13 to 15 years: \%Fat} = (5.119/D_B - 4.688) \times 100 \quad [6]$$

$$\text{Boys aged 15 to 17 years: \%Fat} = (5.033/D_B - 4.592) \times 100 \quad [7]$$

$$\text{Girls aged 15 to 17 years: \%Fat} = (5.075/D_B - 4.639) \times 100 \quad [8]$$

The importance of using the appropriate equations for estimating %Fat from D_B is twofold. The estimation of target body weight at a recommended %Fat depends on an accurate estimation of the FFB. Moreover, the D_B method is the primary method for the calibration and validation of other more clinically useful methods including anthropometry, bioelectric impedance, and infra-red interactance. Thus development of equations for these clinical methods should use the most relevant equation for estimating body composition from D_B for the cohort being assessed.

Clinical Methods for Assessing Body Composition

Whereas densitometry generally offers better accuracy and precision, its application is restricted to a laboratory setting, is limited in availability, and depends on expensive technology. Additionally, it requires considerable subject cooperation and/or a lengthy measurement process. Methods that provide rapid, safe, inexpensive, accurate, and precise body-composition measurements can be useful for testing athletes in the clinical and field-testing settings. In this context, the three most frequently used methods are the body mass index (BMI), anthropometry, and bioelectric impedance analysis (BIA).

Body Mass Index

Although BMI cannot be technically classified as a body-composition measurement method, it has received widespread use with adults for clinical and epidemiologic assessments. The BMI requires measurement only of height (H) and weight (BW). It is defined as BW/H^2 and expressed as kg/m^2. The development of BMI norms from large data bases permits the classification of individuals into categories of underweight, normal weight, overweight, and obese. Use of the BMI has been criticized on grounds that the numerator, BW, is influenced not only by fat but also by the FFB. Indeed, it can be shown that most heavyweight athletes (e.g., weightlifters, football linemen, shot putters) are classified as overweight, if not as obese, by this index, when in fact their %Fat estimates based on body-density measurements are normal for their sport peer group. The same observation has been made for female basketball and volleyball players. Because most athletes have a higher FFB weight, largely because of increased muscle mass, the BMI is of little value in evaluating the athlete and is not recommended.

Anthropometry

Anthropometry, specifically measures of skinfold thickness and circumference, is the most frequently used clinical method to estimate the body composition of athletes. Like BMI, skinfolds are relatively easy and inexpensive to obtain. Standardization of skinfold sites and measurement techniques are described in the *Anthropometric Standardization Reference Manual* (36). Whereas skinfold measurements are relatively easy to obtain, the importance of developing a skillful measuring technique cannot be understated. In theory, subcutaneous fat is believed to make a major contribution to the prediction of total body fat because it composes about 50% of the total body fat, although in the athlete, a significantly lower portion of total body fat may be located subcutaneously. Normally the estimation of body composition from skinfolds, by using either a single site or a combination of sites, is based on the relation to and thereby the prediction of D_B and/or %Fat. The number of equations for estimating D_B from skinfold measures is almost limitless, perhaps because equations derived on one sample often cannot be effectively validated in another independent sample. There are, however, selected equations that have been recognized for broad applicability, have been cross-validated, and are considered generalized equations (37–39). Although these equation have not been developed specifically for athletes, Sinning and colleagues (40,41) found the Jackson and Pollock (38) equation for male subjects and the Jackson, Pollock, and Ward (39) equation for female subjects to be more precise than other equations when tested in both male and female athletic samples, respectively. The prediction errors associated with these equations for estimation of D_b range from 2% to 4% when expressed in terms of %Fat for both male and female subjects. In addition, Withers and colleagues developed and cross-validated generalized equations for male (42) and female (43) subjects in a variety of Australian athletes. These equations have prediction errors similar to those observed for the Jackson equations. Fewer anthropometric equations have generalized characteristics that can be applied to adolescent athletes. Heyward and Stolarczyk (44) recommended the equations of Forsyth and Sinning (45) for male adolescent athletes and those of Jackson and associates (39) for female adolescent athletes. The recommended equations for both adoles-

TABLE 22–1. *Skinfold equations for estimating body density of male and female athletes*

Gender (age)	Equation	Reference
Male (18–29 yr)	$D_B = 1.112 - 0.00043499\ (\Sigma\ 7\ SKF) + 0.00000055\ (\Sigma\ 7\ SKF)^2 - 0.00028826\ (age, yr)^a$	Jackson & Pollock (38)
Male (14–19 yr)	$D_B = 1.10647 - 0.00162\ (SS\ SKF) - 0.00144\ (AB\ SKF) - 0.00077\ (TR\ SKF) + 0.00071\ (MA\ SKF)^b$	Forsyth & Sinning (45)
Female (18–29 yr) (14–19 yr)[d]	$D_B = 1.096095 - 0.0006952\ (\Sigma\ 4\ SKF) + 0.0000011\ (\Sigma\ 4\ SKF)^2 - 0.0000714\ (age, yr)^c$	Jackson, Pollock, & Ward (39)

[a] Σ 7 SKF, the sum of the triceps, subscapular, chest, midaxillary, suprailiac, abdominal, and thigh skinfolds.
[b] The skinfolds are SS, subscapular; AB, abdominal; TR, triceps; MA, midaxillary.
[c] Σ 4 SKF, the sum of the triceps, abdominal, suprailiac, and thigh skinfolds.
[d] This equation is recommended for 14- to 19-year-old female athletes.

cent and adult male and female athletes are provided in Table 22–1.

Bioelectric Impedance Analysis

BIA is a method based on the principle that there is a differential impedance to the flow of an oscillating electrical current in body-composition components of high and low water and electrolyte content. FFB has high water and electrolyte contents, and thus the impedance to the flow of current is low in this component, whereas fat has a substantially higher impedance to current flow because it is relatively low in water and electrolyte content (46). A recent review detailed the fundamental theory, principles, and applications for use of the BIA method (25). A more recent version of BIA is bioelectric impedance spectroscopy (BIS), which differs from BIA in that it measures impedance over an array of oscillating current frequencies as opposed to a fixed frequency as used in the BIA (46a). This allows estimates to be made of intra- and extracellular water in addition to total body water as well as body composition.

Electrical impedance is a function of two electrical properties, resistance (R_C) and reactance (X_C). Resistance has been found to be the most predictive and useful of the two properties for the estimation of body composition (47), although some studies found X_C to add significantly to the estimation of body composition (48). Because the length of the conductor is related to the conducting volume/mass, moreover, height, which is a reasonable approximation of the conductor length, is also an important component and is used in a whole-body-resistance index as follows: height²/resistance (H^2/R_C). Most BIA-prediction equations estimate FFB from a combination of variables including the resistance index, H^2/R_C, and body weight (BW). The H^2/R_C variable has been shown to be related to the conductor volume and hence is related to the volume of FFB and TBW. Because BW is highly related to FFB, the inclusion of BW in the equation substantially lowers the predictive error; in most equations, however, the influence of H^2/R_C dominates the prediction of FFB.

Numerous studies have validated the BIA method to estimate FFB in both adolescent and adult populations by gender, body-composition characteristics, and in various racial groups. Generally, the range of relative error in estimating FFB from BIA is 3.5% to 6% (34). Baumgartner (25), based on reports from several studies, suggested the absolute accuracy of estimating body composition from BIA to be 3.5%Fat to 5%Fat and 2.0 to 3.5 kg FFB when using H^2/R_C and BW as predictor variables. The predictive errors in the BIA method tend to be somewhat lower than observed for anthropometry.

The use of BIA to evaluate body composition in athletes has been somewhat limited at this point. One reason may be the cost of the BIA instrument, which can range from $2000 to $5000. Another reason is that relatively few studies were conducted on athletic samples, leaving some uncertainty about the appropriateness of using equations developed in nonathletic samples for athletes. As with anthropometric equations, the precision of BIA equations to estimate FFB and %Fat is dependent on the characteristics of the sample in which the equation was developed. Thus BIA equations tend to be sample specific; that is, they are typically inaccurate when applied to samples that differ in age, gender, fatness, and racial characteristics from the sample in which they were originally developed. In general, equations provided by manufacturers of BIA instruments, often programmed into the equipment, tend to produce spurious estimates of body composition. Hortobagyi and colleagues (49) and Opplinger and colleagues (50) found that the manufacturers' equations systematically underestimated %Fat in both African-American and Caucasian football players. At present, there is some consensus that the following general equation developed by Lukaski and associates (48) for adult male and female subjects aged 18 to 74 years may provide the most accurate estimates for athletes (44,51). The equation is as follows:

$$FFB = 0.734\,(H^2/R_C) + 0.116\,(BW) + 0.96\,(X_C) + 0.878\,(\text{gender}) \quad [9]$$

where gender is a categoric variable coded as (1) for males and (0) for females. Lukaski and colleagues (52) applied their general equation to 48 male and 46 female athletes from various sports and found that fairly accurate estimates of FFB (standard error of estimate, 2.0 kg) could be obtained. The few studies conducted on adolescent athletes at this time do not allow a recommendation on a general BIA prediction equation for this age group and maturation status, although Oplinger and colleagues (53) developed a BIA equation to estimate FFB in high-school wrestlers.

Clearly this method offers many desirable features for estimating body composition of athletes in the clinical/field setting. It is safe, relatively easy to use, reliable, and typically more accurate than anthropometry. However, it is important to note that, as in other body-composition methods, care must be taken by applying standard measurement techniques and conditions for accurate results to be obtained (25). Furthermore, it is important to consider the range of error associated with the prediction equation used so that appropriate allowance can be made when estimating a target weight for the athlete.

BODY-COMPOSITION CHARACTERISTICS OF ATHLETES

It is evident that the wide array of functional tasks required in sports has influenced the type of physique and body-composition characteristics observed across sport groups, particularly at the elite-performer level. Because of the importance of physique to performance, it is not surprising that there are sport-specific body-composition profiles among various athletic groups. Undoubtedly the unique physical characteristics of elite performers even in various sport groups results largely from a lengthy selection process. It also is important to recognize that there is considerable variability among elite performers within specific athletic groups. As an example, certain sports, particularly team sports in which specialized tasks are performed (e.g., American football), require a wide variety of physique characteristics to perform unique team functions. Thus the use of sport-specific body-composition profiles to estimate a target weight for optimal performance must be considered in the context of the specific physical demands or functional tasks required in the sport.

Use of body-composition profile data to estimate the optimal weight for athletic performance requires at least two assumptions (51): (a) that the range of relative body fatness of the reference group is considered to be the most favorable for the physiologic and biomechanical requirements of the sport; and (b) that these characteristics adequately reflect those of the most superior athletes in the sport. It is important to consider, however, that individual differences in body structure and other factors may alter to some extent the optimal performance body weight and composition on an individual basis. There is some concern about either suggesting or imposing weight and body-composition standards because this may introduce pressure on the athlete to engage in unhealthy practices to achieve perhaps unreasonable goals. This may be particularly troublesome in the female athlete, because there appears to be an increased incidence of eating disorders, amenorrhea, and associated premenopausal osteoporosis. Therefore it is recommended that individualized goals be established and that a range of body-composition values be used in developing target weights for athletes in various sports rather than attempting to get all athletes to a singular goal. Tables 22–2 and 22–3 provide a range of %Fat values for adolescent and young-adult male and female athletes in various sports collated from studies that used reference body-composition methods, either densitometry or total body water. The range of %Fat indicated was computed as ±1 standard deviation (SD) of the reported mean value. Whereas there are limited data on some sport groups, the data reported for most sports were developed from several studies and in some sports included hundreds of athletes.

In general, the athletic population, whether adolescent or adult, is lean, with some of the lowest %Fat values found in the body-composition literature. Most athletic groups are about 1 SD lower in %Fat compared with their nonathletic counterparts. Although the gender-specific differences in %Fat are clearly evident in the athletic population, the lower values in the body-fatness range (−1 SD) indicate that in sports in which translocation of body mass is required, athletes are at

TABLE 22–2. *Body-composition profiles of adolescent athletes in selected sports*

	Males		Females	
Sport	%Fat	FFB/H	%Fat	FFB/H
Ice hockey	7–11	.386		
Gymnastics	6–10	.320	11–19	.265
Swimming	10–14	.352	15–23	.279
Wrestling	10–16	.323		
Track & field				
Jumpers	4–8	.348	10–15	.286
Runners	5–10	.328	10–15	.269
Sprinters	4–8	.359	11–16	.290
Throwers	9–18	.407	19–25	.313

Data from Boileau et al. (186); Thorland et al. (187); Thorland et al. (188); Stager et al. (189).

The range for %Fat is ±SD from the reported mean value.

The FFB/H ratio was computed from the reported mean FFB (kg) divided by the mean height (H).

TABLE 22–3. *Body-composition profiles of young adult athletes in selected sports*

Sport	Males %Fat	Males FFB/H	Females %Fat	Females FFB/H
Ballet			12–22	.269
Baseball/softball	8–15	.423	14–24	.288
Basketball	7–15	.403	14–24	.299
Cycling	8–13	.346		
Football				
Backs/receivers	6–14	.433		
Linebackers	10–19	.465		
Linemen	13–20	.512		
Q'backs/kickers	9–20	.414		
Gymnastics	4–10	.363	11–19	.285
Hockey, ice/field	5–14	.423	14–28	.286
Lacrosse	8–17	.366	14–25	.298
Skiing, nordic	5–9	.373	14–18	.290
Soccer	5–15	.366	16–28	.288
Swimming	6–12	.363	12–20	.280
Tennis	6–17	.364	20–24	.284
Track & field				
Jumpers	6–11	.349	10–16	.285
Runners	4–10	.336	7–15	.251
Sprinters	5–14	.339	7–15	.288
Throwers	12–21	.485	19–35	.340
Triathlon	7–18	.359	15–18	.286
Volleyball	7–13	.379	14–21	.324
Weightlifting				
Olympic	8–12	.458		
Power	8–10	.419	20–23	.343
Wrestling	4–12	.351		

Data from Boileau & Lohman (190), Fleck (191), Sinning (51), Wilmore (192), Withers et al. (42,43). The range for %Fat is ±1 SD from the reported mean value. The reported values were obtained by either densitometry or body water measurements. FFB/H ratio was computed from the reported mean FFB (kg) divided by the mean height (H).

or close to the theoretic minimal body weight estimated at approximately 5%Fat and 12%Fat for male and female subjects, respectively. On the other hand, there are sports in which an exceptionally low relative fatness is not required, as in football line positions and in the throwing field events.

Another aspect to the body composition of the athletic population is the size of the FFB. The FFB consists largely of muscle and to a lesser extent of bone and other connective tissues. Because FFB is related to the stature of an individual, the FFB/H ratio provides an index that allows athletic group and gender comparisons (see Tables 22–2 and 22–3). The difference in FFB/H between male and female subjects across all sport groups is not surprising and likely reflects hormonal influence on the development of both muscle and bone. This morphologic metric may partly reinforce the concept that, in most sports, separate competition between male and female athletes is justified. The range of FFB/H values among sport groups also is interesting. The highest female FFB/H values, as in males, are found in power sports including power weightlifting and in the throwing events of shot putting and discus throwing, whereas the lowest values are observed in distance runners. These observations are consistent with the theoretic influence of this component of body composition on performance in these activities. Football particularly is interesting to analyze in the context of the FFB/H metric because, in general, most football players have a high ratio; however, there also is considerable variability across positions. When comparing the FFB/H values of adolescent and adult athletes, it is not surprising that, in general, the adolescents have lower values. The difference between male adolescents and adults is considerable in most sports, but the difference is not so obvious for female athletes. The difference between adolescence and adulthood seen in male athletes perhaps reflects slower and incomplete physical development, fewer years of training, and perhaps different selection standards; in female athletes, however, physical development occurs earlier, which likely narrows the difference between adolescent and adult female athletes. Thus although the ideal body-size and -composition profile for optimal performance in a specific sport as well as an individual within a sport cannot be precisely estimated, using the characteristics of superior athletes for a specific sport may allow guarded inference about the optimal body weight and composition required for elite performance.

ESTIMATING MINIMAL AND IDEAL WEIGHT

The concept of ideal weight for the athlete encompasses not only the total body weight but also the composition of body weight. As noted previously, optimal body-size and -composition characteristics for a specific sport will vary depending on the physical tasks required to be performed. In several sports, the optimal playing weight may be at or near the theoretic minimal weight for the individual. Minimal weight is derived from the concept that body weight is at its minimum when it contains only the FFB plus essential fat. This definition of minimal weight also is referred to as the lean body mass. Essential fat is the body fat that is necessary for health. Whereas the amount of essential fat for a given individual is not precisely known, it is known that fat associated with the nervous system and cell membranes is essential. It is estimated that essential fat is 2% to 4% of body weight in male and 10% to 12% in female subjects (54). In female subjects, essential fat also includes sex-specific fat, including the mammary tissue.

An accurate measurement of the FFB is essential for the estimation of minimal weight. Because body-composition measurements have both technical and biologic errors, it has been suggested that essential fat values of 5% for male and 12% for female subjects be adopted in the calculation of minimal weight (55). A recent position paper on weight loss in wrestlers (56) suggested that a 7 %Fat value be used in boys 16 years and younger to provide an added margin of safety and to minimize affecting growth in younger athletes. Once FFB has been accurately determined, the minimal weight can be computed by dividing the FFB by the fraction of FFB (fFFB), which represents the respective level of essential fat of 5% and 12% for male and female subjects. Thus for male subjects, the minimal weight is calculated as the FFB/0.95 or FFB/0.93 for adolescent boys and for female subjects as FFB/0.88. It can be noted in Table 22–3 that the lower end of the %Fat range (−1 SD) is near and in some sports below these recommended minimal %Fat levels, indicating that a substantial number of athletes in running, gymnastics, and wrestling may perform at minimal weight.

Most athletes, however, are likely to benefit and perform optimally at a body weight slightly higher than minimal weight, which can be operationally defined as ideal weight. Although a precise definition cannot be given for ideal weight, because of a number of individual factors and considerations, it is normally a body weight at a relative fatness for a specific sport within the range of %Fat values shown in Tables 22–2 and 22–3. The best approach for estimation of a target ideal body weight is to base the estimate on a measured FFB. The choice of the desired %Fat for the ideal weight can be guided by using the range of %Fat values for a specific sport, as presented in Tables 22–2 and 22–3. The %Fat deemed appropriate for a specific sport is then used to calculate the fFFB, which represents the desired %Fat calculated as follows:

$$\text{fFFB} = 1 - \text{\%Fat}/100 \qquad [10]$$

Ideal weight can then be calculated as

$$\text{Ideal weight} = \text{FFB}/\text{fFFB} \qquad [11]$$

Examples of the minimal and ideal weight calculations are presented in Table 22–4.

In summary, the most appropriate estimates of minimal and ideal weight are based on the measurement of FFB. It is essential that accurate and precise measurements of FFB be obtained. It is recommended that body composition be preferentially assessed by densitometry, when possible, because larger errors in estimates of FFB and %Fat have been found with anthropometry and BIA. Because many athletes strive to be as lean as possible, it is important to monitor carefully both body weight and body composition on a regular basis. Furthermore, it is important to consider the implications for both health and performance when body weight is substantially modified in both the short and the long term.

TABLE 22–4. *Examples of minimal and ideal body weight calculations for a male and female athlete*

Variable	Target %Fat	Football lineman male	Target %Fat	Basketball female
Actual BW (kg)		115.1		62.6
Measured FFB (kg)		90.9		49.5
Measured %Fat		17.4		20.8
Est. minimal BW (kg)	@5%	95.7	@12%	56.3
Est target BW (kg)				
	@13%[a]	104.5	@14%[a]	57.6
	@20%[a]	113.6	@24%[a]	65.1

[a]The %Fat used for the target BW estimate was obtained from Table 22–3.

MANIPULATION OF SIZE AND BODY-COMPOSITION STATUS IN THE ATHLETE

Most athletes are interested in optimizing their size and body composition for sport. To this end, certain groups of athletes go to great lengths to manipulate body size and composition with the specific goal of increasing their chances of success in competition. Among the athletes attempting to increase mass, the typical goal is to increase muscle mass in hopes of increasing absolute power and strength. In a few cases such as that of a lineman in football or the shot putter, simply increasing the absolute size regardless of the composition may be justifiable. Those athletes attempting to maintain a constant body weight or those who lose weight before competition generally do so for one of three reasons (57): (a) a requirement to make a specific body-weight class before competition (wrestling, boxing, weightlifting, light-weight rowing); (b) being lighter during the competition is thought to improve their performance (gymnastics, distance runners, ski jumpers); or (c) their appearance of looking lighter and leaner may influence the officials who do the scoring in their sport (dance, diving, figure skating).

Frequently the strategies used by athletes to alter their body mass and composition may put them at risk for certain health problems. With the goal to manipulate size quickly at a minimal distraction to daily training, athletes may reduce energy intake, induce dehydration, or take pharmacologic agents that could ultimately hurt their health. It is even debatable whether the strategies help performance. With prolonged manipulation of body mass, either repeatedly in cycles or sustained for long periods, the athletes may face other risks that affect their performance, growth, and chances of incurring certain diseases. In this section, we examine the effects of manipulating body mass and composition on the physiology, performance, and health of the athlete.

Weight Loss

The most common methods used to reduce body weight in athletes include proper diet and exercise regimens to reduce body fatness, restricted food and fluid intake, exercise-induced sweat, environmentally induced sweating such as sitting in a sauna or hot box, or a combination of these methods (57–60). Additional methods, including use of catharsis (forced vomiting, laxatives) and diuresis through drugs or diet, have been used but to a lesser extent than diet and exercise combinations (60). Some obscure methods include blood letting, in which a volume of blood is withdrawn and reinfused after the weigh-in (61), and standing on one's head. The latter method should have no effect on actual body weight; it may work because the athlete has simply repositioned him or herself on the scale platform and appears to have lost a small amount of body weight.

All methods of weight loss have the potential to affect the nutritional status, physiology, and performance of the athlete. The research involving experimental and descriptive studies is summarized to describe these acute effects as well as the effects of chronic weight loss, either sustained or as weight cycling over a period of months.

Acute Effects

Body Composition/Nutritional Status

The most immediate effects on body composition and nutritional status are reductions in total body water and body glycogen stores. Although total body water has never been assessed in an athlete before and after acute weight reduction, the magnitude of the weight loss in relatively short periods of 2 to 48 hours could be explained only by water loss. Muscle glycogen levels have been assessed. The first published report showed close to a 46% reduction in glycogen concentration in the vastus lateralis (62) in elite wrestlers who reduced weight by 8% in 3 days. This finding was corroborated by a recent study that reported a 54% reduction in glycogen levels in the biceps brachii of wrestlers who lost approximately 5% of body weight (63).

The possibility exists that during acute weight loss in athletes, an increase in fat oxidation and protein breakdown occurs. Although lipid oxidation or protein breakdown has not been measured in athletes during weight reduction, the effects of short-term weight loss has revealed reductions in percentage of body fat and fat-free mass (64). The loss of fat-free mass may be related to negative nitrogen balance, which might be a transient event when the daily protein intake is inadequate (64).

Metabolism/Physiology

Transient reductions in resting metabolic rate of up to 17% have been observed in collegiate wrestlers who have reduced body weight by approximately 7% during their season (65). The reduction paralleled decreases in the FFB mass of the athletes, making it difficult to determine whether the suppression of resting metabolism rate (RMR) was an acute effect of recent food deprivation or a chronic effect due to reduced fat-free mass. In the postseason, when fat-free mass returned to the preseason value, RMR also increased and returned to that of the preseason rates.

Increases in heart rate at submaximal work rate have been reported after short-term weight reduction in collegiate wrestlers (66,67). This response compensates for reduced plasma volume reported to occur in wrestlers (68) and rowers (69). In these athletes, the reduction in plasma volume undoubtedly contributes to reduced stroke volume during sustained, moderate-intensity exercise; with increasing degrees of dehydration, the increase in heart rate is not enough to maintain cardiac output (70). The change in cardiovascular function is transient because once the athletes rehydrate, the heart rate returns to the expected rate for the standard workload (67), and stroke volume returns to the values measured before weight loss (71). It is not clear whether recovery can be made for all degrees of weight loss, however, particularly those observed in the field that tend to be greater than those in controlled studies in the laboratory (62,69).

Health Risks

The most significant health risk with acute weight reduction is that of heat illness, including muscle cramps, heat exhaustion, or heat stroke. Experimental studies examined the effects of dehydration by several means and found increases in electromyogram (EMG) activity that might relate to spasms and cramping in skeletal muscle (72). In the 70-year history of collegiate wrestling as a sport sanctioned by the National Collegiate Athletic Assocation (NCAA), there had never been a published case of heat illness in athletes who achieved rapid weight reduction primarily through dehydration. Nonetheless, in 1997, three collegiate wrestlers died while in the process of exercising to dehydrate and "make weight" for intercollegiate competition (73). The Centers for Disease Control and Prevention (CDC) concluded that the self-imposed heat stress combined with preexisting dehydration were the main factors contributing to their tragic deaths (73).

Case reports suggested that rapid weight loss contributed to pulmonary embolism in one scholastic wrestler (74) and to pancreatitis that occurred with rehydration and refeeding that followed making weight in a collegiate wrestler (75). Subsequent research would be required to clarify the mechanism by which rapid weight reduction acts to produce these pathologies. Experimental evidence reveals that rapid weight reduction may reduce immune function. One study showed that during a 2-week period of weight reduction of 3.7%, female athletes who participated in a variety of sports experienced reduced phagocytic function and a reduction in the stimulation of lymphocyte transformation (76). The significance of these changes remains to be determined. Despite the reduced stimulation, the values for the stimulation index after weight loss remained well above those of the control group. Serum concentrations of prealbumin and retinol-binding protein indices were unchanged in these athletes but have been reported to decrease with sustained weight loss in other athletes (77,78). Thus the effects of sustained or repeated weight reduction over the course of a season of intense training might have an adverse effect on immune status and the ability of the athlete to defend against viral infections.

Performance

As previously reviewed (79,80), rapid weight reduction adversely affects submaximal endurance performance. This is due in part to the reduction in muscle glycogen (62,63), which appears to impair the muscle's ability to sustain contractions at a set workload for long durations (81,82). Rapid weight loss, when accomplished by dehydration, will reduce the plasma volume, which among other factors will reduce cardiac output and thermoregulatory capabilities and will promote higher ratings of perceived exertion than those for the same work completed in a euhydrated state (70,83). These physiologic and psychological changes contribute ultimately to a decrease in endurance capacity (80,84,85).

Rapid weight reduction, despite its profound effects on the physiology and energy reserves in muscle, has a less clear effect on short-duration, high-intensity performance (62,79,85a–89). Generally, among nonathletes, high-power performance may be reduced; however, among athletes who are accustomed to reducing body weight in preparation for competition, single high-power bouts of exertion are unchanged with weight loss (79). Possibly because of the duration of high-intensity efforts that require anaerobic metabolism as a main source of energy production, the muscle is fairly self-sufficient and performs at near-optimal levels. If the efforts are sustained—that is, the athlete executes a high-power effort intermittently or for a duration lasting longer than 30 seconds—the subsequent performance appears to deteriorate more than does the performance with the athlete at his or her normal weight (79,89,90–92). The explanation for this might be that, with repeated bouts, the muscle must rely on external metabolic pathways and systems for recovery. Compromised blood flow to muscle and skin results in deprivation of nutrients and impaired heat dissipation, respectively, both of which will contribute to fatigue in the muscle and will impair subsequent performance.

Chronic Effects

Body Composition, Nutritional Status, and Growth Rate

Studies that have followed wrestlers over the course of their season reveal somewhat consistently that percentage of body fatness and absolute lean body mass decrease (65,87,93–95). The consistency of the findings across several methods of measuring body composition enhances the validity of the changes observed in these athletes. The accuracy of the data in these reports might be challenged because the methods employed in these studies used only the two-component model of measuring body composition. As discussed earlier in this chapter, two component models are subject to bias when certain assumptions are violated. The assumption of normal hydration of the fat-free tissues in athletes who purposely undergo weight reduction is rarely correct. It is questionable over the course of the competitive season whether athletes who purposely dehydrate completely recover to a euhydrated state because of the frequency of having to reduce body weight for each competition (96). Accounting for changes in the hydration state would most likely show that the reductions in lean body mass are slightly greater than previously reported, based on experimental studies in which hydration state was purposely manipulated (97).

The reduction in lean body mass parallels the reductions in plasma proteins, particularly the rapid-turnover proteins that have been used to assess protein nutritional status. Retinol binding protein and prealbumin have been observed to decrease after 7 and 12 weeks, respectively, of the competitive season in high-school wrestlers who reduced their body weight by 6.6% repeatedly over the season (98). These observations were recently confirmed in another study that reported a 22% reduction in prealbumin in high-school wrestlers who had repeatedly reduced body weight by 7.4% over the competitive season and were measured at a time when their body weight was 3.8% lower than in the early season (99). These findings support that the protein nutritional status of these athletes is diminished if not compromised with weight reduction, even when the average protein meets the RDA during the period of weight loss (98,99).

For young athletes who undergo weight reduction as a part of their training, there is a real concern about the effects of this practice on their linear growth rate. For example, some have speculated that participation in sports such as wrestling or gymnastics will stunt growth (100,101). Despite the perpetual concern about growth stunting in such sports, relatively few studies have examined growth rates in the athletes. Studies on young female gymnasts suggested that stunted linear growth may occur. Theintz and colleagues (102) observed that compared with age- and gender-matched swimmers who did not control their weight, female gymnasts had a lower growth velocity. It was difficult to determine whether this is the effect of intense training, in which energy expenditure exceeds intake, or whether the participants are purposely restricting their intake and as a result are not meeting their energy needs (102); the researchers thought that the latter was a contributing factor. These same researchers reported findings to support that the natural-selection process in sports such as gymnastics may draw athletes whose parents are also short (e.g., a naturally small-sized person choosing a sport in which small-sized athletes often excel) (103).

In wrestlers, findings from cross-sectional studies across age groups and longitudinal studies of a group followed up over the course of the season show no change in linear growth rate (99,104). This is somewhat surprising, because reductions of approximately 40% in the daily energy intake of high-school wrestlers have been reported (91,99). In one study that used a cross-sectional design, the slope of the regression lines that describe the relation between height and age of high-school wrestlers was not different from the slope for age- and gender-matched subjects from the National Health and Nutrition Examination Survey (NHANES) data (104). It should be noted, though, that the mean value of the older wrestlers (17 years) falls away from the regression line. Therefore the need exists for a longitudinal study of wrestlers over the course of their career, to determine whether several seasons of participation in weight reduction lead to a decrease in stature or linear growth rate. Short-term longitudinal studies reported no differences in linear growth rate between scholastic wrestlers who had decreased body weight by 3.8% and the linear growth of a control group matched for age, size, and body composition (94). As suggested earlier, a longitudinal assessment of growth rate in young athletes in weight-loss sports is needed before the conclusion can be made that weight loss suppresses growth.

Metabolism/Physiology

Despite the absence of evidence for a change in growth rate in high-school wrestlers, profound changes in plasma hormone concentrations have been observed. Both testosterone and insulin-like growth factor-I (IGF-I) reductions have been reported after several weeks of training in which the athletes reduced their body weight by 3.8% (78). The IGF-I decrease was concomitant with an increase in growth hormone levels but no change in the concentration of IGF binding protein-3. The lack of a change in linear growth rate (94) in the face of what appears to be growth hormone resistance might be explained by two factors. First, the decrease in IGF-I may not have been sustained for a long enough period to stunt growth rate. In fact, IGF-I returned to the baseline levels once the season of competition and weight loss concluded. Second, despite a large reduction in IGF-I and the increase in growth hormone, the concentrations remained within the levels observed for the control group and within the ranges accepted as normal.

In collegiate wrestlers, reductions in IGF-I have been documented after short-term weight loss in experimental studies (105). Low testosterone levels have also been reported for collegiate wrestlers in season compared with postseason values (106); in fact, for some athletes the in-season values were pathologically low. The testosterone levels were directly correlated with changes in the percentage of body fat; the greater the decrease in body fatness, the lower the in-season values for testosterone (106). More recent studies indicate that collegiate wrestlers may have low testosterone levels before the season of competition and subsequent weight reduction (107). This calls into question whether training (e.g., overtraining that can occur because most major-college athletes train year round) or weight reduction is the main factor controlling the change in testosterone. Most longitudinal studies over the course of the competitive season have failed to account for changes in training intensity and volume that will affect body composition and hormone status. For example, once athletes reach the point of perpetual competition events in the season, they often reduce the amount of resistance training. Such a change may contribute to a reduction in body weight or lean body mass regardless of whether the athletes are voluntarily attempting to lose weight.

One cross-sectional study conducted on scholastic wrestlers indicated that those who underwent weight cycling, defined as at least 10 episodes of weight reduction of at least 4.5 kg, had a chronically reduced metabolic rate, reduced 14% of that of the age-matched wrestlers who did not weight cycle (108). The findings in this study are difficult to reconcile with those of collegiate wrestlers whose metabolic rates, even when depressed, were higher than those of the nonwrestling control group (65) or who weight cycled for at least two seasons without a depression in RMR (109). The authors of the study on scholastic wrestlers concluded that the chronically reduced RMR in weight-cycling athletes may contribute to the difficulty of these athletes' ability to maintain body weight and hence promote repeated bouts of weight cycling. In addition, if these effects are sustained after the sports career is complete, the reduced RMR may contribute to increased adiposity for the remainder of life. The data on the collegiate wrestlers (65) showed that the decrease in RMR was transient, and at the lowest value it was still in line with the control group's data.

Endocrine Disorders

A major concern in female athletes who lose weight and experience a perturbation in hormone levels is the possibility of amenorrhea, which precedes the loss of bone mineral content. This concern has immediate implications, such as an increased susceptibility to stress fractures that would shorten the athlete's competitive season and long-term implications that include osteoporosis later in life.

Initially a low body fatness may be the reason for amenorrhea in the female athlete (110), but the current consensus is that body composition was more or less a symptom of the problem, not the cause (111). One of the leading candidates for disrupting the normal hormone cycles in women is an energy imbalance brought about by either excessive expenditure and overtraining, inadequate energy intake due to restrictions or disordered eating, or combination of the two (111,112). One case study of a female runner with amenorrhea and chronic stress fractures used a therapy of reduced training in combination with an increase in total caloric intake (113). After 15 weeks of treatment, the athlete showed increased bone mineral density in the femur and lumbar vertebra by 1.5% and 1.7%, respectively (114) compared with no change in three eumenorrheic women who served as controls. The increase in bone mineral density, though, was within the measurement error of the instrument. The amenorrheic patient also decreased basal cortisol concentrations and increased luteinizing hormone levels during the treatment. Body weight increased by 2.7 kg, and body fatness increased from 8.2% to 14.4%, which is approximately the value considered as the minimum needed to sustain good health and fitness in females (56). Most impressive, but most subjective, was that the running performance times of the patient improved after treatment (56).

Although female subjects have been targeted as the prime candidates for endocrine perturbations resulting from weight reduction and disordered eating, certain male athletes also may be at risk (78,106,115). Elsewhere in this chapter we discussed the observance of reduced testosterone levels in wrestlers. The long-term ramifications of this change are unclear. It is not known whether reductions in muscle mass or bone mineral would result. As a less severe consequence, a reduction in the sexual libido of one collegiate wrestler was documented in parallel with reductions in testosterone level and relative body fatness (116).

Performance

A handful of studies have followed up athletes over the course of their competitive season to determine whether weight reduction has an impact on performance. Most of the studies have been conducted on wrestlers. The main changes observed include reductions in force production (93,94,99), although such decreases have not always been observed (95,117,118). There is some debate as to whether strength loss is explained by a loss of fat-free mass (94) or whether it is some other variable outside of the change in FFB mass such as a reduced ability to recruit motor units (93). The results for power performance are less consistent, with some studies showing no loss of anaerobic power (87), whereas others report a small but significant decrease in anaerobic power (93). The inconsistency might be explained by the methods used. Typically, the resistance setting for testing anaerobic power is based on body weight. As body weight decreases, the resistance setting may be decreased correspondingly, a change that could mask reductions in power performance. In conflict with this explanation is the observation that mean and peak anaerobic power were maintained after a 4.5% weight reduction in wrestlers who were tested by using an isokinetic device (i.e., accommodating resistance established independent of body weight) as opposed to an external resistance predetermined by using body weight (87).

Recommended Methods

Minimal Weight Assessment

With a focus on merely reducing absolute body weight, many athletes lose sight of or are totally unfamiliar with the concept of reducing body fatness while maintaining lean body mass. In some athletic circles, encouragement has been given for several decades to employ safe methods of weight loss (56,119) and objective methods to establish whether athletes can lose weight, and if so, how much weight can be lost safely (120). Until recently, the recommendations have fallen on deaf ears.

In the 1990s, changes have occurred in the sport of wrestling, in which abuses in weight manipulation are the most widely recognized. At the scholastic level for a number of state associations that govern this sport, the protocol of establishing a healthy minimal weight via body-composition assessment has been introduced. The leader in this process has been the Wisconsin Interscholastic Athletic Association (WIAA) (121), with other state associations in Michigan, New York, and California following suit. The WIAA requires that wrestlers be measured for body composition by using skinfold-thickness measurements in the preseason. The results are used to predict a minimal weight at which the wrestler has 7% of body fat. The WIAA program contains a nutritional-education component that encourages slow reduction in weight (2 to 3 lb per week) to achieve the minimal weight if the athlete desires to compete at that weight class.

Dietary Strategies for Nutrition Recovery

There are two issues for athletes who want to prepare nutritionally for competition at the same time that they may become nutritionally unprepared as a consequence of weight loss. For all such athletes, the dietary approach to weekly training across the season is critical. In the discussion, we consider this the chronic approach. For those specific athletes who make weight and have a recovery period between the weigh-in and competition, an acute recovery is another strategy that must be considered.

Acute. Rehydration and the replenishment of body glycogen stores should be the main goals of athletes who have a short recovery period before competition. The extent to which rehydration is achieved is dependent on the duration of the recovery period (79), the volume of fluids consumed (122), and probably the composition of the fluid and foods consumed with the fluids. Concerning the latter variable, if sodium is present in the fluids and food, the likelihood of achieving rehydration is increased (122–125). Sodium is important in helping restore the plasma volume (126,127), which is a critical part of the recovery in athletes who have purposely dehydrated to make weight.

In terms of performance, the macronutrient composition of the food and fluid consumed appear to have an effect on performance recovery when the extent of recovery (weight gain) is controlled. Specifically, under isocaloric treatments, the intake of more carbohydrate tends to restore the performance of high-intensity, anaerobic efforts to those of pre–weight loss values compared with feedings similar in energy density but lower in carbohydrate content (128). More than likely, the foods that have a high glycemic index (i.e., those quickly digested and absorbed to boost blood glucose levels) will stimulate the fastest resynthesis of muscle glycogen (129,130); however, the relationship of specific foods to recovery has yet to be examined in athletes who practice acute weight loss.

Chronic. It has been said that the pre-event meal for athletes who must lose weight is every meal during the competitive season. This statement is largely true because such athletes are likely to have energy and nutrient deficits throughout much of the season; hence great care is needed at every meal to ensure adequate intake of all nutrients. Unfortunately, no published studies have tested these particular athletes over their entire competitive seasons for different diet strategies.

The longest experimental treatments to this point lasted only 1 week. Extrapolating from the results of short-term studies, it would appear that athletes who restrict energy intake must give particular care to obtaining adequate intake of certain macronutrients and micronutrients. In terms of macronutrients, the recommendations are to consume a relatively high carbohydrate diet (i.e., approximately 65% of the total daily energy intake as carbohydrate) and adequate protein (i.e., twice the recommended daily intake, or about 1.6 g per kg body weight). These recommendations are based on observations in wrestlers and weightlifters that a high-carbohydrate diet maintains performance (64,98,105) and that the extra protein prevents a negative nitrogen balance initially seen with the low-protein, high-carbohydrate diet (64,131). The reduction in the total energy intake per day should come from a reduction in fat intake, and the reduction should facilitate a weight loss of approximately 1 to 1.5 kg per week to maximize body-fat reduction and minimize depletion of body glycogen stores or oxidation of muscle proteins.

Micronutrients that typically are low in the weight-loss athlete's diet need special attention. Specifically, intake of vitamins A, C, B_6, and thiamine, and of minerals iron, zinc, calcium, and magnesium may be inadequate, at least in college-age athletes who restrict food intake during their competitive season (132,133). Because athletes now recognize that a diet that maximizes body-fat reduction is one that limits dietary fat intake, it is possible that, with a lower intake of dietary fat, the intake of fat-soluble vitamins could be limiting. Assuming body stores are adequate at the start of the season, however, it is doubtful that the athletes would experience complications due to inadequate intake. Nevertheless, this is something that requires examination.

Weight Gain

Methods Commonly Practiced

Exercise and Diet

Similar to attempts to reduce weight, attempts to gain weight in athletes usually include changes in the training and diet. Specifically, resistance training to stimulate muscle hypertrophy and a diet adjustment to increase energy and protein intake are used. The extent to which muscle mass will increase is controlled by the genetic disposition of the individual, but to some degree almost all individuals can expect an increase in muscle mass as a consequence of initiating a resistance-training program.

At the end of this section, we provide recommendations for the general dietary approach for weight gain in athletes. In the following section, we review several specific supplements and strategies that have been popular among athletes.

Nutritional Supplements

Many athletes will use dietary supplements to help increase muscle mass and strength for their performance. A perusal of any body-building magazine will reveal an extensive list of compounds and supplements marketed with the claims of stimulating muscle growth. The explosion of numbers of compounds is in part due to changes in federal laws in late 1994. The Dietary Supplement Health Education Act (DSHEA) allowed the classification of non–FDA-approved compounds to be sold as dietary supplements rather than as food nutrients or pharmaceutical agents. Restrictions on the claims being made also were relaxed relative to claims allowed for whole foods.

Protein and Amino Acid Supplements. Many athletes attempting to gain weight and strength will consume extra protein or amino acid supplements above the RDA in hopes that the supplements provide the structural components to synthesize additional body protein. Individual amino acids have also been consumed in supplemental amounts in hopes that they will stimulate protein synthesis or inhibit protein breakdown by stimulating the secretion of growth hormone or insulin (134,135). In fact, resistance training may increase protein breakdown, but there appears to be a simultaneous stimulation of protein synthesis with the uptake of amino acids by the muscle cell (136). Although the protein needs are increased over the RDA for both endurance athletes (137) and strength-trained athletes (138), few data suggest that increasing protein intake *per se* increases lean body mass and results in an increase in force production in well-trained athletes (129). For example, one study indicated that in healthy older men an increase in protein intake by 50% of the RDA combined with resistance training for 12 weeks resulted in a 139% increase in thigh-muscle volume ($p < .05$) over that of the control group (exercise only) (139). Both groups showed gains of similar magnitude (19 to 20 kg) for the one-repetition maximum-strength test, however. Others documented the greater increases in body mass (139,140), protein synthesis (140), and nitrogen balance (141) with supplemental protein intake, but none of these studies tested the subjects for changes in strength.

Creatine. Without a doubt, the most popular supplement on the market currently is creatine monohydrate. Loading with doses of 25 g of creatine per day for a 5- to 7-day period followed by a maintenance phase of 2 g per day is pervasive in athletic circles. Initially, researchers hypothesized that, by loading muscle with this intermediate for carrying energy for high-intensity performance, maximal force production could be enhanced (142,143). The performance of repeated sprint intervals in laboratory experiments suggested that an attenuation of fatigue may occur in the latter intervals after creatine loading (142,144). Findings for performance involving a single power effort or short sprint (12 to 30 seconds) (144–146) and longer sprints (90 to 120 seconds) (147) are less than promising for an ergogenic effect. The lone study on endurance performance indicated a significantly slower time by about 26 seconds for a 6-km run open-field running trial after loading with creatine (147). The 0.9-kg average gain in body weight of the runners was suggested as the reason for the impaired performance compared with the placebo group, for which body weight and running time were unchanged after the treatment.

Secondary to the performance outcomes, a fairly consistent observation has been the increase in body mass of approximately 1 to 2 kg during the short, 5-day loading phase (144,148–150). Marketing claims by the supplement distributors stated that the increase is in the lean, muscle tissue, with the implication that contractile protein mass has increased. However, the rapid gain in weight in such a short period has been coupled with a transient reduction in the volume of urine excreted (151). This is highly suggestive of water retention, not an increase in cell protein mass. To this point, none of the short-term studies reporting an increase in fat-free mass (149,152) have used research techniques that overcome the limitations of the two-compartment analysis described earlier in this chapter. A recent preliminary report confirmed that total body water and intracellular fluid volume are expanded after 3 days of creatine loading (153). The study used BIS, which is still in the early stages of being validated for measuring acute alterations in the various compartments that compose the total body water (154). However, concomitant measures of thigh volume by using magnetic resonance imaging were supportive by revealing an expansion of the cross-sectional area for the muscle. Potentially, with prolonged creatine supplementation in combination with resistance training, an increase in lean body mass may occur (154); the true contribution of creatine to stimulating an increase in protein content remains to be determined, however.

To this point, only one study has been conducted on the safety of using creatine. Anecdotal reports from athletic trainers suggests that loading may increase the incidence of muscle cramping, hamstring pulls, and muscle strains (155). A recent report indicated that the reduction in plasma volume associated with voluntary dehydration in weight-classification athletes was magnified if the athletes were loading with creatine (156). Perhaps a disturbance in the plasma volume and extracellular fluid compartment, a disturbance that could alter electrolyte concentrations as well as the fluid volume, might contribute to the increased risk of muscle cramping (155).

There is also speculation that the nitrogenous load produced by ingesting 25 g of creatine per day might be stressful to the kidneys. Excess nitrogen consumed in a high-protein diet produces hyperfiltration and hyperfusion, both of which could result in functional and structural degeneration in the nephrons (157,158). The chance of creatine loading producing a similar stress may be real, based on the observation of an increase in urea excretion in subjects who had loaded with the supplement (154). To test whether renal stress is apparent, five subjects were studied for renal function before and after loading with creatine (159). The findings indicated no increase in urinary protein excretion, nor was creatinine clearance altered. Although the authors concluded that creatine loading for this short-term study did not produce renal stress, it should be noted that total urinary protein excretion was nearly double with creatine loading. Possibly by using a small sample size, the authors were unable to detect a true effect of creatine on kidney function. Further studies over longer periods of time are needed to confirm this conclusion.

Chromium. Another hot supplement among athletes is chromium picolinate. The mineral chromium is recognized as an essential mineral that interacts with insulin as a part of the glucose-tolerance factor (160). The effect is to stimulate the uptake of plasma glucose into the cells of the body. Until recently, most research on supplementation focused primarily on populations that were glucose intolerant, obese, non–insulin-dependent diabetics, or that had a clear long-term, inadequate daily intake of chromium (161–163). In such studies, chronic chromium supplementation appeared to enhance insulin action and improve glucose uptake.

One review paper focused on healthy individuals and presented preliminary findings that suggested that chromium supplementation could stimulate lean body mass accretion (164). This study, the data from which have never been published as a full report in a peer-reviewed journal, has been used to perpetuate the benefits of chromium supplementation among athletes. More recent studies that included appropriate placebo controls and criterion methods of body-composition assessment reveal that, in conjunction with resistance training, chromium offers no added benefit to strength gains or increases in lean body mass (165–167). In fact, most recently, a study on obese women showed an increase in weight of approximately 2 kg without a corresponding increase in lean body mass after 9 weeks of chromium picolinate supplementation (400 μg chromium/day) (168). One study reporting a lack of an anabolic effect of chromium picolinate did reveal a decrease in the iron saturation of transferrin (166). Although the study was done on men and would have minor health ramifications, replication of a similar effect in women would indicate the potential for chromium supplementation to promote anemia in women.

β-Hydroxy-β-Methylbutyrate. β-Hydroxy-β-methylbutyrate (βHβMB) is the latest ergogenic ingredient to arrive on the scene for athletes. This compound is a leucine derivative that has been proposed to have an anabolic effect and will speed recovery after intense resistance training. The theory of how βHβMB might work is yet to be explained, but it may be related to the βHβMB similarity in structure to leucine and the keto-analogue of leucine, ketoisocaproic acid, which are recognized as intermediates that may regulate protein balance during conditions of extreme stress (burns, surgery, sepsis, and fasting) (169). Only one study has been published on the effects of βHβMB as an anabolic agent. The researchers reported a tendency for a dose effect of βHβMB ingestion on lean body mass accretion during a 7-week treatment of supplementation and resistance training (170). Lean body mass was assessed by using the measurement of total body electrical conductivity, which has yet to receive complete validation as criterion method for determining changes in body composition. Interestingly, those subjects receiving βHβMB as opposed to placebo had lower concentrations of plasma creatine kinase, a marker of mechanical trauma to skeletal muscle. If supplemental use of this intermediate increases, βHβMB will likely receive a thorough examination for the efficacy of claims made for its effects on muscle growth and recovery.

Anabolic Steroids

In 1977 and again in 1987, the American College of Sports Medicine issued a position paper warning the sports science community about the dangers associated with using anabolic steroids (171,172). Despite the warning, a survey published 11 years after the first statement revealed that 1 of 15 high-school students experimented with such steroids to enhance size or muscularity (173). This is of particular concern because anabolic steroids use is linked to the likelihood of adolescents' using other illicit drugs (174). As a result of the 1994 DSHEA, the steroids androstenedione and dehydroepiandrosterone (DHEA) can be legally sold over the counter to athletes as dietary supplements for the purpose of attempting to stimulate lean body mass accretion. An anabolic effect of either compound has yet to be demonstrated in healthy athletes, but the medical community has issued a warning about the use of DHEA by young, healthy individuals (175).

Prior reviews on anabolic–androgenic steroid administration and lean body mass accretion and strength development suggest that the effects are inconsistent among human subjects (94,176). The limitation of inferring research findings to the athletic population is that often the dosage used among athletes in the field is higher than that used in research studies. Regardless of the anecdotal reports of the proportive benefits of anabolic steroids, the athletes should recognize the dangers associated with using such compounds. Reductions in the plasma concentration of high-density lipoprotein cholesterol (HDL-C) (177), increases in total serum cholesterol (178), case reports of cerebrovascular events and myocardial infarction (179,180), and inhibition of endogenous testosterone production and atrophy of the testes (181,182) are a few of the side effects that are likely to occur with steroid use.

Recommended Methods

Without a doubt, high-quality resistance training is the greatest stimulus for muscle hypertrophy. The details of training go beyond the scope of this review, but, in general, the closer the resistance or overload is to the maximal effort of the muscle groups for a specific exercise, the greater the recruitment of motor units and, ultimately, the greater the stimulus for muscle adaptations. As the individual adapts, the resistance must be progressively increased to ensure that an overload is maintained for further muscle development.

For the nutritional component to optimize muscle growth, it has been recommended that the athlete seeking to gain strength and lean body mass increase total daily energy intake. The increase must account for calories expended during resistance training, during other physical training, and during protein synthesis (183). The intake of protein should be approximately twice the RDA, or about 1.6 g per kg body weight. There is some evidence in humans that carbohydrate consumed immediately after the resistance training may suppress protein breakdown and thereby contribute to muscle-mass accretion (184). A recent report using an animal model indicates that a protein and carbohydrate feeding may stimulate protein synthesis to a greater extent than carbohydrate alone (185); however, these findings must be replicated in humans. Long-term studies are needed to determine whether any such feedings immediately after training produce a more efficacious accretion of muscle mass.

Acknowledgment

The research for this chapter was supported in part by NIH Grant #AG08513.

REFERENCES

1. Carter JEL. The somatotypes of athletes: review. *Hum Biol* 1970:42:535–569.
2. Cureton TK. *Physical fitness of champion athletes.* Urbana, IL: University of Illinois Press, 1951.
3. Tanner JM. *The physique of the Olympic athlete.* London: Allen & Unwin, 1964.
4. Welham WC, Behnke AR. The specific gravity of healthy men: body weight-volume and other physical characteristics of exceptional athletes and of naval personnel. *JAMA* 1942;118:498–501.
5. Cureton KJ, Boileau RA, Lohman TG. Relationship between body composition measures and AAHPER test performances in boys. *Res Q* 1975;46:218–229.
6. Teeple JB, Lohman TG, Misner JE, Boileau RA, Massey BH. Contribution of physical development and muscular strength to the motor performance capacity of 7 to 12 year old boys. *Br J Sports Med* 1975;9:122–129.
7. Cureton KJ, Boileau RA, Lohman TG, Misner JE. Determinants of distance running performance in children: analysis of a path model. *Res Q* 1977;48:270–277.
8. McLeod WD, Hunter SC, Etchison B. Performance measurements and percent body fat in the high school athlete. *Am J Sports Med* 1983;11:390–398.
9. Boileau RA, Horswill CA, Slaughter MH. Body composition and the young athlete. In: Klish WJ, Kretchmer N, eds. *Report of the 98th Ross Conference on Pediatric Research: body composition measurements in infants and children.* Columbus, OH: Ross Laboratories, 1989:104–111.
10. Leedy HE, Ismail AH, Kessler WV, Christian JE. Relationships between physical performance items and body composition. *Res Q* 1965;36:158–163.
11. Brandon LJ, Boileau RA. The contribution of selected variables to middle and long distance run performance. *J Sports Med Phys Fitness* 1987;27:157–164.
12. Brandon LJ, Boileau RA. Influence of metabolic, mechanical and physique variables on middle distance running. *J Sports Med Phys Fitness* 1992;32:1–9.
13. Lawson DL, Golding LA. Physiological parameters limiting performance in middle distance and sprint running. *Aust J Sports Med* 1978;10:18–24.
14. Cureton KJ, Sparling PB. Distance running performance and metabolic responses to running in men and women with excess

weight experimentally equated. *Med Sci Sports Exerc* 1980; 12:288–294.
15. Forbes RM, Cooper AR, Mitchell HH. The chemical composition of the adult human body as determined by chemical analysis. *J Biol Chem* 1953;203:359–366.
16. Forbes RM, Mitchell HH, Cooper AR. Further studies on the gross composition and mineral elements of the adult human body. *J Biol Chem* 1956;223:969–975.
17. Mitchell HH, Hamilton TS, Steggerda FR, Bean HW. Chemical composition of the adult human body and its bearing on the biochemistry of growth. J *Biol Chem* 1945;158:625–637.
18. Behnke AR, Feen BG, Welham WC. The specific gravity of healthy men. *JAMA* 1942;118:495–498.
19. Brozek J, Grande F, Anderson JT, Keys A. Densitometric analysis of body composition, revision of some quantitative assumptions. *Ann NY Acad Sci* 1963;110:113–140.
20. Keys A, Brozek J. Body fat in adult man. *Physiol Rev* 1953; 33:245–318.
21. Siri WJ. Body composition from fluid spaces and density: analysis of methods. In: Brozek J, Henschel A, eds. *Techniques for measuring body composition.* Washington, DC: National Academy of Sciences, 1961:223–244.
22. Heymsfield SB, Wang Z-M, Withers RT. Multicomponent molecular level models of body composition analysis. In: Roche AF, Heymsfield AB, Lohman TG, eds. *Human body composition.* Champaign, IL: Human Kinetics, 1996:129–147.
23. Forbes GB. *Human body composition: growth, aging, nutrition and activity.* New York: Springer-Verlag, 1987:5–100.
24. Lukaski HC. Methods for the assessment of human body composition: tradition and new. *A J Clin Nutr* 1987;46:537–556.
25. Baumgartner RN. Electrical impedance and total body electrical conductivity. In: Roche AF, Heymsfield AB, Lohman TG, eds. *Human body composition.* Champaign, IL: Human Kinetics, 1996:79–107.
26. Boileau RA. Utilization of total body electrical conductivity in determining body composition. In: *Designing foods: animal product options in the marketplace* Washington, DC: National Research Council/National Academy of Sciences, 1988:251–257.
27. Lohman TG. Dual energy x-ray absorptiometry. In: Roche AF, Heymsfield SB, Lohman TG, eds. *Human body composition.* Champaign, IL: Human Kinetics, 1996:63–78.
28. Conway JM, Norris KH, Bodwell CE. A new approach for the estimation of body composition: infrared interactance. *Am J Clin Nutr* 1984;40:1123–1130.
29. Seidell JC, Bakker CJG, van der Kooy K. Imaging techniques for measuring adipose-tissue distribution: a comparison between computed tomography and 1.5-T magnetic resonance. *Am J Clin Nutr* 1990;51:953–957.
30. Roche AF, Heymsfield AB, Lohman TG, eds. *Human body composition.* Champaign, IL: Human Kinetics, 1996.
31. Akers R, Buskirk ER. An underwater weighing system utilizing "force cube" transducers. *J Appl Physiol* 1969;26:649–652.
32. Wilmore J. A simplified method for determination of residual lung volumes. *J Appl Physiol* 1969;27:96–100.
33. McCrory MA, Gomez TD, Bernauer EM, Mole PA. Evaluation of a new air displacement plethysmograph for measuring human body composition. *Med Sci Sports Exerc* 1995;27:1686–1691.
34. Boileau RA. Body composition assessment in children and youths. In: Bar-Or O, ed. *The child and adolescent athlete.* Oxford: Blackwell Science, 1996:523–537.
35. Lohman TG. Applicability of body composition techniques and constants for children and youth. In: Pandolf KB, ed. *Exercise and sport sciences reviews.* New York: Macmillan, 1986:14; 325–357.
36. Lohman TG, Roche AF, Martorel R, eds. *Anthropometric standardization reference manual.* Champaign, IL: Human Kinetics, 1988.
37. Durnin JV, Womersley J. Body fat assessed from body density and its estimation from skinfold thickness: measurements on 481 men and women aged from 16-72 years. *Br J Clin Nutr* 1974; 32:77–97.
38. Jackson AS, Pollock ML. Generalized equations for predicting body density of men. *Br J Nutr* 1978;40:497–504.
39. Jackson AS, Pollock ML, Ward A. Generalized equations for predicting body density of women. *Med Sci Sports Exerc* 1980;12:175–182.
40. Sinning WE, Wilson JR. Validity of "generalized" equations for body composition analysis in women athletes. *Res Q Exerc Sport* 1984;55:153–160.
41. Sinning WE, Dolny DG, Little KD, et al. Validity of "generalized" equations for body composition analysis in male athletes. *Med Sci Sports Exerc* 1985;17:124–130.
42. Withers RT, Whittingham NO, Norton KI, La Forgia J, Ellis MW, Crockett A. Relative body fat and anthropometric prediction of body density of female athletes. *Eur J Appl Physiol* 1987;56:169–180.
43. Withers RT, Craig NP, Bourdon PC, Norton KI. Relative body fat and anthropometric prediction of body density of male athletes. *Eur J Appl Physiol* 1987;56:191–200.
44. Heyward VH, Stolarczyk LM. *Applied body composition assessment.* Champaign, IL: Human Kinetics, 1996.
45. Forsyth HL, Sinning WE. The anthropometric estimation of body density and lean body weight of male athletes. *Med Sci Sports* 1973;5:174–180.
46. Pethig R. *Dielectric and electronic properties of biological materials.* Chicester: John Wiley, 1979:207–242.
46a. Armstrong LE, Kenefick RW, Castellani JW, et al. Bioimpedance spectroscopy technique: intra-, extracellular, and total body water. *Med Sci Sports Exerc* 1997;29:1657–1663.
47. Van Loan MD, Boileau RA, Slaughter MH, et al. Association of bioelectrical resistance with estimates of fat-free mass determined by densitometry and hydrometry. *Am J Hum Biol* 1990;2:219–226.
48. Lukaski HC, Bolonchuk WW. Theory and validation of the tetrapolar bioelectrical impedance method to assess human body composition. In: Ellis KJ, Yasamura S, Morgan WD, eds. *In vivo body composition studies.* London: The Institute of Physical Sciences in Medicine, 1987:410–414.
49. Hortobagyi T, Israel RG, Houmard JA, O'Brien KF, Johns RA, Wells JM. Comparison of four methods to assess body composition in black and white athletes. *Int J Sport Nutr* 1992;2:60–74.
50. Opplinger RA, Nelson DH, Shetler AC, Crowley ET, Albright JP. Body composition of collegiate football players: bioelectrical impedance and skinfolds compared to hydrostatic weighing. *J Orthop Sports Phys Ther* 1992;15:187–192.
51. Sinning WE. Body composition in athletes. In: Roche AF, Heymsfield AB, Lohman TG, eds. *Human body composition.* Champaign, IL: Human Kinetics, 1996:257–273.
52. Lukaski HC, Bolonchuk WW, Siders WA, Hall CB. Body composition assessment of athletes using bioelectrical impedance measurements. *J Sports Med Phys Fitness* 1990;30:434–440.
53. Oppliger RA, Nelson DH, Hoegh JE, Vance CG. Bioelectrical impedance prediction of fat-free mass for high school wrestlers validated. *Med Sci Sports Exerc* 1991;23:S73.
54. Behnke AR. Comment on the determination of whole body density and a resume of body composition data. In: Brozek J, Henschel A, eds. *Techniques for measuring body composition.* Washington, DC: National Academy of Sciences, 1961:118–133.
55. Lohman TG. *Advances in body composition assessment: current issues in exercise science.* Champaign, IL: Human Kinetics, 1992.
56. American College of Sports Medicine Position Stand: weight loss in wrestlers. *Med Sci Sports Exerc* 1996;28:ix–xii.
57. Fogelholm M. Effects of bodyweight reduction on sports performance. *Sports Med* 1994;18:249–267.
58. Horswill CA. Applied physiology of amateur wrestling. *Sports Med* 1992;14:114–143.
59. Walberg-Rankin JA. Review of nutritional practices and needs of bodybuilder. *J Strength Cond Res* 1995;9:116.
60. Weissinger E, Housh TJ, Johnson GO Evans SA. Weight loss behavior in high school wrestling: wrestler and parent perceptions. *Pediatr Exerc Sci* 1991;3:64–73.
61. Buschschluter S. Games blood-letting. *Swimming technique* 1977;13:99.
62. Houston ME, Marin DA, Green HJ, Thomson JA. The effect of rapid weight loss on physiological function in wrestlers. *Physician Sports Med* 1981;9:73–78.
63. Tarnopolsky MA, Cipriano N, Woodcroft C, et al. Effects of

rapid weight loss and wrestling on muscle glycogen concentration. *Clin J Sport Med* 1996;6:78–84.
64. Walberg JL, Leidy MK, Sturgill DJ, Hinkle DE, Ritchey SJ. Macronutrient content of a hyponenergy diet affects nitrogen retention and muscle function in weightlifters. *Int J Sports Med* 1988;9:261–266.
65. Melby CL, Schmidt WD, Corrigan D. Resting metabolic rate in weight-cycling collegiate wrestlers compared with physically active, noncycling and control subjects. *Am J Clin Nutr* 1990;52:409–414.
66. Herbert WG, Ribisl PM. Effects of dehydration upon physical working capacity of wrestlers under competitive conditions. *Res Q* 1972;43:416–422.
67. Ribisl PM, Herbert WG. Effects of rapid weight reduction and subsequent rehydration upon the physical working capacity of wrestlers. *Res Q* 1970;41:536–541.
68. Vaccaro P, Zauner CW, Cade JR. Changes in body weight, hematocrit and plasma protein concentration due to dehydration and rehydration in wrestlers. *J Sports Med Phys Fitness* 1976;16:45–53.
69. Burge CM, Carey MF, Payne WR. Rowing performance, fluid balance, and metabolic function following dehydration and rehydration. *Med Sci Sports Exerc* 1993;25:1358–1364.
70. Montain SJ, Coyle EF. The influence of graded dehydration on hyperthemia and cardiovascular drift during exercise. *J Appl Physiol* 1992;73:1340–1350.
71. Allen T, Smith DP, Miller DK. Hemodynamic response to submaximal exercise after dehydration and rehydration in high school wrestlers. *Med Sci Sports* 1977;9:159–163.
72. Caldwell JE, Ahonen E, Nousiainen U. Diuretic therapy, physical performance, and neuromuscular function. *Physician Sportsmed* 1984;12:73–85.
73. U.S. Department of Health and Human Services. Hyperthermia and dehydration-related deaths associated with intentional weight loss in three collegiate wrestlers: North Carolina, Wisconsin, and Michigan, November-December 1997. *MMWR* 1998;47:105–108.
74. Croyle PH, Place RA, Hilgenberg AD. Massive pulmonary embolism in a high school wrestler. *JAMA* 1979;241:827–828.
75. McDermott WV, Bartlett MK, Culver PJ. Acute pancreatitis after prolonged fast and subsequent surfeit. *N Engl J Med* 1956;254:379–380.
76. Kono I, Kitao H, Matsuda M, Haga S, Fukushima H, Kashiwagi H. Weight reduction in athletes may adversely affect the phagocytic function in monocytes. *Physician Sportsmed* 1988;16:56–65.
77. Costill DL, Sparks KE. Rapid fluid replacement following dehydration. *J Appl Physiol* 1973;34:299–303.
78. Roemmich JN, Sinning WE. Weight loss and wrestling training: effects on growth-related hormones. *J Appl Physiol* 1997;82:1760–1764.
79. Horswill CA. Weight loss and weight cycling in amateur wrestlers: implications for performance and resting metabolic rate. *Int J Sport Nutr* 1993;3:245–260.
80. Sawka MN. Physiological consequences of dehydration: exercise performance and thermoregulation. *Med Sci Sports Exerc* 1992;24:657–670.
81. Costill DL. Carbohydrates for exercise: dietary demands for optimal performance. *Int J Sports Med* 1988;9:1–18.
82. Costill DL, Hargreaves M. Carbohydrate nutrition and fatigue. *Sports Med* 1992;13:86–92.
83. Sawka MN, Francesconi RP, Young AJ, Pandolf KB. Influence of hydration level of body fluids on exercise performance in the heat. *JAMA* 1984;252:1165–1169.
84. Armstrong LE, Costill DL, Fink WJ. Influence of diuretic-induced dehydration on competitive running performance. *Med Sci Sports Exerc* 1985;17:456–461.
85. Sawka MN, Pandolf KB. Effects of body water loss in physiological function and exercise performance. In: Lamb DR, Gisolfi CV, eds. *Perspectives in exercise science and sports medicine: fluid homeostasis during exercise.* Indianapolis: Benchmark Press, 1990:1–38.
85a. Ahlman K, Karvoner MJ. Weight reduction by sweating in wrestlers, and its effects on physical fitness. *J Sports Med* 1961;1:58–62.
86. Maffulli N. Making weight: a case study of two elite wrestlers. *Br J Sports Med* 1992;26:107–110.
87. Park SH, Roemmich JN, Horswill CA. A season of wrestling and weight loss by adolescent wrestlers: effect on anaerobic arm power. *J Appl Sport Sci Res* 1990;4:1–4.
88. Serfass RC, Stull GA, Alexander JF, Ewing JL. The effects of rapid weight loss and attempted rehydration on strength and endurance of the handgripping muscle in college wrestlers. *Res Q Exerc Sport* 1984;55:46–52.
89. Webster S, Rutt R, Weltman A. Physiological effects of a weight loss regimen practiced by college wrestlers. *Med Sci Sports Exerc* 1990;22:229–234.
90. Hickner RC, Horswill C, Welker J, Scott JR, Costill DL. Test developement for study of physical performance in westlers following weight loss. *Int J Sports Med* 1991;12:557–562.
91. Horswill CA, Hickner RC, Scott JR, Costill DL, Gould D. Weight loss, dietary carbohydrate modification and high intensity, physical performance. *Med Sci Sports Exerc* 1990b;22:470–476.
92. Klinzing JE, Karpowicz W. The effects of rapid weight loss and rehydration on a wrestling performance test. *J Sports Med* 1986;26:149–156.
93. Eckerson JM, Housh DJ, Housh TJ, Johnson GO. Seasonal changes in body composition, strength, and muscular power in high school wrestlers. *Pediatr Exerc Sci* 1994;6:39–52.
94. Roemmich JN, Sinning WE. Weight loss and wrestling training: effects on nutrition, growth, maturation, body composition, and strength. *J Appl Physiol* 1997;82:1751–1759.
95. Song TMK, Cipriano N. Effects of seasonal training on physical and physiological function on elite varsity wrestlers. *J Sports Med* 1984;24:123–130.
96. Steen SN, Brownell KD. Patterns of weight loss and regain in wrestlers: has tradition changed? *Med Sci Sports Exerc* 1990;22:762–768.
97. Girandola RN, Wisewell RA, Romero G. Body composition changes resulting from fluid ingestion and dehydration. *Res Q* 1977;48:299–303.
98. Horswill C, Park S, Roemmich J. Changes in the protein nutritional status of adolescent wrestlers. *Med Sci Sports Exerc* 1990;22:599–604.
99. Roemmich JN, Sinning WE. Sport-seasonal changes in body composition, growth, power and strength of adolescent wrestlers. *Int Sports Med* 1996;17:92–99.
100. Hansen NC. Wrestling with "making weight." *Physician Sportsmed* 1978;6:106–111.
101. Smith NJ. Nutrition in children's sports. In: Micheli LJ, ed. *Pediatric and adolescent sport medicine.* Boston: Little Brown, 1984:134–143.
102. Theintz GE, Howald H, Allemann Y, Sizonenko PC. Growth and pubertal development of young female gymnasts and swimmers: a correlation with parental data. *Int J Sports Med* 1989;10:87–91.
103. Theintz GE, Howald H, Weiss U, Sizonenko PC. Evidence for a reduction of growth potential in adolescent female gymnasts. *J Pediatr* 1993;122:306–313.
104. Housh TJ, Johnson GO, Stout J, Housh DJ. Anthropometric growth patterns of high school wrestlers. *Med Sci Sports Exerc* 1993;25:1141–1150.
105. McMurray RG, Proctor CR, Wilson WL. Effect of the caloric deficit and dietary manipulation on aerobic and anaerobic exercise. *Int J Sports Med* 1991;12:167–72.
106. Strauss RH, Lanese RR, Malarkey WB. Weight loss in amateur wrestlers and its effect on serum testoterone levels. *JAMA* 1985;254:3337–3338.
107. Bemben DA, Walker L, Bemben MG, Fetters N. Influence of preseason training on serum testosterone (T) levels in NCAA I wrestlers [Abstract]. *Med Sci Sports Exerc* 1997;29:S218.
108. Steen SN, Oppliger RA, Brownell KD. Metabolic effects of repeated weight loss and regain in adolescent wrestlers. *JAMA* 1988;260:47–50.
109. Schmidt WD, Corrigan D, Melby CL. Two seasons of weight cycling does not lower resting metabolic rate in college wrestlers. *Med Sci Sports Exerc* 1993;25:613–619.
110. Frisch RE, McArthur JW. Menstrual cycles: fatness as a determi-

nant for minimum weight for height necessary for their maintenance or onset. *Science* 1974;185:949–951.
111. Loucks, AB The reproductive system. In: Bar-Or O, Lamb DR, Clarkson PM, eds. *Perspectives in exercise science and sports medicine. exercise and the female: a life span approach.* Carmel, IN: Cooper Publishing Group, 1996:41–72.
112. Nelson M, Fisher E, Catsos P, Meredith C, Turksoy R, Evans W. Diet and bone mass in amenorrheic runners. *Am J Clin Nutr* 1986;43:910.
113. Dueck C, Matt K, Manore M, Skinner J. Treatment of athletic amenorrhea with a diet and training intervention program. *Int J Sports Med* 1996;6:24–40.
114. Dueck CA, Matt KS, Manore MM, Skinner JS. Effects of a dietary/training intervention on athletic amenorrhea, bone density and body composition: a case study [Abstract]. *Med Sci Sports Exerc* 1995;27:S223.
115. Hackney AC, Sinning WE, Bruot BC. Reproductive hormonal profiles of endurance trained and untrained males. *Med Sci Sports Exerc* 1988;20:60–65.
116. Strauss RH, Lanese RR, Malarkey WB. Decreased testosterone and libido with severe weight loss. *Physician Sportsmed* 1993;21:64–71.
117. Freischlag J. Weight loss, body composition, and health of a high school wrestler. *Physician Sportsmed* 1984;12:121–126.
118. Kelly JM, Gorney BA, Kalm KK. The effects of a collegiate wrestlers on body composition, cardiovasular fitness and muscle strength and endurance. *Med Sci Sports* 1978;10:119–124.
119. American College of Sports Medicine. Postion paper on weight loss in wrestlers. *Med Sci Sports* 1976;8:XI–XIII.
120. Tcheng TK, Tipton CM. Iowa Wrestlng Study: anthropometric measurements and the prediction of a "minimal" body weight in high school wrestlers. *Med Sci Sports* 1973;5:1–10.
121. Opplinger RA, Harms RD, Herrmann DE, Streich CM, Clark RR. Grappling with weight cutting: the Wisconsin wrestling minimum weight project. *Physician Sportsmed* 1995;23:69–78.
122. Shirreffs SM, Taylor AJ, Leiper JB Maughan RJ. Post-exercise rehydration in man: effects of volume consumed and drink sodium content. *Med Sci Sports Exerc* 1996;28:1260–1271.
123. Gonzalez-Alonso J, Heaps CL, Coyle EF. Rehydration after exercise with common beverages and water. *Int J Sports Med* 1992;13:399–406.
124. Maughan RJ, Leiper JB. Sodium intake and post-exercise rehydration in man. *Eur J Appl Physiol* 1995;71:311–319.
125. Wemple RD, Morocco TS, Mack GS. Influence of sodium replacement on fluid ingestion following exercise-induced dehydration. *Int J Sports Med* 1997;7:104.
126. Below PR, Mora-Rodriguez R, Gonzalez-Alonso J, Coyle EF. Fluid and carbohydrate ingestion independently improve performance during 1 h of intense exercise. *Med Sci Sports Exerc* 1995;27:200–210.
127. Carter JE, Gisolfi CV. Fluid replacement during and after exercise in the heat. *Med Sci Sports Exerc* 1989;21:532–539.
128. Walberg Rankin J, Ocel JV, Craft LL. Effect of weight loss and refeeding diet composition on anaerobic performance in wrestlers. *Med Sci Sports Exerc* 1996;28:1292–1299.
129. Burke LM, Collier GR, Hargreaves M. Muscle glycogen storage after prolonged exercise: effect of the glycemic index of carbohydrate feedings. *J Appl Physiol* 1993;75:1019–1023.
130. Coyle EF, Coyle E. Carbohydrates that speed recovery from training. *Physican Sportsmed* 1993;21:111–123.
131. Lemon P. Do athletes need more dietary protein and amino acids? *Int J Sport Nutr* 1995;5:S39.
132. Short SH, Short WR Four-year study of university athletes' dietary intake. *J Am Dietet Assoc* 1983;82:632–645.
133. Steen S, McKinney S. Nutrition assessment of college wrestlers. *Physician Sportsmed* 1986;14:100–116.
134. Elam R, Hardin D, Sutton R, Hagen L. Effects of arginine and ornithine on strength, lean body mass, and urinary hydroxyproline in adult males. *J Sports Med Phys Fitness* 1989;29:52–56.
135. Walberg-Rankin J, Hawkins C, Fild DS, Sebolt DR. The effect of oral arginine during energy restriction in male weight trainers. *J Strength Cond Res* 1994;8:170–177.
136. Biolo G, Maggi SP, Williams BD, Tipton KD, Wolfe RR. Increased rates of muscle protein turnover and amino acid transport after resistance exercise in humans. *Am J Physiol* 1995; 268:E514–E520.
137. Tarnopolsky M, MacDougall J, Atkinson S. Influence of protein intake and training status on nitrogen balance and lean body mass. *J Appl Physiol* 1988;66:187.
138. Tarnopolsky M, Atkinson S, MacDougall J, Chesley A, Philips S, Schwarcz H. Evaluation of protein requirements in trained strength athletes. *J Appl Physiol* 1992;73:1986.
139. Meredith CN, Frontera WR, O'Reilly KP, Evans WJ. Body composition in elderly men: effect of dietary modification during strength training. *J Am Geriatr Soc* 1992;40:155–162.
140. Fern EB, Bielinski RN, Schutz Y. Effects of exaggerated amino acid and protein supply in man. *Experientia* 1991;47:168–172.
141. Lemon P, Tarnopolsky M, MacDougall J, Atkinson S. Protein requirements and muscle mass/strength changes during intensive training in novice bodybuilders. *J Appl Physiol* 1992;73:767–775.
142. Greenhaff PL, Casey A, Short AH, Harris R, Soderlund K, Hultman E. Influence of oral creatine supplementation of muscle torque during repeated bouts of maximal voluntary exercise in man. *Clin Sci* 1998;84:565–571.
143. Harris R, Soderlund K, Hultman E. Elevation of creatine in resting and exercise muscle of normal subjects by creatine supplementation. *Clin Sci* 1992;83:367–374.
144. Balsom PD, Soderlund K, Sjodin B, Ekblom B. Skeletal muscle metabolism during short duration high-intensity exercise: influence of creatine supplementation. *Acta Physiol Scand* 1995; 154:303–310.
145. Cooke WH, Grandjean PW, Barnes WS. Effect of oral creatine supplementation on power output and fatigue during bicycle ergometry. *J Appl Physiol* 1995;78:670–673.
146. Odland LM, MacDougall JD, Tarnopolsky MA, Elorriaga A, Borgmann A. Effects of oral creatine supplementation on muscle [PCr] amd short-term maximum power output. *Med Sci Sports Exerc* 1997;29:216–219.
147. Balsom PD, Harridge SDR, Soderlund K, Sjodin B, Ekblom, B. Creatine supplemenation per se does not enhance endurance exercise performance. *Acta Physiol Scand* 1993;149:521–523.
148. Balsom PD, Ekblom B, Soderlund K, Hultman E. Creatine supplementation and dynamic high-intensity intermittent exercise. *Scand J Med Sci Sports* 1993;3:143–149.
149. Earnest CP, Snell PG, Rodriguez R, Almada,AL, Mitchell TL. The effect of creatine monohydrate ingestion on anaerobic power indices, muscular strength and body composition. *Acta Physiol Scand* 1995;153:207–209.
150. Mujika I, Padilla S. Creatine supplementation as an ergogenic aid for sports performance in highly trained athletes: a critical review. *Int J Sports Med* 1997;18:491–496.
151. Hultman E, Soderlund K, Timmons JA, Cederblad G, Greenhaff PL. Muscle creatine loading in men. *J Appl Physiol* 1996;81: 232–237.
152. Volek JS, Kraemer WJ, Nush JA, et al. Creatine supplementation enhanced muscular performance during high-intensity resistance exercise. *J Am Dietet Assoc* 1997;97:765–770.
153. Ziegenfuss TN, Lemon PWR, Rogers MR, Ross R, Yarasheski KE. Acute creatine ingestion: effects on muscle volume, anaerobic power, fluid volumes, and protein turnover [Abstract]. *Med Sci Sports Exerc* 1997;29:S127.
154. Vandenberghe K, Goris M, Van Hecke P, Van Leemputte M, Vangerven L, Hespel P. Long-term creatine intake is beneficial to muscle performance during resistance training. *J Appl Physiol* 1997;83:2055–2063.
155. Huggins S. Energy supplement stirs debate. *NCAA News* 1996;33:1.
156. Oopik V, Paasuke M, Timpmann S, Medijainen L, Ereline J, Smirnova T. Effect of rapid body weight reduction on metabolism and isokinetic performance capacity in well trained karatekas. Second Annual Congress of the European College of Sports Science. Book of Abstracts II, 1997.
157. Butterfield G. Amino acids and high protein diets. In: Lamb DR, Williams MH, eds. *Perspectives in exercise science and sports medicine: ergogenics-enhancement of performance in exercise and sport.* Indianapolis: Cooper Publishing Group, 1991:87.
158. Klahr S, Levey A, Beck G, et al. The effects of dietary protein

restriction and blood-pressure control on the progression of chronic renal disease. *N Engl J Med* 1994;330:877.
159. Poortmans JR, Auquier H, Renaut V, Durussek A, Saugy M, Brisson GR. Effect of short-term creatine supplementation on renal responses in men. *Eur J Appl Physiol* 1997;76:566–567.
160. Mertz W. Chromium in human nutrition: a review. *J Nutr* 1993;123:626.
161. Anderson RA, Polansky MM, Bryden NA, Bhathena SJ, Canary JJ. Effects of supplemental chromium on patients with symptoms of reactive hypoglycemia. *Metabolism* 1987;36:351–355.
162. Anderson RA, Polansky MM, Bryden NA, Canary JJ. Supplemental-chromium effects on glucose, insulin, glucagon, and urinary chromium losses in subjects consuming controlled low-chromium diets. *Am J Clin Nutr* 1991;54:909–916.
163. Anderson RA. Chromium, glucose tolerance, and diabetes. *Biol Trace Elem Res* 1992;32:19–24.
164. Evans GW. The effect of chromium picolinate on insulin controlled parameters in humans. *Int J Biosoc Med Res* 1989;11: 163–180.
165. Hallmark MA, Reynolds TH, DeSouza CA, Dotson CO, Anderson RA, Rogers MA. Effects of chromium and resistive training on muscle strenght and body composition. *Med Sci Sports Exerc* 1996;28:139–144.
166. Lukaski HC, Bolonchuk WW, Siders WA, Milne DB. Chromium supplementation and resistance training: effects on body composition, strength, and trace element status of men. *Am J Clin Nutr* 1996;63:954–965.
167. Trent L, Thieding-Cancel D. Effects of chromium picolinate on body composition. *J Sports Med Phys Fitness* 1995;35:273.
168. Grant KE, Chandler RM, Castle AL, Ivy JL. Chromium and exercise training: effect on obese women. *Med Sci Sports Exerc* 1997;29:992–998.
169. Nissen SL, Abumrad NN. Nutritional role of leucine metabolite β-hydroxy β-methylbutyrate (HMB). *J Nutr Biochem* 1997; 8:300–311.
170. Nissen S, Sharp R, Ray M, et al. Effect of leucine metabolite β-hydroxy-β-methlbutyrate on muscle metabolism during resistance-exercise training. *J Appl Physiol* 1996;81:2095–2104.
171. American College of Sports Medicine. Position statement on the use and abuse of anabolic-androgenic steroids in sports. *Med Sci Sports* 1977;9:i–iii.
172. American College of Sports Medicine. Position stand on the use of anabolic-androgenic steroids in sports. *Med Sci Sports Exerc* 1987;19:534–539.
173. Buckley W, Yesalis C, Friedl K, Anderson W, Streit A, Wright J. Estimated prevalence of anabolic steroid use among high school seniors. *JAMA* 1988;260:3441–3445.
174. Durant RH, Ashworth CS, Newman C, Rickert VI. Stability of the relationships between anabolic steroid use and multiple substance use among adolescents. *J Adolesc Health* 1998;15: 111–116.
175. Skolnick AA. Scientific verdict still out on DHEA. *JAMA* 1996;276:1365–1366.
176. McCargar LJ, Crawford SM. Metabolic and anthropometric changes with weight cycling in wrestlers. *Med Sci Sports Exerc* 1992;24:1270–1275.
177. Costill D, Pearson DR, Fink WJ. Anabolic steroid use among athletes: changes in HDL-C levels. *Physician Sportsmed* 1984; 12:113–117.
178. Cohen J, Noakes T, Benade A. Hypercholesterolemia in male power lifters using anabolic-androgenic steroids. *Physician Sportsmed* 1988;16:49–56.
179. Frankle M, Cicero,G, Payne J. Use of androgenic anabolic steroids by athletes [Letter]. *JAMA* 1988;252:482.
180. McNutt B, Ferenchick G, Kirlin P, Hamlin N. Acute myocardial infarction in a 22 year old world class weightlifter using anabolic steroids. *Am J Cardiol* 1998;62:164.
181. Kilshaw BH, Harkness RA, Hobson BM, Smith AWM. The effects of large doses of the anabolic steroid, methandrostenolone, on an athlete. *Clin Endocrinol* 1975;4:537–541.
182. Knuth UA, Maniera H, Nieschlag E. Anabolic steroids and semen parameters in bodybuilders. *Fertil Steril* 1989;52:1041–1048.
183. Williams MH. *Nutritional aspects of human physical and athletic performance.* 2nd ed. Springfield: CC Thomas, 1985.
184. Roy BD, Tarnopolsky MA, MacDougall JD, Fowles J, Yarasheski KE. Effect of glucose supplement timing on protein metabolism after resistance training. *J Appl Physiol* 1997;82:1882–1888.
185. Anthony JC, Gautsch TA, Layman DK. Effect of meal composition on skeletal muscle protein synthesis rates (K_s) following prolonged exercise [Abstract]. *FASEB J* 1997;11:A375.
186. Boileau RA, Lohman TG, Slaughter MH. Exercise and body composition in children and youth. *Scand J Sci* 1985;7:17–27.
187. Thorland WC, Johnson GO, Fagot TG, Tharp GD, Hammer RW. Body composition and somatotype characteristics of junior Olympic athletes. *Med Sci Sports* 1981;13:332–338.
188. Thorland WC, Johnson GO, Housh TJ, Retsell MJ. Anthropometric characteristics of elite adolescent competitive swimmers. *Hum Biol* 1983;55:735–748.
189. Stager JM, Cordain L, Becker TJ. Relationship of body composition to swimming performance in female swimmers. *J Swim Res* 1984;1:21–26.
190. Boileau RA, Lohman TG. The measurement of human physique and its effect on physical performance. *Orthop Clin North Am* 1977;8:563–581.
191. Fleck SJ. Body composition of elite American athletes. *Am J Sports Med* 983;11:398–403.
192. Wilmore JH. Body composition in sport and exercise: directions for future research. *Med Sci Sports Exerc* 1983;15:21–31.

Exercise and Sport Science,
edited by William E. Garrett, Jr., and Donald T. Kirkendall.
Lippincott Williams & Wilkins, Philadelphia © 2000.

CHAPTER 23

Exercise Science and the Child Athlete

Thomas W. Rowland

The emergence of the elite young athlete has triggered interest in understanding the anatomic and physiologic responses to exercise in children. Do children have the same exercise physiology as adults? If not, do these differences influence how child athletes should train and compete? Are there particular risks to young athletes based on their physiologic responses to exercise? Attempts to answer these important questions have stimulated considerable research efforts, with books, journals, and scientific organizations specifically devoted to exercise science in children.

Not surprisingly, children do manifest unique features in their responses to exercise that separate them from adults. Children, in contrast to mature individuals, are growing. This growth is both physical (i.e., progressive increases in size of heart, lungs, and muscle) and functional (changes in sweating rate, increases in cellular glycolysis). Many of these changes influence exercise and bear consideration in the care and nurture of young athletes. This is true not only of elite athletes but also of children who participate at all levels of competition.

Currently many questions regarding exercise responses in children and their impact on sports play remain unanswered. This stems largely from the relatively recent development of highly competitive child athletes and the diversity of their participation. Even more so, ethical considerations preclude obtaining certain information in this age group. Major gaps in our knowledge of developmental exercise physiology result from these appropriate constraints (i.e., skeletal muscle enzyme activity by biopsy, responses to extremes of climatic conditions, alterations with pharmacologic intervention).

This chapter reviews current insights into the physiologic responses to exercise in children and their importance to young athletes. The focus is on the prepubertal age group (approximately younger than 12 to 13 years), as changes during early adolescence appear to differentiate characteristics of adults from those of children.

In addition, information is limited to healthy individuals. A discussion follows of the important aspects of exercise physiology in both athletes and nonathletes with chronic disease (i.e., asthma, diabetes mellitus).

PHYSIOLOGIC RESPONSES TO EXERCISE: UNIQUENESS OF THE CHILD

Understanding the physiologic responses to exercise in growing children is fraught with many difficulties. Particularly vexing is the problem of adjusting variables for changes in body size. How, for instance, do we compare the maximal oxygen uptake ($\dot{V}O_2max$) at age 6 years and again in the same child at age 12? Absolute $\dot{V}O_2$ will obviously increase over this time period, but if we are to compare aerobic fitness at the two ages, we need to find some means to "normalize" the absolute value for body size.

The proper denominator to accomplish this is not altogether clear. The traditional use of body mass in kilograms has been challenged as inappropriate, as—in the case cited above—maximal oxygen uptake and body mass do not change proportionately. As a result, $\dot{V}O_2max$ expressed per kilogram body mass is inversely related to body mass. That is, the smaller subject will artifactually be provided a greater value, and the larger subject will be penalized with a lower $\dot{V}O_2max$ per kilogram. The use of allometric scaling techniques may provide more accurate assessment of size-adjusted changes in physiologic variables (1). For example, mass expressed to the 0.75 power may serve as a more accurate denominator for normalizing values of $\dot{V}O_2max$ than mass 1.0.

The difficulty in establishing causal relations between variables during growth of children also is problematic.

T. W. Rowland: Department of Pediatrics, Tufts University School of Medicine, Boston; Baystate Medical Center, Springfield, Massachusetts 01199.

Assume variable A and variable B are in no way related to each other. If both are linked to body size, however, a misleading tight correlation between the two as the child ages will erroneously suggest a causal relation. In the adult model, physiologic responses to exercise have traditionally been divided into strength, short-term or anaerobic work, and endurance or aerobic exercise, based on the energy sources for each of these activities. The following discussion examines each of these areas in the pediatric population. There is some evidence that children are metabolic "nonspecialists"; that is, the child with high fitness in one type of activity will do well in the others (the boy who is fast in the 50-m run is also strong and performs well in distance cycling). This is in contrast to adults, whose fitness is typically limited to a single form of sports (the marathon runner would not make a good defensive linebacker on the football team).

Aerobic Fitness

Maximal oxygen uptake ($\dot{V}O_2$max), the laboratory marker of aerobic fitness, is measured during cycle or treadmill testing in children in the same way as in adults. As $\dot{V}O_2$max indicates the peak capacity of heart, lungs, blood, and skeletal muscle to use oxygen during exercise, it is not unexpected that absolute values should increase with growth of children as the size of these determinants increases.

Average values for $\dot{V}O_2$max increase from approximately 1.0 L/min at age 6 in all children to 2.0 and 2.8 L/min in girls and boys, respectively, at age 15 years (2). Although there is a large overlap in values between genders, average $\dot{V}O_2$max is slightly greater in the boys at all prepubertal ages. When $\dot{V}O_2$max is expressed relative to body mass in kilograms, no significant changes are observed in boys from the ages of 6 to 16 years. The average expected value with treadmill running is approximately 52 mL/kg/min, but $\dot{V}O_2$max is less with cycling or treadmill-walking protocols (3). It has been concluded, then, that the growth of maximal aerobic power in boys is no greater than can be explained by augmented size of the oxygen-delivery system.

Girls, however, show a different pattern. Almost from the ages when it can be first measured, $\dot{V}O_2$max per kilogram steadily declines through the childhood years. Mean treadmill value at age 8 years is approximately 50 mL/kg/min and decreases at age 14 years to 45 mL/kg/min. This phenomenon has been attributed to increases in body fat and social factors causing a more sedentary life style in young girls. There may, however, be gender-specific biologic factors (i.e., smaller cardiac stroke volume) that influence $\dot{V}O_2$max differences in boys and girls as they grow.

Recent investigations using allometric scaling to eliminate the effect of body mass in children have suggested that these descriptions may not be accurate. By expressing $\dot{V}O_2$max to body mass to the 0.75 power, for instance, a pattern of increases in aerobic fitness in boys with increasing age and stable values in girls has been reported (4).

Are children more or less "aerobic" than adults? The answer depends on one's definition of aerobic fitness and how it is expressed. Typical average values of $\dot{V}O_2$max of 52 mL/kg/min in prepubertal boys and 45 to 50 mL/kg/min in girls are higher than those typically described in young adults. This has suggested that, at least in the exercise-testing laboratory, children possess greater aerobic fitness than do adults. Recent investigations in which allometric techniques were used to normalize absolute $\dot{V}O_2$max for body size have failed to support this concept, however. They suggested, instead, that little differences in size-relative maximal aerobic performance exist between pre- and postpubertal subjects and may actually be greater in mature individuals (4).

In field performance, of course, aerobic fitness improves dramatically with age. The average 13-year-old boy can run a mile almost twice as fast as he could when he was 5. The factors responsible for this progressive improvement in endurance fitness during the course of childhood have not been clarified. It is particularly intriguing, and perhaps instructive, that the decrease of the threshold for fatigue in endurance events with age in children is not accompanied by parallel improvements in size-relative $\dot{V}O_2$max. In cross-sectional studies of both adults and children, $\dot{V}O_2$max is linked to endurance performance, an expected association given the reliance of endurance activity on aerobic metabolism. Longitudinal development of endurance fitness in children (which improves with age), however, bears no relation to size-relative maximal aerobic power (which remains stable or declines with age).

In cross-sectional studies of children with the same chronologic age and similar body composition, $\dot{V}O_2$max per kilogram is moderately well correlated with 1-mile run time ($r = 0.60$). What is not accounted for in such analyses is the variability in biologic development in the study sample, which affects performance fitness (but not $\dot{V}O_2$max/kg). It follows that $\dot{V}O_2$max per kilogram cannot serve as a marker of changes in endurance fitness over time in children.

These observations suggest that changes in submaximal factors during growth must be influential in affecting field-endurance performance. Indeed, exercise economy ($\dot{V}O_2$/kg) at a given workload in weight-bearing tasks (i.e., running) steadily improves (i.e., $\dot{V}O_2$/kg decreases) with increasing age. This means that at a given speed of running, for instance, the 13-year-old is working at a lower percentage of maximal metabolic capacity than is the 5-year-old. This translates into better field-endurance performance. *Why* submaximal economy improves during childhood is uncertain, but the roles of decreasing stride frequency, changes in substrate use, altered biomechanics, and elastic recoil have been suggested (5).

Short-Burst Anaerobic Fitness

The evaluation of anaerobic fitness, or capacity for short-burst activities, is handicapped by the lack of a simple physiologic marker such as $\dot{V}O_2max$ for aerobic fitness. Functional laboratory tests, such as performance on an all-out 30-second cycling bout (Wingate test), field performance (50-yard dash), and measurement of blood lactate (an indicator of anaerobic metabolism) have been used to assess anaerobic capacity of children.

These separate approaches all suggest that anaerobic fitness improves in respect to body size during the course of childhood. That is, relative to body dimensions, the child should be expected to perform less well than the young adult. This pattern is most evident in boys, who have been reported to increase size-relative mean power on Wingate testing from 5.4 to 7.5 (watts per kilogram) between ages 8 and 11 years (6) and to decrease 50-yard dash times from 8.4 seconds at age 10 to 7.6 seconds at age 13 (7). Similarly, maximal blood lactate levels during exercise testing progressively increase during childhood, from approximately 5.5 mmol/L at age 4 years in boys to 8.5 mmol/L at age 12 (5). Girls show the same trends.

The reason why anaerobic fitness improves in children at a faster rate than body size may relate to increased enzyme activity within the cellular glycolytic pathways. Alternatively, factors influencing neuromuscular fatigue, fiber type and recruitment, psychological controls, and triggers of anaerobiosis (i.e., catecholamines) may contribute, but these determinants have generally not been evaluated in children.

Although some have concluded that muscle-fiber type does not change with growth, the issue is not fully resolved. There is evidence from cross-sectional studies, for instance, that children possess a higher percentage of slow-twitch (aerobic) fibers compared with fast-twitch (anaerobic) fibers compared with adults (8). This suggests the possibility of a switch to a greater role for anaerobic fiber types with increasing age. Such differences might contribute to the improvements observed in anaerobic fitness during growth.

Strength

By any measure, muscle strength improves as the child grows. The pattern is similar regardless of testing modality or muscle group: strength increases approximately twofold between the ages of 7 and 12 years, with average values slightly greater in boys than in girls. At puberty, the strength of girls plateaus, while, stimulated by androgenic hormones, muscle strength in boys is accentuated (9).

There is no evidence that the tension that can be created by a given amount of muscle tissue changes beyond early infancy in humans. It is logical to assume, then, that most, if not all, gains in strength in children with growth result simply from increases in muscle bulk. Force generated by muscle closely reflects muscle cross-sectional area, and growth in humans is characterized by increases in muscle-fiber size (rather than cell number). Total body muscle mass increases from about 8 kg at age 6 years to 16 to 18 kg at age 12 years.

Research evidence suggests that other factors may play a role, however, as muscle size does not fully account for such changes in strength. Neural influences, particularly, appear to contribute to gains in strength with growth. Possible contributions include increased myelination, improved coordination of muscle synergists and antagonists, and augmented motor-unit activation. The role of these possible determinants, however, remains speculative.

Thermoregulation

Children demonstrate different thermoregulatory responses to exercise than do adults (6). These differences may place the child at greater risk for heat-stress injury, particularly in hot, humid climates. This observation has obvious implications for the child athlete participating in intense competition and training regimens. Means of limiting such exposure when temperature and/or humidity is high and assuring adequacy of fluid intake is important for all athletes, but particularly for children.

To begin with, children expend more energy per kilogram to perform the same work as adults (i.e., they have poorer exercise energy economy). This causes a child to produce a greater amount of heat relative to their body mass than do adults performing the same work. The child compensates by losing heat via a relatively larger body-surface area, but the effectiveness of this compensatory mechanism is lost in hot, humid climatic conditions when environmental temperature approaches skin temperature.

In addition, children sweat less during exercise than do adults, the result of a diminished sweat production per gland. As a result, children must rely more on cutaneous blood flow for convective heat loss during exercise. This may explain why children demonstrate poorer endurance fitness in the heat compared with adults. Such impaired exercise capacity has been attributed not to heat stress itself but to limited cardiovascular reserve (perhaps by shunting of central volume blood to the cutaneous circulation for thermoregulation). When children are placed in unaccustomed conditions of high heat and humidity, they acclimatize over time more slowly than do adults.

RESPONSES TO EXERCISE TRAINING

A program of repeated bouts of exercise is expected to trigger adaptations that improve exercise-specific fitness. Such is the foundation for athletic training. Predictable physiologic changes follow regular exercise of particular intensity, duration, and frequency, and it is expected that these physiologic alterations will be translated into improved performance. Evidence exists that such responses may be quantitatively different in children, particularly regarding aerobic fitness, and these maturational differences in training response may have a biologic basis.

Aerobic Trainability

A young adult who participates in a program of regular endurance exercise of sufficient intensity, frequency, and duration typically demonstrates an improvement in $\dot{V}O_2$max of 15% to 30%. Increases in both maximal stroke volume and arteriovenous oxygen (AVO_2) uptake appear to contribute to this improvement, although the specific triggers for these responses are unknown.

An increasing volume of research indicates that whereas children improve $\dot{V}O_2$max in such training programs, the magnitude of increase in aerobic fitness is considerably less than that demonstrated by adults. Several review articles examined the results of a considerable number of training studies in children over the past 30 years (10–12). Earlier studies, which had several methodologic weaknesses (no documentation of training stimulus, lack of control subjects, small numbers), showed improvements in $\dot{V}O_2$max of 10% to 14% (10,11). More recent, carefully structured studies revealed even less response, some showing no mean increase in $\dot{V}O_2$max at all (13–17). Results of these recent studies are outlined in Table 23–1. The latter conform to the findings of meta-analysis of all training studies in children, which found a mean increase of less than 5% (18).

It appears, then, that most children will show small increases in laboratory-assessed aerobic fitness after endurance training, and such changes are independent of gender. The magnitude of such responses is far less than would be expected in adults, however.

Why should prepubertal subjects be impaired in their "plasticity" of $\dot{V}O_2$max compared with adults? The explanation might be methodologic (i.e., inappropriate training stimulus), related to greater pretraining fitness and activity levels in children, or to biologic factors (hormonal influences at puberty that trigger training responses).

Training Intensity

Evidence exists that intensity of exercise during endurance training may need to be higher in children than that recommended for adults. This concept comes from a consideration of maturity differences in the anaerobic threshold. This threshold is defined as the point in a progressive exercise test at which blood lactate levels are observed to increase. The interpretation of this phenomenon is controversial, but many researchers regard the anaerobic threshold as the point at which aerobic energy sources become limited, with increasing contributions of anaerobic metabolism. If so, the exercise intensity at the anaerobic threshold, usually identified by heart rate, would appear to be an ideal level of exercise during training to improve aerobic fitness. Exercise below this intensity would not sufficiently tax the aerobic system (heart, lungs, skeletal muscle), whereas that above the threshold would not be well tolerated, with progressive lactic acidosis and early fatigue.

The anaerobic threshold, as judged by ventilatory parameters, is higher in children than in adults. This appears to reflect the lower level of anaerobic fitness in prepubertal subjects (see above). Expressed as percentage of $\dot{V}O_2$max, the ventilatory anaerobic threshold is generally 65% to 70% of $\dot{V}O_2$max in prepubertal children and 55% to 60% $\dot{V}O_2$max in young adults. Consequently, the heart rate at the ventilatory anaerobic threshold, which can be used as a target for aerobic-training programs, is higher in children (generally about 170 beats/min) than in adults.

These findings suggest that a group of prepubertal subjects should train at a heart rate of 170 beats/min if changes in $\dot{V}O_2$max are to be expected. This target heart rate may be higher than reported in many pediatric

TABLE 23–1. *Effects of endurance training on $\dot{V}O_2$max in recent studies of children*

Study	Ages, sex	Number	Duration (wk)	Improvement in $\dot{V}O_2$max
Welsman et al. (13)	9–10 F	17	8	0
Rowland & Boyajian (14)	10–12 MF	37	12	+6.5%
Rowland et al. (15)	10–12 MF	31	13	+5.4%
Ignico & Mahon (16)	8–11 MF	18	10	0
Williford et al. (17)	12 M	12	15	+10.3%

training studies. This does not appear to be the answer to the inferior aerobic trainability of children, however, because recent training studies showing few or no changes in $\dot{V}O_2max$ used this high intensity level of exercise (14,15).

Level of Habitual Activity

It is an obvious observation that children are more active in their daily lives than are adults. One of the earliest explanations for the limited aerobic-training response in children, then, was that they "self-train" themselves in their habitual activities. As a consequence, few further gains should then be expected with exercise interventions. A number of observations, however, argue against this idea.

First, the activity level of children, although high, comprises rapid, very-short-burst activities. These are not forms of endurance exercise that would be expected to be necessary to improve $\dot{V}O_2max$. Second, if $\dot{V}O_2max$ is "maximized" in children by their levels of regular activity, one would expect to observe a relation between the two. Studies of children have been equivocal on this point. At least half show no relation between habitual activity and maximal aerobic power measured in the laboratory (19).

Third, if habitual physical activity is a strong determinant of aerobic fitness in children, $\dot{V}O_2max$ would be expected to decline significantly when a child is made sedentary. For ethical reasons, this study has not been performed in children. Studies examining the effect of prolonged bed rest in adults demonstrated a decline of 5% to 28% after 7 to 30 days.

One study in children did provide some insights into this question (20). The $\dot{V}O_2max$ was determined by treadmill testing in five children 7 to 11 years old who were recovering from a fractured femur. The subjects had been nonambulatory and nonweightbearing for an average of 10.6 weeks. During the 3-month recovery period, average value for $\dot{V}O_2max$ increased 13% (from 37.2 to 42.9 ml/kg/min) and then plateaued. Assuming that the plateau $\dot{V}O_2max$ reflected the preaccident $\dot{V}O_2max$, this study suggested that daily activities contribute relatively little to $\dot{V}O_2max$. Moreover, the findings implied that the decrease in $\dot{V}O_2max$ with bed rest in children is not greater than that experienced by adults.

In summary, then, although the idea that children's activities promote physical fitness is intuitively attractive, their habitual activity (a) does not appear to make important contributions to $\dot{V}O_2max$, and (b) cannot easily be implicated as responsible for their dampened aerobic trainability.

Biologic Factors

It is possible that biologic factors that separate mature from immature individuals might be responsible for the low responses of $\dot{V}O_2max$ to endurance training in children. This would presumably involve hormonal influences at the time of puberty, particularly testosterone and growth hormone, which have recognized anabolic effects on components of the oxygen-delivery chain. This is a difficult issue to address, however, because the triggers and mechanisms for improvements in $\dot{V}O_2max$ with training at any age are not well understood. Nonetheless, certain possibilities can be addressed.

According to the Fick principle, $\dot{V}O_2max$ is the product of heart rate × stroke volume × peripheral AVO_2 uptake at peak exercise. Because maximal heart rate does not change appreciably with training, alterations in maximal stroke volume or AVO_2 uptake remain as candidates for increasing $\dot{V}O_2max$. There is evidence in adults, as noted previously, that both contribute. Which of these factors might be limiting in the small responses of $\dot{V}O_2max$ to training in children is difficult to ascertain.

Only one study described AVO_2 uptake in children before and after endurance training (21). That investigation demonstrated an increase in average $\dot{V}O_2max$ from 39 to 45 mL/kg/min in nine 11- to 13-year-old boys after a 16-week aerobic-training program. No significant changes were detected after training in AVO_2 uptake at either rest or maximal exercise, however. This implied that increased maximal stroke volume was the sole mechanism for the 15% increase in $\dot{V}O_2max$.

An inability to improve AVO_2 uptake with training in children might be related to their low arterial oxygen content. Compared with adults, children demonstrate lower blood hemoglobin levels (about 2 g/dL less in the 8-year-old compared with the 16-year-old boy). Children will therefore be handicapped if (a) training increases in AV oxygen difference require reducing venous oxygen content, and (b) adults and children have similar limits to reducing the "floor" of AVO_2 difference.

Increases in maximal stroke volume after a period of endurance training could result from increased preload at rest (i.e., augmented plasma volume), increased cardiac filling during exercise (improved ventricular diastolic function, more effective skeletal muscle pump), improved myocardial contractility (greater adrenergic stimulation), or reduced afterload (reduced peripheral vascular resistance). There is very limited research information to assess how biologic maturation might influence each of these variables, or how biologic differences between adults and children might alter these factors in the course of endurance training. It may be important to note, however, that the actions of growth hormone and testosterone (which both increase at puberty) influence several of these variables, including a stimulation of red blood cell production and hemoglobin concentration, increased skeletal muscle size and strength, and augmented myocardial thickness and contractility.

$\dot{V}O_2max$, Aerobic Trainability, and the Child Endurance Athlete

The foregoing discussion raises pertinent questions regarding aerobic trainability of prepubertal endurance athletes. Is lack of significant response of $\dot{V}O_2max$ to endurance training evident in this group of children as well? If so, is this blunted physiologic response translated into limited improvements in field performance with training as well? The answers to these questions are unknown but deserve further investigation. Clearly the structure of training regimens in child athletes should be influenced by the outcomes expected.

Values for $\dot{V}O_2max$ in highly trained prepubertal male endurance athletes are typically 60 to 65 mL/kg/min, compared with the average value in the general population of about 52 mL/kg/min. Whether the higher levels in the athletes reflect the effects of training or genetic predisposition is not clear. Elite adult endurance athletes, on the other hand, usually demonstrate a $\dot{V}O_2max$ of 70 to 80 mL/kg/min. This discrepancy between child and adult athletes has been cited as evidence for a diminished capacity to improve $\dot{V}O_2max$ with training in the former. Indeed, one author suggested that before puberty, endurance athletes are limited to a "ceiling" of $\dot{V}O_2max$ of approximately 60 mL/kg/min (21a). Alternatively, however, the adult athletes with greater values of $\dot{V}O_2max$ have been training for many more years than the prepubertal athletes.

Whether child endurance athletes should be expected to improve $\dot{V}O_2max$ with training is a difficult issue. Magnitude of response in $\dot{V}O_2max$ with training is recognized to be inversely related to pretraining level of fitness. As would be predicted, then, elite-level adult endurance athletes may show few or no changes in $\dot{V}O_2max$ during their training. Most studies in child athletes have described lack of change in $\dot{V}O_2max$ per kilogram over 2 to 3 years of intensive training, particularly distance runners (22,23).

Similarly, whether training of prepubertal athletes can or cannot produce favorable improvements in endurance performance is problematic. No study has provided any insights into this important question. Endurance fitness normally improves over time as the child grows, and separating normal developmental changes from those resulting from training is challenging. For example, Daniels and Oldridge found no changes in $\dot{V}O_2max$ per kilogram when they trained 10- to 15-year-old male runners for 22 months (23). Average 1-mile run time for the group was 6:10 before training and 5:38 after 13 months. Although this suggests that endurance training in this age group can improve performance without altering $\dot{V}O_2max$, it should be recognized that, in nontraining children of the same age, 1-mile run times on school fitness tests have been reported to improve from 9:06 to 8:20 over a similar time span (7). Whether the improvements in times in the training runners represented expected changes with growth alone is thus obscure.

Research data now suggest that limited improvements in $\dot{V}O_2max$ can be expected with endurance training of prepubertal children. Whether this limitation in aerobic plasticity extends to field performance as well, and whether these findings have implications for aerobic trainability of child endurance athletes, is uncertain.

Anaerobic Trainability

In contrast to aerobic trainability, research data provide no clear indication of whether children can improve laboratory or field markers of anaerobic fitness with training. Part of the difficulty is that while well-recognized criteria exist for the duration, intensity, and frequency of training necessary to increase $\dot{V}O_2max$, no such guidelines are available for improving anaerobic fitness. As a result, comparison of results between studies is difficult.

Evidence for the anaerobic trainability of children depends on the measure considered. In terms of field performance, Mosher and colleagues (24) could find no improvement in 40-yard-dash time after 12 weeks of speed training in 10- to 11-year-old soccer players. However, treadmill endurance time running at 7 mph at 18% grade increased by 20%.

A study of 11- to 13-year-old boys who trained for 6 weeks by high-intensity cycling or sprinting showed small but statistically significant improvements (3.4% and 3.7%, respectively) in mean anaerobic power with Wingate testing (25). Rotstein and co-workers (26) found that mean and peak power by Wingate testing improved 10% and 14% after a 9-week interval training program in 10- to 11-year-old nonathletic boys.

Cross-sectional and longitudinal training studies have consistently shown no effect of athletic training on blood lactate responses to exercise (5). However, a single biopsy study of six 11-year-old boys demonstrated significant increases in glycolytic enzymes with training (27).

More information will be necessary to determine whether child athletes can improve anaerobic performance (i.e., 50-yard dash) with training. By laboratory measures, current research suggests that such improvements might be possible.

Strength Training

For many years, traditional dogma held that, lacking testosterone, prepubertal children were incapable of improving muscle strength through resistance training. This was not an unreasonable expectation, given the recognized anabolic effects of testosterone on muscle size and strength. Over the past 25 years, however, a series of studies have proven this premise to be false. Prepubertal boys and girls are, in fact, capable of safely improving muscle strength with appropriate training regimens. Moreover, the relative magnitude of such responses is comparable to that of postpubertal subjects. [The reader is referred to the extensive reviews of these studies by Sale (28), Weltman (29), and Duda (30).] These findings have implications for injury prevention and enhancement of performance in child athletes.

Resistance-training studies in children have generally used free weights and have been conducted over an 8- to 12-week span. The extent of increases in muscle strength has typically been 20% to 30%, and similar improvements have been observed in boys and girls. Typically, no change in muscle bulk has accompanied increases in strength in these studies.

Several studies compared gains in strength with resistance training in pre- and postpubertal subjects (5). Greater increases in absolute muscle strength were evident in the older subjects, but, when expressed as percentage of strength change, gains were equal or even greater in the children. These investigations with children demonstrated no complications or adverse effects. Considering that optimizing strength may prevent injury and improve performance, a supervised, well-structured strength-training program for child athletes has scientific legitimacy.

By what mechanism can prepubertal children improve muscle strength through training without circulating testosterone or increases in muscle size? Neural influences may be important, as may enhancement of the intrinsic force-producing capacity of muscle (alterations in excitation–contraction coupling, myofibril packing density, and muscle compliance). Studies investigating these possibilities are difficult to perform, and neither of these mechanisms has been adequately assessed.

EFFECTS OF PHYSIOLOGIC AND PSYCHOLOGICAL STRESSES ON CHILD ATHLETES

By its nature, physical training is designed to place stress on body tissues, and the body's adaptations to that stress are expected to improve physiologic function and exercise performance. The dose of such training stress, however, must be wisely chosen, because excessive training will cause tissue damage (i.e., injuries) and reduce performance (i.e., athlete "burnout").

The child athlete differs from his or her adult counterpart by the process of growth. This begs the question: could the high stresses of intensive sports training interfere with the normal physical and psychological development of the child athlete? Such concerns have led to recommendations that limitations be placed on training intensity and level of sports participation in children. This section reviews these concerns and describes the scientific data that do or do not support the need for such restrictions.

The body of such information is not large and has lagged behind the growing number and level of sports involvements of child athletes. Moreover, physical and psychological effects of athletic participation are particularly difficult to characterize. Children are involved in a large number of sports, at various levels of participation. One might expect, for instance, that the physiological impact on a child of participating on a national soccer team would be very different from that of gymnastics at a local school. In addition, the phenomenon of the highly trained child athlete is relatively new, and few long-term follow-up data are available.

There also is the difficulty of selective evaluation. Suppose one evaluates a group of 10-year-old marathon runners and finds no adverse physical or psychological effects. Can it necessarily be concluded that extreme distance running is safe for children this age? No, because only those children who safely and successfully performed such training were evaluated, ignoring those who may not have.

Cardiac

Given the high $\dot{V}O_2max$ of endurance athletes, one would expect that such individuals possess superior cardiac functional capacity. This is clearly true in adults, and recent evidence supports similar findings in children. A study of eight trained male runners aged 9 to 13 years demonstrated an average maximal cardiac index of 13.1 L/min/m^2 compared with a value of 11.1 L/min/m^2 in nontrained controls (31). The difference was accounted for by maximal stroke index (69 vs. 58 mL/m^2), as maximal heart rate was similar in the two groups.

Despite this evidence of high cardiac performance in child athletes, there is still reason for caution. Reports in adults suggest that extremes of endurance competition can transiently reduce myocardial function. For instance, an echocardiographic study of adults participating in a 24-hour ultramarathon run revealed decreases in left ventricular shortening fraction (an index of myocardial contractility) immediately after the race, with full recovery the day after (32). Such findings in humans are consistent with those of animal studies, in which depression of myocardial function has been observed after extended intense bouts of exercise.

Little information is available regarding the effects of acute bouts of intensive training or competition on cardiac function in children. Echocardiographic findings have been described before and after a 4-km road race in trained prepubertal child runners (33). Left ventricular dimensions decreased immediately after the race, a change that was paralleled by decreases in body weight. These findings are consistent with the effects of dehydration, and left ventricular shortening fraction did not change. Left ventricular size and body weight returned to prerace values at repeated assessment 24 hours after the race. Exercise electrocardiograms were normal at all testing sessions. In this study, then, no adverse acute cardiac effects were observed.

The available data regarding long-term effects of training on the hearts of children also are reassuring. Rost (34) studied cardiac chamber size longitudinally in child swimmers by echocardiogram over a 10-year period. Left ventricular sizes were greater than those of nonathletes, and no adverse clinical changes were observed from training.

Cardiac responses to sustained exercise are similar to those of adults. Asano and Hirakoba (35) studied 10- to 12-year-old boys and 20- to 34-year-old men while they cycled for 1 hour at an intensity equivalent to 60% $\dot{V}O_2max$. Average cardiac output did not change appreciably in either group, whereas stroke volume decreased from 58 to 54 mL in the boys and 98 to 86 mL in the men. Similar findings were reported in a comparison of premenarchal girls and adult women (36).

Based on this limited information, then, there is no evidence that intense athletic training impairs normal cardiac development or poses cardiac risk to the child with a normal heart. Continuing monitoring of the cardiac status of child athletes will be important, however, before this conclusion can be drawn with confidence.

Differences have been noted in the anatomic characteristics of the hearts of child and adult athletes. The intensely training adult endurance athlete often demonstrates a set of cardiac findings termed the *athlete's heart*. This include resting bradycardia, mild left ventricular enlargement, increased frequency of heart murmurs and extra sounds, and electrocardiographic changes (left ventricular hypertrophy, conduction delays). As these findings may simulate organic disease, it is important that physicians recognize that the athlete's heart may reflect superior, rather than impaired, heart function in the endurance athlete.

Studies in children, on the other hand, suggest that prepubertal endurance athletes do not typically demonstrate findings of the athlete's heart. Physical examinations of swimmers and runners found no difference in frequency of venous hums, carotid bruits, heart murmurs, or third or fourth heart sounds when compared with those of nonathletic children (37,38). Similarly, electrocardiograms in these athletes have shown no left ventricular hypertrophy or other abnormalities.

All five echocardiographic studies that were performed in highly trained child distance runners demonstrated no increase in left ventricular dimension compared with control subjects when normalized to body size. Two reports in child swimmers, however, indicated mild left ventricular enlargement (38).

The failure of most child athletes to demonstrate features of the athlete's heart may reflect the shorter duration and limited intensity of training compared with that of adult endurance athletes. Alternatively, these findings could indicate that child athletes may be less capable of increasing cardiac dimensions with training compared with adults. This possibility follows logically from the limitations seen in improvements in $\dot{V}O_2max$ observed in children after endurance training.

Musculoskeletal Injury and Growth

The weight-bearing stress of physical activity is an important stimulant for normal bone growth. Sports training, on the other hand, can clearly exceed tolerance limits and cause musculoskeletal damage. Concern has therefore focused on the possible adverse effects of bone growth in children caused by early intense sports participation.

Common overuse injuries such as tendonitis and sprains result from excessive sports training and competition. The growing athlete may be particularly prone to such injuries because of diminished flexibility and muscle–tendon mismatches. Young athletes may also develop osteochondroses (degenerative lesions of ossification centers at points of tendon attachment), which may prevent athletic competition. "Little League elbow" is seen in young baseball pitchers, the result of overhand throwing, which causes damage to the medial epicondyle of the humerus.

The more worrisome concern, however, is the potential for damage to epiphyseal growth centers of long bones from endurance training. These areas of growth are vulnerable to damage from macrotrauma (such as a blow to the knee from a block in football), with resulting limitation of bone growth. The concern is that repetitive microtrauma to epiphyseal centers, as is incurred with the multiple foot strikes in distance running, might have the same effect.

Descriptions of epiphyseal overuse injuries in athletic children have been essentially limited to gymnasts. Caine (39) reported 11 such cases of damage to the wrist bones in highly competitive gymnasts (stress fractures of the distal radial epiphysis, shortening of the radius). Epiphyseal injuries in child distance runners, who should be particularly at risk, are not being reported in sports medicine clinics. Apple (40) has commented that,

> if one theorizes about the compressive loading forces that occur with running, one would expect there to be an increased incidence of pressure injuries to the epiphysis as a consequence of extensive long-distance running prior to epiphyseal closure. Such has not been the case. At the present time, until further evidence is forthcoming, there does not seem to be any adverse effect to pressure on the epiphyses induced by running.

Reassuringly, cross-sectional and longitudinal studies in child athletes have shown no decrement of normal development of stature. The one possible exception is gymnastics (41). Studies, mostly in girls, have indicated that skeletal age may lag behind chronologic age and that stature clusters around the 10th percentile for population norms.

In assessing these data, Malina (42) observed that the anthropologic characteristics of gymnasts

> must be considered in the context of extremely selective criteria applied to this sport, including selection at an early age for small body size and physique, characteristics associated with later maturation. Short stature in gymnasts appears to be frequently familial, and their growth curves indicate that short stature is often evident before the age of onset of intensive training.

Malina (42) concluded that these preselection factors "make it difficult to implicate the stress of training as the causative factor in the slower growth and smaller size of gymnasts."

Sexual Maturation

The observation that athletic girls typically experience onset of menses (menarche) later than nonathletic girls has stimulated concern that sports training might interfere with normal sexual maturation. Menarche in the nonathletic North American girl usually occurs at age 12.3 to 12.8 years, whereas the average menstrual onset in athletes occurs 12 to 24 months later. The explanation for this "delay" is unclear and has sparked a great deal of controversy.

One explanation holds that undernutrition, stress, low body fat, and the "caloric drain" of sports training causes a delay in the hormonal events that normally trigger onset of menses. According to this school of thought, then, athletic training is a direct cause of a true delay in menarche.

Alternatively, the late onset of menarche among athletes might be simply an expression of anthropomorphic preselection. Girls who are slender, with narrow hips and low body fat, have an advantage in many sports, and these same characteristics are associated with later age of menarche. This argument implies, then, that sports training itself is not a causative factor in late menstrual onset in female athletes (43).

It is clear, however, that secondary amenorrhea, or cessation of regular menses after menarche occurs, can be a reflection of intense athletic training. In cases of late menarche or secondary amenorrhea, concerns focus on the possible negative effects of low levels of circulating estrogen on bone mineralization. Estrogen is critical in the accretion of bone mass during adolescence and early adulthood that may protect against osteoporosis and its complications at an older age.

Some studies have suggested that low estrogen levels in amenorrheic athletes predispose to decreases in bone mass. Others are more reassuring, suggesting that the stresses on bone in weight-bearing sports protect against diminished bone mass in these athletes. The true risk of impaired development of bone mass in the amenorrheic training athlete therefore is currently uncertain.

Some authors have recommended an aggressive approach to girls with extended primary or secondary amenorrhea, suggesting reduction of training, improvement in nutrition, and possible estrogen replacement in older adolescents (44). Others have questioned whether "our current understanding of the influence of exercise and caloric restriction on the menstrual cycle warrants interference in an athletic training program" (45).

There is no specific evidence that intensive athletic training delays sexual maturation in boys. In fact, cross-sectional studies indicate advanced levels of sexual and skeletal maturation in young male athletes compared with nonathletes (43). It has been assumed that that is an expression of preselection (i.e., the more rapidly maturing, stronger and larger boy is more likely to be proficient in sports such as football, wrestling, and hockey).

The training process itself does not appear to affect male reproductive hormones. A study showed no significant changes in serum testosterone in a group of high school male distance runners over the course of an 8-week cross-country season (46).

Psychosocial Development

Although this review focuses on anatomic and physiologic aspects, it would be irresponsible not to address—at least briefly—issues regarding the potential negative affects of intensive athletic training on the emotional and social growth of children. Indeed, no other question surrounding the wisdom of such involvement by young athletes has raised greater concern.

Few scientific studies have examined emotional responses to training and the effect of intensive sports competition on social development of child athletes in high levels of competition. Much of the information is anecdotal, raising concerns that may or may not be realistic for the majority of such athletes.

There are concerns that intense training regimens may interfere with normal social relations, educational opportunities, and family structure. The high levels of expectations by coach and family, as well as the stress of competition, may negatively influence mental health in immature athletes. Close coach–athlete relationships may lead to risk of physical, mental, and sexual abuse. Rigid training regimens may predispose to eating disorders and excessive behaviors (drinking, drug abuse) after training is completed. Parents and coaches may vicariously use the child for their own ambitions, leading to unreasonable demands on the young athlete.

It is difficult to determine from published research studies how realistic these concerns actually are. When

Donnelly (47) performed interviews with 45 recently retired elite athletes who had competed as children, many of the aforementioned problems arose. But, in general, their reactions were positive, and more than 90% expressed the thought that they would "do it again." It seems, then, that negative psychosocial responses to intensive training can be experienced by some child athletes, but the limited research suggests that these may be less common than has been feared.

One specific intervention that may be particularly helpful in preventing early burnout, enhancing performance, and reducing injuries is the avoidance of early sport specialization by child athletes. Longitudinal studies in the former East Germany and the Soviet Union found that the child who specializes in a particular sport at an early age had a quick performance peak. Such performance was inconsistent, injuries were common, and athletes tended to drop out of their sport by age 18 years (48).

On the other hand, those who played a variety of sports, with specialization delayed to adolescence, exhibited a greater consistency of performance, had fewer injuries, and experienced a longer duration of sports participation.

Similar findings were described by Carlson in Swedish tennis players (49). He found that those who persisted in competition and reached elite levels of play were more likely to have participated in a well-rounded sports program as children. This was in contrast to those who dropped out of competition early, who had specialized in tennis at a younger age.

In summary, the current level of scientific information does not permit a full realization of the physical and psychological risks of intense sports play by children. For the most part, such data are reassuring. There has been no clear support of concerns that such early involvement in athletics poses serious cardiac, musculoskeletal, growth, endocrine, or reproductive risks. Avoidance of early sports specialization appears wise.

Given our lack of full understanding of such concerns, however, child athletes deserve ongoing medical monitoring. Likewise, they need appropriate coaching by individuals who are knowledgeable in the unique physical, physiologic, and emotional characteristics of young competitors. An understanding of the prevention of heat injury and the need for proper nutrition, which have not been addressed in this review, are also vital for safe participation in sports by children.

CONCLUSION

The increased participation of children in athletics, particularly at the elite level, calls for an improved understanding of the physical, physiologic, and emotional responses to exercise in this age group. Children demonstrate unique exercise responses compared with adults: anaerobic fitness relative to body size is less; they demonstrate lower submaximal energy economy; and their thermoregulatory adjustments are different.

Children have a significantly dampened response of $\dot{V}O_2max$ to endurance training, but it is unclear if this can be translated in similar responses in endurance performance. They can, however, improve strength with resistance training, albeit without increases in muscle bulk.

Such findings have importance for child athletes. These young competitors may tolerate heat less well and need particular attention in maintaining proper hydration. A supervised program of resistance training in children may help prevent injuries and enhance performance. On the other hand, there is evidence to suggest that endurance training in children, at least in distance running, may be less efficacious in improving aerobic fitness as in adults.

Risks from physiological stresses of sports training in child athletes have not been clearly documented, but medical supervision of these children is important. An appreciation of the emotional immaturity of the child athlete and the potential psychological risks of excessive early training and competition must be appreciated.

REFERENCES

1. Winter EM. Scaling: partitioning out differences in size. *Pediatr Exerc Sci* 1992;4:296–301.
2. Krahenbuhl GS, Skinner JS, Kohrt WM. Developmental aspects of maximal aerobic power in children. *Exerc Sport Sci Rev* 1985;13:503–538.
3. Rowland TW. Aerobic testing protocols. In: Rowland TW, ed. *Pediatric exercise testing.* Champaign, IL: Human Kinetics Publishers, 1993:19–42.
4. Welsman JR, Armstrong N, Nevill AM, Winter EM, Kirby BJ. Scaling peak VO_2 for differences in body size. *Med Sci Sports Exerc* 1996;28:259–265.
5. Rowland TW. *Developmental exercise physiology.* Champaign, IL: Human Kinetics Publishers, 1996.
6. Bar-Or O. *Pediatric sports medicine for the practitioner.* New York: Springer Verlag, 1983.
7. American Alliance for Health, Physical Education, Recreation and Dance. *Youth fitness testing manual.* Washington, DC: American Alliance for Health, Physical Education, Recreation and Dance, 1980.
8. Lexell J, Sjostrom M, Norlund A, Taylor CC. Growth and development of human muscle: a quantitative morphological study of whole vastus lateralis from childhood to adult age. *Muscle Nerve* 1992;15:404–409.
9. Blimkie CJR. Age- and sex-associated variation in strength during childhood: anthropometric, morphological, neurologic, biomechanical, endocrinologic, genetic, and physical activity correlates. In: Gisolfi CV, Lamb DR, eds. *Perspectives in exercise science and sports medicine.* Vol 2. Indianapolis: Benchmark Press, 1989:133–166.
10. Rowland TW. Aerobic response to endurance training in prepubescent children: a critical analysis. *Med Sci Sports Exerc* 1985; 17:493–497.
11. Pate RR, Ward DS. Endurance exercise trainability in children and youth. In: Grana WA, Lombardo JA, Sharkey BJ, Stone JA, eds. *Advances in sports medicine and fitness.* Vol 3. Chicago: Year Book Medical, 1990:37–55.
12. Vaccaro P, Mahon A. Cardiorespiratory responses to endurance training in children. *Sports Med* 1987;4:352–363.

13. Welsman JR, Armstrong N, Withers S. Responses of young girls to two modes of aerobic training. *Br J Sports Med* 1997;31:139–142.
14. Rowland TW, Boyajian A. Aerobic response to endurance training in children: magnitude, variability, and gender comparisons. *Pediatrics* 1995;96:654–658.
15. Rowland TW, Martel L, Vanderburgh P, Manos T, Charkoudian N. The influence of short-term aerobic training on blood lipids in healthy 10-12 year old children. *Int J Sports Med* 1996;17:487–492.
16. Williford HN, Blessing DL, Duey WJ, et al. Exercise training in black adolescents: changes in blood lipids and $\dot{V}O_2max$. *Ethn Dis* 1996;6:279–285.
17. Ignico AA, Mahon AD. The effects of a physical fitness program on low-fit children. *Res Q Exerc Sport* 1995;66:85–90.
18. Payne VG, Morrow JR. The effect of physical training on prepubescent $\dot{V}O_2max$: a meta-analysis. *Res Q Exerc Sport* 1993;64: 305–313.
19. Morrow JR, Freedson PS. Relationship between habitual physical activity and aerobic fitness in adolescents. *Pediatr Exerc Sci* 1994;6:315–329.
20. Rowland TW. Effect of prolonged inactivity on aerobic fitness of children. *J Sports Med Phys Fitness* 1994;34:147–155.
21. Eriksson BO. Physical training, oxygen supply, and muscle metabolism in 11-13 year old boys. *Acta Physiol Scand* 1972;suppl 384:1–48.
21a. Koch G. Muscle blood flow in prepubertal boys. In: Borms J, Hebbelink M, eds. *Medicine and sport.* Basel, Switzerland: Karger, 1978:34–46.
22. Van Huss W, Evans SA, Kurowski T, Anderson DJ, Allen R, Stephens K. Physiologic characteristics of male and female age group runners. In: Brown EW, Branta CF, eds. *Competitive sports for children and youth.* Champaign, IL: Human Kinetics Publishers, 1988:143–158.
23. Daniels J, Oldridge N. Changes in oxygen consumption of young boys during growth and running training. *Med Sci Sports* 1971;3:161–165.
24. Mosher RE, Rhodes EC, Wenger HA, Filsinger B. Interval training: the effects of a 12 week programme on elite prepubertal male soccer players. *J Sports Med* 1985;25:5–9.
25. Grodjinovsky A, Inbar O, Dotan R, Bar-Or O. Training effect on the anaerobic performance of children as measured by the Wingate anaerobic test. In: Berg K, Eriksson BO, eds. *Children and exercise IX.* Baltimore: University Park Press, 1980:139–145.
26. Rotstein A, Dotan R, Bar-Or O, Tenenbaum G. Effects of training on anaerobic threshold, maximal aerobic power and anaerobic performance of preadolescent boys. *Int J Sports Med* 1986; 7:281–286.
27. Eriksson BO, Gollnick PD, Saltin B. Muscle metabolism and enzyme activities after training in boys 11-13 years old. *Acta Physiol Scand* 1973;87:485–487.
28. Sale DG. Strength training in children. In: Gisolfi CV, Lamb DR, eds. *Perspectives in exercise science and sports medicine.* Vol 2. Indianapolis: Benchmark Press, 1989:165–222.
29. Weltman A. Weight training in prepubertal children: physiological benefit and potential damage. In: Bar-Or O, ed. *Advances in pediatric sport sciences.* Vol 3. Champaign, IL: Human Kinetics, 1989:101–130.
30. Duda M. Prepubescent strength training gains support. *Physician Sportsmed* 1986;14:157–161.
31. Rowland T, Goff D, Popowski B, DeLuca P, Ferrone L. Cardiac responses to exercise in child distance runners. *Int J Sports Med* 1998;19:385–390.
32. Niemela KO, Palatsi IJ, Ikaheimo MJ. Evidence of impaired left ventricular performance after an uninterrupted competitive 24-hour run. *Circulation* 1984;70:350–356.
33. Rowland T, Goff D, DeLuca P, Popowski B. Cardiac effects of a competitive road race in trained child runners. *Pediatrics* 1997;100:E2.
34. Rost R. *Athletics and the heart.* Chicago: Year Book Medical Publishers, 1987.
35. Assano K, Hirakoba K. Respiratory and circulatory adaptation during prolonged exercise in 10-12 year old children and adults. In: Ilmarinen J, Valimaki I, eds. *Children and sport.* Berlin: Springer Verlag, 1984:119–128.
36. Rowland TW, Rimany TA. Physiological responses to prolonged exercise in premenarcheal and adult females. *Pediatr Exerc Sci* 1995;7:183–191.
37. Rowland TW, Delaney BC, Siconolfi SF. The "athlete's heart" in prepubertal children. *Pediatrics* 1987;79:800–804.
38. Rowland TW, Unnithan VB, MacFarlane NG, Gibson NG, Paton JY. Clinical manifestations of the "athlete's heart" in prepubertal male runners. *Int J Sports Med* 1994;15:515–519.
39. Caine DJ. Growth plate injury and bone growth: an update. *Pediatr Exerc Sci* 1990;2:209–299.
40. Apple DF. Adolescent runners. *Clin Sport Med* 1985;4:641–655.
41. Theintz GE, Howland H, Weiss V, Sizonenko PC. Evidence for a reduction of growth potential in adolescent female gymnasts. *J Pediatr* 1993;122:306–313.
42. Malina RM. Physical growth and biological maturation of young athletes. *Exerc Sport Sci Rev* 1994;22:389–434.
43. Malina RM. Menarche in athletes: a synthesis and hypothesis. *Ann Hum Biol* 1983;10:1–24.
44. American Academy of Pediatrics. Amenorrhea in adolescent athletes. *Pediatrics* 1989;84:394–395.
45. Loucks AB. Athletics and menstrual dysfunction in young women. In: Gisolfi CV, Lamb DR, eds. *Perspectives in exercise science and sports medicine.* Vol 2. Indianapolis: Benchmark Press. 1989:513–538.
46. Rowland TW, Morris AH, Kelleher JF, Haag BL, Reiter EO. Serum testosterone response to training in adolescent runners. *Am J Dis Child* 1987;141:881–883.
47. Donnelly P. Problems associated with youth involvement in high-performance sports. In: Chaill BR, Pearl AJ, eds. *Intensive participation in children's sports.* Champaign, IL: Human Kinetics, 1993:95–126.
48. Bompa T. *From childhood to champion athlete.* Toronto: Veritas Publishing, 1995.
49. Carlson R. The socialization of elite tennis players in Sweden: an analysis of the players' backgrounds and development. *Soc Sport J* 1988;5:241–256.

Exercise and Sport Science,
edited by William E. Garrett, Jr., and Donald T. Kirkendall.
Lippincott Williams & Wilkins, Philadelphia © 2000.

CHAPTER 24

Chronobiology and Physical Performance

Thomas Reilly, Greg Atkinson, and Jim Waterhouse

Biologic rhythms refer to cyclic changes that recur regularly over a given time and are related to underlying physiologic processes. The science concerned with the analysis of biologic rhythms is known as *chronobiology*. It is directed toward understanding the mechanisms of biologic time structures, including the manifestations of life and many aspects of human behavior. In humans the length of the cycles, known as the period, can range from small fractions of a second, such as in neural firing rates, to slower changes that recur every 30 days or so (circamensal), or with seasonal changes that recur once (circannual) or twice a year. Rhythms associated with the solar day are called circadian. Rhythms with periods longer than a day (more than 28 hours) are known as infradian, and those recurring repeatedly within a day (less than 20 hours) are known as ultradian.

Biologic rhythms should not be confused with "biorhythms," a theory without any scientific basis. According to this theory, three independent cycles start for each individual at birth. A physical cycle determines vigor and has a cycle length of 23 days. A cycle of emotion has a period of 28 days, and there is also supposed to be a cycle of intellectual ability with a period of 33 days. Half-way through each cycle, there is a swing across the baseline from positive to negative. The theory suggests that sports performance is benefited when cycles are positive and is adversely affected when they are negative, but it becomes more difficult to interpret a biorhythm profile when the three rhythms are mixed. Proponents of the theory can refer to outstanding sports successes to justify their case, but this is selective evidence, and the theory is easily discredited by retrospective analysis of athletic records. For example, Reilly and co-workers (1) found no relation between the date of the season's best performance and the biorhythms of all the female athletes competing in the European track-and-field championships. They concluded that there is no justification for applying biorhythms theory to strenuous exercise and the scientific preparation of athletes. This contrasts with the acceptance of chronobiology as a respected field of science in its own right.

The classic biologic rhythm has been stylized by a sine wave and its characteristics are often determined by cosinor analysis. The midpoint between the highest and lowest values of a rhythm is termed the "mesor" (midline estimating statistic of a rhythm). The amplitude of a rhythm is half the difference between the highest and lowest point of a fitted cosine curve: the range of a rhythm is the difference between the maximal and minimal values. The location in time of the peak is termed the acrophase, but this strictly refers only to sinusoidal oscillations. The acrophase can be expressed in angular degrees (1 period = 360°) or in absolute units of time (e.g., minutes, hours, days, weeks, or years). In many instances, the cyclic variation may be best fitted by alternative statistical models (such as analysis of variance). There also may be identifiable subharmonics within a major cycle. The term "peak-time" should be used for nonsinusoidal rhythms (2). Once the period or cycle length of a rhythm is known or has been established, the other important characteristics should be determined.

Many human performance measures tend to follow closely the circadian rhythm in body temperature (Fig. 24–1) but are also affected by the sleep–wake cycle and local physiologic conditions within the active tissues. The main physiologic rhythms at rest are considered next so that the consequence for exercise can be appreciated.

HUMAN CIRCADIAN RHYTHMS AT REST

Only in the controlled circumstances of experiments is human activity performed under constant routines. The free-living activity that is typical of everyday life occurs

T. Reilly, G. Atkinson, and J. Waterhouse: Research Institute for Sport and Exercise Sciences, Liverpool John Moores University, Liverpool, England.

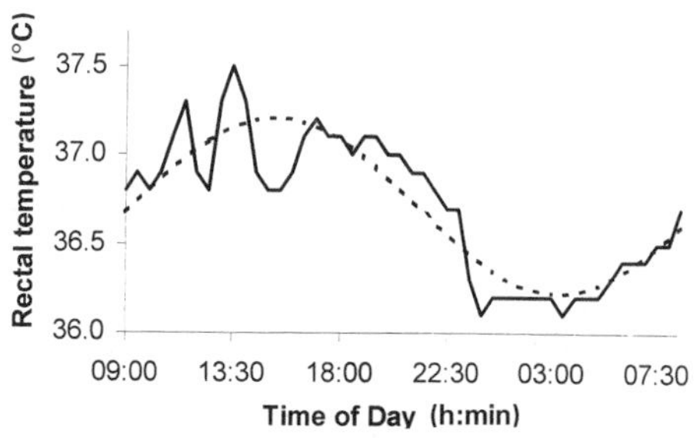

FIG. 24–1. The circadian rhythm in rectal temperature under nychthemeral conditions (*continuous line*) and with the rhythm "purified" by removing the effects of habitual activity and described with cosinor analysis (*broken line*).

under so-called nychthemeral conditions. Thus there is a dynamic effect of active and recovery processes on physiologic functions both during the day and at night.

The Body Temperature Rhythm

Body temperature has been described as the "fundamental variable," and this has led to its use as a marker of circadian rhythms. Generally, body temperature is measured by means of a rectal probe, but more reliable infrared thermometry has made it possible to monitor tympanic temperature safely (3). In field conditions, social circumstance may dictate the use of oral temperature, which is less satisfactory. Midstream urine also may provide a more reliable means for indicating core temperature, but this can have social constraints similar to those for obtaining measurements of rectal temperature.

Body temperature decreases to a minimum during sleep at around 04:00 hours and begins to increase before wakefulness. This increase usually continues until the acrophase of the rhythm is reached at around 18:00 hours. The amplitude of the body-temperature rhythm is 0.4°C to 0.5°C in young adults. The endogenous component of the temperature rhythm is large. In isolation and constant routine studies, the amplitude of the rhythm is not markedly reduced from that observed in normal nychthemeral conditions (see Fig. 24–1). The major exogenous influences on body temperature are sleep and exercise.

Minors and Waterhouse (4) maintained that the circadian rhythm in deep body (rectal) temperature results mainly from fluctuations in heat-loss mechanisms (vasomotor and insensible sweating) rather than heat production (metabolic rate). It seems that it is the set point of thermoregulation that varies with time of day. The peak noradrenergic activity occurs at about 12:00 hours (5). At this time, the dissipation of heat would be counteracted by the resultant vasoconstriction, and deep body temperature would increase as a consequence. Melatonin lowers body temperature, and onset of its secretion from the pineal gland coincides with a sharp decline in core temperature.

Rhythms in Metabolic Variables

The oxygen consumption ($\dot{V}O_2$) at rest displays a circadian rhythm, with a minimum at around 04:00 hours. It seems that the $\dot{V}O_2$ rhythm is partly a result and not a cause of the body-temperature rhythm. The circadian change in core temperature explains only 37% of the range observed in $\dot{V}O_2$ (6). The circadian rhythm in $\dot{V}O_2$ is not attributable to changes in thyroid-stimulating hormone because this variable peaks at the same time as $\dot{V}O_2$ decreases to its nadir (7). Changes in the levels of circulating catecholamines may have some influence over the rhythm in $\dot{V}O_2$.

The blood-glucose level is relatively stable over 24 hours, which may be because the level at any one time is influenced by "multiple metabolic phenomena." A few authors [e.g., Swoyer and colleagues (8)] detected rhythmicity in this variable, albeit with a very low amplitude. It is more usual to find a small-amplitude ultradian rhythm in blood glucose with peak levels corresponding to the three diurnal meals and a fourth increase at the end of sleep (9). Schlierf (10) found that plasma free fatty acids were higher at night than during the day, although this, again, depended greatly on the composition of food ingested.

Rhythms in Ventilation

The forced expiratory volume and peak expiratory flow both vary with time of day, decreasing to minima between 03:00 and 08:00 hours (11). These two variables are indicators of pulmonary airway resistance. Asthmatic patients exhibit markedly greater amplitudes in airway rhythms, depending on the severity of the disease (12). Symptoms of asthma are exacerbated at night and in the early morning, giving rise to the debilitating complaint of "nocturnal asthma" (13). For this reason, asthmatic athletes are advised against performing strenuous training in the early hours of the morning.

Cardiovascular Rhythms

Heart rate varies with an amplitude of 5% to 15% of the 24-hour mean, depending on the extent of the exogenous influences: its acrophase usually occurs around 15:00 hours (6). Similar rhythm characteristics are found for stroke volume, cardiac output, blood flow, and blood pressure (14). Exogenous factors such as sleep, posture, activity, and ingestion of food highly influence the rhythms in heart rate and blood pressure. Given the numerous exogenous influences on blood pressure, its fluctuations over a 24-hour period can be extremely complicated and do not necessarily follow the classic cosine curve of more endogenous rhythms such as body temperature. Zulch and Hossman (15) reported that blood pressure showed a postlunch dip followed by a secondary peak in the afternoon. This phenomenon is clearly evident if individuals nap or have a greater than normal postprandial decrease in blood pressure, such as occurs in aged individuals (16).

Rhythms in Gastrointestinal Function and Excretion

There are circadian rhythms in gastrointestinal motility patterns, intestinal absorption rates, activities of gastrointestinal enzymes, and secretion of gastric acids. Peaks occur diurnally in all these variables (17). Goo and associates (18) reported that rates of gastric emptying for meals administered at 20:00 hours were more than 50% slower than emptying rates for the same meal taken at 08:00 hours. It is not known whether the gastric emptying of carbohydrate drinks during exercise varies with time of day.

Touitou and co-workers (19) reported the peak levels of urinary electrolytes occur in the afternoon at around 16:00 hours (exceptions being urinary chlorides, phosphates, and 17-ketosteroids). Circadian changes in urinary pH mirror those of urinary electrolyte level with the most acidic urine (pH 5.0) observed during the period of sleep, increasing to a maximum of 8.0 in the afternoon (20). Circadian rhythms in urinary pH and excretion of electrolytes should be acknowledged in laboratories concerned with drug testing. Chronopharmacologic studies are needed to ascertain whether an ingested drug would be detected in an athlete's urine at one time of day but not at another.

Rhythms in Hormonal Secretions

Marked peaks in cortisol and growth-hormone levels occur several times during sleep (7). The rhythms in growth hormone and cortisol are strongly influenced by sleep characteristics, which are, in turn, affected by habitual levels of physical activity. Plasma levels of epinephrine and norepinephrine peak in the early afternoon, even during successive days of constant routines (i.e., bed rest with no sleep allowed) (4). The circadian rhythm in blood volume (21) cannot account for these rhythms in hormone levels because the amplitudes are not similar.

Output from endocrine glands, particularly the trophic hormones of the anterior pituitary, exhibit circadian rhythms. Some endocrine secretions (e.g., growth hormone, prolactin, and testosterone) peak during the night. No overall pattern to the rhythms would help to explain the circadian curves in exercise performance to be described later. The rhythms in catecholamines, epinephrine, and norepinephrine are the most closely

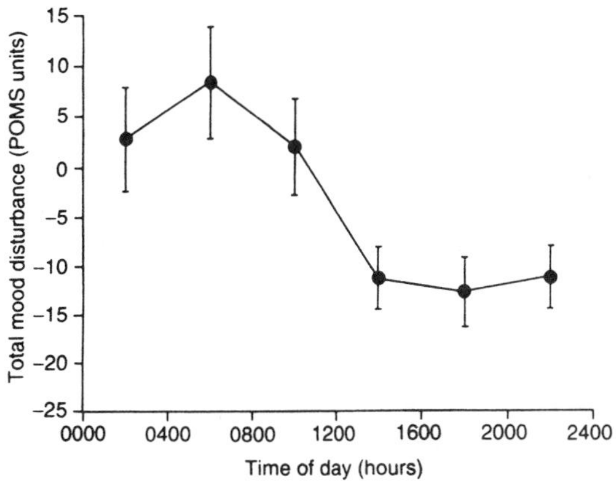

FIG. 24–2. Mood factors vary with circadian rhythms, disturbances being greatest at nighttime and in the morning. From ref. 82, with permission.

related to the performance curve. The excretion of electrolytes also is closely related in phase to the body-temperature and performance rhythms. The diurnal changes in renal function have only marginal impact during exercise because of the relative shutdown of blood flow to the kidneys and the inactive muscles. Angiotensin and aldosterone are linked not only with kidney function but also with the rhythm in blood pressure.

Rhythms in Subjective States

Circadian variation in epinephrine and norepinephrine may mediate fluctuations in arousal or level of alertness. Subjective states of "arousal" have been usually studied in conjunction with other measures in chronobiologic experiments. For example, some researchers used simple visual-analogue scales to measure alertness or the inverse of this, fatigue. Other investigators used recognized inventories such as the Stanford Sleepiness Scale (22) for the measurement of sleepiness or used a questionnaire (Profile of Mood States) (23) for assessment of changes in mood. The research evidence indicates that alertness and positive mood states peak in the waking hours, usually evening. Conversely, mood disturbance is lowest in the afternoon and early evening (Fig. 24–2).

Mood and subjective alertness may be important for human performance because such states can alter an individual's motivation for strenuous physical exercise. Circadian variations in mood states also may affect the "team cohesion" of a sports squad. For example, the ability of individuals to communicate and work together is important for team sports and in coaching contexts.

RHYTHMS IN PERFORMANCE

Sports Performance

There is much indirect evidence that sports-performance capability is highest close to the time that body temperature nears its peak value. Athletic records tend to be set in the late afternoon or evening. This partly reflects the fact that record attempts in track and field events are usually scheduled for evening meetings when the environmental temperature is more favorable for performance than at midday or in the early afternoon. Nevertheless, athletes prefer evening contests and consistently achieve their top performances at this time of day.

The work-rate of male soccer players reflected this preference during indoor five-a-side games sustained for 4 days (24). The pace of play reached its highest intensity at about 18:00 hours and a trough at 05:00 to 06:00 hours on each day. Feelings of fatigue were correlated negatively with levels of activity. The self-paced level of activity conformed closely to the curves in body temperature and in heart rate; this relation persisted throughout successive days. The fact that the freely chosen intensity of exercise is highest at about the time the body-temperature rhythm reaches the top of its diurnal curve has important implications for training as well as for certain competitive sports.

The types of interventions demanded by experimental designs are not feasible in sports competitions. Consequently, research workers have tended to consider the effects of time of day on performance in time trials or simulated contests. Six runners, three weight-throwers, and three oarsmen were found to perform better in the evening than in the morning (25). Swimmers produced faster times over 100 m at 17:00 hours compared with 07:00 hours in three of four strokes studied (26). The speed of running in a 5-minute test also was found to vary in close correspondence to the circadian curve in body temperature (27).

The better performances of swimmers in the evening also apply to multiple efforts. Performances in front crawl were 3.6% and 1.9% faster for 400-m and repeated 50-m swim trials, respectively, at 17:30 hours than at 06:30 hours (28). This time-of-day effect also was observed through 3 successive days of partial sleep deprivation (29). It is clear that evening is best for sprint swimmers, particularly if time-trial results are attributed importance, such as in achieving championship-qualifying standards.

There is a time-band close to the acrophase of body temperature in which optimal performance in sports involving gross motor tasks can be attained. This can extend for 4 to 6 hours, provided that meals and rests are suitably fitted in during the daily routine. Sports requiring fast "explosive" efforts tend to peak earlier and may be related to the sleep–wake cycle rather than to the body-temperature rhythm. In the last 50 years, only in men's shot put and women's javelin have world records been set before noon in track and field events. Practices in which skills have to be acquired should be conducted early in the day or around midday, but more severe training drills and "pressure training" practices are best scheduled for later in the day. It is acknowledged that sports performance is determined by many variables, and there may be multiple performance rhythms. This can be further examined by looking at the existence of rhythms in components of sports performance.

Components Measured Under Controlled Laboratory Conditions

"Performance" is a very broad term, and sports events usually comprise a combination of task components. In the following sections, an attempt is made to isolate components of sports performance and to describe the circadian characteristics of each.

Psychomotor Performance and Motor Skills

Simple reaction time (to either auditory or visual stimuli) is a major component of performances in sprint events. It is an element also of many games skills, such as goalkeeping in soccer or hockey. Reaction time peaks in the early evening at the same time as the maximum in body temperature. This is partly because nerve-conduction velocity increases by 2.4 m/s for every 1°C increase in body temperature. Often there is an inverse relation between the speed and the accuracy with which a simple repetitive test is performed. Therefore accuracy may be worse in the early evening. This illustrates the importance of defining performance because many sports demand accuracy without speed (e.g., golf, darts), and others emphasize power (e.g., first serve in tennis).

Although the effects of time of day on actual performances in these sports have not been examined, their complex nature probably means that they are performed best at times of day when arousal levels are endogenously low. The ability to balance while standing on a "wobble board" represents a task demanding fine motor control, which is performed better in the morning. This is probably because arousal levels are lower than the diurnal peak and closer to the optimal level for performance. Complex aspects of performance such as cognitive operations and short-term memory also peak in the morning rather than in the evening. Rhythms in cognitive variables have relevance to sport in that they influence competitive strategies, decisions, and the delivery and recall of complex coaching instructions.

Circadian rhythms in psychomotor performance, particularly tasks that entail cognitive operations, seem especially prone to a so-called postlunch dip. This phenomenon describes a transient decline in both alertness and performance that occurs early in the afternoon. Some aspects of performance deteriorate at this time without a corresponding decrease in body temperature and occur even if no food is ingested at lunchtime. This time of day should be avoided when the coach is trying to impart new skills or tactics to a group of athletes.

Joint Flexibility and Stiffness

Joint flexibility (range of movement) shows marked rhythmicity across a wide range of human movements. Gifford (30) noted circadian variation in lumbar flexion and extension, glenohumeral lateral rotation, and whole-body forward flexion. Amplitudes of these rhythms can be as high as 20% of the 24-hour mean value. There can be large interindividual differences in the peak times for flexibility.

The rest–activity rhythm present in nychthemeral conditions imposes compressive loading on the spine during the day, leading to the extrusion of water through the invertebral disk wall and a consequent loss of disk height. There is a resultant loss of stature known as "spinal shrinkage" and an increase in the stiffness of the intervertebral disks. This shrinkage is reversed at night during the recumbency of sleeping. Reilly and colleagues (31) provided a comprehensive characterization of the circadian rhythm in human stature. By using a stadiometer accurate to 0.01 mm, they reported that the diurnal variation was 1.1% of overall stature. The circadian variation in the data was better fitted by a power function than by cosinor analysis (32). Peak stature was measured at 07:30 hours, with the greatest rate of shrinkage occurring in the hours immediately after getting up from bed. A period of rest before training or competing in the evening helps to unload the spine and restore its normal responses to compressive loads.

Muscle Strength

Muscle strength, independent of the muscle group measured or the speed of contraction, consistently peaks in the early evening. Grip strength is easy to measure by means of a portable dynamometer, and so it has been frequently used as a marker of the circadian performance rhythm. The rhythm in isometric grip strength peaks between 14:00 and 19:00 hours with an amplitude of about 6% of the 24-hour mean. The grip-strength rhythm is, in part, endogenously controlled because it persists during sleep deprivation and adjusts slowly to changes in sleep–wake regimens. The peak-to-trough variation in grip strength can be 3 times higher than normal in rheumatoid arthritic patients.

It could be important for clinical purposes to know the magnitude of the error associated with determining maximal voluntary contractions (MVCs) in measuring muscle strength at different times of the day. Such errors may be corrected, provided that the cosinor characteristics of the muscle function are known. The MVC_{corr} (corrected for time of day) can be estimated by the equation:

$$MVC_{corr} = \frac{MVC_t}{1 + A \times \cos(15t + 15p)}$$

where t is the time of day at which the test is performed (decimal clock hours), A is the amplitude of MVC as a percentage of the mean divided by 100, and p is the acrophase (peak time). The correction was originally proposed for tests of isometric leg strength, but the equation can be used for other strength tests that display time-of-day effects (33).

There may be a subharmonic within a main circadian rhythm in muscle strength. For example, when the isometric strength of the knee extensors was measured repeatedly during the waking hours of the solar day, two diurnal peaks were noted: one at the end of the morning and another in the late afternoon/evening (34). Performance transiently declined between these times of day. Similarly, there can be a decrease in grip strength between 13:00 and 14:00 hours when the variable is measured every hour for a 24-hour period. This decline was referred to earlier as the postlunch dip.

A true time-of-day effect is not easy to separate from influences resulting from the experimental protocol. The afternoon decline in performance can reflect a decrease in motivation arising from the high number of serial measurements of performance that have been required. Despite this, when isometric strength measures are recorded under the optimal experimental protocol, which allows sufficient recovery between test sessions without disturbing sleep, postlunch declines in performance are still evident. With respect to the isometric strength of other muscle groups, elbow-flexion strength varies with time of day, peaking in the early evening. Back strength also is higher in the evening than in the morning, with an amplitude of around 6% of the 24-hour mean (35).

Both concentric (generation of force while the muscle is shortening) and eccentric (generation of force while the muscle is lengthened) strength values have been obtained at different times of the solar day. A time-of-day effect in these variables was noted with peak isokinetic torque values occurring in the early evening, when measured at slow (between 1.05 and 3.14 rad/s) angular velocities of movement. The test–retest variation of measurements made with computer-controlled isokinetic dynanometers may be as high as 20% at fast angular velocities of greater than 6 rad/s. Unless this error is reduced through multiple trials, any circadian variation may be undetected (36). Inadequate test–retest repeatability of measuring equipment is a problem in chronobiologic research and may explain why rhythms have not been detected in other performance variables.

Short-Term Power Output

Circadian rhythms have been identified in laboratory measures of anaerobic power and conventional tests of short-term dynamic activity. Hill and Smith (37) measured anaerobic power and capacity with a modified version of the Wingate 30-s cycle ergometry test at 03:00, 09:00, 15:00, and 21:00 hours. Peak power in the evening was 8% higher than at 03:00 hours. Similar results were found for mean power over the 30-second test period. Vigorous warm-up procedures that increase both arousal and muscle temperature may "swamp" any existing rhythm in short-term power output. This suggests that proper warm-ups are needed when athletes train or prepare for competitions earlier in the day than they are accustomed to. This warm-up effect, coupled with lack of sensitivity of the ergometry used, may explain the failure in some studies to detect small-amplitude circadian rhythms.

The results of studies that have examined the effects of time of day on fixed-intensity work rates close to maximal oxygen uptake ($\dot{V}O_2max$) seem more conclusive than those that used "supramaximal exercise," such as is required for the Wingate test. Hill and co-workers (38) reported that total work performed at high-intensity, constant-work-rate exercise on a cycle ergometer was significantly higher in the afternoon compared with the morning. These results agree with the findings of Reilly and Baxter (39), who reported longer work times and higher blood lactate levels when a set high-intensity exercise was performed at 22:00 hours compared with 06:30 hours.

With respect to other conventional methods of evaluating short-term explosive activity, Reilly and Down (40) investigated whether performance in jumping shows a circadian rhythm. When individual differences in performances were controlled for, significant circadian rhythmicity was found for length of jump, with an acrophase of 17:45 hours and an amplitude of 3.4% of the 24-hour mean value. Similar rhythm characteristics have been reported by the same authors for anaerobic power output on a stair-run test (41) (see Table 24–1). In view of the fact that margins of victory in competitive jumping events are usually only a few centimetres, time of day should be recognized as a significant factor in competitive attempts or in the ability to meet certain performance standards to qualify for major championships.

The superiority of evening time for swim time trials "in the pool" is likely to be physiologic in origin rather than due to circadian changes in water temperature, because mean and peak power outputs recorded on a swim bench under controlled conditions vary with time of day (42). In this instance, the higher amplitude than normal (Fig. 24–3) is due to the complexity of the simulated arm action of swimming, compared with a grosser movement such as arm cranking.

Physiologic Responses to Exercise

Some circadian rhythms in physiologic responses to exercise are maintained in amplitude, some disappear or are undetectable, whereas others become more marked during exercise. The differing effects of exercise on circadian rhythms could be due to experimental errors such as failure to control prior activity and diet of the study participants. The intensity of exercise and fitness of the individuals involved in the study also may affect the results.

Fluctuations in body temperature are believed to mediate many circadian rhythms in performance. Reilly and Brooks (43) found that the acrophase and amplitude of the rhythm in rectal temperature remained unchanged during exercise despite the exercise-induced elevation in the mean value. Rhythms in skin temperature during exercise were generally in phase with their corresponding resting rhythms but depended on the site of measurement. Skin temperature of the exercising limb did not evidence rhythmicity.

Wahlberg and Åstrand (44) studied responses of 20 men to both submaximal and maximal exercise at 03:00 hours and 15:00 hours. Heart rates during exercise were consistently lower at night, irrespective of work rate, the day–night difference amounting to 3 to 5 beats/min. Cohen and Muehl (45) measured heart rate at rest, during exercise on a rowing ergometer, and in the recovery period of this exercise at 7 times during the solar day. The lowest heart rates were reported to occur be-

TABLE 24–1. *Circadian characteristics of fitness tests, including acrophase of the "standard" rhythms*

Fitness test	Acrophase	Amplitude (% of 24-h mean)	Reference
Whole-body flexibiity	20.12	21.6	(Reilly et al., 1997)
PWC_{150}	3.83	5.2	(Atkinson et al., 1993a)
Standing broad jump	17.45	3.4	(Reilly and Down, 1986)
Anaerobic power (stair-run)	17.26	2.1	(Reilly and Down, 1992)
Leg strength	18.20	9.0	(Coldwells et al., 1993)
Back strength	16.53	10.6	(Coldwells et al., 1993)
Grip strength	20.00	6.0	(Atkinson et al., 1993a)

PWC_{150}, physical working capacity at a heart rate of 150 beats/min. The times for the acrophase are in decimal clock hours.

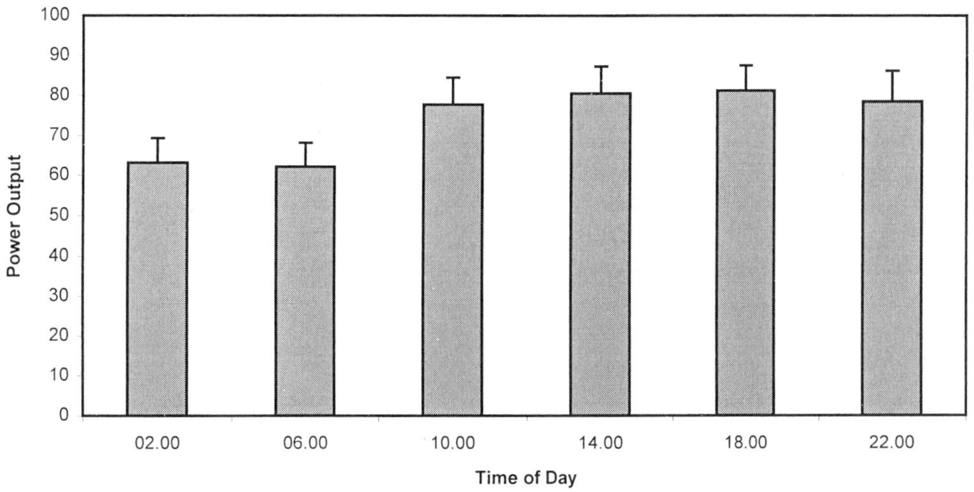

FIG. 24–3. Peak power output in maximal efforts on a swim-bench simulator at different times of day. (Mean ± standard error of the mean.) From ref. 42, with permission.

tween 04:00 and 08:00 hours. This temporal pattern was evident both during and after exercise.

Cohen (46) repeated the latter study but concentrated on an incremental exercise task. The heart-rate responses to maximal exercise just before exhaustion did not vary with time of day, suggesting the absence of a rhythm in maximal heart rate. In many studies of maximal physiologic values, it is often unclear as to whether the ceiling of physiologic capability was reached during the exercise test. In contrast to Cohen's results, Reilly and colleagues (47) found that the rhythm in heart rate persisted during maximal exercise, although it had a reduced amplitude compared with the resting rhythm.

It is difficult to identify the causal nexus of the rhythm in heart rate during exercise complicated by possible metabolic, thermogenic, and sympathetic influences. A circadian variation in cardiac output during exercise has yet to be identified.

Both systolic and diastolic blood pressure measured for 5 minutes after a set exercise regimen were reported by Reilly and co-workers (47) to be unaffected by time of day. Although emphasizing the measurement errors associated with conventional sphygmomanometry, these authors suggested that their preexercise conditions may have swamped any variations in blood pressure. Cable and co-workers (48) concentrated on the phenomenon of postexercise hypotension and reported that the decrease in blood pressure during recovery from exercise was more pronounced in the morning.

Cabri and colleagues (49) measured blood pressure before and after leg exercise on an isokinetic dynamometer at 6 times during the solar day. Whereas systolic blood-pressure responses did not exhibit rhythmicity before or after exercise, diastolic blood pressure (after exercise) did vary with time of day, the rhythm reaching its acrophase between 00:00 and 02:00 hours. It is not known why the acrophase of this rhythm does not coincide with those of other cardiovascular variables at rest or during exercise.

The results of studies that examined circadian variations in metabolic responses to submaximal exercise are not so conclusive as those investigating heart-rate responses. Reilly (50) performed a longitudinal study involving one person in a case study approach. Circadian rhythmicity was observed in $\dot{V}O_2$ (expressed in ml/kg/min) at a power output of 150 W, peaking at 14:40 hours, but this rhythm could be explained fully in terms of circadian variations in body mass (values were slightly lighter in the afternoon). Significant rhythmicity in $\dot{V}O_2$ responses to a lighter work rate than 150 W were evident irrespective of changes in body mass. The time required for $\dot{V}O_2$ to reach steady state (expressed as the fifth minute value) did not vary with time of day. No circadian variations were found for expired carbon dioxide ($\dot{V}CO_2$) or the respiratory-exchange ratio during exercise. This means that no selective use of energy sources for exercise is dependent on time of day and independent of meal times.

The amplitude of the rhythm in minute ventilation ($\dot{V}_E$) is increased during light or moderate exercise. Reilly and Brooks (51) found that the $\dot{V}_E$ response to exercise displayed rhythmicity that was phased similarly to the resting rhythm, but 20% to 40% higher in terms of amplitude. The rhythm in $\dot{V}_E$ may explain the reports of mild dyspnea when exercise is performed in the early morning.

The metabolic responses to exercise at maximal intensities do not demonstrate a circadian rhythm. In both longitudinal and cross-sectional studies, it was found that $\dot{V}O_2max$ is a stable function, independent of the time of day of measurement (60). The amplitude of the resting rhythm in $\dot{V}O_2$ if maintained during maximal exercise would be less than 0.5% of $\dot{V}O_2$max. Such a small amplitude would be difficult to detect, in light of the insensitivity of equipment used to measure $\dot{V}O_2$max (Fig. 24–4).

Circadian variations in the subjective reactions to exercise may be an alternative explanation for rhythms in maximal exercise performance. Faria and Drummond (52) used a crossover-treatment and reverse-sequence design to examine the effects of time of day on ratings of perceived exertion (RPE) during graded exercise on a treadmill. The strength of the relation between RPE and heart rate depended on the time of day. The RPE values were higher during exercise carried out in the early hours of the morning (02:00 to 04:00 hours) than in the evening (20:00 to 22:00 hours). In this study, work rates were set relative to elicited heart rates of 130, 150, and 170 beats/min. As submaximal heart rate at a set work rate is lowest at night, the higher subjective ratings reported at this time would have been due to higher exercise intensities and not to any circadian variation in RPE. Individuals exercised at levels expressed relative to $\dot{V}O_2$max rather than heart rate reported a circadian variation in RPE, only during exercise close to maximal. When performed many times within a solar day, low-intensity exercise may mediate a transient increase in RPE in the early afternoon, consistent with the phasing of the classic "postlunch dip."

Endurance Races and Environmental Temperature

In hot environmental conditions, endurance athletes may have to compete with their body temperatures above the level conducive to optimal performance and close to temperatures normally indicative of heat injury.

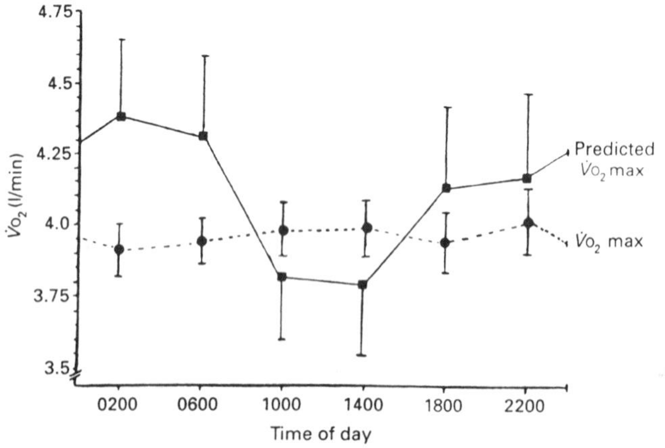

FIG. 24–4. The contrast between results measured for $\dot{V}O_2$max throughout the day and values predicted from heart rate response to submaximal exercise. From ref. 27, with permission.

In training for an attempt at the 1-hour world record, cyclist Chris Boardman's core temperature after a simulation of the effort required for the whole hour was 40°C. If endurance exercise is carried out in the afternoon or evening, there may be a greater risk that such body temperatures are attained, because the rhythm in the body temperature persists during exercise (53). Although a set body-temperature threshold for heat injury has yet to be confirmed, the margin of safety for heat injury can be calculated to be 0.5°C to 0.8°C greater in the morning than the afternoon, when a constant threshold is assumed to apply throughout the day.

Evidence from two sources supports the hypothesis that, in fit individuals, performance in sustained exercise is improved by reduced body temperatures. First, precooling body temperature before 1 hour of submaximal exercise by an amount that corresponds to the amplitude of the circadian rhythm causes a significant increase in work rate (54). Second, there is an interaction between self-selected work rate measured every 10 minutes during 80 minutes of submaximal exercise and the time of day (55,56). In the evening, when body temperature was highest, individuals chose greater work rates at the beginning of the exercise period in the evening compared with the morning. As body temperature increased above optimal levels during the evening exercise, however, the work rate dropped. In the morning, work rate gradually increased as body temperature increased toward optimal levels, until, at the end of the exercise period, individuals chose higher work rates in the morning than in the afternoon. In cold and wet conditions, however, athletes exercising at very low intensities (e.g., charity runners in marathon races) might be at greater risk of hypothermia in the morning. Their low work rate could be insufficient to maintain heat balance because of the high loss of heat to the cold environment. In such conditions, there is a need for appropriate clothing to safeguard against a dangerous decrease in body core temperature.

It has been recognized that environmental temperature may be more favorable for athletes in marathon races in the early morning. Consequently in hot and humid places such as Hong Kong, Singapore, and Penang, marathon races conventionally start at 05:00 to 06:00 hours. In recent years, various competitive marathons have been scheduled at later times of day to coincide with the demands of television audiences. Such scheduling may be disastrous to athletes if environmental temperature is high. This applies when television companies exert their influence over the time of day that sports competitions are held.

TRAINING AND TIME OF DAY

Assuming that athletes are exposed to the external signals that are associated with a diurnal existence, it is unlikely that habitual training in the morning over many weeks (carried out by swimmers, for example) would fully reverse the evening superiority of self-selected training stimuli. This has not yet been fully examined empirically.

Research on the circadian variation in the efficacy of endurance-training programs is equivocal. In one study, the circadian effects of an aerobic-training program in three groups of men who exercised in the morning (09:00 to 09:30), afternoon (15:00 to 15:30), or evening (20:00 to 20:30) were investigated (57). Each group performed exercise for 30 minutes on a cycle ergometer at 60% $\dot{V}O_2max$ (therefore the training stimulus was the same irrespective of time of day) for 4 days per week over a 4-week period. The $\dot{V}O_2max$ was estimated, and adaptive responses of heart rate and blood lactate levels to the training program were recorded. The afternoon group showed the greatest increase in estimated $\dot{V}O_2max$ after 4 weeks, suggesting that aerobic training in the afternoon is the most effective. Other researchers found no significant differences in the training responses to morning and evening exercise.

Improvements in muscle strength after training sessions scheduled at 21:00 hours have been found to be 20% higher than those after training carried out at 09:00 hours (58), although this is with maximal isometric contractions as the training stimuli (which can themselves vary with time of day), and the responses to training of each group of subjects were examined only at the times of day at which they had trained (the group who trained at 21:00 hours was examined at that time after training). Plasma levels of somatotrophin and testosterone have been found to be significantly higher after training in the evening compared with the morning, although, again, maximal muscle contractions, which can be affected by time of day, were used as the training stimuli (59).

There is some evidence to suggest that the learning of motor skills is faster when tasks are performed in the early morning; the greatest improvement in the performance of a pursuit rotor task was evident when the task was performed at 09:00 hours (60). As in the studies on strength, it is difficult to separate a true time-of-day effect on learning/training (the response) from the ability to perform the task (the stimulus) better at certain times of the day. In future, investigators should use sport-specific skills and examine the effect of long-term training in the morning on training responses.

Exercise in the evening may be safer than morning work bouts. For the reasons stated earlier, asthmatic athletes should be discouraged from exercising before or soon after breakfast. Caution also should be exerted in midafternoon by asthmatic athletes who train in urban areas, because this is usually the peak time of day for photochemical smog. Willich and associates (61) reported that the risk of acute coronary events is increased threefold in the morning compared with other times of day. There was a separate effect of physical exertion on cardiac events, the risk being slightly greater in inactive individuals who suddenly perform physical activity. Whereas there may be an interaction between these two effects, it would seem good advice for cardiac patients not to schedule their exercise bouts in the morning.

Delayed-onset muscle soreness (DOMS) is a transient condition of musculoskeletal trauma that can follow vigorous exercise, particularly that involving eccentric muscle contractions. Soreness ratings reach their peak 2 to 3 days after exercise, although any circadian variation within this period has not been researched. The plasma level of creatine kinase (after its leakage from the muscle cell) increases during DOMS and so this enzyme has been used as a marker of muscle damage. Lowest ratings of soreness and plasma levels of creatine kinase have been found after exercise performed in the evening (59). The mechanisms responsible for this finding are unknown.

INDIVIDUAL DIFFERENCES IN PERFORMANCE RHYTHMS

The concept of morning and evening types was first considered by scientists in the early part of the twentieth century. Classification of morning types ("larks"), evening types ("owls"), and intermediate types (neither larks nor owls) is based on the responses to questions regarding sleep and waking times and the phasing of work and habitual activity. Hill and colleagues (62) compared the responses to exercise (at 100 W and also at a work rate corresponding to $\dot{V}O_2max$) on a cycle ergometer between morning and evening types. Diurnal variations in submaximal heart rate, RPE, and $\dot{V}O_2$ were not affected by individual chronotype. In the group of evening types, however, $\dot{V}O_2max$ was best in the evening, whereas in the morning types the $\dot{V}O_2max$ was not affected by time of day. Burgoon and associates (63) claimed that maximal exercise performance on a treadmill at 07:30 and 19:30 hours did not depend on morningness/eveningness scores. Similarly, Reilly and Marshall (42) failed to find a significant influence of chronotype on performance in a swim-bench test. This may reflect the fact that the majority of sports participants are intermediate rather than extreme in chronotype.

Female subjects have higher mean body temperatures than do male subjects over a 24-hour period (64) and smaller rhythm amplitudes in body temperature. Peak temperature also occurs late in the solar day in female subjects, whereas the minimum occurs earlier. There appears to be no research work on gender differences in circadian performance rhythms. Such work should control for the phase of the menstrual cycle, a factor overlooked in previous studies involving female subjects. Body temperature is increased during the luteal phase of the menstrual cycle. The sharp increase in temperature about midway through the menstrual cycle is associated with ovulation.

The rhythm amplitudes in body temperature, arousal, and performance variables of physically fit subjects are around 1.5 times higher than those in sedentary individuals, when studied under standardized laboratory conditions (65,66). The greater rhythm amplitude in body temperature for physically fit subjects is accounted for by a minimum that is 0.4°C lower than that in unfit subjects (35). Although exercise during the day increases body temperature, there is a proportional decrease in body temperature after exercise below the temperature observed during "normal" sleep (i.e., sleep after no activity during the day). This "postexercise thermoregulatory overcompensation" (67) cannot explain the differences in rhythms between fit and unfit subjects because, in the earlier studies, rhythms were compared under controlled conditions with a random order of testing. This implies that the lower nocturnal body temperatures of physically fit subjects may be mediated by endogenous mechanisms (a training effect of habitual physical activity or rhythm characteristics peculiar to athletes). It is plausible that there is an influence of distinct sleep characteristics of athletes, who generally have an increase in "slow-wave sleep" and sleep length, which are, in turn, associated with lower body temperature during sleep.

Circadian timing is altered in elderly individuals. This applies to circadian rhythms in body temperature, hormonal secretions, hematologic parameters, and the urinary excretion of metabolites. Rhythms with a large exogenous component, such as heart rate and blood pressure, also are different in elderly individuals, although probably as a consequence of changes in the sleep–wake cycle and the cardiovascular responses to meals (16). The most consistent age-related circadian differences are a reduction in the amplitudes or a "flattening" of the rhythms, as well as an increase in the variability of rhythm acrophases. Acrophases of the rhythms in elderly subjects often occur earlier than normal in the solar day (66), in agreement with other observations of earlier wake times and increased "morningness" in old age (Fig. 24–5). Veteran cyclists are more likely to be morning-type individuals, scheduling greater amounts of training before 14:00 than do young adults. This is evident before the older cyclists have retired from work (68). The performance of veteran cyclists in time trials is also less affected by setting race starts for the early morning. Laboratory studies have confirmed that, although subjects aged 50 to 60 years still perform best in the early evening, they also perform relatively well in the morning, with age differences in performance being least at this time (68,69). It is still unclear whether such findings reflect age-related changes in the endogenous clock or exogenous influences such as sleep.

THE SLEEP–WAKE CYCLE

Sleep and Exercise

Sleep has been described in terms of a cycle of stages that recurs about every 90 minutes. Use of electroencephalography (EEG) and electrooculography (EOG) provided insights into underlying neurologic events. The two major types of sleep are rapid eye movement (REM) sleep, which composes roughly 20% of total sleep, and non-REM sleep, which is sub-divided into four stages. The waveform of stage 1 closely resembles that of evening drowsiness. Stage 2, the longest of the subdivisions, usually precedes or follows REM, the phase when dreaming occurs. Stages 3 and 4 together constitute slow-wave sleep (SWS), which predominates

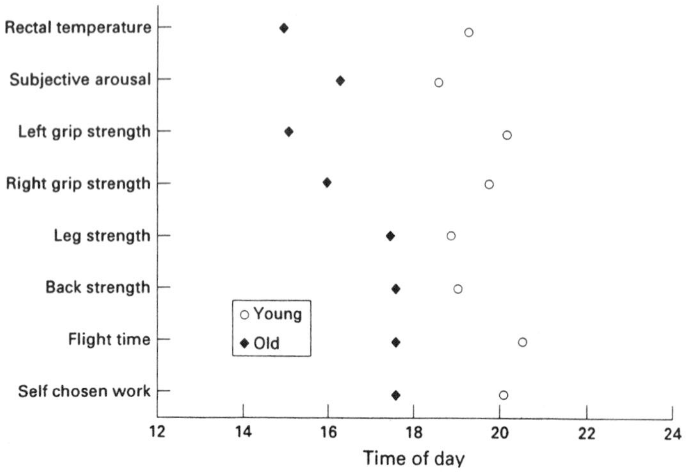

FIG. 24–5. Separation of young (aged 18 to 29 years) and old (aged 47 to 62 years) workers on the basis of acrophases in a range of circadian rhythms. From ref. 66, with permission.

early in sleep, whereas REM sleep predominates later on.

People generally sleep for about 8 hours at night, but there is a large variation between individuals in the amount taken, the coefficient of variation being about 30%. Sound sleep on a regular and habitual basis is assumed to be an essential part of athletes' preparation for performance. Duration is not the only characteristic of a good night's sleep, because restfulness (indicated by relative movements) and latency (indicated by time between lights out and onset of stage 2) are important aspects. Aerobically fit athletes exhibit shorter sleep latencies and longer sleep periods than normal, and they also tend to have greater levels of SWS. To what extent these features reflect contemporary lifestyles of elite athletes rather than aerobic fitness is undetermined.

Sleep patterns of athletes were monitored at times when they were aerobically fit and when they were deemed to be unfit: profiles were compared with sedentary controls (70). Increased stage 3 SWS in the athletes when fit was compensated by opposite changes in stage 4. The biologic significance of this shift is unknown. The athletes tended to have a longer sleep and more non-REM sleep, although the time in bed was similar to that of the inactive controls. The longer REM latency in the athletes was associated with a higher level of SWS in the first cycle of sleep. The differences between the athletes and nonathletes could not be ascribed to aerobic fitness, so it appears that the sleep profiles reflected a trait in athletes rather than an effect of training (71).

Residual fatigue from daytime exercise is believed to alleviate many problems in sleeping. Exercise induces a greater degree of tiredness and sleepiness and, if the exercise is not too vigorous, a better quality of sleep. The intensity and duration of exercise may affect subsequent sleep, as does the interval for recovery before retiring to bed. If vigorous exercise is conducted late in the evening, particularly by unfit individuals, sleep onset may be delayed. Physiologic recovery processes (such as resynthesis of muscle glycogen) can begin once exercise is ended, and the increases in metabolism and body temperature caused by exercise may delay the onset of sleep. Soreness after running on hard surfaces or as a result of physical-contact activities may cause musculoskeletal discomfort to a level that prevents restful sleep. Games players may also find difficulty in getting to sleep after a match because of elevated levels of catecholamines and a tendency to replay in their minds various features of the competitive events.

Sleep is an enigma, and there is not a consensus among sleep researchers about its essential function. One view is that sleep is needed for the restitution of the body's tissues. Tissue-restitution theories have been linked with heightened mitosis during sleep and increased growth-hormone secretion during SWS stages. An alternative view is that the need for sleep is specific to nerve cells. The argument is based on the observations that tissue restitution proceeds during wakefulness, even after exhausting exercise, and convincing evidence such as increased protein turnover in sleep is lacking. It is likely that sleep is needed not only for nerve cells but also for protecting immune functions. Sleep is obviously essential, and this requirement is apparent when we consider how human behavior is altered with severe loss of sleep.

Sleep Deprivation

There is an interaction between sleep loss and circadian rhythms in that impairments in human performance during sleep deprivation are most pronounced at night. In self-paced activity, consisting of four-a-side indoor soccer sustained for 3 to 4 days, the activity level peaked at about 18:00 hours, coinciding with the daily high point of body temperature. Other variables that followed this curve included grip strength and choice reaction time (24). The circadian rhythm persists for as many days as the individual can be kept awake and is superimposed on a day-to-day increase in fatigue. This trend is statistically removed by chronobiologists before establishing circadian rhythm characteristics, for example, by cosinor or Fourier analysis. The trend is not evident in all functions: gross muscular performances, such as isometric strength, are highly resistant to effects of sleep loss, despite the decrease in muscle enzyme activity noted after the first night. In contrast, cognitive functions are easily affected. Complex and challenging tasks are impaired less than monotonous repetitive ones, and strong motivation may help to overcome the effects of sleep loss, at least for short periods. Nevertheless, after 4 days of sustained activity in which only 2 hours sleep was allowed, military subjects were deemed to be ineffective as soldiers (72). This conclusion was based on performance in a 1-km assault course, a shooting test, and a 3-km run; provision of a high-energy diet was unsuccessful in offsetting these impairments. The decline is likely to have been a fatigue effect rather than attributable to sleep loss; soldiers who are deprived of sleep for 2 to 3 nights but not physically fatigued have performed highly demanding tasks at the same work rate as fresh troops (73).

In one study, subjects were kept awake for 64 hours under conditions of isolation from external time cues. Activity was classed as sedentary and was kept as constant as possible, as was intake of food and liquids. Epinephrine secretion showed a pronounced circadian rhythm, with the rhythm in norepinephrine relatively weaker (based on amplitude as a percentage of the mean value). The circadian rhythms in cardiovascular variables (blood pressure, heart rate, contractility, T-wave amplitude, and QRS, PQ, and QT intervals) observed under normal conditions were effectively obliterated, suggesting that alternating between sleeping and waking is their main determinant (74), although the experimental design could not rule out the existence of self-sustained rhythms in cardiovascular variables. Other studies have shown an apparent hemodilution with sleep deprivation, which may be associated with a slight decline in $\dot{V}O_2max$. One difficulty confronting researchers is that subjects may lack the drive to reach a true $\dot{V}O_2max$ when deprived of sleep.

There is also an interaction between sleep loss and environmental stressors, although this effect is not linear. For example, heat compounds the effects of sleep deprivation, whereas noise can offset them. Urinary excretion of melatonin follows a circadian pattern in humans during sleep deprivation when subjects are exposed to light, but excretion levels increase with increased sleep loss.

Subjects deprived of sleep for 1 to 3 nights can exhibit psychotic-like symptoms and bizarre behavior. They also experience temporary visual illusions. In such circumstances, meaningful physical exercise becomes difficult to sustain without error. Sailors will be unreliable on watch duty with such severe sleep loss, and even a minor lapse in motor rally drivers could be disastrous. It has been suggested that naturally occurring brain amines may play a role in the cycles of behavior and mood states associated with prolonged sleep deprivation. A circadian rhythm was found in phenylethylamine levels in the urine of sleep-deprived footballers playing indoors: by the third successive night without sleep, the concentrations of this substance being excreted approached the values typically observed in psychiatric patients (75). Fortunately, such prolonged periods of sleeplessness are experienced only rarely. They may be met by sports medical personnel on hospital duty. In military recruits in whom such regimens are imposed during training, similar trends superimposed on a circadian rhythm in catecholamine excretion have been observed. The curve in catecholamines coincided with the increases and declines in the accuracy of shooting performance (76).

Partial Sleep Loss

Partial sleep disruption and fragmented sleep are more common problems than complete sleep deprivation. Partial loss of sleep can affect athletes who are restless through anxiety, sailors and yachtsmen during prolonged competitions, and athletes with children who themselves have unsettled sleeping patterns. Individuals vary in the usual amount of sleep taken and in their ability to tolerate sleep loss, and so inferences from experimental investigations must be guarded. Besides, there is variation in the sensitivity of laboratory measures of performance to effects of sleep deprivation. Effects of partial sleep loss also depend on motivation, task complexity, stage of sleep most affected, and other factors.

The effects of a nightly ration of only 2.5 hours of sleep on a battery of psychomotor, work-capacity, and mental-state tests were examined over 3 nights of sleep loss and after 1 night of subsequent recovery (77). A 3-day control period was used in a counterbalanced design to eliminate an order effect. Functions that required fast reactions, notably anaerobic power output in a stair run and choice reaction time at rest and while cycling on an ergometer, deteriorated significantly. Physical exercise attenuated the effects of sleep loss on reaction time, suggesting the benefits of manipulating arousal level by means of a warm-up. This beneficial effect is likely to be short lived, and exercise will be less effective in offsetting sleep loss when the disruptions continue over days. Limb speed, as measured by a reciprocal tapping task, also became steadily worse over successive days of partial sleep loss.

Gross physical performance tasks such as grip strength and treadmill run time were unaffected by the restriction of sleep. As the restricted sleep regimen was found to affect the more complex motor-coordination tasks while leaving gross motor functions relatively intact, the data were deemed to support the "nerve cell restitution" theory of sleep.

These effects of partial sleep loss found in male subjects have been replicated in female subjects (78). A group of women was also limited to 2.5 hours of sleep for 3 successive nights in a counterbalanced experimental design: performances were measured each morning (07:00 to 09:00 hours) and each evening (19:00 to 21:00 hours). A diurnal variation was noted in the majority of measures; for gross motor function, this circadian effect was greater than that of sleep loss. The perceived exertion during cycling at 60% of $\dot{V}O_2max$ showed both a diurnal variation and an underlying trend toward increased subjective strain. This coincided with the observations on the sleepiness of subjects, self-rated before exercise.

Observations on the effects of partial sleep deprivation on swimmers further support the view that sleep is needed more for brain restitution rather than for tissue restitution. The sleep ration was restricted to 2.5 hours a night for 3 consecutive nights (29). Performance over 400 m and over four successive 50-m swims was maintained throughout the experimental period. Swimming times were faster in the evening (17:30 hours) compared with the morning (06:30 hours), confirming that the time-of-day effect of gross motor functions exceeds that of sleep loss. Even after disrupted sleep, swimmers can produce maximal efforts, at least if required to do so in the evening. The most notable effects of the restricted sleep regimen were deteriorations in mood throughout the investigation.

Although muscular strength can be retained during consecutive days of partial sleep loss, the quality of training may be adversely affected. This applies to training sessions with repeated or multiple maximal efforts, as occurs in weight-training programs. Thus maximal performances can be reproduced in weight-training exercises executed in the early parts of the session, but the quality of performance declines in the later part (79). Deteriorations in mood with successive nights of deprived sleep can account for this decline.

A paradoxic result of partial sleep loss is that some tasks show an improvement. Hand steadiness, for example, is generally better than usual after loss of sleep. This is attributable to a decrease in spontaneous contraction of involved muscles linked with a reduction in muscle tone. Similarly, tasks with high loadings on short-term memory appear to improve when deprived of sleep owing to a tendency to code information acoustically for mental storage and recall in laboratory tests. Thus care is needed in designing and interpreting sleep-deprivation studies and in drawing inferences about the effects of disrupted sleep on athletic performance. Individuals forced to reduce their normal sleep ration may adapt to their shortened sleep length without any adverse consequences for exercise performance, provided that the reduction does not exceed about 2 hours. Otherwise they may have to reorganize their daily routine to accommodate an afternoon nap. Personal and occupational circumstances will dictate whether this is a practical remedy.

Napping

Ultradian cycles with 90-minute periods are identifiable during sleep and may be latent during wakefulness. This may explain subharmonics within the circadian phase system, as evidenced in the postlunch dip. To what extent this decrease can be offset by napping or reorganization of the work–rest schedule of activity has not been adequately investigated. Individuals on short sleep durations for some days can derive considerable refreshment from brief naps.

Prolonged napping at an inappropriate time can delay the readjustment of rhythms after abrupt circadian phase shifts. A 1-hour nap taken by nocturnal shift workers at 02:00 hours was less effective than caffeine in maintaining performance overnight in a range of tasks (80).

Often people claim that they were unable to sleep during the night, but such accounts may not be true. Short periods of sleep snatched unknowingly during the night do play a restorative role. Individuals deprived of sleep for some time gain considerable benefit from naps, and those deprived of sleep for 2 to 4 days usually recover from their ordeal after one complete night of uninterrupted sleep. A nap could counteract the decrease in arousal underlying any subharmonic in the performance curve linked to ultradian rhythms. There has been no substantive research on the refreshing effects of napping on subsequent exercise performance.

Naps can be described as "recuperative" (the sense used here so far), but also as "appetitive" and "prophylactic." Recuperative naps are taken to relieve fatigue due to lost sleep or activity, or both; appetitive naps are those taken due to habit, even if the subject does not feel sleepy; prophylactic naps are those taken before a period of work to start as refreshed and alert as possible. For the athlete, it is important not to take a nap too close to the start of competition in case of "sleep inertia." This refers to the time it takes to rouse completely after a short nap, and during this period decision making could be impaired. Advocation of a nap before competing in sport depends on factors such as timing of the contest, precompetition feeding, and individual preferences for coping with pre-event anxiety.

Sleeplessness

Although true insomnia is rare, a large number of people—about 10% to 15% of the population—do have difficulty in sleeping. Causes include anxiety, depression, bereavement, stress, overwork, and environmental noise such as motor-vehicle traffic. Some of these problems are transient and self-limiting; others may persist and become chronic.

Exercise is generally thought to promote sleep, and so it is recommended as therapy for individuals having difficulty in sleeping. The effect of physical activity is likely to be indirect, promoting sleep by alleviating the anxieties that prevented it. Strenuous exercise shortly before retiring to sleep is likely to elevate arousal rather than induce drowsiness because of the increased levels of circulating catecholamines. Thus exercise as therapy for sleeping problems should not be strenuous and should be performed early rather than later in the evening.

The usual prescription for insomnia is a sleeping pill. People taking sedatives or hypnotics for a prolonged period develop a dependence on them, and the drugs gradually lose their effectiveness. Minor tranquillizers (the benzodiazepines) are probably now being overprescribed in Europe and North America. Habitual users become dependent on benzodiazepines and suffer severe symptoms if treatment is suddenly stopped. Normal doses also impair reaction time and mental concentration the morning after they have been taken, particularly when the drug has a relatively long half-life. Benzodiazepines also affect muscular performance, notably in movements at high angular velocities. Consequently, their prescription for athletes should be considered only in cases of clear necessity.

Nonpharmacologic methods of treating sleeplessness include hypnotherapy. Biofeedback of skin resistance and EEG also may be used to train the individual to overcome the emotional tension that prevents sleep. Psychological techniques such as visualization of tranquil scenes, concentration on relaxing muscle activity, and deep breathing provide alternative treatments. Stimulus-control therapy refers to a mental training strategy whereby bed and sleeplessness are dissociated: the individual goes to bed only when sleepy, avoids eating, reading, or watching television in the bedroom, and does not "sleep" in the morning. Sensible eating and drinking habits (such as avoiding large meals, heavy alcoholic beverages, or caffeine late at night) also should promote sleep of good quality.

THE BODY CLOCK

The concept of homeostasis, accepted from the mid-nineteenth century and implying that the internal environment within the body is relatively constant, now acknowledges that the internal environment is constantly changing with a regular oscillation. Indeed, the capacity for rhythmic change is accepted as an inherent characteristic of living organisms. Thus when the physiologic responses to exercise assume a so-called steady state, this level may depend on the time of day (6).

Biologic functions and performance of exercise both demonstrate circadian rhythms. The major determinant of the rhythms is the spin of the Earth about its vertical axis. Humans have adapted to this over the ages by timing the alternation of sleep and wakefulness to coincide with the periods of darkness and light, respectively. In turn, this pattern of rest and activity influences many physiologic functions, which slow down at night and accelerate with daylight. Human circadian rhythms have been established at levels ranging from cellular and tissue functions to whole-body activities. The multitude of rhythms in the body interact with each other and also with the environment.

Circadian rhythms in physiologic variables are influenced by rhythmic changes in human behavior and by the environment over a period of 24 hours (81). For example, human society generally exhibits wakefulness and activity diurnally, when the environmental temperature is higher than when it is night and there is natural light rather than darkness. Fluctuations such as these are termed the "exogenous component" of the circadian rhythm. The effect of exogenous stimuli (e.g., exercise) on the parameters of an endogenous rhythm is termed "masking." Eliminating this masking effect to adumbrate the characteristics of the body clock is known as "purifying" the rhythm (82).

The endogenous component of the circadian rhythms is colloquially referred to as the body clock. Rhythmicity persists if an individual remains awake for several days at a constant level of activity or is placed in "temporal isolation." This refers to environmental conditions that do not fluctuate, such as a natural cave or a specially designed isolation chamber. Additionally, during nocturnal shift work or transmeridian travel, circadian rhythms do not adjust immediately to a new sleep–wake schedule.

The most likely site for the circadian body clock is the paired suprachiasmatic nuclei (SCN) located in the anterior hypothalamus, close to the optic chiasm. Other loci of rhythmicity (thus far not conclusively identified) have been postulated because total destruction of the SCN does not disrupt *all* circadian rhythms, and because some circadian rhythms can become "desynchronized" from each other when studied in temporal isolation (4). Nevertheless the fact that many circadian rhythms in resting physiologic functions exist in the absence of any environmental fluctuations and are obliterated after SCN removal suggests that the dominant pacemaker can communicate neurally and/or neurohumerally with other hypothalamic centers and endocrine glands (83). These secondary oscillations, in turn, mediate fluctuations in their respective target tissues in the human, resulting in the myriad circadian rhythms apparent under both resting and exercise conditions.

The inherent *properties* of the body clock have been investigated in isolation studies. When individuals are isolated from all external time signals, the period of circadian rhythms deviates slightly but consistently from 24 hours to about 25 to 26 hours. Therefore the endogenous clock will progressively lag behind exogenous fluctuations as time spent in isolation increases up to 12 days. It thus "free runs." Endogenous rhythms are synchronized or "entrained" to the normal 24-hour environment by *Zeitgebers* (German, meaning "time-givers"), the most important of which are the light–dark cycle and social influences. It is thought that light acts as a *Zeitgeber* to the body clock by transmitting photic information along the retinohypothalamic tract, a neural pathway connecting the retinae with the SCN. Light also entrains and suppresses the production of melatonin by the pineal gland. The hormone melatonin and its precursor serotonin have important roles in sleep regulation, nocturnal secretions being markedly increased after about 21:00 hours or onset by darkness. Such chronobiologic influences of melatonin have led to the theory that administration of bright light or exogenous melatonin has therapeutic applications in the treatment of such rhythm disturbances as jet lag, shift work, seasonal affective disorder (SAD), and insomnia (84). Secretion of melatonin is affected also by the length of the night. Many animals use changes in the length of the daytime to time their seasonal cycles, and consequently, their breeding behavior.

Although environmental and body-temperature changes affect the circadian rhythm in arousal, it is influenced mainly by the sleep–wake cycle and by neural traffic through the reticular activation formation in the brain. Circadian phase systems are not completely isolated from other time structures with different periodicities. Nevertheless, it is by means of environmental signals that rhythms are adjusted to an exact 24-hour period.

The incidence of malaise known as SAD increases when daylight hours are short. The condition is accompanied by decrements in psychomotor performance as well as in mood. Exposure to bright or ultraviolet light may ameliorate the condition. The chronobiologic entity is more prevalent in northern latitudes near and above the Arctic Circle. Increasing the duration and intensity of exposure to daylight does seem to affect the phase of the circadian rhythm: in the northern hemisphere, the peak occurs 55 minutes later in June than in December. Changes in ambient temperature do not appear to alter the rhythm.

The shortened hours of daylight in winter affect the training of some athletes; for example, Scandinavian athletes tend to escape the problem by spending some time during the winter training in southern climates, which are warmer and have longer hours of daylight. Professional soccer players tend to train in the morning, whereas their matches are timed for the afternoon or at night under floodlights in winter. Whether one of the teams would gain an advantage by training at this time for which evening matches are scheduled has not been established.

TRAVEL AND BODY-CLOCK DISRUPTIONS

Travel Fatigue

Travel is now an accepted part of the itinerary of athletes. The habitual activity may entail travel across one's own country for domestic contests as well as travel overseas to training camps or competitive venues. Besides, many athletes may not reside close to good-quality training facilities and so regularly have to travel by car or public transport for the purpose of training. The stresses associated with habitual traveling have been studied in commuters to work, but little is known about the phenomenon of "travel fatigue" in athletes. Detrimental effects may be compounded by subjective feelings of tiredness associated with training and by feelings of boredom. Fatigue also may be precipitated by a failure to allow brief stops in the journey to alleviate stiffness or postural discomfort and to permit drinking and eating if necessary.

Travel fatigue linked with long-distance air flights poses a different range of problems for athletes and team management. These travel stresses apply to all visitors to overseas countries. They include the procedures associated with obtaining and presenting the necessary travel documents and obtaining enough money; checking in and getting through security, passport, and customs screening; and so on. These stresses are common irrespective of direction or distance of travel and can be compounded by delay in boarding at take-off. They call for a positive psychological approach to facing these routines and overriding any negative feelings.

Travel fatigue in long-haul flights may be linked with a gradual dehydration as a result of ambient conditions on board. This is due to the water vapor content of the cabin air, which is low in comparison with fresh air. Headaches also may be linked to a combination of low air pressure and the loss of body water to the dry air within the airplane (85). Caffeine and alcohol are diuretics and so are unsuitable for rehydration purposes.

Spending a long time in a cramped posture can cause stiffness. This can be relieved by simple stretching or by isometric contractions of the muscles affected. These exercises should help to eliminate residual stiffness at the end of the journey.

Flights within the same time zone, such as to South Africa from the United Kingdom or between the east coast of United States and South America, may have residual effects because of the duration of the journey. These are not so disturbing as are flights across multiple time zones. Aftereffects attributable to the flight itself wear off quickly once the destination is reached. Flights eastward or westward that entail travel across time zones additionally lead to a disturbance of the circadian body clock. This desynchronization of biologic rhythms is the cause of "jet lag," but a difficulty in sleeping may accentuate travel fatigue.

Jet Lag

The group of symptoms affecting travelers after rapid journeys to distant places across multiple time zones is referred to as jet lag. There is a general malaise and a sense of feeling and acting "below par" associated with the collective symptoms (see Table 24–2). Physical exercise will appear to be more difficult, and fine skills are likely to be executed less well until the symptoms abate.

Jet lag affects individuals differently, but in general:

- It is more pronounced (that is, it is more severe and lasts longer) after a flight to the east than one to the west through the same number of time zones.
- It is more pronounced the more time zones that are crossed.

TABLE 24–2. *Symptoms associated with the phenomenon of jet-lag*

- Fatigue during the new daytime, and yet inability to sleep at night
- Decreased mental performance, particularly if vigilance is required
- Decreased physical performance, particularly with regard to events that require stamina or precise movement
- A loss of appetite, coupled with indigestion and even nausea
- Increased irritability, headaches, mental confusion, and disorientation

- Younger and fitter people tend to suffer less than do older persons.
- Women may be affected more than men.

The body clock is normally in harmony with the 24-hour changes between daylight and darkness. Because the earth spins on its axis, the sun is at its maximal height above the horizon at any point on the earth's surface once in every 24-hour period. This time is called *local noon*. The world has been divided into 24 time zones in order to standardize all these times. The time zone that all others are related to passes through England [i.e., Greenwich Mean Time (GMT)]. Countries to the east of the United Kingdom have clocks that are ahead of this, because the sun rises earlier, whereas time to the west appears delayed with respect to this reference. Adjusting to a new local time on flying to a new time zone presents difficulties for the endogenous body clock (85).

The body clock is slow to adjust to the change in schedule that is required on traveling to a new country with its own local time. Before adjustment takes place, the player or athlete might train or compete at a time when the body's signal denotes a preference to be asleep, and attempt to sleep when the body clock is directing wakefulness. It is during this period—before adjustment has taken place—that jet lag is experienced. Once the body clock has adjusted, jet lag disappears until the next journey across time zones, usually on the trip home.

Female subjects may be more affected by jet lag than male athletes, as the severity of symptoms can be related to the menstrual-cycle phase at the time of the journey. Disruptions of the menstrual cycle in female travelers have been linked to disturbances in melatonin secretion. In Scandinavia, it has been found that higher melatonin levels in the winter compared with summer values have an inhibiting effect on luteinizing hormone. As a result, ovulation might not occur during that cycle (65). The extent to which the menstrual disturbances accompanying traveling across multiple time zones in themselves alter athletic performance is uncertain.

It takes on average about 1 day for every time zone crossed to recover fully from the effects of jet lag (86), although the recovery is nonlinear. The effects are periodic and can be more intense at particular times of the day. The athlete may be totally unaware of any adverse effects, unless he or she has to do something quickly, make decisions, or perform sports skills.

Local environmental factors can also influence the effects of jet-lag symptoms. Dehydration associated with heat stress, for example, may accentuate difficulties in concentration and mental fatigue. A program of heat acclimatization before departure across multiple time zones can benefit sports participants and was implemented as a formal strategy by British competitors at the 1996 Olympic Games in Atlanta (87).

Adjusting the Body Clock

The body clock, left to itself, would run slow, with a period of 25 to 26 hours rather than the 24-hour day required to remain in time with the alternation of light and dark (4). Under normal circumstances, the body clock is adjusted in the same way as a watch that keeps poor time: by external signals. Several signals adjust the circadian rhythms, and making use of them helps the body to adjust to time-zone transitions.

The main signals are

- Exposure to light, particularly receiving direct sunlight out of doors.
- The pattern of sleep and activity (including exercise).
- The timing and type of meals.
- Exposure to social influences and the alternation of natural daylight and darkness.

Promoting Adjustment of the Body Clock

The Process of Adjustment

Complete adjustment of the body clock takes several days. The aim is to speed up this process as much and as safely as possible, as it is only when fully adjusted to the new time zone that the athlete's performance will be at its peak. This applies to training as well as to competition. Until that time, it will be more difficult for an individual to produce maximal effort. While adjustment is taking place, the shape of the normal rhythm is changed. It displays a lower amplitude, a lower peak value, and a lower average value overall (82).

A practice frequently adopted by athletes before flying overseas in a westward direction is to go to bed 1 to 2 hours later than normal each night and get up 1 to 2 hours later each morning. It might not always be possible to do this, but its main benefit is to promote thinking ahead about times in the country of destination. In contrast, those going eastward bring forward getting to bed and getting up by 1 to 2 hours. It is not useful to try to adjust fully to the time-zone transition before the journey, because this will interrupt training schedules and lifestyle too much and will not alter the body clock very much (88). This advice applies to both a phase delay (getting to sleep later) and a phase advance (getting to bed earlier). Where there is a choice of flight times and airports, the player or team manager should select a schedule that makes planning to adjust all the easier. A flight that gets the European traveler to the U.S. destination in the evening, for example, would be helpful. For trips that entail crossing eight time zones or more, it can be beneficial to plan an overnight stopover midway, which avoids exposure to the symptoms experienced if the journey is done without a break. The ideal travel schedule is seldom available, but at least alternatives that are on offer can be consulted.

Possibilities for Speeding Adjustment

Athletes and coaches must acknowledge the disturbance of the body's circadian rhythms after rapid travel across time zones if they are to take steps to promoting adjustment to the new time zone. Several methods have been suggested (89), differing in their practicality and in their potential side effects. They encompass nutritional, pharmacologic, environmental, and behavioral measures.

Timing and Composition of Meals

It has been suggested that high-protein breakfasts promote alertness and that high-carbohydrate evening meals (vegetables, potatoes, rice, bread, pasta, desserts, and so on) promote sleep (90). The theory is that such meals affect plasma amino acids and, thence, the uptake of the amino acids into the brain, their incorporation into neurotransmitters, and the release of the neurotransmitters. High-protein meals (meat, cheese, eggs, etc.) increase plasma tyrosine, but whether this promotes the release of catecholamines by the activating systems of the brain and so promote alertness is less clear. Similarly, high-carbohydrate meals elevate the concentration of plasma tryptophan, but whether this stimulates the raphe nucleus and sleep is also uncertain (91).

Electroencephalographic waves during sleep have shown some changes in athletes with a carbohydrate-rich diet, but effects on the quality of sleep have not been demonstrated. The two-phase dietary method (alternating feeding and fasting) was promoted in the United States under the title "President Reagan's anti–jet-lag diet."

Only small improvements in sleep and mental performance have been observed when the efficacy of the diet was examined in military personnel (92), but studies have been few and poorly designed. Even so, a variant of this proposal consists of two types of pills, one to be taken in the morning and the other in the evening. Each pill is a mixture of substances, the morning pill containing tyrosine, and the evening one tryptophan. The accompanying marketing literature does not enable a judgment to be made on the scientific evaluation of these preparations. Besides, tryptophan achieved adverse publicity in the early 1990s owing to the finding of impurities in commercially available products, and its use is no longer recommended.

Sleeping Pills

Disturbance of sleep is one of the unwanted corollaries of jet-lag syndrome. Resynchronizing the normal sleep–wakefulness cycle seems to occur first, before restoration of physiologic and performance measures to their normal circadian rhythm (3).

Sports teams traveling on long-haul flights have used sleeping pills to induce sleep while on board (6). Minor tranquillizers (e.g., temazepam) have been used to help get travelers to sleep so as to be refreshed for immediate activities on arrival. Although drugs, such as benzodiazepines, are effective in getting people to sleep, they do not guarantee a prolonged period asleep. Besides, they have not been satisfactorily tested for subsequent residual effects on motor performance, such as sports skills. They may be counterproductive if given at the incorrect time. A prolonged sleep at the time an individual feels drowsy (presumably when he or she would have been asleep in the time zone departed from) simply anchors the rhythms at their former phases and so operates against adjustment to the new time zone (82).

The administration of a low dose of temazepam was found to have no influence on subjective, physiologic, and performance measures after a westward flight across five time zones (3). The circadian rhythms of athletes differed from those of sedentary subjects, although neither group benefited from the sleeping pill. Jet lag and sleep disturbances may be more severe in members of the team management than in athletes, the former being generally older and less fit than the latter. Whether short-acting hypnotics such as zolpidem, which has a shorter half-life than most benzodiazepines, would be effective in their cases and in more extreme phase shifts remains to be clarified.

Melatonin Capsules

In normal circumstances, melatonin from the pineal gland is secreted into the bloodstream between about 21:00 and 07:00 hours. It can be regarded as a "dark pulse" or "internal time cue" for the body clock (2). Some studies have shown that melatonin capsules taken in the evening by local time in the new time zone reduce the symptoms of jet lag (93). This is an important finding, but there are some caveats:

1. Jet lag, as defined in these studies, was concentrated on subjective symptoms. It is not known if there would also be improvements in mental and physical performance and in motivation to train hard, or even if there would be further decrements.
2. It is not clear whether melatonin produces its effect by promoting adjustment of the body clock or by some other means (increasing a sense of well-being or the ability to sleep, for example). Although recent work suggests that melatonin can adjust the body clock, this requires careful timing of ingestion according to whether the need is to advance or delay the clock.
3. Melatonin has a lowering effect on body temperature, and this may account for its hypnotic action.
4. Melatonin is only just becoming commercially available (largely in the United States), and the results from many clinical trials are still awaited.

In summary, more information is required before melatonin can be recommended. Systematic monitoring of athletes voluntarily taking melatonin (freely available in United States but not licensed for Australia or Europe) during long-haul flights and days afterward would help in this respect.

Promoting Alertness

One approach to combating jet lag is to use pharmacologic means of promoting and maintaining alertness. Such drugs include amphetamines, caffeine, modafinil (an α_1-adrenoceptor antagonist) and pemoline (a drug with dopamine-like properties). Although those drugs improve performance in several tasks, they adversely affect the ability to initiate and sustain sleep (94). These effects could be counterproductive after time-zone transitions. Besides, their effects on physical performance relevant to sport have not been adequately addressed, and their use could contravene doping regulations.

Bright-Light Exposure and Exercise

Bright light (that is, of an intensity found naturally but not normally indoors) can adjust the body clock. The timing of exposure is crucially important (95) and is the opposite of that for melatonin ingestion; thus bright light in the morning (05:00 to 11:00 hours) on body time advances the clock, and bright light in the evening (21:00 to 03:00 hours) on body time delays it. Light should be avoided at those times that produce a shift of the body clock in a direction opposite that desired. Table 24–3 gives times when light should be sought or avoided after different time-zone transitions; the timing will vary as the body clock adjusts.

Even though bright light is of an intensity normally not achieved in domestic or interior lighting, light boxes and visors are now available commercially that produce a light source of sufficient intensity. Light visors, in particular, might prove useful.

Because outdoor lighting is the obvious choice, it would be natural, therefore, to consider training outdoors—an easy training session—when light is required, and to relax indoors when it should be avoided. This raises the question of whether physical exercise and inactivity can, in some way, add to the effects of light and dark, respectively. Current evidence is not conclusive.

For the first few days in the new time zone, all-out exercise should be avoided in training. Skills requiring fine coordination are likely to be impaired, which could lead to accidents or injuries if, for example, sports players conducted training sessions or matches too strenuously. Where a series of tournament engagements is scheduled, it is useful to have at least one friendly match during the initial period, that is, before the end of the first week in the overseas country. Subject to these cave-

TABLE 24–3. *The use of bright light to adjust the body clock after time-zone transitions*

	Bad local times for exposure to bright light	Good local times for exposure to bright light
Time zones to the west		
4 h	01:00–07:00[a]	17:00–23:00[b]
8 h	21:00–03:00[a]	13:00–19:00[b]
12 h	17:00–23:00[a]	09:00–15:00[b]
Time zones to the east		
4 h	01:00–07:00[b]	09:00–15:00[a]
8 h	05:00–11:00[b]	13:00–19:00[a]
10–12 h	Treat this as 12–14 h to the west[c]	

[a]Will advance the body clock.
[b]Will delay the body clock.
[c]Note that this is because the body clock adjusts to delays more easily than to advances.

ats, exercise for sports participants is recommended for adjusting the body clock, and it also helps them mentally in their preparations for competition.

In practice, therefore, to combine exposure to bright light and exercise, and to combine dim light and relaxation, would seem practicable. There is very little research evidence to suggest that exercise by itself will alter the speed of adjustment of the body clock in humans.

It might seem that to adjust as fully as possible to the lifestyle and habits in the new zone would be the best remedy. This is not always the case on the first day or so after the flight. Consider a westward flight through eight time zones. To delay the clock requires bright light at 21:00 to 03:00 hours body time and its avoidance at 05:00 to 11:00 hours. By new local time, this becomes equal to 13:00 to 19:00 hours for bright light and 21:00 to 03:00 hours for dim light (see Table 24–3). It can be seen that natural daylight and night would provide this. Consider, by contrast, a flight to the east through eight time zones. Now light is required at 05:00 to 11:00 hours body time (13:00 to 19:00 hours local time) and should be avoided at 21:00 to 03:00 hours body time (05:00 to 11:00 hours local time). That is, morning light for the first day or so *would be unhelpful and tend to make the clock adjust in the wrong direction* (although afternoon and evening light are fine). The timing of exposure to bright light is critical on the first days after the flight. After a couple of days, when partial adjustment has occurred, it is then advised to alter the timing of the light exposure toward that of the local inhabitants, so that the visitors' habits become synchronized with those of locals.

Sleep loss itself is unlikely to have a major adverse effect on exercise performance (see above, the section on The Body Clock). In normal conditions, the effects of substantial sleep disturbances are more pronounced on complex tasks than on gross measures such as muscle strength (79). Indeed the circadian variation in sports performances was found to be greater than that induced by partial sleep deprivation over 3 consecutive nights (29). Difficulties in sleeping after crossing multiple time zones are eventually self-correcting, but disturbances may last longer after eastward compared with westward flights.

Circadian rhythms must be taken into account when traveling across multiple time zones to compete in sport. Deleterious effects of jet lag will be exacerbated if there are additional environmental stressors, such as heat or altitude, to be encountered. Performance can be adversely affected even when flights are within one country, coast to coast in the United States or Australia, for example (96). While jet-lag symptoms persist, even if only periodically during the day, it is recommended that training be light in intensity to reduce possibilities of accidents and injuries occurring. Individuals may be more vulnerable to defeat in the early rounds of tournaments at the hands of home-based players, unless the need for adjustment to the new time zone is considered in the timetable of the tour.

Shift Work and Sports Performance

Altogether, one third of British male manual workers are involved in nocturnal shift work, and an estimated 20 million people in the United States are on some form of shift-work system. Nocturnal shift work entails a disruption of the body clock and affects the normal sleep–wake cycle. The disturbance is not the same as in traveling across time zones, as the external signals maintain their diurnal existence while the rest–work or sleep–wake cycle is altered. In transmeridian travel, the rhythm disturbance is an isolated event, whereas it occurs every time the worker has to rotate shifts.

Many shift workers wish to, but cannot, perform leisure activities at the same times of day as do day workers. For those people participating in team sports or any type of competitive sport, a restriction in leisure time may become one of the major factors in terminating shift work. For people involved in solitary hobbies or those training for (but not competing in) individual sports, this may not be a problem. Atkinson and Reilly (2) noted that 9% of a sample of racing cyclists were shift workers. Participants in individual sports, such as track and field athletics and swimming, may not be as adversely affected by shift work, in terms of the opportunity for training. Although the opportunity to train for some sports may not be hindered by shift work, often this training cannot be scheduled in the early evening, which is the time of day associated with the highest self-paced work rates. The opportunities for the shift worker to participate in sports competitions are undoubtedly hindered, because these are most often scheduled in the early evening and at weekends. At these times, the shift worker may be needing recuperative sleep. Even if the shift worker does manage to arrive at the start of a sports competition, inappropriately phased rhythms and/or marked sleep deprivation may adversely affect performance.

Sport is one of the few leisure activities that may mediate long-term favorable changes in physiologic functions and/or exacerbate the fatigue of the shift worker. Physical activity performed at least twice a week is usually included in guidelines for improving shift-work tolerance. The usefulness of exercise during shift work is poorly understood, and there is evidence that the majority of shift workers do not follow that particular piece of advice. More research is needed regarding not only how leisure interests are affected by shift work, but, conversely, how leisure activities, especially those involving exercise, affect tolerance of shift work.

CONCLUSION

Mostly we are aware of our circadian rhythms only when the various timekeeping mechanisms underlying them are desynchronized. This happens in the cases of nocturnal shift work and long-haul flights. Then there is an obvious impact on athletic performance and on the inclination or ability to train hard. In normal circumstances, the style with which our everyday activities are ordered takes into consideration all the factors that regulate our biologic clocks. Their timing has relevance as far as training and competing in sports events are concerned.

Meticulous planning is the key to combating desynchronization of rhythms, as experienced with jet lag. If at all possible, it is advisable to schedule flights to arrive well in advance of competition. Allowing 1 day for each time zone crossed gives a margin of safety. The time for adaptation may be shortened by exploiting the external factors that reset biologic clocks: rest/exercise, darkness/light, meals, and social influences. It is important to fit in straightaway to the pattern of external influences in the new environment, so that the body time can readjust to local time. Even then, it is important to consider the relation of the restored chronobiologic rhythms to the predisposition for physical performance.

REFERENCES

1. Reilly T, Young K, Seddon R. Investigation of biorhythms in female athletic performance. *Appl Ergon* 1983;14:215–217.
2. Atkinson G, Reilly T. Circadian variations in sports performance. *Sports Med* 1996;21:292–312.
3. Reilly T, Atkinson G, Budgett R. Effects of temazepam on physiological and performanc variables following a westerly flight across five time zones. *J Sports Sci* 1997;15:62.
4. Minors DS, Waterhouse JM. *Circadian rhythms and the human.* Bristol: John Wright, 1981.
5. Akerstedt T. Altered sleep/wake patterns and circadian rhythms. *Acta Physiol Scand* 1979;suppl:469.
6. Reilly T. Human circadian rhythms and exercise. *Crit Rev Biomed Eng* 1990;18:165–180.
7. Veldhuis JD, Johnson ML, Iranmanesh A, et al. Rhythmic and non-rhythmic modes of anterior pituitary hormone release in man. In: Touitou Y, Haus E, eds. *Biological rhythms in clinical and laboratory medicine.* Berlin: Springer-Verlag, 1992:277–291.
8. Swoyer J, Haus E, Lakatua D, et al. Chronobiology in the clinical laboratory. In: Haus H, Kabat H, eds. *Chronobiology 1982–1983.* New York: Karger, 1984:533–543.
9. Mejean L, Kolopp M, Drouin P. Chronobiology, nutrition and diabetes mellitus. In: Touitou Y, Haus E, eds. *Biological rhythms in clinical and laboratory medicine.* Berlin: Springer-Verlag, 1992:375–385.
10. Schlierf G. Diurnal variations in plasma substrate concentration. *Eur J Clin Invest* 1978;8:59–60.
11. Gaultier C, Reinberg A, Girard F. Circadian rhythms in lung resistance and dynamic lung compliance of healthy children: effect of two bronchodilators. *Respir Physiol* 1977;31:169–182.
12. Smolensky MH, Scott PH, Barnes PJ, et al. The chronopharmacology and chronotherapy of asthma. *Annu Rev Chronopharmacol* 1986;2:229–273.
13. Smolensky MH, Alonzo GED. Nocturnal asthma: mechanisms and chronotherapy. In: Touitou Y, Haus E, eds. *Biological rhythms in clinical and laboratory medicine.* Berlin: Springer-Verlag, 1992:453–469.
14. Smolensky MH, Tatar SE, Bergman SA, et al. Circadian rhythmic aspects of human cardiovascular function: a review by chronobiologic statistical methods. *Chronobiologia* 1976;3:337–371.
15. Zulch KJ, Hossman V. 24-hour rhythm of human blood pressure. *Ger Med Mon* 1967;12:513–518.
16. Atkinson G, Witte K, Nold G, Sasse U, Lemmer B. Effects of age on circadian blood pressure and heart rate rhythms in primary hypertensive patients. *Chronobiol Int* 1994;11:35–44.
17. Moore JG. Chronobiology of the gastrointestinal system. In: Touitou Y, Haus E, eds. *Biological rhythms in clinical and laboratory medicine.* Berlin: Springer-Verlag, 1992:210–207.
18. Goo RH, Moore JG, Greenberg E, et al. Circadian variation in gastric emptying of meals in man. *Gastroenterology* 1987;93: 515–518.
19. Touitou Y, Touitou C, Bogdan A, et al. Circadian and seasonal variations of electrolytes in ageing humans. *Clin Chim Acta* 1989;180:245–254.
20. Robertson WG, Hodgkinson A, Marshall DH. Seasonal variations in the composition of urine from normal subjects during a longitudinal study. *Clin Chim Acta* 1977;80:34–55.
21. Wisser H, Breur H. Circadian changes of clinical, chemical and endocrinological parameters. *J Clin Chem* 1981;19:323–328.
22. Hoddes E, Zarcone V, Smythe HR, Dement WC. Quantification of sleepiness: a new approach. *Psychophysiology* 1973;10:431–436.
23. McNair DM, Lorr M, Droppleman LF. *EITS manual for the profile of mood states.* San Diego: Educational and Industrial Testing Service, 1971.
24. Reilly T, Walsh T. Physiological, psychological and performance measures during an endurance record for 5-a-side soccer play. *Br J Sports Med* 1981;15:122–128.
25. Conroy RTWL, O'Brien M. Diurnal variation in athletic performance. *J Physiol* 1974;236:51P.
26. Rodahl A, O'Brien M, Firth PGR. Diurnal variation in performance of competitive swimmers. *J Sports Med Phys Fitness* 1976;16:72–76.
27. Reilly T. Circadian rhythms and exercise. In: McLeod D, Maughan RJ, Nimmo M, Reilly T, Williams C, eds. *Exercise: benefits, limits and adaptations.* London: E and FN Spon, 1987:346–366.
28. Baxter C, Reilly T. Influence of time of day on all-out swimming. *Br J Sports Med* 1983;17:122–127.
29. Sinnerton S, Reilly T. Effects of sleep loss and time of day in swimmers. In: MacLaren D, Reilly T, Lees A, eds. *Biomechanics and medicine in swimming: swimming science VI.* London: E and FN Spon, 1992:399–405.
30. Gifford LS. Circadian variation in human flexibility and grip strength. *Aust J Physiother* 1987;33:3–9.
31. Reilly T, Tyrrell A, Troup JDG. Circadian variations in human stature. *Chronobiol Int* 1984;1:121–126.
32. Wilby J, Linge K, Reilly T, Troup JDG. Spinal shrinkage in females: circadian variation and the effects of circuit weight-training. *Ergonomics* 1987;30:47–54.
33. Taylor D, Gibson H, Edwards RHT, Reilly T. Correction of isometric leg strength tests for time of day. *Eur J Exp Musculoskel Res* 1994;3:25–27.
34. Wit A. *Zagadnienia regulacji w procesie rozwoju sily miesnionej na przykladzi zawodnikow uprawiajacych podnoszenie ciezarow* [in Polish]. Warsaw: Institute of Sport, 1980.
35. Atkinson G, Coldwells A, Reilly T, Waterhouse J. A comparison of circadian rhythms in work performance between physically active and inactive subjects. *Ergonomics* 1993;36:273–281.
36. Atkinson G, Greeves J, Reilly T, et al. Day-to-day and circadian variability of leg strength measured with the LIDO isokinetic dynamometer. *J Sports Sci* 1995;13:18–19.
37. Hill DW, Smith JC. Circadian rhythm in anaerobic power and capacity. *Can J Sports Sci* 1991;16:30–32.
38. Hill DW, Borden DO, Darnaby KM, et al. Effect of time of day on aerobic and anaerobic responses to high intensity exercise. *Can J Sports Sci* 1992;17:316–319.
39. Reilly T, Baxter C. Influence of time of day on reactions to cycling at a fixed high intensity. *Br J Sports Med* 1983;17:128–130.
40. Reilly T, Down A. Circadian variation in the standing broad jump. *Percept Motor Skills* 1986;62:830.

41. Reilly T, Down A. Investigation of circadian rhythms in anaerobic power and capacity of the legs. *J Sports Med Phys Fitness* 1992;32:342–347.
42. Reilly T, Marshall S. Circadian rhythms in power output on a swim bench. *J Swim Res* 1991;7:11–13.
43. Reilly T, Brooks GA. Exercise and the circadian variation in body temperature measures. *Int J Sports Med* 1986;7:358–362.
44. Wahlberg I, Åstrand I. Physical work capacity during the day and at night. *Work Environ Health* 1973;10:65–68.
45. Cohen CJ, Muehl GE. Human circadian rhythms in resting and exercise pulse rates. *Ergonomics* 1977;20:475–479.
46. Cohen CJ. Human circadian rhythms in heart rate response to a maximal exercise stress. *Ergonomics* 1980;23:591–595.
47. Reilly T, Robinson G, Minors DS. Some circulatory responses to exercise at different times of day. *Med Sci Sports Exerc* 1984;16:477–482.
48. Cable NT, Reilly T, Winterburn S, Atkinson G. Circadian variation in post-exercise hypotension [Abstract]. *Med Sci Sports Exerc* 1995;27:566.
49. Cabri J, Clarys JP, De Witte B, Reilly T, Strass D. Circadian variation in blood pressure responses to muscular exercise. *Ergonomics* 1988;31:1559–66.
50. Reilly T. Circadian variation in ventilatory and metabolic adaptations to submaximal exercise. *Br J Sports Med* 1982;16:115–116.
51. Reilly T, Brooks GA. Selective persistence of circadian rhythms in physiological responses to exercise. *Chronobiol Int* 1990;7:59–67.
52. Faria IE, Drummond BJ. Circadian changes in resting heart rate and body temperature, maximal oxygen consumption and perceived exertion. *Ergonomics* 1982;25:381–386.
53. Reilly T, Brooks GA. Investigation of circadian rhythms in metabolic responses to exercise. *Ergonomics* 1982;25:1093–1107.
54. Hessemer V, Langusch D, Bruck K, Bodeker RK, Breidenback T. Effects of slightly lowered body temperature on endurance performance in humans. *J Appl Physiol Respir Environ Exerc Physiol* 1984;57:1731–1737.
55. Atkinson G, Reilly T. Effects of age and time of day on preferred work-rates during prolonged exercise. *Chronobiol Int* 1995;12:121–129.
56. Reilly T, Garrett R. Effects of time of day on self-paced performances of prolonged exercise. *J Sports Med Phys Fitness* 1995;35:99–102.
57. Torii J, Shinkai S, Hino S, et al. Effect of time of day on adaptive response to a 4-week aerobic exercise program. *J Sports Med Phys Fitness* 1992;32:348–352.
58. Hildebrandt G, Gutenbrunner C, Reinhart C, et al. Circadian variation of isometric strength training in man. In: Morgan E, ed. *Chronobiology and chronomedicine.* Vol II. Frankfurt: Peter Lang, 1990:322–329.
59. Gutenbrunner C. Circadian variations in physical training. In: Gutenbrunner C, Hildebrandt G, Moog R, eds. *Chronobiology and chronomedicine.* Frankfurt: Peter Lang, 1993:665–680.
60. Hildebrandt G, Strempel H. Chronobiological problems of performance and adaptional capacity. *Chronobiologia* 1974;4:103–105.
61. Willich SN, Lewis M, Lowel H, et al. Physical exertion as a trigger of acute myocardial infarction. *N Engl J Med* 1993;329:1684–1690.
62. Hill DW, Cureton KJ, Collins MA, Grisham SC. Diurnal variations in responses to exercise of "morning types" and "evening types." *J Sports Med Phys Fitness* 1988;28:213–219.
63. Burgoon PW, Holland GJ, Loy SF, et al. A comparison of morning and evening "types" during maximum exercise. *J Appl Sports Sci Res* 1992;6:115–119.
64. Winget CM, De Roshia CW, Markley CL, Holley DC. A review of human physiological performance changes associated with desynchronosis of biological rhythms. *Aviat Space Environ Med* 1984;54:132–137.
65. Harma M, Laitinen J, Partinen M, Suvanto S. The effect of four-day round trip flights over 10 time zones on the circadian variation in salivary melatonin and cortisol in air-line flight attendants. *Ergonomics* 1994;37:1479–1489.
66. Reilly T, Waterhouse J, Atkinson G. Ageing, rhythms of physical performance and adjustment to changes in the sleep-activity cycle. *Occup Environ Med* 1997;54:812–816.
67. Mermin J, Czeisler C. Comparison of ambulatory temperature recordings at varying levels of physical exertion: average amplitude is unchanged by strenuous exercise. *Sleep Res* 1987;16:253.
68. Atkinson G, Coldwells A, Reilly T, Waterhouse J. Effects of age on diurnal variations in prolonged physical performance and physiological responses to exercise. *J Sports Sci* 1994;12:127.
69. Atkinson G, Coldwells A, Reilly T, Waterhouse J. An age comparison of circadian rhythms in physical performance and mood states. *J Interdisc Cycle Res* 1992;23:186–188.
70. Paxton SJ, Turner J, Montgomery I. Does aerobic fitness affect sleep. *Psychophysiology* 1983;20:320–324.
71. Griffin SJ, Trinder J. Physical fitness, exercise and human sleep. *Psychophysiology* 1978;15:447–450.
72. Rognum TD, Vartdal F, Rodahl K, et al. Physical and mental performance of soldiers on high- and low-energy diets during prolonged heavy exercise combined with sleep deprivation. *Ergonomics* 1986;29:859–867.
73. Myles WS, Romet TT. Self-paced work in sleep-deprived subjects. *Ergonomics* 1987;30:1175–1184.
74. Ahnve S, Theorell T, Akerstedt T, Froberg JE, Halberg F. Circadian variations in cardiovascular parameters during sleep deprivation. *Eur J Appl Physiol* 1981;46:9–19.
75. Reilly T, George A. Urinary phenylethlamine levels during three days of indoor soccer play. *J Sports Sci* 1983;1:70.
76. Akerstedt T, Froberg JE, Froberg Y, Wetterberg I. Melatonin excretion, body temperature and subjective arousal during 64 h of sleep deprivation. *Psychoendocrinology* 1979;4:219.
77. Reilly T, Deykin T. Effects of partial sleep loss on subjective states, psychomotor and physical performance tests. *J Hum Mov Stud* 1983;9:157–170.
78. Reilly T, Hales AJ. Effects of partial sleep deprivation on performance measures in females. In: Megaw ED, ed. *Contemporary ergonomics.* London: Taylor & Francis, 1988:509–515.
79. Reilly T, Piercy M. The effects of partial sleep deprivation in weightlifting performance. *Ergonomics* 1994;37:107–115.
80. Rogers AS, Spencer MB, Stone BM, Nicholson AN. The influence of a 1 h nap on performance overnight. *Ergonomics* 1989;32:1193–1205.
81. Aschoff J. Circadian rhythms in man. *Science* 1965;148:1427–1432.
82. Reilly T, Atkinson G, Waterhouse J. *Biological rhythms and exercise.* Oxford: Oxford University Press, 1997.
83. Haus E, Touitou Y. Principles of clinical chronobiology. In: Touitou Y, Haus E, eds. *Biological rhythms in clinical and laboratory medicine.* Berlin: Springer-Verlag, 1992:6–34.
84. Arendt J. The pineal. In: Toutitou Y, Haus E, eds. *Biological rhythms in clinical and laboratory medicine.* Berlin: Springer-Verlag, 1992:348–362.
85. De Looy A, Minors D, Waterhouse J, Reilly T, Tunstall Pedoe D. *The coach's guide to competing abroad.* Leeds: National Coaching Foundation, 1988.
86. Reilly T, Mellor S. Jet lag in student Rugby League players following a near-maximal time-zone shift. In: Reilly T, Lees A, Davids K, Murphy WJ, eds. *Science and football.* London: E and FN Spon, 1988:249–256.
87. Reilly T, Maughan RJ, Budgett R, Davies B. The acclimatisation of international athletes. In: Robertson SA, ed. *Contemporary ergonomics.* London: Taylor & Francis, 1997:136–140.
88. Reilly T, Maskell P. Effects of altering the sleep-wake cycle in human circadian rhythms and motor performance. Proceedings of the First IOC Congress on Sport Science, Colorado Springs, 1989:106–107.
89. Waterhouse J, Reilly T, Atkinson G. Travel and body clock disturbances. *Sports Exerc Injury* 1997;3:9–14.
90. Graeber R, Sing H, Cuthbert B. The impact of transmeridian flight on deploying soldiers. In: Johnson L, Tepas D, Colquhoun P, eds. *Biological rhythms, sleep and shiftwork.* Lancaster: MTP Press, 1981:513–537.
91. Leathwood P. Circadian rhythms of plasma amino acids, brain neurotransmitters and behaviour. In: Arendt J, Minors D, Waterhouse J, eds. *Biological rhythms in clinical practice.* Bristol: John Wright, 1989:131–159.

92. Graeber RC. Jet lag and sleep disruption. In: Krugger MH, Roth T, Dement C, eds. *Principles and practice in sleep medicine.* Philadelphia: WB Saunders, 1989:324–331.
93. Arendt J, Aldhous M, English J, et al. Some effects of jet-lag and their alleviation by melatonin. *Ergonomics* 1987;30:1379–1393.
94. Akerstedt T, Ficca G. Alertness-enhancing drugs as a countermeasure to fatigue in irregular work hours. *Chronobiol Int* 1997;14:145–158.
95. Minors D, Waterhouse J, Wirz-Justice A. A human phase-response curve to light. *Neurosci Lett* 1991;133:36–40.
96. Jehue R, Street D, Huizenga R. Effect of time zone and game time changes on team performance: National Football League. *Med Sci Sports Exerc* 1993;25:127–131.

Exercise and Sport Science,
edited by William E. Garrett, Jr., and Donald T. Kirkendall.
Lippincott Williams & Wilkins, Philadelphia © 2000.

CHAPTER 25

Ergogenic Aids for Improved Performance

Melvin H. Williams and J. David Branch

Athletic competition is popular worldwide, not only sports involving national and international class athletes, but also local and regional sport competitions for athletes ranging from youth to senior status. No matter what the sport, all athletes want to win. The two key determinants of athletic success are *optimal genetic endowment* with physiologic, psychologic, and biomechanical characteristics that predispose one to success in a given sport, and *optimal training* of those characteristics to achieve one's genetic potential. At the United States Olympic Training Center and similar national centers, sport physiologists, sport psychologists, and sport biomechanists study athletes in order to maximize their physical power, mental strength, and mechanical edge.

Athletes may use ergogenic aids, or ergogenics, however; these are substances used in attempts to enhance physical power, mental strength, or mechanical edge beyond effects attributable to training. Smith and Perry (1) have indicated that athletes view ergogenics as essential components of successful sport performance.

In *The Ergogenics Edge: Pushing the Limits of Sports Performance*, Williams (2) identified various categories of ergogenic aids whereby athletes attempt to enhance either physical power, mental strength, or mechanical edge. *Mechanical* or *biomechanical ergogenics* help modify mechanical aspects of sport to improve energy efficiency (i.e., to maximize mechanical work productivity for any given energy input). Modifications of sportswear, such as lightweight racing shoes, or sports equipment, such as aerodynamic bicycles, can significantly improve performance. Such modifications, however, must be within the regulations of the specific sport. *Psychologic ergogenics* are designed primarily to increase mental strength, and techniques such as imagery, stress management, and hypnosis have been used in attempts to enhance physical performance. Although research findings from group studies are equivocal, psychological ergogenics may benefit individual athletes. *Nutritional ergogenics* include literally dozens of nutritional strategies or supplements designed primarily to enhance energy production. Carbohydrate supplementation has been shown to benefit aerobic endurance athletes, and water-rehydration strategies may help prevent dehydration-induced fatigue. Other than these two nutritional strategies, few data are available to support an ergogenic effect of various nutrients (including protein, amino acids, vitamins, and minerals) or other dietary supplements (such as ginseng, L-carnitine, or yohimbine) on sport performance in a well-nourished athlete.

Two categories of ergogenic aids that have produced the most positive effects on sport performance are the physiologic and pharmacologic ergogenics. *Physiologic ergogenics* are designed to strengthen natural physiologic processes important to sport performance, whereas *pharmacologic ergogenics*, or drugs, are synthetic agents to augment natural neurotransmitter or hormonal functions associated with sport performance. As listed in Table 25–1, numerous physiologic and pharmacologic ergogenics have been used by athletes over the years. Space does not permit a discussion of all these ergogenics, or a detailed evaluation of individual studies. Thus this brief review highlights several physiologic and pharmacologic ergogenics, primarily those that have received the most research attention. For the interested reader, many of the references cited for each ergogenic aid are scientific reviews and provide a more detailed

M. H. Williams and J. D. Branch: Department of Exercise Science, Physical Education, and Recreation, Old Dominion University, Norfolk, Virginia 23529-0196.

TABLE 25–1. *Examples of physiologic and pharmacologic ergogenic aids*

Physiologic ergogenics	Pharmacologic ergogenics
Blood doping	Alcohol
Carnitine	Anabolic steroids
Choline	β-Blockers
Coenzyme Q_{10}	Caffeine
Creatine	Corticosteroids
DHEA (dehydroepiandrosterone)	Diuretics
Erythropoietin	Marijuana
Glycerol	Narcotic analgesics
Human chorionic gonadotropin	Specified β-2 agonists
Human growth hormone	Stimulants
Inosine	Amphetamine
Oxygen	Cocaine
Sodium bicarbonate	Ephedrine
	Testosterone

analysis. Each ergogenic aid is covered relative to theory, effectiveness, health concerns, and legality.

PHYSIOLOGIC ERGOGENICS

Physiologic ergogenics reviewed include blood doping and recombinant erythropoietin (rEPO), sodium bicarbonate, creatine, and glycerol.

Blood Doping and Recombinant Erythropoietin

Blood doping, more technically referred to as induced erythrocythemia, involves either the autologous infusion or homologous transfusion of blood to the athlete. In the autologous infusion, the athlete may receive his or her own blood that has previously been withdrawn, frozen, and saved while normal hemoglobin status was restored. In the homologous transfusion, the athlete receives cross-matched blood from another individual. Amounts of blood used in research range from 500 to 1000 mL.

Erythropoietin (EPO) is a natural hormone produced by the kidney, generally in response to inadequate oxygen delivery. Recombinant EPO (rEPO), a synthetic form, has been derived through recombinant technology. Amounts of rEPO used in research approximate 20 to 40 IU/kg injected three times weekly for 6 weeks. Although technically a drug, rEPO may be considered a physiologic ergogenic, given its similarity to blood doping.

Blood doping has been used as an ergogenic aid since the early 1970s, with rumors that some athletes used it in the 1972 Munich Olympics. rEPO use as an ergogenic is a more recent phenomenon, and at least one athlete was removed from the 1996 Olympics in Atlanta for admitting use of rEPO.

Theoretic Application

Both blood doping and rEPO are used to increase the hematocrit, particularly the red blood cell (RBC) concentration [RBC] and associated hemoglobin concentration [Hb]. Typical blood-doping protocols increase these parameters immediately. Because the hematopoietic effects of rEPO on the bone marrow involve a slower process, however, it may take weeks of rEPO injections to increase [RBC] and [Hb] significantly.

Theoretically, increasing [Hb] increases the oxygen-carrying capacity of the blood. Each gram of Hb transports 1.34 mL oxygen. By increasing the [Hb] 1 g/dL, an athlete with an exercise cardiac output of 25 L/min would increase oxygen transport by 335 mL, which extrapolates to an 8% increase in an athlete with a normal $\dot{V}O_2$max of 4000 mL O_2/min. An increased oxygen delivery should enhance performance in endurance events dependent primarily on oxidative processes, such as distance events like the 10-km race in track athletics.

Effectiveness

Although blood-doping research was conducted as early as 1944, and a few studies were done in the 1960s, it was not until the early 1970s that concerted research efforts were made to investigate its potential to enhance oxygen delivery with a possible application to sport. In an earlier review, Williams (3) noted that the available scientific data were limited and did not provide objective evidence that blood doping enhanced aerobic endurance capacity. However, many of these early studies, by using autologous techniques, did not use frozen blood. Regulations specified that nonfrozen blood must be returned to the donor within 21 days, which may not have provided ample time for the donor to regenerate his or her [Hb] back to normal. Additionally, many of these studies reinfused relatively small amounts of blood, typically 500 mL, an amount not generally shown to improve endurance performance (4).

Several blood-doping studies published in the early 1980s (5,6), with autologous techniques and ample time to restore normal hemoglobin levels, larger amounts of blood (approximately 1,000 mL), highly trained athletes, and better experimental protocols reported rather significant improvements in blood parameters, oxygen use, and exercise performance. Collectively, these studies reported a significant increase in [Hb], about 1 g/dL or 7% (5,6), a 5% increase in $\dot{V}O_{2max}$ (5), a 34% increase in treadmill run time to exhaustion at 95% $\dot{V}O_{2max}$ (5), and 2.5% improvement in 5-mile treadmill run time performance, a 44-second improvement (6).

Numerous studies have been conducted in the intervening years, and two recent reviews (7,8) concluded that appropriate blood-doping protocols will significantly increase total hemoglobin, [Hb], RBC mass, and arterial oxygen content. The increased arterial oxygen content, leading to an increased $\dot{V}O_{2max}$, reduces the stress on the heart during submaximal exercise performance, as indicated by lower heart-rate responses during standardized submaximal exercise tasks. Additionally, the increased oxygen delivery to the muscles decreased blood lactate accumulation, either by enhanced cellular oxidation or an additional buffering effect of hemoglobin. Both the decreased heart rate and serum lactate responses to standardized submaximal exercise tasks were associated with decreased psychological stress, as evidenced by decreased ratings of perceived exertion (RPE) during exercise. Overall, these effects lead to increased endurance performance in submaximal aerobic endurance exercise tasks, such as the 34% increase in treadmill run time to exhaustion at 95% $\dot{V}O_{2max}$ cited earlier (5) and documented in numerous other studies as well (7). Additionally, blood doping has improved endurance performance in several field studies, running events ranging in distance from 1500 to 10,000 m (2).

Only a few studies investigated the effect of rEPO use as a potential ergogenic aid. For example, Ekblom and Berglund (9) reported that rEPO injections (20 to 40 IU/kg, three per week for 6 to 7 weeks) increased hematocrit and [Hb] (about 6% to 11%), $\dot{V}O_{2max}$, and treadmill run time to exhaustion. Although the research data are more limited, the American College of Sports Medicine (7) indicated that the effects of rEPO use are comparable to those seen with blood doping.

Health Concerns

If conducted under appropriate medical supervision, both autologous and homologous blood transfusions are considered safe. Of the two, homologous transfusions pose more health risks, increasing the risk of various infections, such as hepatitis B, hepatitis C, and human immunodeficiency virus [HIV; and acquired immunodeficiency syndrome (AIDS)] and the possibility of receiving an incompatible blood match, which could be fatal. Clerical error and mislabeling or mishandling of blood products also may lead to incompatible transfusions, a possible likelihood if the athlete uses secretive methods to blood dope.

Athletes may self-administer rEPO, which increases health risks dramatically. Use of contaminated needles with rEPO injections may be associated with similar infections, as noted earlier. Additionally, athletes may overdose with rEPO, leading to an exaggerated increase in [RBC] and blood viscosity, with possible thrombosis and myocardial infarction. Unsupervised rEPO use has been associated with the deaths of young European cyclists (10).

Legality

Blood doping was used successfully by American cyclists in the 1984 Los Angeles Olympic games but was placed on the prohibited substances and methods list by the International Olympic Committee (IOC) in 1985. The use of rEPO also is prohibited by the IOC. Unfortunately, however, current drug-testing protocols are unable to detect the use of blood doping, and urine tests may be able to detect rEPO use for only 2 to 3 days after the last administration (11). Such testing is rather useless, as the increase in [Hb] will continue for weeks after the last administration. The International Cycling Union has instituted a blood test, prohibiting competition for athletes with hematocrits greater than 50. Conceivably, the IOC may institute blood testing as a drug-testing protocol in the near future.

Sodium Bicarbonate and Alkaline Salts

Sodium bicarbonate ($NaHCO_3$) is an alkaline salt, a part of the alkaline reserve in the blood that helps to neutralize various metabolic acids; it is more commonly known as baking soda, a popular household commodity. The effect of sodium bicarbonate supplementation on exercise performance has been studied for nearly 70 years, particularly within the past 2 decades. *Buffer boosting, soda loading*, and *soda doping* are terms often used to characterize the use of sodium bicarbonate, and other alkaline salts such as sodium citrate, as an ergogenic aid. Oral supplemental dosages used in research normally have been based on body mass, customarily 300 mg sodium bicarbonate/kg administered 1 to 2 hours before exercise. Some commercial products containing sodium bicarbonate have been marketed to athletes.

Theoretic Application

The increased production of lactic acid, a metabolic byproduct of anaerobic glycolysis, during high-intensity exercise bouts of 1- to 2-minute duration may increase intramuscular [H^+], an effect that may cause fatigue by inhibiting muscle enzyme activity (12) or by impairing the calcium-initiated muscle-contraction process (13). Theoretically sodium bicarbonate supplementation will increase the alkaline reserve, enhancing the efflux of hydrogen ions from the muscle during anaerobic glycolysis and mitigating the development of fatigue. The exact mechanism underlying the ergogenic effect of sodium bicarbonate has not been determined, however.

Effectiveness

Scores of well-controlled double-blind, placebo, crossover laboratory and field studies have investigated the potential ergogenicity of sodium bicarbonate supplementation over the past 20 years. Although not all studies provided evidence of an ergogenic effect, several major reviews of the scientific literature (13–15), including a meta-analysis of 29 of the best studies (16), concluded that sodium bicarbonate supplementation may be an effective ergogenic aid. The following are some of the principal findings emanating from these reviews.

Sodium bicarbonate supplementation increases the resting serum pH before the exercise bout, elicits higher serum pH and lactate concentrations after exercise, and may decrease muscle acidosis.

Sodium bicarbonate supplementation may reduce levels of psychological stress, as measured by RPE, during exercise tasks greater than 80% to 90% $\dot{V}O_{2max}$.

Sodium bicarbonate supplementation may increase performance in laboratory exercise tasks dependent primarily on anaerobic glycolysis, particularly in latter bouts of supramaximal (exercise tasks greater than 100% $\dot{V}O_{2max}$) repetitive exercise tasks with short recovery times. In their meta-analysis, Matson and Tran (16) reported a mean improvement of 27% in exercise time to exhaustion in supramaximal laboratory tests. Sodium bicarbonate supplementation also improved exercise performance in numerous field studies, including 400-m, 800-m, and 1500-m running velocity, 100-m and 400-m swimming velocity, 3-km cycling velocity, and even 1500-m race performance in standardbred horses.

Not all studies showed positive results, however, as noted in several recent reports indicating no significant effect of sodium bicarbonate or sodium citrate supplementation on 600-m run time of trained women or 400-m sprint performance in racing greyhounds (17,18).

Health Concerns

Sodium bicarbonate, a medicinal product, has been used therapeutically for a variety of medical problems, such as excess gastric acidity. When taken in the short term in appropriate dosages, sodium bicarbonate appears to pose no major health risks. In experimental studies, some subjects experienced gastrointestinal distress, primarily bloating, abdominal pain, and diarrhea. Excessive or long-term intake could lead to alkalosis, possibly leading to muscle spasms or cardiac arrhythmias (13,19).

Legality

Although it is interesting to note that some countries ban the use of sodium bicarbonate in race horses, use of sodium bicarbonate by human athletes is not currently prohibited by the IOC, even though its use may be regarded as an artificial means to enhance sport performance.

Creatine

Creatine, a nitrogenous amine, is a natural dietary constituent of animal foods, particularly meat. Creatine also may be synthesized from the amino acids glycine, arginine, and methionine by the liver and kidney. About 2 g daily from either exogenously or endogenously produced sources is needed to replace catabolized creatine, which is excreted by the kidneys as creatinine. Approximately 120 g of creatine is found in the average-sized male subject, 95% in the skeletal muscle. Creatine is not an essential nutrient, so it may be considered a physiologic ergogenic.

Creatine supplementation has become increasing popular in recent years. A standardized supplementation protocol involves ingestion of 20 to 30 g creatine monohydrate, usually taken in multiple 5-g doses throughout the day for 5 to 7 days, but other protocols, such as 3 g/day for 28 days, have been used.

Theoretic Applications

Creatine serves as substrate for the formation of phosphocreatine (PCr), a primary energy source for exercise tasks dependent on the adenosine triphosphate (ATP)–PCr energy system (i.e., maximal exercise tasks of 5- to 10-seconds duration or somewhat longer). Recent research (20,21) has confirmed that oral creatine supplementation increases muscle total creatine (TCr), including free creatine (FCr) and PCr. However, some individuals may be nonresponders, particularly those with normally high muscle creatine levels. Vegetarians appear to respond more than do nonvegetarians. Recent research by Green and colleagues (22,23), however, has shown that combining the creatine with a simple carbohydrate, such as glucose, will increase creatine transport into the muscle, even in subjects with near-normal levels of muscle creatine, possibly via an insulin-mediated effect.

Greenhaff (24) suggested that the increased muscle [PCr] may better maintain ATP turnover during very-high-intensity, short-term exercise bouts. Increased use of PCr as an energy source also could mitigate lactic acid formation and theoretically might enhance performance in exercise tasks dependent primarily on anaerobic glycolysis.

Effectiveness

Serious research efforts evaluating the ergogenicity of creatine supplementation were initiated in the early 1990s. Although not all of these initial studies indicated that creatine was an effective ergogenic, positive results were found in numerous laboratory studies involving maximal isokinetic resistance or cycle ergometer exercise. For example, creatine supplementation significantly increased muscle torque in multiple 10-second stages during five bouts of 30 maximal isokinetic contractions (25) and significantly improved performance in a cycling task involving 10 bouts (6-second) of high-intensity cycling interspersed with 30 seconds of rest (26). Several reviews of these preliminary studies suggested that creatine possessed ergogenic potential for certain sport endeavors (24,27).

Some, but not all, studies conducted subsequent to these reviews also suggested that creatine supplementation may enhance performance in laboratory exercise tests involving very-high-intensity, short-term, maximal, repetitive exercise bouts with relatively short recovery periods. A more recent review (28), although noting that not all studies are in agreement, cited evidence from numerous studies that creatine supplementation may possibly enhance resistance exercise performance (repetitive isometric endurance; isokinetic bench-press endurance; increased isotonic one-repetition maximal bench press) and intense cycle ergometer performance (increased peak power in the last 5 to 6 repetitions of six 10-second cycle sprints; increased peak and mean power output in three 30-second isokinetic cycling tests).

Research suggests, however, that creatine supplementation does not improve performance in field-exercise performance tests involving movement of the body mass, including 25-m, 50-m, or 100-m swim performance in highly trained swimmers (29,30) or run velocities of highly trained athletes during various zones (20 to 30 m; 40 to 50 m; 50 to 60 m) in repetitive 60-m sprints (31). Although field studies do not generally support an ergogenic effect of creatine supplementation, more research is needed concerning the use of creatine in simulated sports tasks and sports events involving multiple high-intensity, intermittent exercise tasks, such as soccer (28).

The effect of creatine supplementation on more prolonged exercise bouts dependent primarily on anaerobic or aerobic glycolysis for energy has received some research attention. In a recent study, Prevost and others (32) found that creatine supplementation significantly improved performance in a variety of exercise tasks dependent on different energy systems. The four exercise protocols involved cycling to exhaustion at 150% of $\dot{V}O_{2max}$ either (a) nonstop, (b) 30-second work/60-second rest, (c) 20-second work/40-second rest, and (d) 10-second work/20-second rest. Although creatine supplementation enhanced performance in all four exercise tasks, the most significant improvement was reported for the fourth protocol. A recent review (28) concluded that although creatine supplementation may benefit performance in exercise events dependent on anaerobic glycolysis, maximal exercise tasks of 30- to 150-second duration, the results of current studies are equivocal. Creatine supplementation is not likely to enhance performance in prolonged endurance events dependent on aerobic glycolysis and may actually be ergolytic (i.e., it may impair performance).

An increase in body mass is a rather consistent finding associated with creatine supplementation. Numerous studies reported increases in body mass ranging from 0.9 to 2.0 kg after 5 to 7 days of supplementation of 20 to 25 g/day for 5 to 7 days (28). However, creatine supplementation decreases urine production during this time frame (21), indicating that the gain in body mass may be increased body-water stores associated with the osmotic effect of creatine in the musculature. This increase in body mass has been associated with impaired aerobic endurance performance in runners (33). If creatine supplementation enhances resistance training, however, the result may be an increased muscle mass, or lean body mass, and associated gains in strength and power.

Health Concerns

No adverse health effects have been associated with short-term creatine supplementation or with longer supplementation of 8 weeks, or even supplementation of from 2 to 5 years, but the possible effects of more prolonged supplementation are not known. Anecdotal reports note muscle cramps and muscle strains after creatine loading, a possibility with increased muscle water stores. However, no scientific data are available to support these reports.

Legality

Creatine is considered to be a dietary supplement, and its use by athletes is not currently prohibited by the IOC.

Glycerol

Glycerol is an alcohol, a sweet, syrupy colorless liquid; it is a natural constituent of triglycerides, the major source of dietary fats. Glycerol may be formed in the body as a by-product of carbohydrate metabolism, but it may also be converted to carbohydrate through liver gluconeogenesis. Glycerol, or glycerin, may be derived commercially from the saponification of fats and oils for use as a solvent or skin emollient. It also may be used medically to reduce ocular tension. Glycerol has been marketed to athletes as Glycerate and has been incorporated into a sports drink, Pro-Hydrator. Glycerol is not an essential nutrient, so it may be considered a physiologic ergogenic.

Theoretic Applications

Serving as a substrate for gluconeogenesis, glycerol at one time was studied for its potential to help maintain blood glucose levels but was found not to have ergogenic potential in this regard (2).

More recently, with various hyperhydration protocols, glycerol was studied as a means to increase osmotic pressure in body fluids and concomitant increases in total body water and plasma volume. The general hyperhydration procedure involves the ingestion of glycerol in amounts approximating 1 g/kg body weight, each gram accompanied by 20 to 25 mL of water. Thus a 60-kg athlete would consume 60 g of glycerol in about 1.2 to 1.5 L of water. Theoretically, from an ergogenic viewpoint, increased body-water stores could increase resistance to fatigue through exercise-induced dehydration, while an increased plasma volume could increase stroke volume and cardiovascular function during aerobic exercise.

Research findings regarding the effects of glycerol-induced hyperhydration, compared with water-induced hyperhydration, are equivocal. Earlier reports from the U.S. Army Research Institute of Environmental Medicine (USARIEM) found that glycerol-induced hyperhydration elicited a greater retention of body fluids compared with water-induced hyperhydration, but there was no significant increase in plasma volume. Later reports from the USARIEM indicated no significant effect of glycerol-induced hyperhydration on total body-water retention. Other reports also provided ambivalent data regarding the efficacy of glycerol-induced hyperhydration to increase either total body water or plasma volume (2).

Effectiveness

Research findings regarding the effects of glycerol-induced hyperhydration, including two studies that provided both glycerol and carbohydrate supplementation, on exercise performance also are equivocal. Several studies have shown that glycerol-induced hyperhydration may reduce the thermal stress of moderate exercise under warm environmental conditions, as evidenced by a lower heart rate and rectal temperature, and may improve cycling endurance performance at 65% $\dot{V}O_{2max}$. Conversely, other studies have shown no effect of glycerol-induced hyperhydration on cardiovascular or body-temperature responses to exercise in a moderate environment, or on cycling performance at exercise intensities ranging from 55% to 75% $\dot{V}O_{2max}$ (34).

Clearly more well-controlled research is needed to help resolve this equivocality. If glycerol-induced hyperhydration does increase total body-water stores, and hence body mass, the increased weight may possibly be detrimental to athletes who must move their body mass as rapidly as possible (i.e., runners). On the other hand, cyclists are less concerned with an additional kilogram or so and may benefit from increased total body-water and plasma volume (35).

Health Concerns

When diluted with water and consumed in appropriate dosages based on body mass, as used in these studies, glycerol supplementation appears to be safe. However, USARIEM researchers noted that larger doses may possibly cause excess fluid retention in the intracellular spaces, leading to abnormal pressures and tissue damage. Headaches and nausea have been observed in some individuals, and individuals with high blood pressure, diabetes, or kidney problems should consult with their physicians before trying glycerol supplementation.

Legality

Glycerol is considered to be a dietary supplement, and its use by athletes is not prohibited by the IOC.

PHARMACOLOGIC ERGOGENICS

Pharmacologic ergogenics reviewed include anabolic–androgenic steroids and human growth hormone, caffeine, amphetamines/sympathomimetics, and β-adrenergic blocking agents.

Anabolic–Androgenic Steroids and Human Growth Hormone

Anabolic–androgenic steroids (AASs) are chemically modified analogues of testosterone, the endogenous gonadal hormone produced by the testes and responsible for development of masculine features (androgyny) and lean-tissue synthesis (anabolism). Testosterone was first isolated and identified in 1935 (36). Many AAS agents have been developed since then, primarily for the treatment of hypogonadism. Use of AAS agents for ergogenic purposes by weightlifters and runners began in the 1950s. Anecdotal reports indicate that AAS agents are currently being used not only by Olympic and professional athletes, but also by younger athletes, bodybuilders, and nonathletes, with black market sales well in excess of $100 million/year (37–39). At present, approximately 30 AAS agents are administered orally (e.g., fluoxymesterone, methenolone, methandrostenolone, methyltestosterone, oxandrolone, stanozolol); injected intramuscularly (i.m.; e.g., boldenone, nandrolone decanoate, testosterone cypionate, testosterone ethanate, testosterone propionate) or combined in concentrations that are 10 to 100 times the recommended pharmacologic doses, a practice known as "stacking" (40).

Human growth hormone (hGH) is a 191-residue, 22-kDa peptide. The secretion of hGH from the anterior pituitary is regulated by the hypothalamic hormones, growth hormone–releasing hormone (hGHrH) and somatostatin. Stimuli for hGH release include sleep, exercise, L-DOPA, and arginine (41). hGH may be obtained from human cadavers, but a more abundant source has become available as recombinant hGH (rhGH), which has been developed by using recombinant technology.

Theoretic Applications

AAS agents are chemical modifications of testosterone, either by alkylation at the 17-α position or by carboxylic acid esterification at the 17-β hydroxyl group on the sterol D ring. Compared with exogenous testosterone, the degradation of the analogue is markedly decreased, resulting in greater anabolic potential due to the higher plasma [analogue]. The *in vivo* physiologic mechanism of AAS action is thought to be similar to that of endogenous testosterone, (i.e., diffusion of the AAS agent across the cell membrane), forming a testosterone analogue/receptor complex that then binds to the nucleus, stimulating *de novo* messenger RNA (mRNA) synthesis and an increase in structural and contractile protein (40). Other possible AAS mechanisms of action include competitive binding to glucocorticoid receptors, inhibiting the catabolic effect of cortisol, and direct neural action through binding to androgen receptors of α-motor neurons and brain tissue (41).

Metabolic actions of hGH are generally anabolic, increasing amino acid uptake, protein synthesis, and the growth of epiphyseal plates of long bones. Although hGH has a short half-life, it stimulates the release of somatomedins (e.g., insulin-like growth factors), which have more prolonged anabolic effects. hGH stimulates renal and hepatic gluconeogenesis as well as lipolysis (41).

Effectiveness

Much of the current understanding of the efficacy of AAS use comes from anecdotal reports and clinical case studies. Compared with controlled clinical trials, greater gains in muscle strength and body mass have been reported in case studies of individuals who undergo "cycling" regimens (i.e., periods of supraphysiologic doses followed by discontinuation) (2).

Of the few well-designed clinical trials, the results are equivocal (40,42). Among studies supporting the efficacy of AAS in improving strength and/or mass, the effects seem to be highly variable and relatively small (43). In addition, the efficacy of AAS appears to be more apparent in trained than in untrained subjects (40,42). A meta-analysis reported a median improvement in strength of 5% (range, 1.2% to 18.7%) across nine studies of trained subjects, with no change in eight studies of untrained subjects. The results of these studies may not be generalizable to the megadose "stacking" regimens that are currently practiced by AAS users (42). To illustrate this point, a recent double-blind placebo control study reported increased strength and muscle size in a group of male subjects receiving intramuscular injections of a supraphysiologic AAS dose (testosterone ethanate; 600 mg/week, i.m.) for 10 weeks while weight training compared with placebo only, AAS only, and placebo/weight-training groups (44).

rhGH supplementation has been shown to increase lean body mass, decrease body fat, and improve skin tone in elderly men who were hGH deficient. Moreover, rhGH supplementation also was shown to increase lean body mass in young men who are not hGH deficient. In a recent review, Yarasheski (45) described his research with several groups of young men with normal hGH levels undertaking strenuous resistance-type exercise training. Although rhGH did increase overall lean body mass in one group of subjects, magnetic resonance imaging revealed that the increase was not muscle mass. Yarasheski suggested that the increased lean body mass might be attributed to fluid retention or increases in other lean tissues, such as the spleen. Moreover, these young subjects experienced no gain in muscular strength, suggesting that rhGH supplementation was not an effective ergogenic in subjects with normal hGH levels.

Health Concerns

AAS use is strongly associated with altered lipid metabolism (decreased serum [HDL-C]), hepatic cellular damage, testicular atrophy, myocardial cellular damage, and cardiomyopathy in humans and animal models (40,46–49). The orally ingested 17α-alkylated AAS agents appear to pose greater health risks than the injected 17β-esters, but use of needles increases the risk of HIV/AIDS, hepatitis, and other infections (48). Other outcomes such as male/female reproductive dysfunction, clitoral enlargement, increased aggressiveness, and acne also are associated with AAS use (41). Ethical considerations preclude the study of megadose AAS regimens on strength gains in a controlled clinical trial. As a result, increased understanding of the health consequences of AAS use will continue to come from anecdotal reports, clinical case studies, and epidemiologic case–control studies. There is an alarming prevalence of AAS use among adolescent and college-aged students (37,50,51). AAS use contributes to a "risk-behavior syndrome," in which AAS use is significantly associated with such high-risk behaviors as drinking and driving, nonuse of seat belts, unsafe sexual practices, and suicidal behavior (38). This tends to support reports of increased aggressiveness among chronic AAS users (40).

hGH use causes acromegaly in adults and gigantism in prepubescent children. Cardiomyopathy and diabetes also are associated with acromegaly (41). hGH must be injected, increasing the risk of infections such as hepatitis.

Legality

AAS agents are prohibited by the IOC and by the governing bodies of all amateur and professional sports. Sensitive quantitative assays have been developed to detect their use (40). The IOC prohibits the use of hGH, but its use cannot be detected by using current drug-testing technology. The IOC plans to have a test available for the year 2000 Olympic games, however.

Amphetamines/Sympathomimetics

Amphetamines represent a pharmacologic class of agents whose parent compound is β-phenylethylamine. Although chemically related to the catecholamines, amphetamines lack the hydroxyl groups at the *meta*- and *para*-positions of the benzene ring that are characteristic of the catecholamines. Amphetamines are unable to interact directly with α- and β-adrenergic receptors, but exert an indirect influence on catecholamine metabolism. Thus amphetamines also are known as sympathomimetic amines (52). Ephedrine is another sympathomimetic amine whose use has been associated with sport. Although a prescribed medication, ephedrine also is present in many over-the-counter medicines, such as Bronkotabs and Co-Tylenol, and dietary supplements such as Ma Huang and herbal weight-control products.

Theoretic Applications

Amphetamines stimulate the release of norepinephrine from sympathetic nerves, resulting in vasoconstriction and increased arterial blood pressure. Amphetamines also stimulate the hypothalamus as well as pleasure centers in the brain, elevating mood and increasing resistance to fatigue by either enhancing the release of dopamine or inhibiting its uptake and/or degradation (52). Other sympathomimetic agents, such as ephedrine, act in a similar fashion.

Effectiveness

Amphetamines have been shown to increase alertness, mask fatigue, and enhance the performance of certain motor tasks. Little research on the ergogenicity of amphetamines has been reported in recent years, mirroring the general decline of amphetamine use (52). In a double-blind placebo-controlled study, improvements in knee-extension strength, acceleration, and anaerobic capacity followed amphetamine ingestion [15 mg dextroamphetamine (Dexedrine)/70 kg]. Although maximal aerobic power ($\dot{V}O_{2max}$) was unchanged, both time to exhaustion and maximal blood [lactate] were increased, suggesting enhanced resistance to fatigue. Considerable interindividual variation in responsiveness also was reported (53).

Although amphetamines are generally believed to possess ergogenic potential, the use of ephedrine has not been associated with enhanced physical performance (2).

Health Concerns

Use of amphetamines has been associated with a host of side effects such as anxiety, tremors, irritability, ventricular dysrhythmias, hypertension, gastrointestinal distress, and hallucinations. Prolonged use may lead to weight loss, addiction, and psychotic behavior (52). Use of needles for injection may increase risk of various infections.

Legality

Amphetamines are considered to be potent stimulants, and their use is prohibited by the IOC and various other sports' governing bodies. Use of related stimulants, such as ephedrine, is also prohibited.

Caffeine

Caffeine (1,3,7-trimethylxanthine) is a common dietary compound found in coffee (60 to 150 mg/6 ounces), tea (25 to 40 mg/6 ounces), cola/soft drinks (15 to 30 mg/6 ounces), chocolate (6 to 15 mg/ounce), and certain over-the-counter medications (e.g., 200 mg/Vivarin tablet). The normal range of caffeine ingested is 100 to 300 mg/day (54,55).

Theoretic Applications

Caffeine facilitates epinephrine release from the adrenal medulla, stimulating vasodilation, lipolysis, glycogenolysis, and bronchodilation. Increasing lipolysis is thought to result in a possible sparing of muscle glycogen, the most studied potential ergogenic mechanism associated with caffeine use. As an inhibitor of the enzyme phosphodiesterase, caffeine may potentiate the action of 3′,5′-cyclic adenosine monophosphate (cAMP), important in the conversion of phosphorylase and hormone-sensitive lipase to their active forms. Caffeine facilitates calcium mobilization from the lateral sacs of the sarcoplasmic reticulum and increases myofibrillar and troponin C subunit sensitivity to calcium (54,56–58). As a known arginine vasopressin [antidiuretic hormone (ADH)] inhibitor, caffeine also increases diuresis (54,55).

Caffeine is a central nervous system (CNS) stimulant and a competitive antagonist of the receptor for adenosine, a CNS depressant. Recent research attention has turned to the neural effect of caffeine, as well as the direct effect of caffeine in muscle force development, as promising ergogenic mechanisms (56).

Effectiveness

Caffeine ingestion of 3 to 13 mg/kg body mass appears to enhance prolonged endurance performance, as well as high-intensity short-duration exercise performed in a laboratory setting (59). Compared with placebo, improvements in endurance times of 22% to 23% have been reported after ingestion of caffeine doses of 3 to 9 mg/kg (60–62), with no evidence of dose–response or ergogenicity by using a higher dose (62). Whereas evidence suggestive of increased lipolysis (i.e., increased [glycerol], [free fatty acids]) and increased β-oxidation (decreased RER) during endurance exercise have been observed after caffeine ingestion, paradoxic increases in blood [lactate] (suggestive of increased glycogenolysis) also were reported (59,61,62).

Although the glycogen-sparing mechanism remains somewhat controversial, well-controlled research by Spriet and others (63) revealed a significant glycogen-sparing effect and improved endurance performance in recreational cyclists, indicating that this may be one of the mechanisms underlying the possible ergogenic effect of caffeine on prolonged aerobic endurance such as running a 42.2-km marathon.

Recent reviews by Graham and Spriet (59,64) also indicated that caffeine may enhance performance in shorter-duration events as well, such as the 1500-m and 5000-m track events. Performance in such events would not appear to be limited by muscle glycogen depletion but possibly by other factors, including neural stimulation. In support of this theory, Cole and others (65) recently reported that caffeine significantly increased cycle ergometer work output when subjects were asked to exercise at a set RPE, a measure of psychological effort during exercise.

A recent report indicated that caffeine did not improve performance in a hyperthermic environment (66). Although caffeine's diuretic effect would be expected to impair thermoregulation, there are no data supporting this viewpoint.

It appears that caffeine may be an effective ergogenic for a variety of exercise tasks, but more research is needed to evaluate its effectiveness under true competitive sport conditions in which athletes may be stimulated naturally by endogenous catecholamine release.

Health Concerns

Controversy exists in the epidemiologic literature concerning the association of caffeine consumption with health-related outcomes. Some possible minor health problems associated with excess caffeine consumption include restlessness, anxiety, irritability, hand tremors, and insomnia. According to a recent Consumers Union report (67), isolated studies over the past few decades have suggested that caffeine use might increase the risk of cancer, coronary heart disease, fibrocystic breast disease, and other disorders, but more recent research refuted most of those possibilities. It is generally agreed that moderate caffeine consumption (i.e., 200 to 300 mg/day/12 to 18 ounces of coffee/day) pose no health risks to most individuals.

In certain susceptible people, however, caffeine may pose some health risks, including elevated blood pressure, abnormal health rhythms, birth and pregnancy problems, ulcers and heartburn, anxiety attacks, and osteoporosis (67).

Legality

Excess amounts of caffeine are prohibited, but, because it is a constituent of many common foods and beverages, use of small amounts of caffeine is not prohibited. However, Spriet (59) noted that enhanced performance has been observed after caffeine doses resulting in urinary [caffeine] excretion *below* the IOC doping limit of 12 μg/mL, and suggested that the ethical implications of this observation demand the attention of sports governing bodies such as the IOC.

β-Adrenergic Blocking Agents (β-Blockers)

Stimulation of cardiac tissue β_1-receptors by norepinephrine results in increased inotropic and chronotropic response, whereas stimulation of adipose tissue β_1-receptors by epinephrine results in increased lipolysis. The β_2-adrenergic receptor is stimulated by epinephrine, resulting in glycogenolysis, bronchodilation, and vasodilation. β-Adrenergic blocking agents, or β-blockers, are a pharmacologic class of medications developed in the 1960s which compete with norepinephrine and epinephrine for binding at β_1 and β_2-adrenergic receptors. More than a dozen β-blockers are currently available. β-Blockers are prescribed primarily as antihypertensives to reduce myocardial afterload and prophylactically after myocardial infarction to reduce myocardial oxygen demand. These agents are either cardioselective (i.e., preferential blocking of the β_1-receptor) or nonselective [i.e., blocking of β_1- and β_2-receptors (68)].

Theoretic Applications

β-Blockers may reduce anxiety, and excess anxiety may be detrimental to performance in sports dependent on neural relaxation. Therefore β-blockers may be ergogenic for athletes involved in certain sports (e.g., golf, marksmanship, archery) or others (e.g., musicians, dancers) for which fine motor control and low-state anxiety are essential for success. Additionally, there is evidence that an upregulation of β_1- and β_2-receptor density can result from β-blockade, supporting the possible ergogenic theory that discontinuation of β-blockade may result in an exaggerated sympathetic response to exercise (69), but this area has received little research attention.

Effectiveness

Studies revealed that β-blockers may decrease anxiety and heart rate in athletes participating in high-stress sports, such as ski jumping (68). Well-controlled studies also showed that β-blockers can decrease anxiety, tension, and heart rate in pistol shooters, improving shooting ability by 13%, a finding attributed to decreased muscle tremor and improved hand steadiness.

However, other physiologic actions of β-blockers may impair sport performance (i.e., elicit ergolytic rather than ergogenic effects). β-Blockers attenuate cardiorespiratory responses (i.e., heart rate, ventilation, peripheral blood flow, and thermoregulation) and impair energy substrate availability (i.e., hepatic and muscle glycolysis, lipolysis) during exercise. Nonselective agents appear to impair maximal oxygen consumption ($\dot{V}O_{2max}$) and glycolysis to a greater extend than cardioselective agents, whereas lipolysis is similarly attenuated with use of both types of agents. β-Blockade may decrease cutaneous blood flow, which adversely affects thermoregulation (68).

Although β-blockers do not appear to impair performance of high-intensity, short-duration (less than 10 seconds) activities requiring strength and anaerobic power, they do impair high-intensity, more prolonged tasks (~30 to 60 seconds) and aerobic endurance events (more than 5 minutes) dependent on, respectively, glycolysis and oxidative process (68).

Health Concerns

β-Blockers may cause drowsiness and fatigue and may also adversely alter serum lipid profiles (i.e., decreased [HDL-C], increased [triglycerides]). β-Blockers are prescription drugs that should be used only under the guidance of a physician.

Legality

β-Blockers are prohibited by the IOC for specific sports events, including pistol and archery competition, and other sports in which excess anxiety could impair performance, such as diving and figure skating.

CONCLUSION

Given the financial and other benefits associated with sports success, athletes have used a variety of ergogenic aids over the years in attempts to gain a competitive edge. They continue to do so, as attested to by the number of incidents of athletes suspended from competition for using prohibited substances. As noted in this brief review, various drugs and doping methods may enhance sport performance, but their use is prohibited by the IOC and other athletic governing organizations. It is hoped that effective drug-testing protocols will help deter their use and provide a level playing field for all athletes.

Nevertheless, use of some effective ergogenic aids, such as sodium bicarbonate and small doses of caffeine, has not been prohibited. Moreover, sport scientists continue to explore effective, safe, and legal ergogenic-aid alternatives (such as creatine and glycerol) to prohibited substances. Some contend that the use of excess amounts of any substance in attempts to enhance performance artificially is unethical, however. For example, the normal daily dietary intake of creatine is 2 g. Is consumption of 20 to 30 g in attempts to enhance performance artificially unethical? Legally, athletes may use an ergogenic aid if its use has not been specifically prohibited (i.e., the IOC or other athletic organization has not listed it as a prohibited substance). Some athletes, because of ethical considerations, may not use such legal ergogenic aids. The issue of ergogenic aid legality has been addressed by the IOC, and we hope that the IOC will address the ethicality issue in the near future.

REFERENCES

1. Smith DA, Perry PJ. The efficacy of ergogenic agents in athletic competition. Part II: other performance enhancing agents. *Ann Pharmacother* 1992;26:653–659.
2. Williams MH. *The ergogenics edge: pushing the limits of sports performance.* Champaign, IL: Human Kinetics, 1998.
3. Williams MH. *Drugs and athletic performance.* Springfield, IL: CC Thomas, 1974.
4. Spriet LL. Blood doping and oxygen transport. In: Lamb DR, Williams MH, eds. *Ergogenics: enhancement of performance in exercise and sport.* Dubuque, IA: Brown & Benchmark, 1991:213–248.
5. Buick FJ, Gledhill N, Froese AB, Spriet LL, Meyers EC. Effect of induced erythrocythemia on aerobic work capacity. *J Appl Physiol* 1980;48:636–642.
6. Williams MH, Wesseldine S, Somma T, Schuster R. The effect of induced erythrocythemia upon 5-mile treadmill run time. *Med Sci Sports Exerc* 1981;13:169–175.
7. American College of Sports Medicine. The use of blood doping as an ergogenic aid. *Med Sci Sports Exerc* 1996;28:i–viii.
8. Simon TL. Induced erythrocythemia and athletic performance. *Semin Hematol* 1994;31:128–133.
9. Ekblom B, Berglund B. Effect of erythropoietin administration on maximal aerobic power. *Scand Med Sci Sports* 1991;1:88–93.
10. Ramotar J. Cyclists' deaths linked to erythropoietin? *Physician Sportsmed* 1990;18:48–49.
11. Wide L, Bengtsson C, Berglund B, Ekblom B. Detection in blood and urine of recombinant erythropoietin administered to healthy men. *Med Sci Exerc Sports* 1995;27:1569–1576.
12. Kirkendall D. Mechanisms of peripheral fatigue. *Med Sci Sports Exerc* 1990;22:444–449.
13. Heigenhauser G, Jones N. Bicarbonate loading. In: Lamb DR, Williams, MH, eds. *Ergogenics: enhancement of performance in exercise and sport.* Dubuque, IA: Brown & Benchmark, 1991:183–212.
14. Linderman JK, Gosselink KL. The effects of sodium bicarbonate ingestion on exercise performance. *Sports Med* 1994;18:75–80.
15. Williams MH. Bicarbonate loading. *Sports Sci Exchange* 1992; 4:1–4.
16. Matson LG, Tran ZV. Effects of sodium bicarbonate ingestion on anaerobic performance: a meta-analytic review. *Int J Sport Nutr* 1993;3:2–28.
17. Tiryaki GR, Atterbom HA. The effect of sodium bicarbonate and sodium citrate on 600 m running time of trained females. *J Sports Med Phys Fitness* 1995;35:194–198.

18. Holloway SA, Sundstrom D, Senior DF. Effect of acute induced metabolic alkalosis on the acid/base response to sprint exercise of six racing greyhounds. *Res Veter Sci* 1996;61:245–251.
19. Reynolds J, ed. *Martindale: the extra pharmacopoeia.* London: The Pharmaceutical Press, 1989.
20. Greenhaff P, Bodin K, Soderlund K, Hultman E. Effect of oral creatine supplementation on skeletal muscle phosphocreatine resynthesis. *Am J Physiol* 1994;266:E725–E730.
21. Hultman E, Soderlund K, Timmons JA, Cederblad G, Greenhaff PL. Muscle creatine loading in man. *J Appl Physiol* 1996;81: 232–237.
22. Green AL, Simpson EJ, Littlewood JJ, MacDonald IA, Greenhaff PL. Carbohydrate ingestion augments creatine retention during creatine feeding in humans. *Acta Physiol Scand* 1996;158:195–202.
23. Green AL, Hultman E, MacDonald IA, Sewell DA, Greenhaff PL. Carbohydrate feeding augments skeletal muscle creatine accumulation during creatine supplementation in humans. *Am J Physiol* 1996;271:E821–826.
24. Greenhaff PL. Creatine and its application as an ergogenic aid. *Int J Sport Nutr* 1995;5:S100–S110.
25. Greenhaff P, Casey A, Short A, Harris R, Soderlund K, Hultman E. Influence of oral creatine supplementation of [sic] muscle torque during repeated bouts of maximal voluntary exercise in man. *Clin Sci* 1993;84:565–571.
26. Balsom P, Ekblom B, Soderlund K, Sjodin B, Hultman E. Creatine supplementation and dynamic high-intensity intermittent exercise. *Scand J Med Sci Sports* 1993;3:143–149.
27. Balsom P, Soderlund K, Ekblom B. Creatine in humans with special reference to creatine supplementation. *Sports Med* 1994;18:268–280.
28. Williams MH, Kreider RB, Branch JD. *Creatine: the power supplement.* Champaign, IL: Human Kinetics, 1999.
29. Burke L, Pyne LD, Telford R. Effect of oral creatine supplementation on single-effort sprint performance in elite swimmers. *Int J Sport Nutr* 1996;6:222–233.
30. Mujika I, Chatard JC, Lacoste L, Barale F, Geyssant A. Creatine supplementation does not improve sprint performance in competitive swimmers. *Med Sci Sports Exerc* 1996;28:1435–1441.
31. Redondo D, Dowling EA, Graham BL, Almada A, Williams MH. The effect of oral creatine monohydrate supplementation on running velocity. *Int J Sport Nutr* 1996;6:213–221.
32. Prevost MC, Nelson AG, Morris GS. Creatine supplementation enhances intermittent work performance. *Res Q Exerc Sport* 1997;68:233–240.
33. Balsom PD, Harridge SDR, Soderlund K, Sjodin B, Ekblom B. Creatine supplementation *per se* does not enhance endurance exercise performance. *Acta Physiol Scand* 1993;149:521–523.
34. American Running and Fitness Association. Glycerol helps fluid balance. *Running Fitness News* 1996;14:1.
35. Legwold G. Hydration breakthrough: a sponge called glycerol boosts endurance by super-loading your body with water. *Bicycling* 1994;35:72–74.
36. Kockakian CD, Murlin JR. Effect of male hormone on protein and energy metabolism of castrate dogs. *J Nutr* 1935;10:437–459.
37. Buckley WE, Yesalis CE, Friedl KE, Anderson WA, Streit AL, Wright JE. Estimated prevalence of anabolic steroid use among male high school seniors. *JAMA* 1988;260:3441–3445.
38. Middleman AB, Faulkner AH, Woods ER, Emans SJ, DuRant RH. High risk behaviors among high school students in Massachusetts who use anabolic steroids. *Pediatrics* 1995;96:268–272.
39. Miller RW. Athletes and steroids: playing a deadly game. *FDA Consumer* 1987;HHS Publication No. 88–3170:2–7.
40. Cable NT. Anabolic-androgenic steroids; ergogenic and cardiovascular effects. In: Reilly T, Orme M, eds. *The clinical pharmacology of sport and exercise.* Amsterdam: Excerpta Medica, 1997: 135–144.
41. Lombardo JA, Hickson RC, Lamb DR. Anabolic/androgenic steroids and growth hormones. In: Lamb DR, Williams MH, eds. *Ergogenics: enhancement of performance in exercise and sport.* Dubuque, IA: Brown & Benchmark, 1991:249–284.
42. Elashoff JD, Jacknow AD, Shain SG, Braunstein GD. Effects of anabolic-androgenic steroids on muscular strength. *Ann Intern Med* 1991;115:387–393.
43. Friedl KE, Dettori JR Hannan CJ, Patience TH, Plymate SR. Comparison of the effects of a high dose of testosterone and 19-nortestosterone to a replacement dose of testosterone on strength and body composition in normal men. *J Steroid Biochem Mol Biol* 1991;40:607–612.
44. Bhasin S, Storer TW, Berman N, et al. The effects of supraphysiologic doses of testosterone on muscle size and strength in normal men. *N Engl J Med* 1996;335:1–7.
45. Yarasheski KE. Growth hormone: effects on metabolism, body composition, muscle mass, and strength. *Exerc Sport Sci Rev* 1994;22:285–312.
46. Melchert RB, Welder AA. Cardiovascular effects of anabolic-androgenic steroids. *Med Sci Sport Exerc* 1995;27:1252–1262.
47. Melchert RB, Herron TJ, Welder AA. The effect of anabolic-androgenic steroids on primary myocardial cell cultures. *Med Sci Sport Exerc* 1992;24:206–212.
48. Welder AA, Robertson JW, Melchert RB. Toxic effects of anabolic androgenic steroids in primary rat hepatic cell cultures. *J Pharmacol Toxicol Methods* 1995;33:187–195.
49. Welder AA, Robertson JW, Fugate RD, Melchert RB. Anabolic-androgenic steroid-induced toxicity in primary neonatal rat myocardial cell cultures. *Toxicol Appl Pharmacol* 1995;133:328–42.
50. Spence JC, Gauvin L. Drug and alcohol use by Canadian university athletes: a national survey. *J Drug Educ* 1996;26:275–287.
51. Yesalis CE, Streit AL, Vicary JR, Friedl KE, Brannon D, Buckley W. Anabolic steroid use: indications of habituation among adolescents. *J Drug Educ* 1989;19:103–116.
52. Conlee RK. Amphetamine, caffeine, and cocaine. In: Lamb DR, Williams MH, eds. *Ergogenics: enhancement of performance in exercise and sport.* Dubuque, IA: Brown & Benchmark, 1991:285–330.
53. Chandler JV, Blair SN. The effect of amphetamines on selected physiological components related to athletic success. *Med Sci Sports Exerc* 1980;12:65–69.
54. Williams JH. Caffeine, neuromuscular function and high- intensity exercise performance. *J Sports Med Phys Fitness* 1991;31:481–489.
55. Williams MH. *Lifetime fitness and wellness.* 4th ed. Dubuque, IA: Brown and Benchmark Publishers, 1996.
56. Dodd SL, Herb RA, Powers SK. Caffeine and exercise performance: an update. *Sports Med* 1993;15:14–23.
57. Nehlig A, Debry G. Caffeine and sports activity: a review. *Int J Sports Med* 1994;15:215–223.
58. Tarnopolsky MA. Caffeine and endurance performance. *Sports Med* 1994;18:109–125.
59. Spriet LL. Caffeine and performance. *Int J Sports Nutr* 1995;5: S84–S99.
60. Jackman M, Wendling P, Friars D, Graham TE. Metabolic catecholamine and endurance responses to caffeine during intense exercise. *J Appl Physiol* 1995;81:1658–1663.
61. Graham TE, LL Spriet. Metabolic, catecholamine, and exercise performance responses to various doses of caffeine. *J Appl Physiol* 1995;78:867–874.
62. Pasman WJ, van Baak MA, Jeukendrup AE, de Haan A. The effect of different dosages of caffeine on endurance performance time. *Int J Sports Med* 1995;16:225–230.
63. Spriet, LL, MacLean DA, Dyck DJ, Hultman E, Cederblad G, Graham TE. Caffeine ingestion and muscle metabolism during prolonged exercise in humans. *Am J Physiol* 1992;262:E891–E898.
64. Graham TE, Spriet LL. Caffeine and exercise performance. *Sports Sci Exch* 1996;9:1–5.
65. Cole, K, Costill DL, Starling R, Goodpaster B, Trappe S, Fink W. Effect of caffeine ingestion on perception of effort and subsequent work production. *Int J Sport Nutr* 1996;6:14–23.
66. Cohen BS, Nelson AG, Prevost MC, Thompson GD, Marx BD, Morris GS. Effects of caffeine ingestion on endurance racing in heat and humidity. *Eur J Appl Physiol* 1996;73:358–363.
67. Consumers Union. What caffeine can do for you—and to you. *Consum Rep Health* 1997;9:97–101.
68. Williams MH. Alcohol, marijuana and beta blockers. In: Lamb DR, Williams MH, eds. *Ergogenics: enhancement of performance in exercise and sport.* Dubuque, IA: Brown & Benchmark, 1991:331–372.
69. Kelly JG. Choice of selective versus nonselective beta blockers: implications for exercise training. *Am J Cardiol* 1985;55:162D–166D.

Exercise and Sport Science,
edited by William E. Garrett, Jr., and Donald T. Kirkendall.
Published by Lippincott Williams & Wilkins, Philadelphia, 2000.

CHAPTER 26

Physical Exercise in Hot and Cold Climates

Michael N. Sawka and Andrew J. Young

Athletes encounter thermal (heat and cold) stress from climatic conditions, insulation worn, and body heat production. Alterations in body temperatures (core, skin, and muscle) above and below "normal" levels can degrade exercise performance. Humans regulate core temperature within a narrow range (35° to 41°C) through two parallel processes: physiologic and behavioral temperature regulation. Physiologic temperature regulation operates through responses that are independent of conscious voluntary behavior, and includes control of (a) rate of metabolic heat production, (b) body heat distribution via the blood from the core to the skin, and (c) sweating. Behavioral temperature regulation operates through conscious behavior, and includes actions such as modifying activity levels, changing clothes, and seeking shelter. For athletes, physiologic thermoregulation is most important during heat stress, and behavioral thermoregulation is most important during cold stress.

HEAT STRESS

Heat stress increases requirements for sweating and circulatory responses to dissipate body heat. When the ambient is warmer than skin, the body gains heat from the climate, and thus increases heat the body must dissipate. In addition, exercise increases metabolic rate and thus increases the rate that heat must be dissipated to keep core temperature from increasing to dangerous levels. Climatic heat stress and exercise interact synergistically, and may push physiologic systems to their limits.

Sports and occupational medicine communities commonly use wet bulb globe temperature (WBGT) to quantitate climatic heat stress (1–3). WBGT is an empirical index of climatic heat stress: outdoor WBGT = 0.7 natural wet bulb + 0.2 black globe + 0.1 dry bulb; indoor WBGT = 0.7 natural wet bulb + 0.3 black globe. (*Natural wet bulb* is the wet bulb temperature under conditions of prevailing air movement; *black globe* is the temperature inside a blackened, hollow thin copper globe whose thermometer is in the center of the sphere.) WBGT is used to decide the permitted physical activity level and strategies to minimize the risk of heat injury. High WBGT values can be achieved either through high humidity (4), as reflected in high wet bulb temperature, or through high air (dry bulb) temperature and solar load (5), as reflected in black globe temperature. WBGT underestimates the risk of heat injury for humid conditions; therefore, different guidance tables must be used in low-, moderate-, and high-humidity climates (1). This index was originally developed for resting comfort and was later adapted for light intensity exercise (6). WBGT does not consider clothing or exercise intensity (metabolic rate), so it cannot predict heat exchange between a person and the climate (1).

Body Temperature Responses

During exercise, core temperature initially increases rapidly and subsequently increases at a reduced rate until heat loss equals heat production and essentially steady-state values are achieved (7). The core temperature increase represents the storage of metabolic heat, which is produced as a by-product of skeletal muscle contraction. At the beginning of exercise, the metabolic rate increases immediately; however, thermoregulatory effector responses for heat dissipation respond more slowly. The thermoregulatory effector responses that enable dry (radiative and convective) and evaporative heat loss increase in proportion to the rate of heat production. Eventually, these mechanisms increase heat loss sufficiently to balance metabolic heat production, allowing a steady-state core temperature to be achieved.

During exercise, the magnitude of core temperature

M. N. Sawka and A. J. Young: U.S. Army Research Institute of Environmental Medicine, Thermal & Mountain Medicine Division, Natick, Massachusetts 01760-5007.

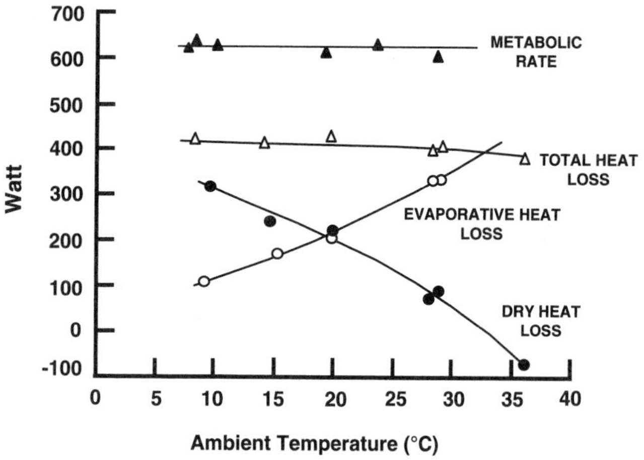

FIG. 26–1. Heat exchange during exercise in a broad range of ambient temperatures. (Adapted from ref. 11.)

increase at steady state is often independent of climatic conditions and proportional to the metabolic rate (8–10). Figure 26–1 illustrates heat exchange data during exercise (cycle ergometer at ~147 W mechanical power output and ~650 W metabolic rate) in a broad range of climatic conditions (5° to 36°C dry bulb temperatures with low humidity) (11). The difference between metabolic rate and total heat loss represents the energy used for mechanical work and the heat storage. The relative contributions of dry and evaporative heat exchange to total heat loss, however, varies with the climatic conditions. As ambient temperature increases, this gradient for dry heat exchange diminishes and evaporative heat exchange becomes more important. When the ambient temperature equals skin temperature, evaporative heat exchange will account for virtually all heat loss.

The idea that the magnitude of core temperature increases during exercise is independent of the climatic conditions may be inconsistent with the personal experience of many athletes. This is because there are biophysical limits to heat exchange between the climate and athlete (12,13). Actually, the magnitude of core temperature increase during exercise is independent of the climate only within a range of conditions or a "prescriptive zone" (8). Figure 26–2 illustrates this by showing steady-state core temperature responses, of a seminude person, during exercise performed at four metabolic intensities in a broad range of climatic conditions (with low humidity) (8). The 250-, 425-, and 600-W metabolic rates represent light-, moderate-, and heavy-intensity exercise for occupational tasks, respectively (14). For athletes, the upper limit for sustained exercise corresponds to a metabolic rate of about 1000 W. Note that, as metabolic rate increases, the prescriptive zone narrows.

Within the prescriptive zone, the core temperature increases proportionally to the metabolic rate during exercise (8–10). The greater the metabolic rate, the higher the steady-state core temperature during exercise (15). The relationship between metabolic rate and core temperature is good for a given person, but it does not always hold for comparisons between different people. The use of relative intensity (percent of maximal oxygen uptake), rather than absolute metabolic rate (absolute intensity), removes most of the intersubject variability for the core temperature elevation during exercise (16–18).

Athletes exercising in hot climates often incur body water deficits (hypohydration) of 2% to 8% of their body weight (19,20). These water deficits develop because of fluid nonavailability or a mismatch between thirst and sweat losses (21). Hypohydration increases physiologic strain, decreases exercise performance, and can cause devastating medical consequences (22). Hypohydration increases core temperature responses during exercise in temperate (23,24) and hot (25) climates. Fluid deficits as small as 1% of body weight can elevate core temperature during exercise (26). As water deficit increases, there is a concomitant graded elevation of core temperature

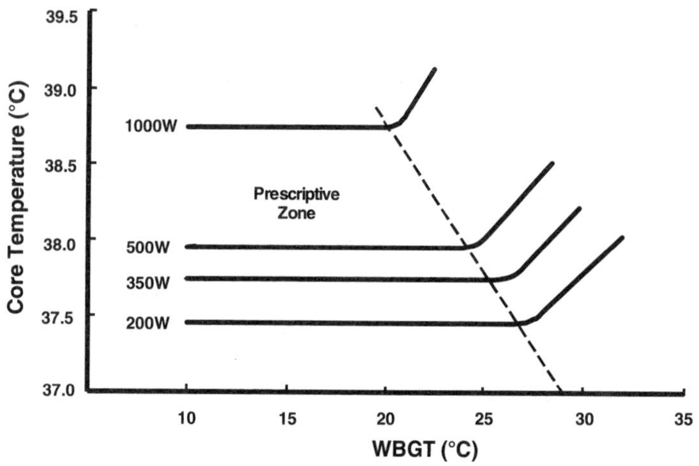

FIG. 26–2. Core temperature response during exercise as related to metabolic rate and heat stress. (Adapted from ref. 8.)

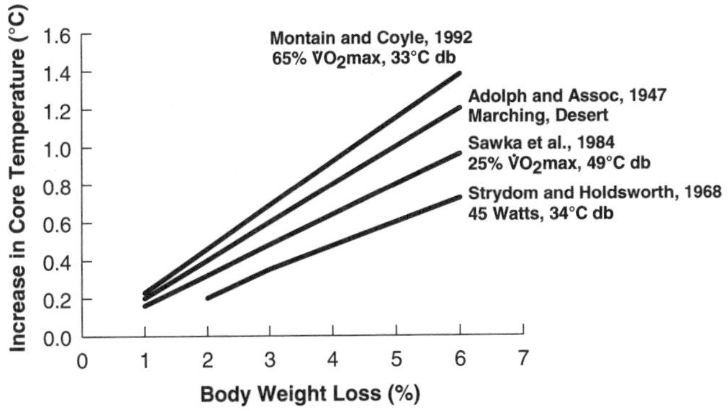

FIG. 26–3. Relationship between body water loss and core temperature elevations. (Adapted from ref. 20.)

during exercise—heat stress (25,27). Figure 26–3 illustrates relationships between body water loss and core temperature elevations as reported in different studies (20). The magnitude of core temperature elevation ranges from 0.1° to 0.23°C for every percent body weight lost (25,27–29). Besides elevating core temperature responses, hypohydration negates the thermoregulatory advantages conferred by high aerobic fitness and heat acclimation (23,30,31).

Exercise Performance

Maximal Exercise

Maximal exercise is achieved by exercising at progressively increasing intensity until physiologic criteria (maximal aerobic power, $\dot{V}O_2max$) or exhaustion (exercise capacity) is achieved. $\dot{V}O_2max$ is the maximal rate at which oxygen is being utilized by body tissues during exercise. High $\dot{V}O_2max$ enables performance of tasks that require sustained high metabolic rates; therefore, a lower $\dot{V}O_2max$ often translates into reduced exercise performance. Most investigators find that $\dot{V}O_2max$ is lower in hot than in temperate climates (32–35). For example, $\dot{V}O_2max$ was 0.25 $L \cdot min^{-1}$ (7%) lower at 49°C than at 21°C in one study, and the state of heat acclimation in this study did not alter the size of the $\dot{V}O_2max$ decrement (36). Several investigators, however, report no effect of ambient temperature on $\dot{V}O_2max$ (37,38).

What physiologic mechanisms might be responsible for such a reduction in $\dot{V}O_2max$? Heat stress, by dilating the cutaneous vascular beds, might divert some cardiac output from skeletal muscle to skin, thus leaving less blood flow to support the metabolism of exercising skeletal muscle. In addition, dilation of the cutaneous vascular bed may increase cutaneous blood volume at the expense of central blood volume, thus reducing venous return and cardiac output. For example, Rowell and colleagues (39) reported that during intense ($\approx$73% $\dot{V}O_2max$) exercise in the heat, cardiac output can be reduced by 1.2 $L \cdot min^{-1}$ below control levels. Such a reduction in cardiac output during heat exposure could account for a 0.25 $L \cdot min^{-1}$ decrement in $\dot{V}O_2max$, assuming each liter of blood delivers $\approx$0.2 L of oxygen (1.34 mL $O_2 \cdot gHb^{-1} \times 15$ $gHb \cdot 100$ mL^{-1} of blood).

Numerous studies have examined the influence of hypohydration on $\dot{V}O_2max$ and exercise capacity (20). In temperate climates, small water deficits (<3% body weight loss) do not alter $\dot{V}O_2max$ (20). With larger water deficits, $\dot{V}O_2max$ has been reported to decrease (30,40,41). In hot climates, Craig and Cummings (42) demonstrated that even small (2% body weight loss) to moderate (4% body weight loss) water deficits produce large reductions of $\dot{V}O_2max$. Likewise, their data indicate a disproportionately larger decrease in $\dot{V}O_2max$ with an increased magnitude of body water deficit. Clearly, climatic heat stress has a potentiating effect on the reduction of $\dot{V}O_2max$ elicited by hypohydration.

Figure 26–4 presents the relationship between hypohydration level and $\dot{V}O_2max$ decrement or exercise capacity decrement during heat exposure (42,43). The exercise capacity (exercise to fatigue without achieving physiologic criteria) for progressive intensity exercise is

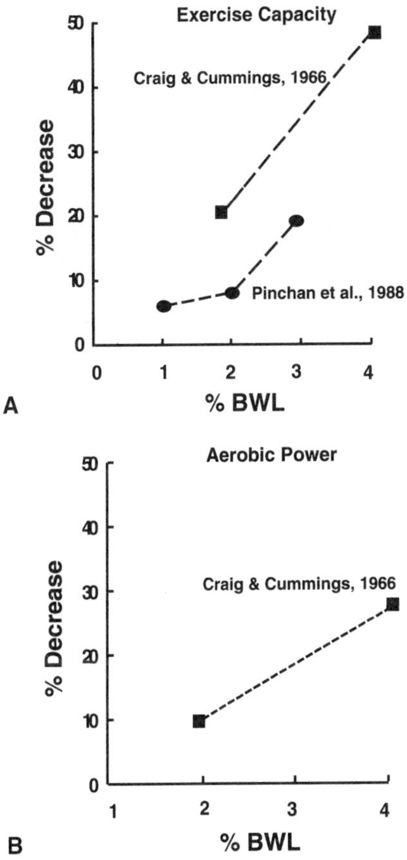

FIG. 26–4. Relationships between hypohydration level with decrements in exercise capacity decrements (**A**) and maximal aerobic power decrements (**B**) during heat exposure. (Adapted from refs. 42,43.)

decreased when hypohydrated (20). Exercise capacity decreased by marginal (1% to 2% body weight loss) water deficits that do not alter $\dot{V}O_2$max (40,44), and the reduction is larger with increasing water deficit. Note that, for a given hypohydration level, greater decrements are observed for exercise capacity than for $\dot{V}O_2$max. Clearly, hypohydration resulted in larger decrements of exercise capacity in hot as compared to temperate climates (44).

It appears that the thermoregulatory system, perhaps via increased body temperatures, has an important role in the reduced exercise performance mediated by a body water deficit (45). A reduced maximal cardiac output might be the mechanism by which hypohydration decreases $\dot{V}O_2$max and exercise capacity. Hypohydration is associated with a decreased blood (plasma) volume during both rest and exercise. A decreased blood volume increases blood viscosity and can reduce venous return. During maximal exercise, viscosity-mediated increased resistance and reduced cardiac filling could decrease both stroke volume and cardiac output. Several investigators (7,46–49) have reported a tendency for reduced cardiac output when hypohydrated during short-term, moderate-intensity exercise.

Submaximal Intensity

Physiologic mechanisms for reduced submaximal exercise performance in the heat include increased thermal and cardiovascular strain, more rapid glycogen depletion, increased metabolite accumulation, and diminished psychologic drive for exercise (7,50,51). The exact mechanisms(s) are unknown, but they probably depend on the specific heat stress, exercise task, and biomedical state of the athlete.

Figure 26–5 demonstrates the effects of air temperature and hypohydration on the submaximal exercise output (28). This analysis is based on heat-acclimated

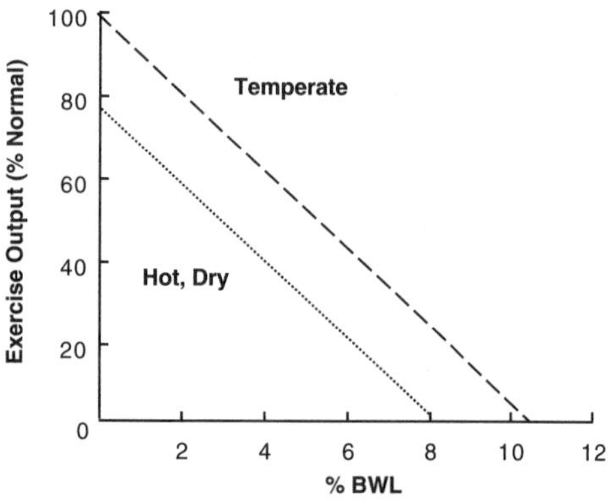

FIG. 26–5. Relationship between air temperature and hypohydration level on submaximal exercise output. (Adapted from ref. 28.)

persons at a metabolic rate of ~650 W and an air temperature of 43°C with low humidity (14). Climatic heat stress reduced submaximal exercise output at all hydration levels. Adolph and associates (28) suggested that for every ~5°C increase in skin temperature, there was a ~10% decrement in submaximal exercise output. In addition, the submaximal exercise output decrements from heat stress and hypohydration were additive (28). For example, exposure to 43°C reduced submaximal exercise output by ≈25% (compared to temperate conditions) and a 2.5% (body weight loss) hypohydration reduced submaximal exercise output (compared to euhydration) by the same amount. With combined heat stress and hypohydration, a person would experience a 50% decrease in submaximal exercise output.

Hypohydration impairs athletic endurance performance. Armstrong and colleagues (44) studied body water deficit effects on competitive distance running performance. They had athletes compete in 1500, 5000 and 10,000 meter races when euhydrated and when hypohydrated. Hypohydration was achieved by diuretic administration (furosemide), which decreased body weight by 2% and plasma volume by 11%. Running performance was impaired at all race distances, but to a greater extent in the longer races (~5% for the 5000 and 10,000 m) than the shorter race (3% for 1500 m). Burge and colleagues (52) examined whether hypohydration (3% body weight loss) affected simulated 2000 m rowing performance. They found that, on average, it took 22 seconds longer to complete the task and average power was reduced 5% when hypohydrated compared to when euhydrated.

Two studies examined hypohydration effects on moderate to intense cycle ergometer performance. In both studies, high-intensity performance tests were conducted immediately after 55 to 60 minutes of cycling during which volunteers either drank nothing or drank sufficient fluid to replace sweat losses. Walsh and colleagues (53) reported that time to fatigue when cycling at 90% $\dot{V}O_2$max was 51% longer (6.5 vs. 9.8 minutes) when subjects drank sufficient fluids to prevent hypohydration. Below and colleagues (54) found that cyclists rode 6.5% faster if they drank fluids during exercise. These studies clearly demonstrate the detrimental effects of hypohydration on submaximal exercise performance.

Heat Tolerance

Uncompensable heat stress is a condition in which the required evaporative cooling (E_{req}) exceeds the climate's maximal evaporative cooling (E_{max}). During uncompensable heat stress, steady-state core temperature cannot be achieved, and body temperature continues to rise until exhaustion occurs. Uncompensable heat stress is associated with exhaustion from heat strain occurring at relatively low core temperatures (55–57). Under these conditions, exhaustion is accelerated because the displacement of blood to skin (cutaneous vasodilation and compliance) causes cardiovascular strain and instability. During compensable heat stress, much higher core temperatures can be tolerated, and exhaustion is usually associated with hypohydration or substrate depletion.

Core temperature provides the most reliable physiologic index to predict the incidence of exhaustion from heat strain (55,56,58,59). Figure 26–6 presents the relationships between core temperature and incidence of exhaustion from heat strain for heat-acclimated persons exercising in uncompensable (56) or compensable heat stress (unpublished data). During uncompensable heat stress, exhaustion was rarely associated with a core temperature below 38°C, and exhaustion always occurred before a temperature of 40°C was achieved (55,56).

Hypohydration, but not aerobic fitness or exercise intensity, appears to modify physiologic tolerance to uncompensable heat stress. In one study, heat-acclimated persons exercised to physical exhaustion when either euhydrated or hypohydrated (8% of total body water) (56). The experiments were designed so that the combined climate [ambient temperature (T_a) = 49°C, relative humidity = 20%] and exercise intensity (47% $\dot{V}O_2max$) would not allow thermal equilibrium and heat exhaustion would eventually occur. Aerobic fitness had no effect on physiologic tolerance to uncompensable heat stress. Hypohydration reduced tolerance time (121 to 55 minutes), but, more important, hypohydration reduced the core temperature that a person could tolerate. Heat exhaustion occurred at a core temperature ~0.4°C lower when hypohydrated than when euhydrated. Another study reported that exercise intensity and climate did not alter the physiologic tolerance to uncompensable heat stress (55).

Nielsen and colleagues (59) studied the effects of heat acclimation in an uncompensable heat stress condition. Highly trained subjects exercised (60% $\dot{V}O_2max$) to exhaustion for 9 to 12 days in a 40°C climate. Final core temperature was consistently 39.7°C at exhaustion and was not changed by heat acclimation. Endurance time was increased, however, probably because the rate of core temperature increase was slowed. The authors also observed increased sweating rate, increased cardiac output, and reduced heart rate at exhaustion after heat acclimation. The state of heat acclimation did not affect the physiologic tolerance to heat strain during uncompensable heat stress in these trained subjects.

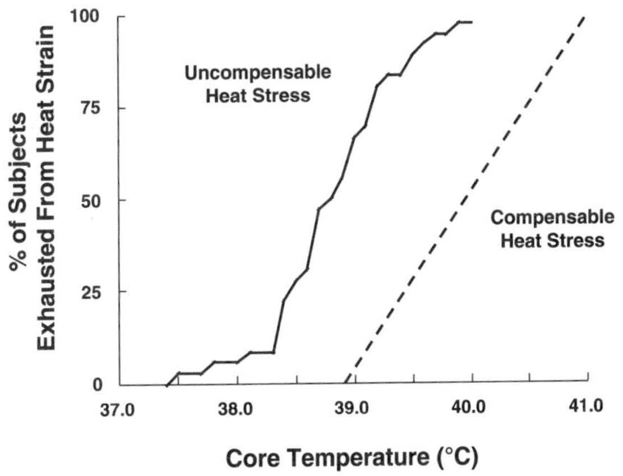

FIG. 26–6. Relationships between core temperature and incidence of exhaustion from heat strain.

Some persons can tolerate core temperatures >40°C and continue to exercise during compensable heat stress. Joy and Goldman (58) reported that 35 of 63 (56%) elite soldiers were still performing military tasks when core temperature reached 39.5°C, their predetermined end-point criteria. Furthermore, some endurance runners can tolerate core temperatures >40°C and continued to perform (60–63). For example, Pugh and colleagues (61) measured the core temperature of 47 runners immediately after a marathon race. Seven finishers, including three of the first five finishers, had core temperatures >40°C (highest value was 41°C). None of the runners who discontinued the race achieved core temperatures as high as 40°C.

Heat Acclimation

Heat acclimation results in biologic adaptations that reduce the negative effects of heat stress. One becomes acclimated to the heat through repeated exposures that are sufficiently stressful to elevate both core and skin temperatures and provoke perfuse sweating. The magnitude of adaptation depends largely on the intensity, duration, frequency, and number of heat exposures. During the initial heat exposure, physiologic strain will be high, as manifested by elevated core temperature and heart rate, but the strain from heat stress will continue to decrease during each day of acclimation. Table 26–1 provides a brief description of the actions of heat acclimation (64). The benefits of heat acclimation are achieved by improved sweating and skin blood flow responses, better fluid balance and cardiovascular stability, and a lowered metabolic rate (7,64,65).

Exercise in the heat is the most effective method for inducing heat acclimation; however, even resting in the heat results in some acclimation, though to a lesser degree (64–67). The full development of exercise-heat acclimation need not involve daily 24-hour exposure. A daily continuous 100-minute exposure produces optimal heat acclimation in dry heat (68). Studies examining heat acclimation have generally used daily heat exposures; however, these are not necessary to produce heat acclimation. Fein and colleagues (69) examined the time course of adaptations to 10 days of heat exposure, when subjects were exposed to heat (47°C, 17% relative humidity) daily or every third day. Therefore, one group

TABLE 26–1. *Actions of heat acclimation*

Thermal comfort—improved	Exercise performance—improved
Core temperature—reduced	Metabolic rate—lowered
Sweating—improved	Cardiovascular stability—improved
Earlier onset	Heart rate—lowered
Higher rate	Stroke volume—increased
Redistribution (tropic)	Blood pressure—better defended
Hidromeiosis resistance (tropic)	Fluid balance—imrpoved
Skin blood flow—increased	Thirst—improved
Earlier onset	Electrolyte loss—reduced
Higher flow	Total body water—increased
	Plasma volume—increased and better defended

Adapted from ref. 64.

completed the acclimation program in 10 days and the other in 27 days. Both methods were equally effective in producing heat acclimation, but with daily heat exposure it took approximately one-third of the total time.

The effect of heat acclimation on performance can be quite dramatic, so that acclimated subjects can easily complete exercise in the heat that earlier was difficult or impossible. During acclimation through daily exercise in a hot climate, most of the improvement in heart rate, skin and core temperatures, and sweat rate is achieved during the first week of exposure, although there is no sharp end to the improvement (7,65). The heart rate reduction develops most rapidly in 4 to 5 days (7,65). After 7 days, the reduction in heart rate is virtually complete, and most of the improvements in skin and core temperature have also occurred. The thermoregulatory acclimation response is generally thought to be complete after 10 to 14 days of exposure (7,65).

Heat acclimation is transient; it gradually disappears if not maintained by repeated heat exposure. The heart rate improvement, which develops more rapidly during acclimation, is also lost more rapidly than thermoregulatory responses. However, there is no agreement concerning the rate of decay for heat acclimation. Lind (70) believed that heat acclimation might be retained for 2 weeks after the last heat exposure, and then be rapidly lost over the next 2 weeks. However, Williams and colleagues (71) report some loss of acclimation in sedentary individuals after 1 week, with the percentage loss being greater with increasing time, and by 3 weeks there were losses of nearly 100% for heart rate and 50% for core temperature. Other authors, however, report longer retention of acclimation in physically trained and aerobically fit persons (72).

Physical Fitness

In addition to improving $\dot{V}O_2max$, endurance training in temperate climates reduces physiologic strain and increases exercise capabilities in the heat (7,44), and endurance-trained individuals exhibit many of the characteristics of heat-acclimated individuals during exercise in the heat. In addition, aerobically fit persons develop heat acclimation more rapidly than less fit persons (72), and high aerobic fitness might reduce susceptibility to heat injury/illness (73). It has been estimated that a person's $\dot{V}O_2max$ accounts for approximately 44% of the variability in core temperature after 3 hours of exercise in the heat, or the number of days required for complete development of heat acclimation. However, endurance training alone does not totally replace the benefits of heat acclimation produced by a program of exercise in the heat (16,74,75).

Some investigators (76,77) believe that for endurance training to improve thermoregulatory responses during exercise in the heat, the exercise training sessions must produce a substantial elevations of core temperature and sweating rate. Henane and colleagues (77) compared thermoregulatory responses of six skiers ($\dot{V}O_2max$ = 66.5 $mL \cdot kg^{-1} \cdot min^{-1}$) with those of four swimmers ($\dot{V}O_2max$ = 65.8 $mL \cdot kg^{-1} \cdot min^{-1}$), and they found that skiers were more heat tolerant and better acclimatized than swimmers; the authors attributed the difference to a smaller increase in the swimmers' core temperature produced during training in cold water. In agreement, Avellini and colleagues (76) found that 4 weeks of training by cycle exercise in 20°C water increased $\dot{V}O_2max$ by 15%, but did not improve thermoregulation during exercise-heat stress. Thus, high $\dot{V}O_2max$ is not always associated with improved heat tolerance.

To achieve improved thermoregulation from endurance training in temperate climates, either strenuous interval training or continuous training at an intensity greater than 50% $\dot{V}O_2max$ should be employed (7,64,78). Lesser training intensities produce questionable effects on performance during exercise-heat stress (79). The endurance training must last at least 1 week (80,81), and some authors show that the best improvements require 8 to 12 weeks of training (78).

Fluid and Electrolyte Replacement

During high-intensity exercise, athletes commonly have sweating rates of 1.0 to 2.5 L/h while in the heat. These high sweating rates, however, are not maintained continuously and are dependent on the person's need to dissipate body heat. Daily fluid requirements range (for sedentary to active persons) from 2 to 4 L/day in temperate climates and from 4 to 10 L/day in hot climates (82).

During exercise in the heat, hypohydration can be avoided by matching fluid consumption to sweat loss. This is difficult because thirst does not accurately track body water requirements (28,83,84). Thirst is probably not perceived until a water deficit of ~2% body weight has been incurred (28,83,85). In addition, ad libitum water intake during exercise in the heat results in an incomplete replacement of body water losses (28,83). Heat-acclimated persons usually replace less than one-half of their fluid deficit when consuming fluid ad libitum (28). As a result, unless forced hydration is stressed, some dehydration will probably occur during exercise in the heat. Humans will usually fully rehydrate at mealtime, when fluid consumption is stimulated by consuming food (28,86). Therefore, active persons need to stress drinking at mealtime to avoid persistent hypohydration.

Athletes can incur significant electrolyte losses during exercise-heat stress. Electrolytes, primarily sodium chloride and, to a lesser extent, potassium, calcium, and magnesium, are contained in sweat. Sweat sodium concentration averages ~35 mEq/L (range 10 to 70 mEq/L) and varies depending on diet, sweating rate, hydration, and heat acclimation level (87,88). Sweat glands reabsorb sodium by active transport, and the ability to reabsorb sodium does not increase with the sweating rate, so at high sweating rates the concentration of sweat sodium increases. Heat acclimation improves the ability to reabsorb sodium, so acclimated persons have lower sweat sodium concentrations (>50% reduction) for any sweating rate (88–90). Sweat potassium concentration averages 5 mEq/L (range 3 to 15 mEq/L), calcium averages 1 mEq/L (range 0.3 to 2 mEq/L) and magnesium averages 0.8 mEq/L (range 0.2 to 1.5 mEq /L) (87). Normal dietary intake will replenish sweat electrolyte losses (91,92), so electrolyte supplementation is not necessary, except occasionally for the first several days of heat exposure (91,92).

"Sports drinks" are used by athletes to replace fluid and electrolyte losses (from sweat) and supplement the body's limited energy stores. If an athlete consumes a normal diet, such drinks are generally not necessary. For heat-acclimated athletes, these drinks are only recommended for use during intense exercise lasting longer than 1 hour (92,93). The composition of these drinks should be 4% to 8% carbohydrate (sucrose, glucose, or maltodextrin), 20 to 30 mEq/L of sodium, 2 to 5 mEq/L of potassium, and chloride as the only anion (91,92).

Hyperhydration, increased total body water, has been suggested to improve thermoregulation during exercise-heat stress above euhydration levels (20). Hyperhydration is not easy to achieve since overdrinking of water or carbohydrate-electrolyte solutions produce a fluid overload that is rapidly excreted by the kidneys (94). Greater fluid retention can be achieved by drinking an aqueous solution containing glycerol while resting in temperate conditions (94,95), but glycerol does not provide a fluid retention advantage over water during exercise-heat stress (96). Glycerol ingestion increases fluid retention by reducing free water clearance (94); however, both exercise and heat stress decrease renal blood flow and free water clearance and negate glycerol's effectiveness as a hyperhydrating agent.

Studies examining thermoregulatory effects of hyperhydration during exercise-heat stress have reported disparate results (20), but hyperhydration probably provides no advantage over euhydration (20,96). One study has reported that glycerol/water hyperhydration had dramatic effects on improving a person's ability to thermoregulate during exercise-heat stress (97). Other studies report similar core temperatures and sweating rates between glycerol and water hyperhydration fluids before exercise in a temperate climate (98), or as rehydration solutions during exercise in warm (99) and hot (96,100) climates.

COLD STRESS

Humans usually rely on behavioral strategies like wearing clothing or remaining in shelters to protect themselves against the cold. The nature of most outdoor wintertime sports and recreational activities, however, requires participants to disregard most behavioral strategies and constrains the effectiveness of others. For example, skiers and skaters eschew heavy insulative garments in favor of clothing less restrictive for freedom of motion. When behavioral thermoregulation provides inadequate protection from the cold, physiologic responses are elicited (101,102). These physiologic responses elicited by cold exposure may influence or be influenced by the physiologic responses to exercise.

Most body heat loss in cold environments occurs via conductive and convective mechanisms. When ambient temperature is colder than body temperature, the resulting thermal gradient favors body heat loss. Besides ambient temperature, wind speed, solar radiation, and humidity also influence the heat loss potential and the associated physiologic strain of defending body temperature during cold exposure. No single cold stress index integrates all these effects with respect to the heat loss potential of the environment, but one, the wind-chill index (WCI), has achieved widespread acceptance and use (103). Wind increases convective heat loss from the body surface (12). The WCI estimates the environmental cooling rate from the combined effects of the wind and air temperature. Typically, the WCI is used to compute tables depicting temperatures of "calm" air having equivalent cooling rates as different combinations of air temperature and wind speed. The tables are divided into zones reflecting the relative risk of freezing tissue injuries (little danger, warmer than −30°C; increasing danger, between −30 and −58°C; great danger, colder than 58°C).

Lacking any better tool, these tables still are useful for guiding decisions concerning the conduct or cancellation of outdoor activities, but some limitations should be appreciated. While the concept of wind chill is sound, the physical and physiologic rationale used to derive the computational formula for the WCI appears flawed (104,105). Wind-chill equivalent temperature tables probably overestimate the effect of increasing wind speed on the risk of tissue freezing, while underestimating the effect of decreasing air temperature (104). Furthermore, the danger zones indicated in wind-chill equivalent temperature tables estimate the risk of tissue freezing only for the exposed skin of sedentary persons. Windproof clothing greatly reduces wind-chill effects (106).

Water has a much higher thermal capacity than air, and the cooling power of the ambient environment is greatly enhanced under cold-wet conditions. During water immersion, conductive and convective heat transfer can be 70-fold greater than in air of the same temperature (12), depending on the water depth or body surface immersed in the water and the individual's metabolic rate (107). Thus, even when water temperatures are relatively mild, long-distance swimmers, triathletes, and fishermen or hunters who wade streams can lose considerable amounts of body heat. Furthermore, when clothing becomes wet due to rain or accidental immersion, its insulative value is compromised, and wetting of the skin facilitates heat loss by conduction, convection, and evaporation.

Physiologic Responses

Cold exposure elicits a peripheral vasoconstriction, resulting in a decrease in peripheral blood flow, which reduces convective heat transfer between the body's core and shell (skin, subcutaneous fat, and skeletal muscle). This effectively increases insulation. Since the exposed body surface loses heat faster than it is replaced, skin temperature declines as illustrated in Fig. 26–7, which shows skin temperature of the finger declining rapidly upon immersion in cold water. During whole-body cold exposure, the vasoconstrictor response spreads throughout the body's peripheral shell. Vasoconstriction begins when skin temperature falls below about 35°C, and becomes maximal when skin temperature is about 31°C or less (108). The vasoconstrictor response to cold exposure retards heat loss and helps defend core temperature, but at the expense of a decline in temperature of peripheral tissue.

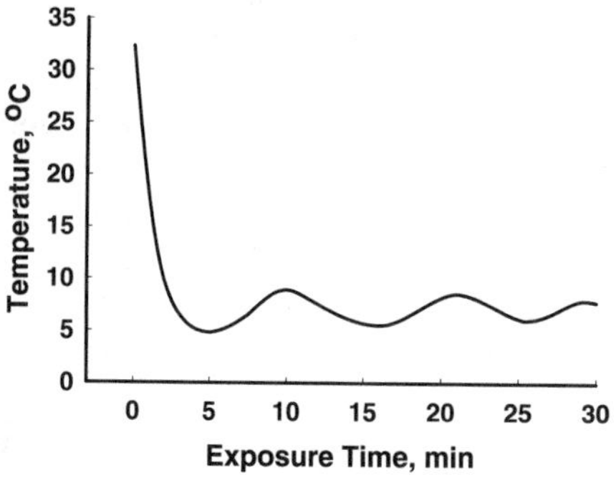

FIG. 26–7. Typical nail-bed temperature response observed during immersion of a finger into cold water.

The vasoconstriction-induced blood flow reduction and fall in skin temperature contribute to the etiology of cold injuries (109,110). Cold-induced vasoconstriction has pronounced effects in the hands and fingers, making them particularly susceptible to cold injury (111) and a loss of manual dexterity (112). In these areas, another vasomotor response, cold-induced vasodilation (CIVD), modulates the effects of vasoconstriction. Figure 26–7 also illustrates this response, first described and termed the Hunting reaction by Lewis (113). Periodic oscillations of skin temperature follow the initial decline during cold exposure, resulting from transient increases in blood flow to the cooled finger. A similar CIVD occurring in the forearm (114,115) appears to reflect vasodilation of muscle as well as cutaneous vasculature (115). Originally thought to be a local effect of cooling (116), evidence now suggests that a central nervous system mechanism mediates CIVD (117).

The other major mechanism elicited to defend body temperature during cold exposure is an increased metabolic heat production, which helps offset heat losses. Muscle is generally the source of the increased metabolic heat production in humans. Certain animals can increase metabolic heat production by noncontracting tissue in response to cold exposure, that is, nonshivering thermogenesis (118), but no clear evidence indicates that humans share this mechanism (119). During muscular contraction, approximately 70% of total energy expended is liberated as heat, with the remainder generating external force.

Shivering, which is involuntarily repeated rhythmic muscle contractions, may start immediately or after several minutes of cold exposure, usually beginning in torso muscles, then spreading to the limbs (120). Shivering intensity increases and more muscles are recruited to shiver as cold stress becomes more severe, causing whole-body oxygen uptake to increase. For example, whole-body oxygen uptake of young men resting in 5°C air with a 1 m/sec wind averaged 600 to 700 mL/min, which corresponded to about 15% of their $\dot{V}O_2max$ (121). Cold-water immersion can elicit even more intense shivering, however. The oxygen uptake of men resting in 18°C water reached about 1 L/min, which corresponded to 25% to 30% of their $\dot{V}O_2max$ (122). Maximal shivering is difficult to quantify, but the highest reported oxygen uptake during shivering is 2.2 L/min in 12°C water, corresponding to 46% $\dot{V}O_2max$ (123).

Another physiologic response sometimes elicited by cold exposure is a diuresis. Termed cold-induced diuresis (CID), this response is actually secondary to the cold-induced vasoconstriction and the resulting redistribution of body fluids from the peripheral to central circulation (124). Exercise minimizes cold-induced vasoconstriction, and the reduction in peripheral blood flow suppresses or blunts CID (124). For this reason, and because the effect is self-limiting (i.e., CID diminishes as body water content falls), this response to cold is not of major physiologic significance.

Modifying Factors

Anthropometric factors can explain much of the variability between individuals in their capability to maintain normal body temperature during cold exposure (125). Since the principal heat loss vector in cold-exposed humans is convective heat transfer at the skin surface, a large surface area favors greater heat loss than a smaller surface area. On the other hand, a large body mass favors maintenance of a constant temperature by virtue of a greater heat content compared to a small body mass (12). In general, persons with a large surface area to mass ratio experience greater declines in body temperature during cold exposure than those with smaller surface area to mass ratios (101).

Both fatty and nonfatty body tissues provide thermal resistance to heat conduction from within the body, but thermal resistivity of fat is greater than that of either skin or muscle (101). Subcutaneous fat provides significant insulation against heat loss in the cold, and insulation is closely correlated with subcutaneous fat thickness. Thus, thermal conductance decreases and insulation increases as the layer of subcutaneous fat thickens. As a result, many studies have confirmed that fat persons shiver less and experience smaller declines in body temperature during cold exposure than lean persons (101).

Most women have greater fat content and thicker subcutaneous fat thickness than men of comparable age or weight, thus accounting for the greater maximal tissue insulation observed in women than men (126). Despite this, women may not have a thermoregulatory advantage over men, at least in terms of maintaining normal heat balance during cold exposure. When women and men of equivalent subcutaneous fat thickness are considered, the women have a greater surface area and smaller total body mass than men. Body heat content is less in the women because of their smaller body mass. Although insulation is equivalent, total heat loss is greater due to the larger surface area for convective heat flux; therefore, body temperature falls more rapidly for any given thermal gradient and metabolic rate (12,127). When men and women whose total body mass is equivalent are compared, women still seem to be at a disadvantage. In this case, surface area differences are less pronounced, and the women's greater fat content enhances insulation. Nevertheless, their smaller lean body mass limits their capacity for heat production, compared to men of comparable total body mass. This disparity may be inconsequential under conditions where metabolism is low. In severely cold conditions that stimulate maximal shivering, however, women's limited thermogenic capacity may allow a more rapid core temperature decline.

Persons chronically exposed to cold can develop adjustments in thermoregulation (102). Habituation is by far the most commonly observed adjustment resulting from chronic cold exposure. Blunting of both shivering and cold-induced vasoconstriction are the hallmarks of habituation (102). These adjustments allow for maintenance of warmer skin during cold exposure, but they could facilitate heat loss, unless clothing is adequate. Beyond habituation, chronic cold exposure can induce two patterns of acclimatization. A more pronounced thermogenic response to cold characterizes metabolic acclimatization (102). An exaggerated shivering response may develop because of chronic cold exposure, and the possibility that humans develop a nonshivering thermogenesis cannot be ruled out. Enhanced heat conservation mechanisms characterize the insulative acclimatization pattern (102). More rapid cutaneous vasoconstriction develops in some chronically cold-exposed persons. This adjustment may reflect an enhanced sympathetic nervous responses (102). Compared to chronic heat stress, physiologic adjustments to chronic cold exposure are less pronounced, slower to develop, and less practical in terms of relieving thermal strain, defending normal body temperature, and preventing cold injury.

Exercise

Exercise can increase metabolic heat production even more than shivering. Figure 26–8 compares the shivering-induced metabolic heat production during cold exposure with the metabolic heat production during moderate and maximal exercise. Thus, during cold exposure, a voluntary increase in physical activity can increase heat production sufficiently to obviate the need

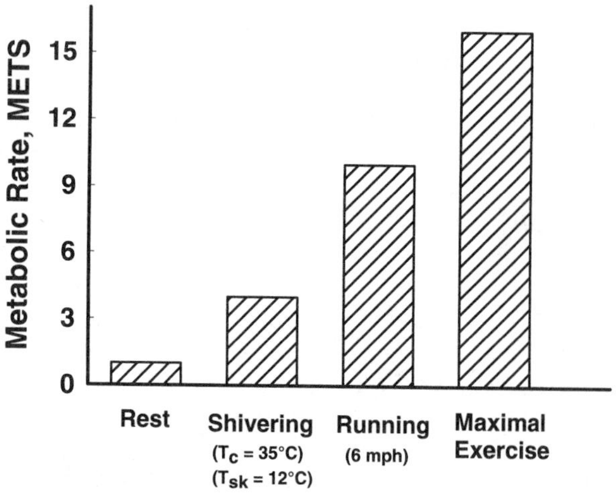

FIG. 26–8. Comparison of metabolic rate (METS) during thermoneutral rest, shivering in cold air, and two levels of exercise. Metabolic rate during shivering estimated from the equation of Hayward and colleagues (157) using core (T_c) and skin (T_{sk}) temperatures shown.

for shivering. Some might consider this an example of behavioral rather than physiologic thermoregulation.

In the cold, oxygen uptake during exercise can be lower than, higher than, or the same as in warm conditions, depending on the exercise intensity (128). During cold exposure, $\dot{V}O_2$max can be, but is not always, reduced (128). Cold stress must be severe enough to markedly reduce core or muscle temperature before $\dot{V}O_2$max is reduced (120,129,130). Exposure to cold conditions that lower core temperature 0.5°C or less do not significantly reduce $\dot{V}O_2$max (131). Low body temperature may impair myocardial contractility (129) and limit maximal heart rate (129,132) sufficiently to limit maximal cardiac output, thus accounting for the reduced $\dot{V}O_2$max.

Figure 26–9 schematically depicts the effect of cold

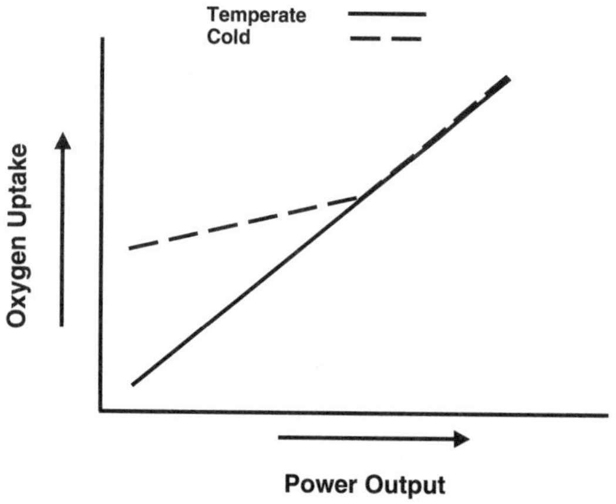

FIG. 26–9. Effect of cold on oxygen uptake during steady-state exercise at different intensities. (Adapted from ref. 133.)

exposure on oxygen uptake during submaximal exercise over a range of intensities (133). At low exercise intensities in the cold, metabolic heat production is not high enough to prevent shivering. Thus, oxygen uptake is higher, with the increased oxygen uptake representing the added requirement for shivering activity. As metabolic heat production rises with increasing exercise intensity, core and skin temperatures are maintained warmer and the afferent stimulus for shivering declines. Thus, the shivering-associated component of total oxygen uptake during exercise also declines. At high intensities, exercise metabolism is high enough to completely prevent shivering, and oxygen uptake during exercise is the same in cold and temperate conditions. The exercise intensity at which metabolic heat production is sufficient to prevent shivering depends on the severity of cold stress.

The effect of inhaling cold air on ventilation during exercise is usually negligible. Upper airway temperatures, which usually remain unchanged during exercise under temperate conditions, fall substantially when extremely cold air is breathed during strenuous exercise, but temperatures of the lower respiratory tract and deep body temperatures are unaffected (134). Pulmonary function during exercise is unaffected by breathing cold air in healthy athletes (135) and nonathletes (136), but in allergy-prone athletes breathing cold air during heavy exercise can cause bronchial spasm and reduced forced expiratory volume (135). This bronchial spasm may actually be triggered by cooling of the facial skin, however, rather than by cooling of the respiratory passages (137). Chronic breathing of cold air can increase respiratory passage secretions and decrease mucociliary clearance, and any resulting airway congestion may impair pulmonary mechanics during exercise (138).

Breathing cold air may exacerbate body fluid loss during exercise. As air temperature decreases, the saturation vapor pressure also declines. Thus, cold air has less water content than warmer air, even if the relative humidity is the same. Each breath of air becomes 100% saturated with water as it passes through the respiratory passages into the lungs. Therefore, more respiratory water is lost in order to humidify the inspiratory air when breathing cold than warm air. It has been calculated that respiratory water loss can be 50% greater when breathing −20°C than 25°C air (139). Respiratory water losses are fairly low during resting ventilation (10 mL/h), so the impact of cold air breathing is negligible for sedentary activities. However, respiratory water loss increases during exercise due to the increase in pulmonary ventilation. During heavy intensity (i.e., 600 W) exercise, respiratory water loss is estimated to be about 60 ml/h while breathing 25°C air, so a 50% increase while breathing −20°C air represent a more important increase (139). Nevertheless, respiratory water loss still represents a relatively small portion of total body fluid loss during exercise in the cold.

Exercise can substantially increase metabolism (see Figure 26–8) and only a small portion of the metabolic energy expenditure results in contractile force; the large remainder results in heat generation. Even in cold environments, metabolic heat production can exceed heat loss, with the resulting heat storage causing body temperature to rise and initiating thermoregulatory responses for heat dissipation, including sweating. Obviously, these sweat losses must be replaced, or dehydration ensues.

The problem, illustrated in Fig. 26–10, is that clothing insulation needed for warmth and comfort in cold environments is much higher during rest and light activity than during strenuous activity (12). Therefore, if one begins exercising vigorously while wearing clothing selected for sedentary activities in the cold, sweating and the resultant drinking fluid requirements can increase substantially (124). Furthermore, sweat can accumulate in clothing, compromising its insulative properties, which will again be necessary when exercise stops. The solution is to dress in multiple clothing layers, which allow insulation to be adjusted according to activity level such that heat storage and sweating can be minimized. It should also be kept in mind that during high-intensity exercise, sweating is usually occurring even when clothing insulation is low and sweat evaporation prevents it from accumulating. Adequate fluids must be ingested to replace these losses, or dehydration will ensue (140).

Cold exposure may also affect muscle energy metabolism during exercise. Blood lactate concentrations during exercise in cold may be higher than in temperate conditions depending on whether experimental conditions allow shivering to occur during exercise (128). Studies in which cold exposure increased blood lactate concentrations during exercise also observed lower core temperatures and higher oxygen uptake during exercise in cold than temperate conditions, indicating that shivering was taking place during exercise. When core temperature and oxygen uptake are similar during exercise in cold and temperate conditions (i.e., no shivering), there is no effect of cold on blood lactate accumulation during exercise. Similarly, muscle glycogen use during low-intensity (e.g., below 25% $\dot{V}O_2max$) exercise has been observed more pronounced in cold than temperate conditions, but no differences are found during high-intensity exercise (141,142). The increased glycogen use during low-intensity exercise was attributed to the added energy cost of shivering (141).

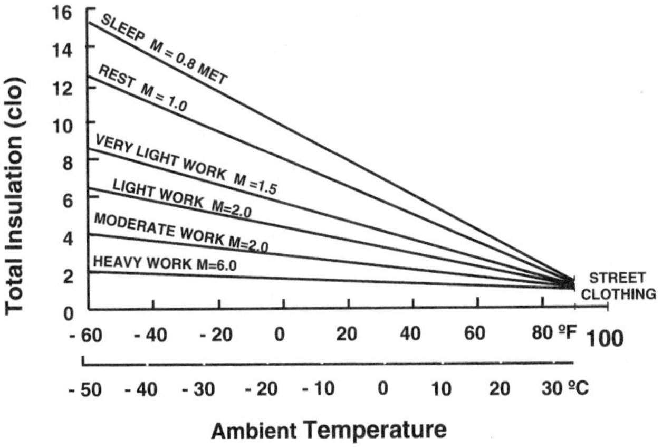

FIG. 26–10. Total insulation (IT, Clo) of clothing plus air necessary for comfort at various metabolic rates (MET = 100 W). (Adapted from ref. 12.)

Muscle force generation can be impaired during cold exposure. Bergh and Ekblom (143) demonstrated that cooling vastus lateralis muscle from 39° to 30°C decreased maximal isometric strength by ~2% per degree C, and it shifted the force-velocity relationship during dynamic muscle contractions such that cooled muscle developed lower force for a given velocity of contraction. Based on that report, Blomstrand and Essen-Gustavsson (144) suggested that the increased muscle glycogen breakdown during short-duration, high-intensity exercise, which they had observed to result from a similar lowering of muscle temperature, could be accounted for by recruitment of an increased number of muscle fibers per unit of force generated. Thus, under extreme conditions in which muscle temperature is reduced (e.g. swimming in cold water), force generation may be compromised, leading to performance deficits. Heat production during sustained dynamic exercise, however, should usually be sufficient to maintain muscle temperature in the normal range and prevent these effects.

Exercise and Thermal Balance

The acute exercise effects on thermal balance, that is, effects on thermal balance apparent while exercise is ongoing, depend on a complex interaction among factors related to exercise intensity, environmental conditions, and mode of activity. Exercise not only increases metabolic heat production, but it also increases blood flow to the skin and muscles, thereby facilitating body heat loss. This enhances convective heat transfer from the central core to peripheral shell. Thus, while metabolic heat production increases progressively as exercise intensity increases, so too does heat loss due to rising muscle and skin blood flow. Also, limb movement increases convective heat loss from the body surface by disrupting the stationary boundary layer of air or water that develops at the skin surface in a still environment.

Arm exercise, as compared to leg exercise, exacerbates the effects of exercise-induced increments in muscle and skin blood flow on convective heat transfer (145). The arms have a greater surface area to mass ratio and a thinner subcutaneous fat layer than the legs, causing a greater heat loss and larger declines in core temperature during arm than leg exercise, both performed at the same absolute metabolic rate (146). The greater convective heat transfer coefficient in water magnifies these effects compared to air. In cold air, metabolic heat production during exercise can be high enough to compensate for increased heat loss and allow core temperature to be maintained even when ambient temperature is extremely cold (101). In contrast, increased heat loss during exercise in cold water can be so great that metabolic heat production during even intense exercise is insufficient to defend core temperature (101).

The possibility that chronic exercise induces adaptations or maladaptations in thermoregulatory responses to cold merits some consideration. Consensus is lacking concerning the effects of influence of training and physical fitness on thermoregulatory response to cold. Bittel and colleagues (147) employed a cross-sectional experimental design to evaluate aerobic fitness effects on responses to cold, and they reported that fit persons maintained warmer skin temperatures than less fit persons during rest in cold air. The effect appeared due to thinner subcutaneous fat thickness and the consequently higher metabolic heat production elicited in fit compared to less fit subjects, rather than to a fitness effect per se (147). Others could demonstrate no relationship between $\dot{V}O_2max$ and skin temperature during rest in cold air (148). Cross-sectional studies do not address endurance training effects very well, however, since factors besides training contribute to a high $\dot{V}O_2max$. Longitudinal investigations indicate that endurance training strengthens the cutaneous vasoconstrictor response to cold. Young and colleagues (142) reported that after 8 weeks of endurance training, subjects exhibited a more rapid decline in skin temperatures during exercise in cold water than before training. In agreement, Kollias and colleagues (149), reported that after 9 weeks of aerobic training there was a more rapid decline in skin temperatures during resting cold air exposure than before training. Therefore, endurance training may provide a thermoregulatory advantage for persons exposed to cold.

As mentioned above, exercise-induced sweating occurs even in cold environments. Just as in the heat, these losses must be offset by drinking, or dehydration will ensue. However, in cold environments a phenomenon called "voluntary dehydration" has been observed (124). In cold weather, thirst is blunted, and persons sometimes restrict their fluid intake to minimize the need to urinate outdoors. The effects of any resulting imbalance between fluid loss and fluid replacement will worsen as duration of cold exposure and chronic exercise are prolonged. The performance impairments associated with hypohydration are likely to be the same in cold as hot environments. It has also been suggested that hypohydration may increase susceptibility to peripheral cold injuries, perhaps by a decrease in peripheral blood flow or an impairment of the CIVD response to cold (150). Hypohydration does not appear to impair shivering during whole-body cold exposure, but it may impair vasoconstrictor responses to cold if exposure is prolonged or severe (151).

Chronic exercise performed without adequate recovery between sessions can lead to exertional fatigue. In addition, when high levels of energy expenditure are sustained for long periods, it is difficult to maintain sufficiently high energy intake to offset expenditure. Both fatigue and underfeeding are thought to impair an individual's ability to maintain thermal balance in the cold. The effects of underfeeding are probably due to hypoglycemia, since depletion of peripheral carbohydrate stores has little effect on shivering (128). Acute hypoglycemia impairs shivering, but this effect appears centrally mediated as opposed to an effect on peripheral substrate availability (152). The anecdotal association between exertional fatigue and susceptibility to hypothermia is well reported (153). Two recent studies attempted to demonstrate the effect of prolonged fatiguing exercise on maintenance of thermal balance in the cold (154,155). Those reports both showed that, as fatigue develops, the intensity of exercise that can be sustained declines; thus, metabolic heat production declines and thermal balance during cold exposure is compromised. With respect to direct fatigue effects on thermoregulation in the cold, the results of those two studies were equivocal, although findings from another recent study indicate that exertional fatigue combined with sleep deprivation may delay the onset of shivering (156).

CONCLUSION

Climatic heat stress and exercise interact synergistically and may push physiologic systems to their limits. Heat stress increases requirements for sweating and circulatory responses to dissipate body heat. Heat stress reduces athletes' ability to achieve maximal metabolic rates and their submaximal endurance performance. Athletes routinely have sweating rates of >1 L per hour during exercise- heat stress and will often underdrink, causing body water deficits (hypohydration). Hypohydration increases core temperature responses during exercise and negates the thermoregulatory advantages conferred by high aerobic fitness and heat acclimation. During heat stress, hypohydration can have devastating effects on exercise performance and heat injury susceptibility.

In the cold, heat balance and requirements for shivering are dependent on the severity of climatic cold stress, effectiveness of vasoconstriction, as well as the intensity and mode of exercise. Cold- induced vasoconstriction decreases blood flow to peripheral tissues and makes them susceptible to cold injury. Reduced muscle temperature degrades finger dexterity and muscular strength, while reduced core temperature can degrade the ability to achieve maximal metabolic rates and submaximal endurance performance. Body composition is the most important physiologic determinant of thermoregulatory tolerance to cold exposure. The clothing insulation required for warmth and comfort is much higher during rest and light activity than during strenuous activity, and overinsulation can cause heat stress that elicits sweating, wet clothing, and hypohydration. Each of those factors can have undesirable affects on athletic performance and cold injury susceptibility.

DISCLAIMER

The views, opinions, and/or findings contained in this report are those of the authors and should not be construed as an official Department of the Army position, policy, or decisions, unless so designated by other official documentation. Approved for public release; distribution is unlimited.

REFERENCES

1. Gonzalez RR. Biophysics of heat exchange and clothing: applications to sports physiology. *Med Exerc Nutr Health* 1995;4: 290–305.
2. National Institute of Occupational Safety and Health. *Occupational exposure to hot environments.* Washington, DC: U.S. Department of Health and Human Services, 1986.
3. Kark JA, Burr PQ, Wenger CB, Gastaldo E, Gardner JW. Exertional heat illness in Marine Corps recruit training. *Aviat Space Environ Med* 1996;67:354–360.
4. Ladell WSS. Terrestrial animals in humid heat: man. In: Dill DB, Adolph EF, Wilber CG, eds. *Handbook of physiology, section 4, adaptation to the environment.* Washington, DC: American Physiological Society, 1964:625–659.
5. Lee DHK. Terrestrial animals in dry heat; man in the desert. In: Dill DB, Adolph EF, Wilber CG, eds. *Handbook of physiology, section 4, adaptation to the environment.* Washington, DC: American Physiological Society, 1964:551–582.
6. Yaglou CP, Minard D. Control of heat casualties at military training centers. *AMA Arch Ind Health* 1957;16:302–316.
7. Sawka MN, Wenger CB, Pandolf KB. Thermoregulatory responses to acute exercise-heat stress and heat acclimation. In: Fregly MJ, Blatteis CM, eds. *Handbook of Physiology, section 4, environmental physiology.* New York: Oxford University Press, 1996:157–185.
8. Lind AR. A physiological criterion for setting thermal environmental limits for everyday work. *J Appl Physiol* 1963;18:51–56.
9. Nielsen B, Nielsen M. Body temperature during work at different environmental temperatures. *Acta Physiol Scand* 1962;56: 120–129.
10. Nielsen M. Heat production and body temperature during rest and work. In: Hardy JD, Gagge AP, Stolwijk JAJ, eds. *Physiological and behavioral temperature regulation.* Springfield, IL: Charles C Thomas, 1970:205–214.
11. Nielsen M. Die Regulation der Körpertemperatur bei Muskelarbeit. *Scand Arch Physiol* 1938;9:193–230.
12. Gagge AP, Gonzalez RR. Mechanisms of heat exchange: biophysics and physiology. In: Fregly MJ, Blatteis CM, eds. *Handbook of physiology, section 4, environmental physiology.* New York: Oxford University Press, 1996:45–84.
13. Eichna LW, Ashe WF, Bean WB, Shelley WB. The upper limits of environmental heat and humidity tolerated by acclimatized men working in hot environments. *J Ind Hyg Toxicol* 1945; 27:59–84.
14. Pandolf KB, Stroschein LA, Drolet LL, Gonzalez RR, Sawka MN. Prediction modeling of physiological responses and human performance in the heat. *Comput Biol Med* 1986;16:319–329.
15. Saltin B, Hermansen L. Esophageal, rectal, and muscle temperature during exercise. *J Appl Physiol* 1966;21:1757–1762.
16. Astrand I. Aerobic work capacity in men and women. *Acta Physiol Scand* 1960;49:64–73.
17. Davies CTM. Influence of skin temperature on sweating and aerobic performance during severe work. *J Appl Physiol* 1979; 47:770–777.
18. Davies CTM, Brotherhood JR, ZeidiFard E. Temperature regulation during severe exercise with some observations on effects of skin wetting. *J Appl Physiol* 1976;41:772–776.
19. Sawka MN, Pandolf KB. Effects of body water loss on physiological function and exercise performance. In: Gisolfi CV, Lamb DR, eds. *Perspectives in exercise science and sports medicine, vol 3: fluid homeostasis during exercise.* Carmel, IN: Benchmark Press, 1990:1–38.
20. Sawka MN, Montain SJ, Latzka WA. Body fluid balance during exercise—heat exposure. In: Buskirk ER, Puhl SM, eds. *Body fluid balance: exercise and sport.* Boca Raton, FL: CRC Press, 1996:143–161.
21. Greenleaf JE. Problem: thirst, drinking behavior, and involuntary dehydration. *Med Sci Sports Exerc* 1992;24:645–656.
22. Hales JRS, Hubbard RW, Gaffin SL. Limitations of heat tolerance. In: Fregly MJ, Blatteis CM, eds. *Handbook of physiology, section 4, environmental physiology.* New York: Oxford University Press, 1996:285–355.
23. Cadarette BS, Sawka MN, Toner MM, Pandolf KB. Aerobic fitness and the hypohydration response to exercise—heat stress. *Aviat Space Environ Med* 1984;55:507–512.
24. Grande F, Monagle JE, Buskirk ER, Taylor HL. Body temperature responses to exercise in man on restricted food and water intake. *J Appl Physiol* 1959;14:194–198.
25. Sawka MN, Young AJ, Francesconi RP, Muza SR, Pandolf KB. Thermoregulatory and blood responses during exercise at graded hypohydration levels. *J Appl Physiol* 1985;59:1394–1401.
26. Ekblom B, Greenleaf CJ, Greenleaf JE, Hermansen L. Temperature regulation during exercise dehydration in man. *Acta Physiol Scand* 1970;79:475–483.
27. Montain SJ, Coyle EF. Influence of graded dehydration on hyperthermia and cardiovascular drift during exercise. *J Appl Physiol* 1992;73:1340–1350.
28. Adolph EF, and associates *Physiology of man in the desert.* New York: Interssciences, 1947.
29. Strydom NB, Holdsworth DL. The effects of different levels of water deficit on physiological responses during heat stress. *Int Z Angew Physiol* 1968;26:95–102.
30. Buskirk ER, Iampietro PF, Bass DE. Work performance after dehydration: effects of physical conditioning and heat acclimatization. *J Appl Physiol* 1958;12:189–194.
31. Sawka MN, Toner MM, Francesconi RP, Pandolf KB. Hypohydration and exercise: effects of heat acclimation, gender, and environment. *J Appl Physiol* 1983;55:1147–1153.
32. Klausen K, Dill DB, Phillips EE, McGregor D. Metabolic reactions to work in the desert. *J Appl Physiol* 1967;22:292–296.
33. Rowell LB, Brengelmann GL, Murray JA, Kraning KK, Kusumi F. Human metabolic responses to hyperthermia during mild to maximal exercise. *J Appl Physiol* 1969;26:395–402.
34. Saltin B, Gagge AP, Bergh U, Stolwijk JAJ. Body temperatures and sweating during exhaustive exercise. *J Appl Physiol* 1972; 32:635–643.
35. Sen Gupta J, Dimri P, Malhotra MS. Metabolic responses of Indians during sub-maximal and maximal work in dry and humid heat. *Ergonomics* 1977;20:33–40.
36. Sawka MN, Young AJ, Cadarette BS, Levine L, Pandolf KB. Influence of heat stress and acclimation on maximal aerobic power. *Eur J Appl Physiol* 1985;53:294–298.

37. Rowell LB, Blackmon JR, Martin RH, Mazzarella JA, Bruce RA. Hepatic clearance of indocyanine green in man under thermal and exercise stresses. *J Appl Physiol* 1965;20:384–394.
38. Cerretelli P, Marconi C, Pendergast DR, Meyer M, Heisler N, Piiper J. Blood flow in exercising muscles by xenon clearance and by microsphere trapping. *J Appl Physiol* 1984;56:24–30.
39. Rowell LB, Marx HJ, Bruce RA, Conn RD, Kusumi F. Reductions in cardiac output, central blood volume, and stroke volume with thermal stress in normal men during exercise. *J Clin Invest* 1966;45:1801–1816.
40. Caldwell JE, Ahonen E, Nousiainen U. Differential effects of sauna-, diuretic-, and exercise-induced hypohydration. *J Appl Physiol* 1984;57:1018–1023.
41. Webster S, Rutt R, Weltman A. Physiological effects of a weight loss regimen practiced by college wrestlers. *Med Sci Sports Exerc* 1990;22:229–234.
42. Craig FN, Cummings EG. Dehydration and muscular work. *J Appl Physiol* 1966;21:670–674.
43. Pinchan G, Gauttam RK, Tomar OS, Bajaj AC. Effects of primary hypohydration on physical work capacity. *Int J Biometeorol* 1988;32:176–180.
44. Armstrong LE, Costill DL, Fink WJ. Influence of diuretic-induced dehydration on competitive running performance. *Med Sci Sports Exerc* 1985;17:456–461.
45. Sawka MN. Physiological consequences of hydration: exercise performance and thermoregulation. *Med Sci Sports Exerc* 1992; 24:657–670.
46. Allen TE, Smith DP, Miller DK. Hemodynamic response to submaximal exercise after dehydration and rehydration in high school wrestlers. *Med Sci Sports* 1977;9:159–163.
47. Sproles CB, Smith DP, Byrd RJ, Allen TE. Circulatory responses to submaximal exercise after dehydration and rehydration. *J Sports Med* 1976;16:98–105.
48. Saltin B. Circulatory response to submaximal and maximal exercise after thermal dehydration. *J Appl Physiol* 1964;19:1125–1132.
49. Montain SJ, Sawka MN, Latzka WA, Valeri CR. Thermal and cardiovascular strain from hypohydration: influence of exercise intensity. *Int J Sports Med* 1998;19:1–5.
50. Bruck K, Olschewski H. Body temperature related factors diminishing the drive to exercise. *Can J Physiol Pharmacol* 1987;65: 1274–1280.
51. Montain SJ, Smith SA, Matott RP, Zientara GP, Jolesz FA, Sawka MN. Hypohydration effects on skeletal muscle performance and metabolism: a ^{31}P MRS study. *J Appl Physiol* 1998;84:1889–1894.
52. Burge CM, Carey MF, Payne WR. Rowing performance, fluid balance, and metabolic function following dehydration and rehydration. *Med Sci Sports Exerc* 1993;25:1358–1364.
53. Walsh RM, Noakes TD, Hawley JA, Dennis SC. Impaired high-intensity cycling performance time at low levels of dehydration. *Int J Sports Med* 1994;15:392–398.
54. Below PR, Mora-Rodríguez R, González-Alonso J, Coyle EF. Fluid and carbohydrate ingestion independently improve performance during 1 h of exercise. *Med Sci Sports Exerc* 1995;27: 200–210.
55. Montain SJ, Sawka MN, Cadarette BS, Quigley MD, McKay JM. Physiological tolerance to uncompensable heat stress: effects of exercise intensity, protective clothing, and climate. *J Appl Physiol* 1994;77:216–222.
56. Sawka MN, Young AJ, Latzka WA, Neufer PD, Quigley MD, Pandolf KB. Human tolerance to heat strain during exercise: influence of hydration. *J Appl Physiol* 1992;73:368–375.
57. Reneau PD, Bishop PA. Validation of a personal heat stress monitor. *Am Ind Hyg Assoc J* 1996;57:650–657.
58. Joy RJT, Goldman RF. A method of relating physiology and military performance: a study of some effects of vapor barrier clothing in a hot climate. *Mil Med* 1968;133:458–470.
59. Nielsen B, Hales JRS, Strange S, Christensen NJ, Warberg J, Saltin B. Human circulatory and thermoregulatory adaptations with heat acclimation and exercise in a hot, dry environment. *J Physiol* 1993;460:467–485.
60. Adams WC, Fox RH, Fry AJ, MacDonald IC. Thermoregulation during marathon running in cool, moderate, and hot environments. *J Appl Physiol* 1975;38:1030–1037.
61. Pugh LGCE, Corbett JL, Johnson RH. Rectal temperatures, weight losses, and sweat rates in marathon running. *J Appl Physiol* 1967;23:347–352.
62. Robinson S. Temperature regulation in exercise. *Pediatrics* 1963;32:691–702.
63. Sawka MN, Knowlton RG, Critz JB. Thermal and circulatory responses to repeated bouts of prolonged running. *Med Sci Sports* 1979;11:177–180.
64. Montain SJ, Maughan RJ, Sawka MN. Heat acclimatization strategies for the 1996 Summer Olympics. *Athletic Therapy Today* 1996;1:42–46.
65. Wenger CB. Human heat acclimatization. In: Pandolf KB, Sawka MN, Gonzalez RR, eds. *Human performance physiology and environmental medicine at terrestrial extremes.* Indianapolis, IN: Benchmark Press, 1988:153–197.
66. Bean WB, Eichna LW. Performance in relation to environmental temperature. Reactions of normal young men to simulated desert environment. *Fed Proc* 1943;2:144–158.
67. Eichna LW, Bean WB, Ashe WF, Nelson N. Performance in relation to environmental temperature. Reactions of normal young men to hot, humid (simulated jungle) environment. *Bull Johns Hopkins Hosp* 1945;76:25–58.
68. Lind AR, Bass DE. Optimal exposure time for development of acclimatization to heat. *Fed Proc* 1963;22:704–708.
69. Fein JT, Haymes EM, Buskirk ER. Effects of daily and intermittent exposures on heat acclimation of women. *Int J Biometeorol* 1975;19:41–52.
70. Lind AR. Physiologic responses to heat. In: Licht S, ed. *Medical climatology.* Baltimore, MD: Waverly Press, 1964:164–195.
71. Williams GG, Wyndham CH, Morrison JF. Rate of loss of acclimatization in summer and winter. *J Appl Physiol* 1967;22:21–26.
72. Pandolf KB, Burse RL, Goldman RF. Role of physical fitness in heat acclimatization, decay and reinduction. *Ergonomics* 1977;20:399–408.
73. Gardner JW, Kark JA, Karnei K, et al. Risk factors predicting exertional heat illness in male Marine Corps recruits. *Med Sci Sports Exerc* 1996;28:939–944.
74. Pandolf KB. Effects of physical training and cardiorespiratory physical fitness on exercise-heat tolerance: recent observations. *Med Sci Sports* 1979;11:60–65.
75. Strydom NB, Wyndham CH, Williams CG, et al. Acclimatization to humid heat and the role of physical conditioning. *J Appl Physiol* 1966;21:636–642.
76. Avellini BA, Shapiro Y, Fortney SM, Wenger CB, Pandolf KB. Effects on heat tolerance of physical training in water and on land. *J Appl Physiol* 1982;53:1291–1298.
77. Henane R, Flandrois R, Charbonnier JP. Increase in sweating sensitivity by endurance conditioning in man. *J Appl Physiol* 1977;43:822–828.
78. Armstrong LE, Pandolf KB. Physical training, cardiorespiratory physical fitness and exercise-heat tolerance. In: Pandolf KB, Sawka MN, Gonzalez RR, eds. *Human performance physiology and environmental medicine at terrestrial extremes.* Indianapolis, IN: Benchmark Press, 1988:199–226.
79. Shvartz E, Saar E, Meyerstein N, Benor D. A comparison of three methods of acclimatization to dry heat. *J Appl Physiol* 1973;34:214–219.
80. Nadel ER, Pandolf KB, Roberts MF, Stolwijk JAJ. Mechanisms of thermal acclimation to exercise and heat. *J Appl Physiol* 1974;37:515–520.
81. Roberts MF, Wenger CB, Stolwijk JAJ, Nadel ER. Skin blood flow and sweating changes following exercise training and heat acclimation. *J Appl Physiol* 1977;43:133–137.
82. Greenleaf JE. Environmental issues that influence intake of replacement beverages. In: Marriott BM, ed. *Fluid replacement and heat stress.* Washington, DC: National Academy Press, 1994:195–214.
83. Hubbard RW, Sandick BL, Matthew WT, et al. Voluntary dehydration and alliesthesia for water. *J Appl Physiol* 1984;57: 868–875.
84. Engell DB, Maller O, Sawka MN, Francesconi RP, Drolet LA,

Young AJ. Thirst and fluid intake following graded hypohydration levels in humans. *Physiol Behav* 1987;40:229–236.
85. Armstrong LE, Hubbard RW, Szlyk PC, Matthew WT, Sils IV. Voluntary dehydration and electrolyte losses during prolonged exercise in the heat. *Aviat Space Environ Med* 1985;56:765–770.
86. Marriott BM. *Nutritional needs in hot environments: application for military personnel in field operations.* Washington, DC: National Academy Press, 1993:
87. Brouns F. Heat-sweat-dehydration-rehydration: a praxis oriented approach. *J Sports Sci* 1991;9:143–152.
88. Allan JR, Wilson CG. Influence of acclimatization on sweat sodium concentration. *J Appl Physiol* 1971;30:708–712.
89. Dill DB, Jones BF, Edwards HT, Oberg SA. Salt economy in extreme dry heat. *J Biol Chem* 1933;100:755–767.
90. Bass DE, Kleeman CR, Quinn M, Henschel A, Hegnauer AH. Mechanisms of acclimatization to heat in man. *Medicine* 1955;34:323–380.
91. Marriott BM. *Fluid replacement and heat stress.* Washington, DC: National Academy Press, 1994.
92. Convertino VA, Armstrong LE, Coyle EF, et al. American College of Sports Medicine Position Stand: exercise and fluid replacement. *Med Sci Sports Exerc* 1996;28:i–vii.
93. Montain SJ, Maughan RJ, Sawka MN. Fluid replacement strategies for exercise in hot weather. *Athletic Therapy Today* 1996;1:24–27.
94. Freund BJ, Montain SJ, Young AJ, et al. Glycerol hyperhydration: hormonal, renal, and vascular fluid responses. *J Appl Physiol* 1995;79:2069–2077.
95. Riedesel ML, Allen DY, Peake GT, Al-Qattan K. Hyperhydration with glycerol solutions. *J Appl Physiol* 1987;63:2262–2268.
96. Latzka WA, Sawka MN, Montain S, et al. Hyperhydration: thermoregulatory effects during compensable exercise- heat stress. *J Appl Physiol* 1997;83:860–866.
97. Lyons TP, Riedesel ML, Meuli LE, Chick TW. Effects of glycerol-induced hyperhydration prior to exercise in the heat on sweating and core temperature. *Med Sci Sports Exerc* 1990; 22:477–483.
98. Montner P, Stark DM, Riedesel ML, et al. Pre-exercise glycerol hydration improves cycling endurance time. *Int J Sports Med* 1996;17:27–33.
99. Murray R, Eddy DE, Paul GL, Seifert JG, Halaby GA. Physiological responses to glycerol ingestion during exercise. *J Appl Physiol* 1991;71:144–149.
100. Latzka WA, Sawka MN, Montain SJ, et al. Hyperhydration: tolerance and cardiovascular effects during uncompensable exercise-heat stress. *J Appl Physiol* 1998;84:1858–1864.
101. Toner MM, McArdle WD. Human thermoregulatory responses to acute cold stress with special reference to water immersion. In: Fregly MJ, Blatteis CM, eds. *Handbook of physiology, section 4, environmental physiology.* New York: Oxford University Press, 1996:379–418.
102. Young AJ. Homeostatic responses to prolonged cold exposure: human cold acclimatization. In: Fregly MJ, Blatteis CM, eds. *Handbook of physiology, section 4, environmental physiology.* New York: Oxford University Press, 1996:419–438.
103. Siple PA, Passel CR. Measurements of dry atmospheric cooling in subfreezing temperatures. *Proc Am Philosoph Soc* 1945; 89:177–199.
104. Danielsson U. Windchill and the risk of tissue freezing. *J Appl Physiol* 1996;81:2666–2673.
105. Holmer I. Work in the cold. *Int Arch Occup Environ Health* 1993;65:147–155.
106. Kaufman WC, Bothe DJ. Wind chill reconsidered, Siple revisited. *Aviat Space Environ Med* 1986;57:23–26.
107. Lee DT, Toner MM, McArdle WD, Vrabas JS, Pandolf KB. Thermal and metabolic responses to cold-water immersion at knee, hip and shoulder levels. *J Appl Physiol* 1997;82:1523–1530.
108. Veicsteinas A, Ferretti G, Rennie DW. Superficial shell insulation in resting and exercising men in cold water. *J Appl Physiol* 1982;52:1557–1564.
109. Purdue GF, Hunt JL. Cold injury: a collective review. *J Burn Cancer Res* 1986;7:331–341.
110. Gamble WB. Perspectives in frostbite and cold weather injuries. *Adv Plast Reconstr Surg* 1994;10:21–72.
111. Boswick JA Jr, Thompson JD, Jonas RA. The epidemiology of cold injuries. *Surg Gynecol Obstet* 1979;149:326–332.
112. Gaydos HF. Effect on complex manual performance of cooling the body while maintaining the hands at normal temperatures. *J Appl Physiol* 1958;12:373–376.
113. Lewis T. Observations upon the reactions of the human skin to cold. *Heart* 1930;15:177–181.
114. Clarke RSJ, Hellon F, Lind AR. Cold vasodilation in the human forearm. *J Physiol* 1957;137:84–85.
115. Ducharme MB, VanHelder WP, Radomski MW. Cyclic intramuscular temperature fluctuations in the human forearm during cold-water immersion. *Eur J Appl Physiol* 1991;63:188–193.
116. Burton AC, Edholm OG. Vascular reactions to cold. In: Bayliss LE, Feldberg W, Hodgkin AL, eds. *Man in a cold environment.* London: Edward Arnold, 1955:129–147.
117. Lindblad LE, Ekenvall L, Klingstedt C. Neural regulation of vascular tone and cold induced vasoconstriction in human finger skin. *J Auton Nerv Syst* 1990;30:169–174.
118. LeBlanc JD, Robinson DF, Tousignant P. Catecholamines and short-term adaptation to cold in mice. *Am J Physiol* 1967;213: 1419–1422.
119. Toner MM, McArdle WD. Physiological adjustments of man to the cold. In: Pandolf KB, Sawka MN, Gonzalez RR, eds. *Human performance physiology and environmental medicine at terrestrial extremes.* Indianapolis: Benchmark Press, 1988:361–399.
120. Horvath SM. Exercise in a cold environment. *Exerc Sport Sci Rev* 1981;9:221–263.
121. Young AJ, Muza SR, Sawka MN, Gonzalez RR, Pandolf KB. Human thermoregulatory responses to cold air are altered by repeated cold water immersion. *J Appl Physiol* 1986;60:1542–1548.
122. Young AJ, Sawka MN, Neufer PD, Muza SR, Askew EW, Pandolf KB. Thermoregulation during cold water immersion is unimpaired by low muscle glycogen levels. *J Appl Physiol* 1989; 66:1809–1816.
123. Golden FSC, Hampton IFG, Hervery GR, Knibbs AV. Shivering intensity in humans during immersion in cold water. *J Physiol (Lond)* 1979;277:48(abst)
124. Freund BJ, Young AJ. Environmental influences body fluid balance during exercise:cold exposure. In: Buskirk ER, Puhl SM, eds. *Body fluid balance: exercise and sport.* New York: CRC Press, 1996:159–181.
125. Toner MM, Sawka MN, Foley ME, Pandolf KB. Effects of body mass and morphology on thermal responses in water. *J Appl Physiol* 1986;60:521–525.
126. Rennie DW, Covino WG, Blair MR, Rodahl K. Physical regulation of temperature in Eskimos. *J Appl Physiol* 1962;17:326–332.
127. McArdle WD, Magel JR, Spina RJ, Gergley TJ, Toner MM. Thermal adjustment to cold-water exposure in exercising men and women. *J Appl Physiol* 1984;56:1572–1577.
128. Young AJ. Energy substrate utilization during exercise in extreme environments. In: Pandolf KB, Hollozsy JO, eds. *Exercise and sport sciences reviews.* Baltimore, MD: Williams & Wilkins, 1990:65–117.
129. Bergh U, Ekblom B. Physical performance and peak aerobic power at different body temperatures. *J Appl Physiol* 1979;46: 885–889.
130. Holmer I, Bergh U. Metabolic and thermal response to swimming in water at varying temperatures. *J Appl Physiol* 1974;37: 702–705.
131. Schmidt V, Bruck K. Effect of a precooling maneuver on body temperature and exercise performance. *J Appl Physiol* 1981; 50:772–778.
132. McArdle WD, Magel JR, Lesmes GR, Pechar GS. Metabolic and cardiovascular adjustment to work in air and water at 18, 25, and 33 degrees C. *J Appl Physiol* 1976;40:85–90.
133. Young AJ, Sawka MN, Pandolf KB. Physiology of cold exposure. In: Marriott BM, Carlson SJ, eds. *Nutritional needs in cold and in high-altitude environments.* Washington, DC: National Academy Press, 1996:127–147.
134. Jaeger JJ, Deal EC, Roberts DE, Ingram RH, McFadden ER. Cold air inhalation and esophageal temperature in exercising humans. *Med Sci Sports Exerc* 1980;12:365–369.
135. Helenius IJ, Tikkanen HO, Haahtela T. Exercise-induced bron-

chospasm at low temperatures in elite runners. *Thorax* 1996; 51:628–629.
136. Chapman KR, Allen LJ, Romet TT. Pulmonary function in normal subjects following exercise at cold ambient temperatures. *Eur J Appl Physiol* 1990;60:228–232.
137. Koskela H, Tukiainen H. Facial cooling, but not nasal breathing of cold air, induces bronchoconstriction: a study of asthmatic and healthy subjects. *Eur Respir J* 1995;8:2088–2093.
138. Giesbrecht GG. The respiratory system in a cold environment. *Aviat Space Environ Med* 1995;66:890–902.
139. Freund BJ, Sawka MN. Influence of cold stress on human fluid balance. In: Marriott BM, Carlson SJ, eds. *Nutritional needs in cold and in high-altitude environments.* Washington, DC: National Academy Press, 1996:161–179.
140. O'Brien C, Freund BJ, Sawka MN, McKay J, Hesslink RL, Jones TE. Hydration assessment during cold-weather military field training exercises. *Arctic Med Res* 1996;55:20–26.
141. Jacobs I, Tiit T, Kerrigan-Brown D. Muscle glycogen depletion during exercise at 9°C and 21°C. *Eur J Appl Physiol* 1985;54: 35–39.
142. Young AJ, Sawka MN, Levine L, et al. Metabolic and thermal adaptations from endurance training in hot or cold water. *J Appl Physiol* 1995;78:793–801.
143. Bergh U, Ekblom B. Influence of muscle temperature on maximal muscle strength and power output in human skeletal muscles. *Acta Physiol Scand* 1979;107:33–37.
144. Blomstrand E, Essen-Gustavsson B. Influence of reduced muscle temperature on metabolism in type I and type II human muscle fibres during intensive exercise. *Acta Physiol Scand* 1987;131: 569–574.
145. Sawka MN. Physiology of upper body exercise. In: Pandolf KB, ed. *Exercise and sport sciences reviews.* New York: Macmillan, 1986:175–211.
146. Toner MM, Sawka MN, Pandolf KB. Thermal responses during arm and leg and combined arm-leg exercise in water. *J Appl Physiol* 1984;56:1355–1360.
147. Bittel JHM, Nonott-Varly C, Livecchi-Gonnot GH, Savourey G, Hanniquet AM. Physical fitness and thermoregulatory reactions in a cold environment in men. *J Appl Physiol* 1988;65:1984–1989.
148. Budd GM, Brotherhood JR, Hendrie AL, Jeffery SE. Effects of fitness, fatness, and age on men's responses to whole body cooling in air. *J Appl Physiol* 1991;71(6):2387–2393.
149. Kollias J, Boileau, Buskirk ER. Effects of physical condition in man on thermal responses to cold air. *Int J Biometeorol* 1972; 16:389–402.
150. Roberts DE, Berberich JJ. The role of hydration on peripheral response to cold. *Milit Med* 1988;153:605–608.
151. O'Brien C, Young AJ, Sawka MN. Hypohydration and thermoregulation in cold air. *J Appl Physiol* 1998;84:185–189.
152. Gale EAM, Bennett T, Green JH, MacDonald IA. Hypoglycaemia, hypothermia and shivering in man. *Clin Sci* 1981;61:463–469.
153. Pugh LGCE. Cold stress and muscular exercise, with special reference to accidental hypothermia. *Br Med J* 1967;2:333–337.
154. Thompson RL, Hayward JS. Wet-cold exposure and hypothermia: thermal and metabolic responses to prolonged exercise in man. *J Appl Physiol* 1996;81:1128–1137.
155. Weller AS, Millard CE, Stroud MA, Greenhaff PL, MacDonald IA. Physiological responses to a cold, wet, and windy environment during prolonged intermittent walking. *Am J Physiol* 1997;272:R226–R233.
156. Young AJ, Castellani JW, O'Brien C, et al. Exertional fatigue, sleep loss, and negative energy balance increases susceptibility to hypothermia. *J Appl Physiol* 1998;85:1210–1217.
157. Hayward JS, Eckerson JD, Collis ML. Thermoregulatory heat production in man: prediction equation based on skin and core temperatures. *J Appl Physiol* 1977;42:377–384.

Exercise and Sport Science,
edited by William E. Garrett, Jr., and Donald T. Kirkendall.
Lippincott Williams & Wilkins, Philadelphia © 2000.

CHAPTER 27

Exercise-Induced Muscle Injury and Inflammation

Lucille L. Smith and Mary P. Miles

EXERCISE-INDUCED MUSCLE INJURY

Soft-tissue sports injuries such as contusions and sprains are a common occurrence and are unquestionably followed by activation of an inflammatory response. This response represents the generalized response of the body to any tissue injury induced by a wide array of stimuli such as chemical or mechanical. The ultimate purpose of inflammation is healing. The extent of inflammation is usually dependent on the extent of the injury, which may be graded as a first-, second-, or third-degree injury corresponding to mild, moderate, or severe, respectively. Treatment of these sport injuries typically involves rehabilitation using a variety of therapeutic modalities (1).

A more insidious, but apparently benign, form of muscle/connective tissue injury may occur in association with certain aspects of training and competing. In this instance, the "injury" appears to be an integral part of the adaptation process and/or an unavoidable consequence of training/competing. In fact, highly trained athletes may constantly experience some degree of muscle damage, which might be viewed as accelerating the normal physiologic state of muscle fiber turnover (2). Mounting evidence suggests activation of acute inflammation in response to these types of injuries (2–5). Unlike the acute sports injuries, however, treatment appears to require nothing more than an appropriate recovery period (1).

Presently, terminology is not sufficiently discriminating to accurately define this type of injury (1). We propose using the term *adaptive microtrauma* (AMT) to suggest that microinjury and regeneration represent a normal progression associated with training, and are integral in the reestablishment of homeostasis at an alternate level.

This adaptive microtrauma appears to be induced via two mechanisms, not necessarily mutually exclusive. First, an abundance of research has verified that *unaccustomed* eccentric muscle action (EMA), an integral part of most movements, during which the muscle lengthens under tension, disrupts muscle architecture (6). Second, although not as clearly characterized, it appears that local muscle ischemia may contribute to tissue injury, inducing injury via metabolic/chemical pathways (7,8). Mounting evidence suggests that injury induced via either mechanism evokes a low-grade acute inflammatory-like response (3,5).

The injury induced by unaccustomed EMA appears as disorganization of myofibrillar material especially at the z-disc and is accompanied by breakage of the myofibrillar cytoskeleton (9). Two theories have been proposed to account for this eccentrically induced soft tissue trauma. The first emphasizes the reduced motor-unit activation that occurs during the eccentric, compared to the concentric, phase of the movement, at the same force output (6). One-third to one-fifth the number of motor units are activated during the negative phase compared to the positive phase of the movement (6). Consequently, fewer fibers are required to sustain higher forces. The increased load per unit fiber supposedly causes the mechanical disruption. An alternate theory emphasizes the lengthening-under-tension aspect of EMA; this suggests that, due to the initial unequal resting length of sarcomeres in series, there is more stress on the shorter units, which are required to elongate relatively more compared to their resting length during an EMA, causing them to "pop" (10).

L. L. Smith: Department of Health, Leisure, and Exercise Science, Appalachian State University, Boone, North Carolina 28608.

M. P. Miles: Department of Health and Human Development, Montana State University, Bozeman, Montana 59717.

The injury induced by unaccustomed EMA is associated with the sensation of muscle soreness referred to as delayed-onset muscle soreness (DOMS) (3,5,6). DOMS is prevalent at the beginning of a season due to the fact that the eccentric phase of the movement is most likely unaccustomed, because many athletes refrain from exercise during the off-season. DOMS is also frequently experienced after an event that demands a dramatic increase in the intensity and or volume of the eccentric phase of the movement, such as a marathon race or a weightlifting competition.

A large body of well-controlled studies using human subjects has demonstrated that there is a significant reduction in force/strength associated with muscle damage and DOMS. From a practical perspective, this suggests that performance will be impaired if athletes compete during this time; appropriate allowances should be made by coaches and trainers.

A curious phenomenon associated with unaccustomed negatives and muscle damage is the "repeated bout effect." After the initial bout of damaging exercise, a subsequent bout at a similar volume and/or intensity, performed at any time within several weeks following the initial bout, will produce significantly less muscle damage and associated DOMS and significantly less decrease in performance. It is generally believed that the healing of the initially damaged tissue results in a more resilient structure (11); this would support the concept of EMA resulting in an adaptive injury, as was proposed earlier.

Although local muscle ischemia/hypoxia is considered a cause of muscle injury (6,12), this mechanism of injury has not been well investigated. If local ischemia does occur during exercise, it could be attributed to a variety of factors. It could be related to the concentric phase of the movement, which is metabolically more demanding due to greater motor-unit activation. Thus, during a bout of high-volume/high-intensity exercise, such as a road race, or during high-intensity resistance training, as well as during high-intensity cycling, the latter involving almost exclusively concentric muscle action, it is possible that all sections of the muscle are not adequately perfused. This results in local ischemia/hypoxia. Reduced perfusion might be attributed to a decrease in plasma volume due to fluid loss (sweating) and redistribution of a portion of blood to the skin, as the body strives to thermoregulate. Reduced perfusion could also be attributed to high-intensity straining-type exercise, such as occurs during power lifting, with increased local pressures impeding circulation, at least temporarily. Additionally, it has been proposed that hypoxic conditions may occur during the early phase of a bout of high force EMA (7). So conceivably, local pockets of transitory ischemia/hypoxia could develop in active muscle, induced by various scenarios.

Although the mechanism inducing hypoxic muscle damage is unclear, considerable research has been directed at elucidating the mechanisms underlying the pathophysiologic alteration of skeletal muscle, due to non–exercise-induced ischemia/hypoxia (13). It was initially believed that this muscle injury process was exclusively due to the ischemia. However, recent studies have found that a variable but substantial portion of the injury occurs at the time of reperfusion/reoxygenation (13), an inevitable consequence of ischemia. Tissue injury during ischemia depends on depletion of tissue oxygen and energy substrates (14). In animal studies, the situation created by ischemic exercise is characterized by the blocking of many of the reactions associated with energy substrate production such as phosphorylations (15). The reperfusion phase, strongly implicated in muscle cell injury, is multifactorial and includes oxidant generation, elaboration of proinflammatory mediators, infiltration of leukocytes, Ca^{2+} overload, phospholipid peroxidation and depletion, impaired nitric oxide metabolism, and reduced adenosine triphosphate (ATP) production (16). In fact, the sequence of events associated with reperfusion injury strongly resembles the acute inflammatory response. Research is needed in this area to clarify the role of ischemia/reperfusion injury that occurs during training/competing.

OVERVIEW OF INFLAMMATION

Inflammation is the generalized response of the body to tissue injury irrespective of the damaging stimulus, with the final purpose of healing. Overt signs and symptoms include swelling, redness, heat, pain, and loss of, or reduced, function; not all clinical manifestations are consistently detectable. There are undoubtedly some variations in the overall inflammatory response, most likely dependent on the nature of the tissue involved and on the extent of the injury. This discussion focuses on inflammation occurring in response to aseptic exercise-induced skeletal muscle injury (17), the type of injury already described. The term *aseptic* implies minimal immune activation (6).

In response to tissue injury, the body mounts an elaborate, carefully synchronized response, with extensive amplification at each step. The overall response is characterized by movement of fluid, plasma protein, and leukocytes into injured tissue. Many of the initial events, manifested within a few hours following injury, are directed toward local recruitment of waves of white blood cells. Neutrophils represent the first wave of infiltrating cells, followed by monocytes. Neutrophils play a predominant role in the initial "cleanup" process, while monocytes/macrophages and to some extent neutrophils synthesize a large variety of inflammatory factors. These inflammatory-related molecules, such as cytokines, chemokines, and cell adhesion molecules, orchestrate the trafficking and activation of white blood cells

(WBCs), and they mediate the local and systemic amplification as well as subsequent termination of inflammation, the latter event being integral to optimal healing. So an elaborate variety of molecules, not normally found in high concentrations in tissue and blood, are synthesized specifically to direct inflammation. The postvenule endothelial lining also participates extensively in the synthesis of these molecules. Several classes of these molecules will now be described.

ACUTE INFLAMMATION AND CYTOKINES

Cytokines are the "emergency" signal molecules that integrate and coordinate local and systemic signaling among various types of cells, including leukocytes, stem cells, progenitor cells, endothelial cells, and hepatocytes (18) during an inflammatory event. They are not stored as preformed molecules but instead are synthesized in response to inflammatory stimuli. They act locally, in an autocrine or paracrine fashion; certain cytokines may be produced in sufficient quantity to circulate and exert endocrine actions. Generally, cytokines are grouped into several families, which include interleukin (IL), tumor necrosis factor (TNF), interferon, colony-stimulating factor, and growth factor.

In general, the effects of individual cytokines on target cells are mediated through specific receptors for each cytokine. Functional redundancy is common among cytokines due largely to homology within the intracellular portions of the receptors with redundant functions. Thus, it is common for more than one cytokine to exert a similar effect on a given target cell. Furthermore, the action of a particular cytokine depends on the type of cell targeted, and the levels of other cytokines that may be exerting synergistic or antagonistic effects on the same target cells. Thus, the cytokine signaling system is complex and difficult to explain in absolute terms (19).

TNF-α, IL-1, and IL-6 are the three cytokines most important for the initiation of an acute inflammatory response. They act in sequence to stimulate proinflammatory events both locally and systemically. TNF-α and IL-1β are the "alarm cytokines," first produced by resident tissue macrophages, stimulated by events directly related to tissue injury or infection (20). The hallmark of the TNF-α and IL-1 response is rapidity; for example, IL-1β messenger ribonucleic acid (mRNA) increases can be measured in monocytes within 15 minutes of exposure to endotoxin. These two cytokines induce production of additional TNF-α, IL-1, and IL-6 by local endothelial cells, fibroblasts, and monocytes. IL-6, being at the temporal end of the cascade, has both pro- and counterinflammatory effects (19).

Locally, all three cytokines are capable of inducing chemokine synthesis, increasing vascular permeability, increasing expression of adhesion molecules on vascular endothelial cells, and attracting various leukocytes to the site of inflammation. Systemically, TNF, IL-1, and IL-6 are capable of inducing fever and synthesis of acute-phase proteins (21).

Activated macrophages account for the vast majority of IL-1 during inflammation. IL-1 has a cell-associated (IL-1α) and a soluble form (IL-1β) (21). These forms are separate gene products, under separate transcriptional control, but they share a common receptor. The soluble IL-1β induces a host of proinflammatory events in many target cells. A few of the key events induced by IL-1 include elevations in body temperature (endogenous pyrogen), activation of endothelial cells, induction of IL-8 to attract neutrophils, increased adhesion molecule expression, increased IL-6 production by monocytes and macrophages, and proteolysis in skeletal muscles (18,21,22). Inhibitors of IL-1β activity include prostaglandin E_2 (PGE_2) and IL-1 receptor antagonist (22).

TNF-α is produced by monocytes and macrophages (23), and by Kupffer cells within the liver (24). Along with IL-1, it is a strong inducer of IL-6 synthesis. Functions of TNF-α, not shared with IL-1 or IL-6, include activation of neutrophils and stimulation of T-cytotoxic cells. During inflammation, IL-6 can be produced in significant quantities by monocytes, macrophages, endothelial cells, and fibroblasts (23), as well as Kupffer cells within the liver (24). In the case of injury to muscle tissue, the IL-6 is produced by local cells, rather than by the cells within the liver (25). IL-6 production is stimulated by PGE_2, and cyclooxygenase inhibitors can reduce IL-6 production (26). Epinephrine can stimulate IL-6 production via β_2- adrenergic receptors. IL-6 stimulates the hypothalamic-pituitary-adrenal (HPA) axis, which leads to release of adrenocorticotropic hormone (ACTH) and then cortisol (19).

Cytokines and Exercise-Induced Muscle Damage

A large portion of the evidence associating strenuous exercise with inflammation is derived from observed elevations in cytokines. The signals for induction of cytokine synthesis have not been identified for microtear injury. Possibilities include free radicals, prostaglandins, and modified proteins (27).

IL-1, TNF-α, and IL-6 have been most extensively investigated in relation to exercise-induced muscle trauma and inflammation. Data from muscle biopsies indicate that IL-1 and IL-6 are produced within skeletal muscle during and after exercise associated with muscle damage (28,29). Inflammatory activity within skeletal muscle may be driven by the local endothelial cells. IL-1β is found near vascular endothelial cells rather than in the myofibrillar portion of the damaged muscle (28). Ultrastructural damage to muscle fibers following downhill running was associated with a slight increase in IL-1β staining intensity at 45 minutes, and a large increase at 5 days postexercise (28). Similarly, the degree of ultrastructural disruption is slight soon after damaging exercise, becoming more extensive in the following days (9,28).

Studies of plasma cytokines during and after exercise indicate that cytokine production is increased in response to strenuous exercise. Light exercise, such as cycling at 60% of $\dot{V}O_2max$ for 60 minutes (30), is not associated with elevations in plasma TNF-α, IL-1β, or IL-6. More intense exercise, such as high-intensity interval running (31) or marathon running (32), induces elevations in plasma IL-6 but not TNF-α or IL-1β. Similarly, exercise with a high-force eccentric component, such as eccentric cycling (33) or eccentric resistance exercise (34), induces elevations in IL-6, while TNF-α and IL-1β are rarely detectable. It could be that TNF-α and IL-1β are only produced locally, that they are not stable in the circulation, or that they are rapidly bound in molecular complexes that render present detection methods ineffective. Regardless, we assume that IL-6 production is preceded by production of TNF-α and IL-1, and we suggest that the IL-6 measured after exercise is indicative of increases in these cytokines.

Inflammatory cytokine production may begin soon after the onset of strenuous exercise, and the time course for resolution is variable. Increased IL-6 was measured at 90 minutes (but not at 15 or 45 minutes), after brief intervals of eccentric exercise (35), and immediately after a 2.5-hour treadmill run (32). Recovery to preexercise plasma levels may occur within hours postexercise (31,33), or may persist for at least 4 days following eccentric exercise when microtearing has been observed (35).

The time course of elevations in IL-6 may correspond to the time course of associated muscle damage processes. For example, peaks in serum creatine kinase (CK) activity, an indirect marker of muscle damage, occur within the first 48 hours following prolonged endurance events (36), and from 3 to 7 days following high-force eccentric exercise (37). Similarly, IL-6 recovery to preexercise levels is more rapid after endurance exercise and more extended after high-force exercise.

A number of cytokines are involved in the termination of the inflammatory response. These include IL-1 receptor antagonist (IL-1ra), IL-4, and IL-10. IL-1ra inhibits the activity of IL-1 by blocking cell surface receptors (38). Among many other functions, IL-4 inhibits monocyte and macrophage synthesis of IL-1, IL-6, and IL-8 (39). Interleukin-10 suppresses production of inflammatory cytokines by macrophages and lymphocytes (40). In accordance with the interleukins' antiinflammatory role, several investigations have measured a delayed increase in IL-1ra, IL-4, and IL-10 after certain inflammatory cytokines, such as IL-1β and IL-6, have peaked (29,32,41). Little is known about the response of these inflammatory control elements to exercise and is just beginning to receive attention in exercise research.

ACUTE INFLAMMATION AND LEUKOCYTES

Neutrophils, as part of the nonspecific arm of the immune system, are the first leukocyte population to respond to tissue injury. A predominant function of the neutrophil is removal of injury-related tissue debris. This involves attachment to particles and debris coated with substances such as complement fragments and immunoglobulins, to which neutrophils have surface receptors. This is followed by phagocytosis. Activated neutrophils also release lysosomal proteases, which degrade local proteins, as well as reactive oxygen species (ROSs), a result of the "oxidative burst." ROSs create a hostile environment and cause tissue destruction or killing. Part of this destruction allows for regeneration of injured tissue. However, this tissue destruction can extend beyond this purpose and, left unchecked, can cause more harm than good (42,43).

Leukocytes and Exercise-Induced Muscle Damage

The response of white blood cells to exercise-induced inflammation can be characterized by the following three ways: (a) changes in circulating concentrations; (b) infiltration into damaged tissue, particularly skeletal muscle; and (c) functional changes in leukocytes.

In regard to circulating leukocyte concentrations, neutrophils are the leukocyte type most responsive to exercise stimuli. The general consensus is that exercise increases circulating neutrophils, with the increase being relative to the intensity and duration of the exercise (42). This neutrophilia is most likely a response to demargination due to increased levels of epinephrine, or possibly due to increased shearing forces associated with increased cardiac output during exercise (42). Other stressors, such as muscle damage and heat, have been shown to enhance the neutrophil response to exercise, with significant elevations in neutrophil count seen between 2 and 3 hours after muscle damage–inducing exercise. This is most likely due to accelerated release from the bone marrow storage pools, typically seen during an inflammatory event (44–47).

Monocytes also respond to exercise stimuli. Circulating monocytes generally increase during exercise, and they often continue to increase in the first few hours after exercise. Total increases are usually 30% to 90% in magnitude (48,49), but severe exercise may elicit increases from 100% to 150% (50,51).

Infiltration of leukocytes into skeletal muscle is a strong indication that microtrauma induces inflammation. Large accumulations of inflammatory cells have been found in human skeletal muscle fibers damaged by high-force eccentric contractions (46,51), and after prolonged endurance events, such as a marathon (52). Neutrophil accumulation may be seen within minutes after the injury and may reside in damaged muscle for 5 to 7 days or longer (46,51,52). Large accumulations of macrophages have been measured as early as 1 day after exercise, with peak accumulations appearing from 3 to 14 days postexercise (51,52).

This time course for cellular infiltration in human subjects after exercise-induced muscle damage is prolonged, compared to what is normally reported after blunt trauma, and compared to rat muscle injury that has been induced by forced lengthening (6,53). Whether this represents a species-related difference, or whether differences are due to methodologic factors, is unclear. The muscle biopsy technique used in human research is limiting due to restrictions placed on what is regarded as a safe biopsy site, as well as the amount of tissue extracted (6). Caution is recommended when generalizing across species.

Functional changes in leukocytes after exercise focus predominantly on phagocytic activity of the neutrophil and the ability of the monocyte to produce cytokines. The capacity of the neutrophil to cause destruction to itself or the local environment has been assessed via analysis of degranulation, the oxidative burst, and the response of proteolytic enzymes. The general consensus of several exercise studies is that phagocytosis is improved following moderate exercise (54), while more intense exercise elicits a decrease in neutrophil oxidative capacity (42). The stimuli responsible for up- or downregulating neutrophil function in response to exercise have not been identified. Although inflammatory cytokines might be able to function in this capacity, this has not been substantiated; factors other than cytokines, possibly certain chemokines (55), are most likely responsible for neutrophil activation.

There is a limited amount of research that has specifically focused on muscle damage and activation of monocytes. Generally, functional changes in monocytes/macrophages focus on the synthesis of cytokines. Circulating monocytes can be divided into immature and mature subsets. During short-duration, high-intensity exercise, mature monocytes increased to a greater degree than immature monocytes (56–58), but decreased during prolonged endurance exercise (59). Furthermore, the mature monocytes produced more TNF-α, IL-1, and IL-6 than immature monocytes (41,59,60). These studies suggest that exercise of a certain intensity and duration increases the mature monocytes, which are most capable of producing inflammatory cytokines. The decrease of mature monocytes and blood cytokine levels seen with prolonged exercise might reflect selective emigration of mature monocytes from the circulation into inflamed tissue.

ACUTE INFLAMMATION AND CHEMOATTRACTANTS

At the onset of inflammation, selective recruitment of neutrophils, which peaks within the first 6 hours, followed by monocytes (47), is a crucial and complex part of the manifestation of inflammation. This event is directed in part by a class of molecules known as chemotactic agents. Chemotactic factors are generated in relatively high concentrations at sites of tissue injury. They are synthesized locally from a number of sources including local tissue cells, infiltrating leukocytes, and the endothelium, stimulated by cytokines and other inflammatory mediators (61,62).

Chemotaxins have a dual function in recruiting leukocytes. They assist in arresting the cell in the inflamed venules, and, once diapedesis has occurred, act to guide the leukocyte to the appropriate area. There are three basic types of leukocyte chemoattractants. The classic chemoattractants act broadly on several cell types including monocytes and neutrophils. These include C5a, a product of complement activation; leukotriene B_4, an arachidonic acid metabolite; and platelet-activating factor, a product of phosphatidylcholine metabolism. Certain cytokines are also classified as chemoattractants and are called chemokines. α-Chemokines, such as IL-8, act on neutrophils and fibroblasts and are involved in wound healing. β-Chemokines include monocyte chemoattractant protein-1 (MCP-1) and monocyte inflammatory protein-1 (MIP-1), and they act on monocyte and lymphocyte subpopulations (61,62). Limited research is presently available on exercise-induced muscle damage and chemoattractants (63).

ACUTE INFLAMMATION AND CELL ADHESION MOLECULES

Vascular endothelium acts as a "gatekeeper" between the circulation and surrounding tissue. Two of its many regulatory functions involve retaining blood-borne molecules and leukocytes within the circulation, and, during an inflammatory event, actively assisting in "capturing" specific leukocytes and directing their movement from the blood into the tissue. The latter is accomplished through the activity of an array of molecules expressed on leukocytes and on activated endothelial cells (EC) in postcapillary venules. These molecules are collectively referred to as cell adhesion molecules (CAMs) (64).

There are several classes of adhesion molecules associated with leukocyte-EC interaction and inflammation (65). The selectins influence the localization of the adhesion response. The immunoglobulin superfamily is characterized by immunoglobulin domains, and includes intercellular adhesion molecule-1 (ICAM-1) and vascular cell adhesion molecule-1 (VCAM-1), which are expressed on activated endothelial cells (64). The integrins represent another class of CAM molecules generally associated with leukocytes, such as very late antigen (VLA)–4 and integrins (64).

If migration of leukocytes is to occur, there are at least three critical sequential steps. The first step, reversible adhesion, involves loose binding of leukocyte adhesion molecules to counterreceptors on endothelial cells, usually involving the selectin family. This loose binding allows rolling along the vessel wall and gives the leukocyte an opportunity to sample the local environment, which will determine whether or not the cell is activated (65). If appropriate signals are present in the form of chemokines or chemoattractants, the cells are arrested. The second event, activation of leukocytes by chemoattractants, triggers a secondary adhesion receptor, an integrin, which interacts with the endothelial counterreceptor. The third step results in strong sustained attachment to the endothelial wall, involving the immunoglobulin (Ig) superfamily of adhesion molecules, and thus completing the process of recognition (65). This is followed by transendothelial and subendothelial migration. The cells then follow a gradient of chemotaxins (65).

The recruitment of specific leukocytes from the circulation is precisely regulated (65). At each step of recruitment from the postcapillary venules, there are multiple choices due to combinations of different cytokines stimulating the expression of different adhesion molecules on endothelium and leukocytes, and different chemoattractants. This differential regulation allows for diversity and selectivity of leukocyte localization. In acute inflammation, the sequence is generally adhesion of neutrophils and then monocytes (66). Monocytes are probably recruited in a similar fashion to neutrophils, the specificity most likely determined by differing responses to assorted chemoattractants.

Cell Adhesion Molecules and Exercise-Induced Muscle Damage

Despite the surge of interest in exercise and immunology, and the importance of cell adhesion molecules, the amount of exercise-related research is limited (67). Decreased proportions of lymphocytes expressing LFA-1 (68) and L-selectin (69,70) suggest that the cells more easily attracted to inflammatory sites may leave the circulation preferentially during strenuous exercise. Increased expression of Mac-1 on circulating neutrophils and lymphocytes was seen for 4 days following exercise (4), and increased soluble VCAM-1 was seen at 6 hours following high-force eccentric exercise that caused muscle damage (71). Baum and colleagues (72) reported that exercise training was associated with an increase in the expression of ICAM-1 on circulating lymphocytes and of soluble ICAM-1 in the plasma. They suggested that these changes, which occurred only in response to the onset of training and not during the regular training season, provided a protective mechanism against infection. A great deal more work is needed to clarify the response of inflammatory adhesion molecules to exercise.

ACUTE INFLAMMATION AND ACUTE-PHASE PROTEINS

At the onset of injury, a sequence of overlapping events begins to unfold, with the common final outcome of healing injured tissue. Many of these events are grouped together and referred to as the acute-phase response (APR), which includes the local activation of the complement system, the synthesis and release of a variety of cytokines and chemoattractants, and an increase in circulating leukocytes, to name a few. Two responses associated with systemic activation of acute inflammation are the febrile response and alteration in gene regulation in the liver, resulting in the production of liver acute-phase proteins (APPs) (20,27,73).

A primary function of APP is to protect the host against excessive damage that might ensue from inflammation. Catabolic enzymes and reactive oxygen species released by phagocytic cells act to clear disrupted host tissue in advance of repair. They do not discriminate between healthy and damaged cells, however, and so aspects of inflammation can lead to destruction of healthy tissue if the process is not controlled. The APPs are the primary mechanism for maintaining control of the inflammatory process (20,27,73).

Most APPs are circulating globulins produced by hepatocytes in response to cytokines, principally IL-6 and IL-1β. Concentrations of several plasma proteins such as C-reactive protein (CRP) and serum amyloid A (SAA), the two major human APPs, may increase more than 1000-fold. Others, such as fibrinogen, may increase modestly. In contrast, there is a decrease of several plasma proteins such as albumin and transferrin.

In all cases there is a lag phase of about 6 hours before the protein concentrations start to rise. The time course for expression of the various APPs differs, with some being significantly changed at 24 hours and others showing significant changes at 5 days after the injury (73). The number of acute-phase reactants and the magnitude of the response are somewhat proportional to the degree of trauma. As with other aspects of the metabolic response to injury, the degree of tissue damage is important in the activation of the APR, though the precise relationship is unclear (27,73). In an experimental situation, it has been shown that increasing the dose of an endotoxin increases the magnitude of each manifestation and increases the number of manifestations such as fever (73).

Acute-Phase Proteins and Exercise-Induced Muscle Damage

In reference to exercise and the APR, postexercise metabolic events of sustained, high-intensity exercise are similar but not analogous to the APR (74–76), with most research conclusions being focused on assessment of C-reactive protein (76). Dufaux and colleagues (75) observed increases in APPs after several days of severe physical activity; they suggested that this represented an exercise-induced inflammatory reaction, possibly as a consequence of nonspecific mechanical tissue damage. Furthermore, there is an apparent distance-related increase in CRP (76). At 24 hours after a 21-km race, only small increases were seen in CRP; however, increases seen after an 88-km ultramarathon were comparable to those found in patients with small myocardial infarctions. It also appears that greater elevations in CRP are seen in untrained versus trained individuals (76). In one study of circulating APPs after bench stepping to produce muscle damage, elevations in CRP but not α_1-acid glycoprotein or α_1-antitrypsin were measured (17).

Presently, there is a consensus concerning the fact that induction of APP requires a considerable dose of exercise, usually greater than 2 hours' duration (76,77), and that APPs are not significantly increased until 24 hours after exercise. The most consistent increase in an APP has been related to measurement of CRP, with increases as high as 300% (17,76,77).

APOPTOSIS AND TERMINATION OF INFLAMMATION

Apoptosis is a method of cell death designed to circumvent the negative effects of cellular necrosis. After necrosis, intracellular contents are released into the local environment, which causes a local inflammatory response (78). In lieu of this, apoptosis is a sequential process involving loss of cell volume, membrane blebbing (zeiosis), disintegration of the nucleus, blebbing off of small apoptotic bodies, and eventually total fragmentation of the cell. In this process, membrane integrity is never lost, and the local environment is protected from harmful intracellular contents, such as the degradative enzymes and toxic proteins in the granules of neutrophils (79–81). Apoptotic bodies and cell fragments are removed by phagocytes without a trace. Part of the resolution of inflammation, particularly the removal of accumulated neutrophils, is because neutrophils are induced to apoptose (43). Neutrophils do not return to the circulation, as do lymphocytes, and they are not disposed of through the lymphatic system. Instead, they are disposable phagocytes, with a short half-life, and apoptosis is the normal mode of elimination (78). There is evidence that IL-6 promotes apoptosis in mature human neutrophils *in vitro* (82). Two additional conditions known to induce apoptosis in neutrophils are aging and withdrawal of inflammatory generated growth factors (83).

There is substantial evidence that the phagocytosis of neutrophils by macrophages has a neutralizing effect on macrophages. Initially, when macrophages are stimulated by proinflammatory cytokines, there is an increased phagocytosis of apoptotic neutrophils (84). Once macrophages have phagocytosed apoptotic cells, however, they no longer release proinflammatory eicosinoids and cytokines (43). Thus, the processes involved in the generation of inflammation become self-limiting and contribute to termination of inflammatory signals. To date, there is no published information on apoptosis as it relates to exercise-induced muscle damage and inflammation.

CORTICOSTEROIDS AND TERMINATION OF INFLAMMATION

Cortisol and inflammatory cytokines influence each other in a feedback loop to control inflammation. Cortisol, the primary active corticosteroid, is considered a potent antiinflammatory, immunosuppressive hormone (85). The degree to which the pharmaceutical analogue of cortisol, hydrocortisone, suppresses production of cytokines is cytokine-specific; the most potent inflammatory cytokines, TNF-α and IL-1β, are the most affected, and IL-6 is the least affected (23).

The HPA axis can be affected by, and can affect, inflammatory cytokines. Both IL-1 and IL-6 are able to stimulate the hypothalamic- pituitary axis to produce ACTH and thus corticosteroid secretion by the adrenal cortex (20,86). Also, it appears that IL-6 may be capable of stimulating the adrenal cortex directly (86). This effect of IL-6 is consistent with its role in controlling inflammation, as this cytokine displays pro- and antiinflammatory properties.

The greatest neutrophilia is often measured a few hours after exercise (4,42,45). This delayed portion of the biphasic neutrophil response is generally considered to be a function of cortisol-induced release of neutrophils from the bone marrow (42). At least two investigations have measured a delayed neutrophilia in the absence of increased cortisol, however (45,87). This suggests that other factors, possibly certain colony-stimulating factors, may be involved in delayed neutrophilia.

PROPOSED SEQUENCE OF EXERCISE-INDUCED ACUTE INFLAMMATION

The following is a simplified proposed sequence of events involved in local initiation, systemic amplification, and subsequent resolution of the acute inflammatory response, keeping in mind that there is an extensive amount of redundancy and pleiotropic activity (Fig. 27–1). The same number assignment to successive list items implies a similarity in temporal sequence.

1. Muscle injury, from EMA or ischemic/reperfusion injury (local).
2. Activation of resident macrophages by some injury-related factor (local).

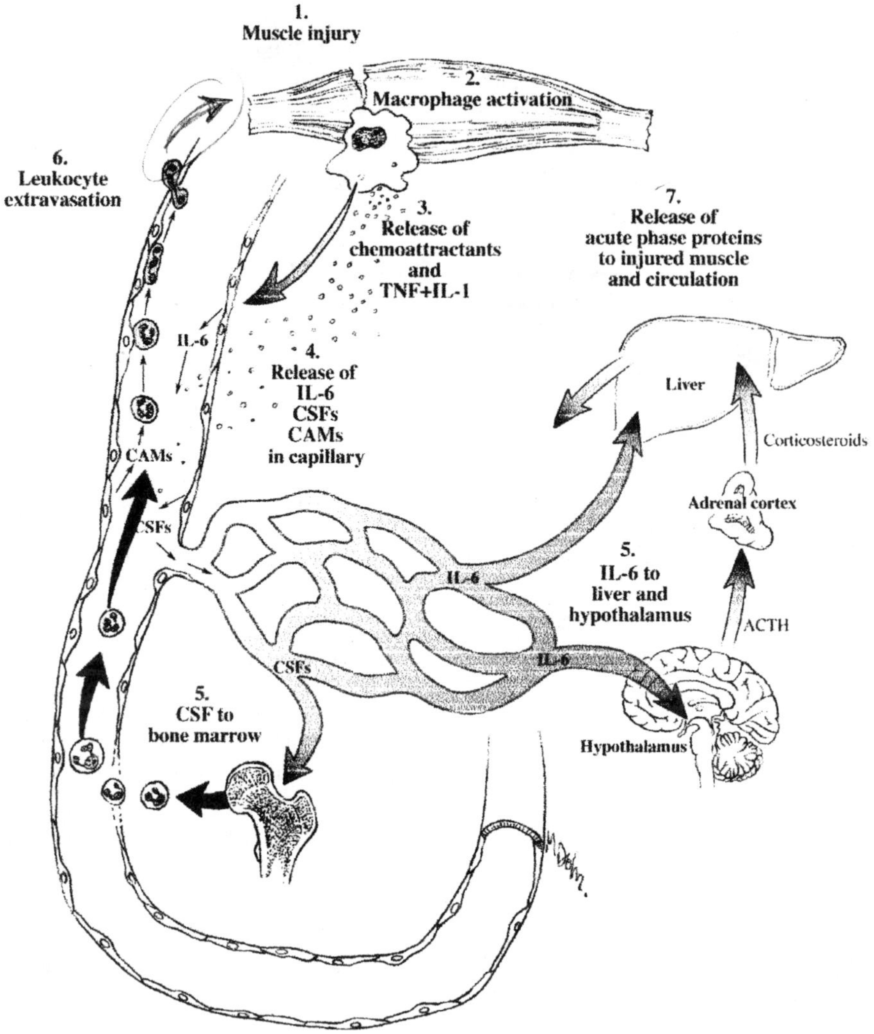

FIG. 27–1. Proposed sequence of events in exercise-induced acute inflammation.

3. Release of cytokines, most likely IL-1β and TNF-α (local).
3. Synthesis of a variety of chemoattractant agents (local). Chemoattractants diffuse into the local post-capillary venules and activate adhesion molecules, resulting in firm adherence of leukocytes to the vessel wall. These agents will subsequently act to guide migrating leukocytes to injured cells (local).
4. Cytokines stimulate local endothelial cells to release IL-6, cell adhesion molecules, and colony-stimulating factors (local).
5. Colony-stimulating factors stimulate release/maturation of leukocytes from bone marrow (systemic).
5. Cytokines stimulate the liver to produce and release acute phase proteins (systemic).
5. Cytokines activate the HPA axis, resulting in release of corticosteroids (systemic).
6. Leukocytes migrate from the circulation into injured tissue (local).
7. Termination is a result of a combination of increased circulating levels of corticosteroids, the activity of certain APPs, the process of apoptosis, and inhibition of proinflammatory factors by molecules such as IL-4, IL-10, and IL-1 receptor antagonist (local and systemic).

QUESTIONING SOME "ANSWERS"

RICE therapy (rest, ice, compression, and elevation) is the recommended treatment for inflammation resulting from all sports-induced soft-tissue injuries (1). The main focus of RICE therapy is to limit swelling, since "the injured area cannot return to normal until swelling is gone" (88). It is recommended for injuries of any severity, although additional therapeutic modalities are suggested for more severe injury (88). It appears that physicians often view sports-related inflammation as a hindrance to athletic performance, assuming that inflammation is an uncontrolled process that, if not contained, may significantly delay recovery. Similarly, albeit to a lesser extent, eccentrically induced muscle damage induces an acute inflammatory response. A considerable amount of research has investigated the use of different modalities for reducing the inflammation and associated DOMS, with varied success (6).

It is a truism that the purpose of inflammation is to promote healing, an ability that from a survival perspective has served us well. The prevalence of RICE therapy begs the following questions: Should we interfere with inflammation? Is inflammation consistently excessive? Has it somehow resisted the finesse acquired by other generalized physiologic responses?

Acute inflammation may be regarded as a double-edged solution to injury. On the one hand, it promotes healing, and in its absence we have failed healing. However, there are aspects of the response that, if excessive, may indeed delay healing. The counterproductive aspect most frequently cited relates to the generation of reactive oxygen metabolites released by activated neutrophils, which invade the injured tissue. In the process of clearing away tissue debris, ROS may inadvertently dismantle healthy host tissue (43,47). Another aspect of inflammation that can become unruly involves the generation of an excess of chemotactic peptides at the site of injury, which induce synthesis of adherence receptors involved in capturing circulating leukocytes. Initially this results in a large efflux of neutrophils into the appropriate area. But then "stickiness" might continue to increase, and the adherent leukocytes remaining in the vessels block the lumen of the smaller vessels and finally cause thrombotic occlusion. This needs to be treated to prevent necrosis of normal tissue. Additionally, excessive production of cytokines can lead to tissue injury or death (89). So it appears that there might be overactive aspects of inflammation that needs to be be curtailed.

Is this excess always present? Probably not. It is generally believed that the inflammatory response is proportional to the stimulus. Anecdotal evidence suggests that with mild injury, healing or regeneration is adequate. Furthermore, research now suggests that there might be overcompensation related to healing, which is implicated in the process of soft tissue hypertrophy. As an injury becomes more extensive, however, it is possible that the amplification at each step is exacerbated, that the process is not contained, and so in this instance inflammation might best be curbed.

In reference to pain associated with injury, it is interesting to note that pain is not always present at the time of tissue injury, such as during execution of unaccustomed EMA (90). The experience of pain has important implications for survival, serving to guide the organism from harmful stimuli, supporting a broad repertoire of avoidance and escape responses. Since pain is generally regarded as a protective/survival mechanism, might the absence of pain at the time of injury serve as an indicator of the severity of the injury, with no pain signaling mild injury and requiring minimal interference? Research is needed to more conclusively answer these questions.

REFERENCES

1. Arnheim DA, Prentice WE. *Principles of athletic training,* 8th ed. Baltimore: Mosby Year Book, 1993:150–183.
2. Evans WJ, Meredith CN, Cannon JG, et al. Metabolic changes following eccentric exercise in trained and untrained men. *J Appl Physiol* 1986;61:1864–1868.
3. Camus G, Deby-Dupont G, Duchateau J, Deby C, Pincemailo J, Lamy M. Are similar inflammatory factors involved in strenuous exercise and spesis? *Intensive Care Med* 1994;20:602–610.
4. Pizza FX, Mitchell JB, Davis BH, Starling RD, Holtz RW, Bigelow N. Exercise-induced muscle damage: effect on circulating leukocyte and lymphocyte subsets. *Med Sci Sports Exerc* 1995;27: 363–370.
5. Smith LL. Acute inflammation: the underlying mechanism in delayed onset muscle soreness? *Med Sci Sports Exerc* 1991;23: 542–551.
6. Armstrong RB. Initial events in exercise-induced muscular injury. *Med Sci Sports Exerc* 1990;22:429–435.
7. Appell H-J, Soares JMC, Duarte JAR. Exercise, muscle damage and fatigue. *Sports Med* 1992;13:108–115.
8. MacIntyre DL, Reid WD, McKenzie DC. Delayed muscle soreness. The inflammatory response to muscle injury and its clinical implications. *Sports Med* 1995;20:24–40.
9. Fridén J, Sjostrom M, Ekblom B. Myofibrillar damage following intense eccentric exercise in man. *Int J Sports Med* 1983;4:170–176.
10. Morgan DL. New insights into the behavior of muscle during active lengthening. *Biophys J* 1990;57:209–231.
11. Ebbeling CB, Clarkson PM. Exercise-induced muscle damage and adaptation. *Sports Med* 1989;7:207–234.
12. Armstrong RB, Warren GL, Warren JA. Mechanisms of exercise-induced muscle fiber injury. *Sports Med* 1991;12:184–207.
13. Troyer-Caudel J. Reperfusion injury. *J Vasc Nurs* 1993:11:76–79.
14. Sabido F, Milazzo VJ, Hobson RW 2nd, Duran WN. Skeletal muscle ischemia-reperfusion injury: a review of endothelial cell-leukocyte interactions. *J Invest Surg* 1994;7:39–47.
15. Authier B, Albramd JP, Decorps M, Reutenauer H, Rossi A. Disruption of muscle energy metabolism due to intense ischaemic exercise: a 31P NMR study in rats. *Physiol Chem Phys Med NMR* 1987;19:83–93.
16. Rubin BB, Romaschin A, Walker PM, Gute DC, Korthuis RJ. Mechanisms of postischemic injury in skeletal muscle: intervention strategies. *J Appl Physiol* 1996;80:369–387
17. Gleeson M, Almey J, Brooks S, Cave R, Lewis A, Griffiths H. Haematological and acute-phase responses associated with delayed-onset muscle soreness in humans. *Eur J Appl Physiol* 1995;71:137–42.
18. Rhind SG, Shek PN, Shephard RJ. The impact of exercise on cytokines and receptor expression. *Exp Immunol Rev* 1995;1: 97–148.
19. Mastorakos G, Chrousos GP, Weber JS. Recombinant interleukin-6 activates the hypothalamic-pituitary-adrenal axis in humans. *J Clin Endocrinol Metab* 1993;77:1690– 1694.
20. Baumann H, Gauldie J. The acute phase response. *Immunol Today* 1994;15:74–80.
21. Dinarello CA. Interleukin-1 and interleukin-1 antagonism. *Blood* 1991;77:1627–1652.
22. Shephard RJ, Rhind S, Shek PN. Exercise and training: influences on cytotoxicity, interleukin-1, interleukin-2 and receptor structures. *Int J Sports Med* 1994;15(suppl):S154–S166.
23. DeRijk R, Michelson D, Karp B, et al. Exercise and circadian rhythm-induced variations in plasma cortisol differentially regulate interleukin-1β (IL-1β), IL-6, and tumor necrosis factor-alpha

(TNF-alpha) production in humans: high sensitivity of TNF alpha and resistance of IL-6. *J Clin Endocrinol Metab* 1997;82:2182–2191.

24. Liao J, Keiser JA, Scales WE, Kunkel SL, Kluger MJ. Role of epinephrine in TNF and IL-6 production from isolated perfused rat liver. *Am J Physiol* 1995;268:R869–R901.
25. Billiar TR, Curran RD, Williams DL, Kispert PG. Liver nonparenchymal cells are stimulated to provide interleukin 6 for induction of the hepatic acute-phase response in endotoxemia but not in remote localized inflammation. *Arch Surg* 1992;127:31–36.
26. Portanova JP, Zhang Y, Anderson GD, et al. Selective neutralization of prostaglandin E2 blocks inflammation, hyperalgesia, and interleukin 6 production in vivo. *J Exp Med* 1996;184:883–891.
27. Koj A, Guzdek A. Modified proteins as possible signals in the acute phase response. *Ann NY Acad Sci* 1995;762:108–119.
28. Cannon JG, Fielding RA, Fiatarone MA, Orencole SF, Dinarello CA, Evans WJ. Increased interleukin 1β in human skeletal muscle after exercise. *Am J Physiol* 1989;257:R451–R455.
29. Rohde T, MacLean DA, Richter EA, Kiens B, Pedersen BK. Prolonged submaximal eccentric exercise is associated with increased levels of plasma IL-6. *Am J Physiol* 1997;273:E85–E91.
30. Smith JA, Telford RD, Baker MS, Hapel AJ, Weidemann MJ. Cytokine immunoreactivity in plasma does not change after moderate endurance exercise. *J Appl Physiol* 1992;73:1396– 1401.
31. Papanicolaou DA, Petrides, Tsigos C, et al. Exercise stimulates interleukin-6 secretion: inhibition by glucocorticoids and correlation with catecholamines. *Am J Physiol* 1996;271:E601–E605.
32. Nehlsen-Cannarella SL, Fagoaga OR, Nieman DC, et al. Carbohydrate and the cytokine response to 2.5 h of running. *J Appl Physiol* 1997;82:1662–1667.
33. Bruunsgaard H, Galbo H, Halkjýr-Kristensen J, Johansen TL, MacLean DA, Pedersen BK. Exercise-induced increase in serum interleukin-6 in humans is related to muscle damage. *J Physiol* 1997;499:833–841.
34. Rohde T, MacLean DA, Richter EA, Kiens B, Pedersen BK. Prolonged submaximal eccentric exercise is associated with increased levels of plasma IL-6. *Am J Physiol* 1997;273:E85–E91.
35. Hellsten Y, Frandsen U, Orthenblad N, Sjødin B, Richter EA. Xanthine oxidase in human skeletal muscle following eccentric exercise: a role in inflammation. *J Physiol* 1997; 498:239– 248.
36. Rogers MA, Stull GA, Apple FS. Creatine kinase isoenzyme activities in men and women following a marathon race. *Med Sci Sports Exerc* 1985;17:679–682.
37. Nosaka K, Clarkson PM, Apple FS. Time course of serum protein changes after strenuous exercise of the forearm flexors. *J Lab Clin Med* 1992;119:183–188.
38. Hannum CH, Wilcox CJ, Arend WP, et al. Interleukin-1 receptor antagonist activity a human interleukin-1 inhibitor. *Nature* 1990;343:336–340.
39. Sugiyama E, Kuroda A, Taki H, et al. Interleukin 10 cooperates with interleukin 4 to suppress inflammatory cytokine production by freshly prepared adherent rheumatoid synovial cells. *J Rheumatol* 1995;22:2020–2026.
40. Howard M, O'Garra A, Ishida H, de Waal A, Malefyt R, de Vries J. Biological properties of IL-10. *J Clin Immunol* 1992;12:239–247.
41. Drenth JPH, van Uum SHM, van Deuren M, Pesman GJ, van der ven-Jongekrijg J, van der Meer JWM. Endurance run increases circulating IL-6 and IL-1ra but down regulates ex vivo TNF-alpha and IL-1β production. *J Appl Physiol* 1995;79:1497–1503.
42. Pyne DB. Regulation of neutropil function during exercise. *Sports Med* 1994;17:245–258.
43. Weiss SJ. Tissue destruction by neutrophils. *N Engl J Med* 1989; 320:365–376.
44. Severs Y, Brenner I, Shek PN, Shephard RJ. Effects of heat and intermittent exercise on leukocyte and sub-population cell counts. *Eur J Appl Physiol* 1996;74:234–245.
45. Smith LL, McCammon M, Smith S, Chamness M, Israel RG, O'Brien KF. White blood cell response to uphill walking and downhill jogging at similar metabolic loads. *Eur J Appl Physiol* 1989;58:833–837.
46. Fielding RA, Manfredi TJ, Ding W, Fiatarone MA, Evans WJ, Cannon JG. Acute phase response in exercise III. Neutrophil and IL-1β accumulation in skeletal muscle. *Am J Physiol* 1993;265: R166–R172.
47. Ryan GB, Majno G. Acute inflammation. *Am J Pathol* 1977;86: 185–284.
48. Gabriel H, Urhausen A, Kindermann W. Mobilization of circulating leucocyte and lymphocyte subpopulations during and after short, anaerobic exercise. *Eur J Appl Physiol* 1992;65:164–170.
49. Nieman DC, Berk LS, Simpson-Westerberg M, et al. Effects of long-endurance running on immune system parameters and lymphocyte function in experienced marathoners. *Int J Sports Med* 1989;10:317–323.
50. Suzuki K, Sato H, Kikuchi T, et al. Capacity of circulating neutrophils after exhaustive exercise. *J Appl Physiol* 1996;81:1213– 1222.
51. Round JM, Jones DA, Cambridge G. Cellular infiltrates in human skeletal muscle: exercise induced damage as a model for inflammatory muscle disease? *J Neurol Sci* 1987;82:1–11.
52. Hikida RS, Staron RS, Hagerman FC, Sherman WM, Costill DL. Muscle fiber necrosis associated with human marathon runners. *J Neurol Sci* 1983;59:185–203.
53. Faulkner JA, Brooks SV, Opiteck JA. Injury to skeletal muscle fibres during contractions: conditions of occurrence and prevention. *Phys Ther* 1993;73:911–921.
54. Rincón EO. Physiology and biochemistry: influence of exercise on phagocytosis. *Int J Sports Med* 1994;15:S172–S178.
55. Cassimeres, Lzigmond SH. Chemoattractant stimulation of polymorphonuclear leukocyte locomotion. *Semin Cell Biol* 1990;1: 125–134.
56. Haahr PM, Pedersen BK, Fomsgaard A, et al. Effect of physical exercise in vitro production of interleukin 1, interleukin 6, tumour necrosis factor-alpha, interleukin 2 and interferon-gamma. *Int J Sports Med* 1991;12:223–227.
57. Lewicki R, Tchórzewski H, Majewska E, Nowak Z, Baj Z. Effect of maximal physical exercise on T-lymphocyte subpopulations and on interleukin 1 (IL-1) and interleukin 2 (IL-2) production in vitro. *Int J Sports Med* 1988;9:114–117.
58. Weinstock C, König D, Harnischmacher R, Keul J, Berg A, Northoff H. Effect of exhaustive exercise stress on the cytokine response. *Med Sci Sports Exerc* 1997;29:345–354.
59. Gabriel H, Urhausen A, Brechtel L, Müller, Kindermann W. Alterations of regular and mature monocytes are distinct, and dependent of intensity and duration of exercise. *Eur J Appl Physiol* 1994;69:179–181.
60. Moyna NM, Acker GR, Fulton JR, et al. Lymphocyte function and cytokine production during incremental exercise in active and sedentary males and females. *Int J Sports Med* 1996;17:585–591.
61. Murphy PM. Blood, sweat, and chemotactic cytokines. *J Leukoc Biol* 1995;57:438–439.
62. Collins T. Adhesion molecules in leukocyte emigration. *Sci Am Sci Med* 1995;12:28–37.
63. Ortega E, Forner MA, Barriga C. Exercise-induced stimulation of murine macrophage chemotaxis: role of corticosterone and prolactin as mediators. *J Physiol* 1997;498:729–734.
64. Elangbam CS, Qualls CW Jr, Dahlgren RR. Cell adhesion molecules—update. *Vet Pathol* 1997;34:61–73.
65. Butcher EC. Leukocyte endothelial cell recognition. *Cell* 1990; 67:1033–1036.
66. Pober J. Cytokines and endothelial cell biology. *Physiol Rev* 1990; 70:427–451.
67. Nehlsen-Cannarella S, Fagoaga O, Foltz J, Grindle S, Hisey C, Thorpe R. Fighting fleeing and having fun: the immunology of physical activity. *Int J Sports Med* 1997;18:S8– S21.
68. Gabriel H, Brechtel L, Urhausen A, Kindermann W. Recruitment and recirculation of leukocytes after an ultramarathon run: preferential homing of cells expressing high levels of adhesion molecule LFA-1. *Int J Sports Med* 1994;15:S148–153.
69. Kurokawa Y, Shinkai S, Torii J, Hino S, Shek PN. Exercise-induced changes in the expression of surface adhesion molecules on circulating granulocytes and lymphocyte populations. *Eur J Appl Physiol* 1995;71:245–252.
70. Miles MP, Leach SK, Kraemer WJ, Dohi K, Bush JA, Mastro AM. Leukocyte adhesion molecule expression during intense resistance exercise. *J Appl Physiol* 1998;84:1604–1609.
71. Smith LL, Anwar A, Fragen M, Rananto CR, Johnson RL, Holbert D. Cytokines and cell adhesion molecules associated with eccentric muscle contractions. *(In review)*.

72. Baum M, Liesen H, Enneper J. Leukocytes, lymphocytes, activation parameters and cell adhesion molecules in middle-distance runners under different training conditions. *Int J Sports Med* 1994;15;S122–126.
73. Fleck CM, Colley AW, Goode AW, Muller BR, Myers APP. Early time course of the acute phase protein in man. *J Clin Pathol* 1983;36:203–207.
74. Weight LM, Alexander D, Jacobs P. Strenuous exercise: analogous to the acute-phase response? *Clin Sci* 1991;81:677–683.
75. Dufaux B, Hoffken K, Hollman W. Acute phase proteins and immune complexes during several days of severe physical exercise. In: Knuttgen GH, Vogel JA, Poortsmans J, eds. *Biochemistry of exercise.* International Series on Sport Sciences, vol 13. Champaigne, IL: Human Kinetics, n.d.
76. Strachan AF, Noakes TD, Kotzenberg G, Nel AE, deBeer FC. C-reactive protein concentrations during long distance running. *Br Med J (Clin Res Ed)* 1984;289:1249–1251.
77. Taylor C, Rogers G, Goodman C, et al. Hematologic, iron-related, and acute-phase protein responses to sustained strenuous exercise. *J Appl Physiol* 1987;62:464–469.
78. Cohen JJ. Apoptosis. *Immunol Today* 1993;14:126–130.
79. Desmouliere A, Badid C, Bochaton-Piallat M, Gabbiani G. Apoptosis during wound healing, fibrocontractive diseases and vascular wall injury. *Int J Biochem Cell Biol* 1997;29:19–30.
80. Squier MK, Sehnert AJ, Cohen JJ. Apoptosis in leukocytes. *J Leukoc Biol* 1995;57:2–10.
81. Ren Y, Savill J. Proinflammatory cytokines potentiate thrombospondin-mediated phagocytosis on neutrophils undergoing apoptosis. *J Immunol* 1995;154:2366–74.
82. Afford SC, Pongracy J, Stockley RA, Crocker J, Burnett D. The induction by human interleukin-6 of apoptosis in the promonocytic cell line U937 and human neutrophils. *J Biol Chem* 1992; 267:21612–21616.
83. Brach MA, de Vos S, Gruss HJ, Hermann F. Prolongation of survival of human polymorphonuclear neutrophils by granulocyte-macrophage colony-stimulating factor is caused by inhibition of programmed cell death. *Blood* 1992;80:2920–2924.
84. Haslett C. Resolution of acute inflammation and the role of apoptosis in the tissue fate of granulocytes. *Clin Sci* 1992;83: 639–648.
85. Weicker H, Werle E. Interaction between hormones and the immune system. *Int J Sports Med* 1991;12:S30–S37.
86. Turnbull AV, Dow RC, Hopkins SJ, White A, Fink G, Rothwell NJ. Mechanisms of activation of the pituitary-adrenal axis by tissue injury in the rat. *Psychoneuroendocrinology* 1994;19: 165–178.
87. Shinkai S, Watanabe S, Asai H, Shek PN. Cortisol response to exercise and post-exercise suppression of blood lymphocyte subset counts. *Int J Sports Med* 1996;17:597–603.
88. Baumert PW. Acute inflammation after injury. *Postgrad Med* 1995;97:35–47.
89. Baxter CR. Management of burn wounds. *Dermatol Clin* 1993; 11:709–714.
90. Newham DJ, Jones DA, Clarkson PM. Repeated high-force eccentric exercise: effects on muscle pain and damage. *J Appl Physiol* 1987;63:1381–1386.

Exercise and Sport Science,
edited by William E. Garrett, Jr., and Donald T. Kirkendall.
Lippincott Williams & Wilkins, Philadelphia © 2000.

CHAPTER 28

Fluids and Electrolytes During Exercise

Ronald J. Maughan, Susan M. Shirreffs, and John B. Leiper

Water is the largest single component of the human body, accounting for about 60% of body mass in the average adult. It also has a high turnover rate; in extreme situations, as much as 25% of the total body water may be exchanged in a single day. If the body water content is reduced by as little as 1% to 2%, however, some aspects of physiologic function are impaired, and serious incapacity occurs when the body water deficit reaches about 10%. This indicates the need for a tight regulation of fluid balance, and—because electrolyte balance is intimately associated with water balance—for the regulation of the intake, distribution, and excretion of the major electrolytes.

Many factors, including a number of disease processes, have a profound influence on the body's fluid and electrolyte balance. For the healthy individual, however, the stress of physical exercise, especially when undertaken in a hot environment, poses the greatest challenge to homeostasis that is likely to be encountered. Heat illness, which may be fatal, is by no means uncommon when physically demanding events take place in warm weather (1). The rise in body temperature that accompanies exercise in the heat can be attenuated by sweating, but large sweat losses result in hypohydration and loss of electrolytes, which may also have serious consequences. There are many military, industrial, and occupational situations that call for men and women to perform hard physical work at extremes of environmental conditions, but the athlete engaged in training or competition is most likely to face extreme conditions on a regular basis. In environments with a combination of high heat and humidity, working capacity is compromised, but the risk to health and well-being is a more serious concern. It has been clearly shown that the same exercise undertaken in different environmental temperatures can be sustained for less time when the environmental temperature is warm (Fig. 28–1). The early onset of fatigue when exercise is undertaken in these conditions may serve to prevent more serious consequences.

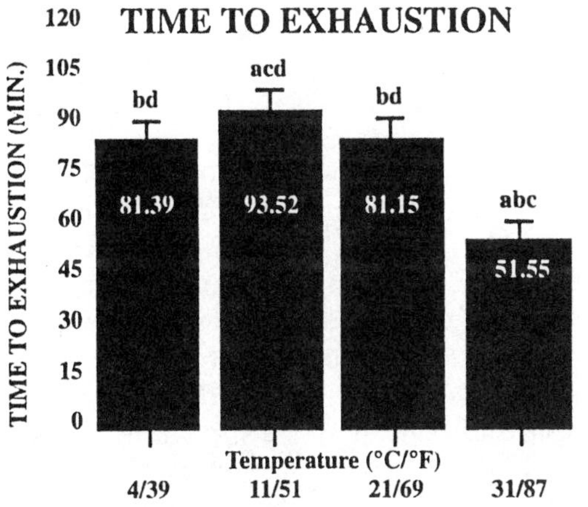

FIG. 28–1. Exercise time to exhaustion under four environmental conditions. (From ref. 78.)

TEMPERATURE REGULATION IN EXERCISE

The catabolic and synthetic reactions involved in metabolism are able to conserve only about 25% of the available energy in stored or ingested fuel substrates. The remainder appears as heat, and this apparent inefficiency is essential to ensure the directionality of these reactions. In homeothermic organisms, this metabolic heat is important in helping to maintain body temperature at an appropriate level, although the resting rate of heat production is rather low.

There are several ways of expressing metabolic rate; in exercise studies it is usual to refer to the oxygen

R. J. Maughan, S. M. Shirreffs, and J. B. Leiper: Department of Biomedical Sciences, University of Aberdeen, Foresterhill, Aberdeen, Scotland.

consumption ($\dot{V}O_2$), which may be expressed in absolute terms (L/min) or related to body mass (mL/kg/min). The typical oxygen consumption of humans at rest is about 4 mL/kg/min, or about 250 to 300 mL/min. When considering thermal balance, however, it is more useful to express the metabolic rate in terms of energy turnover; in this way, the resting metabolic rate is about 60 W.

During exercise, the metabolic rate increases in proportion to the energy demand; in simple locomotor activities such as walking, swimming, or cycling, the energy demand is a function (linear at low speeds, but exponential at higher speeds) of the rate of movement. In most sports situations, as in most daily activities, the exercise intensity is not constant but consists of intermittent activity of varying intensity and duration. In walking or running, where the body mass is moved against gravity at each step, body mass and speed are the two principal determinants of the energy cost, with air resistance becoming a factor at high speeds. The metabolic rate that can be sustained during an event like a 10-km race or a marathon (42.2 km) is determined primarily by the cardiovascular capacity and the availability of substrate, and these issues are covered elsewhere in this volume. Elite athletes can sustain rates of heat production in the order of 1200 W for a little over 2 hours, which is the time it takes to complete a marathon. To prevent a catastrophic rise in body temperature, the rate of heat loss from the body must be increased to match the increased rate of heat production.

Taking the heat capacity of human tissue to be 3.47 kJ/°C/kg, and assuming a body mass of 65 kg, a rate of heat production of 1200 W would cause body temperature to rise by 1°C approximately every 3 minutes, and the runner would exceed the upper limit of the tolerable core temperature within the first 10 to 15 minutes of the race. This does not happen, and core temperature seldom rises above about 40 to 41°C (2). Clearly, however, high running speeds can be maintained only if the capacity for heat dissipation is high.

Heat exchange with the environment occurs by conduction, convection, and radiation; in addition, evaporation of water from the respiratory tract and skin can cause heat to be lost from the body (3). Conduction is important only in water immersion, as air has a low thermal conductivity. Convection and radiation are effective methods of heat loss when the skin temperature is high and ambient temperature is low; under these conditions, convection and radiation will account for a major part of the heat loss even during intense exercise. As ambient temperature rises, however, the gradient from skin to environment falls, and above about 35°C the gradient is reversed so that heat is gained from the environment. Evaporation is therefore the only means of heat loss in hot weather conditions. Ignoring the negligible exchange via conduction, the avenues of heat exchange can be described as follows:

Convective loss: $C = 8.3(T_{sk} - T_a)v$ $\quad$ $W\,°C^{-1}\,m^{-2}$

Radiant loss: $R = 5.2(T_{sk} - T_{mrt})$ $\quad$ $W\,°C^{-1}\,m^{-2}$

Evaporative loss: $E = 124(P_{sk} - P_a)v$ $\quad$ $W\,kPa^{-1}\,m^{-2}$

Where

T_{sk} = mean skin temperature (°C)

T_a = ambient temperature (°C)

T_{mrt} = mean radiant temperature (°C)

P_{sk} = mean skin water vapor pressure (kPa)

P_a = ambient water vapor pressure (kPa)

v = mean air velocity ($m \cdot s^{-1}$)

A high rate of evaporative heat loss is clearly essential when the rate of metabolic heat production is high and where there is little or no loss possible by other means. Although the potential for heat loss by evaporation of water from the skin is high, this will not be the case if the sweating rate is insufficient to wet the skin surface, or if the vapor pressure gradient between the skin and the environment is low. This latter situation will arise if the skin temperature is low or if the ambient water vapor pressure is high; clothing that restricts airflow will also restrict the evaporation of water from the skin surface. A large body surface area and a high rate of air movement over the body surface are also factors that will have a major impact on evaporative heat loss, but these same factors will also promote heat gain by convection when the ambient temperature is higher than skin temperature (3). This may have particular implications for children involved in games or sports taking place in the summer, as their high surface area to volume ratio will impose a large heat stress.

The ability of athletes to complete events such as the marathon, even in adverse climatic conditions, with relatively little change in body temperature indicates that the thermoregulatory system is normally able to dissipate the associated heat load (1). High rates of evaporation require high rates of sweat secretion onto the skin surface, and the price to be paid for the maintenance of core temperature is a progressive loss of water and electrolytes in sweat.

SWEATING: WATER AND ELECTROLYTE LOSSES

Evaporation of 1 L of water from the skin will remove about 2.4 MJ (580 kcal) of heat from the body; variations in electrolyte content within the normal range of sweat composition have a small effect on the latent heat of vaporization, but the effect may become significant as sweat evaporates and the concentration of salt left behind on the skin surface rises over time. In a 2-hour and 30-minute marathon, for a runner with a body mass of 70 kg, to balance the rate of metabolic heat production by evaporative loss alone would require sweat to be evaporated from the skin at a rate of about 1.6 L/h; at such high sweat rates, an appreciable fraction of the sweat secreted will drip from the skin without evaporating, and a sweat secretion rate of about 2 L/h is likely to be necessary to achieve this rate of evaporative heat loss. This is possible, but it would result in the loss of 5 L of body water, corresponding to a loss of more than 7% of body weight for a 70-kg runner. Even in cool conditions, sweat losses may be high when the exercise intensity is high or the duration long; in a marathon held on a cool (12°C) day, mean sweat losses measured on 59 male runners were estimated to be approximately 3.5 L, with a large interindividual variability, even when the running speed was the same (2). In warmer environments, sweat losses can be substantially greater, causing a reduction of as much as 8% in body mass during a marathon (4).

Some water will also be lost by evaporation from the respiratory tract, and this will also contribute to heat dissipation, though this mechanism is much less important in humans than it is in animals such as the dog, which may reflect the limited evaporative capacity resulting from a thick coat of body hair. During hard exercise in a hot, dry environment, respiratory water loss can be significant (5), even though it is not generally considered to be a major heat loss mechanism in humans. The rise of 2 to 3°C in body temperature that normally occurs during marathon running means that some of the heat produced is stored, but the effect on heat balance is minimal; for a 70-kg runner a rise in mean body temperature of 3°C—about the maximum tolerable increase—would reduce the total requirement for evaporation of sweat by less than 300 mL.

The sweat that is secreted onto the skin contains a wide variety of organic and inorganic solutes, and significant losses from the body of some of these components will occur when large volumes of sweat are produced. The electrolyte composition of sweat is variable, and the concentration of individual electrolytes as well as the total sweat volume will influence the extent of losses. The normal concentration ranges for the main ionic components of sweat are shown in Table 28–1, along with their plasma and intracellular concentrations for comparison. A number of factors contribute to the variability in the composition of sweat; methodologic problems in the collection procedure, including evaporative loss, incomplete collection, and contamination with skin cells, account for at least part of the variability, but there is also a large biologic variability.

The sweat composition not only varies among individuals, but it can also vary within the same individual depending on the rate of sweating, the level of fitness, and the state of heat acclimation (3). In response to a standard heat stress, the sweat rate increases with training and in response to acclimation, and the electrolyte content decreases; there is also a redistribution of sweating, with a greater sweat rate on the limbs and relatively less on the trunk. These adaptations are generally considered to allow improved thermoregulation while conserving electrolytes, particularly sodium. An advantage of decreasing the sodium loss is a disproportionate loss of fluid from the intracellular space, thus helping to maintain plasma volume (6). There are, however, some puzzling aspects; where the sweat rate is sufficient to keep the skin wet, further increases in the sweat rate will increase the amount of water that drips from the skin without evaporation but will not further increase the rate of evaporative heat loss.

In spite of the variations that do occur, the major electrolytes in sweat, as in the extracellular fluid, are sodium and chloride (see Table 28–1), although the sweat concentrations of these ions are invariably lower than those in plasma. Contrary to what might be expected, Costill (4) reported an increased concentration of sodium and chloride in sweat content with increased flow; this was attributed to a reduced opportunity for reabsorption in the sweat duct because of the more

TABLE 28–1. *Concentration (mmol/L) of the major electrolytes in sweat, plasma, and intracellular water*

	Sweat	Plasma	Intracellular Water
Sodium	20–80	130–155	10
Potassium	4–8	3.2–5.5	150
Calcium	0–1	2.1–2.9	0
Magnesium	<0.2	0.7–1.5	15
Chloride	20–60	96–110	8
Bicarbonate	0–35	23–28	10
Phosphate	0.1–0.2	0.7–1.6	65
Sulfate	0.1–2.0	0.3–0.9	10

Note: These values are taken from a variety of sources but are based primarily on those reported by Pitts (79), Lentner (80), and Schmidt and Thews (81).

rapid transit through the duct. Verde and colleagues (7), however, found that the sweat concentration of these ions was unrelated to the sweat flow rate. Acclimation studies have shown that elevated sweating rates are accompanied by a decrease in the concentration of sodium and chloride in sweat (8,9) in spite of the increased flow rate. The potassium content of sweat appears to be relatively unaffected by the sweat rate, and the magnesium content is also unchanged or perhaps decreases slightly (see ref. 10 for review). These apparently conflicting results demonstrate some of the difficulties in interpreting the literature in this area. Differences between studies may be due to differences in the training status and degree of acclimation of the subjects used, as well as difference in methodology; some studies have used whole-body wash-down techniques to collect sweat, whereas others have examined local sweating responses using ventilated capsules or collection bags. There may be differences between the composition of sweat from a specific region, such as the hand and forearm, and the whole-body sweat. The use of improved sweat collection techniques will begin to resolve these issues (11).

Because sweat is hypotonic with respect to body fluids, the effect of prolonged sweating is to increase the plasma osmolality, which may have a significant effect on the ability to maintain body temperature. A direct relationship between plasma osmolality and body temperature has been demonstrated during exercise (12,13). Hyperosmolality of plasma, induced prior to exercise, has been shown to result in a decreased thermoregulatory effector response; the threshold for sweating is elevated and the cutaneous vasodilator response is reduced (14). In short-term (30-minute) exercise, however, the cardiovascular and thermoregulatory response appears to be independent of changes in osmolality induced during the exercise period (15). The changes in the concentration of individual electrolytes are more variable, but an increase in the plasma sodium and chloride concentrations is generally observed in response to both running and cycling exercise. Exceptions to this are rare and occur only when excessively large volumes of drinks low in electrolytes are consumed over long time periods; these situations are discussed further, below.

There have been some reports of differences in sweating function and in sweat composition between men and women (see ref. 16 for review), but it is not altogether clear to what extent this apparent sex difference can be accounted for by differences in training and acclimation status. There are some differences between children and adults in the sweating response to exercise and in sweat composition. The sweating capacity of children is low, when expressed per unit surface area, and the sweat electrolyte content is low relative to that of adults (17), but the need for fluid and electrolyte replacement is no less important than in adults. Indeed, in view of the evidence that core temperature increases to a greater extent in children than in adults at a given level of dehydration, the need for fluid replacement may well be greater in children (18).

An extensive review of the literature on sweat composition and sweat electrolyte losses has been completed by Brouns and colleagues (16), who suggested that the upper limit for replacement during exercise of electrolytes lost in sweat can be determined in relation to the losses. It does appear, however, that the variation between individuals and between conditions may be so large as to preclude any meaningful recommendations. It is also not clear that there is any good evidence to show benefits resulting from replacement during exercise of any electrolyte other than perhaps sodium.

SWEAT LOSS: EFFECTS ON EXERCISE PERFORMANCE

It is often reported that exercise performance is impaired when an individual is dehydrated by as little as 2% of body weight, and that losses in excess of 5% of body weight can decrease the capacity for work by about 30% (19). Prior dehydration will impair the capacity to perform high-intensity exercise as well as endurance activities (20,21). Nielsen and colleagues (20) showed that prolonged exercise, which resulted in a loss of fluid corresponding to 2.5% of body weight, resulted in a 45% fall in the capacity to perform high-intensity exercise. A fluid deficit of as little as 1.8% of body mass has recently been shown to impair exercise tolerance (22). It may be that even smaller fluid deficits can adversely affect performance in competitive sport, where the difference between winning and losing is vanishingly small, but that the laboratory methods used to assess performance are not sufficiently sensitive to detect small changes.

Fluid losses are distributed in varying proportions among the body fluid compartments—plasma, extracellular water, and intracellular water. The decrease in plasma volume that accompanies dehydration may be of particular importance in influencing an individual's work capacity; blood flow to the muscles must be maintained at a high level to supply oxygen and substrates, but a high blood flow to the skin is also required to convect heat to the body surface where it can be dissipated (23). When the ambient temperature is high and blood volume has been decreased by sweat loss during prolonged exercise, there may be difficulty in meeting the requirement for a high blood flow to both these tissues. In this situation, skin blood flow is likely to be compromised, allowing central venous pressure and muscle blood flow to be maintained but reducing heat loss and causing body temperature to rise (24).

These factors have been investigated by Montain and Coyle (25,26); their results clearly demonstrate that increases in core temperature and heart rate during prolonged exercise are graded according to the level of hypohydration achieved (25). They also showed, however, that the ingestion of fluid during exercise increases skin blood flow and therefore thermoregulatory capacity, independent of increases in the circulating blood volume (26). Plasma volume expansion using dextran/saline infusion was less effective in preventing a rise in core temperature than was the ingestion of sufficient volumes of a carbohydrate electrolyte drink to maintain plasma volume at a similar level.

CONTROL OF WATER AND ELECTROLYTE BALANCE

Role of the Kidneys

The excretion of some of the waste products of metabolism and the regulation of the body's water and electrolyte balance are the primary functions of the kidneys. Excess water or solute is excreted, and where there is a deficiency of water or electrolytes an attempt is made to conserve them until the balance is restored. Blood volume, plasma osmolality, and plasma sodium concentration seem to be the primary factors regulated. Under normal conditions, the osmolality of the extracellular fluid is maintained within narrow limits. As the major ion of the extracellular space is sodium, which accounts for about 50% of the total osmolality, maintenance of osmotic balance requires that both sodium and water intake and loss are closely coupled.

At rest, about 20% of the cardiac output goes to the two kidneys, and approximately 15% to 20% of the renal plasma flow is continuously filtered out by the glomeruli, resulting in the production of about 170 L of filtrate per day. Most (99% or more) of this is reabsorbed in the tubular system, leaving about 1 to 1.5 L to appear as urine. The volume of urine produced is determined primarily by the action of antidiuretic hormone (ADH), which regulates water reabsorption by increasing the permeability of the distal tubule of the nephron and the collecting duct to water. ADH is released from the posterior lobe of the pituitary in response to signals from the supraoptic nucleus of the hypothalamus; the main stimuli for release of ADH (which is normally present only in low concentrations) are an increased signal from the osmoreceptors located within the hypothalamus, and a decrease in blood volume (which is detected by low-pressure receptors in the atria and by high-pressure baroreceptors in the aortic arch and carotid sinus). An increased plasma angiotensin concentration will also stimulate ADH output.

The sodium concentration of the plasma is regulated by the reabsorption of sodium from the glomerular filtrate, with most of the reabsorption occurring in the proximal renal tubule. Several factors influence the extent to which reabsorption occurs; of particular importance is the action of aldosterone, which promotes sodium reabsorption in the distal tubules and enhances the excretion of potassium and hydrogen ions. Aldosterone is released from the kidney in response to a fall in the circulating sodium concentration or a rise in plasma potassium; aldosterone release is also stimulated by angiotensin, which is produced by the renin-angiotensin system in response to a decrease in the plasma sodium concentration. Angiotensin thus has a twofold action, on the release of aldosterone as well as ADH. Atrial natriuretic factor (ANF) is a peptide synthesized in and released from the heart in response to atrial distention. It increases the glomerular filtration rate and decreases sodium and water reabsorption, leading to an increased loss; this may be important in the regulation of extracellular volume, but it probably does not play a significant role during exercise. Regulation of the body's sodium balance has profound implications for fluid balance, as sodium salts account for more than 90% of the osmotic pressure of the extracellular fluid.

Loss of hypotonic fluid as sweat during prolonged exercise usually results in a fall in blood volume and an increased plasma osmolality; these changes in turn act as stimuli for the release of ADH (27). The plasma ADH concentration during exercise has been reported to increase as a function of the exercise intensity (28). Renal blood flow is also reduced in proportion to the exercise intensity and may be as low as 25% of the resting level during strenuous exercise (29). These factors combine to result in a decreased urine flow during, and usually for some time after, exercise (29). The volume of water conserved by this decreased urine flow during exercise is small, probably amounting to no more than 12 to 45 mL/h (30); compared with water losses in sweat, this volume is trivial.

Exercise normally results in a decrease in the renal excretion of sodium and an increased excretion of potassium, although the effect on potassium excretion is rather variable (30). These effects appear to be largely due to an increased rate of aldosterone production during exercise (29). Although the concentrations of sodium, and more especially of potassium, in the urine are generally high relative to the concentrations in extracellular fluid, the extent of total urinary electrolyte losses in most exercise situations is small.

Fluid Intake: Thirst

In humans, daily fluid intake in the form of food and drink is usually in excess of obligatory water loss, with renal excretion being the main mechanism regulating body water content (31). The ability of the kidneys to conserve water or electrolytes can only reduce the rate of loss, however; it cannot restore a deficit. It is the sensation of thirst, which underpins drinking behavior, that initiates the desire to drink and hence is important in the control of fluid intake and balance. While thirst appears to be a poor indicator of acute hydration status in humans, the overall stability of the total water volume of an individual indicates that the desire to drink is a powerful regulatory factor over the long term (32).

The requirement to drink, which is perceived as thirst, may not be directly involved with a physiologic need for water intake but may be initiated by habit, ritual, and taste, or the desire for nutrients, stimulants, or a warm or cooling effect. A number of the sensations associated with thirst are learned, with signals such as dryness of the mouth or throat inducing drinking, while distention of the stomach can stop ingestion before a fluid deficit has been restored. The underlying regulation of thirst is controlled separately by both the osmotic pressure and volume of the body fluids, however, and as such is regulated by the same mechanisms that affect water and solute reabsorption in the kidneys and control central blood pressure.

Areas of the hypothalamus and forebrain, which are collectively termed the thirst control centers, appear to play a key role in the regulation of both thirst and diuresis. Receptors in the thirst control centers respond directly to changes in osmolality, volemia, and blood pressure, while others are stimulated by the fluid balance hormones that also regulate renal excretion (33). These regions of the brain also receive afferent input from systemic receptors monitoring osmolality and circulating sodium concentration, and from alterations in blood volume and pressure. There may also be a direct neural link from the thirst control centers to the kidneys, which would allow a greater degree of integration between the control of fluid intake and excretion. Changes in the balance of neural activity in the thirst control centers regulated by the different monitoring inputs determine the relative sensations of thirst and satiety, and influence the degree of diuresis. Input from the higher centers of the brain, however, can override the basic biologic need for water to some extent and cause inappropriate drinking responses.

A rise of between 2% to 3% in plasma osmolality is sufficient to evoke a profound sensation of thirst coupled with an increase in the circulating concentration of ADH (34). The mechanisms that respond to changes in intravascular volume and pressure appear to be less sensitive than those that monitor plasma osmolality, with hypovolemic thirst being evident only following a 10% decrease in blood volume (31). As fairly large variations in blood volume and pressure occur during normal daily activity, this lack of sensitivity presumably prevents excessive activity of the volemic control mechanisms. Prolonged exercise, especially in the heat, is associated with a decrease in plasma volume and a tendency for an increase in plasma osmolality, but fluid intake during and immediately following exercise is often less than that required to restore normal hydration status (32). This appears to be due not to a lack of initiation of the drinking response but rather to a premature termination of the drinking response (35).

After developing a water deficit, the drinking response in humans usually consists of a period of rapid ingestion of more than 50% of the total intake followed by intermittent consumption of relatively small volumes of drink over a longer period (36). The initial alleviation of thirst occurs before significant amounts of the beverage have been absorbed and entered the body pools. Therefore, although decreasing osmolality and increasing extracellular volume promote a reduction in the perception of thirst, other preabsorptive factors also affect the volume of fluid ingested. Receptors in the mouth, esophagus, and stomach are thought to meter the volume of fluid ingested, while distention of the stomach tends to reduce the perception of thirst (38). These preabsorptive signals appear to be behavioral learned responses and may be subject to disruption in situations that are essentially novel to the individual. This may partly explain the inappropriate voluntary fluid intake in individuals exposed to an acute increase in environmental temperature or to exercise-induced dehydration.

FLUID AND ELECTROLYTE REPLACEMENT DURING EXERCISE

Limitations to Replacement

The ability to sustain a high rate of work output requires that an adequate supply of carbohydrate substrate be available to the working muscles; in addition to replacing water and electrolytes lost in sweat, drinks consumed during exercise should provide a source of carbohydrate fuel to supplement the body's limited stores. The composition of drinks that can most effectively meet these objectives has been the subject of much debate. Although it is a common belief among athletes that plain water is the best drink during exercise, the scientific evidence does not support this view. There is, however, no single formulation that will best meet the needs of all individuals in all situations.

Increasing the carbohydrate content of drinks will increase the amount of fuel that can be supplied, but it will tend to decrease the rate at which water can be made available (10). Where provision of water is the first priority, the carbohydrate content of drinks will be low, thus restricting the rate at which substrate is provided. The composition of drinks to be taken will thus be influenced by the relative importance of the need to supply fuel and water; this in turn depends on the intensity and duration of the exercise task, on the ambient temperature and humidity, and on the physiologic and biochemical characteristics of the individual athlete. Carbohydrate depletion will result in fatigue and a reduction in the exercise intensity that can be sustained, but it is not normally a life-threatening condition. Disturbances in fluid balance and temperature regulation have potentially more serious consequences, and it may be, therefore, that the emphasis for the majority of participants in endurance events should be on proper maintenance of fluid and electrolyte balance.

In spite of the definitive statement by the American College of Sports Medicine, in its 1984 position stand (38) on the prevention of thermal injuries in distance running, that cool water is the optimum fluid for ingestion during endurance exercise, some of the evidence presented above indicates that there may be good reasons for taking drinks containing added substrate and electrolytes; the emergence of new information has caused the most recent version of this position statement to recognize that plain water is not the best rehydration drink (39). In prolonged exercise, performance is improved by the addition of an energy source in the form of carbohydrate; the type of carbohydrate does not appear to be critical, and glucose, sucrose, and oligosaccharides have all been shown to be effective in improving endurance capacity. Some recent studies have suggested that long-chain glucose polymer solutions are more readily used by the muscles during exercise than are glucose or fructose solutions (40), but others have found no difference in the oxidation rates of ingested glucose or glucose polymer (41,42). Massicote and colleagues (41) also found that ingested fructose was less readily oxidized than glucose or glucose polymers. Fructose in high concentrations is best avoided on account of the risk of gastrointestinal upset. The argument advanced in favor of the ingestion of fructose during exercise, namely that it provides a readily available energy source but does not stimulate insulin release and consequent inhibition of fatty acid mobilization, is in any case not well founded; insulin secretion is suppressed during exercise.

The optimum concentration of sugar to be added to drinks will depend on individual circumstances. High-carbohydrate concentrations will delay gastric emptying, thus reducing the amount of fluid that is available for absorption; very high concentrations will result in secretion of water into the intestine and thus will actually increase the danger of dehydration (43). High sugar concentrations (>10%) may also result in gastrointestinal disturbances. Where there is a need to supply an energy source during exercise, however, increasing the sugar content of drinks will increase the delivery of carbohydrate to the site of absorption in the small intestine.

The available evidence indicates that the only electrolyte that should be added to drinks consumed during exercise is sodium, which is usually added in the form of sodium chloride, but which may also be added as sodium citrate or other salts. Sodium will stimulate sugar and water uptake in the small intestine and will help to maintain extracellular fluid volume (44). Most soft drinks of the cola or lemonade variety contain virtually no sodium (1 to 2 mmol/L); sports drinks commonly contain 10 to 25 mmol/L; oral rehydration solutions (ORS) intended for use in the treatment of diarrhea-induced dehydration have higher sodium concentrations, in the range of 30 to 90 mmol/L. A high sodium content, although it may stimulate jejunal absorption of glucose and water, tends to make drinks unpalatable, and it is important that drinks intended for ingestion during or after exercise should have a pleasant taste in order to stimulate consumption. Effective formulations for specialist sports drinks must strike a balance between the twin aims of efficacy and palatability.

In extreme endurance events lasting more than 3 to 4 hours, there may be advantages in adding sodium to drinks to avoid the danger of hyponatremia, which has been reported to occur when excessively large volumes of low-sodium drinks are taken (45). The fluid intakes of participants in endurance events are generally low, and a progressive fluid deficit is normally observed. It is recognized that failure to ingest an adequate fluid volume may lead to dehydration and heat illness in prolonged exercise when the ambient temperature is high. Accordingly, the advice given to participants in endurance events is that they should drink beyond the level dictated by thirst to ensure sufficient fluid intake to minimize the effects of dehydration. Many of the drinks consumed, whether plain water, soft drinks, or sports beverages, have little or no electrolyte content. Even among the carbohydrate-electrolyte drinks intended for consumption by sports participants during prolonged exercise, most have a low electrolyte content, with sodium concentrations typically in the range of 10 to 20 mmol/L. This is adequate in most situations, but it may not be so when sweat losses and fluid intakes are high.

Hyperthermia associated with dehydration and hypernatremia is relatively common in endurance events held in the heat, often affecting the less well prepared participants. However, it has become clear that a small number of individuals at the end of very prolonged events may be suffering from hyponatremia; this may be associated with either hyperhydration (19,45–47) or dehydration (48). The total number of reported cases is rather small, and the great majority of these have been associated with ultramarathon or prolonged triathlon events; there are few reports of cases of exercise-associated hyponatremia where the exercise duration is less than 4 hours. Noakes and colleagues (45) reported four cases of exercise-induced hyponatremia; race times were between 7 and 10 hours, and postrace serum sodium concentrations were between 115 and 125 mmol/L. Estimated fluid intakes were between 6 and 12 L and consisted of water or drinks containing low levels of electrolytes; estimated total sodium chloride intake during the race was 20 to 40 mmol. Frizell and colleagues (47) reported even more astonishing fluid intakes of 20 to 24 L of fluids (an intake of almost 2.5 L/h sustained for a period of many hours, which is in excess of the maximum gastric emptying rate that has been reported) with a mean sodium content of only 5 to 10 mmol/L in two runners who collapsed after an ultramarathon run and who were found to be hyponatremic (serum sodium concentration 118 to 123 mmol/L).

The dangers of ingestion of excessive volumes of fluid without adding salt has long been recognized in various industrial settings, including foundry workers and ships' stokers. Hyponatremia as a consequence of ingestion of large volumes of fluids with a low sodium content has also been recognized in resting individuals. Flear and colleagues (49) reported the case of a man who drank 9 L of beer, with a sodium content of only 1.5 mmol/L, in the space of 20 minutes; plasma sodium fell from 143 mmol/L before to 127 mmol/L after drinking, although the man appeared unaffected. In these cases, there is clearly a replacement of water in excess of losses with inadequate electrolyte replacement. Noakes (50,51) has suggested that in situations such as this, a significant amount of sodium may move into the volume of unabsorbed fluid in the intestinal lumen, thus resulting in hyponatremia. In competitors in the Hawaii ironman triathlon who have been found to be hyponatremic, however, dehydration has also been reported to be present (48). Fellmann and colleagues (52) reported a small but statistically significant fall in serum sodium concentration, from 141 to 137 mmol/L, in runners who completed a 24-hour run, but food and fluid intakes were neither controlled nor measured.

Some supplementation with sodium chloride in amounts beyond those normally found in sports drinks may be required in extremely prolonged events where large sweat losses can be expected and where it is possible to consume large volumes of fluid. It remains true, however, that electrolyte replacement during exercise is not a priority for most participants in most sporting events. Most collapsed runners will be found to be hypernatremic. Where immediate verification of a collapsed athlete's serum sodium concentration is not possible, it is probably safer to assume that this will be elevated, and intravenous fluid replacement may be warranted.

Early experimental evidence suggested that there is an advantage to taking chilled (4°C) drinks, as this accelerates gastric emptying and thus improves the availability of ingested fluids. The most recent evidence, however, suggests that the gastric-emptying rate of hot and cold beverages is not markedly different (44). In spite of this, there may be advantages in taking chilled drinks, as the palatability of most carbohydrate-electrolyte drinks is improved at low temperatures; this has the effect of stimulating consumption and helps the exercising athlete to feel better. Such effects on the athlete's sense of well-being cannot be ignored.

Cardiovascular, Metabolic, and Performance Effects

There are several potential benefits that can result from the inclusion of electrolytes in beverages used in association with exercise. Their inclusion tends to make the drinks more palatable when consumed by hyperthermic and dehydrated individuals. Adding sodium to drinks also helps maintain the thirst mechanism by preventing the fall in plasma sodium concentration and osmolality that would otherwise occur, thus promoting consumption. The addition of electrolytes, and in particular sodium, also stimulates the absorption of fluids in the small intestine, provided that glucose or another solute that is actively cotransported with sodium is also present. Finally, replacement of sweat sodium losses is also essential for postexercise rehydration.

Many of the published studies investigating the effects of fluid ingestion on exercise performance have used carbohydrate-electrolyte beverages, and therefore it has been difficult to separate the effects of water replacement and substrate provision. One study that did separate these drink components demonstrated an improved exercise performance when plain water was given, over and above that when no fluids were consumed (53), although there were further performance improvements when carbohydrate and electrolytes were also present (Table 28–2). A number of extensive reviews have addressed this issue (10,54–56). Generally, the studies in the literature have reported either no effect of fluid ingestion on exercise performance or a beneficial effect. There seems to be an lessened hyperthermia and cardiovascular drift during prolonged moderate intensity exercise (25,26,57), which is attributed to fluid replacement during the exercise. A better maintenance of blood glucose, which can be used by the exercising muscles with a consequent reduction in the need for mobilization of the limited liver glycogen reserves (58,59), appears to be the major benefit of carbohydrate consumption during exercise. The studies that have reported adverse effects of fluid ingestion on exercise performance have generally been studies in which the fluid ingestion has resulted in gastrointestinal disturbances (60).

One study, however, has attempted to distinguish between the effects of carbohydrate provision from the water replacement properties of a drink. Below and colleagues (61) required eight men to undertake the same cycle ergometer exercise on four separate occasions. After 50 minutes exercise at 80% of $\dot{V}O_2max$, a performance test at a higher exercise intensity (completion of set amount of work as quickly as possible) was completed; this test lasted approximately 10 minutes. On each of the four trials, a different beverage consumption protocol was followed during the 50 minutes of

TABLE 28–2. *Exercise times to exhaustion after consumption of water, an isotonic carbohydrate-electrolyte drink (200 mmol/L glucose, 35 mmol/L sodium), a hypotonic carbohydrate-electrolyte drink (90 mmol/L glucose, 60 mmol/L sodium), and with no drink consumption*

		Drink		
Time (min)	No drink	Water	Isotonic	Hypotonic
Median	80.7	93.1	107.4	110.3
Minimum	64.4	70.7	86.1	80.6
Maximum	133.3	166.6	195.0	139.1

exercise; nothing was consumed during the performance tests. The beverages were electrolyte-containing water in a large (1330-mL) and small (200-mL) volume and carbohydrate-electrolyte solutions (79 g) in the same large and small volumes; the electrolyte content of each beverage was the same and amounted to 619 mg (27 mmol) and 141 mg (3.6 mmol) of sodium and potassium, respectively. The results of the study indicated that performance was 6.5% better after consuming the large volume of fluid in comparison to the smaller volume, and it was 6.3% better after consuming carbohydrate-containing rather than carbohydrate-free beverages; the fluid and carbohydrate each independently improved performance and the two improvements were additive. The mechanism for the improvements in performance with the large fluid replacement versus the small fluid replacement was attributed to a lower heart rate and esophageal temperature when the large volume was consumed. The authors were unable, however, to identify the mechanism by which carbohydrate ingestion improved performance.

PREEXERCISE HYDRATION

Some degree of temporary hyperhydration appears to result when drinks with high-sodium concentrations (100 mmol/L) are ingested, but this does not seem likely to be beneficial for performance carried out in the heat on account of the high osmolality that ensues (14). An alternative strategy that has been the subject of interest has attempted to induce an expansion of the blood volume prior to exercise by the addition of glycerol to ingested fluids. Glycerol in high concentrations has little metabolic effect but exerts an osmotic action; although its distribution in the body water compartments is variable, glycerol will expand the extracellular space, and some of the water ingested with the glycerol will be retained rather than being lost in the urine (62). The elevated osmolality of the extracellular space will result in some degree of intracellular dehydration, and the implications of this are at present unknown (63). It might be expected, however, that the raised plasma osmolality will have negative consequences for thermoregulatory capacity (14,64), although the available evidence at present seems to indicate that this is not the case (65,66). The results of studies investigating the effects on exercise performance of glycerol feeding before or during exercise have shown mixed results; there have been some recent suggestions of improved performance after administration of glycerol and water prior to prolonged exercise (65), but some earlier work clearly indicated that it did not improve the capacity to perform prolonged exercise (63,67).

POSTEXERCISE REHYDRATION

Postexercise replacement of water and electrolyte losses may be of crucial importance when repeated bouts of exercise have to be performed; carbohydrate ingestion at this time is also important when the exercise has resulted in a significant reduction in the body's liver and muscle glycogen stores. The need for replacement of each of these will depend on the extent of the losses incurred during exercise, but will also be influenced by the time and nature of subsequent exercise bouts. Rapid rehydration may also be important in events where competition is by weight category. Competitors in events such as wrestling, boxing, and weightlifting frequently undergo acute thermal and exercise-induced dehydration to make weight. The practice of acute dehydration to make weight should be discouraged, as it reduces exercise performance even when some restoration of the deficit is achieved (68) and increases the risk of heat illness (1), but it will persist and there is a need to find ways to maximize rehydration in the time available.

In an early study in which a moderately severe dehydration (4% of body mass) was induced by heat exposure, fluid consumption over 3 hours in a volume equal to the sweat lost did not restore plasma volume or serum osmolality within 4 hours (69). Ingestion of a glucose-electrolyte solution, however, did result in greater restoration of plasma volume than did plain water; this was accompanied by a greater urine production in the water trial. Where the electrolyte content of drinks is the same, it appears that addition of carbohydrate (100 g/L) or carbonation has no effect on the restoration of plasma volume over a 4-hour period after sweat loss corresponding to approximately 4% of body weight (70).

Gonzalez-Alonso and colleagues (71) have shown that a dilute carbohydrate-electrolyte solution (60 g/L carbohydrate, 20 mmol/L Na^+, 3 mmol K^+) is more effective in promoting postexercise rehydration than either plain water or a low-electrolyte diet cola; the difference between the drinks was primarily a result of differences in the volume of urine produced; there was a suggestion in this study that the caffeine content of the diet cola may have exerted a negative effect because of its diuretic properties.

Ingestion of plain water in the postexercise period results in a rapid fall in the plasma sodium concentration and in plasma osmolality (72). These changes have the effect of reducing thirst and of stimulating urine output, and both of these will delay the rehydration process. In the study of Nose and colleagues (73), subjects exercised at low intensity in the heat for 90 to 110 minutes, inducing a mean dehydration of 2.3% of body mass, and then rested for 1 hour before beginning to drink. Plasma volume was not restored until after 60 minutes when plain water was ingested together with placebo (sucrose) capsules. When sodium chloride capsules were ingested with water to give a saline solution with an effective concentration of 0.45% (77 mmol/L), plasma volume was restored within 20 minutes. In the NaCl trial, voluntary fluid intake was higher and urine output was less; 71% of the water loss was retained within 3 hours compared with 51% in the plain water trial. The delayed rehydration in the water trial appeared to be a result of a loss of sodium, accompanied by water, in the urine caused by reduction in plasma renin activity and aldosterone levels (72).

A systematic evaluation of the effects of replacing a fixed volume of fluid with different sodium concentrations demonstrated that urine output over the few hours following ingestion was inversely related to the sodium content of the ingested fluid (74). In this study, subjects were dehydrated by intermittent exercise in the heat until 2% of body mass was lost, and then consumed a volume of fluid equivalent to 1.5 times the sweat loss; these drinks contained 0, 25, 50, or 100 mmol/L sodium.

These studies make it clear that rehydration after exercise can be achieved only if sodium as well as water is consumed. It might be suggested that rehydration drinks should have a sodium concentration similar to that of sweat, but since the sodium content of sweat varies widely no single formulation will meet this requirement for all individuals in all situations. The upper end of the normal range for sodium concentration (80 mmol/L), however, is similar to the sodium concentration of the ORS recommended by the World Health Organization for rehydration in cases of severe diarrhea (90 mmol/L). By contrast, the sodium content of most sports drinks is in the range of 10 to 30 mmol/L, and the most commonly consumed soft drinks contain virtually no sodium.

The need for sodium replacement stems from its role as the major ion in the extracellular fluid. The inclusion of potassium, the major cation in the intracellular space, should enhance the replacement of intracellular water after exercise and thus promote rehydration (6). The inclusion of potassium has been shown to be as effective as sodium in retaining water ingested after exercise-induced dehydration, in spite of the rather low levels of potassium lost in sweat. Addition of either ion significantly increased the fraction of the ingested fluid retained, over the postexercise period when consumed by subjects who had been moderately dehydrated by exercise in the heat (75). There was no additive effect of including both ions as would be expected if they acted independently on different body fluid compartments, but this may be the result of the rather small volume of fluid ingested and the difficulty in further reducing the urine output; to achieve an effective rehydration, not only should the composition of the fluid be considered, but also the volume ingested should be more than the sweat volume lost if hydration status is to be restored (76). The ingestion of the necessary electrolytes need not come from the beverage itself, however, and if solid food is consumed together with an adequate fluid volume (e.g.. with water or a soft drink), effective rehydration can ensue (77).

REFERENCES

1. Sutton JR. Clinical implications of fluid imbalance. In: Gisolfi CV, Lamb DR, eds. *Perspectives in exercise science and sports medicine, vol 3: Fluid homeostasis during exercise.* Carmel, IN: Brown & Benchmark, 1990:425–448.
2. Maughan RJ. Thermoregulation and fluid balance in marathon competition at low ambient temperature. *Int J Sports Med* 1985; 6:15–19.
3. Leithead CS, Lind AR. *Heat stress and heat disorders.* London: Casell, 1964.
4. Costill DL. Sweating: its composition and effects on body fluids. *Ann NY Acad Sci* 1977;301:160–174.
5. Mitchell JW, Nadel ER, Stolwijk JAJ. Respiratory weight losses during exercise. *J Appl Physiol* 1972;34:474–476.
6. Nadel ER, Mack GW, Nose H. Influence of fluid replacement beverages on body fluid homeostasis during exercise and recovery. In: Gisolfi CV, Lamb DR, eds. *Perspectives in exercise science and sports medicine, vol 3: fluid homeostasis during exercise.* Carmel, IN: Brown & Benchmark, 1990:181–205.
7. Verde T, Shephard RJ, Corey P, Moore R. Sweat composition in exercise and in heat. *J Appl Physiol* 1982;53:1540–1545.
8. Allan JR, Wilson CG. Influence of acclimatization on sweat sodium secretion. *J Appl Physiol* 1971;30:708–712.
9. Kobayashi Y, Ando Y, Takeuchi S, Takemura K, Okuda N. Effects of heat acclimation of distance runners in a moderately hot environment. *Eur J Appl Physiol* 1980;45:189–198.
10. Maughan RJ. Effects of CHO-electrolyte solution on prolonged exercise. In: Lamb DR, Williams MH, eds. *Perspectives in exercise science and sports medicine, vol 4: ergogenics—enhancement of performance in exercise and sport.* Carmel, IN: Cooper, 1991: 35–85.
11. Shirreffs SM, Maughan RJ. Whole body sweat collection in man: an improved method with some preliminary data on electrolyte composition. *J Appl Physiol* 1997;82:336–341.
12. Greenleaf JE, Castle BL, Card DH. Blood electrolytes and tem-

perature regulation during exercise in man. *Acta Physiol Pol* 1974;25:397–410.
13. Harrison MH, Edwards RJ, Fennessy PA. Intravascular volume and tonicity as factors in the regulation of body temperature. *J Appl Physiol* 1978;44:69–75.
14. Fortney SM, Wenger CB, Bove JR, Nadel ER. Effect of hyperosmolality on control of blood flow and sweating. *J Appl Physiol* 1984;57:1688–1695.
15. Fortney SM, Vroman NB, Beckett WS, Permutt S, LaFrance ND. Effect of exercise hemoconcentration and hyperosmolality on exercise responses. *J Appl Physiol* 1988;65:519–524.
16. Brouns F, Saris WHM, Schneider H. Rationale for upper limits of electrolyte replacement during exercise. *Int J Sports Nutr* 1992; 2:229–238.
17. Meyer F, Bar-Or O, MacDougall D, Heigenhauser GJF. Sweat electrolyte loss during exercise in the heat: effects of gender and maturation. *Med Sci Sports Exerc* 1992;24:776–781.
18. Bar-Or O. Temperature regulation during exercise in children and adolescents. In: Gisolfi CV, Lamb DR, eds. *Perspectives in exercise science and sports medicine, vol 2: youth, exercise, and sport.* Indianapolis: Benchmark, 1989:335–362.
19. Saltin B, Costill DL. Fluid and electrolyte balance during prolonged exercise. In: Horton ES, Terjung RL, eds. *Exercise, nutrition, and metabolism.* New York: Macmillan, 1988:150–158.
20. Nielsen B, Kubica R, Bonnesen A, Rasmussen IB, Stoklosa J, Wilk B. Physical work capacity after dehydration and hyperthermia. *Scand J Sports Sci* 1981;3:2–10.
21. Armstrong LE, Costill DL, Fink WJ. Influence of diuretic-induced dehydration on competitive running performance. *Med Sci Sports Exerc* 1985;17:456–461.
22. Walsh RM, Noakes TD, Hawley JA, Dennis SC. Impaired high-intensity cycling performance time at low levels of dehydration. *Int J Sports Med* 1994;15:392–398.
23. Nadel ER. Circulatory and thermal regulations during exercise. *Fed Proc* 1980;39:1491–1497.
24. Rowell LB. *Human circulation.* New York: Oxford University Press, 1986.
25. Montain SJ, Coyle EF. Influence of graded dehydration on hyperthermia and cardiovascular drift during exercise. *J Appl Physiol* 1992;73:1340–1350.
26. Montain SJ, Coyle EF. Fluid ingestion during exercise increases skin blood flow independent of increases in blood volume. *J Appl Physiol* 1992;73:903–910.
27. Castenfors J. Renal function during prolonged exercise. *Ann NY Acad Sci* 1977;301:151–159.
28. Wade CE, Claybaugh JR. Plasma renin activity, vasopressin concentration and urinary excretory responses to exercise in men. *J Appl Physiol* 1980;49:930–936.
29. Poortmans J. Exercise and renal function. *Sports Med* 1984;1: 125–153.
30. Zambraski EJ. Renal regulation of fluid homeostasis during exercise. In: Gisolfi CV, Lamb DR, eds. *Perspectives in exercise science and sports medicine, vol 3: fluid homeostasis during exercise.* Carmel, IN: Benchmark, 1990:247–280.
31. Fitzsimons JT. Evolution of physiological and behavioural mechanisms in vertebrate body fluid homeostasis. In: Ramsay DJ, Booth DA, eds. *Thirst: physiological and psychological aspects.* London: ILSI Human Nutrition Reviews, Springer-Verlag, 1990:3–22.
32. Adolph ED, and associates: *Physiology of man in the desert.* New York: Interscience, 1947.
33. Phillips PA, Rolls BJ, Ledingham JGG, Forsling ML, Morton JJ. Osmotic thirst and vasopressin release in humans: a double-blind crossover study. *Am J Physiol* 1985;248:R645–R650.
34. Hubbard RW, Szlyk PC, Armstrong LE. Influence of thirst and fluid palatability on fluid ingestion. In: Gisolfi CV, Lamb DR, eds. *Perspectives in exercise science and sports medicine, vol 3: fluid homeostasis during exercise.* Indianapolis, IN: Benchmark, 1990:39–95.
35. Rolls BJ, Wood RJ, Rolls ET, Lind W, Ledingham JGG. Thirst following water deprivation in humans. *Am J Physiol* 1980; 239:R476–R482.
36. Verbalis JG. Inhibitory controls of drinking: satiation of thirst. In: Ramsay DJ, Booth DA, eds. *Thirst: physiological and psychological aspects.* London: ILSI Human Nutrition Reviews, Springer-Verlag, 1990:313–334.
37. Vist GE, Maughan RJ. The effect of osmolality and carbohydrate content on the rate of gastric emptying of liquids in man. *J Physiol* 1995;486:523–531.
38. American College of Sports Medicine. Position stand on prevention of thermal injuries during distance running. *Med Sci Sports Exerc* 1984;16:ix–xiv.
39. American College of Sports Medicine. Position stand on exercise and fluid replacement. *Med Sci Sports Exerc* 1996;28(1):i–vii.
40. Noakes TD. The dehydration myth and carbohydrate replacement during prolonged exercise. *Cycling Sci* 1990;23–29.
41. Massicote D, Peronnet F, Brisson G, Bakkouch K, Hillaire-marcel C. Oxidation of a glucose polymer during exercise: comparison with glucose and fructose. *J Appl Physiol* 1989;66:179–183.
42. Rehrer NJ. *Limits to fluid availability during exercise.* Haarlem, The Netherlands: De Vrieseborsch, 1990.
43. Leiper JB, Maughan RJ. Absorption of water and electrolytes from hypotonic, isotonic and hypertonic solutions. *J Physiol* 1986;373:90.
44. Maughan RJ. Physiology and nutrition for middle distance and long distance running. In: Lamb DR, Knuttgen HG, Murray R, eds. *Perspectives in exercise science and sports medicine, vol 7: physiology and nutrition for competitive sport.* Carmel, IN: Cooper, 1994:329–372.
45. Noakes TD, Goodwin N, Rayner BL, Branken T, Taylor RKN. Water intoxication: a possible complication during endurance exercise. *Med Sci Sports Exerc* 1985;17:370–375.
46. Noakes TD, Norman RJ, Buck RH, Godlonton J, Stevenson K, Pittaway D. The incidence of hyponatremia during prolonged ultraendurance exercise. *Med Sci Sports Exerc* 1990;22:165–170.
47. Frizell RT, Lang GH, Lowance DC, Lathan SR. Hyponatraemia and ultramarathon running. *JAMA* 1986;255:772–774.
48. Hiller WDB. Dehydration and hyponatraemia during triathlons. *Med Sci Sports Exerc* 1989;21:S219–S221
49. Flear CTG, Gill CV, Burn J. Beer drinking and hyponatraemia. *Lancet* 1981;2:477.
50. Noakes TD. The hyponatremia of exercise. *Int J Sports Nutr* 1992;2:205–228.
51. Noakes TD. Hyponatraemia during distance running: a physiological and clinical interpretation. *Med Sci Sports Exerc* 1993;24: 403–405.
52. Fellmann N, Sagnol M, Bedu M, et al. Enzymatic and hormonal responses following a 24 h endurance run and a 10 h triathlon race. *Eur J Appl Physiol* 1988;57:545–553.
53. Maughan RJ, Bethell LR, Leiper JB. Effects of ingested fluids on exercise capacity and on cardiovascular and metabolic responses to prolonged exercise in man. *Exp Physiol* 1996;81: 847–859.
54. Coyle EF, Coggan AR. Effectiveness of carbohydrate feeding in delaying fatigue during prolonged exercise. *Sports Med* 1984;1: 446–458.
55. Lamb DR, Brodowicz GR. Optimal use of fluids of varying formulations to minimize exercise-induced disturbances in homeostasis. *Sports Med* 1986;3:247–274.
56. Murray R. The effects of consuming carbohydrate-electrolyte beverages on gastric emptying and fluid absorption during and following exercise. *Sports Med* 1987;4:322–351.
57. Hamilton MT, Gonzalez-Alonso J, Montain SJ, Coyle EF. Fluid replacement and glucose during exercise prevent cardiovascular drift. *J Appl Physiol* 1991;71:871–877.
58. Bosch AN, Dennis SC, Noakes TD. Influence of carbohydrate ingestion on fuel substrate turnover and oxidation during prolonged exercise. *J Appl Physiol* 1994;76:2364–2372.
59. McConell G, Fabris S, Proietto J, Hargreaves M. Effect of carbohydrate ingestion on glucose kinetics during exercise. *J Appl Physiol* 1994;77:1537–1541.
60. Maughan RJ, Fenn CE, Leiper JB. Effects of fluid, electrolyte and substrate ingestion on endurance capacity. *Eur J Appl Physiol* 1989;58:481–486.
61. Below RP, Mora-Rodriguez R, Gonzalez-Alonso J, Coyle EF. Fluid and carbohydrate ingestion independently improve perfor-

mance during 1 h of intense exercise. *Med Sci Sports Exerc* 1995;27:200–210.
62. Riedesel ML, Allen DL, Peake GT, Al-Qattan K. Hyperhydration with glycerol solutions. *J Appl Physiol* 1987;63:2262–2268.
63. Gleeson M, Maughan RJ, Greenhaff PL. Comparison of the effects of pre-exercise feeding of glucose, glycerol and placebo on endurance and fuel homeostasis in man. *Eur J Appl Physiol* 1986;55:645–653.
64. Thecomata A, Nagashima K, Nose H, Morimoto T. Osmoregulatory inhibition of thermally induced cutaneous vasodilation in passively heated humans. *Am J Physiol* 1997;273:R197–R204.
65. Montner P, Stark DM, Riedesel ML, et al. Pre-exercise glycerol hydration improves cycling endurance time. *Int J Sports Med* 1996;17:27–33.
66. Latzka WA, Sawka MN, Matott RP, Staab JE, Montain SJ, Pandolf KB. Hyperhydration: physiologic and thermoregulatory effects during compensable and uncompensable exercise-heat stress. In: *U.S. Army technical report.* 1996;T96–6.
67. Miller JM, Coyle EF, Sherman WM, et al. Effect of glycerol feeding on endurance and metabolism during prolonged exercise in man. *Med Sci Sports Exerc* 1983;15:237–242.
68. Burge CM, Carey MF, Payne WR. Rowing performance, fluid balance, and metabolic function following dehydration and rehydration. *Med Sci Sports Exerc* 1993;25:1358–1364.
69. Costill DL, Sparks KE. Rapid fluid replacement following thermal dehydration. *J Appl Physiol* 1973;34:299–303.
70. Lambert CP, Costill DL, McConnell GK, et al. Fluid replacement after dehydration: influence of beverage carbonation and carbohydrate content. *Int J Sports Med* 1992;13:285–292.
71. Gonzalez-Alonso J, Heaps CL, Coyle EF. Rehydration after exercise with common beverages and water. *Int J Sports Med* 1992; 13:399–406.
72. Nose H, Mack GW, Shi X, Nadel ER. Involvement of sodium retention hormones during rehydration in humans. *J Appl Physiol* 1988;65:332–336.
73. Nose H, Mack GW, Shi X, Nadel ER. Role of osmolality and plasma volume during rehydration in humans. *J Appl Physiol* 1988;65:325–331.
74. Maughan RJ, Leiper JB. Effects of sodium content of ingested fluids on post-exercise rehydration in man. *Eur J Appl Physiol* 1995;71:311–319.
75. Maughan RJ, Owen JH, Shirreffs SM and Leiper JB. Post-exercise rehydration in man: effects of electrolyte addition to ingested fluids. *Eur J Appl Physiol* 1994;69:209–215.
76. Shirreffs SM, Taylor AJ, Leiper JB, Maughan RJ. Post-exercise rehydration in man: effects of volume consumed and drink sodium content. *Med Sci Sports Exerc* 1996;28:1260–1271.
77. Maughan RJ, Leiper JB, Shirreffs SM. Restoration of fluid balance after exercise-induced dehydration: effects of food and fluid intake. *Eur J Appl Physiol* 1996;73:317–325.
78. Galloway SDR, Maughan RJ. Effects of ambient temperature on the capacity to perform prolonged exercise in man. *J Physiol* 1995;489:35–36.
79. Pitts RF. *The physiological basis of diuretic therapy.* Springfield, IL: Charles C Thomas, 1959.
80. Lentner C, ed. *Geigy scientific tables,* 8th ed. Basel: Ciba-Geigy, 1981.
81. Schmidt RF, Thews G, eds. *Human physiology,* 2nd ed. Berlin: Springer-Verlag, 1989.

Exercise and Sport Science,
edited by William E. Garrett, Jr., and Donald T. Kirkendall.
Lippincott Williams & Wilkins, Philadelphia © 2000.

CHAPTER 29

Growth, Maturation, and Performance

Robert M. Malina

The interval between birth and adulthood is customarily divided into infancy, childhood, and adolescence. Infancy is the first year after birth. Childhood is usually subdivided into two phases, early and middle. The former approximates the preschool years, about 1 to 5 years of age, while the latter approximates the elementary school years, about 5 to 6 through 10 to 11 years. The beginning and ending of adolescence are variably defined, as is the beginning of adulthood. Biologically, some girls are sexually mature by 12 to 13 years of age and some boys are sexually mature by 14 to 15 years of age. They are biologically adult, yet they are generally considered adolescents by society. Adulthood is a more socially defined concept, usually in the context of completing high school, and in some instances, completing college.

Growth, maturation, and development are three interacting tasks that dominate approximately the first 2 decades of life. *Growth* refers to the increase in the size of the body as a whole and of its parts. As children grow, they become taller and heavier, they increase in lean and fat tissues, their organs increase in size, and so on. Heart volume and mass, for example, follow a growth pattern like that for body mass, while the lungs and lung functions grow proportionally to height. Different parts of the body grow at different rates and different times, resulting in changes in body proportions.

Maturation refers to progress toward the biologically mature state. It is an operational concept because the mature state varies with body system. Studies of children and adolescents often focus on skeletal, sexual, and somatic maturation. Maturation should be viewed in two contexts—timing and tempo. *Timing* refers to when specific maturational events occur, for example, age at the appearance of pubic hair in boys and girls, or the age at maximum growth during the adolescent growth spurt. *Tempo* refers to the rate at which maturation progresses, for example, how quickly or slowly the youngster passes from initial stages of sexual maturation to the mature state. Timing and tempo vary considerably among individuals.

Development refers to the acquisition and refinement of behaviors expected by society. As children experience life at home, neighborhood, school, church, sports, recreation, and other community activities, they develop intellectually, socially, emotionally, morally, and so on. They develop behavioral competence.

The word *development* is also used to describe the process of differentiation and specialization of embryonic cells into different cell types, tissues, organs, and functional units prenatally. Full differentiation is attained with the onset of function in a particular tissue. Discussion of prenatal development in this context is beyond the scope of this chapter. Emphasis here is on postnatal growth and maturation, although the prenatal period is important because events occurring prenatally may condition postnatal growth and maturation, and perhaps adulthood and aging.

Growth and maturation are biologic processes, while development is a behavioral process. These processes interact to influence the individual's self-esteem, body image, and perceived competence. This chapter, which is based on earlier presentations of this material (1–4), focuses on growth and maturation; behavioral development is not considered. How youngsters cope with their sexual maturation or adolescent growth spurt may influence their behavior, however. It is important, in this context, to recognize that children and adolescents cannot be approached in an exclusively biologic or in an exclusively behavioral manner; rather, a biocultural approach is essential, recognizing the interaction of biologic and societal demands on the growing, maturing, and developing individual.

The processes underlying growth and maturation are cellular. The study of growth and maturation involves

R. M. Malina: Institute for the Study of Youth Sports, Michigan State University, East Lansing, Michigan 48824-1049.

the measurement and observation of the outcomes of these processes, for example, size attained, level of fatness, level of maturity, or the extent to which an individual has progressed to adulthood.

OVERVIEW OF POSTNATAL GROWTH AND MATURATION

The differential course and timing of postnatal growth in various body systems are schematically indicated in Fig. 29–1. The curves of systemic growth, based on Scammon (5), indicate the relative size attained in several body systems expressed as a percentage of adult size (20 years of age is 100%). The four curves illustrate the differential nature of postnatal growth; that is, the human body grows at different rates, at different times, and in different areas or systems. The *neural curve* illustrates extremely rapid growth early in life, so that by 7 years of age the brain and its related structures have attained approximately 95% of their adult size. The *general curve* reflects rapid growth during infancy and early childhood, relatively slow growth during middle childhood, rapid growth once again during the adolescent growth spurt, and a slowing and eventual cessation of growth in late adolescence or early maturity. The *genital curve* shows a slight rise early in life, followed by a latent period through childhood, and then an extremely rapid growth spurt during sexual maturation and the adolescent growth spurt. The *lymphoid curve* is characterized by a rapid rise corresponding to infancy and childhood, indicating that by about 11 to 13 years of age there is, on a relative basis, about twice as much lymphoid tissue as in young adulthood. This relative decrease reflects the gradual involution of the thymus gland and tonsils, whose secretory function is considerably reduced. The amount of lymphoid tissue further decreases during the adult years.

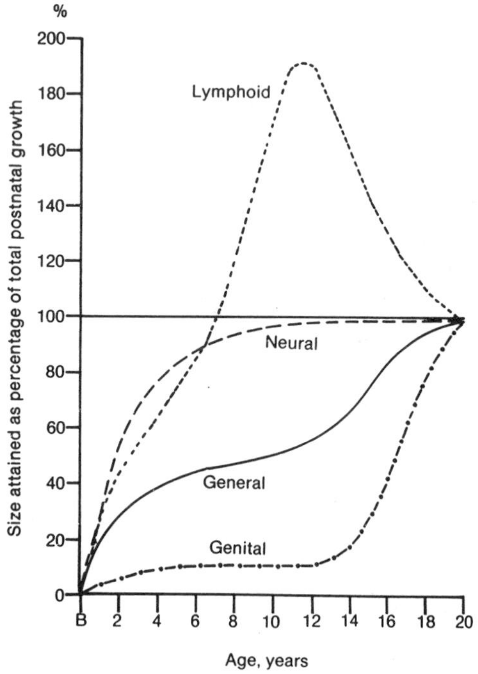

FIG. 29–1. Curves of systemic growth. Each curve is expressed as a percentage of the total gain between birth and 20 years of age. Size at 20 years (young adulthood) is 100%. (From ref. 5, with permission.)

Although these curves are generalized and simplified, they serve to indicate the differential but orderly nature of postnatal growth. Note the rapid growth of the nervous system early in life, the generally quiescent state of the reproductive system until the teen years, the sharp acceleration of the lymphoid system early in life followed by a sharp deceleration, and finally the generally S-shaped curve of overall bodily growth, which is characteristic of most external body dimensions and functions utilized in studies of growth and performance. The differential timing of postnatal growth as reflected in Scammon's curves also serves to emphasize potential sources of variation, for example, the consequences of early undernutrition on growth of neural tissue, or potential impact of heavy training on growth and maturation during adolescence. There are several exceptions to the four curves, for example, the craniofacial skeleton.

THE STUDY OF GROWTH

For the sake of convenience, the study of growth can be summarized in terms of overall body size, body proportions, and body composition.

Body Size

Anthropometry is the traditional and perhaps the basic tool in growth studies. It also has a long tradition of use in the sport sciences (6). Anthropometry refers to systematized measurement techniques that involve specific landmarks and procedures. The number of measurements that can be taken on an individual is almost limitless. Several dimensions commonly used in growth studies are highlighted below (7).

Weight and height are the two most commonly used measurements of growth. *Body weight* or *mass* is a composite of independently varying tissue components, primarily bone, muscle, fat, and viscera. Although body mass should be measured with the individual nude, it is frequently taken with the subject attired in ordinary, indoor clothing without shoes. *Standing height* or *stature* is a linear measurement of the distance from the floor to the vertex of the skull. It is measured with the subject in standard erect posture, without shoes. Stature is a composite of linear dimensions contributed by the lower extremities, trunk, neck, and head. From birth to age 2, height is measured as recumbent length.

Several other dimensions, in addition to mass and height, provide useful information growth status. *Sitting height*, height of the subject while sitting, is measured as the distance from the sitting surface to the top of the head with the subject seated in a standard position. Subtracting sitting height from standing height provides an estimate of *leg* or *subischial length*.

Two of the more commonly used breadth measurements are *biacromial* and *bicristal breadths*. The former measures the distance across the right and left acromial processes of the scapulae and provides an indication of the bony breadth across the shoulders. The latter measures the distance across the most lateral points of the iliac crests and provides an indication of the bony breadth across the hips. Breadths across the condyles of the femur (*bicondylar breadth*) and epicondyles of the humerus (*biepicondylar breadth*) provide information on the robustness of the extremity skeleton.

Measurements of limb circumferences indicate relative muscularity. A circumference includes bone, surrounded by mass of muscle tissue, which is ringed by a layer of subcutaneous tissue and skin. Thus, limb circumferences do not provide a measure of muscle tissue per se. The two more commonly used girth measurements are *arm* and *calf circumferences*.

Proportions

Measurements can be related to each other in the form of an index or ratio. The relationship between body mass and stature is commonly expressed as the *body mass index* (BMI)—mass/stature^2 (kg/m^2). The BMI is related to total body fatness and is widely used as a screening device for the risk of overweight in children and adolescents.

The *ratio of sitting height to stature* (sitting height/standing height × 100) indicates the relative contribution of the trunk and lower extremities to stature. The *ratio of bicristal to biacromial breadths* (bicristal/biacromial × 100) is an indicator of the proportional relationships of shoulders and hips.

Body Composition

Methods for the study of body composition can be arbitrarily grouped into two categories: those that are whole-body oriented and those that are regional or tissue specific. The former indicates the gross composition of the body, most commonly within the context of a two-compartment model:

$$\textit{Body Mass} = \textit{Fat-Free Mass} + \textit{Fat Mass}$$

Measurements of body density, total body water, and potassium concentration in the body have been used most often to estimate body composition in this approach. Advances in technology, specifically in the measurement of bone mineral, have extended the two-compartment model to the four-component model (8):

$$\textit{Body Mass} = \textit{Fat Mass} + \textit{Water} + \textit{Bone Mineral} + \textit{Residual}$$

The whole-body approaches provide important compositional information, but they provide relatively little about the development of the specific body tissues that are responsible for variation in body mass, for example, fat, muscle, bone mineral, and viscera, and regional variation in changes in the specific tissues during growth. Skinfold thicknesses (see below) provide regional information on subcutaneous fat accumulation at specific body sites.

Advances in technology have provided noninvasive methods for estimating bone mineral, skeletal muscle, and adipose tissue. Single- and dual-photon absorptiometry, and dual-energy x-ray absorptiometry provide measures of bone mineral content for the total body or in specific regions, while computed tomography, magnetic resonance imaging, ultrasound, and dual-photon absorptiometry provide measures of skeletal muscle and adipose tissue. Bone mineral has been studied in many samples of children and adolescents, while skeletal muscle and adiposity have been studied with the newer methods primarily in adults (9).

Subcutaneous Fat

A major percentage of fat mass lies immediately beneath the skin in the form of subcutaneous tissue. This tissue, in the form of a double fold of skin and subcutaneous tissue, can be easily measured with skinfold calipers. Skinfold thicknesses can be measured at any number of body sites on the extremities and the trunk. The following skinfolds are commonly used in growth studies: triceps, biceps, and medial calf skinfolds on the extremities, and the subscapular, suprailiac, and abdominal skinfolds on the trunk. Among these, the triceps and subscapular skinfolds have been used most often in growth studies. The sum of skinfolds (sum of four or six skinfolds) is a proxy for overall subcutaneous fat, while the ratio of trunk to extremity skinfolds indicates the relative distribution of subcutaneous fat (9).

Physique or Body Build

Anthropometric dimensions are often used to estimate physique, or body build, using the Heath-Carter protocol (10). Physique refers to the configuration of the entire body rather than specific features. The assessment of physique is expressed in the context of somatotype as conceptualized by Sheldon and colleagues (11). An individual's somatotype is a composite of the contributions of three components: endomorphy (relative roundness and fatness), mesomorphy (relative muscularity and skeletal robustness), and ectomorphy (relative linearity). The technique of Sheldon and colleagues is primarily photoscopic. The Heath-Carter anthropometric protocol utilizes the sum of three skinfolds adjusted for stature to estimate endomorphy; biepicondylar and bicondylar breadths, arm and calf circumferences adjusted for the triceps and medial calf skinfolds, respectively, and stature to estimate mesomorphy; and a height-weight ratio to estimate ectomorphy. The algorithms for estimating each component are given in Carter and Heath (10). Although the same terminology is used, the Heath-Carter and Sheldonian somatotypes are not equivalent. The Heath-Carter anthropometric protocol has reasonably wide application in the sport sciences, largely in the context of characterizing somatotypes of athletes in different sports or events within a sport.

Measurement Variability

Implicit in studies utilizing body measurements is the assumption that every effort is made to ensure reliability and accuracy of measurement and standardization of technique. It is assumed that measurements are made by trained observers. This is essential to obtain reliable and accurate data, and to enhance the usefulness of the data from the comparative perspective. Furthermore, reliable and accurate data are particularly critical in serial studies, short-term or long-term, in which the definition of rather small changes is necessary and errors of measurement can mask the true changes. Therefore, quality control and careful monitoring of the measurement process are essential. Duplicate measurements taken independently on the same individual by either the same technician or by two different technicians can be used to estimate within-observer and between-observer measurement variability (7).

THE STUDY OF MATURATION

The more commonly used maturity indicators include maturation of the skeleton, sexual maturation, and somatic maturation.

Skeletal Maturation

Assessment of skeletal maturation is based on changes in the skeleton that can be easily viewed on standardized radiographs, traditionally of the left hand and wrist. The hand and wrist are placed flat on the x-ray plate with the fingers slightly apart. The bones of the hand and wrist skeleton are observed from the dorsal (posterior) surface. The changes that each bone goes through from initial ossification to adult morphology are fairly uniform. These are *maturity indicators*, specific features of individual bones that can be noted on a hand and wrist x-ray and that occur regularly and in a definite, irreversible order (12). Methods of skeletal maturity assessment are similar in principle. All entail matching a hand and wrist radiograph of a child to a set of criteria. The criteria and methods of scoring differ.

Greulich-Pyle (GP) Method (12)

The GP method entails matching the hand and wrist x-ray of a child as closely as possible with a series of standard x-ray plates, which correspond to successive levels of skeletal maturity expressed as a skeletal age (SA) at specific chronologic ages (CA). The method should be applied by rating the maturity level of each individual bone. Each bone is matched to the standard plates in the atlas, and the one with which the individual bone most closely coincides is noted. The SA of the standard plate is the assigned SA of the bone in question. The process is repeated for all bones that are present in the hand and wrist, and the child's SA is the median of the SAs of each individually rated bone.

Tanner-Whitehouse (TW) Method (13,14)

The TW method requires matching features of 20 individual bones to criteria for stages through which each bone passes from initial appearance on a radiograph to the mature state. The 20 bones include seven carpals (excluding the pisiform) and 13 long bones (radius, ulna, and metacarpals, and phalanges of the first, third, and fifth digits). Each stage is assigned a specific point score, and the scores are summed to give a maturity score. The sum can be converted to an SA, which is referred to as the 20-bone SA. The revised TW method (TWII) provides a carpal SA based on the seven carpals and a radius, ulna, short bone (RUS) SA, in addition to the 20-bone SA.

Fels Method (15)

The Fels method is based on the same 20 bones as the TW method plus the pisiform and adductor sesamoid. Maturity indicators and specific criteria are based on shape changes of individual bones and ratios of the widths of diaphyses and corresponding epiphyses of the long bones. Grades are assigned to the indicators for each bone by matching the film being assessed to the criteria. The assigned grades and ratios are then entered into a microcomputer that calculates the SA and standard error.

Comparison of Methods

The three methods vary in maturity indicators, criteria of assessments, and procedures used to construct a scale of skeletal maturity from which SAs are assigned. The

GP method assigns an SA based on the median of the SAs assigned to each individual bone; sometimes the SA is based on the SA of the standard plate to which the film of a child is most closely matched (thus excluding variation among bones of the hand and wrist). The TW method results in a maturity point score based on the sum of the point scores for each of the 20 bones that are rated, or for the 7 carpals, or the 13 long bones. The score is then converted to an SA. The carpal SA may have more utility in childhood. The carpals are generally mature by 13 years of age, which limits their utility in adolescence. The RUS SA is more useful in adolescence, since the radius, ulna, and short bones continue to mature. The Fels method provides an SA with a standard error; this is a unique feature that is not available with the GP and TW methods. The computation procedure for determining SA in the Fels method weights the contributions of specific indicators depending on age and sex of the child.

Skeletal Age (SA)

All of the methods yield an SA, which corresponds to the level of skeletal maturity attained by a child relative to the reference sample. In the GP method, the reference sample is American children in the Cleveland, Ohio, area studied between 1931 and 1942. In the TW method, the reference sample is British children from several areas of the country studied between 1946 and 1972. TW reference values for American children from the Houston area have been recently proposed (16). In the Fels method, the reference sample is the Fels Longitudinal Study of children from southern Ohio studied between 1932 and 1972. Given the differences in methods and reference samples, the skeletal maturity status of a child rated by all three methods may be different. SAs derived from the GP, TW, and Fels method are not equivalent. It is important that the method used to estimate SA be specified.

The three methods for assessing skeletal maturity have their strengths and limitations. The TW method is more widely used at present. The Fels method is relatively new, and as with other new procedures, acceptance and dissemination take time. The GP method is widely used clinically and is good for identifying individuals who are very advanced or very late in skeletal maturation. It is not as finely tuned as the TW and Fels methods.

SA assessment is basically a method to estimate the level of maturity that a child has attained at a given point in time. SA is expressed relative to CA. It may simply be compared to CA; for example, a child's CA is 10.5 years while his or her SA is 12.3 years. In this instance, the child has attained the skeletal maturity equivalent to that of a child of 12.3 years. Or, a child's CA may be 10.5 years but his or her SA is 9.0 years. The child is chronologically 10.5 years of age, while he or she has only attained the skeletal maturity of a 9.0-year-old child.

Sexual Maturation

The assessment of sexual maturity is based on the appearance and progress of secondary sex characteristics—breasts in girls, penis and testes (genitalia) in boys, and pubic hair in both sexes. Age at menarche is a commonly used indicator in girls. The use of secondary sex characteristics is limited to the pubertal or adolescent phase of growth.

Breasts, Genitalia, and Pubic Hair

The maturation of secondary sex characteristics is ordinarily summarized in scales of five stages for each characteristic. The most commonly used criteria are those specified by Tanner (17), which are based on earlier studies (18–20). Stage 1 indicates the prepubertal state, that is, the absence of development of each characteristic. Stage 2 indicates initial maturation, that is, elevation of the breasts in girls, enlargement of the genitals in boys, and appearance of pubic hair in both sexes. Stages 3 and 4 indicate continued maturation of each characteristic and are somewhat more difficult to evaluate. Stage 5 indicates the adult or mature state for each characteristic. The criteria for the evaluation of breast, genital, and pubic hair development are readily available in textbooks of physical growth (1,17). Excellent color illustrations of the stages are available in the national survey of Dutch children (21).

Ratings of stages of sexual maturation are ordinarily made by direct observation at clinical examination. The method requires extreme sensitivity in application, given the concern of adolescents for privacy. There is also a need for quality control in assessments. How concordant are assessments made by two different examiners or by the same examiner on two independent occasions? The reproducibility of clinical assessments by physicians or other experienced raters is not generally reported.

In practice, ratings are used as follows. A girl, for example, may be rated in stage 2 for the breasts (B 2) and stage 1 for pubic hair (PH 1). Thus, maturation of the breasts has begun, while pubic hair has not yet appeared. This girl is just in the beginning of puberty, since the budding or initial elevation of the breasts (B 2) is most often the first overt sign of sexual maturation in girls. Similarly in males, a boy may be rated in stage 2 of genital maturation (G 2) and stage 1 for pubic hair (PH 1). The boy is likewise just beginning puberty, since the initial enlargement of the testes (G 2) is most often the first overt sign of sexual maturation in boys. In some youngsters, however, pubic hair may appear before breast and genital maturation.

The maturation of secondary sex characteristics is a continuous process upon which the stages are superimposed. The five stages are thus somewhat arbitrary. For example, a boy just entering G 3 is rated the same as a boy nearing the end of G 3. The latter boy is really more advanced in maturation than the former, but, given the limitations of the procedure, both are rated as G 3.

It is common in the pediatric literature to refer to the assessment of secondary sex characteristics as Tanner staging. This is erroneous. Specific characteristics are assessed using the criteria of Tanner (17). The stages are specific to the breasts, genitals, and pubic hair. It is incorrect, for example, to take the average of breast and pubic hair stages to characterize the level of sexual maturation of a girl or group of girls. Individuals should not be rated as being in puberty stage 2 or in Tanner stage 3; the specific secondary sex characteristic and its stage should be noted, that is, genital stage 4 (G 4) or pubic hair stage 3 (PH 3).

A more direct estimate of genital maturation in males is testicular volume. It is estimated with a series of models of known volume that have the shape of the testes (Prader orchidometer). Application of the models requires direct manipulation of the testes at clinical examination as the physician attempts to match the size of the testis with the ellipsoid model that most closely matches it. This procedure, though quite useful, has limited utility in surveys. It is most often used clinically to evaluate boys with extremely late maturation or disorders of growth and sexual maturation.

Self-Assessment of Secondary Sex Characteristics

Given the difficulty in direct assessment of sexual maturation in nonclinical settings, self-assessments by youths are often used. Youngsters are asked to rate their stage of sexual maturation relative to illustrations of the stages. There are limited data on the concordance of self-ratings of youths and those of experienced assessors. Among Brazilian youth, the concordance of self-assessments and physician assessments reached 60% to 70%, with better concordance for pubic hair than for the breasts and genitals (22). Correlations between self and physician ratings are commonly reported; however, given that there are only five stages for each characteristic, the correlations are of limited value. Tendencies to overestimate early stages and underestimate later stages of sexual maturation have been reported (23).

If self-assessments are used, good-quality photographs of the stages with simplified descriptions should be used. They should be done individually in a quiet room after careful explanation of the purpose of the assessment. The timing of genital, breast, and pubic hair maturation in a longitudinal sample of Ohio youths, based on self-assessment, has been reported along with comparative data from other studies based on clinical examination (24).

Menarche

Menarche, the first menstrual period, is the most commonly reported indicator of female puberty. Significant value judgments are associated with the attainment of menarche in many cultures. There are three methods of estimating age at menarche (1,2). The *prospective method* is based on longitudinal studies in which girls are examined at close intervals during adolescence, usually every 3 months. The girl is interviewed as to whether menarche has occurred and when. Given that the interval between examinations is relatively short, age at menarche can be reliably recalled for individual girls. Sample sizes in longitudinal studies, however, are not ordinarily large enough to derive population estimates and may not reflect the normal range of variation.

The *status quo method* is used to estimate age at menarche in a sample of girls. The estimate applies only to the population and not to an individual girl. The method requires a large, representative sample of girls spanning the age range in which menarche normally occurs, 9 to 17 years. Two bits of information are required: the exact age of each girl and whether or not she has attained menarche (simply yes or no). The percentage of girls in each age class who attained menarche is calculated, probits for each percentage are plotted for each age group, and a straight line is then fitted to the points. The point at which the line intersects 50% is the estimated median age at menarche for the sample.

The *retrospective method* requires the individual to recall the age at which she attained menarche. If the interview is done at close intervals as in longitudinal studies, the method is quite accurate. If it is done some time after menarche, it is affected by error in recall. With careful interview procedures, for example, attempting to place the event in the context of a season or event of the school year or holiday, reasonably accurate estimates of the age at menarche can be obtained from most adolescents and young adults. The method should not be used with cross-sectional samples of adolescent girls under 16 or 17 years of age because the resulting estimate will be biased; that is, girls who have not attained menarche will be excluded from the calculations.

Somatic Maturation

Two features of height provide the basis for assessment of somatic maturation: age at peak height velocity and percentage of adult stature attained at a given age.

Age at Peak Height Velocity (PHV)

PHV refers to the maximum rate of growth in stature during the adolescent spurt, and the age when PHV occurs is an indicator of somatic maturity. Longitudinal data are necessary to estimate age at PHV and related parameters of the adolescent growth, for example, age at take-off or initiation of the spurt, PHV, and size at takeoff and PHV. Mathematically fitting individual growth records is used to estimate the timing and magnitude of the spurt, although it is not the only approach to the analyses of longitudinal growth data (25). Several models have been described, primarily for stature. Structural models and polynomials should be distinguished. The former have a preselected form of the growth curve and the parameters or constants of the function have biologic meaning. The Preece-Baines family of growth functions is probably the more commonly used procedure. Although the use of polynomials has been criticized (26), several applications have been useful for describing growth over large age periods and characteristics with no uniform or continuous increase. These applications include moving polynomials, cubic splines, and kernel estimations. Regardless of the model used, curve fitting provides a convenient means of characterizing and comparing individual and/or group differences in adolescent growth in a biologically meaningful manner (27).

Percentage of Adult Stature

Percentage of adult stature attained at a given CA may be used as an indicator of somatic maturity. Children who are closer to adult or mature stature compared to other children of the same CA are advanced in maturity status. For example, two 7-year-old boys have attained the same stature, 122 cm. For one boy this stature accounts for 72% of adult stature, while for the other it accounts for only 66% of adult stature. The former is closer to the mature state, and therefore is maturationally advanced compared to the latter.

Use of the percentage of adult stature attained at a given CA may have utility in the sport sciences if children's stature at the time of examination is expressed as a percentage of their predicted adult stature. This approach may be useful in distinguishing youngsters who are tall at a given CA because they are genetically tall from those who are tall because they are maturationally advanced, that is, they have attained a greater percentage of their predicted adult stature at a given CA.

There are several methods available for the prediction of adult stature, but most incorporate skeletal maturation (SA) into the equation (2). This presents limitations since hand and wrist radiographs are not routinely available. Roche and colleagues (28) provide a method to estimate adult stature when SA is not available. The child's adult stature is predicted from current stature and the measured statures of the parents. Parental statures provide a target range within which the adult stature of the child will likely fall. More recently, Beunen and colleagues (29) provided age-specific equations for the prediction of adult stature in boys 13 to 16 years of age from current stature, sitting height, and the triceps and subscapular skinfolds. These methods need to be evaluated in other samples of children and adolescents. Furthermore, all predictions have an associated error, and the range of error associated with a prediction should be noted.

Interrelationships Among Maturity Indicators

Before the overt manifestation of secondary sex characteristics, skeletal maturation is the primary maturity indicator. With the onset of puberty and the adolescent growth spurt, indicators of skeletal, sexual, and somatic maturation proceed in concert. A question that merits attention is, Do these indicators measure the same kind of biologic maturity? Multivariate analyses of indicators of skeletal (ages at attaining skeletal maturity from 10 to 15 years of age), sexual (ages at attaining stages of genital, breast, and pubic hair maturation), and somatic (ages at peak velocity of height, mass, leg length, and sitting height, and ages at attaining 80% and 90% of adult stature) maturity indicate a general maturity factor that accounts for about 70% to 80% of the variation (30,31). The remaining variation reflects individual differences in the prepubertal or preadolescent tempo of maturation, and methodologic limitations of the scales used to assess biologic maturation.

AGE AND SEX DIFFERENCES IN SIZE, PROPORTIONS, AND BODY COMPOSITION

Body Size

Height and body mass follow a four-phased growth pattern: rapid gain in infancy and early childhood, steady gain in middle childhood, rapid gain during adolescence, and slow increase and eventual cessation of growth at the attainment of adult size or maturity. Body mass usually continues to increase into adult life, while statural growth has ceased. Boys and girls follow the same general course of growth (Fig. 29–2).

Sex differences before the adolescent spurt are minor. Boys tend to be, on average, slightly taller than girls, but there is considerable overlap. During the early part of adolescence, girls are taller and heavier than boys, which indicates the earlier adolescent spurt in girls. Girls, however, soon lose the size advantage as the male adolescent spurt manifests itself. Males catch up and eventually surpass females in height and mass.

The rate of growth in height and mass is different

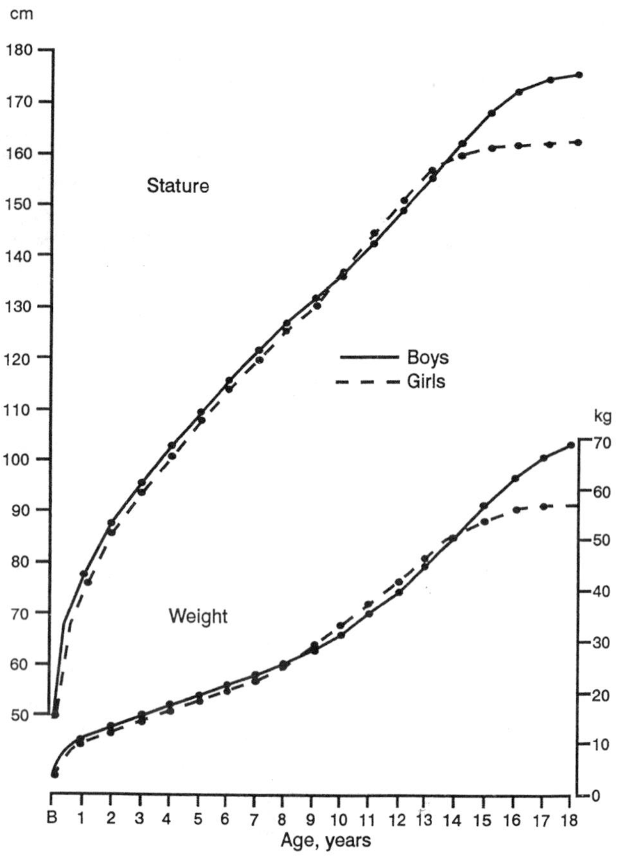

FIG. 29–2. Size attained in stature and weight of American children from birth to 18 years of age. (Data from ref. 32.)

prior to adolescence (1). Growth in height occurs at a constantly decelerating rate, while growth in mass occurs at a slightly but constantly accelerating rate (save for a deceleration in early infancy). Some children show a small growth spurt in stature between 6.5 and 8.5 years of age. Variation in the frequency of measurements in childhood is a factor influencing the detection of this mid-growth spurt. Children are usually measured annually during childhood, and such an interval may not be sufficiently sensitive to detect the change in velocity of growth that defines the mid-growth spurt. This mid-growth spurt occurs, on average, earlier in girls than in boys. During adolescence, growth in height and mass accelerate sharply, indicating the adolescent growth spurt. The adolescent spurts in height and mass occur earlier and are only slightly less intense in girls than in boys.

Most dimensions of the body—for example, sitting height, leg length, skeletal breadths, and limb circumferences—follow the same general pattern as size attained and rate of growth as height and mass (1). Prior to adolescence, sex differences are generally minor; in the early adolescent years, females have a temporary size advantage, on average. With the onset of the male adolescent spurt, males surpass females in size attained.

Body Proportions

Sex differences in proportions, though apparent, are relatively minor during the preadolescent years. Sex differences in the adolescent growth spurt produce the characteristic sexual dimorphism seen in young adults. The growth curve for the ratio of sitting height to stature illustrates the changing proportions of the trunk and legs to stature (Fig. 29–3). The ratio is highest in infancy and declines throughout childhood into adolescence as the legs are growing faster than the trunk. The ratio is lowest during the adolescent spurt, 10 to 12 in girls and 12 to 14 in boys, and is then followed by a slight increase into late adolescence. The late increase is related to late adolescent growth in trunk length at a time when growth in the lower extremities has already decelerated or stopped.

The sitting height/standing height ratio is identical for boys and girls until about 11 years of age, when it becomes slightly higher in girls and remains so through adolescence into adulthood. Thus, prior to the adolescent spurt, both boys and girls are proportionally similar in terms of the contributions of the lower extremities and the trunk to total height. However, during adolescence and in adulthood, females have, for the same stature, shorter legs than males.

Changes in body proportions are also illustrated in the obvious broadening of the shoulders relative to the hips in males, and the broadening of the hips relative to the shoulders in females. The development of these proportional differences is illustrated in the ratio of biacromial to bicristal breadths. Between the ages of 9 and 18, the ratio in boys is almost constant, while in girls it steadily declines. As the hips grow broader relative to the shoulders in girls, the ratio declines since the

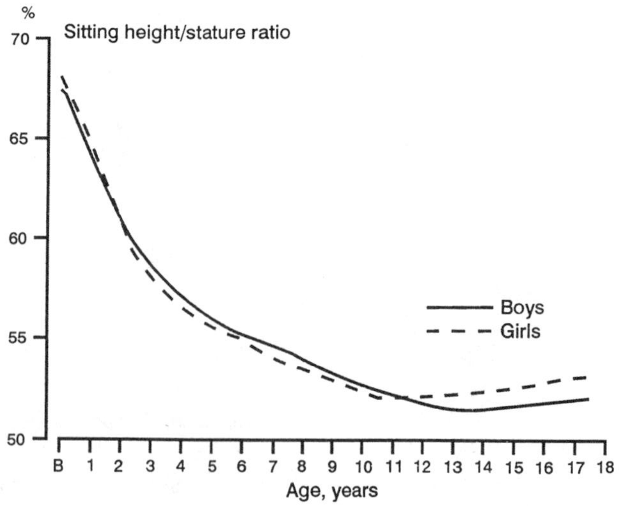

FIG. 29–3. Sitting height/stature ratios of American children from birth through 17 years of age. (Data from ref. 33 for children birth to 5 years, and from ref. 34 for children 6 through 17 years of age.)

denominator increases at a faster rate than the numerator. Both biacromial and bicristal breadths grow at reasonably similar rates during male adolescence, so that the ratio is rather constant.

Body Composition

Changes in estimated fat-free mass, fat mass, and percentage body fat during childhood and adolescence are shown in Fig. 29–4. Fat-free mass has a growth pattern like that for stature and mass, and sex differences become clearly established during the adolescent spurt. Estimated fat mass increases during the first 2 or 3 years of life and then shows little change through 5 or 6 years of age. The sex difference in fatness is negligible at these ages. Subsequently, fat mass increases more rapidly in girls than in boys. Fat mass increases through adolescence in girls, while it appears to reach a plateau or to change only slightly near the time of the adolescent spurt in boys (about 13 to 15 years).

Changes in total body fat as a percentage of body mass are shown in the lower section of Fig. 29–4. Relative fatness increases rapidly in both sexes during infancy and then gradually declines during early childhood. Girls tend to have, on average, a slightly greater percentage of fat than boys at this time, but from 5 to 6 years through adolescence girls consistently have greater relative fatness. The decline in relative fatness during male adolescence is a function of the adolescent spurt in fat-free mass, more specifically muscle mass.

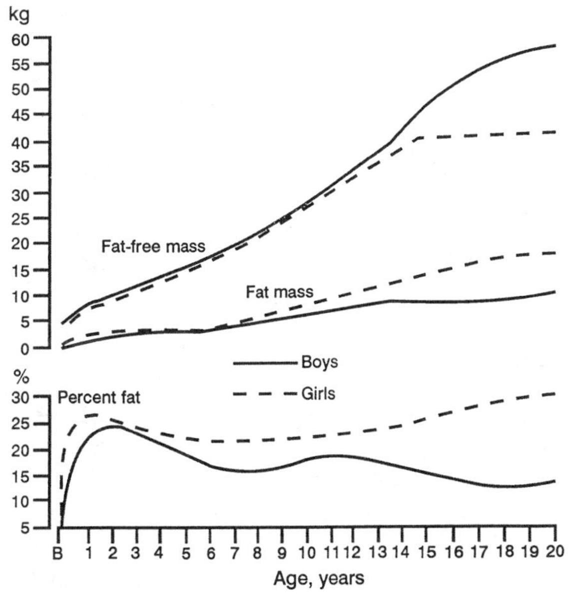

FIG. 29–4. Growth curves for fat-free mass, fat mass, and relative fatness derived from measurements of total body water. (From ref. 1.)

Subcutaneous Fat

Age- and sex-associated variation in a trunk (subscapular) and an extremity (triceps) skinfold are illustrated in Fig. 29–5. The different age trends for the triceps and subscapular skinfolds emphasize the limitation of using a single skinfold as an index of fatness or overweight. Both skinfolds decline in thickness from infancy to about 5 to 6 years of age and then increase in thickness. The subscapular skinfold continues to increase through adolescence into adulthood. In contrast, the triceps skinfold increases with age through adolescence and adulthood in females, but declines in thickness during male adolescence and then increases into adulthood. The sex difference in the triceps skinfold is marked during adolescence compared to the relatively small sex difference in the subscapular skinfold.

Changes in the ratio of trunk (subscapular + suprailiac) to extremity (triceps + biceps) skinfolds are summarized in Fig. 29–6. Shortly after birth, infants have almost equal amounts of subcutaneous fat on the trunk and extremities; the ratio is about 1.0. Subsequently, the ratio decreases through childhood, reaching a low point at about 5 years of age. This suggests proportionally greater accumulation of subcutaneous fat on the extremity than on the trunk. The sex difference in the ratio is negligible. After 5 years of age, the ratio increases gradually through childhood in both sexes and there is no sex difference. Subsequently, the ratio is rather stable in females but increases in males through adolescence. The increasing ratio in males indicates proportionally greater accumulation of subcutaneous fat on the trunk compared to the extremities; in contrast, the stable ratio in females indicates proportionally similar accumulation of subcutaneous fat on the trunk and extremities. Generally similar trends in relative fat distribution from childhood through adolescence are indicated with the ratio of the sum of three trunk (subscapular, suprailiac, abdominal) and three extremity (triceps, biceps, medial calf) skinfolds (9).

Current interest in relative fat distribution focuses largely on abdominal subcutaneous and visceral adipose tissue. Sex differences in abdominal adipose tissue prior to puberty are small, although data are limited. In contrast, young adult males have proportionally more abdominal visceral adipose tissue than young adult females, which suggests that the sex difference has its origin during puberty (9).

Bone Mineral

Bone mineral content and bone mineral density in the total body and several regions based on dual-energy x-ray absorptiometry (DXA) measurements increase with age during childhood. Sex differences are minimal from childhood through midadolescence, are established in later adolescence (about 15 to 17 years), and persist into adulthood (9).

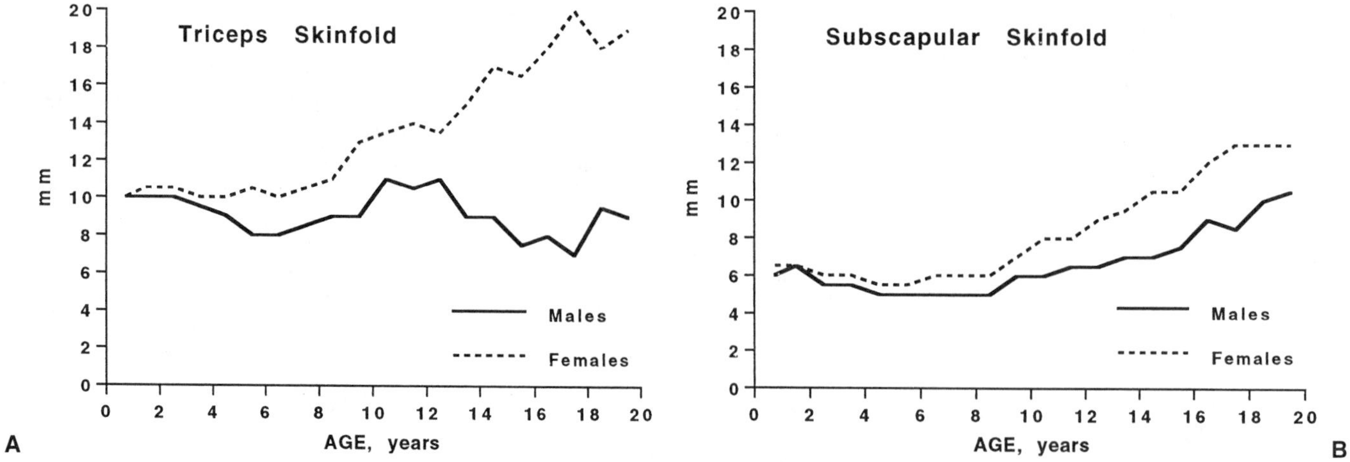

FIG. 29–5. Growth curves for the triceps (**A**) and subscapular (**B**) skinfolds of American youths—infancy to 18 years of age. (Date from ref. 35.)

Skeletal Muscle

The postnatal increase in muscle girth is due entirely to hypertrophy of existing fibers. Muscle fibers increase in diameter with age and body size, but the increase in diameter varies somewhat with the muscle studied (37). The increase in diameter is apparently related to function, but little is known about this phenomenon. During infancy and childhood, muscle fibers of boys and girls do not consistently differ in diameter, and adult diameters are apparently attained during adolescence (37). There is a lack of muscle fiber data for middle childhood and adolescence.

Data derived from standardized radiographs of the arm and calf (38) indicate that muscles of the extremities increase in size during childhood and adolescence and have a growth pattern similar to that for body mass. Sex differences, although apparent, are small during childhood, boys having slightly wider muscles. By about 11 years of age, girls are in their adolescent spurt and have a temporary size advantage in calf muscle width though not in arm muscle width. Boys then have their adolescent spurt and arm and calf muscle widths are especially wider than in females. The sex difference in limb muscle widths, established during adolescence, are more apparent in the upper arm than in the calf (1).

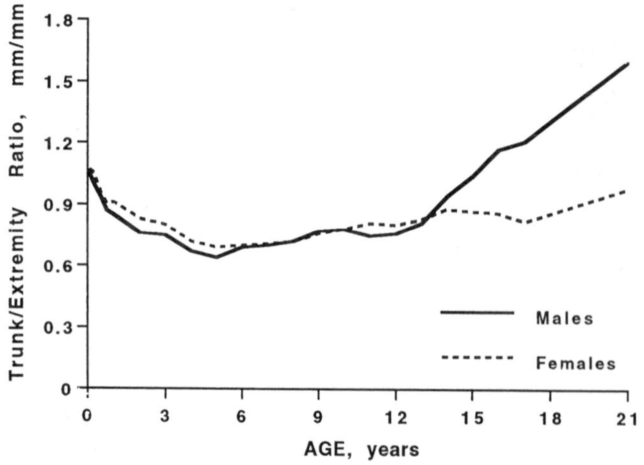

FIG. 29–6. Relative subcutaneous fat distribution expressed as the ratio of trunk (subscapular + suprailiac) to extremity (triceps + biceps) skinfolds from infancy to young adulthood. (Data from ref. 36.)

Physique

Mean values for the three components show rather small differences in somatotype from age to age during childhood and adolescence. With growth, males gain primarily in mesomorphy, while females gain primarily in endomorphy and decline in ectomorphy. The effects of adolescence on physique are such that in young adulthood, as in childhood, there are more endomorphic females than males and more mesomorphic males than females. Females are more concentrated in the endomorphic sector of the somatotype distribution; males tend toward the mesomorphic sector, but are more extensively distributed throughout the somatotype spectrum than are females (1).

MOTOR DEVELOPMENT

The development of proficiency in a variety of movements is a major task of childhood. For the sake of convenience, motor activities can be viewed as patterns and skills. The movement pattern is more general. It refers to the basic elements of specific movement behaviors, for example, walking pattern, running pattern, jumping pattern, and so on. Skill refers to the accuracy, economy, and efficiency of movements. Children learn to run, jump, throw, skip, hop, and so on; however, all children do not perform these movements with the same degree of skill.

During the preschool years and extending into middle childhood, children develop competence in a variety of movement patterns. These movements are the foundation upon which other skills and sport-specific skills are built. With the refinement of the walking pattern, children's control of their locomotor abilities improves so that a considerable amount of independent movement is possible.

Changes involved in the acquisition of basic movement patterns have been described in the context of developmental stages. The process of motor development is continuous. The stages, though arbitrary, provide a convenient means of summarizing developmental sequences for specific movement patterns. The development of movement patterns occurs in a sequential order. Children go through a similar sequence of changes for each movement pattern, but there is considerable variation among individual children in the rate of progress through the sequences.

The ages at which 60% of children in a sample of Michigan children demonstrated specific developmental stages for nine movement tasks are summarized in Fig. 29–7. The numbers on each bar of the figure indicate developmental stages, with 1 denoting the least mature

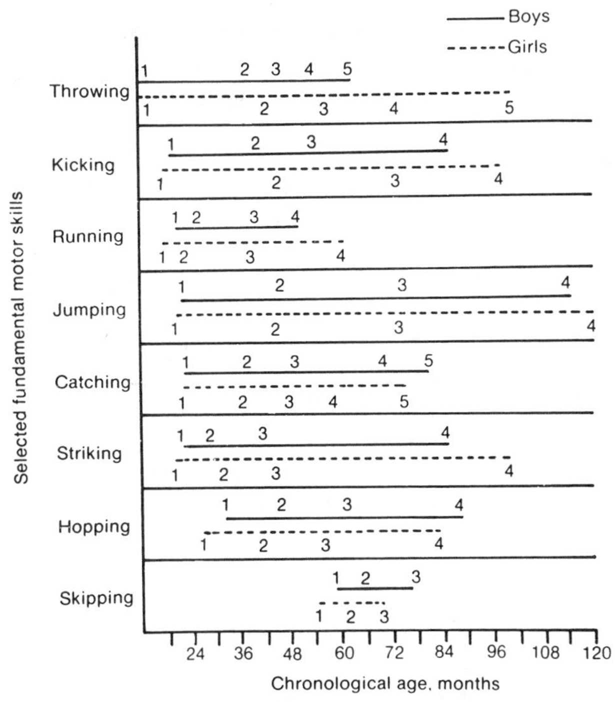

FIG. 29–7. Ages at which 60% of boys and girls were able to demonstrate specific stages of several fundamental movement patterns. *Stage 1* indicates the immature pattern; *stages 4/5* indicate the mature pattern. *Stages 2* and *3/4* are intermediate. (From ref. 39, with permission.)

stage and 4 or 5 denoting the mature stage. The mature stage or pattern simply means that all of the elements of the movement are present. The presence of a mature pattern does not necessarily indicate skillful performance. Skill implies precision, accuracy, and economy of movement. Once the basic pattern is there, guided practice and instruction facilitate the development of skill.

Several trends are suggested in Fig. 29–7. Development of basic movement patterns continues from early childhood (approximately the preschool years) through middle childhood. Boys tend to attain each stage of overhand throwing and kicking earlier than girls. This may relate to emphasis on these skills in activities available to boys more so than to girls in American culture. On the other hand, girls tend to attain each stage of hopping and skipping earlier than boys. This too may relate to emphasis on these skills in activities available to girls more so than to boys, although girls tend to demonstrate slightly better balance than boys in the preschool years. The attainment of stages of the other basic movement skills (running, long jumping, catching, and striking as in batting a ball) shows similarity between boys and girls, although there is some variability in ages at which the final or mature stages are attained. The interval between stages is in part a function of the relative arbitrariness of the definition of each stage for a specific movement pattern. For example, the defined changes from one stage to the next may be too great or the stage demands may be too difficult. There also is, in all likelihood, variation among children in the time required to master the elements of each stage.

As the basic movement patterns are refined through appropriate instruction and practice, performance quality improves and the basic patterns are integrated into more complex movement sequences, such as those required for specific games and sports. The transition from basic movement skills to more complex sports skills depends on experience and quality of instruction and practice. A proficiency barrier may exist for those children who do not have such opportunities for instruction and practice (40).

MOTOR PERFORMANCE

The development of proficiency in basic movement skills is accompanied by improved levels of performance that can be quantified. These are outcomes of the performance of tasks done under specified conditions, for example, the distance or height jumped (power), the distance a ball is thrown (power and coordination), the time elapsed in completing a 30-yard dash (speed) or a shuttle run (speed and agility), the number of sit-ups performed in 20 seconds (abdominal strength), or the force expressed against a fixed resistance (strength).

Data are available for a number of tasks that provide

a good indicator of how performances change with age from childhood through adolescence. Performances on standardized tasks improve with age during childhood. Boys perform, on average, better than girls, but there is considerable overlap between the sexes during early and middle childhood. With the onset of adolescence, the performances of boys show an acceleration or spurt, while those of girls improve linearly to about 13 to 14 years of age and then continue to improve, on average, at a slower rate through later adolescence (41,42). The sex difference in performance is most pronounced for tasks requiring strength, power, and speed.

MATURITY-ASSOCIATED VARIATION

The timing and tempo of maturation influence measures of growth and performance. There is also a clear sex difference in biologic maturation, which is apparent prenatally and persists to the attainment of maturity.

Sex Differences

The sequence of adolescent changes is relatively uniform from individual to individual. In girls, the first sign of impending puberty is, on average, enlargement of the breasts, which is followed in sequence by the appearance of pubic hair, the height spurt, the final stages of secondary sex characteristic maturation, and menarche. In boys, the first sign of impending puberty is, on average, the beginning growth of the testes and scrotum, followed in sequence by the appearance of pubic hair, the height spurt and rapid growth of the penis, and the final stages of secondary sex characteristic maturation (1,17). Although the sequence of maturational events is relatively uniform, youths pass through puberty and adolescence at different CAs; furthermore, rates of progress through the pubertal events also vary considerably.

Girls are advanced, on average, by about 2 years in ages at onset of secondary sex characteristics and of the adolescent growth spurt (age at takeoff), and in age at PHV. Variation, however, is the rule. Among Swiss girls, for example, ages at takeoff and PHV are 9.6 ± 1.1 and 12.2 ± 1.0 years, respectively; corresponding values for boys are 11.0 ± 1.2 and 13.9 ± 0.8 years, respectively. The range of ages at PHV span about 5 years, 9.3 to 15.0 years in girls and 12.0 to 15.8 in boys (43). Similar trends are evident in ages at attaining specific stages of sexual maturation (1). The magnitude of PHV is generally smaller in girls than in boys, and adolescents with an early spurt tend to have a more intense spurt (27).

Youths of Contrasting Maturity Status

Children and adolescents are ordinarily grouped for participation in sports on the basis of CA. Within a given CA group, there are considerable individual differences in overall size, proportions, body composition, and performance. Some of the variation reflects genotypic differences among children, that is, genetic variation in height, proportions, build, and so on, while some of the variation reflects differences associated with the timing and tempo of biologic maturation, which itself is under separate genetic regulation (1,44). Maturity-associated variation, though apparent prior to adolescence, is most pronounced during puberty and the adolescent growth spurt.

Children of the same CA are often categorized as early, average, or late maturing. Criteria for defining maturity groups vary. SA can be expressed as the difference between SA and CA, that is, SA − CA. In the first example given in the section on skeletal maturation (above), SA = 12.3 and CA = 10.5 years, giving a difference of +1.8 years; in the second example, SA = 9.0 and CA = 10.5 years, giving a difference of −1.5 years. Skeletal maturity is advanced in the former by 1.8 years and is later in the latter by 1.5 years relative to CA. If age at menarche is the indicator, one can compare the characteristics of pre- and postmenarcheal girls *within the same CA group*. One can also compare children at different stages of breast, genital, or pubic hair maturation within the same CA group. It must be emphasized that comparisons must be made within the same CA group. It is erroneous to group children by stage of sexual maturation independent of CA. This procedure reduces the variation within the sample somewhat, but variation independently associated with CA is overlooked. A 15-year-old boy in G 4 is quite different in size, physique, strength, and power from a 12-year-old boy in G 4; similarly, a 14-year-old girl in B 4 is quite different from an 11-year-old girl in B 4.

Early-maturing (EM) children are those in whom the maturity indicators are in advance of CA, while late-maturing (LM) children are those in whom the maturity indicators lag relative to CA. Average-maturing (AM) children make up the broad middle range of normal variation, with the normal range in growth studies being defined as plus or minus 1 year of an individual's CA.

Within a given CA group, youngsters of both sexes advanced in biologic maturation (EM) are generally heavier and taller for age from early childhood through adolescence into young adulthood than youngsters later in biologic maturation (LM). EMs and LMs do not differ, on average, in adult stature. EMs also have more mass for height, that is, stockier builds, than LMs. Viewed in somatotype terms, extreme mesomorphy is related to early maturation in boys, while endomorphy and early maturation are related in girls. On the other hand, extreme ectomorphy or linearity of physique is associated with later maturation in both boys and girls. Many of the physique features that characterize EM and LM youngsters are apparent before adolescence.

The differential timing of the growth spurt may alter differences between youths of contrasting maturity status.

EM youths, compared to LM youths, generally have larger amounts of fat, muscle, and bone tissues, and a larger fat-free mass, reflecting to some extent the larger body size of the former. On a relative basis, EM youths are fatter and not as lean as LM; that is, fat accounts for a greater percentage of body mass in EM youths.

Within a given CA group, AMs generally fall between EMs and LMs. However, differences between AMs and LMs are generally not as marked as differences between AMs and EMs and between EMs and LMs.

Maturity-associated variation in performance is more apparent in boys than in girls. EM boys exceed AM and LM boys in performance tasks that place a premium on strength, power, and speed during adolescence. These differences, so evident during adolescence, are not apparent in young adulthood (45), highlighting the transient nature of maturity-associated differences in performance. Girls of contrasting maturity status do not differ greatly in performance, and in many tasks differences in performance are not apparent during adolescence (1).

Maturity Indicators as Landmarks

In longitudinal studies, age at PHV serves as a maturational landmark against which attained size and velocity of other body dimensions and physical performance have been expressed (46). This is done to reduce the time spread across the CA axis during adolescence associated with variation in the timing of maximum growth. Age at menarche can also be used in a similar manner; however, it is a late maturational event that occurs after PHV. Major gains in growth and performance have already occurred.

Changes in other body dimensions and tissues and in performance tasks during adolescence are commonly viewed relative to the time before and after PHV. Data for each individual are plotted relative to his or her PHV, independent of the age at which PHV occurs. On average, maximum velocities of adolescent growth in lower limb dimensions (lengths, breadths, circumferences) precede PHV, while maximum velocities for adolescent growth in body mass, sitting height, and upper limb dimensions follow PHV (47). Peak velocities of growth in arm muscle width (as measured on serial radiographs) occur after PHV; corresponding data are not as clear for calf muscle width (38). Individual skinfolds behave differently during the adolescent growth spurt. In boys, growth velocities for trunk skinfolds (subscapular and suprailiac) tend to remain positive, while those for extremity skinfolds (triceps and calf) tend to become negative prior to or near PHV, and then remain negative for 2 or more years after PHV (47). Corresponding data for girls are limited to only two skinfolds (triceps and subscapular). Accumulation of subcutaneous fat tends to slow near the time of PHV, but velocities do not become negative (27). This differential growth of trunk and extremity skinfolds underlies the sex difference in relative subcutaneous fat distribution, that is, males accumulate proportionally more subcutaneous fat on the trunk during adolescence (9).

Performance during adolescence is also influenced in part by individual differences in the timing of the adolescent growth spurt. In boys, performances in a variety of tasks show well-defined adolescent spurts. Measures of static strength (grip, arm pull), power (vertical jump), and functional strength (flexed arm hang) show peak gains, on average, after PHV. On the other hand, measures of speed and agility (shuttle run), speed of arm movement (as in the number of times two plates, 20 cm in diameter and separated by 60 cm, are tapped in 20 seconds), and lower back flexibility (sit and reach) show peak gains before PHV (47). The trends for measures of strength and power are similar in timing to those for body mass and muscle mass, both of which experience maximum growth after PHV. The earlier adolescent spurts for running speed and lower back flexibility may be related to growth of the lower extremities, which experience maximum growth before the trunk. Thus, boys have relatively longer legs for height early in the adolescent spurt and this may influence running speed and lower trunk flexibility.

Corresponding trends for girls based on mixed-longitudinal data or short-term longitudinal data are reasonably similar. Girls show peak velocities of growth in static strength of the arm (48) and in power (standing long jump, medicine ball throw) after PHV, and in speed and agility (dash, shuttle run) before PHV (49).

GROWTH AND MATURITY STATUS OF YOUNG ATHLETES

Definition and classification of young sport participants as athletes are variable. Many studies of young athletes, however, include youths who can be classified as select, elite, or junior national caliber (3).

Size Attained

The percentile position of mean/median heights and body masses of young athletes in several sports relative to United States reference data (32) are summarized in Table 29–1. Gymnastics is the only sport that consistently presents a profile of short stature in both sexes. More recent samples of elite female gymnasts are, on average, shorter than those of the 1970s (50). Figure skaters of both sexes also present shorter statures, on average, though data are not extensive. Female ballet

TABLE 29–1. *Stature and weight of child and adolescent athletes relative to percentile (P) of United States reference data (32)*

	Males		Females	
Sport	Stature	Weight	Stature	Weight
Basketball	P 50–>P 90	P 50–>P 90	P 75–>P 90	P 50–P 75
Volleyball			P 75	P 50–P 75
Soccer	P 50±	P 50±	P 50	P 50
Ice hockey	P 50±	P 50		
Distance runs	P 50±	≤P 50	≥P 50	<P 50
Sprints	≥P 50	≥P 50	≥P 50	≤P 50
Swimming	P 50–P 90	>P 50–P 75	P 50–P 90	P 50–P 75
Diving	<P 50	≤P 50	≤P 50	P 50
Gymnastics	≤P 10–P 25	≤P 10–P 25	≤P 10–<P 50	P 10–<P 50[a]
Tennis	P 50±	≥P 50	>P 50	P 50±
Figure skating	P 10–P 25	P 10–P 25	P 10–<P 50	P 10–<P 50
Ballet	<P 50	P 10–P 50	≤P 50	P 10–<P 50

[a]More recent samples of gymnasts are closer to P 10.
From refs. 3 and 4.

dancers tend to have shorter statures during childhood and early adolescence, but they catch up to nondancers in late adolescence. Athletes of both sexes in others sports have, on average, statures that equal or exceed reference medians.

Body mass presents a similar pattern. Gymnasts, figure skaters, and ballet dancers of both sexes consistently show lighter body mass. Gymnasts and figure skaters have appropriate mass for height, while ballet dancers have low mass for height. A similar trend in indicated in female distance runners. Young athletes in other sports tend to have body masses that, on average, equal or exceed the reference medians.

Physique

Physique is an important selective factor in some sports, and young athletes in a given sport tend to have physiques similar to those of adult athletes in the sport (10,51).

Maturity Status and Progress

A summary of trends in maturity status of young athletes based upon skeletal maturation and secondary sex characteristics (excluding menarche) is presented in Table 29–2. Maturity differences are most apparent during the transition into adolescence and the adolescent spurt, and they reflect extreme individuality in timing and tempo of maturation. With few exceptions, male athletes in a variety of sports tend to be average or advanced in biologic maturation. Other than gymnasts, who show later skeletal maturation, there is a striking lack of late-maturing boys who are successful in sports during early adolescence. Late-maturing boys are often successful in some sports in later adolescence (16 to 18 years), however, such as track and basketball; this emphasizes the catch-up in skeletal maturation and reduced significance of maturity-associated variation in body size in the performances of boys in late adolescence.

The pubertal progress of boys and girls active in sports suggests no differences in tempo of sexual maturation compared to nonathletes. Mean intervals for progression from one stage to the next or across two stages are similar to those for inactive youths (52), and they are well within the range of normal variation in longitudinal studies of nonathletes (53–56). The interval between ages at PHV and menarche for girls active in sports and inactive girls also does not differ, and it is similar to those for several samples of nonathletic girls, mean intervals of 1.2 to 1.5 years (57).

Limited longitudinal observations for male athletes are generally consistent with the data for SA; that is, age at PHV tends to be average or earlier in male athletes (Table 29–3). PHVs for boys active in sports do not differ from those for inactive boys, and are well within the range of means for boys in longitudinal studies of nonathletes (2). Data for two samples of girls active in sports indicate ages at PHV and PHVs that approximate the means for the general population (2).

Age at Menarche

Most discussions of maturation of female athletes focus on the age at menarche, a late pubertal event. Later mean ages at menarche are reported in athletes in many, but not all, sports (58,59). There is confusion about later ages at menarche in athletes, which is related in part to the methods of estimating age at menarche. Longitudinal data for athletes followed from prepuberty through puberty are ordinarily short term and limited to small,

TABLE 29–2. *Maturity status based on skeletal age and secondary sex characteristics (excluding menarche) in child and adolescent athletes during middle childhood and adolescence, and in late adolescence (indicated ages are approximate)*

Males	Childhood (<11.0 years)	Adolescence (11.0–15.9 years)	Late adolescence (≥16.0 years)
Baseball	*	Advanced	No difference
Football	*	Advanced	No difference
Basketball	No difference	Average/advanced	No difference
Soccer	Average	Average	Advanced
Ice hockey	Average	Average/advanced	Advanced
Distance runs	*	Slightly later/average	No difference
Track and field	*	Advanced	No difference
Swimming	Average/advanced	Advanced	*
Gymnastics	Average	Later	*
Females	**Childhood (<10.0 years)**	**Adolescence (10.0–14.9 years)**	**Late Adolescence (≥15.0 years)**
Basketball	*	*	Average
Volleyball	*	*	Average
Distance runs	*	Slightly later/average	Slightly later/average
Track and field	*	Average	Average
Swimming	Average/advanced	Average/advanced	Average
Gymnastics	Average	Later/average	Later
Ballet	*	Later/average	Later

Note: Characterizing maturity status in late adolescence is influenced by the early attainment of maturity in advanced maturers and catch-up of average and later maturers, that is, all youth eventually reach skeletal and sexual maturity. The upper limit of one skeletal maturity system is 16.0 years (maturity).

*Satisfactory data are not available.

From refs. 3 and 4.

TABLE 29–3. *Estimated ages at peak height velocity (PHV), and peak height velocities in adolescent athletes*

	n	Age at PHV (years)	PHV (cm/yr)
Male athletes			
Soccer	32	14.2 ± 0.9	9.5 ± 1.5
Soccer	8	14.2 ± 0.9	
Basketball	8	14.1 ± 0.9	10.1 ± 1.2
Cycling	6	12.9 ± 0.4	
Rowing	11	13.5 ± 0.5	
Ice hockey	16	14.5 ± 1.0	
Ice hockey	11	12.8 ± 0.5	9.3 ± 3.0
Distance runs	4	12.6	
Several sports[a]	25	13.6 ± 0.9	9.7 ± 1.1
Several sports[b]	21	13.1 ± 1.0	9.3 ± 1.2
Male nonathletes[c]		13.8–14.4	8.3–10.3
Female athletes			
Several sports[a]	12	12.3 ± 0.8	7.8 ± 0.6
Several sports[b]	23	12.0 ± 0.8	8.0 ± 1.3
Female nonathletes[c]		11.6–12.2	7.0–9.0

[a]Several individual and team sports.

[b]Track and rowing with several athletes actively training in swimming.

[c]Range of mean ages at PHV and peak velocities, based on a variety of methods, reported in European longitudinal studies; 18 of the 20 estimated ages at PHV for boys are between 13.9 and 14.2 years, while 14 of 19 estimated ages at PHV for girls are between 11.9 and 12.2 years (2).

From ref. 4.

select samples; a potentially confounding issue is selective dropout. Status quo data for young athletes actively involved in systematic training provide sample or population estimates, but these samples often include athletes of different skill levels and training histories. Nevertheless, only prospective and status quo data deal with maturing athletes. In contrast, the vast majority of data for athletes are retrospective, and are based on samples of mature (postmenarcheal) late adolescent and adult athletes. Also, maturing and mature athletes are quite different.

Prospective and status quo data for young athletes in several sports are summarized in Table 29–4. Mean ages at menarche based on retrospective data are summarized elsewhere (58–60); these mean ages tend to be later than average (61) and vary among athletes in different sports, and they tend to be later in athletes within a sport who are at a higher competitive level.

Prospective and status quo data for gymnasts and ballet dancers, and status quo data for Junior Olympic divers and soccer players, are generally consistent with the retrospective data. The limited prospective and status quo data for tennis players, rowers, and track athletes, and more available data for age-group swimmers indicate earlier mean ages at menarche than retrospective estimates for each sport respectively; that is, late adolescent and young adult athletes (recall data) in these sports tend to attain menarche later than those

TABLE 29–4. *Prospective and status quo ages at menarche (years) in adolescent athletes*[a]

Athletes—prospective		Athletes—status quo	
Gymnasts, Polish	15.1 ± 0.9	Gymnasts, world[c]	15.6 ± 2.1
Gymnasts, Swiss	14.5 ± 1.2	Gymnasts, Hungarian	15.0 ± 0.6
Gymnasts, Swedish[b]	14.5 ± 1.4	Swimmers, age group, US	13.1 ± 1.1
Gymnasts, British[b]	14.3 ± 1.4	Swimmers, age group, US	12.7 ± 1.1
Swimmers, British	13.3 ± 1.1	Divers, Junior Olympic, US	13.6 ± 1.1
Tennis players, British	13.2 ± 1.4	Ballet dancers, Yugoslavia	13.6
Track, Polish	12.3 ± 1.1	Ballet dancers, Yugoslavia	14.1
Rowers, Polish	12.7 ± 0.9	Track, Hungarian	12.6
Elite ballet dancers, US[b]	15.4 ± 1.9	Soccer players, age group, US	12.9 ± 1.1
		Team sports, Hungarian	12.7
Nonathletes[d]	12.1–13.5		

[a]Prospective data report means, while status quo data report medians are based on probit analysis.
[b]Among the British athletes, 13% had not yet attained menarche so that the estimated mean ages will be somewhat later. Small numbers of Swiss and Swedish gymnasts and ballet dancers also had not reached menarche at the time of the studies.
[c]This sample is from the 1987 world championships in Rotterdam. It did not include girls under 13 years of age so that the estimate may be biased toward an older age.
[d]Status quo estimates for European girls from the mid-1960s through the 1980s. All except two of the 39 ages were between 12.5 and 13.5 years. There is a geographic gradient in the distribution of menarcheal ages within Europe; median ages decline from the north to south. The status quo estimate for United States girls is 12.8 years (61).
From ref. 4.

involved in the respective sports during the pubertal years (prospective and/or status quo data). Differences probably represent the interaction of several factors, including the longer growth period associated with later maturation (many do not attain adult body size until the late teens or early 20s), selective success of late-maturing girls in some sports, selective dropout of early-maturing girls, and increased opportunity in sports at the collegiate level or older ages.

Variation among estimated ages at menarche is especially evident among swimmers. Young swimmers, Olympic swimmers, and national-level swimmers from several countries in the 1950s to 1970s attained menarche, on average, at a similar age to nonathletes (about 13.0 years), and there was no difference between younger and older swimmers (58); however, university-level swimmers from elite programs in the United States in the mid-1980s and early 1990s have mean ages at menarche of 14.3 and 14.4 years (60). This trend probably reflects increased opportunities for girls in swimming. It was common for swimmers to retire by 16 to 17 years of age in the 1950s to 1970s. With the advent of Title IX legislation in the United States, many universities added and/or improved swim programs so that more opportunities were available. Also, later-maturing swimmers, catching up to peers in size and strength in late adolescence, probably experienced more success in swimming and persisted in the sport. Another factor may be change in the size and physique of female swimmers associated with the demands of the sport. A comparison of university-level female swimmers in the late-1980s with those in the mid-1970s indicated that the former were taller and more linear, a physique characteristic of later maturers; the more recent swimmers were also significantly more androgynous in build (62).

EFFECTS OF TRAINING FOR SPORTS ON INDICATORS OF GROWTH AND MATURATION

Training refers to systematic, specialized practice for a specific sport or sport discipline for most of the year or to specific short-term experimental programs. Physical activity is not the same as regular training. The measurement, quantification, and specification of training programs by sport needs further attention. Training programs are ordinarily specific (for example, endurance running, strength training, sport skill training, etc.), and they vary in intensity and duration.

Many of the changes attributed to regular training, though not all, are in the same direction as those that accompany normal growth and maturation. It is difficult to partition training effects from those of normal growth and maturation in the presently available data. Many studies of young athletes tend to focus on training per se and overlook other factors that are capable of influencing growth and maturation. An obvious factor is selection; young athletes in many sports are rigorously selected for specific morphologic and maturational features (4). Allowing for these caveats, a discussion of training, growth, and maturation follows.

Growth in Stature

Longitudinal data for young athletes that span childhood and adolescence are extremely limited. Data for active and inactive boys followed from late childhood through adolescence indicate no differences in stature, while corresponding data for boys active in several sports indicate statures consistent with average advanced maturity status (3,52,63). Longitudinal data for girls are less extensive. Girls regularly active in a variety of team and individual sports (track, rowing, swimming, basketball, volleyball) present a pattern of growth that is characteristic of average-maturing individuals (3,53,63). Young female athletes, however, tend to be taller but only slightly heavier than reference data, suggesting a more linear build.

Available short- and long-term longitudinal data indicate mean statures that maintain their position relative to the reference values over time, which suggests that they are not apparently influenced by the regular training for sports. Furthermore, short-term longitudinal studies of male and female athletes in a variety of sports (volleyball, diving, distance running, track, basketball, rowing, cycling, and ice hockey) indicate growth rates within the range expected for nonathletes (3,64).

In the context of these short- and long-term longitudinal observations, and allowing for selective criteria in some sports, regular participation in sports and training for sports has no apparent effect on attained stature and rate of growth in stature.

Adolescent Growth Spurt

Age at PHV is not apparently affected by regular physical activity and training for sports. The data are limited largely to boys, with only few observations for girls (see Table 29–3). The observations for male athletes are consistent with the data for SA, that is, ages at PHV tend to occur early or close to the average in male athletes. Available data for female athletes indicate ages at PHV that approximate the average. Longitudinal data for female athletes in gymnastics, ballet, figure skating, and diving—sports in which later-maturing girls excel during adolescence—are insufficient to estimate ages at PHV. The limited data for gymnasts suggest a later age at PHV and a smaller peak velocity compared to nonathletes (65,66). The parameters of the adolescent spurt in female gymnasts are similar to those for short, normal, late-maturing girls with short parents (66). Samples of ballet dancers show shorter statures during early adolescence, but late adolescent statures that do not differ from nondancers, that is, later attainment of adult stature (3). This is a growth pattern characteristic of late maturers (1).

Skeletal Maturation

Skeletal age (SA) does not differ between active and inactive boys followed longitudinally from 13 to 18 years (67). In boys active in sports, SA and CA show similar gains prior to the adolescent spurt, but SA progresses faster than CA during the growth spurt and puberty in boys, reflecting their advanced pubertal status. In a corresponding sample of girls active in sports, SA and CA progress at the same pace in late childhood through the growth spurt and puberty (63). Although young athletes in several sports, including gymnasts of both sexes, differ in skeletal maturity status, short-term longitudinal observations indicate similar gains in both SA and CA (3). The data thus imply no effect of training for sports on skeletal maturation of the hand and wrist.

Sexual Maturation of Boys

The effects of training for sports on the sexual maturation of boys has not generally been considered. This may not be surprising since early and average maturation are characteristic of the majority of young male athletes. Wrestling is the primary sport among males that has an emphasis on weight regulation. The emphasis on weight control, however, is short term, and longitudinal observations over a season indicate no significant effects on maturation and hormonal profiles (68).

Menarche

Later ages at menarche in young gymnasts, figure skaters, and ballet dancers, and in late adolescent and adult athletes in many sports, are often attributed to regular training for the respective sports. Although some data for gymnasts are prospective, the majority are status quo and retrospective, which renders it difficult to establish causal relationships. Correlations with years of training before menarche are often used to infer that training prior to menarche delays this maturational event. This is erroneous and misleading. Assume that two girls begin training at 6 years of age; one is an early maturer who will attain menarche at 11.0 years, while the other is a late maturer who will reach menarche at 16.0 years. A priori, there will be a correlation between the two events; the early maturer will have 5 years of training before menarche, while the late maturer will have 10 years of training before menarche. Training is not ordinarily quantified in these studies, and distinction between initial training in a sport and systematic, formal training is not made. In some of the analyses, those who take up systematic training after menarche are excluded in discussions of the assumed training effect. Also, it is also important to note that not all athletes experience menarche late.

Menarche is a biologic event. In adequately nourished individuals, age at menarche is a highly heritable characteristic (1,44). There is a familial tendency for later maturation in athletes (69–72). Menarche is also influenced by a number of socially or bioculturally mediated variables. Sports-specific selective factors must be considered as a part of this biocultural matrix in athletes. Number of children in the family is also associated with menarche. Girls from larger families tend to attain menarche later than those from smaller families. The estimated magnitude of the family size effect in athletes, 0.15 to 0.22 years per additional sibling, overlaps that in nonathletes, 0.08 to 0.19 years per additional sibling (73), and athletes tend to be from larger families than nonathletes (73,74). Aspects of the home environment are also implicated in the timing of menarche. Results of several studies suggest a role for household composition and stress as potential factors associated with an earlier age at menarche (75–77).

Dietary concerns are an important factor among athletes (78). Other factors that interact with marginal caloric status and altered eating habits merit closer attention. These may include the psychologic and emotional stress associated with maintaining body mass when the natural course of growth is to gain weight, year-long training (often before school in the morning and after school in the late afternoon), frequent competitions, altered social relationships with peers, and overbearing and demanding coaches.

The mechanisms that link a variety of factors to menarche are not known. The interactions operate along the hypothalamic-pituitary-ovarian axis, which regulates the onset and progress of puberty, including first menstruation. Puberty is a brain-driven event (79), and the brain and central nervous system are the filter through which environmental factors and/or stresses are processed. Given the complexity of factors related to menarche, it is essential that they be considered when inferring causality for training before and/or during puberty as a factor influencing the timing of this maturational event in presumably healthy adolescent athletes (80,81).

Physique

It is difficult to partition potential training effects on physique from those associated with normal growth and maturation. Changes are usually transient and reflect soft-tissue (largely subcutaneous fat) changes (1).

Body Mass and Composition

Regular training influences body mass and specific components of body composition. Males, athletes and nonathletes, show a decline in relative fatness during adolescence, but athletes have less fatness. Relative fatness does not increase as much with age during adolescence in female athletes as it does in nonathletes. Thus, the difference between female athletes and nonathletes is greater than the corresponding trend in males (1).

Training is associated with a decrease in fatness in both sexes and occasionally with an increase in fat-free mass in boys. Changes in fatness depend on continued training (or caloric restriction, which often occurs in sports like gymnastics and ballet in girls and wrestling in boys) for maintenance. When training is significantly reduced, fatness tends to accumulate. On the other hand, it is difficult to partition effects of training on fat-free mass from expected changes associated with growth and sexual maturation.

Skeletal Tissue

Regular physical activity and training during youth are associated with increased bone mineral content, but the osteogenic influence of activity is generally specific to the skeletal sites at which the mechanical strains occur (82). Beneficial effects are also more apparent in weight-bearing than non–weight-bearing activities. Of particular importance is the observation that bone mineral established during childhood and adolescence is a determinant of adult bone mineral status.

Similar trends are apparent both in boys and girls (83,84) and in young athletes from late childhood through young adulthood, although the latter data are derived largely from female athletes in gymnastics, figure skating, ballet, swimming, and running (85–90). The long-term effect of early sports training on skeletal tissue is especially apparent in the dominant compared to the nondominant arms of racket sports athletes. The difference in the mineral content of the humerus and radius of the dominant and nondominant arms of female tennis and squash players who began formal training 3 or more years before menarche was greater than that in athletes who began training near the time of menarche or after menarche (91). The data suggest a dose-response effect.

The concern for skeletal tissue integrity in female athletes is in part related to later sexual maturation. Presumably later sexual maturation is related to reduced total estrogen exposure and in turn potentially less bone mineral content and mass. Adolescent female athletes in several sports tend to have greater bone mineral, however, specifically at the skeletal sites at which mechanical strains occur. Enhanced bone mineral accretion associated with training for sports may offset the reduced estrogen exposure associated with later maturation.

In contrast to the positive influence of training on bone mineralization, excessive training associated with altered menstrual function in some, but not all, postmenarcheal athletes may be associated with loss of bone mineral (92,93). Restrictive diets and/or disordered eating are contributory factors. The interaction of disordered eating, cessation of regular menstrual cycles, and osteoporosis in high-performance athletes is of concern for some, but not all, adolescent athletes, and it may impact the accretion of skeletal mineral during adolescence. A major question is, Can those adolescent athletes at risk be identified and appropriately counseled?

Skeletal Muscle

Information on the effects of training on skeletal muscle tissue is derived largely from short-term studies of small samples. Muscular hypertrophy is associated with high-resistance programs such as weight or strength training in adolescent boys, and does not ordinarily occur in preadolescent boys and girls and in other forms of training. There is no strong evidence to suggest that fiber-type distribution in youths can be changed as a result of training.

Progressive strength training is associated with an increase in the relative area of type II (fast-twitch) fibers, while endurance training is associated with an increase in the relative area of type I (slow-twitch) fibers in young adults. Corresponding data for youths are variable. In 16-year-old boys, 3 months of endurance training were associated with an increase in the areas of both type I and II fibers, while 3 months of sprint training did not affect fiber areas (94).

Data on changes in the metabolic properties of skeletal muscle with training in youths are also limited. Endurance training is associated with increased activities of both succinate dehydrogenase (SDH, oxidative) and phosphofructokinase (PFK, glycolytic) in 11-year-old boys (95). Among 16-year-old boys, in contrast, endurance training results in an increase in SDH but not PFK, while sprint training results in an increase in PFK but not SDH (94). Differences in training protocols may account for the variable results. There is also the possibility of age-associated variation in response to training. Corresponding data for young females are not available.

The limited data suggest that regular training has the potential to modify the metabolic capacity of muscle in youth. After 6 months of no supervised training, however, SDH and PFK activities returned to pretraining levels in the 16-year-old boys (94). This illustrates an important feature of training studies. Changes in response to short-term programs are generally not permanent and depend on regular activity for their maintenance. An important question is, How much training is needed to maintain the beneficial changes?

Adipose Tissue

Cross-sectional data indicate thinner skinfolds in young athletes compared to reference samples (1), but longitudinal data for boys and girls active in sports show skinfold thicknesses that do not differ from reference values (63). The discrepancy may be related to differences in training intensity. More intensive training may be necessary to modify skinfold thicknesses in adolescents.

Data dealing with potential effects of training on subcutaneous fat distribution during growth are presently not available. In young adult males, intensive training for 15 and 20 weeks is associated with a greater reduction in trunk than in extremity skinfolds, while corresponding changes in young adult females are evenly distributed between trunk and extremity sites (96,97).

Information on the effects of regular training on adipose tissue cellularity and metabolism in youths is also lacking. Adipose tissue cellularity increases gradually during childhood and then more rapidly with the onset of puberty. The decrease in fatness associated with training in adults is attributable solely to a reduction in estimated adipocyte size. Trained adults also have increased ability to mobilize and oxidize fat. An increase in lipolysis occurs in sedentary adults exposed to aerobic training, and the increase is greater in males than in females (98).

REFERENCES

1. Malina RM, Bouchard C. *Growth, maturation, and physical activity.* Champaign, IL: Human Kinetics, 1991.
2. Malina RM, Beunen G. Monitoring of growth and maturation. In: Bar-Or O, ed. *The child and adolescent athlete.* Oxford: Blackwell Science, 1996:647–672.
3. Malina RM. Physical growth and biological maturation of young athletes. *Exerc Sports Sci Rev* 1994;22:389–433.
4. Malina RM. Growth and maturation of young athletes: Is training for sport a factor? In: Chang KM, Micheli L, eds. *Sports and children.* Proceedings of the 1997 International Sports Medicine Congress, Hong Kong. Baltimore: Williams & Wilkins, 1998: 33–161.
5. Scammon RE. The measurement of the body in childhood. In: Harris JA, Jackson CM, Paterson DG, Scammon RE. *The measurement of man.* Minneapolis: University of Minnesota Press, 1930:171–215.
6. Malina RM. Anthropometry in physical education and sport sciences. In: Spencer F, ed. *History of physical anthropology: an encyclopedia,* vol 1. New York: Garland, 1997:90–94.
7. Malina RM. Anthropometry. In: Maud PJ, Foster C, eds. *Physiological assessment of human fitness.* Champaign, IL: Human Kinetics, 1995:205–219.
8. Heymsfield SB, Wang Z-M, Withers RT. Multicomponent molecular level models of body composition analysis. In: Roche AF, Heymsfield AF, Lohman TG, eds. *Human body composition.* Champaign, IL: Human Kinetics, 1996:129–147.
9. Malina RM. Regional body composition: age, sex, and ethnic variation. In: Roche AF, Heymsfield AF, Lohman TG, eds. *Human body composition.* Champaign, IL: Human Kinetics, 1996:217–255.
10. Carter JEL, Heath BH. *Somatotyping—development and applications.* Cambridge: Cambridge University Press, 1990.
11. Sheldon WH, Stevens SS, Tucker WB. *The varieties of human physique.* New York: Harper & Brothers, 1940.
12. Greulich WW, Pyle SI. *Radiographic atlas of skeletal development of the hand and wrist,* 2nd ed. Palo Alto, CA: Stanford University Press, 1959.
13. Tanner JM, Whitehouse RH, Marshall WA, Healy MJR, Goldstein H. *Assessment of skeletal maturity and prediction of adult height (TW 2 method).* New York: Academic Press, 1975.
14. Tanner JM, Whitehouse RH, Cameron N, Marshall WH, Healy MJR, Goldstein H. *Assessment of skeletal maturity and prediction of adult height,* 2nd ed. New York: Academic Press, 1983.
15. Roche AF, Chumlea WC, Thissen D. *Assessing the skeletal maturity of the hand-wrist: Fels method.* Springfield, IL: Charles C Thomas, 1988.
16. Tanner JM, Oshman D, Babbage F, Healy M. Tanner-Whitehouse

bone age reference values for North American children. *J Pediatr* 1997;131:34–40.
17. Tanner JM. *Growth at adolescence,* 2nd ed. Oxford: Blackwell, 1962.
18. Greulich WW, Dorfman RI, Catchpole HR, Solomon CI, Culotta CS. Somatic and endocrine studies of puberal and adolescent boys. *Monogr Soc Res Child Dev* 1942;7(serial no. 35).
19. Reynolds EL, Wines JV. Individual differences in physical changes associated with adolescence in girls. *Am J Dis Child* 1948;75: 329–350.
20. Reynolds EL, Wines JV. Individual differences in physical changes associated with adolescence in boys. *Am J Dis Child* 1951;82: 529–547.
21. Roede MJ, Van Wieringen JC. Growth diagrams 1980: Netherlands Third Nationwide Survey. *Tijdschrift Soc Gezonheidszorg* 1985;63(suppl).
22. Matsudo SMM, Matsudo VKR. Self-assessment and physician assessment of sexual maturation in Brazilian boys and girls: concordance and reproducibility. *Am J Hum Biol* 1994;6:451–455.
23. Schlossberger NM, Turner RA, Irwin CE. Validity of self-report of pubertal maturation in early adolescents. *J Adolesc Health* 1992;13:109–113.
24. Roche AF, Wellens R, Attie KM, Siervogel RM. The timing of sexual maturation in a group of US white youths. *J Pediatr Endocrinol Metab* 1995;8:11–18.
25. Goldstein H. *The design and analysis of longitudinal studies.* London: Academic Press, 1979.
26. Marubini E. Mathematical handling of long-term longitudinal data. In: Falkner F, Tanner JM, eds. *Human growth, vol 1: principles and prenatal growth.* New York: Academic Press, 1978: 209–225.
27. Beunen G, Malina RM. Growth and physical performance relative to the timing of the adolescent spurt. *Exerc Sport Sci Rev* 1988; 16:503–540.
28. Roche AF, Tyleshevski F, Rogers E. Non-invasive measurement of physical maturity in children. *Res Q Exerc Sport* 1983;54: 364–371.
29. Beunen GP, Malina RM, Lefevre J, Claessens AL, Renson R, Simons J. Prediction of adult stature and noninvasive assessment of biological maturation. *Med Sci Sports Exerc* 1997;29:225–230.
30. Bielicki T. Interrelationships between various measures of maturation rate in girls during adolescence. *Stud Phys Anthropol* 1975;1:51–64.
31. Bielicki T, Koniarek J, Malina RM. Interrelationships among certain measures of growth and maturation rate in boys during adolescence. *Ann Hum Biol* 1984;11:201–210.
32. Hamill PVV, Drizd RA, Johnson CL, Reed RD, Roche AF. NCHS growth charts for children, birth–18 years, United States. *Vital Health Stat [11]* 1977;165.
33. McCammon RB. *Human growth and development.* Springfield, IL: Charles C Thomas, 1970.
34. Roche AF, Malina RM. *Manual of physical status and performance in childhood,* vol 1. New York: Plenum, 1983.
35. Najjar MF, Rowland M. Anthropometric reference data and prevalence of overweight: United States, 1976–1980. *Vital Health Stat [11]* 1987;238.
36. Rolland-Cachera MF, Bellisle F, Deheeger M, Pequignot F, Sempe M. Influence of body fat distribution during childhood on body fat distribution in adulthood: a two-decade follow-up study. *Int J Obes* 1990;14:473–481.
37. Malina RM. Growth of muscle tissue and muscle mass. In: Falkner F, Tanner JM, eds. *Human growth, vol 2: postnatal growth and neurobiology.* New York: Plenum, 1986:77–99.
38. Tanner JM, Hughes PCR, Whitehouse RH. Radiographically determined widths of bone, muscle and fat in the upper arm and calf from 3–18 years. *Ann Hum Biol* 1981;8:495–517.
39. Seefeldt VD, Haubenstricker J. Patterns, phases, or stages: an analytical model for the study of developmental movement. In: Kelso JAS, Clark JE, eds. *The development of movement control and coordination.* New York: Wiley, 1982:303–318.
40. Seefeldt VD. Developmental motor patterns: implications for elementary school physical education. In: Nadeau CH, Halliwell WR, Newell KM, Roberts GC, eds. *Psychology of motor behavior and sport.* Champaign, IL: Human Kinetics, 1980:314–323.
41. Beunen GP, Simons J. Physical growth, maturation, and performance. In: Simons J, Beunen GP, Renson R, Claessens AL, Vanreusel B, Lefevre J, eds. *Growth and fitness of Flemish girls: the Leuven growth study.* Champaign, IL: Human Kinetics, 1990: 69–118.
42. Haubenstricker JL, Wisner DM, Seefeldt V, Branta CF. Gender differences and mixed-longitudinal reference values for selected motor skills for children and youth. Unpublished report.
43. Largo RH, Gasser Th, Prader A, Stuetzle W, Huber PJ. Analysis of the adolescent growth spurt using smoothing spline functions. *Ann Hum Biol* 1978;5:421–434.
44. Bouchard C, Malina RM, Perusse L. *Genetics of fitness and physical performance.* Champaign, IL: Human Kinetics, 1997.
45. Lefevre J, Beunen G, Steens G, Claessens A, Renson R. Motor performance during adolescence and age thirty as related to age at peak height velocity. *Ann Hum Biol* 1990;17:423–435.
46. Shuttleworth FK. Sexual maturation and the physical growth of girls aged six to nineteen. *Monogr Soc Res Child Dev* 1937;2(serial no. 12).
47. Beunen GP, Malina RM, Van't Hof MA, et al. *Adolescent growth and motor performance: a longitudinal study of Belgian boys.* Champaign, IL: Human Kinetics, 1988.
48. Kemper HCG, Verschuur R. Motor performance fitness tests. In: Kemper HCG, ed. *Growth, health and fitness of teenagers.* Basel: Karger, 1985:66–80.
49. Heras Yague P, de la Fuente JM. Changes in height and motor performance relative to peak height velocity: a mixed-longitudinal study of Spanish boys and girls. *Am J Hum Biol* 1998;10:647–660.
50. Claessens AL. Elite female gymnasts: a kinanthropometric overview. In: Johnston FE, Eveleth P, Zemel B, eds. *Human growth in context.* London: Smith-Gordon, 1999 *(in press).*
51. Carter JEL. Somatotypes of children in sports. In: Malina RM, ed. *Young athletes: biological, psychological, and educational perspectives.* Champaign, IL: Human Kinetics, 1988:153–165.
52. Malina RM. Prospective and retrospective longitudinal studies of the growth, maturation, and fitness of Polish youth active in sport. *Int J Sports Med* 1997;18(suppl 3):S139–S154.
53. Largo RH, Prader A. Pubertal development in Swiss boys. *Helvet Paediatr Acta* 1983;38:211–228.
54. Largo RH, Prader A. Pubertal development in Swiss girls. *Helvet Paediatr Acta* 1983;38:229–243.
55. Marshall WA, Tanner JM. Variations in pattern of pubertal changes in girls. *Arch Dis Child* 1969;44:291–303.
56. Marshall WA, Tanner JM. Variations in the pattern of pubertal changes in boys. *Arch Dis Child* 1970;45:13–23.
57. Geithner CA, Woynarowska B, Malina RM. The adolescent spurt and sexual maturation in girls active and not active in sport. *Ann Hum Biol* 1998;25 *(in press).*
58. Malina RM. Menarche in athletes: a synthesis and hypothesis. *Ann Hum Biol* 1983;10:1–24.
59. Beunen G, Malina RM. Growth and biological maturation: relevance to athletic performance. In: Bar-Or O, ed. *The child and adolescent athlete.* Oxford: Blackwell Science, 1996:3–24.
60. Malina RM. The young athlete: biological growth and maturation in a biocultural context. In: Smoll FL, Smith RE, eds. *Children and youth in sport: a biopsychosocial perspective.* Dubuque, IA: Brown and Benchmark, 1996:161–186.
61. Eveleth PB, Tanner JM. *Worldwide variation in human growth,* 2nd ed. Cambridge: Cambridge University Press, 1990.
62. Malina RM, Merrett DMS. Androgyny of physique of women athletes: comparisons by sport and over time. In: Hauspie R, Lindgren G, Falkner F, eds. *Essays on auxology.* Welwyn Garden City, Hertfordshire: Castlemead, 1995:355–363.
63. Malina RM, Bielicki T. Retrospective longitudinal growth study of boys and girls active in sport. *Acta Paediatr* 1996;85:570–576.
64. Malina RM. Physical activity and training: effects on stature and the adolescent growth spurt. *Med Sci Sports Exerc* 1994;26: 759–766.
65. Theintz GE, Howald H, Weiss U, Sizonenko PC. Evidence for a reduction of growth potential in adolescent female gymnasts. *J Pediatr* 1993;122:306–313.
66. Malina RM. Growth and maturation of elite female gymnasts: Is training a factor? In: Johnston FE, Eveleth P, Zemel B, eds. *Human growth in context.* London: Smith-Gordon, 1999 *(in press).*

67. Beunen GP, Malina RM, Renson R, Simons J, Ostyn M, Lefevre J. Physical activity and growth, maturation and performance: a longitudinal study. *Med Sci Sports Exerc* 1992;24:576–585.
68. Roemmich JN. *Weight loss effects on growth, maturation, growth related hormones, protein nutrition markers, and body composition of adolescent wrestlers.* Doctoral dissertation, Kent State University, Kent, OH, 1994.
69. Baxter-Jones ADG, Helms P, Baines-Preece J, Preece M. Menarche in intensively trained gymnasts, swimmers and tennis players. *Ann Hum Biol* 1994;21:407–415.
70. Brooks-Gunn J, Warren MP. Mother-daughter differences in menarcheal age in adolescent girls attending national dance company schools and non-dancers. *Ann Hum Biol* 1988;15:35–43.
71. Malina RM, Ryan RC, Bonci CM. Age at menarche in athletes and their mothers and sisters. *Ann Hum Biol* 1994;21:417–422.
72. Stager JM, Hatler LK. Menarche in athletes: the influence of genetics and prepubertal training. *Med Sci Sports Exerc* 1988;20:369–373.
73. Malina RM, Katzmarzyk PT, Bonci CM, Ryan RC, Wellens RE. Family size and age at menarche in athletes. *Med Sci Sports Exerc* 1997;29:99–106.
74. Malina RM, Bouchard C, Shoup RF, Lariviere G. Age, family size and birth order in Montreal Olympic athletes. In: Carter JEL, ed. *Physical structure of Olympic athletes: part I. The Montreal Olympic Games Anthropological Project.* Basel: S. Karger, 1982: 13–24.
75. Graber JA, Brooks-Gunn J, Warren MP. The antecedents of menarcheal age: heredity, family environment, and stressful life events. *Child Dev* 1995;66:346–359.
76. Jones B, Leeton J, McLeod I, Wood C. Factors influencing the age at menarche in a lower socioeconomic group in Melbourne. *Med J Aust* 1972;2:533–535.
77. Surbey MK. Family composition, stress, and the timing of human menarche. In: Ziegler TE, Bercovitch FB, eds. *Socioendocrinology of primate reproduction.* New York: Wiley-Liss, 1990:11–32.
78. Sundgot-Borgen J, Larsen S. Preoccupation with weight and menstrual function in female elite athletes. *Scand J Med Sci Sports* 1993;3:156–163.
79. Grumbach MM, Kaplan SL. The neuroendocrinology of human puberty: an ontogenetic perspective. In: Grumbach MM, Sizonenko PC, Aubert ML, eds. *Control of the onset of puberty.* Baltimore: Williams & Wilkins, 1990:1–62.
80. Loucks AB, Vaitukaitis J, Cameron JL, et al. The reproductive system and exercise in women. *Med Sci Sports Exerc* 1992;24: S288–S293.
81. Clapp JF, Little KD. The interaction between regular exercise and selected aspects of women's health. *Am J Obstet Gynecol* 1995;173:2–9.
82. Kannus P, Sievanen H, Vuori I. Physical loading, exercise, and bone. *Bone* 1996;18:1S–3S.
83. Slemenda CW, Miller JZ, Hui SL, Reister TK, Johnston CC. Role of physical activity in the development of skeletal mass in children. *J Bone Miner Res* 1991;6:1227–1233.
84. Slemenda CW, Reister TK, Hui SL, Miller JA, Christian JC, Johnston CC. Influences on skeletal mineralization in children and adolescents: evidence for varying effects of sexual maturation and physical activity. *J Pediatr* 1994;125:201–207.
85. Cassell C, Benedict M, Specker B. Bone mineral density in elite 7- to 9-yr-old female gymnasts and swimmers. *Med Sci Sports Exerc* 1996;28:1243–1246.
86. Grimston SK, Willows ND, Hanley DA. Mechanical loading regime and its relationship to bone mineral density in children. *Med Sci Sports Exerc* 1993;25:1203–1210.
87. Robinson TL, Snow-Harter C, Taaffe DR, Gillis D, Shaw J, Marcus R. Gymnasts exhibit higher bone mass than runners despite similar prevalence of amenorrhea and oligomenorrhea. *J Bone Miner Res* 1995;10:26–35.
88. Slemenda CW, Johnston CC. High intensity activities in young women: site specific bone mass effects among female figure skaters. *Bone Miner* 1993;20:125–132.
89. Taaffe DR, Snow-Harter C, Connolly DC, Robinson TR, Brown MD, Marcus R. Differential effects of swimming versus weight-bearing activity on bone mineral status of eumenorrheic athletes. *J Bone Miner Res* 1995;10:586–593.
90. Young N, Formica C, Szmukler G, Seeman E. Bone density at weight-bearing and non–weight-bearing sites in ballet dancers: the effects of exercise, hypogonadism, and body weight. *J Clin Endocrinol Metab* 1994;78:449–454.
91. Kannus P, Haapasalo H, Sankelo M, et al. Effect of starting age of physical activity on bone mass in the dominant arm of tennis and squash players. *Ann Intern Med* 1995;123:27–31.
92. Drinkwater BL, Nilson K, Chesnut CH, Bremner WJ, Shainholtz S, Southworth MB. Bone mineral content of amenorrheic and eumenorrheic athletes. *N Engl J Med* 1984;311:277–281.
93. Okano H, Mizunuma H, Soda M-Y, Matsui H, Aoki I, Honjo S-I, Ibuki Y. Effects of exercise and amenorrhea on bone mineral density in teenage runners. *Endocr J* 1995;42:271–276.
94. Fournier GB, Ricci J, Taylor AW, Ferguson RJ, Montpetit RR, Chaitman BR. Skeletal muscle adaptation in adolescent boys: sprint and endurance training and detraining. *Med Sci Sports Exerc* 1982;14:453–456.
95. Eriksson BO, Gollnick PD, Saltin B. The effect of physical training on muscle enzyme activities and fiber composition in 11-year-old boys. *Acta Paediatr Belg Suppl* 1974;28:245–252.
96. Despres J-P, Bouchard C, Tremblay A, Savard R, Marcotte M. Effects of aerobic training on fat distribution in male subjects. *Med Sci Sports Exerc* 1985;17:113–118.
97. Tremblay A, Despres J-P, Bouchard C. Alteration in body fat and fat distribution with exercise. In: Bouchard C, Johnston FE, eds. *Fat distribution during growth and later health outcomes.* New York: Liss, 1988:297–312.
98. Despres J-P, Bouchard C, Savard R, Tremblay A, Marcotte M, Theriault G. The effect of a 20-week endurance training program on adipose-tissue morphology and lipolysis in men and women. *Metabolism* 1984;33:235–239.

Exercise and Sport Science,
edited by William E. Garrett, Jr., and Donald T. Kirkendall.
Lippincott Williams & Wilkins, Philadelphia © 2000.

CHAPTER 30

The Effects of Hypo- and Hyperbaria on Performance

Robert F. Chapman and Benjamin D. Levine

Barometric pressure changes as a function of altitude, and the physical features and physiologic effects that accompany changes in pressure, can have a dramatic influence on physical performance. Relative to a normobaric state at sea level (i.e., a standard barometric pressure of 760 mm Hg or 1 atm), *hypobaria* is defined as an environment of reduced pressure. The most simple physical manifestation of hypobaria occurs with travel to increasingly higher altitude, and for the purposes of this chapter hypobaria will be used synonymously with terms such as altitude and elevation. As one descends below sea level, a condition of *hyperbaria*, or increased pressure, exists. The increased pressure of hyperbaria also exists underwater, as the weight of the water above creates additional pressure.

Although the barometric pressure decreases with increasing elevation (Fig. 30–1), the percentages of the individual gases that make up air remain the same. Therefore, with a given change in the barometric pressure, the inspired partial pressure of oxygen (PIO_2) will change in a proportional manner. The density of a gas is also affected by changes in pressure, and it will increase or decrease with hyper- or hypobaria, respectively. Ultimately, exercise performance in hypo- and hyperbaria will be affected by the influence of three factors:

1. The density of the atmosphere and the resultant effect on air resistance, or drag.
2. The partial pressure of oxygen and the resultant effect on oxygen transport and uptake.
3. The process of acclimatization, affecting oxygen transport, metabolism, and acid-base balance.

R. F. Chapman: Human Performance Laboratory, Indiana University, Bloomington, Indiana, 47408.
B. D. Levine: Presbyterian Hospital of Dallas, Institute for Exercise and Environmental Medicine, Dallas, Texas 75231.

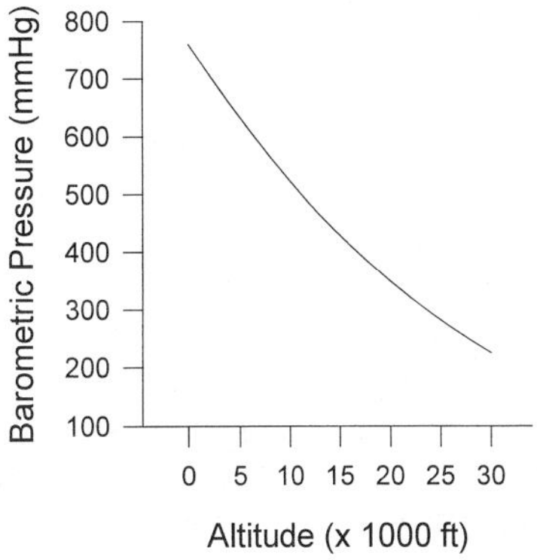

FIG. 30–1. Graph displaying the change in barometric pressure as a function of altitude.

For a given athletic event, the contribution of one of the above factors could be either substantial or insignificant, and the extent of performance change at a given altitude varies widely with the mode of exercise (e.g., swimming, running, cycling, speed skating, etc.) and the event distance (e.g., sprints, middle distance, long distance). Similarly, many athletes show a substantial amount of individual variation in how they are affected by an acute change in PIO_2 (1,2) or how they ultimately acclimatize with chronic exposure to a new atmospheric pressure (3). As a result, it is important to remember the potential for exercise mode, distance, and individual subject variance when discussing the global effects of hypo/hyperbaria on exercise performance in the athletic population.

HYPOBARIA

Sprint Events

To perform well in sprint events, the human body must overcome various resistances to attain as high a speed as possible over a given distance. One of the key resistive components to overcome is the slowing effect of drag (4). Drag is defined as a retarding force acting upon a body in motion through a fluid. The amount of drag faced by an exercising human is dependent on the shape and size of the body, the fluid medium in which the exercise is being performed (i.e., air or water), and the velocity of the body relative to the medium. For motion through air, the amount of drag increases as a function of the square of the velocity. Therefore, for athletic events performed at very high speeds, such as cycling, speed skating, and the sprint events in running, drag has a significant effect on performance. For example, when cycling at speeds >40 km/h, drag is responsible for over 90% of the energy cost needed to maintain that speed (5). With running, the metabolic cost of overcoming air resistance has been measured at 3% to 9% (depending on running speed) of the total energy cost of running in still air (6). At altitude, the reduced density of the air lessens the slowing effect of drag, therefore (a) higher speeds can be generated for a given peak power output, and conversely (b) the energy cost to maintain a given speed is lower (7).

Oxygen transport to the working muscles at altitude is reduced in the sprint athlete, just as it is reduced in the endurance athlete and the untrained individual. For maximal exercise bouts lasting less than 2 minutes in duration, however, the majority of the adenosine triphosphate (ATP) necessary to fuel muscular contraction is derived from substrate-level phosphorylation (i.e., creatine phosphate, free ATP, and glycolysis; although frequently termed anaerobic this is a misnomer). For example, in an event lasting 30 seconds, it is estimated that 80% of the energy requirement is generated glycolytically, and only 20% of the energy requirement is met through oxidative or aerobic sources (8). As a result, the reduction in maximal aerobic power at altitude, being such a small percentage of the overall energy contribution in sprint events, is more than offset by the reduced drag. The end result is that sprint event performances are typically enhanced at moderate altitude, often to the degree that world, Olympic, and national sprint event records have historically been set at altitude. Many sports create special statistical labels, such as an asterisk or an "A," to designate record-setting sprint performances achieved at altitude.

There is one notable exception and a few special cases of the effect of drag on endurance exercise performance at altitude. In swimming, the slowing forces of drag are markedly more substantial than sports that take place in air, due to the special properties of the environmental medium of water (9). Unfortunately for the swimmer, the effect of hypobaria on the density of water is insignificant. Therefore, sprint swimmers do not enjoy the same performance-enhancing effect of reduced drag as "terrestrial" sprint athletes. In the special case of very high speed sports, such as cycling and speed skating, the reduced effect of drag at altitude is beneficial not only for the sprint athlete but for the endurance athlete as well. Although the decline in oxygen transport with increasing hypobaria negatively affects maximal oxygen uptake, a crucial component of success in endurance events, distance cycling, and speed skating performance is typically augmented at moderate altitudes. Due to the high speeds generated, even in the distance events in these sports, the reduced drag at altitude is functionally greater than altitude-induced decline in $\dot{V}O_2max$. As a result, world records for cycling events like the solo 1-hour time trial for distance are often set at moderate altitudes. Mathematical modeling of altitude's combined effects on aerobic power and drag for the 1-hour cycling event suggests that the optimal altitude for this event is between 3400 and 4000 m (11,200 and 13,000 feet) (10–12), compared to sea level, where the distance covered in 1 hour by a top elite cyclist would theoretically increase ~3.9 to 4.8 km (10,12).

The issue of chronic altitude exposure and acclimatization and the effect on sprint performance is controversial. The reduced drag allows higher speeds to be maintained in training, which over time may promote a positive training adaptation. In the longer sprint events (i.e., 1 to 2 minutes), where performance is partially dependent on the ability to tolerate high levels of muscle acidosis (13), the metabolic stimulus generated during sprint training may be altered with altitude exposure and acclimatization. At any given submaximal work load, lactate production is increased; however, during maximal exercise at altitude, the peak accumulation of lactate in the blood and muscles is reduced compared with maximal exercise at sea level, the so-called lactate paradox (14). Thus, it is possible that prolonged sprint training at altitude may ultimately lead to reduced performance for these athletes.

Controversy also surrounds what happens to buffering capacity with chronic exposure to altitude. Ventilation increases in response to altitude, causing a reduction in arterial P_{CO_2} (i.e., respiratory alkalosis). To compensate, the kidneys excrete additional bicarbonate ions, which are the primary acid buffering agent in the blood. What happens to buffering capacity in the muscle is less clear, however, with some studies reporting a decrease in muscle-buffering capacity (15) and others reporting an increase in muscle-buffering capacity with altitude acclimatization (16).

Endurance Events

Although some scientific investigations have examined the effect of altitude on endurance athletes with direct measures of performance (such as 5000-m run time or distance cycled in 1 hour), many more studies have examined hypobaria's effect on maximal oxygen uptake

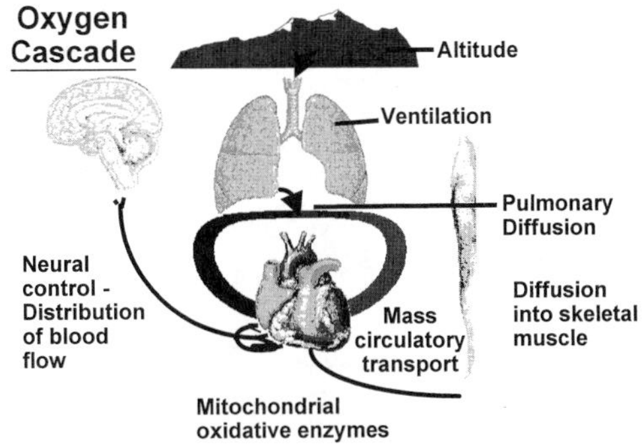

FIG. 30–2. The oxygen cascade.

($\dot{V}O_2$max). This strategy is certainly appropriate in examining the effect of acute altitude exposure on endurance exercise, as success in endurance events is closely linked to the ability to utilize oxygen at a high rate (17).

Since the amount of oxygen transported to the working muscles is a primary determinant of $\dot{V}O_2$max, it becomes important to understand the steps oxygen must follow on its journey from atmosphere to mitochondria—steps known as the *oxygen cascade*. The oxygen cascade refers to the transfer of oxygen from the atmosphere → to the alveoli → the pulmonary capillary and arterial blood → the muscle capillary through the transport of blood → the mitochondria (Fig. 30–2). Oxygen is transported through different portions of the body either through mechanisms of bulk flow (e.g., ventilation, blood flow) or diffusion. The process of diffusion is dependent on a pressure gradient to drive the oxygen from areas of high pressure to areas of lower pressure. As a result, the partial pressure of oxygen (PO_2) always falls as it moves down the cascade. With hypobaric exposure, the initial inlet pressure (i.e., the atmosphere) is reduced; therefore, the PO_2 at each step along the cascade will subsequently be lower compared to that at sea level. The body often attempts to compensate for this reduction in PO_2 at altitude by increasing bulk flow where possible. If the hypobaria is substantial enough, however, less oxygen ultimately reaches the mitochondria and $\dot{V}O_2$max is reduced. With endurance exercise at altitude, the subsequent reduction of performance has been closely linked to the first two steps of the oxygen cascade: the transfer of O_2 from the atmosphere to the alveoli, and the alveoli to the arterial blood.

Oxygen Cascade Step 1—Atmosphere to Alveoli

The first step in the oxygen cascade is the link between the atmospheric or inspired partial pressure of oxygen and alveolar PO_2 (PAO_2). With each inhalation, the bulk flow of oxygen rich air into the lung mixes with the lower oxygen content residual air left in the lung at the end of expiration, resulting in a reduction in PAO_2. For example, at sea level, PIO_2 is 159 mm Hg, but resting PAO_2 is typically between 100 and 110 mm Hg. The magnitude of the fall between PIO_2 and PAO_2 is regulated to a large extent by the process of ventilation. Specifically, the greater the amount of ventilation (or hyperventilation), usually the higher the PAO_2 and the more PAO_2 will resemble the PIO_2.

With acute exposure to altitude, the peripheral chemoreceptors located in the carotid bodies sense the reduction in PO_2 and stimulate the respiratory center in the brain to increase ventilation—a process termed the *hypoxic ventilatory response* (HVR). The magnitude of the HVR is particularly important to one set of endurance athletes who perform at very high altitudes—mountaineers. On the summit of Mt. Everest at 8848 m (29,028 feet), inspired PO_2 is only 49 to 54 mm Hg, depending on climatic conditions. If the magnitude of the oxygen cascade from PIO_2 to PAO_2 on Mt. Everest was similar to the PO_2 change at sea level (as early physiologists hypothesized), PAO_2 would be nearly zero and the summit could not be reached without supplemental oxygen. However, a strong hyperventilatory response to hypoxia maximizes PAO_2 and helps to ensure that the precious little oxygen that is available in the atmosphere finds its way to the arterial blood. One study has confirmed that mountaineers with strong HVRs are able to climb to higher altitudes, versus climbers with reduced HVRs (18). Therefore, the ability to summit Everest is due to not only mountaineering skill (and good luck), but to also a baseline physiologic property that may be beyond the control of the athlete.

As a general group characteristic, endurance athletes have ventilatory responses to hypoxia (19) and exercise (20) that are significantly blunted or reduced compared to untrained individuals and sprint-trained athletes. While this blunted ventilatory response and reduced exercise PAO_2 is generally theorized to be detrimental to endurance exercise performance at altitude, this unique trait may help to minimize the metabolic cost associated with using the ventilatory musculature during heavy exercise (21). Furthermore, the magnitude of the HVR does not correlate well with the decline in distance running performance with acute altitude exposure (Chapman and Levine, unpublished data).

In the highly trained endurance athlete, such as a distance runner or road cyclist, the ventilatory response to exercise at altitude has traditionally been thought to be crucial to performance at altitude (22). Recent scientific data show mixed findings, however. Much of the data from endurance athletes is confounded by the fact that this population often displays varied exercise ventilatory responses to altitude, and many do not possess the compensatory ventilatory reserve necessary to mitigate the fall in PIO_2. As a group, highly trained endurance athletes already have a ventilatory output during maximal exercise at sea level that is 40% to 60%

greater than an untrained individual (23). As a result, a large percentage of endurance-trained athletes reach a mechanical limit to ventilatory flow, despite normal resting pulmonary function (24). When confronted with hypoxic and/or hypercapnic stimuli, these athletes are unable to increase minute ventilation at maximal exercise (24,25). Surprisingly, though, the subset of athletes who do possess a mechanical reserve to increase maximal exercise ventilation in hypoxia show similar declines in $\dot{V}O_2$max compared with athletes with ventilatory flow limitations at maximal exercise (25).

Oxygen Cascade Step 2—Alveolar to Arterial P_{O_2}

Oxygen moves from the alveoli to the arterial blood by dissolving and diffusing through the alveolar membrane and interstitial space. This process of pulmonary gas exchange is extremely rapid, typically occurring in a fraction of a second. In healthy individuals at rest, the difference between alveolar and arterial partial pressures, abbreviated as the A-aD_{O_2}, is small—typically less than 5 mm Hg. During heavy exercise, however, the efficacy of pulmonary gas exchange can become compromised (Fig. 30–3), particularly in the endurance-trained athlete in whom maximal cardiac output can increase with training, but pulmonary mechanics and diffusing capacity are relatively static properties of the lung. As a result, the A-aD_{O_2} in endurance-trained athletes can rise to as high as 50 mm Hg at maximal exercise (20,26). This limitation in pulmonary gas exchange that occurs in many highly trained endurance athletes is due to a combination of two factors: (a) a mismatch between ventilation and blood perfusion within individual alveoli, and (b) a high pulmonary blood flow within a relatively fixed pulmonary capillary blood volume, causing a decrease in the time the erythrocyte is exposed to the gas exchange area of the lung (23). Because many endurance-trained athletes also demonstrate an inadequate hyperventilatory response to heavy exercise (20,26), a reduced Pa_{O_2}, combined with a high A-aD_{O_2}, results in a substantially reduced Pa_{O_2} during heavy exercise.

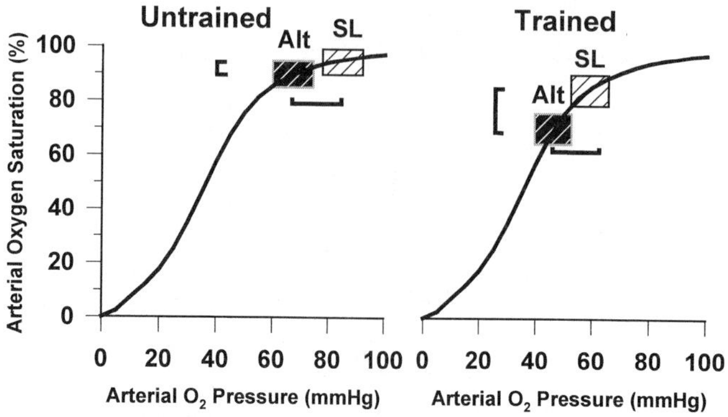

FIG. 30–4. Graphs depicting the change in arterial oxygen saturation for a given change in arterial oxygen partial press (as with altitude) in untrained (*left*) and trained (*right*) subjects. Note the change in arterial oxygen content is much larger in trained subjects.

Because of the unique sigmoidal shape of the oxyhemoglobin dissociation curve, an exercise-induced reduction in Pa_{O_2} in the endurance athlete begins to approach the steeper down-sloping portion of the dissociation curve. At this point, a given change in Pa_{O_2}, as occurs with altitude, has a much larger affect on arterial oxygen saturation and content compared with the flatter portion of the curve (Fig. 30–4). During maximal exercise at sea level, the P_{AO_2} of an untrained individual remains on the upper, flatter portion of the curve, where Sa_{O_2} and arterial oxygen content are relatively unaffected by changes in Pa_{O_2}. Therefore, when the hypoxia of altitude is superimposed on maximal exercise, Pa_{O_2} will fall somewhat uniformly across individuals, but the fall in arterial oxygen saturation can be much more severe in endurance athletes who possess a substantial degree of exercise-induced pulmonary gas exchange limitations. Because at maximal exercise there is little compensatory reserve left in the remaining links of oxygen cascade, total oxygen transport and ultimately $\dot{V}O_2$max are reduced to a greater extent in the athlete compared to more sedentary individuals.

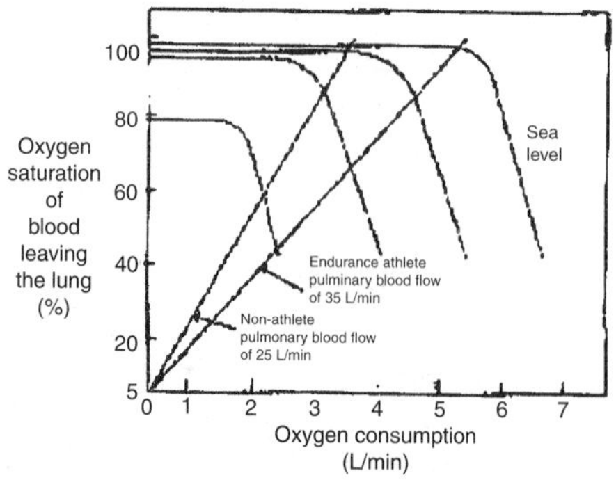

FIG. 30–3. Comparison of the alveolar-arterial oxygen difference between endurance-trained athletes and untrained subjects at maximal exercise.

The Concepts of Susceptibility and Threshold Altitude

Among athletes who live at sea level but regularly compete at altitude, there are often anecdotal accounts of some athletes being more or less affected by altitude than others. Much of the early scientific work investigating the effect of altitude on endurance exercise performance was completed in the late 1960s and early 1970s, coinciding with the Olympic Games of 1968 held in Mexico City (elevation 2290 m, 7550 feet). With acute exposure to altitude, one early study noted that highly trained distance runners demonstrated greater declines in performance, versus lesser trained individuals (27). Since then, several studies have demonstrated a significant correlational relationship between $\dot{V}O_2$max at sea level and the decline in $\dot{V}O_2$max at acute altitude (28–30). Although the individuals with the highest $\dot{V}O_2$max at sea level still have the highest $\dot{V}O_2$max at altitude, these studies do confirm that highly trained endurance athletes are more severely handicapped by acute altitude exposure.

The mechanism behind the relationship between $\dot{V}O_2$max and the decline in $\dot{V}O_2$max at altitude is argued to be the greater pulmonary gas exchange limitations that are present in many elite endurance athletes during heavy exercise (1,28,31,32). Within the highly trained endurance athlete population itself, however, there does not appear to be a relationship between $\dot{V}O_2$max and the decline in $\dot{V}O_2$max at altitude. Although many endurance athletes during heavy exercise at sea level do desaturate (often to $SaO_2 < 92\%$), this phenomenon has been estimated to occur in only about 50% of the endurance athlete population (33). The remaining athletes with similarly high maximal oxygen uptakes are able to maintain SaO_2 at $\dot{V}O_2$max near resting levels (i.e., SaO_2 from 92% to 95%), characteristic of the normal or untrained population. These normoxemic athletes have been documented to have smaller reductions in $\dot{V}O_2$max at a mild altitude, compared to athletes with prominent arterial desaturation at $\dot{V}O_2$max. Moreover, a significant correlation was found between SaO_2 at $\dot{V}O_2$max at sea level and the decline in $\dot{V}O_2$max at altitude (34). This relationship also extends to measures of performance. For example, in a group of 26 elite distance runners, individuals with the highest SaO_2 during maximal exercise at sea level demonstrated the smallest slowing of 3000-m run time from sea level to 2100 m (7000 feet) (Chapman, Stray-Gundersen, and Levine, unpublished data). Taken as a whole, these studies indicate that the ability to maintain arterial oxygen saturation during heavy exercise, and not training status per se, has a strong influence on the ability to maintain $\dot{V}O_2$max and exercise performance at altitude.

Conceptually, as one ascends progressively from sea level, the gradual reduction in inspired PO_2 will be manifested throughout the steps in the oxygen cascade, and exercise performance will ultimately be reduced. However, at very mild altitudes, certain components of the oxygen cascade, such as the oxygen loading of hemoglobin and augmented delivery of blood to working muscles, compensate for the small decline in PIO_2. At some altitude, however, the ability of these oxygen cascade components to compensate for the reduced PIO_2 will be maximized, and any further reduction in PIO_2 will result in a reduction in oxygen transport to the working skeletal muscle. Physiologists have historically referred to this theoretical point as the threshold altitude for aerobic impairment.

The point at which this threshold altitude is believed to occur has undergone debate. Early data published by Buskirk and colleagues (35) in 1967 (35) on moderately trained individuals set the threshold altitude at 1500 m (5000 feet), suggesting that above this point $\dot{V}O_2$max is linearly reduced 1% for every 100 m (330 feet) of elevation. At that time, however, data on the reduction in $\dot{V}O_2$max at milder altitudes was lacking, and several later studies indicated circumstantial evidence for a reduction in $\dot{V}O_2$max at altitudes below 1500 m. Later results indicated a significant reduction in $\dot{V}O_2$max at 4000 feet (1200 m), and a strong linear relationship was present between altitude and $\dot{V}O_2$max (36). As a result, the concept of a threshold altitude may be misleading, and for a group of athletically trained runners $\dot{V}O_2$max may decrease progressively with ascension from sea level. Current theories hold that a threshold altitude is an individual phenomenon, with some athletes impaired immediately with a change in elevation from sea level, and others not impaired until much higher elevations are reached.

The mechanism behind the concepts of threshold altitude and susceptibility to performance declines at altitude are certainly interrelated, both being dependent on a combination of training status and gas exchange limitations. At mild altitudes of 1200 m (31) and 900 m (1), highly trained athletes demonstrated significant declines in SaO_2 and $\dot{V}O_2$max, while untrained subjects did not demonstrate a decline in $\dot{V}O_2$max. Within highly trained athletes themselves, eight athletes with low measures of SaO_2 at $\dot{V}O_2$max at sea level demonstrated significant declines in $\dot{V}O_2$max at 1000 m (3300 feet) (34). In contrast, six athletes who were able to maintain saturation near resting levels during heavy exercise did not have a significant reduction in $\dot{V}O_2$max at mild altitude. Therefore, as a general rule, highly trained endurance athletes (a) demonstrate greater reductions in $\dot{V}O_2$max at altitude compared to nonathletes, and (b) begin to show declines in $\dot{V}O_2$max at very mild altitudes—perhaps immediately upon ascent from sea level. A wide interindividual variability in both altitude susceptibility and threshold altitude are evident across the trained and untrained population, however, with gas exchange abilities in the lung being an important factor. This individual variability will affect not only competitive performance at acute altitude, but also the ability to train at altitude, strongly impacting the level of performance enhancement with chronic altitude exposure.

Training at Altitude for Altitude Performance

Chronic exposure to altitude stimulates the process of acclimatization, which induces a number of physiologic adaptations that improve exercise performance at altitude. A number of the adaptations improve oxygen transfer at various steps along the oxygen cascade, such as an increase in ventilation, hemoglobin concentration, capillary density, mitochondrial number, and tissue myoglobin concentration. Substrate utilization is also altered with chronic altitude exposure, as the mobilization of free fatty acids and dependence on blood glucose are both increased. The result is a sparing of muscle glycogen and a decreased accumulation of lactate and ammonia during submaximal exercise. Taken together, these adaptations dramatically improve submaximal exercise capacity with chronic altitude exposure and training. Maximal exercise capacity is improved over time at altitude, and at moderate altitudes may actually approach sea level values after 1 to 2 weeks of acclimatization.

For competitions that take place at altitude, there is substantial scientific evidence that the processes of acclimatization clearly improve altitude exercise performance. Therefore, it becomes critical to plan an acclimatization period to moderate altitude, if possible, prior to an altitude competition. Most of the short-term acclimatization responses will be obtained after 2 to 3 weeks, a time period that maximizes acclimatization but minimizes the potential for detraining at altitude due to reduced training intensity. If this time period is not available for acclimatization, it has been theorized that arriving at altitude immediately prior to competition may be best. This theory has not been rigorously tested, however.

Training at Altitude for Sea-Level Performance

For altitude training to have a physiologic benefit over training at sea level, performance must be enhanced either through the process of acclimatization to altitude, the adaptations with training in hypoxia, or a combination of the two (37,38). With acclimatization to altitude, the most prominent adaptation that augments endurance exercise performance is an increase in the oxygen-carrying capacity of the blood (39,40). The specific effects of hypoxic training on performance, separate from acclimatization, are less clear. With small-muscle exercise, in which training work rates can be identical in hypoxia or normoxia, hypoxic training has been demonstrated to be accompanied by greater increases in oxidative enzymes compared with normoxic training (15). This adaptation is not conclusive with full-body dynamic exercise such as cycling or running, however. A potential confounding influence is the difference in exercise intensity that is maintained between training at sea level and at altitude. Because of the decline in oxygen transport to working muscles at altitude, training speeds and oxygen uptakes are reduced at altitude, both in low-intensity workouts and high-intensity interval training (38). As a result, the quality of the overall training stimulus is reduced, and many athletes actually detrain with chronic hypoxic exercise (41). Ultimately, the outcome of training at altitude will depend on the delicate balance between the extent of hematologic acclimatization and ability of the athlete to train at a sufficiently high level (3,38).

Historically, studies that have examined the effect of altitude training on sea-level performance have produced contradictory results. A large number of these studies suffer from the following experimental design problems:

1. Controlling for the group training effect. The atmosphere of a training camp has many positive qualities that, in themselves, enhance performance compared to typical training in the athlete's home environment. While at a training camp, the athlete usually does not have the added stressors of work, family, or social responsibilities and can focus solely on training. When athletes gather as a group for a training camp, the quality and quantity of training typically increase over precamp levels (41,42). As a result, performance is often enhanced with a training camp regardless of the location. To adequately control for this phenomenon in altitude-training studies requires a somewhat costly and burdensome step of bringing the athlete cohort together to train at sea level for an extended period of time prior to going to an altitude camp.
2. Uncertain training levels before an altitude camp. In many published studies, the training status of the athletes was not documented prior to altitude training. Therefore, it is not known if an increase (or decline) in $\dot{V}O_2$max or racing performance with altitude training is solely due to the effects of altitude, versus a change in the quantity and quality of training done during an altitude camp. As is needed in controlling for the group training effect, supervised training at sea level can serve as a control, which should ideally be equivalent to the training load completed at altitude.
3. Lack of an independent sea-level control group. While a prealtitude training camp serves as an adequate sea-level control within individuals, it still does not confirm that longitudinal training at sea level is just as effective as altitude training between groups.
4. Controlling for poor iron stores. Iron is a fundamental and required element in the production of hemoglobin and erythrocytes, as well as other heme-containing cytochromes. Unfortunately, a high percentage of highly trained athletes—particularly distance runners—have clinically low levels of iron stored as ferritin (43). With 4 weeks of acclimatization to 2500 m (8000 feet), athletes with low ferritin levels did not increase their total volume of red cells. However, athletes with normal ferritin levels displayed the typical and desired significant increase in red cell volume and $\dot{V}O_2$max (44) (Fig. 30–5). Subse-

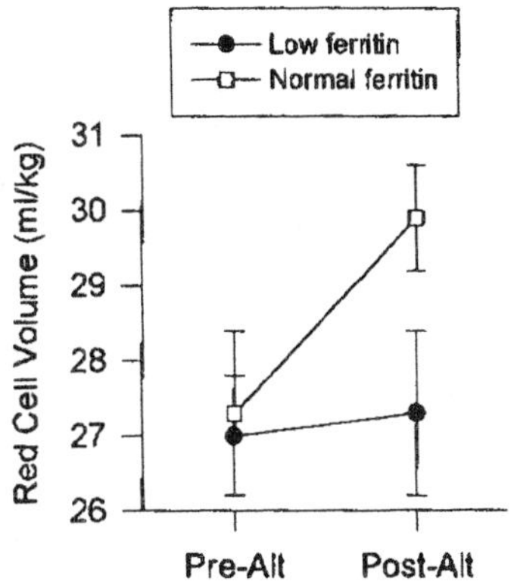

FIG. 30–5. Changes in red cell volume about 4 weeks of exposure to 2500 m (8000 ft) in athletes with normal serum ferritin levels (*open symbols*) and low serum ferritin (*closed symbols*).

quently, if iron-deficient athletes were vigorously supplemented while at altitude (up to 400 mg of elemental iron per day in some athletes), red cell volume increased significantly (43). Many early studies did not realize the importance of proper iron supplementation at altitude and the resultant effect on acclimatization and performance. As a result, the data from many early investigations may be confounded by the status of iron stores in the athlete cohorts being studied.

In the few investigations where substantial effort has been made to establish experimental controls, living and training at altitude has not been proven to be superior to equivalent sea-level training. Arguably the most well-controlled and widely referenced early study on altitude training for sea-level performance was completed by Adams and colleagues in 1975 (45). Twelve well-trained distance runners completed 20 days of training at sea level and 20 days of living and training at 2300 m (7600 feet). Using a crossover design, six athletes trained the first 20 days at sea level while the other six athletes trained at altitude. After 20 days, the two groups switched training locations and continued training for an additional 20 days. After the respective period of training at altitude, $\dot{V}O_2max$ at sea level was 2.8% lower in each group, while 2-mile run time was 7 seconds faster in the altitude/sea-level group and 7 seconds slower in the sea-level/altitude group. The authors concluded that altitude training did not significantly enhance endurance running performance at sea level, over equivalent sea-level training.

Alternative Strategies of Altitude Training for Sea-Level Performance

Perhaps the most promising recent practical application of altitude training for sea-level performance is the alternative theory of live high–train low, as proposed by Levine and Stray-Gundersen (38). The live high–train low model combines living at a moderate altitude of 2500 m (8000 feet) with training at a lower altitude of 1250 m (4000 feet). With the high-low training model, the athlete would theoretically still gain the acclimatization benefit of an increased volume of red cell mass from living at moderate altitude. In conducting training at a lower altitude, however, an altitude-mediated detraining effect may be minimized as training speeds and oxygen uptakes approach sea-level values. The authors investigated this hypothesis by bringing 39 well-trained distance runners to sea level for a 6-week training period prior to a 4-week altitude-training camp (38). This sea-level training period was designed to control for the group training effect, as well as to allow for the normalization of iron stores through gradual and prolonged iron supplementation. The sea-level training period also served as a longitudinal control, with the last 4 weeks of sea-level training designed to match the training conducted during the 4 weeks at altitude. After the sea-level training period, the athletes were randomly divided into three groups, each with nine men and four women: a high-high group that lived at 2500 m (8000 feet) and did all training between 2500 and 3000 m (8000 to 10,000 feet), a high-low group that lived at 2500 m and did all training at 1200 to 1400 m (4000 to 4600 feet), and a low-low group that served as a control by living and training at sea level over hilly terrain. After the 4-week altitude camp, significant increases were found in both red cell mass (~13%) and $\dot{V}O_2max$ (~5%) over prealtitude levels in both the high-high and high-low groups. However, only the high-low group demonstrated a significant 1.5% improvement in sea-level 5000-m run time after the altitude camp. The difference in training between the high-high and high-low groups appears to be a key factor behind this result, as a reduction in training intensity in distance runners has been linked to significantly poorer running performance over 5000 m despite a preservation of $\dot{V}O_2max$ (46). Additionally, the greater training velocities maintained at low altitude are believed to be responsible for the significant increase in the velocity at $\dot{V}O_2max$ and the $\dot{V}O_2max$ at the maximal steady state, shown only by the high-low group.

The high-low group lived in the Park City/Deer Valley area in Utah and was able to reach lower altitude training sites in Salt Lake City, about 30 minutes' driving time. However, despite the advantages of this unique geographic location in implementing the high-low training model, the daily travel burden associated with this approach can be logistically inconvenient. Since the reduction in base or low-intensity training velocity at altitude was unrelated to the change in sea-level 5000-m performance with high-low training, it was proposed that traveling to low altitude only for high-intensity training would be equally as beneficial to sea-level running performance as complete or daily high-low training. Thirteen subjects (nine men, four women) completed the same basic 10-week study design as the high-low subjects, but followed the high-high-low paradigm (live high, base train high, and interval train low) of living at 2500 m, all low-intensity training at elevations between 2200 and 3000 m, and all high-intensity training between 1200 and 1400 m (47). Upon return to sea level, the high-high-low group demonstrated nearly identical mean improvements in $\dot{V}O_2max$ (2.5 mL/kg/min) and 5000 m run time (15 seconds) as the previous high-low group. Because the high-high-low model was just as effective at enhancing performance as the high-low model, it is an attractive method to minimize the burden of travel to low altitude for workouts. Furthermore, in establishing the effectiveness of the high-high-low model, application of this new form of altitude training can be accomplished in more geographic locations—as somewhat longer drives to a sufficiently low altitude for high-intensity training can be tolerated if reduced to 2 to 3 days per week.

The mean improvements in 5000-m performance with the various high-low models, about 14 seconds or 1.5% as seen in United States collegiate level runners, functionally represents about a 60- to 80-m advantage—a substantial amount in competitive terms. For the world-class athlete, who is theoretically nearer to the absolute limit of human performance, there was a concern that an intervention such as the high-low model might not affect performance to the same magnitude as less talented athletes. To test this hypothesis, 22 U.S. national-class distance runners completed 4 weeks of high-high-low training in the same Utah setting as previously studied groups (3). Despite having baseline 3000-m-run performance measures that were, relative to the American record, substantially faster than the collegiate athletes 5000-m-run performances, the national-class group demonstrated similar $\dot{V}O_2max$ and performance responses as the collegiate group to the high-high-low training model (Fig. 30–6). Additionally, the range of

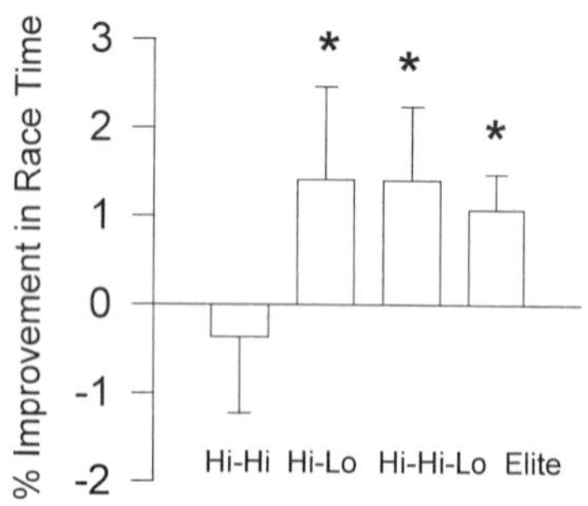

FIG. 30–6. Graph displaying the percentage improvement in 3000- or 5000-m race time after 4 weeks of altitude training. *Hi-Hi,* live high–train high; *Hi-Lo,* live high–train low; *Hi-Hi-Lo,* live high–base train high–interval train low. *Significant improvement, $p < .05$.

responses in performance improvement (−2% to +6%) seen in the national-class group are similar to the range of responses in the collegiate group. Therefore, the degree of performance enhancement with the high-low training model is not dependent on baseline $\dot{V}O_2max$ or performance level.

Individual Variability: Acclimatization Versus Training

What then *does* influence the degree of performance enhancement with altitude training? What accounts for the somewhat wide variation in performance responses with the high-low model? Why do some athletes show improvements with the traditional form of altitude training (i.e., high-high), while others do not improve with the more optimal high-low method? The answer appears to lie in the individual variation of identifiable characteristics in the acclimatization response and the training response to altitude. Thirty-nine collegiate level athletes who lived at a common altitude of 2500 m for 4 weeks and trained either at moderate (2200 to 3000 m) or low (1200 to 1400 m) altitude were retrospectively divided into groups based on the degree of improvement in sea-level 5000-m-run performance (3). Athletes who substantially improved their 5000-m time by 14.1 seconds or more were classified as responders to altitude training (n = 17), while those who ran slower after altitude training were labeled as nonresponders (n = 15). The physiologic responses of each group were then examined to determine what specific characteristics of acclimatization and training influence the degree of performance enhancement with altitude training.

Although both groups demonstrated a significant increase in plasma erythropoietin (EPO) concentration after 30 hours at 2500 m, the responders had a significantly higher EPO concentration versus nonresponders. After 14 days at 2500 m, plasma EPO concentration had declined to near prealtitude levels in nonresponders, but was still significantly elevated in responders. As a result of this strong EPO response to altitude, responders had a significant 7.9% increase in red cell mass and a 6.5% increase in $\dot{V}O_2max$. However, nonresponders did not increase their red cell mass, despite the acute increase in EPO concentration, and $\dot{V}O_2max$ was not changed with altitude training. Since all subjects received iron supplementation before and during the altitude camp, these results suggest that there may be a threshold EPO level that is necessary to stimulate production of additional red cells.

Measures of the training response to altitude also differed between responders and nonresponders. After 14 days at altitude, nonresponders ran a standard 1000-m interval workout at a slower speed and lower oxygen uptake compared to a prealtitude measure. Responders did not have a significant decline in 1000-m interval

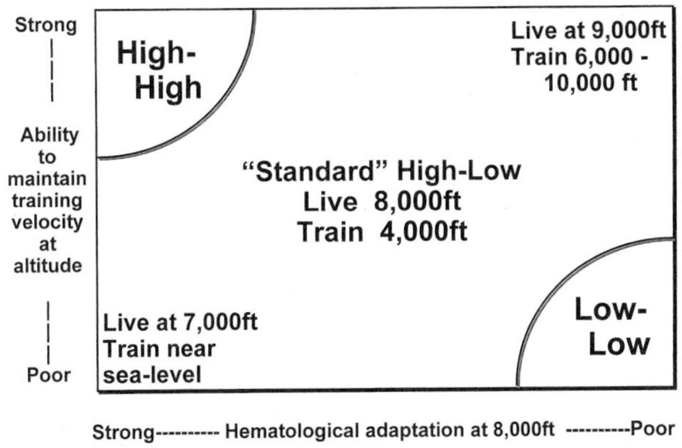

FIG. 30–7. Possible recommendations for altitude training strategy, based on the erythropoietic and training response to altitude.

workout velocity at altitude, and as a result were able to maintain a higher $\dot{V}O_2$ during those intervals compared to nonresponders. In terms of the total weekly running mileage, training duration, and training impulse, however, there was no significant difference between groups. Taken together, these results indicate that the magnitude of performance enhancement will be dependent on a combination of the strength of acclimatization to altitude and the ability to perform high-intensity training at low or moderate altitude. In the future, it may be possible to prescreen the acute EPO response and the acute exercise response to a range of altitudes and subsequently assign an optimized set of living and training altitudes for each individual athlete (Fig. 30–7). Similarly, athletes who have inherently poor responses to altitude, both in the acclimatization and training response, may be identified, and these athletes may be better served (physically and financially) by a sea-level training camp.

Practical Application and Implementation of Altitude Training for Sea-Level Performance

In terms of practical application of altitude training, the key questions most often asked by athletes, coaches, team physicians, and sports scientists are (a) how high to live, (b) how low to train, (c) how long to stay at altitude, and (d) when to return to sea level prior to a major competition.

How High to Live

The EPO response to acute altitude is proportional to the degree of hypoxic stress—the higher the altitude, the more EPO is produced (48). Across individuals, however, the EPO response to a fixed altitude can vary widely (3,43). Furthermore, although most athletes show an increase in red cell mass with 4 weeks of living at 2500 m (8000 feet), some athletes fail to increase red cell mass at this altitude. Athletes who are known to have a poor erythropoietic response to 2500 m (8000 feet) may need to live at a higher elevation to obtain an adequate increase in EPO concentrations and a subsequent increase in the oxygen-carrying capacity of the blood. Although it is logical to presume that if 2500 m is good, then 3000 m must be better in terms of generating an adequate EPO response, living at higher altitudes increases the likelihood that the athlete will experience symptoms of acute mountain sickness: headaches, poor sleep, anorexia, nausea, loss of muscle mass, and possibly pulmonary or cerebral edema. In contrast, athletes with strong EPO responses to altitude may be able to live at elevations lower than 2500 m and still experience increases in red cell mass after an altitude camp. For most individuals, however, cross-sectional data suggest that this threshold altitude is greater than 2000 m, and nearly all studies with exposure to altitudes < 2000 m show no increase in red cell mass.

How Low to Train

Theoretically, the closer to sea level that an athlete trains, the smaller the reduction in training velocity and oxygen flux. However, just as with the acclimatization response, there is a substantial variation in the ability to maintain $\dot{V}O_2$max at mild and moderate altitude among the endurance-trained populations (1,34). The only substantial training data available at this time are at an altitude of 1250 m (4000 feet), which combined with the acclimatization response to 2500 m resulted in an increase in performance (38). Therefore, in terms of a global recommendation, it appears that 1250 m is adequately low enough to preserve the training effect for most individuals. However, some individual athletes may be able to adequately train at higher elevations, while others will need to train even closer to sea level.

How Long to Stay at Altitude

Just as erythropoietin concentration increases within hours of exposure to a significant level of hypoxia or hypobaria, it decreases just as quickly (48). Although reticulocyte levels have been shown to be significantly increased with just 1 day of exposure to 15.3% O_2 (~2500 m or 8000 feet), a substantially longer period of hypoxic residence is necessary to obtain an increase in red cell mass sufficient enough to improve $\dot{V}O_2$max and exercise performance. Because EPO concentration typically peaks between 24 and 48 hours at altitude (49) and gradually declines to normal, prealtitude levels after 21 to 28 days (43), in terms of an erythropoietic response 3 to 4 weeks is the typically recommended altitude camp duration. However, it remains unknown if any additional adaptations (for example, changes in muscle morphology or metabolism) with more prolonged stays at moderate altitude will have a positive or negative effect on sea-level racing performance.

When to Return to Sea Level Prior to a Major Competition

Just as the process of acclimatization to altitude occurs over the time course of minutes to months, the process of deacclimatization occurs upon return to sea level. Some of these responses, such as reestablishment of blood-buffering capacity, should have a beneficial effect on performance. The performance-enhancing effects of an increased volume of red cell mass will eventually fade as the superfluous red cells die, however. In fact, EPO levels are typically reduced below sea-level values on return from altitude, and red-cell survival is substantially shorter than the normal 120 days. Because some given amount of red cells are being removed from the circulation daily, but less are being replaced with the reduced erythropoietic stimulus at sea level, performance should theoretically decline with each day of sea-level residence. Just as performance enhancement with altitude training is dependent on the acclimatization and training response to altitude, however, so does the maintenance of the performance enhancement after altitude training depend on the (de)acclimatization and training responses to sea level. For example, with an increased oxygen-carrying capacity of the blood and improved $\dot{V}O_2max$, higher training work loads can often be maintained upon return to sea level. As a result, an improved postaltitude sea-level training response can potentially offset the negative deacclimatization effects of a reduced O_2-carrying capacity of the blood, prolonging the overall improvement in sea-level race performance. As evidence, after 4 weeks of high-high or high-low training, collegiate athletes did not demonstrate a slowing in 5000-m performance, when measured serially out to 4 weeks of living and training at sea level (38).

Although a substantial amount of research has gone into the process of understanding the process of acclimatization to altitude, much less is known about the deacclimatization process. Still, because of the interaction of deacclimatization with an improved sea-level training response, the ideal time to compete postaltitude camp may depend on the response of the individual athlete and the training design used upon return to sea level. Anecdotally, many athletes prefer not to compete upon their initial return to sea level, which may be related to the gradual normalization of ventilatory work at a given work load or restoration of muscle and blood buffering capacity. Additionally, many runners upon return to sea level kinesthetically sense a lack of foot speed or turnover, which may be less of a factor with high-low training.

The Nitrogen House and Other Simulated Altitude Models

A recent creative application of the high-low training model is the "nitrogen house," primarily in use in lowland northern European nations such as Finland and Norway. With a nitrogen house, a hypoxic living environment is created not through the reduced pressure of hypobaria but rather by decreasing the oxygen content of the inspired air in normobaria. This is done by adding nitrogen in small amounts to the ambient air, decreasing the proportion of oxygen in a small apartment. Through this method, the oxygen content of the inside living environment can be controlled to simulate a moderate altitude. To train at sea level, the athlete can simply walk out the front door of the nitrogen house. To get the desired acclimatization response of an increase in erythropoietin and red cell mass, however, the athlete must stay inside the nitrogen house for a substantial period of time each day. A nearly 100% increase in serum EPO and reticulocytes occurred after 5 days of 18 hours per day residence in a nitrogen house (14.2% O_2, ~3000 m or 9900 feet), in five competitive male cyclists (50). With 14 hours per day residence in 15.3% O_2 (~2500 m or 8000 feet) for 4 days, six female cross-country skiers demonstrated a significant 32% increase in EPO and a 50% increase in reticulocytes (51). However, studies of prolonged use of the nitrogen house have not been completed to determine if the 14 to 18 hours per day dose of hypoxic living results in equivalent increases in red cell mass versus continuous chronic altitude exposure. Continued research is needed to determine the effectiveness of the nitrogen house model in enhancing endurance exercise performance.

Other methods that simulate altitude exposure at sea level are the commercially available hypobaric bag and the hypoxic tent. The hypobaric bag is a long cylindrical tube with just enough room for the athlete to sleep inside. The tube is connected to a vacuum pump that decreases the pressure in the tube, simulating altitude. While effective in changing the environment in the tube to a hypobaric state, safety and logistical concerns are substantially more pronounced than the nitrogen house and high-low training models. The hypoxic tent works on a similar principle to the nitrogen house, but is implemented on a smaller scale. A canopy is placed over an athlete's bed, and hypoxic air is pumped into the air space contained within the canopy. The result is a reduction in the atmospheric oxygen content. The mobility of the athlete is even more limited than the nitrogen house model, however. With these synthetic altitude environment models, the dose of altitude exposure is typically much less than with traditional altitude exposure, and the response has not been well characterized. Also unknown with these simulated altitude environments is how the long-term psychologic effects of these somewhat restrictive living arrangements compare with the more aesthetic mountain environment at altitude, in the face of similar augmentation of red cell mass.

HYPERBARIA

The depth of performance-based research into hyperbaria, or increased atmospheric pressure relative to sea level, is not as extensive as research on the effects of hypobaria on performance. The fact that there are few terrestrial places where significant hyperbaria exists is certainly a major reason for the lack of research on hyperbaria's effect on exercise performance. Additionally, the mild increase in atmospheric pressure at below–sea level sites does not significantly increase arterial oxygen content, due to the flat shape of the oxyhemoglobin dissociation curve at high pressures and the poor solubility of oxygen in blood. However, the arterial oxygen content of the blood can be increased with artificial means of increasing inspired O_2 pressure (e.g., a hyperbaric chamber) or fraction (e.g., a hyperoxic inspirate).

As an intervention, the use of hyperoxia in training may provide a greater training stimulus than normoxic training, particularly when compared to training at low-moderate altitude. Just as the reduced P_{IO_2} at altitude may promote a detraining effect over time, increasing the P_{IO_2} with a hyperoxic inspirate may allow higher training intensities to be maintained and augment the training effect. In a group of national-class junior cyclists, a subset that performed interval training with a hyperoxic inspirate three times per week for 2 weeks maintained a higher intensity during interval training and improved their 120-km performance time 12 seconds more than the athletes who trained in normoxia (J.T. Kearney, personal communication). Interestingly, because the hyperoxic group could achieve a higher work load during the interval sessions, posthyperoxic workout muscle soreness was reported by the athletes to be higher than at any point during the competitive season. Therefore, in terms of practical application of hyperbaric or hyperoxic training, it appears important to plan recovery workouts accordingly and add the appropriate therapeutic interventions to minimize recovery time between high-intensity workouts.

REFERENCES

1. Gore CJ, Hahn AG, Scroop GS, et al. Increased arterial desaturation in trained cyclists during maximal exercise at 580 m altitude. *J Appl Physiol* 1996;80:2204–2210.
2. Stray-Gundersen J, Chapman RF, Levine BD. HiLo training improves performance in elite runners. *Med Sci Sports Exerc* 1998;30:S35.
3. Chapman RF, Stray-Gundersen J, Levine BD. Individual variation in response to altitude training. *J Appl Physiol* 1998;85:1448–1456.
4. Hay JG. *The biomechanics of sports techniques.* Englewood Cliffs, NJ: Prentice Hall, 1985:169–187.
5. McCole SD, Claney K, Conte J-C, Anderson R, Hagberg JM. Energy expenditure during bicycling. *J Appl Physiol* 1990; 68:748–753.
6. Pugh LCGE. Oxygen uptake in track and treadmill running with observations on the effect of air resistance. *J Physiol (Lond)* 1970;207:823–835.
7. Sjogaard G, Neilsen B, Mikkelsen F, Saltin B, Burke ER. *Physiology in cycling.* Ithaca, NY: Movement Publications, 1985.
8. Astrand PO, Rodahl K. *Textbook of work physiology*, 3rd ed. New York: McGraw-Hill, 1986.
9. Holmer I. *Physiology of swimming in man.* Exercise Sports Science Review, vol 7. Philadelphia: Franklin Institute Press, 1980.
10. Peronnet F, Bouissou P, Perrault H, Ricci J. The one hour cycling record at sea-level and at altitude. *Cycling Sci* 1991;3:16–22.
11. Olds TS, Norton KI, Craig NP. Mathematical modeling of cycling performance. *J Appl Physiol* 1993;75:730–737.
12. Capelli C, diPrampero PE. Effects of altitude on top speeds during 1 h unaccompanied cycling. *Eur J Appl Physiol* 1995;71:469–471.
13. Jacobs I, Esbjornsson M, Sylven C, Holm I, Jansson E. Sprint training effects on muscle myoglobin, enzymes, fiber types, and blood lactate. *Med Sci Sports Exerc* 1987;19:368–374.
14. Reeves JT, Wolfel EE, Green HJ, et al. Oxygen transport during exercise at altitude and the lactate paradox: lessons from Operation Everest II and Pikes Peak. *Exerc Sports Sci Rev* 1992; 20:275–296.
15. Terrados N, Jansson E, Sylven C, Kaijser L. Is hypoxia a stimulus for synthesis of oxidative enzymes and myoglobin. *J Appl Physiol* 1990;68:2369–2372.
16. Mizuno M, Juel C, Bro-Rasmussen T, et al. Limb skeletal muscle adaptation in athletes after training at altitude. *J Appl Physiol* 1990;68:486–502.
17. Robinson S, Edwards HT, Dill DB. New records in human power. *Science* 1937;85:409–410.
18. Schoene RB, Lahiri S, Hackett PH, et al. Relationship of hypoxic ventilatory response to exercise performance on Mount Everest. *J Appl Physiol* 1984;56:1478–1483.
19. Byrne-Quinn E, Weil JV, Sodal IE, Filley GF, Grover RF. Ventilatory control in the athlete. *J Appl Physiol* 1971;30:91–98.
20. Dempsey JA, Hanson PE, Henderson KS. Exercise induced arterial hypoxemia in healthy persons at sea level. *J Physiol (Lond)* 1984;355:161–175.
21. Aaron EA, Johnson BD, Seow KC, Dempsey JA. Oxygen cost of exercise hyperpnea: implications for performance. *J Appl Physiol* 1992;72:1818–1825.
22. Sutton JR, Reeves JT, Wagner PD, et al. Tolerable limits of hypoxia for the lungs: oxygen transport. In: Sutton JR, Houston LS, Coates G, eds. *Hypoxia: the tolerable limits.* Indianapolis: Benchmark, 1988:123–130.
23. Dempsey JA. Is the lung built for exercise? *Med Sci Sports Exerc* 1986;18:143–155.
24. Johnson BD, Saupe K, Dempsey JA. Mechanical constraints on exercise hyperpnea in endurance athletes. *J Appl Physiol* 1992; 73:874–886.
25. Chapman RF, Emery M, Stager JM. Degree of expiratory flow limitation influences the ability in increase ventilation in hypoxia. *Respir Physiol* 1998;113:65–74.
26. Harms CA, Stager JM. Low peripheral chemoresponsiveness and inadequate hyperventilation contribute to exercise-induced hypoxemia. *J Appl Physiol* 1995;79:575–580.
27. Dill DB, Adams WC. Maximal oxygen uptake at sea level and at 3,090-m altitude in high school champion runners. *J Appl Physiol* 1971;30:854–859.
28. Lawler J, Powers SK, Thompson D. Linear relationship between maximal oxygen uptake and $\dot{V}O_2$max decrement during exposure to acute hypoxia. *J Appl Physiol* 1988;64:1486–1492.
29. Young AJ, Cymerman A, Burse RL. The influence of cardiorespiratory fitness on the decrement in maximal aerobic power at high altitude. *Eur J Appl Physiol* 1985;54:12–15.
30. Gavin TP, Derchak PA, Stager JM. Ventilation's role in the de-

cline in $\dot{V}O_2max$ and SaO_2 in acute hypoxia. *Med Sci Sports Exerc* 1998;30:195–199.
31. Terrados N, Mizuno M, Andersen H. Reduction in maximal oxygen uptake at low altitudes: role of training status and lung function. *Clin Physiol (Oxf)* 1985;5:S75–S79.
32. Blomqvist G, Johnson RL Jr, Saltin B. Pulmonary diffusing capacity limiting human performance at altitude. *Acta Physiol Scand* 1969;76:284–287.
33. Powers SK, Martin D, Dodd S. Exercise-induced hypoxaemia in elite endurance athletes. *Sports Med* 1993;16:14–22.
34. Chapman RF, Emery M, Stager JM. Degree of arterial desaturation in normoxia influence the decline in $\dot{V}O_2max$ in mild hypoxia. *Med Sci Sports Exerc* 1999;31:658–663.
35. Buskirk ER, Kollias J, Akers RF, Prokop EK, Reategui EP. Maximal performance at altitude and return from altitude in conditioned runners. *J Appl Physiol* 1967;23:259–266.
36. Squires RW, Buskirk ER. Aerobic capacity during acute exposure to simulated altitude, 914 to 2286 meters. *Med Sci Sports Exerc* 1982;14:36–40.
37. Levine BD, Stray-Gundersen J. Exercise at high altitudes. In: *Current therapy in sports medicine,* 3rd ed. St. Louis: Mosby–Year Book, 1995:588–593.
38. Levine BD, Stray-Gundersen J. Living high-training low: effect of moderate-altitude acclimatization with low-altitude training on performance. *J Appl Physiol* 1997;83:102–112.
39. Buick FJ, Gledhill N, Froese AB, Spriet L, Meyers EC. Effect of induced erythrocythemia on aerobic work capacity. *J Appl Physiol* 1980;48:636–642.
40. Weil JV, Jamieson G, Brown DW, Grover RF. The red cell mass-arterial oxygen relationship in normal man. *J Clin Invest* 1968;47:1627–1639.
41. Levine BD, Stray-Gundersen J, Duhaime G, Snell PG, Friedman DB. Living high-training low: the effect of altitude acclimatization/normoxic training in trained runners. *Med Sci Sports Exerc* 1991;23:25.
42. Telford RD, Graham KS, Sutton JR, et al. Medium altitude training and sea level performance. *Med Sci Sports Exerc* 1996;28:S124.
43. Stray-Gundersen J, Mordecai N, Levine BD. O_2 transport response to altitude training in runners. *Med Sci Sports Exerc* 1995;27:202.
44. Stray-Gundersen J, Alexander C, Hochstein A, deLemos D, Levine BD. Failure of red cell volume to increase with altitude exposure in iron deficient runners. *Med Sci Sports Exerc* 1992;24:S90.
45. Adams WC, Bernauer EM, Dill DB, Bomar JB. Effects of equivalent sea-level and altitude training on $\dot{V}O_2max$ and running performance. *J Appl Physiol* 1975;39:262–265.
46. McConnell GK, Costil DL, Widrick JJ, Hickey MS, Tanaka H, Gastin PB. Reduced training volume and intensity maintain aerobic capacity but not performance in distance runners. *Int J Sports Med* 1993;14:33–37.
47. Stray-Gundersen J, Levine BD. Living high–training high and low is equivalent to living high–training low for sea level performance. *Med Sci Sports Exerc* 1997;29:S136.
48. Eckardt K, Boutellier U, Kurtz A, Schopen M, Koller EA, Bauer C. Rate of erythropoietin formation in humans in response to acute hypobaric hypoxia. *J Appl Physiol* 1989;66:1785–1788.
49. Milledge JS, Coates PM. Serum erythropoietin in humans at high altitude and its relation to plasma renin. *J Appl Physiol* 1985;59: 360–364.
50. Mattila V, Rusko H. Effect of living high and training low on sea level performance in cyclists. *Med Sci Sports Exerc* 1996;28:S156.
51. Rusko HK, Leppavuori A, Makela P, Leppaluoto J. Living high, training low: a new approach to altitude training at sea level in athletes. *Med Sci Sports Exerc* 1995;27:S6.

Exercise and Sport Science,
edited by William E. Garrett, Jr., and Donald T. Kirkendall.
Published by Lippincott Williams & Wilkins, Philadelphia, 2000.

CHAPTER 31

Effects of Microgravity on Exercise Performance

Victor A. Convertino

Physical stress imposed by exercise manifests itself by a dramatic elevation in energy exchange that is reflected by such responses as increased oxygen uptake, respiration, heart rate, and sweating. This physiologic strain can be reduced by adaptation with chronically repeated exposure to the exercise stress. Gravity contributes significantly to the magnitude of stress induced by exercise since development of force required by muscles to perform various physical activities such as moving one's body or lifting or throwing objects depends on overcoming forces imposed upon those objects by gravitational acceleration. Since physical exercise on Earth includes gravity as a constant, exercise has traditionally been considered the primary stress factor for performance of physical work by the human body. With the evolution of travel and habitation of humans in space, however, microgravity environments require new adaptations imposed by reduction in hydrostatic pressure gradients within the cardiovascular system, less weight load upon the muscles and bones, and possible lower energy requirement and/or output. It has become clear that the space environment is unique to other environmental stressors in that a given exercise stress is actually reduced due to the absence or reduction of gravity. Travel to space and planets with lower gravitational forces than Earth has provided opportunities to develop new perspectives about exercise stress-strain relationships and unique tools for assessing the influence of gravity on the development and adaptation of our normal physical and physiologic functions.

This chapter presents the available data from space missions regarding human physiologic adaptations to exercise and work in microgravity. Emphasis is placed on human data collected before, during, and after actual spaceflight, with limited reference to supporting ground-based experiments. Although numerous physiologic systems are affected by exposure to space, this review focuses on cardiovascular, metabolic, and muscular adaptations since these systems have the most pronounced impact on the response to acute exercise. Issues regarding bone loss during spaceflight have been excluded from this review since available data do not support the notion that prolonged exposure to microgravity leads to a depleted skeleton that is unable to withstand the stress of exercise. An assessment of the impact of microgravity on bone has been recently reviewed (1). Through comparison and integration of common data generated from various spaceflights, this chapter attempts to generalize the limitations to work and the role of exercise during and after exposures to space, and to present how physiologic adaptations to space impact the stress-strain–adaptation relationship to exercise performance.

EXERCISE PERFORMANCE AFTER ADAPTATION TO SPACE

Maximal Oxygen Uptake

The measurement of maximal oxygen uptake ($\dot{V}O_2max$) provides an integrated index of the functional integrity of the cardiorespiratory system and its regulatory mechanisms during adaptation to chronic exposure to microgravity. $\dot{V}O_2max$ was measured before spaceflight and immediately after return to Earth in six astronauts (four men and two women, ages 35 to 50 years) who participated in two United States Spacelab Life Sciences missions (2). The duration of the spaceflight was either 9 (n = 3) or 14 (n = 3) days. Average $\dot{V}O_2max$ of these six astronauts was reduced by 22% immediately after spaceflight.

Because of the complicating impact of operational constraints and limited data from spaceflight, under-

V. A. Convertino: U.S. Army Institute of Surgical Research, Fort Sam Houston, Texas 78234-6315.

standing the isolated impact of microgravity on $\dot{V}O_2max$ and maximal work capacity has depended primarily on ground-based investigations. It is clear from ground-based studies that when subjects are not exposed to regular exercise, $\dot{V}O_2max$ can be reduced by 5% to 35% following 10 to 30 days' duration of exposure to analogues of spaceflight (3–6). The reduction in $\dot{V}O_2max$ associated with microgravity is dependent on duration of exposure and initial fitness level. Ground-based investigations indicate that the magnitude of reduction in $\dot{V}O_2max$ increases as the duration of exposure to microgravity increases (4). Most of the loss in $\dot{V}O_2max$ occurs rapidly during the initial 3 to 7 days, however, followed by a more gradual decline over the course of exposure (4,7); this suggests that mechanisms of adaptation of systemic aerobic capacity to microgravity involve both fast and slow components. This relationship indicates that the longer an individual is exposed to the absence of gravity in the upright posture, the more physiologic reserve will be lost. In addition, significant negative correlations exist between the initial $\dot{V}O_2max$ and the percent reduction in $\dot{V}O_2max$ following exposure to ground-based analogues of microgravity (4–6), suggesting that fit individuals have a greater reduction in aerobic capacity during adaptation than less-fit individuals. However, percent reduction in $\dot{V}O_2max$ in microgravity appears to be similar across age and gender (5). Therefore, young and older men and women who have adapted to greater exposures to stress on Earth (e.g., athletes) may have greater physiologic consequences when introduced to the space environment where the stress of gravity and/or physical activity is removed or minimized.

The potential operational consequence of reduced aerobic reserve is the inability to maintain given physical work requirements during spaceflight for a given period of time, that is, lower endurance. This notion was supported by poorer endurance to a standardized exercise test (125 W for 5 minutes) in the two crew members during the early part of a 96-day flight aboard the Russian Salyut-6 space station, manifested by increased heart rate, elevated arterial pressure, reduced stroke volume, and an inability to complete the 5-minute exercise bout on the 24th day of flight (8). Clearly, the lower physical stress produced by the space environment manifested itself as greater physiologic strain during the course of the space mission.

Mechanical Efficiency During Submaximal Exercise

Oxygen uptake during 5 minutes of cycle ergometer exercise in spaceflight was less than on Earth at the same absolute work rate (9,10), and postflight exercise $\dot{V}O_2$ lagged appreciably behind the preflight levels (4,11). Also, greater $\dot{V}O_2$ during recovery from exercise was reported after spaceflights (10–12). One explanation for reduced submaximal $\dot{V}O_2$ at equal work output might be increased mechanical efficiency, although this seems unlikely. An alternative hypothesis might be that adaptation to microgravity involves a change in the time constant for the $\dot{V}O_2$ to reach an equilibrium. If the rate change for $\dot{V}O_2$ during the transient phase of exercise were lengthened with microgravity adaptation, then the measured $\dot{V}O_2$ at 3 to 5 minutes of exercise may not reach steady state, and $\dot{V}O_2$ would be lower compared to preexposure levels without a change in mechanical efficiency. This notion is supported by slower $\dot{V}O_2$ kinetics during the transient phase of exercise after exposure of ground-based analogues of microgravity (4), and by greater recovery oxygen uptake following exercise in spaceflight (10,13). These changes in $\dot{V}O_2$ dynamics during and after exercise following exposure to microgravity may reflect a greater requirement for anaerobic metabolism during the transient phase of exercise to provide for adequate energy demand. This notion is further supported by higher blood lactate, ventilation, and respiratory exchange ratios following ground-based simulations of microgravity (5,6,14).

A standardized exercise bout at an intensity of 150 W (2.15 $kcal \cdot min^{-1}$) was performed on a cycle ergometer by Skylab astronauts before and during spaceflight (10). The average energy expenditure required to perform this work was 10.2 ± 0.1 $kcal \cdot min^{-1}$ preflight compared to 9.3 ± 0.1 $kcal \cdot min^{-1}$ inflight. Therefore, the mechanical efficiency of performing cycle ergometer exercise during spaceflight (23%) was not appreciably different from exercising on Earth (21%). The $\dot{V}O_2$ predicted during cycle exercise inflight (160 W) was 2.25 $L \cdot min^{-1}$ compared to the actual measured $\dot{V}O_2$ of 2.31 $L \cdot min^{-1}$ (approximately 20% mechanical efficiency) (4). Since the basal metabolic rate is similar between preflight and inflight (10), gross efficiency of performing exercise on a mechanically stabilized device such as the cycle ergometer is unaltered by microgravity.

The energy cost of locomotion in microgravity may be much higher when the body cannot be stabilized by postural muscles as it is in terrestrial gravity. Exercise was performed on a treadmill at a speed of 120 $m \cdot min^{-1}$ (about 4.5 miles per hour), and a system of bungee cords provided stabilization of the subject on the treadmill; the force on the long axis of the body was estimated at approximately 50 kg (4,15,16). Energy expenditure of treadmill walking/running in Earth gravity would be approximately 5.7 $kcal \cdot min^{-1}$ under these conditions, while the measured energy expenditure of treadmill exercise in space was 7.4 $kcal \cdot min^{-1}$. This difference would reflect a reduction in mechanical efficiency from a predicted 20% on Earth (1*g*) to an actual 15% in space. These findings were corroborated by responses to cycle and treadmill exercise during a 1-year space mission conducted on the Russian Mir space station. During each inflight exercise session, a cosmonaut exercised for about 30 minutes on a treadmill at an average speed of 125 m·min^{-1} (combined walking and running) or for 26.5 minutes on a cycle ergometer at 130 W. Based on prediction equations from 1*g*, subjects would have required an energy expenditure of approximately 570 kcal during treadmill exercise and 500 kcal during cycling. Thus, the total predicted energy expenditure for both exercise sessions would be 1070 kcal (20% mechanical efficiency). An average energy cost of 1460 kcal was actually reported, however, indicating a reduction in mechanical efficiency for both exercise sessions to 15% (15). If we assume that mechanical efficiency of cycle ergometry was not altered from 1*g* as previously indicated (10), then it can be estimated that 960 kcal were required to perform treadmill exercise rather than the predicted 570 kcal, a reduction in mechanical efficiency from 20% to 11%. It therefore appears that some mechanical advantage of using gravity during exercise with the lower extremities is lost in space.

Muscle Function: Strength and Fatigability

The ability to develop and maintain forces with dynamic muscle actions is required for nominal exercise performance. Since skeletal muscles provide the force for moving the body and external objects against Earth's gravity, the absence of gravity removes a major stimulus to maintain normal strength and endurance. Although this may not be detrimental to exercise performance in space, it could significantly limit one's work output upon return to Earth. Indeed, distances of long and high jumps were reduced by an average of 11% and 14%, respectively, after 63 days of spaceflight and were associated with about 10% reduction in force generation in the muscle groups of the lower extremities (4,15). General loss of strength following spaceflight has been measured in postural muscles of the back (4,15), knee flexors and extensors (17), elbow flexors and extensors (17), and ankle flexors and extensors (18).

The average decrease in peak torque for concentric muscle actions was 21% for knee extensors and 8% for knee flexors of the leg in the three Skylab astronauts who were in space for 28 days (15,17). Average body weight loss was 3% and average leg volume was reduced by 10% (19). The general conclusion is that space reduces muscle strength, primarily in the legs, and the magnitude of strength loss is directly associated with body weight and leg volume reduction, and inversely related to volume (duration × intensity × frequency) of exercise performed inflight (19).

Force-velocity relationships of the ankle flexors (anterior tibialis) and extensors (calf muscles) were measured using isokinetic dynamometry before and after short (7 days) and long (110 to 237 days) space missions (18). Static and dynamic strength of these muscle groups were reduced during both durations of exposure. The change in the *in vivo* torque-velocity relationship demonstrated a reduction in force development across all speeds of limb movement during concentric muscle actions (Fig. 31–1) and was qualitatively similar to those changes reported in knee flexor and extensor muscles following exposure to a ground-based analogue of microgravity (20). In addition, ground-based data demonstrated strength loss for eccentric as well as concentric muscle actions and that the reduction of angle-specific peak torque was not significantly influenced by the type or speed of muscle action (20).

The greatest loss of muscular function occurs in the

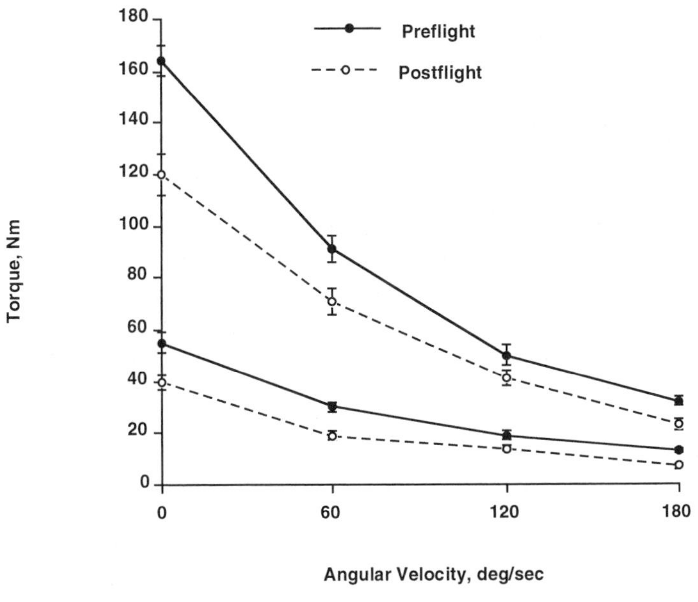

FIG. 31–1. Torque-velocity relationship of the calf (*upper curves*) and anterior tibialis (*lower curves*) muscles before (*closed circles* and *solid lines*) and after (*open circles* and *broken lines*) 110 to 237 days of spaceflight. *Circles* and *bars* represent mean ± standard error (SE) values from six cosmonauts on Salyut-7. (Modified from ref. 18.)

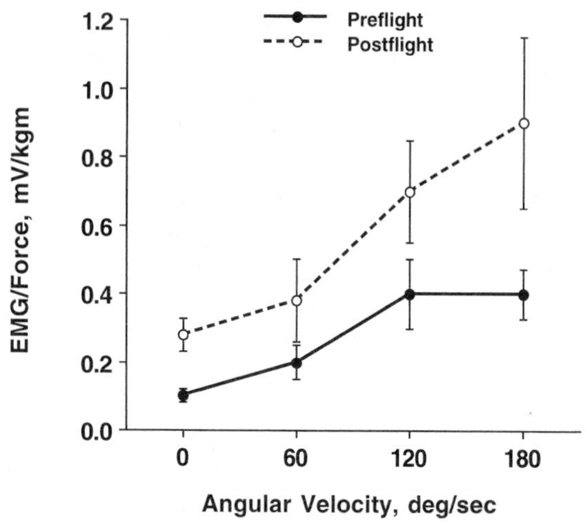

FIG. 31–2. Ratio of electromyography (EMG) activity to force development during maximal ankle extension (calf muscle contraction) performed at four angular velocities before (*closed bars* and *solid lines*) and after (*open bars* and *broken lines*) 7 days of spaceflight. *Circles* and *bars* represent mean ± SE from 11 Salyut-6 cosmonauts. (Modified from ref. 22.)

lower extremities with little change in the upper extremities (15,17). The greater use of arms than legs in space, and the possibility that arm muscles that generate relatively small forces on Earth are less affected by the absence of gravity than antigravity muscles of the lower extremities that generate large forces in 1*g*, could account for smaller strength loss postflight in muscles of the upper compared to the lower extremities.

In addition to loss in muscle strength, there is evidence to suggest that muscle fatigability is increased during exposure to space. Using spectral power analysis from electromyography (EMG) recordings, increased fatigability in the gastrocnemius muscles following flight was evidenced by a shift to lower frequencies in response to maintaining a tension of 50% of maximum voluntary contraction for 1 minute (21). Compared to preflight, increased EMG amplitude per unit of force developed in calf muscles during postflight tests argues for the notion that intensity of contractions of muscles exposed to space is proportionately greater than that of a normal muscle to achieve or maintain a given tension (Fig. 31–2), thus leading to earlier fatigue (22).

Effects of Return to Terrestrial Gravity

Reduction of $\dot{V}O_2$max and exercise capacity may be partly a result of an inability of cardiovascular mechanisms to compensate adequately for the orthostatic challenge of resuming the upright position following adaptation to microgravity. Exercise in the upright posture is much more dependent on venous return from the legs and on the Frank-Starling mechanism to augment stroke volume than is exercise in the supine posture. Mechanisms for control of heart rate and stroke volume become especially sensitive to venous pooling and to underfilling of the heart during upright exercise following changes in vascular volume and compliance. If postural challenges in gravity contribute to reduction in $\dot{V}O_2$max, then changes in the cardiorespiratory response to exercise performed in the upright posture following exposure to microgravity should be greater than those changes during supine exercise, assuming responses to supine exercise are similar to those in microgravity.

Following 6 days of spaceflight, selected physiologic responses to 75 W on a supine and upright (sitting position) cycle ergometer were compared to preflight responses (10). Exercise heart rate was 12% higher in supine and 17% higher in upright cycling compared to preflight responses. These results suggest that higher supine heart rates after flight probably represented the effect of reduced blood volume, while the additional tachycardia in the upright posture probably represented an added influence of the orthostatic effect of 1*g* on end-diastolic filling volume and stroke volume. Furthermore, 84 days of spaceflight reduced average postflight upright exercise stroke volume by 24 mL, while supine stroke volume was decreased by only 5 mL (10). These data support the notion that elevated heart rate during terrestrial exercise following adaptation to microgravity is a compensatory response to reduced stroke volume (2), a response exaggerated in the upright posture compared to the supine position.

The average decrease in $\dot{V}O_2$max after exposure to ground-based analogues of microgravity is about 9% in the supine posture compared to an average 18% reduction during upright exercise testing (4). It appears that the combined reduction of both regular physical activity and venous system fluid shifts induced by absence of gravity contribute nearly equally to the reduction in $\dot{V}O_2$max following adaptation to microgravity.

PHYSIOLOGIC CHANGES ASSOCIATED WITH REDUCED EXERCISE CAPACITY

Pulmonary Function

There is little evidence that changes in minute ventilation or ventilation-perfusion matching in microgravity might limit gas exchange and adversely affect aerobic processes required to support the metabolic demands of exercise in microgravity (e.g., $\dot{V}O_2$max). Vital capacity, residual volume, total lung capacity, tidal volume, alveolar ventilation, forced expiratory volume, maximum voluntary ventilation, and closing volume are not altered with spaceflight (15). Pulmonary function during exercise is well within normal limits in space (13). In fact, pulmonary efficiency during exercise in spaceflight, measured as ventilation volume during exercise at an oxygen uptake of 2.0 L·min^{-1}, was essentially unaltered compared to preflight (10). Average ventilation volume during 75% $\dot{V}O_2$max was reported as 82.4 ± 9.9 L·min^{-1} preflight compared to 83.3 ± 10.8 L·min^{-1} inflight (10,13). These data suggest that pulmonary function probably does not limit gas exchange during exercise in microgravity environments or upon return to Earth's gravity environment.

Blood Volume

One of the most consistent and rapid adaptations to microgravity is the reduction in blood volume. Approximately 8% to 10% (300 mL) of plasma is lost within the initial 24 to 48 hours in microgravity (23–26), while the average hypovolemia is gradually increased with longer spaceflights (13% and 16% for 59 and 84 days, respectively) (27). Therefore, the time course of reduction in blood volume in space indicates an early contraction of plasma followed by a gradual stabilization some time between 30 and 60 days into a mission (Fig. 31–3).

Reduction in circulating plasma volume appears to contribute directly to the limitation of hemodynamic responses required to support adequate blood flow and metabolism during moderate to heavy exercise in microgravity. Using ground-based experiments, a larger percent decrease in plasma volume has been associated with a larger percent reduction in $\dot{V}O_2$max (4). The high correlation coefficient between the relative changes in plasma volume and $\dot{V}O_2$max suggests that microgravity-induced hypovolemia probably contributes to a reduced capacity of the body to transport and utilize oxygen during exercise.

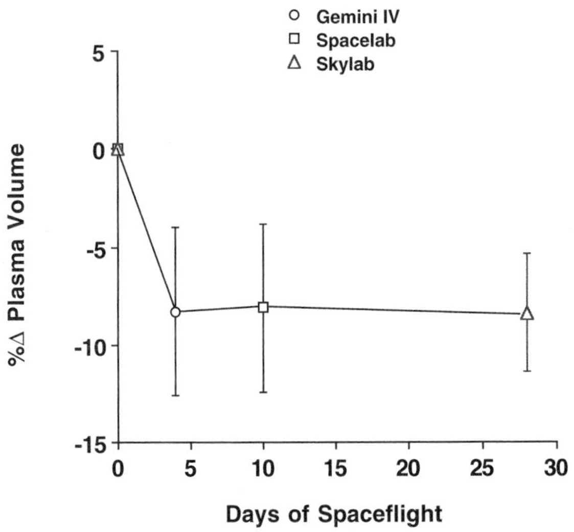

FIG. 31–3. Time course of percent change (%) in plasma volume during adaptation to actual spaceflight. Data are from Gemini IV (ref. 24), Spacelab (ref. 26), and Skylab (ref. 27). (Modified from ref. 23.)

Hypovolemia can contribute to reduced ventricular filling and cardiac output during exercise since it is associated with decreases in mean venous pressure, venous return, and stroke volume. An important impact of microgravity-induced hypovolemia on ventricular filling is supported by a close relationship between reduced plasma volume and elevations in maximal heart rate and reductions in stroke volume, cardiac output, and lower $\dot{V}O_2$max following exposure to ground-based analogues of microgravity (4,6). A rapid 17% to 21% reduction in oxygen uptake during exercise at 160 beats per minute (bpm) within 15 days of spaceflight and its restoration within 24 to 36 hours following return to Earth suggest that changes in vascular volume contribute to reduced $\dot{V}O_2$max following spaceflight (28,29). Plasma volume was reduced by nearly 16% in three astronauts after 84 days in space, however, while inflight $\dot{V}O_2$max was maintained with extensive exercise programs (10). Clearly, reduced vascular volume is only one mechanism that contributes to impaired cardiovascular function and loss of aerobic capacity during exercise with adaptation to microgravity.

Another effect of vascular hypovolemia on the reduction in $\dot{V}O_2$max may be a lower oxygen-carrying capacity of the blood resulting from reduced red cell mass. Indeed, a consistent influence of microgravity has been a reduction in circulating hemoglobin and red cell mass (15,26). Space missions of 7 to 14 days in duration demonstrated that most crew members reduced their red blood cell mass by an average of 6% to 10% (24,26), continuing to 14% and 12% after 28 and 59 days, respectively (25). The magnitude of hemoglobin loss was 13%, 26%, 23%, and 24% at 16, 30, 63, and 96 days of spaceflight, respectively (15). These data suggest an early reduction in red cell mass and hemoglobin with a plateau by 30 days of flight (15,26,27). This represents an approximate 25% reduction in oxygen-carrying capacity of the blood, which could contribute significantly to limiting $\dot{V}O_2$max during and following exposure to microgravity. The relationship between changes in red cell mass and changes in $\dot{V}O_2$max is tenuous, however, since no change in red cell mass following short duration exposure to ground-based analogues of microgravity has been reported despite significant reductions in $\dot{V}O_2$max (3,5,14). It therefore appears likely that the primary effect of microgravity-induced hypovolemia on reducing $\dot{V}O_2$max is due to the contraction of the plasma volume with a lesser contribution from reduced red cell mass.

Cardiovascular Function

Impaired $\dot{V}O_2$max involves changes in central hemodynamics as manifested by elevated heart rate and reductions in stroke and cardiac volumes (10,15,30–32) during exercise after spaceflight. During exercise at 75% $\dot{V}O_2$max after 84 days of spaceflight, mean heart rate increased from 103 bpm preflight to 114 bpm in response to a reduction in stroke volume from 110 mL preflight to 97 mL postflight (32). Despite an average elevated exercise heart rate, the proportionately greater reduction in stroke volume has resulted in consistently lowering cardiac output by approximately 10% during exercise in microgravity (15,16,30,32). Poor postural adaptation, impaired venous return, hypovolemia, or impaired myocardial performance may account for reductions in cardiac output and $\dot{V}O_2$max during and following spaceflight.

There is little evidence from spaceflight data to support the idea that deterioration of myocardial structure and function occurs and contributes to exercise impairment as an adaptation to microgravity. Cardiac responses during spaceflight demonstrated increased pulse wave propagation velocity at rest (28,33) and during exercise (32), an index of greater left ventricular contractility. End-diastolic volume–stroke volume relationships generated on astronauts after 84 days in space demonstrated no change in the slope of the Frank-Starling curve (34). Echocardiographic data collected during rest and exercise on a 237-day spaceflight (30) indicated 30% lower stroke volume in response to graded exercise (125 and 175 W) compared to preflight responses (Fig. 31–4). Average heart rates were 12% and 17% higher at 125 and 175 W, respectively, compared to preflight, but cardiac output remained lower. Left ventricular filling volume (end-diastolic volume) was significantly depressed during rest and did not increase with exercise. Diminution of stroke volume was prevented by greater myocardial contraction as indicated by lesser end-systolic reserve and elevated ejection fraction (see Fig. 31–4). These flight data suggest that myocardial function does not appear to be compromised during exercise following adaptation to microgravity. In fact, augmentation of both left ventricular ejection fraction and heart rate during submaximal and maximal exercise may represent compensatory mechanisms to ameliorate the reduction in cardiac output during and after spaceflight despite lower cardiac end-diastolic volume (preload) and stroke volume. These results suggest that reduction in exercise cardiac output with adaptation to microgravity can be accounted for by lower ventricular filling and end-diastolic volume rather than reduced myocardial function (33). Maintained or improved cardiac performance during exercise, as indicated by increased ejection fractions and aortic pulse wave propagation velocities, refutes the notion that cardiac deconditioning occurs and limits the capacity to perform physical exercise. It appears more likely that reduced stroke volume, cardiac output, and

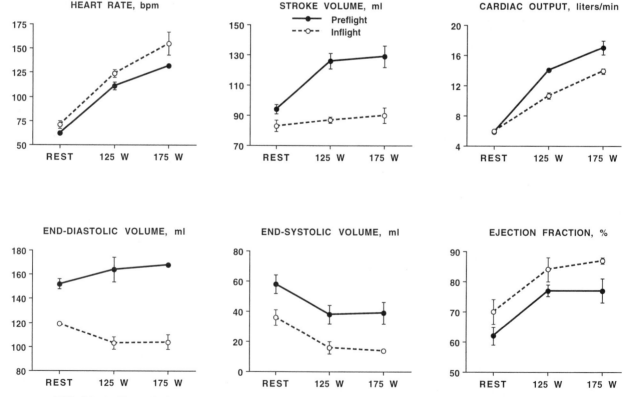

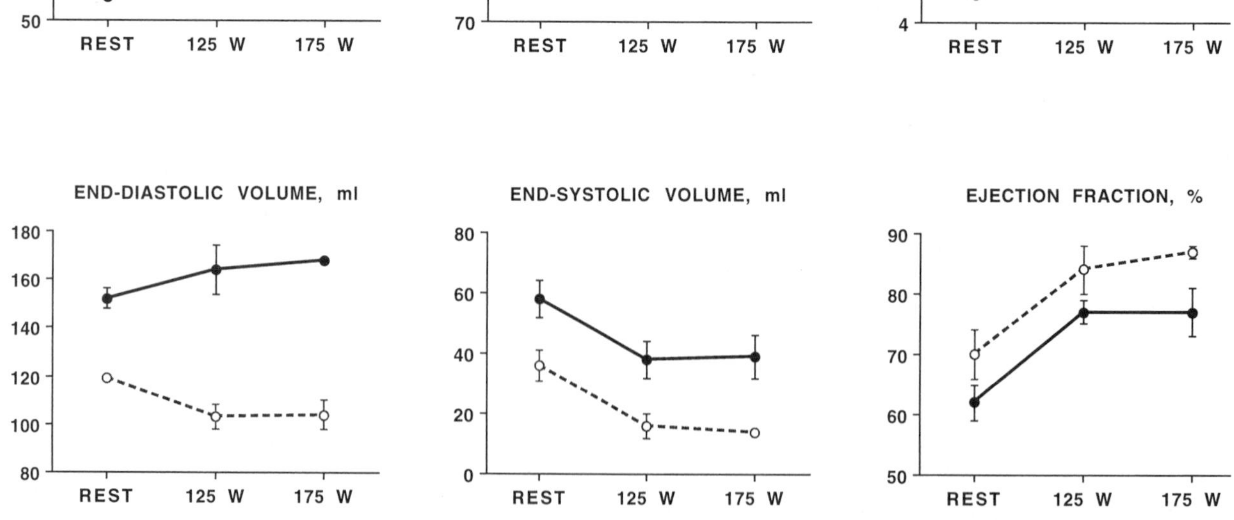

FIG. 31–4. Mean (±SE) cardiac responses of two cosmonauts during rest and at 125 W and 175 W of exercise on a cycle ergometer before (*closed circles* and *solid lines*) and during (*open circles* and *broken lines*) a 237-day space mission. (Modified from ref. 30.)

$\dot{V}O_2max$ can be primarily attributed to reduced circulating plasma volume and its effect on central venous filling pressure and venous return (2,23), ventricular filling, and cardiovascular hemodynamics, rather than on impairment of cardiac function.

Morphologic Changes in Skeletal Muscle

Muscle atrophy resulting from unloading and relative disuse has been proposed as a primary contributing factor to the cause of postflight loss in muscle strength (18,19). This notion was supported by measured reductions of limb size during early spaceflight experiments (19). More recent use of invasive techniques (muscle biopsy) demonstrated that there is significant muscle atrophy in space as evidenced by reduction in the cross-sectional area (CSA) of slow-twitch (type I) and fast-twitch (type II) muscle fibers of the vastus lateralis (35). The relative reduction in muscle fiber CSA tended to be greater in fast-twitch (23% to 36%) compared to slow-twitch fibers (16%) (Fig. 31–5). Crew members from whom these biopsies were taken were among 19 crew members in which the average decline in maximum voluntary concentric force production of ~15% for the knee extensor muscle group compared to the ~20% average reduction in muscle fiber CSA. Additionally, various ultrastructural abnormalities such as disorganized myofibrils, cellular edema, irregular Z-bodies, disrupted fiber membranes and sarcolemma, abnormal mitochondria, disrupted striation patterns, and mitochondria located in the intercellular spaces have occurred in subjects exposed to a ground-based analogue of microgravity (20). It is therefore possible that in addition to muscle atrophy, ultrastructural changes and other factors associated with the control of the contractile apparatus may contribute to loss of muscle force generation with exposure to microgravity.

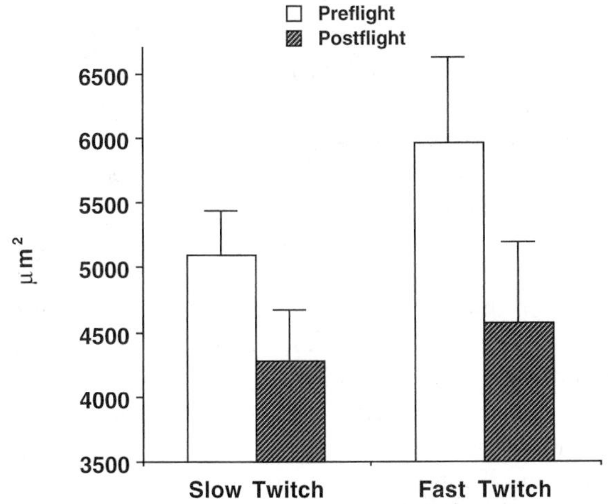

FIG. 31–5. Mean ± SE cross-sectional areas (CSAs) of slow- and fast-twitch muscle fibers of the vastus lateralis before (*open bars*) and after (*hashed bars*) 5 to 11 days of spaceflight. (Data from ref. 35.)

Cellular Metabolism of Skeletal Muscle

In addition to changes in central hemodynamics, reduced $\dot{V}O_2max$ and increased muscle fatigability induced in space may reflect increased metabolic acidosis resulting from a reduced capacity to support oxidative metabolism in skeletal muscle. An elevated acidotic state in exercising muscle fibers is supported by respiratory compensation with elevations in systemic expired carbon dioxide, ventilation volume, and respiratory exchange ratio (9), and increased recovery oxygen uptake associated with fatigue (10,13) during exercise of equal intensities in space compared to preflight. Greater respiratory compensation and blood lactate during steady-state exercise suggests that the rate of oxidation of pyruvate within the muscle has decreased, and a greater proportion of energy demand must rely on anaerobic bioenergetic pathways at the muscle cellular level in space.

Reduced capillary-to-fiber ratio in muscle fibers (35) may decrease the capacity to deliver and diffuse oxygen and substrates to working muscle. Following 11 days of spaceflight, there were 19% to 25% reductions in the mean number of capillaries per fiber in both slow-twitch and fast-twitch muscle fibers. Myofibrillar adenosine triphosphatase (ATPase) activities increased in fast-twitch but not in slow-twitch fibers after flight, while the activity of succinate dehydrogenase (SDH), an enzyme associated with aerobic metabolic pathways, was unaffected by spaceflight. Myofibrillar ATPase/SDH ratios in fast-twitch fibers were higher after spaceflight, however, suggesting that these fibers were more susceptible to fatigue after flight as compared to before flight. In ground-based studies, the activities of two enzymes associated with aerobic metabolic pathways, citrate synthase and β-hydroxyacyl-coenzyme A dehydrogenase, were reduced in slow-twitch muscle fibers after exposure to simulated microgravity (20). These data indicate that in addition to compromised capability to generate force, the effect of prolonged muscle unloading and reduced energy requirements associated with exposure to microgravity may reduce the capacity of oxygen delivery to and utilization by muscle fibers at the cellular level. These adaptations may be underlying mechanisms that contribute to the reduction in exercise endurance and $\dot{V}O_2max$ during and following exposure to microgravity environments.

Venous and Muscle Compliance

Limited venous return during exercise can contribute to reduction in maximal cardiac output and $\dot{V}O_2max$ in microgravity (2,4,6,15,30,31). The increased venous compliance of the lower extremities reported in space (4,15) can compound the effect of hypovolemia on impaired venous return during exercise by providing a greater capacity to pool blood under the same hydrostatic pressure. Increased venous compliance in microgravity is related to reduced size of the muscle compartment so that, when the muscle compartment is reduced, compliance increases (36). Therefore, loss of muscle protein and water that occurs during muscle unloading in microgravity may be important to increased venous compliance of the lower extremities and may ultimately contribute to impairment of venous return, cardiac filling, cardiac output, and $\dot{V}O_2$max due to greater pooling of blood, especially during exercise.

Changes in Thermoregulation

Mean daily values for sweat rate in nine astronauts during an average of 1 hour of daily exercise decreased from 1,750 mL preflight to 1,560 mL during spaceflight (37), suggesting that decreased sweat losses and possibly insensible skin losses are reduced during exercise. The microgravity environment also promotes formation of an observed sweat film on the skin surface during exercise by reducing convective flow and sweat drippage. This results in high levels of sustained skin wetness that acts to suppress sweating (37). In ground-based experiments, body heat storage was increased during external heat loads and exercise of equal work intensities after, compared with before, exposure to simulated microgravity. Increased threshold and reduced responsiveness of thermally induced elevations in vascular conductance after exposure to simulated microgravity indicates a reduced capacity to dissipate heat via conductance (38). Excessive elevation in rectal temperature above ambulatory control levels during 70 minutes of submaximal supine cycle ergometry (~45% $\dot{V}O_2$max) at 22°C ambient temperature was reported without differences in total body sweat production (39). These results suggested that microgravity environments may lower the sensitivity for central control of sweating, that is, inhibition of sweating from the same core temperature stimulus. Thus, data from space and ground-based experiments indicate that exposure to microgravity environments causes some impairment in thermoregulation during exercise, which could limit work performance of extended duration.

FUNCTIONAL IMPACTS OF ADAPTATION TO MICROGRAVITY

Performance During Extravehicular Activity

Regular maintenance of orbiting spacecraft and satellites as well as construction of space stations require the performance of extravehicular activities (EVAs) by humans in the microenvironment of a spacesuit. In the early days of spaceflight, EVAs were marked by two- to threefold elevations in heart rate and respiration, accompanied by profuse perspiration, excessive accumulation of heat, and signs of fatigue (15). It was estimated that performance of operations in space required four to five times more exertion than similar tasks on Earth, resulting in limitation or cancellation of planned operations during these missions due to development of overheating and fatigue. During these EVAs, heart rates were maintained from 130 to 170 bpm while energy expenditure could exceed 500 kcal/hour (O_2 approximately 1.7 $L \cdot min^{-1}$) (15). As a result, progressive elevations in body temperature were observed and work rates had to be limited. Thus, body heat produced from EVAs in the Gemini spacesuit microenvironment represented a limitation to work performance.

With refinement in design of spacesuits, there were decreased cardiorespiratory responses, and average energy expenditure during EVAs was reduced to about 240 kcal/h ($O_2 = 0.8\ L \cdot min^{-1}$) and at no time were EVAs limited by fatigue. However, EVAs during various space shuttle missions have lasted as long as 3 to 6 hours, with $\dot{V}O_2$ during peak work of short duration (minutes) as high as 1.6 L/min. Since EVAs require predominantly arm and upper body activity with $\dot{V}O_2$max of these muscle groups at approximately 1.8 $L \cdot min^{-1}$, astronauts may be functioning for hours at an average intensity of 45% to 50% of $\dot{V}O_2$max, with short periods requiring as much as 80% of their available maximal working capacity. Shuttle astronauts have expressed some degree of fatigue following these long EVAs. Based on these estimations, increased strain on endurance and strength capacities of the arms and upper body may become limiting factors to EVA performance.

Orthostatic Performance Upon Return to Earth

Upon return to Earth, some degree of orthostatic instability has been reported in many individuals who have traveled in space. Orthostatic hypotension induced by microgravity is associated with increased venous compliance in the lower extremities (19,36), reduced plasma and blood volume (4,15,23–25,27,40,41), lower resting venous pressure (42–44), and attenuated cardiac baroreflex response (41,45–47). It became clear to medical personnel that cardiovascular function was compromised on return from space, and that this compromise was most prominent during standing. In some individuals, dramatic tachycardia did not fully compensate for reduced venous return, and stroke volume and syncope could occur during a "stand test." Significant orthostatic hypotension with subsequent syncopal symptoms has been described in 40% to 65% of crew members in the U.S. space program (41,48–50).

Compromised orthostatic performance is of particular operational interest because of its potential impact on the safety of the crew. The use of an aircraft such as the space shuttle requires pilot control during a landing procedure in which there is increased head-to-foot *g* forces. The possibility that a pilot might be significantly less able to tolerate this orthostatic stress and might lose consciousness at a critical time has raised great concern and serious interest in counteracting the problem. In addition, orthostatic intolerance could severely compromise the ability of crew members to effectively egress the aircraft immediately after landing in the event of an emergency. It is clear that increased physiologic strain induced by the orthostatic challenge of return to Earth could significantly compromise the safety and performance of the crew.

EXERCISE AS A COUNTERMEASURE FOR ADAPTATION TO MICROGRAVITY

Effects on Physical Work Capacity

Extensive exercise during spaceflight has been used to ameliorate the reduction in $\dot{V}O_2$max and physical performance. Significant time has been devoted to exercise during long-duration space missions, consisting of work on the cycle ergometer and space treadmill at training intensities of approximately 50% to 75% $\dot{V}O_2$max performed for an average 1.5 hours daily, 6 days per week, for up to 6 month of spaceflight (4). The effectiveness of regular exercise stress on reducing postflight physiologic strain to acute exercise was best demonstrated by the results of the third Skylab mission in which $\dot{V}O_2$max of all three astronauts actually increased by an average of about 8% after 79 to 83 days in space (Fig. 31–6). Ground-based experiments with control groups that received no exercise have corroborated spaceflight data that average reduction in $\dot{V}O_2$max is only about 4% compared to 13% when no exercise is provided (4). These observations clearly indicate that regular performance of exercise in space can protect the stress-strain–adaptation relationship for exercise performance.

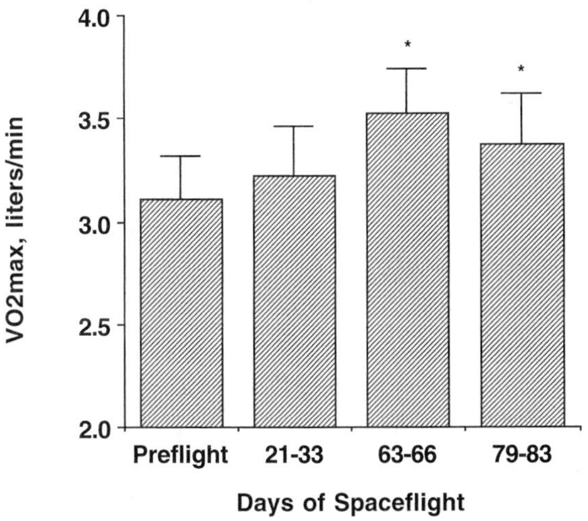

FIG. 31–6. Mean ± SE maximal oxygen uptakes ($\dot{V}O_2$max) of three astronauts before and during an 84-day space mission. *Asterisks* indicate that all crew members demonstrated an increase. (Data plotted from ref. 10.)

Data from human biopsies argue that resistive rather than endurance exercise could be most effective in minimizing muscle atrophy and dysfunction associated with unloading characteristics of space. In the Russian space program, protection of muscle tone, limb circumference, and strength of lower extremity muscles has been associated with inflight use of resistance pulling devices and wearing of spring-loaded suits that provided consistent axial-load resistance up to 50% of body mass to the musculoskeletal system of arms, legs, and torso during waking hours (8 to 12 hours/day). During the U.S. Skylab program, arm and leg strength decreased by 15% to 20% on the initial 28-day space mission despite the use of extensive cycle ergometer exercise (17). After this flight, a device that provided concentric resistive isokinetic exercise for the arms and trunk was added to a subsequent 59-day flight and preserved arm strength (17). Despite the significant increase in volume and mode of exercise during the 59-day mission, however, postflight loss of leg strength was similar to that of the 28-day mission (9,17). On a subsequent 84-day mission, a Teflon-coated plate treadmill was added to the exercise arsenal used on the previous 28- and 59-day flights, and total daily exercise time was increased (17). The tethering harness of the treadmill device was especially used for jumping and toe rises (10). Following flight, the reduction of body weight, leg volume, and leg strength was not eliminated but was less than half that of the previous two missions (17). These observations indicate the possibility of preventing muscle atrophy and dysfunction by replacing resistive stress to specific muscle groups that has been removed by the absence of gravity in the space environment.

Effects on Orthostatic Hypotension After Microgravity Exposure

Since hypovolemia and reduced cardiac filling (central venous) pressure occur during adaptation to microgravity and are associated with orthostatic hypotension following spaceflight (15,41,49), exercise training designed to increase $\dot{V}O_2$max, blood volume, and venous pressure might prove an effective stressor to counter reduced postflight orthostatic performance. Data from spaceflight experiments do not necessarily support this hypothesis. Despite extensive inflight exercise training, crew members have experienced plasma volume reduction, increased venous compliance, and baroreflex malfunction associated with orthostatic instability upon return to Earth (4). These results suggest that an effective prescription of exercise to be used in microgravity must provide specific stimuli to replace the stress to mechanisms associated with blood pressure regulation normally provided by the gravitational environment of Earth.

There is evidence that use of exercise designed to elicit maximal effort can acutely restore various physiologic capacities associated with blood pressure regulation. In ground-based experiments, such exercise reversed attenuated baroreflex responsiveness, plasma volume, and orthostatic intolerance within 24 hours of application (40,46,51). The effectiveness of acute maximal exercise on blood pressure regulation may provide a specific stimulus that acutely replaces the natural stress of gravity on the cardiovascular system.

CONCLUSION

Microgravity environments represent reduced physical stress on cardiovascular and muscle systems (Fig. 31–7). Lower hydrostatic pressure gradients in the cardiovascular system act to reduce the reserve capacities of central (cardiac) and peripheral mechanisms associated with aerobic power ($\dot{V}O_2max$) and orthostatic tolerance. Despite increased heart rate and cardiac contractility during exercise resulting from autonomic adaptations, maximal cardiac output is dramatically reduced by an overwhelming decrease in stroke volume. Since cardiac contractility appears enhanced, the lowered stroke volume must be due to reduced cardiac filling associated with less blood volume and lower central venous pressure. Increased compliance of the veins in leg muscles may also contribute to limited venous return, especially after return to the gravity environment of Earth. In the face of limited cardiac factors, maximal arteriovenous O_2 difference remains constant. However, reductions in blood volume, capillarization, and maximal blood flow in the muscle could limit oxygen delivery and utilization. The ultimate consequence of these alterations in cardiac and vascular functions is the reduction in $\dot{V}O_2max$. In addition, reduced blood volume, cardiac filling, and stroke volume with accompanying venous pooling can contribute to development of orthostatic hypotension.

The unloading of weight and physical activity on skeletal muscles is associated with biochemical, structural, and functional characteristics. There is atrophy of muscle fibers with some evidence of ultrastructural damage to the contractile apparatus; these adaptations are associated with reductions in force development and strength. The diminution of muscle function is depen-

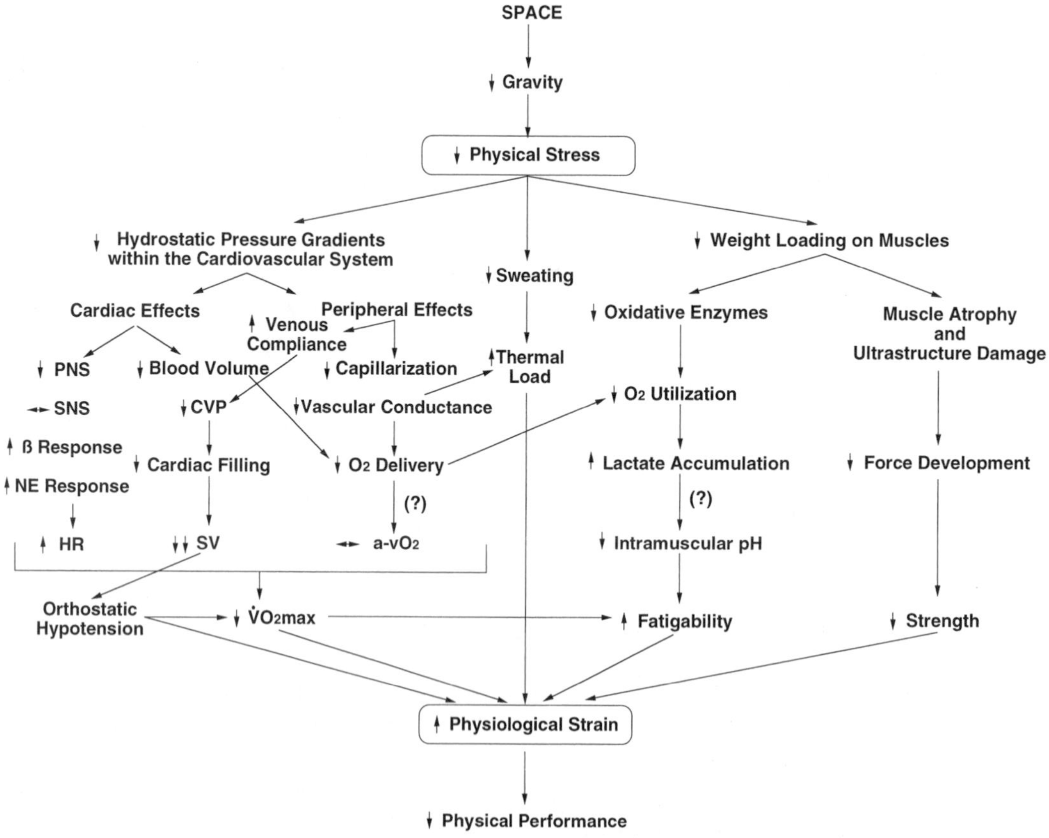

FIG. 31–7. Model of the relationship between physical stress of the space environment and adaptation of cardiovascular and muscular systems to resulting physiologic strain and physical performance.

dent on duration of exposure and is more pronounced for large muscle groups of the lower extremities. Reduction of oxidative enzymes is associated with greater lactate accumulation and fatigability. As a result of these adaptations, increased physiologic strain induced by exercise greatly limits physical performance in space or on return to Earth.

Reduced physical performance can be restored or maintained in space by specific corrective or preventive measures that include regular muscular activity. Effective use of exercise as a replacement stress for the absence of gravity to prevent diminished exercise performance should include an understanding of changes in the physiologic mechanisms involved and an ability to reverse these changes. While conventional endurance exercise training for 1 to 2 hours daily has proven effective in protecting $\dot{V}O_2max$ in space, it has failed to improve postflight orthostatic hypotension. Single bouts of intense exercise designed to elicit maximal stress may be useful in reversing numerous adaptations in physiologic factors associated with reduced exercise performance and postflight orthostatic hypotension. The use of dynamic resistive exercise in space should be given consideration for replacing loading patterns on skeletal muscles normally induced by the gravity environment of Earth. Advantages of incorporating dynamic resistive exercise with a strong emphasis on the use of eccentric muscle actions in addition to concentric actions may prove most effective as a protective measure against muscle atrophy and dysfunction caused by long-duration exposure to microgravity environments.

REFERENCES

1. Bikle DD, Halloran BP, Morey-Holton E. Space flight and the skeleton: lessons for the earthbound. *Endocrinologist* 1997; 7:10–22.
2. Levine BD, Lane LD, Watenpaugh DE, Gaffney FA, Buckey JC, Blomqvist CG. Maximal exercise performance after adaptation to microgravity. *J Appl Physiol* 1996;81:686–694.
3. Convertino VA. Potential benefits of maximal exercise just prior to return from weightlessness. *Aviat Space Environ Med* 1987; 58:568–572.
4. Convertino VA. Exercise and adaptation to microgravity environments. In: Fregly MJ, Blatteis CM, eds. *Handbook of physiology: environmental physiology, vol 3: the gravitational environment.* New York: Oxford University Press, 1995:815–843.
5. Convertino VA, Goldwater DJ, Sandler H. Bedrest-induced peak VO_2 reduction associated with age, gender and aerobic capacity. *Aviat Space Environ Med* 1986;57:17–22.
6. Saltin B, Blomqvist G, Mitchell JH, Johnson RL, Wildenthal K, Chapman CB. Response to exercise after bed rest and after training. *Circulation* 1968;38(suppl 7):1–78.
7. Greenleaf JE, Bernauer EM, Ertl AC, Trowbridge TS, Wade CE. Work capacity during 30-days of bed rest with isotonic and isokinetic exercise training. *J Appl Physiol* 1989;67:1820–1826.
8. Georgiyevskiy VS, Lapshina NA, Andriyako LY, et al. Circulation in exercising crew members of the first main expedition aboard Salyut-6. *Kosm Biol Aviakosm Med* 1980;14(3):15–18.
9. Michel EL, Rummel JA, Sawin CF. Skylab experiment M-171 "metabolic activity"—results of the first manned mission. *Acta Astronautica* 1975;2:351–365.
10. Michel EL, Rummel JA, Sawin CF, Buderer MC, Lem JD. Results of Skylab medical experiment M171—metabolic activity. In: Johnston RS, Dietlein LF, eds. *Biomedical results from Skylab.* Washington, DC: National Aeronautics and Space Administration, 1977:372–387.
11. Beregovkin AV, Vodolazov AS, Georgiyevskiy VS, et al. Reactions of the cardiorespiratory system to a dosed physical load in cosmonauts after 30- and 63-day flights in the Salyut-4 orbital station. *Kosm Biol Aviakosm Med* 1976;10(5):24–29.
12. Vorobyev YI, Gazenko OG, Gurovskiy NN, et al. Experimental Soyuz-Apollo flight. Preliminary results of biomedical investigations carried out during flight of the Soyuz-19 ship. *Kosm Biol Aviakosm Med* 1976;10(1):15–22.
13. Kasyan II, Makarov GF. External respiration, gas exchange and energy expenditures of man in weightlessness. *Kosm Biol Aviakosm Med* 1984;18(6):4–9.
14. Williams DA, Convertino VA. Circulating lactate and FFA during exercise: effect of reduction in plasma volume following simulated microgravity. *Aviat Space Environ Med* 1988;59:1042–1046.
15. Convertino VA. Physiological adaptations to weightlessness: effects on exercise and work performance. *Exerc Sport Sci Rev* 1990;18:119–165.
16. Vorobyov EI, Gazenko OG, Genin AM, Egorov AD. Medical results of Salyut-6 manned space flights. *Aviat Space Environ Med* 1983;54:S31–S40.
17. Thornton WE, Rummel JA. Muscular deconditioning and its prevention in space flight. In: Johnston RS, Dietlein LF, eds. *Biomedical results from Skylab.* Washington, DC: National Aeronautics and Space Administration, 1977:191–197.
18. Grigoryeva LS, Kozlovskaya IB. Effect of weightlessness and hypokinesia on velocity and strength properties of human muscles. *Kosm Biol Aviakosm Med* 1987;21(1):27–30.
19. Thornton WE, Hoffler GW, Rummel JA. Anthropometric changes and fluid shifts. In: Johnston RS, Dietlein LF, eds. *Biomedical results from Skylab.* Washington, DC: National Aeronautics and Space Administration, 1977:330–338.
20. Convertino VA. Neuromuscular aspects in development of exercise countermeasures. *Physiologist* 1991;34(suppl):S125–S128.
21. LaFevers EV, Nicogossian AE, Hursta WN. *Electromyographic analysis of skeletal muscle changes arising from 9 days of weightlessness in the Apollo-Soyuz space mission.* Washington, DC: National Aeronautics and Space Administration, 1976.
22. Kozlovskaya IB, Grigoryeva LS, Gevlich GI. Comparative analysis of effects of weightlessness and its models on velocity and strength properties and tone of human skeletal muscles. *Kosm Biol Aviakosm Med* 1984;18(6):22–26.
23. Convertino VA. Clinical aspects of the control of plasma volume at microgravity and during return to one gravity. *Med Sci Sports Exerc* 1996;28:S45–S52.
24. Fischer CL, Johnson PC, Berry CA. Red blood cell and plasma volume changes in manned spaceflight. *JAMA* 1967;200:579–583.
25. Johnson PC, Kimzey SL, Driscoll TB. Postmission plasma volume and red-cell mass changes in the crews of the first two Skylab missions. *Acta Astronautica* 1975;2:311–317.
26. Leach CS, Johnson PC. Influence of spaceflight on erythrokinetics in man. *Science* 1984;225:216–218.
27. Johnson PC, Driscoll TB, LeBlanc AD. Blood volume changes. In: Johnston RS, Dietlein LF, eds. *Biomedical results from Skylab.* Washington, DC: National Aeronautics and Space Administration, 1977:235–241.
28. Rummel JA, Michel EL, Berry CA. Physiological responses to exercise after space flight—Apollo 7 to Apollo 11. *Aviat Space Environ Med* 1973;44:235–238.
29. Rummel JA, Sawin CF, Buderer MC, Mauldin DG, Michel EL. Physiological responses to exercise after space flight—Apollo 14 through Apollo 17. *Aviat Space Environ Med* 1975;46:679–683.
30. Atkov OY, Bednenko VS, Fomina GA. Ultrasound techniques in space medicine. *Aviat Space Environ Med* 1987;58(suppl 9): A69–A73.
31. Buderer MC, Rummel JA, Michael EL, Maulden DC, Sawin CF. Exercise cardiac output following Skylab missions: the second manned Skylab mission. *Aviat Space Environ Med* 1976; 47:365–372.
32. Yegorov AD, Itsekhovskiy OG, Polyakova AP, et al. Results of

studies of hemodynamics and phase structure of the cardiac cycle during functional test with graded exercise during 140-day flight aboard the Salyut-6 station. *Kosm Biol Aviakosm Med* 1981; 15:18–22.
33. Vorobyev YI, Gazenko OG, Gurovskiy NN, et al. Preliminary results of medical investigations carried out during flight of the second expedition of the Soyuz-4 orbital station. *Kosm Biol Aviakosm Med* 1976;10:3–18.
34. Henry WL, Epstein SE, Griffith JM, Goldstein RE, Redwood DR. Effect of prolonged space flight on cardiac function and dimensions. In: Johnston RS, Dietlein LF, eds. *Biomedical results from Skylab.* Washington, DC: National Aeronautics and Space Administration, 1977:366–371.
35. Edgerton VR, Zhou M-Y, Ohira Y, et al. Human fiber size and enzymatic properties after 5 and 11 days of spaceflight. *J Appl Physiol* 1995;78:1733–1739.
36. Convertino VA, Doerr DF, Stein SF. Changes in size and compliance of the calf following 30 days of simulated microgravity. *J Appl Physiol* 1989;66:1509–1512.
37. Leach CS, Leonard JI, Rambaut PC, Johnson PC. Evaporative water loss in man in a gravity-free environment. *J Appl Physiol* 1978;45:430–436.
38. Crandall CG, Johnson JM, Convertino VA, Raven PB, Engelke KA. Altered thermo-regulatory responses after 15 days of head-down tilt. *J Appl Physiol* 1994;77:1863–1867.
39. Greenleaf JE, Reese RD. Exercise thermoregulation after 14 days of bed rest. *J Appl Physiol* 1980;48:72–78.
40. Convertino VA, Engelke KA, Ludwig DA, Doerr DF. Restoration of plasma volume after 16 days of head-down tilt induced by a single bout of maximal exercise. *Am J Physiol* 1996;270:R3–R10.
41. Convertino VA, Hoffler GW. Cardiovascular physiology: effects of microgravity. *J Fla Med Assoc* 1992;79:517–524.
42. Buckey JC Jr, Gaffney FA, Lane LD, et al. Central venous pressure in space. *J Appl Physiol* 1996;81:19–25.
43. Convertino VA, Doerr DF, Ludwig DA, Vemikos J. Effect of simulated microgravity on cardiopulmonary baroreflex control of forearm vascular resistance. *Am J Physiol* 1994;266:R1962–R1969.
44. Kirsch KA, Rocker L, Gauer OH, Krause R. Venous pressure in man during weightlessness. *Science* 1984;225:218–219.
45. Convertino VA, Doerr DF, Eckberg DL, Fritsch JM, Vernikos-Danellis J. Head-down bedrest impairs vagal baroreflex responses and provokes orthostatic hypotension. *J Appl Physiol* 1990; 68:1458–1464.
46. Convertino VA, Doerr DF, Guell A, Marini JF. Effects of acute exercise on attenuated vagal baroreflex function during bedrest. *Aviat Space Environ Med* 1992;63:999–1003.
47. Fritsch JM, Charles JB, Bennett BS, Jones MM, Eckberg DL. Short-duration spaceflight impairs human carotid baroreceptor-cardiac reflex responses. *J Appl Physiol* 1992;73:664–671.
48. Bungo MW, Johnson PC Jr. Cardiovascular examinations and observations of deconditioning during the space shuttle orbital flight test program. *Aviat Space Environ Med* 1983;54:1001–1004.
49. Hoffler GW. Cardiovascular studies of U.S. space crews: an overview and perspective. In: Hwang NHC, Normann NA, eds. *Cardiovascular flow dynamics and measurements.* Baltimore: University Park Press, 1977:335–363.
50. Buckey JC Jr, Lane LD, Levine BD, et al. Orthostatic intolerance after spaceflight. *J Appl Physiol* 1996;81:7–18.
51. Engelke KA, Doerr DF, Crandall CG, Convertino VA. Application of acute maximal exercise to protect orthostatic tolerance after simulated microgravity. *Am J Physiol* 1996;271:R837–R847.

Exercise and Sport Science,
edited by William E. Garrett, Jr., and Donald T. Kirkendall.
Lippincott Williams & Wilkins, Philadelphia © 2000.

CHAPTER 32

Enhancing Exercise Performance: Nutritional Implications

Jeff S. Volek

Nutrition forms the foundation of an athletic training program. Improper nutrition may negate many of the gains in exercise performance resulting from high-quality research-based training programs. Thus, optimizing nutritional habits should be a high priority in the development of an overall training regimen. While a large body of literature has accumulated over recent years pertaining to endurance activities, there is still a general lack of definitive research in many areas of performance-enhancement nutrition, specifically related to high-intensity and resistance exercise. There are different opinions concerning dietary strategies to enhance performance. To further complicate the issue, many factors contribute to individual nutrient requirements, such as genetics, training goals, phase of training, and training status.

This chapter begins with a brief summary of energy metabolism during exercise; it then discusses the primary energy-providing macronutrients (carbohydrate and fat), emphasizing their influence on coronary artery disease risk. Two primary dietary strategies that have been put forth in the scientific literature as methods to enhance physical performance are presented. An overview of the scientific evidence supporting each method is discussed and distinctions are made between endurance (aerobic-oriented) and high-intensity (anaerobic-oriented) exercise. The effects of different forms of exercise on protein requirements, a general discussion of vitamins and minerals, and the nutritional supplement creatine are also covered. The chapter ends with a summary of the scientific data pertaining to diet and exercise, to provide practical dietary advice to aid athletes in achieving optimal nutrition for sport performance.

There are two primary ways in which diet can enhance exercise performance and the adaptations to physical training. First, dietary intake can influence the synthesis, storage, and mobilization of energy substrates during rest, exercise, and recovery, which can have an impact on performance and, over time, body composition. For example, consuming large amounts of carbohydrate will increase muscle and liver glycogen stores, increase carbohydrate oxidation, and suppress the utilization of fat as a fuel source. Second, dietary intake can influence important recovery processes that are required to maximize physiologic adaptations over a training cycle. For example, adequate protein is required to meet the demands of increased protein synthesis. Central to understanding how nutrition can influence performance is a basic understanding of energy metabolism and the metabolic demands of different types of exercise.

ENERGY METABOLISM

Exercise requires adenosine triphosphate (ATP) for muscular contraction. Resynthesis of ATP in muscle is important for the restoration and maintenance of force-producing capabilities during and following physical activity. Immediate resynthesis of ATP occurs anaerobically (without oxygen) via the high-energy phosphate compound phosphocreatine. Phosphocreatine is rapidly depleted at the onset of high-intensity exercise. As exercise continues, ATP demands are met by metabolic pathways that break down carbohydrates and fats for energy. Some energy sources are located directly in skeletal muscle, whereas others are delivered to skeletal muscle via the circulatory system. The primary energy substrates located within muscle are glycogen and triglycerides. It is well known that glycogen depletion oc-

J. S. Volek: The Human Performance Laboratory, Ball State University, Muncie, Indiana 47306.

curs after various types of exercise. However, the use of intramuscular triglycerides as an energy source may be more important in both endurance and anaerobic high-intensity exercise than previously thought (1,2). Depletion of intramuscular glycogen and triglycerides occurs during both high-intensity/resistance exercise and prolonged endurance activity. Metabolic substrates that can be delivered to the muscle via the circulation include glucose (derived from the diet or the liver), fatty acids (derived from adipose tissue stores), triglycerides (derived from the diet or the liver), and, during certain conditions such as fasting or low carbohydrate intake, ketone bodies (derived from the liver). Circulating blood glucose is balanced between dietary intake and that released by the liver via synthesis from precursors such as alanine, glycerol, pyruvate, lactate, and glutamine (gluconeogenesis) or from breakdown of liver glycogen (liver glycogenolysis); it becomes increasingly important when muscle energy stores become depleted. Glycolysis is the process by which glucose is converted into pyruvate and lactate with concomitant production of ATP. The storage and utilization of energy substrates is influenced to a large extent by dietary intake and is an extremely important aspect regulating the degree to which recovery processes (i.e., glycogen and triglyceride resynthesis, protein accretion, etc.) proceed.

Regulation of carbohydrate and fat metabolism during and after exercise is partially dependent on the intensity of effort and nutritional state (2,3). Although a nice relationship exists between the intensity of exercise and carbohydrate metabolism, the role of fat in providing energy during maximal exercise is more complex (4) and may also be significant (5), especially if the exercise is intermittent in nature (1,6,7). Compared to muscle glycogen, there is much less data on the contribution of intramuscular triglycerides to the energy supply during exercise. The duration of exercise as well as the training status of the individual will also influence the contribution of energy substrates to total energy expenditure.

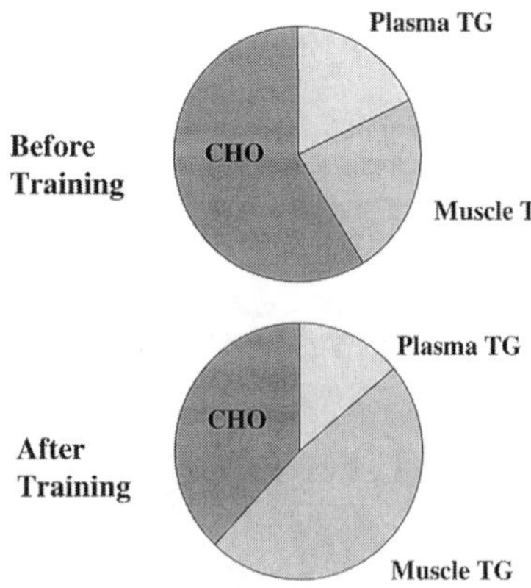

FIG. 32–1. Contribution of different energy sources to total energy expenditure during submaximal exercise before and after endurance training. *TG*, triglycerides; *CHO*, carbohydrate. (Adapted from ref. 8.)

Energy Metabolism During Aerobic Endurance Exercise

During low-intensity exercise (e.g., walking) the majority of energy is derived from fatty acids mobilized from adipose tissue. As the intensity of exercise is increased, proportionally more of the energy is derived from carbohydrate (blood glucose and glycogen) and the contribution of muscle triglycerides is also higher. During moderate-intensity exercise (about 65% $\dot{V}O_2$max) carbohydrate (blood glucose and glycogen) and fat (plasma fatty acids and muscle triglycerides) contribute equally to the total energy expenditure. If exercise is prolonged, muscle substrates (glycogen and triglycerides) contribute less to total energy expenditure and blood glucose and fatty acids become more important. During high-intensity exercise, muscle substrates, primarily glycogen, become the primary sources of energy, and the rate of fat oxidation is lower compared to that during moderate-intensity exercise. There are several potential steps that may limit fat oxidation during high-intensity exercise, including (a) mobilization of fatty acids from adipose tissue, (b) mobilization of fatty acids from plasma triglycerides, (c) transport of fatty acids into the sarcoplasm, (d) uptake of fatty acids by the muscle cell, (e) availability and mobilization of intramuscular triglycerides, (f) activation of fatty acids and transport into the mitochondria, and (g) oxidation of fatty acids in the mitochondria. The extent to which each of these processes limits fat oxidation and the potential for enhancement through chronic dietary intake and/or training is unclear. A well-accepted adaptation to endurance training is an increase in the relative percentage of energy derived from fat (Fig. 32–1) (2). Interestingly, the increase in fat oxidation is not from adipose tissue lipolysis but rather from intramuscular triglycerides (8). Prolonged consumption of a fat-rich diet also results in a similar increase in fat oxidation (9). The exact mechanism(s) that explain the increase in fat oxidation have not been identified.

Energy Metabolism During High-Intensity/Resistance Exercise

Studies examining muscle metabolism during high-intensity and resistance exercise indicate that phosphocreatine breakdown is important in addition to muscle glycogen and triglyceride stores (Fig. 32–2) (1,6,7,10–13). The relative contribution from these sources may be dependent on availability, especially in the case of triglyceride stores (1) and the activity of various enzymes (13). Thus, from a nutritional standpoint it would be advantageous to optimize the use of phosphocre-

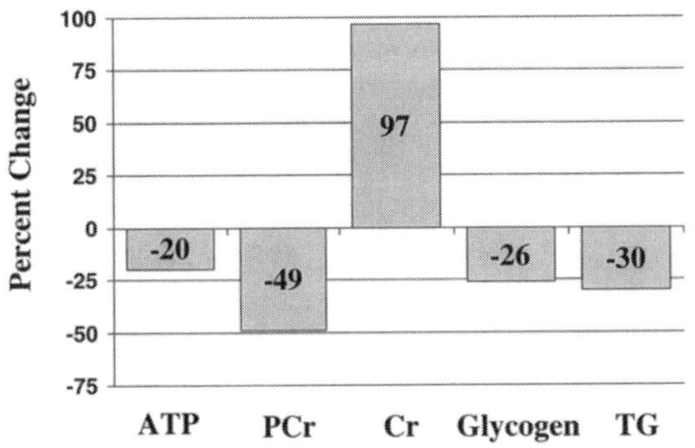

FIG. 32–2. Percent change in muscle metabolites after a resistance training session composed of 20 sets of leg exercises. *PCr*, phosphocreatine; *Cr*, free creatine; *TG*, triglycerides. (Adapted from refs. 1 and 13.)

atine, as this is the most powerful energy system in terms of ATP provision. This is the basis for the currently popular nutritional supplement creatine monohydrate (discussed later). The effects of diet on triglyceride stores and subsequent exercise performance, in particular resistance exercise, are unknown. A high-fat diet does increase muscle triglyceride stores (14) and does not appear to negatively impact high-intensity exercise performance (15).

PRIMARY ENERGY-PROVIDING DIETARY MACRONUTRIENTS

Carbohydrates

An important concept related to the classification of carbohydrates is the glycemic index (GI), which reflects the metabolic effect rather than the structural or chemical characteristics of a particular food. The GI provides a method for classifying foods based on their acute glycemic impact (16). The GI of a food is based on a standard food (usually glucose or white bread), which is given an arbitrary value of 100. The GI of a food is calculated by integrating the 2-hour glycemic-response curve after ingestion of the test food containing 50 g of available carbohydrate. Foods that are digested quickly and appear in the bloodstream rapidly have a high GI, and foods that are more resistant to digestion and appear in the bloodstream at a slower rate have a low GI. Foods with a high GI cause blood sugar and insulin concentrations to rise faster than low GI foods. There is not an obvious correlation between the prevalent chemical classification system of simple or complex carbohydrates and the GI of a food. For example, complex carbohydrates such as white bread and potatoes have a high GI, whereas the simple carbohydrate fructose has a low GI. The main determinant of the GI and the metabolic effect of a food is the rate at which it is digested (17). Factors that influence the digestion of foods and thus the GI include the type of sugar (fructose is lower than sucrose or glucose), the nature of the starch (amylose is lower than amylopectin), fiber content, food portion size, degree of processing, protein and fat in the food, and food preparation method. Table 32–1 lists several foods and their corresponding GI rating.

Fats

Fatty acids contain hydrocarbon chains ranging in length from 4 to 20 carbons. Three fatty acids are esterified with a single glycerol molecule to form triglycerides, the storage form of fat in the body. Compared to carbohydrates, fats are an efficient storage form of energy in the body because they are stored anhydrous (i.e., without water) and they contain more than twice the energy per gram as carbohydrates. Based on the degree of saturation, fatty acids may be classified as saturated (no double bonds), polyunsaturated (more than one double bond), and monounsaturated (one double bond). There are two dietary essential polyunsaturated fatty acids, α-linoleic and γ-linolenic acids. The common name and chemical structure of the most abundant dietary fatty acids including the essential fatty acids are depicted in Fig. 32–3. An overview of the major classes of fatty acids as well as a summary of their influence on various classes of lipoproteins and risk for coronary artery disease is presented.

Saturated Fatty Acids

Saturated fatty acids (SFAs) obtained in the diet contain different lengths of hydrocarbons ranging from short- and medium-chain to the more common longer-chain fatty acids (12:0 myristic, 14:0 lauric, 16:0 palmitic, 18:0 stearic). There are no double bonds in SFAs. Fat contained in animal products (e.g., beef, chicken, dairy products) is predominantly saturated in nature and is solid at room temperature.

Epidemiologic studies strongly indicate that the consumption of SFAs is positively correlated with plasma total and low-density lipoprotein (LDL) cholesterol as well as incidence of coronary artery disease (see ref. 18 for review). These findings derived from epidemiologic data, for the most part, agree with the results obtained from well-controlled feeding studies designed to examine the effect of different classes of fat and individual fatty acids on blood lipids (see ref. 19 for review). Most of the increase in total blood cholesterol from dietary SFAs occurs at the expense of LDL cholesterol; however, most long-chain fatty acids (12:0, 14:0, and 16:0) also raise high-density lipoprotein (HDL) cholesterol slightly. Although most of the attention surrounding SFAs has focused on cholesterol, blood triglycerides may also be negatively impacted. Diets rich in SFAs have been shown to enhance postprandial lipemia (i.e.,

TABLE 32–1. *Glycemic index (GI) of various foods using white bread (GI = 100) as a standard*

Bakery products		Fruit	
Angel food cake	95	Apple	52
Sponge cake	66	Apple juice	58
Croissant	96	Banana	76
Doughnut (cake type)	108	Cherries	32
Muffin (bran)	85	Fruit cocktail (canned)	79
Waffle	109	Grapefruit	36
Breads		Grapefruit juice	69
Bagel	103	Grapes	62
Hamburger bun	87	Orange	62
Kaiser roll	104	Orange juice	74
Wheat bread	99	Pear	47
Cereals		Pineapple	94
All-Bran	60	Plum	34
Cheerios	106	Raisins	91
Corn flakes	119	Watermelon	103
Oat bran	78	Legumes	
Puffed wheat	105	Baked beans	69
Rice Krispies	117	Chick-peas	47
Shredded wheat	99	Kidney beans	42
Cereal grains and pasta		Lentils	41
Barley	36	Lima beans	46
White rice	81	Pinto beans	55
Brown rice	79	Split peas	45
Instant rice	128	Vegetables	
Rye	48	Carrots	101
Wheat	59	Potato (baked)	121
Linguine	65	Sweet potato	77
Spaghetti	59	Peas	68
Dairy foods		Corn	78
Ice cream	87	Soups	
Ice cream (low fat)	71	Lentil	63
Milk (full fat)	39	Split pea	86
Milk (skim)	46	Tomato	54
Yogurt (artificial sweetener)	20	Snack foods	
Sugars		Oatmeal cookies	79
Honey	104	Vanilla wafers	110
Fructose	32	Rice cakes	117
Glucose	138	Jelly beans	114
Sucrose	92	Chocolate	70
Lactose	65	Popcorn	79
Maltose	150	Corn chips	105
		Potato chips	77
		Peanuts	21

Adapted from ref. 128.

the extent and duration of triglyceride elevation after a fat-rich meal) (20,21). Compelling evidence indicates that replacement of certain long-chain SFAs with carbohydrate or unsaturated fat lowers total cholesterol and LDL cholesterol (22,23). Replacing SFAs with unsaturated fat rather than carbohydrate may have several benefits, including improved plasma HDL cholesterol and triglyceride responses (24). While the cholesterol-raising effects of SFAs as a whole are consistently observed, there is also compelling evidence indicating that the individual fatty acids differ in their hypercholesterolemic effect. Controlled clinical trials suggest that myristic is the most potent SFA, followed by lauric and palmitic acids. Stearic acid, rich in beef and chocolate, is unique among the long-chain SFAs in that several studies indicate that it has a neutral effect on blood lipids (25). The mechanism by which SFAs increase LDL cholesterol is not entirely elucidated but is believed to arise via a decrease in the synthesis of hepatic LDL receptors and clearance of LDL cholesterol from the circulation (26).

Polyunsaturated Fatty Acids

Polyunsaturated fatty acids (PUFAs) contain two or more double bonds in their hydrocarbon chain. Depending on where the double bonds are located, PUFAs may be classified as either n-3 or n-6 series. For example,

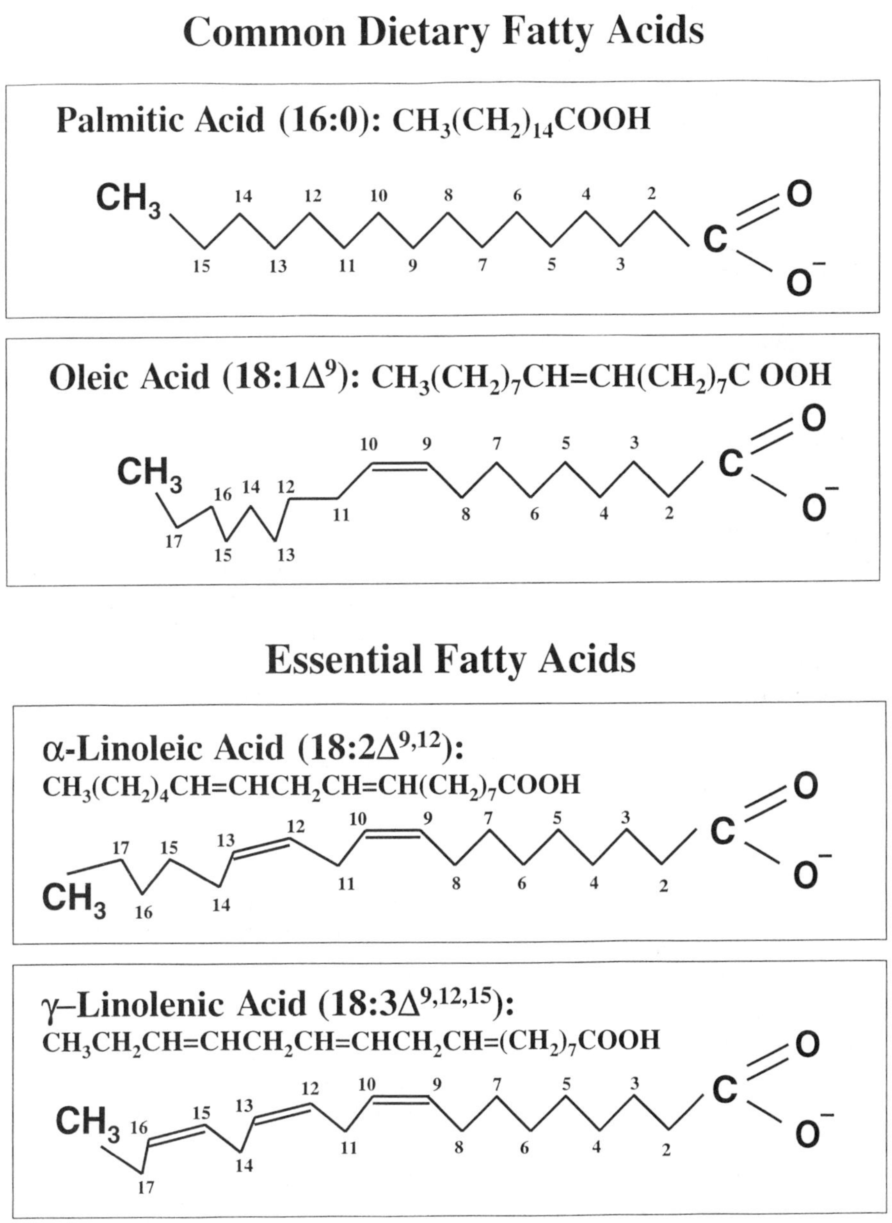

FIG. 32–3. Common names and chemical structures for two abundant dietary fatty acids (palmitic and oleic acids) and the two dietary essential fatty acids (linoleic and linolenic acids). Palmitic acid is a 16-carbon saturated fatty acid and oleic acid is an 18-carbon monounsaturated fatty acid with the double bond located at the ninth carbon from the carboxyl end of the hydrocarbon chain. α-Linoleic acid and γ-linolenic acid are essential 18-carbon polyunsaturated fatty acids with 2 and 3 double bonds, respectively.

an n-3 fatty acid has the first double bond beginning at the third carbon from the terminal methyl group. The most common dietary PUFA from the n-6 series is linoleic acid (18:2n-6), a dietary essential fatty acid. Total, LDL, and HDL cholesterol concentrations decline when PUFAs are substituted for SFAs (27). In contrast, plasma HDL is increased slightly and triglycerides are significantly decreased when dietary carbohydrate is replaced with PUFAs (28,29). Linoleic acid has been shown to lower total and LDL cholesterol concentrations compared to other monounsaturated and saturated fats, including oleic (18:1) and stearic (18:0) acid. There is some indication that linoleic acid–rich diets may increase the susceptibility of certain LDL subclasses to oxidation (30). If this finding is true, PUFAs may be viewed as proatherogenic, as oxidative modification of LDL cholesterol is believed to be a prerequisite for deposition on the artery wall.

Dietary PUFAs with their double bonds beginning at the third carbon from the methyl end of the fatty acid (n-3 series) include linolenic acid (18:3n-3), another dietary essential fatty acid rich in linseed or flaxseed oil, eicosapentaenoic acid (EPA, 20:5n-3) and docosahexaenoic acid (DHA, 22:6n-3) found in tissues of certain organisms of marine origin. Polyunsaturated fatty acids from the n-3 series have been found to have minimal effects on LDL, HDL, and total cholesterol. Fish oils have been shown to possess potent triglyceride-lowering effects, however, and they have received a significant amount of attention due to their potential antiatherogenic properties (31). A recent review of well-controlled human trials examining the effects of n-3 PUFAs on serum lipid and lipoprotein concentrations concluded that supplementation with fish oil reduces fasting serum triglycerides 25% to 30% with minimal effects on other classes of lipoproteins (32). Since n-3 PUFAs have minimal effects on LDL, HDL, and total cholesterol, it is speculated that the cardioprotective effects of diets rich in fish oil observed in certain populations, such as Greenland Eskimos (33), are mediated via alterations in other risk factors related to platelet function, blood pressure, blood flow, and inflammatory and atherogenic processes (34). A significant decrease in the duration and magnitude of postprandial chylomicrons and chylomicron remnants to n-3 PUFA consumption (20,35) indicates a potential role of these fatty acids in either catabolism or synthesis of triglycerides. The triglyceride-lowering effect of n-3 PUFA has been hypothesized to result from increased catabolism via alterations in the size and fatty acid composition of chylomicrons (36) and enhanced post-heparin LDL activity (37), or decreased synthesis of triglycerides in the intestine and liver via inhibition of lipogenic enzymes (38,39).

Monounsaturated Fatty Acids

Monounsaturated fatty acids (MUFAs) contain a single double bond in their hydrocarbon chain; the most common dietary MUFA is oleic acid (18:1n-9), which is rich in olive and canola oils. There is some controversy related to the impact of MUFAs on blood lipoprotein fractions. Substitution for SFAs with MUFAs significantly lowers both LDL and total cholesterol and increases HDL cholesterol. There is also some controversy as to the effects of MUFAs compared to PUFAs on blood lipids and lipoproteins. Recent evidence suggests that MUFAs and PUFAs elicit similar effects on blood lipids when substituted for each other; however, there is some indication that PUFAs may possess a greater total cholesterol-lowering effect (40). Studies examining the lipoprotein responses when MUFAs are substituted for carbohydrate have provided insightful findings. Diets rich in MUFAs (20% to 28% of total energy) and high in total fat (37% to 41%) increase HDL cholesterol (8% to 22%) and decrease triglycerides (0% to 24%), without adversely impacting total cholesterol and LDL cholesterol in healthy subjects (41–45). One advantage to a diet rich in oleic acid compared to n-3 and n-6 fatty acids is a reduction in the susceptibility of LDL cholesterol to oxidative modification (46).

Trans Fatty Acids

During the processing of unsaturated oils and other fats (e.g., margarine), the configuration of the double bonds can be switched from the more common *cis* to the *trans* isomer. The most common *trans* fatty acid is elaidic acid (*trans*-18:1), the *trans* isomer of oleic acid. While *trans* fatty acids make up a relatively small percentage of the human diet (3% to 4%), recent evidence indicates that these fatty acids may have a detrimental effect on blood lipoproteins. The majority of evidence indicates that *trans* fatty acids raise LDL and total cholesterol and, unlike other SFAs, probably lower HDL cholesterol. In addition, *trans* fatty acids have been shown to increase lipoprotein(a), an independent risk factor for coronary heart disease. The LDL cholesterol–raising effects of *trans* fatty acids are slightly less than those of other SFAs (12:0, 14:0, 16:0), similar to those of stearic acid (18:0), and significantly greater than those of 18:1 and 18:2n-6. Plasma triglycerides appear to be unaffected by *trans* fatty acids.

DIETARY STRATEGIES TO ENHANCE PERFORMANCE

During prolonged endurance exercise, exhaustion is accompanied by marked glycogen depletion and hypoglycemia. Two very different dietary approaches have emerged with the intent of preventing or at least delaying the onset of low glycogen and glucose concentrations. Theoretically, glycogen depletion could be delayed by either increasing initial glycogen levels or decreasing the rate of glycogen breakdown. Historically, a carbohydrate-rich diet has been recommended for athletes to increase glycogen, delay glycogen depletion, and thus improve performance. More recent research indicates that a fat-rich diet can also enhance performance by increasing fat utilization, reducing glycogen breakdown, and delaying glycogen depletion. Although very different, both dietary approaches are supported by scientific research. Several excellent review articles have been written that discuss the research pertaining to carbohydrate metabolism (47–50) and lipid metabolism (51–56), emphasizing nutritional implications and the subsequent effects on physical performance.

Carbohydrate-Rich Diets

The importance of dietary carbohydrate on endurance exercise performance has been known for more than 50 years. Early work in this area by Christensen and

Hansen (57) demonstrated that endurance performance was enhanced after 3 days of a carbohydrate-rich diet compared to a normal mixed or high-fat diet. With the advent of the needle muscle biopsy technique in the early 1960s (58), knowledge of substrate storage and utilization in response to various exercise and dietary regimens was vastly improved. Several investigations reported a significant correlation between the amount of muscle glycogen and performance during submaximal exercise performance. Thus, various nutritional interventions to enhance glycogen levels and/or glucose availability were examined with the intent of improving exercise performance. Research has concentrated on the effects of carbohydrate feedings prior to and during exercise (to maximize glucose availability) and carbohydrate loading several days prior to exercise (to maximize glycogen levels). Fewer studies have examined the influence of prolonged carbohydrate-rich diets on exercise training and physical performance.

Carbohydrates Before Exercise

Many of the studies examining the metabolic and performance effects of preexercise carbohydrate feedings have indeed reported that physical performance during prolonged exercise limited by carbohydrate availability can be improved (59,60); however, other studies have shown no effect (60–64). Carbohydrates consumed during the hour prior to exercise generally result in elevated insulin and a decline in blood glucose concentrations at the onset of exercise. In the majority of athletes, this moderate hypoglycemia does not affect performance. There is some debate as to whether carbohydrate feedings prior to exercise should be predominantly high or low GI. Based on data from endurance athletes it may be appropriate to consume pre-event meals with a low glycemic rating (65,66). Low GI foods should provide for a slow release of glucose into the circulation without causing a surge in insulin. By providing a steady source of carbohydrate to exercising muscles when glycogen levels are low, fatigue may be delayed. Additionally, 5 mL/kg body mass of water (~2 cups for a 75-kg athlete) should be consumed during the hour prior to exercise to maintain hydration.

Carbohydrates During Exercise

Exhaustion during prolonged endurance exercise (>2 hours) occurs primarily as a result of hypoglycemia. Carbohydrate feedings during exercise have been utilized to delay fatigue by providing a source of glucose during the later stages of exercise at a time when carbohydrate stores are depleted. Exercise time may be extended by approximately 30 to 60 minutes if the type of carbohydrate and timing of ingestion are appropriate (67–69). A variety of carbohydrates including glucose, sucrose, and maltodextrins in either solid or liquid form have been shown to be effective at maintaining blood glucose late in exercise. Fructose and other low GI foods may not be as effective due to the slower rate of absorption compared to other carbohydrate sources. Carbohydrate feedings should occur early during exercise to ensure enough time for absorption. Generally, 30 to 60 g of a moderate/high GI carbohydrate/hour should be consumed soon after the start of exercise and continued until exhaustion (47,48). If the exercise session is prolonged and glycogen depleting, fluid replacement and carbohydrate ingestion throughout exercise will help to maintain blood glucose levels and improve performance. Surprisingly, during high-intensity exercise lasting 1 hour, both carbohydrate ingestion and fluid replacement independently improved performance (70). Carbohydrate and fluid needs during prolonged intermittent high-intensity exercise can be met by ingesting 600 to 1000 mL/h of a solution containing 4% to 10% carbohydrate (e.g., glucose, sucrose, or maltodextrins).

Prolonged High-Carbohydrate Diets

Compared to the abundance of literature investigating the effects of short-term carbohydrate feedings prior to and during exercise, fewer studies have been performed addressing the contention that long-term carbohydrate-rich diets are superior for optimizing training and performance. High-carbohydrate diets do in fact result in elevated glycogen concentrations compared to low- or moderate-carbohydrate intakes; however, the impact of higher levels of glycogen on the quality of training and performance is less clear. For 1 week, endurance athletes (runners and cyclists) consumed either a moderate-carbohydrate (42% of energy) or high-carbohydrate (84% of energy)—5 or 10 g carbohydrate/kg/day, respectively—eucaloric diet while performing daily training sessions (71). Endurance performance was measured after the 7 days of diet and training. Despite a 30% decline in muscle glycogen by day 5 after moderate-carbohydrate intake, there was no difference in the ability to complete the training sessions and time to exhaustion at 80% $\dot{V}O_2max$ between groups. After 28 days of twice-daily training in rowers, athletes who consumed 10 versus 5 g carbohydrate/kg/day demonstrated significantly increased muscle glycogen and physical performance (72). Surprisingly, athletes consuming the moderate-carbohydrate diet maintained muscle glycogen and performance capabilities. Performance may be affected with moderate-carbohydrate intake, however, when training is intensified if the diet is deficient in total energy (73). These studies suggest that moderate-carbohydrate diets result in lower muscle glycogen compared to high-carbohydrate diets, but the impact on training and performance is variable.

Carbohydrates and High-Intensity Exercise

High-intensity exercise relies heavily on muscular glycogen stores as an energy source, particularly in fast-twitch type II muscle fibers. Furthermore, early depletion of glycogen in these fibers has been implicated as one of many possible causative factors in fatigue (74). Whether initial muscle glycogen levels influence exercise glycogen metabolism and performance is an important question to answer because recommendations for the optimal timing, quantity, and quality of carbohydrate intake are often based on optimizing glycogen levels between successive workouts. Studies designed to investigate this question typically manipulate preexercise glycogen levels by having subjects modify their diet (e.g., either high- or low-carbohydrate diets) and/or perform exhaustive glycogen-depleting exercise hours or days prior to the high-intensity exercise protocol. Although some studies demonstrate that lower-than-normal initial glycogen levels decrease short-term, high-intensity exercise performance (75–77), several reports indicate that lower-than-normal preexercise glycogen levels do not impair performance (78–80). Generally, research shows that higher-than-normal glycogen levels do not offer any additional benefits during high-intensity exercise performance (75,77,81–84); however, a few studies have reported improvements (77,85). These conflicting results most likely reflect one or more of the following methodologic issues: (a) selection of exercise protocol (e.g., continuous versus intermittent), (b) negative effects of prior glycogen-depleting exercise, (c) use of untrained subjects, (d) length of time allowed for adaptation to dietary modification, (e) level of dietary energy intake during low-carbohydrate diet period, and (f) degree of glycogen depletion. Taken together, it appears that increasing glycogen stores by consuming a high-carbohydrate diet does not significantly influence the rate of glycogenolysis (86,87) or short-term, high-intensity exercise performance. Studies demonstrating a negative effect of a lower-than-normal starting glycogen level typically had subjects consume a low-carbohydrate diet for 1 to 3 days (75–77). If subjects were allowed more time to make metabolic and psychologic adaptations to the low-carbohydrate diet, then perhaps high-intensity exercise performance would be maintained despite slightly lower glycogen levels. One factor that may help to spare glycogen depletion and theoretically improve prolonged intermittent high-intensity exercise performance is an increase in the utilization of lipids, especially intramuscular triglycerides, during periods between work bouts (88).

Fat-Rich Diets

Metabolic and Enzymatic Adaptations to High-Fat Diets

Increased capacity to oxidize lipid after adaptation to a fat-rich diet has been documented in several animals and humans. Chronic adaptation to a high-fat diet attenuates glycogen depletion during exercise due to physiologic and metabolic adaptations that enhance the utilization of fat as an energy source at rest and during exercise (9,89–97). These adaptations include decreased muscle glycogen storage (9,15,94), increased storage of intramuscular triglycerides (14,90,92,98), and enzymatic adaptations enhancing mitochondrial oxidative capacity (89,92,93,97,100). Fat-rich diets have been shown to alter the activity of several enzymes including increased carnitine acyl transferase, a key enzyme involved in fatty acid transport into the mitochondria (100); increased β-hydroxyacyl-coenzyme A (CoA) dehydrogenase, a key enzyme in mitochondrial β-oxidation (89,93,97,101); increased lipoprotein lipase, a key enzyme involved in hydrolysis of circulating triacylglycerols (14,102); increased 3-oxoacid CoA thiolase, a key enzyme in ketogenesis (99); increased phosphoenolpyruvate carboxykinase, a key enzyme in gluconeogenesis (103); decreased hexokinase, a key enzyme in glycolysis (100); decreased pyruvate dehydrogenase, an enzyme that controls the flux of glycolysis-derived acetyl-CoA into the citric acid cycle (104,105); and increased branched-chain ketoacid dehydrogenase, a key enzyme in oxidation of branched-chain amino acids (106). These enzymatic adaptations to some extent are fiber-type specific and dependent on the increase in dietary fat intake.

High-Fat Diets and Exercise Performance

The metabolic and enzymatic adaptations to increased fat intake have most likely contributed to the improved endurance capacity after chronic adaptation to fat-rich diets in rats (90,93,97), dogs (91,107,108), horses (91,109–111), and humans (9,15,96,112–114). Lambert and colleagues (15) demonstrated that adaptation to a high-fat diet (70% of energy) for 2 weeks resulted in enhanced endurance during prolonged exercise and no impairment in high-intensity exercise performance, despite significantly reduced starting glycogen levels in a group of trained cyclists. This is the only study that has reported data on the capacity to perform high-intensity exercise after chronic adaptation to a low-carbohydrate, high-fat diet. Recent studies in humans suggest that increasing dietary fat from 15% to 42% increases maximal oxygen consumption and endurance capacity (112, 113) without compromising either immune functioning (115) or blood lipoprotein profiles (112). These data suggest that even moderate increases in dietary fat may be beneficial for overall health and physical performance.

Carbohydrate Loading After Adaptation to a Fat-Rich Diet

Particularly interesting are studies that have chronically adapted human subjects (116) or rats (90,92,98,117) to a high-fat diet to induce favorable changes in muscle fat oxidative capacity and then increased carbohydrate intake for a short period (i.e., carbohydrate loading). Thus, enhanced fat oxidative potential induced by the synergistic effect of a high-fat diet and training, combined with elevated glycogen stores from the acute increase in carbohydrate intake, is hypothesized to optimize physical performance. Taken together, these studies (90,92,98,116,117) indicate that adaptation to a high-fat diet slightly decreases resting muscle glycogen, increases muscle triglycerides, and promotes utilization of fat over carbohydrate as an energy substrate at rest and during moderate-intensity exercise. Short-term change to a high-carbohydrate diet after a habitual high-fat diet increases muscle glycogen above that achieved with a habitual high-carbohydrate diet while still maintaining the enhanced ability to oxidize fat. Saitoh and colleagues (98) demonstrated that short-term carbohydrate feeding to rats adapted to a high-fat diet significantly increased the number of β-adrenergic receptors and *in vitro* lipolysis of adipose tissue. Thus, the increased utilization of fat may be related to adaptations occurring from both peripheral (adipose tissue) and local (skeletal muscle) sites. The effects of adaptation to a high-fat diet followed by short-term carbohydrate intake are mixed, with two studies showing enhanced (90,92) and one study impaired (116) endurance performance compared to performance with a high-carbohydrate diet. Differences in species, training status, and dietary composition probably contribute to these conflicting results. Dietary fat was 65% of total energy in the study by Helge and colleagues (116), whereas dietary fat was 79% in the studies performed in rats (90,92). Thus, the optimal fat intake to induce positive adaptation in energy metabolism and exercise performance of different intensities is not known; however, the potential benefits of short-term change to a high-carbohydrate diet after adaptation to a high-fat diet warrant further investigation.

PROTEIN REQUIREMENTS

Proteins, and their component parts, amino acids, are required or essential dietary nutrients to sustain life. While our body has the capacity to synthesize certain amino acids (nonessential or dispensable amino acids), others must be obtained from the diet (essential or indispensable amino acids). Thus, our actual requirement is not for proteins per se; rather, it is for the nine essential amino acids that, over the course of the evolutionary process, our bodies have lost the ability to synthesize. To promote increases in muscle size (hypertrophy) and increases in strength, it is an absolute requirement that athletes be in a positive nitrogen balance. Nitrogen balance is determined by measuring dietary nitrogen intake (protein is 16% nitrogen) and subtracting nitrogen loss (urine, sweat, feces). A question debated for more than a century is whether large quantities of dietary protein are necessary to maintain nitrogen balance and enhance muscular hypertrophy and strength. The current recommended daily allowance (RDA) for protein is 0.8 g/kg/day, which was derived from both short- and long-term nitrogen balance studies in subjects whose lifestyles were essentially sedentary. Recent data provide a strong indication that athletes can benefit from dietary protein above the RDA. Why should athletes require more protein than their sedentary counterparts? First, exercise causes disruption of the active muscle tissue, which requires additional protein to allow for tissue repair and compensatory hypertrophy. This mechanism is relatively more important for strength and power athletes who perform heavy resistance exercises. Second, exercise enhances the oxidation of amino acids to provide fuel for performance of muscular work, and thus extra protein in the diet is required as an auxiliary fuel source. This mechanism is comparably more important for endurance athletes.

Effects of Heavy Resistance Exercise on Protein Requirements

Amino acids serve as the building blocks for synthesis of proteins into skeletal muscle. Resistance training is a powerful stimulus to increase the rate of amino acid incorporation into muscle proteins. Based on nitrogen balance and metabolic tracer studies examining the optimal protein requirement for strength and power athletes, protein intake should be about 1.7 to 1.8 g/kg/day (118). Consuming protein at levels >2 g/kg/day will cause an increase in amino acid oxidation (119). If insufficient calories are consumed, protein intakes that would normally promote a positive nitrogen balance can induce a negative nitrogen status. Thus, under conditions of inadequate energy consumption, protein requirements may be further increased.

Effects of Endurance Exercise on Protein Requirements

Endurance athletes are not concerned with building large muscles. However, recent data support the notion that protein at the level of the RDA is suboptimal for endurance as well as for strength athletes. Mistakenly, the energy derived from protein is commonly ignored since dietary carbohydrates and fats provide the majority of energy to sustain muscular work. However, oxidation of amino acids does provide a small, but not insignificant, portion of the total energy requirements during exercise. Recent data suggest that the relative contribution of amino acids as an energy source during intense or extended endurance exercise may have been underestimated. While the exact magnitude of the increased requirement of athletes for all amino acids is not known, oxidation of certain amino acids—leucine, for example—

has been shown to increase substantially with endurance exercise. Oxidation of leucine has been shown to be greater as the intensity and duration of exercise increase. Furthermore, one of the physiologic adaptations to chronic endurance training is a proportional increase in the energy derived from amino acids. Based on these findings, the optimal protein intake for endurance athletes is estimated to fall between the current RDA for sedentary individuals and that for strength athletes and is about 1.2 to 1.4 g protein/kg/day.

VITAMINS AND MINERALS

Vitamins and minerals are referred to as micronutrients. Micronutrients act as regulators of metabolic functions and serve as essential components of structures of the body. Unlike macronutrients (protein, carbohydrate, and fat), vitamins and minerals do not supply energy (i.e., they are noncaloric). However, several vitamins and minerals do help convert calories into useful energy for the body.

Vitamins

Vitamins are organic compounds that function as membrane stabilizers, hormones, H^+/e^- donors/acceptors, or coenzymes. Based on certain properties (e.g., absorption and transport), vitamins are classified as either water-soluble or fat-soluble. The water-soluble vitamins include vitamin C and the B-complex group (thiamine, riboflavin, niacin, panothenic acid, folic acid, biotin, pyridoxine, and cyanocobalamin). Water-soluble vitamins function mainly as coenzymes or cofactors in metabolic reactions. Body storage is relatively small for the water-soluble vitamins; thus, ingestion on a regular basis is required. An inadequate intake can result in clinical symptoms of a deficiency in 3 to 7 days. The fat-soluble vitamins include vitamins A, D, and E. These vitamins generally do not function as coenzymes, like the water-soluble vitamins, but instead they act more like hormones.

Minerals

Minerals are inorganic elements that constitute only about 4% of body weight. Their importance is vital for optimal functioning of the body, however. Minerals are generally divided into two categories based on their occurrence in the body. Minerals that are present in smaller quantities (<0.01% of body weight) are called trace elements, and those at higher levels are referred to as macrominerals. A deficiency of either trace elements or macrominerals will produce equally harmful effects. Thus, both are important for attaining optimal health. The macrominerals include calcium, phosphorus, magnesium, and potassium. These minerals play a vital role in such functions as bone metabolism, muscle contraction, nerve impulse transmission, and cell membrane transfer and regulation. The human body only needs a few thousandths of a gram or less for most trace elements, but they are no less important than the macrominerals that are needed in gram amounts. The trace elements for which an RDA has been set are iron, zinc, selenium, and iodine. For copper, manganese, and molybdenum, the committee on dietary allowances has published tentative ranges for safe and adequate daily intakes. Three interrelated concepts are important for optimal nutrition: synergy, amount, and timing of nutrient intake.

The notion that no single nutrient functions alone, but is dependent on multiple interactions with other nutrients to carry out its biologic function, is the underlying principle of synergy. As an example, folic acid requires niacin (B_3), cyanocobalamin (B_{12}), and vitamin C to be converted to its biologically active form. Vitamin D is essential for the absorption of calcium and phosphorus. The B vitamins must all be present to carry out many of their functions. Iron, calcium, manganese, and zinc all compete for absorption in the intestine, and a high intake of any one of these nutrients will decrease the absorption of the others. Thus, self-prescribed single-nutrient supplementation is risky and has the potential to do more harm than good.

The second concept relates to the amount of nutrient consumed. There exists an optimal range of intake for each nutrient that results in maximum biologic function. Any intake below or above this optimal range will yield marginal biologic function. At extremely low and high intakes, the risks of deficiency and toxicity, respectively, are increased and may result in death if not corrected (Fig. 32–4).

The last concept is timing. Macronutrients and micronutrients must be available at precise moments, and in the proper amounts, for physiologic processes to occur

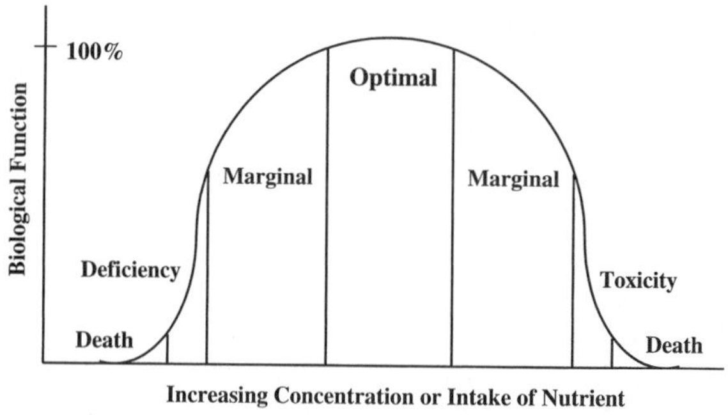

FIG. 32–4. Theoretical continuum describing the relationship between the level of a nutrient and biologic functioning. A narrow range exists that results in maximal biologic functioning of a single nutrient. At low nutrient levels deficiency symptoms are probable, and at high nutrient levels toxicity may result.

at maximum efficiency. This is best exemplified by the enhanced bioavailability of iron in food that occurs when vitamin C is included in the same meal. Vitamin C reduces the ferric form of iron (Fe^{+++}) to the ferrous form (Fe^{++}), creating a stable chelate that is better absorbed in the alkaline environment of the small intestine.

Thus, multiple interactions between nutrients exist and result in maximal biologic function only when the optimal intake of each particular nutrient is present only within a specified range and at a precise time. Even if only one essential nutrient is present in inadequate quantities, other nutrients cannot function properly.

To evaluate the adequacy of vitamin/mineral intake, a common approach is to compare an individual's intake of a micronutrient to the RDA. This must be done with caution because the RDAs are not the optimal amount but represent safe and adequate levels reflecting the state of knowledge concerning a nutrient. It is not possible at this time to establish optimal levels. The RDAs were designed to serve as an aid to design nutrition programs, establish standards for food assistance programs, develop new products, and evaluate the adequacy of food supplies in meeting the general nutritional needs of the population. The RDAs are not designed for special populations but were derived from studies performed on average-size persons with essentially sedentary lifestyles. Therefore, there is some question as to the applicability of using the RDAs to evaluate the nutritional needs of individuals who are significantly larger than the average-size person and/or engage in regular physical exercise.

Athletes are at risk of developing marginal deficiencies for individual micronutrients, which will undoubtedly have an impact on physical performance if left uncorrected for an extended period of time. Several factors may contribute to the development of a micronutrient deficiency. A vitamin or mineral deficiency may originate from inadequate dietary intake or altered dietary composition, loss through urine or sweat, or increased metabolism of a nutrient caused by strenuous exercise.

Athletes' diets may be deficient in several of the micronutrients, especially if calories are being intentionally restricted, for whatever reason. Energy-restrictive diets are common among athletes who participate in sports where a low body weight is necessary to perform well or to compete in a certain weight category (e.g., wrestling, weightlifting, gymnastics, etc.) and in sports where appearance is important (e.g., body building, dancing, etc.). Inadequate micronutrient intakes in various athletes have been reported for folic acid; biotin; pyridoxine (B_6); vitamins A, D, and E; calcium; magnesium; potassium; zinc; selenium; and copper. This is especially true in athletes who obtain a high percentage of their calories from low nutrient–dense foods (e.g., candy, sodas, etc.). Other diet-related factors may also contribute to suboptimal vitamin and mineral status. A diet high in unsaturated fatty acids increases the requirement for vitamin E. A vegetarian diet is likely deficient in iron, zinc, and cyanocobalamin (B_{12}), since the best sources of these micronutrients are foods of animal origin. Furthermore, nutrient losses due to processing, storage, and preparation are significant, especially for some of the minerals and water-soluble vitamins.

CREATINE SUPPLEMENTATION

Creatine is a naturally occurring energy-producing substance in the human body synthesized from amino acids primarily in the liver, pancreas, and kidneys (120). Creatine is also consumed in the diet from the ingestion of animal products. Since our bodies have all the enzymes required for creatine biosynthesis, dietary sources are not an absolute requirement. Thus, creatine is not considered an essential nutrient in the diet. In the human body, creatine exists in both the free and the phosphorylated forms and about 95% of all creatine is contained within skeletal muscle. The normal concentration in muscle is 120 mmol/kg but ranges from about 100 to 140 mmol/kg in the population. Muscle creatine stores break down at a relatively constant rate (approximately 2 g per day) into creatinine. Creatinine is filtered in the kidneys by simple diffusion and excreted in the urine. In a person who consumes a typical Western diet, the 2 g lost daily is made up for by 1 g in the diet and 1 g synthesized. Once in the bloodstream, uptake of creatine into muscle occurs against a concentration gradient via a specific transporter protein on the sarcolemma.

Phosphocreatine has been implicated as a causative factor in the development of muscular fatigue based on data demonstrating correlations between phosphocreatine depletion and reduced force production. In 1992, it was clearly shown that several days of creatine supplementation (i.e., creatine loading) significantly enhance accumulation of both free creatine and phosphocreatine in skeletal muscle (121). Subsequently, numerous studies have examined the acute effects on exercise performance (see ref. 122 for review). Generally, these studies indicate that ingestion of 20 to 25 g creatine per day for 5 to 7 days attenuates the normal decline in force or power production during short-duration, maximal bouts of exercise, especially intermittent protocols. Creatine supplementation has not been shown to improve longer-duration aerobic-type exercise. The mechanism by which elevated muscle creatine enhances exercise performance is an increased ability to match ATP supply to ATP demand. An increase in the rate of phosphocreatine resynthesis during recovery between bouts of exercise, and thus higher phosphocreatine levels at the start of the subsequent exercise bout, is believed to be the primary mechanism explaining the ergogenic effects of

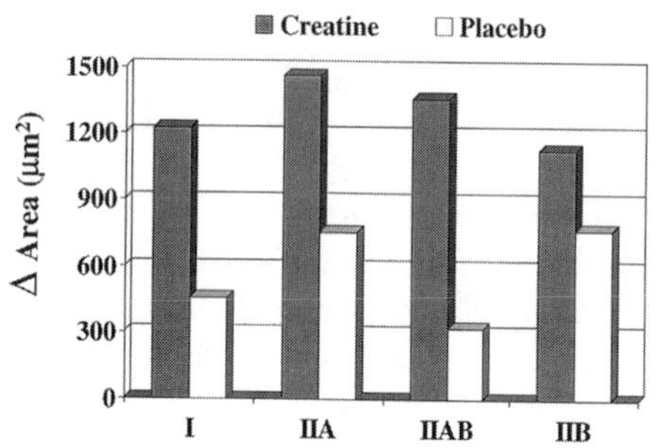

FIG. 32–5. Delta changes in cross-sectional areas of specific skeletal muscle fiber types after 12 weeks of heavy resistance training in men supplemented with creatine or placebo. (Data from ref. 126.)

creatine supplementation during intense intermittent protocols (123). These beneficial effects are related to the extent of creatine loading in muscle. An increase in body mass ranging from 1 to 3 kg is frequently observed after 1 week of creatine supplementation, attributable to an increase in total body water. There are limited data describing the effects of long-term creatine supplementation. Recent data indicate that creatine supplementation may enhance the physiologic adaptations (e.g., muscular strength and fat-free mass) to resistance training in men and women, most likely a result of being able to train more intensely (124–127). Creatine supplementation during resistance training has also been shown to augment skeletal muscle fiber hypertrophy (Fig. 32–5) (126). No adverse side effects associated with creatine supplementation have been documented in the scientific literature. Athletes most likely to gain from creatine supplementation are those who participate in sports or activities that challenge the phosphagen energy system. Nearly all the research examining creatine supplementation has been obtained in the laboratory. Field studies documenting beneficial effects of creatine supplementation during specific sports and competitions are limited.

CONCLUSION

Nutrition is the cornerstone of an athlete's training program. Despite the considerable amount of scientific research examining energy metabolism during various forms of exercise and the nutritional requirements for athletes, there are still many unanswered questions related to the optimal diet to enhance physical performance. Although quite different in practical terms, both carbohydrate-rich and fat-rich diets have been shown to enhance endurance performance. There is less controversy concerning protein requirements for both endurance and strength/power athletes. Whichever dietary approach is adopted, attention should be placed on choosing a wide variety of nutrient-dense foods to ensure an adequate intake of essential vitamins and minerals. Emphasis on polyunsaturated and monounsaturated fat sources, low- to moderate-glycemic index carbohydrate sources, and high-quality protein sources are important to optimize performance and overall health. Once an athlete has attained a sound nutritional program, there may be some advantage to using a daily multivitamin/mineral supplement; and for certain athletes participating in sports/activities that are primarily anaerobic in nature, creatine supplementation may be useful.

REFERENCES

1. Essen-Gustavsson B, Tesch PA. Glycogen and triglyceride utilization in relation to muscle metabolic characteristics in men performing heavy-resistance exercise. *Eur J Appl Physiol* 1990; 61:5–10.
2. Martin WH. Effects of acute and chronic exercise on fat metabolism. *Exerc Sport Sci Rev* 1996;24:203–231.
3. Holloszy JO, Kohrt WM. Regulation of carbohydrate and fat metabolism during and after exercise. *Annu Rev Nutr* 1996;16: 121–138.
4. Romijn JA, Coyle EF, Sidossis LS, et al. Regulation of endogenous fat and carbohydrate metabolism in relation to exercise intensity and duration. *Am J Physiol* 1993;265:E380–E391.
5. Jones NL, Heigenhauser GJF, Kuksis A, Matsos CG, Sutton JR, Toews CJ. Fat metabolism in heavy exercise. *Clin Sci* 1980; 59:469–478.
6. Esseén B. Studies on the regulation of metabolism in human skeletal muscle using intermittent exercise as an experimental model. *Acta Physiol Scand Suppl* 1978;454:1–32.
7. McCartney N, Spriet LL, Heigenhauser GJF, Kowalchuk JM, Sutton JR, Jones NL. Muscle power and metabolism in maximal intermittent exercise. *J Appl Physiol* 1986;60:1164–1169.
8. Martin WH, Dalsky GP, Hurley BF, et al. Effect of endurance training on plasma free fatty acid turnover and oxidation during exercise. *Am J Physiol* 1993;265:E708–E714.
9. Phinney SD, Bistrian BR, Evans WJ, Gervino E, Blackburn GL. The human metabolic response to chronic ketosis without caloric restriction: preservation of submaximal exercise capability with reduced carbohydrate oxidation. *Metabolism* 1983;32:769–775.
10. Pascoe DD, Costill DL, Fink WJ, Robergs RA, Zachwieja JJ. Glycogen resynthesis in skeletal muscle following resistive exercise. *Med Sci Sports Exerc* 1993;25:349–354.
11. Robergs RA, Pearson DR, Costill DL, et al. Muscle glycogenolysis during different intensities of weight-resistance exercise. *J Appl Physiol* 1991;70:1700–1706.
12. Roy BD, Tarnopolsky MA. Influence of differing macronutrient intakes on muscle glycogen resynthesis after resistance exercise. *J Appl Physiol* 1998;72:1854–1859.
13. Tesch PA, Colliander B, Kaiser P. Muscle metabolism during intense, heavy resistance exercise. *Eur J Appl Physiol* 1986; 55:363–366.
14. Kiens B, Essen-Gustavsson B, Gad P, Lithell H. Lipoprotein lipase and intramuscular triglyceride stores after long-term high-fat and high-carbohydrate diets in physically trained men. *Clin Physiol* 1987;7:1–9.
15. Lambert EV, Speechly DP, Dennis SC, Noakes TD. Enhanced endurance in trained cyclists during moderate intensity exercise following 2 weeks adaptation to a high fat diet. *Eur J Appl Physiol* 1994;69:287–293.
16. Jenkins DJA, Wolever TMS, Taylor RH, et al. Glycemic index of foods: a physiological basis for carbohydrate exchange. *Am J Clin Nutr* 1981;34:362–366.
17. Wolever TMS, Jenkins DJA, Jenkins AL, Josse RG. The glycemic index: methodology and clinical implications. *Am J Clin Nutr* 1991;54:846–854.
18. Caggiula AW, Mustad VA. Effects of dietary fat and fatty acids on coronary artery disease risk and total and lipoprotein choles-

terol concentrations: epidemiologic studies. *Am J Clin Nutr* 1997;65(suppl):1597S–1610S.

19. Kris-Etherton PM, Yu S. Individual fatty acid effects on plasma lipids and lipoproteins: human studies. *Am J Clin Nutr* 1997; 65(suppl):1628S–1644S.
20. Demacker PNM, Reijnen IGM, Katan MB, Stuyt PMJ, Stalenhoef AFH. Increased removal of remnants of triglyceride-rich lipoproteins on a diet rich in polyunsaturated fatty acids. *Eur J Clin Invest* 1991;21:197–203.
21. Zampelas A, Murphy M, Morgan LM, Williams CM. Postprandial lipoprotein lipase, insulin and gastric inhibitory polypeptide responses to test meals of different fatty acid composition: comparison of saturated, n-6 and n-3 polyunsaturated fatty acids. *Eur J Clin Nutr* 1994;48:849–858.
22. Morgan SA, Sinclair AJ, O'Dea K. Effect on serum lipids of addition of safflower oil or olive oil to very-low-fat diets rich in lean beef. *J Am Diet Assoc* 1993;93:644–648.
23. Watts GF, Ahmed W, Quiney J, et al. Effective lipid lowering diets including lean meat. *Br Med J* 1988;296:235–238.
24. Kris-Etherton PM, Derr JA, Mustad VA, et al. Effects of a milk chocolate bar per day substituted for a high-carbohydrate snack in young men on an NCEP/AHA step 1 diet. *Am J Clin Nutr* 1994;60:1037S–1042S.
25. Yu SM, Derr J, Etherton TD, Kris-Etherton PM. Plasma cholesterol-predictive equations demonstrate that stearic acid is neutral and monounsaturated fatty acids are hypocholesteremic. *Am J Clin Nutr* 1995;61:1129–1139.
26. Grundy SM, Denke MA. Dietary influences on serum lipids and lipoproteins. *J Lipid Res* 1990;31:1149–1172.
27. Mata P, Garrido J, Ordovas J, et al. Effect of dietary monounsaturated fatty acids on plasma lipoproteins and apolipoproteins in women. *Am J Clin Nutr* 1992;56:77–83.
28. Iacono JM, Dougherty RM. Lack of effect of linoleic acid on the high-density-lipoprotein fraction of plasma lipoproteins. *Am J Clin Nutr* 1991;53:660–664.
29. Katan MJ, Zock PL, Mensink RP. Dietary oils, serum lipoproteins, and coronary heart disease. *Am J Clin Nutr* 1995; 61(suppl):1368S–1373S.
30. Reaven PD, Grasse BJ, Tribble DL. Effects of linoleate-enriched and oleate-enriched diets in combination with α-tocopherol on the susceptibility of LDL and LDL subfractions to oxidative modification in humans. *Arterio Throm* 1994;14:557–566.
31. Dagnelie P, Rietveld T, Swart GR, Stijnen T, van den Berg JWO. Effect of dietary fish oil on blood levels of free fatty acids, ketone bodies and triacylglycerol in humans. *Lipids* 1994;29:41–45.
32. Harris WS. n-e fatty acids and serum lipoproteins: human studies. *Am J Clin Nutr* 1997;65(suppl):1645S–1654S.
33. Kromann N, White A. Epidemiological studies in the Upernavik district, Greenland. Incidence of some chronic diseases 1950–1974. *Acta Med Scand* 1980;208:401–406.
34. Salter AM, White DA. Effects of dietary fat on cholesterol metabolism: regulation of plasma LDL concentrations. *Nutr Res Rev* 1996;9:241–257.
35. Harris WS, Conner WE, Illingworth DR, Rothrock DW, Foster DM. Effect of fish oil on VLDL triglyceride kinetics in man. *J Lipid Res* 1990;31:1549–1558.
36. Levy E, Roy CC, Goldstein R, Bar-On H, Ziv E. Metabolic fate of chylomicrons obtained from rats maintained on diets varying in fatty acid composition. *J Am Coll Nutr* 1991;10:69–78.
37. Zampelas A, Peel AS, Gould BJ, Wright J, Williams CM. Polyunsaturated fatty acids of the n-6 and n-3 series: effects on postprandial lipid and apolipoprotein levels in healthy men. *Eur J Clin Nutr* 1994;48:842–848.
38. Marsh JB, Topping DL, Nestel PJ. Comparative effects of fish oil and carbohydrate on plasma lipids and hepatic activities of phosphatidate phosphohydrolase, diacylglycerol acyltransferase and neutral lipase activities in the rat. *Biochim Biophys Acta* 1987;922:239–243.
39. Rustan AC, Nossen JO, Christiansen EN, Drevon CA. Eicosapentaenoic acid reduces hepatic synthesis and secretion of triacylglycerol by decreasing the activity of acyl-coenzyme A:1,2-diacylglycerol acyltransferase. *J Lipid Res* 1988;29:1417–1426.
40. Howard BV, Hannah JS, Heiser CC, et al. Polyunsaturated fatty acids result in greater cholesterol lowering and less triacylglycerol elevation than do monounsaturated fatty acids in a dose-response comparison in a multiracial study group. *Am J Clin Nutr* 1995;62:392–402.
41. Colquhoun D, Moores D, Somerset S, Humphries J. Comparison of the effects on lipoproteins and apolipoproteins of a diet high in monounsaturated fatty acids, enriched with avocado, and a high-carbohydrate diet. *Am J Clin Nutr* 1992;56:671–677.
42. Grundy SM. Comparison of monounsaturated fatty acids and carbohydrates for lowering plasma cholesterol. *N Engl J Med* 1986;314:745–748.
43. Grundy SM, Florentin L, Nix D, Whelan MF. Comparison of monounsaturated fatty acids and carbohydrates for reducing raised levels of plasma cholesterol in man. *Am J Clin Nutr* 1988;47:965–969.
44. Mensink R, de Groot M, van den Broeke L, Severignen-Nobels A, Demacker P, Katan M. Effects of monounsaturated fatty acid vs complex carbohydrate on serum lipoproteins and apolipoproteins in healthy men and women. *Metabolism* 1989;38:172–178.
45. Mensink RP, Katan MB. Effect of monounsaturated fatty acids versus complex carbohydrates on high-density lipoproteins in healthy men and women. *Lancet* 1987;1:122–125.
46. Reaven PD, Partasararathy S, Grasse BJ, Miller E, Steinberg D, Witztum JL. Effects of oleate-rich and linoleate-rich diets on the susceptibility of low density lipoprotein to oxidative modification in mildly hypercholesterolemic subjects. *J Clin Invest* 1993;91:668–676.
47. Coyle EF. Timing and method of increased carbohydrate intake to cope with heavy training, competition and recovery. *J Sports Sci* 1991;9:29–52.
48. Coyle EF. Substrate utilization during exercise in active people. *Am J Clin Nutr* 1995;61(suppl):968S–979S.
49. Hargreaves M. Carbohydrates and exercise performance. *Nutr Rev* 1996;54:S136–S139.
50. Sherman WM. Metabolism of sugars and physical performance. *Am J Clin Nutr* 1995;62(suppl):228S–241S.
51. Jeukendrup AE, Saris WHM, Wagenmakers AJM. Fat metabolism during exercise: a review. Part I: fatty acid mobilization and muscle metabolism. *Int J Sports Med* 1998;19:231–244.
52. Jeukendrup AE, Saris WHM, Wagenmakers AJM. Fat metabolism during exercise: a review. Part II: regulation of metabolism and the effects of training. *Int J Sports Med* 1998;19:293–302.
53. Jeukendrup AE, Saris WHM, Wagenmakers AJM. Fat metabolism during exercise: a review. Part III: effects of nutritional interventions. *Int J Sports Med* 1998;19:371–379.
54. Lambert EV, Hawley JA, Goedecke J, Noakes TD, Dennis SC. Nutritional strategies for promoting fat utilization and delaying the onset of fatigue during prolonged exercise. *J Sports Sci* 1997;15:315–324.
55. Ranallo RF, Rhodes EC. Lipid metabolism during exercise. *Sports Med* 1998;26:29–42.
56. Saltin B, Astrand PO. Free fatty acids and exercise. *Am J Clin Nutr* 1993;57(suppl):752S–758S.
57. Christensen EH, Hansen O. Arbeitsfähigkeit und ernärung. *Skand Arch Physiol* 1939;81:160–171.
58. Bergström J. Muscle electrolytes in man: determined by neutron activation analysis of needle biopsy specimens. A study in normal subjects, kidney patients and patients with chronic diarrhea. *Scand J Clin Lab Invest* 1962;14(suppl):11–13.
59. Gleeson M, Maughan RJ, Greenhaff PL. Comparison of the effects of pre-exercise feedings of glucose, glycerol and placebo on endurance and fuel homeostasis in man. *Eur J Appl Physiol* 1986;55:645–653.
60. Okano G, Takeda H, Morita I, Katoh M, Mu Z, Miyake S. Effect of pre-exercise fructose ingestion on endurance performance in fed men. *Med Sci Sports Exerc* 1988;20:105–109.
61. Devlin JT, Calles-Escandon J, Horton ES. Effects of preexercise snack feeding on endurance cycle exercise. *J Appl Physiol* 1986;60:980–985.
62. Hargreaves M, Costill DL, Fink WJ, King DS, Fielding RA. Effect of pre-exercise carbohydrate feedings on endurance cycling performance. *Med Sci Sports Exerc* 1987;19:3–36.
63. Keller K, Schwarzkopf R. Preexercise snacks may decrease exercise performance. *Physician Sports Med* 1984;12:89–91.
64. McMurray RG, Wilson JR, Kitchell BS. The effects of fructose

and glucose on high intensity endurance performance. *Res Q* 1983;54:156–162.
65. Thomas DE, Brotherhood JR, Brand JC. Carbohydrate feeding before exercise: effect of glycemic index. *Int J Sports Med* 1991;12:180–186.
66. Thomas DE, Brotherhood JR, Miller JB. Plasma glucose levels after prolonged strenuous exercise correlate inversely with glycemic response to food consumed before exercise. *Int J Sport Nutr* 1994;4:361–373.
67. Coyle EF, Coggan AR, Hemmert MK, Ivy JL. Muscle glycogen utilization during prolonged strenuous exercise when fed carbohydrate. *J Appl Physiol* 1986;61:165–172.
68. Coggan AR, Coyle EF. Carbohydrate ingestion during prolonged exercise: effects on metabolism and performance. *Exerc Sport Sci Rev* 1987;19:1–40.
69. Coggan AR, Coyle EF. Reversal of fatigue during prolonged exercise by carbohydrate infusion or ingestion. *J Appl Physiol* 1991;63:2388–2395.
70. Below PR, Mora-Rodriguez R, Gonzalez-Alonzo J, Coyle EF. Fluid and carbohydrate ingestion independently improve performance during 1 h of intense exercise. *Med Sci Sports Exerc* 1995;27:200–210.
71. Sherman WM, Doyle JA, Lamb DR, Strauss RH. Dietary carbohydrate, muscle glycogen, and exercise performance during 7 d of training. *Am J Clin Nutr* 1993;57:27–31.
72. Simonsen JC, Sherman WM, Lamb DR, Dernbach AR, Doyle JA, Strauss R. Dietary carbohydrate, muscle glycogen, and power output during rowing training. *J Appl Physiol* 1990;70:1500–1505.
73. Costill DL, Flynn MJ, Kirwin JP, et al. Effects of repeated days of intensified training on muscle glycogen and swimming performance. *Med Sci Sports Exerc* 1988;20:249–254.
74. Gollnick PD, Karlsson J, Piehl K, Saltin B. Selective glycogen depletion in skeletal muscle fibers in man following sustained contractions. *J Physiol* 1974;241:59–67.
75. Casey A, Short AH, Curtis S, Greenhaff PL. The effect of glycogen availability on power output and the metabolic response of repeated bouts of maximal, isokinetic exercise in man. *Eur J Appl Physiol* 1996;72:249–255.
76. Jenkins DG, Palmer J, Spillman D. The influence of dietary carbohydrate on performance of supramaximal intermittent exercise. *Eur J Appl Physiol* 1993;67:309–314.
77. Maughan RJ, Poole DC. The effects of a glycogen-loading regimen on the capacity to perform anaerobic exercise. *Eur J Appl Physiol* 1981;46:211–219.
78. Jenkins DG, Hutchins CA, Spillman D. The influence of dietary carbohydrate and pre-exercise glucose consumption on supramaximal intermittent exercise performance. *Br J Sports Med* 1994;28:171–176.
79. Symons DJ, Jacobs I. High-intensity exercise performance is not impaired by low intramuscular glycogen. *Med Sci Sports Exerc* 1989;21:550–557.
80. Wootton SA, Williams C. Influence of carbohydrate-status on performance during maximal exercise. *Int J Sports Med* 1984; 5(suppl):126–127.
81. Bangsbo J, Graham TE, Kiens B, Saltin B. Elevated muscle glycogen and aerobic energy production during exhaustive exercise in man. *J Physiol* 1992;451:205–227.
82. Greenhaff PL, Gleeson M, Whiting PH, Maughan RJ. Dietary composition and acid-base status: limiting factors in the performance of maximal exercise in man. *Eur J Appl Physiol* 1987; 56:444–450.
83. Greenhaff PL, Gleeson M, Maughan RJ. The effects of dietary manipulation on blood acid-base status and the performance of high intensity exercise. *Eur J Appl Physiol* 1987;56:331–337.
84. Vandenberghe K, Hespel P, Vanden Eynde B, Lysens R, Richter EA. No effect of glycogen level on glycogen metabolism during high intensity exercise. *Med Sci Sports Exerc* 1995;27:1278–1283.
85. Pizza FX, Flynn MG, Duscha BD, Holden J, Kubitz ER. A carbohydrate loading regimen improves high intensity, short duration exercise performance. *Int J Sports Nutr* 1995;5:110–116.
86. Ren JM, Broberg S, Sahlin K, Hultman E. Influence of reduced glycogen level on glycogenolysis during short-term stimulation in man. *Acta Physiol Scand* 1990;139:467–474.
87. Spencer MK, Katz A. Role of glycogen in control of glycolysis and IMP formation in human muscle during exercise. *Am J Physiol* 1991;260:E859–E864.
88. Essen B, Hagenfeldt L, Kaijser L. Utilisation of blood-borne and intramuscular substrates during continuous and intermittent exercise in man. *J Physiol* 1977;265:489–506.
89. Cheng B, Karamizrak O, Noakes TD, Dennis SC, Lambert EV. Time course of the effects of a high-fat diet and voluntary exercise on muscle enzyme activity in Long-Evans rats. *Physiol Behav* 1997;61:701–705.
90. Conlee RK, Hammer RL, Winder WW, Bracken ML, Nelson AG, Barnett DW. Glycogen repletion and exercise endurance in rats adapted to a high fat diet. *Metabolism* 1990;39:289–294.
91. Kronfeld DS, Ferrante PL, Grandjean D. Optimal performance for athletic performance, with emphasis on fat adaptation in dogs and horses. *J Nutr* 1994;124(suppl):2745S–2753S.
92. Lapachet RAB, Miller WC, Arnall DA. Body fat and exercise endurance in trained rats adapted to a high-fat and/or high-carbohydrate diet. *J Appl Physiol* 1996;80:1173–1179.
93. Miller WC, Bryce GR, Conlee RK. Adaptations to a high-fat diet that increase exercise endurance in male rats. *J Appl Physiol* 1984;56:78–83.
94. Nakamura M, Brown J, Miller WC. Glycogen depletion patterns in trained rats adapted to a high-fat or high-carbohydrate diet. *Int J Sports Med* 1998;19:419–424.
95. Phinney SD, Bistrian BR, Wolfe RR, Blackburn GL. The human metabolic response to chronic ketosis without caloric restriction: physical and biochemical adaptations. *Metabolism* 1983; 32:757–768.
96. Phinney SD, Horton ES, Sims EAH, Hanson JS. Capacity for moderate exercise in obese subjects after adaptation to a hypocaloric, ketogenic diet. *J Clin Invest* 1980;66:1152–1161.
97. Simi B, Sempore B, Mayet MH, Favier RJ. Additive effects of training and high-fat diet on energy metabolism during exercise. *J Appl Physiol* 1991;71:197–203.
98. Saitoh S, Matsuo T, Tagami K, Chang H, Tokuyama K, Suzuki M. Effects of short-term dietary change from high fat to high carbohydrate diets on the storage and utilization of glycogen and triacylglycerol in untrained rats. *Eur J Appl Physiol* 1996; 74:13–22.
99. Askew EW, Dohm GL, Huston RL. Fatty acid and ketone body metabolism in the rat: response to diet and exercise. *J Nutr* 1975;105:1422–1432.
100. Fisher EC, Evans WJ, Phinney SD, Blackburn GL, Bistrian BR, Young VR. Changes in skeletal muscle metabolism induced by a eucaloric ketogenic diet. In: Knuttgen HG, Vogel JA, Poortmans J, eds. *Biochemistry of exercise*, vol 13. Champaign, IL: Human Kinetics, 1983:497–501.
101. Helge JW, Kiens B. Muscle enzyme activity in man: role of substrate availability and training. *Am J Physiol* 1997;272: R1620–R1624.
102. Jacobs I, Lithell H, Karlsson J. Dietary effects on glycogen and lipoprotein lipase activity in skeletal muscle in man. *Acta Physiol Scand* 1982;115:85–90.
103. Satabin P, Bois-Joyeux B, Chanez M, Guzzennec CY, Peret J. Effects of long-term feeding high-protein or high-fat diets on the response to exercise in the rat. *Eur J Appl Physiol* 1989; 58:583–590.
104. Putnam CT, Spriet LL, Hultman E, et al. Pyruvate dehydrogenase activity and acetyl group accumulation during exercise after different diets. *Am J Physiol* 1993;265:E752–E760.
105. Cutler DL, Gray CG, Park SW, Hickman MG, Bell JM, Kolterman OG. Low-carbohydrate diet alters intracellular glucose metabolism but not overall glucose disposal in exercise-trained subjects. *Metabolism* 1995;44:1264–1270.
106. Shimomura Y, Suzuki T, Saitoh S, Tasaki Y, Harris RA, Suzuki M. Activation of branched-chain α-keto acid dehydrogenase complex by exercise: effect of high-fat diet intake. *J Appl Physiol* 1990;68:161–165.
107. Hammel EP, Kronfeld DS, Ganjam VK, Dunlap HL. Metabolic responses to exhaustive exercise in racing sled dogs fed diets containing medium, low, or zero carbohydrate. *Am J Clin Nutr* 1977;30:409–418.
108. Kronfeld DS, Hammel EP, Ramberg CF, Dunlap HL. Hematological and metabolic responses to training in racing sled dogs

fed diets containing medium, low, or zero carbohydrate. *Am J Clin Nutr* 1977;30:419–430.

109. Harkins JD, Morris GS, Tulley RT, Nelson AG, Kamerling SG. Effect of added fat on racing performance in thoroughbred horses. *J Equine Vet Sci* 1992;12:123–129.
110. Oldham S, Potter GD, Evans WJ, Smith SB, Taylor TS, Barnes WS. Storage and mobilization of muscle glycogen in exercising horses fed a fat supplemented diet. *J Equine Vet Sci* 1990; 10:353–359.
111. Webb SP, Potter GD, Evans WJ. Physiologic and metabolic responses of racing and cutting horses to added dietary fat. *Proc Equine Nutr Physiol Soc* 1987;10:115–120.
112. Leddy J, Horvath P, Rowland J, Pendergast D. Effect of a high or a low fat diet on cardiovascular risk factors in male and female runners. *Med Sci Sports Exerc* 1997;29:17–25.
113. Muoio DM, Leddy JJ, Horvath PJ, Awad AB, Pendergast DR. Effect of dietary fat on metabolic adjustments to $\dot{V}O_2$ and endurance in runners. *Med Sci Sports Exerc* 1994;26:81–88.
114. Pendergast DR, Horvath PJ, Leddy JJ, Venkatraman JT. The role of dietary fat on performance, metabolism, and health. *Am J Sports Med* 1996;24(suppl):S53–S58.
115. Venkatraman JT, Rowland JA, Denardin E, Horvath PJ, Pendergast D. Influence of the level of dietary lipid intake and maximal exercise on the immune status in runners. *Med Sci Sports Exerc* 1997;29:333–334.
116. Helge JW, Richter EA, Kiens B. Interaction of training and diet on metabolism and endurance during exercise in man. *J Physiol* 1996;492:293–306.
117. Saitoh S, Tasaki Y, Tagami K, Suzuki M. Muscle glycogen repletion and pre-exercise glycogen content: effect of carbohydrate loading in rats previously fed a high fat diet. *Eur J Appl Physiol* 1994;68:483–488.
118. Lemon PWR. Is increased dietary protein necessary or beneficial for individuals with a physically active lifestyle? *Nutr Rev* 1996;54(suppl):S169–S175.
119. Tarnopolsky MA, Atkinson SA, MacDougall JD, Chesley A, Philips S, Schwartz HP. Evaluation of protein requirements for trained strength athletes. *J Appl Physiol* 1992;73:1986–1995.
120. Walker JB. Creatine: biosynthesis, regulation, and function. *Adv Enzymol* 1979;50:177–242.
121. Harris RC, Söderlund K, Hultman E. Elevation of creatine in resting and exercised muscle of normal subjects by creatine supplementation. *Clin Sci* 1992;83:367–374.
122. Volek JS, Kraemer WJ. Creatine supplementation: Its effect on human muscular performance and body composition. *J Strength Cond Res* 1996;10:198–208.
123. Greenhaff PL, Bodin K, Söderlund K, Hultman E. Effect of oral creatine supplementation on skeletal muscle phosphocreatine resynthesis. *Am J Physiol* 1994;266:E725–E730.
124. Kreider RB, Ferreira M, Wilson M, et al. Effects of creatine supplementation on body composition, strength, and sprint performance. *Med Sci Sports Exerc* 1998;30:73–82.
125. Vandenberghe K, Goris M, Van Hecke P, Van Leemputte M, Vangerven L, Hespel P. Long-term creatine is beneficial to muscle performance during resistance training. *J Appl Physiol* 1997; 83:2055–2063.
126. Volek JS, Duncan ND, Mazzetti SA, et al. Performance and muscle fiber adaptations to creatine supplementation and heavy resistance training. *Med Sci Sports Exerc* 1999;31:1147–1156.
127. Volek JS, Kraemer WJ, Bush JA, et al. Creatine supplementation enhances muscular performance during high-intensity resistance exercise. *J Am Diet Assoc* 1997;97:765–770.
128. Foster-Powell K, Miller JB. International tables of glycemic index. *Am J Clin Nutr* 1995;62:871S–893S.

Exercise and Sport Science,
edited by William E. Garrett, Jr., and Donald T. Kirkendall.
Lippincott Williams & Wilkins, Philadelphia © 2000.

CHAPTER 33

Overtraining and Overreaching: Causes, Effects, and Prevention

Laurel T. Mackinnon and Sue L. Hooper

Overtraining is a process of excessive training in high-performance athletes that may lead to persistent fatigue, performance decrements, neuroendocrine changes, alterations in mood states, and frequent illness, especially upper respiratory tract infection (URTI) (1–5). Overtraining syndrome is a neuroendocrine disorder that may result from the process of overtraining and reflects accumulated fatigue during periods of excessive training with inadequate recovery.

At an international conference on overtraining in Memphis, Tennessee, in 1996, a definition of overtraining was proposed:

> an accumulation of training and/or nontraining stress resulting in long-term decrement in performance capacity with or without related physiological and psychological signs and symptoms of overtraining in which restoration of performance capacity may take several weeks and/or months (3).

The term *overreaching* also was adopted to describe qualitatively similar symptoms (fatigue, performance decrements, mood-state changes), but of a more transitory nature. Thus, overreaching is resolved with short periods of rest or recovery training, whereas overtraining may require weeks to months (3–5). Other terms previously used to describe overtraining syndrome include *burnout* and *staleness*.

Overtraining is an important issue for elite and professional sports. Prolonged periods of inconsistent performance and/or recuperation needed for recovery may lead to loss of income or government funding and even premature retirement in the elite athlete.

L.T. Mackinnon: Department of Human Movement Studies, The University of Queensland, Brisbane, Queensland, Australia.

S.L. Hooper: Centre for Physical Activity and Sport Education, The University of Queensland, Brisbane, Queensland, Australia.

SIGNS AND SYMPTOMS OF OVERTRAINING

Myriad signs and symptoms are associated with overtraining syndrome (2,4,6), although few of these have been clearly documented as reliable and valid indicators of the syndrome (discussed in more detail below). Among purported indicators of overtraining syndrome are physiological variables including

- performance decrements despite continued training
- decreased economy of effort during exercise or decreased work rate at lactate threshold
- persistent fatigue
- cardiovascular changes such as increased early morning heart rate (EMHR) or resting blood pressure
- hematologic changes such as decreased serum ferritin concentration
- hormonal changes such as decreased catecholamine production or alterations in the ratio of serum free testosterone to cortisol
- frequent illness such as URTI
- persistent muscle soreness
- loss of body mass

Psychological and behavioral variables often associated with overtraining syndrome include

- mood-state changes as shown by the Profile of Mood States (POMS)
- apathy, lack of motivation
- loss of appetite
- sleep disturbances
- high self-reported stress levels
- irritability or depression

At present, the only parameters consistently associated with overtraining/overreaching are

- performance decrements (7–11)
- persistent high fatigue ratings (8–14)

- decreased maximal heart rate (15–17)
- changes in the blood lactate threshold, lactate concentration at a given work rate, or maximal blood lactate level (4,15–18)
- neuroendocrine changes such as elevated resting plasma norepinephrine levels (8,9,15,16) and decreased norepinephrine excretion (11,14–16)
- high self-reported stress levels and sleep disturbances (8–10,12,17,18)

Each of these variables is discussed in detail below.

MODELS TO STUDY OVERTRAINING

There are two general models for studying overtraining. In one model, athletes are followed over the course of a normal training season, usually 3 to 8 months' duration. Performance and other physiological or psychological variables are sampled at several times corresponding with periods of low- and high-intensity training. These variables may then be compared across the season within the same athletes, or between athletes showing symptoms of overtraining with those considered well trained (i.e., not overtrained). This model provides information about the responses during prolonged periods of intense training in the athlete's natural environment, that is, during normal training and competition. Not all studies include appropriate controls to account for seasonal variability, however. Moreover, it is not always possible to control for other potentially confounding factors such as psychological stress, competition, travel, diet, and changes in training programs. In addition, illness or injury may require an athlete to reduce or stop training before overtraining syndrome can be identified.

In the second model, training is intensified over a specific period, usually 1 to 4 weeks' duration; for ethical reasons, 4 weeks has been considered the maximal time that elite athletes can tolerate significant increases in already high training loads (10,14,19–21). Because of the relatively short time (i.e., less than 4 weeks), athletes cannot be considered overtrained by using this model, and, in the more recent literature, they are classified as overreached. Performance and other variables are then compared from before to after intensified training, or less commonly, between overreached and well-trained athletes. Although it may be possible to control the volume and intensity of training in this model, there is individual variation in the response to increased training (i.e., some athletes quite easily tolerate increased training loads, whereas others may exhibit poor adaptation). Moreover, the increases in training volume/intensity often used (e.g., doubling of volume within a few weeks) do not reflect normal training regimens, which involve more gradual increases in volume/intensity, as performed by elite athletes. Despite these limitations, by combining data from both models it has been possible to gain an understanding of the physiological and psychological responses to overtraining in athletes.

PREVALENCE OF OVERTRAINING AND OVERREACHING

It is difficult to estimate the prevalence of overtraining and overreaching in elite athletes. To do so requires extensive surveying of large groups of athletes over considerable periods. Moreover, only recently have clear definitions of overtraining and overreaching been accepted (3,4); earlier reports used a variety of operational definitions. In addition, the term *overtraining* evokes quite strong reactions from elite coaches, who may be reluctant to classify their athletes as overtrained.

At any given time, about 7% to 20% of elite athletes may show symptoms of overtraining (8,22–24). For example, Hooper and colleagues (8,9) followed a group of 14 elite swimmers over a 6-month season and reported that 3 (or 21%) exhibited clear signs and symptoms of overtraining syndrome, such as performance decrements, high fatigue ratings, sleep disturbances, and persistent muscle soreness. The prevalence varies by sport, and overtraining is thought to occur most frequently in endurance sports involving high-volume intense training such as swimming, road cycling, distance running, and rowing. Overtraining syndrome has been reported in athletes from diverse sports including distance running (14,20,25–28), swimming (8,9,22), cycling (29), rowing (30), speed skating (31), boxing (32), basketball (24), and wrestling (22).

Because more studies used the short-term (1 to 4 weeks) model, the prevalence of overreaching can be more clearly discerned from the research literature. Costill and co-workers (7) intensified training over 10 days in eight collegiate swimmers and reported that four were unable to maintain training loads and exhibited symptoms of overreaching. In a group of military special services officers who performed very intense running interval training for 10 days, all athletes showed symptoms of overreaching, such as mood-state changes, excessive fatigue, and muscle soreness (12,13). Lehmann and associates (14–16,20) doubled training volume over 4 weeks in elite middle-distance runners and reported that all athletes showed symptoms as indicated on a "complaints index." In a study of elite swimmers who progressively increased training volume for 4 weeks, 33% exhibited signs and symptoms of overreaching such as poor performance, sleep disturbances, persistent fatigue, and lower norepinephrine excretion (10,11). These latter studies showed that, given a sufficiently rigorous training regimen, most if not all well-performing athletes will experience symptoms of overreaching over the short term (up to 4 weeks). It is difficult, however, to gauge the prevalence of overtraining from short-term studies because, as discussed above, these studies induced artificially high training loads.

PHYSIOLOGICAL CHANGES DURING OVERTRAINING AND OVERREACHING

Overtraining and overreaching are, by definition, associated with performance decrements, which may in turn reflect changes in any number of physiological or psychological variables. As mentioned above, the accepted physiological indicators of overtraining, besides performance decrements and persistent fatigue, include changes in maximal heart rate and lactate variables. Other purported physiological indicators have generally not been supported by empirical research, including changes in EMHR or resting heart rate (RHR), body mass or body fat levels, aerobic power ($\dot{V}O_2max$), and blood pressure.

Performance Changes

Performance decrements constitute the most obvious objective indicator of overtraining/overreaching and have been documented in a variety of sports. Decrements in competitive and training performance of 10%, as well as an inability to maintain training loads, are not unusual (9,10,25). In a study of the largest performance decrements documented to date, training pace decreased 11% to 15%, competition pace 6% to 17%, and training distance 43% to 71% in overtrained distance runners (25). Performance decrements in laboratory testing and competition appear to be of similar magnitude. For example, in a study of internationally ranked swimmers, overtrained swimmers exhibited performance declines of 0.7% and 2.4% in experimental testing (time trial) and competition, respectively, whereas corresponding performances improved 3.1% and 1.1% in well-trained swimmers (9). Although deterioration in performance is an essential criterion for the diagnosis of overtraining, it is not sufficient as a single marker of the syndrome, because performance also may be adversely affected by short-term fatigue.

Heart-Rate Changes

Although EMHRs or RHRs are often monitored by athletes and coaches, the majority of empirical evidence suggests that these variables do not change during overreaching or overtraining in endurance athletes (8,9,15–19,33). For example, Hooper and colleagues (8) found no significant changes in EMHR in elite swimmers followed over a 6-month period, nor were there significant differences at any time between overtrained and well-trained swimmers. Unchanged RHRs were reported in runners and swimmers during 3 weeks of intensified training (19) and in competitive cyclists who performed 7 days of normal training followed by 15 days of intensified training and 7 days of recovery training (18).

In contrast, there is good evidence that maximal heart rate (measured at maximal work rate in a progressive exercise test) decreases by 5 to 10 beats per minute during overreaching/overtraining in endurance athletes (7,15–18,20). For example, heart rate during a maximal 366-m swim declined significantly after 10 days of intensified training in competitive swimmers (7). In distance runners, 4 weeks of increased training volume resulted in a significant decrease in maximal heart rate during an incremental exercise test (15). In cyclists, heart rate was significantly lower at all work rates during an incremental exercise test to maximum during 15 days of intensified training compared with values obtained during normal training (17).

Decreased maximal heart rate is consistent with suggestions that overtraining syndrome is a neuroendocrine disorder related primarily to catecholamine depletion and/or reduction in sympathetic drive (discussed further below) (14,20,24,27).

Changes in Lactate Variables

Although resting blood lactate concentration may not change appreciably (8,17,18,34), decreases in blood lactate concentration at maximal work rate have been consistently noted in overreached/overtrained athletes (15–18,34,35). Snyder and colleagues (17,18) studied male cyclists during 14 to 15 days of intensified training followed by 6 to 14 days of recovery training; all subjects exhibited symptoms of overreaching by the end of the intensified training period. In a graded cycle ergometer test, blood lactate concentrations were significantly lower at all work rates including the maximum. During the overtraining period, the ratio of blood lactate level to rating of perceived exertion (RPE; HLa/RPE) declined more than 25% in all cyclists, reflecting the lower blood lactate concentration despite unchanged RPE scores at each work rate (Fig. 33–1). The HLa/RPE ratio returned to normal levels after 6 to 14 days of recovery training, indicating that changes in the ratio are temporary and are sensitive to changes in training loads. In a 1996 study on swimmers (36), slower recovery of blood lactate levels after brief maximal interval exercise was correlated with performance decrements and symptoms of overtraining.

There are several possible mechanisms to explain decreased maximal blood lactate concentration during overreaching/overtraining. First, lower submaximal and maximal lactate levels may reflect enhanced lactate clearance. This seems unlikely, however, because of the magnitude of changes (e.g., 50% reduction in maximal lactate level) during overtraining/overreaching. Moreover, enhanced lactate removal should be associated with improvements rather than decrements in perfor-

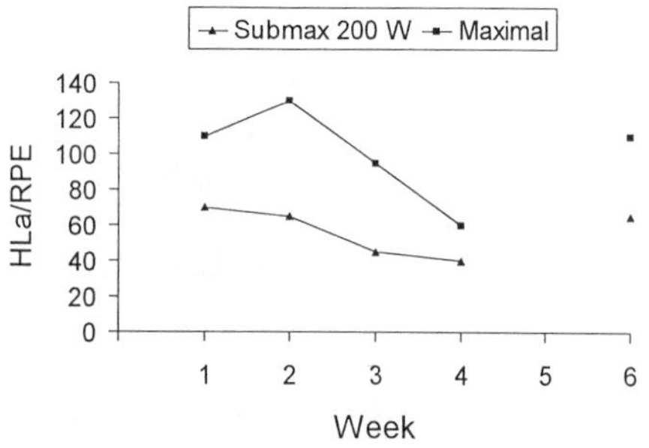

FIG. 33–1. Ratio of blood lactate concentration to rating of perceived exertion (HLa/RPE) during submaximal exercise at 200 W and maximal exercise in seven well-trained cyclists. Weeks 1 to 2 were during normal (moderate) training, weeks 3 to 4 during overtraining (high-intensity interval training), and weeks 5 to 6 during recovery (normal) training. HLa/RPE ratios declined during intensified training and returned to normal values during recovery training. From ref. 18.

mance. Second, skeletal muscle glycogen depletion may limit substrate available for lactate-generating anaerobic glycolysis. This too seems unlikely, because overreaching and decreased HLa:RPE ratio have been shown to occur despite maintenance of normal muscle glycogen levels (discussed further below) (17). Third, and most likely, reduced catecholamine production and/or sensitivity (discussed further below) may be responsible. Catecholamines mediate part of the exercise-induced activation of glycogenolysis (37), and reduced stimulation may limit glycogen availability for anaerobic glycolysis and thus lactate production.

Muscle Glycogen

Skeletal muscle glycogen depletion has been associated with fatigue and inability to train during overreaching/overtraining. For example, of eight collegiate swimmers who doubled training volume over a 10-day period, the four who could not maintain increased training also exhibited significantly greater declines in skeletal muscle (m. posterior deltoid) glycogen concentration compared with the four who tolerated increased training (7). However, a more recent study refuted the role of muscle glycogen depletion as a contributing factor to overreaching. Snyder and co-workers (17) intensified training over a 15-day period in eight cyclists who consumed a liquid carbohydrate (CHO) supplement during the 2 hours after each training session; usual total dietary CHO intake was maintained during this time. All subjects displayed symptoms of overreaching such as decreased maximal work capacity, lactate/RPE ratio, and self-reported symptoms. Resting skeletal muscle (m. vastus lateralis) glycogen content increased nonsignificantly over the 15-day period, indicating that symptoms of overreaching may occur despite maintenance of normal muscle glycogen concentration.

Muscular Strength and Endurance

Although most studies have focused on endurance athletes, overtraining and overreaching also occur in power and strength athletes such as weightlifters (34,38) and judo athletes (39). In these athletes, increased training volume and/or intensity may produce performance decrements and signs of overtraining/overreaching, including fatigue, hormonal changes, and decreases in muscular strength and muscular endurance (reviewed in ref. 40).

For example, Fry and associates (34) increased training volume and intensity in experienced weightlifters who performed maximal lifts daily for 2 weeks. Compared with a control group of similarly trained lifters who did not overtrain, these lifters experienced significant decreases in several measures of leg-extension strength including 1 repetition maximum (RM) strength, low- and high-velocity isokinetic strength, stimulated maximal isometric strength, and muscular endurance (total work performed in repeated contractions at 70% of 1 RM to exhaustion). Moreover, maximal blood lactate concentration declined significantly after the 2 weeks of overtraining. Callister and colleagues (39) studied a group of elite judo athletes during 10 weeks of intensified training, which included 50% to 100% increases in resistance, interval (running and cycling), and judo training volume; athletes trained 4 to 7 hours, 6 days per week. Upper- and lower-body isokinetic muscular strength at several velocities and 300-m sprint performance declined significantly during intensified training, although athletes did not show other signs of overreaching (e.g., maximal heart rate and blood lactate levels did not change significantly).

Decreases in muscular strength and endurance accompanying overtraining/overreaching may adversely affect performance in many sports, from pure strength/power (e.g., weightlifting, sprinting) to games (e.g., soccer, basketball) to endurance activities (e.g., rowing, swimming, cycling, distance running). On the other hand, there is a paucity of well-controlled studies on muscular strength changes during overtraining/overreaching (40). It is unclear whether such changes reflect short-term muscular fatigue resulting from the last training sessions before testing or longer-term fatigue attributable to overtraining/overreaching. For example, it was recently demonstrated that full-strength recovery may require up to 72 hours after resistance training (41).

HORMONAL CHANGES DURING OVERTRAINING AND OVERREACHING

Overtraining has been associated with alterations in blood concentrations or urinary excretion of several hormones including norepinephrine, cortisol, testosterone, and growth hormone (reviewed in refs. 5,40). Although the levels of these hormones may change during periods of intense training, only changes in norepinephrine levels appear to be consistently associated with symptoms of overtraining/overreaching syndrome (5,8, 11,15,16,20).

Catecholamines

Higher resting and lower maximal plasma norepinephrine concentrations have been reported after 4 weeks of intensified training (doubling training volume) in middle-distance runners (15,16). Higher resting plasma norepinephrine levels also were reported in overtrained compared with well-trained elite swimmers (8). The higher resting levels may reflect the physical stress of intense training. For example, Hooper and co-workers (8) attributed the increasing plasma norepinephrine concentration during the taper (2 to 3 weeks of reduced training before competition) to the maintenance of high training loads in the overtrained swimmers who, in actuality, did not reduce training volume during the taper period.

The lower plasma norepinephrine concentration observed during maximal exercise in some studies has been attributed to adrenal exhaustion, or the so-called parasympathetic form of overtraining. This form of overtraining is associated with impaired catecholamine secretion, resulting in many of the symptoms of overtraining syndrome such as persistent fatigue, lower maximal heart rate and blood lactate levels, and impaired performance (5,15,16,27).

Excretion of catecholamines in the urine has been suggested to be an integrative indicator of total production and excretion of catecholamines (42). Thus, a decline in urinary excretion of norepinephrine is consistent with the concept of adrenal exhaustion. Lehmann and associates (15,16,27) observed progressively decreasing urinary excretion of norepinephrine in various athletes over a 4-week period of intensified training during which most subjects exhibited symptoms of overreaching (Fig. 33–2). Moreover, the decrease in norepinephrine excretion was significantly correlated with self-reported symptoms on a complaints index. In a recent study of competitive swimmers, 4 weeks of intensified training was associated with significantly lower urinary excretion of norepinephrine in overreached swimmers (11) (Fig. 33–3). Compared with well-trained swimmers, overreached athletes exhibited significantly lower urinary norepinephrine excretion at the start of and throughout the study. This difference was apparent before the onset of symptoms, such as persistent fatigue or poor performance. It was suggested that the lower norepinephrine concentration may have reflected physical stress accumulated before the onset of the study (which began in midseason), and that low levels may predispose an athlete to develop symptoms of overreaching/overtraining during subsequent increased training. These data suggest that impaired catecholamine production may precede and possibly contribute to overreaching/overtraining.

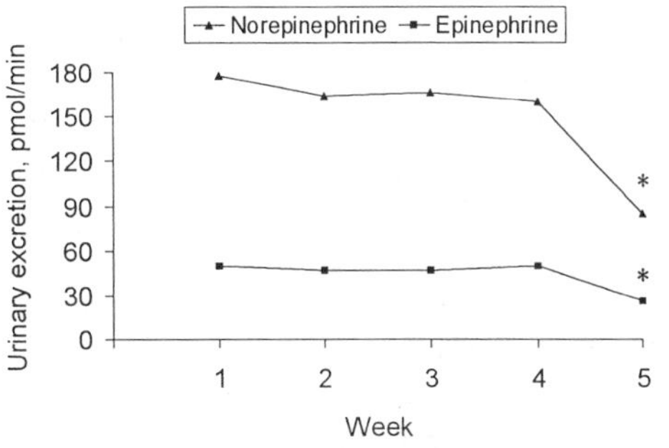

FIG. 33–2. Median overnight urinary norepinephrine and epinephrine excretion in male distance runners during 4 weeks of intensified training in which training volume was doubled. *Significantly lower at week 5 compared with week 1. From ref. 16.

Testosterone, Cortisol, and the Free Testosterone/Cortisol Ratio

Testosterone and cortisol are thought to have opposing effects on muscle metabolism, protein synthesis, and growth (i.e., anabolic and catabolic effects, respectively). The ratio of free testosterone to cortisol in the blood (FTCR) has been suggested to reflect the balance of positive and negative adaptations to exercise training (43). Although some studies have shown changes in these hormone concentrations or their ratio during peri-

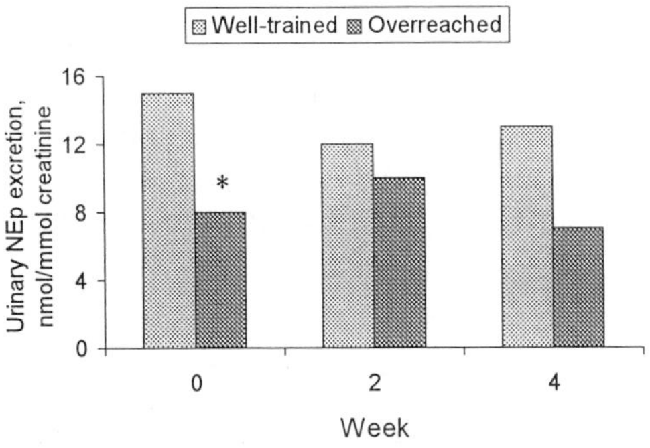

FIG. 33–3. Overnight urinary norepinephrine (NEp) excretion in well-trained and overreached competitive swimmers during 4 weeks of intensified training. Overreaching was identified in eight of 24 swimmers, based on decrements in performance, high fatigue ratings, and subjective comments in daily log books indicating poor adaptation to training. *Significantly lower in overreached compared with well-trained. From ref. 11.

ods of intense training (33,43–45), most studies indicate that such changes are not consistently associated with overreaching/overtraining (12,19,44–47). Many studies report no changes in the plasma concentrations of these hormones or the FTCR during overtraining and overreaching in a variety of athletes including male distance runners (12,19,21,27), male and female swimmers (8,11, 19,33,44), and junior male weightlifters (48). In two prospective studies of swimmers, the ratio remained unchanged over time and was normal in overtrained (8) and overreached (11) compared with well-trained swimmers. Moreover, the same training program may elicit dissimilar responses in different athletes (45,46); that is, the FTCR may decrease in some athletes while remaining unchanged in others. Furthermore, relatively large increases in training volume are needed to elicit changes in the FTCR (19).

A recent study suggested that the ratio of these two hormones may yield important information about the athlete's adaptation to training stress (44). Plasma total testosterone (TT), non–sex hormone binding globulin-bound testosterone (NSBT), and cortisol (C) were measured at various times over a training season in competitive swimmers. Although the TT/C and NSBT/C ratios did not significantly change over the season, these ratios were negatively correlated with training volume, and changes in these ratios were highly positively correlated with performance changes. Thus, although blood concentrations of testosterone and cortisol, and their ratio, do not appear to be good markers of overtraining, if followed over time in individual athletes, the ratio of these hormones may give an indication of the athlete's adaptive response to short-term physiological strain (5,44).

IMMUNOLOGICAL CHANGES DURING OVERTRAINING AND OVERREACHING

Overtraining is associated with frequent illness, mainly viral URTI (1,2). As shown in Chapter 12, athletes are at high risk of URTI during intense training and competition. Intense exercise may suppress immune function immediately after a single exercise session and for a long time during periods of intense training (reviewed in ref. 49).

Illness Rates in Overtrained Athletes

Despite the widely held belief among exercise scientists, coaches, and athletes that frequent illness is a symptom or outcome of overtraining (1,2,4,50), surprisingly few studies have directly addressed this issue (10,51). In a recent study, training was intensified over a 4-week period in 24 elite swimmers, 8 of whom were identified as overreached (10). Of the 24 swimmers, 10 (42%) exhibited URTI during the 4 weeks. Surprisingly, the incidence of URTI during the 4 weeks was higher in the well-trained [9 of 16 (56%)] compared with overreached [1 of 8 (12.5%)] swimmers. It was suggested that increased risk of URTI may not necessarily be associated with overreaching but may occur as a consequence of intense training in all athletes.

Immune Cells

Immune cells are the major effectors of host resistance to infectious disease. These cells can directly kill foreign organisms or infected cells and also may produce soluble mediators that activate other immune cells and induce killing of pathogenic microorganisms. Resting leukocyte number is generally clinically normal even during intense training (8,12,13,52), although counts at the low end of the clinically normal range have been reported in distance runners during 4 weeks of intensified training (16). In a related study, low leukocyte counts were associated only with increased training volume and not increased intensity for 4 weeks (20). A recent study also has suggested that lymphocyte count may decline during 4 weeks of intensified training in swimmers (11). Thus, resting leukocyte and lymphocyte counts are generally normal in well-trained athletes, but cell numbers may decline to the low end of the clinically normal range during periods of very intense, high-volume training. Whether such declines impair immune function has yet to be determined.

Neutrophils, the most prevalent leukocytes, are phagocytic cells that provide an essential first line of defense in the early stages of infection. Lower resting and postexercise neutrophil function was reported in trained cyclists (53), distance runners (54), and swimmers (51) compared with nonathletes. In swimmers, neutrophil oxidative activity decreased significantly during a 12-week intense training period; lowest values were observed during the peak training phase, and activity recovered partially during a rest phase at the end of the intense training period (51). Despite the marked decrease in neutrophil oxidative activity, however, there was no correlation with the appearance of URTI during the 12-week intense training, suggesting that such changes may not always compromise immune function in athletes.

Natural killer (NK) cells are a lymphocyte subset important in early defense against viral infection. Data suggest that NK cell number declines during both short (10 days; 12) and longer (7 months; 52) periods of intense training, despite no changes in other immune cell numbers. NK cell number and cytotoxic activity both at rest and after exercise decreased after 4-week intensified training in elite swimmers (55). These data suggest that intense training may influence NK cell number and function, which may possibly compromise immunity to viral infection in athletes. Other immune cell functions such as lymphocyte proliferation and activation do not appear to be adversely affected by intense exercise training (12,21,52).

Immunoglobulin

Clinically low serum immunoglobulin (Ig) levels have been reported in elite swimmers (52), although the ability to produce antibodies in response to an immunological challenge does not appear to be suppressed in these athletes (56). Secretory IgA is an important effector of resistance to pathogens causing URTI. Clinically low IgA levels have been reported in elite swimmers (52), and lower IgA concentration was reported in overtrained compared with well-trained swimmers (57). These data suggest that mucosal immunity may be compromised in overtrained athletes and/or during prolonged periods of intense training.

Plasma Glutamine

Glutamine, the most prevalent amino acid in the body, is required for normal function by immune cells and serves a dual role as a nitrogen source for nucleotide synthesis as well as a carbon source for energy production (58). It has been suggested that low plasma glutamine levels associated with overtraining may compromise lymphocyte function and possibly contribute to an increased incidence of infectious illness in competitive athletes (28,58–60).

Parry-Billings and colleagues (28) reported a 9% lower plasma glutamine concentration in 40 overtrained compared with nonovertrained athletes. The lower resting plasma glutamine concentration in overtrained athletes was not reflected in impaired lymphocyte function, however. In endurance-trained male soldiers, plasma glutamine concentration decreased during 10 days of intensified interval training, resulting in clear signs of overreaching (59). Despite the decreasing plasma glutamine concentration during intensified training and recovery, however, there was no evidence of immunosuppression. In a recent study of swimmers in which training volume was increased over a 4-week period, plasma glutamine concentration increased significantly in the well-trained swimmers, remaining unchanged in the overreached swimmers (10). However, plasma glutamine concentrations were not significantly different between swimmers exhibiting URTI and those who did not.

Rowbottom and co-workers (61) noted that plasma and skeletal muscle glutamine concentrations were the only biochemical or immunological parameters that distinguished athletes showing symptoms of chronic fatigue syndrome from healthy athletes or clinical norms. Although 26 weeks of glutamine supplementation increased plasma and skeletal muscle glutamine concentrations to clinically normal levels in these athletes, however, there were no improvements in self-reported symptoms, nor were there any changes in the incidence of URTI or lymphocyte and subset counts (62). Taken together, these data indicate that, although plasma glutamine concentrations may be lower in overtrained/overreached compared with well-trained athletes, no direct link has been established between plasma glutamine level and overtraining symptoms, prognosis, or immune function.

PSYCHOLOGICAL CHANGES DURING OVERREACHING AND OVERTRAINING

Overtraining syndrome is characterized by negative affective states such as anxiety, depression, apathy, lack of motivation, irritability, inability to relax, and lack of self-confidence (22,25). Research showed mood states to fluctuate with training volume and intensity (13,22, 23,63), and mood-state disturbances coincided with increased training loads over both the short (days to weeks) and long term (weeks to months) (13,19,22,64). Moreover, well-being ratings (discussed further below) showed significant deterioration with overtraining (14, 65).

Mood States

In athletes, mood states have been quantified by the Profile of Mood States (POMS) (66), which is a 65-item inventory assessing measures of tension, depression, anger, confusion, vigor, and fatigue; a composite of these items provides an indication of total mood disturbance (TMD). TMD scores for athletes identified as overtrained have been reported in the range of 155 to 231 (22,64,67) compared with a nonathlete-population average of 150 (22) and a nonovertrained-athlete range of 80 to 224 (64,67).

The specific POMS measures of tension and depression have shown measurable changes with overtraining. For example, tension and depression scores were consistently higher during a 6-month training season in overtrained compared with well-trained elite swimmers (67). A significant increase in tension scores with increasing training intensity also was observed over a competitive season in swimmers (64). Depression may not always accompany overtraining syndrome, however. For example, in the study by Hooper and associates (67), one swimmer who showed clear symptoms of overtraining syndrome had a depression score similar to those of well-trained swimmers.

Ratings of Well-Being

In a number of studies, self-reported measures such as fatigue, quality of sleep, muscle soreness, nontraining

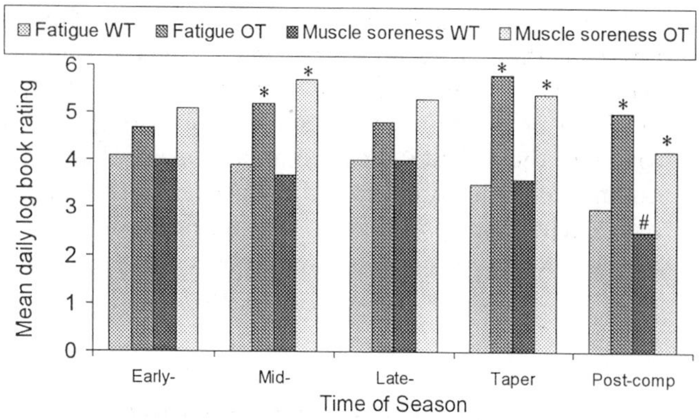

FIG. 33–4. Self-ratings of well-being in elite swimmers studied over a 6-month season. Swimmers rated fatigue and muscle soreness on a 1 to 7 scale (1, very very low; 7, very very high) in daily log books. Weekly means were obtained for each rating at 5 times in the season: early-, mid-, and late-season, during the taper before, and within 4 days after major competitions. Swimmers were diagnosed as well-trained (*WT*) or overtrained (*OT*) based on performance decrements, high fatigue ratings, and subjective comments in daily log books indicating poor adaptation to training. *Significantly higher rating in OT compared with WT swimmers at times designated. #Significantly lower rating after competition compared with early-season. From ref. 9.

stress, and other indicators of well-being have been monitored to assess adaptation in athletes during periods of intense training (8–10,14,68,69). For example, in distance runners, increases in training volume over a 4-week period were reflected in a self-rated complaints index (14). In elite swimmers, daily self-ratings of well-being, such as stress, quality of sleep, fatigue, and muscle soreness predicted overtraining syndrome several weeks before the appearance of symptoms or performance decrements (Fig. 33–4) (9). These ratings were quantified on a 1 to 7 scale; the higher the score on a particular item, the poorer the adaptation to training loads. Self-ratings were also able to predict by 1 to 2 weeks subsequent performance decrements and appearance of overreaching in a short-term (4-week) study of swimmers (10).

MONITORING, PREVENTING, AND TREATING OVERTRAINING SYNDROME IN ATHLETES

Identifying Overtraining Syndrome

Two main observations are critical to the diagnosis of overtraining syndrome: poor performance despite continued training and persistent, high fatigue levels. Unfortunately, these have been quantified in only a few reports. A stagnancy or decrement in training or competitive performance is a minimum requirement. Published reports suggest performance decrements of 1% to 15% (8,25,26), but any stagnancy in performance when improvement is expected may be critical to the athlete. The level of fatigue is more difficult to assess because of its subjectivity. Fatigue is more accurately assessed by long-term, daily self-ratings recorded on a standardized qualitative and/or quantitative scale, as described below. This allows the degree of change to be assessed somewhat objectively for each athlete and identifies any trends toward high fatigue levels. Because some level of fatigue is expected to accompany intense training, long-term records (i.e., over months) are required to differentiate normal from abnormal responses. Moreover, such records permit the coach and athlete to discern whether high levels of fatigue are easily dissipated by a few days rest or recovery training, or whether longer periods are needed. Other behavioral and psychological signs and symptoms such as high stress levels, poor sleep, or mood disturbances may help support the diagnosis. These cannot be used without other supporting evidence, however, because they have not been clearly and consistently shown to occur with overtraining syndrome (13,50).

Any unexpected change in an athlete's performance warrants investigation, but it does not necessarily indicate overtraining. Performance may be adversely affected over the short term by changes in training volume, intensity, or mode; diet; travel; or the introduction of new techniques or movement patterns. Before overtraining can be implicated, it is first necessary to consider and discount other possible causes including illness, injury, emotional upset, inadequate sleep or dietary intake, dehydration, and menstruation.

Preventing Overtraining Syndrome

Because poor performance resulting from overtraining syndrome may adversely affect an athlete's career for some time and may lead to premature retirement, preventing overtraining is of utmost importance. Several key issues must be addressed by the coach to ensure the athlete's welfare (Table 33–1). Many of these issues

TABLE 33–1. *Preventing overtraining*

- Identify susceptible athletes for monitoring
- Minimize known causes such as
  - Sudden increases in training load
  - Inadequate dietary carbohydrate
  - Stresses unrelated to training
  - Heavy competition schedules
  - Inadequate recovery after competition or between seasons
- Individualize training in recognition of individual differences in overtraining threshold
- Systematically periodize training
- Program recovery as integral component of training
- Monitor athletes for early-warning signs
  - Fatigue, mood state changes

relate to the need for a scientifically based training program incorporating principles such as periodization and individualization of training (covered elsewhere in this text). The following section, therefore, discusses the important consideration of monitoring athletes for indications of overtraining.

Monitoring Athletes

Based on the plethora of factors that may be related to overtraining, it is not surprising that there are, as yet, no confirmed reliable markers to identify overtraining syndrome clearly (reviewed in refs. 2,4,65). Part of this problem relates to the relative paucity of well-controlled long-term studies monitoring athletes because of the inherent difficulties in such an approach (discussed above). In addition, varying demands of different types of athletic performance (e.g., sprint/power compared with endurance) make it likely that different markers are required. Based on the current level of understanding of overtraining syndrome, the following suggestions can be made for monitoring athletes.

Physiological Measures

Blood parameters such as red and white blood cells, hemoglobin, hematocrit, urea, and ammonia are not usually abnormal during overtraining/overreaching and are thus not effective indicators of overtraining syndrome (4,11,19,65). Although changes in exercise blood lactate concentration and the blood lactate threshold are often accepted as good indicators (discussed above), these data must be used with caution to diagnose the syndrome. Inconsistent changes have been reported with overtraining (9,15,16,27,70), possibly because blood lactate levels may be influenced by factors unrelated to overtraining, including diet, previous exercise, ambient temperature, and phase of the training season. To be used as an effective indicator of overtraining syndrome, blood lactate variables must be assessed repeatedly over time (i.e., weeks to months) and under strictly controlled exercise and environmental conditions. There are many ways to assess lactate profiles in athletes, and decreases in blood lactate concentration at maximal work rate or the HLa/RPE ratio seem to be most closely related to overtraining (15–18,36). Time, cost, and the invasive nature of blood sampling may preclude use of this measure for routine monitoring of all athletes, although these variables may be relevant for research studies and for athletes with access to such testing.

For routine monitoring, reduced maximal heart rate and prolonged heart rate recovery after a standardized submaximal exercise appear to be more viable and easily administered. Heart-rate measurement is inexpensive, noninvasive, and easily incorporated into training, because athletes are familiar with heart-ra
Although maximal heart rate and heart r
appear to be good indicators in endurance a
ever, there are insufficient data to deterr
such monitoring is effective in other types

Psychological Measures

The POMS questionnaire has been successfully used to identify athletes predisposed to overtraining (23,67,71). For example, TMD scores were predictive of the subsequent appearance of overtraining several weeks later in elite swimmers (67). Because TMD represents a synthesis of the six specific mood states measured in the POMS (anger, depression, tension, confusion, vigor, and fatigue), it may be of value in monitoring some athletes for early signs of overtraining. The POMS should be used with caution, however, because it does not always identify overtrained athletes; that is, some athletes may exhibit clear signs of overtraining but have normal TMD scores (67). It is also not yet clear whether the POMS can predict overtraining in all types of athletes, or whether it is effective during competition phases when mood states may reflect impending competition stress (71). Moreover, because significant mood-state changes may occur in athletes who are not overtrained (64,72), the POMS cannot be used alone to identify overtrained athletes.

Self-Analysis Measures

Several investigators have suggested that overtraining is best monitored by athletes themselves by using self-analysis tools (5,9,69). Daily documentation by athletes including sources and ratings of stress, fatigue, muscle soreness, quality of sleep, irritability, and perceived exertion during training or standardized exercise may be effective in predicting and identifying overtraining (65,69,73). As described above, self-ratings of well-being have been shown to predict the subsequent appearance of overtraining before deterioration of performance and the onset of other symptoms in swimmers (9). Moreover, self-analysis measures (complaints index) were shown to be significantly correlated with decreases in urinary catecholamine excretion (15,16), suggesting that self-analysis measures may provide an inexpensive, noninvasive method of estimating physiological responses to intensive training or overtraining. Although further work is required to determine whether self-analysis accurately and reliably predicts overtraining in different types of athletes and under varying circumstances, it appears prudent for athletes to keep a daily diary of self-analysis measures, as shown in Table 33–2. This method of monitoring is simple, inexpensive, time efficient, and noninvasive; however, athletes' distortions of their responses and the need for interpretation by the reviewer also must be considered as possible sources of bias.

TABLE 33–2. *Recommended items for daily log book self-analysis by athletes*

- Training details
  - Distance, duration, pace, perceived intensity, heart-rate responses, resistance work
- Space for athletes' comments on training
  - Enjoyment, coping
- Well-being ratings on a quantifiable scale (e.g., 1–7)
  - Fatigue, stress, quality of sleep, muscle soreness, irritability
- Causes of stress/dissatisfaction
- Illness, injury, menstruation (for female athletes)

Certainly some type of monitoring to prevent overtraining is an important component of effective management of athletes during intense training. Comprehensive, invasive testing (e.g., blood analysis) has yet to be shown to be more effective than less expensive, simpler, and noninvasive testing (e.g., performance, heart-rate responses to standardized exercise, self-analysis by athletes). Table 33–3 presents an example of a monitoring program that may be adapted for particular athletes.

Treating the Overtrained Athlete

Once diagnosed as overtrained, the athlete should be regularly monitored for physiological and psychological responses to recovery. Clinical diagnosis is necessary to document and treat any illness, infection, or other medical disorders secondary to overtraining or that may contribute to symptoms. Causal and contributing factors, such as nontraining stress, frequent competition, and training and recovery practices should be systematically analyzed. This information is essential for designing effective recovery programs and preventing recurrence of overtraining syndrome. Rehabilitation should include substantially reduced training loads or complete rest (determined by the severity and duration of symptoms); increased recovery time within and between workouts; introduction of variety in training, such as cross-training; and regeneration techniques such as massage or hydrotherapy.

TABLE 33–3. *Example of monitoring program over a season*

Time frame	Monitoring
Daily	Training logs
Microcycle	Recovery after standardized submaximal exercise test (e.g., heart rate, blood lactate concentration)
Macrocycle	POMS
	Response to standardized maximal-effort exercise (e.g., heart rate, blood lactate)
Seasonal	Biochemical, hormonal, and immunological profiles

POMS, profile of mood states.

MECHANISMS UNDERLYING OVERTRAINING

It is unlikely that a single mechanism may explain such diverse physiological and psychological changes affecting so many different types of athletes. As mentioned above, neuroendocrine changes are likely to underlie many of the symptoms of overtraining, such as poor performance, alterations in mood states, inability to maintain training loads, lower maximal heart rate and lactate production, and decrements in muscular strength (4,40). Urhausen and colleagues (5) recently proposed a neuroendocrine model of overtraining in which physical and psychological stress associated with intense training initially causes elevation of stress hormone levels, catecholamines and cortisol in particular. It is further proposed that persistently elevated stress hormone levels lead to a variety of other effects including decreased sensitivity and number of adrenergic receptors and disturbances in other hormones (e.g., insulin, pituitary hormones, sex steroids). These in turn may influence metabolic activity (e.g., impaired glycogen synthesis and glycogenolysis, increased protein degradation). It is thought that persistent stimulation of adrenergic activity over time may, through an as-yet-unidentified mechanism, lead to autonomic dysfunction or the so-called parasympathetic form of overtraining reflected in decreased catecholamine production. Physiological changes and symptoms associated with overtraining, such as fatigue and decreases in maximal heart rate, lactate levels, muscular strength, and overnight norepinephrine excretion, are consistent with this proposed pathway. This model awaits further experimental testing before it can be conclusively linked to the phenomenon of overtraining, however.

REFERENCES

1. Fitzgerald L. Overtraining increases the susceptibility to infection. *Int J Sports Med* 1991;12(suppl):S5–S8.
2. Fry RW, Morton AR, Keast D. Overtraining in athletes: an update. *Sports Med* 1991;12:32–65.
3. Kreider RB, Fry AC, O'Toole ML. Overtraining and overreaching in sport: terms, definitions, and prevalence. In: Kreider RB, Fry AC, O'Toole ML, eds. *Overtraining and overreaching in sport: physiological, psychological, and biomechanical considerations.* Champaign, IL: Human Kinetics Publishing, 1997:vii–ix.
4. Lehmann M, Foster C, Keul J. Overtraining in endurance athletes: a brief review. *Med Sci Sports Exerc* 1993;25:854–862.
5. Urhausen A, Gabriel H, Kindermann W. Blood hormones as markers of training stress and overtraining. *Sports Med* 1995; 20:251–276.
6. Stone MH, Keith RE, Kearney JT, Fleck SJ, Wilson GD, Triplett N. Overtraining: a review of the signs, symptoms and possible causes. *J Appl Sport Sci Res* 1991;25:35–50.
7. Costill DL, Flynn MG, Kirwan JP, et al. Effects of repeated days of intensified training on muscle glycogen and swimming performance. *Med Sci Sports Exerc* 1988;20:249–254.
8. Hooper S, Mackinnon LT, Gordon RD, Bachmann AW. Hor-

monal responses of elite swimmers to overtraining. *Med Sci Sports Exerc* 1993;25:741–747.
9. Hooper S, Mackinnon LT, Howard A, Gordon RD, Bachmann AW. Markers for monitoring overtraining and recovery in elite swimmers. *Med Sci Sports Exerc* 1995;27:106–112.
10. Mackinnon LT, Hooper SL. Plasma glutamine and upper respiratory tract infection during intensified training in swimmers. *Med Sci Sports Exerc* 1996;28:285–290.
11. Mackinnon LT, Hooper SL, Jones S, Gordon RD, Bachmann AW. Hormonal, immunological and hematological responses to intensified training in swimmers. *Med Sci Sports Exerc* 1997; 29:1637–1645.
12. Fry RW, Morton AR, Crawford GPM, Keast D. Cell numbers and in vitro responses of leucocytes and lymphocyte subpopulations following maximal exercise and interval training sessions of different intensities. *Eur J Appl Physiol* 1992;64:218–227.
13. Fry RW, Grove JR, Morton AR, Zeroni PM, Gaudieri SD, Keast D. Psychological and immunological correlates of acute overtraining. *Br J Sports Med* 1994;28:241–246.
14. Lehmann M, Dickhuth HH, Gendrisch G, et al. Training-overtraining: a prospective, experimental study with experienced middle- and long-distance runners. *Int J Sports Med* 1991; 12:444–452.
15. Lehmann M, Baumgartl P, Wiesenack C, et al. Training-overtraining: influence of a defined increase in training volume vs training intensity on performance, catecholamines and some metabolic parameters in experienced middle- and long-distance runners. *Eur J Appl Physiol* 1992;64:169–177.
16. Lehmann M, Gastmann U, Petersen G, et al. Training-overtraining: performance, and hormone levels, after a defined increase in training volume versus intensity in experienced middle- and long-distance runners. *Br J Sports Med* 1992;26:233–242.
17. Snyder AC, Kuipers H, Cheng B, Servais RM, Fransen E. Overtraining following intensified training with normal muscle glycogen. *Med Sci Sports Exerc* 1995;27:1063–1070.
18. Snyder AC, Jeukendrup AE, Hesselink MKC, Kuipers H, Foster C. A physiological/psychological indicator of over-reaching during intensive training. *Int J Sports Med* 1993;14:29–32.
19. Flynn MG, Pizza FX, Boone JB Jr, Andres F, Michaud TA, Rodriguez-Zayas JR. Indices of training stress during competitive running and swimming seasons. *Int J Sports Med* 1994;15:21–26.
20. Lehmann MH, Mann U, Gastmann J, et al.. Unaccustomed high-mileage vs intensity training-related changes in performance and serum amino acid levels. *Int J Sports Med* 1996;17:187–192.
21. Verde T, Thomas S, Shephard RJ. Potential markers of heavy training in highly trained endurance runners. *Br J Sports Med* 1992;26:167–175.
22. Morgan WP, Brown DR, Raglin RS, O'Connor PJ, Ellickson KA. Psychological monitoring of overtraining and staleness. *Br J Sports Med* 1987;21:107–114.
23. Raglin JS, Morgan WP. Development of a scale for use in monitoring training induced distress in athletes. *Int J Sports Med* 1994; 15:84–88.
24. Verma SK, Mahindroo SR, Kansal DK. Effect of four weeks of hard physical training on certain physiological and morphological parameters of basketball players. *J Sports Med* 1978;18:379–384.
25. Barron JL, Noakes TD, Levy W, Smith C, Miller CP. Hypothalamic dysfunction in overtrained athletes. *J Clin Endocrinol Metab* 1985;60:803–806.
26. Costill DL. *Inside running.* Indianapolis: Benchmark Press, 1996: 123–134.
27. Lehmann M, Schnee W, Scheu R, Stockhausen W, Bachl N. Decreased nocturnal catecholamine excretion: parameter for an overtraining syndrome in athletes. *Int J Sports Med* 1992; 13:236–242.
28. Parry-Billings M, Budgett R, Koutedakis RY, et al. Plasma amino acid concentrations in the overtraining syndrome: possible effects on the immune system. *Med Sci Sports Exerc* 1992;24:1353–1358.
29. Kuipers H, Keizer HA. Overtraining in elite athletes. *J Sports Med* 1988;6:79–92.
30. Wenger HA, Belcastro AN, Daillaire J, Schutz RW, Smith M. C.A.S.S. overstress study: maximal tests and recovery heart rates. *Med Sci Sports Exerc* 1990;22:S131.
31. Foster C, Pollock M, Farrell P, Maksud M, Anholm J, Hare J. Training responses of speed skaters during a competitive season. *Res Q* 1982;53:243–246.
32. Wolf WA. Contribution to the question of overtraining. In: Larson LA, ed. *Health and fitness in the modern world.* Chicago: Athletic Institute, 1961:291–301.
33. Kirwan JP, Costill DL, Flynn MG, et al. Physiological responses to successive days of intense training in competitive swimmers. *Med Sci Sports Exerc* 1988;20:255–259.
34. Fry AC, Kraemer WJ, van Borselen F, et al. Performance decrements with high-intensity resistance exercise overtraining. *Med Sci Sports Exerc* 1994;26;1165–1173.
35. Jeukendrup AE, Hesselink MK. Overtraining—what do lactate curves tell us? *Br J Sports Med* 1994;28:239–240.
36. Pelayo P, Mujika I, Sidney M, Chatard J-C, Blood lactate recovery measurements, training, and performance during a 23-week period of competitive swimming. *Int J Sports Med* 1996;74;107–113.
37. Brooks GA, Fahey TD, White TP. *Exercise physiology: human bioenergetics and its applications.* 2nd ed. New York: Macmillan, 1996.
38. Warren BJ, Stone MH, Kearney JT, et al. Performance measures, blood lactate and plasma ammonia as indicators of overwork in elite junior weightlifters. *Int J Sports Med* 1992;13:372–376.
39. Callister R, Callister RG, Fleck SJ, Dudley GA. Physiological and performance responses to overtraining in elite judo athletes. *Med Sci Sports Exerc* 1990;22:816–824.
40. Fry AC, Kraemer WJ. Resistance exercise overtraining and overreaching: neuroendocrine responses. *Sports Med* 1997;23:106–129.
41. Logan PA. The inter-session recovery interval in heavy resistance training. PhD thesis, The University of Queensland, Australia, 1996.
42. Esler M, Jennings G, Korner P, et al. Assessment of human sympathetic nervous activity from measurement of norepinephrine turnover. *Hypertension* 1988;11:3–20.
43. Aldercreutz H, Harkonen M, Kuoppasalmi K, et al. Effect of training on plasma anabolic and catabolic steroid hormones and their response during physical exercise. *Int J Sports Med* 1986; 7:27–28.
44. Mujika I, Chatard J-C, Padilla S, Guezennec CY, Geyssant A. Hormonal responses to training and its tapering off in competitive swimmers: relationship with performance. *Int J Sports Med* 1996; 74:361–366.
45. Vervoorn C, Quist AM, Vermulst IJM, Erich WBM, deVries WR, Thijssen JHH. The behaviour of the plasma free testosterone/cortisol ratio during a season of elite rowing training. *Int J Sports Med* 1991;12:257–263.
46. Alen M, Pakarinen A, Hakkinen K, Komi PV. Responses of serum androgenic-anabolic and catabolic hormones to prolonged strength training. *Int J Sports Med* 1988;9:229–233.
47. Hakkinen K, Pakarinen B, Alen M, Komi PV. Serum hormones during prolonged training of neuromuscular performance. *Eur J Appl Physiol* 1985;53:287–293.
48. Fry AC, Kraemer WJ, Stone MH, Warren BJ, et al. Endocrine responses to overreaching before and after 1 year of weightlifting. *Can J Appl Physiol* 1994;19:400–410.
49. Mackinnon LT. Effects of overtraining and overreaching on immune function. In: Kreider RB, Fry AC, O'Toole ML, eds. *Overtraining and overreaching in sport: physiological, psychological, and biomechanical considerations.* Champaign, IL: Human Kinetics Publishing, 1997:219–241.
50. Hackney A, Pearman AN, Nowacki J. Physiological profiles of overtrained and stale athletes: a review. *Appl Sports Psychol* 1990;2:21–33.
51. Pyne DB, Baker MS, Fricker PA, McDonald WA, Telford RD, Weidemann MJ. Effects of an intensive 12-wk training program by elite swimmers on neutrophil oxidative activity. *Med Sci Sports Exerc* 1995;27:536–542.
52. Gleeson M, McDonald WA, Cripps AW, Pyne DB, Clancy RL, Fricker PA. The effect on immunity of long term intense training in elite swimmers. *Clin Exp Immunol* 1995;102:210–216.
53. Smith JA, Telford RD, Mason IB, Weidemann MJ. Exercise, training, and neutrophil microbicidal activity. *Int J Sports Med* 1990;11:179–187.
54. Hack V, Strobel G, Weiss M, Weicker H. PMN cell counts and

phagocytic activity of highly trained athletes depend on training period. *J Appl Physiol* 1994;77:1731–1735.
55. Gedge VL, Mackinnon LT, Hooper SL. Effects of 4 wk intensified training on natural killer (NK) cells in competitive swimmers. *Med Sci Sports Exerc* 1997;29:S158.
56. Gleeson M, Pyne DB, McDonald WA, et al. Pneumococcal antibody response in elite swimmers. *Clin Exp Immunol* 1996; 105:238–244.
57. Mackinnon LT, Hooper S. Mucosal (secretory) immune system responses to exercise of varying intensity and during overtraining. *Int J Sports Med* 1994;15:S179–S183.
58. Newsholme EA. Biochemical mechanisms to explain immunosuppression in well-trained and overtrained athletes. *Int J Sports Med* 1994;15:S142–S147.
59. Keast D, Arstein D, Harper, Fry RW, Morton AR. Depression of plasma glutamine concentration after exercise stress and its possible influence on the immune system. *Med J Aust* 1995; 162:15–18.
60. Rowbottom DG, Keast D, Morton AR. The emerging role of glutamine as an indicator of exercise-stress and overtraining. *Sports Med* 1996;21:80–97.
61. Rowbottom DG, Keast D, Goodman C, Morton AR. The haematological, biochemical and immunological profile of athletes suffering from the overtraining syndrome. *Eur J Appl Physiol* 1995; 70:502–509.
62. Rowbottom DG, Keast D, Pervan Z, et al. The role of glutamine in the aetiology of the chronic fatigue syndrome: a prospective study. *J Chronic Fatigue Syndrome* 1988;4:3–22.
63. Raglin JS, Morgan WP, O'Connor PJ. Changes in mood states during training in female and male college swimmers. *Int J Clin Lab Investigation* 1991;39:407–413.
64. O'Connor PJ, Morgan WP, Raglin JS, Barksdale CM, Kalin NH. Mood state and salivary cortisol levels following overtraining in female swimmers. *Psychoneuroendocrinology* 1989;14:303–310.
65. Hooper SL, Mackinnon LT. Monitoring overtraining in athletes: recommendations. *Sports Med* 1995;20:321–327.
66. McNair DM, Lorr M, Droppelman LF. *EDITS manual for the profile of mood states.* San Diego: Educational and Industrial Testing Service, 1971.
67. Hooper SL, Mackinnon LT, Hanrahan SJ. Mood states as an indication of staleness and recovery. *Int J Sport Psychol* 1997;28:1–12.
68. Collins D. Early detection of overtraining problems in athletes. *Coaching Forum* 1995;28:17–20.
69. Rushall BS. A tool for measuring stress tolerance in elite athletes. *Appl Sport Psychol* 1990;2:51–66.
70. Kindermann W. Overtraining: expression of a disturbed autonomic regulation. *Dtsch Z Sportsmed* 1996;8:238–245.
71. Berglund B, Safstrom H. Psychological monitoring and modulation of training loads of world-class canoeists. *Med Sci Sports Exerc* 1994;26:1036–1040.
72. Morgan WP, Costill DL, Flynn MG, Raglin JS, O'Connor PJ. Mood disturbance following increased training in swimmers. *Med Sci Sports Exerc* 1988;20:408–414.
73. Morgan WP. Psychological components of effort sense. *Med Sci Sports Exerc* 1994;26:1071–1077.

Exercise and Sport Science,
edited by William E. Garrett, Jr., and Donald T. Kirkendall.
Lippincott Williams & Wilkins, Philadelphia © 2000.

CHAPTER 34

Periodization of Training

David G. Rowbottom

Coaches and athletes are constantly seeking new methods to improve performance, even by the slightest of margins. Despite innovations in clothing (1) and equipment design (2), modern trends in nutrition (3) and supplementation (4) for athletes, and the genesis of drug taking in sports (5), the major factor influencing athletic performance is still training. Many of the coaching practices and training techniques that have been developed over the years owe more to the observations of outstanding coaches than to breakthroughs from sports scientists (6). Indeed, some training regimens have been immortalized by the record-breaking achievements of the athletes who used them (7). The pendulum still appears to swing perpetually between schools of coaching thought. The speed emphasis versus endurance emphasis of training distance runners is a good case in point. This chapter does not propose to enter into any such long-standing debates, but instead it focuses on the structure, rather than the specific content, of the training program. Specifically, we consider the systematic planning of athletic training that has become known as periodization.

Misconceptions remain about the role of periodization in training programs and about the scientific basis of the coaching theory. This chapter looks at periodization from four different perspectives. First, a historical perspective traces the origins of periodization as a coaching practice. Second, a coaching perspective looks at the proposed structure of a periodized training program, as well as the advantages and possible problems of periodization. A scientific perspective investigates the evidence in support of the current coaching practice, and finally a research perspective looks at future direction and the possible role that research investigation could have in improving the current recommendation of training strategies to elite-level athletes.

D.G. Rowbottom: School of Human Movement Studies, Queensland University of Technology, Kelvin Grove, Queensland, Australia.

A HISTORICAL PERSPECTIVE

Some authors have suggested that the practice of periodization of training has been used in an unrefined form for an unknown period, perhaps dating back to the early Greek Olympians (8). It may surprise the modern coaching fraternity to learn that what appears to be a recent coaching innovation has such early origins. The modern structure, terminology, and ideas were coined among Soviet sports scientists in the 1960s but perhaps owe much to the earlier work of Hans Selye (9) and his ideas on stress and adaptation in the human body. The work of the Soviet professor L. P. Matveyev, published in Moscow in 1965, appears to be the earliest published summary of the ideas of periodization (10). These concepts were developed further by other Eastern European coaches and sports scientists (11–15). Even as early as the mid-1970s, Western European coaches also were promoting the use of periodized training plans for their athletes (10,16). The sporting successes of the Eastern European nations during the 1960s through the 1980s may have helped to kindle the widespread popularity of periodization in many parts of the world (17).

In recent years, numerous sports scientists and coaches have emphasized the benefits to athletes in structuring training programs in accordance with the principles of periodization (8,18–25). The periodization of athletic training is a concept that now forms the basis of most modern coaching theory and practice. Coaches and athletes have applied the principles of periodization to such diverse sporting applications as swimming (17), distance running (7), strength training (26), basketball (27), kayaking (28), triathlon (25), Australian football (24,29) and rugby union (30).

A COACHING PERSPECTIVE

The role of the modern athletic coach has two conflicting demands. On the one hand, coaches are required to design and implement training programs to maximize the performance potential of the athletes under their charge. There is now increasing emphasis on the long-term planning process to bring young athletes to optimal performance at some stage in the future, for either Olympic or world championship competition. On the other hand, a coach needs to be keenly aware of the risk of overtraining athletes. The problems associated with overtraining are becomingly increasingly known, including the potential to end the career of a promising athlete. It is probably fair to say that most coaches and athletes are now aware of the competing nature of these demands. What may be absent, however, are effective means to meet them. Periodization of training is a process that has the potential, if used correctly, to assist coaches and athletes to optimize athletic performance while minimizing the very real risk of overtraining.

The Periodization Plan

In many senses, it would be true to say that the key to optimal athletic performance is effective planning. It is widely recognized that elite-level athletic performance is not an attribute with which an individual is born but is at least in part a result of a long-term development process. Planning an athlete's career development toward an ultimate goal is now an integral part of the coaching role. Clearly the long-term goal of the training plan forms the foundation on which the plan itself is designed. Even with the keenest sense of long-term vision, however, it is essential for both coach and athlete to break down the planning process into discrete, manageable units, incorporating both short-term and intermediate goals. This partitioning of the training plan enhances the systematic organization of training for the athlete (8).

It has been suggested by some authors that training should be structured in terms of Olympic cycles, that is, cycles lasting 4 years each (12,22,31). Although there are conceivable benefits from this planning process, it has not been developed to any great extent in the published literature. Instead, the current trend is to structure training plans around an annual training cycle (7,8,22,24). Performance and development goals can be set on an annual basis, and the major championship, whether it is national, world, or Olympic, may be the focus of the training year.

Yet even at an annual level, it would be hard for an athlete to remain focused on a championship goal that may be up to 10 months away. Periodization of training is therefore a process that divides a complete training year into distinct, smaller periods of training of more manageable size, each with specific performance or development targets. As will become evident, periodization works on the basis of "building blocks" that make up the whole training structure. For instance, at the highest level of division, an Olympic cycle may be divided into four yearly building blocks. Unfortunately, the use of terminology to describe the phases and cycles of training within the periodization structure has varied somewhat among authors (7,8,12,17,22,23,25). For the purposes of this chapter, the terminology follows that laid out in the original periodization structure by Matveyev (12). The basic building block of the training structure, usually the training week, is referred to as a *microcycle* (literally "small cycle"). Microcycles form the building blocks for a discrete unit of training, usually a few weeks in duration, termed a *mesocycle* (literally "medium cycle"). A number of repeated mesocycles make up a *macrocycle* (literally "large cycle"), usually lasting a number of months. Finally, three or more macrocycles make up the training year or annual plan (Fig. 34–1). The rationale behind these subdivisions is best understood when the training program is broken down, starting at the highest level.

Macrocycles

Even in the most unrefined form of periodization, there is an obvious distinction between different stages of the training program. Each year, part of the training program is dedicated to preparation, part of the year is given over to competitions and the major championship goals, and part is used for rest and recovery before the next training year. These three macrocycles naturally have been given the names *preparatory*, *competitive*, and *transition* (12). The division of the training program in this rudimentary way ensures that training is focused toward certain general targets.

First, the preparatory macrocycle is used for basic or foundation training, upon which later performance targets will be based. Many coaches have emphasized the importance of this stable foundation of training (6,7, 24,30). In practice, this macrocycle cannot be shorter than the time necessary to produce an acceptable level of fitness. The recommended length of the preparatory macrocycle is determined by the nature of the sporting event, but in annual training cycles a period of 5 to 7 months has been suggested (12). Other coaches have included the subdivision of the preparatory macrocycle into "general preparatory" and "specific preparatory" to highlight shifts in training emphasis during the preparation of the athlete (8,24). In the structure proposed here, this distinction would probably be better addressed at the mesocycle level.

The competitive macrocycle is the phase during which basic fitness is converted into competition performance. Here the emphasis shifts from increasing an athlete's

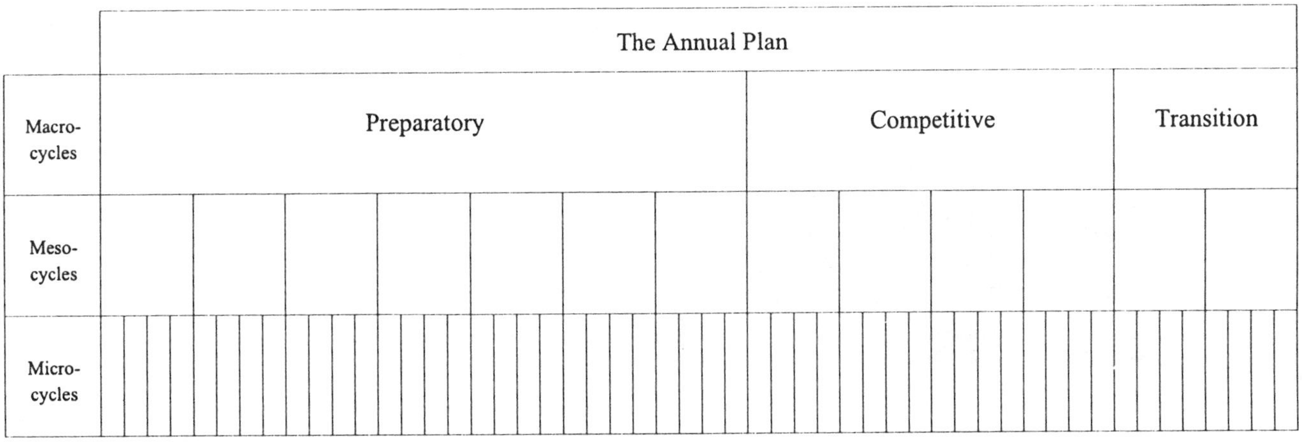

FIG. 34–1. A schematic illustration of the division of the annual training plan into macrocycles, mesocycles, and microcycles. From ref. 19.

fitness level to peaking for competition and maintaining a certain level of performance (8). The length of this phase is determined by how long an acceptable level of performance can be maintained, and 2 to 4 months has been recommended (12). Once again, Bompa (8) suggested that this macrocycle could be divided into a "precompetition" phase and a "competition" phase.

Finally, the transition phase provides a period of rest and regeneration at the end of a training year before the subsequent one begins. It is generally accepted that there may be a temporary loss of fitness during this macrocycle (12), but others have included "active rest" to minimize this possibility (8). The recommendation has usually been that the transition macrocycle should be long enough to allow complete rehabilitation of the athlete (7,12,17,22), usually 2 to 4 weeks (12). Unfortunately, too much emphasis has been placed on the transition macrocycle, at the conclusion of a training year, as the time for recovery and regeneration of the athlete. Athletes need regularly scheduled recovery periods throughout the training year, not just at its conclusion, to avoid the problems associated with overtraining (23,32). The division of each macrocycle into smaller blocks of training (mesocycles) provides a structure for the inclusion of these recovery periods in the training program.

Mesocycles

Whereas macrocycles may provide a rudimentary division of the training year, the mesocycle is arguably the crucial building block within the multitiered framework of training. Potentially, the mesocycle structure has major roles in both minimizing the risk of overtraining (23,32) and improving athletic performance (8). A large number of review articles on overtraining in athletes have highlighted an imbalance between training and recovery as a major causative factor (21,32–36). Mesocycles are designed to be discrete blocks of training, each incorporating a period of intensive training as well as a period of reduced training for recovery and regeneration (Fig. 34–2). It is encouraging to note that most prospective research studies that have used 2 to 4 weeks of increased training to bring about an overtrained state (37–41) have only been able to induce the short-term effects of overreaching (32,38). The implication seems to be that the long-term effects of overtraining can be avoided if an athlete restricts intensive training to between 2 and 4 weeks before scheduling a period of recovery. Therefore it is recommended that each mesocycle should be between 3 and 6 weeks long, with a preference given to approximately monthly cycles (12,22). In this way, the accumulation of fatigue in athletes may be controlled (12) and potential problems from overtraining recognized at an early stage (32).

It is strongly recommended that an athlete not begin the next mesocycle until demonstration of complete recovery from the previous one (12,22). This process can be monitored by performance and other tests, commonly achieved through appropriate race scheduling, time trials, or laboratory-based tests (21). Without an effective recovery period before these types of assessment, however, it is unlikely that the test results will give a reasonable indication of the athlete's fitness level (22,32). These benchmarks of progress also are important to verify to both coach and athlete that they are still on target for preplanned goals. A particularly good performance may require refinement of the training load in the planning of the next mesocycle. Conversely, a poor performance may require an extension of the recovery period before beginning the next phase of training. In this way, the training plan can be frequently reviewed and appropriate adjustments made to both training and performance targets. The potential for re-

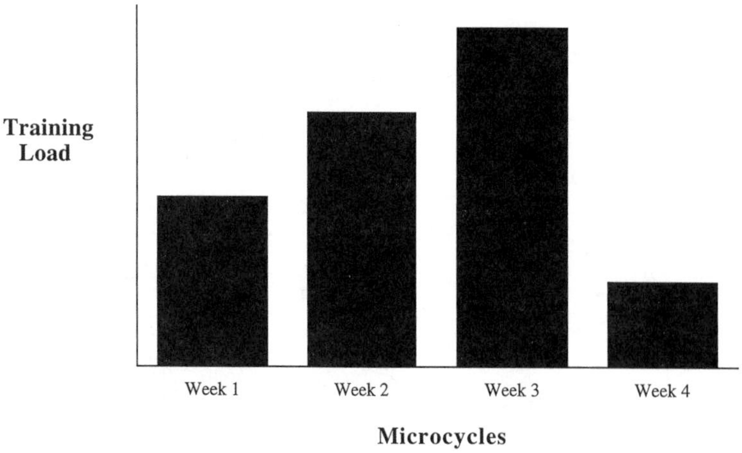

FIG. 34–2. The proposed structure of a 4-week mesocycle.

fining optimal peaking strategies also is apparent (22). Essentially, though, a coach needs to ensure that an athlete has fully recovered from each mesocycle, before beginning the subsequent cycle of training.

Another essential consideration is the logical sequence for the development of fitness components [strength, speed, endurance, skill, etc. (8)] in recognition that the development of some abilities is a prerequisite to the development of others (22). Each mesocycle should be designed with the aim of eliciting significant improvements in a particular aspect of fitness (17), whereby each cycle is designed to build on the previous one. Unfortunately, coaches and sports scientists have tended to disagree as to the precise sequence of required development (6,8,11,12,15,22). The traditional progression from predominantly endurance/aerobic training, through anaerobic threshold and interval/transition training, to speed and power training has perhaps been established more by coaching experience than by systematic research (6). Nevertheless, a training program should be designed to effect a progression toward the season's goal, and the mesocycle building blocks provide a structure for this progression. The majority of these recommendations for periodization of training are of a qualitative nature. Fewer recommendations have been made regarding the quantitative aspects of periodization, and particularly the distribution of training volume within the mesocycle (12,42). It may be at the level of the individual microcycle that this shortfall can be addressed.

Microcycles

In most periodization structures, the microcycle is associated with a weekly training plan (8,12,13,22), and it is at this level that the cyclic nature of any program is most evident. It has been pointed out that some training objectives may not fit within a 7-day structure (12), and more flexible training plans have been promoted (17). Nevertheless, the advantages of weekly microcycles to the nonprofessional athlete who is trying to balance training with other commitments, or to team-sport players with weekly playing commitments, are clear. Whereas a 7-day microcycle may not fully correspond to the optimal structure of the training process, it is important for coaches to try to dovetail the training regimens of their athletes with other aspects of life and work (12).

Despite the repetitive nature of the weekly training plan, it is apparent from the description of the mesocycle that not all microcycles have the same training content or objectives. Clearly the type of microcycle will depend on its place within the larger, mesocycle structure (see Fig. 34–2). A number of particular microcycles have been suggested with specific functions in mind (8,11–14,22,31). A frequent recommendation is that a mesocycle should consist of four microcycles in a specific order: "ordinary" → "development" → "shock" → "rehabilitation" (8,12,22). As shown in Fig. 34–2, there is a gradual progression of increasing training load through the first three microcycles, culminating in what has been termed a *shock microcycle.* As the name suggests, this is designed to contain a substantially increased training load during which cumulative overload is maximized (12,13). The mesocycle is completed with a rehabilitation microcycle, intentionally placed to follow the shock microcycle immediately. During the rehabilitation microcycle, training load and intensity are dramatically reduced, allowing adaptation and overcompensation to occur and fatigue to be eliminated (8,12,13,43).

One aspect of this structure that is readily apparent is that complete recovery is not achieved either between each training session or even between each microcycle (22). An athlete will experience an accumulation of fatigue during the three intensive-training weeks (13,14), with complete recovery expected only after each mesocycle (22). A possible consequence is that an athlete may be less capable of completing high-intensity speed, power, or even interval-training sessions toward the end of this period. It may, therefore, be appropriate to follow the lead of some Eastern European coaches and schedule speed training early in the mesocycle and predominantly muscular and cardiovascular endurance during the shock microcycle (11).

Advantages of Periodization

It has already been shown how periodization of training may benefit athletes both by maximizing performance improvements and by minimizing the risk of overtraining. A number of other legitimate reasons for the use of a periodized training structure also need to be considered. For instance, female athletes have been reported to experience significant changes in performance through the menstrual cycle (44). The use of a monthly mesocycle format would allow this variation to be taken into account when planning training (12).

A number of researchers have identified the potential for athletes to become "stale," not through a training overload, but from the boredom of regular, monotonous training (21,33). Coaches have observed motivational problems when athletes feel they are on a "never-ending training treadmill" (7), committed to week after week of daily hard training. Athletes can avoid becoming "bogged down" in long preparation training programs if a periodization approach is used. It allows the athlete to have regular changes in training format and content, as well as the added motivation of seeing regular improvements in athletic performance.

An athlete is exposed not just to physical stress from the training program; other stresses from life events in school, work, relationships, finances, social activities, and health must be considered (45). The cumulative nature of stress has been recognized for some time (9) but has often been overlooked in the management of training programs (22,32,46). Although coaches can prescribe an athlete's training stress, they may be unaware of the nature and extent of additional life stresses. If left unchecked, this cumulative stress could lead to poor training adaptation and even overtraining. In such circumstances, a periodized training structure would be beneficial. The proposed regular assessment of an athlete's performance may highlight such problems at an early stage and allow the training load to be reduced accordingly, until other life stresses have been reduced or eliminated.

Potential Problems

The benefits of periodization of training are equally applicable to both team and individual sports. It is therefore unfortunate that so few authors have addressed the issue of training periodization in team sports (24,27, 29,30). In the main, these efforts have concentrated on the progressive development of fitness components at a macrocycle level (27,29,30) rather than the conflict of interests between training periodization and weekly competition (24). In many team sports, a regular playing season may last as long as 6 to 8 months (24), with players expected to compete at or near their peak every weekend or even every day. In some respects, it is extraordinary that these demands continue to be placed on professional team-sport athletes, when modern coaching practice almost universally accepts the theory of periodization. Dawson (24) highlighted the problem for team-sport athletes in achieving a "minipeak" each weekend, having to combine postgame recovery, midweek training, and a pregame taper all within the 5- to 8-day break between games.

There is good reason to suggest that the current administrative system in most of the major team sports does not lend itself to a periodized training structure. A complete mesocycle of cumulative overload and recovery would be difficult to implement in a team-sport environment. Compromising the player's performance on particular weekends within the cycle is almost inevitable. This conflict of interests, particularly in professional team sports, opens up a minefield of potential controversy. How many team managers would be accepting of the fact that multimillion-dollar star players would not be available to compete on every fourth weekend during a rehabilitation microcycle? Similarly, how many sports fans would be understanding of players producing below-average performances, as a result of accumulated fatigue, during a shock microcycle?

Changes at an administrative level have the potential to reconcile accepted coaching practice with the demands of professional team sports. Playing schedules could easily allow clubs to have periodic rest weekends throughout a playing season, whether on a universal basis or by rotation. One could argue that the major obstacle to such a plan would be the clubs and organizing bodies themselves. Would they be prepared to accept the inevitable cuts in revenue through lost ticket sales and television rights? It is more probable that financial pressures will win the day over any advances in coaching recommendations. Unfortunately, it is the athlete who "is relegated to the role of a short-lived tool in corporate machinations" (7).

A SCIENTIFIC PERSPECTIVE

The application of both basic and applied science to the field of elite sports has had a tremendous impact in recent years. The efficiency of coaching the top-level athlete has been greatly improved by this interaction between sports and science. When the field of periodization of training is viewed from a scientific perspective, however, the availability of research data is lamentable. The recommendations for periodization of training, as laid out by many authors (8,12–14,16), have an excessively speculative character. In their earlier review of periodization, Fry and colleagues (22) concluded that "most of the information contained in the literature . . . is conjectural or experiential and not supported by research," and they strongly suggested that "there is a need for systematic research in this area to test present opinions" (22). It has been argued by others that recommendations are being made to athletes without a precise knowledge of the effects of these training interventions on athletic performance (6). That is not to say, however, that the foundations of periodization of training are not based on scientific principles.

The Scientific Rationale

Underlying the theory of periodization are the documented effects of overload and regeneration on an organism. In brief, an exercise stress or overload will displace the homeostasis of the body (9,12), resulting in a number of catabolic events. These may include the breakdown of structural and functional proteins (47) and use of endogenous energy stores (48). Consequently, a single exercise bout will result in a certain level of fatigue and a loss of performance capacity for an athlete. After overload, the body then works to reestablish homeostasis (9,46), including the replenishment of endogenous energy stores and the synthesis of new protein (31). The length of time required for regeneration depends mainly on the degree of the initial overload and the displacement of homeostasis (8,9,13), but it will also be influenced by any further overload imposed during the recovery period.

An observation in a number of different biologic systems has been that this process does not simply restore, but may in fact surpass, the initial level of functional capacity (8,13,14). If the same stress or overload were to be imposed again, homeostasis would be displaced to a lesser degree. Consequently the body is capable of doing more work for the same displacement of homeostasis (9). This process has been termed *overcompensation* or *supercompensation* (8,13,14,49). In practice, this would mean an improvement in performance for the athlete (Fig. 34–3).

It has been argued that the degree of overcompensation achieved depends on the magnitude of the overload imposed (13,22,46). Based on this thesis, a series of training sessions undertaken by an athlete, without sufficient recovery time between every two sessions, would result in an accumulation of overload or fatigue. This has been termed the *valley of fatigue* (50). Periodization of training is founded on the assumption that this cumulative overload would produce a more powerful stimulus for subsequent overcompensation during a prolonged regeneration phase (8,12,13). A schematic diagram of this theory is presented (Fig. 34–4*B*). It is still open to debate whether this periodized training structure has benefits, solely from a performance perspective, over an even distribution of training load, by using a "train–recover–train" cycle of events (Fig. 34–4*A*).

Research Evidence

A number of authors have commented that a performance change of as little as 1% to 2% can make the difference between a world champion and a nonqualifier for the event (37,51). Considering this small margin between success and failure, it is quite remarkable that so little systematic research has been conducted to support directly or to refute the current coaching practice of periodization. It has been pointed out that the published work of Matveyev (12) was based on a systematic investigation of top Soviet athletes (8), but little of the content of those investigations has been published. In the absence of such studies, it is necessary to review some of the research evidence from related fields that lends support to the theory of periodization.

There would appear to be three important assumptions that spring from the scientific rationale of periodization. First, an increase in training load would produce

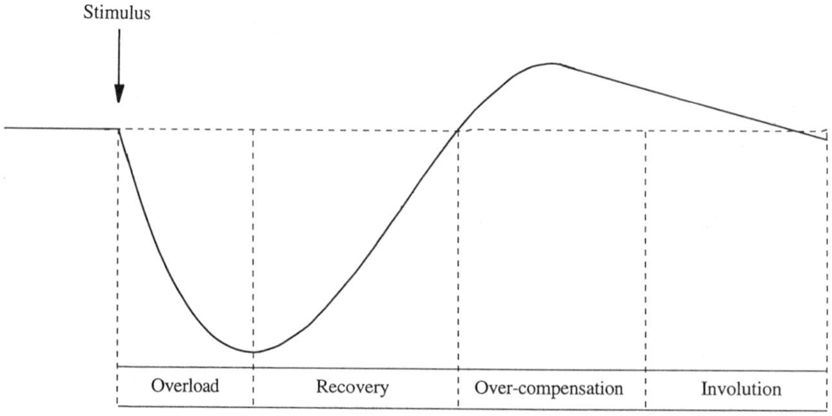

FIG. 34–3. The cycle of overcompensation after training. From ref. 49.

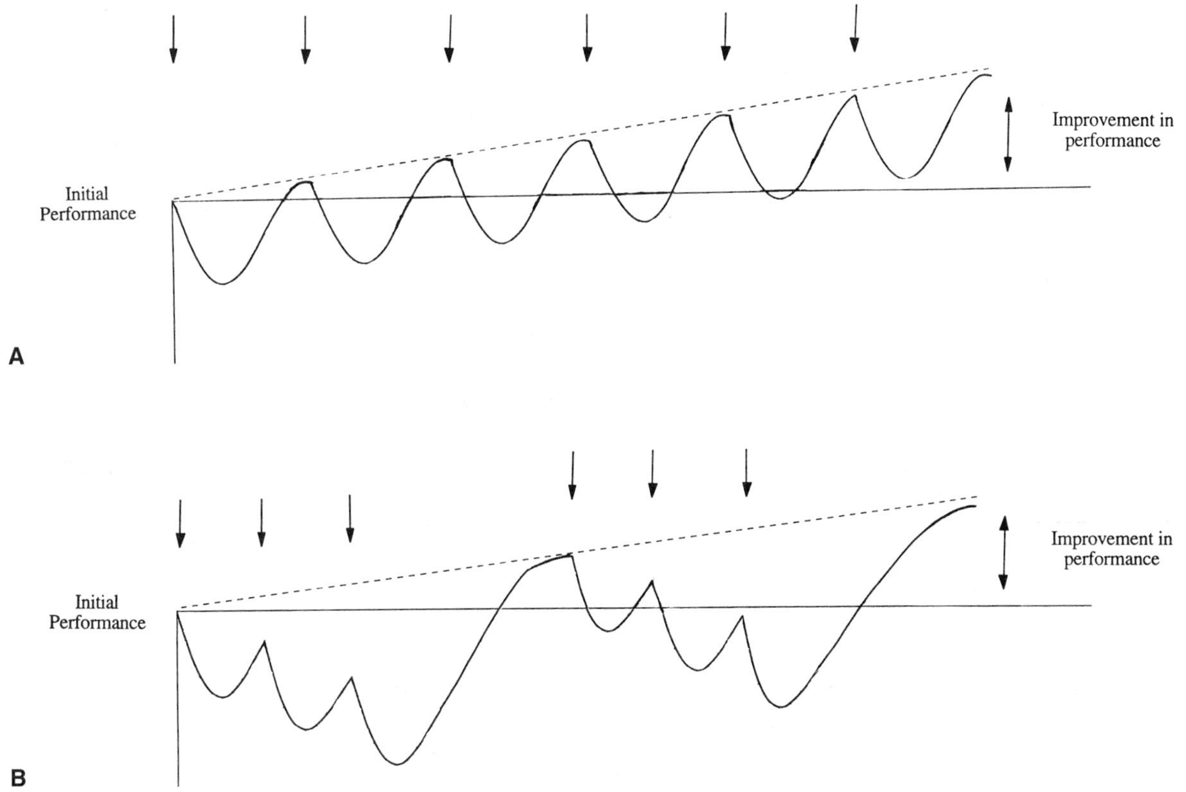

FIG. 34–4. A schematic comparison of two strategies for overcompensation. The train–recover–train cycle (**A**), and the periodization structure of cumulative overload and prolonged recovery (**B**). From refs. 13 and 46.

an increase in adaptation or performance, even in well-trained athletes. Second, there should be a point at which this increased load can no longer be tolerated, or at which adaptation ceases to occur. Third, a period of enforced recovery or rest should result in an increase in adaptation (overcompensation) and consequently improved performance. Research data in support of each of these assumptions will be examined.

Increased Training Load

In well-trained athletes, there is evidence to support a positive association between performance and both training volume and training intensity (52–56). In marathon and ultramarathon runners, Scrimgeour and colleagues (52) reported that those athletes who trained in excess of 100 km/week had significantly faster running times than those runners whose training did not exceed the 100km/week threshold. Similarly, performance variables in well-trained triathletes have been reported to correlate positively with training load (53,54). However, the theory of periodization suggests that a further short-term increase in training overload, if appropriately managed, would eventually result in improved performance even in well-trained athletes.

A number of studies have observed performance improvement after short-term increases in the training load of already well-trained athletes. This is usually achieved by the introduction of high-intensity interval training into an athlete's program, replacing a portion of aerobic training. Acevedo and Goldfarb (57) reported a significant 3% improvement in 10-km time-trial performance in male long-distance runners after 8 weeks of increased-intensity running on 3 days/week. This performance improvement was accompanied by a significant decrease in blood lactate concentration at running speeds equivalent to 85% and 90% of maximal aerobic capacity ($\dot{V}O_2$max). Two similar studies in endurance cyclists replaced 15% of their aerobic training with high-intensity interval training over a 4-week period (58) and a 6-week period (59), respectively. Laboratory-simulated 40-km time-trial performance was improved by approximately 2.5% in both studies.

With a slightly different protocol, Mikesell and Dudley (60) replaced the predominantly aerobic training programs of well-trained distance runners with a reduced-volume, high-intensity regimen for 6 weeks. Runners completed 40-minute runs at 90% $\dot{V}O_2$max and interval-training sessions on alternate days. After 5 weeks of training, significant improvements were reported in

10-km race time and $\dot{V}O_2max$ (60). These data suggest that short-term increases in training load, particularly training intensity, may produce significant performance increments. A sixth week of training resulted in decreased performance, however, suggesting that this level of increased training load could not be maintained indefinitely (60).

Plateaus in Performance Improvement

A number of research studies reported plateaus or decrements in performance after 2 to 4 weeks of intensive or increased training (6,37–41,60,61). In untrained individuals, Hickson and co-workers (61) reported that improvements in measures of aerobic capacity reached a plateau after 3 weeks of training. A similar plateau was observed in a second period of training at an increased intensity. In trained cyclists, the introduction of high-intensity training sessions on 2 days/week resulted in significant improvements in peak power output and 40-km time-trial performance after only 2 to 3 weeks (58). Extending this training regimen from 3 weeks to 6 weeks did not result in any further performance improvements, despite routine adjustment of training intensity relative to new performance levels (6).

Other studies have implemented considerable increases in training volume and intensity over a 2- to 4-week period to elicit an overtraining response (37–41). Stagnated or decreased performance was a consistent observation. For example, in trained cyclists, a 2-week period of intensified training resulted in a 5% decrement in time-trial performance (38). In the same study, a subsequent 2 weeks of reduced training resulted in time-trial performances 3% above preoverload levels (Fig. 34–5). These data suggest that a mesocycle training structure has the potential to produce significant performance improvements. Unfortunately, few researchers have extended overtraining studies to observe the time-course and extent of subsequent recovery (37,38,40). If the practice of periodization is to be supported, it would have to be consistently shown that cumulative overload of this nature produces performance benefits after such a period of recovery and regeneration.

Reduced Training and Tapering

A reasonable amount of work has been undertaken on the potential benefits of reduced training or "tapering" at the conclusion of a training season to produce optimal performance at the time of major competitions. The practice of tapering has been used by coaches for many years, and a number of studies have reported a positive impact on performance and related physiologic variables (62–70). Mujika and associates (68) found that two tapering periods during a competitive swimming season among elite athletes resulted in approximately 3% improvements in performance on both occasions. Similar performance improvements (3%) were reported in collegiate swimmers after a 10- to 14-day taper (62,64), and racing performance (5 km) has been found to improve in endurance runners after a 7-day (66), a 10-day, and a 13-day taper (69). Trained strength athletes may also benefit from a period of reduced-volume training (70). The consistency of these results across a variety of different athletes, sporting events, and racing distances would support the wide-ranging benefits of tapering.

Although tapering may produce increases in athletic performance, some studies have shown little concomitant effect on related physiologic indicators (65,66). On the other hand, muscle-biopsy studies in endurance runners and cyclists have reported increases in muscle oxi-

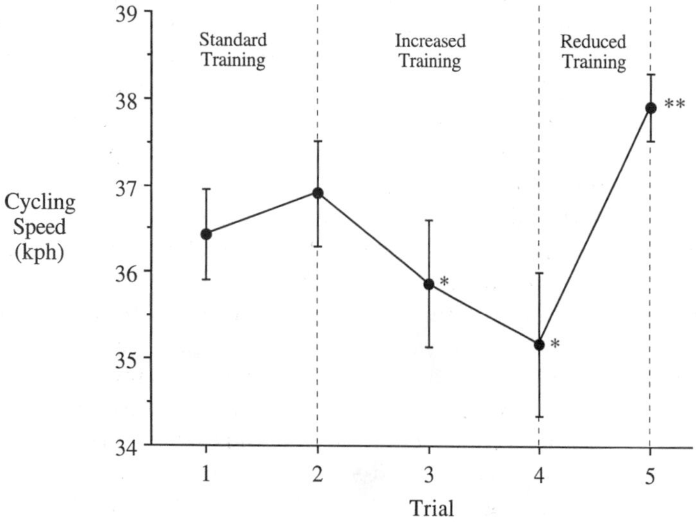

FIG. 34–5. Average cycling speed of competitive cyclists for an 8.5-km time trial during standard training load (trials 1 and 2), during 2 weeks of increased training load (trials 3 and 4), and after 2 weeks of reduced training load (trial 5). From ref. 38.

dative enzymes and muscle glycogen levels (15% to 35%) after tapering protocols (65,71). These adaptations may exert a positive effect on endurance performance and explain the observed benefits of tapering.

Studies have indicated that training volume needs to be substantially reduced to have any observable effect, whereas training intensity may need to be maintained to bring about performance improvements (65,66). In distance runners, a 62% reduction in training volume for 7 days did not improve performance, whereas a 90% reduction in training volume over the same period resulted in a 22% increase in exercise time to exhaustion (65). In swimmers, tapering programs involving 60% to 90% reductions in weekly training volume were shown to improve performance (67). In terms of the duration of reduced training, significant improvements in performance were reported with tapers lasting from 7 to 21 days (62,63,65,67,72). Undoubtedly the optimal taper duration would be influenced by the volume and intensity of training completed beforehand.

In summary, there is substantial research evidence for the beneficial effects of a period of reduced training or tapering on athletic performance. Many coaches are now aware of this research evidence and usually incorporate a tapering period at the conclusion of a period of training, before the major competitions. In essence, the proposed periodization plan systematically and routinely schedules periods of reduced training or tapering throughout the training program, at the conclusion of each mesocycle. The significant benefits observed after tapering protocols would equally support the practice of periodization. Although periodized training plans have not been systematically tested in well-designed research studies, there is considerable evidence to warrant further investigation.

Theoretic Aspects

Since the late 1970s we have witnessed the development of a more theoretic approach to the study of physiologic adaptation and the training–performance relation. This work may have important implications for the theory and practice of periodization of training. Mathematical models have been proposed that assume a dose–response relationship between training input and two theoretic, antagonistic responses of the human system: fitness and fatigue (73–76).

In brief, a quantifiable "dose" of training is assumed to give rise to two physiologic "responses": an increase in "fitness," a positive factor, and an increase in "fatigue," a negative factor. Without further training input, both responses would decay, albeit at different rates; the assumption is that fatigue would decay faster than fitness. A subsequent dose of training, of course, would add to both the fitness and fatigue levels. At any time, a predicted performance may be calculated from the difference between fitness and fatigue levels (42,74). Fundamentally, the model's fitness component is a performance potential, attainable only when fatigue is eliminated. Likewise, the model's fatigue component could be considered as the difference between a potential performance level (fitness) and the actual performance level (76).

A number of studies have attempted to validate the predictive power of the model by using empiric data from different training situations: recreational runners (74), elite swimmers (68), and a hammer thrower (76). Invariably, predicted and actual performance were shown to be reasonably well correlated (68,74,76). This mathematical model approach to training adaptation has been used in a number of ways to calculate the optimal combination of training and recovery required for peak performance (42,74,77).

It has been shown that a reduction in training, or complete training cessation, would theoretically produce a transient improvement in performance (78), an observation well documented from tapering studies (63,67). Influence curves have suggested that there is a critical period before competition during which training actually has a negative effect on performance. Similarly, there is an earlier period during which training has its greatest positive effect (77,78). With the model, it was predicted that training undertaken during the last 12 to 14 days before competition has a net negative effect, whereas training undertaken 6 weeks before competition has the greatest positive influence on performance (77). An application of these data might lead to the suggestion that an optimal periodization structure would combine 4 weeks of intensive training followed by 2 weeks of recovery.

Morton (42) modeled a number of different training structures over a 300-day training period. This analysis revealed that maximal performance would be produced by a training structure that is triangular in shape, is negatively skewed, and involves daily, high-intensity training. When this pattern of training-load distribution is plotted over a 30-day mesocycle (Fig. 34–6), the hypothetical program would involve a stepwise increase in training load followed by a shorter period of dramatically reduced training, something akin to the proposed periodization structure (12,21,22) and to current coaching practice (8).

Perhaps more direct evidence for the potential benefits of periodization can be gained from modeling a periodized 30-week training structure (Fig. 34–7*A*), compared with a flat, continuous 30-week regimen (Fig. 34–7*B*) in which the same total training load is completed. By using the proposed model (74), peak performance can be predicted for both training programs, assuming complete training cessation at the end of the 30-week program. Predicted peak performance is dependent on the default values used for the model con-

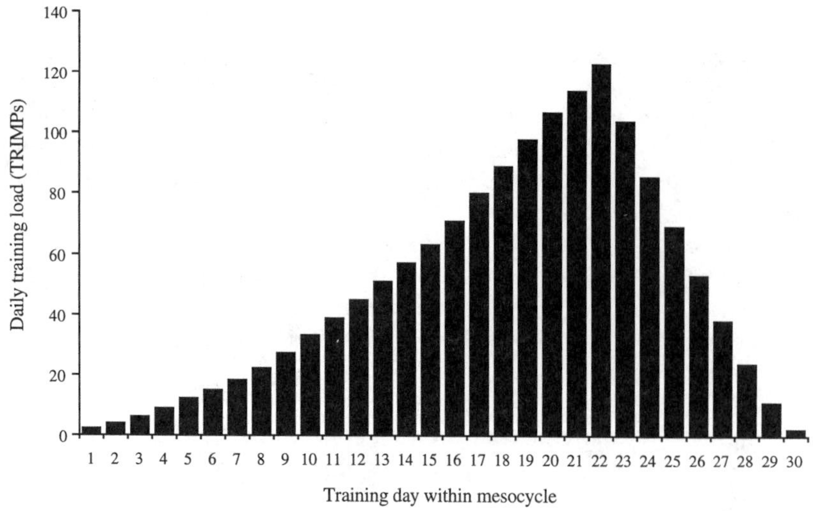

FIG. 34–6. A schematic diagram of a 30-day mesocycle training profile, triangular in shape, negatively skewed, and involving daily training of high intensity. From ref. 42.

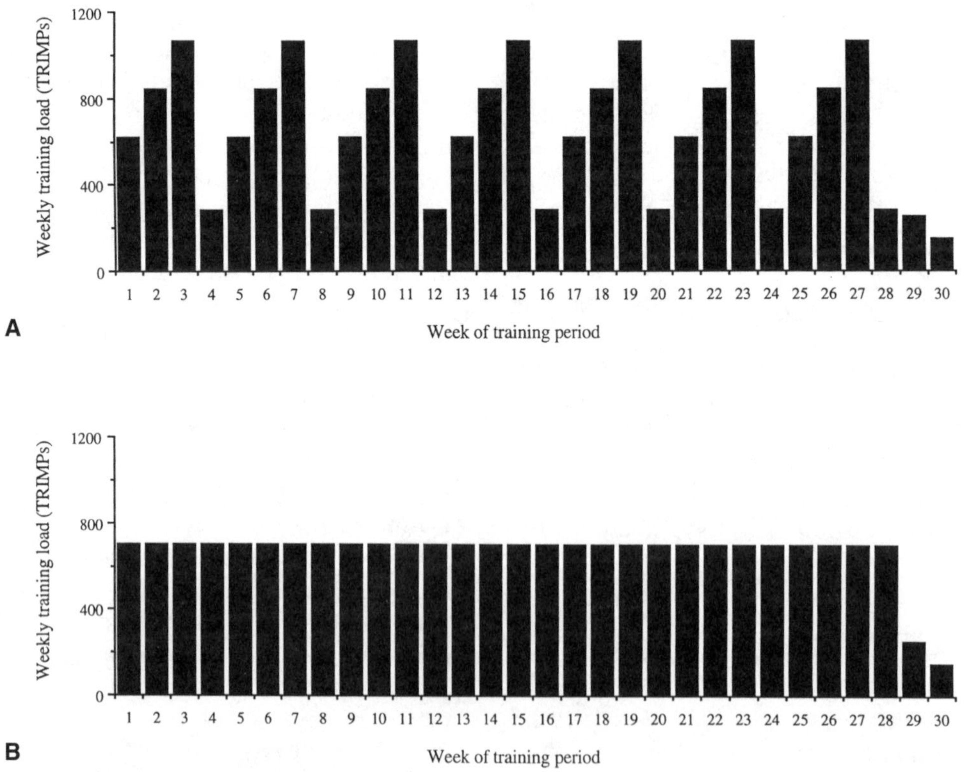

FIG. 34–7. A comparison of two hypothetical 300-day training seasons. A distributed training load in accordance with the proposed periodization structure (**A**), and an evenly distributed training load throughout the season (**B**). In both training regimens, the same total training load is completed.

stants (42), but in all cases the model predicted a 3% to 5% difference in performance improvements after the periodized training structure (Rowbottom, unpublished observations). Future research efforts must establish whether periodization of an athlete's training provides the benefits that can be predicted from the mathematical model.

There is obvious appeal in using a mathematical model to aid in the planning of a training program to produce optimal performance. However, caution should be exercised while there are still some discrepancies between model prediction and physiologic data (67). For instance, the model would predict performance improvements after short-term training cessation, whereas research studies have suggested that maintaining low-volume, high-intensity training is required for optimal performance gains (67). Furthermore, it has been recognized that studies to date have been only observational in nature (42). There is still a need for controlled research studies, whereby training structure is deliberately manipulated in accord with modeled predictions.

A RESEARCH PERSPECTIVE

It has been suggested that much of modern coaching theory is based on experience and observation rather than on systematic research (6,22). Periodization of training is a prime example of a theory, without direct scientific support, being adopted by coaches and athletes in a variety of different sports (7,17,24–30). If further advances are to be made in the detailed recommendation of training strategies to elite-level athletes, there is a real need for systematic research studies either to support or to refute these currently accepted training paradigms.

On the other hand, it should be emphasized that the experiential origin of a coaching practice does not make it erroneous. A reasonable case can be argued, by using related scientific evidence, that periodization is based on solid foundations. From a research perspective, it seems unlikely that sports scientists are going to rewrite the coaching handbook with completely innovative training techniques. Perhaps the refinement of present coaching practice, to optimize an athlete's performance potential, may be more productive. While there is a general need for research in the field of periodization of training, particular areas may warrant future research attention.

Optimizing Training Overload

One of the ongoing challenges of any training program is to optimize the training stimulus, whereby maximal performance gains are achieved and overtraining is avoided (32). Periodization of training has the potential to aid in this process, but unanswered questions remain. The precise point at which the training overload should be removed and the recovery phase initiated has always been a subjective decision. Similarly, the line that separates the benefits of recovery and overcompensation from the negative effects of detraining has not been clearly established (68,79). At present, coaches can rely only on intuition to schedule these aspects of a training program (80).

Recommendations by coaches for microcycle and mesocycle duration (8,12,17,21,22) have not been substantiated by systematic research as the optimal combinations of overload and recovery. Manipulating these variables in experimental settings may help to refine the current coaching recommendations. Researchers previously used mathematical models to predict the optimal duration for precompetition taper (68,70,77), and an application of these techniques may be a first step in determining the optimal balance of overload and recovery within a mesocycle.

Quantification of Training Load

Quantification of training load should be an essential component of any research into the periodization of training. A research study, designed to investigate the cause-and-effect relationship among overload, recovery, and performance, cannot be practically implemented by the coach without a quantitative indication of training load (81). Furthermore, for the coach to determine whether an athlete is complying with a training prescription, some means of training quantification must be used.

Simple data acquisition has been achieved in the past by having an athlete maintain a diary of training sessions completed, detailing durations and intensities. Unfortunately, it has not been clearly established whether exercise intensity is best recorded in terms of heart rate, oxygen uptake, power output, blood lactate level, or a rating of perceived exertion. Whether these variables should be recorded as absolute levels or relative to an individual maximum also is debatable. Another confounding factor may be the intermittent nature of some sporting activities such as tennis and other racket sports, field and ice hockey, football, volleyball, and basketball. The quantification of training load in these sports has not been adequately addressed.

The integration of individual training sessions into an overall measure of training load is another area that has received relatively little research attention. This becomes an important issue in sports that require multidisciplinary training, such as triathlon (53), and in sports that combine weight training in their preparation programs (76). Some efforts have been made to quantify training sessions of different durations and intensities (73–76), in which a short-duration, high-intensity session might rate equally with a long-duration, low-intensity session in terms of "training impulse" (74). This process has not yet taken into account the observable fact that some types of training may be more beneficial than others to performance in a particular event (56–60) and should be weighted accordingly. There is clearly scope for further research in this area before a thorough insight into the quantitative relation between training and performance can be gained (34).

Indicators of Overload and Recovery

Athletic performance has often been promoted as the measure of choice in both experimental and coaching settings (7,8,12,21–23,37,38,63–68,74–76). It has been assumed that performance measures will give a valid and reliable indication of the degree of overload and the extent of recovery during a training program. Although periodic performance assessment is essential for monitoring athletic development, it may not be the most suitable measure in all situations (32). During a shock microcycle performance tests may be inappropriate, and during rehabilitation they may be detrimental to recovery.

As an alternative indicator of overload and recovery, certain biochemical variables have been reported to fluctuate in response to changes in both performance and fatigue levels. After a single prolonged period of endurance exercise, an inverse relationship between serum enzyme activities and aerobic performance was reported (82). Other studies have demonstrated that fatigue levels, predicted from the mathematical model, correlate with various biochemical measures (80,83–85). These included various serum enzyme activities (83), iron status in female long-distance runners (84), and hormonal responses in weightlifters (80,85). Overtraining research has suggested that performance decrements may be associated with changes in serum levels of testosterone, cortisol (33,86), catecholamines (39,41), and glutamine (87). It may be possible to exploit these observations as a means of identifying the point of optimal overload and recovery, without subjecting an athlete to repeated performance tests. Ideally, when the biochemical indicator reaches a critical level, training overload is withdrawn and recovery initiated. Research work is still some way from this utopia of guiding the coach and athlete to optimal performance strategies.

CONCLUSION

As a structured approach to planning training, periodization has many advantages in optimizing athletic development and minimizing the risk of overtraining. Modern coaching practice has embraced the theory of periodization of training in a variety of different sporting settings, but perhaps with insufficient emphasis on training-load distribution within the mesocycle. Team-sport athletes, in particular, may be less able to implement these aspects of periodization. Although the theory of periodization is based on the principles of overload and overcompensation, there is still a need for systematic research to support or refute the coaching practice. Particular areas that should be addressed include the quantification of training load, the optimization of overload and recovery durations, and the use of indicators other than performance for monitoring development.

REFERENCES

1. Cordain L, Kopriva R. Wetsuits, body density and swimming performance. *Br J Sports Med* 1991;25:31–33.
2. Kyle CR. Energy and aerodynamics in bicycling. *Clin Sports Med* 1994;13:39–73.
3. Deakin V, Inge K. Training nutrition. In: Burke L, Deakin V, eds. *Clinical sports nutrition.* Sydney: McGraw-Hill, 1994.
4. Balsom PD, Söderlund K, Ekblom B. Creatine in humans with special reference to creatine supplementation. *Sports Med* 1994; 18:268–280.
5. Catlin DH, Murray TH. Performance-enhancing drugs, fair competition, and Olympic sport. *JAMA* 1996;276:231–237.
6. Hawley JA, Myburgh KH, Noakes TD, Dennis SC. Training techniques to improve fatigue resistance and enhance performance. *J Sports Sci* 1997;15:325–333.
7. Martin DE, Coe PN. Developing running with periodisation of training. In: Martin DE, Coe PN, eds. *Better training for distance runners.* 2nd ed. Champaign, IL: Human Kinetics, 1997:167–252.
8. Bompa TO. *Theory and methodology of training.* Dubuque: Kendall/Hunt, 1983.
9. Selye H. *The stress of life.* London: Longmans Green, 1957.
10. Kruger A. Periodisation, or peaking at the right time. *Track Techn* 1973;56:1720–1724.
11. Ozolin NG. *Sovremennaia systema sportivnoi trenirovky* [Athletes' training system for competition]. Moscow: Phyz. I. Sport, 1971.
12. Matveyev L. *Fundamentals of sports training.* Moscow: Progress Publishers, 1981.
13. Harre D. The formulation of the standard of athletic performance. In: Harre D, ed. *Principles of sports training.* Berlin: Sportsverlag, 1982:A7–A68.
14. Kukushkin G. *The system of physical education in the USSR.* Moscow: Radugi Publishers, 1983.
15. Bondarchuk A. Periodisation of sports training. *Legkaya Atletika* 1986;12:8–9.
16. Dick FW. Periodisation: an approach to the training year. *Track Techn* 1975;62:1968–1970.
17. Pyne D. The periodisation of swimming training at the Australian Institute of Sport. *Sports Coach* 1996;18:34–38.
18. Costill DL. *Inside running: basics of sports physiology.* Indianapolis: Benchmark Press, 1986.
19. Bompa TO. Periodisation as a key element of planning. *Sports Coach* 1987;11:20–23.
20. Noakes T. *Lore of running.* Cape Town: Oxford University Press, 1989.
21. Fry RW, Morton AR, Keast D. Overtraining in athletes: an update. *Sports Med* 1991;12:32–65.
22. Fry RW, Morton AR, Keast D. Periodisation of training stress: a review. *Can J Sports Sci* 1992;17:234–240.
23. Fry RW, Morton AR, Keast D. Periodisation and the prevention of overtraining. *Can J Sports Sci* 1992;17:241–248.
24. Dawson B. Periodisation of speed and endurance training. In: Reaburn P, Jenkins D, eds. *Training for speed and endurance.* Sydney: Allen & Unwin, 1996:76–96.
25. Evans M. Training volume and periodisation. In: Evans M, ed. *Endurance athlete's edge.* Champaign, IL: Human Kinetics, 1997:35–60.
26. Poliquin C. Applied strength training: part 1: short term periodisation. *Sports Coach* 1992;15:25–28.
27. Stapff A. The art and science of sports performance. *Sport Health* 1996;14:6–7.

28. Aitken D. Periodisation of the kayak program. *Canoe Coach* 1994;6:7–9.
29. Woodman L, Pyke F. Periodisation of Australian football training. *Sports Coach* 1991;14:32–39.
30. Jenkins D. Fitness testing and periodisation of training. In: *Preparing to play rugby.* Sydney: Australian Sports Commission, 1995: 24–34.
31. Bompa TO. Physiological intensity values employed to plan endurance training. *Track Techn* 1989;108:3435–3442.
32. Rowbottom DG, Keast D, Morton AR. Monitoring and prevention of overreaching and overtraining in endurance athletes. In: Kreider R, Fry AC, O'Toole M, eds. *Overreaching and overtraining in sport.* Champaign, IL: Human Kinetics 1998:47–66.
33. Kuipers H, Keizer HA. Overtraining in elite athletes: review and directions for the future. *Sports Med* 1988;6:79–92.
34. Lehmann M, Foster C, Keul J. Overtraining in endurance athletes: a brief review. *Med Sci Sports Exerc* 1993;25:854–862.
35. Hooper SL, MacKinnon LT. Monitoring overtraining in athletes. *Sports Med* 1995;20:321–327.
36. Hooper SL, MacKinnon LT, Howard A, Gordon RD, Bachmann AW. Markers for monitoring overtraining and recovery. *Med Sci Sports Exerc* 1995;27:106–112.
37. Fry RW, Morton AR, Garcia-Webb P, Crawford GPM, Keast D. Biological responses to overload training in endurance sports. *Eur J Appl Physiol* 1992;64:335–344.
38. Jeukendrup AE, Hesselink MCK, Snyder AC, Kuipers H, Keizer HA. Physiological changes in male competitive cyclists after two weeks of intensified training. *Int J Sports Med* 1992;13:534–541.
39. Lehmann M, Dickhuth HH, Gendrisch G, et al. Training-overtraining: a prospective, experimental study with experienced middle- and long-distance runners. *Int J Sports Med* 1991;12:444–452.
40. Snyder AC, Jeukendrup AE, Hesselink MKC, Kuipers H, Foster C. A physiological/psychological indicator of over-reaching during intensive training. *Int J Sports Med* 1993;14:29–32.
41. Hooper SL, MacKinnon LT, Gordon RD, Bachmann AW. Hormonal responses of elite swimmers to overtraining. *Med Sci Sports Exerc* 1993;25:741–747.
42. Morton RH. The quantitative periodisation of athletic training: a model study. *Sports Med Train Rehabil* 1991;3:19–28.
43. Goletz VI, Osadchy VP. The complex use of restorative means in different stages of the annual training cycle. *Velosipedniy Sport* 1986;1:23–26.
44. Zaharieva E. Survey of sportswomen at the Tokyo Olympics. *J Sports Med Phys Fitness* 1965;5:215–219.
45. Miller TW, Vaughn MP, Miller JM. Clinical issues and treatment strategies in stress-orientated athletes. *Sports Med* 1990;9: 370–379.
46. Kipke L. The importance of recovery after training and competitive efforts. *N Z J Sports Med* 1985;13:120–128.
47. Viru A. Mobilisation of structural proteins during exercise. *Sports Med* 1987;4:95–128.
48. Costill DL, Bowers R, Branam G, Sparks K. Muscle glycogen utilization during prolonged exercise on successive days. *J Appl Physiol* 1971;31:834–838.
49. Yakovlev NN. *Sports biochemistry.* Leipzig: Deutsche Hochschule für Korperkultur (German Institute for Physical Culture), 1967.
50. Counsilman JE. *The science of swimming.* Englewood Cliffs, NJ: Prentice Hall, 1968.
51. Levin S. Overtraining causes Olympic-sized problems. *Physician Sportsmed* 1991;19:112–118.
52. Scrimgeour AG, Noakes TD, Adams B, Myburgh K. The influence of weekly training distance on fractional utilisation of maximum aerobic capacity in marathon and ultra-marathon runners. *Eur J Appl Physiol* 1986;55:202–209.
53. Rowbottom DG, Keast D, Garcia-Webb P, Morton AR. Training adaptation and biological changes among well-trained male triathletes. *Med Sci Sports Exerc* 1997;29:1233–1239.
54. O'Toole ML. Training for ultraendurance triathlons. *Med Sci Sports Exerc* 1989;21:S209–S213.
55. Foster C, Daniels JT, Yarbrough RA. Physiological and training correlates of marathon running performance. *Aust J Sports Med* 1977;9:58–61.
56. Krebs PS, Zinkgraf S, Virgilia SJ. Predicting competitive bicycling performance with training and physiological variables. *J Sports Med Phys Fitness* 1986;26:323–330.
57. Acevedo EO, Goldfarb AH. Increased training intensity effects on plasma lactate, ventilatory threshold, and endurance. *Med Sci Sports Exerc* 1989;21:563–568.
58. Lindsay FH, Hawley JA, Myburgh KH, Schomer HH, Noakes TD, Dennis SC. Improved athletic performance in highly-trained cyclists after interval training. *Med Sci Sports Exerc* 1996;28:1427–1434.
59. Westgarth-Taylor C, Rickard S, Myburgh KH, Noakes TD, Hawley JA, Dennis SC. Metabolic and performance adaptations to interval training in endurance trained cyclists. *Eur J Appl Physiol* 1997;75:298–304.
60. Mikesell KA, Dudley GA. Influence of intense endurance training on aerobic power of competitive distance runners. *Med Sci Sports Exerc* 1984;16:371–375.
61. Hickson RC, Hagberg JM, Ehsani AA, Holloszy JO. Time course of the adaptive responses of aerobic power and heart rate to training. *Med Sci Sports Exerc* 1981;13:17–20.
62. Costill DL, King DS, Thomas R. Effects of reduced training on muscular power in swimmers. *Physician Sportsmed* 1985; 13:94–101.
63. Houmard JA. Impact of reduced training on performance in endurance athletes. *Sports Med* 1991;12:380–393.
64. Johns RA, Houmard JA, Kobe KW, et al. Effects of taper on swim power, stroke distance, and performance. *Med Sci Sports Exerc* 1992;24:1141–1146.
65. Sheply B, MacDougall D, Cipriano N, Sutton JR, Tarnopolsky MA, Coates G. Physiologic effects of tapering in highly trained athletes. *J Appl Physiol* 1992;72:706–711.
66. Houmard JA, Scott BK, Justice CL, Chenier JC. The effects of taper on performance in distance runners. *Med Sci Sports Exerc* 1994;26:624–631.
67. Houmard JA, Johns RA. Effects of taper on swim performance: practical implications. *Sports Med* 1994;17:224–232.
68. Mujika I, Chatard JC, Busso T, Geyssant A, Barale F, Lacoste L. Effects of training on performance in competitive swimming. *Can J Appl Physiol* 1995;20:395–406.
69. Gibala MJ, MacDougall JD, Sale DG. The effects of tapering on strength performance in trained athletes. *Int J Sports Med* 1994;15:492–497.
70. Zarkadas PC, Carter JB, Banister EW. Modelling the effect of taper on performance, maximal oxygen uptake, and the anaerobic threshold in endurance triathletes. *Adv Exp Med Biol* 1995; 393:179–186.
71. Neary JP, Martin TP, Reid DC, Burnham R, Quinney HA. The effects of a reduced exercise duration taper programme on performance and muscle enzymes of endurance cyclists. *Eur J Appl Physiol* 1992;65:30–36.
72. Costill DL, Thomas R, Robergs RA, Pascoe D, Lambert C, Barr S, Fink WJ. Adaptations to swimming training: influence of training volume. *Med Sci Sports Exerc* 1991;23:371–377.
73. Banister EW, Calvert TW, Savage MV, Bach T. A systems model of training for athletic performance. *Aust J Sports Med* 1975; 7:57–61.
74. Morton RH, Fitz-Clarke JR, Banister EW. Modeling human performance in running. *J Appl Physiol* 1990;69:1171–1177.
75. Busso T, Carasso C, Lacour JR. Adequacy of a systems structure in the modelling of training effects on performance. *J Appl Physiol* 1991;71:2044–2049.
76. Busso T, Candau R, Lacour JR. Fatigue and fitness modelled from the effects of training on performance. *Eur J Appl Physiol* 1994;69:50–54.
77. Fitz-Clarke JR, Morton RH, Banister EW. Optimizing athletic performance by influence curves. *J Appl Physiol* 1991;71:1151–1158.
78. Morton RH. Modelling training and overtraining. *J Sports Sci* 1997;15:335–340.
79. Neufer PD. The effect of detraining and reduced training on the physiological adaptations to aerobic exercise training. *Sports Med* 1989;8:302–321.
80. Busso T, Hakkinen K, Pakarinen A, et al. A systems model of training responses and its relationship to hormonal responses in elite weightlifters. *Eur J Appl Physiol* 1990;61:48–54.

81. Hopkins WG. Quantification of training in competitive sports: methods and applications. *Sports Med* 1991;12:161–183.
82. Galun E, Burstein R, Tur-Kaspa I, Assia E, Epstein Y. Prediction of physical performance through muscle enzymes activity. *Eur J Appl Physiol* 1988;57:597–600.
83. Banister EW, Morton RH, Fitz-Clarke J. Dose/response effects of exercise modelled from training: physical and biochemical measures. *Ann Physiol Anthropol* 1992;11:345–356.
84. Banister EW, Hamilton CL. Variation in iron status with fatigue modelled from training in female distance runners. *Eur J Appl Physiol* 1985;54:16–23.
85. Busso T, Hakkinen K, Pakarinen A, Kauhanen H, Komi PV, Lacour JR. Hormonal adaptations and modelled responses in elite weightlifters during 6 weeks of training. *Eur J Appl Physiol* 1992;64:381–386.
86. Adlercreutz H, Härkönen M, Kuoppasalmi K, et al. Effect of training on plasma anabolic and catabolic steroid hormones and their response during physical exercise. *Int J Sports Med* 1986;7:S27–S28.
87. Rowbottom DG, Keast D, Morton AR. The emerging role of glutamine as an indicator of exercise stress and overtraining. *Sports Med* 1996;21:80–97.

PART V

Sports Biomechanics

Exercise and Sport Science,
edited by William E. Garrett, Jr., and Donald T. Kirkendall.
Lippincott Williams & Wilkins, Philadelphia © 2000.

CHAPTER 35

Biomechanics of Cycling

Robert J. Gregor

Cycling is a popular form of exercise used for aerobic conditioning, as a competitive sport, and as a rehabilitation modality in physical therapy. In competition, the major focus is on maximal performance, in which the rider assumes an aerodynamic position designed to minimize wind drag and maximize energy input to the crank. Research on elite competitive cyclists usually focuses on factors such as (a) the physiologic and mechanical response to changes in work load and/or power output, and (b) the effects of body position and frame setup on performance. When the bicycle is used as aerobic exercise, the primary focus is on comfort, safety, and the ability to regulate resistance in accommodating a broad range of individual demands. The stationary bicycle is commonly used as a form of aerobic exercise for weight loss and cardiac rehabilitation, and the rider can often be in a recumbent position. In rehabilitation, a major focus is on providing a safe environment that adequately challenges each patient or athlete recovering from injury. In designing a rehabilitation program, the physical therapist or trainer must have specific knowledge of the injury or disability as well as a good understanding of cycling mechanics to regulate, appropriately, the demands placed on the patient to maximize the rehabilitation program and to limit further trauma. The bike uniquely combines lower-extremity strengthening, range of motion, and cardiovascular conditioning in addition to controlling joint, tendon, and ligament stress. Bicycle components can be adjusted to meet the requirements of an individual at his or her stage of training or rehabilitation. The extent of lower-limb loading, which can be regulated by the resistance setting, pedaling cadence, and seat-height changes, also offers the potential for objective measurements to document progress. This benefit can then be applied to both exercise/training and rehabilitation.

R.J. Gregor: Department of Health and Performance Sciences, and Center for Human Movement Studies, The Georgia Institute of Technology, Atlanta, Georgia 30332-0110.

The primary focus of this chapter is to provide information related to the mechanics of the rider/bicycle interface with emphasis on the lower extremities as they assume the primary role in transmission of power to the bicycle. Major sections of information include common chronic injuries, cycling kinematics, muscle-activity patterns with electromyography, and lower-limb kinetics related to human power output and mechanical work.

COMMON CYCLING OVERUSE INJURIES

Several factors might contribute to overuse injuries in repetitive endurance sports such as cycling. They include insufficient warm-up and cool-down and abrupt changes in exercise duration, intensity, and frequency, leading to muscle and tendon strain. Appropriate training programs should provide gradual increases in duration, intensity, and frequency. Lack of strength and flexibility also appear to be related to injury and can be a significant factor in overuse injuries in cycling. For example, if an individual goes on a long ride that involves hill climbs and high-power outputs and maintains a seated position, there will be concentrated loading of hip, knee, and ankle joints in a limited range of joint motion. Because the exercise involves high intensity in this limited range, it would be important for the rider to stretch both before and after this long bout of exercise to improve flexibility and minimize cumulative trauma.

Cycling-specific parameters, which increase risk of injury, include poor riding habits, excessive hill training, excessive early-season mileage, pushing big gears at low revolutions/minute, incorrect bike size, and cleat malalignments (1,2). In the past, corrective techniques for cyclists with chronic lower-extremity ailments have been limited to trial-and-error modifications in areas of training intensity, rider–bicycle geometry adjustment, shoe-cleat adjustment, and in-shoe orthotics. Baker (3) cites several contributors to overuse injuries, with a major concern focused on position adjustment on the bicycle. Adjusting seat, crank, and handlebars is important in minimizing the accumulation of trauma resulting in overuse injuries. Many general anatomic classifications of overuse injuries that have been reported in the literature include tendonitis, bursitis, compression neuropathy, neck pain, scapula syndrome, cyclists' palsy (ulnar neuropathy), carpal tunnel syndrome, and low-back pain (3). There also have been reports of neck and back pain, especially when assuming aero and advanced-aero positions on the bicycle, with numerous studies documenting ulnar neuropathy and saddle-related ailments, pudendal neuropathies, and perineum irritations (4). Low-back and neck pain become apparent for obvious reasons, but most of the major overuse injuries involve the hip, knee, and ankle. This is not to minimize proper back support and training and the use of proper neck exercises to minimize loads on the neck in these aero positions, but most of the most profound injuries occur in the lower extremities, which obviously produce the highest loads and experience the greatest amount of load on connective tissue structures and muscle.

Foot and Ankle Injuries

Incidence of serious overuse injuries to the ankle and foot appears to be low. Compression of the digital nerves of the foot as a result of excessively tight shoes and/or toe clips and straps has been known to cause numbness and temporary paraesthesia. Management of this problem usually entails periodically loosening the shoes and straps, while cycling, as a method of relief. Modern clipless (float) pedals eliminate the pressure of the toe-clip and strap on the top surface of the forefoot, which may have contributed to the design of the clipless pedal systems.

Pedal size is another factor, especially when related to the high levels of force acting on the foot. Increased localized pressure from the pedal through the shoe also can be a problem and is related to the stiffness of the sole of the shoe. There is a trade-off between the need for a stiff sole to distribute pressure and the need to maintain enough compliance to allow some natural foot movement. Sanderson (5) recognized the importance of shoe design to ensure safety, comfort, and effective transmission of force to the crank. Size and weight appear to be important performance parameters, but concentrated areas of pressure during long rides do little to benefit the cyclist and can lead to chronic injury problems. Pressure distribution on the sole of the shoe during cycling is presented in the section on Cycling Kinetics, page 525.

Baker (3) also discussed several overuse injuries in the foot and ankle and listed, specifically, tibialis anterior (TA) tendonitis, Achilles tendonitis, Achilles bursitis, plantar fasciitis, and foot or toe numbness as major problems from prolonged overuse in cycling. Length of crank, position of the foot on the pedal, and saddle height all affect these various chronic problems associated with ankle and foot function during cycling.

Mellion (4) also suggested that ankle tendonitis may be relieved through adjustments of the shoe–pedal interface (consideration was also given the floating-pedal system). He further suggested that Achilles tendonitis and plantar fasciitis can develop if the saddle is too low, forcing pronounced dorsiflexion. In addition, Francis (6) described foot structural malalignments, including forefoot and rearfoot varus and valgus, but inferred that these problems may have greater influence on knee kinematics and subsequent knee pain. Francis (6) did not discuss the implications of pedal design, but only the potential for orthotics placed in the shoe to benefit knee function. Orthotics, as they relate to different types of float designs, also warrant attention because the foot–pedal interface receives the highest forces from the environment as they enter the leg. The potential influence of pedal-reaction forces and torsional moments at the pedal are discussed on page 525 in the section on Cycling Kinetics.

Knee Injuries and Knee Pain

Knee pain, resulting from improper mechanics and repetitive loading, remains the most common overuse problem at all levels of cycling (1,7,8,9). Knee injuries in cycling include chondromalacia patella, quadriceps tendonitis, patellar tendonitis, iliotibial band syndrome, retropatellar or prepatellar bursitis, pes anserinus bursitis, infrapatellar fat-pad syndrome, medial capsule strain and inflammation of the synovial plica, and medial or lateral collateral ligament sprain; a more detailed review is available in the literature (3,8).

The primary factor influencing knee mechanics and the subsequent potential for tissue damage is the interface between the rider and bicycle, which includes shoe-cleat alignment, seat height and fore–aft adjustment, crank length, and trunk position designed to minimize wind drag. Secondary factors relate to individual pedaling technique, structural variations between cyclists, and anatomic asymmetries between right and left sides. Structural asymmetries result in individual variations in bike setup and selective modifications of equipment components.

Holmes and colleagues (1) studied 134 cyclists over a 5-year period for complaints of chronic knee pain. All were evaluated by using standard clinical orthopedic examinations including radiographs when needed. The most common form of knee pain (64%) was reported as anterior knee pain, specifically chondromalacia patella and patellar tendonitis. In a survey of cycling and knee pain, Gregor and Wheeler (8) reported overuse injuries and shoe/pedal-type data collected from 168 riders. Sixty percent of the respondents to a detailed questionnaire were experienced racers and reported anterior knee pain, especially retropatellar, to be the most frequently identified location of pain. These complaints were followed by complaints of lateral knee pain and then pain on the medial side of the knee.

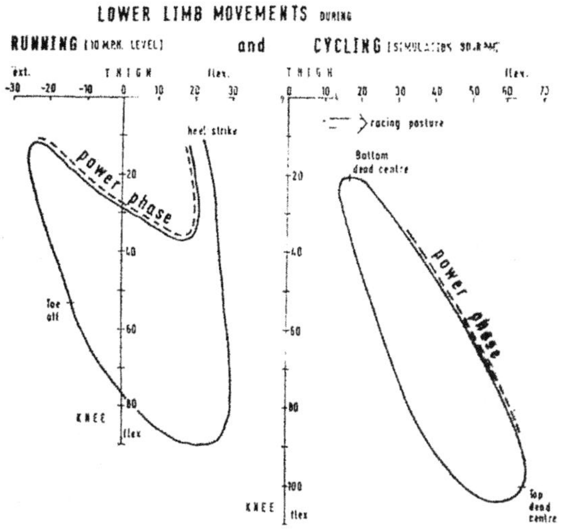

FIG. 35–1. Angle/angle diagram for the thigh and knee during running and cycling. Power phase is from 0 degrees to 180 degrees of the pedaling cycle and from heel strike to toe-off during running.

Hip Injuries

Overuse hip injuries from cycling are rare and consequently not well documented in the literature. Mellion (4) suggested that trochanteric bursitis and iliopsoas tendonitis may develop when the seat is set too high. Apparently very few cyclists are set up with excessively high seat positions for extended periods, which may partially account for the lack of reported cases of chronic hip ailments. Chronic hip problems may relate more to high-load pedaling in limited ranges of motion, lack of joint flexibility, and joint stiffness.

CYCLING KINEMATICS

Discussion of the kinematic patterns of the lower extremities during cycling usually focuses on the rhythmic, alternating movement of the legs, operating in some "optimal" range of motion designed to yield maximal benefit from the mechanical properties of the muscles involved (i.e., skeletal muscles in the lower extremities used to energize the bicycle). In some cases, individuals consider cycling to be very similar to other tasks (e.g., running) that also involve rhythmic alternating movement of the legs. To highlight the unique demands imposed by the cycling task on the legs, discussion of cycling kinematics begins with a simple comparison with running (Fig. 35–1). These data show distinct differences in the range of motion and relative position of the thigh and leg between these two tasks. These differences are of special interest during the power phase (between 0 degrees and 180 degrees of crank rotation for cycling and the stance phase between foot contact and toe-off in running). Among the many differences noted in these data, two are considered significant. They are (a) the thigh never extends beyond a vertical position in cycling but definitely extends well beyond the vertical position in running (the vertical position is 0 degrees), and (b) the knee continuously extends during the power phase in cycling, as the hip extends, but experiences a distinct "yield" phase during running in which the knee flexes during weight acceptance in early stance. The fundamental differences in kinematics are a result of the constrained versus unconstrained nature of cycling and running, respectively, and the very different kinetics during the power phases of these two activities. For example, as discussed in the section on muscle activity during cycling, the quads are active early in the power phase in both activities but are placed in stretch during running but not during cycling. The result is a very different experience for the leg musculature and is discussed below as we explore the unique kinetics of the cycling task.

Most reports on cycling kinematics are limited to the sagittal plane: hip and knee flexion and extension and ankle dorsiflexion and plantar flexion. In this limited setup, displacements, velocities, and accelerations of the thigh, leg, and foot appear to be most affected by cadence and bicycle setup (e.g., seat height, fore–aft position on the seat, crank length, and foot position on the pedal). In general, trunk inclination appears to have little effect on leg kinematics (effects of the aero and advanced-aero positions on cycling kinetics are discussed on page 525, in the section on Cycling Kinetics). The complex interactions between bicycle geometry and rider performance and attempts to "optimize" the bicycle–rider system have been the subjects of many studies that evaluate changes in kinematic output resulting from systematic variation in bicycle configuration (10). One fact, however, is relatively clear: once the constrained cyclic movement of the lower extremity is established at a seat position and crank length comfortable to the rider, lower-extremity kinematic patterns remain relatively constant. Pushing extreme gears on high load may further modify rider kinematics, but for the most part, in a seated position across a range of loads, rider kinematics are relatively stable.

Limiting their analysis to the sagittal plane, Faria and Cavanagh (11) reported a total excursion during one pedaling cycle of 45 degrees for the thigh, 75 degrees for the knee, and 20 degrees for the ankle. Data from our own laboratory (12) (see Fig. 35–1) demonstrate the effect of seat-height changes on hip and knee range of motion as seat height varied from 100% to 115% of pubic symphysis height (height measured from the pubic symphysis, or crotch, to the floor). Related to these data, it appears that many road riders choose between 106% and 109% of pubic symphysis height as their most comfortable seat position.

As observed in Fig. 35–2, the general pattern for hip- and knee-angle changes remained relatively constant across the four seat-height conditions. Whereas peak knee extension increased as seat height increased to a greater degree than peak hip extension, peak hip flexion and extension always seemed to occur at approximately 10 degrees and 180 degrees of the pedaling cycle, respectively. In contrast, peak knee flexion and extension seemed to occur at approximately 350 degrees and 170 degrees of the pedaling cycle. Other studies in our laboratory at lower seat-height conditions (96% to 108% of pubic symphysis height) provided results identical to the patterns described in Fig. 35–2. In addition, all data indicated that the knee joint was most affected by changes in seat height, with other joints less affected.

The profound effects of seat-height changes on knee-joint range of motion are supported by results from Ericson and colleagues (13). Data from their study show knee-joint range of motion to be at least 20 degrees greater than either the hip or the ankle at a "low" seat height, and almost 50 degrees greater than either the hip or the ankle at the "high" seat-height condition. In addition, it appears that the knee flexes to a greater degree at the low seat-height condition and extends to a greater degree at the high seat-height condition (13). Although hip range of motion changed less dramatically, the thigh was generally more extended at the high seat height, placing muscles that cross both the hip and the knee in a potentially different range of length than when they function at lower seat-height conditions. Although we discuss kinematics with respect to hip, knee, and ankle joints in this section, it is important to remember the potential effects these kinematic changes may have on the surrounding musculature. The range of joint motion will affect the range of shortening and/or lengthening of individual muscles, but the absolute range within which they shorten or lengthen (e.g., with respect to resting muscle length) also will be affected by the angles through which each joint proceeds during the cyclic movement of the lower extremity. The obvious result is an effect on force-production capabilities of these individual muscles as it relates to their length–tension curve, both active and passive, and their individual force–velocity curves. These considerations are discussed again in later sections of this chapter related to muscle-length change and joint kinetics.

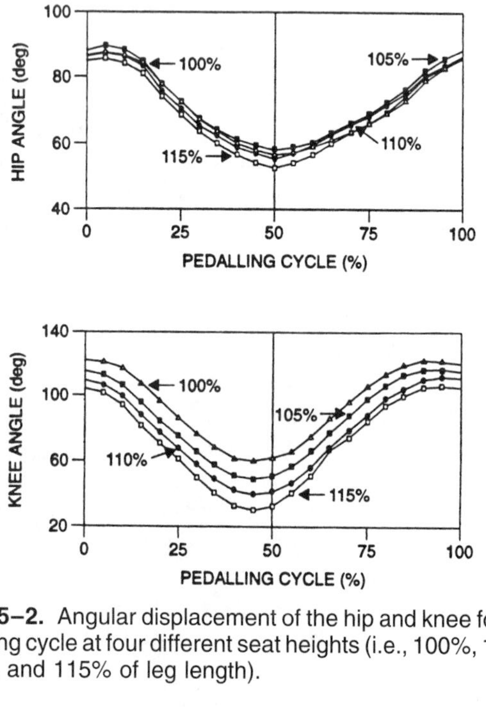

FIG. 35–2. Angular displacement of the hip and knee for one pedaling cycle at four different seat heights (i.e., 100%, 105%, 110%, and 115% of leg length).

Although the cycling task has been considered, historically, a planar movement, over the past several years significant information has been presented related to the three-dimensional nature of the cycling task. For example, information concerning internal and external rotation of the tibia about its long axis, translation of the knee in the frontal plane, and movement of the lower extremity outside the sagittal plane have all been reported (9). Movement of the knee in the frontal plane has been reported by McCoy (14), Ruby and colleagues (15), and Boutin and co-workers (16), with results indicating that the knee may move as much as 6 cm in the frontal plane during one pedaling cycle. Movement of the knee in the sagittal and frontal planes is presented in Fig. 35–3 for a single subject pedaling at 90 rpm at 250 W. These data show considerable movement of the knee in the frontal plane. It appears that at the beginning of the pedaling cycle (0 degrees), the femur adducts as the lower extremity proceeds through the power phase. The knee moves medially with respect to the pedal, while the tibia rotates inwardly as the foot pronates. Rotational components about the long axis of each segment are considerably more difficult to measure than are translateral ones, but allowing these natural rotational movements to take place with minimal constraint (i.e., at the pedal) will have a marked effect on joint forces and tissue stresses. The evolution of the floating pedal, for example, is testimony to the need to allow normal kinematic movement of the limb, especially during the power phase, when joint loads and pedal forces are high.

Cycling is an individual activity, and the concept of

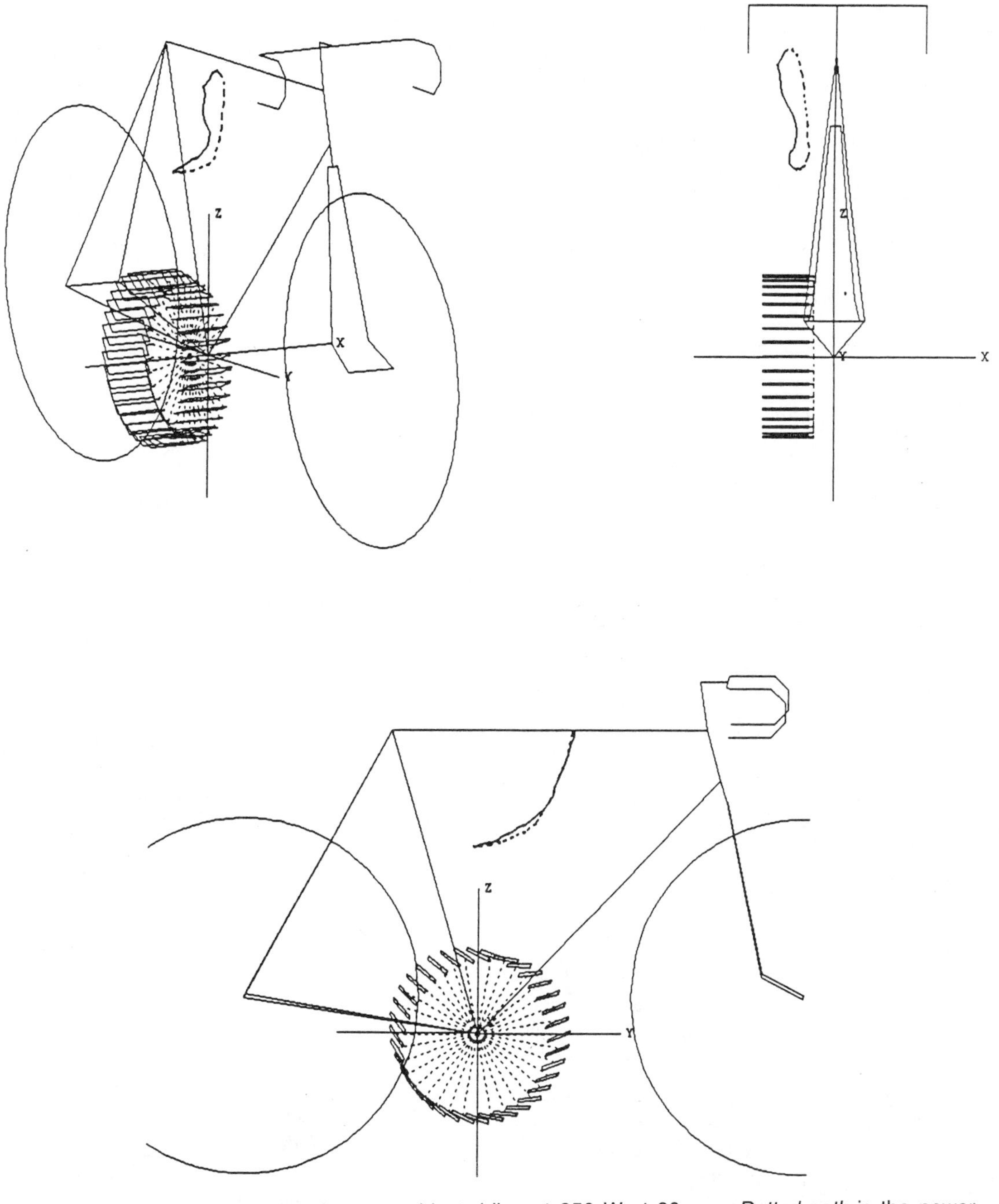

FIG. 35–3. Knee-joint pattern for one subject riding at 250 W at 90 rpm. *Dotted path* is the power phase, whereas the *solid line* is the recovery phase.

knee pain is vague. With recent improvements in cycling equipment and knowledge of cycling mechanics, however, injuries and trauma to the lower extremities are, we hope, becoming less profound. Kinematics and subsequently kinetics are affected by bike geometry and work load, with questions related to how much movement should be allowed to minimize unnecessary loads on muscle and connective tissue structures remaining open to discussion. Hannaford and associates (9) reported that subjects without knee problems showed less transverse and frontal plane movement than did riders who had reported a history of knee pain. In support of these findings, Francis (6) reported less movement in the frontal plane in elite cyclists using in-shoe orthotics. Trial-and-error adjustments in pedal cant, together with video feedback, reduced frontal plane movement and seemed to reduce knee pain in elite cyclists (6). Although these data are interesting, the solution to these issues remains unclear. The actual fit-and-function test performed by the riders themselves when "setting up"

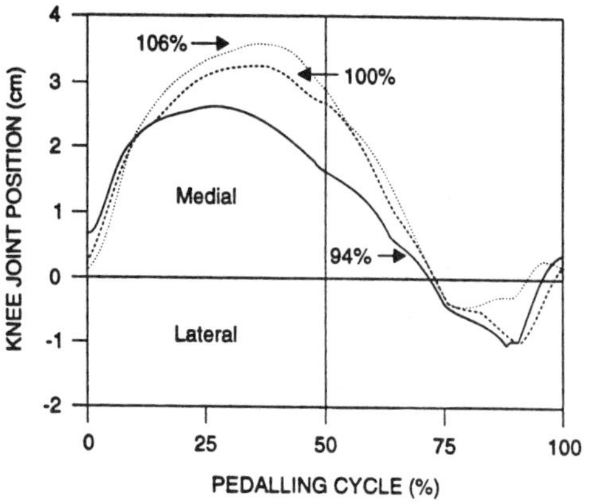

FIG. 35–4. Position of the knee, midknee joint, during the pedaling cycle with respect to the pedal center of pressure at three different seat heights (i.e., 94%, 100%, and 106% of leg length). Each curve is an average of 150 pedal revolutions (10 subjects × five trials) at 200 W and 80 rpm. From ref. 14, with permission.

their bicycle is probably the most important phase of injury prevention. In addition, the continuous updating of bicycle geometry to accommodate variation in training and/or rehabilitation protocols for injured athletes is also a major feature of performance, injury prevention, and injury rehabilitation.

In further support of the evidence that work load increases the frontal plane movement of the knee joint, McCoy (14) investigated the effects of different seat positions on lower-extremity frontal plane kinematics. Seat height varied from 94% to 106% of leg length, with the greatest magnitude of knee-joint excursion observed at approximately 90 degrees of crank rotation at the low seat height and 150 degrees of crank rotation at the medium and high seat heights. Data presented in Fig. 35–4 show knee-joint position with respect to the pedal center of pressure in the frontal plane. (The concept of center of pressure and the details of this type of analysis, as well as its significance to joint kinetics, are presented later in this chapter.) The importance of these data lies in the fact that the knee joint is medial to the center of pressure during the entire power phase, and that the degree to which the knee deviates medially increases as seat height increases. These results suggest that knee-joint excursion in the frontal plane is always medial to the center of pressure during the power phase, and that the range of motion in the frontal plane for the knee joint increases as seat height increases. Although their measurements were referenced to the center of the pedal and not the center of pressure, Ruby and colleagues (17) reported data similar to those presented in Fig. 35–4.

Muscle-Length Changes

Understanding kinematics of cycling with specific reference to the effects of bicycle geometry on lower-extremity movement is only the first step in understanding how the human body energizes the bicycle. It is obvious that bicycle geometry affects limb trajectories and that muscles within the limbs are affected by ranges of motion (i.e., kinematic patterns). To begin to understand the interface between the rider and the bicycle and the demands placed on the rider, we must understand how muscles in the legs function during the cycling task. Furthermore, we must understand how changes in bicycle geometry and limb trajectory influence the length change and velocity patterns and subsequently the muscles' ability to produce a force. Muscle length, velocity, architecture, activation, and history all affect their ability to produce force. Although we have little to do with the architecture of the muscle, changes in bicycle geometry will definitely affect the length and velocity through which muscles move as they produce force to energize the bike. Indeed, understanding muscle function is the bridge to understanding joint kinetics.

Range of motion information and hence knowledge of muscle-length and velocity changes are important to our understanding of muscle injury as well. Knowledge of environmental demands imposed on the muscle, or, more specifically, the operating conditions under which the muscle must produce force to energize the bike, is important when understanding muscle injury and chronic trauma. For example, after acute injuries, rehabilitation should begin with exercises that minimize muscle-length changes, especially when muscle is active, as muscle-length changes will increase tension on the healing structures.

With angular kinematics and lower-extremity anatomy, estimates of length changes of all major lower-extremity muscle-tendon units were reported previously (10,12,16). Exemplar data for different seat-height conditions are presented in Figs. 35–5 and 35–6 for the vastii and hamstring muscle groups, respectively, at seat heights between 100% and 115% of leg length (12). The zero line in each case is referenced to the hip and knee positioned at 90 degrees, a different convention from that reported in Fig. 35–1, in which cycling was compared with running. Results on the vastii and hamstring muscles clearly indicate that changes in seat height markedly affect muscle-length patterns and further support the fact that as seat height increases, muscle-tendon unit shortening and lengthening velocities increase. For example, as seat height increases at a constant cadence, the vastii muscles experience greater shortening as the knee extends toward total limb extension. In contrast to the knee extensors, the hamstring muscles show initial lengthening before shortening, less shortening in the 115% versus 100% condition, and qualitatively similar velocities in each condition. Furthermore, the velocities of the single joint vastii are usually higher in similar conditions than are those of their flexor antagonists, the biarticular hamstrings. The general patterns for the

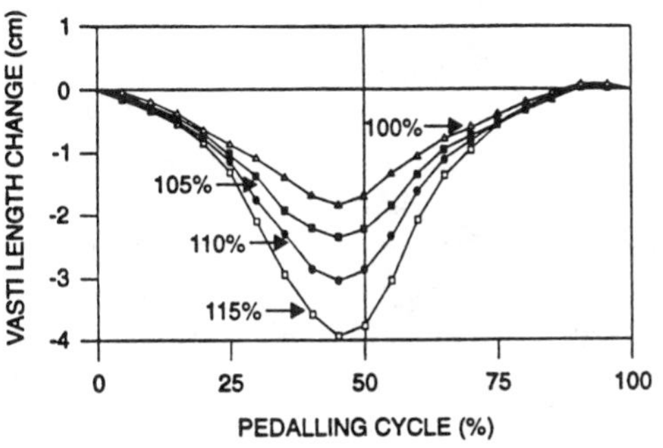

FIG. 35–5. Patterns of muscle-tendon unit length change during the pedaling cycle for the vasti group (vastus lateralis and medialis) at four different seat heights (i.e., 100%, 105%, 110%, and 115% of leg length). The *zero line* represents the muscle length with the hip and knee at 90 degrees. *Negative slopes* indicate muscle-tendon unit shortening.

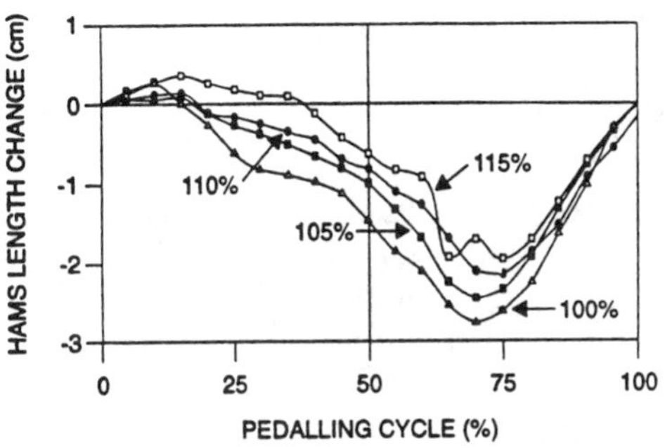

FIG. 35–6. Patterns of muscle-tendon unit length change during the pedaling cycle for the hamstring group (all biarticular muscles) at four different seat heights (i.e., 100%, 105%, 110%, and 115% of leg length). The *zero line* represents the length with the hip and knee at 90 degrees. *Negative slopes* indicate muscle-tendon unit shortening.

hamstring muscles presented in Fig. 35–6 are supported in the literature (18–20).

Muscle-length change patterns for both the gastrocnemius and soleus muscles are presented in Figs. 35–7 and 35–8, respectively, and indicate that changes in seat height affect the magnitude of length change in the soleus more than in the gastrocnemius; the soleus muscle lengthens up to about 90 degrees in the pedaling cycle, but shows marked differences in shortening patterns for the remainder of the power phase as seat height increases. The velocities of shortening markedly increase in the 108% condition above both the 96% and 102% conditions. Differences in subsequent shortening for the remainder of the recovery phase are all quite different for the three seat heights and indicate that, whatever increases in the range of motion take place at the ankle, these changes markedly affect the length and velocity changes of the soleus muscle and ultimately its force-production capability.

In contrast to the soleus muscle, we see quite similar patterns of lengthening for the gastrocnemius, but subsequent changes in shortening affected by seat height. Because the gastrocnemius length change is dictated by both the knee and the ankle, the only real differences between seat-height conditions lie at the end of the power phase and the beginning of the recovery phase, with the most marked difference, again, at the 108% pubic symphysis height condition. These patterns of muscle-length change also are supported in the literature (18–20).

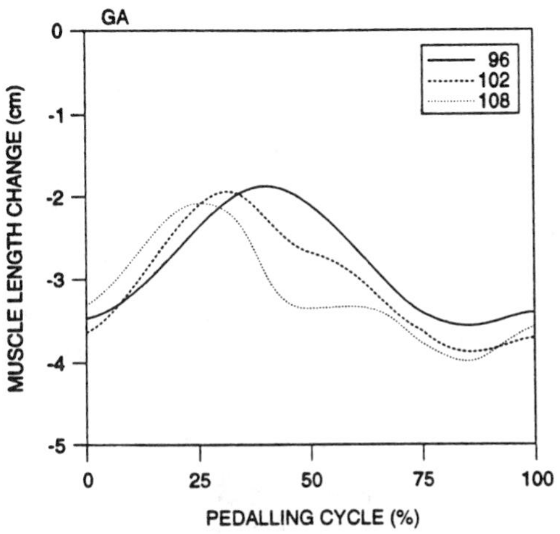

FIG. 35–7. Patterns of muscle-tendon unit length changes during the pedaling cycle for the gastrocnemius muscle (both medial and lateral head) at three different seat heights (i.e., 96%, 102%, and 108% of pubic symphysis height. The *zero line* represents the length in the anatomic position. *Negative slopes* indicate muscle-tendon unit shortening.

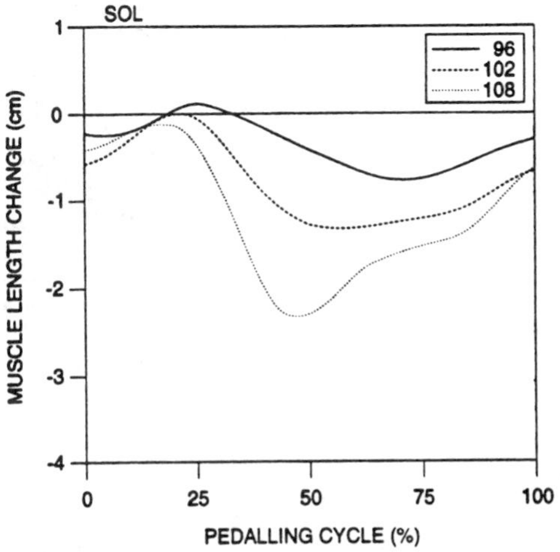

FIG. 35–8. Patterns of muscle-tendon unit length changes during the pedaling cycle for the soleus muscle at three different seat heights (i.e., 96%, 102%, and 108% of public symphysis height. The *zero line* represents the length in the anatomic position. *Negative slopes* indicate muscle-tendon unit shortening.

MUSCLE ACTIVITY DURING CYCLING

Patterns of muscle activation (electromyography; EMG) provide information about how the central nervous system controls movement. These data are important to our understanding of movement sequences. Muscle-recruitment patterns during cycling have been reported for major lower-extremity muscles by using both surface and fine-wire EMG (21–25). Activity patterns are most commonly described relative to crank angle, where, in general, the greatest activity seems to occur during the propulsive phase, when almost all of the energy needed to drive the bicycle is imparted to the crank.

Data presented in Fig. 35–9 represent 15 pedaling cycles from each of 18 experienced cyclists (270 pedaling cycles) riding a racing bicycle at 90 rpm and 250 W. The bicycle was set up to mimic the conditions for their own bicycles and, consequently, minimized adjustments required by the rider in the laboratory. The patterns represent 10 major muscles, but few data are available in the literature on muscles such as adductors, single-joint hip flexors, the tensor fasciae latae, or sartorius. For the most part, muscles are studied with respect to single and biarticular functions primarily as flexors and extensors of the joints.

In reviewing the data in Fig. 35–9, several observations become clear. First, single-joint extensors [i.e., gluteus maximus, soleus, vastus lateralis (VL) and vastus medialis (VM)] generate the greatest electrical output during the power phase (0 degrees to 180 degrees). In fact, data from our laboratory (25) indicate that the single-joint knee extensors (VM and VL) are temporally identical across this population of cyclists. A second feature of these patterns is that the single-joint flexors [i.e., the tibialis anterior (TA)] show the greatest activity during the recovery phase. This increased activity is obviously in preparation for the subsequent power phase, which begins at 0 degrees of the pedaling cycle. A third observation is that the hamstring muscles, presented as a group, show their greatest activity between 90 degrees and 135 degrees of the pedaling cycle. In short, the hamstring muscles are coactive with the knee and hip extensors, but have a phase lag in time of their peak activity.

All biarticular muscles appear to have patterns that are more variable than those of single-joint muscles. For example, the rectus femoris, which acts at both the knee and the hip, shows a great deal of activity in the power phase as a knee extensor acting with the vastii muscles. A large amount of activity, however, also is observed during recovery, which indicates its importance to hip flexion during the recovery phase in preparation for the subsequent power phase. The final interesting feature relates to the biarticular gastrocnemius muscle, which, although active during the power phase, has a phase lag to the maximal activity seen in the soleus. The reasoning behind this phase lag in peak activity of the gastrocnemius will become apparent when we discuss joint moments in the subsequent section.

In summary, the major points regarding muscle activation during the cycling task are: (a) coactivation of knee flexors and extensors appears during the first 90 degrees of the pedaling cycle, whereas the hamstrings and gastrocnemius muscles continue activation through the second quadrant and actually past bottom dead center; (b) single-joint muscle activity is much more consistent across subjects than is biarticular muscle activity; and (c) almost all muscles begin activity during a muscle-stretch phase of the pedaling cycle. That is, activity begins before top dead center when muscles are typically being stretched, and activity typically ends before the muscle has completed its shortening during the power phase.

Differences between EMG patterns reported in the literature and those shown in Fig. 35–9 may result from variations in electrode preparation and placement, individual differences within and between rider populations (experienced vs. novice riders), differences in rider–bicycle configuration, and the various methods of data collection and reduction, which include use of surface electrodes and/or fine-wire electrodes. For example, Ryan and Gregor (25) reported patterns of muscle activity in the hamstring muscles by using fine-wire electrodes. Data were compared with those of Ericson and colleagues (22), Jorge and Hull (24), and Gregor and co-workers (26), with specific reference to the output of the biceps femoris muscle. Two distinct patterns were reported in this muscle regardless of different electrode preparations. In other words, whether fine-wire or surface electrodes were used, two patterns emerged for the biceps femoris, supporting the fact that individual differences do exist.

Electromyography and Seat Height

The effect of seat height on EMG patterns in selected lower-extremity muscles has received a great deal of attention (21–24). Although it is difficult to compare directly the effects of seat-height changes across different studies, it is generally agreed that muscle activity increases as seat height decreases, especially in the quadriceps and hamstring muscle groups. For example, Houtz and Fischer (23) reported that a higher seat height allowed the subjects to pedal with greater ease, particularly at higher work loads.

Ericson and associates (22), in contrast to the general opinion that high seat heights reduce muscle activity, reported that the gluteus medius, semimembranosus, and medial gastrocnemius increased activity at high seat heights, with insignificant changes in the remaining muscles studied. An accurate comparison of seat-height measurement technique, referenced to specific anatomic

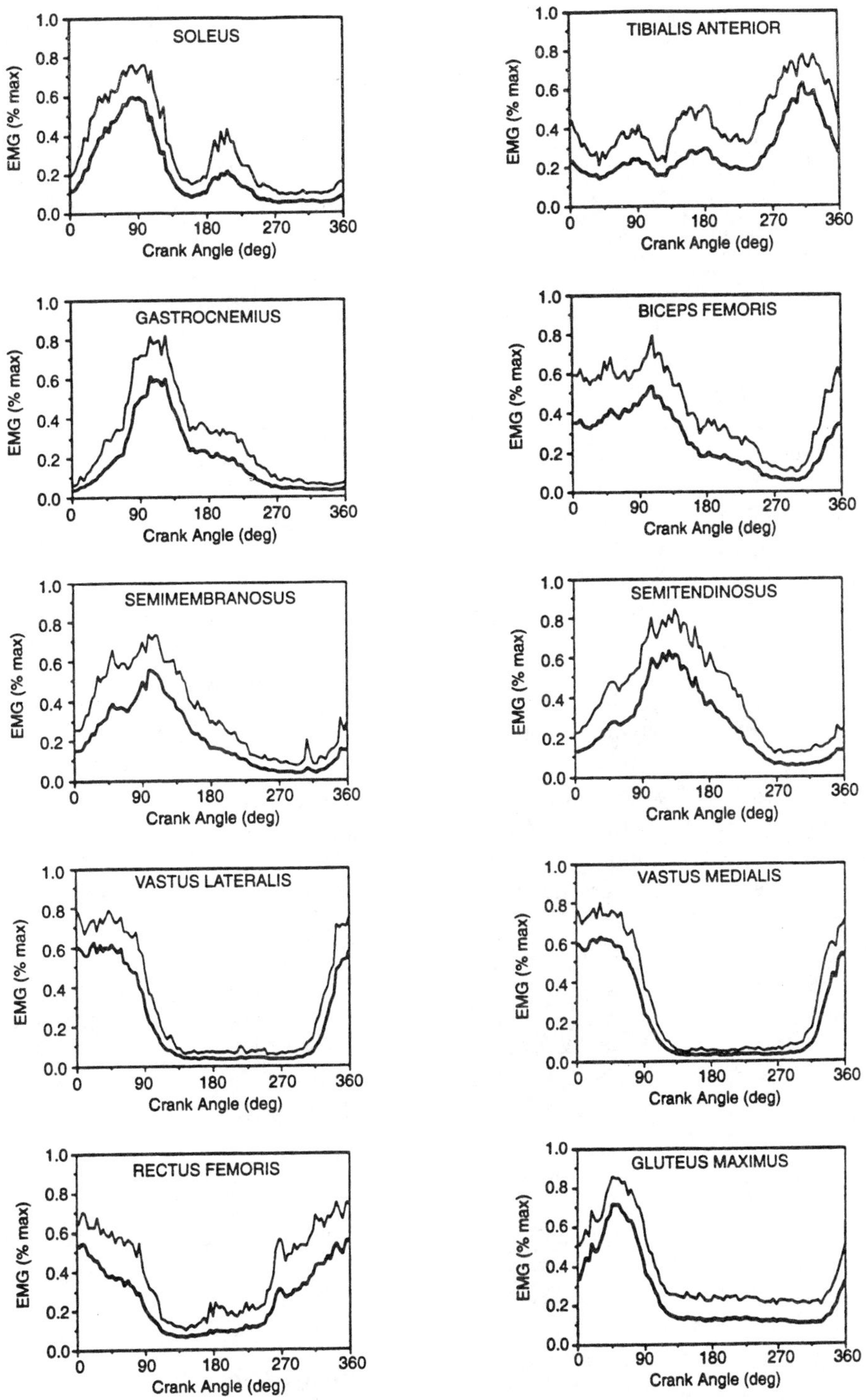

FIG. 35–9. Mean patterns of muscle activation during the pedaling cycle for 10 muscles in the lower extremities. The *darker lower curve* is the average pattern from 15 pedaling cycles across 18 subjects (270 cycles), and the *lighter upper curve* is one standard deviation above the mean. Magnitudes are normalized to maximal activation. From ref. 25, with permission.

features, may be required to resolve the reported differences. Phase shifts in muscle activation resulting from changes in seat height also were reported by Desipres (21), but other researchers (22–24) described no phase changes in EMG.

Electromyography and Cadence

Patterns of muscle activity in major flexors and extensors in the lower extremities are expected to change with modifications in cadence. Ericson and colleagues

(22) and Goto and co-workers (27) reported increased muscle activity in the gluteus maximus, VL, semitendinosus, semimembranosus, gastrocnemius, soleus, and TA as cadence increased from 40 rpm to 100 rpm. Although the rectus femoris (RF) and biceps femoris (BF) muscles exhibited similar increased activity at higher cadence, the changes were not significant. Additionally, Suzuki and colleagues (28), studying EMG patterns between 12 rpm and 60 rpm, reported that RF and BF activity began progressively earlier in the pedaling cycle as cadence increased, each exhibiting double bursts of activity at the higher cadences generally attributed to the muscle's biarticular function. The medial gastrocnemius shifted in phase as cadence increased, but little change in timing was observed in the VM and TA. Suzuki (29) suggested that a preferential and selective activation of faster-twitch fibers occurs as cadence increases. This observation is supported by Duchateau and associates (30) in a study on the contribution of slow and fast muscles of the triceps surae to a cyclic movement. Studying changes in magnitude and phase of the soleus and medial gastrocnemius muscles, this group of investigators observed a linear increase in soleus integrated EMG, with increasing load at a constant speed of 60 rpm, with no change noted in the medial gastrocnemius integrated EMG below 40 N of force. In contrast, when the pedaling speed was increased from 30 rpm to 170 rpm at a constant load, medial gastrocnemius integrated EMG displayed the largest increase. In addition, although both muscles' EMGs appeared earlier in the movement, with increases in load and/or speed, the delay between the onset of both EMGs remained unchanged at constant speed, and synchronization of the medial gastrocnemius and soleus was observed only when the speed was increased above 140 rpm. The conclusion suggests that different muscles in the triceps surae make different contributions to the development of mechanical tension required to maintain or increase the speed of movement and that this is related to the muscle-fiber type of the two different muscles.

Recently there has been considerable interest in acceleration pedaling and the effects this might have on the timing of EMG output in major muscles in the lower extremities. Welter and co-workers (31) and Neptune and colleagues (32) reported the effect of pedaling rate on the coordination in cycling. Both studies concluded that, as pedaling rate increased, EMG activity in major muscles in the lower extremities began earlier in the pedaling cycle. Welter and co-workers (31) thought these activity changes were aimed at exploiting inertial effects. It appeared that movements were regulated by the continuously changing flow of proprioceptive information, but it appeared unlikely that feedback was used in triggering and shaping activity on an ongoing basis. Neptune and colleagues (32) thought that large increases observed in EMG activity represented a pedaling-rate sensitivity possibly related to coping with increasing magnitude of velocity-dependent interaction forces (inertial effects) arising either between individual limb segments or at the crank. In summary, both studies concluded that during acceleration pedaling, the high-velocity inertial dependence created a situation in which muscle activity was needed earlier in the cycle to control limb movement.

Electromyography and Work Load

Most studies reported increasing work load by increasing resistance at a constant cadence. At higher loads, EMG magnitudes are expected to be greater, with timing of activation remaining relatively constant. Houtz and Fischer (23) supported this finding in nine major lower-extremity muscles. Ericson and associates (22) varied ergometer work load from 0 to 240 W at constant cadence (60 rpm) and also found EMG magnitudes in 10 major lower-extremity muscles increased with increased work loads, whereas Goto and co-workers (27) reported similar findings for the gluteus maximus, VL, gastrocnemius, and TA. There was no reference in either of these studies, however, to the effect of work load on activation timing.

Jorge and Hull (24) assessed EMG differences as work load changed by varying gear ratios at a constant pedaling rate on a laboratory bicycle on rollers. At lower power levels (83 and 100 W), timing and magnitude of activity appeared insensitive to changes in work load (17 W). Hamstrings and the TA displayed greater activity at 83 W than at 100 W. Their data were averaged for six subjects and, consequently, these trends may not represent individual pattern sensitivity to work load. Interestingly, Jorge and Hull (24) state that the greatest variability between subjects, most noticeable in the hamstring group and TA, could be attributed to differences in pedaling technique. As work load increased to 125 W the magnitude of activity in all muscles except the gastrocnemius increased substantially. These data support those of Houtz and Fisher (23), Ericson and co-workers (22), and Goto and colleagues (27).

Electromyography and Shoe–Pedal Interface

Cleated shoes and toe clips (or clipless pedals and associated shoes) permit the application of productive pedal forces through bottom dead center (pulling back) and into recovery (pulling up). Consequently, shoe–pedal interfaces may affect muscle-activation patterns. Ericson and associates (22) compared cycling with and without toe clips and found that muscle activity increased significantly in the RF, BF, and TA muscles when toe clips were used. In contrast, toe clips produced significantly lower activity levels in the vastii and soleus muscles, although the gluteal muscles and the gastrocnemius and medial hamstring muscles were not significantly different between conditions. Ericson and colleagues (22), however, did not evaluate the effect of cleated shoes on muscle activation, because only soft-soled shoes were used in their study.

The effects of cleated shoes with toe clips versus soft-soled shoes without toe clips were evaluated by Jorge and Hull (24), who reported that single-joint knee extensors (vastii and hamstring muscles) increased muscle activity during normal regions of peak activity with soft-soled shoes. Associated decreases in activity were reported in the gastrocnemius and the RF muscles. Although the isolated effect of the cleated cycling shoe in the toe–clip interface configuration is not known, current reports suggest that the addition of toe clips and cleated cycling shoes modifies the load-sharing distribution of lower-extremity muscles. The effect of the new clipless shoe–pedal interface on muscle-activity patterns, including those with rotational freedom about their vertical axes, has not been studied and warrants further investigation.

CYCLING KINETICS

Environmental Loads: Equation of Motion

In a complete biomechanical analysis of cycling, one becomes interested in the optimal integration between the rider and the bicycle. This integration involves muscular output from the cyclist and a complete understanding of the external forces and interactive forces from the bicycle that act on the rider. An equation of motion for each rider would reveal a balance between external forces and muscular output. The equation presented below describes the relationship between rider work and bicycle speed and was developed by considering five principal resistive elements: drive-train friction, inertial forces associated with acceleration of the bicycle, gravitational forces (e.g., climbing), tire-rolling resistance, and aerodynamic drag. The functional equation of motion for bicycle riding accounting for these five elements was presented by Broker (33) and takes the form:

$$P_{cyc} = P_{dt} + mVA_{cyc} + WV_{sin}\,(\text{ArctanG}) + WVCrr_1\cos\,(\text{ArctanG}) + NCrr_2V^2 + 1/2\,C_dA_pV(V = V_w)^2$$

where:
- P_{cyc} = the net instantaneous mechanical power produced by the rider
- P_{dt} = the power to overcome drive-train friction
- m = the mass of the rider and bicycle
- V = bicycle velocity
- A_{cyc} = instantaneous acceleration or deceleration of the bicycle/rider system
- W = the weight of the bicycle and rider
- G = the grade
- Crr_1 = the coefficient of static rolling resistance
- N = the number of wheels (in case a tricycle is analyzed)
- Crr_2 = the coefficient of dynamic rolling resistance
- C_d = the coefficient of aerodynamic drag
- A = the frontal surface area of the rider and bicycle
- D = the air density
- V_w = the velocity of the headwind or tailwind (positive for headwind)

In examining this equation, Broker (33) highlighted several important points. First, the mass of the rider and the bicycle is linearly related to the second, third, and fourth elements of the equation. In addition, power to offset dynamic rolling resistance is related to the fifth term in the equation, appears independent of rider and bicycle mass, and increases as the square of bicycle velocity. Finally, power to overcome aerodynamic drag increases as the third power of velocity, so doubling bicycle speed increases power to overcome aerodynamic drag forces by a factor of 8. We will not discuss further the general equation of motion involving the rider and the bicycle, but will instead focus our attention on the interactive and propulsive forces at contact points between the rider and the bicycle.

Interactive Forces: The Seat and Handlebars

To understand rider–bicycle interface completely, reaction forces at the handlebars, seat, and pedals must be measured. Several reports are available in the literature related to pedal forces, but few data are available on forces generated at the handlebars and seat. Soden and Adeyefa (34) and Bolourchi and Hull (35) have presented data on seat and handlebar forces. Soden and Adeyefa (34) were interested, primarily, in assessing the strength and performance of bicycle frames and made measurements on handlebar, seat, and pedal forces during starting, climbing, and steady-level cycling. These authors reported a net pull applied to the handlebars of 0.64 body weight (BW) during starting, with a maximal pull of 1.08 BW with one arm and a maximal push of 0.44 BW with the contralateral arm. These asymmetric forces offset the asymmetric loads applied to the pedals in an effort to begin forward movement of the bicycle. During climbing, a pulling force of 0.36 BW and a pushing of 0.27 BW were reported and compared with 0.11 BW reported during pulling and 0.17 BW during pushing, during steady-level cycling. The authors verified these estimates in the laboratory and on the road by using specially constructed pedals, with the differences between the theoretic values and the measured values typically less than 20% (34).

Bolourchi and Hull (35) measured the effect of pedaling rate on rider-induced loads. Varying cadence from 63 rpm to 110 rpm at a constant resistance, these authors reported handlebar and seat-load profiles independent of subject and cadence. It appears that handlebar forces peaked at 140 degrees of the pedaling cycle, and average horizontal seat forces were significantly related to cadence. Although reactive to pedal forces, other load components of the handlebars and seat were not significantly related to cadence. These studies are some of the few that report rider/bicycle interaction at the seat and the handlebars. Because most of the power is generated by the legs, however, the primary interactive forces reported in the literature involve pedal forces. The next section focuses on instrumentation and pedal-force profiles as our initial link to the power output of the rider.

Propulsive Forces: Pedal Forces

The earliest account of instrumentation used to measure pedal-reaction forces was presented by Sharp (36) in a book that described many features of the bicycle that are applicable to current developments in cycling technology. A review of the different types of pedals reported in the literature designed specifically to measure pedal-reaction loads is presented by Gregor and colleagues (10). The pedal designed in our laboratory and currently used in our cycling research is presented in Fig. 35–10. It includes two piezoelectric load cells and a surface that can be adapted to both a regular cleat and toe-strap configuration and to the current clipless float designs. Exemplar data describing the three components of the pedal-reaction force, the magnitude of the moment about an axis through the center of pressure

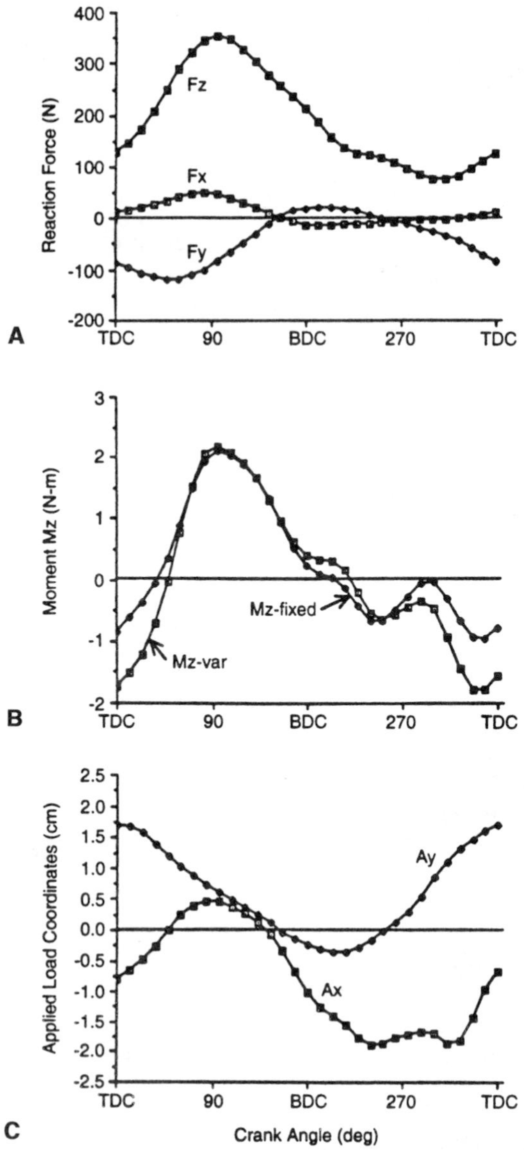

FIG. 35–11. Mean patterns for five pedal revolutions for the pedal-reaction force (**A**), applied moment (**B**), and center of pressure patterns during one pedaling cycle [top dead center 0 degrees (TDC) to top dead center 360 degrees (TDC)]. **A**: F_z is the component orthogonal to the pedal surface, F_y is A/P shear, and F_x is medial/lateral shear. **B**: The applied moment (M_z) about an axis orthogonal to the pedal surface when this axis is through the center of pressure ($M_{z\text{-var}}$) or through the center of the pedal ($M_{z\text{-fixed}}$), and (**C**) coordinates of the applied load in the x (A_x) and y (A_y) directions. From ref. 10, with permission.

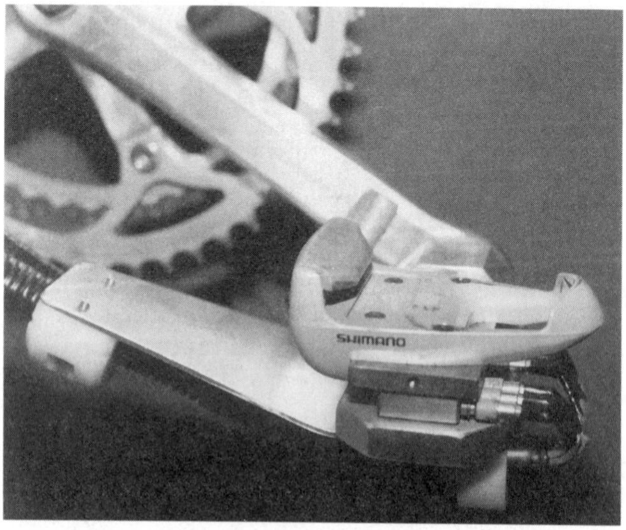

FIG. 35–10. Specially designed pedal capable of measuring three components of the pedal-reaction force and center of pressure on the pedal surface.

as well as through a fixed point in the center of the pedal, and the excursion of the two components of the center of pressure on the pedal are presented in Fig. 35–11. F_z is the component orthogonal to the pedal surface, F_y is the anterior/posterior shear component, whereas F_x is the medial lateral component of shear on the pedal surface. These force profiles have been reported by several other authors (10).

As observed in Fig. 35–11, peak force perpendicular to the pedal surface is approximately 350N or 60% of the subject's BW. This percentage is about the same for all seated cyclists under steady-state conditions and will increase only if the rider stands or attempts to accelerate the bicycle for some consistent period. These reaction forces will, of course, increase as resistance increases, but they will rarely exceed BW again unless the rider stands or pulls on the handlebars. In addition, although riders often feel that they pull up on the pedal during recovery, this is rare. Pulling up on the pedal is not essential to efficient cycling technique, and competitive riders reserve this action for climbing or sprinting. Symmetry in pedaling also is rare, and we will quite often see unequal loading on the right and left sides. This is true for most other forms of locomotion (e.g., walking) and appears to be the same in cycling. This is apparently true for both highly competitive cyclists and recreational cyclists and depends on power-output requirements, individual conditioning, and bike setup.

Although the magnitude of the pedal-reaction force is important, orientation of the result vector (F_r) with respect to the lower extremities also is important and will markedly influence how leg muscles respond to varying work load demands. An exemplar pattern of the resultant pedal-reaction force measured every 30 degrees during the pedaling cycle is presented in Fig. 35–12. In the center of the figure, we see data at 250 W at a constant pedaling speed of 90 rpm. This figure shows data from the right sagittal-plane view with pedaling occurring in a clockwise direction. One can readily see the changing orientation of the pedal and the changing orientation of the resultant force in the bicycle and pedal reference system. The right-hand figure shows the same data in the frontal plane for the first 180 degrees of the pedaling cycle, whereas the left-hand figure shows data in the frontal plane for the resultant force from 180 degrees to 360 degrees of the pedaling cycle. Pedal-reaction force magnitude and orientation change constantly throughout the pedaling cycle, as does the position of the leg above the pedal. As a consequence, the dynamics of cycling become quite complex when considering the true three-dimensional movement of the limbs and the varying orientation of the resultant vector coming from the pedal. It is the reaction to this vector that requires effort on the part of the musculature in the lower extremities, and this vector represents the summation of the interactive components in the legs and the environment in describing the true nature of rider/bicycle interaction.

The angle of the pedal-reaction force with respect to each segment (e.g., the knee) in the frontal plane is important, and several published reports (14,15,37) indicate, for example, that a varus load is applied to the knee during the power phase. This pattern becomes apparent in Fig. 35–13, which shows data for three separate seat heights. The convention in the figure indicates that the measurements on the vertical axis represent the deviation in degrees between the pedal-reaction force and the knee position during a complete pedaling cycle. What becomes obvious is that during the power phase, despite the fact that the reaction force is medial to a vertical line, it is also medial to the knee. In the recovery phase, a time when pedal-reaction forces are much lower, the orientation of this force appears lateral to the knee for each of the three seat-height conditions. An additional interesting feature of these data lies in the fact that the center of pressure, as shown in Fig.

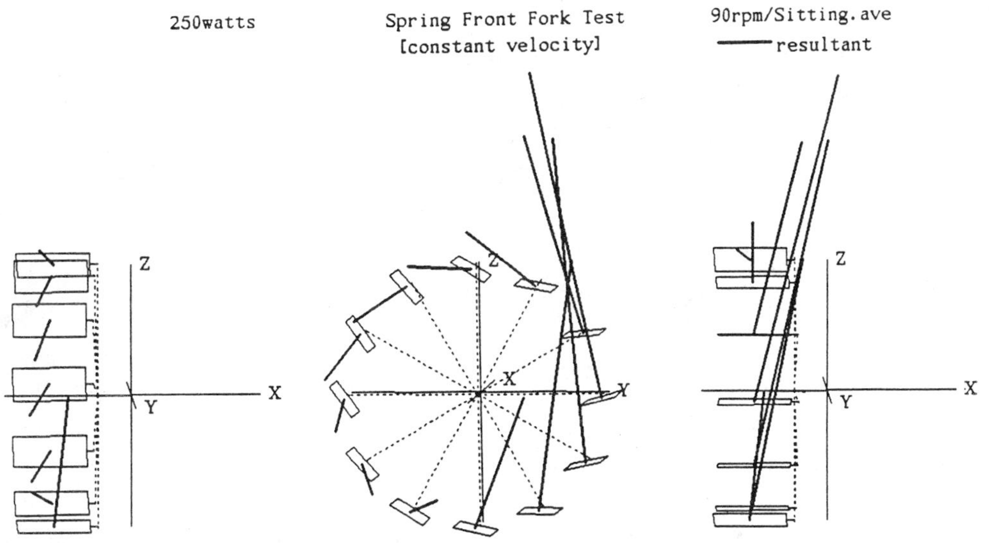

FIG. 35–12. Resultant force profile of one subject at 250 W and 90 rpm. Center is the sagittal-plane view, right is 0 degrees to 180 degrees in the cycle, and left is 180 degrees to 360 degrees in the cycle.

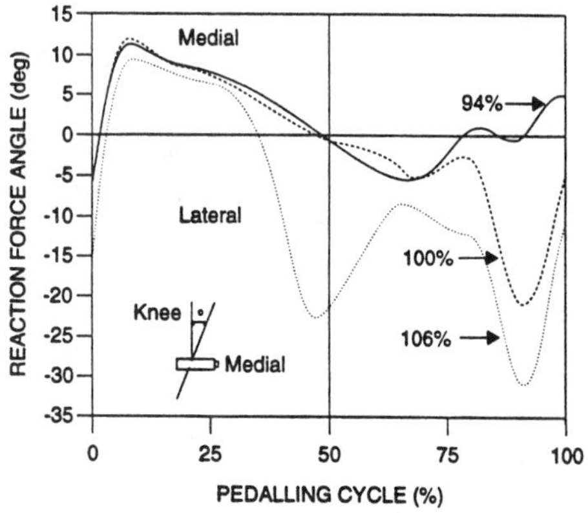

FIG. 35–13. Position of the pedal-reaction force with respect to the knee during the pedaling cycle in the frontal plane. Each curve is an average of 150 pedal revolutions (10 subjects × five trials) at 200 W and 80 rpm. Separate patterns are an average at three seat conditions (i.e., 94%, 100%, and 106% of leg length). From ref. 14, with permission.

35–11, changes during the pedaling cycle, and the data presented in Fig. 35–13 show a deviation that takes into account the moving center of pressure. In other words, the center of pressure moves medially and laterally during the pedaling cycle, the knee moves medially and laterally during the pedaling cycle, and the vector orientation in the frontal plane moves medial to lateral during the pedaling cycle. The net effect of these three elements moving continuously during both power and recovery phases is presented in Fig. 35–13. The effect this force has on the knee, for example, is described in a subsequent section that discusses joint kinetics and moments in the frontal plane. The data are consistent and supported by the literature (15,37) that the force vector is medial to the knee during the power phase and, although markedly affected by high seat heights, is, in general, lateral to the knee during recovery.

Whereas the orientation of the vector with respect to the leg is important, orientation of the vector with respect to the crank also is important and provides information of how "effective" the rider is in imparting energy to the crank. Data from a single rider at 250 W at a constant pedaling speed of 90 rpm, showing both the resultant pedal force and the effective force resolved to the crank, are presented in Fig. 35–14. The effective force with respect to the crank is that component calculated orthogonal to the crank throughout the pedaling cycle. Resolving the pedal resultant force to both effective (orthogonal to the crank) and ineffective (parallel to the crank) components requires knowledge of pedal and crank orientation. With these two parameters, it becomes clear that the effective force against the crank is positive and large during the power phase and negative and small during recovery. Figure 35–15 shows the average pattern for an effective force during one pedal revolution, describing the "productive region" during the power phase and a "counterproductive region" during the recovery. LaFortune and Cavanagh (38) were the first to describe pedaling effectiveness, with the data shown in Figs. 35–14 and 35–15 consistently supported in the literature.

Browning (39) examined the "index of effectiveness" when elite triathletes assumed an aerodynamic versus an advanced-aerodynamic position on the bike and concluded that there was no change in force effectiveness between the two positions. It seems that as the riders assumed a more forward *advanced* aerodynamic position, one in which they are in a very low position out over the handlebars, the "effective force" pattern simply

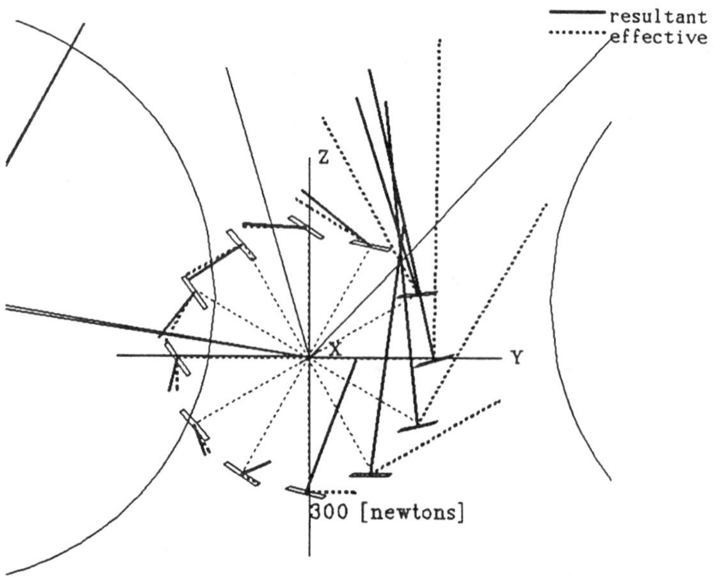

FIG. 35–14. Resultant pedal-reaction force (*solid lines*) and the effective crank force (*dashed lines*) for one subject at 250 W and 90 rpm.

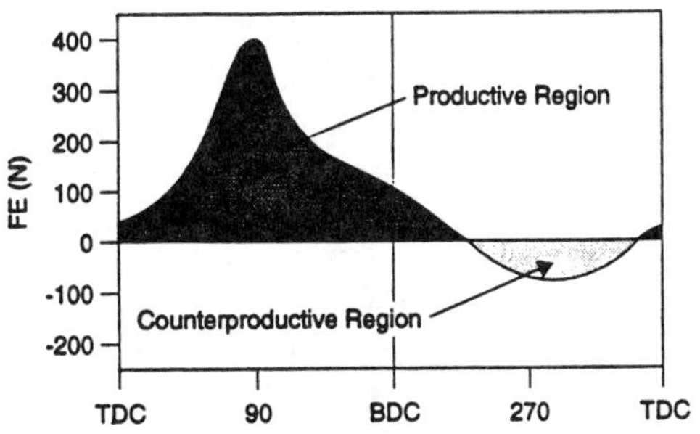

FIG. 35–15. Effective force profile during one pedal revolution. Productive region is positive work done to drive the crank, whereas the counterproductive region during recovery represents an extra load that the contralateral limb must work against during its power phase (*TDC* to *BDC*).

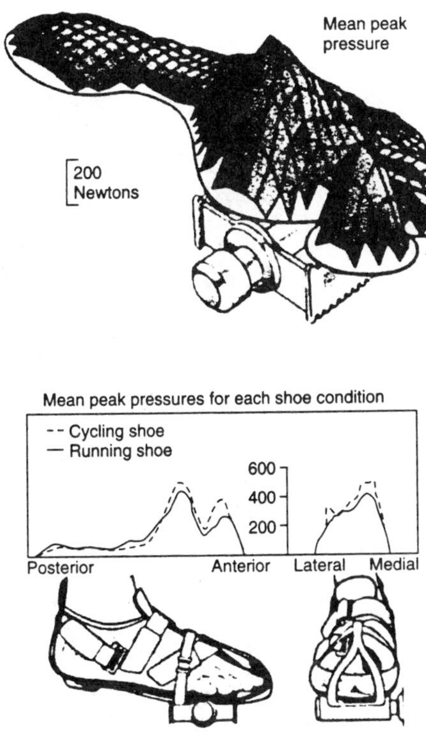

FIG. 35–16. Pattern of pressure distribution on the sole of the cycling shoe, including data from a subject using a cycling shoe and a running shoe. From ref. 5, with permission.

rotated forward, or clockwise, offering the same mechanically efficient kinetics regardless of the rider's position. These results are of great practical value and support the conclusion that, as the rider assumes an aerodynamic position to minimize wind drag, there are minimal losses in cycling efficiency with very similar patterns of effective force on the crank. Wheeler and colleagues (40) reported that regardless of the pedal design (toe-strap and cleat, clipless fixed, or clipless float), power transmitted to the bike, as measured by effective crank-force patterns, was not compromised. These results also are significant because there has been some speculation that clipless pedal designs permitting "float" result in a reduction in power transferred to the bike.

Pressure Distribution on the Shoe

As we discussed earlier, knowledge of the forces acting on the bottom of the foot and pressures on different regions of the foot are useful in examining injuries related to the interface between the foot and the pedal. Sanderson (41) studied the variations in pressure distribution throughout the pedaling cycle by using a specially designed insole with 256 discrete force-measuring elements (Fig. 35–16). He reported that the majority of foot pressure was localized in the forefoot directly over the pedal and especially over the head of the first metatarsal and hallux. More recently, Sanderson and Hennig (42) used a specialized shoe insert to measure the distribution during steady-state cycling and found more evenly distributed pressures across the sole of rigid cycling shoes when compared with running shoes (Fig. 35–16). Amoroso and co-workers (43) also measured pressure distributions across different cadences; Hennig and Sanderson (44), across different power outputs, found an increased relative pressure assumed by the anterior/medial structures of the forefoot, first metatarsal, and hallux, with increased resultant pedal force. The implications for injury and rehabilitation were not addressed in these reports.

Pedal Torsion Measurements

As stated previously in this chapter, our interest in the interactive forces between the pedal and the foot are important because the rider experiences the greatest forces coming into the leg at this interface, and it is indeed at this interface that the bike is energized. We also discussed, in the section on injuries, that the movement of the leg is truly three dimensional and must be allowed to proceed in three dimensions to energize the bike effectively, as well as to minimize injuries to the legs (i.e., chronic overuse injuries). We looked at the pedal-reaction forces in three dimensions, the center of pressure, and the general pressure distribution at the shoe–pedal interface. The final component to discuss now focuses on the rotation of the foot, or the tendency to rotate the foot, on the pedal. It is important to understand this rotational component because, if it is unnecessarily constrained, it may cause significant injury.

The applied moment at the pedal surface about an axis perpendicular to the pedal surface (M_z) is a kinetic parameter that has been reported to be directly related to knee loads and subsequent chronic knee pain (8,15,45). A sketch of this moment with the pedal pre-

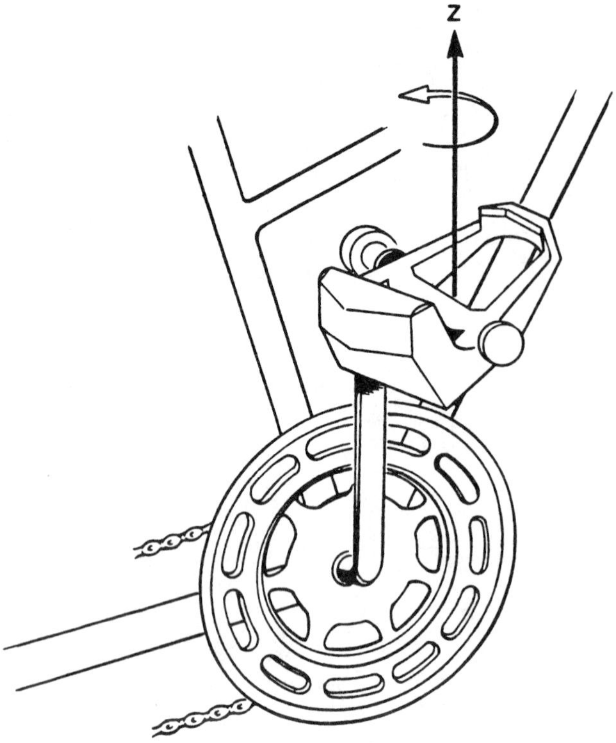

FIG. 35–17. Sketch of the applied moment (M_z) about an axis orthogonal to the pedal surface.

sented in Fig. 35–10 is presented in Fig. 35–17. The average patterns of this moment with three different types of shoe–pedal interface are presented in Fig. 35–18. Because the center of pressure and force magnitudes change during the pedaling cycle, clearly M_z changes as well. In fact, Ruby and associates (15) calculated knee loads from force-pedal data, sagittal plane kinematics, and frontal plane knee motion, and reported that the moment, M_z, about the axis orthogonal to the pedal surface was a significant contributor to M_z' at the knee, or the twisting moment at the knee.

The twisting moment M_z at the pedal also directly relates to the "float" pedal designs currently on the market because the claim of many of these designs is that if movement is allowed, forces are minimized and the risk of injury is reduced. The dual-transducer force pedal system was adapted for compatibility with several popular pedal systems (toe-clip and strap, Shimano and Time) with and without float features. Data showed that individual peak M_z applied to the pedal surface was attenuated with the use of clipless float designs (Fig. 35–18). Applied internal moments ($+M_z$) about the z-axis correspond to a shoe force exerted onto the pedal surface tending to rotate the toe in and heel out. Applied external moments ($-M_z$) correspond to a shoe force onto the pedal surface tending to rotate the toe out and heel in (see Fig. 35–17). Gregor and Wheeler (8) concluded that (a) the applied moment M_z was external for approximately the first 60 degrees of the pedaling cycle, with an internally applied moment dominating the remainder of the power phase; (b) an externally applied moment occurred throughout the recovery phase (180 to 360 degrees); (c) the peak internally applied moment ($+M_z$) increased significantly with increased workload (e.g., an increase from 150 W to 350 W nearly doubled the magnitude of peak $+M_z$ value, whereas externally applied moments ($-M_z$) changed very little with work load; (d) the use of clipless float systems markedly decreased both the internal and external M_z peaks; (e) asymmetric moment patterns were observed throughout their subject population; and (f) cyclists with chronic anterior knee pain, the most common type reported by cyclists, demonstrated exaggerated internally applied peak moments, increased rates of loading (dM_z/dt), and longer duration of the applied internal moment during the power phase of the pedaling cycle (0 degrees to 180 degrees; Fig. 35–19).

Further to these results, Wooten and Hull (46) presented another pedal system designed to study the shoe–pedal interface and its effect on overuse injuries at the knee. Their pedal setup permitted an evaluation of inversion/eversion and abduction/adduction, either separately or in combination. By using the same system, Ruby and Hull (47) investigated the significance of permitting relative motion between the shoe–pedal interface with regard to the effects on three-dimensional knee loads as modeled by Ruby and colleagues (15). Ruby and Hull (47) found that, relative to the fixed-platform condition, (a) permitting medial–lateral translation did not significantly decrease intersegmental knee-load quantities, (b) both rotation platforms sig-

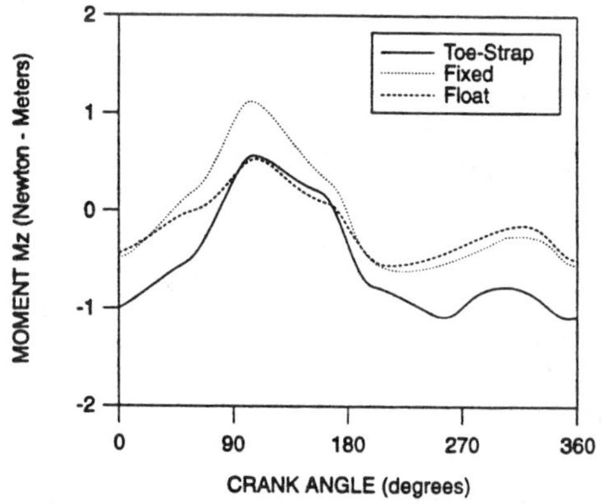

FIG. 35–18. The applied moment (M_z) pattern during the pedal cycle averaged across 27 subjects with three separate shoe/pedal interface designs (i.e., a standard toe-strap and cleat, a clipless fixed design, and a clipless float design). A positive moment indicates an inwardly applied moment against the pedal surface (heel out). From ref. 40, with permission.

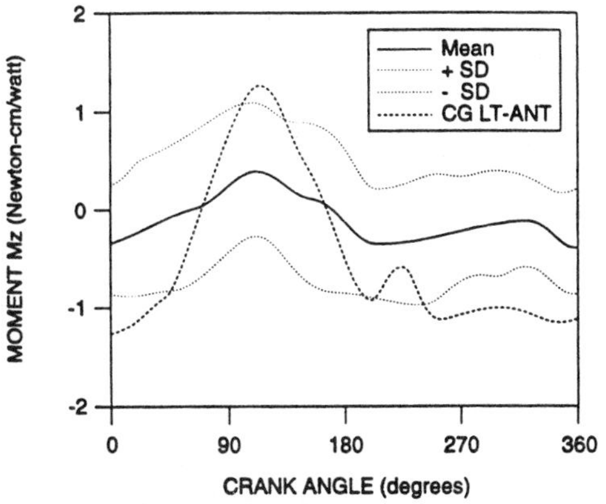

FIG. 35–19. The mean applied moment (M_z) pattern (±1 SD) during the pedaling cycle for 27 subjects with a clipless float shoe/pedal interface design and the mean pattern for one knee-pain patient. A positive moment indicates an inwardly applied moment against the pedal surface (heel out). From ref. 40, with permission.

nificantly decreased many of the predicted knee-load quantities and did not significantly increase any of the knee loads, (c) permitting abduction/adduction significantly reduced axial and varus/valgus knee moments, and (d) permitting inversion/eversion decreased varus/valgus knee moments. Specifically, the internal axial knee moments ($+M_z$) exerted by the tibia onto the femur were attenuated during the power phase (0 degrees to 180 degrees) of the pedaling cycle when rotational movements were permitted at the pedal surface. These data, in conjunction with the exaggerated M_z patterns demonstrated by cyclists with knee pain (8), make a strong argument for the benefits of pedal-float systems with regard to reducing knee load and injury prevention. It also seems that regardless of the pedal design (toe-clip and strap, fixed, or float), energy imparted to the bike, as measured by the force-effectiveness pattern, is not compromised. Browning (39) reported that elite riders and triathletes maintained the ability to impart power effectively to the bike by using a range of pedal systems and aerodynamic riding positions.

Lower-Extremity Joint Kinetics: Joint-Reaction Forces

As a consequence of modeling the lower extremities as rigid bodies, reactive forces at the pedal result in calculated joint-reaction forces at the hip, knee, and ankle. These are not bone-on-bone forces, but rather are calculated values describing segment interactions during the pedaling cycle. Knowledge of joint-reaction forces is significant to our understanding of lower-extremity function, but few data are available on these calculated values for the cycling task. What data are available, for the most part, describe knee-joint loads because the knee is the most widely studied joint of the lower extremity. Vector components specific to the knee joint are schematically presented in Fig. 35–20, with a positive Fy_k (the tensile component) along the long axis of the tibia and positive Fx_k (the anterior component) along the tibial plateau. Ft_k represents the anterior/posterior shear component corrected for the inclination of the tibial plateau. Any medial/lateral shear component would be orthogonal to the anterior/posterior shear component.

McCoy and Gregor (48) reported knee-joint reaction forces from 10 male cyclists riding at 200 W at a cadence of 80 rpm. Results presented in Fig. 35–21 show that at seat-height conditions of 94%, 100%, and 106% of leg length, the vector calculated along the tibial shaft was compressive throughout the entire pedaling cycle and reached a similar value (approximately 208N) at 92 degrees in the pedaling cycle for the 106% condition and at 110 degrees in the pedaling cycle at both the 94% and 100% conditions. The most noticeable effect of seat height was the rapid change in compressive load at the 106% condition. After reaching its peak value, the load decreased to about 15N while the riders were still in the power phase. In contrast, the pattern of compressive loading was essentially the same for the other two seat-height conditions and did not reach the minimal values until the recovery phase.

The anterior/posterior shear-force component was anteriorly directed during the power phase, with peak

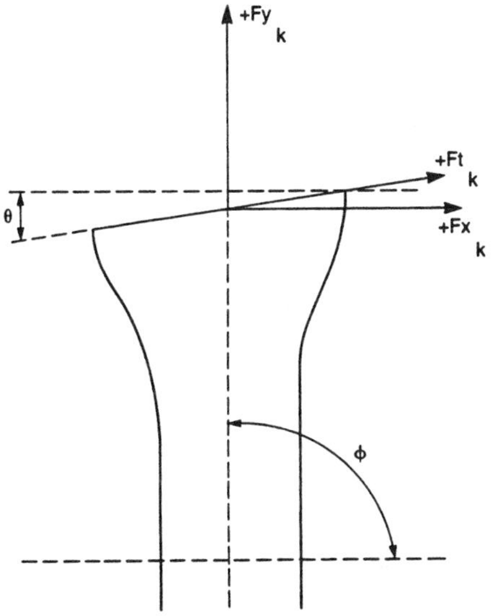

FIG. 35–20. Sagittal-plane view of the proximal tibia and the orientation of the posterior tilt angle of the tibial plateau with respect to the horizontal axis of the tibia. Ft_k is the A/P shear joint-reaction force component, Fx_k is the horizontal shear component, Fy_k is the vertical knee-reaction force component, 0 is the posterior tilt angle, and 0 is the shank angle.

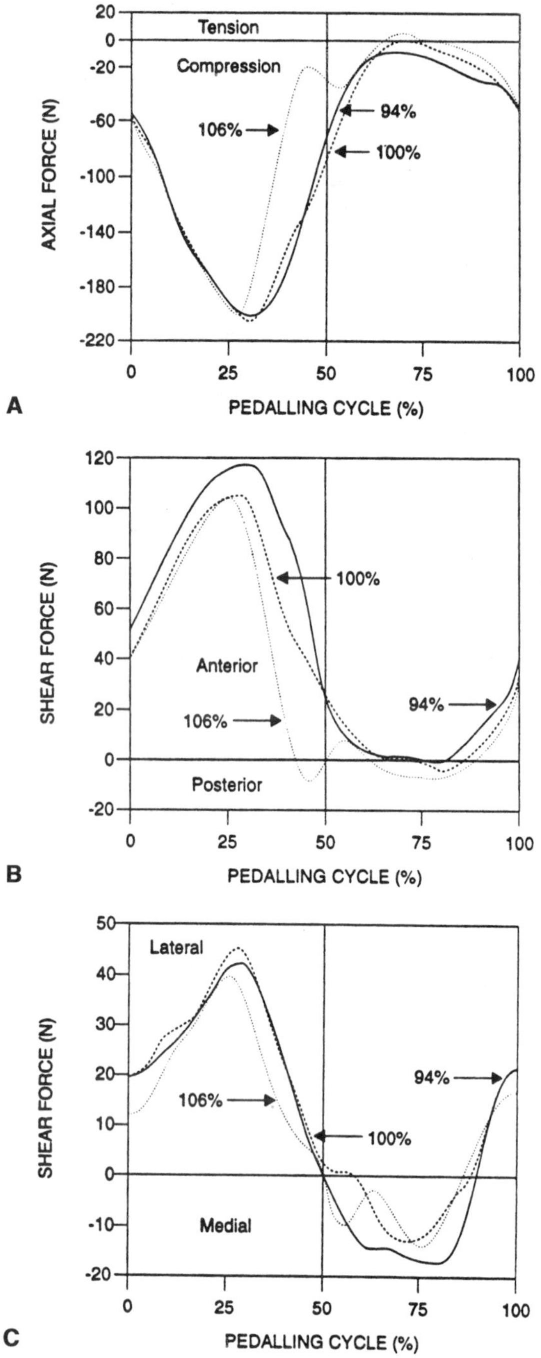

FIG. 35–21. Knee-joint reaction force components averaged for 150 pedal revolutions (10 subjects × five trials) at 200 W and 80 rpm for three seat-height conditions (i.e., 94%, 100%, and 106% of leg length). **A**: The axial component along the shaft of the tibia. **B**: The anterior/posterior shear force component. **C**: The medial/lateral shear force component. From ref. 14, with permission.

values observed near 90 degrees for all seat-height conditions (see Fig. 35–21). Peak magnitudes at the 94% seat-height condition, however, were significantly larger ($p < .05$) than the values obtained at either the middle or highest seat-height conditions (a difference of approximately 15N). Similar to the compressive joint-reaction force, the anterior joint-reaction force decreased at a greater rate at the 106% seat-height condition than at either the 94% or 100% conditions, and it actually became posteriorly directed late in the power phase. The appearance of a posteriorly directed shear-force component at this phase of the pedaling cycle is consistent with the data presented by Ericson and associates (37) and supports the hypothesis that changes in seat height have a marked effect on the direction of the shear-force component at the knee. This finding is extremely important when considering, for example, rehabilitation of anterior cruciate ligament (ACL)–deficient patients. The obvious question is where to place the seat to maximize the benefits of the rehabilitation program yet not place too high a demand on the ligament repair.

The medial/lateral joint-reaction force was laterally directed during the power phase with peak values observed just after 90 degrees into the pedaling cycle for all seat-height conditions (see Fig. 35–21) (48). Values obtained during the highest seat-height condition were significantly smaller ($p < .05$) than the peak lateral force calculated at both the middle and lowest seat-height conditions. Absolute differences were approximately 4N to 6N. Medially directed forces occurred during the recovery phase of the pedaling cycle with values smaller and more variable than the laterally directed forces and significantly larger at the 94% condition than at the 100% seat-height condition.

Ericson and co-workers (49) calculated anterior/posterior shear forces in noninjured tibiofemoral joints during ergometer cycling and found that they reflected both an external joint-reaction force and an estimated force component due to extensor activity at the knee. Tests were conducted at 60 rpm, 120 W of power, and a seat height of 113% ischial tuberosity to medial malleolus length (a bit different from the one previously described). By using a position in which the lateral malleolus was over the pedal spindle, Ericson and co-workers (49) reported shear forces posteriorly directed for the first 80 degrees of the pedaling cycle at a time when the knee was extending from approximately 110 degrees to 75 degrees (remember that 0 degrees is full extension). Shear forces then became anteriorly directed from 80 degrees to 140 degrees of crank rotation as the knee continued to extend from 75 degrees to 48 degrees. The peak anterior shear force was only 37N (0.05 BW) and occurred at about 104 degrees of the pedaling cycle and at a knee angle of approximately 68 degrees. Shear forces then shifted posteriorly between 135 degrees and 180 degrees in the pedaling cycle. Finally, these authors found that use of a posterior foot position (the ball of the foot over the pedal spindle) as well as increased pedaling speed increased the magnitude of the anteriorly directed shear-force component, whereas changes in seat height had little effect on the shear-force component.

Ruby and associates reported patterns of three-dimensional knee-joint loading during seated cycling for 11 male subjects cycling at their chosen seat height at 90 rpm and 225 W (15). Data agree with McCoy and Gregor (48) and show a compressive load during the entire pedaling cycle, with a peak value of about 240N between 80 degrees and 100 degrees in the pedaling cycle. Shear forces were anteriorly directed for the entire pedaling cycle, reaching a peak of about 125N at about 70 degrees and laterally directed during the first half of the pedaling cycle, peaking at approximately 50N around 90 degrees.

Finally, the patellofemoral joint-reaction force is critical to knee function during cycling, and Ericson and Nisell (50) estimated patellofemoral joint forces by using a bicycle ergometer. Six male subjects were studied at 0, 120, and 240 W, pedaling at 40, 60, 80, and 100 rpm at three different seat heights. Two foot positions on the pedal were used, and all data supported previous statements that cycling is an excellent form of exercise and rehabilitation because of the low loads and tissue strains imposed on the knee. Magnitudes of patellofemoral joint forces appeared to be independent of BW, pedaling rate, and foot position, but they were greatly influenced by load and seat height. These data may be specifically useful for knee-pain patients and patients with chondromalacia patella.

Lower-Extremity Joint Kinetics: Muscle Moments

External demands placed on each lower extremity must be met by internal moments produced by muscle and/or connective tissue forces acting about the axis of rotation of each joint. For example, when an external flexor muscle moment is produced about the knee joint, an internal knee-joint extensor muscle moment, presumed to be dominated by the quadriceps muscles, must be generated. In the case of an external knee abductor muscle moment, an internal knee adductor muscle moment, dominated by the medial collateral ligament and VM, must be generated. This internal muscle moment represents the integration of *all* active and passive structures acting about a joint producing moments in response to external demands. An internal knee-flexor muscle moment, for example, does not mean that the knee-extensor muscles are not active but that the net result of all forces results in a flexor muscle moment and a tendency to move into flexion.

Moments in the Sagittal Plane

Sagittal plane muscle moments, in particular large hip and knee-extensor moments, create crank rotation during the propulsive phase of cycling. During the recovery phase, flexor moments may act to unload the pedal, potentially minimizing resistance to the contralateral limb. Hip, knee, and ankle-extensor and flexor moments are the most significant in powering the bicycle. Investigations using a force pedal system to evaluate lower-extremity kinetics during cycling have produced a great deal of information on muscle moment patterns during normal, steady-state cycling. Although first reported by Gregor (51) (Fig. 35–22*A*), many investigators have shown similar results (26,49,52–55). It seems that the muscle moments at the hip, knee, and ankle have *fairly repeatable patterns* despite variations in loading conditions, subject population, and bike setup. Magnitudes may increase in response to increased demands, and some timing features may be affected by cadence, but in almost all cases the general patterns shown in Fig. 35–22*A* remain the same.

The data presented in Fig. 35–22*A* show the hip and knee performing very different actions during the propulsive phase of cycling (i.e., the hip produces an extensor moment while the knee produces an extensor and then a flexor moment before attaining bottom-dead-center (BDC) in the pedaling cycle. This switch from a knee-extensor to a knee-flexor moment during knee extension in the power phase is unique to cycling. Gregor and colleagues (26) discussed the moment reversal at the knee during propulsion with specific reference to the behavior of biarticular muscles (i.e., a two-joint muscle may act as an extensor of the joint of which it is also a flexor). The muscles to study here are the hamstrings and quadriceps, antagonists at the hip and knee. Van Ingen Schenau (56) further described the potential role of flexors and extensors in the distribution of energy between adjacent segments during the cycling task. He essentially concluded that the uniarticular muscles are "power producers" and that the biarticular muscles are "power distributors" in the coordinated action of the lower-extremity segments during cycling. In other words, the vastii muscles and gluteus maximus probably provide a great deal of the power needed for propulsion, whereas the rectus femoris and hamstring muscles apparently distribute energy to the joints unable to meet the power demands during certain portions of the cycling task.

In an effort to understand the extent to which individual muscles contribute to the joint moment, Gregor and colleagues (57) presented data on Achilles tendon forces, gastrocnemius and soleus EMG, and muscle-length changes, as well as EMG activity in the VM and TA muscles. In an additional article, Gregor and coworkers (58) described the contribution made by the triceps surae to the joint moment at the ankle during cycling at three separate power outputs. Results indicated that Achilles tendon forces increased as external resistance increased. As power was increased by increas-

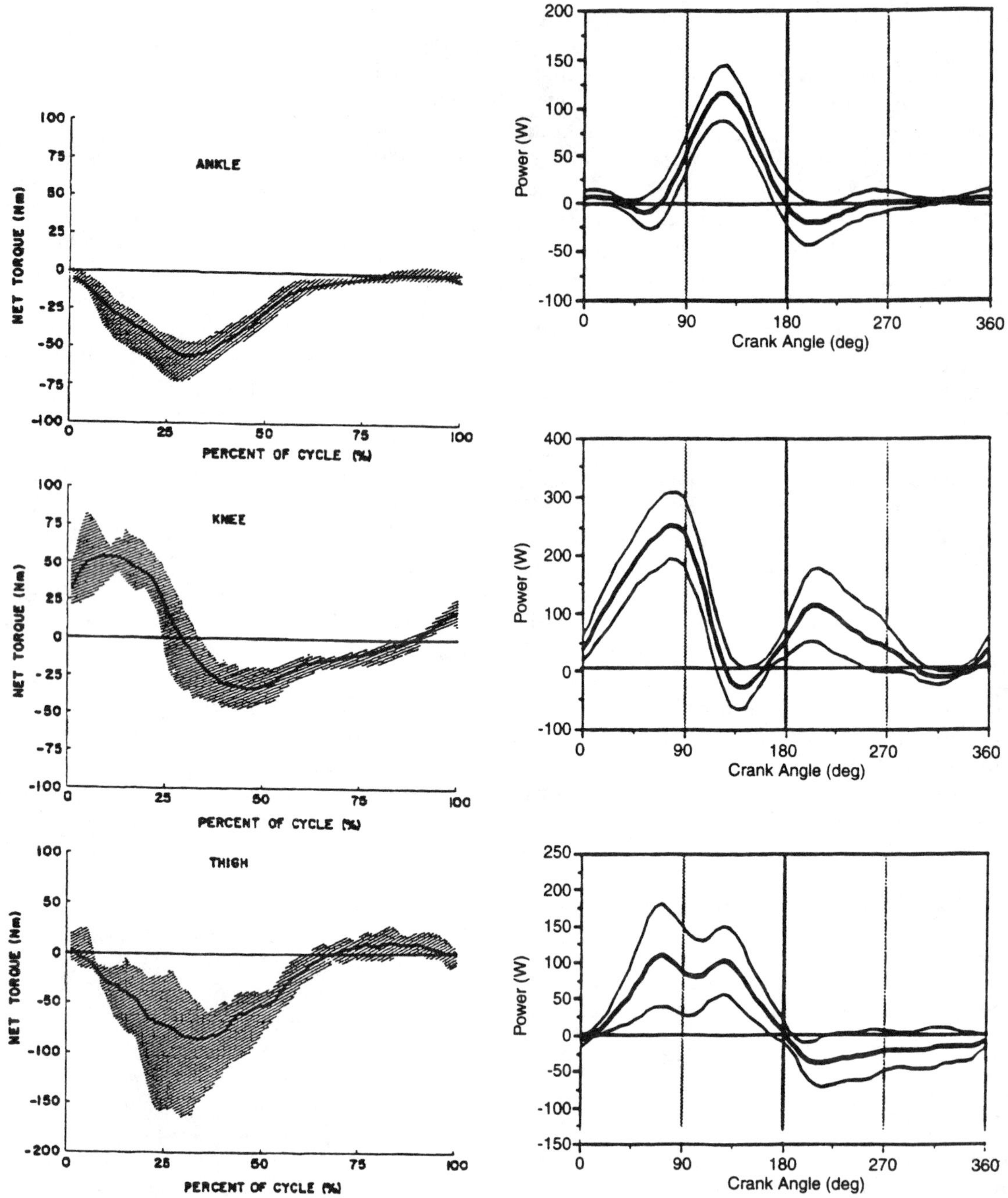

A B

FIG. 35–22. **A**: Muscle-moment (torque) patterns for the ankle, knee, and thigh (hip) during the pedaling cycle. Patterns represent the average of 25 pedaling cycles (five subjects × five trials) at approximately 260 W and 84 rpm (left). From ref. 26, with permission. **B**: Muscle-power patterns (calculated as the product of the muscle moment and angular velocity for each joint) during the pedaling cycle for 12 subjects riding at 250 W and 100 rpm. The top trace is the ankle, the middle trace is the knee, and the bottom trace is the hip. From ref. 59, with permission.

ing cadence alone (at constant work load), peak Achilles tendon force did not change. In addition, the impulse generated by the triceps surae muscles consistently represented about 65% of the impulse calculated by using the *muscle moment* at the ankle at all power levels studied. EMGs and muscle-length changes recorded by Gregor and associates (58) further support a division of effort between the gastrocnemius and soleus in their contribution to the Achilles tendon force. In short, the soleus muscle appears to contribute to the muscle moment early in the power phase, whereas the contribution by the gastrocnemius peaks a bit later in the power phase, near the time the knee moment changes from an extensor moment to a flexor moment.

Browning and colleagues (53) reported that the ankle-muscle moment increased in peak magnitude as seat height decreased from 108% to 96% of pubic symphysis height. Additionally, seat height affected the magnitude of peak knee-extensor moments, with higher peak magnitudes reported at the 96% than at 108% pubic symphysis condition. Browning and associates (53) also reported that knee-flexor moments occurred earlier in the pedaling cycle (approximately 100 degrees) at 108% pubic symphysis height and later in the pedaling cycle (approximately 145 degrees) at 96% pubic symphysis height. Furthermore, peak knee-flexor magnitudes were higher at 108% than those reported at either 96% or 102% pubic symphysis height, a finding also supported by McCoy and Gregor (48). Finally, seat height also affected the peak hip moment with higher peak-extensor magnitudes reported at the higher seat-height conditions.

Muscle Moments in the Frontal Plane

As previously discussed, motion in the frontal plane occurs to varying degrees at the hip, knee, and ankle during cycling and appears most influenced by bike setup, rider position, and load. Frontal-plane muscle moments generated at the knee in response to the varus load from the pedal force oriented medial to the knee begin as valgus moments with values ranging between 6 and 7 Nm across seat-varying positions (14,48) (Fig. 35–23). Magnitudes then appear to increase and reach a peak value near 90 degrees of crank rotation for all three seat heights (48). The lowest valgus moment (−16 Nm) was observed at the highest seat height (106% of leg length). The valgus muscle moment at the knee

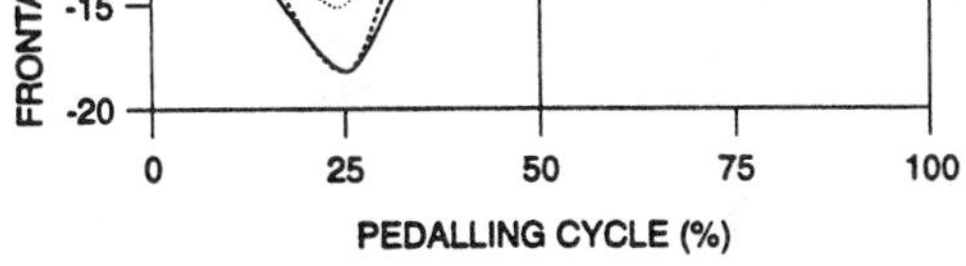

FIG. 35–23. Knee-muscle-moment patterns in the frontal plane averaged for 150 pedal revolutions (10 subjects × 5 trials) at 200 W and 80 rpm for three seat height conditions, that is, 94%, 100%, and 106% of leg length. (From ref. 45, with permission.)

subsequently decreased to zero near BDC (180 degrees in the pedaling cycle), where it became a varus muscle moment for most of recovery. The peak varus muscle moment was significantly smaller ($p < .05$) for the middle seat position (4 Nm at 100% of leg length) when compared with the lowest (6 Nm at 94% of leg length) and highest (7 Nm at 106% of leg length) seat-height conditions (48). In addition, Ruby and co-workers (15, 17) suggested that because external loads are applied to the foot during pedaling, anatomic variations of the foot may contribute to the loads transmitted to the knee and subsequently to joint injury.

In total, these findings suggest that the bicycle is a relatively benign environment for some structures in the knee while placing potentially significant demands on others. With loads lower than those observed during walking, a varus moment applied to the knee as a result of a medially directed pedal-reaction force places strain on the lateral structures of the knee, especially during the power phase. A valgus muscle moment generated in response to the pedal loads, however, is also lower than those observed during walking. With proper supervision and control, the bicycle appears to offer a valuable exercise paradigm designed to meet specific demands imposed in a rehabilitation setting.

Lower-Extremity Joint Kinetics: Mechanical Work and Power

In the final analysis, the lower extremities are responsible for transmitting power to the bicycle. Whereas this mechanical transmission contains information relative to the bicycle (e.g., gear selection, crank length), the focus of this final section is on the "human" machine and how effectively it operates within the constraints created by a personalized bicycle setup. Mechanical work and power are variables traditionally of interest to both biomechanists and exercise physiologists because they are related to mechanical power transmission to the bike as well as the physiologic cost of cycling at selected work loads. In an effort to address how muscles might function effectively and as groups in "total" lower-extremity function (not just considering each muscle and joint but looking from the perspective of the whole limb), Broker (59) used a clipless force pedal design to study the management of mechanical energy and the "load-sharing" among the hip, knee, and ankle joints in the lower extremities of 12 elite cyclists. Newtonian equations were developed by using a sagittal-plane model of the right lower extremity to calculate joint muscle powers (the product of the muscle moment and angular velocity for each joint) and hip-joint force power (the product of the hip-joint reaction force and velocity of the estimated center of rotation of the hip) for the 12 elite cyclists at work loads of 200, 250, and 300 W and 90, 100, and 110 rpm. It was suggested by

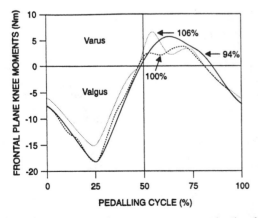

Ericson and colleagues (49) and Van Ingen Schenau (56) that greater than 80% of the energy generated at the joints in the lower extremities can, in fact, be delivered to the pedals as useful energy to drive the bicycle. This is in contrast to the results of similar analyses on running and walking, in which the mechanical efficiency of the task is much lower. In his analysis, Broker (59) used three energy models to study the issue of energy production and transmission during cycling. Because it is now generally considered that single-joint muscles produce energy and biarticular muscles can transfer, or distribute, energy from one joint to another, the three models ranged from one in which only hypothetical single-joint muscles acted (no transfer) to a hypothetical model in which multijoint muscles acted and permitted unlimited transfer. The major result was that during the cycling task, a third model, one that had a sound basis in anatomic function and consistency with reported EMG patterns in the lower extremities during cycling, resulted in the appropriate transfer of energy across two-joint muscles and limited the energy dissipated to nontransferable sources to less than 6 joules per limb during cycling. The muscles primarily responsible for the appropriate transfer of energy were the hamstrings, modeled as a group, and the gastrocnemius muscle. Joint muscle powers are presented in Fig. 35–22*B*, and regions in the pedaling cycle where energy transfers are possible are summarized here:

1. Energy absorbed at the knee during the second quadrant (90 degrees to 180 degrees) can potentially be transferred to the ankle by the active gastrocnemius and to the hip by the active hamstrings.
2. Energy absorbed at the ankle and hip during the third quadrant can be potentially transferred to the knee by the active gastrocnemius and active hamstring muscles, respectively.

CONCLUSION

In conclusion, the cycling task presents a unique opportunity to study the lower extremities as a total system whose purpose is to deliver power effectively to the bicycle. Evaluation of lower-extremity kinetics at the level of intersegmental dynamics, "load sharing" among all segments (thigh, leg, and foot) responsible for the coordination of energy delivery to the crank, is important and can provide information useful to biomechanists, physiologists, orthopedic surgeons, physical therapists, and physicians in physical medicine and rehabilitation. For example, it appears that unlike walking and running, the stretch–shorten cycle of muscle action in cycling is not necessary to reduce mechanical energy expenditure. Broker (59) reported that this can be accomplished based on logic in limb mechanics. The presence of the active stretch–shorten cycle in many muscles of the lower extremities, then, appear most important to the metabolic and physiologic function of the muscle and not necessarily its mechanical output. Understanding total system dynamics also is important in rehabilitation. For example, how does the contralateral leg adapt to the loss of the involved leg in a unilateral stroke patient in energizing the bicycle during rehabilitation? How do the hip and knee adapt in a unilateral below-knee amputee? And how does each lower extremity adapt in a patient after ACL reconstruction? Certainly a great deal of work is needed to apply existing biomechanical-analysis procedures to exercise as well as clinical and rehabilitation problems.

REFERENCES

1. Holmes JC, Pruitt AL, Whalen NJ. Cycling knee injuries. *Cycling Sci* 1991;June:11–14.
2. Pruitt AL. The cyclist's knee: anatomical and biomechanical considerations. In: Burke ER, Newsom B, eds. *Medical and scientific aspects of cycling*. Champaign, IL: Human Kinetics Books, 1988:17–24.
3. Baker A. *Smart cycling: successful training and racing*. San Diego: Argo Publishing, 1996.
4. Mellion MB. Common cycling injuries: management and prevention. *Sports Med* 1991;11:52–70.
5. Sanderson DJ. The biomechanics of cycling shoes. *Cycling Sci* 1990:27–30.
6. Francis PR. Injury prevention for cyclists: a biomechanical approach. In: Burke ER, ed. *Science of cycling*. Champaign, IL: Human Kinetics Books, 1986:145–185.
7. Bohlmann JT. Injuries in competitive cycling. *Physician Sports Med* 1981;9:117–124.
8. Gregor RJ, Wheeler JB. Knee pain: biomechanical factors associated with shoe/pedal interfaces: implications for injury. *Sports Med* 1994;17:117–131.
9. Hannaford DR, Moran GT, Hlavac HF. Video analysis and treatment of overuse knee injury in cycling: a limited clinical study. *Clin Podiatr Med Surg* 1986;3:671–678.
10. Gregor RJ, Broker JP, Ryan MM. The biomechanics of cycling. *Exerc Sport Sci Rev* 1991;19:127–169.
11. Faria E, Cavanagh PR. *The physiology and biomechanics of cycling ACSM series*. New York: John Wiley, 1978.
12. Rugg SG, Gregor RJ. The effect of seat height on muscle lengths, velocities and moment arm lengths during cycling. *J Biomech* 1987;20:899.
13. Ericson MO, Nisell R, Nemeth G. Joint motions of the lower limb during ergometer cycling. *J Orthop Sports Phys Ther* 1988;9:273–278.
14. McCoy RW. The effect of varying seat position on knee loads during cycling. Unpublished doctoral dissertation, University of Southern California Department of Exercise Science, 1989.
15. Ruby P, Hull ML, Hawkins D. Three-dimensional knee loading during seated cycling. *J Biomech* 1992;25:41–53.
16. Boutin RD, Rab GT, Hassan IAG. Three dimensional kinematics and muscle length changes in bicyclists. In: Pope M, ed. *Proceedings of the 13th Annual Meeting ASB*. Burlington, VT: UVM Conferences, 1989:94–95.
17. Ruby P, Hull ML, Kirby KA, Jenkins DW. The effect of lower-limb anatomy on knee loads during seated cycling. *J Biomech* 1992;25:1195–1207.
18. Prilutsky BI, Gregor RJ, Albrecht AA. Strategy of muscle coordination in cycling: pushing and pulling the pedal. *J Neurophysiol* (in review).
19. van Ingen Schenau GJ, Darssers WMM, Welter TG, Beeben A, deGroot G, Jacobs R. The control of mono-articular muscles in

multijoint leg extensions in man. *J Physiol (Lond)* 1995; 484:247–254.
20. Hull ML, Hawkins DA. Analysis of muscular work in multisegmental movements: application to cycling. In: Winters J, Woo L-Y, eds. *Multiple muscle systems: biomechanics and movement organization*. Berlin: Springer-Verlag, 1990:302–311.
21. Desipres M. An electromyographic study of competitive road cycling conditions simulated on a treadmill. In: Nelson RC, Morehouse C, eds. *Biomechanics IV*. Champaign, IL: Human Kinetics Publishers, 1974:349–355.
22. Ericson MO, Nisell R, Arborelius UP. Muscular activity during ergometer cycling. *Scand J Rehabil Med* 1985;17:53–61.
23. Houtz SJ, Fischer FJ. An analysis of muscle action and joint excursion during exercise on a stationary bicycle. *J Bone Joint Surg Am* 1959;41:123–131.
24. Jorge M, Hull ML. Analysis of EMG measurement during bicycle pedaling. *J Biomech* 1986;19:683–694.
25. Ryan MM, Gregor RJ. EMG profiles of lower extremity muscles during cycling at constant workload and cadence. *J Electromyogr Kinesiol* 1992;2:69–80.
26. Gregor RJ, Cavanagh PR, LaFortune M. Knee flexor moments during propulsion in cycling: a creative solution to Lombard's paradox. *J Biomech* 1985;18:307–316.
27. Goto S, Toyoshima S, Hoshikawa T. Study of the integrated EMG of leg muscles during pedaling of various loads, frequency, and equivalent power. In: Asmussen E, Jorgensen K, eds. *Biomechanics VI-A*. Baltimore: University Park Press, 1976:246–252.
28. Suzuki S, Watanabi S, Homma S. EMG activity and kinetics of human cycling movements at different constant velocities. *Brain Res* 1982;240:245–258.
29. Suzuki Y. Mechanical efficiency of fast- and slow-twitch muscle fibers in man during cycling. *J Appl Physiol Respir Environ Exerc Physiol* 1979;47:263–267.
30. Duchateau J, LeBozec S, Hainaut K. Contributions of slow and fast muscles of triceps surae to a cyclic movement. *Eur J Appl Physiol* 1986;55:476–481.
31. Welter TG, Darssers WMM, Beelen A, van Ingen Schenau GJ. Coordination in cycling at increasing pedaling rates is not compatible with invariant relative timing models. In: Miyashita M, Fukunaga T, eds. *Proceedings XVIth Congress of the International Society of Biomechanics*. Tokyo, August 25–29, 1997:270.
32. Neptune RR, Hull ML, Kawtz SA. The effect of pedaling rate on coordination in cycling. In Miyashita M, Fukunaga T, eds. *Proceedings XVIth Congress of the International Society of Biomechanics, Tokyo,* August 25–29, 1997:271.
33. Broker JP. Equations of motion. In: Gregor R, Conconi F, eds. *Cycling biomechanics, handbook of cycling, IOC Medical Commission*. Oxford: Blackwell Science (in press).
34. Soden PD, Adeyefa BA. Forces applied to a bicycle during normal cycling. *J Biomech* 1979;12:527–541.
35. Bolourchi F, Hull ML. Measurement of rider induced loads during simulated bicycling. *Int J Sports Biomech* 1985;1:308–329.
36. Sharp A. *Bicycles and tricycles*. Cambridge, MA: MIT Press, 1977:267–270.
37. Ericson MO, Nisell R, Ekholm J. Varus and valgus loads on the knee joint during ergometer cycling. *Scand J Sports Sci* 1984; 6:39–45.
38. LaFortune MA, Cavanagh PR. Effectiveness and efficiency during bicycle riding. In: Matsui H, Kobayashi K, eds. *Biomechanics VIII-B*. Champaign, IL: Human Kinetics Publishers, 1983: 928–936.
39. Browning RC. Lower extremity kinetics during cycling in elite triathletes in aerodynamic cycling. Unpublished masters thesis, University of California at Los Angeles, 1991.
40. Wheeler JB, Gregor RJ, Broker JP. The effect of clipless float design on shoe/pedal interface kinetics: implications for overuse injuries during cycling. *J Appl Biomech (in press)*.
41. Sanderson DJ, Cavanagh PR. An investigation of the in-shoe pressure distribution during cycling in conventional cycling shoes or running shoes. In: Jonsson B, ed. *Biomechanics X-B*. Champaign, IL: Human Kinetics Publishers, 1987:903–907.
42. Sanderson DJ, Hennig EM. In-shoe pressure distribution in cycling and running shoes during steady-rate cycling. *Proceedings of the Second North American Congress on Biomechanics*. Chicago, August 24–28, 1992:247–248.
43. Amoroso AT, Hennig EM, Sanderson DJ. In-shoe pressure distribution for cycling at different cadences. *Proceedings of the Second North American Congress on Biomechanics*. Chicago, August 24–28, 1992:249–250.
44. Hennig EM, Sanderson DJ. In-shoe pressure distribution for cycling at different power outputs. *Proceedings of the Second North American Congress on Biomechanics*. Chicago, August 24–28, 1992:251–252.
45. Wheeler JB, Gregor RJ, Broker JP. A dual piezoelectric bicycle pedal with multiple shoe/pedal interface compatibility. *Int J Sports Biomech* 1992;8:251–258.
46. Wooten D, Hull ML. Design and evaluation of a multi-degree-of-freedom foot/pedal interface for cycling. *Int J Sports Biomech* 1992;8:152–164.
47. Ruby P, Hull ML. Response of intersegmental knee loads to foot/pedal platform degrees of freedom in cycling. *J Biomech* 1993;26:1327–1340.
48. McCoy RW, Gregor RJ. The effect of varying seat position on knee loads during cycling. *Med Sci Sports Exerc* 1989;21:S79.
49. Ericson MO, Bratt A, Nisell R, Nemeth G, Ekholm J. Load moments about the hip and knee joints during ergometer cycling. *Scand J Rehabil Med* 1986;18:165–172.
50. Ericson MO, Nisell R. Patellofemoral joint forces during ergometric cycling. *Phys Ther* 1987;67:1365–1369.
51. Gregor RJ. A biomechanical analysis of lower limb action during cycling at four different loads. Unpublished doctoral dissertation, Pennsylvania State University, 1976.
52. Andrews JG. The functional roles of the hamstrings and quadriceps during cycling: Lombard's paradox revisited. *J Biomech* 1987;20:565–575.
53. Browning RC, Gregor RJ, Broker JP, Whiting WC. Effects of seat height changes on joint force and moment patterns in experienced cyclists. *J Biomech* 1988;21:871.
54. Jorge K, Hull ML. Biomechanics of bicycle pedaling. In: Terauds J, Barthels K, Kreighbaum E, Mann R, Crakes E, eds. *Sports Biomechanics*. Del Mar, CA: Research Center for Sports, 1984: 233–246.
55. Redfield R, Hull ML. On the relation between joint moments and pedaling rates at constant power in bicycling. *J Biomech* 1986;19:317–329.
56. van Ingen Schenau GJ. From rotation to translation: constraints on multi-joint movements and the unique action of bi-articular muscles. *Hum Mov Sci* 1989;8:301–337.
57. Gregor RJ, Komi PV, Jarvinen M. Achilles tendon forces during cycling. *Int J Sports Med* 1987;8(suppl 1):S9–S14.
58. Gregor RJ, Komi PV, Browning RC, Jarvinen M. Comparison between the triceps surae and residual muscle moments at the ankle during cycling. *J Biomech* 1991;24:287–297.
59. Broker JP. Mechanical energy management during constrained human movement. Unpublished doctoral dissertation, University of California at Los Angeles, 1991.

Exercise and Sport Science,
edited by William E. Garrett, Jr., and Donald T. Kirkendall.
Lippincott Williams & Wilkins, Philadelphia © 2000.

CHAPTER 36

Biomechanics of Landing

Kathy J. Simpson, Teri Ciapponi, and He Wang

During any movement whereby the body is projected into the air, the landing phase starts at contact with the landing surface (henceforth referred to as the ground) and ends when the falling performer has no momentum. It has been surmised that bone stress–reaction problems (e.g., stress fractures) are related to force loading that occurs during the landing phase of events such as long jumping, running, dancing, and so on. Many factors can modulate force loading during landing, but it has been difficult to prove direct relations between injury etiology with these factors (1).

Figure 36–1 is a hypothetical biomechanical model of selected factors that may increase the loading on lower-extremity tissues and, hence, also increase the likelihood of impact-related injuries (e.g., bone stress–reaction injuries such as stress fractures). It is likely that lower-extremity problems due to repetitive impact with the ground have a multifactorial origin. Furthermore, we recognize that impact-related injuries related to landing activities are likely to be dependent on other factors not mentioned here (e.g., number of repetitions). Therefore, in the section on Ground-Reaction Forces, we discuss a selected few factors related to force loading on tissues during landings. Before examining these factors, however, it will be helpful to understand the actions that occur during typical landing activities during which the foot contacts the ground.

THE LANDING PHASE

After the descent phase, in which the performer is airborne, the landing phase begins at contact with the ground and ends when the center of mass of the body stops moving downward. The landing phase can be further broken down into two subphases. The passive subphase consists of the first 50 to 80 milliseconds (2). It is so named because Nigg (2) surmised that no additional muscular activation can occur in response to the sudden, high-frequency impact forces that are applied to the foot within this time frame. During the subsequent active phase, however, additional eccentric muscle activity is thought to be generated to resist the lower-extremity flexion that occurs and thereby bring the body's motion to zero.

When the predominant direction of movement during the descent is vertical (e.g., a basketball rebound or a drop landing) at contact with the ground, the forefoot generally contacts the floor first, although there are individuals who land more flat-footed and even a small number of individuals who land on their heels first. During forefoot landings, rapid dorsiflexion occurs. During any foot-landing style, knee and hip flexion also occurs. Flexion of the lower extremity serves several purposes, as it (a) reduces the amount of body mass that is involved in the initial collision with the ground (the effective mass), (b) allows tissues of the lower extremity to act collectively as a dampened spring to absorb impact forces and/or to prepare the body for a subsequent propulsive movement, and (c) may serve to reduce the forces acting on the body by increasing the distance that the center of mass travels while these forces act on the body. Later, we explore how landing technique influences the external impact forces as well as forces acting internally on the lower extremity.

GROUND-REACTION FORCES

To understand the internal force loading that is applied to tissues during any landing movement, the influence of external forces that act on a performer must first be examined. When the performer contacts the ground, thereby applying forces to the ground, the ground applies equal and opposite force to the performer, called

K.J. Simpson, T. Ciapponi, and H. Wang: Department of Exercise Science, University of Georgia, Athens, Georgia 30602-6554.

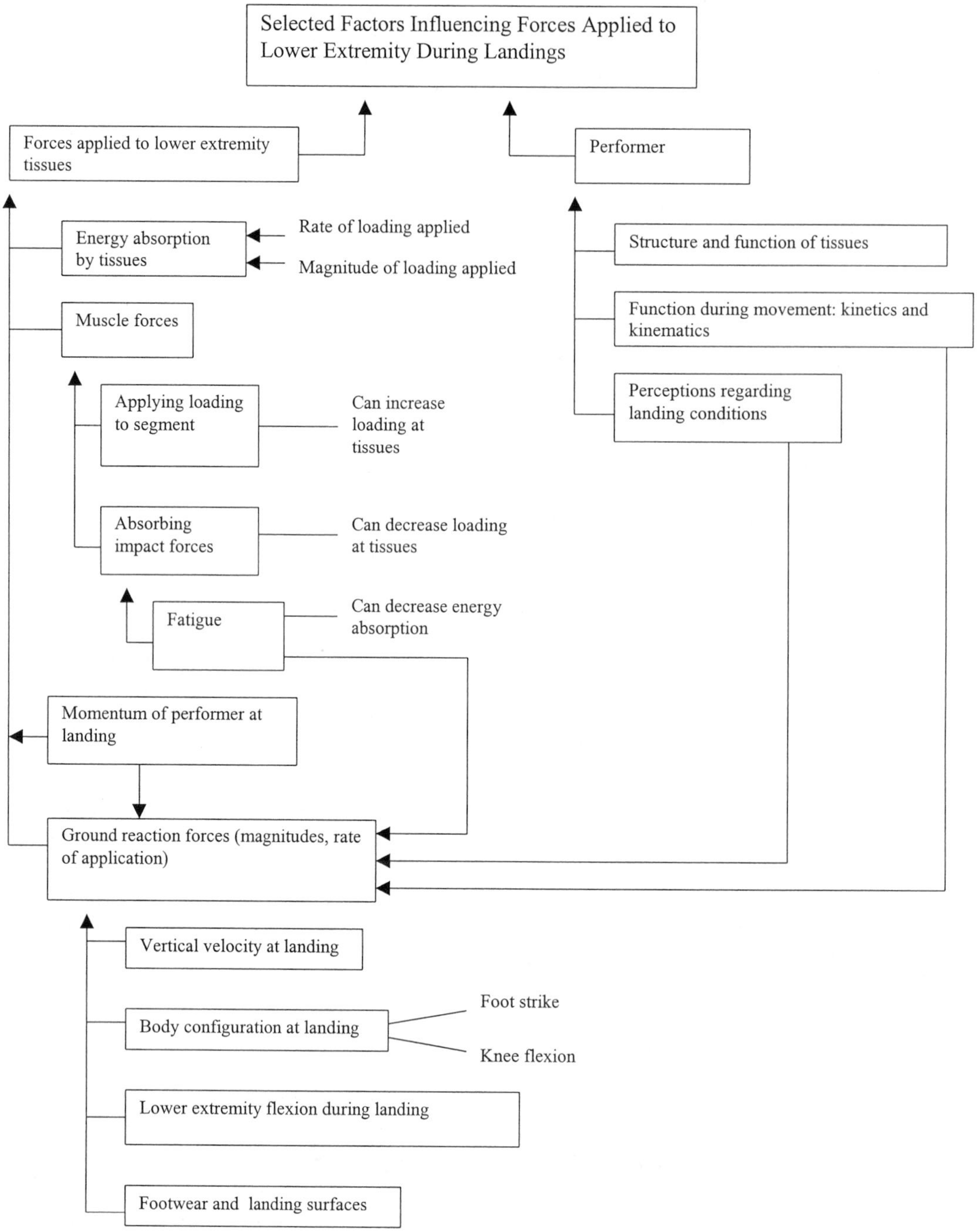

FIG. 36–1. A model of selected factors influencing forces applied to the lower extremity during landings.

grounds-reaction forces (GRFs). Vertical GRFs (VGRFs) are of most interest, as the magnitude and rate of application of VGRFs have been most closely associated with bone stress–reaction injuries (3–6).

There often are two maxima associated with the VGRF–time curve (see Fig. 36–1). The first maximum (F_1) occurs during the passive phase. F_1 is believed by some (4–6) to be related to bone stress–reaction injuries because it is indicative of impulsive loading, which has been shown in animal experiments to be related to changes in subchondral bone and articular cartilage that occur during the osteoarthritic process (4–6). The second maximum (F_2) occurs during the active phase and involves a lower frequency of loading than the passive phase (2). F_2 may occur during some movements because of active muscular effort being used to finish slowing the body's momentum to zero. For other movements, such as midfoot landings during running or low-

TABLE 36–1. *Examples of maximum vertical ground-reaction force magnitudes for the first peak (F_1), second peak (F_2), or the overall peak magnitude that are exhibited during various landing activities*

Activity	Max. vertical magnitudes (BW)	Author
Simulated basketball rebound	F_1, 1.3 F_2, 4.1 F_1 only, 6.0 Peak, 2.3–7.1	Valiant and Cavanagh (33) (forefoot landings exhibit F_1 and F_2 peaks; flat-footed landings have only one peak)
Bench-step aerobic movements	Low impact, 1.74 High impact, 3.14	Johnson et al. (77)
Dance landing	1.4–2.8	Simpson et al. (60)
Double back somersault	F_1, 12.3 F_2, 15.1	Panzer (8,9) (values may be underestimated because of various surfaces on f. platform)
Running	F_1, 1.5–3.0	For a review, see Williams (78)
Volleyball block	3.7 BW, F_1	Adrian and McLaughlin (76)
Walking		For a review, see Nigg (2)

Force is normalized to body weight (BW).

velocity impacts during dance landings, only one impact peak may occur. Magnitudes for either F_1 or maximal VGRFs for a single leg range from 1.25 times body weight (BW) for walking (7) to 15.1 BW for a double back handspring vault (8,9) (see Table 36–1 for other selected examples). For some movements, another maximum also may be exhibited during the passive phase after F_1 during very-high-impact landings (Fig. 36–2 shows a drop landing).

Also of interest in regard to loading is the rate at

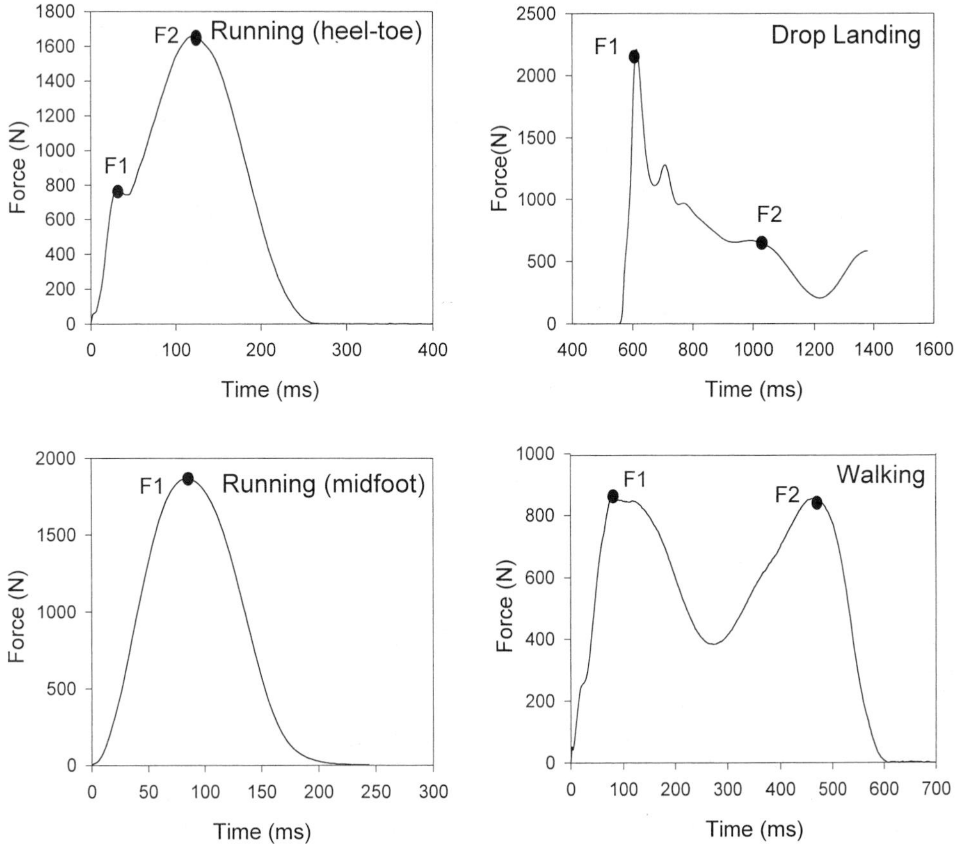

FIG. 36–2. Vertical ground-reaction force curves for various movements. The two most common maxima reported in the literature also are shown. F_1 occurs during the passive phase, and F_2 occurs during the active phase. From refs. 2 and 58, with permission.

which VGRFs are applied to the foot. Because the tissues responsible for absorbing force (e.g., bone, heel pad, and muscle) are viscoelastic, these tissues are sensitive to the rate of loading. As the rate of loading increases, the stiffness of these tissues increases to be able to absorb more force/unit deformation. Thus the rate at which impact forces are applied may influence the stiffness of these tissues. Furthermore, the rate of impulsive loading has been suggested to be the critical variable relative to stimulating degenerative changes to the cartilage (3,4,6,10). The rate of VGRF application is reported as either (a) the maximal slope of the VGRF curve between the time of surface contact and F_1, or (b) the value of the first maximal VGRF divided by the time to the first maximal VGRF.

FACTORS INFLUENCING GRF ATTENUATION DURING LANDINGS

In Fig. 36–1, several of the factors proposed to be related to impact loading and injury are shown. Some of these factors may be modified to reduce (or increase) VGRFs. How important is footwear in reducing impact forces? Do harder surfaces mean greater impact forces or rates of loading? Can a performer's technique mediate such influences as hard landing surfaces or high-velocity landings?

Attenuation of VGRFs by Footwear and Surfaces

Let us start with investigating the role of cushioning material in footwear for attenuating GRFs. There is a surprising amount of debate over whether softer midsole material changes any relevant GRF variables compared with harder materials. Lafortune and Hennig (11) reported that softer versus harder midsoles produced less impact force and lower shank shock during running. Other investigators (12–16) have reported conflicting results, however. Based on the results of 10 male recreational runners who ran across a force platform during nine footwear conditions, Snel and co-workers (12) concluded that maximal impact force did not differ significantly among various midsole hardnesses. The rate of force application and time to maximal force did vary among the shoes, however. The authors concluded that the magnitude of the impact forces was not influenced by either the model or the perceived quality of the footwear. Gross and Nelson (13) also observed that for countermovement jumps (CMJs), when landing on a force platform that was uncovered (aluminum surface) or covered with a 9.0-mm thick tartan rubber gymnasium flooring or a 13.0-mm thick midsole material commonly found in running shoes, peak impact forces and ankle-joint motion varied little among the participants. They interpreted these findings to mean that entrenched kinematics of landing overrode any adaptation to surface conditions. However, it also is possible that kinematic adjustments did occur that were not detected, that there was not enough statistical power to detect any existing differences among the surface conditions, or that individuals adapted differently from one another to various surface conditions.

In addition, there is evidence that softer midsoles may actually increase impact forces compared with harder or less protective plantar surface coverings. Nigg (14) reported that softer-midsole-material running shoes actually demonstrated significantly greater impact forces than harder-midsole-material shoes.

Stacoff and associates (15,16) suggested that this phenomenon may occur because of a cushioning effect that transpires when the foot pronates during impact. It has been observed that pronation increases with increased midsole hardness (16), but the peak impact force decreases; hence the proposition that greater pronation cushioning causes reduced peak impact forces (15).

Robbins and colleagues, in a series of investigations (17–19), provided limited evidence to support a different explanation for the lack of attenuation of VGRFs provided by softer midsole materials. They believe that individuals can modulate impact-moderating behavior (17,18). Robbins and colleagues (17) hypothesized that footwear use diminishes plantar sensation, triggering a reduction of impact-moderating behavior. Such behavior would include the modulation of temporal-load control (by intrinsic foot-shock absorption and hip flexion) and load-magnitude control (through factors causing diminished vertical movement of the body or otherwise reducing impact forces). However, Robbins and colleagues have used very controlled, somewhat static experiments. Participants were either seated with the leg stationary at a 90-degree knee angle with the foot supported by a plate (18) or lying supine with the leg extended and supported by a table (17). For seated studies, loads were applied to the knee that caused the foot to be pushed down against the foot plate. Subsequent plantar-avoidance behavior was assumed to be produced by hip flexor–force production in response to the applied load. Thus the force measured from the load cell at the base of the plantar-surface plate was believed to reflect avoidance behavior. For the supine studies, a penetrometer (a slender, rod-shaped device) was used to press various loads against various plantar regions. In support of the impact-moderating behavior premise, Robbins and associates (19) determined that wearing athletic footwear compared with not wearing footwear caused perceptions of the magnitude of plantar loading to be reduced. In another study (18), however, Robbins and associates did not observe a reduced magnitude of hip-flexor force production when athletic footwear was worn compared with the responses observed when participants were unshod but subjected to different-textured surfaces at the plantar surface of the foot.

In further support that individuals can moderate their impact-loading behavior relative to perceptions about the foot–surface interface, Robbins and Waked (20) covered the force platform with the same material but made the surface look different for three surface conditions. The 15 participants were then told deceptive information about the impact-absorption ability of the three surface conditions: The material provided either (a) superior impact absorption and injury protection, (b) poor impact absorption and high injury risk, or (c) unknown impact-absorption ability and safety. When the participants ran across the force platform, greater impact forces were demonstrated during conditions when the participants perceived the surface to have superior or unknown impact-force absorption compared with the perceived unsafe surface or to running across an uncovered platform. The authors concluded that perception of impact absorption and safety directly influences impact-moderating behavior negatively.

It is difficult to ascertain how participants respond biomechanically to perceptions of varying cushioning properties. Gross and Nelson (13) detected no significant differences for peak VGRFs or accelerations of the calcaneus and tibia during landings onto a force platform either covered by tartan or a common midsole material or uncovered (aluminum plate). The authors also could not detect any kinematic differences for different surface conditions. However, it is possible that individual participants responded differently to surface changes from other participants, thereby masking kinematic differences that could have existed.

Other investigators (21,22) found evidence that participants could accurately detect differences in high-frequency forces (F_1) among shoes of varying midsole hardnesses when asked to rate perceived "impact shock." The softest midsoles exhibited the greatest F_1 force. It is unknown how the participants were able to distinguish impact shock, as the correlation between peak pressure on the heel (which would support Robbins and co-workers' plantar sensory-feedback hypothesis) and perceived impact shock showed mixed results among the studies.

Contrary to the notion that soft cushioning reduces plantar sensory feedback, producing high-impact forces and thus more injury, a prospective study of military recruits showed that soft cushioning can decrease fatigue fractures of the lower extremity (23). Although impact forces were not measured, only 10.7% of recruits developed a fatigue fracture when a soft orthotic (an insert inside the shoe) was worn, compared with 26.8% of the control recruits.

The authors of these studies, therefore, raised an important question: What influences a given individual to respond differently compared with another individual to various landing conditions (e.g., varied footwear designs)? It has been very difficult to tease apart the factors of anatomic structure and function, participant perceptions, sensory feedback, and so on. For example, for a study of 10 aerobic-dance instructors (24), four movements that involved an impact landing onto the forefoot (including continuous aerobic dance and single drop-landing movements) were performed during four footwear conditions (court, running, aerobic, and walking shoes). A greater number of significant differences among the VGRF variables existed among the participants than among the footwear conditions. Furthermore, for any given movement, the footwear that exhibited the lowest F_1 peak and maximal rate of application varied among the participants. The sources of the interparticipant variability were not apparent.

The results from the Dufek and Bates (25) study support the observation that individual participants uniquely adapt to various footwear designs. A 25-trial, single-subject design was used to evaluate F_1 and F_2 differences among four court shoes for five subjects who performed 0.60-m drop landings onto a force platform. Individuals and the group tended to minimize F_1 and F_2 for particular shoes.

Wright and colleagues (26) measured kinematics and kinetics of nine runners. Simulations also were performed for each participant to determine whether various factors would influence impact-force magnitudes and loading. Between a hard- and a soft-shoe condition, no differences for VGRF magnitudes were detected, although a greater rate of application was observed for the hard-shoe condition. However, individual participants responded somewhat uniquely to changes in shoe hardness in regard to impact forces and kinematics.

In summary, the role of footwear and surfaces for attenuating the magnitude, timing, and rate of application of VGRFs is not well understood (27). Few studies have independently verified Robbins and colleagues' (18) hypothesis that current athletic footwear reduces impact-avoidance behavior via dampened plantar sensation. It is apparent that individual participants respond uniquely to particular landing conditions for reasons not known. However, there is a substantial body of evidence to suggest that performers do moderate their technique in response to various landing conditions.

Use of Landing Technique to Attenuate Impact Force

It has been suggested that interparticipant differences in landing technique may be a factor influencing injury potential (3,28,29). During limited testing of axial impact loading and the coupled motions of the pelvic girdle and the vertebral column, Recknagel and Witte (30) noted that during the first few milliseconds of landing, the lumbar region of the spine tends to straighten, perhaps leading to high loading in the vertebral arches. Therefore, they suggested that by landing incorrectly, excessively high vertebral loading could occur. Furthermore, high vertebral loading could perhaps promote spondylolysis and spondylolisthesis, although this was not investigated or proven.

Radin and co-workers (3) observed that the loading rate of the VGRFs during walking by individuals who had activity-related knee pain was 37% greater than that of the control group. The authors speculated that because these individuals with knee pain demonstrated less knee flexion and eccentric quadriceps action, they were exhibiting ineffective neuromuscular control before and during the initial landing phase of gait. They related this "microklutziness" to the progression of osteoarthritis. It is not clear, however, whether a greater loading rate was due to microklutziness or to existing pain.

Based on self-report, most dancers (84%) experience an injury that affects their dancing at some time, and chronic injuries are estimated to afflict 47% of ballet and modern dancers (31). Chronic dance injuries have been related to improper landing techniques by Gans (29), who observed that dancers with a history of shin splints demonstrated a different foot-landing pattern from that of injury-free dancers. However, it could not be determined whether the landing technique caused the injury, or if the injury caused the differences in landing technique.

In regard to how technique influences VGRFs, several investigations showed that for vertical movements (e.g., basketball rebound or drop landings), landing on the forefoot first rather than landing flat-footed produces significantly less peak-impact force (32–34). For example, Valiant and Cavanagh (33) observed that of 10 participants performing a simulated basketball rebound, eight chose to land by using a forefoot landing, exhibiting a mean of 1.3 BW and 4.1 BW for F_1 and F_2, respectively. The other two participants self-selected a flat-footed landing that produced a single vertical peak of 6.0 BW.

Further attenuation may be possible if forefoot contact occurs and the heel does not contact the ground (13). Nonheel-contact landers were shown by Gross and Nelson to eliminate the F_1 associated with heel contact, thereby reducing exposure to high-frequency forces by 50%. Thus some investigators (34,35) suggested that drop heights for activities such as plyometric exercises should not exceed the height at which participants can avoid landing onto their heels, perhaps a height of 40 cm (35). Barrier and associates (34) observed that heel–toe landings primarily load the knee and hip extensors, whereas toe–heel landings primarily load the ankle plantarflexors. Thus it is premature to suggest that people should land only on the balls of the feet, as other unanticipated kinetic and kinematic changes may occur.

Using joint flexion of the lower extremity has been suggested as a method to attenuate VGRFs during landings (28,32). Mizrah and Suzak (32) surmised that preprogrammed nonreflex muscle action and lower-extremity flexion were responsible for the increased VGRF attenuation observed during drop-landing conditions requiring greater joint flexion. At a higher versus lower landing height (1.0 m vs. 0.5 m), individuals of Mizrah and Suzak's study chose to increase the range of flexion at all joints. On inspection of the individual participant data, however, it is evident that when comparing the higher height values to the lower height values, there was a mixture of individual participant responses. Some participants increased the range of motion (ROM) at only one or two joints, whereas others even exhibited decreased ROM at some joints.

For gymnastic movements, Panzer and associates (8,9) observed that knee flexion reduced vertical-impact values slightly, but the time of the peak value was of more importance. McNitt-Gray (36) observed greater peak forces at greater versus lower heights for recreational athletes and gymnasts. The gymnasts exhibited greater peak forces (11.0 BW) and earlier times to peak force at the highest height than did the recreational athletes (9.1 BW), however, findings that were not true at the lower heights. McNitt-Gray concluded that gymnasts were less sensitive to changes in landing height than were the other athletes.

As most studies showed that participants reduced impact forces if greater flexion was used (28,37), it is not surprising that participants tend to use greater joint flexion at higher heights than at lower heights (28,37), as the velocity at touchdown is greater during high versus low heights. For a study in which participants were required to perform drop landings for three knee-flexion conditions (low, natural, and high knee flexion) at two heights (0.45 m and 0.70 m), Jameson and associates (28) observed that individuals self-selected a maximal degree of knee flexion that was intermediate to the constrained flexion conditions at a given height and chose to flex more at the higher height. Consequently, the maximal impact force also was intermediate to the low and high knee-flexion values of impact forces. Not surprisingly, the low-flexion peak impact value at the highest height was the greatest of all the flexion-height conditions. At the low height, time to maximal impact force and average rate of application also were related to the magnitude of knee flexion.

Observations regarding individual performances also were made by Jameson and co-workers (28). Some individuals exhibited natural knee-flexion values that were closer to the those of the low-flexion condition than the high-flexion condition and, therefore, also tended to display maximal impact forces that were closer to the low-flexion-condition values. One participant exhibited the greatest rate of force application during the natural landing condition at both heights. Although many participants self-selected greater knee flexion at the high height than at the low height, there was much interparticipant variability for time to maximal force and rate of application at the high height. This suggests that at higher heights there was more variability in movement kinematics and kinetics among participants than at lower heights.

Similarly, Dufek and Bates (37) also observed that among various heights, horizontal-landing distances and knee-flexion conditions (slight, low, and high) tested for drop landings, the most demanding landing condition (greatest height and horizontal distance and least knee flexion) produced the greatest F_2 values. However, F_1 exhibited significant interactions among landing height, distance, and individual landing technique.

Can force attenuation be taught by encouraging greater lower-extremity joint ROM during landings? Tant and associates (38) first had 30 young gymnasts drop land from 25 cm and 30 cm. Then, during a practice period, the gymnasts practiced landing as softly as possible, by using the vertical-force curves as feedback. Based on the postpractice data, gymnasts were able to reduce maximal VGRFs by 50% and 63% for the lower and higher heights, respectively. This was accomplished through kinematic alterations that included greater forward trunk flexion and increased hip and knee flexion. Therefore, individuals can be taught to attenuate forces more effectively, but it is not known at this time whether these alterations would be permanent or would create other problems (e.g., increased musculoskeletal internal force loading or reduced performance).

There is some other limited evidence that impact forces can be reduced with training (39). Female athletes involved in jumping activities underwent a 6-week neuromuscular training program involving plyometrics, during which time they were taught neuromuscular control of the lower limb during landing and were trained to increase vertical jumping height. At the end of the training period, peak VGRFs exhibited during a volleyball block were reported to decrease by 22%, while knee adduction and abduction muscle moments also decreased. Vertical-jump performance increased by 9.2%. The control group consisted of untrained male subjects, however, which may not have been an appropriate group to match with trained female athletes.

Not only may the final knee-flexion angle influence GRFs, but the joint angles of the ankle and knee at touchdown also appear to be related to impact-force attenuation (40,41). By using a four-segment model and a direct dynamics simulation technique to predict the impact phase during heel-strike running, Gerritsen and associates (40) investigated the influence of surface properties and various muscle-activation dynamics, position, and velocities of body segments at touchdown on impact forces. They determined that for initial plantarflexion angles of 8 degrees to 12 degrees, increasing plantarflexion by 1 degree would decrease the maximal impact force by 85N as well as reduce the rate of VGRF application. At the knee joint, for initial angles ranging from 92 degrees to 96 degrees, for every degree of greater knee flexion at touchdown the impact force would decrease by an average of 68N. This latter finding was supported by Lafortune and colleagues (41). Participants were placed in a pendulum apparatus with the knee angle constrained until contact with a force platform mounted vertically on a wall. A greater degree of knee flexion at contact reduced impact forces, but greater lower-leg acceleration that reflected increased tibial shock also occurred. Modulating the initial rate of knee flexion may be one method participants use to decrease F_1, possibly by decreasing the effective mass of the leg and consequently, VGRFs (26).

ROLE OF MUSCLES DURING LANDING

It has been hypothesized that during landings, eccentric muscle activity of lower-extremity extensor muscles serves as a dampening element to absorb some of the energy of the collision and to allow the body to be lowered to the ground in a smooth manner by controlling the rate of lower-extremity flexion. As it has been suggested that additional muscular activation cannot occur during the passive phase in response to the collision with the ground, activation of muscles occurs before contact with the ground (42–44). Furthermore, if muscles serve as anatomic shock absorbers (7), then how might fatigue influence impact forces? There are three aspects of the roles of muscles: (a) how do individuals adjust precontact muscle activity for different landing situations (e.g., harder surfaces); (b) what might be the role of elastic energy for movements that involve a jumping movement subsequent to a landing movement; and (c) what effect does fatigue have on impact forces?

Muscle Activation Before Landing

It was previously discussed how individuals choose to flex the lower extremity to a greater degree when landing on surfaces perceived to produce more impact force than on surfaces perceived to produce less force (e.g., a higher vs. a lower drop height). For various lower-extremity muscles, there is some evidence that precontact muscle activity exhibited during low-knee-flexion landings is less than activity demonstrated during high-knee-flexion landings, although not all extensor muscles show this effect (43,45,46). This ensures that the lower extremity can flex only to the desired degree. Later in this chapter, we show that low- versus high-flexion landings, therefore, increase the internal compressive loading on joints due to not only high-impact force loading but also increased muscle forces.

Precontact activity of the lower-extremity muscles may be related to the task demands. Precontact activity of the quadriceps muscles appears to be greatest when the movement requires a jump subsequent to the landing phase. Viitasalo and Aura (44) reported that the greatest precontact muscle activity occurred during a high jump, compared with a long horizontal hop, running hop, or drop jump. The drop jump exhibited the lowest precontact activity. They concluded that performers could modulate the preparatory activity of the neuromuscular system under varying landing/jumping conditions. In support of these observations, it appears that during a landing-only movement (e.g., drop landing), the muscles serve only as dampening elements, whereas during movement also involving projecting the body upward again (e.g., hopping), the musculotendinous units serve as springs; hence the differences in precontact muscle activation between these two types of movements (42).

Muscle force has been believed to be enhanced during jumping movements by performing a countermovement (e.g., lowering the body or performing a downward landing movement) just before the takeoff phase. One mechanism proposed to explain this phenomenon is the use of elastic energy. Another mechanism is enhanced muscle-force production due to neural responses to muscle stretch. Much of what is known about these mechanisms, however, does not come from investigating jumping movements preceded by landing movements. Knowledge of these mechanisms instead comes from comparing countermovement vertical jumps with squat jumps (SJs). Therefore, as we discuss the mechanisms, the reader should be aware that these mechanisms may work quite differently during a landing movement.

Role of Elastic Energy

During a CMJ, the person starts from a standing position and then quickly flexes the lower extremity just before the takeoff phase. In comparison, an SJ requires the participant to hold a squat position until the signal to jump as high as possible is given. Typically, an individual can jump higher when using a CMJ than an SJ (47–49). One explanation for this finding is based on storing elastic energy in musculotendinous tissues during the countermovement phase. This stored energy then is used during the takeoff phase to produce more musculotendinous force. Thus it is surmised that during the countermovement phase, lower-extremity extensor muscles are eccentrically loaded, and elastic elements of the muscles are stretched, resulting in elastic energy being stored. This elastic energy is then used to augment contractile force generated by the lower-extremity flexors during the takeoff phase (48,50).

However, some investigators (47,51,52) do not believe that greater jump height occurring during CMJ versus SJ is due to the storage and reuse of elastic energy, per se. These researchers have developed simulation models that are verified by using data from actual jump performances. In this manner, the effects of manipulating the properties of the musculotendinous tissues (e.g., tendon compliance) can be artificially determined. It is difficult, however, to verify whether the body uses the optimal strategies of muscle activation that their models predict (52). Bobbert and co-workers (52) attributed the greater jump height achieved during CMJ versus SJ by male volleyball players and by the simulation models primarily to the ability of the extensor muscles to build up active state and force before the jumping phase; hence the generation of greater muscle moments during the early takeoff phase.

Zajac (51) agreed that energy storage and use is very important during jumping but believed that there is a tradeoff between using stored energy and being able to generate active force. Therefore, he postulated that using energy storage may be an effective method of reducing the magnitude of active contractile force without compromising jump performance. Thus the benefit of a CMJ is not greater height as much as reducing the amount of contractile force required.

Based on the results of their simulation model, Anderson and Pandy (47) agreed that energy storage and reuse decreased the amount of actively generated muscle force. In addition, they found that as much strain energy was stored during the SJ as during the CMJ, but that more elastic energy was lost to heat in the CMJ. Energy also was stored differently for the two types of jumps. More energy was stored during the SJ than the CMJ via contractile elements as they worked to stretch the tendons and the series elastic elements.

Countermovements also were suggested to enhance muscle-force production during CMJ because of increased muscle stimulation compared with SJ. Lower-extremity extensor muscles are presumed to be stretched during the countermovement phase, thereby triggering spinal reflexes and/or longer-latency muscle responses that increase muscle stimulation beyond the stimulation that occurs without prior stretch (52). Bobbert and colleagues (52) questioned whether we can even determine if this mechanism explains improved jump performance, as the time period of the takeoff phase during which the enhanced muscle force would occur is not known. For the study comparing the kinetics of CMJ and SJ described above, however, Bobbert and associates acknowledged that this phenomenon could have contributed to the high level of active state and muscle force occurring during the CMJ.

Fatigue

It has been hypothesized that the ability of muscles to serve as anatomic shock absorbers (7) may be reduced by muscle fatigue or flexibility. McPoil and Cornwall further conjectured that a reduced ability to absorb impact energy may explain bone-stress reactions or fractures, although no evidence was provided to support this premise. Few studies have investigated the influence of fatigue on GRFs during actual landing activities. Dickinson and associates (53) had six participants run across a force platform barefoot for three trials before and at various times during the fatigue phase (15, 30, and 45 minutes). At the end of the fatigue phase, only a 0.08 BW difference between the unfatigued and fatigued state existed. No other variables demonstrated any significant differences for time, suggesting that fatigue had little influence on vertical GRFs. However, others have observed that fatigue affects muscle activity, F_1, and the rate of application of VGRFs during running (54) and drop landings (55). Participants in the study of James and co-workers (55) were fatigued by performing maximal-effort vertical jumps. Muscle activity decreased during the fatigue condition, whereas the F_1 and loading rate of VGRFs increased.

In another study investigating how fatigue may influence VGRFs during a short training interval, Sigg and colleagues (56) had well-trained runners reduce their weekly training by 80% for 2 weeks. Then one group of runners increased its weekly running distance by 200% for 10 days, while the control group ran at 100% of its normal mileage and performed cycling training. Although there was no differences between the groups for tibial acceleration representing impact shock, both groups exhibited greater tibial acceleration and reported increased leg fatigue and muscle soreness.

One study found that fatigue actually decreased impact forces applied to the heel region during a 45-minute run (57). It was not reported, however, whether the participants changed their step length or frequency during the running bout. With fatigue, increased variability for kinematic touchdown parameters and greater maximal pronation also were demonstrated.

JOINT KINETICS AND ENERGETICS

The net muscle moment (a *moment* is the effect of a force causing rotation) at a joint represents the net effect of all the moments created by muscle forces and other passive structures acting across a joint. Let's say that a 10-Nm knee-extensor moment was exhibited at some instant in time during a landing movement. This means that the knee extensors were the predominant knee-muscle group and that the knee extensor muscles produced 10-Nm more muscle moment than the knee flexors. With this in mind, the use of net muscle moments and power (net muscle moment × joint angular velocity) can provide some insight, albeit somewhat limited, into predominant muscle activity during landings and the mechanisms by which individuals effectively and safely land (58,59).

DeVita and co-workers (46) surmised that during the descent phase before landing, hip-flexor moments serve to rotate the trunk and thigh forward in preparation for landing. During the late descent phase, eccentric hip-extensor moments reduce hip-flexion velocity. At contact, while the lower extremity performs flexion, the muscle moments are extensor for the ankle (60) and predominantly extensor for the knee. For the hip joint, flexor moments occur during the initial contact [e.g., within the first 25 to 35 milliseconds (58,61)] and then become predominantly extensor thereafter (35,58,61). However, others have observed extensor dominance throughout the landing phase for all lower-extremity joints (62,63). DeVita and co-workers (46) observed that the general landing strategy was first to control ankle plantarflexion and knee flexion while actively flexing the trunk, thereby rotating the trunk forward and down. Hip flexion was controlled last.

At greater landing heights, when the participant has more momentum at landing, increased extensor-muscle moments about the hip and knee (62,64) and ankle joints (28) occur. The same response does not occur when little knee flexion is used during landing, however.

Participants were asked to land in such a way that the maximal amount of knee flexion required during the landing phase varied from low to high knee flexion. DeVita and Skelly (61) observed that the muscle moments at the hip and knee that were generated just before landing were preset to prepare the participants for low or high knee-flexion landings. Furthermore, as maximal knee flexion decreased, DeVita and Skelly observed that the relative contribution of the ankle plantarflexors increased, but that of the knee and hip extensors decreased.

The latter observation was supported by Jameson and associates (28). Ankle-joint moments increased as the degree of maximal knee flexion displayed during drop landings decreased. For natural landings, Jameson and colleagues also observed that the magnitude of ankle-muscle moments was intermediate to those at the low- and high-flexion landings. It was surmised that high internal contact forces would be generated at the ankle joint during low-flexion landings due to high impact forces and muscle forces. As muscles appear to absorb more energy during high-flexion landings (61,65), DeVita and Skelly also believed that other tissues, most likely the skeletal system, would be exposed to greater forces during landings when little knee flexion occurred.

INTERNAL LOADING

As noted by Cole and co-workers (10), external loading conditions do not necessarily reflect loading of internal structures. It is of interest to investigate internal loading that occurs during landing activities. To date, it is very difficult to estimate internal loading on various tissues accurately during actual landing movements, and the results of such studies should be viewed cautiously.

During landings, bone is subjected to loading in a variety of directions. For axial loading (i.e., loading that occurs in the direction parallel to the long axis of the tissue), forces can act to produce compression or tension. By using a simple Newtonian model of the foot and leg, Simpson and Kanter (60) investigated the compressive loading acting on the talus and on the proximal tibia during dance landings called traveling jumps (a two-footed takeoff to a one-footed landing with the lead leg flexed) at varying jump distances. Whereas the maximal-impact VGRF values ranged from 1.4 BW to 2.8 BW, the greatest single jump value for axial loading at the proximal tibia was 16.8 BW, produced by the femur. The quadriceps muscle group produced a maximal axial-loading value of nearly 14 BW. GRF magnitudes and rates of application for the vertical and anteroposterior directions were not correlated to the ankle axial-force magnitudes and rates of loading, whereas the compressive effects of the triceps surae were highly correlated. The knee axial force also was most sensitive to muscle forces. It was concluded that axial loading was highly affected by the amount of axial loading produced by muscles.

By using a simple model of the lower leg and foot to calculate internal loading, Skelly and DeVita (61) required participants to land with a low amount of knee flexion (mean, 117 degrees) and a high amount of knee flexion (mean, 77 degrees). Peak axial loading at the ankle was equal to 15.8 BW during the low-flexion landings and was significantly greater than loading demonstrated during high-flexion landings. This suggests that high axial loading may occur when individuals land with little knee flexion.

For running at an undisclosed speed, Scott and Winter (66) estimated peak ankle axial forces of 10.3 to 14.1 BW and Achilles tendon forces of 6.1 to 8.2 BW. At the hip joint, van den Bogert and co-workers (67) estimated that for running at 3.5 m/s, a contact force at the hip joint of 5.2 BW was produced during the propulsive phase, but only 2.5 BW was generated during walking. They concluded, therefore, that walking was safer than running for a patient with a hip prosthesis.

For another running study, Cole and associates (10) used a six-segment model of the foot to determine whether midsole hardness of running shoes affected the bone-on-bone (axial) force created at each of the joints separating the six segments of the foot. Although the amount of intertrial and interparticipant variability and possible sources of methodologic error may have masked internal force differences among footwear, Cole and associates concluded that midsole hardness had little effect on the magnitude or rate of loading of the bone-on-bone force at the subtalar and ankle joints during the impact phase of running.

Patellofemoral Loading During Landings

Knee injuries are a significant problem for dancers and become more prevalent with age (68). Of 1055 dancers treated at a sports medicine clinic during a 5-year period, 22% had knee problems (68). Patellofemoral dysfunctions, predominantly chondromalacia or patellar tendinitis, accounted for most of these knee injuries. Silver (69) reported that approximately 40% of dancers may have knee problems.

Clippinger-Robertson and colleagues (70) investigated landing technique and anatomic and structural factors to determine their relations to patellofemoral pain. Of the 362 ballet and modern dancers, 65% had experienced knee pain previously; 36% to 39% of this group reported three or more symptoms characteristic of chondromalacia patella. The authors hypothesized that high patellofemoral compression forces occurred because of the quadriceps activity that occurs to control the magnitude and rate of knee flexion during landing. Some indication of greater electromyogram (EMG) quadriceps amplitudes suggesting greater quadriceps force was demonstrated by the dancers with symptoms of chondromalacia compared with healthy dancers. Other technique-related differences between the healthy participants and those with symptoms of chondromalacia also appeared to occur. These findings should not be construed as proving that these factors caused chondromalacia, however.

Simpson and co-workers (71) also explored the role of the quadriceps in producing high patellofemoral forces during landings. For traveling jumps, we observed that as the jump distance increased, so did the quadriceps force, and, consequently, so did patellofemoral forces, ranging from an estimated 1.8 BW to 15.8 BW. To estimate patellofemoral pressure, we had to account for the complex interaction between knee flexion, contact surface area, patellofemoral force, and patellofemoral pressure (72–74). Contact area increases with greater knee flexion (up to 70 degrees to 80 degrees) or patellofemoral force, although this increased area is constrained by the increased resistance of the cartilage at high loads (73,75). Therefore, even though the patellofemoral forces increased during landings at greater versus lesser jump distances, the estimated increase in peak patellofemoral pressure was likely mediated to some degree by increased contact area and increased knee flexion. It also was concluded that the eccentrically generated quadriceps muscle forces that occurred during the landing phase were highly influential in producing high patellofemoral pressure.

CONCLUSION

In summary, landings occur during many movements. It is evident that the relations between impact-related injuries and factors believed to influence injury still must be explored. It is apparent that differences among individuals regarding footwear, technique, and their perceptions about the safety of footwear and landing surfaces make it difficult to ascertain the role of each of these factors in reducing loading on the lower extremities. In addition, other factors not discussed here (e.g., training, anatomy, and shock absorption mechanics of various tissues) are likely to play important roles in determining the magnitude and rate of lower-extremity loading as well.

Individual participants respond somewhat uniquely to different footwear–surface interfaces and landing velocities, which is, in part, influenced by their loading techniques. However, flexion of the lower extremity appears to benefit the performer during situations in which high-impact loading is anticipated, as it serves to reduce internal loading due to high-impact forces and muscle forces. Having more flexion at the knee at contact has been shown to be important in reducing impact forces and internal loading, perhaps to allow a greater range of flexion to occur during the impact phase.

Musculotendinous tissues play several important roles. They serve as anatomic shock absorbers during the landing phase. Precontact activation of muscles is necessary to prepare for the contact phase, as additional muscle activity cannot occur during the initial impact phase. To effectively perform movements that also include jumping, precontact activation is important during the flight phase. During the landing phase, activation during the active phase is surmised to occur, which may enhance the muscle force generated during the jump phase. The storage of elastic energy before jumping via eccentric loading of the lower-extremity extensor muscles is purported to be regained during the jumping phase, but whether the regained energy adds to the contractile muscle force or causes less contractile force to be generated is still controversial.

REFERENCES

1. Nigg BM, Bobbert M. On the potential of various approaches in load analysis to reduce the frequency of sports injuries. *J Biomech* 1990;23(suppl 1):3–12.
2. Nigg BM. Loads in selected sport activities: an overview. In: Winter DA, Norman RW, Wells RP, Hayes KC, Patla AE, eds. *Biomechanics IX-B.* Champaign, IL: Human Kinetics, 1985:91–96.
3. Radin EL, Yang KH, Riegger C, Kish VL, O'Connor JJ. Relationship between lower limb dynamics and knee joint pain. *J Orthop Res* 1991;9:398–405.
4. Radin EL, Paul IL. Response of joints to impact loading. *Arthritis Rheum* 1971;13:356–362.
5. Radin EL, Parker HG, Pugh JW, Steinberg RS, Paul IL, Rose RM. Response of joints to impact loading: III. *J Biomech* 1973;6:51–57.
6. Radin EL, Martin RB, Burr DB, Caterson B, Boyd RD, Goodwin C. Mechanical factors influencing cartilage damage. In: Peyron JG, ed. *Osteoarthritis: current clinical and fundamental problems.* Paris: CIBA-Geigy, 1985:90–99.
7. McPoil TG, Cornwall MW. Biomechanics in rehabilitation: running. In Zachezewski JE, Magee DJ, Quillen WS, eds. *Athletic Injuries.* Philadelphia: WB Saunders (*in press*).
8. Panzer VP. Dynamic assessment of lower extremity loading characteristics during landing. Unpublished doctoral dissertation, University of Oregon, 1987.
9. Panzer VP, Wood GA, Bates BT, Mason BR. Lower extremity loads in landings of elite gymnasts. In: DeGroot G, Hollander AP, van Ingen Schenau GJ, eds. *Biomechanics XI-B.* Amsterdam: Free University Press, 1988:727–735.
10. Cole GK, Nigg BM, Fick GH, Morlock MM. Internal loading of the foot and ankle during impact in running. *J Appl Biomech* 1995;11:25–46.
11. LaFortune MA, Hennig EM. Cushioning properties of footwear during walking: accelerometer and force platform measurements. *Clin Biomech* 1992;7:181–184.
12. Snel JG, Delleman NJ, Heerkens YF, van Ingen Schenau GJ. Shock-absorbing characteristics of running shoes during actual running. In: Winter DA, Norman RW, Wells RP, Hayes KC, Patla AE, eds. *Biomechanics XI-B.* Champaign, IL: Human Kinetics, 1985:133–137.
13. Gross TS, Nelson RC. The shock attenuation role of the ankle during landing from a vertical jump. *Med Sci Sports Exerc* 1988;20:506–514.
14. Nigg B. Factors influencing kinetic and kinematic variables in running. In: Nigg B, ed. *Biomechanics of running shoes.* Champaign, IL: Human Kinetics, 1983:139–160.
15. Stacoff A, Denoth J, Kaelin X, Sutessi E. Running injuries and shoe construction: some possible relationships. *Int J Sport Biomech* 1988;4:342–357.
16. Maeda A, Ebashi H, Nishizono H, Shibayama H. Lower extremity function for shock attenuation during landing on one leg. *Jpn J Phys Fitness Sports Med* 1994;43:219–227.
17. Robbins SE, Gouw GJ, Hanna AM. Running-related injury prevention through innate impact-moderating behavior. *Med Sci Sports Exerc* 1989;21:130–139.
18. Robbins SE, Hanna AM, Gouw GJ. Overload protection: avoidance response to heavy plantar surface loading. *Med Sci Sports Exerc* 1988;21:130–139.
19. Robbins SE, Hanna AM, Jones L. Sensory attenuation induced by modern footwear. *J Test Eval* 1988;16:412–416.
20. Robbins SE, Waked EG. Hazard of deceptive advertising of athletic footwear. *Br J Sports Med* 1997;31:299–303.
21. Hennig EM, Valiant GA, Liu Q. The relationship between biomechanical variables and the perception of cushioning for running in various types of footwear. *Clin Biomech* 1996;12:294–300.
22. Kimmeskamp S, Milani TL, Hennig EM. Relationships between perception scores and biomechanical variables for running in different footwear constructions. In: McGill S, Gross M, Patla A, eds. *Proceedings of the Third North American Congress on Biomechanics Waterloo, Ontario.* Waterloo, Ontario: University of Waterloo, 1998:327–328.
23. Finestone A, Simkin A, Milgrom C. The effect of custom biomechanical shoe orthotics on the incidence of fatigue fractures in infantry recruits. In: Kaneko Y, Shorten M, eds. *Third Symposium on Footwear Biomechanics, Tokyo, Japan.* Tokyo: Tokyo Metropolitan University, 1997:42–43.
24. Bates BT, Simpson KJ, Panzer VP. The evaluation of subject, shoe, and movement variability. In: Jonsson B, ed. *Biomechanics X-B.* Champaign, IL: Human Kinetics, 1989:909–913.
25. Dufek JS, Bates BT. Dynamic performance assessment of selected sport shoes on impact forces. *Med Sci Sports Exerc* 1991;23:1062–1067.
26. Wright IC, Neptune RR, van den Bogert AJ, Nigg BM. Passive regulation of impact forces in heel-toe running. In: Kaneko Y, Shorten M, eds. *Third Symposium on Footwear Biomechanics, Tokyo, Japan.* Tokyo: Tokyo Metropolitan University, 1997: 16–17.
27. Grau S. Sports shoes and injury: wish and reality of preventing injuries through sport-shoes. In: Kaneko Y, Shorten M, eds. *Third Symposium on Footwear Biomechanics, Tokyo, Japan.* Tokyo: Tokyo Metropolitan University, 1997:44–45.
28. Jameson EG, Simpson KJ. Effect of knee joint stiffness on ankle mechanics during a drop landing. In: Vaughan K, ed. *Proceedings of the 21st Annual Meeting of the American Society of Biomechanics.* Clemson, SC: Clemson University, 1997:91–92.
29. Gans A. The relationship of heel contact in ascent and descent from jumps to the incidence of shin splints in ballet dancers. *Phys Ther* 1985;65:1192–1196.
30. Recknagel S, Witte H. Landing procedures after jumps: wrong performance supports spondylolysis. *Z Orthop Grenzgebiete* 1996;134:214–218.
31. Bowling A. Injuries to dancers: prevalence, treatment, and perceptions of causes. *Br Med J* 1989;298:731–734.
32. Mizrah J, Suzak Z. Analysis of parameters affecting impact force attenuation during landing in human vertical free fall. *Eng Med* 1982;11:141–147.

33. Valiant G, Cavanagh PR. Drop landing from a jump: implications for the design of a basketball shoe. In: Winter DA, Norman RW, Wells RP, Hayes KC, Patla AE, eds. *Biomechanics IX-B.* Champaign, IL: Human Kinetics, 1985:117–122.
34. Barrier J, Kovacs I, Racz L, Tihanyi J, DeVita P, Hortobagyi T. Differential effects of toe versus heel landing on lower extremity joint kinetics [Abstract]. *Med Sci Sports Exerc* 1997;29(suppl): S233.
35. Bobbert MA, Huijing PA, van Ingen Schenau GJ. Drop jumping II: the influence of dropping height on the biomechanics of drop jumping. *Med Sci Sports Exerc* 1987;19:339–345.
36. McNitt-Gray JL. Kinematic and impulse characteristics of drop landings from three heights. *Int J Sport Biomech* 1991;7:201–224.
37. Dufek JS, Bates BT. The evaluation and prediction of impact forces during landings. *Med Sci Sports Exerc* 1990;22:370–377.
38. Tant CL, Wilkerson JD, Browder KD. Technique comparisons between hard and soft landings of young female gymnasts. In: Gregor RJ, Zernicek RF, Whiting WC, eds. *Proceedings of the XIIth International Congress of Biomechanics.* Los Angeles, CA: UCLA, 1989:Abstract 118.
39. Hewett TE, Stroupe AL, Nance TA, Noyes FR. Decreased impact forces and increased hamstrings torques in female athletes with plyometric training [Abstract]. *Med Sci Sports Exerc* 1996;28:S54.
40. Gerritsen KGM, van den Bogert AJ, Nigg BM. Direct dynamics simulation of the impact phase in heel-toe running. *J Biomech* 1995;28:661–668.
41. Lafortune MA, Hennig EM, Lake MJ. Dominant role of interface over knee angle for cushioning impact loading and regulating initial leg stiffness. *J Biomech* 1996;29:1523–1529.
42. Dyhre-Poulsen P, Simonsen ER, Voigt M. Dynamic control of muscle stiffness and H reflex modulation during hopping and jumping in man. *J Physiol (Lond)* 1991;437:287–304.
43. Irvine DME, McNitt-Gray JL, Munkasy BA, Barbieri C, Welch MD. Muscle activity and kinetics during landings with reduced vertical reaction forces. *J Biomech* 1993;26:359.
44. Viitasalo JT, Aura O. Myoelectrical activity of the leg extensor musculature before ground contact in jumping. In: Jonsson B, ed. *Biomechanics X-B.* Champaign, IL: Human Kinetics, 1987: 695–700.
45. Fukuda H, Misyashita M, Fukuoka M. In: Jonssen B, ed. *Biomechanics X-A.* Champaign, IL: Human Kinetics, 1987:301–305.
46. DeVita P, Dolan T, Skelly WA. Identification of a general mechanism of impact absorption in the lower extremity [Abstract]. *J Biomech* 1993;26:358.
47. Anderson FC, Pandy MG. Storage and utilization of elastic strain energy during jumping. *J Biomech* 1993;26:1413–1427.
48. Bosco C, Tarka I, Komi PV. Effect of elastic energy and myoelectrical potentiation of triceps surae during stretch-shortening cycle exercise. *Int J Sports Med* 1982;3:137–140.
49. Hudson JL. Coordination of segments in the vertical jump. *Med Sci Sports Exerc* 1986;18:242–251.
50. Brooks G, Fahey T. *Fundamentals of human performance.* New York: Macmillan, 1987.
51. Zajac FE. Muscle coordination of movement: a perspective. *J Biomech* 1993;26:109–124.
52 Bobbert MF, Gerritsen KGM, Litjens MCA, Van Soest AJ. Why is countermovement jump height greater than squat jump height? *Med Sci Sports Exerc* 1996;28:1402–1412.
53. Dickinson JA, Cook SD, Leinhardt TM. The measurement of shock waves following heel strike while running. *J Biomech* 1985;18:415–422.
54. Christina K, White S, McCrory J. The effects of dorsiflexor fatigue on kinetic measures during running. In: McGill S, Gross M, Patla A, eds. *Proceedings of the Third North American Congress on Biomechanics, Waterloo, Ontario.* Waterloo, Ontario: University of Waterloo, 1998:311–312.
55. James CR, Dufek JS, Bates BT. Fatigue accommodation during running [Abstract]. *Med Sci Sports Exerc* 1994;26(suppl):S100.
56. Sigg J, Flynn MG, Pizza FX, Armstrong CW, Brolinson PG. Excessive training and foot impact shock in competitive distance runners [Abstract]. *Med Sci Sports Exerc* 1992;24(suppl):S130.
57. Brueggemann GP, Arndt A. Fatigue and lower extremity function. In: Shorten MR, ed. *Symposium on the biomechanics of functional footwear, Calgary, Alberta.* Calgary, Alberta: University of Calgary, 1994:4–5.
58. Dufek JS, Bates BT. Biomechanical factors associated with injury during landing in jump sports. *Sports Med* 1991;12:326–337.
59. Winter DA. Kinematic and kinetic patterns in human gait: variability and compensating effects. *Hum Mov Sci* 1984;3:51–76.
60. Simpson KJ, Kanter L. Jump distance of dance landings influencing internal joint forces: I. axial forces. *Med Sci Sports Exerc* 1997;29:916–927.
61. DeVita P, Skelly WA. Effect of landing stiffness on joint kinetics and energetics in the lower extremity. *Med Sci Sports Exerc* 1992;24:108–115.
62. McNitt-Gray JL. Landing strategy adjustments to impact speed [Abstract]. *Med Sci Sports Exerc* 1989;S21:S89.
63. Fukuda H. Biomechanical analysis of landing on surfaces with different stiffnesses. In: DeGroot G, Hollander AP, van Ingen Schenau GJ, eds. *Biomechanics XI-B.* Amsterdam: Free University Press, 1988:102–106.
64. Dufek JS, Bates BT. The relationship between maximum ground reaction forces and lower extremity extensor joint moments during landing. In: *Proceedings of the 14th Annual American Society of Biomechanics.* Miami, FL, 1990:14–16.
65. Tsiorsky VM, Prilutsky BI. Soft and stiff landing. In: Jonsson B, ed. *Biomechanics X-B.* Champaign, IL: Human Kinetics, 1987:739–743.
66. Scott SH, Winter DA. Internal forces at chronic running injury sites. *Med Sci Sports Exerc* 1990;22:357–369.
67. van den Bogert AJ, Read L, Nigg BM. An analysis of hip joint loading during walking, running and skiing. In: Williams KR, ed. *Proceedings of the Nineteenth Annual Meeting for the American Society of Biomechanics, Stanford, CA.* Stanford, CA: Stanford University, 1995:203–204.
68. Garrick J. Ballet injuries. *Med Prob Perform Artists* 1986; 1:123–127.
69. Silver DM. Knee problems and solutions in dancers. *Kines Dance* 1985;8:9–10.
70. Clippinger-Robertson K, Hutton R, Miller D, Nichols T. Mechanical and anatomical factors relating to the incidence of etiology of patellofemoral pain of dancers. In: Shell C, ed. *The 1984 Olympic Scientific Congress Proceedings.* Vol 8. Eugene, OR: University of Oregon, 1986:53–72.
71. Simpson KJ, Jameson EG, Odum S. Estimated patellofemoral compressive forces and contact pressures during dance landings. *J Appl Biomech* 1996;12:1–14.
72. Zidorn T. Intramedullary patel pressure measurement dependent on the functional position of the knee joint. *Z Orthop* 1991; 129:488–491.
73. Hehne HJ. Biomechanics of the patellofemoral joint and its clinical relevance. *Clin Orthop* 1990;258:73–85.
74. Huberti HH, Hayes WC. Patellofemoral contact pressures: the influence of Q-angle and tendofemoral contact. *J Bone Joint Surg Am* 1984;66:715–724.
75. Reithmeier E, Plitz W. A theoretical and numerical approach to optimal positioning of the patellar surface replacement in a total knee endoprosthesis. *J Biomech* 1990;23:883–892.
76. Adrian MJ, Laughlin CK. Magnitude of ground reaction forces while performing volleyball skills. In: Matsui H, Kobayashi K, eds. *Biomechanics VIII-B.* Champaign, IL: Human Kinetics, 1983: 903–914.
77. Johnson BF, Rupp JC, Berry SA, Rupp DA. Peak vertical ground reaction forces (PVGRFs) and time-to-peak force (TTPFs) in bench-step aerobics [Abstract]. *Med Sci Sports Exerc* 1992; 24(suppl):S131.
78. Williams KR. Biomechanics of running. In: Terjung RL, ed. *Exercise and sport sciences review.* Vol 13. New York: Macmillan, 1985:389–439.

Exercise and Sport Science,
edited by William E. Garrett, Jr., and Donald T. Kirkendall.
Lippincott Williams & Wilkins, Philadelphia © 2000.

CHAPTER 37

Biomechanics of Kicking

William R. Barfield

The development of all skilled behavior, as described by Bernstein (1), can be divided into two successive stages. Initially the learner must organize the degrees of freedom within the neuromuscular system into units that are functional and useful for the learner. The process can be simplified by reducing movement in the joints and through the introduction of strong temporal coupling between joint complexes. In the second stage, economic organization allows enhancement of the movement through effective use of the active forces generated by the musculature.

Anderson and Sidaway (2) suggested that kicking patterns classified as skilled movement will be enhanced, organized, and more economic with training, particularly if the objective is to maximize foot velocity, and, in turn, resultant ball velocity. The authors attributed increased improvement to changes in coordination rather than to simple increases in the speed of the entire movement pattern. Summation of speed from the hip to the knee appears to be less effective at the initiation of practice and is demonstrated in the movement through greater contributions to linear velocity of the foot from linear and angular movements at the hip. As skill develops, linear foot velocity becomes greater through an increase in angular velocity at the knee without a concomitant increase in hip angular velocity, which suggests that practice provides economic organization for the learner by effectively reducing the numbers of degrees of freedom (2). Data from Anderson and Sidaway (2) further suggest that effective summation of speed occurs when the distal segment initiates the extension movement slightly before maximal velocity of the proximal segment, although, as this chapter points out, this has not been conclusively shown.

W.R. Barfield: College of Charleston; Department of Orthopaedic Surgery, Medical University of South Carolina, Charleston, South Carolina 29425.

Of the skills necessary to participate in soccer, none has received more biomechanical research attention than kicking. From a historical perspective, the act of organized kicking had simple beginnings in games such as *tsc chu* in China around 3000 B.C. Other games such as *kemari* (Japan), *harpaston* (Italy), and *episkiyros* (Greece) involved kicking and were early versions of soccer that involved the kicking movement (3).

Kicking is a complex motor movement and therefore follows generally predictable stages. When Elliott and colleagues (4) analyzed punting by young boys between the ages of 2 and 12 years, they found that chronologically young children often struck the ball with body parts other than the foot, but by age 9 they had developed a well-defined kicking pattern. Although chronologic age was shown not necessarily to be an accurate predictor of skill development, it appears that skill develops rapidly between the ages of 4 and 6 years (4,5). For boys and girls, there appears to be a linear relationship between age and mature kicking skill between kindergarten and grade 4 (6). With skilled soccer players between the ages of 9 and 18, however, the timing pattern does not appear to differ significantly (7).

Differences between skill levels and within skill levels have been examined. When elite athletes are evaluated, the general consensus is that they exhibit less mechanical variability and therefore perform more consistently than less-skilled athletes. Rodano and Tavana (8) lend evidence to support the fact that differences exist in motor performance from one trial to the next, which will consequently influence intratrial variability. When they evaluated professional soccer players, they found increased correlations between foot speed and ball speed between their best performances and mean values. This finding led them to the conclusion that even among subjects with high technical expertise in kicking, minimal variations in motor performance can negatively influence the motor characteristics of movement, when within-subject variability is considered. Phillips (9) pointed out that lack of variability is indicative of a more acutely refined motor program, whereby muscle contractions are temporally distinct. The alternative view is that in kicking, the variability and adaptability of the neuromuscular system and the mechanical interrelations of skilled behavior are demonstrated best. When a skilled kicker was compared with a club player, the skilled kicker demonstrated less variability, based on the magnitude of standard deviations. This was seen particularly with respect to angular positions during the kicking movement. There were no significant differences in resultant ball velocities between the skilled player and the club player, and consistency of kicking by the skilled player was likely attributable to the two-step approach as opposed to the unrestricted approach used by the club player. The club player failed to use a consistent approach, which subsequently led to more inconsistent kicking velocities (9).

FRACTIONIZATION OF KICKING

The process of ball kicking, which is a variation of bipedal locomotion, has been fractionated in a number of different ways. One set of authors chose three phases: (a) approach, (b) ball strike, and (c) follow-through (10). Another chose four major movements. They were (a) initial stance, (b) approach, (c) placement of the support foot and leg adjacent the ball, and (d) swing of the kicking foot and leg (11). For our purposes, the following divisions of movement are used because these divisions of motion best describe and define kicking from a biomechanical perspective: (a) angle of approach, (b) forces on the support foot, (c) loading of the swing limb, (d) swing-limb movement during flexion at the hip and extension at the knee, (e) ball contact, and (f) follow-through. Within these areas, the muscular and mechanical components that commonly are termed *biomechanics of kicking* are addressed. The muscular component primarily concerns the effect of strength development, age, and gender differences. Mechanically, kinematics and kinetics of the swing limb, transfer of momentum, and kicker approach speed on ball velocity are discussed within each of the six components listed.

Major differences between skilled and unskilled players are based on the relative percentage of movement that is devoted to each of the components. In unskilled players, ball-kicking movement is dominated by the approach phase; skilled players, however, use approach movements, backswing, and forward-swing movements to define the kicking movement, which leads to the conclusion that with less skill, the movement is more poorly coordinated (12–14). Skilled athletes also appear to take longer strides as they approach the ball, and the temporal proximity of selected events during the kicking movement (i.e., maximal hip extension and knee flexion) is more closely associated (15).

ANGLE OF APPROACH

Developmentally, differences in the approach to the ball when attempting to kick are seen from the earliest ages. Children from ages 3.75 to 4.67 years do not take any steps to the ball, and at earlier ages simply walk into the ball. As children mature chronologically, a paced run-up is used, and the angle of the approach becomes more diagonal. Efficient segmental timing for the kick reveals that maximal angular velocity at the knee progressively increases with age during the preadolescent years, and the timing of maximum angular velocity at the knee corresponds more closely with ball contact (15). One of the most surprising findings from Bloomfield and associates (5) is the wide range of abilities from the subjects tested between the ages of 3.75 and 11.17 years. Despite differences exhibited between children in similar age groups (intragroup variability), the authors believe that there is a general developmental trend that most children tend to follow. It is important to note, however, that all children do not follow traditional stages of development (5).

Several authors have emphasized that the diagonal approach, as opposed to the straight approach, results in greater swing-limb velocity (16–19). Plagenhoff (19) reported that the side approach (30°–40°), when compared with the straight-ahead approach, generated greater ball velocities (28.9 m/s vs. 25.0 m/s) because of greater "effective mass of the foot." Plagenhoff believed that the two primary factors in determining ball velocity were (a) effective mass of the foot, and (b) foot velocity immediately before ball contact. His findings provided evidence that foot velocity before impact is similar with straight and angled approaches, yet the angled approach yielded greater ball velocity; this led to the conclusion that the primary differences in ball velocity are based on greater effective striking mass with an angled approach, rather than foot velocity at ball contact (11,19).

Isokawa and Lees (17) showed that peak ball velocity is greatest at an approach angle of 45 degrees, although peak ankle velocity is greatest at a 30-degree approach angle. Peak velocity at the hip was greatest at a 15-degree approach angle, and peak knee velocity was greatest with the straight approach (0°/s). The authors attributed these notable differences to increased striking mass and greater knee and ankle fixation at the 45-degree approach angle. In the straight-ahead approach, there is limited rotation of the leg about the vertical axis through the body. As the approach angle increases, however, the leg must rotate about a vertical axis to kick the ball straight. The resistance torque that is imparted to the vertical axis through the body by the ground-reaction force (GRF) is reduced by the torque actively generated by the swing limb as the approach angle is increased. At an approach angle of 45 to 60 degrees, the active torque created by the swing limb completely balances the resistance torque generated by body motion (17). The 45- to 60-degree angled approach enables the player to take advantage of the development of significant translational and rotational components, thereby increasing leg and foot momentum at ball contact (20). When the approach angle is greater than 60 degrees, the active torque applied to the leg creates a negative torque, and therefore should be considered when assessing methods for sound technique development and prevention of injury (17).

Certainly, in the game of soccer, there are times when the objective in kicking is not to strike the ball as hard as possible; therefore, if ball placement is a crucial variable, particularly with mature players, the approach angle may be dictated by the objective (21).

The position of the plant foot from a mediolateral perspective with respect to the ball is well defined, because if support-foot position is located too far from the ball, the direction of the kick and the kicker's body balance will be negatively compromised. Most investigators are in general agreement and believe that the optimal support-foot position is 5 to 10 cm to the left of the ball, assuming the kicker is kicking with the right foot (11). Placement of the support foot alongside and adjacent the ball, perpendicular to an imaginary line drawn through the ball center, appears to provide the most appropriate environment for a successful instep-kick performance (15). When skilled and unskilled players were compared, the skilled athletes placed the support foot alongside and closer to the ball, whereas unskilled players tended to position the support foot behind the ball (22).

The position of the support foot from an anterior/posterior position is less well defined, primarily because foot position will dictate ball flight. That is, the farther behind the center of the ball the kicking foot is placed, the greater the likelihood that the ball will become flighted, which may or may not meet the kicker's objective (11).

When a conventional American football kicker was compared with a soccer-style kicker, the findings supported later studies that concluded that the soccer-style kicker, with an angled approach, displayed faster angular velocities at the knee (3560°/s) than the conventional-style kicker (2200°/s). This led the authors to conclude that the soccer-style kicker demonstrated superior kinematic variables when compared with the conventional straight ahead–style kicker (18).

FORCES ON THE SUPPORT FOOT

The relationship between GRF on the support foot and predicted distance of the punt kick has been investigated. Kermond and Konz (23) found a significant inverse relationship between vertical GRF and punt distance. The implication in this finding is that greater distance in the punt can be generated through less GRF. Based on the authors' conclusions, maximizing the force transfer to the ball while minimizing the forces on the plant foot leads to a better outcome, when ball distance is the objective.

GRFs on the plant foot also were studied with skilled and unskilled soccer populations. When compared in a ball-kicking task to determine how fast they could kick the ball, as expected, skilled players kicked faster than unskilled (25.9 m/s vs. 23.4 m/s) and the GRFs the skilled players exhibited vertically, anteroposteriorly, and laterally were greater than those among unskilled players, which is different from the conclusions drawn by Kermond and Konz (23). It is worth noting that kicking style and objective in the kick were markedly different in the two experimental procedures. Kermond and Konz's research objective was to change the ball's vertical position, whereas the objective of the study of Dos Anjos and Adrian (24) was to change the horizontal position of the ball. Dos Anjos and Adrian (24) concluded that some of the variance in greater speed of kicking among skilled players could be attributed to greater GRFs being generated in these subjects.

Isokawa and Lees (17) reported that as approach angle moved from zero to 90 degrees, peak vertical force varied minimally; however, peak frontal force and peak lateral force showed an anticipated inverse relation, with frictional force oriented increasingly in a lateral direction as the approach angle neared 90 degrees. In a later study, Barfield (13) found six mediolateral force variables [(a) maximal mediolateral force, (b) time of maximal mediolateral force, (c) mediolateral force at ball contact, (d) mean mediolateral force from support-foot contact to maximum force, (e) mean mediolateral force from support-foot contact to ball contact, and (f) time between ball contact and maximal mediolateral force] to be positively correlated with resultant ball velocity in dominant-side kicking, yet none of the same variables, at the same approach angle, were correlated on the nondominant side. As demonstrated by the graphs in Fig. 37–1, peak mediolateral force occurred before peak anteroposterior force, which is not an unexpected finding; because of the angled approach, body momentum will initially be blocked laterally. Mediolateral forces in Barfield (13) [1.07 × body weight (BW)] and Rodano and co-workers (8) (1.24 × BW) were similar in magnitude, yet Rodano and colleagues (8) found no significant correlations between GRFs and ball velocity. If the GRFs can be extrapolated without reaching a ceiling, evidence would suggest that greater mediolateral forces will enhance resultant ball velocity. Subjects have been shown to exert greater forces vertically than mediolaterally or anteroposteriorly; in Abo-Abdo's study (15),

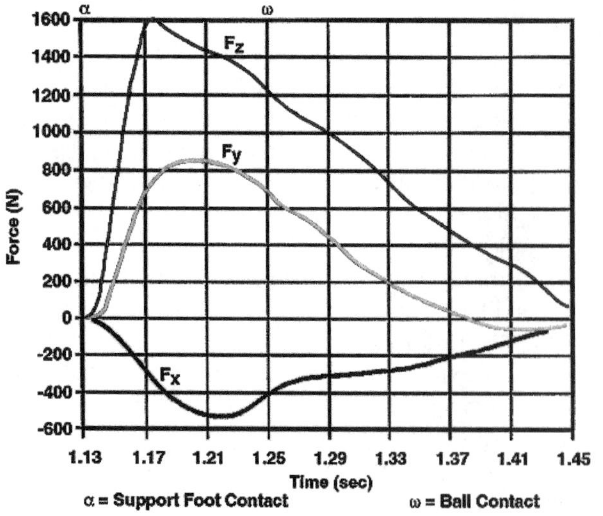

FIG. 37–1. A representative trial depicting force platform data. *Fz*, vertical; *Fy*, mediolateral; *Fx*, anteroposterior. From ref. 13, with permission.

force exerted during movement in vertical and horizontal thrusting directions was significantly correlated with "level of performance," although level of performance was not quantified (15).

The application point from these findings is that with an angled approach, when instep kicking for maximal effort, momentum that is generated from the approach path and plant-foot position can and does influence the channeling of forces that eventually are used in propelling the ball.

LOADING OF THE SWING LIMB

Consistent temporal patterning of the lower-limb segments seems to be an essential component of successful instep-kicking motion (15). The initiation of forward movement begins with the kicking-limb knee flexed and the kicking foot at approximately hip height, but well behind the coronal plane through the body. The extent of swing limb and foot placement, during the loading phase, before flexion at the hip and extension at the knee, is a function of age, skill level, ability, and the kicker's distance and path to the ball (11). As the support foot strikes the ground adjacent to the ball, the swing limb is concurrently involved in extension at the hip and flexion at the knee. During "loading" of the swing limb, the kicker's eyes are focused on the ball and not the direction the ball will travel, because ball direction is dictated by support-foot position and ultimately by hip position at ball contact (25). The loading of the swing limb allows the primary hip flexors (iliopsoas and rectus femoris) and the knee extensors (rectus femoris and vastii) to be eccentrically stretched (loaded) in preparation for the forward movement of the limb into position to strike the ball.

As demonstrated in Fig. 37–2 from Robertson and Mosher (26), the hip flexors and knee extensors show negative power (power at each articulation was calculated by using the respective product of net muscle moment and angular velocity at the hip and knee joints) between 0.00 and 0.07 s to halt the swing limb's backswing. The activity of hip flexors and knee extensors becomes concentric, yielding positive power during the forward movement in kicking (26).

Before ball contact, a large extension torque at the knee (230 Nm) is produced to provide a rapid extension rate; however, the flexion torque (280 Nm) produced at or immediately after ball contact is larger than the extensor moment. If flexion torque is initiated too early in the kicking movement, the limb and kicking foot are slowed before contact, which subsequently decreases eventual ball velocity. Obviously, to achieve optimal performance, the energy that is generated before ball contact should not be reduced. Limiting the time avail-

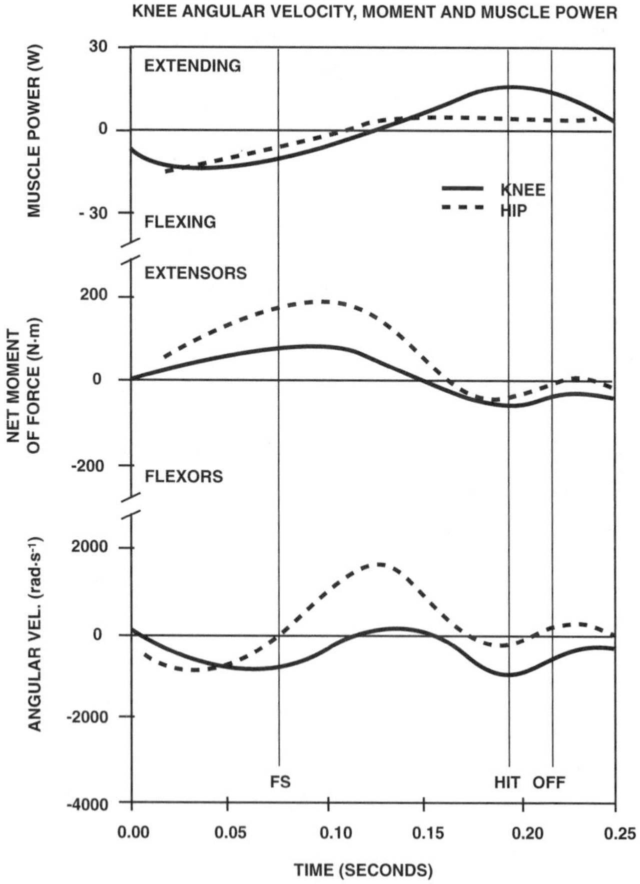

FIG. 37–2. Hip (*dashed lines*) and knee (*solid lines*) angular velocity, net moment of force, and power during a soccer kick. *FS*, contralateral leg footstrike; *HIT*, ball contact; *OFF*, start of ball flight. From ref. 26, with permission.

able to dissipate stored energy increases the muscle forces required eventually to slow the limb, however (27). Findings from Gainor and colleagues (27) indicated that in kicking, 15% of the kinetic energy is transmitted to the ball; however, the balance must be expended by other mechanisms including activation of the knee flexors. Immediately after the kick, the kicker appears to be in greatest danger of injury because additional loads placed on the knee can create an environment in which soft-tissue structures already under tension can readily rupture.

When slow kicks (15.24 m/s) were compared with medium (21.34 m/s) and fast kicks (27.42 m/s), knee-extensor torque increased gradually with slow kicks and was maintained throughout knee extension. In medium and fast kicks, more effective coordination was required; as one link decelerated, a more distal link showed significant accelerations, although knee-extensor torque decreased quickly a few milliseconds before or at the initiation of knee extension (28,29). Immediately before ball contact, the hamstrings (knee flexors) become dominant, which results in negative power (see Fig. 37–2).

SWING-LIMB MOVEMENT DURING FLEXION AT THE HIP AND EXTENSION AT THE KNEE

As the hip flexors forcefully contract to swing the thigh forward and downward, the leg (defined from knee to foot) and foot maintain a constant relationship and rotate as a unit. As thigh angular velocity decreases, the leg and foot begin to accelerate because of support from elastic and contractile components in the knee extensors in anticipation of striking the ball (11). The exact biomechanics of movement between the thigh and the leg and foot are a source of considerable research, which is discussed throughout this section.

The sequential segmental motion and concomitant decrease in angular velocity of the proximal segment of the leg while the distal segment increases is thought to play a critical role in kicking (7,19,30,31). Plagenhoff (19) pointed out through his research on the straight-ahead versus the angled approach to the ball that kicks with the lowest thigh deceleration showed the greatest knee extension. This points to the influence of one segment on another. The greater the muscle force used at one articulation, the less will be required at an adjacent joint to attain equal velocity at a terminal point, in this case, the foot.

Generally, there is a high degree of relationship between linear foot velocity and resultant ball velocity, and faster lower-limb angular velocity before ball contact leads to greater resultant ball velocity (13,15,32), although, as previously stated, this has not been conclusively demonstrated. As seen in the two graphs on linear and angular velocity (Figs. 37–3 and 37–4, respectively), linear velocity at the ankle is close to maximum at ball

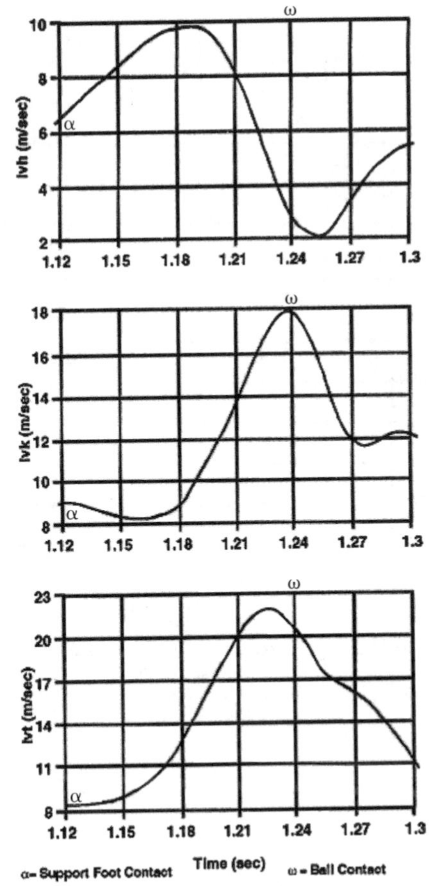

FIG. 37–3. A representative trial depicting linear velocity of the toe (*lvt*), knee (*lvk*), and hip (*lvh*). From ref. 13.

contact, as is angular velocity at the knee. Evidence to support these two graphs was previously provided by Gainor and colleagues (27) when they found that, toward the end of the kicking movement, at ball contact, the flexion moment was greater than the extension moment at the knee to prevent hyperextension.

Roberts and Metcalfe (33) found that the primary factors that influence swing-limb velocity are hip rotation initially, followed by hip flexion and knee extension before impact. There appears to be an exchange in angular velocities between proximal and distal segments in kicking, which would indicate a transfer of momentum from the more massive thigh to the less massive leg (34). Such claims, however, have not been substantiated, and there is evidence, based on segmental interaction analysis, that decreasing thigh angular velocity in kicking creates a less effective environment for an increase in leg angular velocity. The decrease in thigh angular velocity is thought by some to be the result of the leg's motion on the thigh (31,35).

There are conflicting findings as to whether this effect is the result of assistance from the eccentric role played by hip extensors (26), or whether action from the hip

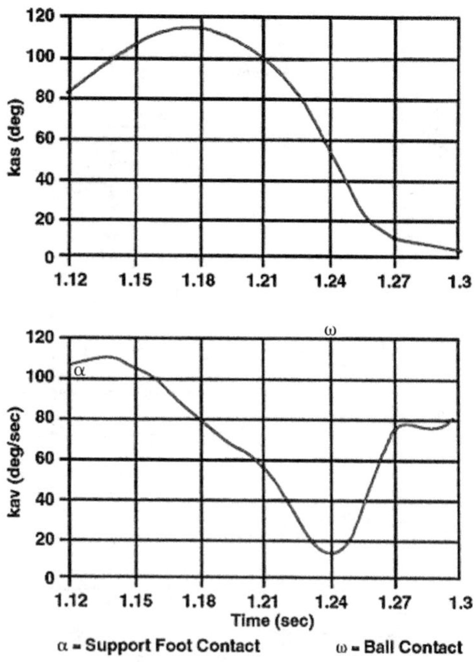

FIG. 37–4. A representative trial depicting angular displacement (*kas*) and velocity (*kav*) at the knee. From ref. 12, with permission.

flexors counters the decrease in thigh angular velocity (31,35). In a related sport activity, Joris and colleagues (36) found that the slowing of the proximal segment in handball resulted from a "pushing off" by the distal segment, which resulted in an energy flow from proximal to distal segments. The hip-extensor moment in the final phase of kicking also was given responsibility for the transfer of momentum. However, when reduced by 25%, the effect was minimal, thereby keeping the role of the hip extensors unclear (37). Putnam (31) showed that a decrease in thigh angular velocity results from a large hip-flexor moment, which counteracts the effect of the leg on the thigh, thereby limiting the loss of positive thigh angular velocity. The generally accepted thought that negative angular acceleration of a proximal segment leads to positive acceleration of an adjacent distal segment through the summation of speed principles (larger proximal muscle work continued to smaller muscles of the distal segment) cannot be supported by evidence from Putnam (31). These apparent contradictions with speed and moments relate to the fact that motion of a single segment within a linked system cannot be attributed solely to muscle forces and moments working on that one segment. Because the relationship between resultant joint moments and single-segment movement is nonlinear, quantification of segmental roles is difficult to ascertain (31).

For example, the intended speed of ball movement may be a factor in determining the roles that muscles play while kicking. Zernicke and Roberts (38) found that in slow kicks (15.24 m/s), knee-extensor action was initiated and maintained throughout the movement; however, in medium (21.34 m/s) and fast (more than 27.42 m/s) kicks, knee-extensor activity decreased immediately before or at the instant of the initiation of knee extension.

At the point of ball impact, the thigh slows, and the lower-leg velocity increases to a range of values between 20 and 30 rads/s (1100 to 1700°/s); however, the dominant impulsive moment often occurs at the hip, which indicates flexor activity (39).

When a running kick (six to eight steps) was compared with a standing kick, as expected, the linear and angular velocities of the three leg segments were greater in the running kick. When the speed of body movements was factored out, however, movement velocities for the three lower-limb segments were greater in the standing kick. Based on angular-acceleration profiles (Fig. 37–5), the data suggest that muscular effort applied to the lower limb is greater in the standing kick (40).

There is ample research demonstrating that strength development improves performance. The stretch-shortening cycle of strength training when combined with soccer training will result in greater functional kicking performance (41). The research that has been published to date, however, has been characterized by varying protocols, subject groups, ages, and ability levels. We also do not know, in most cases, whether torque values have been corrected for gravity. Despite differences in research protocols, the following is a summary of germane findings in this area.

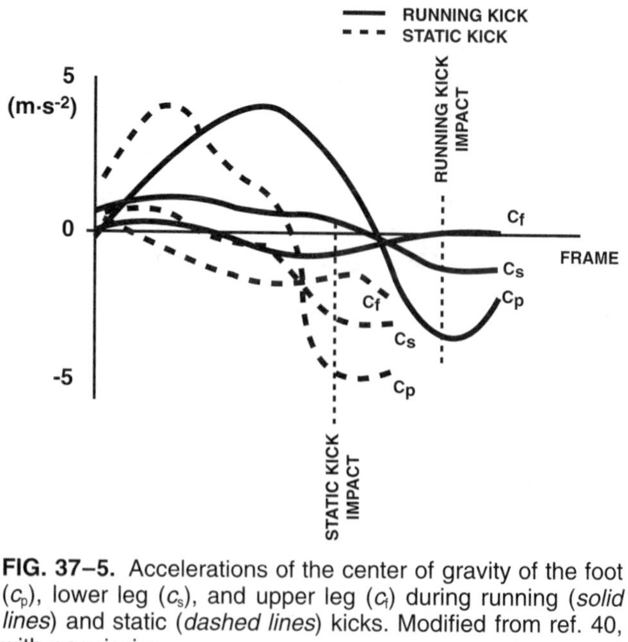

FIG. 37–5. Accelerations of the center of gravity of the foot (c_p), lower leg (c_s), and upper leg (c_f) during running (*solid lines*) and static (*dashed lines*) kicks. Modified from ref. 40, with permission.

DeProft and colleagues (42) examined the extent of agonist and antagonist muscle function during a soccer kick. They reported that the knee extensors were likely to be most active during flexion, when they are antagonist to the movement, and that skilled soccer player antagonist muscle activity was greater when compared with that of nonskilled players. On the other hand, nonskilled players appear to have greater agonist muscle action.

DeProft and co-workers (43) found that adult and youth (average age, 15.5 years) soccer players demonstrated significant increases in concentric hip-flexor and eccentric hip-extensor strength, eccentric hamstring strength (77%), and concentric quadriceps strength (25%), as measured isokinetically at 210°/s, in a study that evaluated the efficacy of a strength-training program. They also found that functional explosive muscle-power tests (long jump, vertical jump, and single-legged triple jump) were significantly correlated with kick distance. These findings lend support for a soccer-training program that is enhanced with a strength program when the objective is to improve kick distance and functional power ability in youth and adult soccer players.

Although the hip flexors have been examined less than the knee flexors, hip-flexion torque has been estimated, through ballistic movement, to be approximately three times greater than that found in the knee flexors (34). This finding has not been conclusively shown isokinetically. Discrepancies may be based on (a) the constrained, artificial environment of isokinetic testing (ballistically peak torque in hip flexion occurs with the hip extended between 29 and 46 degrees); (b) the contribution from the elastic component in the hip flexors that is not accounted for in isokinetic conditions; and/or (c) the damping effect from the isokinetic testing device, which may result in an underestimation of hip-flexion torque (44).

Research protocols also differ in the assessment of hip-flexion torque. For example, in a study that examined youth players (mean age, 17.3 years), hip-flexion torque at 180°/s was shown to be 139 Nm (mean of dominant and nondominant) (44), whereas among elite professional Greek players, hip-flexion torque was shown to be 95 Nm (45). The lower value for hip-flexion torque from elite players was probably more a function of the method of testing (no countermovement) than significant strength differences between youth players, who would normally be expected to demonstrate less torque than a group of professionals. Among youth players, the hip was extended before initiation of the movement, which allowed the countermovement to assist with the development of torque.

Oberg and associates (46) found that knee flexor/extensor strength was significantly higher in soccer players than in nonsoccer players. However, there appear to be conflicting data among populations with different research protocols. For example, when young adult male soccer players (mean age, 22 years) were compared with a control group, no significant differences existed in hamstring/quadriceps torque when they were measured at 60°/s; however, soccer players demonstrated values that were 5% to 10% greater than those of the controls. The concentric/eccentric ratio between quadriceps and hamstrings was slightly lower for soccer players than for the controls, which would indicate that the acceleration and deceleration demands of the game provide a suitable stimulus that allows development of the hamstring and quadriceps groups. During the deceleration movement, the hamstrings act eccentrically to slow extension at the knee, and the quadriceps act eccentrically to control the lowering of body weight when players approach a stop. No differences existed between dominant and nondominant sides, which would seem to indicate that among soccer players, training and matches provide sufficient bilateral exercise to prevent muscle imbalance (47). Symmetry, which is an important aspect in soccer, appears to be developed through proper arrangement of training sessions. That is, reasonably equal amounts of time are spent developing motor skills and strength, which in turn provides the stimulus necessary to produce relatively equal levels of torque in preferred and nonpreferred limbs (48).

When prepubescent male (mean age, 9.6 years) soccer players were compared with an untrained group for force and power, findings were similar to those proposed by Brady and colleagues (47) and Capranica and associates (48). Young soccer players performed, statistically, at a significantly higher level than did nonplayers. The authors surmised that soccer training enhances lower-limb muscle function without strength training (47,48). They also found no significant differences between preferred and nonpreferred limbs, which supported an earlier study that was subsequently confirmed with other studies examining preadolescent muscle dominance (47–49).

Barfield, when testing mature, skilled soccer players, found no significant differences between dominant and nondominant limbs in isokinetic testing at the hip and knee when subjects were evaluated at 180°/s. Wyatt and Edwards (50) had earlier reported no differences in knee extensor torque between dominant and nondominant limbs in non–soccer players.

Mognoni and colleagues (44) found that peak knee extension torque on the nondominant side was greater than that on the dominant side. The authors attributed this seemingly paradoxic finding to the role the nondominant knee extensors play through eccentric support of body weight and torque generated by the swing limb.

As would be expected, demonstration of muscle torque in soccer players increases with age, with the largest gains occurring between the ages of 16 and 17 years, particularly at low angular velocities (51). Differences between age groups appear to be mainly in magnitude of force production; among all age groups, however, the pattern of skilled kicking movement appears to be similar in type and timing (7).

Narici and colleagues (52) measured isokinetic torques for extension at the knee and flexion at the hip at angular speeds that closely approximated the speed of kicking and then correlated the findings with ball velocity. They varied the method of data collection so that the isokinetic movement more closely approximated actual kicking motion (i.e., hip flexion was preceded by a countermovement). They recorded peak torque and values at angles that corresponded with peak ballistic torque (ballistic peak torque of knee extensors was estimated at 90 Nm at 450°/s). Among junior players (mean age, 17.3 years), the peak torque of knee extension on the dominant side was 107 Nm, which could have been attributable to (a) the fact that torque was measured at a lower angular velocity (300°/s), and/or (b) the constrained effect of isokinetic testing (44).

Narici and co-workers (52) found when examining levels of torque at the hip and knee at 180°/s and 300°/s, respectively, that peak torque values always occurred, time wise following values calculated for peak ballistic torque. Although no differences existed between dominant and nondominant sides, there was a significant difference in ball velocities between the two sides. The authors concluded that this may have been due to an increased ability for the dominant limb to produce higher torque ballistically (52).

Cabri and colleagues (53) examined isokinetic strength at the hip and knee at 210°/s, which corresponded with angular velocities that more closely approximated the speed of dynamic limb movement in kicking, and correlated their findings with kicking a soccer ball for distance. With a three-step approach, soccer players and controls kicked a soccer ball as far as possible. With kick performance standardized, soccer players kicked the ball significantly farther than did controls, although isokinetic concentric strength at the knee was not significantly greater in soccer players when compared with the control group. However, isokinetic strength was positively correlated with kick performance eccentrically in the hamstrings and concentrically in the quadriceps. The authors concluded that soccer players have better ability to use their muscular system, thereby generating greater force in a shorter period, which is an asset when kicking for distance. Isokinetic findings from Barfield (13) are similar to those found by Cabri and co-workers (53), which indicated higher correlations between ball velocity and flexion/extension at the knee than with ball velocity and the same two isokinetic movements at the hip. Findings from Barfield (13) and Cabri and colleagues (53) are different than those from Tant (54), who found no significant relationship between torque at the knee and hip and ball velocity. Tant did, however, report that as the speed of isokinetic Cybex testing approached the speed of limb movement, a stronger relationship was observed. Isokinetic values from Barfield (13) were greater than those found by Cabri and associates (53); however, the speed of testing by Cabri and colleagues was 210°/s, and Barfield (13) tested at 180°/s. As expected, peak torque will decrease linearly on a semilogarithmic scale as angular velocity increases (55). The ratio of hamstring torque to quadriceps torque increases as the angular speed of movement increases (50).

Barfield (12) found that flexion and extension at the knee at 180°/s was correlated with maximal ball velocity on dominant and nondominant sides, which is similar to findings by Cabri and co-workers (53). Barfield (12) also found that hip-extension torque was correlated with ball velocity on the nondominant side, which would seem to provide evidence of greater variability in movement on the nondominant side.

Subject weight has a significant effect on the production of peak torque in the quadriceps in soccer and basketball players. That is, the heavier one is, the greater the torque production. However, when torque is expressed as a percentage relative to body weight, the differences between sports (basketball and soccer) and between levels of play are insignificant (28). Kamimukai and Hasegawa (56) lent further evidence in support of kicking power being a function of relative strength and torque production when they found that among female soccer players, peak isokinetic torque at 300°/s in knee extension was positively correlated with one-step kicking distance.

When soccer players were compared with nonplayers, the electromyogram (EMG) patterns of the agonist and antagonist muscles involved in kicking showed remarkably similar patterns. The single greatest discriminator was that in nonplayers, the agonists were always more active than the antagonists, which may have been indicative of a less-coordinated, less-well-defined movement. At ball contact, which is a critical point in the kicking movement, nonplayers demonstrated only 50% maximal voluntary contraction (MVC) in the antagonists, which was less than that seen in soccer players during this phase of the movement. When the entire linear-movement envelope was considered, non–soccer players showed more muscle activity than did soccer players, yet they did not kick the ball as far. Therefore, soccer players kick the ball farther with less muscle activity, but greater eccentric antagonistic activity, which may be indicative of more synergistic control in skillful movement. The message here is that soccer players may need to train the knee extensors to act concentrically at ball contact and the flexors eccentrically for kicking motion to be fluid and well controlled (42).

At the point of ball contact, the knee extensors and hip flexors are agonists and therefore need to be trained concentrically (57). At other points during the kicking movement, these same muscles act eccentrically as antagonists and follow "Lombard's paradox," which means that flexor activity is dominant during extension, and extensor activity dominates during flexion [Lombard's paradox (58) was originally used in 1903 in the description of the movement of "standing from a chair"].

Later the pattern of muscle recruitment was demonstrated in an EMG study to evaluate differences between the punt and the drop-kick. The "soccer paradox," which is another author's way of describing Lombard's paradox, as defined by DeProft and colleagues (43), showed that quadriceps activity was greatest during the loading phase when they were antagonistic to the movement. During the forward swing of the leg, the hamstrings were most active when they were antagonistic to the movement (59).

Macmillan (60), when analyzing kicks used in Australian Rules Football, found that maximal foot velocity before ball contact was primarily a function of angular velocity during knee extension. Robertson and Mosher (26) reported no knee-extensor activity immediately before ball contact. In fact, eccentric activity from the knee flexors dominated the end of the kicking motion, which subsequently reduced angular velocity at the knee. The authors offered two possible explanations for lack of knee-extensor activity. First, the hamstrings act eccentrically to reduce the possibility of hyperextension at the knee. Second, due to the velocity of knee extension (1200°/s), concentric extensor activity is inhibited because of the force–velocity relationship first proposed by Hill (61). Robertson and Mosher (26) concluded by stating that the hip muscles are the most important component of kicking because 90% of the work in kicking is attributed to thigh motion and extension at the knee. A weak and insignificant positive correlation between ball speed and angular velocity at the hip and knee (8) was similar to findings reported by Barfield (13), who found that angular velocity at the knee was not significantly correlated with ball velocity, yet the maximal value for angular velocity at the knee did occur in close proximity with ball contact.

When comparing differences in kicking between dominant and nondominant sides, Barfield (13) found that maximal angular velocity at the knee occurred in close proximity with ball contact in the dominant limb, which is a desirable finding when the objective is generation of maximal resultant ball velocity. It has, however, been shown that the maximal extending moment at the knee occurs very early in the kicking movement, before ball contact, and that the flexion moment at the knee is dominant as ball contact approaches. Figure 37–4 demonstrates that although angular velocity at the knee is close to maximum at ball contact, there is some slowing of knee extension, which is an expected finding.

Based on EMG studies, peak activity occurs in the hamstrings near the time of ball contact, which will retard a strong kick (62). Equilibrium and balance between the flexors and extensors is likely to reduce the incidence and frequency of injury, improve the neuromuscular kick pattern and generally improve kick performance (57).

Generally, when skilled and novice soccer players are compared, the muscular activity for all phases of the kicking movement, based on EMG studies, shows that skilled players demonstrate greater relaxation in the swing phase and less overall muscle activity than recreational players. For skilled players, peak quadriceps activity is seen at the end of the loading phase (flexion), which confirms the paradoxic muscular activity in soccer kicking. The fact that recreational players exhibit greater muscle activity throughout the kicking movement supports the concept that skilled players have more efficient use of their muscular system, thereby reinforcing the importance of the development of technical motor skills (63).

Despite the importance of the contributions that research on kinematics and kinetics of swing-limb motion in kicking have provided, there are conflicting studies. The reader will be left to his or her own devices to determine the validity of each finding.

BALL CONTACT

The kicker's support-foot position and contact-foot position at the time the foot makes ball contact, however brief, is of critical importance in determining the result. The time for foot/ball contact has been determined to be between 6 and 16 milliseconds (19,33,39,64,65). Plagenhoff (19) reported the lowest contact times (6 milliseconds). The apparent inconsistency of foot/ball contact may be attributable to changes in the laws of soccer, which allowed the lowering of pressure in the ball in 1975 from 1.0 to 0.6 to 0.7 kg/m^2. With lower ball pressure, the ball is likely to deform more, thereby increasing the time the foot and ball are in contact with each other. Contact time in tennis is 4 to 5 milliseconds (66), and in golf, the contact time is 0.45 milliseconds (67), both of which, by comparison, are short compared with kicking in soccer. The obvious difference is the nature of the colliding bodies and the fact that the mass of a soccer ball is significantly greater than that of a tennis or golf ball (65).

At ball contact, the knee is slightly flexed, and the foot is moving in a forward and upward arching direction. The foot is in contact with the ball during the final few degrees of extension, and angular velocity at the knee 15 milliseconds before contact is between 1500 and 2000°/s (33). Estimated impact force is between 1.0 and 1.1 kN (64,65).

The hip of the kicking limb is flexed at approximately 140 degrees as contact is made; therefore angular velocity of the thigh is minimal and provides a limited contribution to the kick at this point during the movement. Several investigators have examined the relationship between foot speed and ensuing ball speed. Roberts and Metcalfe (33) reported that foot speed 15 milliseconds before ball contact was 18 to 24 m/s, and the resultant ball velocity immediately after ball impact was 5 to 7 m/s faster than foot speed. Asami and Nolte (64) reported that foot speed decreased from 28.3 to 15.5 m/s, which differed radically from Plagenhoff (19), who earlier reported that deceleration of the foot at contact was only 3 m/s (24.1 to 21.0 m/s). This may have been attributable to (a) differences in ball inflation, which would have influenced the coefficient of restitution between balls used in the two projects, and/or (b) differences in technologies used in the projects. The Asami and Nolte (64) study used a camera speed of 500 Hz, whereas Plagenhoff likely filmed at a significantly slower rate, although the author provided no indication of film speed. Differences in foot deceleration in turn influenced striking mass, with Asami and Nolte (64) reporting a mean of 1.02 kg, which was lower than the striking mass reported by Plagenhoff (19) (3.90 kg).

Most authors have modeled the ball/foot impact as classic Newtonian mechanics; that is, the sum of the impulses (FΔt) generated by external forces on the two bodies (in this case, the foot and ball) during the time of impact will equal the change in momentum (mv) during the interval of contact. Although the time of impact is brief (6 to 16 milliseconds), magnitude changes, displacement of the ball/foot collision, and the work accomplished by active muscle force must be considered when evaluating the ball/foot-contact period during the kicking movement. Tsaousidis and Zatsiorsky (65) offered three points, which lead to the conclusion that the collision phase of kicking cannot be analyzed as a classic elastic impact event during which conservation of momentum occurs. First, during contact, there is substantial ball–foot displacement (26.0 $\pm$ 2.3 cm). Second, at the instant of peak deformation, ball speed is 54% (13.4 m/s) of ball speed when the foot is no longer in contact with the ball (24.9 m/s). Therefore, more than 50% of resultant ball speed occurs without any contribution from the potential strain energy that resulted from deformation of the ball. Finally, during the time that the ball regains its shape (recoil), foot deceleration does not occur, despite the recoil force from the ball. The authors attributed this finding to the mechanical work of muscles during this period. There is some loss of energy during impact because of hysteresis and friction between the ball/ground interface and between the foot and ball (65).

Greater foot velocity at ball impact does not always correspond with greater ball velocity. Plagenhoff (19), after finding a poor relationship between foot speed and ball speed, concluded that placement of the foot on the ball was a greater variable in attaining resultant ball velocity than maximal foot velocity. Similar findings were reported later by Aitchison and Lees (68) when they examined rugby union football. Rodano and Tavana (8), when evaluating instep kicking by professional soccer players, surprisingly found a relatively poor correlation (r = 0.49) between linear speed of the distal end of the kicking foot at the fifth metatarsal and resultant ball velocity. The indications of this finding are that other factors, such as rigidity of the limb at impact and position of the foot relative to the ball, play meaningful roles, which influence resultant ball velocity. This finding was earlier confirmed by Ben-Sira (22) when he evaluated ball velocity after ball contact among collegiate and professional soccer players (skilled athletes). He found that manner of contact between the player and ball appeared to be a major distinguishing factor between skilled and unskilled athletes, and that no significant differences exist between the professionals and collegians when assessing the postimpact ball velocity.

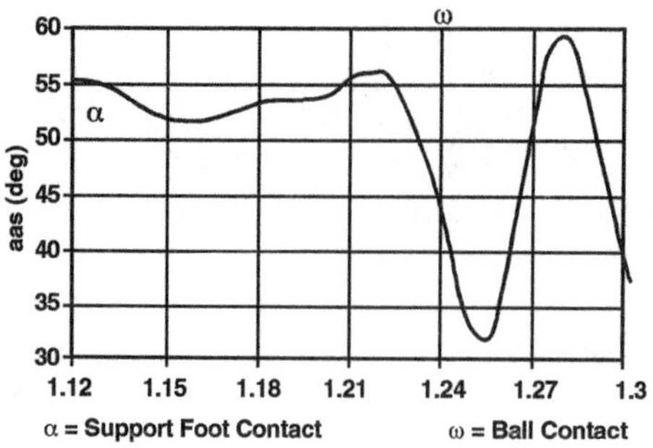

FIG. 37–6. A representative trial depicting angular displacement of the ankle at ball impact. From ref. 13, with permission.

Zernicke and Roberts (38), however, found a close positive relationship between foot speed and ball speed when testing skilled players. Ben-Sira (22) found that skilled players contact the ball closer to the ankle and display less "give" at ball contact, although forced plantar flexion has been shown to occur in a skilled population, as demonstrated in Fig. 37–6. As can be seen, at ball contact, the foot is forced into extended plantar flexion.

Therefore, firmness of the foot at ball impact is an important factor that contributes to forceful kicking. At ball contact, in instep kicking, the foot is forced into plantar flexion. Asami and Nolte (64) found that change in the ankle-joint angle did not negatively influence ball velocity, but the angle change at the metatarsophalangeal articulations correlated with decreased ball velocity.

FOLLOW-THROUGH

The follow-through after execution of a kick, as in all ballistic movements, has a twofold purpose. First, one of the primary objectives in kicking is for the kicker to keep the contacting body part (the foot in this case) in touch with the ball for as long as possible. In tennis, baseball, and other sporting activities, the implement (racquet/bat) provides a lever effect, thereby increasing the force that can be generated because of the length of the lever. In kicking, the longer the foot can keep contact with the ball, the greater the momentum that can be imparted. Second, follow-through protects the body from injury, in particular the swinging limb. The muscle and elastic forces that have been generated during other phases of the kick are dissipated during the follow-through (11). The follow-through increases the time component of the impulse side of the impulse–momentum equation, thereby reducing injury possibility.

Recent findings by Tsaousidis and Zatsiorsky (65) provide convincing support for the recommendations that have been provided to athletes for many years to follow through in completing an athletic movement such as kicking. Based on their findings, follow-through increases the mechanical work the muscles provide for the ball, thereby improving the resultant ball velocity. Follow-through is best characterized by concentric hip-flexor activity initially followed closely by eccentric knee-extensor activity. Toward the end of follow-through, concentric activity of the hip extensors dominates (26).

CONCLUSION

Kicking will continue to be a topic that will bear much discussion and research in the field of biomechanics because there continue to be a number of unresolved issues; these include: (a) the influence forces on the plant foot play in dictating ball velocity, (b) more definitive fractionization of moments and forces at the hip and knee, and (c) the relative contributions each makes to kicking.

With increased participation in soccer from every area of society from young to old, men and women, and different races, there will continue to be a need for active ongoing research to improve training, to prevent injury, and to assist with rehabilitation techniques.

REFERENCES

1. Bernstein N. *The coordination and regulation of movement.* New York: Pergamon, 1967.
2. Anderson DI, Sidaway B. Coordination changes associated with practice of a soccer kick. *Res Q Exerc Sport* 1994;65:93–98.
3. Schmid IR, McKeon JL, Schmid MR. *Skills and strategies of successful soccer.* Englewood Cliffs, NJ: Prentice-Hall, 1968.
4. Elliott BC, Bloomfield J, Davies CM. Development of the punt kick: a cinematographical analysis. *J Hum Mov Stud* 1980:6: 142–150.
5. Bloomfield J, Elliott B, Davies C. Development of the soccer kick: a cinematographical analysis. *J Hum Mov Stud* 1979; 3:152–159.
6. Butterfield SA, Loovis EM. Influence of age, sex, balance, and sport participation on development of kicking by children in grades K-8. *Percept Mot Skills* 1994;79:691–697.
7. Luhtanen P. Kinematics and kinetics of maximal instep kicking in junior soccer players. In: Reilly T, Lees A, Davids K, Murphy WJ, eds. *Science and football.* New York: E & FN Spon, 1988: 441–448.
8. Rodano R, Tavana R. Three-dimensional analysis of instep kick in professional soccer players. In: Reilly T, Clarys J, Stibbe A, eds. *Science and football II.* New York: E & FN Spon, 1993:357–361.
9. Phillips SJ. Invariance of elite kicking performance. In: Winter DA, Norman RW, Wells RP, Hayes KC, Patla AE, eds. *Biomechanics IX-B.* Champaign, IL: Human Kinetics, 1985:539–542.
10. Lohnes JH, Garrett WE, Monto RR. Soccer. In: Fu F, Stone DA, eds. *Sports injuries: mechanisms, prevention, treatment.* Baltimore: Williams & Wilkins, 1994:603–624.
11. Hay JG. *The biomechanics of sports techniques.* 4th ed. Englewood Cliffs, NJ: Prentice Hall, 1996.
12. Barfield WR. Effects of selected biomechanical variables on a coordinated human movement: instep kicking with dominant and nondominant feet. Unpublished doctoral dissertation. Auburn University, Alabama, 1993.
13. Barfield WR. Effects of selected kinematic and kinetic variables on instep kicking with dominant and nondominant limbs. *J Hum Mov Stud* 1995;29:251–272.
14. Nishijima T, Tasaki E, Noda Y, Tanaka K. Development of principal motor movements controlling ball kicking performance [Abstract]. *ACSM National Meeting Proceedings. Med Sci Sports Exerc.* 1996;28(suppl).
15. Abo-Abdo HE. Kinematic and kinetic analysis of the soccer instep kick. Unpublished doctoral dissertation. Indiana: Indiana University, 1981.
16. Asai T, Kobayashi K, Oshima Y. Biomechanical analysis of instep kick in soccer [Abstract]. In: *Proceedings of Japanese Physical Education.* 1980:139.
17. Isokawa M, Lees A. A biomechanical analysis of the instep kick motion in soccer. In: Reilly T, Lees A, Davids K, Murphy WJ, eds. *Science and football.* New York: E & FN Spon, 1988:449–455.
18. Kaufmann DA, Stanton DE, Updyke WF. Kinematical analysis of conventional-style and soccer style place kicking in football [Abstract] *Med Sci Sports Exerc* 1975;7:77–78.
19. Plagenhoff S. *Patterns of human motion: a cinematographic analysis.* Englewood Cliffs, NJ: Prentice-Hall, 1971.
20. Olson JR, Hunter GR. Anatomic and biomechanical analyses of the soccer style free kick. *Nat Strength Cond Assoc J* 1985:7:50–53.
21. Levy M. The effect of target locations and kicking techniques on approach angle in soccer [Abstract]. *ACSM National Meeting Proceedings. Med Sci Sports Exerc.* 1996;28(suppl).
22. Ben-Sira D. A comparison of the mechanical characteristics of the instep kick between skilled soccer players and novices. Unpublished doctoral dissertation. University of Minnesota, 1980.
23. Kermond J, Konz S. Support leg loading in punt kicking. *Res Q* 1978;49:71–79.
24. Dos Anjos LA, Adrian MJ. Ground reaction forces during soccer kicks performed by skilled and unskilled subjects [Abstract]. *Rev Bras Cienias Esporto* 1986;8:129–133.
25. Chyzowych W. *The official soccer book of the United States Soccer Federation.* New York: Rand McNally, 1979.
26. Robertson DGE, Mosher RE. Work and power of the leg muscles in soccer kicking. In: Winter DA, Norman RW, Wells RP, Hayes KC, Patla AE, eds. *Biomechanics IX-B.* Champaign, IL: Human Kinetics, 1985:533–538.
27. Gainor BJ, Piotrowski G, Puhl JJ, Allen WC. The kick: biomechanics and collision injury. *Am J Sports Med* 1978:6:185–193.
28. Zakas A, Mandroukas K, Vamvakoudis E, Christoulas K, Aggelopoulou N. Peak torque of quadriceps and hamstring muscles in basketball and soccer players of different divisions. *J Sports Med Phys Fitness* 1995;35:199–205.
29. Zernicke RF. Human lower extremity kinetic parameter relationships during systematic variation in resultant limb velocity. Unpublished doctoral dissertation. University of Wisconsin, Madison, 1974.
30. Putnam CA. Interaction between segments during a kicking motion. In: Matsui H, Kobayashi K, eds. *Biomechanics VIII-B.* Champaign, IL: Human Kinetics, 1985:688–694.

31. Putnam CA. A segment interaction analysis of proximal-to-distal sequential segment motion patterns. *Med Sci Sports Exerc* 1991; 23:130–144.
32. Barfield WR. Biomechanics of kicking. In: Garrett WE, Kirkendall DT, eds. *Textbook of sports medicine*. Baltimore: Williams & Wilkins, 1997:86–94.
33. Roberts EM, Metcalfe A. Mechanical analysis of kicking. In: Wartenweiler J, Jokl E, Hebbelinck M, eds. *Biomechanics I*. Baltimore: University Park Press, 1968:315–319.
34. Huang TC, Roberts EM, Youm Y. Biomechanics of kicking. In: Ghista DJ, ed. *Human body dynamics: impact, occupational, and athletic aspects*. New York: Clarendon Press & Oxford University Press, 1982:409–443.
35. Dunn EG, Putnam CA. The influence of lower leg motion on thigh deceleration in kicking. In: deGroot G, Hollander AP, Huijing PA, van Ingen Schenau GJ, eds. *Biomechanics XI-B*. Amsterdam: Free University Press, 1988:787–790.
36. Joris HJ, Edwards van Muyen AJ, van Ingen Schenau GJ, Kemper HCG. Force, velocity and energy flow during the overarm throw in female handball players. *J Biomech* 1985;18:409–414.
37. Marshall RN, Wood GA. Movement expectations and simulations: segment interactions in drop punt kicking. In: Adrian M, Deutsch H, eds. *Biomechanics: the 1984 Olympic Scientific Congress Proceedings*. Eugene, OR: Microform Publications, 1986: 111–118.
38. Zernicke RF, Roberts EM. Human lower extremity kinetic relationships during systematic variations in resultant limb velocity. In: Komi PV, ed. *Biomechanics V-B*. Baltimore: University Park Press, 1976:20–25.
39. Lindbeck L. Impulse and moment of impulse in the leg joints by impact from kicking. *J Biomech Eng* 1983;105:108–111.
40. Opavsky P. An investigation of linear and angular kinematics of the leg during two types of soccer kick. In: Reilly T, Lees A, Davids K, Murphy WJ, eds. *Science and football*. New York: E & FN Spon, 1988:456–459.
41. Jelusic V, Jaric S, Kukolj M. Effects of the stretch-shortening strength training on kicking performance in soccer players. *J Hum Mov Stud* 1992;22:231–238.
42. DeProft E, Clarys JP, Bollens E, Cabri J, Dufour W. Muscle activity in the soccer kick. In: Reilly T, Lees A, Davids K, Murphy WJ, eds. *Science and football*. New York: E & FN Spon, 1988: 443–440.
43. DeProft E, Cabri J, Dufour W, Clarys JP. Strength training and kick performance in soccer players. In: Reilly T, Lees A, Davids K, Murphy WK, eds. *Science and football*. New York: E & FN Spon, 1988:108–113.
44. Mognoni P, Narici MV, Sirtori MD, Lorenzelli F. Isokinetic torques and kicking maximal ball velocity in young soccer players. *J Sports Med Phys Fitness* 1994;34:357–361.
45. Poulmedis P. Isokinetic maximal torque power of Greek elite soccer players. *J Orthop Sports Phys Ther* 1985;6:293–295.
46. Oberg B, Moller M, Gillquist J, Ekstrand J. Isokinetic torque levels for knee extensors and knee flexors in soccer players. *Int J Sports Med* 1986;7:50–53.
47. Brady EC, O'Regan M, McCormack B. Isokinetic assessment of uninjured soccer players. In: Reilly T, Clarys J, Stibbe A, eds. *Science and football II*. New York: E & FN Spon, 1993:351–356.
48. Capranica L, Cama G, Fanton F, Tessitore A, Figura F. Force and power of preferred and non-preferred leg in young soccer players. *J Sports Med Phys Fitness* 1992;32:358–363.
49. Burnie J, Brodie DA. Isokinetic measurement in preadolescent males. *Int J Sports Med* 1986;7:205–209.
50. Wyatt MP, Edwards AM. Comparisons of quadriceps and hamstring torque values during isokinetic exercise. *J Orthop Sports Phys Ther* 1981;3:48–56.
51. Rochcongar P, Morvan R, Jan J, Dassonville J, Beillot J. Isokinetic investigation of knee extensors and knee flexors in young French soccer players. *Int J Sports Med* 1988;9:448–450.
52. Narici MV, Sirtori MD, Mognoni P. Maximal ball velocity and peak torques of hip flexor and knee extensor muscles. In: Reilly T, Lees A, Davids K, Murphy WJ, eds. *Science and football*. New York: E & FN Spon, 1988:429–433.
53. Cabri J, DeProft E, Dufour W, Clarys JP. The relation between muscular strength and kick performance. In: Reilly T, Lees A, Davids K, Murphy WJ, eds. *Science and football*. New York: E & FN Spon, 1988:186–193.
54. Tant CL. Segmental interactions of a three-dimensional soccer instep kick. Unpublished doctoral dissertation; Texas Women's University, 1990.
55. Ingemann-Hansen T, Halkjaer-Kristensen J. Force-velocity relationships in the human quadriceps muscles. *Scand J Rehabil Med* 1982;11:85–89.
56. Kamimukai C. Hasegawa Y. The relationship between ball kicking distance and isokinetic strength of the trunk and knee in female soccer players [Abstract]. *ACSM National Meeting proceedings*. 1996.
57. Clarys JP, Cabri J. Electromyography and study of sports movement: a review. *J Sports Sci* 1993;11:379–448.
58. Lombard WP. The action of two-joint muscles. *Am Phys Educ Rev* 1903:8:141–145.
59. McCrudden M, Reilly T. A comparison of the punt and the drop-kick. In: Reilly T, Clarys J, Stibbe A, eds. *Science and football II*. New York: E & FN Spon, 1993:362–366.
60. Macmillan MB. Determinants of the flight of a kicked football. *Res Q* 1975;47:48–57.
61. Hill AV. The heat of shortening and dynamic constants of muscle. *Proc R Soc B* 1938:126:136–195.
62. Wahrenberg H, Lindbeck L, Ekholm J. Knee muscular moment, tendon tension force and EMG during a vigorous movement in man. *Scand J Rehabil Med* 1978;10:99–106.
63. Bollens EC, DeProft E, Clarys JP. The accuracy and muscle monitoring in soccer kicking. In: Jonsson B, ed. *Biomechanics X-A* Champaign, IL: Human Kinetics, 1987:283–288.
64. Asami T, Nolte V. Analysis of powerful ball kicking. In: Matsui H, Kobayashi K, eds. *Biomechanics VIII-B*. Champaign, IL: Human Kinetics, 1983:695–700.
65. Tsaousidis N, Zatsiorsky V. Two types of ball-effector interaction and their relative contribution to soccer kicking. *Hum Mov Sci* 1996;15:861–876.
66. Baker JAW, Putnam CA. Tennis racket and ball responses during impact under clamped and freestanding conditions. *Res Q* 1979; 50:164–170.
67. Gobush W. Impact force measurements on golf balls. In: Cochran AJ, ed. *First World Scientific Congress of Golf*. London: E & FN Spon, 1990:219–224.
68. Aitchison I, Lees A. A biomechanical analysis of place-kicking in rugby union. In: Brodie DA, Burnie J, Eston RG, Sanderson F, Thornhill JJ, eds. *Proceedings of sport and science*. Liverpool: University of Liverpool, 1983:1–7.

Exercise and Sport Science,
edited by William E. Garrett, Jr., and Donald T. Kirkendall.
Lippincott Williams & Wilkins, Philadelphia © 2000.

CHAPTER 38

Biomechanics of Overhead Sports

Glenn S. Fleisig, Eugene G. Jameson, Charles J. Dillman, and James R. Andrews

Biomechanics typically uses kinematics and kinetics to quantify human movement. Kinematics quantifies the motion of a system (i.e., the linear and angular displacement, velocity, and acceleration), whereas kinetics quantifies the forces and torques that cause those motions. By using kinematics and kinetics, the overhead arm motions during various sports can be quantified and compared to determine the relative risks and injury potential of each.

Some of the most demanding activities on the arm result from sports requiring overhead motions. These sports include those involving the throwing motion as well as tennis, volleyball, team handball, badminton, water polo, swimming, and even diving. The prevalence of overuse injury due to throwing and other overhead movements is well documented and typically occurs as a result of repeated loading at the shoulder and elbow (1). Proper understanding and application of the principles of mechanics can help to reduce the potential for injury resulting from faulty mechanics, while helping to maximize the performance of the athlete. Because most of the overhead motions in their respective sports resemble the overarm throwing motion, and because the mechanics involved in overarm throwing have been well documented, the mechanics of overhead sports are explained relative to the throwing motion. The biomechanics of each phase of the throwing motion are presented in detail by using baseball pitching and football passing as examples. Those ideas are then applied to the specific movements and/or conditions unique to each of the other overhead sports discussed. Finally, common injuries due to overhead motions are presented, followed by rehabilitation methods and the research behind those methods.

THE KINETIC CHAIN

The concept of the kinetic chain refers to energy being created with the larger segments and muscles and then the transfer of that energy up through the trunk, out to the throwing arm, wrist, and ultimately the ball. The motion of each of the segments in the chain helps not only to maintain the energy transferred but also to build on it (2,3). The more body segments that sequentially contribute to the total force output, the greater the potential velocity at the distal end where the object is released. Proper execution of the kinetic chain in an overhead motion increases the efficiency of the movement by displacing less energy.

During throwing activities, movements are initiated from the larger muscles of the base segments and terminate with the smaller distal segments (Fig. 38–1). Previous researchers have concluded that there are primarily seven segments that have both angular and linear movements during overhead sports activities: (a) lower extremity, (b) pelvis, (c) spine, (d) shoulder girdle, (e) upper arm, (f) forearm, and (g) hand (3–8). These segments rotate about the ankle, knee, hip, intervertebral, sternoclavicular, shoulder, elbow, radioulnar, and wrist joints, which serve as the axes of rotation.

Moment of Inertia

To rotate a body segment, an athlete applies a torque, or angular force, at a joint. The amount of angular acceleration of a body segment caused by an applied torque is inversely related to that segment's moment of inertia, or the segment's resistance to rotation. The moment of inertia is related to how much mass a body segment has and the distribution of that mass from its axis of rotation. For any given muscle torque, the greater

G.S. Fleisig, E.G Jameson, and J.R. Andrews: American Sports Medicine Institute, Birmingham, Alabama 35205.
C.J. Dillman: Orthofix International Inc., Huntersville, North Carolina 28078.

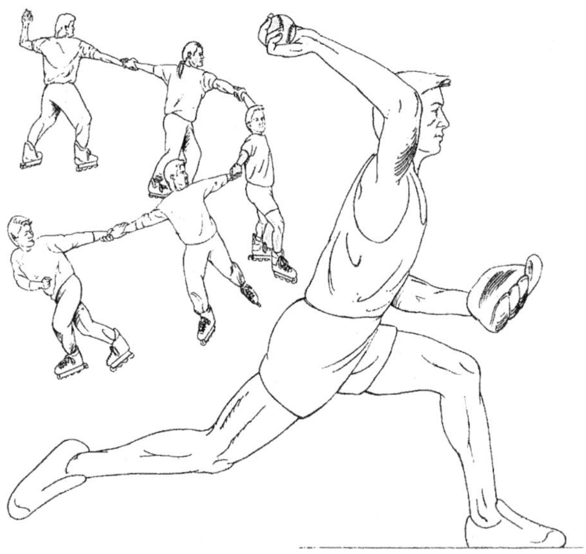

FIG. 38–1. Illustration of baseball pitcher. The larger lower-body segments are used to initiate the movement and transfer their energy up to the trunk and to the throwing arm. From ref. 9, with permission.

the mass of a segment and the farther that mass is distributed away from its rotational axis, the greater that segment's moment of inertia. This can be shown in the equation, $\alpha = T/I$, where α is the angular acceleration, T is torque, and I is the moment of inertia (Newton's Second Law). Consequently, as a segment's moment of inertia increases, angular acceleration of that segment will decrease proportionately.

In throwing, the lower extremity, pelvis, and trunk are the larger segments that produce the muscular torques that accelerate the smaller distal segments (i.e., the shoulder girdle, upper arm, forearm, and hand). These base segments have greater moments of inertia; thus they exhibit smaller angular velocities as they rotate. The smaller distal segments have smaller moments of inertia, however; therefore, they move with greater angular velocities.

Conservation of Angular Momentum

The law of conservation of angular momentum can be used to further describe the kinetic-link principle. This law states that the total angular momentum (the product of moment of inertia, I, and angular velocity, ω) of a system remains constant if there is no net torque acting on the system (i.e., $I\omega$ = constant). Figures 38–2*A* and *B* show an ice skater to illustrate this principle; for simplicity, we assume friction between the ice and skater to be nominal. With both arms abducted, a skater can rotate about a vertical axis through the body. In this case, moment of inertia is high and angular velocity is low, because mass is being distributed farther away from the axis of rotation (Fig. 38–2*A*). To generate more angular velocity, the skater can bring both arms in closer to the axis of rotation, thus reducing moment of inertia (Fig. 38–2*B*). Because there is no net torque acting on the body (remember, ice friction is negligible), angular momentum is conserved. Therefore, a decrease in moment of inertia corresponds with an increase in angular velocity and vice versa.

Fleisig and colleagues (9) used a three-segment throwing model of the pelvis, trunk, and arm to illustrate how angular momentum is conserved in throwing. When the athlete applies force to the ground, an equal but opposite force is applied by the ground to the athlete (Newton's First Law). This external force applies force and torque to the athlete, accelerating the athlete and adding both linear and angular momentum to the system. The trunk flexors and trunk rotators also impart an internal torque between the pelvis and trunk segments, thus decelerating the pelvis segment and accelerating the trunk segment. Because angular momentum is conserved, the trunk segment gains the angular momentum lost by the pelvis segment. Similarly, the intersegmental muscles between the trunk and arm impart an internal torque between these two segments, thus decelerating the trunk segment and accelerating the arm segment. Angular momentum is conserved; thus the angular momentum lost by the trunk is gained by the arm. As this process is continued, angular momentum is finally transferred to the hand segment, which releases the ball. As angular momentum is transferred from the larger base segments to the smaller distal segments, moment of inertia decreases and angular velocity in-

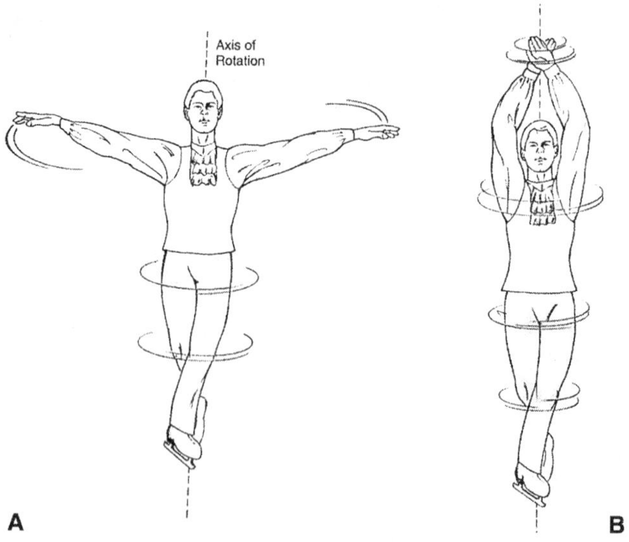

FIG. 38–2. Angular velocity of an ice skater varying with changes in moment of inertia: (**A**) slow velocity due to large inertia; and (**B**) large velocity due to small inertia. From ref. 9, with permission.

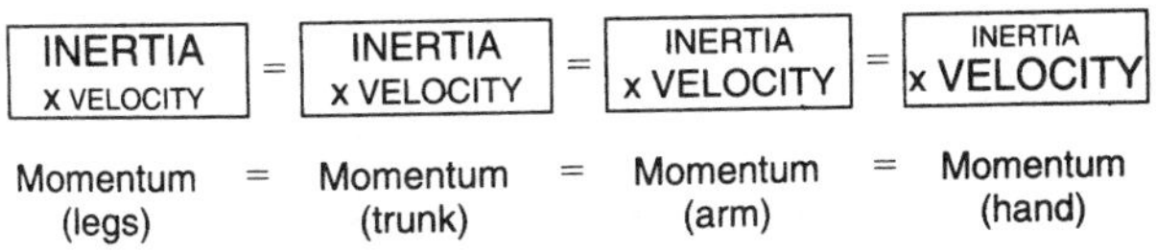

FIG. 38–3. Conservation of angular momentum.

creases, thus conserving angular momentum (9). This conservation is illustrated schematically in Fig. 38–3. In this situation, the moment of inertia is large in the more massive base segments and becomes smaller as angular momentum is transferred to the smaller distal segments. Alternatively, angular velocity is small in the larger base segments and increases as angular momentum is transferred to the distal segments.

The analysis of human movement is complex; however, the simplistic example given above should provide greater understanding of the concepts involved. It also is important to note other factors that can contribute to total joint torques. Among these are muscle-activation patterns and the related temporal characteristics, as well as the physical and mechanical properties of the muscles and other soft tissue surrounding the involved joints. It is currently not possible to accurately model the muscles' contribution to total joint forces and torques during highly dynamic activities such as throwing. Through the process known as inverse dynamics, we can estimate the net moment about a joint, but generalizations as to the amount of internal force involved must be made and interpreted with caution.

THE THROWING MOTION

The general throwing motion is similar among various sports including baseball, softball (except underhand pitching), football, team handball, javelin, water polo, and so on. The serve and overhead in tennis, the badminton smash, the serve or spike in volleyball, and even the freestyle stroke in swimming have very similar mechanics. To rehabilitate athletes and minimize injury potential, a thorough understanding of the biomechanics of overhead motions is needed.

Fleisig and colleagues used baseball pitching and football passing (Table 38–1) to represent a general model for overhead motions (9). Kinematic and kinetic ranges presented throughout this section are primarily for baseball pitching, with some ranges also presented for football passing. Baseball-pitching and football-passing parameters are compared in Table 38–1. Ranges given throughout this chapter are those values measured from high school, college, and professional baseball pitchers and football quarterbacks.

The throwing motion can be divided into six phases

TABLE 38–1. *Mean values of baseball pitching and football passing kinematic parameters*

	Baseball pitching ($n = 26$)	Football passing ($n = 26$)
Foot-contact parameters (deg)		
Elbow flexion[a]	98 ± 18	77 ± 12
Shoulder external rotation[b]	67 ± 24	90 ± 33
Shoulder abduction	93 ± 12	96 ± 13
Shoulder horizontal adduction[a]	−17 ± 12	7 ± 15
Lead knee flexion[a]	51 ± 11	39 ± 11
Delivery parameters		
Angular variables (deg)		
Max elbow flexion[a]	100 ± 13	113 ± 10
Max external rotation[b]	173 ± 10	164 ± 12
Angular velocity parameters (deg/s)		
Max elbow extension[a]	2340 ± 300	1760 ± 210
Max internal rotation[a]	7550 ± 1360	4950 ± 1080
Max upper torso[a]	1170 ± 100	950 ± 130
Max pelvis[a]	660 ± 80	500 ± 110
Release parameters (deg)		
Elbow flexion[a]	22 ± 6	36 ± 8
Shoulder horizontal adduction[a]	7 ± 7	26 ± 9
Lead knee flexion[a]	40 ± 12	28 ± 9
Trunk tilt forward[b]	58 ± 10	65 ± 8
Trunk tilt lateral[a]	124 ± 9	116 ± 5
Ball velocity (mph)[b]	35 ± 3	21 ± 2

[a]Significant difference $p < .001$.
[b]Significant difference $p < .01$.
From ref. 20, with permission.

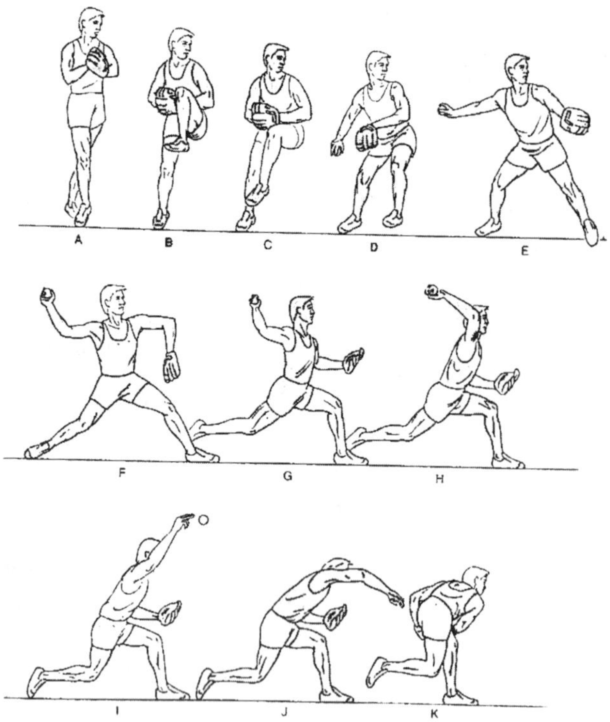

FIG. 38–4. The six phases of throwing, shown for a baseball pitcher: wind-up (**A–C**); stride (**C–F**); arm cocking (**F–H**); arm acceleration (**H–I**); arm deceleration (**I–J**); and follow-through (**J–K**). From ref. 7, with permission.

(Fig. 38–4): wind-up, stride, arm cocking, arm acceleration, arm deceleration, and follow-through (6,8).

Wind-up

The wind-up begins when the athlete initiates the first motion and ends with maximal knee lift of the stride leg. For pitching, the time from when the stance foot pivots to when the knee has achieved a maximal height and the pitcher is in a balanced position is typically between 0.5 and 1.0 seconds.

In pitching, the athlete typically begins with the weight evenly distributed on both feet. The stance foot then pivots to a position parallel with the rubber (Fig. 38–4*A*). The lead leg is lifted by concentric contractions of the hip flexors (rectus femoris, iliopsoas, sartorius, pectineus), and the lead side (left side for a right-handed thrower) faces the target. Except during pitching, the leg lift is usually not very high. The stance leg bends, slightly controlled by eccentric contractions from the quadriceps muscles, and remains in a fairly fixed position because of isometric contractions of the quadriceps until a balanced position is achieved (Fig. 38–4*B*). The hip abductors (gluteus medius, gluteus minimis, and tensor fascia latae) of the stance leg also must contract isometrically to prevent a downward tilting of the opposite-side pelvis, and the hip extensors of the stance leg contract both eccentrically and isometrically to stabilize hip flexion (10). The shoulders are partially flexed and abducted and held in this position by the anterior and medial deltoids, supraspinatus, and the clavicular portion of the pectoralis major (11,12). In addition, elbow flexion is maintained by isometric contraction of the elbow flexors (biceps brachii, brachialis, and brachioradialis) (1,10). Normally, low forces, torques, and muscle activity occur in the throwing arm during this phase.

Stride

The stride phase begins at the end of the wind-up, when the lead leg begins to fall and move toward the target and the two arms separate from each other (Fig. 38–4*C*). This phase, which ends when the lead foot first contacts the ground (Fig. 38–4*E*), lasts between 0.50 and 0.75 seconds during pitching (Fig. 38–5), and between 0.25 and 0.50 seconds during the throwing of a football.

As the phase begins, the lead leg strides toward the

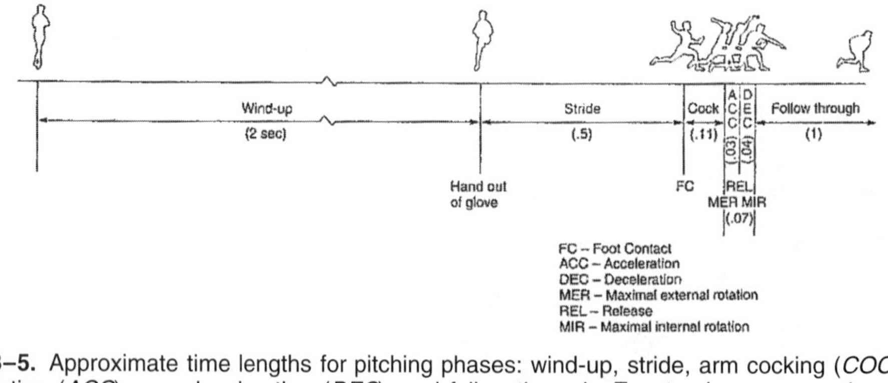

FIG. 38–5. Approximate time lengths for pitching phases: wind-up, stride, arm cocking (*COCK*), arm acceleration (*ACC*), arm deceleration (*DEC*), and follow-through. Events shown separating phases: hand out of glove, foot contact (*FC*), maximal shoulder external rotation (*MER*), ball release (*REL*), and maximal internal rotation (*MIR*). From ref. 9, with permission.

target as the stance leg remains in contact with the ground. Eccentric contraction of the hip flexors controls the lowering of the lead leg, while concentric contraction from the stance-leg hip abductors helps lengthen the stride. In pitching, it is still unclear how much of the stride is due to pushing off the rubber and how much is simply from "falling" off the rubber. In either case, the forward movement is probably initiated to some degree by hip abduction, followed by knee and hip extension from the stance leg. As the lead leg falls downward and forward, the lead hip begins to rotate externally (initiated by the gluteus maximus, sartorius, and the six deep external hip rotators), while the stance hip begins to rotate internally (initiated by the gluteus medius, gluteus minimis, and tensor fascia latae) (13). The stance hip also extends because of concentric contractions from the hip extensors (gluteus maximus and hamstrings) (10). Throughout the stride phase, the trunk is tilted slightly sideways, away from the target.

The stride length, when measured from ankle to ankle at lead-foot contact, varies considerably depending on the type of throw. In pitching, it is approximately 70% to 80% of the athlete's height, whereas a quarterback's stride during the throw is approximately 55% to 65% of the height. At foot contact, the lead foot should be pointed slightly inward (i.e., closed). For a right-handed pitcher, the left foot would point to the right, and for a left-handed pitcher, the right foot would point to the left. This closed-foot position is usually between 5 and 25 degrees deviation from the foot pointing straight ahead toward home plate (Fig. 38–6). This position helps the lead leg to act as a stable brace over which the upper body can rotate. The lead knee is flexed approximately 45 to 55 degrees at foot contact. The placement and position of the lead foot is very important in throwing. The lead foot should land directly in front of the rear foot toward the direction of the throw, or a few centimeters closed (lead foot to the right of stance foot in right-handed throwing) or open (lead foot to the left of stance foot in right-handed throwing). If it is positioned excessively closed, however, pelvis rotation can be impeded, and the athlete ends up "throwing across the body," which will minimize the contribution of the lower body to the force of the throw. Conversely if the foot is positioned excessively open, pelvis rotation occurs too early. This results in improper timing, causing energy from pelvis rotation to be applied to the upper trunk too early. Consequently, one ends up throwing with "too much arm," because the energy generated from the pelvis rotation is dissipated instead of being applied to the arm. The elastic energy generated in the legs, trunk, and arms during the stride phase is transferred to subsequent phases of the throw.

During the stride, both shoulders abduct, externally rotate, and horizontally abduct because of concentric muscle action (Fig. 38–4*E*). At lead-foot contact, throwing shoulder abduction is approximately 80 to 100 degrees. The deltoid and supraspinatus are responsible for abducting and holding the arm in this position, while maintaining the humeral head in the glenoid fossa. The upper trapezius and serratus anterior rotate upwardly and position the glenoid for the humeral head; this action is extremely important because an improperly positioned scapula can lead to impingement and shoulder-control problems (14). Muscular activity during the stride phase is shown in Table 38–2.

During the stride phase, the throwing arm is positioned slightly behind the trunk (i.e., horizontally abducted) during pitching, and slightly in front of the trunk during football passing. The posterior deltoid, latissimus dorsi, teres major, and posterior rotator-cuff muscles (infraspinatus and teres minor) are responsible for horizontally abducting the shoulder, while the rhomboids and middle trapezius retract the scapula (15).

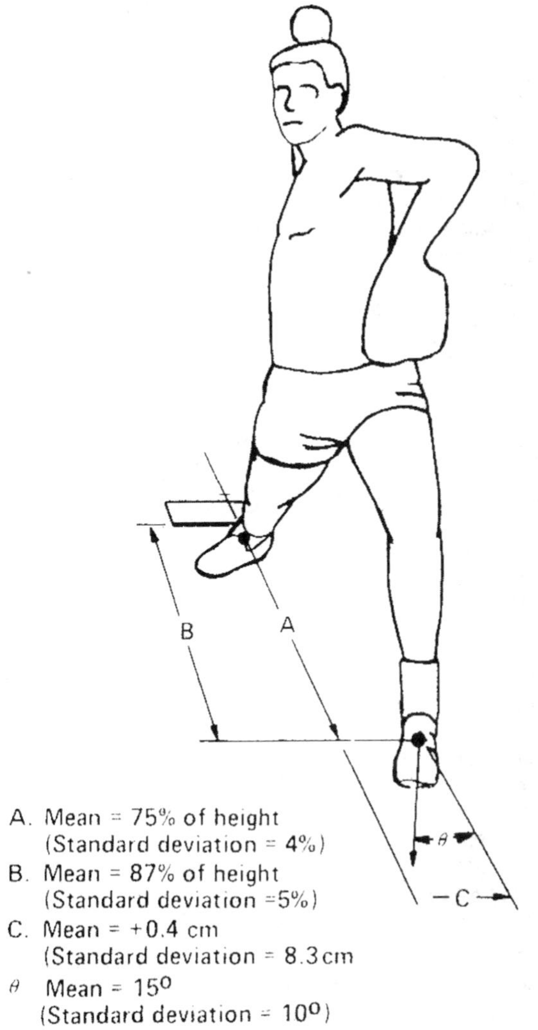

FIG. 38–6. The stride during baseball pitching. From ref. 6, with permission.

TABLE 38–2. *Muscle activity during pitching*

	N	Windup	Stride	Arm cocking	Arm accel.	Arm decel.	Follow-through
Scapular muscles							
Upper trapezius	11	18 ± 16	64 ± 53	37 ± 29	69 ± 31	53 ± 22	14 ± 12
Middle trapezius	11	7 ± 5	43 ± 22	51 ± 24	71 ± 32	35 ± 17	15 ± 14
Lower trapezius	13	13 ± 12	39 ± 30	39 ± 29	76 ± 55	78 ± 33	25 ± 15
Serratus anterior (sixth rib)	11	14 ± 13	44 ± 35	69 ± 32	60 ± 53	51 ± 30	32 ± 18
Serratus anterior (fourth rib)	10	20 ± 20	40 ± 22	106 ± 56	50 ± 46	34 ± 7	41 ± 24
Rhomboids	11	7 ± 8	35 ± 24	41 ± 26	71 ± 35	45 ± 28	14 ± 20
Levator scapula	11	6 ± 5	35 ± 14	72 ± 54	77 ± 28	33 ± 16	14 ± 13
Glenohumeral muscles							
Anterior deltoid	16	15 ± 12	40 ± 20	28 ± 30	27 ± 19	47 ± 34	21 ± 16
Middle deltoind	14	9 ± 8	44 ± 19	12 ± 17	36 ± 22	59 ± 19	16 ± 13
Posterior deltoid	18	6 ± 5	42 ± 26	28 ± 27	68 ± 66	60 ± 28	13 ± 11
Supraspinatus	16	13 ± 12	60 ± 31	49 ± 29	51 ± 46	39 ± 43	10 ± 9
Infraspinatus	16	11 ± 9	30 ± 18	74 ± 34	31 ± 28	37 ± 20	20 ± 16
Teres minor	12	5 ± 6	23 ± 15	71 ± 42	54 ± 50	84 ± 52	25 ± 21
Subscapularis (lower third)	11	7 ± 9	26 ± 22	62 ± 19	56 ± 31	41 ± 23	25 ± 18
Subscapularis (upper third)	11	7 ± 8	37 ± 26	99 ± 55	115 ± 82	60 ± 36	16 ± 15
Pectoralis major	14	6 ± 6	11 ± 13	56 ± 27	54 ± 24	29 ± 18	31 ± 21
Latissimus dorsi	13	12 ± 10	33 ± 33	50 ± 37	88 ± 53	59 ± 35	24 ± 18
Elbow and forearm muscles							
Triceps	13	4 ± 6	17 ± 17	37 ± 32	89 ± 40	54 ± 23	22 ± 18
Biceps	18	8 ± 9	22 ± 14	26 ± 20	20 ± 16	44 ± 32	16 ± 14
Brachialis	13	8 ± 5	17 ± 13	18 ± 26	20 ± 22	49 ± 29	13 ± 17
Brachioradialis	13	5 ± 5	35 ± 20	31 ± 24	16 ± 12	46 ± 24	22 ± 29
Pronator teres	14	14 ± 16	18 ± 15	39 ± 28	85 ± 39	51 ± 21	21 ± 21
Supinator	13	9 ± 7	38 ± 30	54 ± 38	55 ± 31	59 ± 31	22 ± 19
Wrist and finger muscles							
Extensor carpi radialis longus	13	11 ± 8	53 ± 24	72 ± 37	30 ± 20	43 ± 24	22 ± 14
Extensor carpi radialis brevis	15	17 ± 17	47 ± 26	75 ± 41	55 ± 35	43 ± 28	24 ± 19
Extensor digitorum communis	14	21 ± 17	37 ± 25	59 ± 27	35 ± 35	47 ± 25	24 ± 18
Flexor carpi radialis	12	13 ± 9	24 ± 35	47 ± 33	120 ± 66	79 ± 36	35 ± 16
Flexor digitorum superficialis	11	16 ± 6	20 ± 23	47 ± 52	80 ± 66	71 ± 32	21 ± 11
Flexor carpi ulnaris	10	8 ± 5	27 ± 18	41 ± 25	112 ± 60	77 ± 42	24 ± 18

Means and standard deviation, expressed as a percentage of the maximal manual muscle test.
From ref. 19, with permission.

Elbow flexion of the throwing arm at foot contact is approximately 80 to 100 degrees, while the forearm is rotated up approaching a vertical position (Fig. 38–4*F*). Quarterbacks have slightly greater elbow flexion and shoulder external rotation at lead-foot contact as compared with pitchers (see Table 38–1). In both cases, the elbow-flexor muscles of the throwing arm contract eccentrically and isometrically in controlling elbow flexion, while the supinator and biceps brachii muscles supinate the forearm as the shoulder abducts and externally rotates. Electromyography has shown that the wrist and finger extensors (extensor carpi radialis, extensor carpi ulnaris, and extensor digitorum) have very high activity during this phase, causing the wrist to move from a position of slight flexion to a position of hyperextension (15). These muscles contract concentrically as they work against gravity, with the throwing palm and ball facing downward and the shoulder abducting. Consequently, they must overcome the mass of both the hand and the ball.

Arm Cocking

Arm cocking begins at lead-foot contact and ends at maximal shoulder external rotation. In the arm-cocking phase, which lasts between 0.10 and 0.15 seconds (see Fig. 38–5), the upper body is rotated to face the target. The quadriceps of the lead leg initially contracts eccentrically to decelerate knee flexion and then contracts isometrically to stabilize the lead leg during the arm-cocking phase. At this time, the thrower's body should be extended in the direction of the target. In pitching, the ankle of the stance leg plantarflexes as it leaves contact with the rubber. This motion usually occurs concurrent with pelvis rotation, just after lead-foot contact.

The pelvis continues its transverse rotation as both hips now internally rotate. In baseball pitching, the pelvis achieves a maximal rotation of approximately 400 to 700 degree/s. Maximal pelvis rotation occurs approximately 0.03 to 0.05 seconds after foot contact, which is approximately 30% into the arm-cocking phase. As the pelvis rotates to face the target, the trunk rotators are placed on stretch, producing a recoil effect for the subsequent shoulder rotation. Shortly after the pelvis begins its rotation, the upper torso begins transverse rotation about the spinal column (Fig. 38–4*G*); consequently, the anterior trunk faces the target. Maximal upper-torso angular velocity of approximately 900 to 1300°/s (approximately twice as large as pelvis angular velocity) is achieved (see Table 38–1). This action occurs 0.05 to 0.07 seconds after lead-foot contact, which is approximately 50% into the arm-cocking phase. The abdominal and oblique musculature are placed on stretch because of the hyperextension of the lumbar trunk that occurs as the upper torso rotates.

As the larger base segments of the pelvis and upper torso rotate about the longitudinal vertebral axis, a great deal of energy is imparted to the system. Subsequently, this energy is transferred to the smaller, more distal segments if the motion is done correctly. The sequence of attaining maximal pelvic rotation before maximal upper-torso rotation is important in establishing proper timing and coordination for subsequent portions of the throw.

As the trunk rotates to face the target, the throwing shoulder horizontally adducts, moving from a position of 20 to 30 degrees of horizontal abduction at lead-foot contact to a position of 15 to 20 degrees of horizontal adduction at the time of maximal shoulder external rotation (Fig. 38–7*C*) (6). During this time, a maximal shoulder horizontal adduction velocity (relative to the trunk) of approximately 500 to 650°/s is obtained. The pectoralis major and the anterior deltoid are the primary shoulder horizontal adductors. These muscles initially contract eccentrically as the trunk rotates to face the target, thus limiting shoulder horizontal abduction. It is still unclear how much these muscles act isometrically as arm stabilizers to allow the arm to move with the trunk, and how much they function concentrically to provide dynamic horizontal adduction at the shoulder. Undoubtedly, both functions are performed in varying degrees throughout this phase.

The shoulder-girdle muscles (levator scapulae, serratus anterior, trapezius, rhomboids, and pectoralis minor) also are important during the arm-cocking phase. The serratus anterior is the most active, as it provides both stabilization and protraction to the scapula (15). The middle trapezius and rhomboids, which oppose the scapular motion created by the serratus anterior, have been shown to be quite active as well (see Table 38–2). The levator scapulae displays high muscle activity (see Table 38–2). These muscles work together in helping to stabilize the scapula and provide the position of the glenoid for subsequent action of the humeral head. Dysfunction of these scapula muscles may induce additional stress to the anterior shoulder stabilizers. During arm cocking, the serratus anterior is important in providing upward

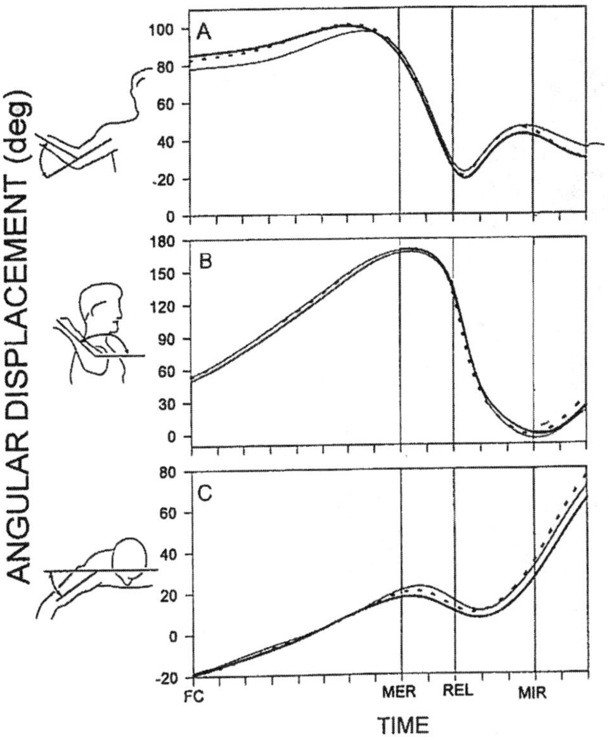

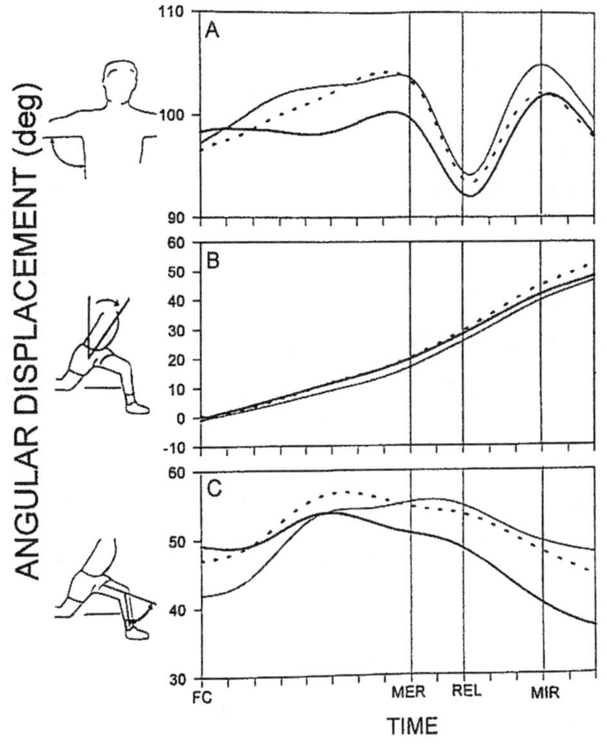

FIG. 38–7. Shoulder abduction, external/internal rotation, and horizontal adduction. *FC*, time of foot contact; *MER*, maximal shoulder external rotation; *REL*, ball release; *MIR*, maximal internal rotation. From ref. 57, with permission.

rotation and protraction of the scapula, allowing the scapula to move with the horizontally adducting humerus.

Throughout the arm-cocking phase, the shoulder remains abducted approximately 80 to 100 degrees (see Fig. 38–7*A*). The forearm and hand segments lag behind the rapidly rotating trunk and shoulder, producing a maximal shoulder external rotation of approximately 165 to 180 degrees (Figs. 38–7*C* and 38–8). The forearm now lies in a horizontal position approximately 90 degrees backward from its vertical position obtained at or just after lead-foot contact. Because of how shoulder external rotation is measured in biomechanical research, this apparent abnormal position of the throwing arm is not totally the result of external rotation at the glenohumeral joint. Some of the "external rotation" measurement is from shoulder-girdle movement at the scapulothoracic interface, and some is due to hyperextension of the lumbar trunk. Nevertheless, shoulder external rotation appears to be very important in throwing, for this parameter influences the range of motion that ensues during the rapid-acceleration phase.

Throwers with inadequate shoulder flexibility may need to perform various shoulder-stretching and -strengthening exercises to improve the range of motion and the motion available in the trunk and shoulder. Repetitive throwing tends to increase shoulder-capsule laxity and shoulder flexibility. It is not unusual for a baseball pitcher to possess 10 to 15 degrees more external rotation in the throwing shoulder compared with the nonthrowing shoulder (16,17). This extra range of motion may help both to maximize performance and to minimize injury potential at the shoulder by allowing a greater range of motion in which force can be generated, but having too much shoulder flexibility can be detrimental as well. Excessive stretching may exacerbate shoulder-capsule laxity, which over time may lead to shoulder instability. Injuries to the capsulolabral complex and rotator-cuff muscles often accompany shoulder instability. Stretching the shoulder complex should therefore be closely monitored by the trainer or therapist and should be individualized after shoulder flexibility has been properly assessed.

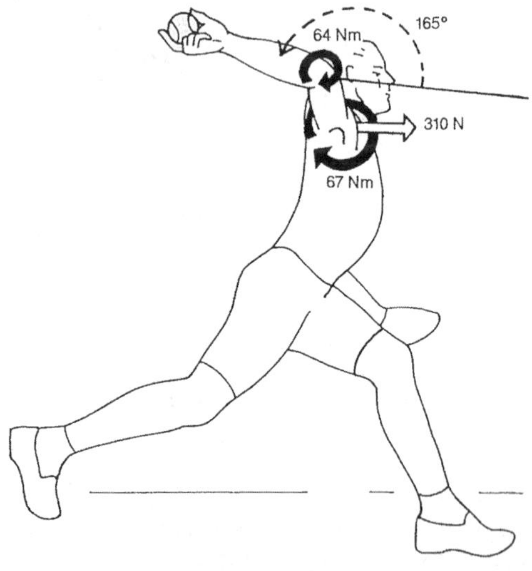

FIG. 38–8. Shortly before maximal external rotation is achieved, a critical instant occurs; at this instant, a pitcher's shoulder is externally rotated 165 degrees, and the elbow is flexed 95 degrees. Among the loads generated at this time are 67 Nm of internal rotation torque, 310 N of anterior force at the shoulder, and 64 Nm of varus torque at the elbow. From ref. 8, with permission.

In a study comparing amateur pitchers with professionals, Gowan (18) showed that the muscle activity of the subscapularis during arm cocking is approximately twice as great in professional pitchers as that observed in amateur pitchers. However, muscle activity of the biceps, serratus anterior, and supraspinatus exhibited approximately 50% greater muscle activity in the amateur pitchers. The pectoralis major exhibited approximately 50% greater muscle activity in the amateur pitchers. This may be due to better throwing efficiency by professional pitchers; thus less muscle recruitment is needed.

Shoulder-joint forces and torques generated during the arm-cocking phase are quite high. A maximal compressive force of approximately 550 to 770 N (approximately 80% body weight) is produced to resist distraction due to centrifugal force generated by rapid pelvis and upper-torso rotation (8). This compressive force is generated largely by high activity from the rotator-cuff muscles (supraspinatus, infraspinatus, teres minor, and subscapularis; Table 38–2), which help to keep the humeral head properly centered within the glenoid fossa. Furthermore, the posterior rotator-cuff muscles apply a posterior force to the humeral head to resist anterior humeral head translation that occurs as the shoulder externally rotates (11,19). Eccentric internal-rotation torque is produced to decelerate shoulder external rotation. In pitching, a peak shoulder internal-rotation torque of approximately 55 to 80 Nm is generated just before maximal shoulder external rotation (see Fig. 38–8) (8) because of strong eccentric contractions from the shoulder internal rotators (pectoralis major, latissimus dorsi, anterior deltoid, teres major, and subscapularis). In addition, a maximal shoulder anterior shear force of approximately 290 to 470 N (Fig. 38–9) and a shoulder horizontal adduction torque of approximately 80 to 120 Nm (Fig. 38–10) are produced at the shoulder to resist posterior translation at the shoulder and keep the arm moving with the trunk (8). A baseball pitcher's shoulder anterior force is greatest when throwing a fastball (Table 38–3). Football passing generates significantly less shoulder-joint forces and torques compared with baseball pitching (20).

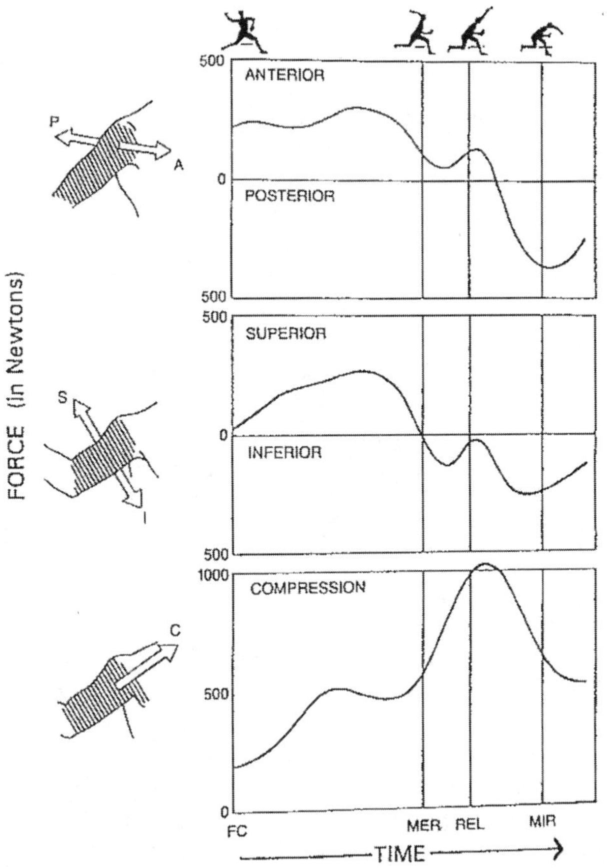

FIG. 38–9. Forces applied to a pitcher's arm at the shoulder in anteroposterior (*AP*), superoinferior (*SI*), and compression (*C*) directions. The instants of foot contact (*FC*), maximal shoulder external rotation (*MER*), ball release (*REL*), and maximal shoulder internal rotation (*MIR*) torque are shown. From ref. 8, with permission.

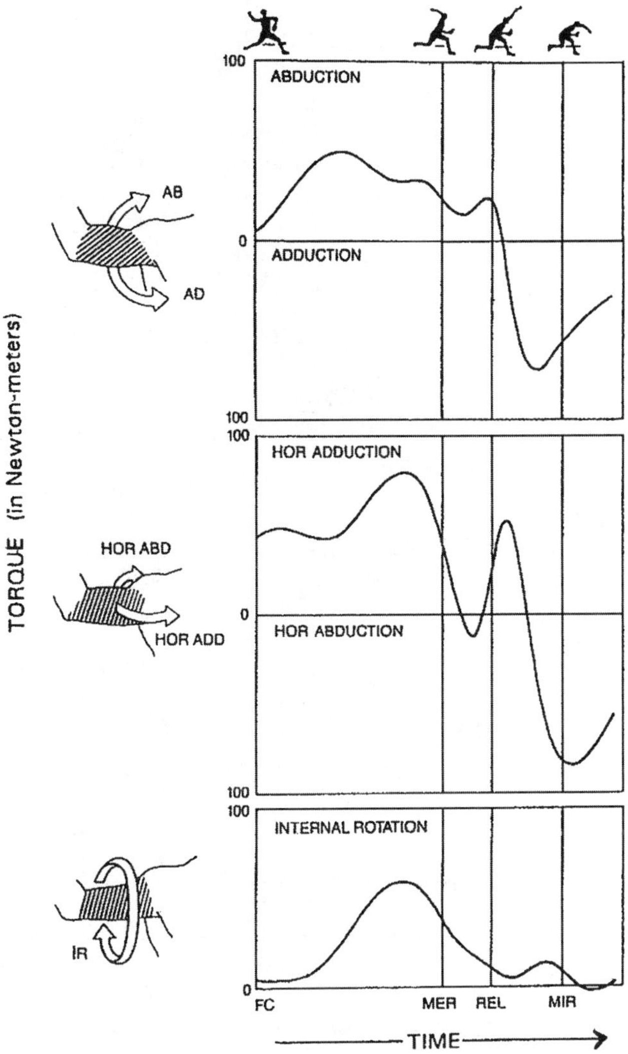

FIG. 38–10. Torques applied to a pitcher's arm at the shoulder in abduction–adduction (*AB-AD*), horizontal adduction–abduction (*HOR ABD, HOR ADD*), and internal rotation (*IR*) directions. The instants of *FC, MER, REL,* and *MIR* torque are shown. From ref. 8, with permission.

Elbow-joint forces and torques are generated throughout the arm-cocking phase. Maximal elbow-extensor torques of approximately 20 to 40 Nm have been reported during the arm-cocking phase (Fig. 38–11) (7,8,21). Consequently, the elbow flexors show some activity, primarily during the middle third of the arm-cocking phase (1,7,15). A large valgus torque is produced at the elbow, caused in part by the large amount

TABLE 38–3. *Elbow and shoulder biomechanics compared between different pitches*

	Fastball	Curveball	Change-up	Slider
Arm cocking				
Elbow medial force (N)	290	270	240	240
Shoulder anterior force (N)	370	330	320	330
Arm acceleration				
Elbow-extension velocity (deg/s)	2400	2400	2100	2400
Shoulder internal rotation velocity (deg/s)	7700	7000	6400	7300
Arm deceleration				
Elbow compressive force (N)	790	730	620	780
Shoulder compressive force (N)	890	820	760	920

From ref. 61, with permission.

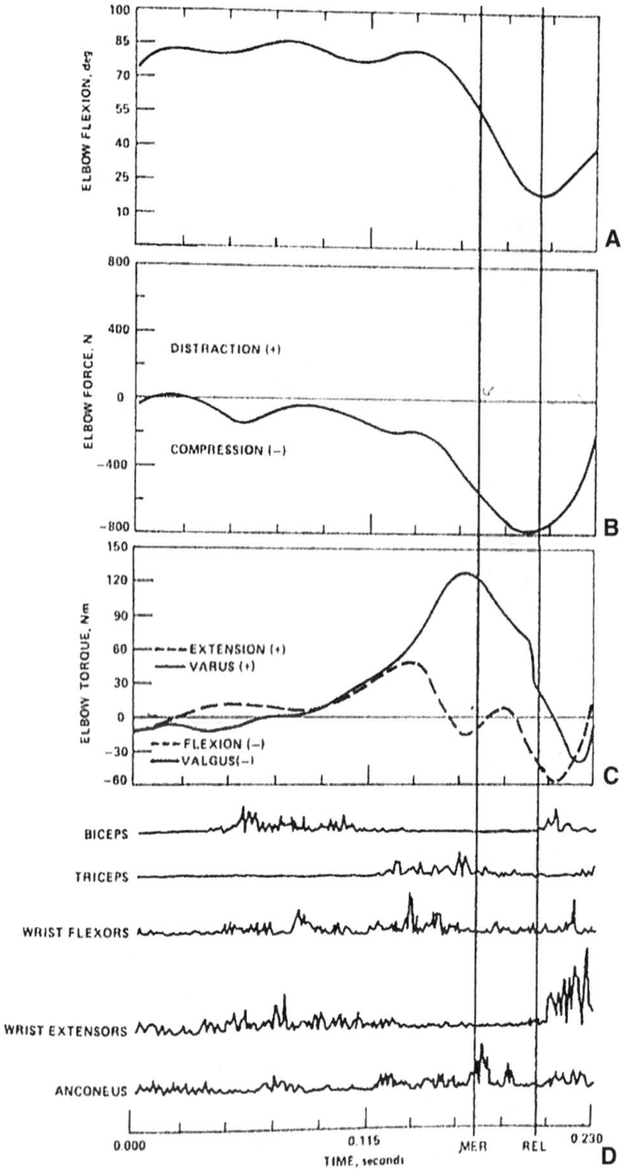

FIG. 38–11. Time-matched measurements during the baseball pitch: (**A**) elbow flexion, (**B**) force applied at the elbow, (**C**) torque applied at the elbow, and (**D**) electromyographic muscle activity. From ref. 7, with permission.

of shoulder external rotation. To resist valgus torque, a maximal varus torque of approximately 50 to 75 Nm is generated shortly before maximal shoulder external rotation (see Fig. 38–8) (8). The flexor and pronator muscle mass of the forearm display moderate to high activity, which contributes to varus torque (see Table 38–2) (15). Because these muscles originate at the medial epicondyle, they contract to help stabilize the elbow. Large tensile forces on the medial aspect of the elbow result from the valgus torque placed on the arm. Repetitive valgus loading may eventually lead to tensile injury to the ulnar collateral ligament (UCL); furthermore, inflammation of the medial epicondyle or adjacent tissues also may occur (i.e., medial epicondylitis).

Other forces are produced at the elbow during arm cocking. A maximal anterior elbow force of approximately 100 to 220 N is applied by the upper arm onto the forearm to resist posterior translation of the forearm at the elbow (Fig. 38–12). In addition, a maximal elbow compressive force of approximately 250 to 350 N is applied by the upper arm to the forearm to resist distraction of the forearm at the elbow (see Fig. 38–12).

The elbow achieves a maximal flexion of approximately 80 to 90 degrees about 0.03 seconds before maximal shoulder external rotation (Fig. 38–11*A*) (7,8). Maximal elbow flexion appears to be controlled by the triceps muscle, which shows moderate activity during the last third of the arm-cocking phase (7,15). This hypothesis is supported by data from Roberts, which show that if the triceps muscle is paralyzed by a radial nerve block, the elbow "collapses" and continues flexing near its limit (approximately 145 degrees) (22). This collapse is caused by a centripetal flexion torque at the elbow, which is created by the rapidly rotating upper torso and arm. The triceps muscle apparently contracts eccentrically and then isometrically in resisting the centripetal elbow-flexion torque that occurs during late arm cocking. At about the time that the elbow reaches maximal elbow flexion, the triceps contract concentrically to aid in elbow extension (7,8). The interaction between muscle activity, elbow-joint torque, and elbow extension can be seen in Fig. 38–12.

Arm Acceleration

The arm-acceleration phase begins at maximal shoulder external rotation (Fig. 38–4*H*) and ends at ball release (Fig. 38–4*I*). The acceleration phase is very rapid, lasting approximately 0.03 to 0.04 seconds (see Fig. 38–5). The acceleration phase has been shown to have fairly low muscle activity, even though the arm accelerates forward both linearly and angularly (11,12).

Just before maximal shoulder external rotation, elbow extension begins. This movement is followed immediately by the onset of shoulder internal rotation. The initiation of elbow extension before shoulder internal rotation allows the thrower to reduce the moment of inertia about the arm's longitudinal axis, therefore allowing greater internal-rotation velocity to be generated. The shoulder internal rotators contract concentrically to help produce an extremely high maximal internal rotation velocity of approximately 7000 to 8000 degree/s in pitching and 4000 to 5000°/s in football passing (see Table 38–1). Maximal shoulder internal-rotation angular velocity, which occurs at approximately ball release, is greatest during the fastball and least during the change-up (see Table 38–3) (58,59). Studies of myoelectric activity show that the subscapularis is the most

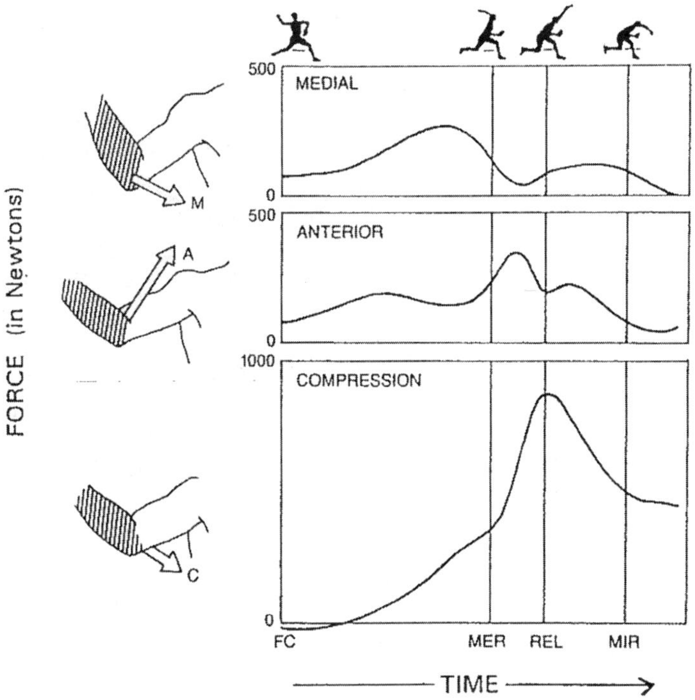

FIG. 38–12. Forces applied to a pitcher's forearm at the elbow in the medial (*M*), anterior (*A*), and compression (*C*) directions. The instant of *FC, MER, REL,* and *MIR* torque are shown. From ref. 8, with permission.

active of the shoulder internal rotators, followed by the latissimus dorsi and pectoralis major (14,15,18,23).

As the elbow extends and the shoulder internally rotates, the trunk flexes forward from its hyperextended position to a neutral position at ball release. High muscle activity from the trunk flexors (rectus abdominals and obliques) has been demonstrated during the acceleration phase (23). Forward trunk tilt achieves a maximal angular velocity of approximately 300 to 450°/s for pitchers and 200 to 325°/s for quarterbacks (see Table 38–1). Forward flexing of the trunk is enhanced by the lead knee beginning to straighten, providing a stable base about which the trunk can rotate. At ball release, the lead knee has approximately 30 to 40 degrees of flexion, which is slightly less than that seen at foot contact (see Table 38–1). This is due to a straightening of the lead leg, which occurs during the latter portion of the acceleration phase. Forward trunk tilt may be hindered if the lead knee continues flexing and moving forward. At release, the trunk of a baseball pitcher is normally flexed forward from a vertical position approximately 25 to 40 degrees, with quarterbacks usually having less forward flexion than pitchers (see Table 38–1). The throwing shoulder remains abducted approximately 80 to 100 degrees throughout the acceleration phase (see Fig. 38–7), which implies that this is a strong position for the shoulder. This is true regardless of the type of throwing pattern that occurs: sidearm, three-quarters, or overhand (24,25). It is the trunk tilt that changes with varying types of deliveries, with an overhand thrower tilting the trunk sideways (away from the throwing arm) more than a sidearm thrower, whose trunk is close to vertical (Fig. 38–13). In throwing, trunk tilt normally deviates from a vertical position 20 to 30 degrees away from the throwing arm (see Table 38–1).

The rotator-cuff muscles, trapezius, serratus anterior, rhomboids, and levator scapula have all demonstrated high levels of activity during the acceleration phase (15). This implies that humeral head control and scapula stabilization are crucial during this phase. However, Gowan (18) demonstrated that rotator-cuff activity is significantly different between professional and amateur pitchers. Muscle activity of the infraspinatus, teres minor, supraspinatus, and biceps was 2 to 3 times higher in amateur pitchers. In contrast, the muscle activity of the subscapularis, serratus anterior, and latissimus dorsi was much greater in professional pitchers. These findings may imply that professional pitchers coordinate the movements of their body segments better, to increase their throwing efficiency. This improved efficiency may minimize glenohumeral instability during the arm-cocking and acceleration phases; thus less rotator-cuff muscle activity is needed. These findings also seem to support the results of previous electromyographic studies (11,12).

Maximal elbow angular velocity during pitching occurs approximately halfway through the acceleration phase and reaches a peak of approximately 2100 to 2400°/s (see Tables 38–1 and 38–3) (7). This rapid elbow extension may be due primarily to centrifugal force act-

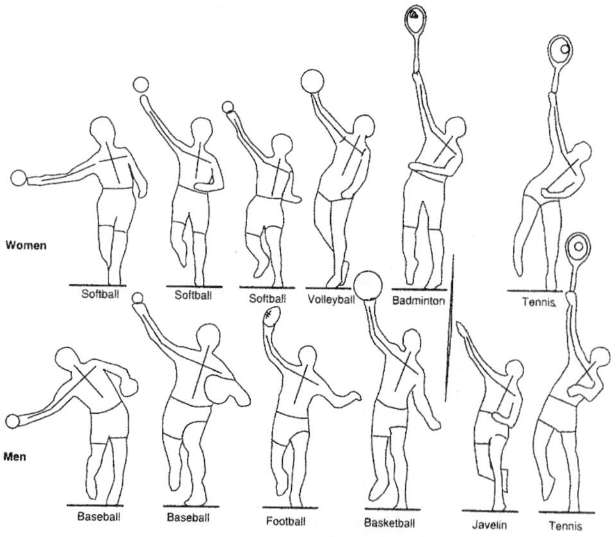

FIG. 38–13. Release/contact positions for a variety of unilateral throwing and striking skills for women and men. The most extreme overhead sports motions are on the *right*, and the less severe side/underarm motions are on the *left*. Note that the spatial orientation of the arm at release in all skills (whether near the vertical or horizontal) is determined primarily by lateral trunk flexion toward or away from the throwing arm, rather than by shoulder-joint action. From ref. 4, with permission.

ing at the elbow as the trunk and arm rotate, for it is unlikely that the elbow extensors can shorten fast enough to generate the high angular velocity measured at the elbow.

Several studies have examined the role of the triceps in extending the elbow during the acceleration phase of throwing. Roberts (22) reported that a pitcher with a paralyzed triceps due to a differential nerve block was able to throw a ball more than 80% of the speed attained before paralysis. This seems to support the concept that triceps contraction does not generate all of the elbow-extension velocity, and that centrifugal force is a major factor. Electromyography has shown high triceps and anconeus activity during the arm-acceleration phase, suggesting that the triceps probably does initiate or contribute to some of the angular velocity generated during this phase (1,7,12,15). The anconeus muscle may function more as an arm stabilizer than as an accelerator, however (21).

Toyoshima and colleagues (26) compared average overarm throwing, incorporating motions of the entire body, with throwing by using only the forearm to extend the elbow. The forearm throw involved a maximal voluntary effort to extend the elbow with the upper arm immobilized. If it is assumed that the triceps muscle shortened voluntarily as fast as possible during the forearm throw, then the resulting elbow angular velocity would be the maximum that could be generated with maximal triceps contraction alone. The results from this study showed that normal throwing generated more than twice the elbow angular velocity that could be achieved during the forearm throw. It was concluded that the elbow was swung open like a whip when the entire body was involved in the throw, and that the elbow angular velocity that occurred during normal throwing was due more to the rotary actions of other parts of the body, such as the hips, trunk, and shoulder, than to the elbow-extending capabilities of the triceps. It was further stated that, in normal throwing, the elbow contributed less than 43% to ball velocity, and that a larger percentage of ball velocity resulted from body rotation. An optimization study by Ahn (27) showed similar results, in that the conclusion was that ball velocity was created primarily by body segments other than the upper extremity, principally by the legs, pelvis, and trunk.

At ball release, the elbow is almost fully extended and positioned slightly anterior to the trunk. In baseball pitching, the elbow is flexed approximately 20 to 30 degrees at release, whereas shoulder horizontal adduction is approximately 5 to 20 degrees (see Table 38–1). In football passing, the elbow is flexed more at ball release and positioned more anterior to the trunk.

Shoulder internal-rotation torque and elbow varus torque decrease during the arm-acceleration phase as the arm begins rotating forward and generating speed. By the time the arm has reached its maximal velocity, near the time of ball release, low forces and torques are generated at the shoulder and elbow joints (see Figs. 38–9, 38–10, 38–11, and 38–12) (7,24,28,29). However, resisting valgus stress at the elbow can result in a wedging of the olecranon against the medial aspect of the trochlear groove and the olecranon fossa. This impingement leads to osteophyte production at the posterior and posteromedial aspects of the olecranon tip and can cause chondromalacia and loose-body formation (29). Figure 38–11*C* shows that substantial varus torque is generated throughout the arm-cocking and arm-acceleration phases to resist valgus torque. During these phases, the elbow extends from approximately 85 degrees of elbow flexion to 20 degrees of elbow flexion (see Fig. 38–11*A*) (8). This combination of elbow extension and resistance to valgus torque supports the "valgus extension overload" mechanism described by Wilson and colleagues (29). In addition, Campbell and associates (30) found greater valgus torque (normalized by body weight × height) in 10-year-old pitchers than in professional pitchers at the instant of ball release, which they thought may be related to "Little League elbow" syndrome in young pitchers. However, Fleisig and coworkers (31) found a decrease in resistance to valgus torque in children.

A maximal elbow compressive force of approximately 600 to 900 N is produced at the elbow to prevent distraction of the forearm due to the centrifugal force acting on the forearm (see Fig. 38–12) (7). In addition, a maximal elbow-flexor torque of approximately 50 to 60 Nm is generated by low to moderate activity from the elbow flexors (see Fig. 38–11) (1,7,8,15). Contraction of the elbow flexors in this phase adds compressive force for joint stability and also controls the rate of elbow extension. The final segment to impart force to the ball is the hand, which moves from a hyperextended wrist position at maximal shoulder external rotation to a neutral wrist position at ball release. The wrist flexors (flexor carpi radialis, flexor carpi ulnaris, and flexor digitorum) have been shown to be active during this phase of throwing (see Table 38–2). Their activity may initially be eccentric to slow the hyperextending wrist at the beginning of the acceleration phase; however, as they continue to fire, they concentrically contract and flex the wrist as ball release is approached. In addition, the pronator teres is active during this phase to pronate the forearm. Mean ball velocity for college and professional football passers is approximately 45 to 55 miles/h, whereas college and professional pitchers average approximately 75 to 85 miles/h (see Table 38–1).

Arm Deceleration

This phase, which lasts between 0.03 and 0.05 seconds (see Fig. 38–5), goes from ball release to maximal shoulder internal rotation (Fig. 38–4*J*). The trunk and hips continue to flex, and the lead knee and throwing elbow continue to extend until almost full extension is reached. The stance leg now starts moving upward in reaction to the flexing trunk and hips. Internal shoulder rotation continues until approximately 0 degrees (i.e., neutral position). Pronation occurs at the radioulnar joint during this phase, but the extent of the pronation is somewhat dependent on the type of pitch. For example, Barrentine and associates (32) found that during arm deceleration, forearm pronation can be as great as 58 degrees during a fastball pitch. Other motions that occur at the wrist include approximately 19 degrees of radial deviation and 2 degrees of wrist flexion during deceleration. The moving of the hand and arm forward, down, and across the body is a natural occurrence in throwing to minimize injury potential at the wrist, elbow, and shoulder (33).

Large eccentric loads are needed at both the elbow and the shoulder joints to decelerate the arm. Fisk (34) demonstrated that the pronator teres is quite active as the forearm pronates during the deceleration phase. The biceps and supinator muscles are eccentrically loaded to decelerate the rapidly pronating forearm. Table 38–2 shows that the brachialis also is active during this phase. The similar firing patterns of the biceps and brachialis suggest that the primary function of the biceps during this phase is to decelerate elbow extension. Elbow extension terminates when the elbow is flexed approximately 15 to 25 degrees. The triceps has been shown to be active after ball release (12). Because all three heads of the triceps fire in similar sequence and activity, the triceps may affect the elbow more than the shoulder, because only the long head crosses both joints.

The posterior muscles of the shoulder have been identified as playing a very important part in resisting shoulder distraction and anterior subluxation forces (10,12, 14,19,25,28,35,36). Specifically, these muscles include the infraspinatus, supraspinatus, teres major and minor, latissimus dorsi, and posterior deltoid (10). Contraction of the teres major, latissimus dorsi, and posterior deltoid helps to decelerate the shoulder abduction that occurs during this phase. The lower trapezius, rhomboids, and serratus anterior have all been shown to be quite active, thus providing stability to the scapula (see Table 38–2). The teres minor, which is often an isolated source of rotator-cuff pain, demonstrated the highest activity of all the glenohumeral muscles during this phase, providing a posterior restraint that may limit humeral-head anterior translation, horizontal adduction, and shoulder internal rotation (11,14,15). In comparing professional and amateur pitchers, Gowan (18) found that amateur pitchers had more than twice as much muscle activity in the biceps and posterior deltoid. This may imply that amateur pitchers are subjected to greater posterior shoulder stress because of a less efficient throwing pattern.

The wrist and finger flexors have very high muscle activity during this phase (see Table 38–2). These muscles continue contracting and flexing the wrist. In addition, the wrist and finger extensor muscles demonstrate low to moderate activity, perhaps being eccentrically active to decelerate the flexing wrist and fingers.

Large shoulder and elbow forces and torques are needed during arm deceleration to slow the rapidly moving arm. Maximal compressive forces of approximately body weight are needed at both the elbow (800 to 1000 N) and shoulder (1000 to 1200 N) to prevent distraction at these joints (Figs. 38–9, 38–12, and 38–14) (8). These compressive forces, which are 2 to 3 times greater than other shoulder and elbow forces generated during throwing, are greatest during a fastball or slider, and least during a change-up (see Table 38–3). Compressive forces are 15% to 20% greater in pitchers than in quarterbacks.

A maximal shoulder posterior force of approximately 310 to 490 N and a maximal shoulder horizontal abduction torque of approximately 75 to 125 Nm are applied to the arm to resist shoulder anterior humeral-head translation and horizontal adduction (see Figs. 38–9 and 38–10) (8). In addition, a maximal shoulder inferior force of approximately 230 to 390 N and a maximal shoulder adduction torque of approximately 60 to 110 Nm are produced to resist shoulder abduction and supe-

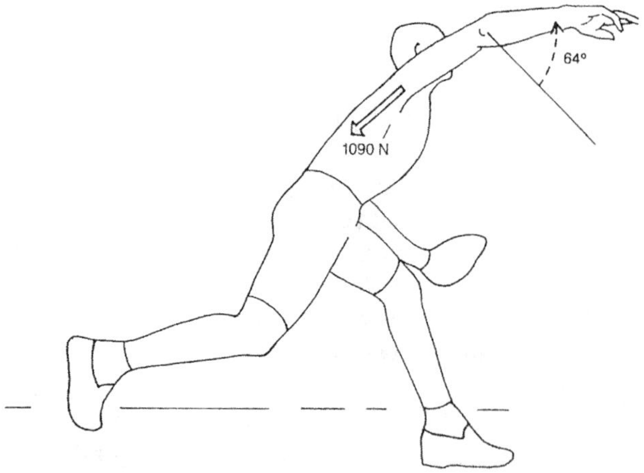

FIG. 38–14. Shortly after ball release, a second critical instant occurs; at this instant, a pitcher's shoulder is externally rotated 64 degrees, and the elbow is flexed 25 degrees. Among the loads generated at this time are 1090 N of compressive force at the shoulder. From ref. 8, with permission.

rior humeral-head translation (see Figs. 38–9 and 38–10) (8).

Follow-Through

The follow-through phase begins at the time of maximal shoulder internal rotation and ends when the arm completes its movement across the body and a balanced position is obtained. In the follow-through phase, energy in the throwing arm continues to be dissipated back through the kinetic chain. A long arc of deceleration from the throwing arm, as well as sufficient forward tilting of the trunk, allows energy to be absorbed by the large musculature of the trunk and legs. This absorption helps reduce the stress placed on the throwing arm. All of the body's weight is now borne by a straight or almost straight lead leg. The trunk and hips continue flexing, and the stance leg continues moving upward (Fig. 38–4*K*).

As in the deceleration phase, the posterior shoulder muscles continue to be eccentrically active throughout the follow-through, thus continuing to decelerate the horizontally adducting shoulder. Shoulder- and elbow-joint forces and torques generated during the follow-through are generally lower than joint forces and torques generated during the deceleration phase.

The serratus anterior has demonstrated the highest activity of all scapular rotators in this phase, contracting either concentrically or isometrically (see Table 38–2); however, the middle trapezius and rhomboids are eccentrically loaded to decelerate scapula protraction. As in the deceleration phase, electromyography has shown that the wrist and finger extensor muscles had low to moderate activity during the follow-through, implying that they are eccentrically loaded to decelerate the flexing wrist (Table 38–2).

OTHER OVERHAND SPORTS

Water Polo

Recently, researchers have investigated the kinematics and kinetics experienced during the penalty throw in water polo (37,38). The obvious difference between the water polo penalty throw and the football pass and baseball pitch is that the latter two are initiated with a stride approximating 60% to 75% of the athlete's body height. The penalty throw is executed while the athlete treads water to keep the throwing arm above the surface. This prohibits the water polo athlete from benefiting from the kinetic chain as much as the pitcher and quarterback, as the larger muscles of the lower body have little effectiveness in generating momentum. One other main difference concerns the projectile being thrown. The water polo ball weighs approximately 3 times more than the baseball and about the same as an American football.

The kinematic study by Feltner and colleagues (37) shows that the variables associated with the shoulder are fairly similar for the water polo delivery as for the baseball pitch and football pass. Ball speed at release for the penalty throw was 16.5 m/s compared with 21 and 33 m/s for the football and baseball, respectively. During the penalty throw, maximal external rotation was 155 degrees, less than both passing and pitching. The related internal-rotation velocity was significantly lower for the penalty throw than for either of the other two throws at 1980°/s. Maximal horizontal-adduction angular velocity for the penalty throw also was lower than the passing and pitching values at 490°/s. At the elbow, the extension angular velocity reached 1034°/s.

Feltner and co-workers (38) went on to investigate the kinetics involved in the penalty throw of water polo and found that many of the resultant joint torques were similar to those seen in baseball pitching and football passing. The maximal internal-rotation torque was 59 Nm for the penalty throw. This is less than that seen in pitching but more than that in passing. The maximal horizontal-abduction torque for the penalty throw was 64 Nm compared with 100 Nm and 78 Nm for the baseball pitch and football pass, respectively. At the elbow, the torque results for the penalty throw are very close to those exhibited during pitching. The maximal elbow-flexion torque was 23 Nm, less than seen in pitching and passing. The maximal elbow-varus torque during the penalty throw reached 62 Nm, which is very similar to that in both pitching and football passing.

It is clear that the water polo throw is without much of the kinetic-chain properties that throwing on land uses. The penalty throw does not benefit from the stride and pelvic rotation that the pitch and pass use. Therefore, much of the momentum at the shoulder is produced at the shoulder through muscle activation. This is, most likely, why the resultant joint torques for the water polo penalty throw are similar in magnitude to the football pass but impart less velocity to the ball.

Javelin

Although the physical aspects of a javelin and a ball are quite different, the throwing motions are very similar. The biggest difference is that whereas most ball-throwing motions are initiated from a stationary wind-up, the javelin throw begins with a running approach. The linear velocity of an elite javelin thrower is 5.6 ± 0.7 m/s at the beginning of the stride phase, and 3.1 ± 0.9 m/s at the moment of release (39). As the javelin thrower decreases linear velocity, linear momentum of the body is converted into linear momentum (and consequently distance) of the javelin (40). Although a javelin throw does not have a wind-up phase as described in the general throwing description above, it does include stride, arm cocking, arm acceleration, arm deceleration, and follow-through phases similar to those of other throws.

At the time of lead-foot contact, a javelin thrower has less elbow flexion and more external rotation than a baseball pitcher or football quarterback. The javelin thrower also has less lead-knee flexion (see Table 38–1). Near the time of lead-foot contact, the "stance foot" leaves the ground or starts to be dragged along the ground by the forward-moving body (40). Rotational motions appear to play an important role in javelin throwing, as both the athlete's center of mass and the javelin grip move on pathways to the right of the lead foot (for a right-hander thrower), producing centripetal force used to generate javelin velocity (39).

At the instant of release, the javelin and its velocity vector are pointed approximately 30 degrees above the horizontal (39,40). Release velocity (39) and aerodynamic conditions (40) affect the distance of a javelin throw.

Kinetic parameters for javelin throwing have not been reported, because of difficulty in modeling the javelin itself. Although biomechanists can assume reasonable accuracy by modeling a ball as a point mass, inertial and vibrational forces cannot be neglected for a javelin.

Tennis

The tennis serve is an overhead activity that subjects the shoulder and elbow to large ranges of motion, as well as movements. The upper-limb segment rotations during a tennis serve were investigated by Elliot and colleagues (41), who found that peak shoulder internal-rotation velocity during a power serve reached approximately 2100°/s. This amounts to a 54.2% contribution to the linear velocity of the racket head. In addition, elbow-extension velocity and forearm pronation during the serve can reach approximately 1200°/s and 940°/s, respectively (41). Motions and forces in tennis can, over time, lead to injuries of the elbow and shoulder (42,43).

Other Overhead Sports

Other sports require a great deal of overhead motion (see Fig. 38–11) that cannot be overlooked simply because it does not involve throwing. Volleyball spikes and overhead serves, as well as freestyle swimming, are all movements very similar to the throwing motion. The kinetic factors associated with these movements have not been documented. Based on the motion itself and its dynamic characteristics, we must assume that these sports subject the shoulder and elbow to forces and movements that can lead to overuse injuries in these athletes just as they do throwing athletes.

INJURIES ASSOCIATED WITH THROWING AND OTHER OVERHEAD MOTIONS

Shoulder

Most shoulder injuries in throwing involve soft tissues, including muscles, tendons, ligaments, capsule bursae, and fibrocartilaginous tissue. Both static (capsulolabral complex) and dynamic stabilizers (rotator cuff and scapular rotators) control the movement and stability of the humeral head within the glenoid cavity. Subacromion impingement syndrome, in which the rotator-cuff muscles and long biceps tendon are intimately involved, is a common soft-tissue injury seen in throwing. The rotator-cuff muscles generate shear and compressive forces to depress, rotate, and center the humeral head within the glenoid fossa. Consequently, they help prevent superior translation of the humeral head caused largely by deltoid activity. When these muscles function abnormally, such as when a partial or complete rotator-cuff thickness tear occurs, or because of muscle fatigue and weakness, superior translation of the humeral head occurs, and the upper surfaces of the rotator-cuff muscles and tendons are abraded against the undersurface of the acromion. Because of its intimate relation with the rotator-cuff muscles, the long biceps tendon also is often impinged.

Anterior shoulder instability is also common in throwers, especially baseball pitchers. Glousman (44) reported that muscle activity between pitchers with normal and abnormal shoulder stability differed significantly during each pitching phase (Figs. 38–15 through 38–21). The greatest differences in muscle activity were seen during the arm-cocking, acceleration, and follow-through phases. The muscle-activity pattern of pitchers with normal shoulder stability is very similar to muscle

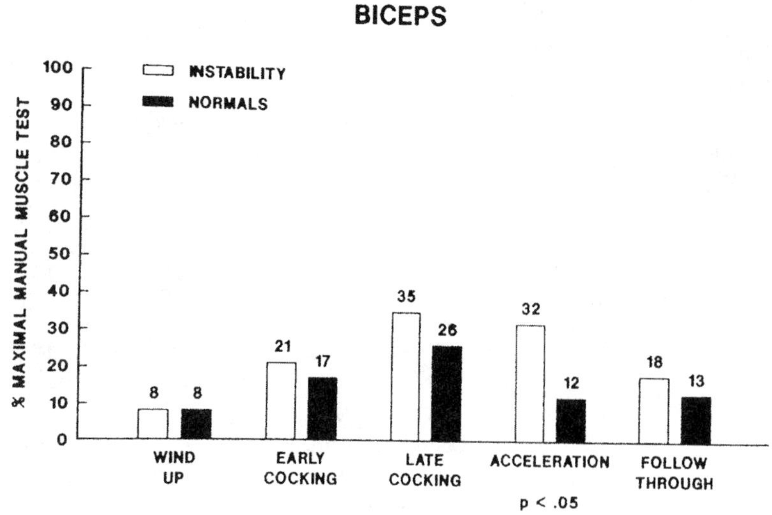

FIG. 38–15. Comparison of activity in the biceps brachii in an unstable shoulder as compared with a normal shoulder. A statistically significant difference between the groups ($p < .05$) is indicated. From ref. 44, with permission. NOTE: Wind-up, early cocking, late cocking, acceleration, and follow-through in Figs. 38–15 through 38–21 correspond to wind-up, stride, arm cocking, arm acceleration, and arm deceleration in this chapter, respectively.

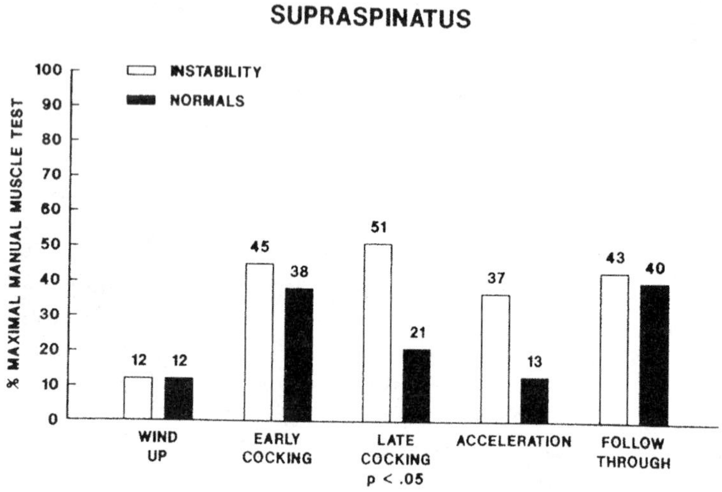

FIG. 38–16. Comparison study in the supraspinatus in an unstable shoulder as compared with a normal shoulder. A statistically significant difference between the groups ($p < .05$) is indicated. From ref. 44, with permission.

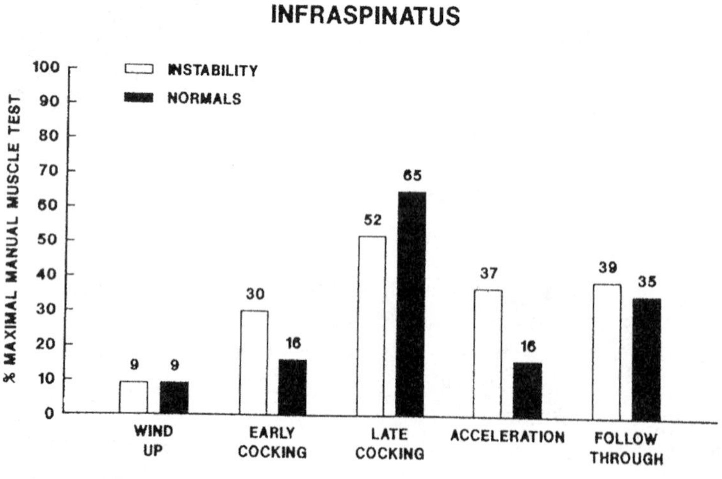

FIG. 38–17. Comparison of activity in the infraspinatus in an unstable shoulder as compared with a normal shoulder. From ref. 44, with permission.

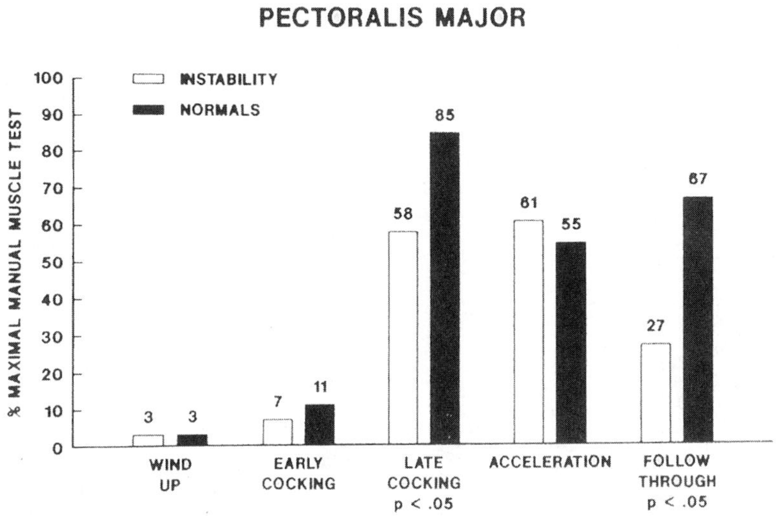

FIG. 38–18. Comparison of activity in the pectoralis major in an unstable shoulder as compared with a normal shoulder. A statistically significant difference between the groups ($p < .05$) is indicated. From ref. 44, with permission.

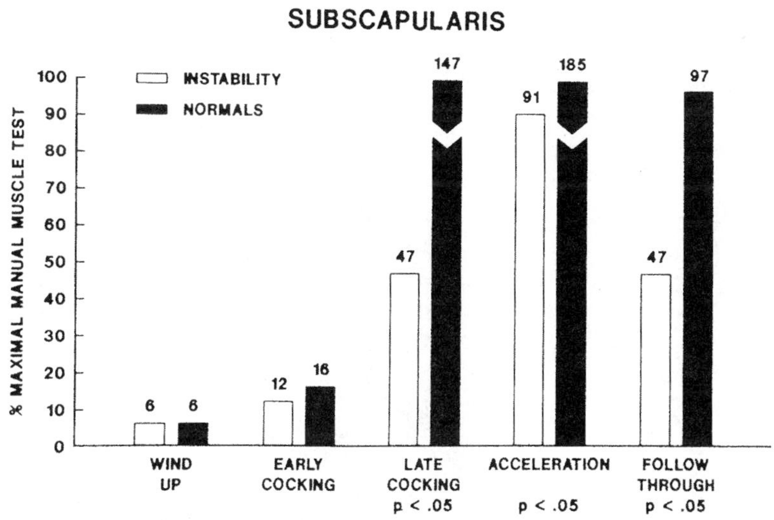

FIG. 38–19. Comparison of activity in the subscapularis in an unstable shoulder as compared with a normal shoulder. A statistically significant difference between the groups ($p < .05$) is indicated. From ref. 44, with permission.

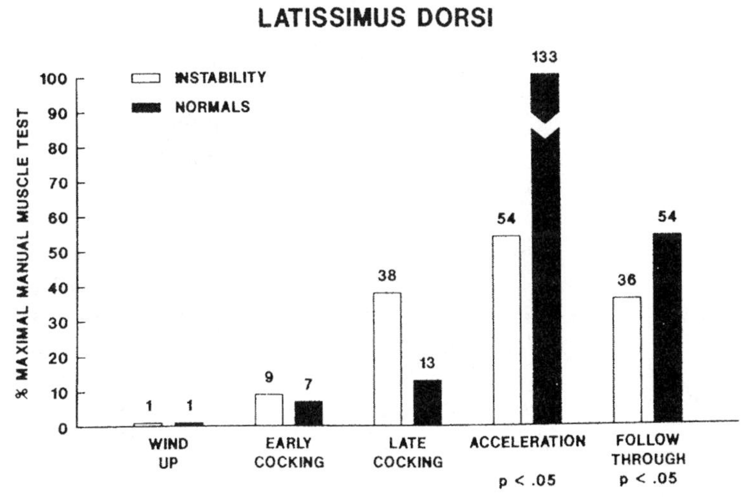

FIG. 38–20. Comparison of activity in the latissimus dorsi in an unstable shoulder as compared with a normal shoulder. A statistically significant difference between the groups ($p < .05$) is indicated. From ref. 44, with permission.

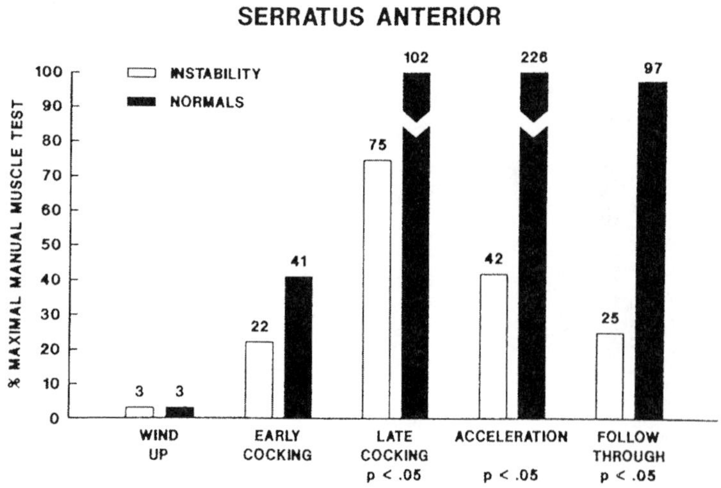

FIG. 38–21. Comparison of activity in the serratus anterior in an unstable shoulder as compared with a normal shoulder. A statistically significant difference between the groups ($p < .05$) is indicated. From ref. 44, with permission.

activity patterns observed in the professional pitchers studied by Gowan (18). Furthermore, pitchers with abnormal shoulder stability exhibited muscle-activity patterns similar to those observed in amateur pitchers.

Muscle imbalances between the anterior–posterior shoulder rotator muscles can exacerbate the impingement problem. This is true for at least two reasons: (a) the internal rotators of the shoulder are greater in both number and strength than in the shoulder external rotators; and (b) most weight-training programs emphasize muscles that horizontally adduct the shoulder and de-emphasize those muscles that horizontally abduct the shoulder.

Impingement also can occur as the subacromion space becomes smaller. An inflamed subacromion bursae or swollen rotator-cuff muscles and biceps tendon can decrease the volume of the subacromion space. The subacromion space also can diminish as the shoulder-joint musculature hypertrophies. These latter conditions often are the result of an overload response that occurs in muscles and connective tissue. Baseball pitchers, for example, may throw several thousand pitches per year. Consequently, this repetitive microtrauma can increase injury potential.

Different phases of the throw affect shoulder structures differently. During the wind-up and stride, the stresses and muscle activity generated at the shoulder are fairly low; however, shoulder stress is much greater during the arm-cocking, arm-acceleration, arm-deceleration, and follow-through phases.

The rotator-cuff muscles are very active during the arm-cocking phase to stabilize the humeral head within the glenoid fossa and to control the large external rotation of the shoulder that occurs. Because of the rapid transverse rotation of the trunk, eccentric muscle loading by the horizontal adductors and internal rotators of the shoulder is very high. As the shoulder proceeds into horizontal abduction and external rotation, the humeral head tends to sublux posteriorly first and then anteriorly against the anterior capsule; consequently, tendinitis of the anterior muscle tendons (especially the pectoralis major and latissimus dorsi) is quite common (19,45,46). Muscle imbalances, such as overpowering anterior shoulder muscles and weak posterior shoulder muscles, can also contribute to the humeral head being pulled forward within the glenoid. Repeated stretching of the anterior capsule can further stress the joint, leading to chronic inflammation and damage to the anterior capsular structures and anterior labrum. Hyperlaxity or laxity within the joint can exacerbate this problem, resulting in further anterior shoulder instability. In the study by Glousman and co-workers (44) comparing anterior shoulder instability with normal shoulder stability, they found that the supraspinatus showed significantly greater muscle activity in pitchers with anterior shoulder instability (see Fig. 38–16).

Distraction and translation of the humerus during the arm-acceleration or -deceleration phases introduces an increased risk of labrum degeneration. This is due to humeral motion coupled with rapid internal rotation of the humerus, causing a "shoulder-grinding factor" (47). If the stability of the shoulder is breached because of fatigue or trauma, the glenoid labrum becomes more vulnerable to injury and could be torn by either the traction of the biceps tendon or the impingement between the humeral head and the glenoid cavity (47).

When compared with pitchers with normal shoulder stability, significant increases in the muscle activity of the biceps were observed in pitchers with anterior shoulder instability (see Fig. 38–15). In contrast, pitchers with normal shoulder stability produced significantly greater muscle activity in the subscapularis, latissimus dorsi, and serratus anterior (see Figs. 38–15, 38–20, and 38–21).

Because of the large eccentric loads during the deceleration and follow-through phases, posterior shoulder muscles are frequently injured during throwing. If the rotator-cuff muscles and other posterior shoulder muscles are weak, fatigued, or injured, the humeral head may distract and anteriorly translate out of the glenoid fossa. This action can place abnormal stress on the posterior capsule and lead to "posterior capsule syndrome" (45,46). Repeated abrasions of the posteroinferior capsule structures have been described as creating an exostosis of the posteroinferior glenoid (48,49).

Although the biceps has been considered to function primarily at the elbow, the biceps also contributes to shoulder abduction and flexion, especially when the shoulder is externally rotated and the forearm is supinated (50,51). Biceps activity, especially the long head, has been shown to be a significant contributor to shoulder abduction and flexion in a compromised shoulder, such as that with a torn rotator cuff (44). Because the long head of the biceps originates at the anterosuperior glenoid labrum, its contraction could abnormally stress this portion of the labrum. This is especially true in throwing, because the biceps has been shown to contract eccentrically in decelerating the rapidly extending elbow. Andrews and associates (52) arthroscopically observed 73 throwing athletes who had labrum tears in the throwing shoulder. The long head of the biceps tendon appeared to have pulled the anterosuperior portion of the labrum off the glenoid. This condition, called a slap lesion, was verified arthroscopically by electrically stimulating the biceps muscle. When stimulated, the tendinous portion became taut near its attachment to the labrum and actually lifted the labrum off the glenoid (52).

Another injury that occurs during the deceleration and follow-through phases is a "snapping scapula." This pathology, which can be quite painful, is the result of an inflamed bursa located beneath the medial border of the scapula. This bursa provides lubrication as the scapula moves in relation to the thorax. During repeated and overuse conditions, bursitis can develop, resulting in both pain and a "snapping" sound as the swollen tissue impinges on the thorax. A good follow-through can help minimize the injury potential of the shoulder. A long arm arc of deceleration and sufficient forward trunk tilt (trunk approximately in a horizontal position) both help minimize stress on the shoulder complex.

The pectoralis major, subscapularis, latissimus dorsi, and serratus anterior muscles are all active during arm deceleration. Muscle activity is significantly greater in pitchers with anterior shoulder instability (see Figs. 38–18 to 38–21).

Elbow

Medial Compartment

An *in vitro* study by Morrey and An (53) showed that the UCL contributes approximately 54% of the resistance to the valgus. Assuming that the UCL produces 54% of a 64-Nm varus torque generated by an elite pitcher, the UCL would then provide 35 Nm of the varus torque (8). This is similar to the 32-Nm failure load of the UCL reported by Dillman and associates (54); thus, during baseball pitching, the UCL appears to be loaded near its maximal capacity (8). This result is only an approximation of the UCL's contribution in throwing, however, because the cadaveric research does not account for muscle contributions. Muscle contraction during this phase may reduce the stress on the UCL by compressing the joint and adding stability (7).

Valgus torque also can cause high compressive force on the lateral elbow, which can lead to lateral elbow compression injury (8). Specifically, valgus torque can cause compression between the radial head and humeral capitellum (4). According to the *in vitro* study by Morrey and An (53), 33% of the varus torque needed to resist valgus torque applied by the forearm is supplied by joint articulation. Thirty-three percent of the 64-Nm maximal varus torque generated during pitching is 21 Nm. Assuming that the distance from the axis of valgus rotation to the compression point between the radial head and the humeral capitellum is approximately 4 cm, then the compressive force generated between the radius and humerus to produce 21 Nm of varus torque is approximately 500 N (8). Muscle contraction about the elbow or loss of joint integrity on the medial side of the elbow can cause this compressive force to increase. Excessive or repetitive compressive force can result in avascular necrosis, osteochondritis dissecans, or osteochondral chip fractures (4).

In addition to a varus torque, a 240- to 360-N medial force is applied by the upper arm onto the forearm to resist lateral translation of the forearm at the elbow (see Fig. 38–12). This force is significantly greater when throwing a fastball or curveball compared with throwing a slider or change-up (see Table 38–3). The greater medial force during arm cocking in the curveball compared with the change-up or slider may put the medial elbow at greater risk when throwing the curveball. More research is needed to address this issue further. The forearm is supinated more during the arm-cocking phase for a curveball than for a fastball, which also may be related to the risk of injury (55).

Medial musculotendinous injuries are quite common, especially involving the muscles that originate at the medial epicondyle (medial epicondylitis). These muscles, which are collectively referred to as the flexor–pronator mass, comprise primarily the pronator teres, flexor carpi radialis, flexor digitorum superficialis, and flexor carpi ulnaris. During throwing, pain and tenderness can occur in the medial epicondyle region. The flexor–pronator mass is greatly stressed as a result of tensile force during the arm-cocking and acceleration phases of throwing. These dynamic contractile structures must apply a varus torque to the forearm to resist the valgus stress created by the throwing motion. An excessive or repetitive valgus stress also can create abnormal tension on the medial capsule.

Capsular and ligamentous tensile stress on the ulna and humerus may lead to osteophyte formation. These osteophytes usually form distally at the ulnar attachment. Because the ulnar nerve lies near the medial capsule and UCL, these osteophytes may compress the nerve. Furthermore, the repetitive valgus stress of the medial elbow during throwing can excessively stretch the ulnar nerve, contributing to ulnar neuritis. The UCL, which also originates at the medial epicondyle, helps reinforce the medial elbow capsule. The UCL is most susceptible to injury when the flexor–pronator muscle mass weakens and fatigues due to repetitive throwing and overuse.

To protect a previously injured elbow, an athlete may try to alter his or her mechanics; specifically he or she may "lead with the elbow" (i.e., increase elbow flexion and shoulder horizontal adduction). Such modification in throwing mechanics may indeed reduce the load on the medial aspect of the elbow, but it may increase the load and injury probability at other locations, such as the shoulder complex. Leading with the elbow also may decrease performance by reducing ball velocity. Leading with the elbow, however, was not found to be significantly more prevalent in Little League pitchers as previously believed, but it may still be seen in pitchers who have injured their arms and may be afraid to throw 100%. Fleisig and colleagues (31) found no difference in horizontal adduction values for Little League through professional baseball pitchers.

Anterior Compartment

The anterior elbow is the least commonly injured region; however, anterior capsular sprains, flexor–pronator strains, bicipital tendinitis, and intraarticular loose bodies are problems that may occur in the anterior elbow (56). In the throwing athlete, these pathologies can lead to incomplete elbow extension, especially during the acceleration phase of the throw.

Anterior pain also can result from neural injuries, such as radial nerve entrapment. Repetitive supination and pronation movements, such as those occurring during the throwing motion, can lead to entrapment. For example, anterior pain can occur when the median nerve is entrapped between the two heads of the pronator teres. This is referred to as pronator teres syndrome and occurs because of repetitive forearm pronation, which is seen during throwing.

Posterior Compartment

Because of overuse, the triceps tendon can be injured (triceps tendinitis) at its insertion on the olecranon. Furthermore, it may partially avulse off the olecranon. After repetitive extension of the elbow during throwing, the olecranon is continually and forcefully driven into the olecranon fossa. Consequently, a stress fracture of the olecranon or a hypertrophic olecranon may develop. Valgus stress that occurs during late arm cocking and early acceleration may exacerbate the problem by forcing the olecranon against the medial olecranon fossa (i.e., valgus extension overload) (29). Because of the repetitive trauma of the olecranon against the olecranon fossa, osteophytes may form and migrate anteriorly. Loose bodies also can arise as a result of a shearing off of osteocartilaginous fragments.

Lateral Compartment

Converse to medial musculotendinous injuries, lateral musculotendinous injuries involve the wrist and finger extension musculature. These muscles, which all originate at or near the lateral epicondyle, can cause lateral epicondylitis when abnormally stressed. These muscles are rapidly stretched and eccentrically loaded during the deceleration and follow-through phases in pitching.

Whereas the medial elbow is subject to high tensile stresses, the lateral region is subject to high compressive forces. These compressive forces occur between the radial head and the humeral capitellum. Degenerative changes in the articular cartilage of these structures can result from the repetitive compressive stress across the radiocapitellum joint. Consequently, loose-body formations can occur as the articular cartilage fragments break off into the joint. Osteochondrosis of the radiocapitellum joint also may occur in preadolescent athletes before physeal closure.

REHABILITATION FOR THE OVERHEAD ATHLETE

Because of the involvement of the full body in the throwing motion, it is important to condition the musculature of both the upper and lower body to maximize performance and minimize the risk of injury. The principle of the kinetic chain implies that weakness in any segment may result in a deficiency in performance. When an athlete with a deficiency in one section of the kinetic chain tries to compensate by increasing the demands on other segments, injury can result.

It is especially important to evaluate a thrower's mechanics after rehabilitation from an injury. Improper mechanics may be related to either the cause of the initial injury or modifications resulting from the initial injury. In either case, improper mechanics should be corrected to prevent reinjury.

Joint flexibility and high-speed controlled motion are essential for throwing and should be emphasized in a rehabilitation program. Constrained exercises that include limited ranges of motion and joint speeds are useful during rehabilitation but have certain limitations. Another important concept in the design and selection of a rehabilitation program for the throwing athlete is that joint loads in throwing be largely eccentric. These eccentric loads occur primarily in the arm-cocking, acceleration, and deceleration phases. Exercises emphasizing eccentric contractions should therefore be performed with appropriate ranges of motion and speeds of movement (57). The best exercise for throwing rehabilitation is throwing. Under the guidance of a therapist or trainer, an athlete should include throwing in rehabilitation as soon as possible. An interval throwing program or other moderate throwing program may be appropriate. Joint loads do not reach maximal values during the acceleration phase, where velocity is at its maximum, but rather during the arm-cocking and deceleration phases of the throw. In accordance with Newton's Second Law of Motion, it is the acceleration and deceleration of a segment, not the velocity, that is proportional to the net force acting on that segment. An analogy of a cyclist can be used to illustrate this. A cyclist who wishes to ride a short distance needs to generate significant force to start the motion, but minimal force to maintain the motion.

CONCLUSION

Because throwing is a highly dynamic activity in which body segments move through large arcs of motion and high speeds of movement, large joint forces and torques are generated at the elbow and shoulder. A proper understanding of the throwing mechanism is necessary for physicians, therapists, trainers, and coaches to prescribe appropriate treatment and conditioning protocols.

REFERENCES

1. Sisto DJ, Jobe FW, Moynes DR. An electromyographic analysis of the elbow in pitching. *Am J Sports Med* 1987;15:260–263.
2. Feltner ME, Dapena J. Three-dimensional interactions in a two-segment kinetic chain. Part I: general model. *Int J Sport Biomech* 1989;5:403–419.
3. Dillman CJ. Proper mechanics of pitching. *Sports Med Update* 1990;5:15–18.
4. Atwater AE. Biomechanics of overarm throwing movements and of throwing injuries. *Exerc Sport Sci Rev* 1979;7:43–85.
5. Feltner ME, Dapena J. Three-dimensional interactions in a two-segment kinetic chain. Part II: application to the throwing arm in baseball pitching. *Int J Sport Biomech* 1989;5:420–450.
6. Dillman CJ, Fleisig GS, Andrews JR. Biomechanics of pitching with emphasis upon shoulder kinematics. *J Orthop Sports Phys Ther* 1993;18:402–408.
7. Werner SL, et al. Biomechanics of the elbow during baseball pitching. *J Orthop Sports Phys Ther* 1993;17:274–278.
8. Fleisig GS, et al. Kinetics of baseball pitching with implications about injury mechanisms. *Am J Sports Med* 1995;23:233–239.
9. Fleisig GS, et al. Biomechanics of throwing. In: Zachazewski JE, Magee DJ, Quillen WS, eds. *Athletic injuries and rehabilitation.* Philadelphia: WB Saunders, 1996:332–353.
10. Jacobs P. The overhand baseball pitch: a kinesiological analysis and related strength-conditioning programming. *NCSA J* 1987; 9:5–13.
11. Jobe FW, et al. An EMG analysis of the shoulder in throwing and pitching: a preliminary report. *Am J Sports Med* 1983;11:35.
12. Jobe FW, et al. An EMG analysis of the shoulder in pitching: a second report. *Am J Sports Med* 1984;12:218–220.
13. Fleisig GS, Dillman CJ, Andrews JR. Proper mechanics for baseball pitching. *Clin Sports Med* 1989;1:151–170.
14. Bradley JP. Electromyographic analysis of muscle action about the shoulder. *Clin Sports Med* 1991;10:789–805.
15. DiGiovine NM. An electromyographic analysis of the upper extremity in pitching. *J Shoulder Elbow Surg* 1992;1:15–25.
16. Bigliani LU, Codd TP, Connor Levine WN, Littlefield MA, Hershon SJ. Shoulder motion and laxity in the professional baseball player. *Am J Sports Med* 1997;25:609–613.
17. Brown LP, Niehues SL, Harrah A. Upper extremity range of motion and isokinetic strength of internal and external shoulder rotators in major league baseball players. *Am J Sports Med* 1988; 16:577–585.
18. Gowan ID. Comparative electromyographic analysis of the shoulder during pitching. *J Sports Med* 1987;15:586–590.
19. Cain PR. Anterior stability of the glenohumeral joint. *Am J Sports Med* 1987;15:144–148.
20. Fleisig GS, et al. Kinematic and kinetic comparison between baseball pitching and football passing. *J Appl Biomech* 1996;12: 207–224.
21. Feltner M, Dapena J. Dynamics of the shoulder and elbow joints of the throwing arm during a baseball pitch. *Int J Sport Biomech* 1986;2:235–259.
22. Roberts TW. Cinematography in biomechanical investigation. Selected topics in biomechanics. In: Cooper JM, ed. *CIC Symposium on biomechanics.* Chicago: The Athletic Institute, 1971:41–50.
23. Moynes DR. Electromyography and motion analysis of the upper extremity in sports. *Phys Ther* 1986;66:1905–1911.
24. Dillman CJ, et al. Biomechanics of the shoulder in sports: throwing activities. In: *Postgraduate studies in sports physical therapy.* Berryville, Virginia, Forum Medicum, 1991:1–9.
25. Fleisig GS, et al. Biomechanics of the shoulder during throwing. In: Andrews JR, Wilk KE, eds. *The athlete's shoulder.* New York: Churchill Livingstone, 1994:355–368.
26. Toyoshima S, et al. Contributions of the body parts of throwing performance. In: Nelson RC, Morehouse CA, eds. *Biomechanics IV.* Baltimore: University Park Press, 1974:169–174.
27. Ahn BH. *A model of the human upper extremity and its application to a baseball pitching motion.* Unpublished dissertation, Michigan State University, 1991.
28. Fleisig GS, et al. A biomechanical description of the shoulder joint during pitching. *Sports Med Update* 1991;6:10–15.
29. Wilson FD. Valgus extension overload in the pitching elbow. *Am J Sports Med* 1983;11:83–88.
30. Campbell KR, et al. Kinetic analysis of the elbow and shoulder in professional and little league pitchers. *Med Sci Sports Exerc* 1994;26:S175.
31. Fleisig GS, et al. Kinematic and kinetic comparison of baseball pitching among various levels of development. *J Biomech (in press).*
32. Barrentine SW, et al. Kinematic analysis of the wrist and forearm during baseball pitching. *J Appl Biomech* 1998;14:24–39.
33. Dillman CJ, et al. Biomechanics of the shoulder in sports: throwing activities. In: Matsen FA, ed. *The shoulder: a balance of mobility and stability.* Rosemont: American Academy of Orthopaedic Surgeons, 1993:621–633.
34. Fisk CS. *Dynamic function of skeletal muscles of the forearm: an*

electromyographical and cinematographical analysis. Unpublished dissertation. Indiana University, 1976.
35. Tullos HS, King JW. Throwing mechanism in sports. *Orthop Clin North Am* 1973;4:709–720.
36. Howell SM, Kraft TA. The role of the supraspinatus and infraspinatus muscles in glenohumeral kinematics of anterior shoulder instability. *Clin Orthop* 1991;263:128–134.
37. Feltner ME, Nelson ST. Three-dimensional kinematics of the throwing arm during the penalty throw in water polo. *J Appl Biomech* 1996;12:359–382.
38. Feltner ME, Taylor G. Three-dimensional kinetics of the shoulder, elbow, and wrist during a penalty throw in water polo. *J Appl Biomech* 1996;13:347–372.
39. Mero A, et al. Body segment contributions to javelin throwing during final thrust phases. *J Appl Biol* 1994;10:166–177.
40. Best RJ, et al. A three-dimensional analysis of javelin throwing technique. *J Sports Sci* 1993;11:315–328.
41. Elliot BC, et al. Contributions of upper limb segment rotations during the power serve in tennis. *J Appl Biomech* 1995;11:433–442.
42. Kibler WB. Clinical biomechanics of the elbow in tennis: implications for evaluation and diagnosis. *Med Sci Sports Exerc* 1994; 26:1203–1206.
43. Kibler WB. Biomechanical analysis of the shoulder during tennis activities. *Clin Sports Med* 1995;14:79–85.
44. Glousman R, et al. Dynamic electromyographic analysis of the throwing shoulder with glenohumeral instability. *J Bone Joint Surg Am* 1988;70:220–226.
45. Jobe F, Kvitne R. Shoulder pain in the overhand or throwing athlete; the relationship of anterior instability and rotator cuff impingement. *Orthop Rev* 1989;18:963–975.
46. McLeod WD, Andrews JR. Mechanisms of shoulder injuries. *Phys Ther* 1986;66:1901–1904.
47. McLeod WD. The pitching mechanism. In: Zarins B, Andrews JR, Carson WG, et al., eds. *Injuries to the throwing arm.* Philadelphia: WB Saunders, 1985:2229.
48. Colachis SC, Strohn BR. Effects of suprascapular and axillary nerve blocks on muscle force in upper extremity. *Arch Phys Med Rehabil* 1971;52:22–29.
49. Dvir Z, Berme N. Shoulder complex in elevation of the arm: a mechanism approach. *J Biomech* 1978;11:219–225.
50. Basmajian JV. Integrated actions and functions of the chief flexors of the elbow: a detailed electromyographic analysis. *J Bone Joint Surg* 1957;39:1106–1118.
51. Furlani J. Electromyographic study of the m. biceps brachii in movements of the glenohumeral joint. *Acta Anat* 1976;96:270–284.
52. Andrews JR. Glenoid labrum tears related to the long head of the biceps. *Am J Sports Med* 1985;13:337–341.
53. Morrey BF, An KN. Articular and ligamentous contributions to the stability of the elbow joint. *Am J Sports Med* 1983;11:315–319.
54. Dillman C, et al. Valgus extension overload in baseball pitching. *Med Sci Sports Exerc* 1991;23(suppl):S135.
55. Sakurai S, Ikegami Y, Okamoto A, et al. A three-dimensional cinematographic analysis of upper limb movement during fastball and curveball baseball pitches. *J Appl Biomech* 1993;9:47–65.
56. Andrews JR. Common elbow problems in the athlete. *J Orthop Sports Phys Ther* 1993;17:289–295.
57. Jameson EG, et al. Muscle activity during shoulder rehabilitation exercises. *Proceedings of the North American Congress on Biomechanics*, Waterloo, Ontario, 1998.
58. Escamilla RF, et al. Kinematic comparisons of throwing different types of baseball pitches. *J Appl Biomech* 1998;14:1–23.
59. Escamilla RF, et al. A kinematic and kinetic comparison while throwing different types of baseball pitches. *Med Sci Sports Exerc* 1994;26:S175.

Exercise and Sport Science,
edited by William E. Garrett, Jr., and Donald T. Kirkendall.
Lippincott Williams & Wilkins, Philadelphia © 2000.

CHAPTER 39

Biomechanics of Powerlifting and Weightlifting Exercises

Rafael F. Escamilla, Jeffrey E. Lander, and John Garhammer

This chapter examines select biomechanical variables during exercises that comprise the sports of powerlifting (squat, bench press, and deadlift) and weightlifting (snatch, and clean and jerk). These exercises are commonly performed by strength and power athletes, and they are an integral part of strength and conditioning programs for many sports that require high levels of strength and power, such as football, track and field (sprints and field events), powerlifting, and weightlifting. In addition, since these exercises constitute a closed kinetic chain, some may be appropriate in rehabilitation settings. Several studies have demonstrated the favorable use of the squat and other closed kinetic chain exercises during knee rehabilitation (1–7), such as after cruciate ligament reconstructive surgery. Consequently, knee biomechanics of the squat may be helpful to therapists, trainers, sports medicine physicians, and researchers who are interested in closed kinetic chain exercises or knee rehabilitation.

Athletes in many sports or activities utilize some of these exercises in their training regimens. The squat primarily strengthens hip, thigh, and back musculature, which are very important muscles in running, jumping, and lifting. The deadlift exercise develops the same muscles as the squat, with a greater emphasis on back development. Like the squat, the deadlift is a closed kinetic chain exercise. While the squat and deadlift exercises develop the lower extremities and posterior trunk, the bench press develops the upper extremity and anterior trunk, primarily the chest, shoulder, and triceps. Although the squat, deadlift, and bench press make up the sport of powerlifting, the name is somewhat of a misnomer since only moderate power outputs are produced during maximal efforts (8). In contrast, some of the highest human power outputs recorded are from the clean and jerk and snatch exercises (9,10). These exercises produce total body development and enhance an athlete's ability to generate power.

The first section of this chapter reviews the biomechanics of the squat, deadlift, and bench press, with its primary focus on squat biomechanics since relatively few studies have examined biomechanical parameters during the deadlift and bench press. Because the knee has been the focus of most squat studies, a review of knee biomechanics of the dynamic squat is presented, specifically tibiofemoral shear and compressive forces, patellofemoral compressive force, knee muscle activity, and knee stability. The second section presents biomechanical profiles during the clean and jerk and snatch exercises. The third section examines the role and effects of weight belts and intraabdominal/intrathoracic pressures during lifting.

KNEE BIOMECHANICS OF THE DYNAMIC SQUAT

Tibiofemoral Shear and Compressive Forces

Excessive shear forces can be injurous to the cruciate ligaments, while excessive compressive forces can be deleterious to the menisci and articular cartilage. Eight studies have quantified tibiofemoral shear and compressive forces during the dynamic squat (6,11–17). Seven of these articles studied the barbell squat with an external load, and one article (12) studied the body weight

R. F. Escamilla: Department of Surgery, Duke University Medical Center, Durham, North Carolina 27710.

J. E. Lander: Department of Sport Health Science, Life University, Marietta, Georgia 30060.

J. Garhammer: Department of Kinesiology & Physical Education, California State University, Long Beach, California 90840.

(BW) squat. All squats were performed at maximum knee flexion (0 degrees, defined as full knee extension), and the thighs were parallel or below parallel with the ground. Comparing tibiofemoral compressive and shear forces among these studies is difficult, since only five studies modeled both external (e.g., gravity, ground reaction) and internal (e.g., muscle, bone, ligament) forces (11–15). The remaining three studies modeled external forces only (6,16,17). To quantify the actual shear and compressive forces across the articulating surface of the knee, muscle force from those muscles that cross the knee must be determined. The primary muscles that cross the knee are the quadriceps, hamstrings, and gastrocnemius, which compose ≈98% of the total cross-sectional area of all the muscles that cross the knee (18). When the quadriceps, hamstrings, and gastrocnemius contract, they produce additional compressive and shear force components within the knee. For example, consider a 115-kg lifter standing upright with a 200-kg barbell across his back. Since ≈100 kg of the lifter's mass is above his knees, there is a total of 300 kg of mass (m) above the lifter's knees on which gravity will act in a downward direction to compress the tibiofemoral joint. Therefore, the tibiofemoral compressive force (F) generated due to these two external forces (lifter and barbell) is derived as $F = ma = (300\ \text{kg})\ (\approx 10\ \text{m}\cdot\text{s}^{-2}) \approx 3000\ \text{N}$. [Note: If the acceleration (a) constant 10 is used instead of 9.81, newtons can easily be converted to kilograms by dividing by 10; thus, 3000 N ≈ 300 kg. Similarly, a rough estimate for converting newtons of force to pounds of force is to remember that 1 N is a little less than $\frac{1}{4}$ lb; hence, 3000 N of force is a little less than 750 lbs of force.] Now consider the same lifter, load, and position, but this time with quadriceps, hamstrings, and gastrocnemius activity. The additional compressive forces generated by muscle forces will cause tibiofemoral compressive forces much higher than the 3000 N produced by external forces only. In fact, it has been demonstrated that during a maximum voluntary contraction of the quadriceps the force generated ranges from 2000 to 8000 N, depending on knee flexion angle (19). Consequently, it is hypothesized that studies that model both external and muscle forces will show greater tibiofemoral compressive and shear forces compared to studies that model external forces only. However, developing mathematical models that estimate knee muscle and ligament forces can be difficult, and potentially inaccurate, depending on the variables measured and the methodology employed.

Throughout this chapter, anterior shear forces are defined as forces restrained primarily by the anterior cruciate ligament (ACL), and posterior shear forces will be defined as forces restrained primarily by the posterior cruciate ligament (PCL). This is reasonable, since Butler and colleagues (20) have reported that the ACL provides 86% of the total restraining force to anterior drawer, and the PCL provides 95% of the total restraining force to posterior drawer.

A biomechanical comparison of seven studies that quantified shear and compressive forces is shown in Table 39–1. Only three studies specified the direction of the tibiofemoral shear force (6,13,15), making it difficult to determine which cruciate ligament was loaded. All three of these studies reported posterior shear forces and PCL loading throughout the movement, although Nisell and Ekholm (15) did show minimum anterior shear forces and ACL loading between 0- and 60-degree knee flexion. Since the loads lifted varied greatly among

TABLE 39–1. *Comparison of tibiofemoral compressive and shear forces among squat studies*

Study	Mean subject weight (N)	Mean barbell load lifted (N)	Knee flexion range (°)	Shear force direction	Mean peak shear force (N) @ knee flexion angle (°)	Normalized mean peak shear force %(BW + load)	Mean peak compressive force (N) @ knee flexion angle (°)	Normalized mean peak compressive force %(BW + load)
Escamilla et al. (13)	912 ± 145	1437 ± 383	0–95	Posterior	1868 ± 878 @ 63	79.5 ± 37.3	3134 ± 1040 @ 53	133 ± 44.3
Stuart et al. (6)	798 ± 75.5	223 ± 0.0	0–90	Posterior	295 ± 32 @ 93	28.9 ± 3.1	550 ± 50 @ 80	53.9 ± 4.9
Nisell and Ekholm (15)	1079 ± 0.0	2453 ± 0.0	0–130*	Posterior Anterior	1800* ± 0.0 @ 130* 500* ± 0.0 @ 20*	51.0* ± 0.0 14.2* ± 0.0	7000* ± 0.0 @ 130*	198* ± 0.0
Ariel (11)	888 ± ?	1982 ± ?	0–117*	?	1593 ± 106* @ 48*	55.5 ± 3.7*	7928 ± 1965* @ 106*	276 ± 68.5*
Dahlkvist et al. (12)	732 ± 78.5	0	0–140*	?	2652 ± 290 @60*	362 ± 39.6	4018 ± 1230 @ 60*	549 ± 168
Hattin et al. (17)	790 ± 109	1129 ± 212	0–90*	?	963 ± 561 @ 90*	50.2 ± 29.2	5220 ± 1461 @ 90*	272 ± 76.1
Andrews et al. (16)	?	?	0–110*	?	1000* ± ? @ 110*	?	?	?

*Value estimated from graphs and data in study.
?Variable unknown.
BW, body weight.

studies, mean peak shear and compressive force were normalized by the sum of BW and load lifted and were expressed as a percent. Although normalized results vary, values from Dahlkvist and colleagues (12) appear inordinately high. Discounting these values, normalized shear forces ranged from ≈30% to 80% of the total weight lifted, while normalized compressive force ranged from ≈50% to 275% of the total weight lifted.

Since the ultimate strength of the PCL has been estimated up to 4000 N for active young people (21), the peak PCL forces observed during the squat (Table 39–1) are probably not of great enough magnitude to be injurious to the healthy PCL. The results of these studies suggest that the squat may be a safe and effective rehabilitation exercise to perform for those who wish to minimize tensile loading of the ACL (e.g., after ACL reconstruction), assuming the PCL and other knee structures are healthy. The peak 500 N anterior shear force reported by Nisell and Ekholm (15) should not be injurious to the healthy ACL, since two independent studies have calculated its ultimate failure load to be between 1725 and 2160 N (22,23). The greater strength of the PCL compared to the ACL is primarily due to a 20% to 50% greater cross-sectional area (24).

Peak compressive forces from Table 39–1 ranged from ≈550 to 8000 N. It is difficult to know at what magnitude compressive force becomes injurious to knee structures, such as menisci and articular cartilage. Excessive loading of the menisci and articular cartilage can lead to degenerative changes. However, compressive forces have been demonstrated to be an important factor in knee stabilization by resisting shear forces and minimizing tibia translation relative to the femur (25–28).

Studies have shown that expert squatters (i.e., competitive and experienced) have more favorable kinematics (joint positions) and kinetics (joint forces and torques), and perform better, than do novice squatters (29,30). Escamilla and colleagues (13) chose 10 male powerlifters and bodybuilders experienced in performing the barbell squat, because they were considered experts in knowing how to perform the squat exercise correctly. The subjects had a mean height of 176.5 ± 8.9 cm, mass of 93.0 ± 14.8 kg, and age of 29.2 ± 6.4 years. Each subject performed three repetitions with their 12 repetition maximum (12 RM) load, lifting a mean load of 1.6 times BW (Table 39–1). Four video cameras collected 60-Hz kinematic data, while two force platforms were utilized to collect 960-Hz kinetic data. Electromyography (EMG), inverse dynamics, mathematical knee modeling, and computer optimization techniques were employed to estimate internal muscle and ligamentous forces. Muscle forces (F_{mi}) from the quadriceps, hamstrings, and gastrocnemius were estimated from the equation $F_{mi} = c_i k_i A_i \sigma_{mi}(EMG_i/MVC_I)$, where c_i is a weight factor adjusted in a computer optimization program to minimize errors in muscle force estimates, k_i is a muscle force-length factor as a function of knee and hip flexion, A_i is the physiologic cross-sectional area (PCSA) of the ith muscle, σ_{mi} is the maximum voluntary isometric contraction force (MVIC) per PSCA, and EMG_i and MVC_i are EMG window averages during the squat and MVIC, respectively. Additional descriptions of this analytical knee model are available elsewhere (31).

Tibiofemoral compressive forces, ACL tensile forces, and PCL tensile forces are shown in Fig. 39–1. These forces progressively increased with knee flexion and decreased with knee extension. Forces were slightly greater during the ascent compared to the descent. Although these forces were estimated and not measured directly, it is interesting that there were no ACL tensile forces (i.e., anterior shear forces) measured throughout the squat exercise. These data are similar to the results of Stuart and colleagues (6). The absence of ACL forces during the squat may in part be due to moderate hamstring activity, since several studies have demonstrated that the hamstrings help unload the ACL by producing a posteriorly directed force to the leg throughout the knee movement (3,32–38). In contrast, the quadriceps, via the patella tendon, exert an anteriorly directed force on the leg between ≈0- and 60-degree knee flexion, and a posteriorly directed force when the knee is flexed greater than ≈60 degrees (39). When posteriorly directed shear forces acting on the leg exceeds anteriorly directed shear forces, the net result will be a posterior shear force, which is restrained primarily by the PCL. During the squat ascent, a mean peak PCL tensile force of 1868 ± 878 N occurred at 63-degree knee flexion,

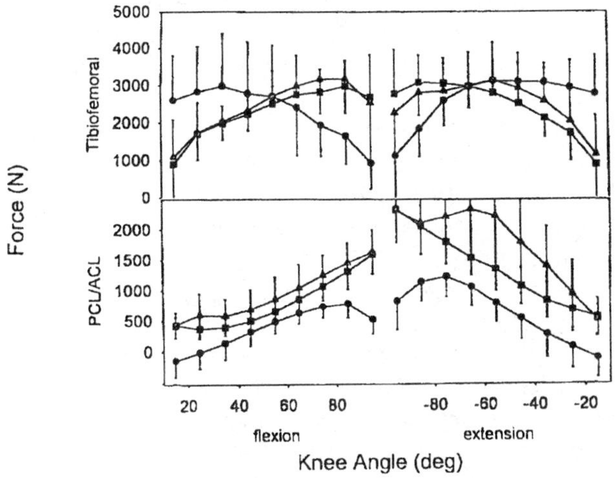

FIG. 39–1. Mean and standard deviation (n = 10) of tibiofemoral compressive force and posterior cruciate ligament (*PCL*) (+) and anterior cruciate ligament (*ACL*) (−) tensile forces during the squat (*triangles*), leg press (*squares*), and leg extensions (*circles*). (From ref. 13, with permission.)

while a mean peak compressive force of 3134 ± 1040 N occurred at 53-degree knee flexion. During the descent, a mean peak PCL tensile force of 1635 ± 369 N occurred at 95-degree knee flexion, while a mean peak compressive force of 2192 ± 930 N occurred at 81-degree knee flexion.

Using the same methods as in their previous study reported above (13), Escamilla and colleagues (14) compared the effects of technique variations (stance width and foot angle) on shear and compressive forces. Their subjects performed a narrow stance (distance between medial malleoli equals distance between anterior superior iliac spines) and wide stance (twice the narrow stance distance) squat with the feet parallel (i.e., pointing straight ahead) with each other and with the feet turned outward 45 degrees. Their preliminary data show that the effects of foot angle on shear and compressive forces are generally insignificant, with few significant differences in ACL and PCL tensile forces observed between stance widths. A wide stance squat generates significantly greater compressive forces compared to the narrow stance, however. The authors conclude that the greater compressive forces generated during the squat may help protect the knee against excessive shear forces. The role of compressive forces in resisting shear forces are discussed below.

Nisell and Ekholm (15) did a two-part study. They first examined knee joint loads in three world-class powerlifters during the ascent portion of the powerlifting squat. The subjects had a mean height of 173 ± 8.5 cm, mass of 95.0 ± 18.0 kg, and age of 27.3 ± 6.5 years. Each subject was filmed (4 Hz) with a one-camera motion system in the sagittal plane of movement. Using quasi-static two-dimensional biomechanical knee models by Nisell (40) and Nisell and colleagues (41), external and muscle forces acting on the leg were estimated.

Compressive and shear forces were reported for a 110-kg subject squatting 250 kg. The quadriceps tendon force and tibiofemoral compressive force were approximately the same magnitude from 130- to 60-degree knee flexion. A maximum value of ≈8,000 N occurred at ≈130-degree knee flexion, and slowly declined to ≈5500 N at ≈60-degree knee flexion. At 30-degree knee flexion, compressive force was ≈3500 N, while quadriceps tendon force dropped down to ≈2000 N. Although these force magnitudes are quite high, most rehabilitation patients and athletes training in the squat will experience considerably smaller forces, since the loads lifted in this study are much greater than what most athletes or rehabilitation patients will utilize.

Patellar tendon force was ≈6,000 N at ≈130-degree knee flexion, and slowly decreased to ≈2,000 N at ≈30-degree knee flexion. Although a peak patellar tendon force of 5000 N at 60-degree knee flexion was calculated by van Eijden and colleagues (19) during MVIC of the quadriceps femoris the strength of the patellar tendon in the healthy knee is probably much higher than 5000 N. Cooper and colleagues (42) have quantified the ultimate strength of the central third of the patellar tendon (a 15-mm bone–patellar tendon–bone composite) to be 4389 ± 708 N. Zernicke and colleagues (43) reported a ruptured patellar tendon in a 82.2-kg weightlifter who was performing a rapid squat descent (see Fig. 39–8*A,B*) during a 175-kg clean and jerk. A rapid downward acceleration was followed by tremendous forces being generated in the quadriceps to decelerate the weight in preparation to press the barbell overhead (see Fig. 39–8*C,D*). Large decelerations during the squat generate tremendous forces across the knee structures, which is why the squat descent should be performed in a slow, controlled manner. A 14,500-N tensile force (17.5 times BW) was calculated in the patellar tendon at the time of rupture. Extrapolating these data, the ultimate strength of the patellar ligament in the healthy knee is probably somewhere between 10,000 and 15,000 N, which is ≈13 to 19 times BW for an 80-kg individual. The peak quadriceps tendon force observed was the same as the 8000 N peak force reported by van Eijden and colleagues (19). How much force the quadriceps tendon can generate before rupture is unclear. However, since Nisell and Ekholm (44) found the thickness and breadth of the quadriceps tendon to be 35% to 40% greater than the thickness and breadth of the patellar tendon, it is likely that the ultimate strength of the quadriceps tendon is greater than the 10,000- to 15,000-N estimate for the ultimate strength of the patellar tendon.

Nisell and Ekholm (15) reported a peak posterior shear force of ≈1800 N at ≈130-degree knee flexion, which is similar to the 1863 N peak PCL tensile force calculated by Escamilla and colleagues (13), who also used powerlifters as subjects and quantified muscle forces. At ≈60-degree knee flexion, the posterior shear force changed to an anterior shear force. This force increased fairly linearly throughout the remainder of the ascent, peaking at ≈500 N at ≈20 degrees. It is interesting that even though tremendous muscle forces were generated in the three subjects due to the large loads lifted, tensile forces in the PCL and ACL were only ≈50% and ≈25%, respectively, of the estimated ultimate tensile strength in these ligaments. The presence of anterior shear forces during the second half of the ascent is in agreement with data from Beynnon and colleagues (45), who inserted strain transducers into the anteromedial bundle of the ACL in eight subjects immediately after arthroscopic knee menisectomies and debridements. After the strain transducers were inserted into the ACL, the experimental procedures began. Under local anesthesia, the subjects were asked to squat down from an upright position to ≈90-degree knee flexion and then ascend back to an upright position. The subjects were then asked to repeat the squat using an elastic resistance cord, which generated 136 N of force at full knee extension, and 34 N of force at 90-degree knee flexion. Minimal ACL strain (<4%) was observed at knee flexion angles less than 70 degrees during both the squat descent and ascent, with no significant differences observed in ACL strain between the two squat conditions. ACL strain was greatest at full extension, and progressively decreased as the knee flexed to 90 degrees. There were several limitations to this study that would make it difficult to extrapolate these results to the barbell squat as performed by athletes in training. First, Markolf and colleagues (27) have reported that lateral and medial knee menisectomies significantly increase anteroposterior knee laxity in the unloaded knee. Since most of Beynnon and colleagues' subjects had lateral and medial menisectomies, this may have caused higher ACL strain than if the menisectomies had not been performed. Because the knee was loaded when ACL strain was recorded, however, anteroposterior translation due to the menisectomies may be insignificant, as concomitant compressive force may resist this anteroposterior translation. However, compressive force magnitudes would be low due to a small external load (i.e., BW only) and low muscle force production from the quadriceps and hamstrings. Second, hamstring activity was probably minimal due to the minimal load lifted and the squatting technique employed in the experimental setup. Third, how the patients normally would perform the squat was probably affected by the knee surgery they had a few hours prior. Nevertheless, the results of this study may be applied to patients who just had ACL reconstructive surgery, and they should be helpful to therapists, trainers, and orthopedists who work with these patients in early postoperative rehabilitation programs.

The second part of the study by Nisell and Ekholm (15) involved a force analysis of a bilateral complete rupture of the quadriceps tendon (at its insertion into the superior patella) in a world-class powerlifter injured in competition while lifting a 382.5-kg load. The rupture occurred where the quadriceps tendon inserts into the patella. Although the injury was filmed, a biomechanical analysis of the injured subject was not able to be conducted, since the filming was not perpendicular to the lifter's sagittal plane of motion. Since the injury occurred at the deepest portion of the squat just prior to beginning the ascent, knee joint forces were calculated in this position during a simulated squat using the three healthy subjects and the 382.5-kg load. Estimated quadriceps tendon force for the three subjects ranged from 10,900 to 18,300 N (12 to 20 times BW), while the force in the patellar tendon ranged from ≈8000 to 13,000 N. Estimated compressive force ranged from ≈10,200 to 15,800 N, while estimated posterior shear force ranged from ≈1500 to 2500 N.

Knee joint biomechanical models and anthropometric data used to estimate knee forces in the study by Nisell and Ekholm (15) were based on 10 healthy male subjects with a mean height of 180 cm and a mean body mass of 75 kg (40,41). This is one limitation to this study, since the three healthy subjects used in this study had a mean body mass of 95.0 ± 18.0 kg and a mean height of 173 ± 8.5 cm. Another limitation in this study was that the effect of co-contraction of the hamstring musculature was not considered. Since the calculated knee torque was the resultant torque (i.e., sum of all flexor and extensor torques), hamstring activity, which generates a knee flexor torque, would cause greater quadriceps activity and extensor torque. Consequently, all calculated knee forces in this study would be underestimated, since these forces are functions of quadriceps tendon and patellar tendon forces. Because the quadriceps tendon thickness is significantly greater than the patellar tendon thickness, it should be able to withstand a higher load before rupture. High magnitudes of compressive force and stress (force/area) between the femoral intercondylar notch and the quadriceps tendon may increase the injury potential of the quadriceps tendon, however. Tendofemoral compressive force between the quadriceps tendon and the femoral intercondylar notch began high at 6,000 N at ≈130-degree knee flexion, but quickly decreased to ≈1750 N at 90-degree knee flexion, and ≈0 N at ≈60-degree knee flexion. Assuming a 3.4 cm^2 tendofemoral contact area when the knee is flexed ≈130 degrees (46), tendofemoral compressive stress would be 17.6 MPa (6000 N/0.00034 m^2). This large stress applied repetitively over time may cause degenerative changes in the tendofemoral complex. Hence, performing the squat at low to moderate knee flexion angles (e.g., 0 to 90 degrees) will minimize tendofemoral stress, and minimize injury potential to the tendofemoral complex.

Ariel (11) used 12 experienced weightlifters to investigate forces acting about the knee joint during a deep knee barbell squat with a mean load of 202 kg. The subjects had a mean height of 181.5 cm and mass of 90.5 kg, and an age range between 21 and 25 years. A computer program was written that took inertial (i.e., acceleration), external, and muscle forces into account. Three of the 12 subjects were used during the kinetic analyses, since their performances were thought to be representative of the other lifters. Subject one bounced at the bottom, subject two lifted the greatest load (295 kg), and subject three exhibited the greatest forward knee movement. Shear forces were generally greatest at knee flexion angles less than 60 degrees, ranging from ≈600 to 1600 N. Shear force direction was not stated. Contrary to findings from several studies (6,12,13,15–17), shear forces progressively decreased at knee flexion angles greater than ≈60 degrees, with minimum shear values occurring at ≈90- to 120-degree knee flexion. Minimum shear values were ≈600 N for the subject that bounced at the bottom, ≈120 N for the subject that lifted the most weight, and ≈1120 N for the subject that had the greatest forward knee movement. Bouncing at the bottom of the squat increased shear force by ≈33%. Interestingly, the subject that lifted the most had the smallest shear forces, and the lifter that had the greatest forward knee motion had the greatest shear forces. The results of this study indicate that forward knee movement, as well as bouncing at the bottom, both contributed to high shearing forces. Beyond 90-degree knee flexion, the knee was thought to be more vulnerable, and the author suggested that shear forces may adversely affect knee ligaments. For all three subjects, an inverse relationship was observed between compressive and shear forces. This is contrary to the findings of several other studies (12,13,15,17), which found that both shear and compressive forces increase as knee flexion increases. Compressive forces were generally highest at higher knee flexion angles, and ranged from ≈6720 to 10,390 N.

Dahlkvist and colleagues (12) used six male subjects to perform the deep BW squat during regular, slow, and fast descents and ascents. The subjects had a mean height of 180.0 ± 5.0 cm, mass of 74.6 ± 8.0 kg, and age of 20.7 ± 0.52 years. Kinematic data were recorded with one camera system filming at 50 Hz in the sagittal plane of motion. A force platform was used to quantify kinetic data, while EMG was used to estimate knee muscle forces. Cadence rates for the ascent and descent phases were not reported. The force in the patellar ligament was higher during the descent phase of the squat compared to the ascent. This was assumed to be due to greater deceleration needed during the descent to slow down the body. Mean compressive and shear (direction not stated) forces during the descent of the fast squat were 4110 N and 2521 N, respectively. Mean compressive and shear forces during the ascent of the fast squat were 3564 N and 2056 N, respectively. Mean compressive and shear forces during the descent of the slow squat were 3834 N and 2913 N, respectively. Finally, mean compressive and shear forces during the ascent of the slow squat were 3413 N and 2126 N, respectively. Mean compressive forces were greatest during the fast squat descent, while mean shear forces were greatest during the slow squat descent. The general pattern observed was that, as knee flexion increased, compressive and shear forces also increased.

Hattin and colleagues (17) examined the effect of load, cadence, and fatigue on tibiofemoral joint force during the parallel squat. Ten male subjects volunteered for this study, lifting a mean 1 RM of 115.1 ± 21.6 kg. The subjects had a mean height of 177.5 ± 5.3 cm, mass of 80.5 ± 11.1 kg, and age of 22.6 ± 2.2 years. Three load conditions were used—15%, 22%, and 30% of each subject's 1 RM. Two different cadences were used: a slow cadence, where the descent and ascent phases lasted 2 s each; and a fast cadence, where the descent and ascent phases lasted 1 s each. To test for fatigue, 50 continuous repetitions were completed for each load and cadence, and were subdivided into initial, middle, and final phases. Kinematic data were captured at 50 Hz by a three-camera motion system, while a force platform was used to collect kinetic data. Inverse dynamics and external forces were used to calculate knee joint forces. For each load condition, shear (direction not stated) and compressive forces significantly increased as the subjects progressed through each of the three phases, with shear forces being most affected by fatigue. Hence, fatigue may increase loading of the cruciate ligaments. Fatigue became most apparent when the subjects were approximately halfway through their 50 repetitions.

Knee forces were quite symmetrical between knee flexion angles during the descent and ascent. Maximal shear and compressive forces occurred at maximum knee flexion. Mean values for anteroposterior shear, compressive, and mediolateral shear forces were 869 N, 4740 N, and 79 N, respectively, for the 15% of 1 RM condition; 711 N, 4424 N, and 79 N, respectively, for the 22% of 1 RM condition; and 869 N, 4661 N, and 79 N, respectively, for the 30% of 1 RM condition. Mediolateral shear forces were small throughout all conditions and squat phases, and can be discounted. Anteroposterior shear, compressive, and mediolateral forces were 711 N, 4266 N, and 79 N, respectively, for the slow cadence, and 948 N, 4898 N, and 79 N, respectively, for the fast cadence. Consequently, performing the squat at a faster cadence significantly increased shear and compressive forces. During the initial phase, before fatigue became a factor, shear forces increased 50% from a slow to a fast cadence, while compressive forces increased 28%.

Stuart and colleagues (6) had six male subjects perform the barbell squat with a 22.7-kg load. Four 60-Hz cameras were used to collect kinematic data, and a force platform was used to collect kinetic data. The subjects had a mean height of 181 ± 7.7 cm, mass of 81.3 ± 7.7 kg, and age of 26.6 ± 5.1 years. External and inertial forces were considered in quantifying compressive and shear forces. Compressive forces between 500 and 600 N remained fairly constant through the descent and ascent phases of the squat. The considerably less compressive and shear forces in this study compared to other studies (11–13,15–17) is primarily due to less weight being lifted and the omission of muscle force contributions. Posterior shear forces were observed for all subjects throughout the descent and ascent phases. These shear forces increased with knee flexion and decreased with knee extension, which is consistent with data from other studies (12,13,15–17). Mean peak posterior shear forces were 295 ± 32 N at 93-degree knee flexion during the ascent, and 295 ± 33 N at 97-degree knee flexion during the descent. The authors concluded that the shear force magnitudes calculated were unlikely to be detrimental to the injured or reconstructed PCL. Furthermore, since no anterior shear forces were observed, performing the squat may be appropriate for ACL patients.

Andrews and colleagues (16) calculated knee shear forces while their subjects performed the barbell and machine squat exercises. Cadence and lifting loads were comparable during both types of squats. Three males with extensive lifting experience were studies, each utilizing the barbell squat and the universal leg-squat. Three load conditions (40%, 60%, and 80% of their 4 RM) and three lifting ascent speeds (slow, 3 s; medium, 2 s; and fast, 1 s) were performed by each subject. The descent was 2 s for all conditions. A two-dimensional lifting model utilized external forces and inverse dynamics. During the barbell squat slow lifting rate, shear force was ≈300 N at the beginning and end of the lift, and reached a maximum ≈1,000 N at the lowest position (≈110 knee flexion). During the barbell squat fast lifting rate, shear force was ≈350 N at the beginning of the lift, reached a maximum of ≈1,200 N at the lowest position of the squat, and was ≈200 N at the end of the lift. Shear force curves for the machine squat (slow and fast cadences) were more irregular in shape. During the slow lifting rate, shear force was ≈300 N at the beginning of the lift, reached a maximum of ≈900 N at ≈110-degree knee flexion, and remained at ≈600 N during most of the ascent. During the machine squat fast lifting rate the shear force was ≈600 N near the beginning of the lift, reached a maximum of ≈1,000 N at ≈110-degree knee flexion, and remained at ≈600 N during most of the ascent. For both the barbell and machine squat exercises, peak shear force occurred at the lowest position of the squat. Shear forces were similar between the barbell and machine squats, but they stayed at maximum values longer during the machine squat exercise. The authors concluded that shear forces were ≈30% to 40% greater during the machine squat compared to the barbell squat. Furthermore, the fast lifting rate produced greater shear force than the slow lifting rate. Hence, injury potential to the cruciate ligaments may be greater during the machine squat and during fast lifting rates.

Patellofemoral Compressive Forces

Patellofemoral compressive force produces stress (compressive force divided by contact area) on the articular cartilage of the patella. Excessive compressive force and stress, or repetitive occurrences of lower magnitude force and stress, may contribute to patellofemoral degeneration and pathologies, such as patella chondromalacia and osteoarthritis. Three forces act on the patella during the squat: (a) quadriceps tendon force; (b) patellar tendon force; and (c) patellofemoral compressive force. During the squat, all these forces are affected by knee flexion angle. Mathematically, compressive force is greatest at higher knee flexion angles, since there are larger force components from the quadriceps tendon and patellar tendon in the compressive direction.

Patellofemoral compressive forces arise from contact between the undersurface of the patella and the femoral condyles. From full extension to full flexion, the patella moves caudally approximately 7 cm, with femoral contact on the patella moving cranially as the knee flexes. Patellofemoral contact has been reported to occur initially between 10- and 20-degree knee flexion (46,47), which is when the patella begins to glide onto the articular surface of the femoral intercondylar notch. The femur makes contact with the medial and lateral inferior facets between ≈20- and 30-degree knee flexion, with the medial and lateral middle facets between ≈30 and 60 degrees, with the medial and lateral superior facets between ≈60 and 90 degrees, and with the medial vertical "odd" facet and lateral superior facet between ≈90 and 135 degrees (46,47). At ≈90-degree knee flexion, the "odd" facet for the first time makes contact with the lateral margin of the medial condyle (47). Since contact is increased as the knee continues into full flexion, this area is a common site of osteochondritis dissecans.

Six studies quantified patellofemoral compressive forces during the dynamic squat (12–15,48,49). Four of these studies involved the barbell squat (13–15,48), and two involved the BW squat (12,49). Escamilla and colleagues (13) employed a mathematical model of the patella (44,50,51) to calculate patellofemoral compressive forces as a function of knee angle. Compressive forces increased with knee flexion and decreased with knee extension, and were slightly greater during the descent compared to the ascent (Fig. 39–2). During the descent a peak compressive force of 4548 ± 1395 N occurred at 85-degree knee flexion, while during the ascent a peak compressive force of 4042 ± 955 N occurred at 95-degree knee flexion (13). When normalized by the sum of the subjects' BW and load lifted, and expressed as a percent, peak compressive force was 194% during the descent and 172% during the ascent.

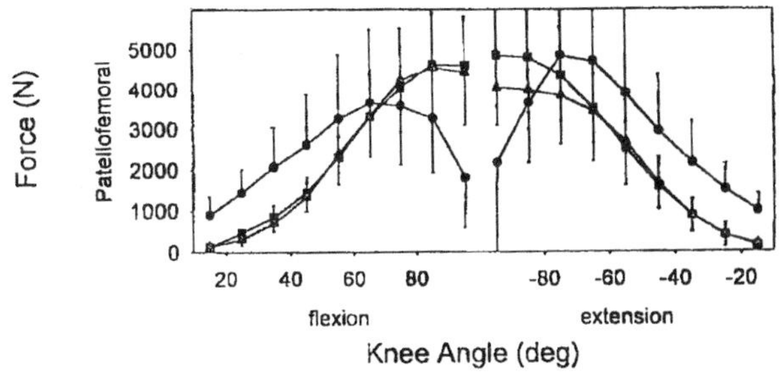

FIG. 39–2. Mean and standard deviation (n = 10) of patellofemoral compressive force during the squat (*triangles*), leg press (*squares*), and leg extensions (*circles*). (From ref. 13, with permission.)

A follow-up study was conducted by these authors (14) to examine the effects of stance width and foot angle on patellofemoral compressive forces. Their preliminary data show no significant differences in compressive forces between a narrow and wide stance squat.

Analyzing the squat ascent, Nisell and Ekholm (15) found a patellofemoral compressive force pattern similar to that of Escamilla and colleagues (13), with a peak force of ≈6750 N occurring near maximum knee flexion (≈130 degrees), and then progressively decreasing as the knee extended. When normalized by the sum of the subjects' BW and the load lifted (see Table 39–1), and expressed as a percent, peak compressive force was 191%, which is similar to 172% value from Escamilla and colleagues (13).

Wretenberg and colleagues (52) used eight weightlifters with a mean height of 177 ± 7.56 cm, mass of 81.6 ± 11.0 kg, and age of 18.9 ± 3.00 years, and six powerlifters with a mean height of 171 ± 10.1 cm, mass of 87.3 ± 20.4 kg, and age of 30.8 ± 3.13 years. The powerlifters employed a low-bar squat position, in which the bar was positioned across the back ≈3 to 5 cm below the level of the acromion. The weightlifters employed a high-bar squat position, in which the bar was positioned across the back at approximately the level of the acromion. All subjects lifted 65% of their 1 RM, with the weightlifters lifting a mean load of 66.3 ± 17.9 kg, and the powerlifters lifting a mean load of 100 ± 13.7 kg. Patellofemoral compressive forces generally increased as knee flexion increased. Mean peak patellofemoral compressive forces were 4700 ± 590 N for the weightlifters and 3300 ± 1700 N for the powerlifters, and occurred at ≈90- to 120-degree knee flexion. When normalized by the sum of the subjects' BW and load lifted, and expressed as a percent, peak compressive forces were 324% for the weightlifters and 180% for the powerlifters. The large disparity in these normalized values between weightlifters and powerlifters is probably due to technique variations, such as low and high bar positions. Powerlifters typically employ a low-bar squat position and greater forward trunk lean compared to weightlifters. The primary reason for this is to lift more weight, since powerful trunk (e.g., erector spinae) and hip (e.g., gluteus maximus and hamstrings) musculature are more involved in this position compared to the high-bar squat position employed by weightlifters, in which the trunk remains more upright. Consequently, the low-bar squat position produced greater hip extensor torque and less knee extensor torque compared to the high-bar squat. Mean peak knee extensor torques are typically between 100 and 300 N·m during the barbell squat (6,11,13, 15,30,48,52–54). Since these torques are resultant (i.e., net) torques, they represent the sum of all flexor and extensor knee torques. For example, a 500 N·m extensor torque and a 300 N·m flexor torque yields a 200 N·m resultant torque. Hence, it cannot be deduced that lower knee extensor torque equates to less quadriceps force being produced in the powerlifters, although it is enticing to do so. Less quadriceps force would indeed explain why peak patellofemoral compressive force was less in powerlifters, since quadriceps tendon force and patellar tendon force would also be less. However, EMG data from Wretenberg and colleagues (52) show greater quadriceps and hamstring activity in the low-bar squat compared to the high-bar squat. Since the hamstrings produce a knee flexor torque, a greater knee extensor torque would be needed. Hence, greater quadriceps force would be needed to generate this force. In addition, gastrocnemius force can also cause the quadriceps to generate more force during the squat, since the gastrocnemius also generates a knee flexor torque by their duel role as knee flexors and ankle plantar flexors. Moderate gastrocnemius activity and force have been observed during the squat (12,13), which is needed during the squat to control ankle dorsiflexion during the descent and cause ankle plantar flexion during the ascent.

Many strength and power athletes train the low-bar squat to develop the hip and trunk extensors primarily. In contrast, many athletes use the high-bar squat to elicit more quadriceps development and less hip and trunk extensor development. Also, since the high-bar squat is more similar to the squat movement performed during the clean and jerk, it is preferred by weightlifters. The low-bar squat technique may be desirable for athletes or rehabilitation patients who want to perform the squat, but minimize patellofemoral compressive force. Moreover, the low-bar squat position of greater forward trunk lean has been reported to decrease potential ACL strain, in part due to greater hamstring activity and less quadriceps activity (4). Hence, squatting with greater forward trunk lean may be appropriate for those wanting to minimize ACL stress. Furthermore, greater forward trunk lean also minimizes forward knee movement, which has been shown to increases knee shear force (11). Unfortunately, a greater forward trunk lean increases the injury risk to the back musculature and ligamentous structures.

The final two studies that quantified patellofemoral compressive force were by Dahlkvist and colleagues (12) and Reilly and Martens (49), whose subjects performed the BW squat. Like the three previous studies, compressive forces increased with knee flexion, peaking near maximum knee flexion (≈130 degrees). Dahlkvist and colleagues found peak compressive forces were 5455 ± 260 N during the descent and 5124 ± 676 N during the ascent. When normalized by the subjects' BW (Table 39–1) and expressed as a percent, peak compressive force was 745% during the descent and 700% during the ascent. Similar results were observed from Reilly and Martens, who found a peak compressive force of 6377 N, with a normalized value of 765%. These normalized values from Dahlkvist and colleagues and Reilly and Martens were approximately four times greater than the normalized values from the other three studies above. These large disparities in normalized values are probably due to methodologic differences.

From the above studies, patellofemoral compressive force generated during the squat can reach five to six times BW when training with moderate (70% to 85% of 1 RM) to heavy (85% to 100% of 1 RM) loads. While these loads are higher than most rehabilitation patients will experience, they are typical loads for strength and power athletes, such as football players. Unfortunately, it is currently unknown how much compressive force and stress is detrimental to the patellofemoral joint. Patellofemoral joint contact area has been reported to be 2.6 ± 0.4 cm^2 at 20-degree knee flexion, 3.1 ± 0.3 cm^2 at 30 degrees, 3.9 ± 0.6 cm^2 at 60 degrees, 4.1 ± 1.2 cm^2 at 90 degrees, and 4.6 ± 0.7 cm^2 at 120 degrees (46). Using these contact areas and squat ascent compressive force data from Escamilla and colleagues (13), patellofemoral joint stress at 20-, 30-, 60-, and 90-degree knee flexion would be ≈1.15 MPa, ≈2.42 MPa, ≈7.69 Mpa, and ≈11.6 Mpa, respectively. Consequently, during the squat, patellofemoral compressive force and stress both increase with knee flexion, reaching peak values at ≈90- to 100-degree knee flexion. Beyond 90- to 100-degree knee flexion, compressive force has been shown to remain relatively constant (13,15). Hence, stress may decrease at larger knee flexion angles, since patellofemoral contact area continues to increase.

From Fig. 39–2, one can see that the rate of increase (i.e., the slope at any given point on the curve) in patellofemoral force is maximum between ≈50- and 80-degree knee flexion, thus generating proportionately greater patellofemoral force compared to lower knee flexion angles. Therefore, performing the squat within the functional knee range of 0 to 50 degrees will minimize patellofemoral joint force and stress, and may be effective for athletes or patients with patellofemoral pathologies. For athletes with healthy knees, performing the squat at higher knee flexion angles (i.e., ≈90 to 110 degrees) should not be problematic, as long as heavy loads are not used excessively. This can be a potential problem for powerlifters and football players, who often train with heavy loads for long periods of time. Periodization techniques should be employed when performing the squat, in which training is divided into light, medium, and heavy intensity cycles throughout the year.

Muscle Activity

In order to determine which muscles are developed during the squat, and to what degree, it is helpful to quantify muscle activity through the use of electromyography. Ten studies have quantified muscle activity about the knee during the dynamic squat (6,12,13,48,52,55–59). In eight of these studies, subjects performed the barbell squat with an external load, and in two studies the subjects performed the BW squat. The primary knee muscles are the quadriceps, hamstrings, and gastrocnemius, and co-contractions among these muscles are believed to enhance knee stability.

Escamilla and colleagues (13) quantified quadriceps, hamstring, and gastrocnemius activity using a 12-RM load for 10 male subjects experienced in the squat. Quadriceps activity increased with knee flexion, with peak activity at ≈80- to 90-degree knee flexion (Fig. 39–3).

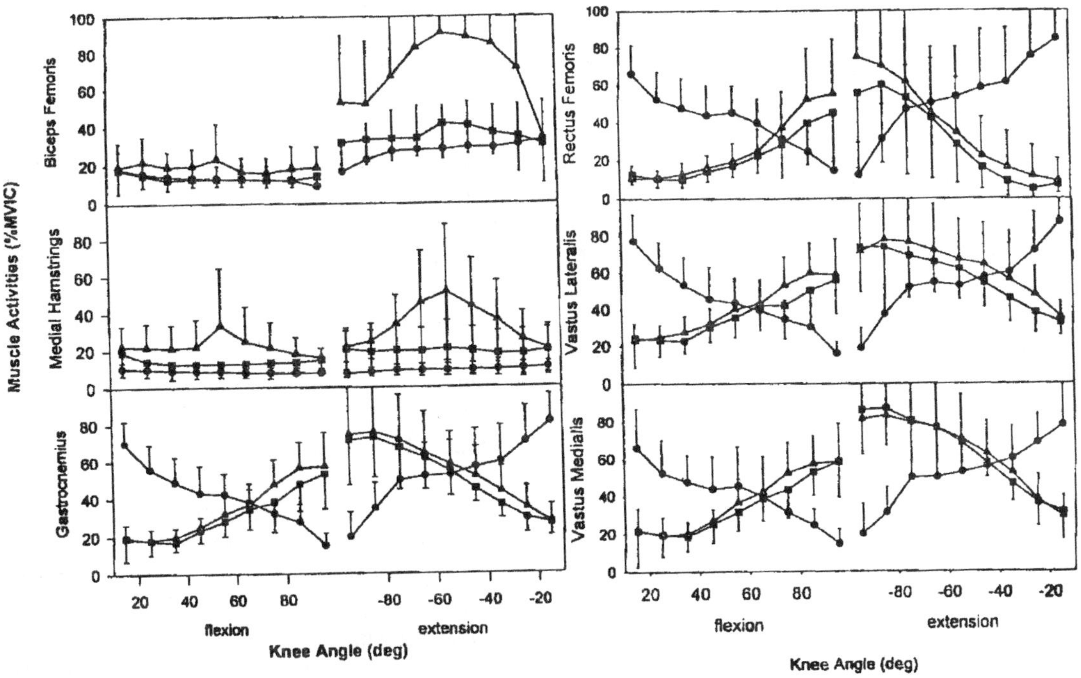

FIG. 39–3. Mean and standard deviation (n = 10) of quadriceps, hamstrings, and gastrocnemius muscle activity during the squat (*triangles*), leg press (*squares*), and leg extensions (*circles*). (From ref. 13, with permission.)

Similar results were observed in several other studies (6,48,56–58). Quadriceps activity remained fairly constant beyond 80- to 90-degree knee flexion, which has also been observed in other studies (6,48,52). Hence, descending beyond 90-degree knee flexion, which is near the parallel squat position, may not enhance quadriceps development.

Escamilla and colleagues (13) reported that the two vasti muscles produce ≈50% more activity than the rectus femoris, which is in agreement with squat data from Wretenberg and colleagues (48,52) and Isear and colleagues (56). The lower activity observed in the rectus femoris compared to the vasti muscles may be due to its biarticular function as both a hip flexor and knee extensor. Increased activity from the rectus femoris would increase hip flexor torque, with a concomitant increase in the amount of hip extensor torque needed from the hamstrings, gluteus maximus, and adductor magnus (ishial fibers) to extend the hip. The rectus femoris is probably more effective as a knee extensor during the squat when the trunk is more upright, since it is in a lengthened positioned compared to when the trunk is tilted forward in hip flexion. Compared to each other, the vastus medialis and lateralis produced approximately the same amount of activity, which is in agreement with data from Signorile and colleagues (58), who had 10 experienced lifters perform the squat with a 10-RM load.

Hamstring activity from Escamilla and colleagues (13) was highest during the squat ascent, with the biceps femoris showing greater overall activity than the medial hamstrings (see Fig. 39–3). Peak hamstring activity was 50% to 80% of a MVIC, and occurred near 50-degree knee flexion. In contrast, peak hamstring activity from Isear and colleagues (56), Ninos and colleagues (57), and Stuart and colleagues (6) were ≈12% MVIC, ≈15 MVIC, and ≈20% MVIC, respectively, with peak values occurring between 10- and 60-degree knee flexion. The lower hamstring activity in these studies is probably due to their subjects' lifting a lower percentage of their 1 RM. Isear and colleagues' subjects used no external lifting loads; Ninos and colleagues' subjects and Stuart and colleagues' subjects used lifting loads of 25% BW and 28% BW, respectively; and Escamilla and colleagues' subjects lifted 158% BW. Several studies have reported greater overall hamstring activity during the ascent compared to the descent (6,13,56,57). Since the hamstrings are biarticular muscles, it is difficult to delineate these muscles during the squat as performing eccentric work during the descent and concentric work during the ascent. They may actually be working near isometrically during both the squat descent and ascent, since they are concurrently shortening at the knee and lengthening at the hip during the descent, and lengthening at the knee and shortening at the hip during the ascent. If they are indeed working eccentrically during the descent and concentrically during the ascent, as is traditionally believed, then data from the above studies would be in accord with data from Komi and colleagues (60), who reported decreased activity during eccentric work and increased activity during concentric work. In any case, the hamstrings probably do not change length much throughout the squat. Hence, in accordance with the length-force relationship in skeletal muscle, a constant length in the hamstrings will allow them to be more effective in generating force throughout the entire squatting movement.

Three studies have reported gastrocnemius activity and force during the squat (12,13,56). Moderate gastrocnemius activity was observed during the squat, increasing with knee flexed and decreasing with knee extension (see Fig. 39–3). Escamilla and colleagues (13) and Isear and colleagues (56) reported peak gastrocnemius activity between 60- and 90-degree knee flexion. Since the ankle dorsiflexes during the descent and plantar flexes during the ascent, it is a common belief that the gastrocnemius contracts eccentrically during the descent to help control the rate of ankle dorsiflexion, and concentrically during the ascent to aid in ankle plantar flexion. Since the gastrocnemius is a biarticular muscle, however, its length may not change much throughout the squat; it shortens at the knee and lengthens at the ankle during the descent, and lengthens at the knee and shortens at the ankle during the ascent.

Three studies have investigated the effects of varying foot angles on quadriceps and hamstrings activity (14,57,59). Escamilla and colleagues (14) had 10 male experienced lifters perform the parallel squat with their 12 RM with their feet parallel with each other and with their feet turned outward 45 degrees. No significant differences were observed. Signorile and colleagues (59) had 10 male subjects perform the parallel squat with an 8- to 10-RM load using three different foot angles: (a) feet parallel with each other, (b) toes pointed outward as far as possible (≈80 degrees from parallel position), and (c) toes pointed inward ≈30 degrees from parallel position. They found no significant differences in vastus medialis, vastus lateralis, and rectus femoris activity among the three foot positions. Ninos and colleagues (57) had 25 male and female subjects perform the squat (0- to 60-degree knee flexion) with a 25% BW load using two different foot angles: (a) self-selected neutral position, and (b) foot turned outward 30 degrees from the neutral position. No significant differences were observed in quadriceps (vastus medialis and lateralis) or hamstrings (semimembranosus, semitendinosus, and biceps femoris) activity between the two foot angles. Hence, data from these studies show that varying foot angles do not appear to affect quadriceps or hamstrings activity during the squat.

Only one known study has investigated the effects of stance width (narrow stance vs. wide stance) during the squat (55). The wide stance produced 10% to 30% more medial and lateral hamstring activity than the narrow stance, while gastrocnemius activity was 10% to 15% greater in the narrow stance squat. There were generally no significant differences in quadriceps activity between the narrow and wide stance squats.

Knee Stability

Eight studies have examined how the dynamic squat affects knee stability (1,5,45,61–65). Klein (62) examined the effects that the "deep" squat exercise had on knee ligaments. The deep squat was defined as when the posterior thigh came in contact with the calf, which typically occurs between ≈130- and 150-degree knee flexion. This is typically how competitive weightlifters perform the squat, since this is what occurs during the "clean" portion of the clean and jerk exercise. This type of squatting is usually not recommended, however; rather, the parallel squat is advocated by most strength and conditioning specialists. Klein suggested that normal tibial internal rotation in knee flexion and tibial external rotation in knee extension changes during closed kinetic chain exercises such as the squat. Instead, the femur tends to rotate externally during knee flexion (i.e., the descent) and internally during knee extension (i.e., the ascent). As the femur externally rotates during the descent, the tibia also attempts to externally rotate. This observation is supported Costigan and Reid (66), who demonstrated that during the deep squat the tibia generated an external rotation torque against the ground during knee flexion and an internal rotation torque during knee extension. As the femur rotates externally during the descent, the menisci are forced to move posteriorly (especially the medial meniscus), causing the posterior portions of the menisci to be compressed between the tibial and femoral condyles. As the femur rotates internally at the beginning of the ascent, this forces the posterior medial meniscus toward the center of the joint space. This can place strain on the inner medial meniscus, causing it to tear. The medial meniscus also can tear due to a twisting strain applied to the medial collateral ligament (MCL), especially with severe internal rotation of the femur relative to the tibia. Since the MCL attaches to the medial meniscus, a twisting stain to the MCL may tear or detach the medial meniscus from its adjacent fibrous capsule. Part of this torn meniscus can become displaced toward the center of the joint space and become lodged between the femoral and tibial condyles. This can "lock" the knee in a flexed position, preventing full extension.

Using 64 cadaver cases, Klein (62) found that the MCL stretched a mean of ≈8% of its original length, while the lateral collateral ligament (LCL) stretched a mean of ≈13% of its original length. From these data he concluded that both the LCL and MCL are susceptible to injury and abnormal stretch during the deep squat. Klein also investigated the stress on the collateral and cruciate ligaments during the deep squat, comparing a deep squat group to a control group. The deep squat group was composed of 128 competitive weightlifters, all of whom practiced the deep squat exercise in training and competition. The control group was composed of 386 subjects from beginning weight training, basketball, and gymnastic classes from local universities. None of them had ever performed the deep squat. Comparing the results within the deep squat group, the LCL was stretched to a greater extent than the MCL, thus verifying the results from the cadaveric study. Furthermore, there was 19.4% more right LCL instability compared to right MCL instability, and 12% more left LCL instability compared to left MCL instability. Compared to the control group, the deep squat group showed (a) 61% greater instability in two of more ligaments of both legs; (b) 46% and 58%, respectively, greater MCL instability in the right and left legs; (c) 67% and 59%, respectively, greater LCL instability in the right and left legs; and (d) 16% and 25%, respectively, greater ACL instability in the right and left legs. Unfortunately, the PCL was not investigated in this study. Klein (62) hypothesized that the PCL could be abnormally stressed during the deep squat due to the "jacking apart" action that occurs within the joint due to the posterior thigh musculature coming in contact with the calf muscle at the bottom position of the squat. In effect, this changes the center of rotation from somewhere within the knee joint to the point of contact between the thigh and calf musculature. From these data, it was suggested that the parallel squat be used in place of the deep squat, since the greater ligamentous loading during the deep squat may have deleterious effects.

Meyers (63) reproduced the deep squat study by Klein (62), using the same mediolateral collateral ligament testing instrument to measure collateral ligament stability. Sixty-nine male subjects were randomly assigned to eight different treatment groups involving variations of the deep and parallel squat consisting of low and high lifting loads and speeds. All subjects trained on alternating days 3 days per week for 8 weeks. For each training session, each subject performed one set of 10 repetitions, for a total of 240 repetitions for the 8 weeks. All subjects were pretested 1 week prior to beginning their training program, and posttested 1 week following the end of training. No significant differences were found within any of the eight treatment groups in collateral ligament instability and knee joint flexibility, although the amount of stretch in the LCL decreased from the pretest to the posttest in both the deep squat and parallel squat. Contrary to Klein's results, these data imply that increased knee stability may occur following a squat training program, and that the squat is not detrimental to knee stability.

Henning and colleagues (1) measured ACL elongation using an *in vivo* instrumentation during a one-legged half squat between 20- and 90-degree knee flexion. Two subjects were used in this study, both with a grade II sprain of their ACL. ACL elongation was expressed relative to fiber elongation using a force of 357 N during a Lachman test. The one-legged squat produced 21% as much elongation as the Lachman test. In contrast, normal walking produced 36% as much elongation as the Lachman test, jogging 2.24 m/s on a level treadmill produced 63% as much elongation as the Lachman test, and partial knee extension exercises produced over 100% as much elongation as the Lachman test. Since the squat generated lower ACL strain compared to walking or jogging, it was concluded that the squat was a low-risk exercise in rehabilitation of the ACL. As previously discussed, Beynnon and colleagues (45) also reported minimal *in vivo* ACL strain during the squat at knee flexion angles less than 70 degrees.

Steiner and colleagues (65) used a commercial knee laxity testing device to measure anteroposterior knee laxity just before and after performing the squat, playing basketball, and running. Four groups of subjects (37 males and 18 females) with healthy knees were used; the groups were sedentary controls, squat powerlifters, basketball players, and distance runners. Nine sedentary controls were measured before and after a 2-hour time interval. Twenty-four athletes performed the powerlifting squat, lifting an average of 1.6 times BW for a mean of 24 repetitions. Ten basketball players were tested before and immediately after a strenuous 1.5-hour practice, and 12 distance runners were measured 30 minutes before and immediately after a sanctioned 10-km run. The percent changes between the pretest and posttest for anterior laxity, posterior laxity, and total anteroposterior laxity, respectively, were 1%, 4%, and 3% for the control group, 5%, −3%, and 2% for the powerlifters, 19%, 18%, and 19% for the basketball players, and 20%, 19%, and 19% for the distance runners. Significant increases in anteroposterior laxity were observed in the basketball players and distance runners (average increase of 0.5 mm in anterior laxity and 0.6 mm increase in posterior laxity), but not in the powerlifting and control groups. The powerlifters had the smallest percent change in total anteroposterior laxity, with a decrease in posterior laxity from pretest to posttest. Resting anteroposterior laxity among the groups was also recorded. Distance runners had significantly less anterior laxity than all other groups, while powerlifters had significantly less posterior laxity than all other groups. Since the greatest anteroposterior laxity was found in basketball players and distance runners, it was deduced that high compressive loads in the knee during the powerlifting squat might have facilitated the low anteroposterior laxities observed.

Chandler and colleagues (61) examined how the squat exercise affected knee stability. This study was composed of two parts: an 8-week squat training study, and a descriptive study of powerlifters and weightlifters. In part one, 100 males and females volunteered to be subjects. They were divided into three groups: (a) half-squat group, (b) parallel-squat group, and (c) control group. All subjects had no previous history of ligament or cartilage injuries. Twenty-seven powerlifters and 28 weightlifters composed two additional groups for part two of this study. The parallel-squat and half-squat groups were the only groups that performed a periodization weight training program. All subjects were tested for knee stability with a knee ligament arthrometer at 30- and 90-degree knee flexion. Measurements were taken at pre-, mid-, and posttraining intervals. Anterior drawer (69 to 88 N applied force), posterior drawer (88 N applied force), maximum manual drawer, and the quadriceps active drawer tests were used to quantify knee stability.

For part one of this study, the only significant difference across trials at 30-degree knee flexion was in posterior drawer. All groups tested demonstrated significantly greater posterior drawer knee displacement measurements in the posttest compared to the pretest. For 90-degree knee flexion, male subjects showed significantly less displacement in both the anterior and posterior drawer tests. For part two of this study comparing the lifting groups with a control group, the powerlifters and weightlifters showed tighter knees for the 90-degree quadriceps active drawer test. For the anterior drawer at 90 degrees, powerlifters showed tighter knees than the control group, while the weightlifting group showed no significant difference compared to powerlifters and controls. When groups were subdivided by skill, low-skilled weightlifters had significantly tighter knees than the controls for the quadriceps active drawer at 90-degree knee flexion. Since the significant differences seen were all less than 2 mm, perhaps the 8-week program two to three times per week was not long enough to elicit meaningful changes. This places more importance on the findings in part two, however. The weightlifters and powerlifters were all successful competitive lifters, and had been lifting heavy loads for many years. Interestingly, the control subjects, who had very little or no squatting experience, consistently had the loosest knees. Furthermore, powerlifters had tighter knees than the controls on seven of the nine measurements, while weightlifters were tighter than the controls for four of the nine measurements. The authors concluded that the squat did not have negative effects on knee stability, and may be considered safe in terms of not causing permanent stretching of the ligaments.

Shelbourne and Nitz (5) examined the effect of an accelerated rehabilitation program on ACL healing and strengthening after ACL reconstruction. Progress in ACL recovery was compared between 247 subjects in an accelerated program and 138 subjects in a nonaccelerated program. The nonaccelerated group had their leg splinted in slight flexion and were allowed to bear partial weight with crutches during the first 6 weeks. An agility program began after 7 to 8 months, while by 9 months a return to all activities with a knee brace was permitted. The accelerated subjects did not have their leg immobilized, and began continuous passive motion and weight-bearing exercise the day after surgery. The patient usually returned to light sports activities in 2 months, and full activity 4 to 6 months after reconstruction. Decreased postoperative anterior knee pain and an increased subjective feeling of knee stability were noted in the accelerated group. Mini-squats, leg press, step-ups, and other types of weight-bearing exercises were a big part of the accelerated program. The accelerated group achieved full knee extension and flexion quicker than the nonaccelerated group. The accelerated group also achieved higher quadriceps strength scores and less anteroposterior knee translations at all four testing sessions done during the first year after reconstruction. The authors surmised that the knee joint compression that occurred during the closed kinetic chain exercises used in the accelerated group provided inherent joint stability and minimized anteroposterior knee shear forces. They added that the closed kinetic chain exercises were also are more functional in terms of many athletic movements, such as running and jumping.

Panariello and colleagues (64) examined the effect of the squat exercise on anteroposterior knee translation in professional football players. Thirty-two subjects with normal knees participated in a 21-week off-season conditioning program involving the parallel squat. Two periodization training cycles were utilized during the 21 weeks. The first cycle was 12 weeks in duration, immediately followed by a 9-week cycle. The squat was performed twice a week, with subjects performing an average of 32 repetitions per session, and lifting an average of 130% to 200% BW. A knee ligament arthrometer (KT-1000) was used to measure anteroposterior knee stability. Subjects were tested prior to the start of the training program, at the end of the 12-week cycle, and at the end of the 9-week cycle. Of the 2440 individual tests conducted, only eight pairs of tests showed increased excursions of greater than 2 mm. There were no significant differences between any pair of pre- and postexercise measurements, and no significant differences in anteroposterior knee translations in athletes using the squat as part of their training regimen. Hence, it was deduced that the squat is a safe exercise to include in an athlete's training program.

Conclusion

This section examined select biomechanical variables during the dynamic squat. Low to moderate posterior shear force is generated throughout the squat, restrained primarily by the PCL. In addition, low anterior shear force may occur between 0- and 60-degree knee flexion, restrained primarily by the ACL. Hence, the squat is an effective exercise to employ after an ACL injury or reconstruction, and it can also be used with light loads after PCL injury or reconstruction. Moderate to high tibiofemoral and patellofemoral compressive forces are produced during the squat. Tibiofemoral compressive force helps resists anteroposterior shear forces and translation. Excessive patellofemoral compressive force can lead to patellofemoral pathologies, such as chondromalacia or osteoarthritis. Patellofemoral and tibiofemoral compressive forces and shear forces all increased as knee flexion increased, reaching peak values near maximum knee flexion. Hence, training the squat in the functional range between 0- and 50-degree knee flexion may be appropriate for many knee rehabilitation patients. For athletes with healthy knees, performing the parallel squat is recommended over the deep squat, since injury potential to the menisci and cruciate and collateral ligaments may increase with the deep squat. The squat does not compromise knee stability and may enhance stability if performed correctly. Finally, the squat can be effective in developing hip, knee, and ankle musculature, since moderate to high quadriceps, hamstrings, and gastrocnemius activity is produced during the squat. Muscle activity generally increased as knee flexion increased, which supports athletes' performing the parallel squat over the half squat. Since the hip, knee, and ankle extensors are among the strongest and most powerful muscles in the body, and important in functional activities such as running and jumping, the squat is an excellent choice for strength and power athletes.

BIOMECHANICS OF THE DEADLIFT

Like the squat, the deadlift is one of the three exercises that compose the sport of powerlifting. Football players and other strength athletes also use the deadlift in their training regimen. The deadlift, which is an excellent total body exercise, primarily develops the hips, thighs, and back. Compared to the squat, lower back musculature is involved to a greater extent. The deadlift is similar to the squat in that the lifter squats down and then returns to an upright position. In the deadlift, however, the lifter squats down to grip a bar that is ≈22 cm above the ground in front of the lifter's feet. An alternating grip is usually employed, with one hand gripping under the bar (supinated) and the other hand gripping over the bar (pronated). From this starting position, the lifter then stands to an upright position (arms remain straight throughout movement) with the knees and hips fully extended and the shoulders pulled back. Hence, unlike the squat, the deadlift has only an ascent phase, since the deadlift descent is simply to grip the bar and establish a starting position and to lower the weight at the completion of the lift.

Two techniques are employed to perform the deadlift—sumo and conventional. The primary differences between these two styles are that the feet are further apart in the sumo style, and the hands grip the bar inside the thighs during the sumo deadlift and outside the thighs during the conventional deadlift. The inside heel to inside heel distance is approximately three times greater in the sumo style (≈80 to 100 cm) compared to the conventional style (≈25 to 35 cm). In both styles, the grip width is similar (inside hand to inside hand distance of ≈30 to 40 cm), although the sumo grip is typically slightly less wide than the conventional grip. The feet are typically parallel with each other during the conventional deadlift, and they are turned outward ≈30 to 45 degrees during the sumo deadlift.

The conventional deadlift is used by the majority of powerlifters (≈65% to 75%), especially among lifters in the heavier weight classes. For example, from observational data from the 1991 American Drug Free Powerlifting Association National Masters Powerlifting Championships (Daytona Beach, FL), 45% of the male lifters (n = 56) in the lighter weight classes (52 to 82 kg) used the sumo style, while only 15% of the male lifters (n = 54) in the heavier weight classes (90 to 125+ kg) employed the sumo style. Compared to male lifters, there appears to be more female lifters who employ the sumo style deadlift.

Although more than 100 studies have quantified biomechanical variables during lifting activities (e.g., 67–72), only seven studies have examined biomechanical variables during the barbell deadlift (73–79). Brown and Abani (73) performed the first biomechanical examination of the deadlift during actual powerlifting competition. Twenty-one adolescent lifters were analyzed (two-dimensional) while lifting maximum or near maximum loads during the 1981 Michigan Teenage Powerlifting Championships. These lifters were then subdivided into a skilled group (best lifters in each BW class) and an unskilled group (worst lifters in each BW class). A kinematic comparison between skilled and unskilled groups is shown in Table 39–2. Trunk, thigh, and shank angles were defined relative to the right horizontal measured at the hip, knee, and ankle, respectively, from a sagittal view of a lifter's right side. Hip and knee angles were relative angles between the trunk and thigh and between

TABLE 39–2. *Kinematic, temporal, and antropometric comparisons between sumo and conventional deadlifts*

	Sumo (M ± SD): McGuigan and Wilson (76)	Conventional (M ± SD)		
		McGuigan and Wilson (76)	Brown and Abani (73)	
			Skilled	Unskilled
	(n = 10)	(n = 19)	(n = 10)	(n = 11)
Liftoff				
Hip (°)	77 ± 9**	67 ± 5**	69 ± 5*	64 ± 5*
Knee (°)	127 ± 8	120 ± 10	123 ± 6*	111 ± 8*
Trunk (°)	25 ± 8*	17 ± 7*	23 ± 6	25 ± 10
Thigh (°)	136 ± 6	137 ± 5	134 ± 4*	141 ± 8*
Shank (°)	63 ± 11	59 ± 5	76 ± 3*	72 ± 4*
Knee passing				
Hip (°)	130	122	134 ± 18	132 ± 10
Knee (°)	168	165	165 ± 6	167 ± 4
Trunk (°)	48	43	59 ± 14	55 ± 8
Thigh (°)	106	107	105 ± 4	103 ± 2
Shank (°)	70	63	90 ± 3	91 ±2
Liftoff to knee: passing range				
Hip (°)	51 ± 9	56 ± 11	65 ± 14	68 ± 9
Knee (°)	41 ± 11	45 ± 10	42 ± 7*	57 ± 10*
Trunk (°)	23 ± 5	26 ± 12	37 ± 13	29 ± 9
Thigh (°)	29 ± 8	29 ± 5	28 ± 5*	38 ± 9*
Shank (°)	7 ± 3*	4 ± 3*	14 ± 4*	19 ± 4*
Maximum load lifted (kg)	218.0 ± 32.1	215.0 ± 33.2	230.3 ± 32.1+	168.5 ± 18.9+
Body mass (kg)	83.3 ± 15.6	84.8 ± 15.8	79.1 ± 18.4+	85.3 ± 20.9+
Age (y)			17.9 ± 1.1+	16.3 ± 0.73+
Total lift time (s)	2.1 ± 1.1	1.9 ± 0.3		
Time from liftoff to knee passing (s)	1.71 ± 0.49*	1.34 ± 0.20*		
Distance to lockout (% of height)	26.8 ± 4.2**	32.9 ± 2.3**		
Sticking region (% lift time)	45.6 ± 15.1	37.8 ± 18.2		

+Not statistically analyzed.
*$p < .05$; **$p < .01$.

the thigh and shank, respectively. At liftoff (when barbell disks first left the ground), the skilled subjects had greater hip and knee angles (i.e., less hip and knee flexion), and they maintained their thigh and shank in a more vertical position. From liftoff to knee passing (when bar passed the knee joint center), the unskilled subjects extended their knees at a greater rate and over a larger range.

At liftoff, mean hip, knee, and ankle extensor torques were 437 N·m, 44.0 N·m, and 190 N·m, respectively, for the skilled group, and 335 N·m, 4.7 N·m, and 166 N·m, respectively, for the unskilled group. At knee passing, mean hip, knee, and ankle extensor torques were 306 N·m, 157 N·m, and 168 N·m, respectively, for the skilled group, and 204 N·m, 111 N·m, and 118 N·m, respectively, for the unskilled group. Although spinal (trunk) extensor torques were not quantified, data from a similar study (75), whose subjects lifted a mean load of 186 kg, found spinal extensor torques near liftoff to range between 300 and 400 N·m. These values are similar to the hip extensor torques generated in this study. The larger hip extensor torques compared to knee and ankle extensor torques were due to greater hip moment arms (perpendicular distance from hip joint to line of action of bar) compared to knee and ankle moment arms. At liftoff, mean hip, knee, and ankle moment arms were 34.1 cm, 5.8 cm, and 15.7 cm, respectively, for the skilled group; they were 34.1 cm, 4.3 cm, and 17.2 cm, respectively, for the unskilled group. At knee passing, mean hip, knee, and ankle moment arms were 24.5 cm, 14.3 cm, and 14.5 cm, respectively, for the skilled group, and 22.6 cm, 12.7 cm, 12.5 cm, respectively, for the unskilled group. From these data, it can be deduced that the hip extensors (gluteus maximus, hamstrings, adductor magnus) and spinal extensors (e.g., erector spinae) are heavily involved during the deadlift to overcome relatively large hip and spinal flexor torques, which are primarily due to the barbell load and hip and spinal moment arms. The very small knee extensor torque generated at liftoff is due to the small knee moment arm at liftoff. A similar amount of knee and ankle extensor torques at knee passing were generated since knee and ankle moment arms were approximately the same.

McGuigan and Wilson (76) performed a kinematic analysis that was similar to that of Brown and Abani (73), except that they compared the sumo deadlift to the conventional deadlift during two 1992 regional New Zealand powerlifting championships (see Table 39–2). The only significant differences observed were that the sumo group had a more upright trunk and less hip flexion at liftoff, and the shank range from liftoff to knee passing was greater in the sumo group. One limitation of this study is that it was a two-dimensional analysis. This is fine for the conventional deadlift, but motion occurs in three dimensions during the sumo deadlift. Hence, to more accurately compare sumo and conventional deadlift kinematics, a follow-up study should be performed using a three-dimensional analytical model.

Granhed and colleagues (79) calculated L3 compressive loads and bone mineral content (BMC) in eight Swedish powerlifters, who were filmed while performing the deadlift (≈285 kg mean load) at the 1983 Powerlifting World Championships (Göteborg, Sweden). Mathematical models were utilized to calculate lumbar compressive loads (80,81), while BMC was quantified with dual-photon absorptiometry. Although not stated directly, it was implied that all lifters performed the conventional-style deadlift. Peak compressive loads on L3 ranged from 18,800 to 36,400 N, which is two to three times greater than the ultimate compressive strength of the lumbar spine, which has been reported *in vitro* to have a maximum value less than 11,000 N (82). These peak compressive loads occurred just after liftoff, when the barbell disks were less than 30 cm above the ground. Since all lifters wore a weight belt, the increase in intraabdominal pressure (IAP) due to the weight belt may help unload the spine and decrease spinal compressive loads. In fact, Harman and colleagues (78) have demonstrated that while subjects lifted a 90% 1-RM load during the deadlift, peak IAP was 12.5% greater when they wore a weight belt compared to when they did not. Abdominal muscle contractions have also been shown to increase IAP (83), and they may also help decrease compressive loads. In addition, forced expiration against a closed glottis during lifting increases intrathoracic pressure (ITP), which may also help unload the spine stabilize the trunk. The role and effects of weight belts and IAP/ITP during lifting will be discussed in greater detail in the final section of this chapter.

The L3 moment arm (perpendicular distance from L3 to line of action of the bar) is the most important factor in affecting L3 compressive loads. The authors noted that two of the lifters who lifted the same weight had a 10,000 N difference in L3 compressive loads. This occurred because one lifter had a 29.1-cm moment arm, and the other lifter had a 45.0-cm moment arm. Keeping the weight as close to the body as possible minimizes the moment arm and compressive load, while moving the bar away from the body increases the moment arm and compressive load.

A direct relationship has been demonstrated between BMC and the ultimate compressive strength of the lumbar spine (82). Compared to 39 control subjects who were age and weight matched with the powerlifters, the powerlifting group had 36% greater BMC. BMC has been reported to be greater among active individuals, especially strength athletes, who are typically involved in weight training (84–87). The lifters in this study had extremely high BMC, and it was highly correlated (r^2 = 0.82) to the amount of weight lifted during their annual training regimen. The lifter's annual total weight lifted in training ranged from 300 to 5000 tons. The authors concluded that strenuous weight training over time would increase BMC to an extent that the spine will be able to tolerate extraordinary loads.

Cholewicki and colleagues (74) examined the relationship between lifting style (sumo vs. conventional) and spinal load (L4/L5 torque, L4/L5 disc shear and compression) using a two-dimensional analysis of the subjects' lifting extremely heavy weights. Since L4/L5 torques have been shown to be greatest near the beginning of a lifting activity (69), this analysis was performed just after liftoff when the barbell disks were 5 cm off the ground. Male and female sumo ($n = 21$) and conventional ($n = 36$) lifters were filmed during the 1989 Canadian Powerlifting National Championships. Mean loads lifted were 205.5 kg for the sumo group and 208.5 kg for the conventional group. The conventional group had significantly greater L4/L5 torque (626 N·m vs. 566 N·m) and L4/L5 load shear (2602 N vs. 2397 N). L4/L5 disc compression and shear were 10,405 N and 1530 N, respectively, for the sumo group, and 10,738 N and 1643 N, respectively, for the conventional group. The 11% greater L4/L5 torque generated by the conventional deadlift group implies that injury risks to the L4/L5 area may be greater with the conventional style.

The final deadlift study was performed by Cholewicki and McGill (75), who examined lumbar ligament (interspinous, supraspinous, capsular, ligamentum flavum, intertransverse, and posterior and anterior longitudinal) and disc contributions in subjects' resisting trunk flexion torques while lifting extremely heavy weights. Four Canadian national-caliber powerlifters performed two trials each of the conventional style deadlift (186 kg mean load) while a lateral radiologic view of their lumbar spine was recorded with a videofluoroscope. Each subject was also recorded in full lumbar flexion using BW only. Mean lumbar flexion just after liftoff was 4.6 degrees less than the mean value obtained from the full lumbar flexion trials, with only one of the eight lifting trials slightly exceeding full lumbar flexion. Interestingly, for the trial in which full lumbar flexion was slightly exceeded, the subject complained of mild low back discomfort during the lift. This suggests that lower back injury risk during lifting may be greatest near full lumbar flexion, especially when lifting extremely heavy loads. Resultant ligament lengths (measured indirectly) at the beginning of the lift ranged from 56.1% to 99.8% of their lengths during full lumbar flexion, which supports the findings that full lumbar flexion was not achieved during the lifting trials. The interspinous and supraspinous ligaments underwent the greatest elongation. The interspinous ligament has been shown to provide 95% of the ligamentous contribution in resisting lumbar flexion (88).

There were no measurable shearing or compressive translations of the vertebral discs during any of the trials. Since the angular range of motion of the intervertebral joints was considerably smaller in the lifting trials compared to the full lumbar flexion trials, the authors concluded that the spinal column remained moderately flexed and fairly rigid throughout the motion, except near the end of the lift. This implies that most of the lifting motion occurred at the hips and knees. Compared to a fully flexed and nonrigid lumbar spine, the moderately flexed and rigid lumbar spine may be an advantageous lifting position, since the lumbar spine is stronger under compressive loads when it is moderately flexed (89). These spinal compressive loads can exceed 10,000 N (over 10 times BW) during extremely heavy lifting (74). In fact, it has been shown that the osteoligamentous spine is unstable with compressive loads less than BW (90,91). The rigid and moderately flexed spine is especially important during the beginning of the lift, where lumbar spinal loads are maximum. Since the line of action of the erector spinae is primarily in the compressive direction of the spine, strong contractions from these muscles help stabilize and maintain spinal rigidity, and they are primarily responsible for the large spinal compressive forces that are generated (unfortunately, these large compressive forces may have deleterious effects on the spinal disc). Furthermore, in accordance with the length-force relationship of muscle tissue, the erector spinae is more effective in generating force when the lumbar spine is partially flexed and rigid throughout its motion. This is because a partially flexed spine lengthens the erector spinae, causing a more optimal interdigitization between the myosin cross-bridges and actin myofilaments. Also, in accordance with the force-velocity relationship of muscle, an isometric contraction of the erector spinae (needed to maintain spinal rigidity) is more effective in generating force than a concentric contraction, which occurs more at the end of the lift (when spinal loads are less) to extend the spine.

Although other studies have shown that the lumbar spine has a safety margin in forward bending (92,93), achieving full lumbar flexion with extremely heavy loads increases lumbar injury risk. However, the most important finding from this study is that the lumbar ligaments "did not strain sufficiently to significantly resist the extremely heavy loads placed on the lumbar spine, suggesting that it is not their primary role to assist the musculature but, more likely, to limit the range of motion" (75). While studies have shown that the osteoligamentous spine provides ≈50% of the spinal extensor torque needed to help resist spinal flexor torque due to gravity during full lumbar flexion (93,94), the powerlifters used by Cholewicki and McGill (75) fell short of full lumbar flexion by several degrees. Since studies have shown that only a few degrees of extension from the fully flexed lumbar position can cause a dramatic decrease in tension in the lumbar ligamentous structures (88,95), lower back muscle strength appears to be of paramount importance during lifting. Therefore, it is very important to have strong spinal extensors (e.g., erector spinae), since these muscles are largely responsible for generating the spinal extensor torques needed to extend the spine. Increased IAP and ITP can also help resist spinal extensor torques, and thus unload the spine. As previously mentioned, IAP can be increased by wearing a weight belt and by having strong abdominal musculature.

In conclusion, there is a sparcity of data in the literature concerning the barbell deadlift, especially during the sumo style. Furthermore, since the two studies that analyzed the sumo deadlift used a two-dimensional model, a three-dimensional analysis is needed to corroborate these data, since motion during the sumo style clearly occurs in three dimensions. Moreover, no known deadlift studies have examined knee biomechanics or muscle activity. Hence, research needs to be initiated in these areas. Finally, the importance of having strong trunk musculature is paramount in minimizing injury risks during lifting.

BIOMECHANICS OF THE BENCH PRESS

Strength and power athletes commonly perform the bench press to develop strength and size in chest, shoulder, and triceps musculature. The type of equipment used (e.g., machines vs. free weights) and the lifting techniques and methods employed can affect muscle development, force production, and performance (96–100). The bench press starts in a supine position on a flat bench while holding a barbell (grip is typically slightly wider than shoulder width) above the shoulders with straight arms. From this position, the bar is slowly brought down to the chest (a few centimeters superior to the xiphoid process), and then returned back to the starting position. Although the rules of powerlifting requires the bar to pause momentarily at the chest (≈0.5 to 1.0 s) before pressing the bar upward, most strength athletes not competing in powerlifting train the bench press with a smooth but continuous stretch-shortening transition between lowering and raising the bar. Not only is a rapid stretch-shortening transition more sports specific, but studies have shown that more elastic strain energy can be utilized and transferred from the eccentric descent phase to the concentric ascent phase (101–103).

Bouncing the bar off the chest and "bridging" (i.e., arching the back with the buttocks coming off the bench) are common occurrences among athletes. However, since these bouncing and bridging techniques increase injury risk to the sternum, ribs, and lower back, they should be avoided. Although injuries to the ribs (104) and shoulders (105) have been reported during the bench press, the most common injury reported in the literature involves a rupture of the pectoralis major muscle (106–109) while using heavy weights (85% to 100% of 1 RM). These injuries often occur near the bottom of the descent when the pectoralis major is contracting eccentrically and being stretched. The combination of high muscle tension and excessive muscle lengthening causes the rupture to occur at the muscle's insertion into the humerus.

Although numerous studies have quantified biomechanical variables during the bench press (77,96–102,110–114), Madsen and McLaughlin (110,111) were the first researchers to examine bench press kinematics and kinetics. Comparing 17 recreational weightlifters (novice group) to 19 national- and world-caliber powerlifters (expert group), several differences were observed between these two groups: (a) the expert group lowered the bar more slowly; (b) the expert group used a bar path that was closer to the shoulder and followed a different path between lowering and raising the bar (Fig. 39–4); and (c) although the expert group lifted 79% more weight, the peak normalized force the expert group exerted on the bar was only 43% greater during

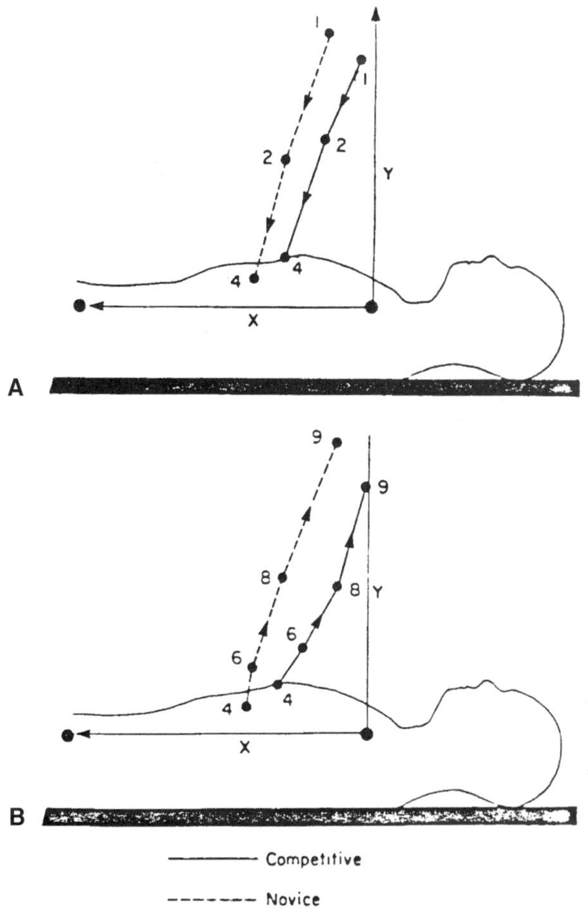

FIG. 39–4. **A:** Comparative bar paths: lowering the bar. *1,* start; *2,* peak bar velocity during descent; *4,* bar at chest. **B:** Comparative bar paths: raising the bar. *4,* bar at chest; *6,* peak bar velocity during ascent; *8,* minimum bar velocity during ascent. (From ref. 110, with permission.)

the downward phase and 45% greater during the upward phase. In addition, the forces exerted on the bar throughout the downward and upward phases were more uniform in the expert group.

To help evaluate injury potential during the bench press, it is important to understand the relationship between vertical bar velocity, acceleration, and force. First, bar direction can be determined by observing whether the velocity is positive or negative. Negative velocities were arbitrarily chosen to represent the descent (between events 1 and 4), while positive velocities were chosen to represent the ascent (between events 4 to 9) (Fig. 39–5). Accelerations are more difficult to interpret, since unlike velocity, a negative or positive acceleration does not provide any information regarding whether the bar is moving up or down. A negative acceleration implies that the bar is speeding up during the descent or slowing down during the ascent. Conversely, a positive acceleration implies that the bar is slowing down during the descent or speeding up during the ascent.

Now we will examine the relationship between velocity and acceleration using typical values that are generated from expert lifters (see Fig. 39–5). Note that the slope (i.e., line tangent to the curve) at any given point on the velocity-time curve is the acceleration value at that corresponding time on the acceleration-time curve. For example, consider events 2, 6, and 8 on the velocity-time curve, whose slopes are clearly zero (a horizontal line). Notice that the corresponding acceleration values at events 2, 6, and 8 are also zero. In addition, note that the slopes of the velocity-time curve are negative between events 1 to 2 and 6 to 8, which correspond to negative acceleration values on the acceleration-time curve between these same events. Similarly, the slopes of the velocity-time curve are positive between events 2 and 6, which correspond to positive acceleration values on the acceleration-time curve between events 2 and 6.

Next we will examine the relationship between acceleration and force. Newton's second law of motion states that the acceleration (a) of the barbell is directly proportional to net force (ΣF) acting on the barbell: $\Sigma F = ma$, where m is the mass of the barbell. Hence, the shape of the force-time curve will be the same as the shape of the acceleration-time curve shown in Fig. 39–5. Two forces compose the net force acting on the barbell; first, the downward (arbitrarily chosen as negative) force due to gravity (g), which is commonly known as the barbell weight (w), and second, the upward (positive) force (F) exerted by the hands. Therefore, $\Sigma F = ma \rightarrow F - w =$

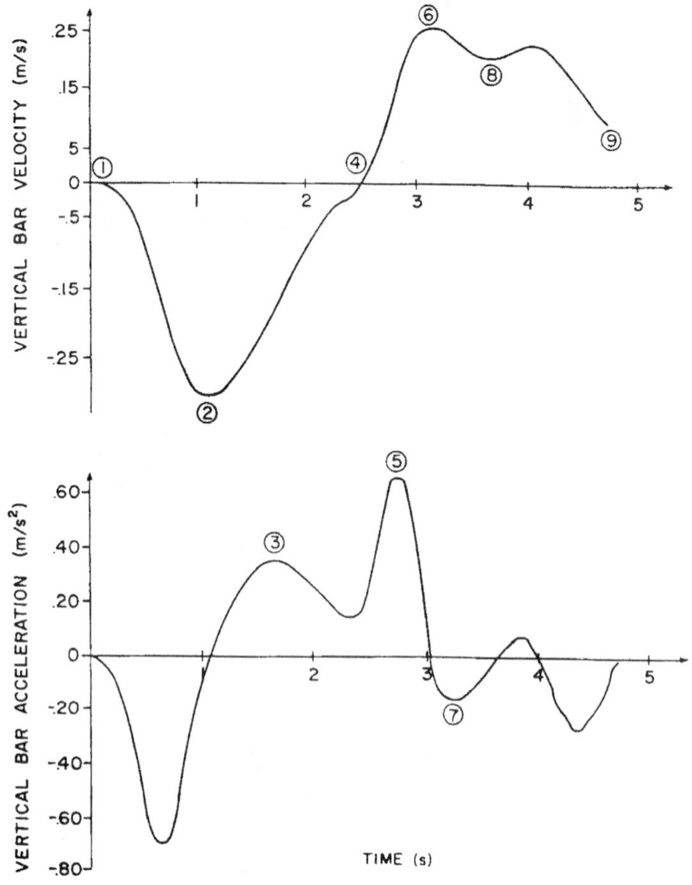

FIG. 39–5. Typical vertical bar movement with identification of instants used in quantifying bench press: *1,* start; *2,* peak bar velocity during descent; *3,* peak bar acceleration during descent; *4,* bar at chest; *5,* peak bar acceleration during ascent; *6,* peak bar velocity during ascent; *7,* first minimum bar acceleration during ascent; *8,* first minimum bar velocity during ascent; *9,* end. (From ref. 110, with permission.)

$ma \rightarrow F = w + ma$. From this equation, notice that when there is no acceleration ($a = 0$), then $F = w$. Similarly, when $a < 0$, $F < w$, and when $a > 0$, $F > w$. This implies the following: (a) the force that the hands exert against the bar is equal to the barbell weight when bar acceleration is zero (i.e., at the start and end of the lift); (b) the force that the hands exert on the bar is less than the barbell weight when bar acceleration is negative (i.e., when the bar speeds up during the descent or slows down during the ascent); and (c) the force that the hands exert on the bar is greater than the barbell weight when bar acceleration is positive (i.e., when the bar slows down during the descent or speeds up during the ascent). The relationship between acceleration and force presented for the bench press can also be applied to the squat, which has the same descent and ascent phases. The only difference is that the bar force is applied by the upper back during the squat instead of by the hands.

Now consider a lifter performing a bench press with a 1500 N (≈340 lbs) load. Since $m = w/g$ and $g = 9.81$ $m \cdot s^{-2}$, $m = 1500$ N/9.81 $m \cdot s^{-2} = 152.9$ kg. Since the bar is not moving at the start of the lift (event 1 in Fig. 39–5), $a = 0 \rightarrow F = w = 1500$ N. By Newton's third law of motion, this 1500 N force exerted on the bar by the hands is equal in magnitude but opposite in direction to the force exerted on the hands by the bar. This force applied by the bar on the hands is transmitted down to the elbows and shoulders. From the starting position, the bar progressively increases in speed until event 2 is reached. Notice that the slope of the velocity-time curve is greatest at a point approximately halfway between events 1 and 2, which means acceleration will also be greatest at this point (≈−0.70 $m \cdot s^{-2}$ from the graph). Hence, the force that the bar exerts against the hands is $F = 1500$ N + (152.9 kg) (−0.70 $m \cdot s^{-2}$) = 1393 N, or 7.1% less force than the 1500 N weight of the barbell. Since the bar continuously speeds up (i.e., accelerates downward) between events 1 and 2, forces applied to the hands by the bar will be less than the barbell weight. The greater the barbell initially accelerates downward, the smaller the forces applied to the hands. Greater upward accelerations and forces are needed to slow down the rapid moving bar as it approaches the chest, however. This is the primary reason why the barbell should be lowered in a slow and controlled manner.

Between events 2 and 4, the barbell is still being lowered, but it is slowing down with a peak upward acceleration (event 3) of ≈0.35 $m \cdot s^{-2}$. (Note: the acceleration is directed upward, not downward, in order to slow the downward moving bar.) Hence, $F = 1500$ N + (152.9 kg) (0.35 $m \cdot s^{-2}$) = 1554 N, or 3.6% greater force than the barbell weight. The bar will now begin moving up between events 4 and 9. The bar accelerates upward between events 4 to 6, with a peak acceleration (event 5) of ≈0.65 ms^2. Hence, $F = 1500$ N + (152.9 kg) (0.65 $m \cdot s^{-2}$) = 1599 N, or 6.6% greater force than the barbell weight. The upward moving bar slows down between events 6 and 8, with a peak downward acceleration (event 7) of ≈−0.15 $m \cdot s^{-2}$. Hence, $F = 1500$ N + (152.9 kg) (−0.15 $m \cdot s^{-2}$) = 1477 N, or 1.5% less force than the barbell weight. Since the region between events 6 and 8 produces minimum bar force, it has been defined by Lander and colleagues (98) as the "sticking region" and is the most difficult portion of the lift. The sticking region, which occurs when the bar is between ≈30% and 50% of its vertical ascent displacement, is thought to be due to muscles being in poor mechanical force–producing positions (e.g., force-length relationship), and decreased utilization of stored elastic strain energy (largely from eccentric muscle contractions at the end of the descent) in myosin cross-bridges and tendons (97). From this example, it is clear that the greatest forces generated during the bench press occurred at event 3, which are needed to slow down the weight during the descent, and at event 5, which are needed to upwardly accelerate the weight during the ascent. Using these velocity and acceleration data from Fig. 39–5, peak forces applied to the hands by the bar are only ≈5% to 10% greater than the barbell weight. However, bench press peak vertical force data from novice and less skilled lifters have been reported to be 30% to 60% greater than the barbell weight (115).

Since forces exerted by the bar on the hands are transmitted to the elbow and shoulder, lowering and raising the weight in a slow and controlled manner is important in minimizing shoulder and elbow stress. To further illustrate this point, consider a former world-champion powerlifter who ruptured his pectoralis major while performing the bench press in the 1978 Senior National Powerlifting Championships. While bench pressing 2332 N (523 lbs), the injury occurred ≈0.8 s into the descent just prior to the bar reaching the chest. A peak upward-directed bar acceleration of ≈9 $m \cdot s^{-2}$ was quantified by McLaughlin (115) just prior to the injury. Hence, the force (F) applied by the bar to the hands at the instant of this peak acceleration is calculated using $F = w + ma$: $m = w/g = 2332$ N/9.81 $m \cdot s^{-2}$ = 227.5 kg. Hence, $F = w + ma = 2332$ N + (227.5 kg) (9 $m \cdot s^{-2}$) = 4380 N (≈1000 lbs), which is almost twice the barbell weight! It is not difficult to understand why this lifter was injured. Interestingly, this same lifter competed 1 year later in the 1979 Senior National Powerlifting Championships. Lifting almost the same barbell weight (2359 N, or 529 lbs), a peak upward bar acceleration of ≈1.2 $m \cdot s^{-2}$ occurred at ≈1.3 s into the descent, which implies that he lowered the weight much more slowly compared to when he was injured. In fact, using the above equations to calculate the force at the instant of this peak acceleration yields ≈2648 N (593 lbs), or ≈12% greater force than the barbell weight.

BIOMECHANICS OF WEIGHTLIFTING EXERCISES

A form of weightlifting was included in the 1896 Olympic Games, but it was not until 1932 that the sport matured into a consistent three-lift format. In 1972 the sport was economized by eliminating the clean and press lift, so that only the snatch and clean and jerk lifts remained part of regular competitions. The sport of weightlifting, often referred to as Olympic weightlifting due to its inclusion in the Olympic Games, continues to this day to include only these two lifts. In competition, each athlete is permitted three attempts at each of the two lifts. The athlete with the highest total lift, a combination of his or her best successful snatch and clean and jerk lift, is the winner in each BW division. Currently there are eight men's and seven women's BW divisions. World records in the snatch lift average about 2.1 times BW for men and 1.6 times BW for women. In the clean and jerk, these factors increase to about 2.6 for men and 2.0 for women. Athletes in the heavier divisions lift less relative to BW than those in the lighter divisions.

Descriptions of the Snatch and Clean and Jerk Lifts

The snatch must be executed by lifting a barbell from the floor to straight arm's length overhead in one continuous motion. To minimize the height to which the barbell must be elevated, a wide hand spacing is used and the bar is caught at arm's length overhead in a deep squat position (Fig. 39–6). Use of this common "squat snatch" technique requires considerable flexibility in the shoulder and lower extremity joints.

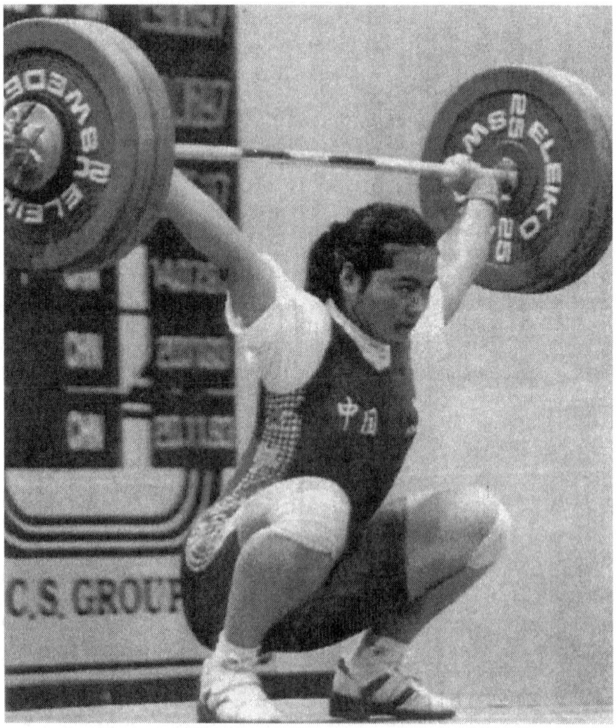

FIG. 39–6. Catch position for the squat snatch lift. Photo by Klemen/Reno.

The clean phase of the clean and jerk lift is similar to the snatch but is executed with a narrower hand grip spacing, with the bar caught at shoulder level resting on the clavicles, deltoids, and hands rather than the overhead position. As in the snatch lift, the height to which the barbell must be lifted is minimized by catching the bar in a deep squat position (Fig. 39–7*E*). After a successful squat clean, the athlete must rise and stand erect with the bar held at shoulder level. A shallow "dip" via knee and hip flexion then occurs, followed immediately by a rapid and forceful upward thrust from knee and hip extension and ankle plantar flexion to propel the barbell overhead, where it must be caught with straight arms. The height to which the barbell must be thrust overhead is reduced by athletes, in most cases, by splitting their feet forward and backward when catching the bar overhead before standing erect to complete the lift (Fig. 39–8). Some athletes catch the barbell overhead by executing a partial or full squatting motion rather than using the split movement. This less commonly used technique requires great shoulder flexibility.

Biomechanical and Injury Considerations for Weightlifting

The biomechanical characteristics of performing the above lifting movements help to explain why these and related exercises are frequently used in training by athletes from other sports that require fast and forceful muscle exertions, as well as to indicate when injury potential during each lift is greatest.

The pulling motion used to lift the barbell from the floor, and to accelerate it upward, is very similar for both the snatch and clean lifts. The main difference is that during the snatch pull a wider hand grip spacing is used, causing the athlete's hips to be lower and or the torso to be inclined more forward at the start of the pull compared to the clean. Fig. 39–7 illustrates the sequence of key positions that occur during the complete "pulling" phase for a clean. At the start or "lift off" (Fig. 39–7*A*) the arms and back are straight, while considerable flexion exists at the hip and knee joints. During the initial movement or "first pull," the barbell is lifted from the floor to knee height (Fig. 39–7*A,B*) by hip and knee extension and slight ankle plantar flexion while the back and arms remain straight. A very high level of isometric tension is required in the extensor muscles of the spine during the first pull to maintain a straight torso posture while it is inclined forward due to the long lever arm lengths from the bar and upper body center of mass to the lumbar joint centers. The term *straight back* is used to indicate maintenance of the

FIG. 39–7. Squat clean technique. **A:** Lift-off, start of first pull. **B:** End of first pull. **C:** Near finish of transition and start of second pull. **D:** End of second pull. **E:** Catch position. Photo by Klemens/Reno.

normal spinal curvatures during the entire pull, although some athletes maintain a slightly hyperextended lumbar spine.

As the bar rises above knee level the first pull ends and a transitional movement occurs in preparation for the second pull. This transition (Fig. 39–7*B,C*) is often referred to as the second knee bend, since as the athlete's hips move forward toward the bar as it slides upward along the thighs, and the torso rotates to a more vertical position, the knees rebend (flex) slightly and move under the bar. This maneuver is responsible for a complete pull of this type being called the double

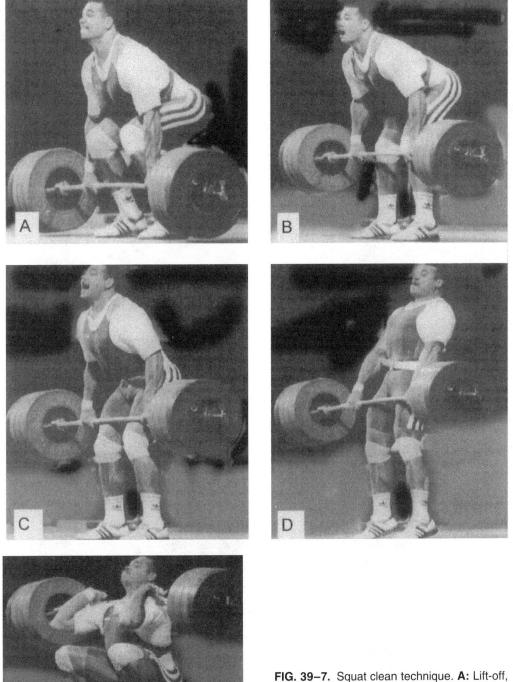

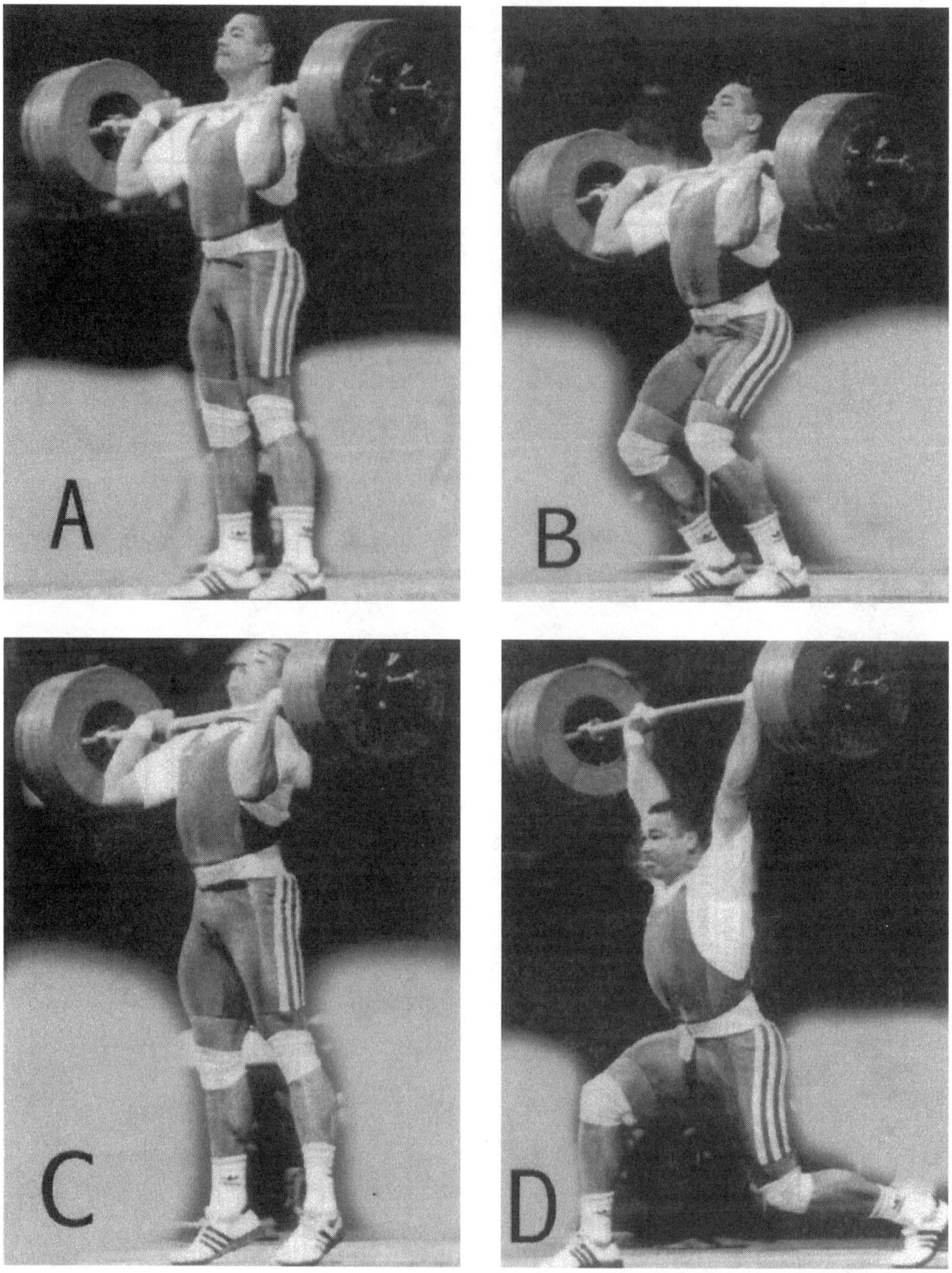

FIG. 39–8. Split jerk technique. **A:** Start. **B:** Lowest point of dip. **C:** End of thrust. **D:** Catch. Photo by Klemens/Reno.

knee bend technique. Enoka (116) has shown that this transitional movement reduces the tension requirement of the spinal extensor muscles considerably due to a large reduction in the above-mentioned lever arm lengths. It also produces a sudden forceful stretch on the quadriceps femoris, which may permit elastic energy recovery and elicit a stretch reflex facilitation of the immediately ensuing increased recruitment to produce a rapid knee extension during the second pull.

The second pull (Fig. 39–7*C,D*) is a very short duration (0.1 to 0.2 s) vertical jumping motion that quickly accelerates the barbell to its maximum velocity. The upward propulsion is derived from hip and knee extension, ankle plantar flexion, and rapid elevation of the shoulder girdle (shrugging the shoulders). The arms and torso should remain straight during the entire pulling motion to this point. Elbow flexion is employed at the end of the second pull to help accelerate movement of the body downward to position it under the bar in preparation for the catch at arm's length overhead for the snatch (Fig. 39–6), or at the shoulders for the clean (Fig. 39–7*E*). Despite the large mechanical stresses placed on the joints when catching the bar in a low squat position for both of these lifts, the frequency of injury in weightlifting is no greater than for other sports (117).

During the first pull the barbell moves upward and toward the athlete's body as his or her balance shifts from midfoot toward the heels. Balance shifts forward to the balls of the feet during the transition phase of the pull as the barbell moves forward. It then moves straight upward or upward and slightly backward during the second pull. Typical patterns for bar trajectory and velocity increase during the entire pull of a snatch lift are shown in Fig. 39–9. The maximum bar height and velocity for a clean pull is about 80% of that for a snatch lift, but the trajectory and pattern of velocity increase are very similar for a given athlete. Note that the rate of increase of bar velocity is greater during the second pull compared to the first pull. A slight decrease in velocity during the transition phase of the pull is seen for most athletes who use the double knee bend pulling technique. Force applied to the bar during the pull is closely related to the vertical ground reaction force (VGRF), that is, the force applied to the feet of the athlete in response to gravity acting on the body mass and the barbell, and from muscle forces. Typical VGRF patterns show a phase between the first and second pull where the force level falls below the combined weight of the athlete and barbell, accounting for the decrease in bar velocity during the transition phase of the pull (Fig. 39–10). This decrease in VGRF prior to the high force thrust phase is comparable to that which occurs during the countermovement prior to the thrust phase of a vertical jump (118,119).

After rising from a squat clean the barbell must be "jerked" overhead, as illustrated in Fig. 39–8, to complete the clean and jerk lift. The rapid and forceful stretch of knee and hip extensor muscles, which occurs near the lowest point of the "dip" or countermovement phase of the jerk, can produce a stretch reflex facilitation of the immediately following concentric contraction of these muscles to thrust the barbell upward via a jumping motion. Recovery of elastic strain energy may also contribute to the upward thrust forces. This very forceful stretch-shortening cycle movement is analogous to the common plyometric exercise called a depth or drop jump, with the stopping of the downward momentum during the jerk dip or drop jump landing being followed by a maximal effort upward jumping action in both cases. For sports highly dependent on jumping ability, the jerk lift and its variations are very productive training exercises due to exercise specificity. As mentioned above, the transition phase of a snatch or clean pull also generates this type of high-tension, stretch-shortening activity for the hip and knee extensors, but to a lesser extent. The change of downward to upward body and barbell motion during the jerk requires a rapid increase in tension in the knee and hip extensor muscles and produces large load forces on the joints and associated

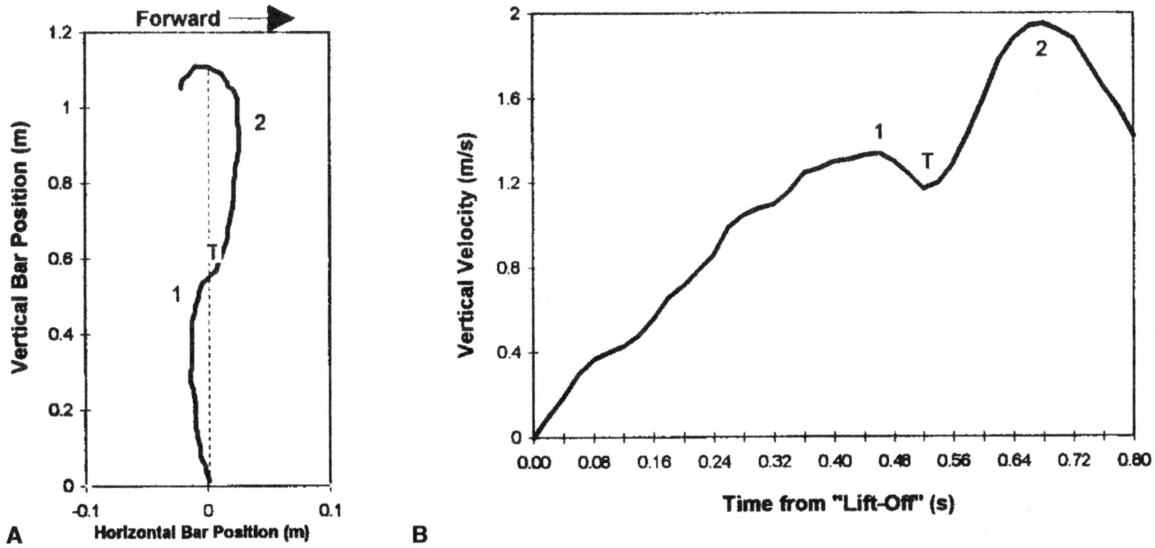

FIG. 39–9. **A:** Typical barbell trajectory for a snatch lift from a side view (100-kg athlete facing forward). **B:** Typical barbell velocity profile for the same athlete. *1*, end of first pull; *2*, end of second pull; *T*, transition.

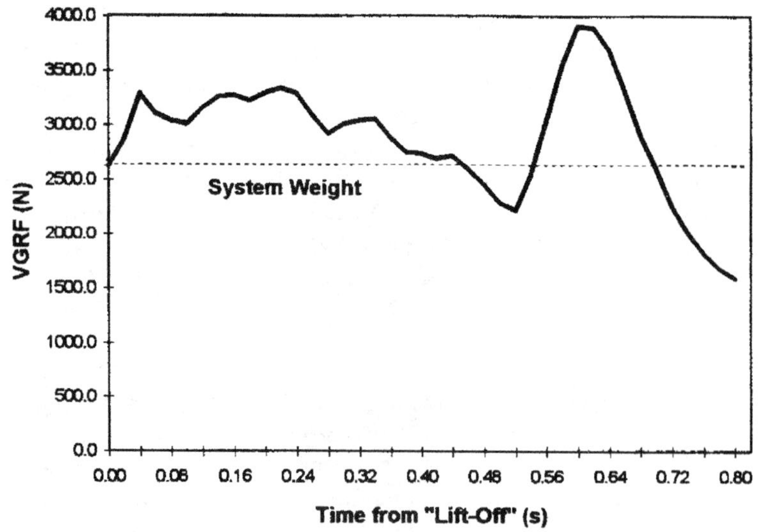

FIG. 39–10. Vertical ground reaction force (VGRF) on the athlete's feet during a snatch pull. *System weight* = barbell weight plus body weight.

connective tissues. A number of tendon or ligament ruptures have occurred at the knee joint in national and international weightlifting competitions, mostly in the 1970s, near the position shown in Fig. 39–8*B*. These injuries may have been connected with the use of specific anabolic steroids at that time and related effects on the mechanical properties of connective tissues. As previously mentioned, one biomechanical analysis of such an injury *in vivo* determined the patellar ligament tension to be ≈17 times BW at failure (43).

Mechanical Power Output

One of the most unique biomechanical characteristics of the snatch and clean and jerk lifts, and related training lifts, is the very high mechanical power output that must be generated for their proper execution. In world-championship competitions, male and female weightlifters have been documented producing, on average, more than 52 and 39 watts per kilogram (W/kg) of body mass, respectively, during the second pull for snatch and cleans lifts and during the jerk thrust (9,10). As discussed above, these are the phases of the complete lifts that are analogous to a vertical jump. Ongoing research is likely to show that current maximal power output values are somewhat higher due to increases in world-record lifts, particularly for women, in the 10 to 20 years since the values quoted were determined. These values are considerably higher than those produced in high-level powerlifting competitions, where 12 W/kg is representative for elite male athletes performing maximal squats and deadlifts. Power output values for bench presses are only about 4 W/kg due to the muscle mass involved being limited to the upper body (8,120). The main reason why power outputs are so much lower for these "power" lifts is that the very heavy weights lifted are moved slowly. It is important to point out, however, that these quoted values are for maximal effort lifts. It is known that power output can double for these powerlifts if the weight lifted is reduced to about 90% of maximum (121). The power output increase with reduced load is not as great in weightlifting, but it is likely to be 10% to 20% higher if the weight lifted in the snatch or clean and jerk is reduced 5% to 20% from maximum (8). Athletes in these and other sports that are highly dependent on muscle power capabilities for elite performance train most frequently with weights in the 70% to 90% of maximum range. Thus, the highest muscle power outputs are developed when performing snatch, clean, jerk, and related exercises, although the powerlifts also involve high power outputs when common submaximal training weights are used.

THE ROLE AND EFFECTS OF WEIGHT BELTS AND INTRAABDOMINAL/INTRATHORACIC PRESSURES DURING LIFTING

Weight belts are becoming more prevalent in everyday life. It's difficult to find even a discount store without employees wearing some type of weight belt. Weightlifters have long known and researchers have verified some of the likely benefits of wearing weight belts for short periods of time during their lifting routines. However, researchers have yet to demonstrate conclusively the effectiveness of using weight belts in industry for long periods of time with loads that are generally much smaller than a typical weightlifter would encounter.

While injuries during weightlifting are not common, the large forces that occur on the various structures of the trunk can exceed recommended levels for safe performance (74,79). The strength of the structures involved in the stability of the lumbosacral joint for example have been rated as weak, strong, and moderate for skeletal, ligament, and muscle components, respectively. Research has shown that compressive forces acting on the spine have reached 36,400 N during heavy lifting (79), while cadaver studies have shown damage to the vertebrae with only 3698 N for elderly female subjects and up to 12,981 N for a formerly healthy 46-year-old man (92).

It has been shown that weight belts can increase the IAP and thereby possibly reduce the forces acting on the spine. A tightly worn weight belt can help to pressurize the abdominal cavity, enabling it to bear up to 50% of the load normally placed on the spinal column and associated structures (53,122,123).

Types of Weight Belts

There are three sizes of weight belts that are the most popular for various types of weight training: (a) regular—a weight belt that is a single layer of leather or fabric that is 10 cm wide in the rear and ≈6.5 cm wide in front; (b) wide—same as a regular weight belt in the front, but 15 cm wide in the rear; and (c) power—a weight belt made of several layers of material that is 10 cm wide all around and is typically worn by powerlifters. Other types of weight belts resemble a girdle or corset and are made of rather light and stretchable fabric and are typically used in industrial settings. Since the mechanism of increasing IAP seems to be how a weight belt operates, this latter type of weight belt may not provide much protection, especially during athletic weightlifting.

Most weight belts are made of leather, consisting of either one or multiple layers, sometimes with a suede covering. Over the last few years, some manufacturers have marketed weight belts made of fabric. Leather has the advantage of being long-wearing, but some leather weight belts tend to be overly stiff and can cause cuts and bruises. Fabric weight belts are more flexible and comfortable due to their ability to mold better to the body contours. It is difficult to say how long some of the fabric weight belts will last because of their recent introduction. Some fabric weight belts also have the advantage of being washable, unlike the leather versions.

Weight belts typically have a either a single- or double-prong buckle to secure it. Newer designs feature different closure devices to speed up the tightening and loosening of the weight belt and include Velcro fasteners. Most of the weight belts described above, regardless of material or fastener, can increase IAP and help to relieve spinal structures.

Several points should be considered when making a decision on what type of weight belt is best for a particular individual. The most important factor is the width of the front of the weight belt, because a weight belt works by pressurizing the abdominal contents, as described in the next section. The width of the weight belt in the rear is of little value, and a weight belt that is 10 cm wide all around is recommended. Research has shown the tighter the weight belt, the better it potentially acts (122–126). If a 10 cm wide weight belt cannot be tightened properly due to the distance between the crest of the ilium and the lower ribs, it may be necessary to use a narrower weight belt, or a more flexible fabric weight belt, or cut down a leather weight belt only where it binds on the sides of the body.

Mechanism of Intraabdominal Pressure and Intrathoracic Pressure

Many questionable devices are available that promise to enhance performance or help provide an extra measure of protection. A properly utilized weight belt, however, is a device that can help a training regimen both in safety and performance. It has been suggested that the human spine without its muscular support can withstand only 20 N of force before it will topple over (122). The muscles that run up and down the spine act as guy wires, stabilizing this inherently unstable structure. This, however, is not the only way that the spine receives support.

The Valsalva maneuver consists of taking a deep breath and holding it just prior to lifting a very heavy weight. When the thoracic spine region is inflated, it creates an increase in ITP. Forced expiration against a closed glottis will further increase ITP. From biomechanical models, this pressurized air-filled ball or cavity can now support up to 50% of the load placed on the entire trunk. Increasing ITP is achieved rather easily because the rib cage provides a firm enclosure for the thoracic cavity. The only weak links (the glottis and the diaphragm) are readily controlled. Since a deep breath will cause the diagram to contract and descend into the abdominal cavity, an increase in IAP ensues. The downfall of using this protective maneuver is that venous blood flow in the thoracic cavity is impeded. Therefore, it is very important to remember to breathe between repetitions to allow blood to flow through the thoracic cavity.

A weight belt does not work primarily as a brace but more as a corset. A back brace, for example, works by directly transmitting the load on the shoulders to pelvic girdle by way of a metal and plastic structure. Weight belts that are 15 cm wide in the rear provide little extra support over a 10 cm wide weight belt, since a thin piece of leather is too flexible and does not run the entire length of the spine.

Increasing IAP is accomplished in a similar manner as increasing ITP. It is valuable to picture the abdominal cavity as a semi–fluid-filled ball instead of an air-filled ball (Fig. 39–11). The top of the cavity is the diaphragm and its stability is dependent on the amount of ITP. The bones of the pelvic girdle provide a stable base for the ball to rest on. Similarly, the spinal column and the

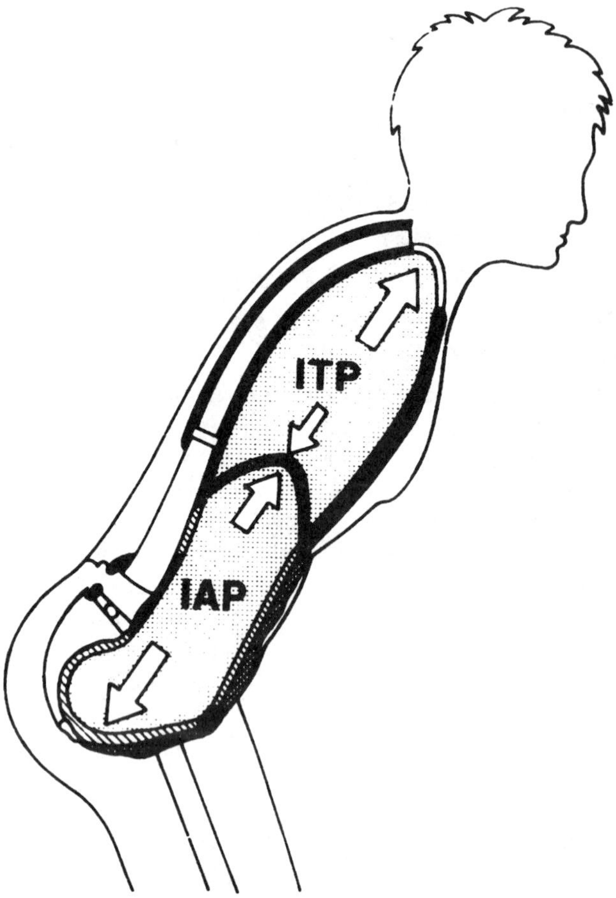

FIG. 39–11. Illustration of the action of intraabdominal pressure (*IAP*) and intrathoracic pressure (*ITP*).

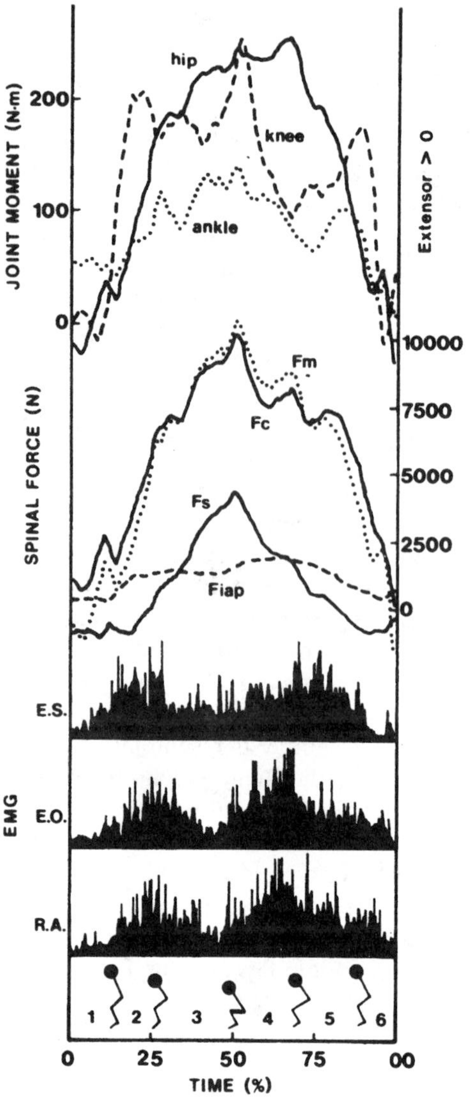

FIG. 39–12. Top: Sample trial of joint moments. Hip (*solid line*); knee (*dashed line*); ankle (*dotted line*). **Middle**: Sample trial of spinal forces. F_m, back muscle force (*dotted line*); F_c, compression force (*solid line*); F_s, shear force (*solid line*); F_{iap}, intraabdominal relieving force (*dashed line*). **Bottom**: Sample trial of electromyography. *E.S.*, erector spinae group; *E.O.*, external oblique; *R.A.*, rectus abdominus. (From ref. 125, with permission.)

muscles of the low back provide for a stable rear of the cavity. The only weak links are the muscles on the sides and front of the abdominal cavity. The only way to pressurize the abdominal cavity is to constrict the contents, and this is accomplished in everyday life by the rectus abdominus, transverse abdominus, and internal and external obliques.

Even strong abdominal muscles cannot increase IAP as well as a weight belt. Several studies have shown an increase in IAP from 13% to 40% when a weight belt was used (78,124,125,127). This means that even a lifter with very strong abdominals will benefit from wearing a weight belt. As with the Valsalva maneuver, wearing a weight belt increases the IAP and decreases the forces acting directly on the lumbar spine by up to 50%. This is important because the compressive force on the lower spine has been shown to exceed 10,000 N during a 150-kg squat (125) (Fig. 39–12).

IAP is typically greater than ITP during lifting. Since the liquid and solid composition of the abdominal cavity is only slightly compressible, high pressures can be generated without appreciably affecting its volume. In contrast, the largely gas-filled thoracic cavity must be reduced considerably to substantially increase pressure, since pressure in the thoracic cavity is inversely related to its volume. Harman and colleagues (77) quantified IAP and ITP during the lifting and jumping exercises using a 4-RM load. During the deadlift, peak IAP was 21.5 ± 5.5 kPa and peak ITP was 13.5 ± 4.4 kPa. IAP was also greater in the leg press, slide row, box lift, vertical jump, drop jump, and Valsalva maneuver. However, during the bench press peak ITP was greater (12.8

± 5.0 kPa) than peak IAP (10.7 ± 5.9 kPa). This is not surprising since during the bench press the weight from the barbell is transmitted through the arms to the thoracic cavity.

The degree to which biomechanical models reflect reality is equivocal, but studies have shown that the use of weight belts and the concomitant rise in IAP increases the stiffness of the trunk (128,129). Studies that directly measure intradiscal pressure during lifting are rare, but one study found a 25% decrease of intradiscal pressure when using an inflatable corset (126). Other research has demonstrated a decrease in spinal shrinkage (130) and an increase in muscle strength and endurance in the industrial setting from the use of athletic weight belts (131).

Physiologic Factors

Although IAP can exist without ITP, the most effective way to unload the spine is to use both mechanisms in concert with each other. The diaphragm forms the top of the abdominal cavity; by increasing ITP, a firm top can be accomplished regardless of the strength of the diaphragm. Numerous studies have examined the physiologic effects of increasing ITP by performing the Valsalva maneuver, but few studies have shown these effects in concert with a weight belt (132).

Four phases of the Valsalva maneuver have been identified. In the first phase (onset of straining) there is an immediate increase in systemic arterial pressure and a sudden decrease in heart rate (HR). These changes are a reflex action from the sudden rise in blood pressure due to the blood being forced from the lungs to the periphery. The second phase (sustained straining) begins 2 to 3 seconds after the onset. In this phase blood is dammed back in the venous system, causing a slow and gradual increase in the venous pressure. Concurrently, the arterial pressure falls causing an increase in HR. During the third phase (immediate poststrain), the blood pressure drops with the sudden cessation of straining, causing the HR to increase. In the fourth phase (bradycardia), the blood again enters the right heart to be pumped, and results in an overshoot in blood pressure inducing reflex bradycardia.

The use of ITP with IAP combined can have profound physiologic effects. An increase in IAP above venous pressure will inhibit vena cava blood flow back to the heart and force blood from the abdominal cavity. As with the Valsalva maneuver alone, there is a considerable decrease in cardiac output (up to 50%) and rapid oxygen debt ensues.

As intracavity pressures increase, so do the negative effects on blood flow and the stresses on the heart. For this reason, weight belts should be tightened only for limited periods of time. Fig. 39–13 shows how IAP varies from small values at the start and end of the lift to rather

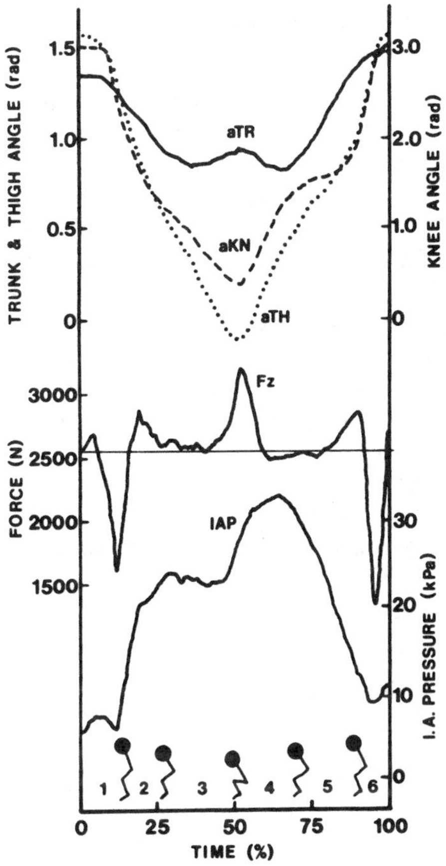

FIG. 39–13. **Top**: Sample trial of kinematic data. a_{TR}, trunk angle (*solid line*); a_{KN}, knee angle (*dashed line*); a_{TH}, thigh angle (*dotted line*). **Bottom**: Sample trial of vertical ground reaction force (F_z) and intraabdominal pressure (*IAP*). (From ref. 125, with permission.)

large values during the up phase of a squat. It has been suggested that if performed properly, the variations in IAP can act as an "abdominal pump" and encourage blood flow back to the heart. Unfortunately, this probably does not occur when the thoracic cavity is already highly pressurized, as is often the case in heavy weightlifting. To maximize IAP and ITP during heavy lifting (e.g., squat and deadlift), a power weight belt should be tightened maximally, and the lifter should inhale deeply during the descent, perform the Valsalva maneuver during the "sticking region" (i.e., the most difficult portion of the lift) by forced expiration against a closed glottis, and push against the weight belt by strongly contract the abdominal musculature. Although this will maximize trunk stability and stiffness, the Valsalva maneuver should be performed for only a few seconds maximal, which is usually sufficient time to get through the sticking region and complete the lift. Once beyond the sticking region, the lifter should slowly exhale until the lift is completed. Proper breathing between repetitions should allow for a more normal flow of blood.

Athletic Versus Industrial

Controversy still surrounds the effectiveness of weight belts in the industrial setting. Several critical differences exist between athletic and industrial settings. Athletes typically lift heavy weights for very short periods of time and use a stiff, heavy-duty weight belt. In contrast, workers typically lift light weights over longer periods of time and use a very flexible light-duty elastic weight belt. The effectiveness of weight belts in athletic movements appears to relate directly to the mechanism of their corset-like action in increasing IAP and ITP. However, due to the type of weight belt typically used in industry and the physiologic consequences of constricting the abdominal and thoracic cavities for prolonged period of time, industrial weight belt studies have shown little or no effect. Several review articles address the current situation in industry and expound upon the differences between the industrial and athletics settings (133–136).

When a Weight Belt Should be Used

A weight belt will be of the greatest benefit during lifts that heavily load the trunk. Squats and deadlifts are two exercises that fit into this category. There are some exercises in which wearing a weight belt will have little effect, such as the bench press. During a flat bench press the Valsalva maneuver is utilized to increase ITP and stabilize upper spine region. Since a weight belt stabilizes the lower spine, it is of limited value during the bench press. However, during the incline bench press more stress falls on the lower lumbar area, so a weight belt may be beneficial. In some exercises, wearing a weight belt actually prevents proper execution of the lift. For example, a weight belt is often not worn during the snatch and clean and jerk, since it physically can impede the path of the bar.

Wearing a weight belt is most beneficial when lifting moderate (70% to 85% of 1 RM) to heavy (85% to 100% of 1 RM) loads (125). These percentages correspond to a 6 to 12 RM for moderate loads and a 1 to 6 RM for heavy loads. Some caution should be employed when lifting lighter loads so as not to detrain the muscles and other structures involved in support of the spine. Even if the loads are not heavy, weight belts may still provide protection during the later repetitions of a set when fatigue sets in. One study showed no increased benefit across repetitions of weight belt usage during an eight-repetition set (≈80% of 1 RM) (124). However, this does not negate the possibility of increased benefit when performing more than eight repetitions, or when fatigue is a greater factor.

Several recommendations can be made concerning the proper use of weight belts. For illustrative purposes, the following recommendations refer to a heavy, deep squat, but with some modifications they apply to other lifts (e.g., deadlift) where the spine is loaded heavily and a weight belt is employed: (a) Use a weight belt that is 10 cm wide all around. This assumes that the trunk is long enough to allow for proper tightening. (b) Just prior to performing a set, tighten the weight belt as much as possible. (c) Take a breath and close the glottis to increase ITP and stabilize the thoracic spine. (d) Tighten the abdominal muscles and push against the weight belt as needed throughout the lift. This will increase the IAP and help to protect the lumbar spine. (e) Lower the weight while maintaining a normal spinal curvature. This is especially important at the bottom of the lift where the stresses on the spine are the greatest. (f) Raise the weight under control and begin to exhale after passing through the most difficult part of the lift (i.e., the sticking region). (g) By the completion of the repetition, all air should have been exhaled. Inhale and reestablish proper trunk posture in preparation for the next repetition. This is a natural way of breathing and should not take much practice.

Conclusion

Weight belts appear to provide a beneficial effect when lifting heavy weights, but the literature is not in total agreement. Two studies utilizing traditional weight belts have shown little or no effect (137,138), while other studies reviewed earlier have shown positive but conflicting results. Due to the extreme invasiveness of measuring intradiscal pressure, many studies relied on biomechanical models to predict vertebral compression and shear forces. Therefore, our knowledge is limited by the accuracy of these models and may or may not stand the test of time. Further research is needed to quantify when the use of a weight belt is warranted, and under what conditions there may be negative consequences.

REFERENCES

1. Henning CE, Lynch MA, Glick KR Jr. An in vivo strain gage study of elongation of the anterior cruciate ligament. *Am J Sports Med* 1985;13:22–26.
2. Lutz GE, et al. Comparison of tibiofemoral joint forces during open-kinetic-chain and closed-kinetic-chain exercises. *J Bone Joint Surg* 1993;75A:732–739.
3. More RC, et al. Hamstring—an anterior cruciate ligament protagonist. An in vitro study. *Am J Sports Med* 1993;21:231–237.
4. Ohkoshi Y, et al. Biomechanical analysis of rehabilitation in the standing position. *Am J Sports Med* 1991;19:605–611.
5. Shelbourne KD, Nitz P. Accelerated rehabilitation after anterior cruciate ligament reconstruction. *Am J Sports Med* 1990;18:292–299.
6. Stuart MJ, et al. Comparison of intersegmental tibiofemoral joint forces and muscle activity during various closed kinetic chain exercises. *Am J Sports Med* 1996;24:792–799.
7. Yack HJ, Collins CE, Whieldon TJ. Comparison of closed and open kinetic chain exercise in the anterior cruciate ligament-deficient knee [see comments]. *Am J Sports Med* 1993;21:49–54.
8. Garhammer J. A review of power output studies of olympic and

powerlifting: methodology, performance prediction, and evaluation tests. *J Strength Cond Res* 1993;7:76–89.
9. Garhammer J. Power production by Olympic weightlifters. *Med Sci Sports Exerc* 1980;12:54–60.
10. Garhammer J. A comparison of maximum power outputs between elite male and female weightlifters in competition. *Int J Sport Biomech* 1991;7:3–11.
11. Ariel BG. Biomechanical analysis of the knee joint during deep knee bends with heavy loads. In: Nelson R, Morehouse C, eds. *Biomechanics*, vol 4. Baltimore: University Park Press, 1974:44–52.
12. Dahlkvist NJ, Mayo P, Seedhom BB. Forces during squatting and rising from a deep squat. *Eng Med* 1982;11:69–76.
13. Escamilla RF, et al. Biomechanics of the knee during closed kinetic chain and open kinetic chain exercises. *Med Sci Sports Exerc* 1998;30:556–569.
14. Escamilla RF, et al. The effects of technique variations on knee biomechanics during the squat and leg press. *Med Sci Sports Exerc* 1997;29:S156.
15. Nisell R, Ekholm J. Joint load during the parallel squat in powerlifting and force analysis of in vivo bilateral quadriceps tendon rupture. *Scand J Sports Sci* 1986;8:63–70.
16. Andrews JG, Hay JG, Vaughan CL. Knee shear forces during a squat exercise using a barbell and a weight machine. In: Matsui H, Kobayashi K, eds. *Biomechanics,* vol 8B. Champaign, IL: Human Kinetics, 1983:923–927.
17. Hattin HC, Pierrynowski MR, Ball KA. Effect of load, cadence, and fatigue on tibio-femoral joint force during a half squat. *Med Sci Sports Exerc* 1989;21:613–618.
18. Wickiewicz TL, et al. Muscle architecture of the human lower limb. *Clin Orthop* 1983:275–283.
19. van Eijden TM, et al. Forces acting on the patella during maximal voluntary contraction of the quadriceps femoris muscle at different knee flexion/extension angles. *Acta Anat* 1987;129:310–314.
20. Butler DL, Noyes FR, Grood ES. Ligamentous restraints to anterior-posterior drawer in the human knee. A biomechanical study. *J Bone Joint Surg* 1980;62A:259–270.
21. Race A, Amis AA. The mechanical properties of the two bundles of the human posterior cruciate ligament. *J Biomech* 1994;27:13–24.
22. Noyes FR, et al. Biomechanical analysis of human ligament grafts used in knee-ligament repairs and reconstructions. *J Bone Joint Surg* 1984;66A:344–352.
23. Woo SL, et al. Tensile properties of the human femur-anterior cruciate ligament-tibia complex. The effects of specimen age and orientation. *Am J Sports Med* 1991;19:217–225.
24. Harner CD, et al. The human posterior cruciate ligament complex: an interdisciplinary study. Ligament morphology and biomechanical evaluation. *Am J Sports Med* 1995;23:736–745.
25. Hsieh HH, Walker PS. Stabilizing mechanisms of the loaded and unloaded knee joint. *J Bone Joint Surg* 1976;58A:87–93.
26. Shoemaker SC, Markolf KL. Effects of joint load on the stiffness and laxity of ligament-deficient knees. An in vitro study of the anterior cruciate and medial collateral ligaments. *J Bone Joint Surg* 1985;67A:136–146.
27. Markolt KL, et al. The role of joint load in knee stability. *J Bone Joint Surg* 1981;63A:570–585.
28. Yack HJ, Washco LA, Whieldon T. Compressive forces as a limiting factor of anterior tibial translation in the ACL-deficient knee. *Clin J Sports Med* 1994;4:233–239.
29. McLaughlin TM, Dillman CJ, Lardner TJ. A kinematic model of performance in the parallel squat by champion powerlifters. *Med Sci Sports* 1977;9:128–133.
30. McLaughlin TM, Lardner TJ, Dillman CJ. Kinetics of the parallel squat. *Res Q* 1978;49:175–189.
31. Zheng N, et al. An analytical model of the knee for estimation of internal forces during exercise. *J Biomech* 1998;31:963–967.
32. Aune AK, et al. Hamstrings and gastrocnemius co-contraction protects the anterior cruciate ligament against failure: an in vivo study in the rat [see comments]. *J Orthop Res* 1995;13:147–150.
33. Draganich LF, Jaeger RJ, Kralj AR. Coactivation of the hamstrings and quadriceps during extension of the knee. *J Bone Joint Surg* 1989;71A:1075–1081.
34. Draganich LE, Vahey JW. An in vitro study of anterior cruciate ligament strain induced by quadriceps and hamstrings forces. *J Orthop Res* 1990;8:57–63.
35. Durselen L, Claes L, Kiefer H. The influence of muscle forces and external loads on cruciate ligament strain. *Am J Sports Med* 1995;23:129–136.
36. O'Connor JJ. Can muscle co-contraction protect knee ligaments after injury or repair? *J Bone Joint Surg* 1993;75B:41–48.
37. Yasuda K, Sasaki T. Exercise after anterior cruciate ligament reconstruction. The force exerted on the tibia by the separate isometric contractions of the quadriceps or the hamstrings. *Clin Orthop* 1987;220:275–283.
38. Yasuda KT, Sasaki T. Muscle exercise after anterior cruciate ligament reconstruction. Biomechanics of the simultaneous isometric contraction method of the quadriceps and the hamstrings. *Clin Orthop* 1987;220:266–274.
39. Herzog W, Read LJ. Lines of action and moment arms of the major force-carrying structures crossing the human knee joint. *J Anat* 1993;182(pt 2):213–230.
40. Nisell R. Mechanics of the knee. A study of joint and muscle load with clinical applications. *Acta Orthop Scand Suppl* 1985;216:1–42.
41. Nisell R, Nemeth G, Ohlsen H. Joint forces in extension of the knee. Analysis of a mechanical model. *Acta Orthop Scand* 1986;57:41–46.
42. Cooper DE, et al. The strength of the central third patellar tendon graft. A biomechanical study. *Am J Sports Med* 1993;21:818–823; discussion: 823–824.
43. Zernicke RF, Garhammer J, Jobe FW. Human patellar-tendon rupture: a kinetic analysis. *J Bone Joint Surg* 1977;59A:179–183.
44. Nisell R, Ekholm J. Patellar forces during knee extension. *Scand J Rehabil Med* 1985;17:63–74.
45. Beynnon BD, et al. The strain behavior of the anterior cruciate ligament during squatting and active flexion-extension. A comparison of an open and a closed kinetic chain exercise. *Am J Sports Med* 1997;25:823–829.
46. Huberti HH, Hayes WC. Patellofemoral contact pressures. The influence of q-angle and tendofemoral contact. *J Bone Joint Surg* 1984;66A:715–724.
47. Hungerford DS, Barry M. Biomechanics of the patellofemoral joint. *Clin Orthop* 1979;144:9–15.
48. Wretenberg P, et al. Joint moments of force and quadriceps activity during squatting exercise. *Scand J Med Sci Sports* 1993;3:244–250.
49. Reilly DT, Martens M. Experimental analysis of the quadriceps muscle force and patello-femoral joint reaction force for various activities. *Acta Orthop Scand* 1972;43:126–137.
50. van Eijden TM, et al. A mathematical model of the patellofemoral joint. *J Biomech* 1986;19:219–229.
51. van Eijden TM, Kouwenhoven E, Weijs WA. Mechanics of the patellar articulation. Effects of patellar ligament length studied with a mathematical model. *Acta Orthop Scand* 1987;58:560–566.
52. Wretenberg P, Feng Y, Arborelius UP. High- and low-bar squatting techniques during weight-training. *Med Sci Sports Exerc* 1996;28:218–224.
53. Lander JE, Bates BT, Devita P. Biomechanics of the squat exercise using a modified center of mass bar. *Med Sci Sports Exerc* 1986;18:469–478.
54. Wilson JM, Robertson DGE. Analysis of biomechanical principles in weighted deep knee bends. Paper presented at the Fifth Biennial Conference and Human Locomotion Symposium of the Canadian Society for Biomechanics, Ottawa, Ontario, Canada, 1988.
55. Escamilla RF. The effects of technique variations on tibiofemoral forces and muscle activity during the squat and leg press. Unpublished dissertation, Auburn University, 1995.
56. Isear JA Jr, Erickson JC, Worrell TW. EMG analysis of lower extremity muscle recruitment patterns during an unloaded squat. *Med Sci Sports Exerc* 1997;29:532–539.
57. Ninos JC, et al. Electromyographic analysis of the squat performed in self-selected lower extremity neutral rotation and 30 degrees of lower extremity turn-out from the self-selected neutral position. *J Orthop Sports Phys Ther* 1997;25:307–315.
58. Signorile JF, et al. An electromyographical comparison of the

squat and knee extension exercises. *J Strength Cond Res* 1994;8:178–183.
59. Signorile JF, et al. Effect of foot position on the electromyographical activity of the superficial quadriceps muscles during the parallel squat and knee extension. *J Strength Cond Res* 1995; 9:182–187.
60. Komi PV, Kaneko M, Aura O. EMG activity of the leg extensor muscles with special reference to mechanical efficiency in concentric and eccentric exercise. *Int J Sports Med* 1987;8(suppl 1):22–29.
61. Chandler TJ, Wilson GD, Stone MH. The effect of the squat exercise on knee stability. *Med Sci Sports Exerc* 1989;21:299–303.
62. Klein KK. The deep squat exercise as utilized in weight training for athletes and its effects on the ligaments of the knee. *JAPMR* 1961;15:6–11.
63. Meyers EJ. Effect of selected exercise variables on ligament stability of the knee. *Res Q* 1971;42:411–422.
64. Panariello RA, Backus SI, Parker JW. The effect of the squat exercise on anterior-posterior knee translation in professional football players. *Am J Sports Med* 1994;22:768–773.
65. Steiner ME, et al. The effect of exercise on anterior-posterior knee laxity. *Am J Sports Med* 1986;14:24–29.
66. Costigan PA, Reid JG. Radial torque of the tibia during a deep knee bend. In: Winter DA, ed. *Biomechanics,* vol 9B. Champaign, IL: Human Kinetics, 1985:420–423.
67. Anderson CK, et al. A biomechanical model of the lumbosacral joint during lifting activities. *J Biomech* 1985;18:571–584.
68. Ekholm J, et al. Load on knee joint structures and muscular activity during lifting. *Scand J Rehab Med* 1984;16:1–9.
69. McGill SM, Norman RW. Dynamically and statically determined low back moments during lifting. *J Biomech* 1985;18:877–885.
70. McGill SM, Norman RW. Partitioning of the L4-L5 dynamic moment into disc, ligamentous, and muscular components during lifting [see comments]. *Spine* 1986;11:666–678.
71. McGill SM, Norman RW. Potential of lumbodorsal fascia forces to generate back extension moments during squat lifts. *J Biomed Eng* 1988;10:312–318.
72. Holmes JA, Damaser MS, Lehman SL. Erector spinae activation and movement dynamics about the lumbar spine in lordotic and kyphotic squat-lifting. *Spine* 1992;17:327–334.
73. Brown EW, Abani K. Kinematics and kinetics of the deadlift in adolescent powerlifters. *Med Sci Sports Exerc* 1985;17:554–566.
74. Cholewicki J, McGill SM, Norman RW. Lumbar spine loads during the lifting of extremely heavy weights. *Med Sci Sports Exerc* 1991;23:1179–1186.
75. Cholewicki J, McGill SM. Lumbar posterior ligament involvement during extremely heavy lifts estimated from fluoroscopic measurements. *J Biomech* 1992;25:17–28.
76. McGuigan MRM, Wilson BD. Biomechanical analysis of the deadlift. *J Strength Cond Res* 1996;10:250–255.
77. Harman EA, et al. Intra-abdominal and intra-thoracic pressures during lifting and jumping. *Med Sci Sports Exerc* 1988; 20:195–201.
78. Harman EA, et al. Effects of a belt on intra-abdominal pressure during weightlifting. *Med Sci Sports Exerc* 1989;21:186–190.
79. Granhed H, Jonson R, Hansson T. The loads on the lumbar spine during extreme weightlifting. *Spine* 1987;12:146–149.
80. Schultz AB, Andersson GB. Analysis of loads on the lumbar spine. *Spine* 1981;6:76–82.
81. Schultz A, et al. Loads on the lumbar spine. Validation of a biomechanical analysis by measurements of intradiscal pressures and myoelectric signals. *J Bone Joint Surg* 1982;64A:713–720.
82. Hansson T, Roos B, Nachemson A. The bone mineral content and ultimate compressive strength of lumbar vertebrae. *Spine* 1980;5:46–55.
83. Tesh KM, Dunn JS, Evans JH. The abdominal muscles and vertebral stability. *Spine* 1987;12:501–508.
84. Karlsson MK, Johnell O, Obrant KJ. Bone mineral density in weightlifters. *Calcif Tissue Int* 1993;52:212–215.
85. Suominen H. Bone mineral density and long term exercise. An overview of cross-sectional athlete studies. *Sports Med* 1993;16:316–330.
86. Tsuji S, Akama H. Weight training may provide a better stimulus for increasing bone mineral content (BMC) than run and swimming training [letter; comment]. *Med Sci Sports Exerc* 1991;23:882–883.
87. Wittich A, et al. Professional football (soccer) players have a markedly greater skeletal mineral content, density and size than age- and BMI-matched controls. *Calcif Tissue Int* 1998;63:112–117.
88. McGill SM. Estimation of force and extensor moment contributions of the disc and ligaments at L4-L5. *Spine* 1988;13:1395–1402.
89. Adams MA, Hutton WC. The effect of posture on the lumbar spine. *J Bone Joint Surg* 1985;67B:625–629.
90. Bergmark A. Stability of the lumbar spine. A study in mechanical engineering. *Acta Orthop Scand Suppl* 1989;230:1–54.
91. Crisco JJ, Panjabi MM. Postural biomechanical stability and gross muscular architecture in the spine. In: Winters JM, Woo SL-Y, eds. *Multiple muscle systems.* Berlin: Springer, 1990:438–450.
92. Hutton WC, Adams MA. Can the lumbar spine be crushed in heavy lifting? *Spine* 1982;7:586–590.
93. Adams MA, Hutton WC. Has the lumbar spine a margin of safety in forward bending? *Clin Biomech* 1986;1:3–6.
94. Adams MA, Hutton WC, Stott JR. The resistance to flexion of the lumbar intervertebral joint. *Spine* 1980;5:245–253.
95. Shirazi-Adl A, Ahmed AM, Shrivastava SC. A finite element study of a lumbar motion segment subjected to pure sagittal plane moments. *J Biomech* 1986;19:331–350.
96. Barnett C, Kippers V, Turner P. Effects of variations of the bench press exercise on the EMG activity of five shoulder muscles. *J Strength Cond Res* 1995;9:222–227.
97. Elliott BC, Wilson GJ, Kerr GK. A biomechanical analysis of the sticking region in the bench press. *Med Sci Sports Exerc* 1989;21:450–462.
98. Lander JE, et al. A comparison between free-weight and isokinetic bench pressing. *Med Sci Sports Exerc* 1985;17:344–353.
99. Rosentswieg J, Hinson M, Ridgway M. An electromyographic comparison of an isokinetic bench press performed at three speeds. *Res Q* 1975;46:471–475.
100. Wagner LL, et al. The effect of grip width on bench press performance. *Int J Sport Biomech* 1992;8:1–10.
101. Wilson GJ, Elliott BC, Wood GA. The effect on performance of imposing a delay during a stretch-shorten cycle movement. *Med Sci Sports Exerc* 1991;23:364–370.
102. Wilson GJ, Wood GA, Elliott BC. Optimal stiffness of series elastic component in a stretch-shorten cycle activity. *J Appl Physiol* 1991;70:825–833.
103. Wilson GJ, et al. Stretch shorten cycle performance: detrimental effects of not equaling the natural and movement frequencies. *Res Q Exerc Sport* 1996;67:373–379.
104. Goeser CD, Aikenhead JA. Rib fracture due to bench pressing. *J Manipulative Physiol Ther* 1990;13:26–29.
105. Cresswell TR, Smith RB. Bilateral anterior shoulder dislocations in bench pressing: an unusual cause. *Br J Sports Med* 1998;32:71–72.
106. Kretzler HH Jr, Richardson AB. Rupture of the pectoralis major muscle. *Am J Sports Med* 1989;17:453–458.
107. Rijnberg WJ, van Linge B. Rupture of the pectoralis major muscle in body-builders. *Arch Orthop Trauma Surg* 1993;112:104–105.
108. Urs ND, Jani DM. Surgical repair of rupture of the pectoralis major muscle: a case report. *J Trauma* 1976;16:749–750.
109. Wolfe SW, Wickiewicz TL, Cavanaugh JT. Ruptures of the pectoralis major muscle. An anatomic and clinical analysis. *Am J Sports Med* 1992;20:587–593.
110. Madsen N, McLaughlin T. Kinematic factors influencing performance and injury risk in the bench press exercise. *Med Sci Sports Exerc* 1984;16:376–381.
111. McLaughlin TM, Madsen NH. Bench press techniques of elite heavyweight powerlifters. *Natl Strength Cond Assoc J* 1984;6:44, 62–65.
112. Murphy AJ, Wilson GJ. The assessment of human dynamic muscular function: a comparison of isoinertial and isokinetic tests. *J Sports Med Phys Fitness* 1996;36:169–177.
113. Wilson GJ, Elliott BC, Wood GA. Stretch shorten cycle performance enhancement through flexibility training. *Med Sci Sports Exerc* 1992;24:116–123.

114. Murphy AJ, et al. Isometric assessment of muscular function: the effect of joint angle. *J Appl Biomech* 1995;11:205–215.
115. McLaughlin TM. *Bench press more now: breakthroughs in biomechanics and training methods.* Marietta, GA: Biomechanics, 1984:85.
116. Enoka RM. The pull in olympic weightlifting. *Med Sci Sports* 1979;11:131–137.
117. Stone MH. Muscle conditioning and muscle injuries. *Med Sci Sports Exerc* 1990;22:457–462.
118. Garhammer J, Gregor R. Force plate evaluations of weightlifting and vertical jumping. *Med Sci Sports Exerc* 1979;11:106.
119. Garhammer J, Gregor R. Propulsive forces as a function of intensity for weightlifting and vertical jumping. *J Appl Sport Sci Res* 1992;6:129–134.
120. Garhammer J. Weightlifting and training. In: Vaughan CL, ed. *Biomechanics of sport.* Boca Raton, FL: CRC, 1989:169–211.
121. Garhammer J, McLaughlin T. Power output as a function of load variation in olympic and powerlifting. *J Biomech* 1980;3:198.
122. Morris JM, Lucas D, Bresler B. Role of the trunk in stability of the spine. *J Bone Joint Surg* 1961;43A:327–351.
123. Eie N. Load capacity of the low back. *J Oslo City Hosp* 1966;16:73–98.
124. Lander JE, Hundley JR, Simonton RL. The effectiveness of weight belts during multiple repetitions of the squat exercise. *Med Sci Sports Exerc* 1992;24:603–609.
125. Lander JE, Simonton RL, Giacobbe JK. The effectiveness of weight belts during the squat exercise. *Med Sci Sports Exerc* 1990;22:117–126.
126. Nachemson A, Morris JM. In vivo measurements of intradiscal pressure: discometry, a new method for the determination of pressure on the lumbar discs. *J Bone Joint Surg* 1964;46A:1077–1092.
127. McGill SM, Norman RW, Sharratt MT. The effect of an abdominal belt on trunk muscle activity and intra-abdominal pressure during squat lifts. *Ergonomics* 1990;33:147–160.
128. Cholewicki J, et al. Can an abdominal belt and/or intra-abdominal pressure increase spine stability? Paper presented at the North American Congress on Biomechanics, Waterloo, Ontario, Canada, 1998.
129. McGill S, Seguin J, Bennett G. Passive stiffness of the lumbar torso in flexion, extension; lateral bending, and axial rotation. Effect of belt wearing and breath holding. *Spine* 1994;19:696–704.
130. Bourne ND, Reilly T. Effect of a weightlifting belt on spinal shrinkage. *Br J Sports Med* 1991;25:209–212.
131. Holmstrom E, Moritz U. Effects of lumbar belts on trunk muscle strength and endurance: a follow-up study of construction workers. *J Spinal Disord* 1992;5:260–266.
132. Hunter GR, et al. The effects of a weight training belt on blood pressure during exercise. *J Appl Sport Sci Res* 1989;3:13–18.
133. Hodgson EA. Occupational back belt use: a literature review. *AAOHN J* 1996;44:438–443.
134. McGill SM, Norman RW. Low back biomechanics in industry: the prevention of injury through safer lifting. In: Grabnier M, ed. *Current issues in biomechanics.* Champaign, IL: Human Kinetics, 1993:69–120.
135. Minor SD. Use of back belts in occupational settings. *Phys Ther* 1996;76:403–408.
136. Quinet RJ, Hadler NM. Diagnosis and treatment of backache. *Semin Arthritis Rheum* 1979;8:261–287.
137. Woodhouse ML, et al. Selected isokinetic lifting parameters of adult male athletes utilizing lumbar/sacral supports. *J Orthop Sports Phys Ther* 1990;11:467–473.
138. Woodhouse ML, et al. Effects of back support on intra-abdominal pressure and lumbar kinetics during heavy lifting. *Hum Factors* 1995;37:582–590.

Exercise and Sport Science,
edited by William E. Garrett, Jr., and Donald T. Kirkendall.
Lippincott Williams & Wilkins, Philadelphia © 2000.

CHAPTER 40

Biomechanics of Alpine and Nordic Skiing

Serge P. von Duvillard, Kenneth W. Rundell, Bernard Bilodeau, and David W. Bacharach

BIOMECHANICS OF ALPINE SKIING

Since the development of ski schools in alpine countries and until very recently, studies of alpine skiing technique have been merely descriptions of posture. The major reason for this has not been a lack of interest in, but rather a lack of technical expertise in, measuring forces acting on a skier. Even with improvements in modern biomechanical equipment and methods (1), two problems continue to plague researchers in this area: (a) it is difficult to assign objective criteria to the components of a skiing action; and (b) the very small displacements of body segments needed to distinguish technique differences can only be measured with extreme effort, time, and cost.

Given the limiting external factors involved, it is understandable that the data are limited. To compound the problem, motor control processes executed by the skier under varying external forces are known only in general terms. New information regarding the stretch-shortening cycle has helped; however, we are a long way from fully understanding the complexity of skiing's demands on the body. Laboratory simulators or small portable data loggers capable of generating kinetic data have been combined with kinematic (video) data to provide us with a glimpse of the complexity involved in alpine skiing. This chapter discusses the current state of biomechanical information relative to alpine skiing.

S. P. von Duvillard: Department of Physical Education and Exercise Science, Human Performance Laboratory, University of North Dakota, Grand Forks, North Dakota 58202-8235.

K. W. Rundell and B. Bilodeau: Sports Science and Technology Division, U.S. Olympic Committee, Lake Placid, New York 12946.

D. W. Bacharach: Department of Health, Physical Education, Recreation, and Sport Science, Human Performance Laboratory, St. Cloud State University, St. Cloud, Minnesota 56301.

Basic Principles of Alpine Skiing

There are several key forces that act on a skier. The weight of the skier acts in a vertical direction through the skier's center of mass. Altering a skier's mass will also affect forces as well as velocity. Ground reaction force is the force the snow is exerting against the skier at any given point in time. When standing or gliding on a flat surface this force is equal to the person's mass times the force of gravity (9.8 N). As skiers increase velocity and/or change direction by turning, they increase the ground reaction force.

For example, a person with a mass of 100 kg (person plus equipment) has a ground reaction force of 980 N (100 kg × 9.8 N). If that same person were to ski down a smooth slope for a vertical distance of 500 m, then the work could be calculated as follows:

$$980 \text{ N} \times 500 \text{ m} = 490{,}000 \text{ joules (490 kilojoules)}$$

If this same skier were to encounter a dip in the hill, ground reaction force will be altered (2). Table 40–1 shows how the radius of a dip in a hill or how velocity can affect ground reaction force.

The same concept holds true for turning. With no change in velocity, as the radius of a turn decreases, force increases. If velocity increases without a change

TABLE 40–1. *Variations in ground reaction force for dips in the hill*

Radius of dip (m)	Velocity (m/s)	Force (N)
20	11.1	616
10	11.1	1232
20	22.2	2464
10	22.2	4928

TABLE 40–2. *Variations in ground reaction force during turns*

Radius of turn (m)	Velocity (m/s)	Force (N)
5	8.3	1378
4	8.3	1722
20	16.6	1378
10	16.6	2756

in the turn radius, force increases (Table 40–2). As one can see from Table 40–2, more force is required to complete a short radius turn at 30 km/h (8.3 m/s) compared to a longer radius turn at 60 km/h (16.6 m/s).

Air resistance represents another force that acts on a skier. Combinations of velocity and body position that relates to body surface area can both influence the downhill speed of the skier.

Basic kinesiologic considerations for skiing include body stance and initiating, controlling, and exiting turns. Body stance is similar to that in most sports—a slight crouch where the center of gravity is low, slightly forward of the ankle joint, and balanced between the feet. There should be a line perpendicular to the skis that bisects the ball of the foot and runs through the shoulders and head. With no rotary forces acting on the body, this position is used for straight run gliding.

Initiation of a turn is characterized by an up or down unweighting followed by a weight shift and rotary or steering motions. The control phase of a turn is made up of edging, pressure control, and steering with a maximal ground reaction force. The completion or exiting phase of a turn entails pressure control and regaining a neutral body position to allow a new weight shift to occur.

Figure 40–1 (3) shows the potential edging, steering, and pressure of a ski turn. Without proper alignment, additional force must be exerted or absorbed by the legs. Fig. 40–2 (3) depicts an ideal alignment for the knee over the ski boot. An ideal range for alignment is between 1 and 2.5 degrees inside of center of alignment. Many ski boot manufacturers offer various adjustments for proper alignment. Foot beds can be raised or lowered, and cuffs can be canted in or out and adjusted for a proper forward lean. If the skier cannot be aligned with simple boot adjustments, canting the soles of the boots or the skis is recommended.

Movement Regulation

The most important objective of sound alpine ski technique is to achieve a dynamic equilibrium (1). All other factors are incidental to the ability to remain balanced over the skis. Displacement of body segments cannot be regarded as changes in posture. Body movements while skiing are more a regulation of movement frequencies relative to body mass. Berg and colleagues (4)

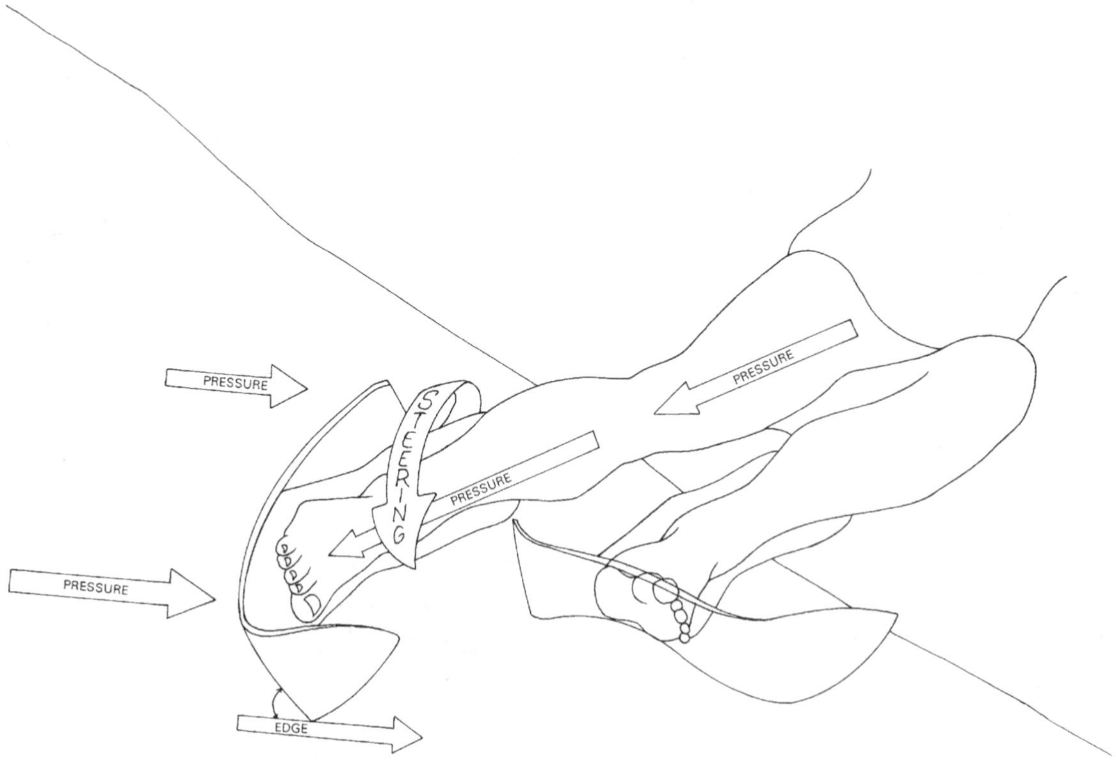

FIG. 40–1. To control a ski in the snow, you can edge it, pressure it, and steer it. (From ref. 3.)

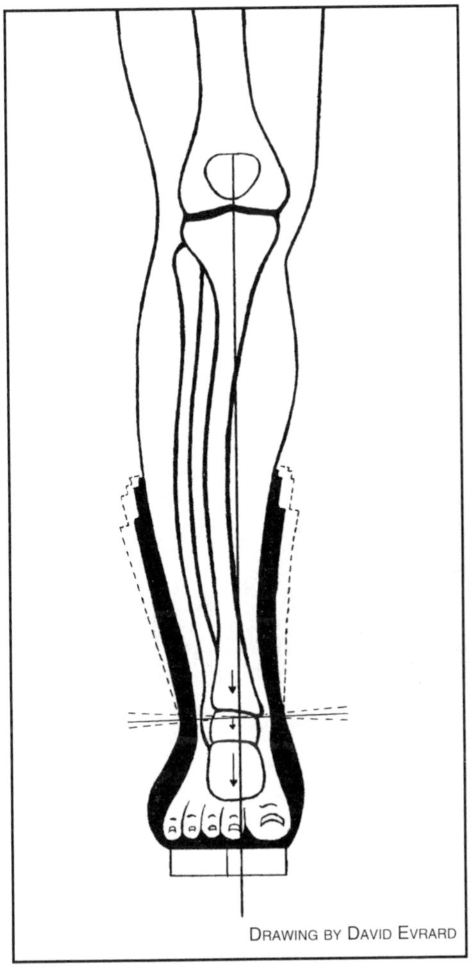

FIG. 40–2. Cuff adjustment. (From ref. 3.)

and Mester (1) have identified several control frequencies during alpine skiing. Ground reaction force frequencies of 1 to 3 Hz have been shown to be important for balance and are often referred to as "body sway" (Fig. 40–3). Eccentric activation of the quadriceps via electromyography (EMG) also revealed activity in the range of 1 to 6 Hz. A second peak range of ground reaction force frequencies has been identified at around 15 to 20 Hz. This range has been associated more closely with physiologic mechanisms.

It has been suggested that ski vibrations along with muscle activation to control forces in the leg occur in this frequency range. From a physiologic perspective, the closer the vibrations of skiing get to this faster range of frequencies, the better the neuromuscular regulation of movement.

Involvement of Muscle Action

Electromyography

Portable data acquisition and telemetry systems have facilitated the study of muscle activation during a ski turn. Hintermeister and colleagues (5) compared inside and outside leg activity during slalom (SL) and giant slalom (GS) turns. By synchronizing video and EMG recordings, they were able to quantify muscle activity during the initiation, turning, and completion phases of a turn for the inside and outside leg. For SL turns, they reported similar EMG activity between the inside and outside leg. A more upright body position during SL turns was assumed to be responsible for the similar EMG activity between the inside and outside leg. During GS turns, similar results were observed for the long turning phase. Greater unilateral activity was observed for GS during both the initiation and turning phases. In the completion phase of the GS turn, differences were noted for trunk and anterior thigh muscles. Trunk muscles were most active during the latter portion of the completion phase, suggesting deceleration under eccentric conditions.

These results are supported by data from Berg and colleagues (4), who measured joint angle and eccentric muscle action in GS racing. Elite alpine skiers have exhibited variations in muscle action. Ski turns have isometric, concentric, and eccentric components. Berg and colleagues hypothesized that eccentric muscle use is the dominant component of adaptations to strength for an alpine skier. They measured joint angles of the hip and knee along with EMG of quadriceps muscles and found not only an increase in eccentric EMG with a decrease in knee angle, but also a greater total time component of eccentric activity compared with the concentric portion of the turn (Fig. 40–4). The predominant notion of unilateral muscle activity was supported in this study's finding of an interesting biphasic pattern of the rectus femoris. It was suggested that the rectus femoris has two roles during a GS turn: (a) to assist in knee extension of the outside leg, and (b) to act as a hip flexor for the inside leg.

Kinematic and Kinetic Analysis

A combination of new technologies has provided researchers with a variety of options to assess kinematic and/or kinetic data. Procedures developed by Drenk (6) to record video data using a panned, tilted, and/or zoomed camera can accurately measure displacement. Research by Raschner and colleagues (7) utilized Drenk's technique to combine video with pressure distribution measurements of the sole of the foot. Kinematic and kinetic data were synchronized, and after lengthy calculations a variety of data presentations were available to researchers and coaches (Table 40–3). Figure 40–5 shows a racer during data collection.

Using these data, two training devices were built from the following perspectives on training:

1. Selection of exercise(s) should approximate the competition requirements as closely as possible.

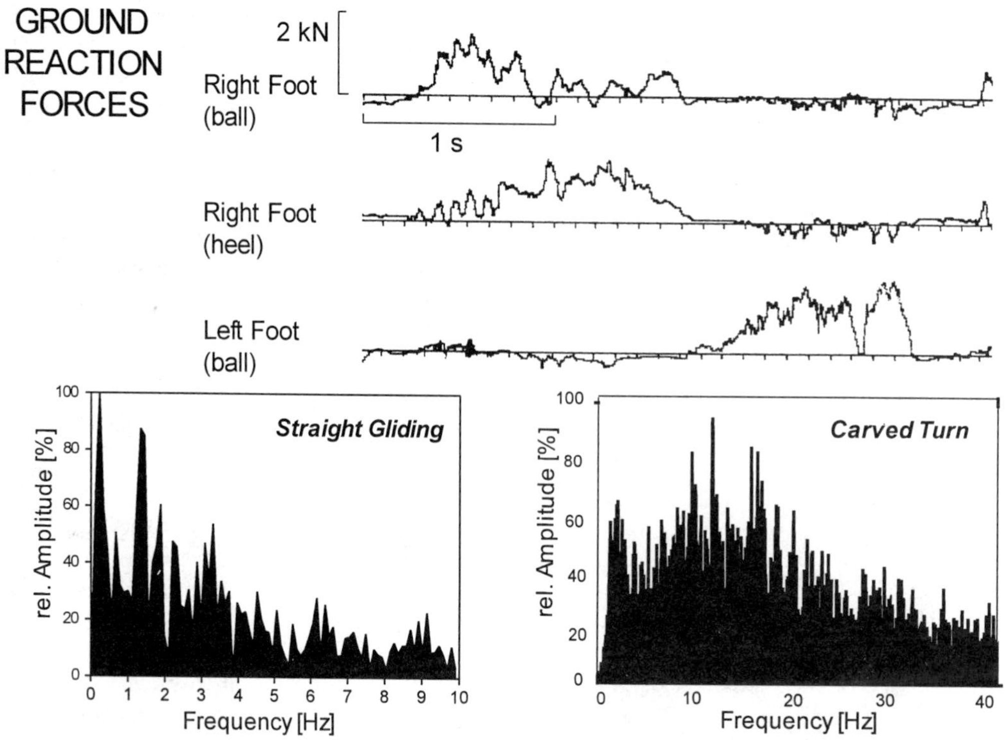

FIG. 40–3. Foot curves and frequency analyses of ground-reaction forces. (From ref. 1.)

2. Resistance encountered during the exercise(s) should match that in competition.
3. Energy demands and movement frequency should mimic that in competition.
4. Duration of exercise(s) should evoke fatigue while allowing for full recovery in a short period of time.

The first training tool was named the "ski-power home trainer" (Fig. 40–6). Its validity was checked using the same equipment as the on-snow trials and it was determined to be accurate for inside and outside edging patterns. Slight variations were noted for the outside leg when landing on the home trainer. Force-time curves exhibited double-peaked force-time durations that were not seen on snow.

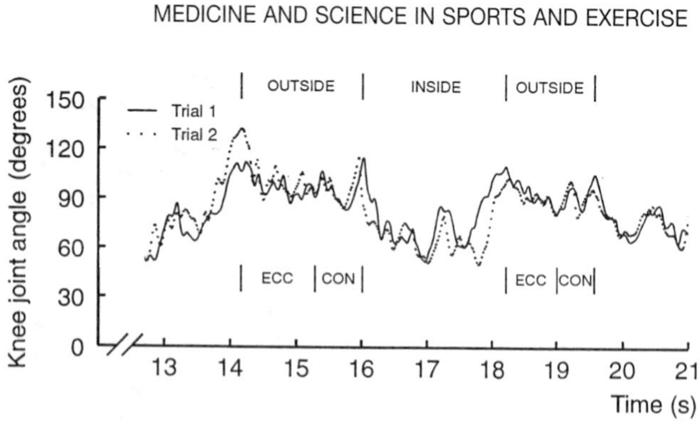

FIG. 40–4. Raw knee joint angle signal of the right leg from one subject in two consecutive trials in the giant slalom course. Two complete movement cycles are displayed. A left turn where the right leg controls the outside ski is denoted *OUTSIDE*. The intermediate turn is denoted *INSIDE*. (From ref. 4.)

TABLE 40–3. *Selected kinematic and kinetic parameters*

Kinematic parameters	Kinetic parameters
Knee angle	Ground reaction force from the outer leg
Hip angle	Ground reaction force from the inner leg
Inward leaning angle	Just the force of the heel
Angle of the skis to the movement direction	Just the force of the forefoot
Angle of the shoulder and hip axis to the movement direction	Force of the inside edge
Edging angle	Force of the outside edge
Velocity of the center of gravity	Movement of the weak point under the foot

From ref. 7.

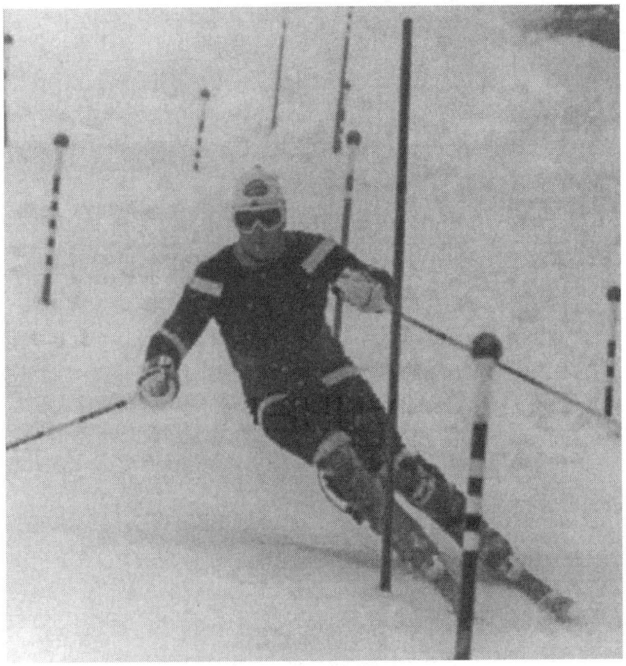

FIG. 40–5. Racer during a test run. (From ref. 7.)

The second device, the "ski-power simulator"(Fig. 40–7), was tailored for high-performance athletes in schools and academies. Its main purpose is to establish the optimal levels of strength and stamina necessary for skiing. Data derived from the simulator compared well with data from on-snow slalom skiing (Fig. 40–8). Figure 40–9 compares the knee angle in the simulator and in on-snow slalom skiing. The temporal aspects and the dynamic structure of the ski turn were maintained using the simulator. What remains to be determined is how well the use of such devices can transfer to ski-specific strength.

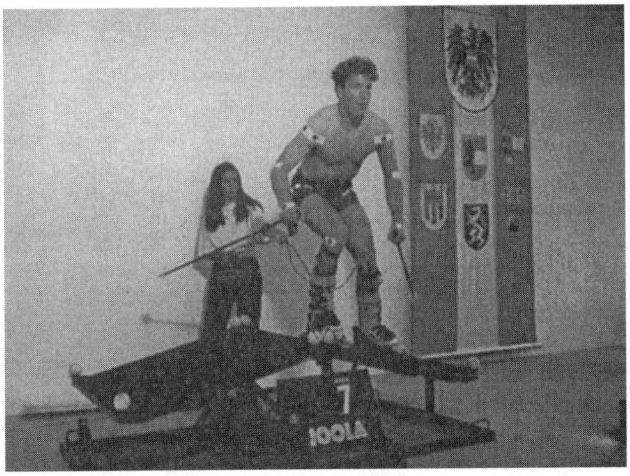

FIG. 40–6. Ski-power home trainer. (From ref. 7.)

Frick and colleagues (8) used video and foot pressure distribution measurements to determine what types of muscle actions are utilized by skiers during slalom skiing. Seven elite skiers were filmed while the authors measured pressure distribution under the soles of the feet inside the boots. Force-time curves were generated and matched to kinematic data. The authors found that the outside hip joint is flexed, and the hip extensors are working eccentrically. This suggests that during a slalom turn, the muscle of the outside leg does not utilize the stretch-shortening cycle. In contrast, kinematics and force-time curves revealed that extensor muscles of the inside leg acted eccentrically (flexion) followed by a concentric (extension) phase, which would clearly utilize the stretch-shortening cycle. Frick and colleagues concluded that the muscle action of the inside and outside leg along with the skill sequence of the movement should be taken into consideration when designing training exercises for alpine skiers.

Because of the limitations of humidity and temperature resistance inside a ski boot, only capacitive or piezoresistive methods can be used. A number of studies have utilized either a capacitive or piezoresistive method to measure pressure distribution inside a ski boot. As recently as the early 1980s, this type of measurement was not feasible. Recently, miniaturization of electronics has made it not only feasible but also economically possible. The capacitive systems of 100 Hz have limited use with high-frequency tasks such as elite alpine ski racing. The piezoresistive devices are able to sample frequencies up to 1000 Hz, with the primary range of 200 to 250 Hz being of greatest interest for the ski researcher.

For pressure distribution mapping, three areas on the sole of the foot are of primary concern: the big toe, the ball of the foot, and the heel (Fig. 40–10). An important key to performance in downhill, super giant slalom (super-G), and GS is having proper equalized pressure distribution when gliding, and specific periods of increased heel pressure during steering in the turn.

Schaff and colleagues (9) incorporated a 64-contact point measuring sock in which pressure could be distributed not only to the sole of the foot but throughout the boot itself (Figs. 40–11 and 40–12). Such a system detects changes in pressure along the medial forefoot, ankle, and lower tibia. Pressures in these areas relate more closely to steering compared to fore/aft pressure characterized by foot sole pressure.

From specialized systems such as the measuring sock, a simple feedback mechanism was developed. The Swingbeep System is a biofeedback system utilizing two pressure-sensitive switches, with one located inside each boot and under the heels of the skier. The Swingbeep can be adjusted for pressure sensitivity; it emits a visual

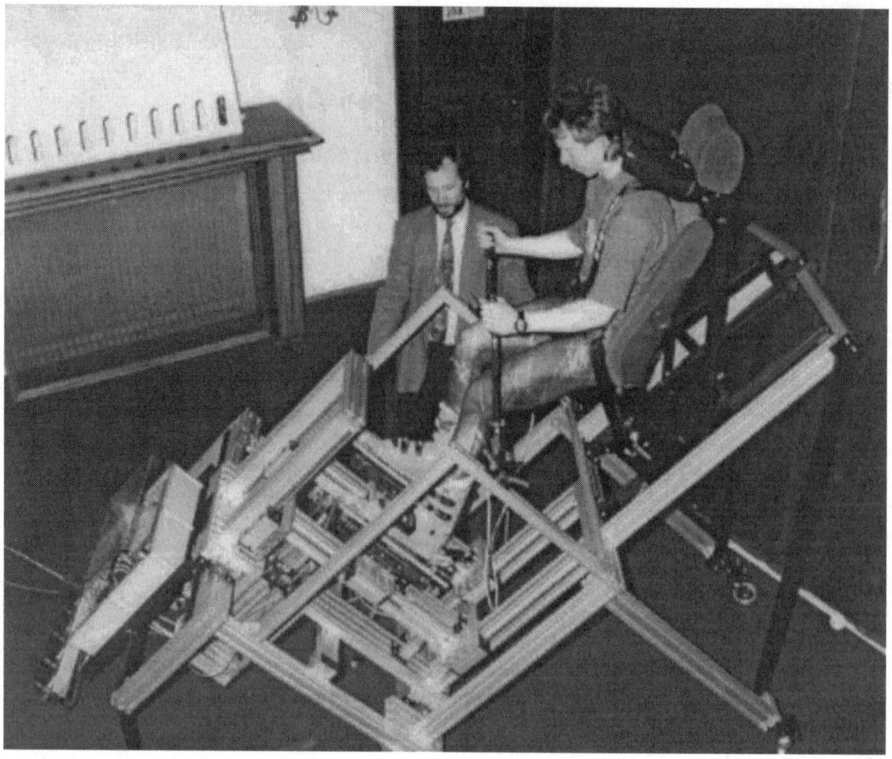

FIG. 40–7. Ski-power simulator. (From ref. 7.)

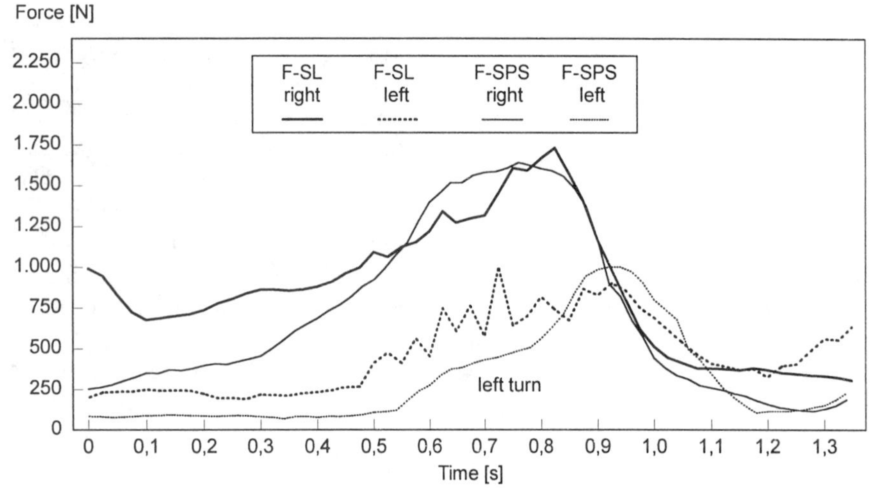

FIG. 40–8. Comparison of the ground-reaction forces from the elite athlete: slalom vs. ski-power simulator simulation exercise. (From ref. 9.)

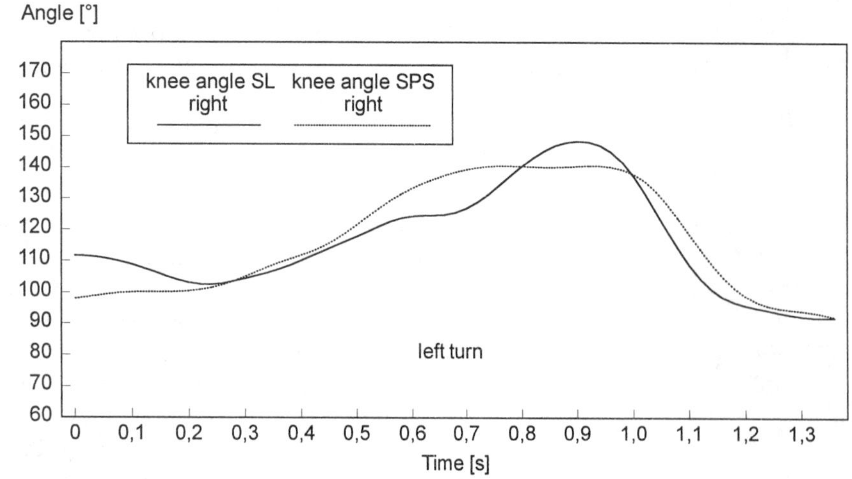

FIG. 40–9. Comparison of the knee angle from the elite athlete: slalom vs. ski-power simulator simulation exercise. (From ref. 9.)

and auditory signal when heel pressure does not reach or exceeds a preset level. Conceptually, too much or too little heel pressure or improper timing of heel pressure results in poor skiing performance. In the early 1980s, measuring pressure distribution within a ski boot was not feasible, but today it is; further progress in in-boot pressure measurements with real-time feedback will continue to be made.

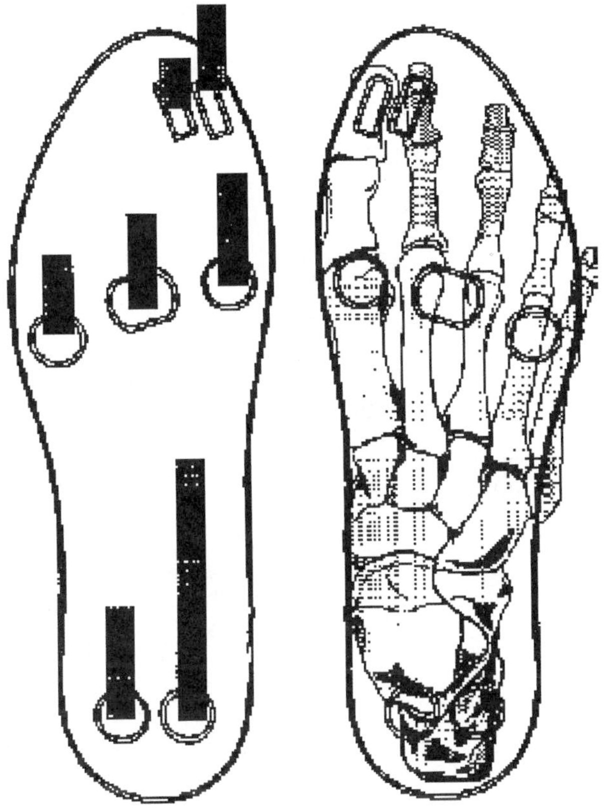

FIG. 40–10. Location of the pressure transducers used by elite skiers. (From ref. 9.)

BIOMECHANICS OF CROSS-COUNTRY SKIING

Modern-day cross-country skiing incorporates two distinct styles, traditional (classic) and freestyle (skating), with separate races held for each. The skiing movement in both techniques can be distinguished by two distinct phases—propulsion and gliding. These phases are often difficult to delineate, since cross-country skiing is a dynamic movement in which one phase flows into another. A third phase, recovery, is sometimes described within the gliding phase. Variables such as displacement cycle velocity, cycle length, cycle rate, duration of different phases, and joint and segment angular displacement and velocity are discussed in this section. The kinetic variables of ski and pole forces, measures of power, work, and energy are also addressed.

Classic Cross-Country Skiing

Movement Phases of the Diagonal Stride

The diagonal stride is the backbone of classic technique and consists of alternating kick and gliding with a single pole movement from the arm opposite the kicking leg in tracks parallel to the direction of travel. The movement

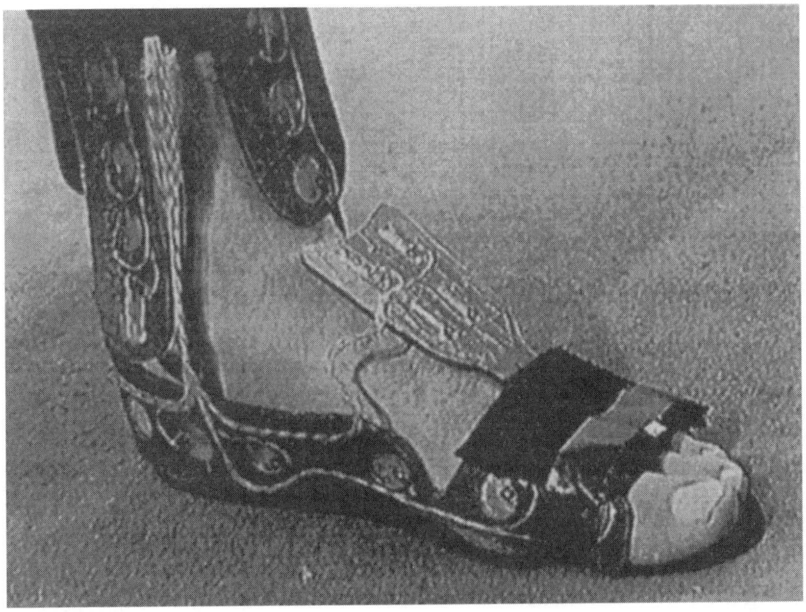

FIG. 40–11. The measuring sock mounted on the foot. (From ref. 9.)

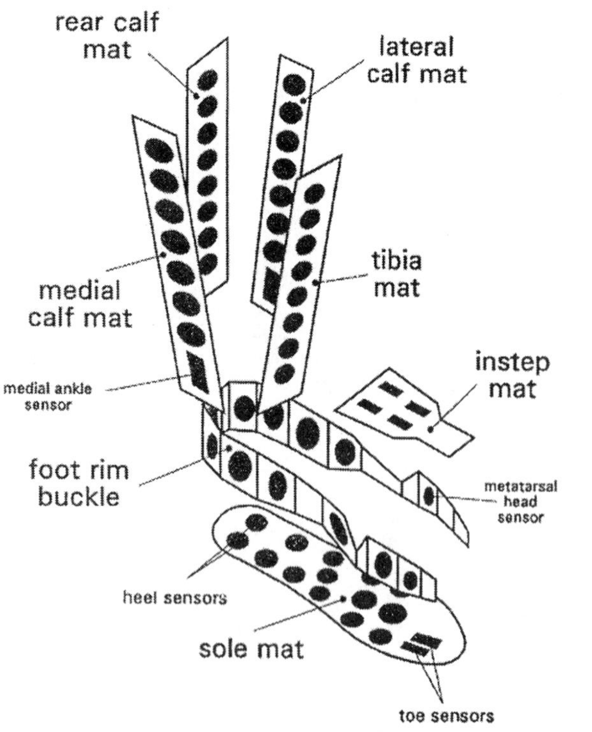

FIG. 40–12. The different parts of the measuring sock, with location of the 64 transducers. (From ref. 9.)

coordination is similar to walking with an arm swing. Several studies have quantified this technique as a percentage of each phase in a cycle. Roy and Barbeau (10) reported values for the propulsive phase (simultaneous arm and leg propulsions) varying between 22% and 27% of the full cycle, depending on skiing speed (Fig. 40–13).

Norman and Roy (11) reported values of 24% for the same phase on some world-class skiers. Bilodeau and colleagues (12) reported a value of 26% for the propulsive phase on flat terrain, and a value of 36% on uphill (5%). Dufek and Bates (13) reported values of 26% on flat terrain and 32% on an uphill section for the propulsive phase of two elite skiers. However, Marino and colleagues (14), Komi and colleagues (15), and Gagnon (16) obtained higher values. Marino and colleagues obtained values of 50% for the propulsive phase. Unfortunately, this phase was not well defined in their study. Komi and colleagues reported values varying between 36% and 48% of the cycle, while Gagnon (16) reported a propulsive phase of 44% of the cycle. This wide variation among these reported values could be due to the lack of consensus among researchers about the duration of the propulsive phase.

The gliding phase, during which no propulsion occurs, includes the skier's recovery from the previous push of the arm and/or the leg. In theory, a longer gliding phase will permit the skier to recover physiologically for a longer period of time (17). Norman and Roy (11) reported the gliding phase duration to be 30% of a full cycle and Komi and colleagues (15) reported a gliding phase lasting 27% of the cycle. Bilodeau and colleagues (12) observed a gliding phase of 30% on flat terrain and 16% on a slight uphill (5%). Others have reported values of 12% to 17% (14,16). Waser (18) noted that among world-class skiers participating at the 1978 World Championships in Lahti, Finland, the fastest skiers had a longer gliding phase than their slower counterparts. Again, the wide variability between the reported values may be due to the different definitions of the pure gliding phase among researchers, and to a lesser extent the difference in performance levels between skiers of these studies, as well as variable snow conditions between studies.

The moment between the pole plant and the beginning of the propulsion of the contralateral leg has been called the pole-assisted glide. In that period, only one pole propels the skier in the forward direction. In some studies, this phase of pole-assisted glide represented 46% of the full cycle (11,16). Bilodeau and colleagues (12) reported a value of 44% on flat terrain and 49%

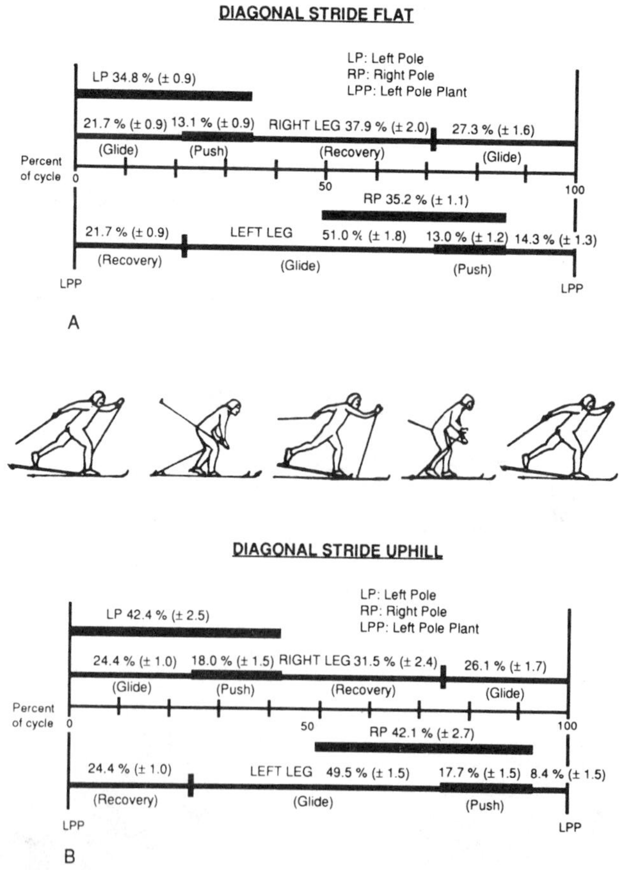

FIG. 40–13. Schematic illustration of the diagonal stride on flat **(A)** and uphill **(B)** terrain. The *thick lines* represent the propulsive phases; the *narrow lines* represent the glide on each leg. All values are mean ± SD. (From ref. 12.)

on uphill. Komi and colleagues (15) did not cite the duration of this propulsion, but from their data it can be estimated at around 46% of the total cycle. Marino and colleagues (14) obtained a phase of pole-assisted glide of 33%. It is important to note that the faster skiers during the 1978 World Championships in Finland had a shorter pole plant phase than slower skiers (18). The small variation in this phase may be accounted for by a more generally agreed upon definition of this phase among researchers.

Velocity, Cycle Length, and Cycle Rate in Classic Skiing

Diagonal Stride on Flat Terrain

Some of the earlier biomechanical studies of cross-country skiing originated from Switzerland and used films of world-class skiers during races. These studies investigated the relationships between cycle length and/or cycle rate with velocity. Cycle length is defined as the distance the body travels during each complete cycle of movement, while cycle rate is the number of times the body moves through a complete cycle during 1 second. Soliman (19) analyzed the diagonal stride technique on flat terrain and found a high correlation between cycle length and velocity. He suggested that increasing the cycle length would improve performance. Waser and Denoth (20) also observed that faster skiers had longer cycle lengths than slower skiers, and noted that fast skiers had greater forward lean than slow skiers, similar to the results of Waser (18). Dillman and colleagues (21) also observed that cycle length was more highly correlated with performance than cycle rate.

Similar analyses were also performed during racing. During the 1978 World Championships 15-km race, Norman and Komi (22) analyzed world-class cross-country skiers on flat terrain (an incline of 1.6%). Results demonstrated that the top 10 skiers were about 4.7% faster than those ranked between the 30th and 60th positions. The first group achieved this faster speed with an 8.2% longer cycle length and 3.4% lower cycle rate. Comparing world-class and recreational skiers, Norman and colleagues (23) observed that skilled skiers skied at a 16.3% faster velocity than the unskilled and achieved this velocity with a 26.0% longer cycle length and a 7.7% lower cycle rate. It was concluded that elite skiers consistently obtained longer glide per stride and greater cycle length, probably due to higher leg swing and greater use of gravitation force as a supplement to muscle force in the leg swing. In another study, Bilodeau and colleagues (12) also proposed that all skiers should focus on skiing with long cycle length instead of increasing tempo on flat or slightly uphill terrain. The correlation between cycle length and velocity on flat terrain was $r = 0.90$, and between cycle rate and velocity $r = -0.45$. Roy and Barbeau (10) noted that both cycle length and cycle rate increased by 16% while increasing speed. It was the increased pure gliding phase (85%) that contributed most to the increase in cycle length, however. The same conclusion appears to apply for female skiers, as India (24) observed that faster skiers used longer cycle lengths and lower cycle rates than slower skiers. Marino and colleagues (14) studied the different phases of the diagonal stride in nine international-caliber female cross-country skiers, during the 10-km race of the 1979 North American Championships. Once again, cycle length was highly correlated to velocity while cycle rate was not ($r = 0.84$ and $r = 0.14$, respectively).

Diagonal Stride on Uphill Terrain

Studies on uphill terrain show a consistent relationship between cycle length, but not cycle rate, and performance and/or cycle velocity. Haberli (25) found that cycle length was the crucial factor determining ski performance on uphills. The best skiers exhibited longer cycle length than slower skiers. Martin (26) also found a high correlation between cycle length and performance, and suggested that cycle length would best result from emphasis on lengthening pole and thrust phase distances. Furthermore, Bilodeau and colleagues (12) proposed that all skiers should focus on skiing with a long cycle length instead of increasing tempo on a slight uphill (5%). The correlation coefficient between cycle length and cycle velocity on uphill terrain was $r = 0.70$, while the correlation coefficient between cycle rate and velocity was $r = 0.56$. Bilodeau and colleagues (27) also obtained significant correlations between race velocity and cycle length on an incline of 7% uphill over several laps, while the relationships between race velocity and cycle rate were not significant. On a slightly steeper uphill (incline of 9%), Norman and Komi (22) observed a good correlation between cycle length and performance. The fastest skiers were 12% faster than the second group, with a 9% longer stride and a 3% faster cycle rate. For both groups on the uphill, the average velocity was slower, the cycle length shorter, and the cycle rate faster than observed on flat terrain.

The same type of analysis was performed by Norman and colleagues (28) on 13 world-class cross-country skiers on an 11.8% uphill during the 30-km classic race of the 1988 Calgary Olympic Games. The correlation coefficient between velocity and cycle length was $r = 0.78$, and $r = 0.57$ between velocity and cycle rate. A longer cycle length during uphill skiing is thought to result from a wider range of motion in the hip as well as numerous arm angular positions identified with the fastest skiers (29). These variables were not statistically different between fast and slow groups on flat terrain. Although these studies have shown higher correlations between cycle length and performance (or velocity) than cycle rate and performance (or velocity), cycle rate is the main mechanism used by all skiers in adjusting velocity (30,31).

Double-Pole Technique

Only a few studies have investigated double-pole and kick double-pole techniques. The scarcity of studies pertaining to these techniques is puzzling, since they are often many times faster than the diagonal stride, especially on flat or gradual downhill course sections. The double-pole technique employs the arms and trunk compression for propulsion and is more dependent on cycle rate for higher velocity than diagonal striding (Fig. 40–14). Roy and Barbeau (32) showed an increase in velocity by 20% while double poling resulted in increased cycle rate by 24% and decreased cycle length by 4%. An investigation by Hoffman and colleagues (33) showed that submaximal velocities were controlled by cycle rate; at maximal velocity, velocity was controlled by an increase in cycle rate and a decrease in cycle length. Moreover, Smith (30,31) proposed that faster skiers were double poling at higher tempo than slower skiers. These results suggest that to increase velocity with the double-pole technique, a skier must increase cycle rate. This is in contrast to the diagonal stride, where increases in skiing velocity are primarily accomplished by increasing cycle length.

Kick Double-Pole Technique

The kick double-pole technique, which is a combination of the double-poling motion of the arms and the kick from the diagonal stride, has also been shown to be cycle rate dependent for velocity increases. Andres (34) observed that performance was positively associated with cycle rate; faster skiers were doing the kick double pole at a higher tempo than slower skiers. Smith (35) also observed that elite skiers tend to perform this technique with a relatively constant cycle length, but increased cycle rate across a range of speeds. He also showed a significant correlation coefficient of $r = 0.61$ between cycle rate and velocity and a nonsignificant correlation coefficient of $r = -0.09$ between cycle length and velocity. Roy and Barbeau (32) showed that with a 32% increase in speed, cycle length was increased by only 6%, while cycle rate increased by 23%. These results showed that to increase speed with this technique, a skier must try to increase cycle rate. Smith (30,31) suggested that for the kick double pole, it was cycle rate that was significantly related to performance.

Only two studies have compared the double-pole and kick double-pole techniques under the same experimental conditions. Hoffman and colleagues (33) reported that cycle rate was higher and cycle length shorter for the double pole than for the kick double pole. Maximal velocity was 6% faster with double poling than with kick double pole. Roy and Barbeau (32) also showed that double poling has a higher tempo (faster cycle rate), but a shorter cycle length than the kick double pole, at several velocities. Results of the duration of the various phases and of velocity cycle length and cycle rate for the classic techniques are summarized in Table 40–4.

Ski and Pole Forces in Classic Techniques

The measurements of forces applied to skis and poles are important elements in understanding skiing locomotion patterns. Two instrumentation approaches for determining ski and pole forces during skiing have been reported by Komi (36). The first procedure uses an instrumented platform set under the snow surface, while the second approach uses the mounting of a force plate system attached between the binding and the upper surface of the ski while poling forces are determined with strain gauge instrumented poles.

Most studies have shown that the axial force exerted by the pole represents between 10% and 24% of the skier's body weight, while leg vertical force may be from 1.5 to 2.5 times the skier's body weight (37–40), even though leg propulsion is very short (0.02 to 0.03 s) (37). Ekström (37) also measured a horizontal breaking force of the ski, which represented about 10% of the skier's body weight when the skier glides over the ski, as well as a 10% body weight horizontal propulsive force when the skier initiates the kick.

Komi and Norman (39) examined the phenomenon

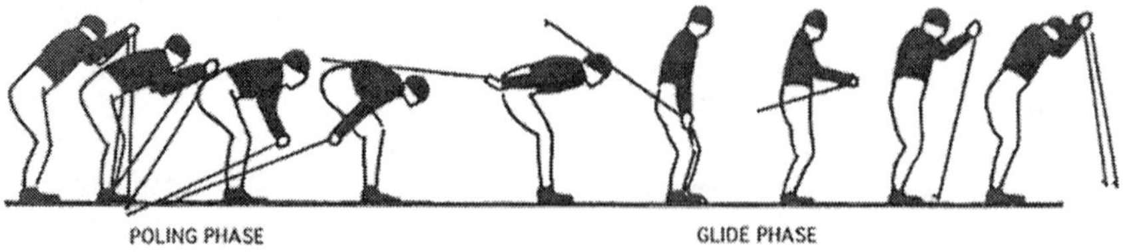

FIG. 40–14. The double-poling cycle began at the pole plant and continued until the next pole plant. The cycle was composed of a poling phase and a glide phase in which the arms and pole swing forward in recovery and preparation for the next poling. Cycle length was determined from the displacement of the body center of mass during the cycle. (From ref. 70.)

TABLE 40–4. *Comparison among different studies of classic cross-country skiing techniques*

Techniques	Propulsion (%)	Gliding (%)	Pole-assisted glide (%)	Velocity (m · s^{-1})	Cycle length (m)	Cycle rate (Hz)
Diagonal stride on flat						
Dillman et al. (1979)	—	25	—	4.64	5.76	0.81
Gagnon (1980)	44*	12	46	—	—	—
Marino et al. (1980)	50*	17	33	3.78	3.82	0.99
Komi et al. (1982)	36–48*	27	46	4.81	5.92	0.82
Norman and Roy (1985)	24	30	46	—	—	—
Dufek and Bates (1987)	26	—	—	—	—	—
Norman and Komi (1987)	—	—	—	4.81	5.60	0.86
Roy and Barbeau (1990)	22	—	—	4.78	5.96	0.81
Bilodeau et al. (1992)	26	30	44	4.75	5.95	0.80
Diagonal stride on uphill						
Dufek and Bates (1987)	32	—	—	—	—	—
Norman and Komi (1987) (5°)	—	—	—	3.93	3.03	1.30
Norman et al. (1989) (12°)	—	—	—	2.57	2.36	1.09
Bilodeau et al. (1992) (5°)	36	16	49	3.79	4.47	0.85
Double-poling						
Roy and Barbeau (1991)	—	—	—	4.84	6.22	0.78
Kick double-poling						
Smith (1985)	42	58	—	5.43	6.81	0.81
Roy and Barbeau (1991)	—	—	—	4.90	7.11	0.69

*Propulsion of arm and leg, until the leg starts its recovery.

of stretch-shortening in cross-country skiing with major emphasis on the phase preceding the leg (ski) thrust in the diagonal stride technique. The skiers were four athletes filmed during the Lahti World Championships in 1978. Based on hip, knee, ankle, and elbow angular velocity curves and observed muscular activity patterns, the authors found that the end of the preloading phase coincided with the peak vertical and propulsive force. Similar results have been observed by Candau and colleagues (41) with the skating technique.

Selection of Techniques During Classic Races

Only one study has looked at technique selection of world-class skiers during a classic race (42). This study analyzed a transition zone from flat terrain to a moderate uphill, during the men's 30-km race at the 1992 Winter Olympic Games. The skiers were divided into three groups depending on their technique at the transition zone video sector. Five skiers used the double pole to make a direct transition to diagonal stride, nine skiers used an early change to diagonal stride, and four skiers involved "casting" (double pole kick) forward with one pole between double poling and diagonal striding. During the transition, mean cycle velocity for double-poling was 5.23 m·s^{-1} compared to 4.24 m·s^{-1} for diagonal striding and 4.58 m·s^{-1} for casting. Cycle rates were similar for each technique, but mean cycle length for double poling was 5.87 m compared to 4.88 m for diagonal striding and 5.27 m for casting. Mean center of mass height change was 0.26 m for double poling, 0.10 m for diagonal striding, and 0.12 m for casting. The authors suggested that the energy cost of double poling may be greater than for the other techniques, but it is probably advantageous to use because of the greater average velocity through the transition zone.

CROSS-COUNTRY SKI SKATING

Since the advent of the skating technique, the race pace of the world's best skiers during classic skiing has remained fairly constant at about 2:50 min·km^{-1}, while skating pace has improved to 2:30 min·km^{-1} (43). Several investigations have been conducted to explain the speed differences between these techniques. The overwhelming number of studies pertaining to the biomechanics of the skating techniques of cross-country skiing are temporal or kinematic studies.

Several skating techniques have been employed and refined over the years. For the purpose of this review, each technique is described. The three most commonly used skating techniques are the V-1, the V-2, and the V-2 alternate, while the marathon skate and the diagonal V-skate are not used with regularity. The V-1 skating technique (also called "offset" or "paddle dance") has nonsymmetrical leg strides with asymmetric pole plants every other ski stride and is typically used on moderate to steep uphills, or on flat terrain when snow drag is high (such as in cold temperature conditions). The V-2 technique (also called "1-skate" or "double dance") has a double symmetrical pole plant for each leg stride, and is used on a cross-section of flat terrain and slight uphills. The V-2 alternate technique (also called "2-skate," "open-field skate," "gunde skate," or "single dance") has a double symmetrical pole plant for two leg strides, and is used on flat terrain, slight downhill, and, in fast snow conditions, slight uphills. The timing of the pole plant is the primary distinguishing characteristic between techniques. With V-1, the pole plant is in time with the skating step, while the pole plant precedes the skating step in the V-2 and V-2 alternate.

Within the technical bag of tricks of elite skiers there are intermediate techniques within the continuum between V-1 and V-2 alternate. These hybrid techniques are often employed in slow snow conditions or on course inclines where either technique (V-1 or V-2 alternate) would not be the fastest choice. One such technique, which is not discussed here, is the Alsgaard skate, a hybrid between V-1 and V-2 alternate developed by Thomas Alsgaard. This technique times the pole plants much closer to the first skate step and has a much more upright position than the V-2 alternate.

The first technique to appear on the ski scene was the marathon skate (also called the Siitonen step), which involves skiing with one ski in the tracks while simultaneously pushing laterally with one ski and double poling. This technique is used primarily on flat and slightly downhill terrain, when the set diagonal tracks are faster than the skating track. The diagonal V-skate is used only for very steep uphills and involves skating with a single pole plant for each leg stride. This technique is not used too frequently because the velocity that can be attained with this is too low for high-level competition.

Movement Phases

Marathon Skate

This technique was first used at the end of the 1960s by Pauli Siitonen of Finland during ultramarathon ski races. The marathon skate did not appear on the World Cup circuit until 1982, however, when American skier Bill Koch used that technique to win 4 of the 10 World Cup races. Only one study has investigated the propulsive and gliding phases of the marathon skate technique. In this study, Smith (35) observed that the poling phase across four different effort levels varied between 25% and 28% of the cycle, while the skating phase varied between 12% and 15% of the cycle. The gliding phase varied between 59% and 63% of the cycle.

V-1

Several studies have examined the temporal phases of the V-1 technique. Due to a lack of consensus among researchers about the beginning and the end of the phases, however, interpretation across studies is difficult. Many studies define the skating phase as the time period when the skate is in contact with the snow, while others have tried to distinguish between glide and actual propulsion. Since ski skating is a dynamic movement, this distinction is difficult to make without force measurements. The phases of each study discussed below are defined.

The first study to analyze the V-1 technique was by Pinchak and colleagues (44), who measured two phases (recovery and gliding/propulsive phases) during snow skiing and roller skiing on pavement. The recovery phase lasted from the moment the ski was lifted from the snow/ground until it regained contact with the snow/ground, while the gliding/propulsion phase was the moment the ski was in contact with the snow/ground. The authors reported a recovery phase for the V-1 on snow between 48% and 54% of the cycle, while the gliding/propulsion phase lasted between 46% and 52% of the cycle. These values changed to 41% to 43% for the recovery phase, and to 57% to 59% for the gliding/propulsion phase on roller skis. The values were significantly different between snow skiing and roller skiing.

Smith and co-workers (45–48) performed several investigations on uphill terrain. The first study found that world-class skiers had slightly shorter gliding/propulsive phases than slower skiers (45). The strong- and weak-side poles were involved in propulsion (contact with snow) for 47% and 44% of the cycle, while the total time the strong- and weak-side legs were in contact with the snow represented 46% and 53%, respectively, of the cycle (Fig. 40–15).

In subsequent studies, Smith (46,47) found that cycle times consistently decreased as velocity increased, results that he confirmed the following year. Smith (47) also reported that the poling phase remained relatively constant across velocities, involving 47% and 43% of full cycle, while the skating motion covered 62% and 66% of the cycle (strong- and weak-sides, respectively). Furthermore, Smith and Nelson (48) found that cycle phase percentages were relatively constant across the three intensities, even though cycle times were significantly shorter.

The function of the legs in V-1 skating appears to be primarily to support the body and to induce lateral motion, while the function of the upper body is primarily propulsive in the forward direction. Smith (47) calculated a propulsive value of the arms and trunk of 66% for the total propulsive forces in the forward direction during uphill V-1 skiing. A study performed by Street (49) examined the forces generated by cross-country skiers during performance of the V-1 technique on roller skis. He found that propulsive forces existed throughout 90% of the cycle as a result of the staggering of the poling and skating phases. He also observed that the skating thrust was about 70% longer than in diagonal stride, and the skating forces remained unchanged across velocities.

Smith and colleagues (50) analyzed the V-1 technique during Olympic competitions on moderate and steep uphills, to examine changes occurring with slope. The

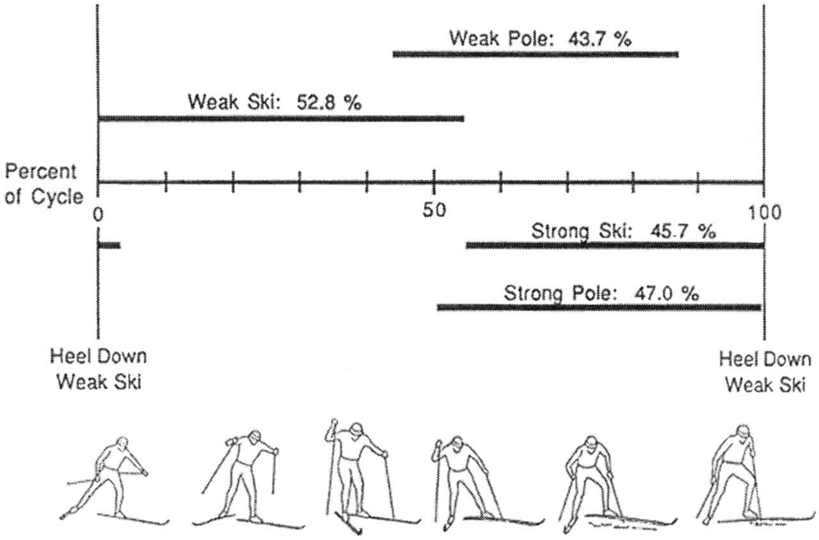

FIG. 40–15. The V-1 skating cycle begins with heel-down of the weak-side skate and continues with poling and strong-side skate phases. Completion of the cycle occurs with the subsequent weak-side heel-down. (From ref. 45.)

two filming sites were a moderate uphill of about 6% to 7% and a steeper uphill of about 10% to 11%. On the moderate hill, they observed that the weak-side arm pushed for 38% of the cycle, while the strong-side arm pushed for 40%. They obtained values of 60% and 53% for the gliding/propulsive phase of the cycle for the weak- and strong-sides legs. On the steeper uphill, they obtained 48% and 49% for the weak- and strong-side arms, while the relative duration for the weak- and strong-side legs were 60% and 57% of the cycle. Similar results have been observed on steep uphill by female skiers during the 20-km skating race, with the exception that females skiers used their strong-side pole more extensively than their male counterparts. It was thus concluded that for male skiers, on the steeper hill, the poling phases (as percentage of the cycle) tended to be longer, whereas the skating phases (legs) tended to be either equal or longer. The recovery phases on the steeper terrain tended to be shorter than on the moderate uphill.

The study by Bilodeau and colleagues (12) is unique in the way the authors calculated the total propulsion coming from both legs. In most studies, it was assumed that leg propulsion was taking place as soon as the ski was set on the snow. The total time a ski is in contact with the snow contains both a gliding as well as a propulsive phase, however. Bilodeau and colleagues defined the gliding phase as the moment the ski touched the snow until the beginning of the knee extension, while the propulsive phase was considered to last from that moment until the ski was lifted from the snow. Using these definitions, they reported relative durations of the total propulsive and gliding phases on flat terrain of 48% and 46%; on a slight uphill, these values were 54% and 36%, respectively. The strong- and weak-side arms were involved for 25% and 24% on flat, while on uphill, arm involvement reached 35% and 29%, respectively. The strong- and weak-side legs were in contact with the snow for 57% and 61% for level skiing, and for 60% for both strong- and weak-side legs on uphill terrain (Fig. 40–16).

The estimates using this technique must be interpreted with caution because the skating movement is dynamic; to distinguish between gliding and propulsion without actual force measurements may underestimate the propulsive phase. Additionally, Humphreys and colleagues (51) compared the movement patterns of successful and unsuccessful female Olympic competitors. Ten female participants in the 1992 Winter Olympic Games were filmed V-1 skating on a gradual uphill during the 30-km race. Five of these skiers finished in the top 12 positions, while the other five finished in the bottom 15. It was observed that the best skiers used the trunk and the weak-side leg more extensively than the slower five skiers. From this study, it was concluded that the most successful female Olympic competitors were able to maintain a higher race velocity by achieving a substantially longer cycle length, which was accomplished in part by a more extensive involvement of the trunk and the weak-side leg.

V-2

Two studies have investigated the relative proportion of recovery and gliding/propulsion phases of the V-2

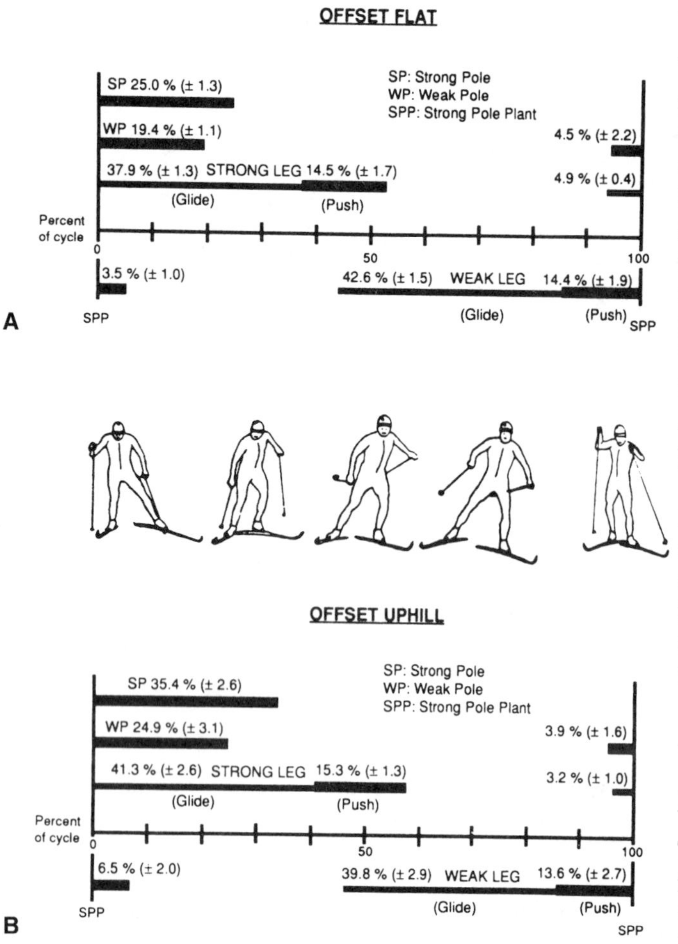

FIG. 40–16. Schematic illustration of the offset on flat (**A**) and uphill (**B**) terrain. (From ref. 12.)

technique. Pinchak and colleagues (44) analyzed the basic differences between the various phases during a complete cycle with the V-2 technique skiing on snow and roller skiing. On snow, the recovery period lasted 45% and the gliding/propulsion phase lasted 55%, while on roller skis these phases represented 46% and 54%, respectively. Bilodeau and colleagues (12) compared the relative duration of the propulsive and gliding phases between the three most commonly used skating techniques (V-1, V-2, V-2 alternate). At approximately 80% of maximal skiing speed on flat terrain, the phases for the V-2 did not show any significant difference with the V-2 alternate; the propulsive phase of the V-2 was significantly shorter than the corresponding phase of the V-1, while the pure gliding phase was slightly longer than the same phase of V-1. The propulsive and the gliding phases for the V-2 represented 45% and 55% of the cycle on flat terrain, while on a slight uphill the same phases were 52% and 48% of the cycle.

V-2 Alternate

The relative proportion of the propulsive and gliding phases with the V-2 alternate has been found to be quite similar to that found with the V-2 technique. Bilodeau and colleagues (12) found that the propulsive and gliding phases with the V-2 alternate on flat terrain represented 46% and 54% of the full cycle, respectively, values not statistically different from those of the V-2. On uphill terrain, the corresponding phases for the V-2 alternate were both equal to half the duration of the cycle. When comparing the V-2 alternate and the V-1 on both flat and uphill terrain, the propulsive phase was not different between the techniques, while the gliding phase was longer for the V-2 alternate.

Smith and Heagy (52) studied the V-2 alternate technique of Olympic cross-country skiers on flat terrain during the 50-km skating race. They reported that the skating phase represented about 55% of the cycle, while the poling phase represented about 20% of the full cycle; that last value is quite similar to the poling value obtained by Bilodeau and colleagues (12).

Velocity, Cycle Length, and Cycle Rate

Marathon Skate

The first study to investigate the marathon skate examined kinematic characteristics at four intensities (35). Observations demonstrated relatively constant cycle lengths across a range of speeds whereby increases of speed were produced by higher tempo skiing; in fact, cycle length decreased slightly at higher intensities. The author observed that the correlation between cycle length and velocity was nonsignificant ($r = 0.19$), whereas the correlation coefficient between cycle rate and velocity was 0.59. Later, Gervais and Wronko (53) investigated the similarity in the marathon skate technique with two dry-land training devices (roller skates and skating roller skis) and skating on snow. They showed that significant differences were found between the means for the roller skis and skis for both cycle length and time. The data revealed that the roller skis covered a proportionally greater distance during propulsion when compared to skis and roller skates. It was also observed that both dry-land devices failed to simulate skiing on all the movement characteristics investigated.

V-1

The V-1 technique, used across a wide variety of terrain, has been the most dominant skating technique in cross-country skiing (45,54). For this reason, several studies have been devoted to V-1.

Several studies have shown a strong relationship between V-1 cycle length and velocity or performance (12,27,45,48,51,55–57). Thus, faster skiers have longer cycle lengths than slower skiers when using V-1. Correlation coefficients between cycle length and velocity for flat and slightly uphill terrain range between $r = 0.76$ and $r = 0.92$ (12,27,45,56,57). Humphreys and colleagues (51) found a high correlation between cycle length and velocity for female Olympic skiers. They demonstrated that the fastest skiers used the weak-side leg to a greater extent that slower skiers, as measured by the range of motion (ROM) at the knee. Weak-side knee extension was greater, and a more complete flexion of the trunk during propulsion was observed on the faster skiers. Supporting this observation, Gregory and colleagues (58) also observed greater trunk flexion, weak-side elbow flexion, and weak-side knee flexion in faster female skiers. Faster and slower skiers typically have a similar tempo; hence, V-1 cycle rates are not highly associated with velocity.

Some studies have shown that cycle rate can be a major factor in increasing velocity under certain circumstances (33,47–49). For example, Street (49) reported that at slow to moderate velocities, the subjects tended to ski faster by increasing both cycle length and cycle rate. This was similar to the results obtained on roller skis by Hoffman and colleagues (33). At maximal velocities, however, cycle length reached a plateau, and any further increases in velocity were generally accomplished by increasing cycle rate. It is interesting to note that Smith and colleagues (50) found that for male skiers in uphills, increases in velocity were performed by increasing both cycle length and cycle rate, while for females only cycle rate seemed to govern velocity.

Velocities, cycle lengths, and cycle rates have also been studied over different terrains and/or uphill grades. From flat to uphill terrain, velocities are diminished, cycle lengths are shorter, and cycle rates tend to increase (12,50,59). Boulay and colleagues (56) also found a decrease in velocity and a shorter cycle length as grade increases, but thetdid not find any change in cycle rate as the hill gets steeper. Velocities of skiers in that study were approximately a 5-km race pace.

V-2

To date, little emphasis has been given to kinematics of the V-2 technique, even though V-2 is thought to be best suited to flat and slightly uphill terrain. It has been noted that the V-2 technique is the most predominant skating technique for biathlon ski racing, while the V-1 is greatly emphasized in cross-country skiing (54,60,61). These researchers proposed that the discrepancy between the techniques and ski disciplines is probably due to the rifle carried during biathlon races. With the V-2 technique, little direction and speed change is observed compared to the V-1 technique, which would result in reduced energy cost of rifle carriage (61). Cycle rate of V-2 was lower (0.55 Hz) than for V-1 (0.83 Hz).

Bilodeau and colleagues (12) investigated the biomechanical parameters of several skating techniques. Correlation coefficients for velocity and cycle length on flat terrain was $r = 0.91$, and $r = -0.57$ for velocity and cycle rate. On a slight uphill (5%), the corresponding correlation coefficients were $r = 0.68$ for velocity and cycle length, and $r = 0.23$ for velocity and cycle rate. Boulay and colleagues (56) also found a strong relationship between cycle length and velocity ($r = 0.96$), and no correlation between cycle rate and velocity.

V-2 Alternate

The first study to look at this technique was by Bilodeau and colleagues (12). The authors measured velocity, cycle length, and cycle rate. On flat terrain, they found a good correlation ($r = 0.97$) between velocity and cycle length, and a significant negative correlation between velocity and cycle rate ($r = -0.74$). On a slight uphill of 5%, the correlation coefficient between velocity and cycle length was $r = 0.96$, while it was only $r = -0.53$ between cycle rate and velocity. This suggests that skiers should try to focus on skiing with long cycle lengths instead of increasing tempo on flat and slightly uphill terrain when using the V-2 alternate. Smith and Heagy (52) also showed that for Olympic cross-country skiers during the 50-km race of the Albertville Games in 1992, velocity during V-2 alternate skiing was strongly related to cycle length ($r = 0.76$), but not to cycle rate. The authors concluded that faster skiers skated with longer cycle length and more knee extension during the skating stroke than did slower skiers. A strong correlation ($r = 0.97$) between cycle length and velocity, but not cycle rate, was also found by Boulay and colleagues (56).

Comparisons Between the Skating Techniques

Only a few studies have compared skating techniques under similar experimental conditions. The first study performed was by Bilodeau and colleagues (12), who compared the V-1, V-2, and V-2 alternate techniques on flat and slightly uphill terrain. For all techniques and for both terrains, it was found that cycle length was the major determinant of velocity, while cycle rate had almost no relation to velocity. No significant difference in velocity was observed between the techniques at the same perceived effort. The longest cycle lengths were observed with the V-2 technique, while V-1 had the fastest cycle rates; these results are in accordance with those of Boulay and colleagues (56) (Fig. 40–17).

Street (54) also found that the V-2 had a lower cycle rate than V-1, but the upper body was found to have a slightly longer (by 23%) recovery period for the V-1 technique. Recovery time between pole phases were approximately 0.78 s for the V-1, and only 0.63 s for the V-2. Boulay and colleagues (56) also found no sig-

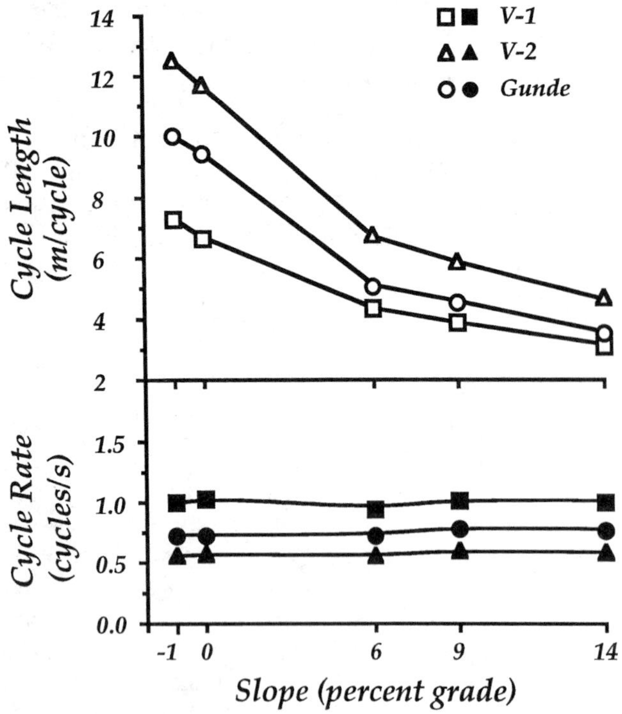

FIG. 40–17. Evolution of cycle length and cycle rate with slope variation. Cycle length and cycle rate were always different between techniques ($p < .01$). Across terrain, cycle length differences were significant ($p < .01$) except between 6% and 9% (all techniques) and between −1% and 0% (Gunde and V-2). Across terrains, cycle rates were similar. (From ref. 56.)

nificant differences in velocity between the V-1, V-2, and V-2 alternate on a slight downhill (−1%), flat, and uphill (6%) terrains. At steeper inclines (9% to 10%), however, the V-1 technique was significantly faster than the other two techniques. Results of the duration of the various phases and of velocity, cycle length, and cycle rate for the skating techniques are summarized in Table 40–5 for flat terrain, and in Table 40–6 for uphill terrain.

OTHER BIOMECHANICAL ASPECTS OF SKATING TECHNIQUES

Aro and colleagues (59) compared the V-1 skating technique of Olympic skiers on moderate (5% to 6%) and steep (10% to 11%) uphill terrain during the men's 50-km and women's 20- km events at the 1988 Calgary Olympics. They found that on the steeper grade, both men and women significantly increased cycle rate, strong-side ski edging angle, strong- and weak-side ski angle (with respect to the forward direction), stance width, and forward step displacement. Both groups decreased lateral displacement of the center of mass, cycle length, and velocity. Several studies of V-2 alternate during Olympic competitions from the 1992 Albertville Games were done by Smith and co-workers. On the first project, Smith and Heagy (52) studied the V-2 alternate on flat terrain and found that the technique involved substantial trunk flexion as well as arm and knee extension. They observed that the fastest skiers skated with more knee extension during the skating stroke than did slower skiers. They also proposed that a flat ski during the early part of each skating stroke would be advantageous, because a flat ski will glide with less drag than when it is edged. This feature is more easily attained while skiing on flat than on uphill terrain. Contrary to the belief that maintaining the skis flat to the snow surface is advantageous for enhancing glide, however, Smith and Heagy (62) found that the skis were set down on the snow nearly flat and immediately began increasing their angle with respect to the surface until the completion of the skating stroke. Mean set-down angles were similar for both fast and slow skiers. Contrary to conventional understanding of the skating stroke, no flat ski gliding was observed for any skier in this study. These results suggested that factors other than ski edging are primary determinants of ski glide.

A final study from the same group investigated if aligning the toe, knee, and nose (a common coaching suggestion) would help in flat ski placement, thus enhancing glide and ski speed (63). From a frontal plane, the authors found that no significant differences were found between fast and slow skiers on several angles measured (ski edging angles, toe-head, toe-shoulder, toe-knee-shoulder, toe-knee-head, toe-center of mass, and toe-knee-hip). The skiers were significantly more vertical in their head-toe alignment on the poling side (2.3%) than on the nonpoling side (5.1%), with both angles indicating lean toward the nongliding side. At ski set-down, a vertical line rises from the toe to a point between the shoulder and the head. This indicates that elite skiers are not quite vertically aligning toe to head at glide initiation, but instead they are leaning slightly toward the nongliding side. This may be associated with less lateral motion, perhaps in an attempt to minimize center of mass motion or to increase cycle rate. These findings suggest that a reevaluation of the toe-knee-head-alignment coaching suggestion may be in order. These measurements were made at a velocity close to maximal, however, and in a situation where the athletes tried to ski as fast as possible; during training at slow velocity, the toe-knee-head alignment should probably be enforced to improve stability and help increase the length of the gliding phase.

Candau and colleagues (41) examined the occurrence of the stretch-shortening cycle in the V-2 alternate technique. They found that the stretch-shortening cycle occurred during a skating cycle in the knee and ankle joints. These stretch-shortening cycles are more economical than activities including pure concentric contractions. Similar observations have been reported for the diagonal stride technique by Komi and Norman (39).

TABLE 40–5. *Comparison among different studies of cross-country skiing skating techniques on flat terrain*

Techniques	Propulsion arm (%)	Propulsion leg (%)	Propulsion total (%)	Gliding (%)	Velocity ($m \cdot s^{-1}$)	Cycle length (m)	Cycle rate (Hz)
V-1							
Street (1990)	—	—	—	—	6.14	6.60	0.93
Bilodeau et al. (1992)	19	32	48	46	5.84	7.19	0.81
Gregory et al. (1994)[a]	25	59	—	—	5.60	6.67	0.84
Gregory et al. (1994)[b]	27	59	—	—	5.30	6.46	0.82
Boulay et al. (1995)	—	—	—	—	6.76	6.61	1.02
Boulay et al. (1995) (−1°)	—	—	—	—	7.15	7.27	0.98
V-2							
Bilodeau et al. (1992)	29	27	45	55	5.89	8.69	0.98
Boulay et al. (1995)	—	—	—	—	6.68	11.70	0.57
Boulay et al. (1995) (−1°)	—	—	—	—	6.99	12.51	0.56
V-2 alternate							
Bilodeau et al. (1992)	19	33	46	54	5.79	8.18	0.71
Smith and Heagy (1994)	20	55	—	—	6.32	9.41	0.67
Boulay et al. (1995)	—	—	—	—	6.68	9.44	0.71
Boulay et al. (1995) (−1°)	—	—	—	—	7.03	10.02	0.70
Marathon skating							
Smith (1985)	—	—	—	—	6.06	6.63	0.91

[a]Fast skiers (top 26).
[b]Slow skiers (28th to 49th).
Arm propulsion = average propulsion for both arms.
Leg propulsion = average propulsion for both legs.

TABLE 40–6. *Comparison among different studies of cross-country skiing skating techniques on uphill terrain*

Techniques	Propulsion arm (%)	Propulsion leg (%)	Propulsion total (%)	Gliding (%)	Velocity ($m \cdot s^{-1}$)	Cycle length (m)	Cycle rate (Hz)
V-1							
Smith et al. (1988) (7°)	45	49	53	37	3.23	3.84	0.84
Smith and Nelson (1988) (7°)	39	60	—	—	4.08	4.34	0.95
Smith (1989) (ref. 47) (8°) 45	64	—	—	—	—	—	
Smith et al. (1989) (10–11°)	49	58	61	31	2.40	2.99	0.81
Aro et al. (1990) (5–6°)	—	—	—	—	3.15	4.23	0.75
Aro et al. (1990) (10–11°)	—	—	—	—	2.50	3.11	0.81
Bilodeau et al. (1992) (5°)	25	35	54	36	4.62	5.19	0.89
Boulay et al. (1995) (3°)	—	—	—	—	4.23	4.52	0.94
Boulay et al. (1995) (4°)	—	—	—	—	3.85	3.87	0.99
Boulay et al. (1995) (6°)	—	—	—	—	3.11	3.09	1.01
Rundell and McCarthy (1996) (11–12°)	—	—	—	—	2.13	2.58	0.83
V-2							
Bilodeau et al. (1992) (5°)	37	36	52	48	4.58	6.19	0.74
Boulay et al. (1995) (3°)	—	—	—	—	4.25	7.73	0.55
Boulay et al. (1995) (4°)	—	—	—	—	3.46	5.85	0.59
Boulay et al. (1995) (6°)	—	—	—	—	2.81	4.71	0.60
V-2 alternate							
Bilodeau et al. (1992) (5°)	28	35	50	50	4.45	5.87	0.76
Boulay et al. (1995) (3°)	—	—	—	—	4.08	5.69	0.72
Boulay et al. (1995) (4°)	—	—	—	—	3.42	4.51	0.76
Boulay et al. (1995) (6°)	—	—	—	—	2.74	3.54	0.77

Arm propulsion = average propulsion for both arms.
Leg propulsion = average propulsion for both legs.

In another study examining economy of rifle carriage in biathlon skiing, Rundell and Szmedra (61) found that a longer cycle length resulted in lower energy cost of rifle carriage. Additionally, Kammermeier and colleagues (64) demonstrated that ski skating economy was related to upper body power as well as cycle length.

During the 1985 World Cup freestyle (skating) race in Biwabik, Minnesota, Street and colleagues (65) examined world-class skiers to determine whether the absolute and relative uphill velocities of two groups of skiers (top 20 skiers and skiers between 30th and 50th place) were different. This group examined uphill velocity on three laps to determine whether the faster and slower skiers paced themselves differently across the three race laps. Results indicated that the faster skiers skied up the hill at a higher absolute velocity (5.08 $m \cdot s^{-1}$) than the slower skiers (4.77 $m \cdot s^{-1}$). However, both groups ascended the hill at the same relative velocity, 78% to 79% of average race velocity. As a group, all skiers had both a higher absolute (5.00 $m \cdot s^{-1}$) and relative velocity (79.7%) on lap 1 than on lap 3 (4.86 $m \cdot s^{-1}$ and 77.6%). When the skiers were divided into fast and slow groups, it became evident that the faster skiers maintained a relatively uniform velocity across all three laps, while the slower skiers ascended the hill at a faster velocity on lap 1 than on the last two laps. Thus, elite skiers all decreased their velocities by the same relative amount for a given uphill; within these top 50 skiers, however, the faster skiers ascended the uphill at higher absolute velocities.

Gregory and colleagues (58) filmed several female Olympic skiers on flat terrain using the V-1 technique and then divided the skiers according to their performance levels: eight skiers in the top 26 (group 1), and eight skiers placed between 28th and 49th (group 2). They found that cycle rate was not different between the groups (0.84 Hz for group 1 and 0.82 Hz for group 2). Cycle length for both groups was 6.67 and 6.46 m, and cycle velocity was 5.60 vs 5.30 $m \cdot s^{-1}$, respectively. Several kinematic differences were found between groups. Weak-side elbow angles at pole plant and pole release from the snow were different; however, no difference was observed for ROM for the weak-side elbow between the groups or for strong-side elbow positions and ROM. There were no differences in strong-side knee angles between groups, but there was a tendency for the faster skiers to have greater strong-side knee flexion during the initial kick phase of the skating motion. A significantly smaller angle in the mean minimum weak-side knee angles for the faster skiers was evident, and ROM for both strong- and weak-side knees were similar for both groups. The minimum knee angles observed in group 1 confirmed the qualitative observation that faster skiers were in a lower, more crouched body position at the beginning of the skating motion. Although the faster and slower skiers were in a similar upright position at the beginning of the poling motion, the faster skiers ended up in a position of greater trunk flexion during the poling motion. Also, though not significantly different, there was a trend toward greater trunk ROM in the faster skiers. Gregory and colleagues (58) suggested that a greater propulsive force or propulsion for a longer period of time explained the greater skiing velocities. They found that the length of the poling and skating phases, when expressed in time or in percentage of the full cycle, were not different for both groups. Therefore, the difference in the impulse produced between the groups of skiers would be the result of producing a larger force rather than applying that force for a longer period of time. The greater trunk, weak-side elbow, and weak-side knee flexions observed in group 1 might be indicative of this suspected force difference.

Ragache and Thievenaz (66) observed skiers on different sections of the race course during the 1987 World Championships in Oberstdorf, Germany, and they did not find any consistency between skiers in the utilization of the different skating techniques. They concluded that technique selection was based on individual choice. This observation was confirmed by Bilodeau and colleagues (67), who did not find any significant physiologic differences between the three most commonly used skating techniques on several types of terrains. This interpretation, however, should be viewed with caution, because ski technology and refinement of ski technique has improved since these studies were completed.

POLING AND SKIING FORCES WITH THE SKATING TECHNIQUES

Measurements of forces applied to skis and poles during skating have also used the same methods discussed by Komi (36) for the evaluation of the classic techniques. The first study performed on the skating technique was by Pierce and colleagues (40), who measured the forces between the bindings and skis and those applied through the poles of different levels of skiers using the marathon skate. Using this technique, the pole forces represented 18% of body weight, while the forefoot vertical forces reached 125% of body weight. Street (49) and Street and Frederick (68) also examined the forces generated by cross-country skiers during the V-1 technique. A portable force measurement system was installed in both ski poles and one roller ski (Fig. 40–18).

Force data were collected on four skiers as they skated a 7% uphill grade at three different velocities. Results showed that the poles played an important role in propulsion, such that the average peak resultant poling force was 0.45 times the body mass, 2 to 3.5 times larger than those reported for the diagonal stride (36–38,40). Furthermore, the poling forces provided a larger com-

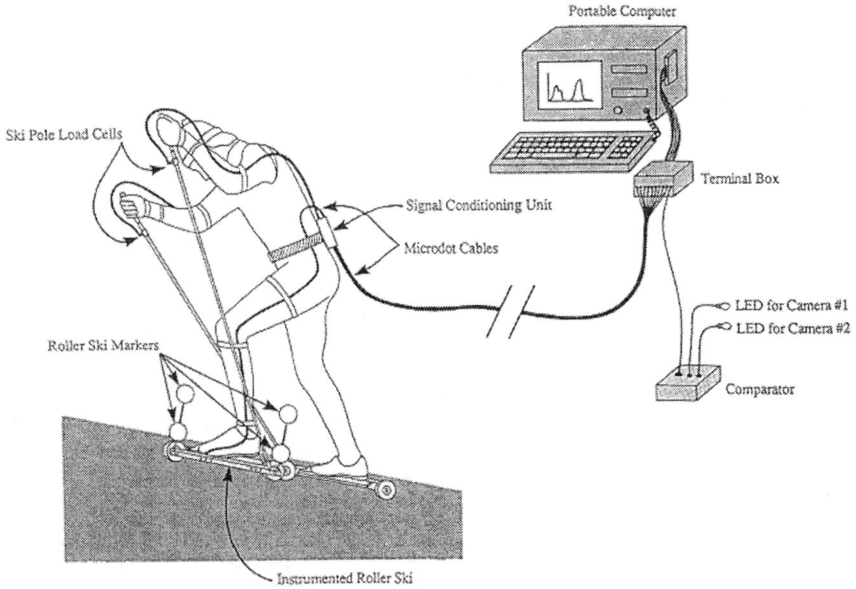

FIG. 40–18. Schematic of the force measurement system. (From ref. 68.)

ponent in the forward direction than the skating forces, even though the resultant skating force was seven times larger than the resultant poling force (Fig. 40–19). This study also indicated that a major function of the skating forces was to support the weight of the skier. The duration of the skating thrust was about 70% longer than in diagonal stride. Additionally, across velocities, poling forces increased and the skating forces remained fairly unchanged, suggesting that poling was the major contributor to forward velocity during V-1. Similar observations have been reported by Smith (46), who analyzed forces generated during a cycle with the V-1 technique. The technique was performed by six skiers on a 9% and a 14% uphill grades at four chosen velocities. Center of mass motion tended to be oriented in a more forward direction at higher velocities and the 9% uphill grade. The peak resultant force of the arms were 0.58 and 0.50 times body mass (strong and weak sides, respectively). Skating peak forces (vertical forces) were 1.48 and 1.27 times body mass for strong and weak legs, respectively. Total propulsive force tended to increase with velocity and also with grade. Smith concluded that the function of the legs in V-1 skating appears to be primarily as support for the body and to induce lateral motion, while the function of the arms is primarily propulsive, as shown by a propulsive value of the arms and trunk representing 66% of the total propulsive forces in the forward direction.

The center of pressure of the skating force was also determined throughout the V-1 skating cycle by Smith (30). He observed that centers of pressure were individually consistent across velocities but exhibited some characteristic differences between skiers and between strong- and weak-side skis. The typical pattern involved an initial center of pressure approximately centered on the ski in the mediolateral direction and near midfoot. As the skating phase progressed, the center of pressure migrated medially in sequence with ski edging and anteriorly during the plantar flexion of the foot near the end of the skating stroke. The center of pressure on the strong-side ski was typically forward by about 10% to 15% of foot length compared with that observed for the weak-side ski. Leppävuori and colleagues (69) tested the forces generated by the legs during a cycle of the V-1 technique on a platform covered by snow. The skier was asked to maintain a constant speed and to adjust his steps to the platform, so that no pole plant was taken while on the platform. Results showed that the maximal force component of the skating kick was about 1.3 times the skier's body weight.

CONCLUSION

The general conclusion from both classic and skating cross-country skiing studies is that, with most techniques (diagonal stride, V-1, V-2, and V-2 alternate), the fastest skiers can generally travel a longer distance during each cycle, while cycle rate is similar between fast and slow skiers. For double poling, kick double poling, and the marathon skate techniques, cycle rate is more important and generally distinguishes skiers of different level of performance better than cycle length.

Comparisons of movement phases of skating and diagonal stride show that the skating techniques have substantially longer phases of propulsion than diagonal stride, and this may partly explain the difference in velocity between these techniques. Additionally, the poling forces are more important with skating, while

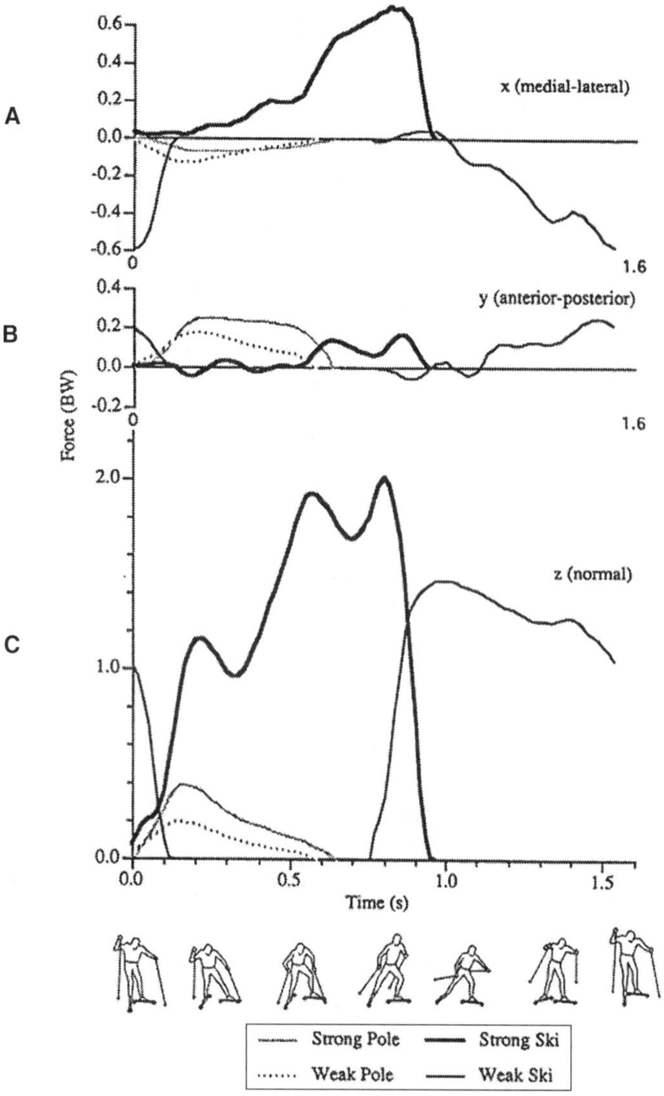

FIG. 40–19. Sample force tracing of the strong- and weak-side poling and skating forces in the (**A**) medial-lateral, (**B**) anterior-posterior (forward direction of progression), and (**C**) superior-inferior (normal to road surface) direction. (From ref. 68.)

skiing forces (leg propulsion) are usually greater with classic skiing.

REFERENCES

1. Mester J. Movement regulation in alpine skiing. In: Müller E, Schwameder H, Kornexl E, Raschner C, eds. *Science and skiing.* London: E & FN Spon (Chapmann & Hall), 1997:333–348.
2. Karlsson J, Erikson A, Forsberg A, Kallberg L, Tesch P. Force development and maximal muscular strength. In: *Physiology of alpine skiing.* Park City, UT: United States Ski Coaches Association, 1978:16–17.
3. Witherell W, Evrard D. *The athletic skier.* Salt Lake City: Athletic Skier, 1978:42–74.
4. Berg HE, Eiken O, Tesch PA. Involvement of eccentric muscle actions in giant slalom racing. *Med Sci Sports Exerc* 1995;27(12):1666–1670.
5. Hintermeister RA, Lange GW, O'Connor DD, Dillamn CJ, Steadman JR. Muscle activity of the inside and outside leg in slalom and giant-slalom skiing. In: Müller E, Schwameder H, Kornexl E, Raschner C, eds. *Science and skiing.* London: E & FN Spon (Chapmann & Hall), 1997:141–149.
6. Drenk V. *Planning, documentation of the supplemental program for using panned, tilted and zooming cameras in peak 3D.* Leipzig, Germany: 1993.
7. Raschner C, Müller E, Schwameder H. Kinematic and kinetic analysis of slalom turns as a basis for the development of specific training methods to improve strength and endurance. In: Müller E, Schwameder H, Kornexl E, Raschner C, eds. *Science and skiing.* London: E & FN Spon (Chapmann & Hall), 1997:151–261.
8. Frick U, Schmidtbleicher D, Raschner C, Müller E. Types of muscle action of leg and hip extensor muscles in slalom. In: Müller E, Schwameder H, Kornexl E, Raschner C, eds. *Science and skiing.* London: E & FN Spon (Chapmann & Hall), 1997:262–271.
9. Schaff P, Senner V, Kaiser F. Pressure distribution measurements for the alpine skier—from the biomechanical high tech measurements to its application as swingbeep-feedback system. In: Müller E, Schwameder H, Kornexl E, Raschner C, eds. *Science and skiing.* London: E & FN Spon (Chapmann & Hall), 1997:159–172.
10. Roy B, Barbeau L. Facteurs d'efficacité dans certaines techniques classiques en ski de fond: le pas alternatif. *STAPS* 1990; 11:43–50.
11. Norman RW, Roy B. *Investigation of biomechanical variables which distinguish elite from less skilled cross country skiers.* Technical Report. Ottawa, Ontario: Cross-Country Canada, 1985.
12. Bilodeau B, Boulay MR, Roy B. Propulsive and gliding phases in four cross-country skiing techniques. *Med Sci Sports Exerc* 1992;24:917–925.
13. Dufek JS, Bates BT. Temporal gait characteristics of cross-country skiers. In: Jonsson B, ed. *Biomechanics,* vol 10B. Champaign, IL: Human Kinetics, 1987:729–732.
14. Marino GW, Titley B, Gervais P. A technique profile of the diagonal stride patterns of highly skilled female cross-country skiers. In: Nadeau CH, Holliwell WR, Newell KM, Roberts GC, eds. *Psychology of motor behavior and sport—1979.* Champaign, IL: Human Kinetics, 1980:614–621.
15. Komi PV, Norman RW, Caldwell G. Horizontal velocity changes of world-class skiers using the diagonal technique. In: Komi PV, Nelson RC, Morehouse CA, eds. *Exercise and sport biology.* Champaign, IL: Human Kinetics, 1982;12:166–175.
16. Gagnon M. Caracteristiques dynamiques du pas alternatif en ski de fond. *Can J Appl Sport Sci* 1980;5:49–59.
17. Eisenman PA, Johnson SC, Bainbridge CN, Zupan MF. Applied physiology of cross-country skiing. *Sports Med* 1989;8:67–79.
18. Waser J. Technique under study: diagonal stride and one-step double pole. *Ski Coach* 1983;6:79–86.
19. Soliman AT. Cross-country skiing: the diagonal stride in flat. Unpublished thesis, Swiss Federal Institute of Technology, Laboratory of Biomechanics, Zurich, Switzerland, 1977.
20. Waser J, Denoth J. Biomechanical analysis of the diagonal stride on the flat. Proceedings of the International Symposium on Sport Biology, Vierumaki, Finland, 1979.
21. Dillman C, India DM, Martin PE. Biomechanical determination of effective cross-country skiing techniques. *J US Ski Coaches Assoc* 1979;3:38–42.
22. Norman RW, Komi PV. Mechanical energetics of world class cross-country skiing. *Int J Sport Biomech* 1987;3:353–369.
23. Norman RW, Caldwell G, Komi PV. Differences in body segment energy utilization between world-class and recreational cross-country skiers. *Int J Sport Biomech* 1985;1:253–262.
24. India DM. Mechanical analysis of female world class cross-country skiers performing the diagonal stride on a flat terrain. Unpublished thesis, University of Illinois, Urbana, Illinois, 1979.
25. Haberli R. *Cross-country skiing: a film analysis of the diagonal stride during elevation.* Zurich, Switzerland: Swiss Federal Institute of Technology, Laboratory of Biomechanics, 1977.
26. Martin PE. Multiple regression analysis of the diagonal stride of cross-country skiing on uphill terrain. Unpublished thesis, University of Illinois, Urbana-Champaign, Illinois, 1979.
27. Bilodeau B, Rundell KW, Roy B, Boulay MR. Kinematics of cross-country ski racing. *Med Sci Sports Exerc* 1996;28:128–138.

28. Norman RW, Ounpuu S, Fraser M, Mitchell R. Mechanical power output and estimated rates of nordic skiers during Olympic competition. *Int J Sport Biomech* 1989;5:169–184.
29. Norman RW, Ounpuu S. *Towards the identification of biomechanical indices which distinguish successful from less successful high performance cross-country skiers executing the diagonal stride.* Unpublished manuscript, University of Waterloo, Occupational Biomechanics Laboratories, Waterloo, Ontario, 1987.
30. Smith GA. Biomechanics of cross-country skiing. *Sports Med* 1990;9:273–285.
31. Smith GA. Biomechanical analysis of cross-country skiing techniques. *Med Sci Sports Exerc* 1992;24:1015–1022.
32. Roy B, Barbeau L. Facteurs d'efficacit<aae> dans certaines techniques classiques en ski de fond: le pas de un et la poussee simultanee. *STAPS* 1991;12:37–43.
33. Hoffman MD, Clifford PS, Bender F. Effect of velocity on cycle rate and length for three roller skiing techniques. *J Appl Biomech* 1995;11:257–266.
34. Andres P. *Cross-country skiing: a film analysis for the ascertainment of parameters which determine performance in conjunction with the double pole with thrust.* Zurich, Switzerland: Swiss Federal Institute of Technology, Laboratory of Biomechanics, 1977.
35. Smith GA. Perceived exertion and kinematic characteristics of cross-country skiers using the marathon skate and double pole with stride techniques. Unpublished thesis, University of Illinois, Urbana, Illinois, 1985.
36. Komi PV. Force measurements during cross-country skiing. *Int J Sport Biomech* 1987;3:370–381.
37. Ekström H. Force interplay in cross-country skiing. *Scand J Sports Sci* 1981;3:69–76.
38. Roy B, Voyer B. *Le ski de fond: technique, biomecanique et preparation physique.* Quebec: Les Editions de l'Homme, 1983.
39. Komi PV, Norman RW. Preloading of the thrust phase in cross-country skiing. *Int J Sports Med* 1987;8:48–54.
40. Pierce JC, Pope MH, Renstrom P, Johnson RJ, Dufek J, Dillman C. Force measurement in cross-country skiing. *Int J Sport Biomech* 1987;3:382–391.
41. Candau R, Belli A, Carrez G, Chatard J-C, Lacour J-R. *Stretch shortening cycle in alternate stride skating of cross-country skiing.* Grenoble, France: Congress Scientifique International: Sport et Montagne, 1992.
42. Orendurff MS, Smith GA. Transition techniques used by Olympic cross-country skiers. *Med Sci Sports Exerc* 1993;25:S170.
43. Street GM. Technological advances in cross-country ski equipment. *Med Sci Sports Exerc* 1992;24:1048–1054.
44. Pinchak AC, Hancock DE, Hagen JF, Hall FB. Biomechanical differences between cross-country snow skiing and roller skiing: analysis of some kinematic measurements. In: Rekow ED, Thacker JG, Erdman AG. eds. *Biomechanics in sport: a 1987 update.* New York: American Society of Mechanical Engineers, 1987a:55–60.
45. Smith GA, Mcnitt-Gray J, Nelson RC. Kinematic analysis of alternate stride skating in cross-country skiing. *Int J Sport Biomech* 1988;4:49–58.
46. Smith GA. The effect of velocity and grade on the kinematics and kinetics of V1 skating in cross country skiing. Unpublished dissertation, Pennsylvania State University, 1989.
47. Smith GA. Kinetic analysis of the V1 skate in cross-country skiing. In: *Proceedings of the First IOC World Congress on Sport Sciences, Colorado Springs, Colorado.* Colorado Springs: IOC, 1989: 281–282.
48. Smith GA, Nelson RC. Effects of increased velocity on the kinematics of V1 skating in cross-country skiing. In: Kreighbaum E, McNeil A, eds. *Biomechanics in sports*, vol 6. Bozeman, MT: International Society of Biomechanics in Sports, 1988:429–438.
49. Street GM. Kinetic analysis of the V1 skate technique during roller skiing. *Med Sci Sports Exerc* 1989;21:S79.
50. Smith GA, Nelson RC, Feldman A, Rankinen JL. Analysis of V1 skating technique of Olympic cross-country skiers. *Int J Sport Biomech* 1989;5:185–207.
51. Humphreys SE, Street GM, Smith GA. Kinematics analysis of female Olympic cross-country skiers. *Med Sci Sports Exerc* 1993;25:S170.
52. Smith GA, Heagy BS. Kinematic analysis of skating technique of Olympic skiers in the men's 50-km race. *J Appl Biomech* 1994;10:79–88.
53. Gervais P, Wronko C. The marathon skate in nordic skiing performed on roller skates, roller skis, and snow skis. *Int J Sport Biomech* 1988;4:38–48.
54. Street GM. Biomechanics of cross-country skiing. In: Casey MJ, Foster C, Hixson EG, eds. *Winter sports medicine.* Philadelphia: FA Davis, 1990:284–301.
55. Dillman C, Schierman G. *Biomechanical features of uphill "ski skating" on cross-country skis.* Colorado Springs: Biomechanics Laboratory, United States Olympic Committee, 1986.
56. Boulay MR, Rundell KW, King DL. Effect of slope variation and skating technique on velocity in cross-country skiing. *Med Sci Sports Exerc* 1995;27:281–287.
57. Rundell KW, McCarthy JR. Effect of Kinematic variables on performance in women during a cross-country race. *Med Sci Sports Exerc* 1996;28:1413–1417.
58. Gregory RW, Humphreys SE, Street GM. Kinematic analysis of skating technique of Olympic skiers in the women's 30-km race. *J Appl Biomech* 1994;10:382–392.
59. Aro TA, Smith GA, Nelson RC. An analysis of male and female Olympic skiers: effect of slope on V-1 skate kinematics. *Med Sci Sports Exerc* 1990;22:S18.
60. Frederick EC, Street GM. Nordic ski racing: biomedical and technical improvements in cross-country skiing. *Sci Am* 1988; 258:T20–T22.
61. Rundell KW, Szmedra L. Energy cost of rifle carriage in biathlon skiing. *Med Sci Sports Exerc* 1998:30:570–576.
62. Smith GA, Heagy BS. Ski edging and skating performance of Olympic cross-country skiers. *Med Sci Sports Exerc* 1994;26:S194.
63. Fewster JB, Smith GA, Heagy BS. Body alignment in ski-skating of Olympic cross-country skiers. *Med Sci Sports Exerc* 1994;26:S100.
64. Kammermeier P, Blegen M, Rundell KW. Upper body power relates to ski skating economy of elite biathlon skiers. *Med Sci Sports Exerc* 1996;28:S796.
65. Street GM, Mcnitt-Gray J, Nelson RC. *Timing study World Cup cross-country ski race, Biwabik, Minnesota.* Technical report. University Park, PA: Pennsylvania State University, Biomechanics Laboratory, 1986.
66. Ragache J-C, Thievenaz R. Ski nordique: analyse de l'utilisation des pas de la technique de patinage. *STAPS* 1988;9:31–45.
67. Bilodeau B, Roy B, Boulay MR. A comparison of three skating techniques and the diagonal stride on heart rate responses and speed in cross-country skiing. *Int J Sports Med* 1991;12:71–76.
68. Street GM, Frederick EC. Measurement of skier-generated forces during roller-ski skating. *J Appl Biomech* 1995;11:245–256.
69. Leppavuori AP, Karras M, Rusko H, Viitasalo JT. A new method of measuring 3-D ground reaction forces under the ski during skiing on snow. *J Appl Biomech* 1993;9:315–328.
70. Smith GA, et al. *J Appl Biomech* 1996;12:88–103.

Exercise and Sport Science,
edited by William E. Garrett, Jr., and Donald T. Kirkendall.
Lippincott Williams & Wilkins, Philadelphia © 2000.

CHAPTER 41

Biomechanics of Swimming

Huub M. Toussaint, A. Peter de Hollander, Coen van den Berg, and Andrei R. Vorontsov

In competitive swimming, world-level performances require years of hard training, training that is devoted to improvement of determinants of performance like technique, coordination, strength, and aerobic capacity. It may be argued that training time will be especially efficient when it is devoted to the enhancement of those performance factors that are weak links in the performance chain, that is, that represent the phase of the process where the performance system first becomes insufficient. These are known as limiting or determining factors, because they are the first to reduce, and hence determine, performance (1). This could lead to the conclusion that the most specific form of training is to swim races, because then the greatest stress is put on the weakest factor needing the most improvement. However, this will only stress one factor, albeit a dominant one, sufficiently to produce a maximum training effect. The other factors may not be stressed optimally and will therefore not improve as much as they might with another form of training (2). Therefore, it might make more sense to train several factors in a somewhat isolated manner and overload them maximally without interference from other processes, such that each would improve separately to a greater extent and then contribute more to performance when integrated with the other factors during a race. Thus, it is necessary to identify the relevant performance factors and design the optimal training programs to improve them. Competitive swimming events differ in stroke employed (breaststroke, backstroke, butterfly, and front crawl) and distance swum (50 to 1500 m). Swimming a 50-m sprint in 23 seconds requires considerable strength, power, and technique; whereas the 1500 m takes at least 14 minutes and 40 seconds to complete and thus calls for a high endurance capacity. It is obvious that these different events will place different demands on the swimmer's body and that performance factors will depend on the specific event the swimmer is training for. Still, some important performance factors are involved in all competitive swimming events. An analysis of these factors is useful in designing training programs, taking into consideration whatever deficiencies there may be in the swimmer's resources or capabilities.

This chapter starts with an analysis of the resistance encountered during swimming, as resistance is thought to be a major performance factor. The hydrodynamic basis of this velocity-dependent force is discussed and the different attempts to measure drag are presented. This is followed by an overview of the different theories that relate the kinematics of the propelling surfaces to the produced propulsive forces. A common characteristic of swimming propulsion is that, apart from the start and turns, it cannot be generated by pushing-off from a fixed object. Therefore, a thorough analysis of the mechanics of the swimmer's body and of the surrounding water involved in the generation of propulsion is presented, with emphasis on fluid dynamics. The mechanics (and especially the propulsion technique) of swimming is intimately tied to the energetics of swimming, and thus this chapter discusses the link between the biomechanical and physiologic bases of performance, with an emphasis on swimming the front crawl. Other competitive strokes and techniques are not covered. Special attention is given to the role of the arms, since it is generally agreed that the arms provide more than 85% of the total thrust in the crawl stroke (3–6).

DRAG

When swimming, the body undergoes a retarding force of resistance, or drag, due to the viscosity of the water and, at high speeds, to turbulence behind the swimmer.

H. M. Toussaint, A. P. Hollander, and C. van den Berg: Faculty of Human Movement Sciences, Vrije Universiteit, Amsterdam, The Netherlands.

A. R. Vorontsov: Department of Sport Swimming, Russian State Academy of Physical Education, Moscow, Russia; National Performance Center Bath, Bath University, Bath, Somerset, England.

Furthermore, when movement occurs at the water surface, additional resistance occurs due to gravitational forces on the waves set up by the motion. Each of these three components will be discussed from a basic hydrodynamic point of view.

Friction Drag

Viscosity is the property that makes syrup difficult to stir. It is essentially a frictional force between different layers of water as they move past one another. The viscosity of water (or any fluid) can be expressed by the coefficient of viscosity η ($0.897 \cdot 10^{-3}$ N·s·m^{-2} for water at 26°C). The water layer directly in contact with the swimmer is held to the skin by adhesive forces (this is known as the no-slip condition). Thus, this fluid layer moves with the same velocity v as the swimmer. The fluid velocity will diminish with distance from the body. Fluid far in front of the body, far at either side of it, and far behind it is at rest. Thus, the layer of water close to the body will be retarded by the layer just beside it; this layer is retarded by the next layer, and so on. It is found that this friction or viscous force is proportional to the total surface area of the swimmer (the wetted surface) and to the speed v. As long as the water around the swimmer is neatly arranged in layers (the flow is then called laminar), the total drag force exerted by the water will equal this viscous force.

Above a certain speed, the flow may become turbulent. Turbulent flow is characterized by erratic movement of fluid elements, compared to the orderly behavior in the laminar domain. At what speed and where on the body turbulence first becomes apparent depends on the shape and size of the swimmer. The onset of turbulence is often abrupt and occurs at a critical value of the so-called Reynolds number, *Re* (a dimensionless scaling number):

$$Re = \frac{vL\rho}{\eta} \qquad [1]$$

where ρ and η are the density and viscosity of water, v is the swimming velocity, and L is a characteristic length of the swimmer. Depending on the shape of the object, the critical value of *Re* will be in the order of 500,000 (7). For a competitive swimmer, with $v = 2$ m·s^{-1}, $L = 2$ m, $\rho = 1000$ kg·m^{-3}, and $\eta = 0.897 \cdot 10^{-3}$ N·s·m^{-2}, *Re* will be about 4.5×10^6 for the swimmer body. This implies that in competitive swimming turbulence will probably always play a role.

Pressure Drag

The orderly flow over the swimmer's body may separate at a certain point, depending on the shape, size, and velocity of the swimmer. Behind the separation point, the flow reverses and may roll up into distinct eddies (vortices). As a result, a pressure differential arises between the front and the rear of the swimmer, resulting in pressure drag, which is proportional to the pressure differential times the cross-sectional area of the swimmer. In general, pressure drag D_p will be dependent on the square of the swimming speed v, a dimensionless drag coefficient C_D accounting for form effects (e.g., bluff versus torpedo-shaped), the cross-sectional area A_p, and ρ, the density of water:

$$D_p = \tfrac{1}{2}\rho A_p v^2 C_D \qquad [2]$$

Wave Drag

For swimming near the water surface, a third component of the total resistance is due to the so-called wave-making resistance. When a swimmer is near the surface, water tends to pile up in front of him and to form hollows behind, thus creating a wave system. With increasing velocity both the wave length (the crest to crest distance) and the wave amplitude increase. At a certain speed the wave length equals the water-line length of the swimmer, which is presumably proportional to the height of the swimmer. This swimming speed is called the *hull speed*, a term from shipbuilding introduced into competitive swimming by Miller (8). At that velocity the swimmer is trapped in a self-created hollow between crests of waves. More effort will lead to a higher wave amplitude, leading to a deeper hollow, and thus any further attempts to increase swimming speed will be extremely difficult as most energy is used to "climb out of the hollow" (9). In practice, this means that it is impossible to swim faster than the hull speed. The relative speed that, together with the form of the swimmer, determines the magnitude of the wave drag is defined as the Froude-number (*Fr*, another dimensionless number):

$$Fr = \frac{v}{\sqrt{gL}} \qquad [3]$$

where g is the acceleration of free fall (9.81 m·s^{-2}). Swimmers with equal body form, but differing in height, will create an identical wave system (relative to body dimensions) when their Froude number is equal. For the shorter swimmer this corresponds to a lower velocity (see below).

MEASUREMENT OF DRAG

A considerable part of the energy expenditure in swimming is utilized to overcome drag (10), which is one of the factors that may limit swimming performance. Throughout the history of swimming research, attempts have been made to measure this resistance. As early as 1905, Dubois-Reymond (11) towed people behind a rowing boat, measuring resistance using a dynamometer. Liljestrand and Stenstrom (12) towed swimmers by means of a windlass on shore. Amar (13) was the first to assume that the resistance is related to the square of the swimming velocity (14,15) according to the following equation (compare Eq. 2):

$$D = \mathrm{K} \cdot v^2 \qquad [4]$$

in which D denotes drag force, and K is a constant incorporating ρ, C_D, and A_p. Karpovich (15) used a "natograph" to register drag dependent on velocity. Both Amar (13) and Karpovich used measurement techniques determining the resistance of swimmers gliding passively through the water. The relation between resistance (N) and velocity ($m \cdot s^{-1}$) based on their experiments was approximately $D = 29 \cdot v^2$. The body is, of course, never in a stable prone position when swimming, however, since propulsive forces need to be generated. It was conjectured that the movements necessary to create propulsion could induce additional resistance (16–18). This led to attempts to determine the drag of an active swimming person.

Determination of Active Drag

Techniques to determine this active drag were developed by several groups in the 1970s (19–23). In the method used by Holmér (21), Prampero and colleagues (22), and Rennie and colleagues (23), the variation in oxygen consumption as a result of small additional forces applied to the swimmer is extrapolated. In the method introduced by Clarys and colleagues (19), variations in external forces applied on a moving carriage as a function of imposed speed variations are extrapolated. Both methods yielded comparable results and, as expected, higher drag values (150% to 300%) than the previously reported values for passive drag.

Schleihauf (24) developed a new approach (see below) that did not rely on extrapolation. His technique was based on the balance of propulsive and resistive forces that, according to Newton's law, must exist when swimming at a constant speed. Hence, by determining the propulsive forces, drag can be estimated. In the mid-1980s, Hollander and colleagues (25) developed another approach to *m*easure *a*ctive *d*rag (MAD system, Fig. 41–1). The technique relies on the direct measurement of the push-off forces on a swimmer doing the front crawl. Kolmogorov and Duplisheva (26) designed yet another method to determine the active drag. In their so-called velocity perturbation method, subjects are asked to swim a 30-m lap twice at maximal effort: first swimming free, and then swimming with a hydrodynamic body attached that created additional resistance. For both trials the average velocity is calculated. Under the assumption that in both swims the power output is maximal and constant, active drag can be calculated as power equals force times speed:

$$D_1 \cdot v_1 = D_2 \cdot v_2 \qquad [5]$$

where the subscript numbers refer to the swims. Using Eq. 4 this can be expanded:

$$\mathrm{K}v_1^3 = \mathrm{K} \cdot v_2^3 + F_b \cdot v_2 \qquad [6]$$

where F_b represents the added drag due to the hydrodynamic body. Since the hydrodynamic properties of this added body were calibrated previously, it was possible to compute F_b at any velocity. Then, K can be solved and, since $D_1 = K \cdot v_1^2$, D_1 is defined as follows:

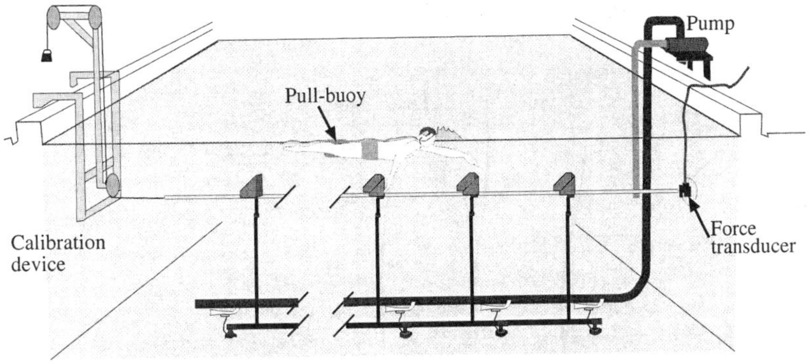

FIG. 41–1. Schematic drawing of the measure active drag (MAD) system mounted in a 25-m pool. The MAD system allows the swimmer to push off from fixed pads with each stroke. These push-off pads are attached to a 22-m-long rod. The distance between the push-off pads can be adjusted (normally 1.35 m). The rod is mounted 0.8 m below the water surface. The rod is connected to a force transducer enabling direct measurement of push-off forces for each stroke. Subjects use their arms only for propulsion; their legs are floated with a small buoy. If a constant swimming velocity is maintained, the mean propelling force equals the mean drag force. Hence, swimming one lap on the system yields one data-point for the velocity-drag curve. (Note: the cord leading to the calibration device is detached during drag measurement.)

$$D_1 = K \cdot v_1^2 = \frac{F_b \cdot v_2 \cdot v_1^2}{v_1^3 - v_2^3} \qquad [7]$$

The interesting aspect of this approach is that it can be applied to measure active drag in all four competitive strokes, while the MAD system and indirect methods are applicable only to the front crawl. The approach yields only one drag estimate at maximal speed, however.

When these more recent techniques were used to estimate active drag (18,26–29), considerably lower values were found than values reported earlier (20). Except for the velocity perturbation method, the values were comparable to values reported earlier for passive drag (i.e., $D = 26 \cdot v^2$). Kolmogorov and Duplisheva's (26) approach yielded even lower values: $D = 16 \cdot v^2$. It was established that active drag is related to the square of the swimming velocity (v in $m \cdot s^{-1}$) according to $D = K \cdot v^2$ (Eq. 4). A complicating factor in this drag dispute was the fact that methods were never compared using the same subjects (30). To finally resolve this issue, Hollander and colleagues (31) compared active and passive drag in 13 elite male swimmers. Active drag was determined using Schleihauf and colleagues' (27) technique and using the MAD-system, while passive drag was determined during towing experiments in a swimming flume. The two methods yielded similar active drag values ($r = 0.76$); again drag was related to velocity according to $D = 26.5 \cdot v^2$. Values for passive drag ($F_{passive}$) were much lower than the active drag values ($F_{passive} = 14.5 \cdot v^2$) and lower than older estimates for passive drag (13,15). It was demonstrated that passive drag values are extremely dependent on body position during the measurements (see also ref. 9). In particular, small variations of head position could induce drag values differing by ± 100%, a phenomenon previously observed by Miyashita and Tsunoda (32). Given this discrepancy, active drag measurements probably result in the most reliable values for drag during swimming.

Factors Determining Active Drag

Using the MAD-system, we found that mean values for K are about 30 for males and about 24 for females in front crawl swimming (28). These results are similar to the values previously reported by Karpovich (15). It is interesting to unravel what factors could determine the exact value of K. In the literature it was more than once suggested that body build could be such a factor. For instance, Cureton (33) reported that the "tall, slim type has been shown to glide better through the water." In addition, several others noted that swimmers are taller than the mean population, suggesting a performance advantage related to height (34–38). In line with these suggestions, Clarys (14,19,39) proposed using form indices derived from ship-building technology to study the relationship between body build and drag. In a collaboration between Clarys and the MAD system, the relationship between morphology and active drag was evaluated (40). It was established that drag is determined to a great extent by the maximal body cross-sectional area ($r^2 = 0.76$). Furthermore, the difference in mean body cross-sectional area (0.091 m^2 for males versus 0.075 m^2 for females) could explain the difference in mean drag between male and female swimmers (K = 30 for males versus K = 24 for females). The effect of height on drag became apparent from a longitudinal study [2.5 years (41)] of a group of children (mean age at the start: 12.9 years). In this study the body cross-sectional area of the children increased by 16%, while no differences in total drag were found (start: 30.1 N ± 2.37 versus end: 30.8 N ± 4.50; both drag values determined at a swimming velocity of 1.25 $m \cdot s^{-1}$). As we have indicated above, total drag (D) is determined not only by pressure drag (D_p) but also by friction drag (D_f) and wave-making resistance (D_w):

$$D = D_p + D_f + D_w \qquad [8]$$

Pressure drag is dominant at the prevailing high Reynold's number Re of $2.2 \cdot 10^6$ to $2.5 \cdot 10^6$, and at equal swimming speed is determined mainly by the body cross-sectional area. The friction drag (D_f), being dependent on total surface area (see above), could increase somewhat since the total skin surface will increase due to growth (but see also ref. 42). Hence, changes in D_p and D_f cannot explain the lack of increase in total drag at the end of the study.

The wave-making resistance (D_w) relates to the Froude number. One of the effects of growth is increase in height. Thus, swimming at the same absolute speed would imply a decrease of the Froude number when height increases (see Eq. 3), with consequent reduced formation of waves leading to a lower wave-making resistance. Thus, in children the increase of height (from 1.52 to 1.69 m) resulted in a decrease of F_r (from 0.324 to 0.308 at a swimming velocity of 1.25 $m \cdot s^{-1}$). In Fig. 41–2*A* the mean drag curves for the entire group are related to speed. Again it is clear that the drag has not changed. When the same drag data are presented with respect to the Froude number (Fig. 41–2*B*), hence correcting for the change in height, it appears that the drag had increased. If the drag is calculated for a Froude number of 0.324 ($v = 1.25\ m \cdot s^{-1}$), it gives a drag of 30.1 N. After 2.5 years drag at the same Froude number yields a value of 34.6. The increase of 15% is about the increase in size of the body cross-sectional area (see also ref. 43). The suggestion that the increase in pressure drag was compensated for by a decrease in wave-making resistance is in line with the common notion that taller swimmers seem to have an advantage in front crawl swimming performance. Furthermore, form indices derived from ship-building technology revealed changes

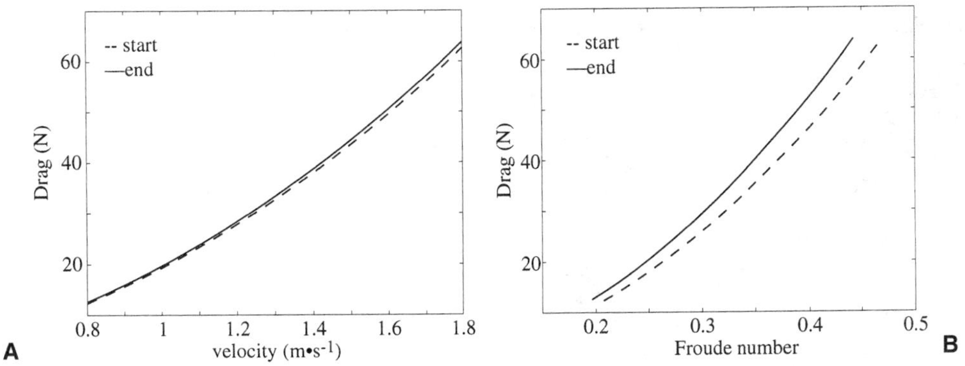

FIG. 41–2. Drag is presented for children at the beginning (mean age 12.9 years, *dotted line*) and after 2.5 years (*solid line*), dependent on velocity (**A**) and dependent on the Froude number (**B**).

that fostered a more streamlined body. For example the length-thickness ratio [equal to (height)^2/body cross-sectional area] significantly increased from 36.5 to 39.4 (41). Therefore, during growth a complex process takes place in which different drag-determining factors, such as height, body shape, and body cross-sectional area, change in directions that have opposite effects on drag.

Recently, Vorontsov (9) examined the interesting problem of determining the depth at which the wave-making resistance would be negligible. He reasoned that at a certain depth the hydrostatic pressure is higher than the pressure created by the moving swimmer that sets up a wave system. This wave-equilibrium depth appears to be between 0.7 and 1.2 m, depending on the wave-making characteristics of the swimmer. The practical follow-up problem is whether total resistance will be less when swimming below the wave-equilibrium depth. According to Vorontsov, the wave-making resistance is related to the swimming velocity cubed. Consequently, this component rises sharply and becomes significant at high speeds ($>1.8\ m \cdot s^{-1}$). Such high velocities are indeed attained after the start and turns. A glide below the wave-equilibrium depth would evade this high wave-making resistance, and thus a much smaller propulsive force is required to maintain a high speed. So far, experimental results are controversial. However, some excellent swimmers showed outstanding results in competition by covering up to 50% of the competitive distance under water using the butterfly kick only. This suggests that there may be a performance advantage when the swimmer dives under the wave-making resistance at the short competitive distances where a high swimming speed can be developed.

Several authors have suggested that the drag forces encountered while swimming at the surface may be diminished by improving the swimming technique (1,44,45). If true, this would lead to the hypothesis that elite swimmers have lower resistance at high swimming velocities than poorer ones. To test this hypothesis, Hollander and colleagues (46) determined the relationship between drag and maximal swimming performance. Active drag was determined in 12 male and 12 female elite swimmers at high velocities (mean velocity per group 1.86 and 1.63 $m \cdot s^{-1}$, respectively). As no significant relationships were found (males $r = -0.27$, females $r = 0.07$; Fig. 41–3), it was concluded that drag per se is not a determining factor of maximal swimming speed. In an experiment in which triathletes were compared to swimmers (47), however, a considerable difference in drag was found: K (see Eq. 4) was 30.5 for the competitive swimmers and 41.6 for the triathletes. In part this difference could explain the difference in performance between the two groups of athletes. The different values for K could be interpreted as being a result of the poorer technique of the triathletes causing superfluous body movements in the vertical and horizontal plane perpendicular to the swimming velocity (1,44,45). In other words, competitive swimmers seem to be able to use a better stroking pattern resulting in a more stable body position and hence a smaller value of K.

The question of whether drag is a major performance-determining factor cannot be entirely resolved on the basis of the research presently available. It seems as if drag is determined by anthropometric dimensions (e.g., body cross-sectional area and height) in groups of elite swimmers who are homogeneous with respect to swimming technique. Probably a small reduction in drag can be achieved by stretching the arm in the glide phase of the stroke, as was suggested by Holmér (48). The body cross-sectional area is especially reduced when the shoulder is stretched behind the arm. Furthermore, in all descriptions of active drag, it is implicitly assumed that K is constant during the stroke cycle. Most probably this is not the case. This could, for example, explain why despite the large oscillations in the propulsive force, rather small intracyclic velocity oscillations are reported (49). It could be conjectured that skilled swimmers are

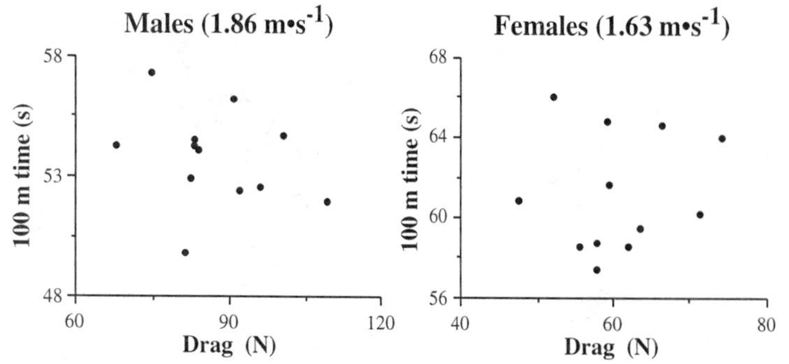

FIG. 41–3. Performance expressed as 100 m time is presented as a function of drag measured at a velocity of 1.63 $m \cdot s^{-1}$ for females (n = 12) and 1.86 $m \cdot s^{-1}$ for males (n = 12).

able to synchronize the propulsive peaks with the phases in which the body cross-sectional area (and consequently pressure drag) is at a maximum. Hence, the oscillations in propulsion coincide with oscillations in drag, such that the resultant force on the swimmer (about zero at constant speed) shows much less variation. In line with this suggestion is the fact that reduced velocity oscillations are observed in the more proficient swimmers (49–51). Another as yet unresolved issue is the function of the glide. It could be theorized that the forward stretched arm increases the length of the "hull," with consequent reduction of the Froude number and wave-making resistance. Also, the gliding arm could reduce the pressure above it and in front of the head, thereby reducing the amplitude of the bow wave, that is, similar to the function of the cone-shaped nose below the water line in large ships (52). It has been suggested that proficient swimmers have a lower wave-making resistance. Whether this is the result of technique or anthropometry is another unresolved issue (see ref. 53).

PROPULSION IN HUMAN SWIMMING

The mechanics involved in the generation of propulsive forces received scarce attention until the late 1960s, when Counsilman (45) published his famous kinematic analysis of the swimming strokes and began to speculate on the fluid dynamic mechanism of propulsion. Previously, propulsive forces on the surface of the hand were thought to be created in a similar fashion to those on the surface of an oar. It was reasoned that the drag forces generated by moving the hand backward would propel swimmers forward as a direct application of Newton's third law (action = −reaction; Fig. 41–4). Counsilman modified this view by pointing out that instead of pushing water backward in a straight line, the hand follows a curvilinear path continuously to find still water to push against and thus gain more resistance than it would by pushing against water that had already been accelerated. In part this description of the involved hydrodynamics could explain the curved paths of actions observed and reported in swimmers and frequently referred to as S-shaped or inverted question-mark pulls (Fig. 41–5).

Shortly thereafter, Counsilman also drew attention to the importance of lift forces, which act perpendicular to the direction of hand movement. He stated that both lift and drag forces are important for propulsion. This modified theory could explain the sculling movements

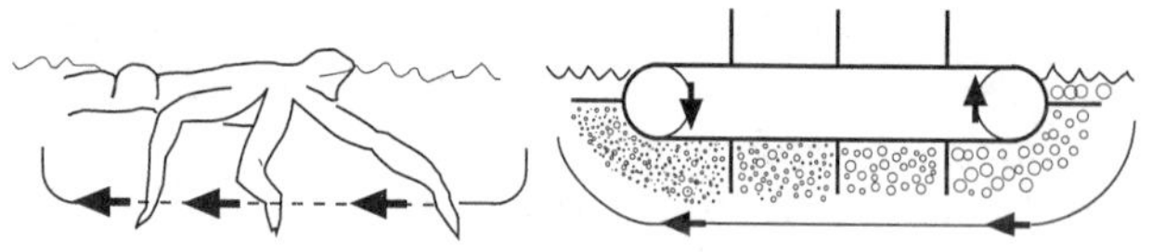

FIG. 41–4. Early view of the mechanics of propulsion. The hand is used as an oar. The hand is pulled straight back, creating a high-pressure zone on the palm and a low-pressure zone on the back of the hand. The resulting propulsive drag force would propel swimmers forward corresponding to the caterpillar paddle-wheel (*right*). However, in reality this form of propulsion is rather ineffective, because turbulence from one blade affects the ability of the following blade to create drag. Also, a relative small mass is given a rather large velocity change, leading to large losses of kinetic energy to the water.

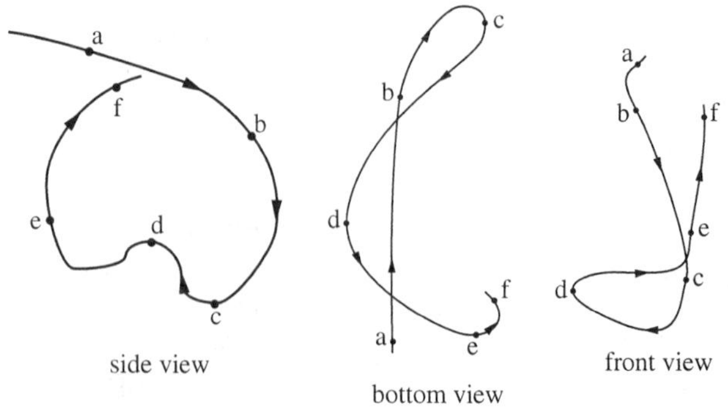

FIG. 41–5. Front crawl stroke pattern of the right hand in three dimensions. *a–b,* entry; *b–c,* entry scull; *c–d,* inward pull or insweep; *d–e,* outward pull; *e–f,* exit or upsweep. (From ref. 54.)

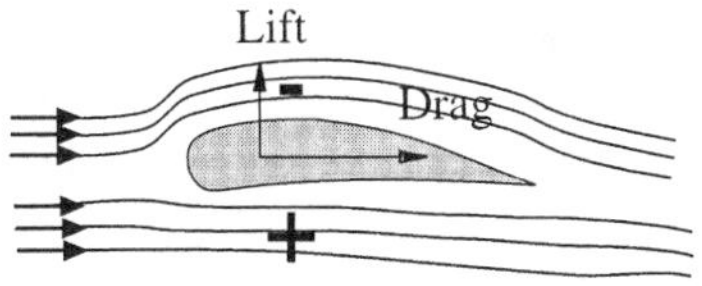

FIG. 41–6. Movement through water is resisted by the water immediately in front and around the hydrofoil. This water resistance is called *drag.* Drag force always acts in the direction of flow. Due to its shape the water speed above the hydrofoil is greater than below. The pressure above the hydrofoil is less than below, resulting in a net upward force called *lift.* By definition, lift acts perpendicular to drag.

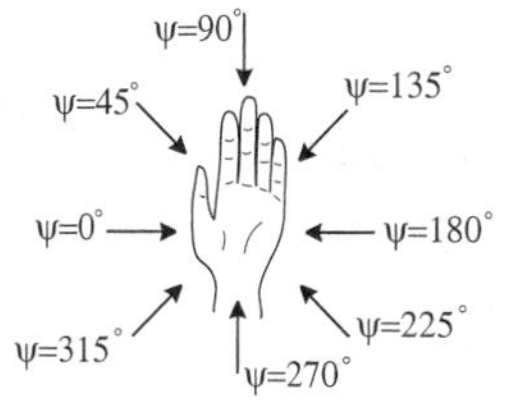

FIG. 41–8. Sweepback angle convention. (From ref. 24.)

during the arm pull observed with underwater cinematography (Fig. 41–5).

The nature of the lift force is similar to that experienced by an aircraft wing. As Counsilman (55) explained: "A wing provides aerodynamic lift through the camber (curvature) of its surfaces. Because the upper surface is more highly cambered than the lower surface, the air moving over the top surface is forced to move more quickly. This results in a lower pressure on the upper surface as compared with the lower surface and results in aerodynamic lift (Bernoulli's principle)" (p. 61). Thus, the pressure differential results in a lift force directed at right angles to the line of motion of the propelling surface (Figs. 41–6 and 41–7). Subsequently, numerous articles were published to support the notion that the total propelling force acting on the hands is composed of both a lift and drag component (56–61).

The suggested hydrofoil behavior of the hand was investigated in depth by Schleihauf and colleagues (24,27,60,62–64). According to hydrodynamic theory the drag and lift force can be derived using the following equations (compare Eq. 2):

$$L = \tfrac{1}{2}\rho\, u_h^2\, C_l S \qquad [9]$$

$$D = \tfrac{1}{2}\rho\, u_h^2\, C_d S \qquad [10]$$

where L = lift force, D = drag force, ρ = density of water, u_h = hand velocity, C_l = lift coefficient, C_d = drag coefficient, and S = propelling surface of the hand. Values of C_l and C_d for the human hand as a function of angle of attack and sweep-back angle were determined in a fluid lab using hand models (24). Similar data were obtained by Wood (65), who measured the lift properties of plaster casts of swimmers' hands and forearms in a wind tunnel. Both Schleihauf and Wood, and more recently Berger and colleagues (66) and Payton and Bartlett (67), demonstrated that the propulsive forces generated by the hand are indeed composed of both drag and lift forces. The values of the lift coefficient (C_l) and drag coefficient (C_d) are dependent on the angle of attack and the sweep-back angle. The angle of attack is the angle formed by the inclination of the propelling surface to its direction of motion (Fig. 41–7). The sweep-back angle defines the leading edge of the hand (Fig. 41–8).

The coefficients of lift and drag are strongly dependent on the angle of attack. Small changes in the angle of attack can significantly change the resulting propelling force, which is the vector product of the lift and drag force. Thus the propelling force can be steered in the desired forward direction by varying the lift and drag component by means of the angle of attack. This implies that, instead of one optimal line of motion straight backwards, numerous solutions exist to combine lift and drag force components to provide propulsion in a straight, forward direction (Fig. 41–9). For an optimal propulsive force, the orientation of the hand must be constantly fitted to ever-changing directions of hand movement during the pull (60). To select the angle of attack that gives the optimal combination of drag and lift forces at every moment of a pull, the swimmer has to have a feel for the water, which is one aspect of a talent for swimming.

The propulsive forces generated by the hand during a pull may now be estimated given the values of C_l and C_d for the hand and the velocity and orientation of the hand during the stroke. In his more recent experiments

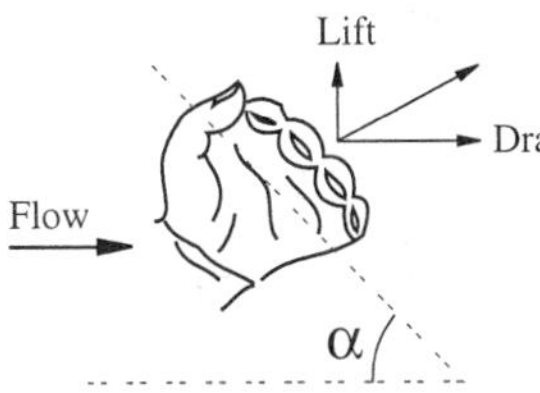

FIG. 41–7. The angle of attack (α). (From ref. 55.)

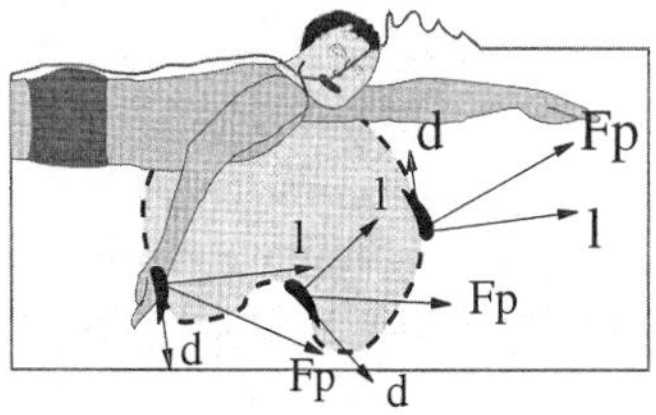

FIG. 41–9. The direction of the hand velocity changes during the pull. The angle of attack is continuously adapted to direct the propulsive force F_p forward.

Schleihauf used two battery-operated video cameras (30 Hz) in underwater housings to simultaneously collect front and side views of the swimmer. Eight points on the swimmers body were studied frame by frame from both front and side view. The body landmarks were middle fingertip (I), center of the wrist joint (W), index finger metacarpophalangeal joint (T), little finger distal metacarpal end (P), elbow joint, shoulder joint, and anterior superior iliac spine. The plane of the hand is defined by the vectors IW and TP. The angle of attack is defined as the angle between the line of motion of the hand and the plane of the hand. The sweep-back angle defines the leading edge of the hand (see Fig. 41–8). (For a more extensive description, see ref. 27.) Using this technique, Schleihauf has presented detailed analyses of stroke mechanics and hydrodynamic forces of elite swimmers representing all stroke techniques (24,64). The analyses reveal that swimmers use complex sculling motions of the hands (compare Fig. 41–5). By changing the angle of attack of the hand, they successfully combined lift and drag forces in a resultant propulsive force in the direction of motion (see Fig. 41–9). Furthermore, it was demonstrated that highly skilled swimmers utilized the most rapid hand actions (high velocity v, implying high propulsive forces; see Eqs. 9 and 10) in the side-to-side and up-and-down dimensions of motion, rather than in the front-to-back direction, which would have been expected for purely drag-based propulsion. It may be concluded that lift forces play an important role in propulsion.

Although the presented lift-drag approach can explain the complex sculling underwater movements of the hand, recent experiments yield observations suggesting that the lift-drag approach sketched above has some deficiencies (31,68). In these experiments a comparison was made between the propulsive forces using Schleihauf's approach and those measured directly on the MAD system (see Fig. 41–1). In general, a reasonable degree of agreement between the two methods was observed ($\bar{F}_{mad} = 34$ N, $\bar{F}_{Schlei} = 30$ N,$_{,r} = 0.76$). Schleihauf's approach yielded on average 10% lower values, however (31). Different explanations can be given for this discrepancy. An important assumption of Schleihauf's quasi-steady approach is that the coefficient of lift and drag of the underarm and hand obtained using stationary flow in a flow tank can be applied for modeling hydrodynamic forces in front crawl swimming. It can be questioned whether the steady flow conditions in the lab can be extrapolated to the flow conditions that are experienced during swimming. The hand in skilled front crawl swimming constantly changes its angle of attack and sweep-back angle with respect to the water and also accelerates and decelerates; the flow conditions are highly unsteady. In fluid mechanics there are two important dynamic effects associated with an immersed accelerating segment. These are the vortex shedding and dynamic stall (or delayed stall) effects (69,70). These effects are ignored, or assumed to be negligible, in the quasi-static approach. Therefore, the in essence two-dimensional (2D), quasi-static approach to determine lift and drag coefficients has been questioned (70,71). Could it be that the quasi-steady assumption fails?

Until recently, a similar situation was present in the study of insect flight. Careful quasi-steady analyses, combining kinematics and wind-tunnel force measurements of isolated wings, similar to Schleihauf's analysis above, led to the paradoxical result that many flying insects cannot generate enough force to carry their own weight (72). The implication was that the quasi-steady assumption fails and that unsteady lift-enhancing mechanisms must play an important role. To better understand the problems and peculiarities of unsteady flow, some more fluid dynamic background is needed.

As shown above, a wing will experience an upward lift force when the average air pressure above the wing is lower that the pressure under the wing (see Fig. 41–6). According to Bernoulli's principle (inverse relationship between pressure and velocity), this is the case when the average air velocity at the upper surface of the wing is higher than that beneath the wing. The total airflow around the wing may be decomposed in a circulating flow around the wing with velocity v and a uniform flow at velocity u passing the wing (Fig. 41–10). The velocity of the air above the wing will be $u + v$, and beneath it $u - v$. The pressure difference is then approximated by

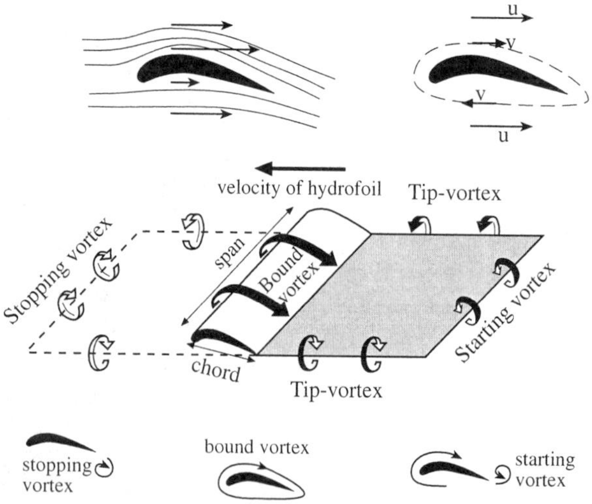

FIG. 41–10. Streamlines round a wing, which is shown in section. The flow past the wing can be decomposed in uniform flow with velocity u with a circulation around the wing with velocity v. The 3D vortex wake created by a rapid acceleration of a wing is shown at the *top*. The *shaded area* indicates air given a downward impulse. *Dashed lines* and *unshaded* vortices indicate future events. Creation of the starting, bound, and stopping vortices is shown below in a 2D view, depicting the vertical plane. (From ref. 72.)

$\rho(u + v)^2/2 - \rho(u - v)^2/2 = 2\rho uv$. This pressure difference acting across a wing of area A_p gives a lift-force of $2\rho uvA_p$.

The circulating flow around the wing is called a bound vortex (Fig. 41–10). The strength or circulation of the bound vortex is proportional to v. Aerodynamics texts such as Prandtl and Tietjens (73) give a formal definition of circulation. In the case presented in Fig. 41–10 it may be approximated by the circumference of the wing (twice the chord, c) multiplied by v, hence $\Gamma = 2cv$ (74). The lift on a wing of span s with circulation Γ must be equal to that given in Eq. 9 and is given by ($c \cdot s = S$):

$$L = \rho u \Gamma s = \tfrac{1}{2}\rho u^2 C_l c\, s = \tfrac{1}{2}\rho u^2 C_l S \qquad [11]$$

Circulation and lift are constant for a wing moving at a constant speed (steady state). When the wing accelerates impulsively from rest to a certain speed, however, the circulation needs time to build up. At the start of the motion, air swirls around the trailing edge and vortices are shed into the wake (see Fig. 41–10). This buildup of the so-called starting vortex continues until a constant circulation is reached. During this period the bound vortex will develop to the final steady-state value. This gradual buildup of the bound vortex is called the Wagner effect. Even after six chord lengths of travel, the circulation and lift are only 90% of the final values (72). Since the chord of a hand is about 0.1 m, the steady-state value of circulation (requiring >0.6 m of travel at constant velocity) may not be reached at all during swimming.

It is a fundamental rule of fluid dynamics that no vortex can be created unless a vortex of the opposite sense and strength is set up simultaneously (Kelvin's circulation theorem). Thus, the starting vortex is equal in magnitude but opposite in sense of rotation to the bound vortex. Tip vortices join up the starting and bound vortices. They are created as air swirls around the tips from the higher pressure zone below the wing to the lower pressure zone above. Accidental entrapment of air in the water often produces visible evidence of tip vortices trailing behind a swimmer's hands in the early stages of the stroke (51). Thus, the accelerating wing (or a hand) generates a vortex "ring," enclosing air (water) that has been blown downward. When the wing motion stops, the bound vortex then swirls off the trailing edge and forms the stopping vortex, closing the vortex ring, which subsequently moves downward into the wake (or backward in the case of a swimmer). Whether the water flow associated with swimming propulsion is unsteady or quasi-steady, the reaction force to the lift must impact momentum to the fluid. With a periodic propulsion, as in insect flight and swimming, the formation of start, tip, and stop vortices is unavoidable. As argued above, this may well result in a vortex ring left behind in the wake during each halfstroke (in swimming, a pull may be divided in substrokes, dependent on the movement direction of the hand, e.g., change from insweep to upsweep, point d in Fig. 41–5). The momentum of this ring must correspond to the lift force generated during the halfstroke. Thus, in principle, propulsive forces can be estimated by analyzing the wake of the propelling surfaces (75).

The lift coefficient of a wing is generally roughly proportional to the angle of attack, up to a certain limit. The limit is due to the phenomenon called stalling, and the angle of attack at which stalling occurs is known as the stalling angle. When the angle of attack is less than the stalling angle, the flow is attached to the surface of the wing. When it is greater than the stalling angle, the flow separates from the upper surface of the wing and large eddies form leading to a sudden drop in lift force and hence of $C_l(\alpha)$. It was shown that the lift forces needed to support the weight of insects during hovering is greater than the peak lift forces the wing can generate before it stalls in steady motion (72). The problem is even worse because the quasi-steady analysis ignores past history and therefore the Wagner effect. Circulation and lift will not grow to steady-state values on each half stroke because the wing moves only three to four chord lengths during hovering. Thus, the quasi-steady estimate of lift is overly optimistic, and the discrepancy with actual forces produced is even greater. As observed above, this crisis forced insect flight researchers to look for unsteady lift-enhancing mechanisms. Several mechanisms have been proposed (reviewed in ref. 72).

Weis-Fogh (76) proposed two novel mechanisms of lift generation that explained the flight mechanism for certain groups of insects. The lift produced by these mechanisms depends on events during the rotational phases (pronation and supination) at either end of the wingbeat, when the wing rapidly rotates about its long axis through about 120 degrees in preparation for the next half stroke. These rotations might be comparable to what happens in the front crawl during the transition from insweep to outward pull (see Fig. 41–5). It is hardly surprising that these mechanisms were new to aerodynamics; conventional wings are never operated in this extreme manner (72). Another class of unsteady mechanisms seems more applicable to swimming and is discussed next.

Delayed Stall or Dynamic Stall

We have seen that if the angle of attack is slowly increased to values above the stalling angle, separation of flow from the wing surface occurs. However, if the angle of attack is suddenly increased above the stall angle, or if the wing is accelerated quickly with a high angle of attack, separation of flow is delayed and the wing may move for several chords, generating lift that exceeds the maximum steady-state value. The growth of lift beyond the values observed during steady state

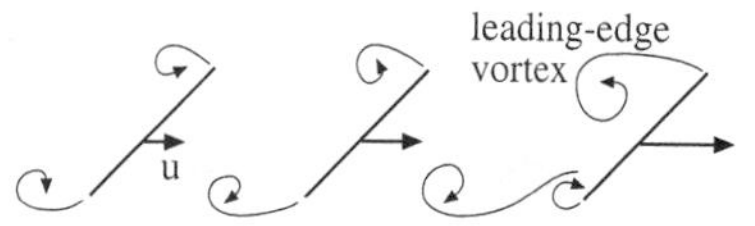

FIG. 41–11. Leading- and trailing-edge vortex shedding from a flat wing moving with increasing speed. Maximum lift is produced when the leading-edge vortex is located above the wing (dynamic stall). (From ref. 72.)

are associated with the formation of a leading-edge vortex (Fig. 41–11). The leading-edge vortex is formed when the flow separates from the wing at the onset of stalling. As long as the leading-edge vortex is above the wing, circulation around the wing is enhanced, leading to significantly increased lift forces. However, the problem with accelerating wings in translation is that the leading-edge vortex breaks away rather quickly (within two chords of travel), and lift will reduce sharply. In other words, the leading-edge vortex is rather unstable.

In one study, the airflow around flapping wings was visualized, using smoke released from the leading edge of a scaled-up robotic model of a hawkmoth (77). Analysis showed that a strong leading-edge vortex was present during the down stroke, which was stabilized by a strong axial flow (i.e., from wing base to wing tip). Thus, in a flapping wing that rotates around the shoulder, the leading-edge vortex was stable enough to remain attached along the wing for approximately three-fourths of the wing length during most of the downstroke. At the tip it separates and blends into a wide, tangled-tip vortex. The leading-edge vortex is stabilized by a strong axial flow, originating from a pressure differential that is caused by the velocity gradient between wing base and wing tip (the tip moves faster than the base). The velocity gradient is due to the rotation of the wing about its shoulder joint, such that the up and down velocity at the base is small but increases toward the tip. (In the front crawl stroke a similar situation occurs; the velocity of the hand relative to the water is higher than the velocity of the elbow.)

The extra lift force generated by this vortex alone was sufficient to carry two-thirds of the hawkmoth's weight, while the impulse of the two ring vortices left in the wake corresponded to about 1.5 times its body weight (78,79). This new lift-enhancing mechanism seems promising to explain the high lift forces produced by a range of insects. It also showed that the conventional quasi-steady approach failed for two reasons: (a) dynamic stall cannot occur in (quasi-)steady conditions; and (b) the axial flow component, which turned out to be large and crucial for stability of the vortex, is ignored in the 2D quasi-steady approach. A similar leading-edge vortex with strong axial flow is observed in delta-winged airplanes and is responsible for the high lift forces generated by such wings.

Could similar unsteady, lift-enhancing mechanisms be operative in the generation of propulsion in competitive swimming? A first step to identify the hydrodynamic mechanisms underlying propulsion is flow visualization. Surprisingly enough, few attempts have been reported to visualize the flow around the arms during swimming (80). We conducted a pilot study in which the direction of the flow around the hand and lower arm was visualized using 20 woolen tufts (10 cm long) attached to the hand and lower arm. In the glide phase, the flow wraps around the arm from tip to base in a gently spiraling fashion. During the transition to the insweep, the flow detaches from the surface of the hand and later also from that of the arm. During the insweep the flow is approximately perpendicular to the arm axis, as had been expected from conventional hydrofoil theory (Fig. 41–12). However, during the upsweep the flow over the back of the hand showed a strong axial component (in the direction of the fingertips), which, at the level of the hand, was at more than 45 degrees with the direction of the hand movement. The flow behind the trailing edge (as shown by the twisted tuft on the thumb and the little finger; Fig. 41–12) seemed to show a tip vortex at the finger tips and also at the tip of the extended thumb and was in the general direction of the arm movement. This axial flow over the hand surface is very suggestive in the light of the three-dimensional (3D) leading-edge vortex observed in insect flight. It is possible that a similar 3D leading-edge vortex is formed along the leading edge of the hand (i.e., the side of the little finger) during the upsweep. The ulnar abduction of the hand during the upsweep suggests that the hand may be used as a delta wing in this phase of the stroke. More detailed visualization studies are needed to substantiate this hypothesis. Whatever the propulsive mechanism, however, this study

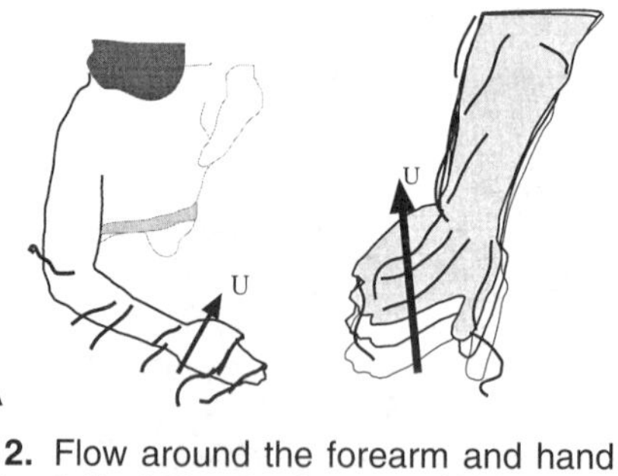

FIG. 41–12. Flow around the forearm and hand visualized using woolen tufts during the insweep (**A**) upsweep (**B**). Outlines of the swimmer and tufts are traced from an underwater video. The *arrow* indicates the movement direction of the hand (*U*). During the insweep a flow pattern compatible with conventional (Schleihauf's) stroke mechanics is observed (**A**) During the upsweep, however, the tufts on the hand are arranged in a direction almost perpendicular to the direction of hand motion. This suggests a strong axial component in the direction of the fingertips not compatible with Schliehauf's 2D approach.

clearly demonstrates that the flow pattern during the upsweep is very different from that expected.

ENERGETICS

The discussion has focused thus far on the forces involved with swimming. It is obvious, however, that in swimming the aerobic and anaerobic capacities codetermine success. Thus, the question is not simply how to maximize the propulsive force and minimize resistance, but rather how to accomplish this with finite metabolic capacities. Hence, it is also important to analyze the energetics of swimming. We will first discuss the measurement of the total rate of energy expenditure and some of its determining factors such as velocity, drag, and buoyancy, and then look at the measurement of energetics involved with the propulsion mechanics.

Different procedures have been used to determine the energy expenditure of swimming. The measurement of oxygen uptake during and immediately after swimming offers an indirect method to approximate energy expenditure. The oxygen uptake is only directly related to the intensity of the effort, however, as long as the swimmer is performing in steady state and at less than 50% to 70% of the maximum oxygen uptake ($\dot{V}O_2max$). A variety of techniques were developed to assess the oxygen uptake during swimming. Karpovich and colleagues (81,82) had the swimmers hold their breath during 50-yard swims. The expired gas of the swimmers was collected for 20 to 40 minutes after the completion of the swim to determine the so-called oxygen-debt (83). This same procedure was adopted by Adrian and colleagues (84) and by Klissouras (85). Another approach was introduced by Montpetit and colleagues (86) for swims of longer duration (>5 minutes). The technique relies on the backward extrapolation of the O_2-recovery curve to determine the $\dot{V}O_2$ during swimming. The swimmers are instructed to take a breath approximately one stroke before the finish of a 400-m swim and to exhale the breath into a breathing mask as soon as it is sealed over the face immediately after the swim. Expired air is continuously collected for the first 20 or 40 seconds after the swim (2,87). This procedure has the major advantage that the swimmer can perform without restrictions presented by the instrumentation used (breathing valve and hoses). Direct measurements of energy expenditure have also been performed during tethered swimming (88–90), flume swimming (21,38,91–95), swimming in an annular pool (16,22,23), and free swimming (47,89,96–101).

Energetics Related to Buoyancy and Drag

Almost all studies find that women require a 30% lower rate of energy production than men to maintain a given velocity (10,16,22,23,87,94,102,103). It was suggested that women did not need to expend as much energy in staying afloat, because of their higher mean percentage of fatty tissue (8,104,105). Furthermore, the distribution of adipose tissue along the head-feet axis is more favorable in women than in men, so that the tendency for the feet to sink is lower (10,16,105). Thus, women may need less energy to keep the body in a horizontal position (102), while it is also likely that a more horizontal position reduces drag (48). Thus, the question can be raised whether increased buoyancy or reduced drag has the most effect on the energy expenditure.

During constant speed swimming, a considerable fraction of the energy expenditure is utilized to overcome drag (10). As was indicated previously, drag is related to the square of the swimming velocity (Eq. 4). Consequently, the power to overcome drag (P_d) is related to the velocity cubed and a drag factor K: $P_d = K \cdot v^3$ (28). When we related the rate of energy expenditure to the power to overcome drag, no differences between males and females were found (10). In other words, the males do not expend additional energy to stay afloat. The 30% difference in energy expenditure at a velocity of 1 $m \cdot s^{-1}$ reported by Pendergast and colleagues (16) and di Prampero and colleagues (22) can be explained by the 29% lower resistance reported for female swimmers at this velocity. The lower drag values were related to the difference in frontal area (106); see also Eq. 2. This is in line with the observations of Montpetit and colleagues (102), who demonstrated that the difference in energy expenditure between males and females disappears when correcting for body size. Still, it is interesting to study the interrelationship between drag and buoyancy. The effect of a triathlon wet suit on drag was studied in eight male and four female competitive swimmers swimming at a velocity of 1.25 $m \cdot s^{-1}$ (42). A 14% reduction in drag (from 48.7 N to 41.8 N) was found. The effect of the reduction was probably due to increased buoyancy inducing less frontal resistance. Since the effect of the suit on the lower-density female swimmers was not different from the effect on the high-density male swimmers, however, the true relationship among buoyancy, drag, and energy expenditure remains to be determined.

ENERGY LOSSES IN PROPULSION

It seems obvious that the generation of the propulsive force in swimming is different from the propulsion generated during on-land activities. On land the push-off is performed against the Earth. Due to the large mass, the Earth will endure an undetectable (and therefore negligible) acceleration. Similarly, in the aquatic environment propulsion is generated by accelerating water. In this case, however, the acceleration of the water cannot be ignored. Or more formally, by Newton's second law of motion, the force F required to give a mass m an acceleration du/dt is given by

$$F = m\, du/dt \qquad [12]$$

Since the momentum of a mass of water m traveling with velocity u is $m \cdot u$, Eq. 12 states that the force applied to the mass of water equals the rate of change of momentum. Irrespective of the fluid dynamic mechanism of propulsion (drag, lift, or vortex; see above), the thrust that propels the swimmer forward is generated by giving a mass of water backward momentum (Fig. 41–13). Suppose a swimmer obtains the thrust F required to swim with velocity v, by giving some of the water a backward velocity $-u$. Thus, a mass of fluid will acquire a change of momentum (action = −reaction). Consequently, the kinetic energy ($0.5\, m \cdot u^2$) given to the water in unit time equals the force acting on the mass of water (F) times the velocity (u): $F \cdot u$. This is the power (P_k) consumed in driving water backward, in giving it a kinetic energy change, which is wasted power (107). Suppose that the swimmer swims at constant speed. In that case the resistive forces must equal the propulsive forces. The power required to drive the swimmer through the water equals $F \cdot v$. This can be denoted as useful power. Now we can define an efficiency, known as the Froude efficiency, or propelling efficiency (e_p) (107,108):

$$\textit{Propelling Efficiency} = \frac{\textit{Useful Power}}{\textit{Useful Power} + \textit{Power Lost to Water}} = \frac{v}{v + u} \qquad [13]$$

From Eq. 13 it follows (since u will not be much smaller than v) that the generation of propulsion in a fluid always will lead to the loss of mechanical energy of the swimmer that will be transferred in the form of kinetic energy to the fluid. Two aspects of this analysis are important for human swimming: (a) the power losses are considerable ($e_p << 100\%$), and (b) the power losses to the water are highly dependent on technique.

The first aspect is underlined by the propelling efficiency values observed in fish swimming. For trout, values range from e_p of 15% (swimming at 20% of maximum speed) up to e_p of 80% at maximal speed (109). Even if it is assumed that humans could use a swimming technique as efficient as that of trout, still 20% of the available mechanical power would be lost to moving water backward instead of moving the swimmer forward. Hence, a considerable amount of mechanical power is not transferred into forward speed of the swimmer. In fact, e_p is even lower in human swimmers (see below).

The magnitude of the propelling efficiency depends on the propulsion mechanism. The efficiency is higher if the swimmer accelerates a large mass of water per unit time to a low velocity, than if he obtains the same propulsion by accelerating a small mass to a high velocity (see Eq. 13). Or, as already stated by Counsilman (56), the technique should be such that the amount of water against which the push-off takes place is as large as possible. Thus, swimming at the same speed requiring the same propulsive force can have different associated energy costs depending on the technique that is employed. Consequently, maximal swimming speed can be achieved by a swimming technique in which optimal propelling force is obtained with an optimal propelling efficiency and a minimal body drag (110). Hydrodynamics applied to fish swimming shows that these requirements of a high propulsive force with limited wasted power can be met, in part, by a proper use of lift forces on the propelling surfaces (107,111). This implies that the analyses of lift and drag forces acting on the lower arm and hand can be related to propelling efficiency (27,66,67). Again, it is emphasized that basic mechanics of propulsion in swimming reveal that thrust and loss of mechanical energy to pushed-away masses of water are two sides of one coin. For a true understanding of the performance-determining factors, both aspects should be incorporated in the analysis.

In the 1970s several authors noted that the power lost to water (P_k) should be incorporated in the power bookkeeping or power balance. For example, Holmér (21) commented on the energy for propulsion: "Not all mechanical energy is useful in overcoming drag. Part of it is lost in the creation of turbulence, and in vertical and lateral displacement of water." Charbonnier and colleagues (112) stated, "The speed with which the swimmer can move depends on the energy he can furnish to push towards the rear masses of water with his limbs, and the resistance opposing his forward progress in the water." Miyashita (113) observed,

> An efficiency (work output/chemical energy used) in land exercises was approximately 20 to 25%. On the contrary, efficiency in swimming was 0.5 to 2.2%. Therefore, the swimmer must produce more external work than that estimated from the speed variations and water resistance. Propulsive force which drives the swimmer forward is created by the swimmer's arms and legs as

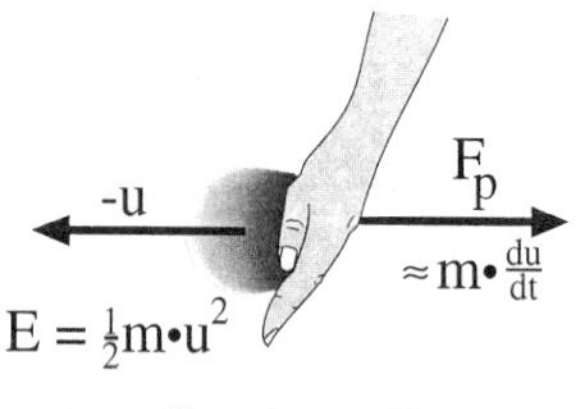

FIG. 41–13. The propelling force F_p is generated by giving a mass of water m a velocity change du/dt. Consequently, the pushed-away mass of water acquires a kinetic energy ($0.5\, m \cdot u^2$). This kinetic energy is the result of the work done by the swimmer on the pushed-away mass of water. Hence, part of the total mechanical work the swimmer delivers is converted into kinetic energy of the water, rather than forward speed of the swimmer.

they push the water backwards. This means that some parts of chemical energy may be transformed into kinetic energy of water.

Nevertheless, in numerous articles on the energetics of swimming, P_k was not acknowledged, leading to questionable conclusions with respect to the estimated values for active drag and mechanical efficiency (16,22,23,114,115). (For a more extensive discussion, see ref. 116.)

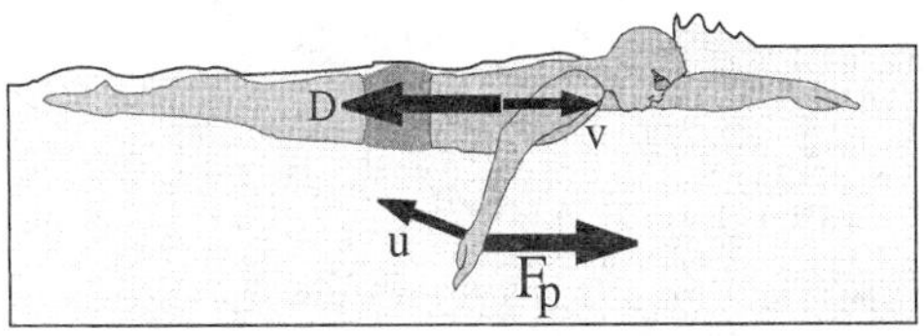

FIG. 41–14. "Free-body" diagram of swimmer. When swimming at constant speed (arms only), propulsion (F_p) equals drag (D). Thus two major forces act on the swimmer in the swimming direction, whereby the point of application of each force has a velocity. Since power equals the dot product of F and v, the diagram shows that one "energy flow" relates to drag and one to propulsion.

Measurement of Energetics Involved with the Propulsion Mechanics

The total mechanical work a swimmer produces is apportioned to work to overcome the total resistance and work to generate the propulsion. Since in competition the swimming velocity is to be optimized, it is more relevant to look at the time derivative of the work produced by the swimmer, which is the mechanical power production. Power (P) is defined as the rate at which energy is transferred from one system to the other (from swimmer to the aquatic environment), and equals the dot-product of the force-vector **F** and the velocity of the point of application **v**:

$$P = \mathbf{F} \cdot \mathbf{v} \qquad [14]$$

where **F** equals a force vector (i.e., drag or propulsion) and **v** the velocity vector of the point of application of the force (i.e., the swimming velocity or hand velocity). The two dominant forces in front crawl swimming (propulsion and drag) are indicated in Fig. 41–14 (ignoring gravity and the buoyant force) with their respective velocity of application. This free-body diagram emphasizes that two major power components can be discerned in competitive swimming: power necessary to overcome drag (P_d), and power expended in giving a kinetic energy change to pushed-away mass of water (P_k).

The mechanical power required to overcome drag is thus defined as follows (101,117):

$$P_d = \mathbf{D} \cdot \mathbf{v} = \mathrm{K} \cdot v^2 \cdot v = \mathrm{K} \cdot v^3 \qquad [15]$$

The mechanical power lost in the generation of propulsion (P_k) is less obvious to calculate. At least three approaches can be used: (a) Estimate the transfer of kinetic energy to the water on the basis of measured kinematics and estimated kinetics of the propelling surfaces, whereby the propelling force ($\mathbf{F}_p$) and its velocity of application (**u**) are estimated (68), hence:

$$P_k = \mathbf{F}_\mathbf{p} \cdot \mathbf{u} \qquad [16]$$

(2) Quantify the rate of kinetic energy change of the water (see below). And (c), estimate the difference in rate of total energy expenditure between swimming in which the push-off is made against water, and swimming in which the push-off is made against fixed points (P_k = 0) (108). This approach is shown in Fig. 41–15. When the push-off is made against fixed push-off points swimming on the MAD system, no kinetic energy is lost to the water (P_k = 0). Hence, the difference in rate of energy expenditure, when swimming at the same velocity, is proportional to P_k. The magnitude of P_k is esti-

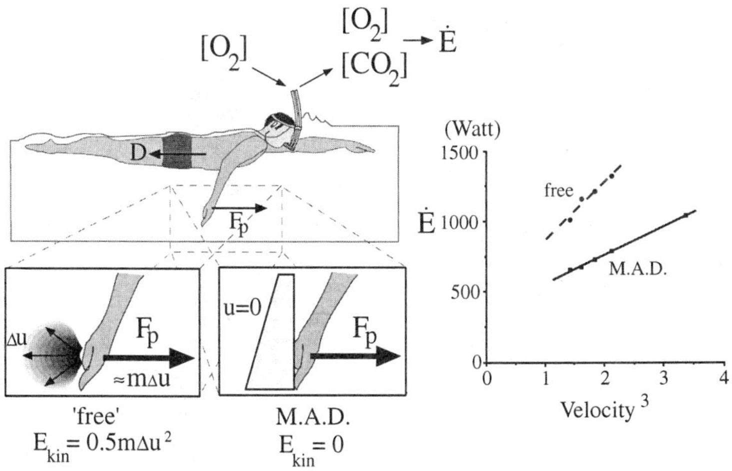

FIG. 41–15. The power lost in the generation of propulsion is estimated by comparing the oxygen uptake during free swimming to the oxygen uptake during MAD swimming at the same velocity. In the free swimming condition the rate of oxygen uptake reflects the power necessary to overcome drag plus the power necessary to generate the propulsive force, whereas during MAD swimming the oxygen uptake reflects the power necessary to overcome drag only.

mated by multiplying the difference in rate of energy expenditure ($\dot{E}$) with the gross-efficiency. This is the ratio of the mechanical power produced swimming on the MAD system (**D**·**v**) and $\dot{E}$ (101). With this approach it was established that P_k is a considerable part of the total mechanical power output (P_o) of the swimmer. The ratio between the useful mechanical power spent to overcome drag and the total mechanical power output (P_o) is defined as the propelling efficiency e_p (see Eq. 12):

$$e_p = \frac{P_d}{P_o} = \frac{P_d}{P_d + P_k} \qquad [17]$$

For a group of highly trained swimmers, e_p values of 61% were found (108). Hence, even in highly skilled swimmers (among them an Olympic champion), still 39% of the total mechanical power is lost to P_k. In well-trained but not so skilled swimmers (triathletes), a value for e_p of 44% was found, emphasizing the importance of technique (i.e., optimizing the propelling efficiency) as a performance determinant (47).

Values for propelling efficiency quantified on the basis of measured kinematics and estimated kinetics of the propelling surfaces yielded values for e_p of about 35% versus an e_p of 56% for the same group of swimmers using oxygen uptake measurements (68). Berger and colleagues (68) could not give a satisfactory explanation for the large difference in values. As indicated above, however, the kinematics method is based on a 2D, quasi-static approach to determine lift and drag forces. As indicated above, this approach fails in at least part of the stroke (i.e., the upsweep).

FACTORS DETERMINING PROPELLING EFFICIENCY

Propulsion Mechanics

The propulsive force is caused by momentum flow. This fluid momentum is convected by vortex action, as was explained above. Irrespective of the kind of propulsion (i.e., lift or drag), the propulsive system generates wake vortices. The strength or circulation (Γ) of the wake vortex is determined in a similar way as the strength of the bound vortex around the wing and is roughly proportional to the rotation velocity (ω) times the radius of the vortex. In 3D, the center of a vortex forms a line. The strength of a vortex line is constant along its length, and a vortex line cannot end in a fluid. It must extend to the boundaries of the fluid or form a closed path, for example, a ring vortex (Helmholtz's vortex theorem). As explained above, vortex rings transport momentum. The magnitude of the momentum carried by a ring vortex is proportional to the product of its area and the vortex strength (circulation). This implies that the vortex ring will also carry kinetic energy. Thus, energy is transferred from the swimmer to the water in the form of kinetic energy whenever a vortex is shed. The amount of energy of a vortex lost to the water is proportional to the strength squared divided by the square root of the vortex area. Thus, the most efficient vortex with given momentum is large in size and has low vortex strength. According to Lighthill (118), vortices of approximately circular shape carry a large amount of momentum in relation to their energy. This type of vortex is created by propelling surfaces (tails) with a special lunate shape. The visualization of flow in swimming propulsion might shed more light on this interesting issue, as was indicated in the preceding discussion and as was previously suggested by Ungerechts (119,120). Hence, a true quantification of the kinetic energy of the pushed-away masses of water might resolve the divergent values obtained for e_p using the methods described previously. As a first approximation to solve this problem, it is interesting to note that a ring vortex moves at a so-called self-induced velocity, which is proportional to its kinetic energy. Hence, a first-order estimate of the kinetic energy of the wake may be obtained if the diameter and the self-induced velocity of the ring vortex can be estimated (compare ref. 78).

Hand Surface Area

A factor that will affect P_k and thereby e_p is the size of the propelling surfaces. It can be conjectured that small propelling surfaces (small hand area) will push-off from a small mass of water, while larger hands will push-off from larger masses. This implies that for the same propulsive force and with the same technique, the swimmer with smaller hands must give a larger velocity (u) to the water. Consequently, the loss of kinetic energy to the pushed-away water will be larger when pushing off with smaller hands. This suggests that large propelling surfaces (a large hand area) give a performance advantage in swimming (e.g., one can swim much faster with flippers on the feet). This can be derived mathematically by expanding Eq. 13:

$$e_p = \frac{P_d}{P_d + P_k} = \frac{\mathbf{D} \cdot \mathbf{v}}{\mathbf{D} \cdot \mathbf{v} + \mathbf{F}_p \cdot \mathbf{u}} \qquad [18]$$

If, for the sake of simplicity, only drag forces are generated by the hand, then $\mathbf{D} = \mathbf{F}_p$. Equation 18 can be developed using Eqs. 2 and 4 in a similar, but slightly more complicated, formula that can be derived if lift forces are also taken into consideration:

$$e_p = \frac{\frac{1}{2} \cdot \rho \cdot v^3 \cdot C_{db} A_p}{\frac{1}{2} \cdot \rho \cdot v^3 \cdot C_{db} \cdot A_p + \frac{1}{2} \cdot \rho \cdot u^3 \cdot C_{dh} \cdot S} = \frac{1}{1 + \sqrt{\dfrac{C_{db} \cdot A_p}{C_{dh} \cdot S}}} \qquad [19]$$

with C_{db} the coefficient of drag of the body, A_p the frontal area of the whole body, C_{dh} the coefficient of drag of the hand, and S the frontal area of the hand. In this formula, an increased propelling surface size S directly leads to an increase of the propelling efficiency e_p. To test whether swimming with an enlarged propelling surface will increase e_p, $\dot{E}$ was measured at equal speeds of swimming with and without paddles (attached to the hands) (121). At the same average velocity the effect of swimming with paddles was an increase of e_p of 8%. This is in line with other studies that showed that swimmers of a high performance level have a significantly larger hand and arm surface than swimmers of lower performance level (122,123). This finding has some practical implications for swim training. Although for obvious reasons the use of hand paddles in competition is not allowed, they may be useful during training. If maximal performance is taken into account, at an equal power output a higher swimming velocity can be attained, due to the higher propelling efficiency. Hence, a higher propulsive force must be applied, since the drag forces will increase at higher swimming speed, and again at constant speed the average propulsion must equal the average drag. In this sense paddle swimming might be a rather specific form of strength training. Paddles significantly reduce backward hand velocity and reduce the rotation of the upper arm, however (124). If both movement pattern and movement speed specificity are deemed important, the efficacy of paddle swimming as a specific resistance training exercise can be questioned. Apart from the practical implications for training, the paddle study did show that P_k and e_p are important and may be changed by improving technique.

Power Balance Applied to Swimming

Several aspects of the mechanics and energetics of swimming are hotly debated. For example, discussion persists about whether the rate of oxygen uptake is linearly related to velocity (87,102) or to the cube of the velocity (101). Another issue is whether active drag differs from passive drag (17). It is also debated whether the mechanical efficiency of proficient swimmers is much better than their less speedy counterparts (10,16,35,94). Is there a way to more or less resolve the debated issues? A fundamental approach is to use the first law of thermodynamics: Energy can be neither created nor destroyed, it can only change in form (125). The swimmer converts metabolic energy to heat, to energy for internal organs (heart, lungs, brain, etc.), and to mechanical energy necessary to generate the propulsion and overcome the resistive forces of the water. Energy conservation implies that a balance must exist among these various forms of energy. Also, the rate of energy conversion must be in balance. Hence, a power balance should also exist. If a consistent power balance can be formulated, it provides evidence, albeit circumstantial, for the correctness of the incorporated elements.

The power balance during steady state swimming can be described as:

$$P_o = e_g \cdot \dot{E} \qquad [20]$$

where e_g equals the gross efficiency and reflects that not all metabolic power is converted to mechanical power; part of it is converted to heat or is necessary to support other body functions. In the transformation process, part of the chemical power present in foodstuff is converted to heat; e_g is quantified by the total mechanical power output (P_o) divided by the rate of energy expenditure. The average regression equation describing the process of converting $\dot{E}$ into P_o while swimming was estimated with the MAD system and appears to be the following (47,101):

$$P_o = 0.093 \cdot \dot{E} - 16 \qquad [21]$$

Since P_o equals P_d/e_p (see Eq. 17), Eq. 19 develops into the following (using Eq. 14):

$$\dot{E} = \frac{P_d}{e_p \cdot e_g} = \frac{K \cdot v^3}{e_p \cdot e_g} \qquad [22]$$

This suggests that the rate of energy expenditure is determined by the swimming velocity, the drag factor K, and the gross and propelling efficiencies. This equation holds as long as the energy spent in accelerating the body is negligible. Holmér (48) showed that this is the case in the front and back crawl. In general, data in the literature provide support for the presented relationship; the energy expenditure rate was shown to increase with velocity cubed when swimming at velocities above 1 $m \cdot s^{-1}$ (82,84,85,94,96). At the same speed, the more proficient swimmer (higher e_p) swims at a lower $\dot{E}$ than the less skilled (16,22,23,47,82,93,94,96). This is only true if the gross efficiency is similar for the groups that are compared. This seems to be the case, as no differences in gross or mechanical efficiency are observed when comparing elite and less skilled swimmers (47,101,112,123).

Equation 22 can more or less be substantiated from results in the literature. All of these studies used oxygen uptake measures to quantify $\dot{E}$. The majority of the competitive distances is equal to or shorter than 200 m, however, thus lasting less than 2 minutes and 30 seconds (200 m breaststroke for women). Therefore, a considerable part of the total power production will be from the immediate adenosine triphosphate creatine phosphate (ATP-CP) and the short-term (anaerobic glycolysis) rather than the long-term (oxidative or aerobic system) power production systems (126). Each of these systems has its own time constant, and therefore the rate at which $\dot{E}$, or metabolic power, is produced is dependent on the duration of the exercise. For example, Costill (127; see also ref. 128) estimates the relative contribu-

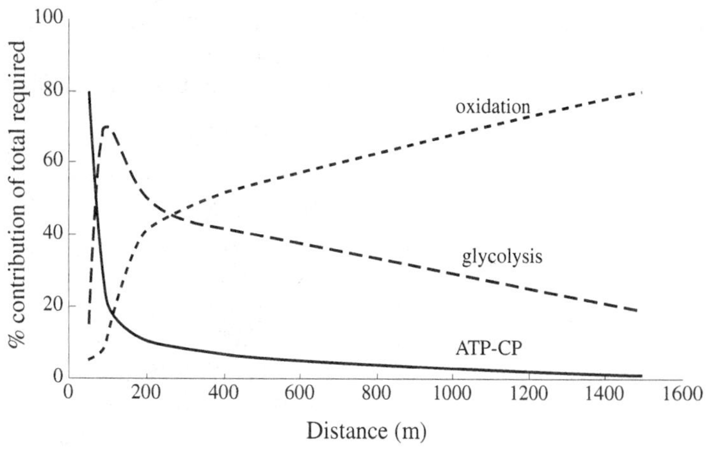

FIG. 41–16. The relative contribution of the ATP-CP, glycolytic, and oxidative energy system dependent on race distance. (From ref. 126)

tion of the different power contribution systems dependent on the distance swum (Fig. 41–16). The ATP-CP system relies on the phosphocreatine and ATP stores that are present in the muscle. The amount of ATP and phosphocreatine in the muscle is rather limited, and at intense levels of exercise this power production system is exhausted in a few seconds.

Modeling of the Aerobic and Anaerobic Power Production in Swimming

Studies of ice skating (129,130) and running (131) have shown that the power production of the aerobic and anaerobic systems can be modeled and related to the mechanical power output. It seems justified to assume that the metabolic power production in swimming (both anaerobic and aerobic system) will obey a power-time curve similar to those modeled for speed-skating or running:

$$P_{aer} = P_{aer,\max}(1 - e^{-\lambda t}) \text{ and } P_{an} = P_{an,\max}e^{-\lambda t} \quad [23]$$

where P_{aer} equals the metabolic power liberated aerobically, and P_{an} the metabolic power liberated anaerobically. In words, the anaerobic system immediately has its peak activity and activity decays exponentially over time, while the aerobic system kicks in gradually and approaches its peak asymptotically in time. $P_{aer,\max}$ and $P_{an,\max}$ equal the maximal aerobic and anaerobic power, while λ denotes a time constant defining the rate of increase and decrease of aerobic and anaerobic power, respectively. Following Margaria (132) and Ward-Smith (133), it is assumed that the power production of the anaerobic and aerobic pathways can be described with one time constant, suggesting a causal relation between them. The total amount of aerobic and anaerobic energy over a certain amount of time τ can be calculated by integration of the P_{aer} and P_{an} functions:

$$E_{aer} = \int_0^\tau P_{aer,\max}(1 - e^{-\lambda t})dt$$

$$= P_{aer,\max}\tau + \frac{P_{aer,\max}}{\lambda}(e^{-\lambda\tau} - 1) \quad [24]$$

$$E_{an} = \int_0^\tau P_{an,\max}e^{-\lambda t}dt = \frac{P_{an,\max}}{\lambda}(1 - e^{-\lambda\tau}) \quad [25]$$

An Energy Balance Applied to Front Crawl Swimming

The energy production of the aerobic and anaerobic system is used to swim a specific event. The required metabolic power ($\dot{E}$) swimming at a specific velocity can be quantified using the power balance equation (Eq. 21). Integration of this equation gives the energy expenditure necessary to swim a certain distance (d) at a specific constant speed (v) or in a certain time (τ):

$$\dot{E} = \frac{K \cdot v^2 \cdot d}{e_p \cdot e_g} = \frac{K \cdot d^3}{\tau^2 \cdot e_p \cdot e_g} \quad [26]$$

The energy generated should balance the energy necessary to swim a distance in a certain time. In other words, ($E_{an} + E_{aer}$) at time t must equal the total metabolic energy expended to swim a distance d in a time τ (i.e., with velocity d/t). This equality can be used to predict the performance times over different distances, hence:

$$\frac{K \cdot d^3}{\tau^2 \cdot e_p \cdot e_g} = P_{aer,\max}\tau + \frac{P_{aer,\max}}{\lambda}(e^{-\lambda\tau} - 1)$$

$$+ \frac{P_{an,\max}}{\lambda}(1 - e^{-\lambda\tau}) \quad [27]$$

The magnitude of λ can be estimated from repeated oxygen uptake measurements during one maximal exercise bout. Data were available from a group of eight male college swimmers (weight: 65.74 ± 8.23 kg, and $\dot{V}O_2max_{(swimming)}$: 3.54 ± 0.67 l·min^{-1}) that had performed a 60-second all-out swim in a swimming flume. Every

10 seconds the oxygen uptake was determined. The data were least square fitted to the function $P_{aer} = P_{aer,max} (1 - e^{-\lambda t})$, where $P_{aer,max}$ was set equal to the individual power equivalent of the $\dot{V}O_2max$.

The estimation of $P_{an,max}$ relies on a method to measure the total anaerobic energy production, which was described by Medbø and colleagues (134) for running. This method was applied in the context of swimming by Troup and colleagues (135) and Ogita and colleagues (136,137). In a series of submaximal swims the relation between oxygen consumption and the cube of the swimming velocity was determined. From this regression equation the oxygen consumption was estimated ($\dot{V}O_{2(100m)}$) to swim at the speed equal to the individual 100-m best performance. The subject was then invited to swim at this specific speed for 60 seconds in the swimming flume. During this (maximal) exercise, all oxygen consumed is measured by integrating the measured $\dot{V}O_2$. The accumulated oxygen deficit can then be calculated from the integrated amount of oxygen necessary to swim at this speed (duration · $\dot{V}O_{2(100m)}$) minus the total oxygen consumed. This deficit reflects the total anaerobic energy production (134,135). Data derived from the literature for K, e_g, and e_p were used to estimate E of the front crawl dependent on v. The results of the model were compared to the actual swimming times. The coefficients of correlation were, for the 50-yard distance, 0.94 (adjusted coefficient of determination: 0.86) and for the 100-yard distance 0.91 (adjusted r^2: 0.80) (138). The coefficients of correlation indicate that reasonable predictions of individual swim performances can be made with a power equation model based on the individual kinetics of the anaerobic and aerobic pathways. Thus, although for all subjects the same mean values were used for the gross efficiency (9.2%) and propelling efficiency (60%), and drag was estimated on the basis of subject mass, more than 80% of the variance in sprint performance could be explained with the model. Even better predictions can be expected when individually determined values for these parameters are incorporated in the model. Apart from the mass-dependent drag coefficient, the subject-specific input of the model related only to the metabolic factors. This suggests that these factors determine sprint performance for reasonably skilled swimmers (i.e., a propelling efficiency equal to 60%) given their drag profile. The success of the model in explaining variance of sprint performance provides support for the validity of the model. As stated above, however, individual data concerning K, e_g, e_p, and performance times at the longer distances were not available for the group; thus, the final verification of this approach remains to be determined (see also ref. 139). The outcome also underlines the importance for the training practice of determining the capacity of the aerobic and anaerobic energy systems.

Another practical test to determine the capacity of the aerobic and anaerobic metabolic pathways was developed by Wakayoshi and colleagues (140,141). The test estimates the swimming velocity that theoretically can be maintained forever without exhaustion. This so-called critical swimming velocity is the slope of the regression line between swimming distance and time. This equation (distance = critical velocity · time + anaerobic swimming capacity) is used to determine the capacity of the aerobic and anaerobic metabolic pathways. There is, however, uncertainty that critical velocity and anaerobic swimming capacity are fitness measures that truly separate aerobic and anaerobic components. Therefore, Eq. 27 was used to predict the critical velocity and the anaerobic swimming capacity (Fig. 41–17) (139). The

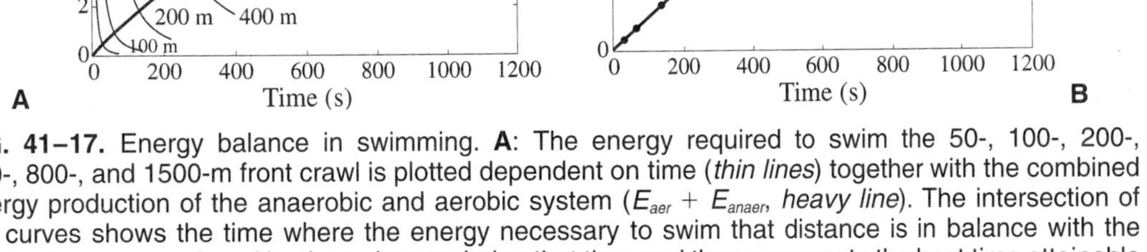

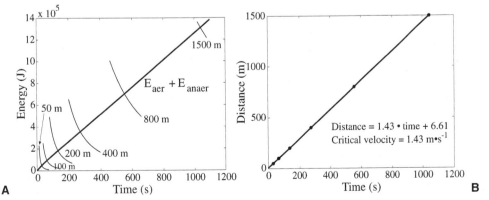

FIG. 41–17. Energy balance in swimming. **A**: The energy required to swim the 50-, 100-, 200-, 400-, 800-, and 1500-m front crawl is plotted dependent on time (*thin lines*) together with the combined energy production of the anaerobic and aerobic system ($E_{aer} + E_{anaer}$, *heavy line*). The intersection of the curves shows the time where the energy necessary to swim that distance is in balance with the maximal energy produced by the swimmer during that time and thus represents the best time attainable for that distance. **B**: The predicted best times for the 50, 100, 200, 400, 800, and 1500 m together with the linear fit between swimming distance and time.

effect of a 20% increase and decrease for $P_{aer,max}$ and $P_{an,max}$ on the performance for the 50, 100, 200, 400, 800, and 1500 m and on the regression equation of distance on time was determined. The 20% decrease and increase in $P_{aer,max}$ resulted in a 5.7% decrease and 6.2% increase, respectively, of the critical velocity. This suggests that changes in $P_{aer,max}$ are reflected in critical velocity albeit to a considerable lesser extent than the 20% variation in $P_{aer,max}$. The changes in $P_{an,max}$ had no influence on the critical velocity, but strongly affected the y-intercept of the regression equation (−54.7% and 48.5%, respectively). This is in line with Hill and colleagues (142), who suggested that the y-intercept is a measure of the anaerobic capacity. However, it also became apparent that besides $P_{an,max}$, variations in $P_{aer,max}$ have an influence on the y-intercept. Thus the model calculations suggest that variations in the y-intercept can not be attributed to variations in $P_{an,max}$ only. This agrees with previous observations in which the test-retest reliability of the anaerobic capacity was qualified as ambiguous (143).

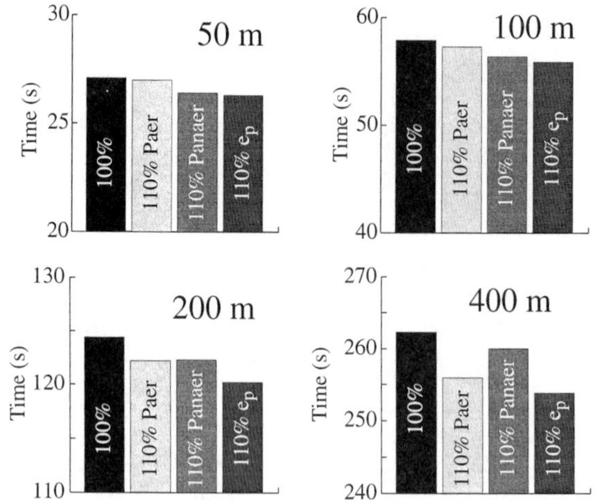

FIG. 41–18. Estimated best times for the 50-, 100-, 200-, 400-m front crawl. The distances were adapted to incorporate the effect of the dive, turns, and final touch with the hands (116). The *black bar* gives the result if $P_{aer,max}$, $P_{an,max}$, and E_p are set to 100%.

CONCLUSION

The model calculations illustrate that the critical swimming velocity is a measure of swimming endurance and thus reflects the aerobic capacity of the swimmer. However, the y-intercept of the regression line between swimming distance and time was influenced by both $P_{aer,max}$ and $P_{an,max}$. This suggests that the anaerobic swimming capacity does not truly reflect $P_{an,max}$.

Equation 22 can also be used to answer questions such as, What if the aerobic power increases 10%? or What if the anaerobic power or technique (propelling efficiency) improves by 10%? Results of model predictions regarding these questions are presented in Fig. 41–18.

For the shorter distances (50 and 100 m), performance is predicted to benefit from gain in the anaerobic capacity, whereas on the 400 m a clear effect is seen when improving the aerobic power. For all distances, a 10% improvement of technique gives the highest performance gain. This emphasizes the importance of technique improvement in training and the need for a better understanding of the fluid dynamics of swimming propulsion such that guidelines aimed at improving thrust while reducing energy losses (P_k) can be applied. In our opinion this is the true challenge of swimming research into the twenty-first century (52).

For an optimal use of training time and for an optimal use of the capacities of the swimmer, it is important to determine both the mechanical parameters (technique, drag) and the parameters describing the energy production ($P_{aer,max}$, $P_{an,max}$, and the time constant λ). The analysis techniques described here can help to estimate these parameters for each swimmer. From such an inventory of weak and strong points, it can be decided what the optimal distance is to train for, and what performance factors are the weakest and most likely to improve with training.

REFERENCES

1. Maglischo EW. *Swimming faster.* Palo Alto: Mayfield, 1982:472.
2. Costill DL, Maglischo EW, Richardson AB. *Handbook of sports medicine and science. Swimming.* Oxford: Blackwell Scientific, 1992:214.
3. Bucher W. The influence of the leg kick and the arm stroke on the total speed during the crawl stroke. In: Clarys JP, Lewillie L, eds. *Swimming* II. Baltimore: University Park Press, 1975:180–187.
4. Faulkner JA. Physiology of swimming. *Res Q* 1966;37:41–54.
5. Hollander AP, Groot G de, Ingen S, van GJ, Kahman R, Toussaint HM. Contribution of the legs in front crawl swimming. In: Ungerechts BE, Reischle K, Wilke K, eds. *Swimming*, vol 5. Champaign, IL: Human Kinetics, 1988:39–43.
6. Watkins J, Gordon AT. The effect of leg action on performance in the sprint front crawl stroke. In: Hollander AP, Huijing PA, Groot G de, eds. *Biomechanics and medicine in swimming.* Champaign, IL: Human Kinetics, 1983:310–314.
7. Anderson JD. *Fundamentals of aerodynamics*, 2nd ed. Aerospace Science Series. New York: McGraw-Hill, 1991.
8. Miller DI. Biomechanics of swimming. In: Wilmore JH, Keogh JF, eds. *Exercise and sport sciences reviews.* New York: Academic Press, 1975:219–248.
9. Vorontsov A. Propulsion and drag in swimming. In: eds. *IOC encyclopedia of sports. In press.*
10. Prampero PE. The energy cost of human locomotion on land and in water. *Int J Sports Med* 1986;7:55–72.
11. Dubois-Reymond R. Zum Physiologie des Schwimmens. *Arch Anat Physiol (Abt Physiol)* 1905;29:252–279.
12. Liljestrand G, Stenstrom N. Studien uber die Physiologie des Schwimmens. *Skand Arch Physiol* 1919;39:1–63.
13. Amar J. *The human motor.* London: G. Routledge, 1920.
14. Clarys JP. Human morphology and hydrodynamics. In: Terauds J, Bedingfield EW, eds. *Swimming*, vol 3. Baltimore: University Park Press, 1979:43.
15. Karpovich PV. Water resistance in swimming. *Res Q* 1933;4:21–28.

16. Pendergast DR, di Prampero PE, Craig AB, Wilson DR, Rennie DW. Quantitative analysis of the front crawl in men and women. *J Appl Physiol* 1977;43:475–479.
17. Clarys JP. Relationship of human body form to passive and active hydrodynamic drag. In: Asmussen E, Joergeusen K, eds. *Biomechanics,* vol 6B. Baltimore: University Park Press, 1978:120–125.
18. Kolmogorov SV, Rumyantseva OA, Gordon BJ, Cappaert JM. Hydrodynamic characteristics of competitive swimmers of different genders and performance levels. *J Appl Biomech* 1997; 13:88–97.
19. Clarys JP, Jiskoot J, Rijken H, Brouwer PJ. Total resistance in water and its relation to body form. In: Nelson RC, Morehouse CA, eds. *Biomechanics,* vol 4. Baltimore: University Park Press, 1974:187–196.
20. Clarys JP, Jiskoot J. *Total resistance of selected body positions in the front crawl.* Baltimore: University Park Press, 1975.
21. Holmér I. Efficiency of breaststroke and freestyle swimming. In: Clarys JP, Lewillie L, eds. *Swimming,* vol 2. Baltimore: University Park Press, 1975:130–136.
22. Prampero PE di, Pendergast DR, Wilson DW, Rennie DW. Energetics of swimming in man. *J Appl Physiol* 1974;37:1.
23. Rennie DW, Pendergast DR, Prampero PE di. Energetics of swimming man. In: Clarys JP, Lewillie L, eds. *Swimming,* vol 2. Baltimore: University Park Press, 1975:97–104.
24. Schleihauf RE. A hydrodynamic analysis of swimming propulsion. In: Terauds J, Bedingfield EW, eds. *Swimming,* vol 3. Baltimore: University Park Press, 1979:70–109.
25. Hollander AP, Groot G de, Ingen Schenau GJ van, et al. Measurement of active drag forces during swimming. *J Sports Sci* 1986;4:21–30.
26. Kolmogorov SV, Duplisheva A. Active drag, useful mechanical power output and hydrodynamic force coefficient in different swimming strokes at maximal velocity. *J Biomech* 1992;25:311–318.
27. Schleihauf RE, Gray L, DeRose J. Three-dimensional analysis of swimming propulsion in the sprint front crawlstroke. In: Hollander AP, Huijing PA, Groot G de, eds. *Biomechanics and medicine in swimming.* Champaign, IL: Human Kinetics, 1983:173–184.
28. Toussaint HM, Groot G de, Savelberg HHCM, Vervoorn K, Hollander AP, Ingen Schenau GJ van. Active drag related to velocity in male and female swimmers. *J Biomech* 1988;21:435–438.
29. Vaart AJM van der, Savelberg HHCM, Groot G de, Hollander AP, Toussaint HM, Ingen Schenau GJ van. An estimation of active drag in front crawl swimming. *J Biomech* 1987;20:543–546.
30. Hay JG. The status of research on the biomechanics of swimming. In: Ungerechts BE, Wilke K, Reischle K, eds. *Swimming science,* vol 5. Champaign, IL: Human Kinetics, 1988:3–14.
31. Hollander AP, Troup JP, Schleihauf RE, Toussaint HM. The determination of drag in front crawl swimming. *J Biomech* (*in press*).
32. Miyashita M, Tsunoda T. Water resistance in relation to body size. In: Eriksson B, Furberg B, eds. *Swimming medicine,* vol 4. Baltimore: University Park Press, 1978:395–401.
33. Cureton TK. Factors governing success in competitive swimming: a brief review of related studies. In: Clarys JP, Lewillie L, eds. *Swimming,* vol 2. Baltimore: University Park Press, 1975:9–39.
34. Andrew GM, Becklake MR, Guleria JS, Bates DV. Heart and lung functions in swimmers and nonathletes during growth. *J Appl Physiol* 1972;32:245–251.
35. Faulkner JA. Physiology of swimming and diving. In: Falls HB, eds. *Exercise physiology.* New York: Academic Press, 1968:415–446.
36. Kunski H, Jegier A, Maslankiewicz A, Rakus E. The relationship of biological factors to swimming performance in top Polish junior swimmers aged 12 to 14 years. In: Ungerechts BE, Wilke K, Reischle K, eds. *Swimming science,* vol 5. Champaign, IL: Human Kinetics, 1988:109–113.
37. Marconnet P, Spinel W, Gastaud M, Ardisson JL. Evaluation of some physiological parameters in swimming school students during a two year period. In: Eriksson B, Furberg B, eds. *Swimming medicine,* vol 4. Baltimore: University Park Press, 1978:161–169.
38. Nomura T. The influence of training and age on $\dot{V}O_2$max during swimming in Japanese elite age group and Olympic swimmers. In: Hollander AP, Huijing PA, Groot G de, eds. *Biomechanics and medicine in swimming.* Champaign, IL: Human Kinetics, 1983:251–257.
39. Clarys JP. Doelgerichte antropormetrie voor een hydrodynamisch onderzoek. *Bull Soc R Belge Anthrop Prehist* 1978;89:53–73.
40. Huijing PA, Toussaint HM, Clarys JP, et al. Active drag related to body dimensions. In: Ungerechts BE, Reischle K, Wilke K, eds. *Swimming science,* vol 5. Champaign, IL: Human Kinetics, 1988:31–37.
41. Toussaint HM, Looze M de, Rossem B van, Leijdekkers M, Dignum H. The effect of growth on drag in young swimmers. *Int J Sport Biomech* 1990;6:18–28.
42. Toussaint HM, Bruinink L, Coster R, et al. Effect of a triathlon wet suit on drag during swimming. *Med Sci Sports Exerc* 1989;21:325–328.
43. Chatard JC, Padilla S, Cazorla G, Lacour JR. Influence of body height, weight, hydrostatic lift and training on the energy cost of the front crawl. *NZ J Sports Med* 1985;13:82–84.
44. Bober T, Czabanski B. Changes in breaststroke techniques under different speed conditions. In: Clarys JP, Lewillie L, eds. *Swimming,* vol 2. Baltimore: University Park Press, 1975:188–193.
45. Counsilman JE. *Science of swimming.* Englewood Cliffs, NJ: Prentice-Hall, 1968.
46. Hollander AP, Toussaint HM, Groot G de, Ingen Schenau GJ van. Active drag and swimming performance. *NZ J Sports Med* 1985;13:110–113.
47. Toussaint HM. Differences in propelling efficiency between competitive and triathlon swimmers. *Med Sci Sports Exerc* 1990;22:409–415.
48. Holmér I. Physiology of swimming man. In: Hutton RS, Miller DI, eds. *Exercise and sport sciences reviews.* Philadelphia: Franklin Institute Press, 1979:87–123.
49. Holmér I. Analysis of acceleration as a measure of swimming proficiency. In: Terauds J, Bedingfield EW, eds. *Swimming,* vol 3. Baltimore: University Park Press, 1979:118–125.
50. Kornecki S, Bober T. Extreme velocities of a swimming cycle as a technique criterion. In: Eriksson BO, Furberg B, eds. *Swimming medicine,* vol 4. Baltimore: University Park Press, 1978:402–407.
51. Colwin CM. *Swimming into the 21st century.* Champaign, IL: Human Kinetics, 1992.
52. Larsen OW, Yancher RP, Bear CLH. Boat design and swimming performance. *Swimming Tech* 1981;18:38–44.
53. Takamoto M, Ohmichi H, Miyashita M. Wave height in relation to swimming velocity and proficiency in front crawl stroke. In: Winter DA, Norman RW, Wells RP, Hayes KC, Patla AE, eds. *Biomechanics,* vol 9B. Champaign, IL: Human Kinetics, 1985:486–491.
54. Svec O. Biofeedback for pulling efficiency. *Swimming Tech* 1982;19:38–46.
55. Counsilman JE. The application of Bernoulli's principle to human propulsion in water. In: Lewillie L, Clarys JP, eds. *Swimming,* vol 1. Brussels: Universite Libre de Bruxelles, 1971:59–71.
56. Barthels K, Adrian MJ. Three dimensional spatial hand patterns of skilled butterfly swimmers. In: Clarys JP, Lewillie L, eds. *Swimming,* vol 2. Baltimore: University Park Press, 1974:154–160.
57. Hay JG. *The biomechanics of sports techniques.* Englewood Cliffs, NJ: Prentice Hall, 1973.
58. Rackham GW. An analysis of arm propulsion in swimming. In: Clarys JP, Lewillie L, eds. *Swimming,* vol 2. Baltimore: University Park Press, 1975:174–179.
59. Reischle K. A kinematic investigation of movement patterns in swimming with photo-optical methods. In: Terauds J, Bedingfield EW, eds. *Swimming,* vol 3. Baltimore: University Park Press, 1979:127–136.
60. Schleihauf RE. A biomechanical analysis of freestyle. *Swimming Tech* 1974;11:89–96.
61. Ungerechts BE. Optimizing propulsion in swimming by rotation

of the hands. In: Terauds J, Bedingfield EW, eds. *Swimming,* vol 3. Baltimore: University Park Press, 1979:55–61.
62. Schleihauf RE. 3-D computer stroke analysis. *Swimming Tech* 1982;19:20–25.
63. Schleihauf RE. Swimming skill: a review of basic theory. *J Swimming Res* 1986;2:11–20.
64. Schleihauf RE, Higgins JR, Hinrichs R, et al. Propulsive techniques: front crawl stroke, butterfly, backstroke, and breaststroke. In: Ungerechts BE, Wilke K, Reischle K, eds. *Swimming science,* vol 5. Champaign, IL: Human Kinetics, 1988:53–59.
65. Wood TC. A fluid dynamic analysis of the propulsive potential of the hand and forearm in swimming. In: Terauds J, Bedingfield EW, eds. *Swimming*, vol 3. Baltimore: University Park Press, 1979:62–69.
66. Berger MAM, Groot G de, Hollander AP. Hydrodynamic drag and lift forces on human hand/arm models. *J Biomech* 1995;28:125–133.
67. Payton CJ, Bartlett RM. Estimating propulsive forces in swimming from 3-dimensional kinematic data. *J Sport Sci* 1995;13:447–454.
68. Berger MAM, Hollander AP, Groot G de. Technique and energy losses in front crawl swimming. *Med Sci Sports Exerc* 1997;29:1491–1498.
69. Childress S. *Mechanics of swimming and flying.* Cambridge, England: Cambridge University Press, 1981.
70. Pai YC, Hay JG. A hydrodynamic study of the oscillation motion in swimming. *Int J Sport Biomech* 1988;4:21–37.
71. Lauder MA, Dabnichki P. A proposed mechanical model for measuring propulsive forces in front crawl swimming. In: Haake S, eds. *Engineering of sport.* Rotterdam, Netherlands: Balkema, 1996:257–262.
72. Ellington CP. Unsteady aerodynamics of insect flight. *Symposia of the Society for Experimental Biology* 1995;49:109–129.
73. Prandtl L, Tietjens OG. *Applied hydro- and aerodynamics,* 2nd ed. New York: Dover, 1957.
74. Alexander RM. *Animal mechanics.* Oxford: Blackwell Scientific, 1983.
75. Rayner JMV. Dynamics of the vortex wakes of flying and swimming vertebrates. *Symposia of the Society for Experimental Biology* 1995;49:131–155.
76. Weis-Fogh T. Quick estimates of flight fitness in hovering animals, including novel mechanisms for lift production. *J Exp Biol* 1973;59:169–230.
77. Ellington CP, Berg C van der, Willmott AP, Thomas ALR. Leading-edge vortices in insect flight. *Nature* 1996;384:626–630.
78. Berg C van der, Ellington CP. The vortex wake of a "hovering" model hawkmoth. *Philos Trans R Soc Lond [Biol]* 1997;352:317–328.
79. Berg C van der, Ellington CP. The three-dimensional leading-edge vortex wake of a "hovering" model hawkmoth. *Philos Trans R Soc Lond [Biol]* 1997;352:329–340.
80. Hay JG, Thayer AM. Flow visualization of competitive swimming techniques: the tufts method. *J Biomech* 1989;22:11–19.
81. Karpovich PV, Pestrecov K. Mechanical work and efficiency in swimming crawl and back strokes. *Arbeitsphysiologie* 1938/39;10:504–514.
82. Karpovich PV, Millman N. Energy expenditure in swimming. *Am J Physiol* 1944;142:140–144.
83. Åstrand P-O, Rodahl K. *Textbook of work physiology.* New York: McGraw-Hill, 1977.
84. Adrian MJ, Singh M, Karpovich PV. Energy cost of leg kick, arm stroke, and whole crawl stroke. *J Appl Physiol* 1966;21:1763–1766.
85. Klissouras V. Energy metabolism in swimming the dolphin stroke. *Int Z Angew Physiol Einschl Arbeitsphysiol* 1968;25:142–150.
86. Montpetit RR, Leger LA, Lavoie JM, Cazorla G. $\dot{V}O_2$ peak during free swimming using the backward extrapolation of the O_2 recovery curve. *Eur J Appl Physiol* 1981;47:385–391.
87. Costill DL, Kovaleski J, Porter D, Kirwan J, Fielding R, King D. Energy expenditure during front crawl swimming: predicting success in middle-distance events. *Int J Sports Med* 1985;6:266–270.
88. Bonen A, Wilson BA, Yarkony M, Belcastro AN. Maximal oxygen uptake during free, tethered, and flume swimming. *J Appl Physiol* 1980;48:232–235.
89. Magel JR, Faulkner JA. Maximum oxygen uptakes of college swimmers. *J Appl Physiol* 1967;22:929–938.
90. Magel JR. Comparison of the physiologic response to varying intensities of submaximal work in tethered swimming and treadmill running. *J Sport Med* 1971;11:203–212.
91. Barzdukas AP, Franciosi P, Trappe S, Letner C, Troup JP. Adaptations to interval training at common intensities and different work:rest ratios. In: MacLaren D, Reilly T, Lees A, eds. *Biomechanics and medicine in swimming, swimming science,* vol 6. London: E & FN Spon, 1992:189–194.
92. d'Acquisto LJ, Bone M, Takahashi S, Langhans G, Barzdukas AP, Troup JP. Changes in aerobic power and swimming economy as a result of reduced training volume. In: MacLaren D, Reilly T, Lees A, eds. *Biomechanics and medicine in swimming, swimming science,* vol 6. London: E & FN Spon, 1992:201–206.
93. Holmér I. Oxygen uptake during swimming in man. *J Appl Physiol* 1972;33:502–509.
94. Holmér I. Physiology of swimming man. *Acta Physiol Scand Suppl* 1974;407:1–55.
95. Holmér I. Energy cost of arm stroke, leg kick, and the whole stroke in competitive swimming styles. *Eur J Appl Physiol* 1974;33:105–118.
96. Andersen KL. Energy cost of swimming. *Acta Chir Scand Suppl* 1960;253:169–174.
97. Åstrand PO, Eriksson BO, Nylander I, Engstrom L, Karlberg P, Saltin B. Girl swimmers with special reference to respiratory and circulatory adaptation and gynaecological and psychiatric aspects. *Acta Paediatr Suppl* 1963;147:43–70.
98. Chatard JC, Lavoie JM, Lacour JR. Analysis of determinants of swimming economy in front crawl. *Eur J Appl Physiol* 1990;61:88–92.
99. Handel PJ van, Katz A, Morrow JR, Troup JP, Daniels JT, Bradley PW. Aerobic economy and competitive performance of U.S. elite swimmers. In: Ungerechts BE, Wilke K, Reischle K, eds. *Swimming science*, vol 5. Champaign, IL: Human Kinetics, 1988:219–227.
100. McArdle WD, Glaser RM, Magel JR. Metabolic and cardiorespiratory response during free swimming and treadmill walking. *J Appl Physiol* 1971;30:733–738.
101. Toussaint HM, Knops W, Groot G de, Hollander AP. The mechanical efficiency of front crawl swimming. *Med Sci Sports Exerc* 1990;22:402–408.
102. Montpetit RR, Cazorla G, Lavoie JM. Energy expenditure during front crawl swimming: a comparison between males and females. In: Ungerechts BE, Reischle K, Wilke K, eds. *Swimming science*, vol 5. Champaign, IL: Human Kinetics, 1988:229–235.
103. Pugh LGC, Edholm OG, Fox RH, et al. A physiological study of channel swimming. *Clin Sci* 1960;19:257–273.
104. Dobeln VW, Holmér I. Body composition, sinking force, and oxygen uptake of man during water treading. *J Appl Physiol* 1974;37:55–59.
105. Pendergast DR, Craig AB. Biomechanics of floating in water. *Physiologist* 1974;17:305.
106. Huijing PA, Clarys JP, Toussaint HM, et al. Active drag related to body dimensions. In: Ungerechts B, eds. *Abstracts—5th international symposium of biomechanics and medicine in swimming.* Bockenem: Fahnemann, 1986:48.
107. Alexander RM. Swimming. In: Alexander RM, Goldspink G, eds. *Mechanics and energetics of animal locomotion.* London: Chapman and Hall, 1977:222–249.
108. Toussaint HM, Beelen A, Rodenburg A, et al. Propelling efficiency of front crawl swimming. *J Appl Physiol* 1988;65:2506–2512.
109. Webb PW. The swimming energetics of trout II: oxygen consumption and swimming efficiency. *J Exp Biol* 1971;55:521–540.
110. Groot G de, Ingen Schenau GJ van. Fundamental mechanics applied to swimming: technique and propelling efficiency. In: Ungerechts BE, Wilke K, Reischle K, eds. *Swimming science,* vol 5. Champaign, IL: Human Kinetics, 1988:17–30.
111. Lighthill MJ. *Mathematical body fluid dynamics.* Philadelphia: Society for Industrial and Applied Mathematics, 1975.
112. Charbonnier JP, Lacour JR, Riffat J, Flandrois R. Experimental

study of the performance of competition swimmers. *Eur J Appl Physiol* 1975;34:157–167.

113. Miyashita M. Method of calculating mechanical power in swimming the breast stroke. *Res Q* 1974;45:128–137.
114. Capelli C, Zamparo P, Cigalotto A, et al. Bioenergetics and biomechanics of front crawl swimming. *J Appl Physiol* 1995;78:674–679.
115. Pendergast DR, Tedesco M, Nawrocki DM, Fisher NM. Energetics of underwater swimming with scuba. *Med Sci Sport Exerc* 1996;28:573–580.
116. Toussaint HM, Hollander AP. Energetics of competitive swimming—implications for training-programs. *Sports Med* 1994;18:384–405.
117. Toussaint HM, Groot G de, Hollander AP, et al. Measurement of efficiency in swimming man. In: Ungerechts BE, Reischle K, Wilke K, eds. *Swimming science,* vol 5. Champaign, IL: Human Kinetics, 1988:45–52.
118. Lighthill MJ. Hydromechanics of aquatic animal propulsion. *Annual Review of Fluid Mechanics* 1969;1:413–445.
119. Ungerechts BE. On the relevance of rotating water flow for the propulsion in swimming. In: Jonsson B, eds. *Biomechanics,* vol 10B. Champaign, IL: Human Kinetics, 1987:713–716.
120. Ungerechts BE. The relation of peak body acceleration to phases of movements in swimming. In: Ungerechts BE, Wilke K, Reischle K, eds. *Swimming science,* vol 5. Champaign, IL: Human Kinetics, 1988:61–66.
121. Toussaint HM, Janssen T, Kluft M. Effect of propelling surface size on the mechanics and energetics of front crawl swimming. *J Biomech* 1991;24:205–211.
122. Grimston SK, Hay JG. Relationships among anthropometric and stroking characteristics of college swimmers. *Med Sci Sports Exerc* 1986;18:60–68.
123. Toussaint HM, Helm FCT van der, Elzerman JR, Hollander AP, Groot G de, Ingen Schenau GJ van. A power balance applied to swimming. In: Hollander AP, Huijing PA, Groot G de, eds. *Biomechanics and medicine in swimming.* Champaign, IL: Human Kinetics, 1983:165–172.
124. Payton CJ, Lauder MA. The influence of hand paddles on the kinematics of front crawl swimming. *J Hum Movement Stud* 1995;28:175.
125. Brandt RA, Pichowsky MA. Conservation of energy in competitive swimming. *J Biomech* 1995;28:925–933.
126. Serresse O, Loertie G, Bouchard C, Boulay MR. Estimation of the contribution of the various energy systems during maximal work of short duration. *Int J Sports Med* 1988;9:456–460.
127. Costill DL. Lactate metabolism for swimming. In: MacLaren D, Reilly T, Lees A, eds. *Biomechanics and medicine in swimming, swimming science,* vol 6. London: E & FN Spon, 1992:3–11.
128. Ogita F, Onodera T, Tabata I. The effect of hand paddles on anaerobic energy release during supramaximal swimming. *Med Sci Sports Exerc* 1999;31:729–735..
129. Ingen Schenau GJ van, Koning JJ de, Groot G de. Optimisation of sprinting performance in running cycling and speed skating. *Sports Med* 1994;17:259–275.
130. Koning JJ de, Ingen Schenau GJ van. On the estimation of mechanical power in endurance sports. *Sport Sci Rev* 1994; 3:34–54.
131. Péronnet F, Thibault G. Mathematical analysis of running performance and world running records. *J Appl Physiol* 1989;67:453–465.
132. Margaria R. *Biomechanics and energetics of muscular exercise.* Oxford: Clarendon Press, 1966.
133. Ward-Smith AJ. A mathematical theory of running based on the first law of thermodynamics and its application to the performance of world class athletes. *J Biomechanics* 1985;18:337–350.
134. Medbø JI, Mohn A-C, Tabata I, Bahr R, Vaage O, Sejersted OM. Anaerobic capacity determined by maximal accumulated O_2 deficit. *J Appl Physiol* 1988;64:50–60.
135. Troup JS, Hollander AP, Bone M, Trappe S, Barzdukas AP. Performance related difference in the anaerobic contribution of competitive freestyle swimmers. In: MacLaren D, Reilly T, Lees A, eds. *Biomechanics and medicine in swimming, swimming science,* vol 6. London: E & FN Spon, 1992:271–277.
136. Ogita F, Taniguchi S. The comparison of peak oxygen-uptake between swim bench exercise and arm stroke. *Eur J Appl Physiol Occup Phys* 1995;71:295–300.
137. Ogita F, Hara M, Tabata I. Anaerobic capacity and maximal oxygen-uptake during arm stroke, leg kicking and whole-body swimming. *Acta Physiol Scand* 1996;157:435–441.
138. Toussaint HM, Hollander AP. Mechanics and energetics of front crawl swimming. In: Miyashita M, Mutoh Y, Richardson AB, eds. *Medicine and science in aquatic sports.* Basel: Karger, 1994:107–116.
139. Toussaint HM, Wakayoshi K, Hollander AP, Ogita F. Simulated front crawl swimming performance related to critical speed and critical power. *Med Sci Sports Exerc* 1998;30:144–151.
140. Wakayoshi K, Yoshida T, Udo M, et al. A simple method for determining critical speed as swimming fatigue threshold in competitive swimming. *Int J Sports Med* 1992;13:367–71.
141. Wakayoshi K, Ikuta K, Yoshida T, et al. The determination and validity of critical speed as swimming performance index in the competitive swimmer. *Eur J Appl Phys* 1992;64:153–157.
142. Hill DW, Steward RP, Lane CJ. Application of the critical power concept to young swimmers. *Pediatr Exerc Sci* 1995;7:281–293.
143. Morton RH. A 3-parameter critical power model. *Ergonomics* 1996;39:611–619.

Exercise and Sport Science,
edited by William E. Garrett, Jr., and Donald T. Kirkendall.
Lippincott Williams & Wilkins, Philadelphia © 2000.

CHAPTER 42

Biomechanics of Walking and Running

Philip E. Martin and David J. Sanderson

Walking and running are two highly complex motor skills that incorporate input from multiple levels of the nervous system, involve muscular contributions throughout the body, and require the coordination of many skeletal degrees of freedom. Nevertheless, under nonpathologic conditions, an individual can produce a highly stable and repeatable gait pattern without conscious control of the process.

A substantial body of research literature on the biomechanical aspects of walking and running already exists and is rapidly growing. A simple search of the computer-based Medical Literature Analysis and Retrieval System (MEDLINE) of the United States National Library of Medicine yields more than 1000 references written since 1966 for both biomechanics of walking and biomechanics of running. Given the extensive and diverse literature base and the complexity of the motor skills, developing a comprehensive review of the biomechanics of walking and running in a single chapter is a daunting, if not impossible, task.

There already exist many published review articles and books that focus broadly on the biomechanical nature of walking and/or running (e.g., 1–14) as well as many more focused reviews on the subject (e.g., 15–22). Therefore, we have not attempted to produce a comprehensive review of walking and running biomechanics in this chapter, but rather we have chosen a small subset of topics that we feel are interesting and timely and that complement existing reviews. These include the relationships between gait biomechanics and economy, age-related changes in walking mechanics, amputee locomotion, the role of elastic mechanisms in gait, and the adaptability of gait. The reader is encouraged to seek other original and review sources for alternative perspectives on gait biomechanics.

P. E. Martin: Department of Exercise Science and Physical Education, Arizona State University, Tempe, Arizona 85287-0404.

D. J. Sanderson: School of Human Kinetics, University of British Columbia, Vancouver, British Columbia, Canada.

RELATIONSHIPS BETWEEN GAIT BIOMECHANICS AND ECONOMY

Considerable research has focused on the aerobic demand and energy cost of walking and running, and their associations with biomechanical features of gait. Economy, defined as the steady-state aerobic demand for a given submaximal task, has performance implications for the runner seeking to maximize distance running performance as well as for special clinical populations that have heightened energy cost demands and relatively low physical working capacities. Research has demonstrated that gait economy tends to vary widely among individuals, and that this variation exists in the absence of neurologic and musculoskeletal deficiencies and disease that can increase energy cost substantially. As an example, Daniels and colleagues (23) reported aerobic demands for 13 competitive distance runners ranging from 39.5 to 45.1 mL/kg/min for graded walking at 1.78 m/s, 43.2 to 53.8 mL/kg/min for level running at 4.13 m/s, and 33.2 to 43.0 mL/kg/min for a 30-cm step test. Interestingly, Daniels and colleagues also observed that the economy measures for different forms of exercise were not strongly associated with one another. They suggested that economy "is not a function of inherent muscular metabolic economy" (p. 613) but rather may be related to either skill level or anatomic differences that contribute to different muscle mechanical advantages about joints. The question then is whether selected biomechanical and/or structural factors explain economy differences between individuals.

Gait Speed

The speed at which one locomotes is perhaps the simplest and most fundamental descriptor of gait kinemat-

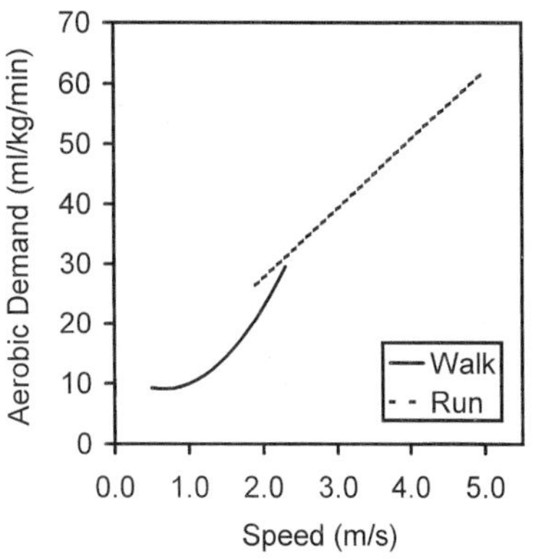

FIG. 42–1. The aerobic demands (mL/kg/min) for walking and running increase systematically as speed increases. A curvilinear relationship between aerobic demand and speed is apparent for walking but not for running.

ics. Altering gait speed is also one of the most common ways of manipulating exercise intensity, in both research and recreational exercise settings. Aerobic demands expressed per unit of time (mL/kg/min) for both walking and running increase systematically as speed, and thus exercise intensity, increases (Fig. 42–1). When the aerobic demand or energy cost is considered relative to the distance traversed (e.g., mL/kg/km), it becomes apparent that walking and running economy responses are substantially different from one another (Fig. 42–2). The mass- or weight-specific aerobic demand to cover a given distance varies little with running speed, indicating that the total energy cost to run a given distance is nearly the same whether a leisurely pace or a high speed is used. It should be noted that the data for running in Fig. 42–2 are for treadmill locomotion for which wind resistance effects are negligible. Aerobic demand for overground running at 5 m/s is 5% to 7% higher than that for treadmill running (24). Because wind resistance is proportional to speed squared (25), the tendency for the aerobic demand to decline subtly with increasing running speed, as shown in Fig. 42–2, would be diminished for overground running. Thus, it is reasonable to conclude that there is no clearly defined most economical speed of running. In contrast, there is considerable variation in walking aerobic demand per unit of distance traveled as speed changes, and a readily apparent most economical speed of walking (1.3–1.4 m/s) emerges (26,27). Martin and colleagues (26) have shown that this most economical walking speed is quite insensitive to the age and physical activity status of the subjects. Young and elderly, active and sedentary adults had very similar most economical speeds.

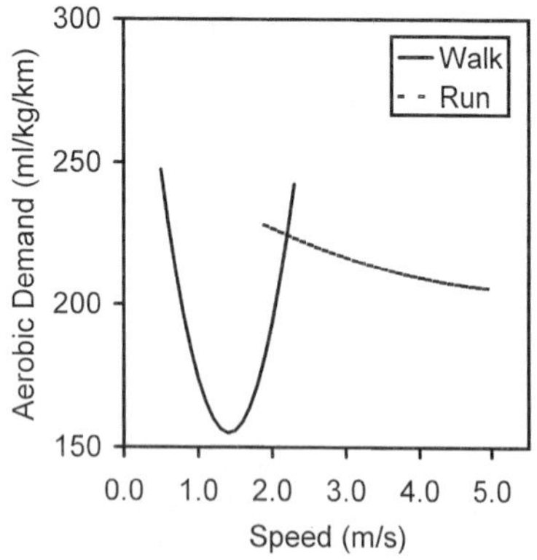

FIG. 42–2. The aerobic demands of walking and running reflect substantially different responses to increases in speed when expressed per unit of distance traveled (mL/kg/km). A most economical speed of walking is apparent for walking but not for running.

In a cross-species assessment of the energy cost of running, Kram and Taylor (28) noted that the energy consumed to move a unit of body weight or mass a given distance (i.e., cost of transport, e.g., J/N/m) changes little with running speed. The running aerobic demand data for humans reflected in Fig. 42–2 fit well with this observation. Kram and Taylor further proposed that the cost of transport for running is inversely proportional to support distance (i.e., the distance the body moves forward during single limb support), and they showed that support distances changed little across a range of running speeds for multiple species. Running support distances for humans, however, increase as running speed increases (29,30), and thus they are not consistent with Kram and Taylor's model.

The absence of a speed-independent cost of transport for walking (Fig. 42–2) appears to be associated with two factors. At the slow end of the walking speed continuum (i.e., <1.3 m/s), the relative contribution of the cost of resting or maintenance metabolism to the total energy cost increases as speed decreases (26). This results in a relatively high cost of transport at very slow walking speeds despite a low exercise intensity. As walking speed increases, both stride length and rate increase. At the fast end of the walking speed continuum (>1.4 m/s), lower-extremity musculature must not only produce higher forces to generate longer stride lengths but also must produce those forces at higher speeds as stride rate rises. Hill (31) demonstrated that muscle efficiency is a function of shortening velocity such that a most efficient velocity exists. Thus, fundamental force-velocity and associated power-velocity properties of muscle likely contribute to less efficient production of force at very high walking speeds (26).

Stride Rate/Length

The aerobic demand of walking and running at any given speed is a function of stride rate (SR) and length (SL), such that aerobic demand increases curvilinearly as SR is either increased or decreased (and thus, SL is either shortened or lengthened, respectively) from the preferred SR (Fig. 42–3) (32–37). An individual's preferred SR/SL combination usually is in close agreement

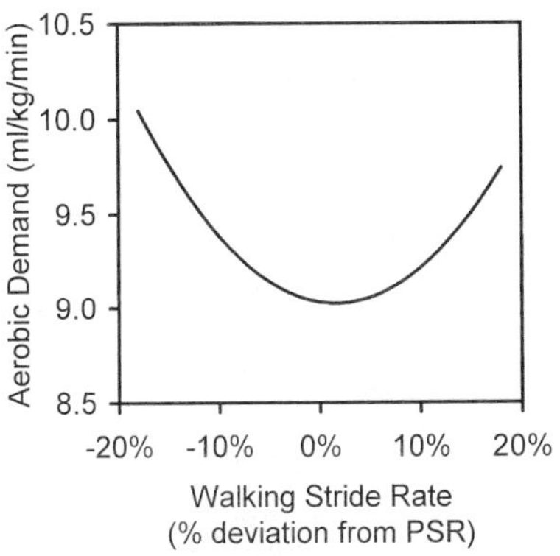

FIG. 42–3. The aerobic demand of walking (mL/kg/min) at an intermediate walking speed changes systematically as stride rate and length are manipulated. For most individuals, their preferred stride rate and length combination coincides closely with their most economical stride rate and length. Running aerobic demand responds similarly to stride rate and length manipulation.

with his or her optimal or most economical SR/SL. Morgan and colleagues (37) observed that only 20% of a sample of 45 recreational runners used a preferred SR/SL combination that deviated by 5% or more from their most economical SR/SL. The specific mechanisms underlying the U-shaped SR/SL–aerobic demand response is again linked to fundamental muscle force and power-generating capabilities. Changes in SR and SL require concomitant changes in the rates of muscle lengthening and shortening and rate of force development that ultimately affect aerobic demand (28,38).

Holt and colleagues (39) suggest that stride rate rather than stride length is the critical factor that determines the muscular effort required to generate the gait cycle, and that stride rate is strongly influenced by the inertia characteristics of the swinging limbs. They propose that walking can be modeled as a force-driven harmonic oscillator (FDHO) and that the resonant frequency of the FDHO model, which is dependent on the anthropometric and inertia properties of the legs, corresponds to the preferred rate of walking. Their results supported their hypothesis that "the resonant frequency of a harmonic oscillator can accurately predict that chosen by subjects when appropriate adjustments are made to the formula based on an optimization criterion of minimum force" (p. 64). They concluded that stride rate or stride time is effectively a motor control parameter that is determined by the physical attributes of the system, namely its inertia characteristics. In subsequent research, Holt and colleagues (40) confirmed that preferred stride rate was not different from that predicted from their FDHO model. When stride rate was manipulated during constant speed treadmill walking, both preferred and FDHO-predicted stride rates resulted in minimal aerobic demand, lending additional support to the association between SR/SL and gait economy. Recent research examining preferred and FDHO predicted stride rates for backward walking (41) and for children (42) lends some support for the generalizability of the notion that the body tends to self-optimize gait such that muscular effort and energy cost are minimized. This phenomenon needs to be examined further for other cyclic, submaximal tasks.

Ground Reaction Forces

Although various features of the ground reaction force (GRF) have been studied extensively, the association between GRF characteristics and gait economy is not well documented. In their cross-species research involving mammals ranging in mass from 30 g to 140 kg, Kram and Taylor (28) confirmed their hypothesis that the rate of energy consumption per unit of body weight is inversely proportional to the weight-specific rate of force application to the ground, and ultimately to the time of force application, during each stride. Thus, they suggested that simple knowledge of single limb stance time and body weight allows for a good approximation of an animal's rate of energy consumption during running. In contrast with Kram and Taylor's hypothesis, Williams and Cavanagh (43,44) found a direct relationship between support time and running aerobic demand in humans (r=0.49), indicating that longer support times were associated with higher rates of energy consumption. While Kram and Taylor's principle provides a powerful first approximation of the energy cost of running in humans and animals, the utility of this principle for explaining interindividual differences in running economy in humans is unsubstantiated. Williams and Cavanagh (43) also noted that more economical runners are more likely to display lower first peaks in the vertical GRF, smaller anteroposterior and vertical peak forces, and a rear-foot striking pattern. They suggested forefoot strikers place greater demands on the musculature, particularly the plantar flexors, to assist with impact absorption in early stance, whereas rear-foot strikers rely more heavily on footwear and skeletal structures to cushion and support the body in early stance.

Mechanical Power

Aerobic demand represents a global descriptor of the physiologic demand of walking or running, whereas mechanical power output reflects a global expression of muscular effort or output. Assuming that a substantial portion of the metabolic demands of walking and running is attributed to muscles doing work (i.e., actively shortening or lengthening), then mechanical power should be an effective predictor of gait economy. When considered across a wide range of walking or running speeds, mechanical power is directly and strongly related ($r > 0.79$) to walking or running speed (e.g., 45–47) and aerobic demand (45,47). At any given speed, however, the power-economy relationship is substantially weaker. Taylor and colleagues (38,48) concluded that mechanical work or power does not satisfactorily explain economy variations among species of animals varying widely in body size.

A major limitation of mechanical power computations is their inability to account for isometric contributions of muscles during gait, which recent research suggests may be substantial. In a creative assessment of tendon forces and muscle fiber length changes in running turkeys, Roberts and colleagues (49) reported that most of the muscular force and activity in level running occurs when muscles experience little change in length during the support phase. Operating under near isometric conditions allows a muscle to function in the high force region of its force-velocity curve and thereby tends to maximize force per cross-sectional area of active muscle. Thus, "the demands of support may be met most economically by muscles that produce force while minimizing mechanical work" (p. 1115).

Segment Mass Distribution

The energetic cost of locomotion has been hypothesized to be an important factor influencing the evolution of limb structure in terrestrial animals (e.g., 50–52). This hypothesis is based on the debatable assumption that a major portion of metabolic demand during walking and running is associated with accelerating the limbs with each stride (49). It suggests that those animals that rely on economical locomotion for survival are more likely to reflect a limb structure that presents a smaller inertia load to the musculature, either because less mass is concentrated in the limbs or because limb mass is concentrated more proximally (53). Support for the association between limb inertia characteristics and gait economy comes primarily from segment loading studies in which segment inertia has been modified artificially (e.g., 54–56). The cost of carrying load on the distal aspect of the lower extremities is significantly greater than that when load is carried more proximally on the limb or on the trunk. For example, the relative increase in running aerobic demand produced by adding a given load to the feet is twice as great as that produced by thigh loading (7.0% per kg vs. 3.5% per kg of added load) (54,55), and approximately seven times greater than the increase produced by trunk loading (57). Myers and colleagues (58), however, suggest the mass distribution factor may be of only modest significance. In an assessment of the independent effects of speed, stride rate, and body mass distribution (1.8 kg of mass added to the trunk vs. 0.9 kg of mass added to each shank) on running aerobic demand, they reported that mass distribution accounted for less than 3% of the explained variance in aerobic demand. In contrast, speed and stride rate accounted for 70% and 15% of running aerobic demand variation, respectively. Thus, while the mass distribution hypothesis is theoretically sound, the significance of this factor is not well substantiated or understood.

Joint and Muscular Flexibility

A commonly held belief is that a high level of flexibility is important for optimal running performance. A hypothesis that improved flexibility contributes to less passive resistance about the joints and thereby reduces the demands placed on the musculature is also intuitively appealing. Consistent with this notion, Godges and colleagues (59) reported a reduction in aerobic demand of running following an acute bout of stretching that resulted in increased hip flexion-extension range of motion. In contrast, Gleim and colleagues (60) observed that individuals who displayed poorer flexibility based on a series of 11 static trunk and lower extremity flexibility measures were more economical runners. Their least flexible subjects were as much as 12% more economical than the most flexible individuals. Craib and colleagues (61) reported similar findings. Running aerobic demand was significantly related to maximum passive ankle dorsiflexion angle (r=0.65) and standing external hip rotation (r=0.53), indicating more economical runners showed more limited ranges of motion for these two joint actions. These two flexibility measures explained 47% of the variance in running economy. Decreased need for activation of posture-stabilizing musculature about the hip and increased elastic energy reutilization about the ankle were speculated to be two mechanisms contributing to more economical running (60,61). Because of the limited empirical research on the association between joint flexibility and gait economy, additional research on the specific effects of flexibility and other structural features on the economy of motion is needed.

GAIT BIOMECHANICS OF SPECIAL POPULATIONS

Gait Adaptations Associated with Aging

There is an extensive body of research literature focusing on changes in gait patterns with advancing age. While the majority of this literature simply describes age-related changes in walking mechanics, there is increasing interest in the potential causes underlying gait changes and in the efficacy of intervention strategies for improving gait mechanics in older adults. The most consistently reported and robust age-related change in gait is a decrease in the preferred or freely chosen speed of walking (e.g., 26,62–67). Preferred walking speeds for elderly adults are typically 10% to 30% lower than those of younger adults. The rate at which walking speed declines, however, is not constant across adulthood. In an investigation of 438 adults ranging in age from 19 to 102, Himann and colleagues (63) demonstrated that preferred walking speed declines modestly (0.11% to 0.20% per year) until age 60 to 65, at which time the rate of decline of preferred walking speed increases by a factor of 10 (1.24% to 1.60% per year).

Other commonly reported age-related changes in the walking pattern include decreases in stride length and the ratio of swing-to-stance time, and increases in stance width and double support time. An increase in variability of the gait pattern has also been suggested as a possible age-related phenomenon, although this may be a trait linked more specifically with older adults who have a history of falling (68–70). Because many gait parameters are speed dependent and because the majority of research has not contrasted older and younger adults under controlled walking speeds, it is less apparent whether these various temporal and kinematic changes are independent of the decrease in preferred walking speed (64,67). Larish and colleagues (64) reported that older adults demonstrated shorter relative stride lengths than young adults (1.56 vs. 1.66 times leg length, respectively) when both groups were studied at a common intermediate walking speed (1.34 m/s). Thus, their results suggest that age-related changes in gait kinematics are affected by more than just the decline in walking speed.

The underlying causes of the observed slowing of walking with age are less clear. Age-related declines in musculoskeletal function are well documented in the gerontology literature (e.g., 71,72). For example, both dynamic muscle strength and joint range of motion decrease with advancing age (e.g., 73–76). Several studies have reported positive relationships between various expressions of lower extremity muscular strength or power, particularly that pertaining to the ankle plantar flexors, and walking speed in older adults (65,67,77–80). Correlation expressions, however, are typically on the order of 0.4 or lower, indicating that the associations between strength and walking speed are not especially strong. Maximal aerobic capacity has also been positively associated with preferred walking speed (78,81), suggesting that individuals who are more fit aerobically tend to have faster self-selected walking speeds. Similarly, preferred walking speed has also been associated with physical activity status of elderly adults such that those who are more physically active tend to self-select higher speeds (26).

Results of exercise-based intervention programs on gait parameters have been mixed. For example, Cunningham and colleagues (82) reported that 60- to 65-year-old men showed significant increases in both maximal aerobic capacity (9.5%) and preferred walking speed (1.29 to 1.43 m/s) following participation in a 1-year walking or jogging aerobic training program. Using a 20-week multifaceted exercise program (e.g., aerobic, balance, coordination, and strength exercises), Lord and colleagues (83) observed strength improvements (9% to 21%) in several lower extremity muscle groups and a concomitant 6% improvement in preferred walking speed for a community-based cohort of 160 women aged 60 to 83. Similarly, Judge and colleagues (84) reported that 12 weeks of balance and lower extremity resistance training by elderly adults residing in life-care communities produced strength improvements of approximately 30% as well as an 8% increase in preferred walking speed. Other recent investigations, however, have shown no gait improvements in elderly adults following strength and/or endurance training (85–87). Sipila and colleagues (86), for example, reported improvements in both strength and walking velocity in elderly adults following 18 weeks of strength and endurance training. Control subjects, however, reflected similar improvements in walking speed despite the absence of strength gains.

The preceding exercise and aging discussions have focused entirely on physical changes that may be linked to changes in gait. Maki (70) provides an alternative perspective for considering gait changes. He found that slower walking speeds, shorter stride lengths, and a prolonged period of double support were associated with a preexisting fear of falling, but not necessarily with previous history of falling nor subsequent rate of falling. He suggests that age-related changes in gait may actually reflect a strategy to improve stability. This only serves to underscore the importance of examining decrements of gait performance and the efficacy of intervention strategies from multiple perspectives.

Amputee Locomotion

In biomechanical analyses of human locomotion, left-to-right symmetry in all biomechanical variables is typically assumed. The normal variations in segment dimensions (such as girth and strength) appear to have minimal effect on the kinematic and kinetic events associated with either walking or running (88,89). However, for the unilateral below-knee amputee this situation is quite different because the structural asymmetry arising from the amputation results in a concomitant loss of muscle and sensory feedback. The amputee has the substantial challenge of adapting motor control strategies to compensate for the functional loss of significant locomotor musculature and the altered structural properties of the supporting limb. These adaptive processes must incorporate prosthetic limb motion with those of the intact limb to develop a reasonably symmetrical gait (90).

The role of the ankle and foot to functional locomotion is complex. The 52 bones, multiple muscles, and ligaments serve to provide the body with a means to interact with the ground during the support phase. Prior to 1985 the most common prosthetic foot type was a relatively simple single-axis cushioned heel (SACH) device. More recent prosthetic designs attempt to mimic the motion of an intact foot and lower extremity more effectively, particularly the contributions of the plantar flexors. Winter (91) confirmed the importance of the plantar flexors when he observed that more than 80% of the mechanical power during walking is generated by the plantar flexors during push off. In 1985 the first so-called dynamic energy returning (DER) prosthesis, the Seattle Foot, was released commercially (92). This prosthesis was designed to store energy during early and mid-stance, when the prosthesis was deformed due to normal loading, and to return a portion of that strain energy to the lower extremity during push off. Since the introduction of the Seattle Foot, many other DER prostheses have become available to amputees.

Despite the intuitive appeal of DER designs, research evidence suggests that these prostheses produce only modest effects on biomechanical features of gait. Not surprisingly, these effects appear to be stronger for running than walking because of the higher loading that occurs with running. Gitter and colleagues (93) contrasted walking biomechanics for amputees wearing the Seattle and SACH prostheses. They reported increased energy generation during push-off for the Seattle Foot, but no significant differences in the pattern or magnitude of knee and hip power outputs compared to the SACH foot. Torburn and colleagues (94) reported no differences in gait symmetry nor in preferred and fast overground walking speed when contrasting several DER prostheses with the SACH foot; they concluded, "There are no advantages of the dynamic elastic response feet for the amputee who is limited to level walking" (p. 383). Czerniecki and colleagues (103) examined the effect of energy-storing prostheses on lower-extremity joint moments and muscle power outputs during the stance phase of running. While there were individual differences in response to wearing a so-called dynamic prosthesis, amputees generally showed improvement in power characteristics of the lower extremity when using DER compared to passive prostheses. That is, the dynamic prostheses contributed to power profiles that were more similar to those of nonamputees.

There is little evidence suggesting that DER prostheses lead to substantial metabolic energy savings. Both Torburn and colleagues (94) and Colborne and colleagues (95) reported no differences in walking aerobic demand when contrasting amputees using DER prostheses and the SACH foot. Postema and colleagues (96) suggested that DER feet would lead to a maximum saving of 3% of metabolic energy during walking. They considered it unlikely that the subjects would notice this difference, and concluded that differences in energy expenditure of this magnitude were probably not clinically relevant.

From a motor control perspective, one of the interesting questions is how unilateral amputees adapt control strategies to offset the substantial losses of structural, motor, and sensory function. Young, active unilateral amputees are capable of generating reasonably symmetrical walking and running patterns from temporal and kinematic perspectives (97–99). Returning to a symmetrical gait pattern following amputation is typically an important goal of the rehabilitation process. Enoka and colleagues (97) observed some differences in running kinematics between their amputee group and previously published data on nonamputees, but they suggested that 60% of the amputee runners exhibited temporal and kinematic patterns that were similar to nonamputees. Furthermore, they showed that the remaining 40% had differences that would have been removed with prosthetic adjustment or training. Sanderson and Martin (98,99) reported marked asymmetries in underlying ankle, knee, and hip moment profiles, but reasonably symmetrical temporal and kinematic features of walking and running gaits. Joint moment asymmetries were particularly notable at the knee and to a lesser extent at the ankle and hip. The contribution of the prosthetic limb knee extensor musculature to the overall support function was substantially reduced or missing, presumably because of an apparent necessity to reduce loading on and about the knee. To offset this reduced extensor function, the prosthetic limb hip generally reflected a higher extensor contribution. Miller (100) and Miller and colleagues (101) reported similar adaptations in lower extremity joint kinetics during running.

Not surprisingly, there has been little attention paid to the nonprosthetic leg. Nevertheless, research suggests that intact limb mechanics are altered along with prosthetic limb responses during the motor control adaptation process. Powers and colleagues (102) showed that intact limb loading, as reflected by ground reaction force profiles, was dependent on the type of prosthesis used. Specifically, intact limb loading was reduced with the Flex-foot compared to the SACH foot. Sanderson and Martin (98,99) showed that there were different responses on the intact side compared to the prosthetic side and concluded that there was some modulation of the intact leg to match the prosthetic leg rather than to maintain a pattern similar to the normal. Results suggested that there was no need to develop completely new patterns of joint moments, but rather that it was sufficient to retune the current moment patterns to account for new segmental properties and thus retain internal timing characteristics. Czerniecki and colleagues (103) presented data showing that there was energy transfer between the swing leg and the trunk that may reflect an adaptive strategy to allow energy redistribution to the trunk, which may, in turn, compensate for the reduced power output of the prosthetic limb late in the stance phase.

One of the more recent research emphases relating to prosthetic design and amputee locomotion has focused on the effect of prosthetic limb inertia manipulation on gait biomechanics and energetics. In general, lower extremity prosthetic limbs tend to be much lighter than the limbs they replace, resulting in a substantial inertia asymmetry. This trend toward light prostheses has been driven in part by advances in light-weight materials used in construction of prosthetic limbs and by clinical opinion that prostheses should be as light as possible, presumably to reduce the muscular effort needed for prosthetic control. Data supporting such a prescription, however, are limited. In an early computer modeling effort of the swing leg in which lower-extremity inertia properties were manipulated, Mena and colleagues (104) concluded, "Leg motion was less sensitive to increases in the [segment inertial properties] than to decreases." They suggested further that "a 'lightweight' prosthesis would be less desirable than a 'heavy' prosthesis, while a prosthesis that had the same inertial properties of the removed limb may be most desirable" (p. 831). This raises the question of whether inertial modifications of prosthetic limbs may lead to a more effective (e.g., faster preferred walking speeds, more symmetrical walking pattern) and more economical gait pattern.

Czerniecki and colleagues (105) demonstrated that the addition of up to 1.34 kg of mass near the location of the shank center of mass produced no increases in the aerobic demand of above-knee amputees during walking under multiple controlled speeds. Mean data suggested that aerobic demand tended to decrease subtly with the addition of mass. Similarly, Gailey and colleagues (106) reported no significant change in walking aerobic demand when nearly 1 kg of mass was evenly distributed over the length of the prosthetic limb of below-knee amputees. These results provide encouraging data suggesting that heavier prosthetic limbs do not necessarily lead to higher energy costs. Hale (107) and Gitter and colleagues (108) reported no changes in walking speed and temporal characteristics of the gait cycle as the mass of the prosthetic shank was increased as much as 3.37 kg in above-knee amputees. Both studies showed that increases in shank mass resulted in increases in hip muscular effort during the swing phase, however. Despite this increased demand, four of Hale's six subjects preferred an intermediate loading condition; that is, one that increased their shank mass, but not to the point such that the prosthetic shank mass matched that of the intact limb. Furthermore, Gitter and colleagues suggested amputees have the ability to self-optimize their gait pattern across a range of prosthetic masses without adverse affects, and that further research needs to be conducted "to determine the psychobiologic underpinnings of changes in perceived exertion associated with alterations in prosthetic mass" (p. 120).

ELASTIC MECHANISMS DURING WALKING AND RUNNING

The Stretch-Shortening Cycle and Musculotendinous Elasticity

Many human movements, particularly those produced at high speeds and requiring high levels of muscle power, reflect patterns whereby concentric actions of muscle are immediately preceded by eccentric phases. This sequence of active lengthening of muscle followed by active shortening is referred to as the stretch-shortening cycle (SSC) of muscle (109), and it normally results in enhanced muscle performance (e.g., increased muscle work, higher power production) in explosive movements (e.g., maximal vertical jumping). Although this phenomenon is often referred to as a process involving storage and reutilization of elastic energy, it is important to recognize that a variety of mechanisms may contribute to the enhanced performance (see ref. 110 for a review). These include (a) a reflex mechanism in which muscle stretch during the eccentric phase heightens muscle stimulation during the concentric phase (111,112); (b) a heightened level of activation and muscle force present at the initiation of the concentric phase when preceded by eccentric action (113–115); (c) a force-enhancement mechanism whereby stretching of the muscle fibers during the eccentric phase temporarily enhances force-velocity properties (116,117); and (d) an elastic mechanism whereby strain energy is temporarily stored in the musculotendinous unit during the eccentric phase of a movement and then reutilized during the concentric phase (118–121).

Both walking and running reflect SSC behavior in multiple muscle groups, suggesting that muscle output may be enhanced by the mechanisms noted in the preceding paragraph. Neither walking nor submaximal running require maximal production of work or power by active musculature, however. For movements involving repetitive SSCs under submaximal, steady-state conditions, it is more appropriate to consider the benefits of the SSC, particularly the role of elasticity of the musculotendinous unit, in terms of the economy or efficiency of muscle power production rather than work or power generation (110). More specifically, the contractile elements of a muscle do not have to produce all of the necessary increases in mechanical energy during a movement cycle if elastic structures conserve some mechanical energy during an SSC. It should be further noted that only certain musculotendinous units can provide significant elastic energy contributions. Those muscles that have relatively slender and compliant tendons that are substantially longer than the muscle fascicles offer the greatest potential for elastic energy storage and return (122). Ankle plantar flexors are an example. In addition, Alexander and Ker (122) noted that significant metabolic energy savings will occur only if these relatively compliant tendons undergo large strains (on the order of 4% of their length) under high loading conditions. The need for high stresses to produce these strains is a primary reason that elastic energy contributions in walking are substantially lower than those in running. Hof (123) estimates elastic energy contributions of 13 to 23 J for walking (0.75–1.75 m/s) and 47 to 51 J for running (2.0–2.75 m/s).

There has been some debate on whether the ability of a muscle to store elastic energy can be altered with training and, indeed, whether there is an optimal compliance for effective return of energy. Wilson and colleagues (124) concluded that performance enhancement was increased as a consequence of flexibility training that caused increased compliance, which in turn resulted in an increased utilization of elastic strain energy. The authors further suggested that augmentation of performance from the SSC was dependent on the relationship between the resonant frequency of the movement and the frequency of the SSC itself. In a later study, however, Wilson and colleagues (125) suggested that the rate of force development is a more critical factor for athletic performance than elastic energy contributions, diminishing the value of training-induced changes in elastic response.

Footwear and Surface Elasticity

There is a limited body of research on how elastic properties of running footwear and surfaces influence running performance. The possibility that running shoes have the potential to store strain energy when the viscoelastic materials of the shoe are deformed in early stance and then return some portion of that strain energy to the runner during push-off in late stance has not received significant research support. For a sport shoe to provide a significant return of elastic strain energy to a runner, Nigg and Segesser (126) argued that several conditions must be met. First, the energy must be returned at the location where forces acting at the shoe/foot interface are centered. Second, the energy must be returned at the right time; that is, it must be well synchronized with the push-off at the end of the stance phase. Finally, the energy return must occur at a rate consistent with the rate of development of push-off force by the runner. Using a simple spring model, Nigg and Segesser estimated that under ideal conditions the maximum possible energy return from a sport shoe per step is approximately 5 J or 1% of the total energy per step. Shorten (127) used a much more sophisticated multiple-element, nonlinear viscoelastic model of a running shoe to estimate energy dissipation, storage, and return during the stance phase. Under typical running and footwear conditions, he estimated that 6 to 12 J may be recovered from the shoe. Although he suggested that this amount of energy is potentially significant, he noted that energy storage and return from lower-extremity musculotendinous structures are likely to be more than 10 times greater than that provided by the shoe. Shorten further noted that it may be possible to increase the energy returned to the runner by shifting toward a more resilient sole, which might compromise the cushioning property of the shoe.

McMahon and Green (128) introduced the concept of a "tuned" running surface in which the compliance properties of the surface were tuned to biomechanical characteristics of an individual during the stance phase of running. Their theoretical assessment demonstrated that running surfaces of intermediate compliance can result in a slight enhancement of running speed. Their analysis formed the basis of design characteristics of a new indoor running track at Harvard University. Anecdotal evidence suggested that performance improvements following the installation of the track were modest (approximately 2%), which was consistent with their theoretical prediction. Perhaps equally impressive was the suggestion that running surfaces of intermediate compliance potentially reduce the initial impact peak force, which may contribute to a reduction in injury incidence.

More flexed knee angles at heel strike have also been implicated as an important kinematic mechanism of initial impact shock attenuation. Lafortune and colleagues (129), however, demonstrated that the knee joint does not regulate initial leg stiffness and provided only partial support for their hypothesis that a more flexed knee at impact improves cushioning. Using a human pendulum experimental setup to control impact conditions, they found that greater knee flexion at contact reduced impact force but increased the shock traveling throughout the shank. The impact surface had a larger effect on shock attenuation. More compliant interfaces produced substantial reductions in both initial leg stiffness and severity of the shock experienced by the lower limb. The high correlation ($r = 0.95$) between the rate of lower extremity loading and limb stiffness (defined by the heel fat pad and interface deformations) suggested that interface interventions are more likely to protect the locomotor system against impact loading than neuromuscular strategies involving knee angle at impact.

GAIT ADAPTABILITY

One can consider locomotion to be the translation of the center of mass with the least expenditure of energy possible. Motions of the limbs can be considered to act in harmony to achieve this aim. Saunders and colleagues (130) developed a unifying model that permitted these movements to be classified and in so doing developed the so-called six determinants of gait: pelvic rotation, pelvic tilt, knee flexion, hip flexion, knee and ankle interaction, and lateral pelvic displacement. They argued that while the body could comfortably account for the loss of one of these determinants, it was much more difficult to do so when two (or more) were lost, due to injury or disease. Loss of two determinants would make effective compensation impossible and the associated metabolic costs would increase to the point that locomotion would not be achievable. We have already seen that with amputee locomotion there is a level of adaptation occurring. Persons who walk with a prosthetic device have shown that they can accommodate many different devices while maintaining overground locomotion (e.g., 94). Furthermore, it seems that an important factor in determining the motion is the desire for symmetrical motion of the lower limbs. Sanderson and Martin (98,99) and Czerniecki and colleagues (103) have shown that the external kinematic features and timing information appear to be retained at the expense of changes within the internal environment. That is, joint moment and powers change but the end result is a temporal or kinematic pattern of motion that is remarkably similar to normal gait.

Adaptations to Surface Constraints

An area of continuing interest concerns the nature of the accommodation individuals make to changes in the terrain over which they are walking or running. Much effort has been expended examining the importance of vestibular information for balance and postural control (131,132) as well as the visual system for environmental feedback (133–137). Warren (138), Warren and Whang (139), and Patla (140) have focused on identifying specific movement adaptations that are based on features of the environment, such as stair riser heights and obstacles to step over. Patla and colleagues (136) further stressed the importance of the kinesthetic system as one that actively monitors angular displacement of the knee joint and adjusts toe elevation accordingly to ensure obstacle clearance. Specific obstacle clearance strategies were observed, including clearance strategies to go over obstacles of different sizes and shapes safely, implementation of obstacle avoidance strategies within the same step cycle in which the obstacle is presented, and necessary direction changes for avoiding an obstacle, which must be planned in the previous step (135,141). Sanderson and colleagues (142) and Patla and colleagues (143) have observed that when changes to the gait cycle are forced within a step, the adaptation will be made in such a way as to preserve the overall timing of the gait cycle. This appears to be related to the observations made on amputee locomotion, in which adjustments are made to the internal moments and powers to preserve the symmetry of external kinematics.

Gait Plasticity to Biomechanical Training

Based on the information that has been presented for kinematic and kinetic descriptors of gait, one may conclude that the association between biomechanical descriptors of walking and running patterns and gait economy is complex and elusive. Nevertheless, a close examination of published data demonstrates that some individuals clearly do not display economical movement patterns. A particular runner, for example, may tend to significantly over- or understride with each stride. From an energy-conserving standpoint, such individuals may clearly benefit from changes in their pattern of motion. Unfortunately, only a few researchers have attempted to consider whether lasting changes in gait mechanics that significantly affect economy can be produced through biomechanical training.

Results from five recent studies fail to reflect a consensus on the effects of biomechanical training on gait economy and technique. Petray and Krahenbuhl (144) found that the running economy, stride length, and vertical displacement of 10-year-old boys were not significantly improved by an 11-week instruction program that consisted of 5 minutes of instruction per week on various aspects of running technique, including "reducing unnecessary vertical displacement, awareness of stride rate and length, and general suggestions regarding posture and relaxation" (p. 252). Messier and Cirillo (145) reported significant but generally modest changes in gait descriptors, but no significant changes in either oxygen consumption or rating of perceived exertion for female adult novice runners after fifteen 20-minute treadmill training runs during which subjects received visual and verbal feedback on trunk inclination, arm swing, lower extremity mechanics, and vertical oscillation. Miller and colleagues (146) provided visual feedback for a single technique factor to four uneconomical runners during 10 days of 20-minute training sessions. These four subjects displayed reductions in aerobic demand greater than those observed in control subjects, but changes were not statistically significant. Morgan and colleagues (37) provided audio and visual feedback in an attempt to shift nonoptimal stride lengths toward an optimal stride length. Their experimental group showed a significant shift in their freely chosen stride length toward the optimal stride length relative to a control group without feedback. Furthermore, they also showed a marked reduction in the oxygen uptake from that recorded at the freely chosen stride length. Finally, Williams and colleagues (147) evaluated the effect of training at a longer than optimal stride length on numerous running technique descriptors and aerobic demand. Posttraining technique descriptors were generally intermediate to those of the pretraining and imposed training values, but most kinematic adaptations were not significant. Posttraining aerobic demand was significantly less than pretraining values, a change opposite to that which would be expected. The O_2 decline also was not specific to the training stride length but rather occurred across all tested stride length conditions.

From these analyses, it appears that both economy and gait technique factors are resistant to change due to training programs such as those described. Perhaps these mixed results should not be surprising considering the brief duration of the training programs, differences in experimental design, the highly complicated nature of the interrelationships among various technique factors, and our relatively poor understanding of factors believed to be primary determinants of interindividual differences in economy of motion. The question regarding our ability to improve economy significantly through biomechanical training remains unanswered and warrants further research.

Gait Transitions

One of the most basic locomotor adaptations made by humans and animals is the transition from one mode of gait to another (e.g., walk to run, trot to gallop) in response to changes in speed. Numerous investigations have attempted to identify critical factors that trigger transitions from one mode to another. Proposed mechanisms have focused on minimization of energy cost, minimization of musculoskeletal stress, limitations in the stride pattern imposed by anatomic or biomechanical constraints, minimization of mechanical energy or power generation, and changes in the stability of the stride pattern.

Hoyt and Taylor (148) demonstrated that the energy cost per unit of distance traveled for horses reflects a U-shaped, curvilinear response within each mode of gait (walk, trot, gallop) such that the highest costs were observed at the extreme speeds for a given mode of gait. They also observed that preferred speeds within each gait mode coincided with the energetically optimal speed. Although they did not systematically quantify gait transition speeds in their analysis, they concluded that changes in gait occur in an effort to minimize energy demand. In tests on human subjects, both Hreljac (149) and Brisswalter and Mottet (150) questioned the importance of energy cost minimization when they found that the predicted transition speed based on minimization of energy cost (2.24 and 2.19 m/s for Hreljac and Brisswalter and Mottet, respectively) was significantly greater than the observed walk-to-run transition speed (2.11 and 2.13 m/s, respectively). Whether this difference between the preferred and the energetically optimal transition speeds is of physiological significance remains open to interpretation and debate.

Farley and Taylor (151) discounted the role of energy cost in triggering gait transitions and proposed that musculoskeletal forces were a more reasonable triggering mechanism in part because of the availability of biologic transducers for detecting and communicating loading information to the central nervous system. Focusing on the trot-to-gallop transition in horses and using vertical ground reaction force data to predict forces of distal extensor muscles, they concluded that the gait transition occurred when musculoskeletal forces reached a critical level. This same mechanism, however, does not explain the walk-to-trot transition in quadrupeds nor the walk-to-run transition in humans because contact forces, and thus musculoskeletal loading, tend to increase with these transitions (152,153).

Several investigators have considered whether anatomic (e.g., leg length) or biomechanical (e.g., stride length) constraints affect gait transition (e.g., 154–156). Minetti and colleagues (156) concluded that the angle of lower limb spread (i.e., maximum inter-thigh angle) is an important anatomic constraint that limits walking step length and thereby stimulates a walk-to-run transition. This conclusion, however, was not generalizable to the run-to-walk transition during which inter-thigh angle increased, nor to walk-to-run transitions under different incline conditions where maximum inter-thigh angle changed as incline changed. Hreljac (152) proposed that fatigue or exertion levels in the ankle dorsiflexors trigger the walk-to-run transition. Under different incline conditions, he observed that the walk-to-run transition speed decreased as incline increased. The maximum ankle dorsiflexion velocity, however, reached the same peak value under the different incline and transition speed conditions. Hreljac proposed that perceptions of localized discomfort in the dorsiflexors is a plausible source of feedback to the central nervous system that prompts a gait transition. Unfortunately, the run-to-walk transition cannot be explained by this same mechanism.

Using a simple inverted pendulum model of walking (157), Kram and colleagues (153) suggested that the walk-to-run transition may occur in an effort to minimize the demand for mechanical power generation. At preferred walking speeds, substantial exchanges between kinetic and gravitational potential energy components from a pendulum-like mechanism minimize the need for power generation by musculature to sustain walking. As walking speed increases, however, the effectiveness of this mechanical energy exchange diminishes. Under running conditions, minimization of mechanical power generation is associated with an elastic spring mechanism, rather than a pendulum energy exchange mechanism. Thus, it can be suggested that the walk-to-run transition occurs at a speed at which the energy-conserving characteristic of the elastic mechanism exceeds that of a pendulum mechanism. Theoretically, the only major force affecting the inverted pendulum-like movements during walking is gravity. By supporting the body vertically at varying levels and thereby simulating reduced gravity conditions, Kram and colleagues found support for their hypothesis that the walk-to-run transition occurs at slower absolute speeds as the gravitational effect is reduced. The effects of reduced gravity on the relative effectiveness of pendulum-like and elastic spring mechanisms at conserving mechanical energy was not tested in these experiments, and is unclear.

A final potential mechanism underlying gait transitions deals with the stability of the gait pattern. Dynamical systems theory (158) predicts that complex systems, such as the locomotor process in humans and animals consisting of a high number of degrees of freedom, are self-organized into a small number of simple and distinctive patterns (e.g., walking and running). Based on dynamical systems theory, it would be predicted that preferred speeds of walking and running reflect stable attractor states of the motor system. Increases in walking speed or decreases in running speed from the preferred states should result in less stable and more variable kinematic and kinetic attractor states of gait that trigger a transition. The majority of research to date on dynamical systems theory has focused on simple upper extremity movements. From a gait perspective, researchers are still attempting to identify those collective variables that most effectively encompass multiple degrees of freedom. Nevertheless, using relative phase differences between hip, knee, and ankle peak extensions near the end of the stance phase, Dietrich and Warren (159) effectively manipulated attractor state stability through inertial and incline or grade manipulations and correspondingly altered the walk-run transition speed. In addition, Brisswalter and Mottet (150) observed an increase in stride duration variability as walking speed approached gait transition speed. With a further increase in speed and a shift to running, stride duration variability abruptly dropped.

The preceding discussion of gait transition reflects many perspectives from which the phenomenon has been investigated, and it perhaps underscores the complexity of the locomotor process. It may also leave the reader with the mistaken impression that the various perspectives are mutually exclusive. Rather, it is more likely that gait transition is a multifactorial issue and that some of the energetic, biomechanical, and anatomic factors discussed as important determinants of gait transition are interrelated. As one example, Dietrich and Warren (159) speculated that gait stability and metabolic energy cost are closely linked, suggesting that the "metabolic cost reflects the consequences of driving the system away from its attractor states" (p. 61).

CONCLUSION

This chapter provided an overview of our current state of knowledge on a limited number of topics, in part because a broader review would lead to a more superficial consideration of topics and because many other reviews already exist on various topics associated with walking and running biomechanics. It is hoped that our discussion has reinforced the notion that walking and running are extremely complex movements that are best understood only when investigated thoroughly from multiple perspectives that include, but are not limited to, kinematic, kinetic, metabolic, neurobiologic, and psychobiologic assessments.

REFERENCES

1. Cavanagh PR. *Biomechanics of distance running.* Champaign, IL: Human Kinetics, 1990.
2. Inman VT, Ralston HJ, Todd F. *Human walking.* Baltimore: Williams & Wilkins, 1981.
3. Winter DA. *The biomechanics and motor control of human gait: normal, elderly, and pathological,* 2nd ed. Waterloo, Ontario: University of Waterloo Press, 1991.
4. Adelaar RS. The practical biomechanics of running. *Am J Sports Med* 1986;14:497–500.
5. Cappozzo A. The mechanics of human walking. In: Patla AE, ed. *Adaptability of human gait.* New York: Elsevier, 1991:167–186.
6. Farley CT, Ferris DP. Biomechanics of walking and running: center of mass movements to muscle action. *Exerc Sport Sci Rev* 1998;26:253–285.
7. Miller DI. Biomechanics of running—what should the future hold? *Can J Appl Sports Sci* 1978;3:229–236.
8. Oonpuu S. The biomechanics of walking and running. *Clin Sports Med* 1994;13:843–863.
9. Putnam CA, Kozey JW. Substantive issues in running. In: Vaughan CL, ed. *Biomechanics of sport.* Boca Raton, FL: CRC Press, 1989:2–33.
10. Thordarson DB. Running biomechanics. *Clin Sports Med* 1997;16:239–247.
11. Vaughan CL. Biomechanics of running gait. *CRC Crit Rev Biomed Eng* 1984;12:1–48.
12. Vaughan CL, Sussman MD. Human gait: from clinical interpretation to computer simulation. In: Grabiner MD, ed. *Current issues in biomechanics.* Champaign, IL: Human Kinetics, 1993:53–68.
13. Williams KR. Biomechanics of running. *Exerc Sport Sci Rev* 1985;13:389–441.
14. Williams KR. Biomechanics of distance running. In: Grabiner MD, ed. *Current issues in biomechanics.* Champaign, IL: Human Kinetics, 1993:3–31.
15. Czerniecki JM. Foot and ankle biomechanics in walking and running. A review. *Am J Phys Med Rehabil* 1988;67:246–252.
16. Davis BL, Cavanagh PR. Simulating reduced gravity: a review of biomechanical issues pertaining to human locomotion. *Aviat Space Environ Med* 1993;64:557–566.
17. Komi PV, Fukashiro S, Jarvinen M. Biomechanical loading of Achilles tendon during normal locomotion. *Clin Sports Med* 1992;11:521–531.
18. Martin PE, Morgan DW. Biomechanical considerations for economical walking and running. *Med Sci Sports Exerc* 1992;24:467–474.
19. Nigg BM. *Biomechanics of running shoes.* Champaign IL: Human Kinetics, 1986.
20. Patla AE. *Adaptability of human gait: implications for the control of locomotion.* New York: Elsevier Science, 1991.
21. Rodgers MM. Dynamic foot biomechanics. *J Orthop Sports Phys Ther* 1995;21:306–316.
22. Winter DA, McFadyen BJ, Dickey JP. Adaptability of the CNS in human walking. In: Patla AE, ed. *Adaptability of human gait.* New York: Elsevier Science, 1991:127–144.
23. Daniels JT, Scardina NJ, Foley P. $\dot{V}O_2$ submax during five modes of exercise. In: Bachl N, Prokop L, Sucket R, eds. *Proceedings of the World Congress on Sports Medicine.* Vienna: Urban and Schwartsenberg, 1984:604–615.
24. Jones AM, Doust JH. A 1% treadmill grade most accurately reflects the energetic cost of outdoor running. *J Sports Sci* 1996;14:321–327.
25. Kyle CR, Caiozzo VJ. The effect of athletic clothing aerodynamics upon running speed. *Med Sci Sports Exerc* 1986;18:509–515.

26. Martin PE, Rothstein DE, Larish DD. Effects of age and physical activity status on the speed-aerobic demand relationship of walking. *J Appl Physiol* 1992;73:200–206.
27. Ralston HJ. Energy-speed relation and optimal speed during level walking. *Arbeitsphysiologie* 1958;17:277–283.
28. Kram R, Taylor CR. Energetics of running: a new perspective. *Nature* 1990;346:265–267.
29. Grillner S, Halbertsma J, Nilsson J, Thorstensson A. The adaptation to speed in human locomotion. *Brain Res* 1979;165:177–182.
30. Nilsson J, Thorstensson A, Halbertsma J. Changes in leg movements and muscle activity with speed of locomotion and mode of progression. *Acta Physiol Scand* 1985;123:457–475.
31. Hill AV. The maximum work and mechanical efficiency of human muscles, and their most economical speed. *J Physiol* 1922;56:19–41.
32. Cavanagh PR, Williams KR. The effect of stride length variation on oxygen uptake during distance running. *Med Sci Sports Exerc* 1982;14:30–35.
33. Heinert LD, Serfass RC, Stull GA. Effect of stride length variation on oxygen uptake during level and positive grade treadmill running. *Res Q Exerc Sport* 1988;59:127–130.
34. Högberg P. How do stride length and stride frequency influence the energy output during running? *Arbeitsphysiologie* 1952; 14:437–441.
35. Knuttgen HG. Oxygen uptake and pulse rate while running with undetermined and determined stride lengths at different speeds. *Acta Physiol Scand* 1961;52:366–371.
36. Morgan DW, Martin PE. Effects of stride length alteration on race-walking economy. *Can J Appl Sports Sci* 1986;11:211–217.
37. Morgan DW, Martin PE, Craib M, Caruso C, Clifton R, Hopewell R. Effect of step length optimization on the aerobic demand of running. *J Appl Physiol* 1994;77:245–251.
38. Taylor CR. Force development during sustained locomotion: a determinant of gait, speed and metabolic power. *J Exp Biol* 1985;115:253–262.
39. Holt KG, Hamill J, Andres RO. The force-driven harmonic oscillator as a model for human locomotion. *Hum Movement Sci* 1990;9:55–68.
40. Holt KG, Hamill J, Andres RO. Predicting the minimal energy costs of human walking. *Med Sci Sports Exerc* 1991;23:491–498.
41. Schot PK, Decker MJ. The force driven harmonic oscillator model accurately predicts the preferred stride frequency for backward walking. *Hum Movement Sci* 1998;17:67–76.
42. Jeng S-F, Liao H-F, Lai J-S, Hou J-W. Optimization of walking in children. *Med Sci Sports Exerc* 1997;29:370–376.
43. Williams KR, Cavanagh PR. Relationship between distance running mechanics, running economy, and performance. *J Appl Physiol* 1987;63:1236–1245.
44. Williams KR, Cavanagh PR. Biomechanical correlates with running economy in elite distance runners. In: *Proceedings of the North American Congress on Biomechanics,* Montreal, 1986; 287–288.
45. Burdett RG, Skrinar GS, Simon SR. Comparison of mechanical work and metabolic energy consumption during normal gait. *J Orthop Res* 1983;1:63–72.
46. Cavagna GA, Saibene FP, Margaria R. Mechanical work in running. *J Appl Physiol* 1964;19:249–256.
47. Shorten MR, Wootton SA, Williams C. Mechanical energy changes and the oxygen cost of running. *Eng Med* 1981;10:213–217.
48. Taylor CR, Heglund NC, McMahon TA, Looney TR. Energetic cost of generating muscular force during running. *J Exp Biol* 1980;86:9–18.
49. Roberts TJ, Marsh RL, Weyand PG, Taylor CR. Muscular force in running turkeys: the economy of minimizing work. *Science* 1997;275:1113–1115.
50. Gray J. *Animal locomotion.* New York: Norton, 1968.
51. Hildebrand M. Walking, running, and jumping. *Am Zool* 1962;2:151–155.
52. Howell AB. *Speed in animals.* Chicago: University of Chicago Press, 1944.
53. Taylor CR, Shkolnik A, Dmi'el R, Baharav D, Borut A. Running in cheetahs, gazelles, and goats: energy cost and limb configuration. *Am J Physiol* 1974;227:848–850.
54. Martin PE. Mechanical and physiological responses to lower extremity loading during running. *Med Sci Sports Exerc* 1985;17:427–433.
55. Myers MJ, Steudel K. Effect of limb mass and its distribution on the energetic cost of running. *J Exp Biol* 1985;116:363–373.
56. Steudel K. The work and energetic cost of locomotion. I. The effects of limb mass distribution in quadripeds. *J Exp Biol* 1990;154:273–285.
57. Keren G, Epstein Y, Magazanik A, Sohar E. The energy cost of walking and running with and without a backpack. *Eurp J Appl Physiol* 1981;46:317–324.
58. Myers MJ, Steudel K, White SC. Uncoupling the correlates of locomotor coss: a factorial approach. *J Exp Zool* 1993;265:211–223.
59. Godges JJ, MacRae H, Longdon C, Tinberg C. The effects of two stretching procedures on hip range of motion and gait economy. *J Orthop Sports Phys Ther* 1989;7:350–357.
60. Gleim GW, Stachenfeld NS, Nicholas JA. The influence of flexibility on the economy of walking and jogging. *J Orthop Res* 1990;8:814–823.
61. Craib MW, Mitchell VA, Fields KB, Cooper TR, Hopewell R, Morgan DW. The association between flexibility and running economy in sub-elite male distance runners. *Med Sci Sports Exerc* 1996;28:737–743.
62. Murray MP, Kory RC, Clarkson BH. Walking patterns in healthy old men. *J Gerontol* 1969;24:169–178.
63. Himann JE, Cunningham DA, Rechnitzer PA, Paterson DH. Age-related changes in speed of walking. *Med Sci Sports Exerc* 1988;20:161–166.
64. Larish DD, Martin PE, Mungiole M. Characteristic patterns of gait in the healthy old. *Ann NY Acad Sci* 1988;515:18–32.
65. Bendall MJ, Bassey EJ, Pearson MB. Factors affecting walking speed of elderly people. *Age Ageing* 1989;18:327–332.
66. Ferrandez A-M, Pailhous J, Durup M. Slowness in elderly gait. *Exp Aging Res* 1990;16:79–89.
67. Kerrigan DC, Todd MK, Croce UD, Lipsitz LA, Collins JJ. Biomechanical gait alterations independent of speed in the healthy elderly: evidence for specific limiting impairments. *Arch Phys Med Rehabil* 1998;79:317–322.
68. Gabell A, Nayak USL. The effect of age on variability of gait. *J Gerontol* 1984;39:662–666.
69. Hausdorf JM, Edelberg HK, Mitchell SL, Goldberger AL, Wei JY. Increased gait unsteadiness in community-dwelling elderly fallers. *Arch Phys Med Rehabil* 1997;78:278–283.
70. Maki BE. Gait changes in older adults: predictors of falls or indicators of fear? *J Am Geriatr Soc* 1997;45:313–320.
71. Larsson L. Aging in mammalian skeletal muscle. In: Mortimer JA, Pirozzolo FJ, Maletta GJ, eds. *The aging motor system.* New York: Praeger, 1982.
72. Faulkner JA, Brooks SV, Zerba E. Skeletal muscle weakness and fatigue in old age: underlying mechanisms. *Annu Rev Gerontol Geriatr* 1990;10:147–166.
73. Aniansson AG, Grimby G, Rundgren A. Isometric and isokinetic quadriceps muscle strength in 70-year old men and women. *Scand J Rehabil Med* 1980;12:161–168.
74. Larsson L, Grimby G, Karlsson J. Muscle strength and speed of contraction in relation to age and muscle morphology. *J Appl Physiol* 1979;46:451–456.
75. Murray MP, Gardner GM, Mollinger LA, Sepic SB. Strength of isometric and isokinetic contractions: knee muscles of men aged 20–86. *Phys Ther* 1980;60:412–419.
76. Murray MP, Duthie EH, Gambert SR, Sepic SB, Mollinger LA. Age-related differences in knee muscle strength in normal men. *J Gerontol* 1985;40:275–280.
77. Bassey EJ, Bendall MJ, Pearson M. Muscle strength in the triceps surae and objectively measured customary walking activity in men and women over age 65 years of age. *Clin Sci* 1988;74:85–89.
78. Buchner DM, Cress ME, Esselman PC, et al. Factors associated with changes in gait speed in older adults. *J Gerontol* 1996;51A:M297–M302.
79. Judge JO, Davis RB, Oonpuu S. Step length reductions in advanced ages: the role of ankle and hip kinetics. *J Gerontol* 1996;51A:M303–M312.
80. Rantanen T, Avela J. Leg extension power and walking speed

in very old people living independently. *J Gerontol* 1997;52A:M225–M231.
81. Cunningham DA, Rechnitzer PA, Pearce ME, Donner AP. Determinants of self-selected walking pace across ages 19 to 66. *J Gerontol* 1982;37:560–564.
82. Cunningham DA, Rechnitzer PA, Donner AP. Exercise training and the speed of self-selected walking pace in men at retirement. *Can J Aging* 1986;5:19–26.
83. Lord SR, Lloyd DG, Nirui M, Raymond J, Williams P, Stewart RA. The effect of exercise on gait patterns in older women: a randomized controlled trial. *J Gerontol* 1996;51A:M64–M70.
84. Judge JO, Underwood M, Gennosa T. Exercise to improve gait velocity in older persons. *Arch Phys Med Rehabil* 1993;74:400–406.
85. Topp R, Mikesky A, Wigglesworth J, Holt W, Edwards JE. The effect of a 12-week dynamic resistance strength training program on gait velocity and balance of older adults. *Gerontologist* 1993;33:501–506.
86. Sipila S, Multanen J, Kallinen M, Era P, Suominen H. Effects of strength and endurance training on isometric muscle strength and walking speed in elderly women. *Acta Physiol Scand* 1996;156:457–464.
87. Buchner DM, Cress ME, de Lateur BJ, et al. The effect of strength and endurance training on gait, balance, fall risk, and health services use in community-living older adults. *J Gerontol* 1997;52A:M218–M224.
88. Hamill J, Bates BT, Knutzen KM. Ground reaction force symmetry during walking and running. *Res Q Exerc Sport* 1984;55:289–293.
89. Herzog W, Nigg BM, Read LJ, Olsson E. Asymmetries in ground reaction force patterns in normal locomotion. *Med Sci Sports Exerc* 1989;21:110–114.
90. Brouwer BJ, Allard P, Labelle H. Running patterns of juveniles wearing SACH and single-axis foot components. *Arch Phys Med Rehabil* 1989;70:128–134.
91. Winter DA. Energy generation and absorption at the ankle and knee during fast, natural and slow cadences. *Clin Orthop Rel Res* 1983;197:147–154.
92. Michael J. Energy storing feet: a clinical comparison. *Clin Prosth Orthot* 1987;11:154–168.
93. Gitter A, Czerniecki JM, DeGroot DM. Biomechanical analysis of the influence of prosthetic feet on below-knee amputee walking. *Am J Phys Med Rehabil* 1991;70:142–148.
94. Torburn L, Perry J, Ayyappa E, Shanfield SL. Below-knee amputee gait with dynamic elastic response prosthetic feet: a pilot study. *J Rehabil Res Dev* 1990;27:369–384.
95. Colborne GR, Nauman S, Longmiur PE, Berbrayer D. Analysis of mechanical and metabolic factors in the gait of congenital below knee amputees. *Am J Phys Med Rehabil* 1992;71:272–278.
96. Postema K, Hermens HJ, de Vries J, Koopman HFJM, Eisma WH. Energy storage and release of prosthetic feet. Part 1: biomechanical analysis related to user benefits. *Prosth Orthot Int* 1997;21:17–27.
97. Enoka RM, Miller DI, Burgess EM. Below-knee amputee running gait. *Am J Phys Med* 1982;61:66–84.
98. Sanderson DJ, Martin PE. Joint kinetics in unilateral below knee amputees during running. *Arch Phys Med Rehabil* 1996;77:1279–1285.
99. Sanderson DJ, Martin PE. Lower extremity kinematic and kinetic adaptations in unilateral below knee amputees during walking. *Gait Posture* 1997;6:126–136.
100. Miller DI. Resultant lower extremity joint moments in below-knee amputees during running stance. *J Biomech* 1987;20:529–541.
101. Miller DI, Enoka RM, McCulloch RG, Burgess EM, Frankel VH. Vertical ground reaction force time histories of lower extremity amputee runners. In: Asmussen E, Jorgensen K, eds. *Biomechanics,* vol 6. Baltimore: University Park Press, 1981:453–460.
102. Powers CM, Torburn L, Perry J, Ayyappa MD. Influence of prosthetic foot design on sound limb loading in adults with unilateral below-knee amputations. *Arch Phys Med Rehabil* 1994;75:825–829.
103. Czerniecki JM, Gitter AJ, Beck JC. Energy transfer mechanisms as a compensatory strategy in below knee amputee runners. *J Biomech* 1996;29:717–722.
104. Mena D, Mansour JM, Simon SR. Analysis and synthesis of human swing leg motion during gait and its clinical applications. *J Biomech* 1981;14:823–832.
105. Czerniecki JM, Gitter A, Weaver K. Effect of alterations in prosthetic shank mass on the metabolic costs of ambulation in above-knee amputees. *Am J Phys Med Rehabil* 1994;73:348–352.
106. Gailey RS, Nash MS, Atchley TA, et al. The effects of prosthetic mass on metabolic cost of ambulation in nonvascular trans-tibial amputees. *Prosth Orthot Int* 1997;21:9–16.
107. Hale SA. Analysis of the swing phase dynamics and muscular effort of the above-knee amputee for varying prosthetic shank loads. *Prosth Orthot Int* 1990;14:125–135.
108. Gitter A, Czerniecki J, Meinders M. Effect of prosthetic mass on swing phase work during above-knee amputee ambulation. *Am J Phys Med Rehabil* 1998;76:114–121.
109. Shorten MR. Muscle elasticity and human performance. In: van Gheluwe B, Atha J, eds. *Current research in sports biomechanics.* Basel: Karger, 1987:1–18.
110. Ingen Schenau GJ van, Bobbert MF, Haan A de. Does elastic energy enhance work and efficiency in the stretch-shortening cycle? *J Appl Biomech* 1997;13:389–415.
111. Bosco C, Viitasalo JT, Komi PV, Luhtanen P. Combined effect of elastic energy and myoelectric potentiation during stretch-shortening cycle exercise. *Acta Physiol Scand* 1982;114:557–565.
112. Dietz V, Schmidtbleicher S, Noth J. Neuronal mechanisms of human locomotion. *J Physiol* 1978;238:139–155.
113. Bobbert MF, Gerritsen KGM, Litjens MCA, Soest AJ van. Why is countermovement jump height greater than squat jump height? *Med Sci Sports Exerc* 1996;28:1402–1412.
114. Chapman AE, Caldwell GE, Selbie WS. Mechanical output following muscle stretch in forearm supination against inertial loads. *J Appl Physiol* 1985;59:78–86.
115. Walshe AD, Wilson GJ, Ettema GJC. Stretch-shorten cycle compared with isometric preload: contributions to enhanced muscular performance. *J Appl Physiol* 1998;84:97–106.
116. Edman KAP, Elzinga G, Noble HIM. Enhancement of mechanical performance by stretch during tetanic contractions of vertebrate skeletal muscle fibres. *J Physiol* 1978;281:139–155.
117. Edman KAP, Elzinga G, Noble HIM. Residual force enhancement after stretch of contracting frog single muscle muscle fibers. *J Gen Physiol* 1982;80:769–784.
118. Asmussen E, Bonde-Petersen F. Storage of elastic energy in skeletal muscles. *Acta Physiol Scand* 1974;91:385–392.
119. Bosco C, Komi PV. Potentiation of the mechanical behavior of the human skeletal muscle through prestretching. *Acta Physiol Scand* 1979;106:467–472.
120. Cavagna GA, Dusman B, Margaria R. Positive work done by a previously stretched muscle. *J Appl Physiol* 1968;24:21–32.
121. Cavagna GA, Saibene FP, Margaria R. Effect of negative work on the amount of positive work performed by an isolated muscle. *J Appl Physiol* 1965;20:157–158.
122. Alexander RMcN, Ker RF. The architecture of leg muscles. In: Winter JM, Woo SL-Y, eds. *Multiple muscle systems, biomechanics and movement organization.* New York: Springer-Verlag, 1990:568–577.
123. Hof AL. Effects of muscle elasticity in walking and running. In: Winter JM, Woo SL-Y, eds. *Multiple muscle systems, biomechanics and movement organization.* New York: Springer-Verlag, 1990:591–607.
124. Wilson GJ, Elliott BC, Wood GA. Stretch shortening cycle performance enhancement through flexibility training. *Med Sci Sports Exerc* 1992;24:116–123.
125. Wilson GJ, Murphy AJ, Pryor JF. Musculotendinous stiffness: its relationship to eccentric, isometric, and concentric performance. *J Appl Physiol* 1994;76:2714–2719.
126. Nigg BM, Segesser B. Biomechanical and orthopedic concepts in sport shoe construction. *Med Sci Sports Exerc* 1992;24:595–602.
127. Shorten MR. The energetics of running and running shoes. *J Biomech* 1993;26(suppl 1):41–51.
128. McMahon TA, Green PR. The influence of track compliance on running. *J Biomech* 1979;12:893–904.
129. Lafortune MA, Hennig EM, Lake MJ. Dominant role of inter-

face over knee angle for cushioning impact loading and regulating initial leg stiffness. *J Biomech* 1996;29:1523–1529.
130. Saunders J, Inman V, Eberhart H. The major determinants in normal and pathological gait. *J Bone Joint Surg* 1953;35A:543–558.
131. Nashner LM. Balance adjustments of humans perturbed while walking. *J Neurophysiol* 1980;44:650–664.
132. Patla AE. Adaptation of postural responses to voluntary arm raises during locomotion in humans. *Neurosci Lett* 1986;68:334–338.
133. Georgopoulous AP, Grillner S. Visuomotor coordination in reaching and locomotion. *Science* 1989;245:1209–1210.
134. Bardy BG, Baumberger B, Fluckiger M, Laurent M. On the role of global and local visual information in goal directed walking. *Acta Psychol (Amst)* 1992;81:199–210.
135. Patla AE, Rietdyk S. Visual control of limb trajectory over obstacles during locomotion: effect of height and width. *Gait Posture* 1993;1:45–60.
136. Patla AE, Rietdyk S, Martin C, Prentice S. Locomotor patterns of the leading and trailing limb while going over solid and fragile obstacles: some insights into the role of vision during locomotion. *J Motor Behav* 1994;28:35–47.
137. Berg WP, Wade MG, Greer NL. Visual regulation of gait in bipedal locomotion: revisiting Lee, Lishman, and Thomson (1982). *J Exp Psychol [Hum Percept]* 1994;20:854–863.
138. Warren WH. Perceiving affordances: visual guidance of stair climbing. *J Exp Psychol [Hum Percept]* 1984;10:683–703.
139. Warren WH, Whang S. Visual guidance of walking through apertures: body scaled information for affordances. *J Exp Psychol [Hum Percept]* 1987;13:371–383.
140. Patla AE. Neurobiomechanical bases for the control of human locomotion. In: Bronstein A, Brandt TH, Woollacott M, eds. *Clinical aspects of balance and gait disorders.* London: Edward Arnold, 1995.
141. Patla AE, Prentice SD, Robinson C, Neufeld J. Visual control of locomotion: strategies for changing direction and going over obstacles. *J Exp Psychol [Hum Percept]* 1991;17:603–634.
142. Sanderson DJ, Franks IM, Elliott D. The effects of targeting on the ground reaction forces during level walking. *Hum Movement Sci* 1993;12:327–337.
143. Patla AE, Robinson C, Samways M, Armstrong CJ. Visual control of step length during overground locomotion: task-specific modulation of the locomotor synergy. *J Exp Psychol [Hum Percept]* 1989;15:6.
144. Petray CK, Krahenbuhl GS. Running training instruction on running technique, and running economy in 10-year old males. *Res Q Exerc Sport* 1985;56:251–255.
145. Messier SP, Cirillo KJ. Effects of a verbal and visual feedback system on running technique, perceived exertion and running economy. *J Sports Sci* 1989;7:113–126.
146. Miller TA, Milliron MJ, Cavanagh PR. The effect of running mechanics feedback training on running economy. *Med Sci Sports Exerc* 1990;22:S17.
147. Williams KR, Jones JE, Snow RE. Mechanical and physiological adaptations to alterations in running stride length. *Med Sci Sports Exerc* 1991;23:S6.
148. Hoyt DF, Taylor CR. Gait and the energetics of locomotion in horses. *Nature* 1981;292:239–240.
149. Hreljac A. Preferred and energetically optimal gait transition speeds in human locomotion. *Med Sci Sports Exerc* 1993;25:1158–1162.
150. Brisswalter J, Mottet D. Energy cost and stride duration variability at preferred transition gait speed between walking and running. *Can J Appl Physiol* 1996;21:471–480.
151. Farley CT, Taylor CR. A mechanical trigger for the trot-gallop transition in horses. *Science* 1991;253:306–308.
152. Hreljac A. Determinants of the gait transition speed during human locomotion: kinetic factors. *Gait Posture* 1993;1:217–223.
153. Kram R, Domingo A, Ferris DP. Effect of reduced gravity on the preferred walk-run transition speed. *J Exp Biol* 1997; 200:821–826.
154. Hreljac A. Determinants of the gait transition speed during human locomotion: kinematic factors. *J Biomech* 1995;28:669–677.
155. Hreljac A. Effects of physical characteristics on the gait transition speed during human locomotion. *Hum Movement Sci* 1995; 14:205–216.
156. Minetti AE, Ardigo LP, Saibene F. The transition between walking and running in humans: metabolic and mechanical aspects at different gradients. *Acta Physiol Scand* 1994;150:315–323.
157. Alexander RMcN. Mechanics and scaling of terrestrial locomotion. In Pedley TJ, ed. *Scale effects in animal locomotion.* New York: Academic Press, 1977:93–110.
158. Kelso JAS, Schoner G. Self-organization of coordinative movement patterns. *Hum Movement Sci* 1988;7:27–46.
159. Dietrich FJ, Warren WH. The dynamics of gait transitions: effects of grade and load. *J Motor Behav* 1998;30:60–78.

Exercise and Sport Science,
edited by William E. Garrett, Jr., and Donald T. Kirkendall.
Lippincott Williams & Wilkins, Philadelphia © 2000.

CHAPTER 43

Biomechanics of Ice Hockey

David J. Pearsall, René A. Turcotte, and Stephen D. Murphy

THE GAME OF ICE HOCKEY

The origins of ice hockey date back to the 1880s in Canada, when it was a recreational winter activity. The cold winter environment provided the ice. The cultural influence of English, Scottish, and Irish immigrants in the French milieu led to the organization of play and to the founding of the rules of ice hockey. The game of ice hockey attributes many of the aspects of early stick games, such as bandy, shinny, and hurley, to lacrosse, with its set goal zones, posts, and goalies, and to rugby, with its contact and such rules as no forward pass allowed (1).

Since the 1880s, the evolution of the game has proceeded at a fast pace and it is played worldwide, in environments far from natural ice. Along with the increase in the popularity of the sport, ice hockey has become more sophisticated and expensive to play due to technical innovations in equipment design and facilities as well as improvement in training, coaching, and game strategies. The game of ice hockey retains strong cultural roots, and it is played by children and seniors and by men and women. The sport of ice hockey is highly organized, with community, national, and international leagues promoting participation and attracting spectators. Ice hockey research has focused primarily on the physiology of training and conditioning (2), skill development, and safety and injury prevention (3,4). In comparison, very little attention has been paid to the biomechanics of ice hockey. This chapter summarizes the current knowledge of the biomechanics of ice hockey, specifically skating and stick skills, and identifies areas for future study.

D. J. Pearsall and R. A. Turcotte: Department of Physical Education, McGill University, Montreal, Quebec, Canada.
S. D. Murphy: Department of Kinesiology, Faculty of Applied Health Sciences, University of Waterloo, Waterloo, Ontario, Canada.

HOCKEY SKILLS

Classification of Skills

Because the game of ice hockey is played under specialized conditions, that is, on a surface of low friction, it involves a unique set of skills distinctive from other team sports. The skills are primarily goal oriented, with the timing and organization of movements a secondary function of the pursuit. Thus, it is necessary to consider both the objectives and the player's movements, so as to determine the person's skill level.

To understand the mechanics of ice hockey, the various tasks required of the player must be categorized. Some skills of hockey may be considered "closed," in that certain features of the environment are constant, for example, rink dimensions, equipment and set drill courses. More often the skills are considered "open," however, with the performance of a skill varying according to the changing surroundings, for example, position of opponents and team members, whether one is standing or moving, and level of competition. The skills are not always performed in a predictable way. Given the open conditions, a player's perception, decision making, and reaction times are as important as the movements in defining skill level (5). The athlete must be able to discriminate among a multitude of internal and external cues to choose the most appropriate response in an appropriate period of time (6). Thus, to define the level of hockey skill possessed by a player, several qualities describing the efficiency of movement may be noted, such as timing, anticipation, direction, balance, accuracy, rhythm, speed, versatility, agility, and reaction time.

Hockey skills include the general movement patterns of skating, stick handling, and checking. These movement patterns are characterized by a series of voluntary movements in time and space. Within each of these groupings exists several variations or subsets of the movement pattern (Fig. 43–1). Depending on the influence of various factors, skills may be executed individu-

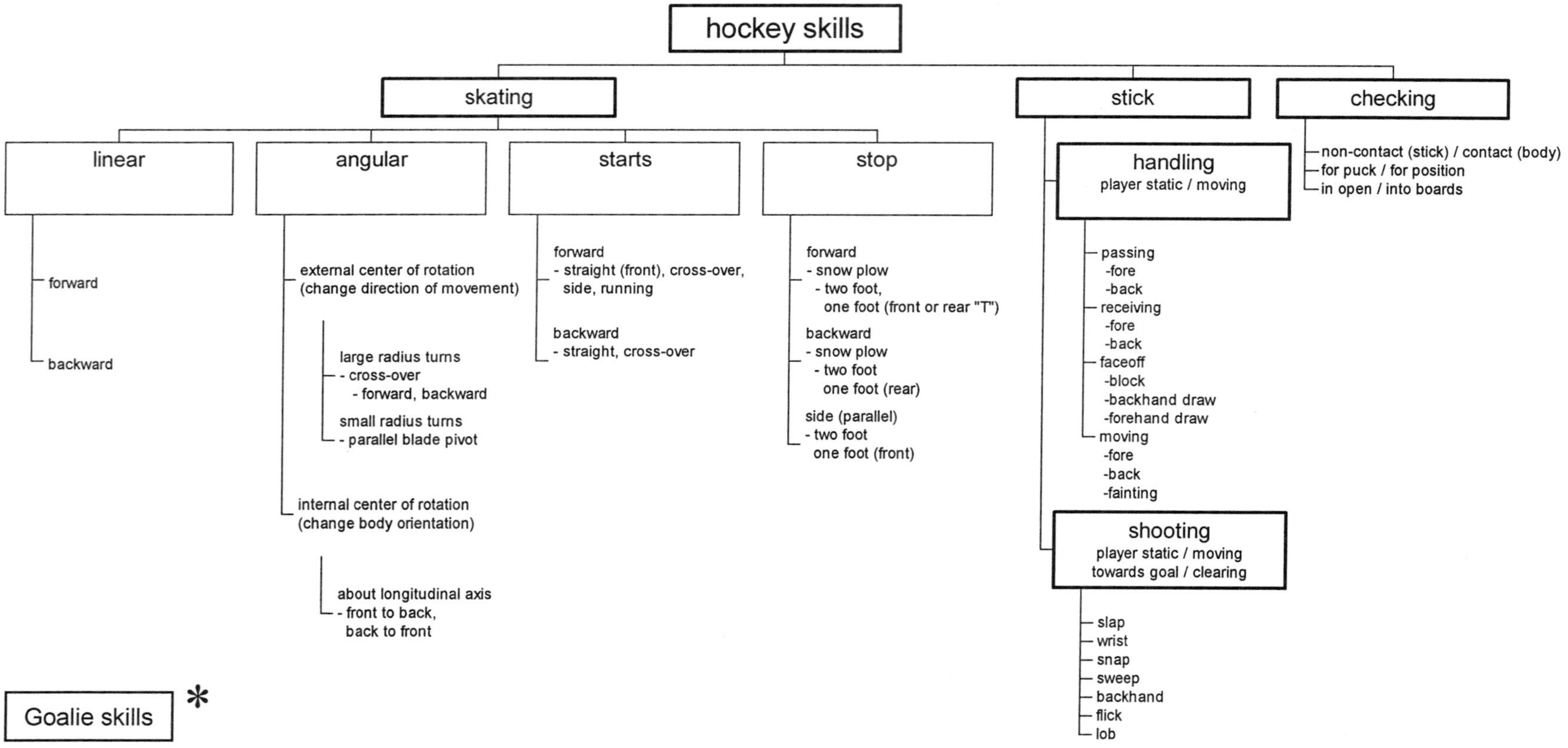
hockey skills
skating
linear
forward
backward
angular
external center of rotation
(change direction of movement)
large radius turns
- cross-over
- forward, backward
small radius turns
- parallel blade pivot
internal center of rotation
(change body orientation)
about longitudinal axis
- front to back,
back to front
starts
forward
- straight (front), cross-over,
side, running
backward
- straight, cross-over
stop
forward
- snow plow
- two foot,
one foot (front or rear "T")
backward
- snow plow
- two foot
one foot (rear)
side (parallel)
- two foot
one foot (front)
stick
handling
player static / moving
passing
-fore
-back
receiving
-fore
-back
faceoff
-block
-backhand draw
-forehand draw
moving
-fore
-back
-fainting
shooting
player static / moving
towards goal / clearing
slap
wrist
snap
sweep
backhand
flick
lob
checking
non-contact (stick) / contact (body)
for puck / for position
in open / into boards
Goalie skills
*

ally and in combination or sequentially with other skills. The variety of techniques and combinations of skills employed by players within an ever-changing environment leads to unpredictable outcomes and is extremely complex to analyze. These factors make ice hockey an exciting sport to play and watch, as well as a challenge for coaches to understand the mechanics of ice hockey.

Factors Affecting Performance

As implied above, the performance of skills depends on the interaction of factors related to the individual, the environment, and the equipment utilized (Fig. 43–2). These factors are mutually interdependent. For instance, changes in the environment such as rink dimensions for Olympic hockey (30 m wide by 60 m long) versus for North American hockey (26 m wide by 60 m long) can have a profound effect on the skills required in the game. Changes in team organization can affect performance; for instance, the increase, since the 1970s, in the number of players on a team has reduced playing shifts to approximately 45 seconds in the National Hockey League, thus permitting athletes to execute skills with higher intensity than previously. The player's position on the team (goalie, offensive, defense, center, wings, referee) will emphasize different skills; for instance, forward and defensive players will need to excel at forward and backward skating, respectively, more than other players. In turn, changes in players' desires to skate faster and check harder has catalyzed innovations in both skate and protective equipment design. Thus, to understand the mechanics of hockey skills, one needs to consider each of these three factors. The challenge remains to link research with practice to augment both the level and safety of ice hockey.

SKATING MECHANICS

The unique combination of an ice surface and skates allows hockey players to move with great agility and speeds. Ice surfaces possess mechanical properties that permit skating motion to be achieved. At one extreme, ice surfaces must provide a sufficiently low coefficient of friction in order to allow a player to glide. On the other extreme, it must provide sufficiently high friction at a different point in time for players to push off during starts and strides (7). The skates provide the tools by which the diverse frictional properties of the ice surface can be elicited and controlled by the player. It is this unique marriage of ice and equipment that makes the game of hockey dynamic and fast paced. The following discussion focuses on these two components.

Ice Surfaces

Recreational ice hockey is played on frozen rivers, ponds, and outdoor rinks, whereas higher levels of organized play and competitive leagues rely more on indoor arenas where ice surface conditions can be controlled by refrigeration systems. Several factors affect the quality of ice surfaces for skating. The ice surface must be level, free of slopes and irregular contours or cracks. Commonly, the smooth indoor ice surface is achieved by using resurfacing machines (Zamboni) that remove a thin layer of ice from the surface and deposit a thin layer of hot water.

The surface of ice has a low coefficient of friction closely tied to its temperature. Koning and colleagues (8) measured coefficients of friction that varied between 0.003 and 0.007 with optimal temperatures at between −6° and −9°C. Kobayashi (9) had determined a higher

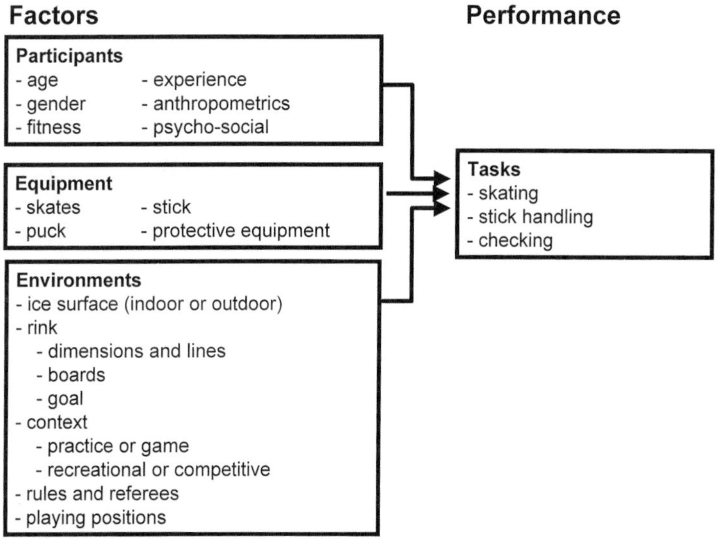

FIG. 43–2. Factors affecting the performance of specific ice hockey tasks.

← **FIG. 43–1.** Ice hockey skill inventory. Identification of categories of related skills, excluding goaltending skills.

optimal temperature of −2.2°C, but this was based on lightly weighted skates drawn on a sled. Ice hockey players often comment on whether ice is hard or soft, with the latter being "slower." At colder temperatures the ice becomes less fluid, making it easier for the puck to slide and for players to glide along the ice more quickly as they skate. Thus, the refrigeration systems used to control the ambient temperature and humidity are crucial components for achieving optimal ice conditions. Indeed, high air temperature, humidity, and accumulated cuttings and shavings on ice can result in a 0.001 to 0.002 change in the coefficient of friction (9). In addition to environmental conditions, if ice conditions are unmonitored, they may vary topographically in terms of surface water and in density, which in turn may influence fatigability, speed, performance of power movements, agility, and puck control (10).

Studies of the physical properties of ice and of how ice interacts with a skate blade may lead to innovative methods for the preparation and standardization of ice surfaces (10) and to the development of products that may enhance the quality of playing surfaces (11). Several theories describing the mechanics of ice surfaces and skating have been suggested (8,10–15). Early reports suggested that the low frictional coefficient during ice skating is a result of high pressure causing the ice adjacent to the blade to melt, producing a thin, fluid layer between the blade and the ice, and thus reducing friction. Recent studies, however, have calculated that the friction and pressures needed to achieve such conditions would cause the ice to fracture (12). Additionally, at speeds of 5 m/s a liquid layer of less than 0.1 μm thickness would exist over only a 15 μm length, which appears much too short a distance to produce skate gliding. Alternatively, using modern surface science technology (11,15), it has been conjectured that the surface of ice has a constant, thin semiliquid layer producing low frictional interfaces. These conditions would preclude the need to melt the ice to provide a liquid lubricant layer to reduce friction, given that at −157°C a liquid layer one molecule thick exists. The number of liquid layers present increases as ice is warmed, which is a likely explanation for the difference between the faster (less water) colder ice and the warmer (more water) slower ice (11).

Skates

A number of factors affect the interaction of the skate with the ice including the characteristics of the skate design and construction. The skate boot consists of an outer covering of leather or composite material, ankle support, toe box, heel counter, rigid sole, skate blade housing, and blade (Fig. 43–3). The design of skate blades has evolved from those that existed in the 1880s. Early skates had the metal blade attached to the boot by means of a wooden support. Eventually, a pure metal blade assembly was used, adding considerable weight to the skate and reducing skating speed; however, the metal assemblies offered improved control and durability. The development of tubular skate blades in the 1950s helped decrease this weight. By the 1960s and 1970s added safety features (e.g., covered blade end) and the use of composite plastics (e.g., polyethylene resins, carbonates, fiber glass) with metal blade assemblies further reduced skate mass, facilitating improvement in skating speed and maneuverability (16). The specific effects of these design changes on the actual kinematics and kinetic performance characteristics of skating have not been thoroughly investigated. The work of Lamontagne and colleagues (17) suggested that force transmission in all-metal versus plastic housings is drastically different. Further investigation must examine the nature of the mechanical response of these types of skates on ice and the relationship to skating performance.

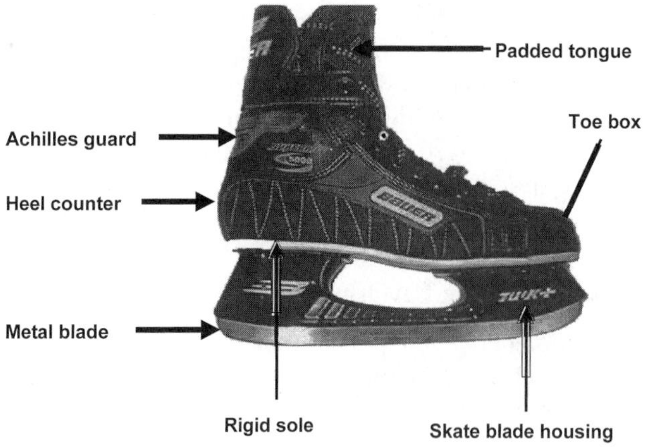

FIG. 43–3. Identification of structural components of the ice hockey skate.

Several other skate design features are known to influence skating performance. A consensus from research on figure skates suggests that edge sharpness, blade thickness, blade taper, radius of curvature (rocker radius), and the boot-to-blade angle are variables identified as those that impact on skating performance (18). Little research has been done, however, to determine the relative importance of each of these characteristics to on-ice performance. With respect to ice hockey, changes in skate feature may affect a skater's balance in such a way as to alter linear skating, cross-overs, turning, stopping, passing, and/or shooting. Important characteristics include the radius of curvature (rocker) of the blade, its center of curvature, and the alignment of the blade with the boot and foot (Fig. 43–4) (4).

Players continually strive to maintain optimally sharp blade edges to maximize skating control. Sharper edges

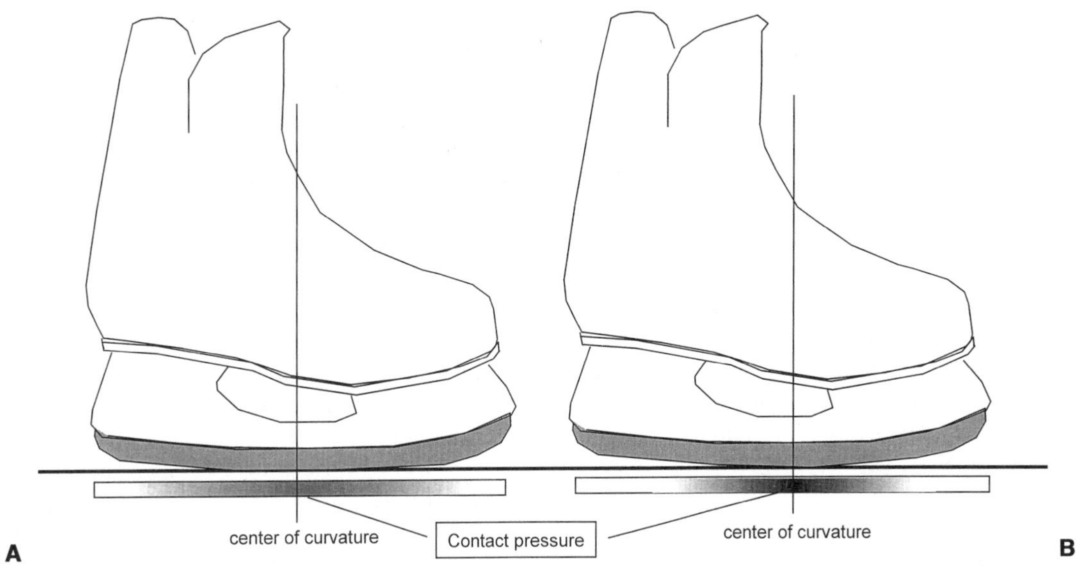

FIG. 43–4. Radius of curvature and its effect on surface contact. Radii vary from 3 m (**A**) to 2 m (**B**).

enable the blade to cut into the ice, which is necessary for push-off; however, sharper blades make smooth stops more difficult (4). If the blade has a duller edge, the skater has more difficulty digging in and pushing off. Blade sharpness must be optimized so that an acceptable trade-off among smooth stopping, turning, and pushing-off is achieved. The runner of the blades (the portion of blade in contact with the ice) has both inside and outside edges with an intermediate shallow channel or hollow to accentuate the sharpness of the edges. During the gliding phase, either one or both of the edges may be in contact with the ice. During the push-off phase, the blade is angled acutely to the ice surface, permitting primarily the inside edge to cut into the ice (Fig. 43–5). During turns such as pivots or crossovers and stops, the outer edge of the skate blade is important in applying force to the ice surface.

Boot construction parameters have an important impact on skating performance. For example, different materials (e.g., leather, polyethylene shells, lacing) and construction (e.g., sewing, gluing, material orientation, and layers) used in making the skate boot can alter its stiffness characteristics. The high-cut boots provide essential lateral and medial support to the ankle during sharp turns but restrict plantar flexion and dorsiflexion during striding and push-off. Regional variation of stiffness characteristics in the boot may help optimize skate design for performance needs (19). The performance trade-off between support and flexibility needs to be determined.

Identification of desirable design skate features specific for ice hockey may be delineated from time-motion studies that have ranked the importance of different skating tasks executed in the game situation. Hansen and Reed (20) provide a detailed inventory of skating tasks required based on interviews with professional players, scouts, coaches, and managers. They delineate a high specificity of skills with given playing positions (i.e., forwards, center, wingers, defense, and goalies), which suggests that different design components may be needed for players at different positions. Renger (21) found similar specialization of skills by position when he surveyed 16 professional scouts to ranks task require-

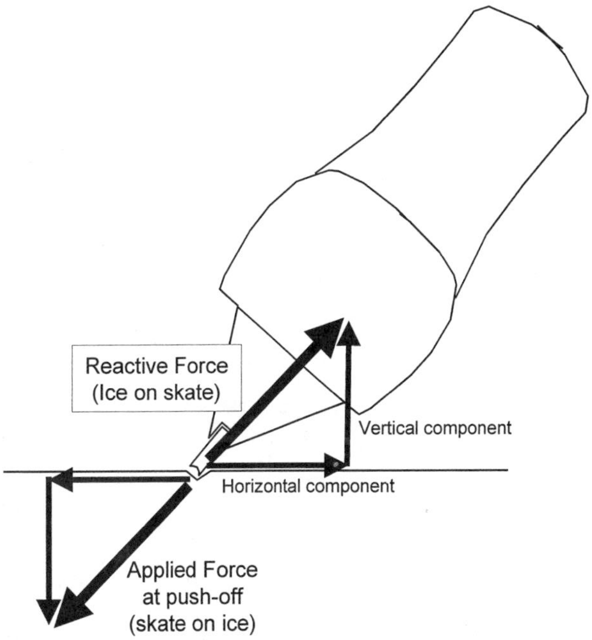

FIG. 43–5. Orientation of skate to ice surface to optimize reactive force at push-off.

ments. The prevalence of specific skating tasks during games, however, needs to be further delineated.

Skating Skills

Skating is the single most important skill for an ice hockey player. Similar gross motor patterns are exhibited in speed and figure skating; however, the context of the game and tasks are fundamentally different, requiring specific skate designs. For instance, a player must start, accelerate, decelerate, stop, change direction, or turn in response to game cues, with decisions on the appropriate action often being made in an instant. Skating performance is determined by numerous interacting mechanical factors (22) (Fig. 43–6). The extent to which each factor influences the resulting performance is not well known given the limited research specific to ice hockey. Thus, many inferences need to be drawn, with caution, from studies of speed and figure skating, given the fundamental differences in skating contexts and blade design.

Skating is a novel form of locomotion for humans in that the reactive push-off force cannot be elicited in the backward direction. Due to the relatively low coefficient of friction between the skate blade runner and ice, little force can be elicited by pushing off parallel to the long axis of the skate blade. Skaters rely on the reactive force that is elicited perpendicular to the skate blade. In forward skating, by externally rotating at the hip, setting the blade on edge through pronation, and pushing laterally, skaters are able to elicit the large reactive forces necessary to propel the body forward. For optimal push-off, the blade is oriented approximately 45 degrees to the ice plane (see Fig. 43–5).

As a result of the alternating directions of lateral impulses, substantial movement of the body occurs in the frontal plane while attempting to move forward. Consequently, the center of mass follows a sinusoidal trajectory over the course of the stride (Fig. 43–7) (23). The amplitude of displacement varies from approximately 25 cm at higher stroke frequencies to 50 cm at lower stroke frequencies as the result of a prolonged glide phase. As the skater pushes off, the center of mass displaces orthogonal to the longitudinal axis of the skate blade. The center of mass leans away continually from the single supporting limb to permit forward movement. The laterally directed kinetic energy of the body must be steered forward during the glide (23) (Table 43–1).

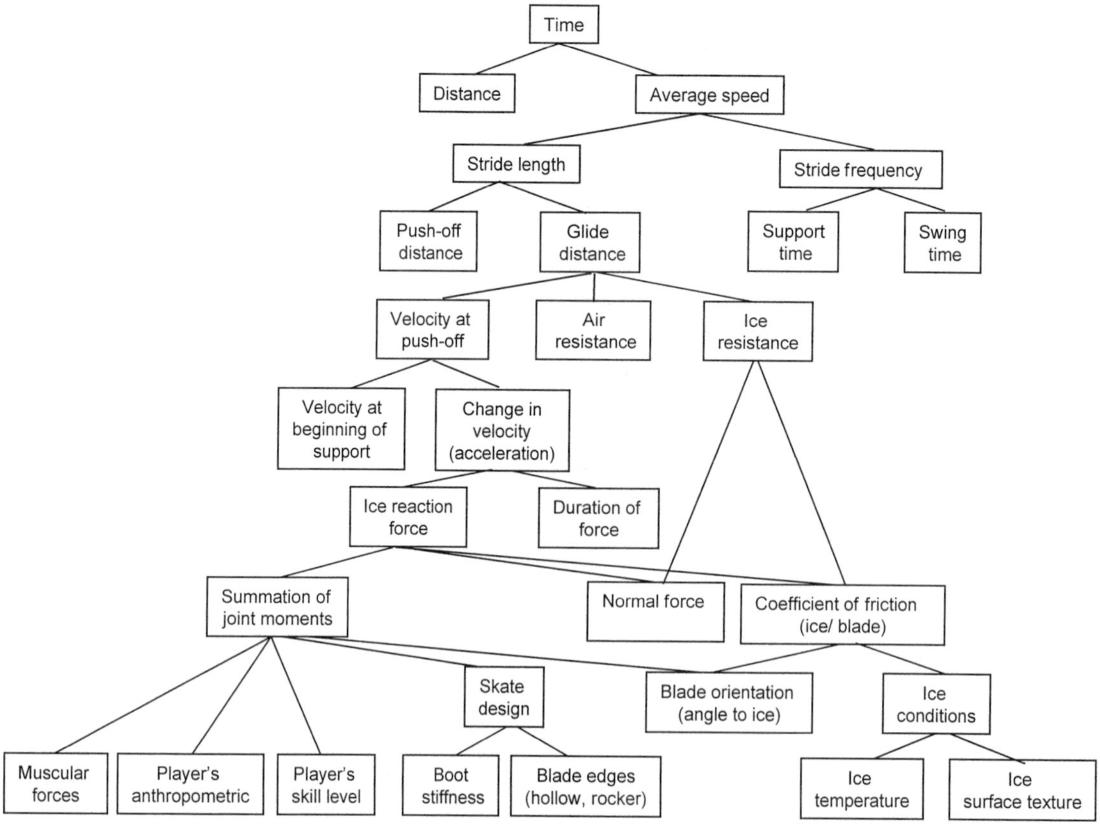

FIG. 43–6. Relationship between skating performance and determining mechanical and physical factors.

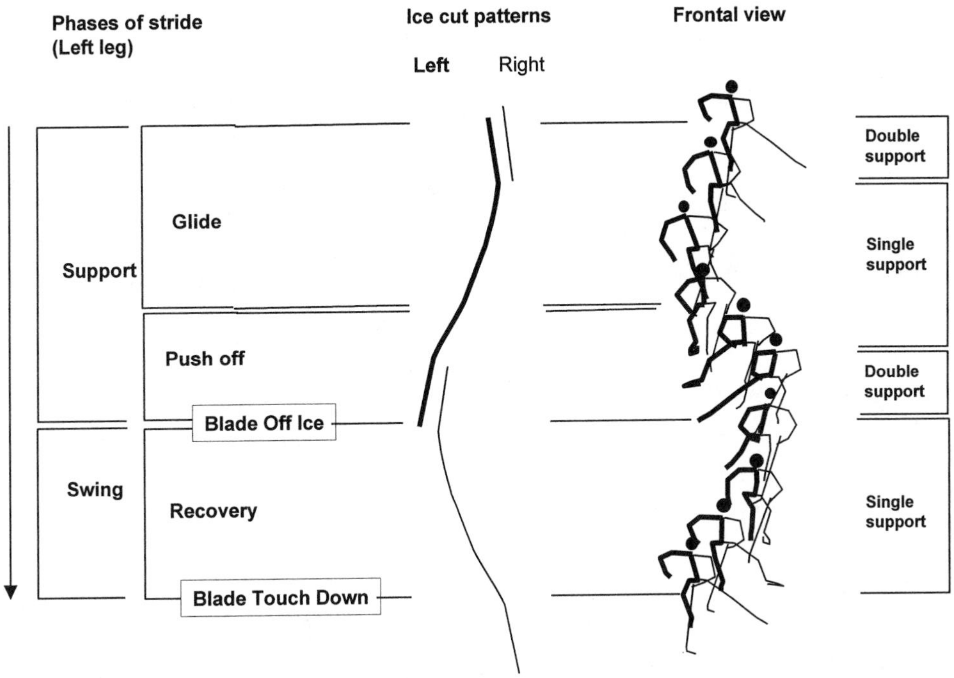

FIG. 43–7. Lateral displacement of body during forward skating. Ice cuts depict sinusoidal skating pattern in the transverse plane.

Linear Movement Paths

Forward Skating

A player must stride as efficiently and as quickly as possible to reach a target location. This may entail positioning oneself to accept a pass, to check an opponent on a fore-checking or a back-checking assignment, or to shoot on the net. Several studies have attempted to understand the most efficient means of forward striding. Early reports described static characteristics of starting and finishing positions while striding with little reference to actual dynamics (24). Subsequent studies have attempted to identify kinematic measures that correlated with the skating stride in ice hockey (25–28). The linear and angular kinematics of the body provides a means of quantifying the technique of skating movement patterns.

The skating stride at constant velocity is essentially biphasic, composed of the support phase and the swing phase (Fig. 43–8). Support may be subdivided into single- and double-support phases (28,29) occupying approximately 18% and 82%, respectively, of the total support time. However, the percentage of time for each phase can vary substantially when the player is accelerating, decelerating, or merely coasting. Propulsion may occur in both the double- and single-support phases of the stride (28). Generally, propulsion begins halfway through the single-support period after the outward rotation of the thigh and coincides with the initial extension of the hip and the knee. As the contralateral skate

TABLE 43–1. *Summary of the position of the skater's center of mass (CM) while forward ice skating*

Phases	Glide: Early support (blade contact)	Glide: Middle support	Glide: Late support (push-off)	Swing recovery
Position of CM				
In sagittal plane	Anterior to ipsilateral ankle	Further anterior to ipsilateral ankle	Anterior to contralateral ankle	Anterior to contralateral ankle
In frontal plane	Above ipsilateral ankle	Mid-body	Above contralateral ankle	Above contralateral ankle

Adapted from ref. 4.

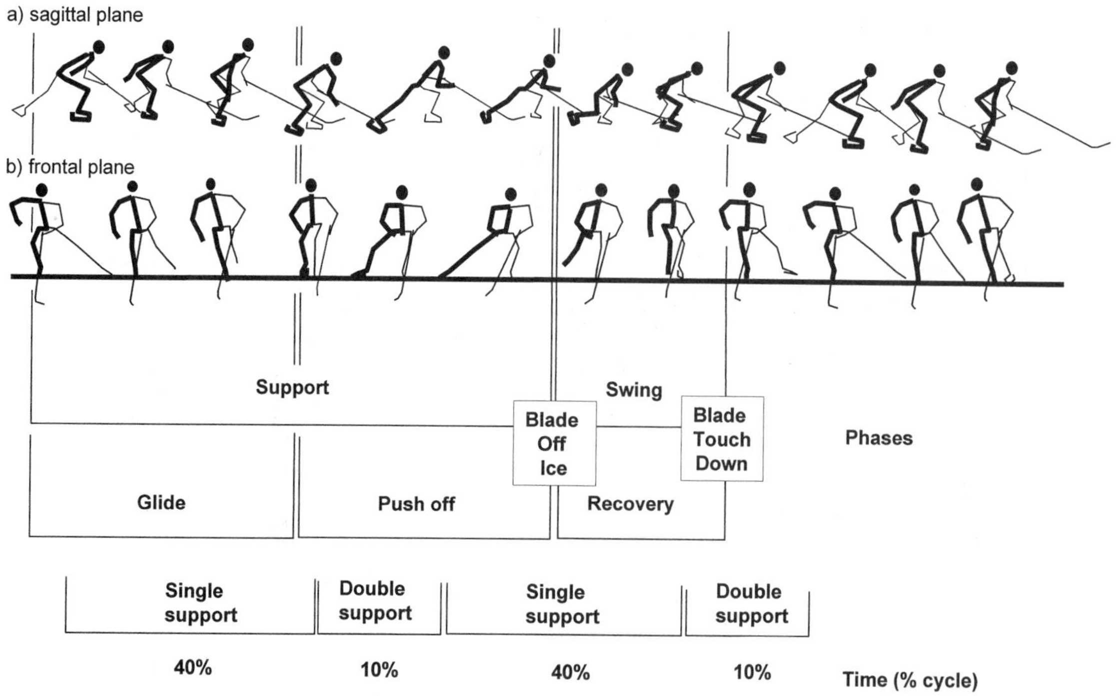

FIG. 43–8. Forward skating sequences in the sagittal (**A**) and frontal (**B**) planes. The skating stride may be subdivided into phases identified by support and swing.

touches down, the propulsive limb pushes off by summating extension of the knee, hyperextension, and abduction of the hip and plantar flexion of the ankle.

The activity patterns of muscle groups during the movements of the leg in the different phases of the stride can be inferred from speed skating studies of elite and trained athletes on 400- and 1500-m rinks (30,31). Activity of primary muscles in the lower limb in conjunction with kinematic analysis documents the gross movement pattern coordination (Fig. 43–9, Table 43–2). These measures indicate that concentric contraction of the gluteus maximus is primarily responsible for the generation of power during the push-off (30). The hamstring muscles (semitendinosus and biceps femoris) are active during the gliding phase but do not contribute to the generation of power due to eccentric contraction. Power generation at the knee joint occurs as an explosive burst of activity of the quadriceps (vastus medialis and the rectus femoris) from about 200 ms before the end of the push-off. This coincides with a decrease in activity of the biceps femoris and the gastrocnemius (both extensor antagonists). Previous to this period, during the gliding phase both the knee extensors and flexors are active to optimize leg position prior to push-off. The short burst in the last 100 ms of the push-off at the ankle might be due to contraction of the soleus (30). Plantar flexion activity is minimal in ice hockey, however, due to the restriction of ankle range of motion by the high-cut boot and rigid sole. Technical innovations in the skate designs similar to recent changes in speed skating could increase the ankle dorsiflexion and plantar flexion to permit potentially greater propulsion and an increase in skating velocity (32).

Marino (25) identified important features of the kinematics of skating strides by observing skaters of different ability at various speeds. The stride frequency plus glide and propulsive phases were correlated to speed rather than stride length. Specifically, velocity increases correlated positively with increases in stride frequency and decreases in double-support time. These results indicate that more power at higher velocities is achieved. Later studies confirmed this trend, with double-support times accounting for only 15% of the stride time (26,28,33,34). Similar findings have been seen in speed skating where higher stroke frequency contributed more to forward velocity than full extension of the limbs. In addition, Koning and colleagues (35) noted that the push-off in these first few strides was primarily straight back. Other variables that have been related to acceleration include increased trunk lean (low hip flexion angle near 40 degrees and center of mass forward), positioning of the skate under the hip at push-off, a low blade surface angle to 45 degrees, and full range of motion of the knee with rapid extension.

Some research has been done in an attempt to relate selected strength and anthropometric determinants to skating speed. For example, Song and Reid (36) examined the relationship of lower-limb flexibility, strength,

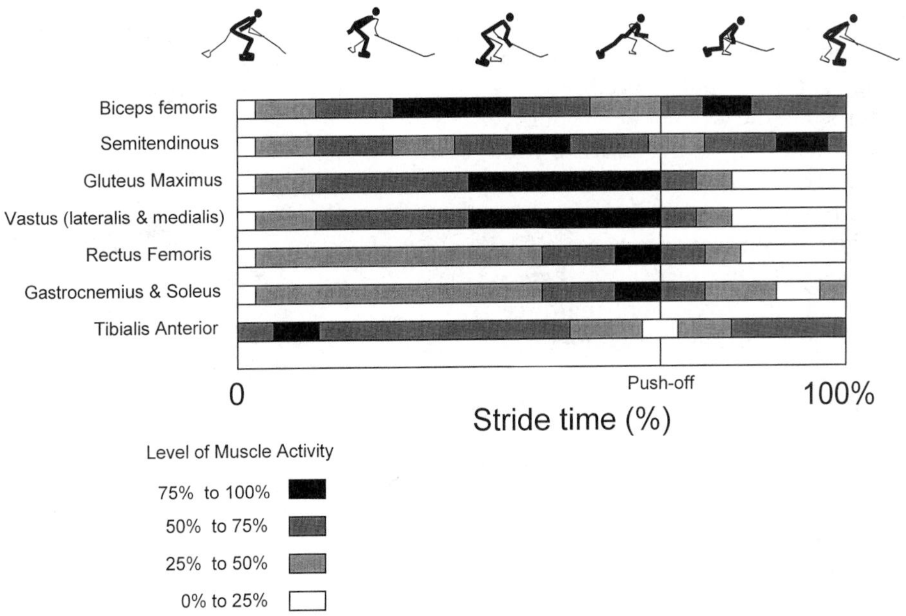

FIG. 43–9. Level of muscle activity in the lower limb during the forward skating stride (31).

and anthropometric measures to skating speed in ice hockey players. Of the measures taken, hip flexion strength, ankle dorsiflexion, hip adduction-abduction flexibility, and knee flexion-extension flexibility were the most important for predicting 25-m skating speed from a standing start. Ankle flexion-extension was negatively correlated with skating speed, suggesting that plantar flexion may not be desirable during a start. It is worthy of note that two different regression equations were developed for players skating with and without a stick. Song and Reid suggest that the emergence of two separate equations demonstrates that the biomechanics of skating with and without a stick are quite different. Thus, the use of the hockey stick should be mandatory when studying kinematic patterns of skating in ice hockey.

While skating, the player must strive to increase or maintain forward velocity. Within a fixed amount of time for a particular stride, the skater must maximize the transverse impulse applied to the ice to increase the kinetic energy of the center of mass (37). This horizontal impulse depends on the magnitude and direction of the ice reactive force and the time during the stride the force is applied. To maximize the time spent applying force, the propulsive limbs should be moved through as large a range of motion as possible without compromising stride rate. Given the relationship between velocity and stride rate, the power generated while skating is the product of the stroke frequency and the mechanical work per stroke.

Acceleration occurs throughout the double-support phase and for 50% of the single-support (glide) phase (28). During the glide phase, there is a period of deceleration caused by a lack of propulsive forces and the presence of air and ice friction. Only after 1.75 seconds from the start did negative acceleration occur. Following

TABLE 43–2. *Summary of lower limb movements while forward skating*

	Glide			
Phases	Early support (blade contact)	Middle support	Late support (push-off)	Swing recovery
Joint position				
Hip	45°	100° and external rotated	180° and external rotated	180 to 40° and internal rotated
Knee	90°	160°	180°	180° to 90°
Ankle and foot	Dorsiflexed and pronated	Neutral and pronated	Plantarflexed and pronated	Dorsiflexion and supinated

Adapted from ref. 4.

that point, it was hypothesized that a skater exhibits alternate periods of acceleration and deceleration during full-speed striding. The glide phase occurs as the recovered skate is returned to the ice and the propulsive skate reaches the end of its range of motion. The glide phase continues during the recovery of the rear skate. One of the main difficulties is recovering the propulsive leg rapidly enough to begin a subsequent push-off. The glide subphase continues until the recovered skate is laterally rotated and begins effectively applying force.

Little work has been done to evaluate the kinetics of ice skating in hockey and, therefore, inferences may be drawn from speed skating. From glide to push-off, the center of pressure shifts from the rear to front edge of the blade. The amount of weight borne by the blade during glide and push-off varies from 95% to 130% of body weight, respectively, within 400 ms of the end of the stroke (23). Similar patterns of loading can be observed during forward skating in ice hockey. For instance, equivalent magnitudes of force have been measured in our lab using pressure sensors placed within the boot during skating (Fig. 43–10).

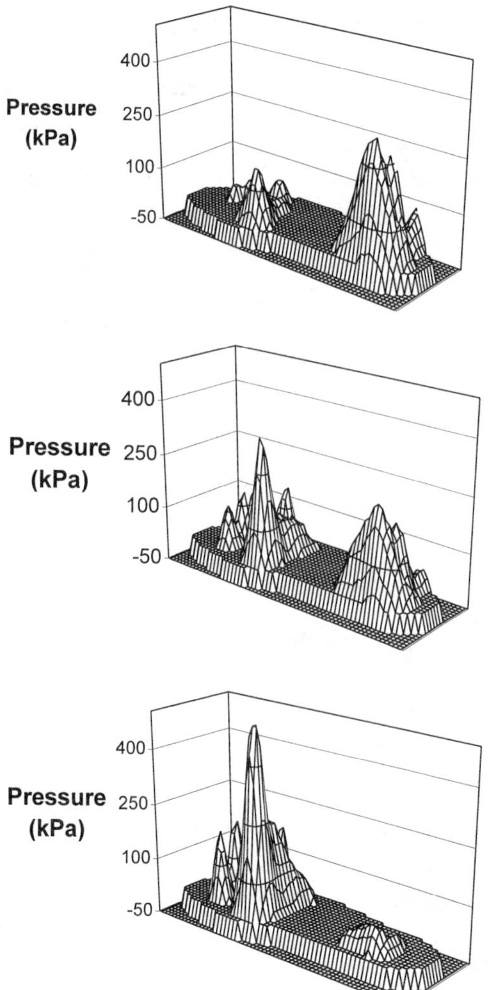

FIG. 43–10. Pressure patterns on sole of the skate during forward skating as shown in initial support (**A**), middle support (**B**), and late support (**C**) phases.

Backward Skating: Starts and Stops

Though backward movement is a predominant component of ice hockey, its mechanics have not been investigated. Various forms of backward skating, starts, and stops are part of the game (Fig. 43–11). This is another movement skill unique to ice hockey and absent in speed skating. Consequently, this helps to explain the differences in blade geometry used in these two sports. Speed skate blades are typically flat, while ice hockey blades require a curved base (rocker). In ice hockey, the high-cut boot design is needed for medial and lateral ankle stability, but this reduces the range of motion at the ankle in dorsiflexion and plantar flexion, which in turn reduces the ability of the ankle to accommodate a different body orientation for backward skating. The curved blade aids weight transfer from the front to the back of the skate by permitting the body to "rock." This permits balance to be maintained and greater power while skating backward.

In skating backward, trunk lean in the direction of movement is not possible as seen in forward skating. Thus, the player must adopt a deeper hip and knee flexed posture and lead with one's buttocks. Similar mechanics for propulsion are required in that the force is applied perpendicular to the edge of the blade. To produce backward movement requires the force to be applied in the lateral and anterior (forward) direction with respect to the player's view. To generate this force requires the push-off leg to be internally rotated in contrast to external rotation as observed with forward skating. Similar sinusoidal patterns of the body's center of

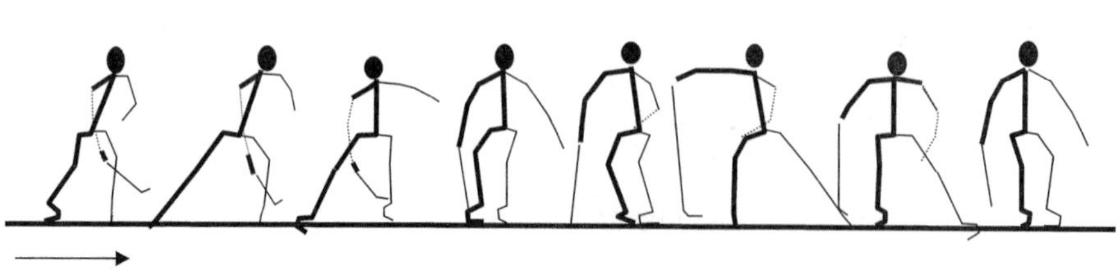

FIG. 43–11. Backward skating sequence in the frontal plane. Stride sequence proceeds from left to right.

mass will be observed. In addition to the above differences, a smaller range of motion at the hip and knee will occur compared to forward skating. These obstacles result in reduced maximal speeds compared to forward skating. Consequently, defensive players often start forward to accelerate rapidly, then turn to skate backward in response to the opposing player's movements. Alternatively, instead of skating straight backward, a player may choose to cross over to gain speed as well as move laterally (29). Unfortunately, this restricts the player mobility while starting, permitting the opponent to pass on the noncommitted side (i.e., the side opposite to crossover). Further research needs to address this category of skills.

Starts and Stops

Perhaps the most important predictor of skating success is the player's ability to change pace rapidly and appropriately. In game situations a player must make transitions in movement direction rapidly. These transitions require high power to attain maximum speed in as short a time span as possible in a variety of offensive and defensive game situations. Fundamental to the agility of the player is the ability to start and stop partially or fully in order to make quick and frequent directional changes. This is a skill executed by players at all positions including goaltenders retrieving or playing loose pucks behind the net. Few studies have evaluated the effectiveness of the hockey starts and stops.

There are three basic ice hockey starts: straight forward start, crossover side start, and thrust/glide "T" start. Disagreement in the literature exists as to the most effective start. The backward skating stride and start, the forward skating crossovers, and backward and forward starts have not been evaluated in the academic literature.

The forward start has been studied in speed skating at distances of 500 m. Fifty percent of the variability in final times is attributable to the acceleration of the first second of the start of the race (38). It is rare that ice hockey players will sprint distances greater than 60 m given the confines of the rink. Players are more likely to sprint part of this distance, stop, change direction, and sprint again. Nonetheless, effective stops/starts/stops are essential skills for ice hockey players.

The angle of push-off in the forward start is almost perpendicular to the direction of skating. Koning and colleagues (35) also noted that the rotational velocity (i.e., the rapidity of turnover of the recovery leg to a propulsive phase) contributed more to the horizontal velocity of the center of mass than did velocity produced by the extension of the leg during push-off.

Specific to ice hockey, Naud and Holt (39) compared three starting techniques: the front start, the crossover, and the thrust/glide. Twenty-four professional and amateur skaters were filmed at 60 frames/second and timed with photoelectric cells while they started and then skated a distance of 20 feet. The thrust/glide start was the quickest for all groups ($p < .05$) except in the case of professionals, who showed no differences between techniques. Film analysis revealed a greater initial acceleration of the center of gravity over the first two strides with the thrust/glide start. The slower starts using the crossover were attributed to a longer air time. With the front start technique, the push-off angle was 45 degrees, whereas it was 90 degrees in relation to the direction of travel with the thrust/glide start. Despite these findings, the crossover and front starts are much more popular than the thrust/glide start in ice hockey since a greater time is required for positioning the body prior to executing the thrust and glide start.

Naud and Holt (40) extended their studies with the same group of subjects to examine various stop/reverse, and start strategies. Two stops were examined. A parallel stop and a skates in-line stop followed by either crossover with the two stops or a thrust/glide start after a parallel stop. As in the previous study, the use of the thrust/glide after a parallel stop was superior to both of the other strategies ($p < .05$). Naud and Holt explained that stopping at 90 degrees and maintaining that angle with the rear foot during the initiation of the subsequent start made the parallel stop followed by a thrust/glide start the quickest way to stop and change directions. This is noteworthy, since this set of skills is important and often executed during a game of ice hockey. With the other two strategies, players also tended to glide sideways further (14 and 9 inches compared to 7 inches) when stopping.

Marino (33) examined acceleration-time relationships using a front skating start. Four subjects varying in skill level were timed and filmed in one plane. Subjects required four full strides to complete the 20 feet in a mean time of 1.87 s. The least skilled subject had a lower velocity and a lower average acceleration over the 20 feet. Stride time and single-support and double-support time ratios were similar in all subjects. Acceleration-time curves revealed high initial accelerations, with lower acceleration at the 20-foot mark, while deceleration occurred after approximately 1.75 s (range = 1.64–1.80 s). Thus, acceleration was noted to occur even during the single support phase in the first few strides. Marino suggested that this was made possible by an outward rotation of the hip, and knee and ankle flexion in the recovery leg during double support and lasted for the entire stride.

The mean angles of propulsion during the initial strides decrease from 70 to 40 degrees for the first to fourth acceleration strides, respectively (29). As the angle of propulsion decreases, the forward component of the reactive force also decreases. In addition, a number of kinematic variables were found to be important during the acceleration phase of striding. These included high stride rate, significant forward lean, a low takeoff angle, and placement of the recovery foot under the body at the end of the single-support phase. In adolescent skaters, a lower angle of takeoff at the end of the propulsive phase (69 and 60 degrees for faster and slower skaters, respectively) was associated with higher velocities of skating (34). During acceleration just after the start, the angle of propulsion was 40.5 degrees (26).

Marino and Dillman (27) developed regression models to predict the important determinants of a successful front start using 69 volunteers of varying skating ability. The factors identified were high stride rate, significant forward lean, a low takeoff angle, and placement of the recovery foot under the body at the end of the single-support phase. These findings concur with speed skating data (35).

Other studies have attempted to identify the dynamics of the skate start. Roy (41) compared the side, front, and crossover starts in eight adults. Forces on the starts and during the initial stride were measured by a force platform on a synthetic surface. The coefficients of friction on this surface were 0.114 for the static and 0.067 for the dynamic friction, respectively. The forward impulses ranged from 166.6 to 174 N·s, while lateral impulses were only 6.9 to 32.3 N·s. The crossover and side starts produced the greatest vertical and forward impulses, respectively. In a similar study, Simm and Chao (42) reported that during front starts with roller skates, vertical forces ranged from 1.5 to 2.5 times body weight. Posterior and lateral forces were approximately 681 N and 363 N, respectively.

Another study was undertaken to examine forces generated by parallel stops in two skilled subjects (17,43). Angular kinematics revealed that at the beginning of the stop there was a horizontal rotation and a quick lateral flexion of both skates to achieve a quick perpendicular orientation in relation to the direction of displacement. These factors allowed subjects to develop large braking forces while maintaining balance. A small anteroposterior angle of inclination was observed at the beginning of the braking period while the interior skate flexion angle was much lower (i.e., remains more vertical than the outside skate). Due to technical difficulties, force transducers did not yield reliable or valid representations of the forces.

Angular Movement Paths

Angular skating and turns are equally important skills to skating forward and backward, and often represent a transition from one mode of skating to another. Angular movements can occur about external points of rotation or about an axis internal to the player (i.e., turns about one's longitudinal axis).

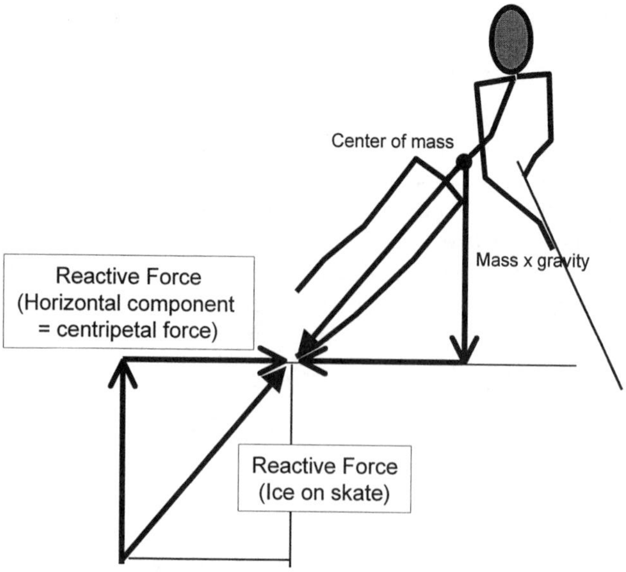

FIG. 43–12. Generation of centripetal force in skating turns.

To produce angular movements about an external axis requires centripetal force that will alter the path of body (Fig. 43–12). The greater the centripetal force, the smaller the radius of curvature of the player's path. This centripetal force can be accommodated by leaning the trunk in toward the desired direction of the turn, that is, leaning in toward the center of the turn where the axis of rotation resides. This lean while skating will position the player's center of mass outside and lateral to the base of support defined by the skate blade contact on the ice. To counteract the tendency for gravity to cause the player to topple over, countermoments are generated from lateral reactive forces at the blade ice interface. The reactive force on the blades will then press upward (i.e., equal and opposite the gravitational force) and in toward the center of rotation (i.e., a force that can generate an equal and opposite gravitational moment) with the player maintaining balance. The horizontal component of the reactive force provides the needed centripetal force, thus generating a turn. Turns of this nature can be accomplished on either the inside or outside edge of the blade. This angular path may be followed with blades parallel as in pivots or by a series of crossover steps (Fig. 43–13). With the latter, propulsion can be generated while skating. The outside leg (away from the center of rotation) will press with the inside blade edge as typical of forward skating. The inside leg (closed to the center of rotation) will press with the outside blade edge as it scissors under the body (29). In speed skating, during the crossover both stroke time and peak force at push-off are reduced, and there is an absence of a middle phase with sub-body weight loads in comparison to forward skating (23,44). These

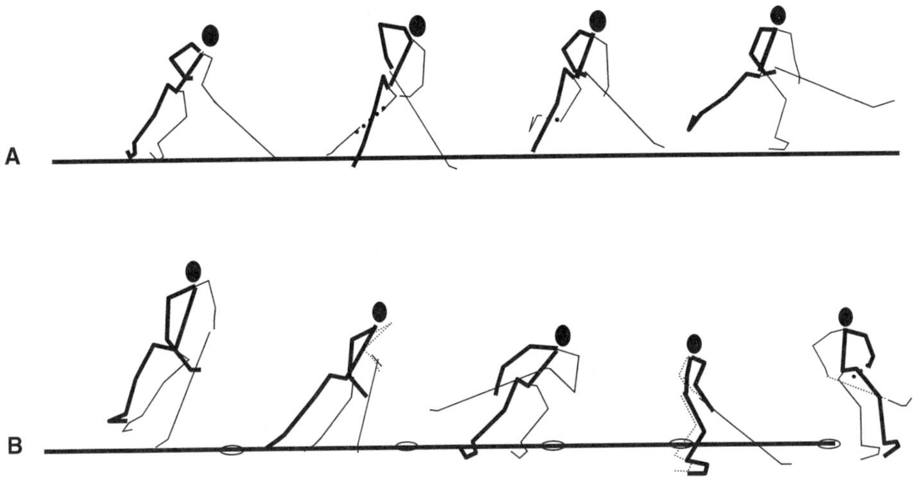

FIG. 43–13. Angular skating sequence during crossover (**A**) and pivot (**B**) turns.

decreased stride times may relate to decreased glide time and smaller radius of curvatures.

The tightness of the turn can be modulated by the extent of body lean. Extreme turns or pivots of small curvature radius are an important skill; for instance, as possession of the puck changes, the player must rapidly change direction to shift into defensive or offensive modes. Similarly, agile changes in direction are fundamental to getting past opponents or in tracking opponents. Blade-ice angles greater than 45 degrees and up to 60 degrees can be achieved. Blade sharpness is crucial to maintaining control so that the blades can cut into the ice surface at these extreme acute angles. Too extreme an angle will result in lateral slipping of the blade, reducing the reactive force and potentially causing the player to fall. Again the blade's rocker facilitates the ice hockey player by allowing the skate blade to maintain contact with the ice as weight is shifted from front to back or vice versa.

Angular movement about an internal axis of rotation is evident in ice hockey. Often, players have little room to maneuver and need to turn direction in pursuit of the puck or opponent. These rotations are mediated by an off-center force created with one skate blade pressing perpendicular to the ice surface while the skate blade of the opposite foot will act as the fulcrum for rotation. Alternatively, a player with linear momentum from skating may drag or cut one skate blade into the ice surface to act as the rotation point while the momentum is redirected.

STICK AND PUCK MECHANICS

Biomechanical studies of hockey sticks have not been widely published. Descriptions of sticks and stick tasks have generally been treated qualitatively, often tending to focus on shooting with little attention to puck handling or passing. Even less attention has been given to quantifying the mechanics of using the hockey stick. Most studies have focused on shooting, with little regard to other stick-handling skills.

Hockey Sticks and Pucks

The hockey stick is an implement used as an extension of one's arms to create a longer lever and thus generate greater velocities on projection of the puck. Sticks are used for controlling the puck position while skating, passing and receiving, and shooting at a net. Skills using the stick, particularly shooting, are determined by numerous mechanical factors that interact (Fig. 43–14) (45–47). The extent to which each factor influences the resulting performance is not well known given the limited research specific to ice hockey.

As with skates, hockey sticks have evolved considerably since the game's beginnings. The original hockey sticks were made entirely from a single piece of wood. By the 1950s, separate shaft and blades were constructed and then joined. In the late 1960s, the stick was modified with curvature applied to the blade that led to increased maneuverability of the puck during forehand stick handling as well as significantly increased shooting velocity. The trend by the 1970s was to envelop the wood core of the blade with fiberglass and plastics, thereby reducing wood use and weight. In the 1980s, manufacturers added plastic inserts to the bottom of the blade to increase durability. In the 1990s, alternative materials for stick construction include aluminum alloys, carbon plastics, and fiberglass in various combinations.

Hockey sticks have various geometric, static, and dynamic characteristics (48,49). The geometric characteristics include length, minor axis dimension, major axis dimension, length of blade, thickness of blade, curvature of blade, lie (angle between shaft and blade), and center

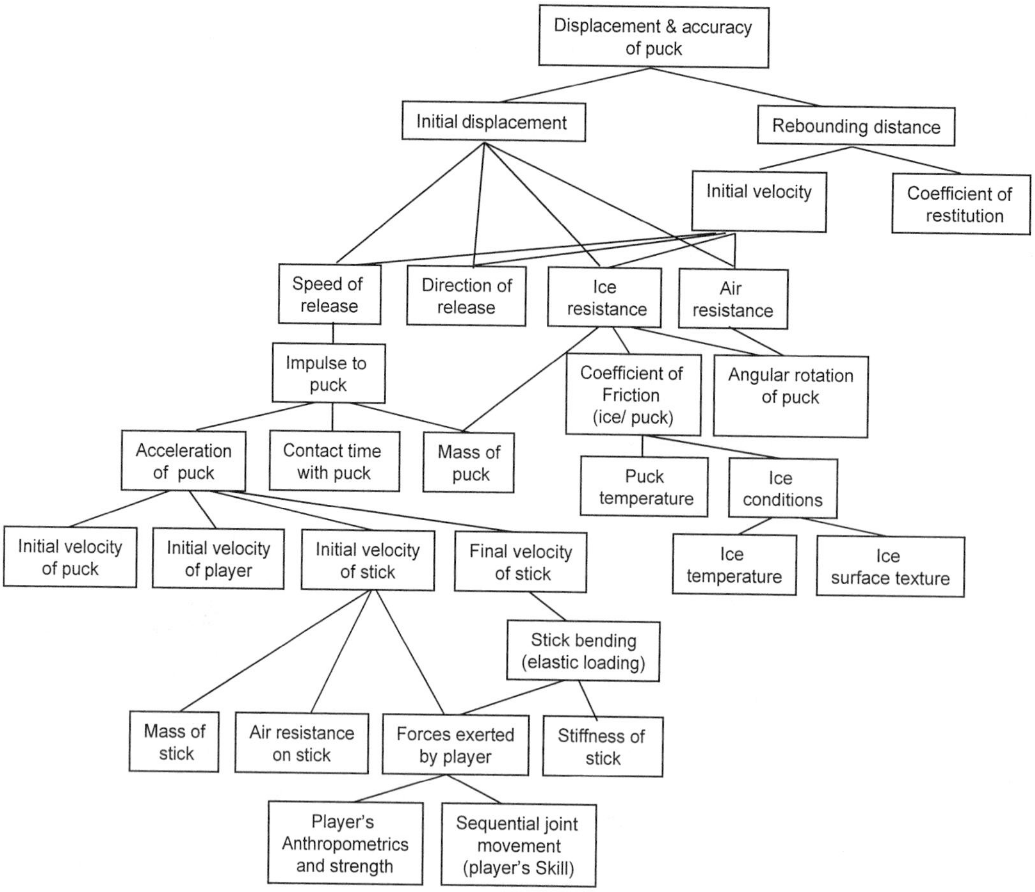

FIG. 43–14. Relationship between shooting performance and determining mechanical and physical factors.

of mass. The static characteristics include the following stiffness measurements: blade stiffness, stiffness of the shaft through the minor axis, stiffness of the shaft through the major axis, and the torsional stiffness of the shaft. Certain dimensions of the stick have been standardized for the National Hockey League, such as its minimum length, 25 cm (63 inches); maximum blade length, 5 cm (12.5 inches); and maximum blade curvature in deflection, 0.2 cm (0.5 inches) (1).

Puck dimensions and properties have been standardized as well. The puck is cylindrical in shape with a thickness of 2.5 cm (1 inch) and a diameter of 7.5 cm (3 inches). The pucks must be kept in frozen condition. Typically the puck has a mass of 5.5 to 6 ounces and is composed of reclaimed hydrocarbon with filler carbon black, ash, and softener. The puck has a Shore D hardness of approximately 90, with a coefficient of restitution of 0.25 that decreases with temperature and speed of impact by an additional 0.05 (50). Warmed pucks rebound more due to an increased elastic coefficients; thus, game rules dictate that pucks must be kept frozen (1).

Shooting

The ability to shoot the puck with optimal velocity and precision is a decisive factor in the overall performance of a player (51). Using the puck velocity data as a guideline and depending on the caliber of the adult player, today one would expect to record puck velocities for the standing slap shot that fall within 100 to 115 km/h. Higher velocity values could be expected due to the improvements in the constructions of hockey sticks, coaching, and hockey-specific training programs since the original studies were undertaken. Table 43–3 summarizes the puck velocities recorded for the various types of shots that have been studied. At least five different approaches were used to calculate puck velocities: impact velocity (52,53), average velocity (41,54–56), instantaneous velocity (7,42), and maximal velocity (46) and radar (46a).

Initial attempts at describing the mechanics of slap shots were qualitative. For instance, Hayes (57) outlined the proper execution of the slap shot as well as common faults that should be avoided. Furthermore, the author

TABLE 43–3. *Summary of puck velocities [mph (Km/h)] reported by various studies*

Studies	Method	Velocity	Age	Slap Skate	Slap Stand	Wrist Skate	Wrist Stand	Sweep Skate	Sweep Stand	Backhand Skate
Alexander et al. 1963	Ballistic	Impact	Adult	127 (79)	111 (69)	117 (73)	97 (60)			
Alexander et al. 1964	Ballistic	Impact	Varsity	121 (75)		114 (71)				
Cotton 1966			Adult	100 (62)	90 (56)	90 (56)	81 (50)	90 (56)	83 (51)	
Furlong 1968	Stop watch	Avg	Pro's	175 (108)		163 (102)				
Chau et al. 1973	Cine	Instant	Adult	132 (82)	110 (68)	143 (99)	132 (92)			
Roy et al. 1974	Cine	Avg	Junior B	89 (55)	92 (57)	81 (50)	64 (40)	85 (53)		64 (40)
Roy and Doré 1976	Sound	Avg	Pee-wee		69 (43)					
			Adult		96 (60)					
Doré and Roy 1976	Sound	Avg	Adult	104 (65)	97 (60)					
Simm and Chau 1978	Cine	Max	High school	150 (90)						
			Adult	200 (120)						
Rothsching 1997	Radar	Max	Varsity		108 (67)					

noted that a heavier stick would increase the striking mass but decrease the velocity at contact; thus, lighter sticks should be chosen. A later report by Emmert (58) provided a description of the slap shot motion and recommended an overall training program that would improve the player's performance. The slap shot was described as being composed of distinct phases: backswing (preparatory), action (downswing, preload, load, and release), and the follow-through phases. Though the above studies described the required actions, no quantitative data were supplied to support the hypotheses.

In the late 1950s and early 1960s, as the use of the slap shot increased in popularity, differences concerning the speed and accuracy of the wrist shot and slap shot as well as the effect of grip strength were studied (52). Thirty players from professional and amateur teams of varying caliber were the subjects. The maximum shot velocity was obtained from the skating slap shot (122–138 km/h), while the minimum velocity was obtained from the standing wrist shot (87–101 km/h). The mean velocity of the skating slap shot (127 km/h) was greater than the mean skating wrist shot (117 km/h), whereas the corresponding mean velocities while standing were 111 km/h and 97 km/h, respectively. The skating wrist shot was the most accurate. A low correlation between static grip strength and the speed of the shot was observed, indicating the importance of technique when executing slap shots or wrist shots in hockey.

A subsequent study investigated the effect of strength development on the speed of shooting (53). Four players were photographed using a high-speed camera three times from the front and side positions while performing skating slap and wrist shots. Resistance training emphasizing upper body strength resulted in an increased shot velocity mean compared to controls. The players recorded skating slap shot velocities between 113 and 121 km/h, while the skating wrist shot velocities were between 105 and 113 km/h. The isometric training program significantly improved the shot velocity by 6.7 km/h for the skating slap shot and by 8.7 km/h for the skating wrist shot.

In comparison, Cotton (59) found higher velocities of the wrist and slap shots while skating (average 90 and 100 km/h, respectively) than standing. The sweep shots were recorded with velocities of 82 to 138 km/h, which were similar to the wrist shot velocities from the same study. Using manual stop watches, Furlong (60) found that professional players had greater velocities for skating wrist and slap shots (164 km/h and 174 km/h, respectively).

With more precise instrumentation, Chau and colleagues (7) and Simm and Chao (42) used high-speed cinematography to obtain kinematic information of various hockey activities of two adult players and one juvenile player. These included puck velocities, stick kinematics, push off kinematics and kinetics, various skating speeds (forward, backward, and sliding speed) as well as impact forces due to a puck when different absorption materials were used. One Photosonic camera was used to record shooting speed at frame rates of 400 Hz, while a second camera was used to record the shooting speed using frame rates of 750 to 1000 Hz. Puck velocities were calculated at 6.1 m (20 feet) from the player.

The peak skating slap shot puck velocity recorded was 132 km/h, while the peak skating wrist shot puck velocity was 143 km/h. Comparison of puck velocities indicated that the skating wrist was greater than the slap shot, contradicting Alexander and colleagues (52) finding, but it may be explained by the small sample size and caliber of the players. The above puck velocities were based on one subject since the shot velocities were only recorded for a chosen player. The peak forward skating velocity was 43 km/h, while the peak backward skating velocity was 27 km/h. The sliding speed was 24 km/h.

In a study of four junior B caliber players, Roy and colleagues (56) used high-speed film (200 to 500 Hz) to calculate puck velocity data. Additional stick kinematic information included the impulse duration while the puck was in contact with the blade, deflection duration, maximal deflection, deflection velocity, maximal angular velocity, horizontal blade linear velocity, and percentage of velocity of the puck. Both the slap shot and wrist shot with the players standing or skating were investigated. Additionally, the sweep and backhand shots were recorded while the players were skating only.

The maximal velocity for a slap shot was 89 km/h, which compared favorably with Cotton (59) and was noticeably lower than Alexander and colleagues (52). The four junior B caliber players had a slap shot impulse duration of 35 ms. The deflection duration was 63 ms and 82 ms while the angular velocities were 17 to 13 radians per second for standing and skating slap shots, respectively. It is interesting to note that the puck left the blade when the angular deflection velocity had reached its maximum. The angular velocity results did not compare well with those of Chau and colleagues (7). For the slap shot, 40% to 50% of the velocity of the puck was attributable to the deflection of the shaft, while 25% to 34% and 8% to 10% were the corresponding percentages for the wrist shot and backhand (and sweep), respectively. The authors suggested that the stick deformation is mainly due to friction between the blade and the ice rather than the blade and the puck.

The horizontal velocity of the blade reached a maximum of 20 m/s prior to making contact with the ice, at which time the horizontal blade velocity decreased. The blade reached a maximum of 20 m/s when the strain energy stored due to the deflection of the shaft was released. Though the graphed data provided some useful comparisons and insight into the various shots studied, they were noticeably smooth and none of the events were identified. From their study Roy and colleagues (56) recommended that since both the sweep and backhand shots used little deflection of the stick to transmit velocity to the puck, stiff sticks were suitable for these shots. Conversely, the proper stiffness was considered an important factor for the slap shot. Thus, younger players (midget and below) should use a more flexible stick to better perform slap and wrist shots without adversely affecting backhand and sweep shots, though shaft stiffness recommendations should be adjusted for the player's morphology and level of play. The authors further recommended that the shots should be synchronized to yield the maximal angular deflection velocity near the end of the shot.

In another study, Roy and Doré (55) recorded puck velocities, morphologic and functional parameters of the standing slap shot for males from three age groups: 11 to 12 years (peewee), 15 to 16 years (midget), and 17 years and older (adult). The average puck velocities were determined with a digital time counter triggered by a magnetic cell embedded in the ice and stopped by the impact sound recorded by a microphone. The peewee group had standing slap shot velocities of 69 km/h, while the midget and adult group had average velocities of 93 km/h and 97 km/h, respectively. The midget and adult results corresponded fairly closely to those of Cotton (59) and Roy and colleagues (56). As expected, the peewee group differed significantly from the two older age groups in morphologic and strength measures as well as in puck velocity. Since the younger players had higher correlations between puck velocity and morphologic and strength measurements, it seemed that the younger players relied more heavily on these attributes to execute the slap shot than the older players. These results seem to confirm that the younger players should choose a suitably flexible hockey stick (56).

Roy (41) reviewed the puck velocity data that were available and attempted to identify interactions between factors affecting shooting, such as the stick design, type of shot, and skill level. Roy and Doré (55) investigated the effects of sticks with two different stiffnesses on the velocity and accuracy of slap and sweep shots of peewee-level players (11 years old). Forty-eight players from three teams were used in the study. Twenty-four players used a senior stiff stick (24.1 lb/in), and 24 players used a senior flexible stick (17.1 lb/in) that was 29% less stiff than the senior stiff model. Use of a flexible stick produced a slight increase in velocity [from 54.4 km/h to 56.8 km/h (4%)] and in accuracy. Based on industry averages, current junior models are approximately 40% less stiff than a current senior medium-stiff model. One may be able to anticipate a further increase in the slap shot velocity when the current junior models are used.

Roy and Doré (55,61,62) performed the first kinetic evaluations of the slap shot, wrist shot, sweep shot, and backhand. The dynamic characteristics of the stick were obtained by using high-speed film (200 frames/second) cinematography and strain gauges located on the shaft and blade. From the high-speed film the following values were obtained: impulse phase, deflection of the shaft during the impulse phase, puck velocity, and the velocity of the blade during the impulse phase. Several strain gauges were placed on the long shaft to calculate the forces exerted by the top and bottom hands as well as the back side of the blade during the various shots. The results provided force time histories calculated from the equilibrium equations. Six peewee players aged 12.3 years old executed two sweep shots and two slap shots using both a stiff and flexible stick (34.3 N/cm and 22.3 N/cm, respectively). The maximum forces exerted occurred approximately when the puck left the blade at the top and bottom hand locations through the minor axis. Forces at these locations were from 13% to 33% lower for the flexible stick (40 to 61 N for stiff sticks and 27 to 53 N for flexible sticks, respectively, for top and bottom hands). From these results, the authors again suggested that flexible sticks should be used by younger players, since lower forces are required to achieve the same puck velocity recorded with stiffer sticks. A lighter and more flexible junior stick used by a peewee player may have provided even higher puck velocities.

In a recent study, Rothsching (63) evaluated the slap shot of six varsity hockey players with sticks of different stiffness (13 to 19 KN/m). Ground reaction forces were monitored using a force plate in conjunction with high-speed video (480 frames/second) and tracking radar gun. Puck velocities ranged from 105 to 112 Km/h. Vertical forces ranged from 120 to 130 N (approximately one-fifth body weight), while anterior forces were much less (16 to 25 N). Total contact lasted about 60 ms compared to 90 ms found by Roy and Doré (55). Peak stick deflection angle reached 20 degrees. Noticeable interactions between subjects and stiffness values were evident. Though the more flexible stick achieved the highest puck velocities overall, substantial variation between subjects occurred, emphasizing the greater importance of player technique and strength.

The above studies are the first attempts at comprehensive analysis of the mechanics of shooting with hockey sticks. Given the complex interactions, much remains to be understood. Future studies will need to address and identify the significance of the factor determining shooting accuracy and speed velocity for various shot types and stick handling (manipulation) skills.

CONCLUSION

Further study of the interactions among the equipment, the environment, and the players is necessary to understand the mechanics of ice hockey skills and performance. Biomechanical research needs to focus on more than forward skating, starts, and slap shots. Many other skills fundamental to ice hockey, such as backward skating, turning, lateral displacement strategies, stick maneuvering tasks, and checking, must be addressed. With the sophisticated measurement tools available today, there is the potential for improved precision to record kinematic and kinetic parameters within three dimensions of movement. Ultimately, this research can lead to enhanced performance.

REFERENCES

1. Duplacey A. *The rules of hockey.* Toronto: Dan Diamond, 1996.
2. Montgomery DL. The physiology of ice hockey. *Sports Med* 1988;5:99–126.
3. Bishop PJ. Protective equipment: biomechanical evaluation. In: Renstroem PA, ed. *Sports injuries: basic principles of prevention and care.* Boston: Blackwell Scientific, 1993:355–373.
4. Minkoff J, Varlotta GP, Simonson BG. Ice Hockey. In: Fu FH, Stone D, eds. *Sports injuries: mechanisms, prevention and treatment.* Baltimore: Williams & Wilkins, 1994:397–444.
5. Connolly KJ. The nature of motor skill development. *J Hum Movement Stud* 1977;3:123–143.
6. Marteniuk RG. Motor skill performance and learning: considerations for rehabilitation. *Physiother Can* 1979;31(4):187–202.
7. Chau EG, Sim FH, Stauffer RN, Johannson KG. Mechanics of ice hockey injuries. In: Bleustein JL, ed. *Mechanics and sport.* Detroit: American Society of Mechanical Engineers, 1973:143–154.
8. Koning JJ de, Groot G de, Ingen Schenau J van. Ice friction during speed skating. *J Biomech* 1992;25(6):565–571.
9. Kobayashi T. Studies of the properties of ice in speed skating rinks. *ASHRAE J* 1973;73:51–56.
10. Montebell GM. Ice skating surfaces. *ASTM Standardization News* 1992;20:54–59.
11. Somorajai GA. Modern surface science and surface technologies: an introduction. *Chem Rev* 1996;96:1223–1235.
12. Colbeck SC. Pressure melting and ice skating. *Am J Phys* 1995;63:888–890.
13. Evans DCB, Nye JF, Cheeseman KJ. The kinetic friction of ice. *Proc R Soc Lond [A]* 1976;347:493–512.
14. Mendelson KS. Why is ice so slippery? *Am J Phys* 1985;53:393.
15. Stanners CD, Gardin D, Somorjai GA. Correlations of atomic structure and reactivity at solid-gas and solid-liquid interfaces. *J Electrochem Soc* 1994;141:3278–3290.
16. Couture G. Safety factors in the modern ice hockey skate blade. In: Castaldi CR, Hoerner EF, eds. *Safety in ice hockey.* ASTM STP 1050. Philadelphia: American Society for Testing and Materials, 1989:117–140.
17. Lamontagne M, Gagnon M, Doré R. Développement, validation et application de systèmes de patins dynamométriques. *Can J Appl Sport Sci* 1983;8(3):169–179.
18. Broadbent S. Skateology: the science and technology of the edge/ice interface. USOC/SETC Conference, Colorado Springs, CO, December 8–9, 1989.
19. Hoshizaki TB, Kirchner G, Hall K. Kinematic analysis of the talocrural and subtalar joints during the hockey skating stride. In: Castaldi CR, Hoerner EF, eds. *Safety in ice hockey.* ASTM STP 1050. Philadelphia: American Society for Testing and Materials, 1989:141–149.
20. Hansen H, Reed A. Functions and on-ice competencies of a high calibre hockey player: a job analysis. In: Terauds J, Gros HJ, eds. *Science in skiing, skating and hockey.* Del Mar, CA: Academic Publishers, 1979:107–115.
21. Renger R. Identifying the task requirements essential to the success of a professional ice hockey player: a scout's perspective. *J Teaching Phys Ed* 1994;13: 180–195.
22. Hay JG. *The biomechanics of sports techniques,* 4th ed. Englewood Cliffs, NJ: Prentice-Hall, 1993.
23. Ingen Schenau GJ van, Boer RW de, Groot G de. Biomechanics of speed skating. In: Vaughan CL, ed. *Biomechanics of sports.* Boca Raton, FL: CRC Press, 122–167, 1989.
24. Lariviere G, Lavalle H. Evaluation du niveau technique de joueurs de hockey de categorie moustique. *Mouvement* 1972;7:101–111.
25. Marino GW. Kinematics of ice skating at different velocities. *Res Q Exerc Sport* 1977;48(1):93–97.
26. Marino GW. Selected mechanical factors associated with acceleration in ice skating. *Res Q Exerc Sport* 1983;54(3):234–238.
27. Marino GW, Dillman CJ. Multiple regression models of the mechanics of the acceleration phase of ice skating. In: Landry F, Orban W, eds. *Biomechanics of sport and kinanthropology: Proceedings of the International Congress of Physical Activity Sciences.* Quebec City, Miami: Symposia Specialist, 1978:193–201.
28. Marino GW, Weese RG. A kinematic analysis of the ice skating stride. In: Terauds J, Gros HJ. eds. *Science in skiing, skating and hockey.* Del Mar, CA: Academic Publishers, 1979:65–74.
29. Stamm L. *Power skating,* 2nd ed. Champaign, IL: Human Kinetics, 1989.
30. Boer RW de, Cabri J, Vaes W, et al. Moments of force, power and muscle coordination in speed-skating. *Int J Sports Med* 1987;8(6):371–378.
31. Koning JJ de, Groot G de, Ingen Schenau GJ van. Coordination of leg muscles during speed skating. *J Biomech* 1991;24(2):137–146.
32. Ingen Schenau GJ van, Groot GG de, Scheurs AW, Meester H. Koning JJ de. A new skate allowing powerful plantar flexion improves performance. *Med Sci Sports Exerc* 1996;28(4):531–535.
33. Marino GW. Acceleration-time relationships in an ice skating start. *Res Q Exerc Sport* 1979;50(1):55–59.
34. Marino GW. Analysis of selected factors in the ice skating strides

of adolescents. *J Can Assoc Health Phys Ed Recreation* 1984(Jan-Feb):4–8.

35. Koning JJ de, Thomas R, Berger M, Groot G de, Ingen Schenau GJ van. The start in speed skating from running to gliding. *Med Sci Sports Exerc* 1993;27(12):1703–1708.
36. Song TMK, Reid R. Relationship of lower limb flexibility, strength and anthropometric measures to skating speed. In: Terauds J, Gros HJ, eds. *Science in skiing, skating and hockey.* Del Mar, CA: Academic Publishers, 1979:83–98.
37. Boer RW de, Schermerhorn P, Gademan Jl, Groot G de, Ingen Schenau GJ van. Characteristic stroke mechanics in elite and trained male speed skaters. *Int J Sport Biomech* 1986;2:175–186.
38. Koning JJ de, Groot G de, Ingen Schenau GJ van. Mechanical aspects of the sprint start in Olympic speed skating. *Int J Sport Biomech* 1989;5:151–168.
39. Naud RL, Holt LE. A comparison of selected hockey skating starts. *Can J Appl Sports Sci* 1979;4(1):8–10.
40. Naud RL, Holt LE. A comparison of selected stop, reverse start (SRS) techniques in ice hockey. *Can J Appl Sports Sci* 1980;5(2):94–97.
41. Roy B. Les lancers au hockey: rétrospective et prospective biomécanique. *Mouvement* 1974;9:85–89.
42. Simm FH, Chao EV. Injury potential in modern ice hockey. *Am J Sports Med* 1978;6(6):378–384.
43. Gagnon M, Doré R, Lamontagne M. Development and validation of a method for determining tridimensional angular displacements with special applications to ice hockey motions. *Res Q Exerc Sport* 1983;54(2):136–143.
44. Ingen Schenau GJ van, Groot GJ de, Boer RW de. The control of speed in elite female speed skaters. *J Biomech* 1985;18(2):91–96.
45. Doré R, Roy B. Dynamometric analysis of different hockey shots. In: *Biomechanics,* vol 5B. Proceedings of the Fourth International Congress of Biomechanics. Baltimore: University Park Press, 1973:277–285.
46. Doré R, Roy B. *Influence de la rigidité des batons sur al cinématique et al cinétique des tirs au hockey sur glace.* Technical report no. EP 78-R-5. Montreal: Ecole Polytechnique de Montréal, 1978.

46a. Rothsching N. The effect of shaft stiffness on the performance of the ice hockey slap shot. MA thesis. Department of Physical Education, McGill University, Montreal, Quebec, Canada, 1997.

47. Hoerner EF. The dynamic role played by the ice hockey stick. In: Castaldi CR, Hoerner EF, eds. *Safety in ice hockey.* ASTM STP 1050. Philadelphia: American Society for Testing and Materials, 1989:154–163.
48. Roy B, Delisle G. Caracteristiques geometriques et dynamique des batons de hockey en regard de leur performance. *Can J Appl Sport Sci* 1984;9(4):214–219.
49. Therrien RG, Bourassa PA. Mechanics application to sports equipment: protective helmets, hockey sticks and jogging shoes. In: Ghista DN, ed. *Human body dynamics: impact, occupational and athletic aspects.* Oxford: Clarendon Press, 1982:498–523.
50. Smith TA, Bishop PJ. *Static and dynamic characteristics of ice hockey pucks. A report for Cooper, Canada.* 1986:106–121 (unpublished).
51. Lariviere G, Bournival G. *Hockey: the right start.* Montreal: Holt-Rinehart, 1973.
52. Alexander JF, Haddow JB, Schultz GA. Comparison of the ice hockey wrist and slap shots for speed and accuracy. *Res Q Exerc Sport* 1963;34:259–256.
53. Alexander JF, Drake CJ, Rechenbach PJ, Haddow JB. Effect of strength development on speed of shooting of varsity ice hockey players. *Res Q Exerc Sport* 1964;35:101–106.
54. Doré R, Roy B. Results on a kinetic analysis of hockey shots. In: Komi PV, ed. *Proceedings of the Fifth International Congress on Biomechanics, Biomechanics,* vol 5B. Baltimore: University Park Press, 1976:277–285.
55. Roy B, Doré R. Kinematics of the slap shot in ice hockey as executed by players of different age classifications. In: Komi PV, ed. *Biomechanics,* vol 5B. Proceedings of the Fifth International Congress on Biomechanics. Baltimore: University Park Press, 1976:287–290.
56. Roy B, Doré R, Parmentier PH, Deroy M, Chapleau C. Facteurs biomécaniques caractéristiques de différents types de lancers au hockey sur glace. *Mouvement* 1974;9:169–175.
57. Hayes D. A mechanical analysis of the hockey slap shot. *J Can Assoc Health Phys Ed Recreation* 1965;31(2):17.
58. Emmert W. The slap shot—strength and conditioning program for hockey at Boston college. *Natl Strength Conditioning Assoc J* 1984;6(2):4.
59. Cotton C. Comparison of ice hockey wrist, sweep and slap shots for speed. Master's thesis, University of Michigan, Ann Arbor, 1966.
60. Furlong WB. How science is changing hockey: 80 mph mayhem on ice. *Popular Mechanics* 1968(February);110–114.
61. Roy B, Doré R. Kinematics of the slap shot in ice hockey as executed by players of different age classifications. In: *Biomechanics,* vol 5B. Proceedings of the Fourth International Congress of Biomechanics. Baltimore: University Park Press, 1973;286–290.
62. Roy B, Doré R. Incidence des caractéristique des bâtons de hockey sur l éfficacite gestuelle des lancers. *Ingénieur* 1975;306:13–18.

PART VI

Applied Sports Physiology

Exercise and Sport Science,
edited by William E. Garrett, Jr., and Donald T. Kirkendall.
Lippincott Williams & Wilkins, Philadelphia © 2000.

CHAPTER 44

Physiology of Alpine Skiing

Robert A. Hintermeister and Gene R. Hagerman

Skiing had its origin in Scandinavia thousands of years ago when skis were used for transportation, hunting, and waging war (1). This form of skiing is known today as nordic or cross-country skiing. In the late nineteenth century, slalom or downhill skiing was developed in Norway (2) and spread to the alpine regions of central Europe. English sportsmen, who traditionally summered in the Alps and were persuaded to contrast the sunny alpine winter with the dreary English weather, became the early ambassadors of winter resort life and skiing, spreading its popularity to other parts of Europe (1).

Winter resort life, and the popularity of skiing in North America, had its roots in the village of Lake Placid. The Lake Placid Club, in upstate New York's Adirondack Park, first remained open for the winter in 1905. For the following season they purchased 40 pairs of skis from Norway for their guests. From this capricious beginning, and as host of the 1932 and 1980 Olympic Winter Games, Lake Placid has etched its place in winter sports and skiing history.

Alpine skiing is embodied by the timeless sensation of speed and rhythm that is combined with the allure of nature's winter wonderland. Today, millions of skiers worldwide participate in this enticing winter pastime on both a recreational and competitive level. This chapter discusses the applied physiology of competitive skiing, including the events, the physiologic demands, a profile of the competitive skier, and current concepts for training.

THE SPORT

Alpine skiing events are contested annually on the World Cup circuit and every 4 years as part of the Olympic Winter Games. The rules and regulations for international competition are under the jurisdiction of the Federation Internationale de Ski (FIS) and can be found in a handbook that is updated periodically (3). In the United States, the U.S. Ski Association (USSA) is the major governing body for ski racing.

Competitive alpine skiing consists of four events: slalom, giant slalom, super giant slalom, and downhill. Because downhill is the name of a specific discipline, alpine skiing is the preferred terminology when referring to the sport in general. The events differ in terms of vertical drop from start to finish, radius of and distance between turns, terrain, and speed. The standards for each event also differ according to gender and age classifications (Table 44–1).

Age group competition is popular, but categories are not standardized worldwide. The FIS distinguishes five general categories, while in the United States there are typically many more divisions for youth and masters competitors (Table 44–2).

In competition, skiers follow a course down the slope marked with gates (poles with colored flags or panels) that they must pass through. The gates are set to dictate the types of turns specified by the particular event and to help control speed, and should incorporate the natural flow of the terrain. The time it takes to negotiate the course correctly determines the order of finish.

Slalom is the shortest event, lasting 45 to 60 seconds. It is distinguished by short radius turns with emphasis on quickness and precision, with rapid completion of all turns. The terrain can be steep (a 33- to 45-degree slope is required for Olympic and FIS championships), but speed is controlled and usually does not exceed 30 mph. The course should be a "clever composition" of turns suited to the terrain, with gates set both down and across the fall line (3). The fall line is the path a free-rolling ball would most likely follow down the slope. The total time is combined from two runs on different courses, set on the same slope.

Giant slalom is characterized by mostly medium ra-

R. A. Hintermeister: Avon, Colorado 81620.
G. R. Hagerman: Topper Sportsmedicine, Edwards, Colorado 81632.

TABLE 44–1. *Course characteristics for Alpine skiing events*

Event	Men	Women	Children I	Children II	Gate spacing (m)
Slalom					$0.75 \leq d \leq 15$
Vertical drop (m)	140–220	120–200	140	180	
No. of gates	55–75	45–60	32–45	38–60	
Giant slalom					$d \geq 10$
Vertical drop (m)	250–400	250–350	300	350	
No. of gates	— 12%–15% of VD (m) —		— 15% of VD (m) ± 3 —		
Super G					$d \geq 25$
Vertical drop (m)	500–650	350–600	250–350	280–400	$d \geq 15$ with combinations
Max. no. of gates	— 10% of VD (m) —				
Min. no. of gates	35	30	25	28	
Downhill					Not specified
Vertical drop (m)	800–1100	500–800	—	400	

d, distance in meters; VD, vertical drop in meters.

dius turns with some variety. The course typically lasts 60 to 75 seconds and covers undulating terrain that utilizes the width of the slope. The number of gates ranges from 12% to 15% of the vertical drop in meters, so 60 gates would be the maximum for men. Speeds usually do not exceed 45 mph. Giant slalom is also a two-run, combined-time event.

Super giant slalom, or super G as it is known, was added as an FIS event in 1983, and as an Olympic event for the 1988 Calgary Games. Super G is a hybrid of giant slalom and downhill, consisting of a variety of long- and medium-radius turns, with some gates set out of the fall line. The course lasts 75 to 90 seconds, with speeds reaching up to 60 mph, and is contested in one run. The maximum number of gates is equal to 10% of the vertical drop, with a minimum of 35 for men and 30 for women.

The downhill is perhaps the most glamorous of the alpine disciplines. According to the FIS, it consists of five components: technique, courage, speed, risk, and condition. It is distinguished by fast speeds (up to 90 mph), large radius turns mostly in the fall line, and a variety of terrain changes such as steeps, flats, jumps, and compressions. The downhill is the longest one-run event, lasting 90 to 140 seconds. Three days of training and timed trials are scheduled and are compulsory for competitors at the international level. At least 2 days of training are required if inclement weather disrupts the schedule.

THE DEMANDS OF SKIING

The demands of any sport are a result of the participants' attempting to deal with the forces acting on them while trying to accomplish the specified task. Fundamentally, alpine skiing requires maintaining balance while sliding down a snow-covered slope on skis, and turning to change direction and control speed. The competitive skier must accomplish this while negotiating a race course as fast as possible. More precisely, therefore, the goal of the competitive skier is to minimize friction and deceleration while skiing the fastest line within his or her physical capabilities.

Forces Acting on the Skier

The main forces that act on a skier are gravity, friction, wind, and centrifugal force (4,5). Gravity is constant

TABLE 44–2. *FIS* and United States age group classifications for competition*

FIS		U.S.	
Category	Age (y)	Category	Age (y)
Children I	12–13	J5	10 and younger
Children II	14–15	J4	11–12
Juniors	16–19	J3	13–14
Licensed competitors	16 and older	J2	15–16
Masters		J1	17–19
Masters A	Men 30–54	Seeded competition	20 and older
Masters B	Men 55 and older	Masters	Varies with region
Masters C	Women 30 and older		

*FIS, International Skiing Federation.

and pulls all objects toward the center of the earth. The steepness of a slope determines the component of gravitational force that accelerates the skier downhill. Friction between the skis and snow, and wind resistance also influence the skiers speed or velocity. Centrifugal force acts on the skier when turning and pulls the skier away from the center of the turn. The skier counteracts this force with angulation and muscular effort mainly from the legs.

Centrifugal force (F_c) is directly proportional to the skiers mass (m) and velocity squared (v^2), and inversely proportional to the turn radius (r):

$$F_c = \frac{m * v^2}{r}$$

Centrifugal force is therefore greater for heavier skiers, and it increases as the skier goes faster and the turn radius gets smaller. For example, an 80-kg skier traveling at 20.31 m/s (45 mph) with a turn radius of 15 m would have to resist 2200 N of centrifugal force. Indeed, Nachbauer and Rauch (6) have measured reaction forces between the boot and ski as large as 2717 N (610 lbs) during slalom skiing. Forces of this magnitude clearly demonstrate why good skeletal alignment and considerable leg strength are important for competitive alpine skiing.

Motor Control

The demands of skiing also require precise motor control for balance and application of pressure to the ski at fast speeds. The dynamic aspects of balance that a skier must master include lateral movements that primarily affect edging and weight transfer, and fore-aft movements that modify pressure distribution over the ski. Lateral movements start with subtle adjustments of the foot and ankle, and are magnified by knee and hip angulation and total body inclination. Fore-aft adjustments are typically accomplished through flexion and extension of the ankles, knees, and hips. Movements in both planes serve to edge the ski and hold a turn. All of these movements are initiated from a basic symmetrical stance and must be implemented over a wide range of speeds, varying terrain, and snow conditions.

Muscle Activity and Movement Patterns

Studying muscle activity patterns can also help us understand the demands of any sport. Muscle contraction is a biochemical event, caused by depolarization of the muscle, and can be measured with electrodes. Such electromyographic (EMG) recordings can provide valuable information about the amplitude, duration, and timing of muscle contractions, and with qualitative and quantitative movement analysis can help us understand the resulting motion.

Skiing consists of a series of turns with a transition between each. The ski turn has been partitioned into various phases based on visual analysis (7–9) and from force data (6). Phases based on force patterns are probably the most meaningful. A fundamental working definition simply includes the more static turning phase and the highly dynamic transition phase.

Results of muscle activity experiments in competitive skiers (8–12) include coactivation of the quadriceps and hamstring muscles at levels that exceed maximal voluntary isometric contractions (MVCs). Muscle activity greater than MVC is possible due to the inherent momentum of the skier. High levels of coactivation occur in the turning phase, typically peaking after the skier passes the fall line. This coincides with the portion of the turn where the external forces on the skier are greatest. Centrifugal force and the component of gravity accelerating the skier are both acting in the same direction—down the hill (4). Substantial EMG activity indicates that the leg muscles are resisting large forces, and equal coactivation suggests that it is being accomplished by stabilizing the hip, knee, and ankle with opposing muscle groups and little movement.

Although speeds in alpine skiing can reach upward of 60 miles per hour, hip and knee angular velocities are rather slow, 20 to 40 degrees per second (9,10), in comparison to sport activities such as baseball pitching where angular velocities of 6000 degrees per second have been reported for internal rotation of the shoulder (13). This evidence helps substantiate the stabilizing function of the lower extremity musculature and suggests a quasi-static component to skiing. This is most evident in the turning phase, as the skier utilizes eccentric, isometric, and concentric muscle actions to resist gravity and centrifugal force and to fight for the best line.

In general, flexion of the legs under load (eccentric muscle action) allows the skier to angulate and get the appropriate edge angle for the turn, and absorb variations in the terrain. Concentric muscle actions enable the skier to extend the legs and resist (isometric muscle action) the increasing forces with a greater contribution from skeletal support (12). The undulating patterns of knee angle recordings (9) and coactivation of the knee musculature suggest that rapid alternating bursts of all three muscle actions occur throughout the turn as the skier resists centrifugal force and negotiates the irregularities of, and vibrations from, the terrain.

In addition to balance, speed of movement, and the forces that accompany turning, duration of the events plays an important role in determining the overall physiologic demands of skiing. Because alpine skiing events range in duration from 45 to 140 seconds and take place over a variety of terrain, the metabolic demands for movement are similarly mixed, requiring significant contributions from aerobic and anaerobic sources. These and other physiologic factors that result from the demands of competitive skiing are considered in the next section.

PHYSIOLOGIC REQUIREMENTS OF SKIING

From a physiologic perspective, the relative involvement of the metabolic systems that provide energy for alpine skiing are of primary interest. The anaerobic and aerobic energy pathways work simultaneously, providing energy in proportion to the demands of exercise. Flexibility is also important for functional proficiency over an adequate range of motion.

Anaerobic Capacity

Competitive alpine skiing is considered more anaerobic than aerobic (14–18), with increasing contributions of aerobic metabolism to the total energy demand as the event duration gets longer. Events typically last from 45 seconds to less than $2\frac{1}{2}$ minutes, so anaerobic energy sources provide a substantial amount of the total energy utilized.

The enhanced leg strength required to resist large forces at relatively slow angular velocities of joint motion can be evaluated in terms of maximal force and power, with an endurance component as the duration of activity increases. Maximal force is important for resisting the large centrifugal forces that occur when turning at fast speeds or with small radius turns. Maximal force is more standardized when measured isometrically at a specific joint angle or dynamically at a specific speed of movement. Power is defined as force times velocity, and is maximized in situations where large forces are applied with fast speeds of movement. Muscular endurance, the ability to maintain a certain level of muscle force for repeated contractions over time, is important not only for a series of turns or over the course of a day, but also for endurance over a whole season.

Maximal Force

Not surprisingly, elite skiers demonstrate enhanced quadriceps strength. Thorstensson and colleagues (19) reported that elite Swedish male alpine skiers had the greatest peak torque [3.9 Newton meters (Nm)/kg] for isometric leg extension compared with track sprinters and jumpers (3.8 Nm/kg), race walkers (3.4 Nm/kg), sedentary men (3.2 Nm/kg), and orienteers (3.1 Nm/kg). At angular velocities of 180 degrees per second, however, the track athletes produced significantly greater mean peak torque (2.7 Nm/kg) compared to the skiers (2.3 Nm/kg). The authors attributed this difference to the specific adaptation of the skiers to the large static forces in skiing.

Karlsson and colleagues (10) reported that male (2874 N) and female (1844 N) elite Swedish skiers had notable isometric strength in leg press (knee angle = 90 degrees), the males exceeding the strength of most other sportsmen, including volleyball players and sprinters. They also reported a correlation of $r = 0.86$ between static and dynamic leg strength in the elite skiers, and suggested that training dynamic muscle strength favorably influences static strength. The authors characterized skiing as "relatively slow dynamic muscle work with static components in the loading phase" and more dynamic actions necessary for correcting movements.

Haymes and Dickinson (20) compared knee extensor strength isometrically (included knee angle = 115 degrees) and isokinetically (at 30 and 180 degrees/s) in alpine, cross-country, and nordic combined U.S. Ski Team members. Within gender, isometric leg strength was greatest in male (3078 N) and female (2194 N) alpine skiers. Knee extensor torque at 30 degrees/s, scaled for body weight, was significantly greater for male (3.53 Nm/kg) versus female (3.23 Nm/kg) alpine skiers.

Brown and Wilkinson (21) evaluated isokinetic leg extension and flexion strength in 42 Canadian national, regional, and club skiers. The national skiers had similar torque (3.98 Nm/kg) to regional skiers (3.88 Nm/kg) and significantly greater torque than club skiers (3.44 Nm/kg) at 30 degrees per second. All three groups were similar at 180 degrees per second. National skiers also had a smaller hamstring-to-quadriceps torque ratio that was due to significantly greater quadriceps strength. The authors concluded that alpine ski racers typically have superior slow concentric knee extension strength and emphasized its importance in skiing.

The significance of eccentric muscle actions in alpine skiing has been emphasized by several authors (2,9,16,18,22). Abe and colleagues (23) compared eccentric, isometric (included knee angle = 100 degrees), and concentric leg extension and flexion strength in nine elite and 10 collegiate female skiers. Absolute eccentric extensor (234 vs. 201 Nm) and flexor (115 vs. 100 Nm) torque was significantly greater for the elite group. Extensor torque, scaled for body mass, was also greater for the elite group (3.77 vs. 3.31 Nm/kg). There were no differences in isometric or concentric measures. The authors suggested that eccentric muscle strength was more predictive than other muscle actions in the performance of alpine ski racers.

Power

Tests of power that have been used to evaluate skiers are the vertical jump, 60-second repeated jump, the Margaria-Kalamen stair run, and the Wingate cycle ergometer test. The duration of the test reflects the energy systems that are utilized. The vertical jump and the Margaria-Kalamen stair run typically require less than a second and rely on creatine phosphate stores, whereas the repeated jumps and Wingate tests require 30 to 90 seconds and rely on creatine phosphate and glycolysis for muscle contraction. These tests of longer duration are more frequently referred to as tests of anaerobic power to differentiate them from tests of instantaneous power.

Vertical Jump

The vertical jump tests instantaneous power of the lower extremity. Karlsson and colleagues (10) reported average vertical jump heights of 66 cm for male and 50 cm for female elite skiers and noted that these values did not change appreciably over several seasons despite increases in static strength. These authors noted that volleyball and basketball players and sprinters and jumpers in track and field had better jumping ability and greater dynamic strength than skiers. The faster movement speeds required in these sports and utilization of the calf musculature were given as explanations of specific adaptations that result in greater jumping ability.

The vertical jump has also been used with moderate success to differentiate skier ability. Haymes and Dickinson (20) detected a significant correlation ($r = 0.64$) between FIS giant slalom points and vertical jump (60.5 cm) for 12 male U.S. Team skiers. Andersen and colleagues (24) reported a significant correlation between giant slalom time and vertical jump height ($r = -0.57$). Brown and Wilkinson (21) and Andersen and colleagues (24) compared Canadian national/provincial, divisional, and club skiers and reported similar results. National/provincial skiers jumped significantly higher than club skiers, but they were not different from divisional skiers. White and Johnson (25) reported that absolute power from the vertical jump was the second best predictor of international, national, or regional group competitive status in 61 skiers.

Margaria-Kalamen Stair Run

The Margaria-Kalamen stair run was used by Haymes and Dickinson (20) to evaluate power in alpine skiers. Men had significantly greater power than women. For men, power correlated significantly with FIS slalom ($r = 0.64$) and giant slalom ($r = 0.80$) points.

Repeated Vertical Jumps

White and Johnson (25) also reported that the average work from a 60-second repeated vertical jump test was the best discriminator of skier ranking for men and women. Bosco and colleagues (15) reported a significant 17.5% improvement in mechanical power over a 4-month period for a 30-second repeated vertical jump test. Preparatory training for the 12 internationally ranked male Italian skiers consisted of squat and leg press exercises in addition to specific speed endurance bouncing and jumping exercises.

Wingate Test

The Wingate test has been used to evaluate average and peak power and anaerobic endurance, and as a fatigue index in skiers. Song (26) used a 30-second Wingate test with 5.5 kpm resistance to test nine junior racers. He reported a significant correlation of -0.63 between anaerobic power and downhill performance but no correlation with giant slalom performance. Andersen and colleagues (24) used a 60-second Wingate test with 75 grams/kg of resistance and reported a significant correlation of -0.73 between absolute mean power and giant slalom race times in Canadian club, divisional and provincial skiers. White and Johnson (25) used a 30-second Wingate test with 75 grams/kg of resistance and reported that the third best discriminator of skier ranking for men was anaerobic endurance and for women it was relative average power. The international caliber skiers were significantly better than national and regional skiers.

Stark and colleagues (27) compared slalom and downhill skiers in a 90-second Wingate test. The slalom skiers had greater peak power and a faster rate of fatigue than the downhill skiers, who had better average power over the 90 seconds. The mean power of the slalom skiers fell below that of the downhillers about 40 seconds into the test, leading the authors to recommend a 90-second Wingate test for skiers.

Bacharach and Duvillard (17) compared 30- and 90-second Wingate tests with 75 g/kg of resistance in 18 racers. Minimum power and a fatigue index were significantly correlated with racing points in the women for both the 30- and 90-second tests, and for the men in just the 90-second test. Additionally, mean power was also correlated with the 90-second test for the men. The authors also concluded that the 90-second Wingate test was better than the 30-second test for alpine skiers.

Duvillard and Knowles (28) varied the length and resistance of Wingate tests in junior male ($n = 12$) and female ($n = 14$) racers. Duration ranged from 30 to 120 seconds and resistance ranged from 0.05 to 0.09 kg/kg. The 60-, 90-, and 120-second tests at 75, 50, and 50 g/kg, respectively, provided the best correlations between variables of power output and body composition. Absolute power output measures accounted for less than 25% of the variance in USSA points for the four alpine disciplines.

Anaerobic Endurance

In addition to the longer Wingate tests, only a few strength tests with an endurance component have been used to evaluate skiers. Karlsson and colleagues (10) tested isometric endurance in elite Swedish skiers by having them maintain 50% of their maximal isometric strength for as long as possible during a leg press with a 90-degree knee angle. Overall, times for the men (92.5 seconds) were not different from those for the women (89.3 seconds). Subjects with great maximal strength had shorter endurance times than subjects with less maximal strength, however.

Haymes and Dickinson (20) measured the number of rapid isokinetic leg extensions U.S. Ski Team members could perform in several seconds before the torque fell below 50% of the initial value. There was no difference in the number of contractions—37—performed by men and women. There were significant correlations between 50% peak torque decrement and FIS points in slalom for men ($r = -0.80$) and women ($r = -0.78$), and for men ($r = -0.75$) in giant slalom.

Muscle and Blood Lactate

Muscle and blood lactate are important indicators of anaerobic metabolism that have been used to evaluate the contribution of anaerobic energy sources to the total energy cost of skiing. Anaerobic metabolism and lactate production may be enhanced during skiing due to occlusion of blood flow, which occurs with static muscle contractions exceeding 30% to 50% MVC (29). This is more likely in less skilled skiers who have more static muscle activity patterns than skilled skiers (2,10,11). Lactate concentrations in the blood of greater than 2 to 4 mM/L indicate an active contribution to total energy demand from anaerobic sources. In trained athletes, lactic acid concentration can exceed 20 mM/L in the blood and 30 mM/kg (wet weight) in the muscle during maximal exercise (30). Methodologically, fingertip blood samples are typically obtained 5 minutes postexercise to measure peak plasma lactate. Only a few investigators have employed the muscle biopsy technique to measure lactate accumulation in the muscle during skiing (10,14).

Tesch and Larsson (14) took biopsies of the vastus lateralis in five male skiers after 1 minute of maximal slalom skiing and reported a mean muscle lactate of 13 mmol/kg (wet weight), ranging from 9 to 24 mmol/kg (wet weight). Interindividual differences were large, but individual responses were similar for the two trials. Muscle lactate concentration and the percentage of fast-twitch fibers were highly correlated ($r = 0.99$) in this small sample. Blood lactates were also assessed and ranged from 6 to 13 mmol/L in skilled skiers during giant slalom interval training.

Karlsson and colleagues (10) measured blood lactate in competitive skiers during racing and training. Values ranged from 8 to 16 mmol/L in 20 men (mean = 13.0) and 13 women (mean = 10.1) participating in a giant slalom race. There was no correlation between lactate concentration and order of finish. During training, mean lactate concentration for three skiers was 8.5 mmol/L in slalom and 7.5 mmol/L in giant slalom. In another study, the lactic acid values were higher in all four skiers in timed slalom runs (11.6 mmol/L) versus untimed runs (10.0 mmol/L). The authors emphasized the use of timed training runs, especially as the competitive season nears.

Veicsteinas and colleagues (31) tested eight top-ranked male skiers; six performed slalom and five performed giant slalom. Mean blood lactate was 12.4 mmol/L after a 70-second giant slalom and 11.7 mmol/L after a 55-second slalom. A control group of five less skilled skiers had blood lactate levels of 8.8 mmol/L after a 78-second giant slalom. The authors calculated that lactate production accounted for 40% of the total energy cost of skiing. In another experiment, total energy expenditure was 23% greater in slalom versus giant slalom for a course of the same duration. Lactate accumulation for the 50-second course was 14 mmol/L in slalom and 10 mmol/L in giant slalom.

Saibene and colleagues (32) measured blood lactate in eight national-level skiers during a simulated giant slalom competition. Mean blood lactate was 6.8 ± 0.9 mmol/L after the 82-second giant slalom. The authors calculated that lactate production accounted for 25.3% of the total energy cost of skiing.

Richardson and colleagues (33) measured blood lactate in five female U.S. Ski Team members. Lactate samples were taken 1 minute postexercise following three consecutive downhill training runs lasting an average of $1\frac{1}{2}$ minutes each. Lactate increased significantly from the first to second run and averaged 6.0 ± 1.7 mmol/L. The authors suggested that active recovery between runs would facilitate lactate removal and increase the quality of training.

Measurements of blood lactate following strenuous exercise tests in the laboratory have also been used to evaluate the anaerobic capacity of skiers. In running tests to measure oxygen consumption ($\dot{V}O_2$) on the treadmill, Karlsson and colleagues (10), reported mean lactates of 15.5 mmol/L in male and 13.9 mmol/L in female ski racers. A maximal treadmill run to exhaustion did not differentiate between 10 Canadian National (12.0 mmol/L) and seven club (12.4 mmol/L) male ski racers (21). However, in tests that are more anaerobic—a 60-second Wingate test and a 90-second high box jumping test—provincial skiers accumulated significantly more lactate (~19 mmol/L) than either divisional (~14 mmol/L) or club (~11 mmol/L) racers (24). Lactate measures from the shorter anaerobic tests seem more relevant to the requirements of skiing than the $\dot{V}O_2max$ tests.

Aerobic Capacity

Aerobic capacity regulates exercises that rely upon the assimilation of oxygen to produce adenosine triphosphate (ATP). These are primarily endurance exercises of low-intensity muscle contraction and long duration, or many repetitions. Running and biking at moderate exertion are primarily aerobic, and so are resistance exercises done with light loads and many repetitions.

The relative importance of aerobic capacity to skiing performance has been the subject of varying opinion over the years (2,10,15,16,18,22,26,34–36). Initial emphasis on the importance of aerobic capacity to competitive skiers can be traced to the impressive test results of the Swedish National Team in the mid-1970s. The average oxygen consumption for nine males was 68 mL/kg and 53 mL/kg for seven females. Even more noteworthy, however, is the fact that the dominant skier on the World Cup at the time, Ingemar Stenmark, had the highest $\dot{V}O_2max$ (71 mL/kg) ever reported in a skier (10). For many, the perception that aerobic capacity was correlated to performance was easy to justify in light of Stenmark's dominance.

Evidence that aerobic capacity is related to skiing performance, however, is slight and the results are mixed. Several authors have reported moderate correlations with performance (20,26), while others have concluded that aerobic capacity does not differentiate between skiers of varying ability (21,25).

Treadmill running tests of aerobic capacity on National Team skiers have resulted in average values ranging from 52.7 to 68 mL/kg for males and 53.1 mL/kg for females (10,20,31,34,37). These results demonstrate the intermediate capabilities of alpine skiers in comparison to athletes at the extremes of the aerobic continuum, such as cross-country skiers or sprinters (80 to 55 mL/kg for males). Although the value for alpine skiers is quite respectable, it indicates that aerobic capacity is less important than for endurance events (16).

Several investigators have actually measured oxygen consumption during skiing using the Douglas-bag technique to collect expired air. Swedish researchers measured $\dot{V}O_2$ in three male racers during the latter half of an 85-second giant slalom and reported values ranging from 75% to 100% of maximal (10,11). The average of several runs for the skiers was equivalent to 88% of their $\dot{V}O_2max$ measured during treadmill running. In the last run, when the skiers went all out, $\dot{V}O_2$ averaged 95% of maximal.

Two Italian groups have examined the total energy cost of skiing using oxygen consumption in addition to the blood lactate assessments mentioned previously (31,32). Oxygen consumption measured during exercise and recovery was added to an oxygen equivalent for blood lactate [3.2 mL O_2/kg of body weight (38)] to estimate the total energy cost. In the slalom and giant slalom racers studied by Veicsteinas and colleagues (31), the overall aerobic contribution to energy metabolism was approximately 30% to 35%. In slalom, the racers utilized 64% of $\dot{V}O_2max$ compared to 54% in giant slalom. In another experiment, total energy expenditure was 23% greater in slalom versus giant slalom when the duration of both courses was similar (50 seconds).

In the simulated giant slalom competition staged by Saibene and colleagues (32), oxygen consumption from exercise, recovery, and the lactate equivalent averaged 89.4 mL/kg, corresponding to 120% of the mean oxygen consumption. Aerobic energy sources accounted for 46.4% of the total energy cost. While skiing, the racers utilized 82% of their $\dot{V}O_2max$, also measured during treadmill running. The authors suggested that alpine skiers would be better served by concentrating on strength and neuromuscular coordination rather than aerobic conditioning.

Although aerobic capacity was at one time touted as an essential factor in top-level alpine skiing (10), it has received less attention since the mid-1980s. It has been suggested that the higher aerobic capacities reported for some competitive alpine skiers might really represent training adaptations rather than the actual demands of the sport (2). The relatively high percentage of oxygen utilization measured during skiing does promote the benefits of some endurance training, however. Good aerobic fitness does provide an essential base for the demands of skiing, which often includes training and competing in hypoxic conditions at altitude. Improvements in aerobic capacity also provide potential for further increases in the absolute lactate threshold with anaerobic training. Improved aerobic conditioning may also provide some protection against fatigue-related injury. As a single parameter, however, aerobic capacity is an unlikely determinant of success in competitive alpine skiing (18).

Heart Rate

During endurance exercise the heart rate accurately reflects the rate of oxygen delivery. Since competitive skiing is predominantly anaerobic, however, the high heart rate only confirms that large forces are involved (16). Heart rates in the range of 130 to 160 bpm have been monitored in ski racers in the starting gate and are most likely due to anticipation, anxiety, and psychologic stress (10,16). Several investigators have measured heart rate (HR) during skiing and reported rates of 180 to 190 bpm, or approximately 95% of maximal, at the end of giant slalom (10,31) and downhill training runs (33). These values are somewhat higher than the 141 to 143 bpm (85% HRmax) mean reported for a group of 51-year-old men during 6 days of recreational skiing at altitude (39).

Fiber Type and Glycogen Utilization

In sports that depend mainly on the utilization of either aerobic or anaerobic energy, the fiber-type composition of skeletal muscle can be an important factor for success. Elite athletes in endurance sports such as long-distance running and nordic skiing have muscles containing predominantly slow-twitch fibers, while sprinters and weightlifters have a large percentage of fast-twitch fibers (40). For the majority of sports that fall between these extremes, the muscular profile of participants is widely variable.

Alpine skiers, who rely on great technical skill and a combination of aerobic and anaerobic energy sources, are no exception and do not have a distinct fiber-type profile. Most fiber-type assessments in the skiing literature date back to the late 1970s and consist of biopsies of the vastus lateralis and small sample sizes. The mean slow-twitch fiber percentage reported in these studies ranges from 47% to 63%, with considerable variability, and it does not differ from aged-matched physically active individuals (10,14,19,37,41).

In conjunction with muscle biopsies, Tesch and Larsson (14) and Karlsson and colleagues (10) reported on the pattern of glycogen depletion observed during skiing. In a group of five skilled skiers, muscle glycogen levels dropped by an average of 32 mmol/kg (wet muscle) over 2 days of training, 34 mmol in the first day of giant slalom training, and 21 mmol after the second day of slalom training. The unskilled skiers had greater depletion in the fast-twitch fibers compared to the skilled skiers, who seemed to rely more on the slow-twitch fibers.

In terms of appropriate nutrition, glycogen depletion should not be a problem in competitive skiers due to the short duration of the events (18). Both competitive and recreational skiers would be well advised to eat meals high in carbohydrate content following strenuous training or skiing, however. This maximizes the replenishment of muscle glycogen and may delay muscle fatigue in subsequent days of skiing.

Flexibility

Flexibility is important for obtaining adequate joint range of motion and enables an athlete to assume functional positions without undue strain on tendons, ligaments, and joints. Good flexibility may also enhance optimal alignment, sparing muscular effort with bone-on-bone forces. In alpine skiing, sufficient hip extension in the turn, while keeping the trunk countered, is such an example. In fact, Song (26) reported that in tests of shoulder, trunk, hip, knee, and ankle flexibility in nine male junior skiers, only hip flexibility was greater than for age-matched controls. Good flexibility may also provide some protection from injury in situations where the range of motion exceeds normal joint tolerances.

The demands of skiing require large forces to be generated and absorbed by the legs and trunk. Therefore, flexibility and muscular balance of the prime movers surrounding the knee, hip, and trunk are a priority for the ski racer. Key muscles include the quadriceps, hamstrings, hip flexors and extensors, abdominals, obliques, and erector spinae. With the rotational requirements of skiing, support of the spine through balanced strengthening and flexibility of the pelvic region is critical for optimal function and injury prevention (42).

THE ATHLETE

Several authors have compiled information about the physical characteristics of alpine skiers, including age, height, mass, and percent body fat (34,43). Kornexl (44,45), who studied the 15 best alpine ski racers over 11 years, concluded that downhillers tend to be heavier (77 to 78 kg) than slalom or giant slalom skiers (69 kg). Karlsson (2) noted that alpine skiers had traditionally been of average height and mass, but the successful alpine skier had gotten taller and heavier. This statement was based on anthropometric data collected in 1965 and 1975 by Eriksson and colleagues (46). The average height and mass of male Swedish Ski Team members had increased from 168 to 178 cm and 64 to 76 kg. It has been suggested that elite performance in many sports is related to height and mass since both features are related to endurance and strength (30). It has also been suggested that the increased size of today's alpine skiers is related to the use of breakaway poles and changing technique (36).

More recent studies suggest that the trend in increasing mass has continued, with eight Swedish Ski Team males averaging 81 kg (9) and five female members of the U.S. Ski Team averaging 66.1 kg (33). The ranges of average age, height, mass, and percent body fat of competitive alpine skiers listed in Table 44–3 are expanded from those compiled by Andersen and Montgomery (34) to include information from Eriksson and colleagues (46), Orvanová (43), White and Johnson (25), Richardson and colleagues (33), Bosco and colleagues (15), Berg and colleagues (9), and Duvillard and Knowles (28).

A few authors have identified moderate correlations between anthropometric variables and performance. Haymes and Dickinson (20) reported that smaller and leaner U.S. skiers were better in slalom, and those with a greater percent body fat were better in downhill. Percent body fat ($r = 0.78$), mass ($r = 0.76$), and lean body weight ($r = 0.64$) correlated significantly with FIS slalom points in males. Percent body fat was correlated with

TABLE 44–3. *Physical characteristics of competitive Alpine skiers*

	Male	Female
Age (y)	15.7–24.1	16.6–21.8
Height (cm)	168–180	159–169
Mass (kg)	64–81	56.7–66.1
Body Fat (%)	6.1–11.0	13.1–23.8

FIS downhill points for males ($r = -0.67$) and females ($r = -0.74$). Song (26) reported that lower leg length was correlated with downhill performance ($r = 0.72$) in nine junior male racers. Unfortunately, these relationships do not seem to be consistent across different studies over the years.

Differences in mass and body composition have also been identified between racers of varying ability. Nationally ranked male Canadian racers had significantly greater mass than divisional or club racers (21), and international male U.S. racers had significantly greater mass than regional racers (25). Fat-free mass was significantly greater for U.S. International males than either national or regional level racers, whereas for females international and national racers had more fat-free mass than regional racers. The trend of increasing body mass is related to physical maturation, however, since significant increases in average age for the different performance categories existed in both studies. The trend of increasing fat-free mass is probably more meaningful, since it relates to the strength and power demands of skiing.

Gender Differences

If an athlete has adequate strength to withstand the forces encountered in skiing, further gains in body mass, for the sake of increasing lean mass, may have diminishing returns on performance. Increases in mass require increased energy expenditure for movement and may reduce quickness. The appropriate body composition for each athlete may be evaluated objectively by tracking performance both on and off snow, and subjectively by how the athlete feels.

Anatomic and physiologic differences between the sexes do exist and can influence skiing (47). However, individual variability is often greater than specific gender characteristics, so it is difficult to generalize. On average, the main anatomic differences are a lower center of mass (CoM), a wider pelvis resulting in a greater "Q" angle at the knee, and shorter bone lengths for women versus men. The difference in CoM is less than 1% in the college-aged population, 56.2% of standing height for males versus 55.4% for females (48). Twardokens (7) has estimated that the addition of skis, boots, and bindings further lowers the CoM in skiers by about 10%, rendering the 1% difference in CoM between the sexes of questionable practical significance. In addition to individual differences, the anatomic variations that result from a wider pelvis and increased Q angle may dramatically influence medial-lateral and fore-aft alignment issues, the proper fitting of equipment, and individual strength requirements necessary to compensate for deviations in optimal alignment.

Physiologically, strength and body composition are the main differences between the sexes. In terms of absolute strength, women are about 66% as strong as men (49). Most of this disparity is a result of less muscle mass, with the greatest differences stemming from upper body development. The average female also has a greater percentage of fat (27%) than the average male (15%). The discrepancy is primarily attributable to more essential fat in the female that is necessary for reproduction (49).

TRAINING THE ATHLETE

The Season

The FIS competitive alpine ski racing calendar starts on July 1st and finishes the following June 30th. In the Northern Hemisphere, the competitive season typically lasts 5 months, from November 15th through April 15th. Recently, the World Cup schedule has started in the western United States in November and is completed by mid-March, but many national and regional championships take place through April.

The number of races that a competitive skier chooses to participate in is highly individual and varies by age. Recommended guidelines for competition starts, issued by the U.S. Ski Coaches Association, are listed in Table 44–4.

Sports-Specific Training

Four general components—aerobic capacity, anaerobic capacity, movement skills, and flexibility—encompass most aspects of physical training for alpine skiing. Emphasis is mainly on the lower extremities and trunk, with the chest, upper back, and arms being secondary. This section deals with on- and off-snow training activities that are specific to skiing.

On Snow

Movement skills and anaerobic capacity are two of the four general components of alpine skiing that benefit the most from on-snow training. Increases in aerobic capacity require 20 minutes or more of continuous light-to moderate-intensity exercise. Although long uninterrupted ski runs are helpful, they rarely exceed 5 to 10 minutes and do not provide adequate aerobic training stimulus. Flexibility exercises can certainly be done in ski boots and skis on snow, but they are probably best suited to a warm, relaxing indoor environment.

Technical proficiency and choice of line are perhaps the most influential factors for skiing performance and benefit the most from on-snow training. The acquisition and implementation of movement skills by the skier is the domain of the coach. There are numerous technical and gate drills for improving skiing technique and choosing an appropriate line (7,50–54).

TABLE 44–4. *Number of recommended starts by skier's age and skiing event*

Age	10	11–12	13–14	15–16	17–18	19–20	≥21
Level/Focus	Club/YSL	Club/YSL Division	Divisional/ Regional	Divisional/ Regional/ National/Int.	Regional/ National/ International	National/ International	International
GS	1–3	3–5	4–8	7–10	9–12	7–14	personal
SL	1–2	1–3	2–5	3–6	6–9	4–12	personal
SG	0	0–2	2–4	3–6	6–9	4–12	personal
DH	0	0	0–2	2	2–6	2–9	
Total	2–5	4–10	8–19	15–24	20–30	25–35	personal

Starts do not include race simulation starts or competitions used as race simulation. In the 19- to 20-year-old age group, there is a wide range due to specialization.

GS, giant slalom; SL, slalom; SG, Super G; DH, downhill.

From ref. 78, with permission.

Quality training of specific movement skills with repetition in variable and adverse conditions is critical to solidify fundamentals and to build a repertoire of effective movement patterns. The coach must also be cognizant of individual anatomic and specific equipment characteristics that influence the proper execution of technique (55–57). Constant testing and timing must be a part of training, so changes in technique and equipment may be objectively evaluated. From a physiologic perspective, attention to proper movement training and equipment adjustments should result in reduced energy expenditure. The skier becomes more efficient, resistant to fatigue, and can attack the second half of the course with ample energy.

Free skiing with emphasis on balance, fundamental movement patterns, and basic racing technique is a good way to start on-snow training. Ski racing requires extraordinary one-footed balance with the ability to ski on both edges of each ski. Drills for balance include skiing on one ski, both inside and outside edges, skiing without poles, with one pole, in bumps, over jumps, and in obstacle courses. Skiing fast in bumps, flush drills, rhythm changes, and practicing starts are all good for quickness and coordination.

A general progression from free skiing to giant slalom, which provides the technical basis for all the alpine disciplines, is characteristic. Emphasis is on choosing the fastest line, effective movement patterns in the transition, and turning phases and independent foot action, in all kinds of conditions. Over- and underlength courses may be utilized with various gate combinations and rhythm changes.

At this time, the athlete should also become familiar with a prescribed level of effort. The athlete should know what is required for a certain level of performance. What kind of effort and risks are necessary to ski all out versus 90% or 95% of ability? This is a relative and dynamic scale. As the athlete improves, the scale is reset to reflect new capabilities. Training such keen self-awareness will pay off in gauging how to ski each new course with confidence.

Mastery of giant slalom technique provides the fundamentals for slalom, super G, and downhill. Slalom training incorporates perhaps the widest variety of turns and combinations, and like all the disciplines, utilizes gates and the terrain to emphasize specific tactical and technical proficiencies. Progression from shorter to longer courses in training is typical.

Super G and downhill athletes also spend a good deal of time training a variety of turns and working in varied terrain such as compressions and jumps and fall-away and banked turns. Aerodynamics and gliding are critical to the speed events, so time is spent practicing various body positions to best negotiate flats, steeps, and jumps. Experimenting with and evaluation of various lines is critical, as well as letting the skis run to maximize speed. As training progresses, timed runs under competitive conditions are routine for all the disciplines.

Off Snow

Since most skiers do not have access to snow on a year-round basis, conditioning for skiing requires participation in other activities. Cross-training can improve performance with exercises that imitate the movement patterns of skiing—the principle of specificity. There are many innovative types of dry-land training that can mirror on-snow movement patterns.

Motocross, mountain biking, in-line skating, ice skating, water skiing, jet skiing, and horseback riding are activities with skill components similar to skiing (58). All these activities demand dynamic balance starting from a symmetrical stance, lateral movements with weight transfer, and flexion and extension of the ankles, knees, and hips to absorb and generate force. Additionally, many require selection of the appropriate line at varying speeds through undulating terrain, with vibrations similar to skiing. Selecting exercises with specific attributes required for alpine skiing is the key to an appropriate cross-training program.

Other exercises with components of specificity have also been recommended in the skiing literature. Karlsson and colleagues (10) emphasized uphill, forward and backward lateral jumps with ankle motion restricted, as if in a ski boot, for push-off and landing. Also, walking backward in a downhill tuck position is recommended because it utilizes the entire foot for push-off, eliminates plantar flexion, and therefore requires more force generation from the quadriceps muscles.

Skiing performance has also been evaluated with several dryland performance tests (24,59–62). Andersen and colleagues (24) reported good correlations between giant slalom performance and the hex obstacle (r = 0.82), five jumps ($r = -0.86$), and high box ($r = -0.80$) tests. Piper and colleagues (60), using recreational student skiers, reported a multiple correlation of r = 0.61 between slalom performance and a lateral vault, hex jumps, triceps skinfolds, and body weight. As mentioned by White and Johnson (36), many of these dry-land skills tests are complex tasks and it is difficult to identify exactly what they are evaluating. Since they have not resulted in consistent predictive capability across studies, their value for discriminating among competitive skiers is questionable.

Supplemental Training

Many aspects of physical training for alpine skiing can be addressed through supplemental, or non–sports-specific, training. Traditional methods of improving aerobic and anaerobic capacity, movement skills, and flexibility can be utilized. Emphasis is placed on the major muscle groups involved in skiing. The U.S. Ski Team's Physical Fitness Medals Test (63) has been designed for evaluating preseason physical conditioning.

As discussed previously, the importance of aerobic capacity in conditioning programs for skiing has been emphasized (22,64,65) and de-emphasized (15,66). Endurance exercises of low-intensity muscle contraction and long duration, such as running and biking, or many repetitions, such as resistance exercises done with light loads, build aerobic capacity. In-line skating and roller skiing are more specific to skiing. A good aerobic base complements enhanced anaerobic fitness and helps an athlete maintain fitness over a whole season.

The general consensus in the training literature suggests that anaerobic capacity is the most important physiologic aspect of skiing (15,64,66–70), playing a predominant role in strength and power activities. For the legs, sprint and jumping drills, plyometrics, and resistance exercises with heavy to medium loads have all been recommended. Exercises, such as squats, that emphasize strength, power, and eccentric muscle actions are key (15,22,64,67,69). Running or biking intervals, from 30 seconds to 2 minutes in duration, help train more extended anaerobic capabilities. For powerful starts, triceps extensions and pull-downs for the latissimus dorsi condition the arm extensors (69).

Bosco and colleagues (15) implemented a training program of squat jumps and continuous jumping exercises in 12 international male Italian racers during the off-season. They were evaluated in June, July, October, and April. Squat jump heights and continuous jumping power increased with training and were maintained over the competitive season. The authors concluded that the demands of competition provided adequate stimulus to maintain the improvements induced by training, implying the specificity of strength and power training to skiing. Unfortunately, no correlations were reported between jumping parameters and skiing performance.

Movement skills require balance, appropriate movement patterns, and their coordination in a variety of circumstances. Quickness and agility drills, such as cariocas, that are common in other sports have also been recommended to improve lower extremity balance and coordination in skiing (64,65,67).

Flexibility of the major muscle groups surrounding the knee, hip, and trunk (71) are most important for the skier. Stretches for the knee (quadriceps and hamstrings), hip (psoas, rectus femoris, gluteus, adductors, and abductors), abdomen (rectus abdominis and obliques) and low back (erector spinae, psoas, hamstrings) will benefit the functional requirements of the skier and may help prevent injury.

A general source that contains some suggestions for supplemental training is the U.S. Ski Team's "Alpine Athlete Competencies" (72). This special journal issue outlines a progression of technical, tactical, physiologic, motor, psychologic, and social skills deemed beneficial by the U.S. Ski Team staff for skier development.

Periodization of Training

Periodization is a systematic approach to training that attempts to organize and optimize training to achieve a desired goal in a definitive amount of time (73,74). General and sports-specific physical training and skill acquisition are among the many components incorporated into the athlete's program. A progression of stress and adaptation cycles within a training phase, over a season and over an athlete's career, form the basis of periodization. The English-language literature on the periodization of training for alpine skiing is mixed in terms of nomenclature and specific timing (7,35,67,75–77). Much of the following information is a synthesis of the material cited above.

It is well recognized that skiing at the World Cup level requires year-round training (7,69,75,77). The training calendar can be partitioned into five phases: general preparation, specific preparation, precompetitive, competitive, and transition. Typically the training plan is established by working backward from the competitive phase and allocating adequate time to accomplish the goals of each phase (74).

In alpine skiing, the four training components—aerobic capacity, anaerobic capacity, movement skills, and flexibility—are addressed with varying emphasis in each phase. For physical training, the emphasis progresses from initial base preparation with concentration on aerobic endurance activities, to more anaerobic strength and power-related exercises. The athlete's goal is to acquire and maintain adequate endurance, strength, power, and flexibility to execute skiing movements and deal with the external forces encountered. In terms of movement skills, the emphasis begins with refining fundamentals and progresses to specific skills and individual problems, with competence in a variety of terrain and conditions. The dry-land training is most effective if it parallels the on-snow progression.

The general preparation phase for skiing lasts about 3 months (May to July). Substantial volume with low intensity is the modus operandi. For physical training, the major emphasis is on aerobic endurance activities with some anaerobic strength and power exercises. This translates into running, biking, in-line skating, roller skiing, and high repetition resistance training, with gradual incorporation of some interval training. The more sports specific the exercises, the greater opportunity for skill crossover. On-snow opportunities are dominated by free skiing, concentrating on balance and fundamental movement patterns, and some rhythmical gate training. Basic racing technique and tactics are addressed along with equipment testing and alignment. There is a gradual transition to more strength and power exercises in the latter part of this phase.

The specific preparation phase also lasts about 3 months (August to October). The overall volume of work increases. Development of anaerobic capacity (strength and power) is the predominant emphasis of this stage, with maintenance of aerobic endurance capacity. Dry-land exercise sets employ more intensity but are of shorter duration. Interval training and plyometrics are used along with strength and power resistance training. On-snow training incorporates long nonstop free skiing runs, technical exercises, and gate drills for timing, quickness, and selected movement skills with emphasis on individual racing technique.

The precompetitive phase lasts about 4 weeks (in October or November). Emphasis remains on anaerobic capacity (strength and power) with maintenance of aerobic capacity. On-snow training includes simulating race situations with full-length timed runs and emphasis on finishing and speed. Technical gate drills for combinations, timing, and line are utilized. Initially the work volume may increase, but then it is reduced with a recovery period leading into the first races.

The competitive phase may last up to 6 months (November to April). Careful planning of training geared to specific competitions and adequate rest and recovery are the hallmarks of this phase. Technical exercises and gate drills for individual problems are utilized. Maintenance of physical conditioning is important, and proper mental preparation becomes critical.

The transition phase lasts approximately 4 to 6 weeks (April to May). Training should be recreational in nature with personal sports activities. It is a time for the athlete to reflect on the competitive season, establish new goals, and become physically and mentally regenerated for a new cycle.

REFERENCES

1. Howe N. The boys who invented winter. In: Needham R, ed. *Warren Miller's ski fever.* Del Mar, CA: Tehabi, 1995:144–155.
2. Karlsson J. Profiles of cross-country and alpine skiers. *Clin Sports Med* 1984;3(1):245–270.
3. Federation Internationale de Ski (FIS). *The international ski competition rules.* Berne: International Ski Federation, 1996.
4. Howe JG. *Skiing mechanics.* Laporte, CO: Poudre Press, 1983.
5. McMurtry JG. Biomechanics of alpine skiing. In: Casey MJ, Foster C, Hixson EG, eds. *Winter sports medicine.* Philadelphia: FA Davis, 1990:344–350.
6. Nachbauer W, Rauch A. Biomechanische Analysen der Torlaufund Riesentorlauftechnik. In: Fetz F, Müller E, eds. *Biomechanik des alpinen Skilaufs.* Stuttgart: Enke Verlag, 1991:50–100.
7. Twardokens G. Skiing biomechanics. *United States Ski Team Alpine training manual.* Park City, UT: United States Ski Coaches Association, 1985:283–302.
8. Hintermeister RA, O'Connor DD, Dillman CJ, Suplizio CL, Lange GW, Steadman JR. Muscle activity in slalom and giant slalom skiing. *Med Sci Sports Exerc* 1995;27(3):315–322.
9. Berg HE, Eiken O, Tesch PA. Involvement of eccentric muscle actions in giant slalom racing. *Med Sci Sports Exerc* 1995; 27(12):1666–1670.
10. Karlsson J, Eriksson A, Forsberg A, Kallberg L, Tesch P. *Physiology of alpine skiing.* Park City, UT: The U.S. Ski Coaches Association, 1977.
11. Eriksson A, Forsberg A, Nilsson J, Karlsson J. Muscle strength, EMG activity, and oxygen uptake during downhill skiing. In: Asmussen, Jorgensen, eds. *Biomechanics,* vol 6A. Baltimore: University Park, 1978.
12. Hintermeister RA, Lange GW, O'Connor DD, Dillman CJ, Steadman JR. Muscle activity of the inside and outside leg in slalom and giant slalom skiing. In: Müller E, Schwameder H, Kornexl E, Raschner C, eds. *Science and skiing.* London: E & FN Spon, 1997:141–149.
13. Feltner M, Dapena J. Dynamics of the shoulder and elbow joints of the throwing arm during a baseball pitch. *Int J Sports Biomech* 1986;2:235–259.
14. Tesch P, Larsson L. Muscle glycogen depletion and lactate concentration during downhill skiing. *Med Sci Sports* 1978;10(2):85–90.
15. Bosco C, Cotelli F, Bonomi R, Mognoni P, Roi GS. Seasonal fluctuations of selected physiological characteristics of elite alpine skiers. *Eur J Appl Physiol* 1994;69:71–74.
16. Physiology. In: Leach RE, Fritschy D, Steadman JR, eds. *Handbook of sports medicine and science: alpine skiing.* Oxford: Blackwell Scientific, 1994:17–29.
17. Bacharach DW, Duvillard SP. Intermediate and long-term anaerobic performance of elite alpine skiers. *Med Sci Sports Exerc* 1995;27(3):305–309.
18. Tesch PA. Aspects on muscle properties and use in competitive alpine skiing. *Med Sci Sports Exerc* 1995;27(3):310–314.

19. Thorstensson A, Larsson L. Muscle strength and fiber composition in athletes and sedentary men. *Med Sci Sports* 1977;9(1):26–30.
20. Haymes EM, Dickinson AL. Characteristics of elite male and female ski racers. *Med Sci Sports Exerc* 1980;12(3):153–158.
21. Brown SL, Wilkinson JG. Characteristics of national, divisional, and club male alpine ski racers. *Med Sci Sports Exerc* 1983;15(6):491–495.
22. Steadman JR, Swanson KR, Atkins JA, Hagerman GR. Training for alpine skiing. *Clin Orthop Rel Res* 1987;216:34–38.
23. Abe T, Kawakami Y, Ikegawa S, Kanehisa H, Fukunaga T. Isometric and isokinetic knee joint performance in Japanese alpine ski racers. *J Sports Med Phys Fitness* 1992;32(4):353–357.
24. Andersen RE, Montgomery DL, Turcotte RA. An on-site test battery to evaluate giant slalom skiing performance. *J Sports Med Phys Fitness* 1990;30(3):276–282.
25. White AT, Johnson SC. Physiological comparison of international, national and regional alpine skiers. *Int J Sports Med* 1991; 12:374–378.
26. Song TMK. Relationship of physiological characteristics to skiing performance. *Phys Sports Med* 1982;10(12):97–102.
27. Stark R, Reed A, Wenger H. Power curve characteristics of elite slalom and downhill skiers performing a modified 90 seconds Wingate test (abstract). *Can J Sport Sci* 1987;12(3):24.
28. Duvillard S, Knowles WJ. Relationship of anaerobic performance tests to competitive alpine skiing events. In: Mu ller E, Schwameder H, Kornexl E, Raschner C, eds. *Science and skiing.* London: E & FN Spon, 1997.
29. Kilbom A, Persson J. Leg blood flow during static exercise. *Eur J Appl Physiol* 1982; 48:367–377.
30. Åstrand P, Rodahl K. *Textbook of work physiology,* 2nd ed. New York: McGraw-Hill, 1977.
31. Veicsteinas A, Ferretti G, Margonato V, Rosa G, Tagliabue D. Energy cost of and energy sources for alpine skiing in top athletes. *J Appl Physiol Respir Environ Exerc Physiol* 1984;56(5):1187–1190.
32. Saibene F, Cortilli G. Energy sources in alpine skiing (giant slalom). *Eur J Appl Physiol* 1985;53:312–316.
33. Richardson RS, White AT, Seifert JD, Porretta JM, Johnson SC. Blood lactate concentrations in elite skiers during a series of on-snow downhill ski runs. *J Strength Conditioning Res* 1993;7(3):168–171.
34. Andersen R, Montgomery D. Physiology of alpine skiing. *Sports Med* 1988;6:210–221.
35. Plisk S. Physiological training for competitive alpine skiing. *Natl Strength Coaches Assoc J* 1988;10(1):30–33.
36. White A, Johnson S. Physiological aspects and injury in elite alpine skiers. *Sports Med* 1993;15(3):170–178.
37. Rusko H, Havu M, Karvinen E. Aerobic performance capacity in athletes. *Eur J Appl Physiol* 1978;38(2):151–159.
38. DiPrampero, PE. Energetics of muscular exercise. *Rev Physiol Biochem Pharmacol* 1981;89:143–222.
39. Kahn JF, Jouanin JC, Esprito-Santo J, Monad H. Cardiovascular responses to leisure alpine skiing in habitually sedentary middle-aged men. *J Sport Sci* 1993;11:31–36.
40. Gollnick PD, Armstrong RB, Saubert CW IV, Piehl K, Saltin B. Enzyme activity and fiber composition in skeletal muscle of untrained and trained men. *J Appl Physiol* 1972;33:312–319.
41. Bergh U, Thorstensson U, Sjödin B, Hulten B, Piehl K, Karlsson J. Maximal oxygen uptake and muscle fiber types in trained and untrained humans. *Med Sci Sports Exerc* 1978;10(3):151–154.
42. Roalstad M, Watkins R. Spine injuries and issues in skiers. *Am Ski Coach* 1995;17(2):21–25.
43. Orvanová E. Physical structure of winter sports athletes. *J Sports Sci* 1987;5(3):197–248.
44. Kornexl E. Anthropometrische Untersuchungen in alpinen Schirennlauf (I Teil). *Leibesübungen-Leibeserziehung* 1975; 29:196–201.
45. Kornexl E. Anthropometrische Untersuchungen in alpinen Schirennlauf (II Teil). *Leibesübungen-Leibeserziehung* 1976; 30:5–8.
46. Eriksson A, Ekholm J, Hulten B, Karlsson E, Karlsson J. Anatomical, histological, and physiological factors in experienced downhill skiers. *Orthop Clin North Am* 1976;7(1):159–165.
47. Suplizio CL, Hintermeister RA. Do anatomical and physiological differences between genders affect skiing. *Professional Skier* 1993; 19–20,62–63.
48. Atwater AE. Biomechanics of the Female Athlete. In: Puhl J, Brown CH, Voy RO, eds. *Sport science perspectives for women.* Champaign, IL: Human Kinetics, 1988.
49. McArdle WD, Katch FI, Katch VL. *Exercise physiology: energy, nutrition and human performance.* Philadelphia: Lea & Febiger, 1981.
50. *U.S. Ski Team alpine fundamentals* (video). Park City, UT: United States Ski Coaches Association, 1990.
51. *Dryland training and skiing fundamentals featuring the Norwegian National Alpine Ski Team* (video). Park City, UT: Nordic Equipment, 1992.
52. *U.S. Ski Team speed elements training* (video). Park City, UT: United States Ski Coaches Association, 1992.
53. *U.S. Ski Team free skiing and advanced elements of alpine ski technique* (video). Park City, UT: United States Ski Coaches Association, 1993.
54. Post-Foster E. *Race skills for alpine skiing.* Edwards, CO: Turning Point Foundation, 1994.
55. Witherall W. *How the racers ski.* New York: Norton, 1972.
56. Witherell W, Evrard D. *The athletic skier.* Salt Lake City, UT: Athletic Skier, 1993.
57. Harb HR. *Anyone can be an expert skier.* Dumont, CO: Harb Ski Systems, 1997.
58. Hintermeister R, Holden M. Anatomy and conditioning. In: Ayers RW, ed. *Alpine manual.* Lakewood, CO: Professional Ski Instructors of America Education Foundation, 1996:122–124.
59. Kornexl E. *Das sportmorische Eigenschaftsniveau des alpinen Schirennläufers.* Innsbruck, Austria:Inn-Verlag, 1980.
60. Piper FC, Ward CHT, McGinnis PM, Milner EK. Prediction of alpine ski performance based upon selected anthropometrical and motor dexterity parameters. *J Sports Med Phys Fitness* 1987;27(4):478–482.
61. Kipp RW, Reid, RC. The high box test. *Am Ski Coach* 1994;16(3):8–10.
62. Kipp RW, Reid, RC. The hexagonal obstacle test and its use in training. *Am Ski Coach* 1994;16(4):2–6.
63. United States Ski Coaches Association. U.S. Ski Team physical fitness medal test. *Am Ski Coach* 1989;12(4):21–25.
64. Atkins J, Hagerman G. Formula for success (a conditioning guideline for potential U.S. Ski Team athletes). *Am Ski Coach* 1989;12(4):3–9.
65. Hagerman GR. Physiology of alpine skiing. In: Casey MJ, Foster C, Hixson EG, eds. *Winter sports medicine.* Philadelphia: FA Davis, 1990:338–343.
66. Johnson S. Alpine physiology project. *Am Ski Coach* 1989; 12(4):37–38.
67. O'Shea P, Larsson O. Ski racing-the giant slalom turn. *National Strength Coaches Assoc J* 1990;12(1):4–8,84–87.
68. Egan B. Plyometrics and skiing: an essential link. *Am Ski Coach* 1992;15(3):30–35.
69. Lavallee T. Physical preparation for the collegiate alpine skier. *Natl Strength Conditioning Assoc J* 1992;14(4):58–69.
70. White A. A review of skiing physiology. *Am Ski Coach* 1992;15(3):7–8.
71. Tiefel L, Brown C. U.S. Ski Team trunk routine. *Am Ski Coach* 1989;12(4):26–28.
72. Johnson SJ, Keller L, Kipp R, LaMarche T, Radamus A, Reid R, Ross T. Alpine athlete competencies. *Am Ski Coach* 1997;18(2):1–53.
73. Matveyev L. *Fundamentals of sports training.* Moscow: Progress Publishers, 1981.
74. Sands WA. Periodization and planning of training. *Am Ski Coach* 1992;15(3):9–17.
75. Atkins JW, Hagerman GR. Alpine skiing. *Natl Strength Coaches Assoc J* 1984;5(6):6–8.
76. Kallerud T. Planning of on-snow preparation period for alpine ski racers. *Am Ski Coach* 1992;15(3):22–26.
77. Roalstad M. Periodized year-round training for alpine skiing. *Am Ski Coach* 1992;15(3):18–21.
78. U.S. Ski and Snowboard Association, Alpine athlete competencies. *Am Ski Coach* 1997;18(2):53.

Exercise and Sport Science,
edited by William E. Garrett, Jr., and Donald T. Kirkendall.
Lippincott Williams & Wilkins, Philadelphia © 2000.

CHAPTER 45

Physiology of Baseball

Kevin E. Wilk

The overhead throwing athlete is a highly skilled individual. To perform the overhead throwing motion successfully, the athlete must exhibit significant flexibility, muscular strength, coordination, synchronicity of muscle firing, and neuromuscular efficiency. In some instances, the thrower may be throwing a baseball at velocities up to 97 to 100 mph. In other instances, the thrower may be throwing a pitch, such as a curve ball or slider, that requires the same arm speed but creates much different, and in some instances, higher stresses at the elbow and shoulder joints.

The overhead throwing motion produces excessively high stresses because of the unnatural movements frequently performed by the overhead thrower. The thrower's shoulder must be flexible enough to allow the excessive external rotation required to throw a baseball. However, the thrower's shoulder also must be stable enough to prevent the shoulder joint from subluxation. Therefore there appears to exist a paradox when describing the thrower's shoulder: the thrower's shoulder must be "loose enough to throw" but stable enough to prevent humeral head subluxation. Hence the thrower's shoulder is in delicate balance between mobility and stability.

The surrounding musculature of the thrower's shoulder must exhibit sufficient muscular strength, power, and neuromuscular control efficiency. The thrower's shoulder musculature must be strong enough to assist in arm acceleration but must also exhibit neuromuscular efficiency to enhance dynamic functional stability. The surrounding musculature works synergistically with the glenohumeral joint capsule to provide functional stability. The overhead throwing motion places tremendous demands on the shoulder and elbow-joint complex musculature to produce functional stability, especially the shoulder joint. The musculature must function and react while the arm and shoulder joint are moving at incredibly high angular velocities. Furthermore, the shoulder musculature must function effectively throughout the entire range of motion, especially at end ranges, which are usually much greater than normal motions, all of which are occurring at tremendously fast speeds.

In this chapter, the biomechanics of the overhead baseball throwing motion is briefly discussed, and key physiologic aspects are highlighted. Additionally, the physical requirements (such as range of motion, muscular strength, ligamentous stability, and neuromuscular control) are thoroughly described. Those physical requirements are then applied to a conditioning program to prevent injuries to the shoulder and elbow joint in the overhead thrower. Finally, some suggestions and guidelines are presented for the rehabilitation of common throwing injuries.

THE SPORT

Physical Requirements

The Biomechanics of the Overhead Throw

At its most basic level, baseball involves throwing, catching, and hitting. The biomechanics of throwing are covered in detail in Chapter 38. The overhead throwing motion is a highly skillful, extremely stressful, and violent activity. In general, the throwing motion for throwing a baseball is similar to, but not exactly the same as, that of throwing a football or javelin. To understand the physical requirements for throwing a baseball, one must understand the biomechanics of the overhead throwing motion.

The overhead pitching motion can be divided into five distinct phases (Fig. 45–1). These phases include the wind-up, early cocking, late cocking, acceleration,

K. E. Wilk: Tampa Bay Devil Rays Baseball Organization, St. Petersburg, Florida 33705; Marquette University, Milwaukee, Wisconsin 33201; and HealthSouth Rehabilitation Corporation, Birmingham, Alabama 35205.

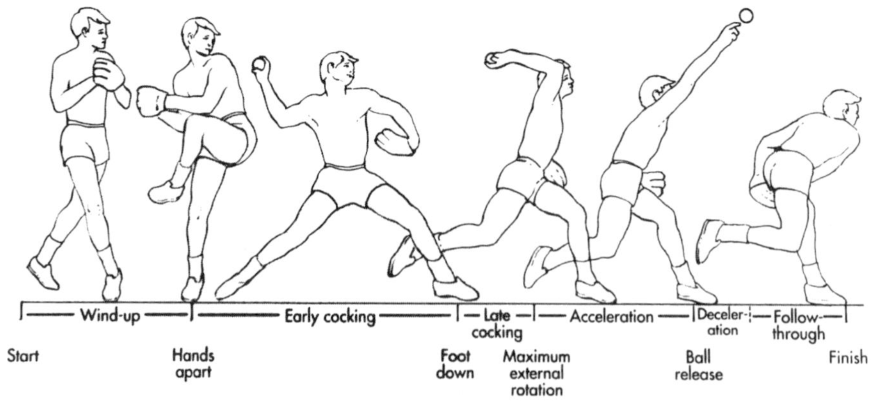

FIG. 45–1. The five phases of the overhead pitching motion. These phases include the wind-up, early cocking, late cocking, acceleration, and deceleration. (From ref. 3, with permission.)

and deceleration follow-through (1). During the throw, the kinetic energy is generated from the legs and trunk and is transferred upward to the shoulder and arm (Fig. 45–2). At ball release and follow-through, the generated energy is transferred downward and back through the legs. It has been estimated that more than 55% of the kinetic energy and momentum necessary to throw a ball is generated from the legs and lower trunk (2).

The Wind-up Phase

The wind-up begins when the pitcher initiates the first motion and ends with the ball being removed from the glove. During the pitching motion, the athlete will pivot on the stance foot to a parallel position with the pitching rubber. The lead leg is then lifted concentrically by the hip flexors while the stance leg is slightly flexed to support the athlete's body weight. This position is referred to as the "balanced position" (Fig. 45–3). The pitcher must exhibit significant muscular strength not only in the stance leg but also in the pelvis and lower trunk to maintain this difficult balanced position. The quadriceps femoris of the stance leg performs an eccentric and isometric contraction to maintain the flexed knee posture, while the hip abductors and extensors co-contract to stabilize the pelvis. This balanced position is a very important position in the overhead pitching motion. The body must be vertical; thus balance, proprioception, and kinesthesia are important attributes in maintaining this posture. Young throwers often mistakenly attempt to gain arm speed and ball velocity by propelling themselves toward the target too soon, and never accomplish the balance position. This omission

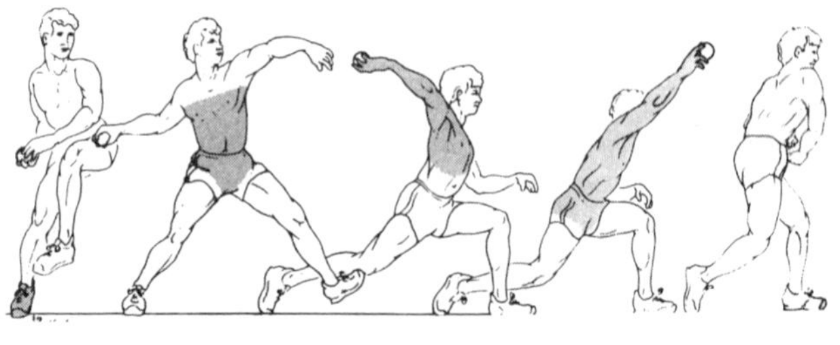

FIG. 45–2. During the pitch, the transfer of kinetic energy is generated from the legs and transferred upward. (From ref. 1, with permission.)

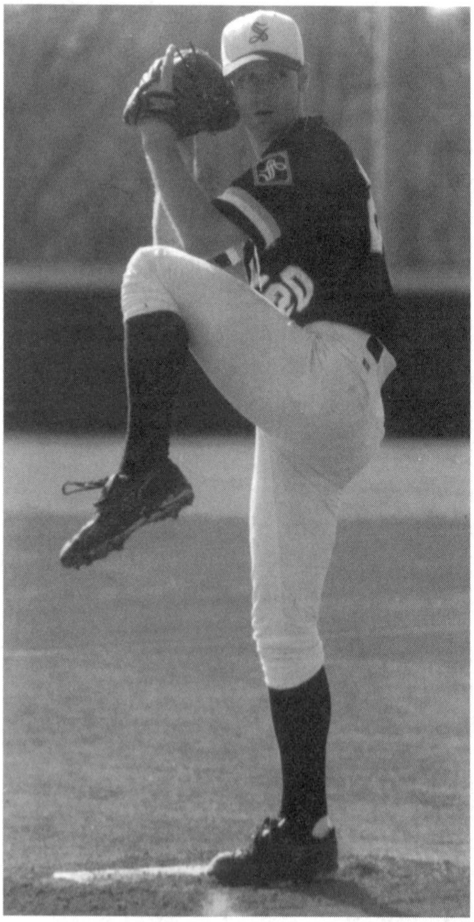

FIG. 45–3. The "balanced position" during the wind-up of the overhead pitch.

can lead to significant injuries to the shoulder from the shoulder's turning to the target too early. The main purpose of the wind-up phase is to place the thrower in an advantageous starting position to maximize the effort and perhaps to act as a distraction to the batter.

The Cocking Phase

The early cocking phase begins as the two arms separate (the ball being taken out of the glove). During this phase, the pitcher pushes off the pitching rubber by using a concentric contraction of the stance leg's hip extensors, hip abductors, knee extensors, and plantar flexors. The stride leg is lunged forward, with the lead foot pointed at the target. Usually the lead foot is turned slightly inward (approximately 5 to 25 degrees). The lead leg's knee is flexed to approximately 45 to 55 degrees at foot contact. This position allows the body to rotate on this fixed and stable base of support. In addition, during this phase, the shoulder is abducted, externally, and is horizontally abducted. During early cocking, the upper trapezius, supraspinatus, deltoid, and serratus anterior muscles exhibit moderately high to moderate levels of electromyographic (EMG) activity, respectively (Table 45–1) (3). The upper trapezius and serratus anterior musculature work synchronously to rotate the scapula upward, while the deltoid muscle is elevating the arm and the rotator cuff muscles are co-contracting to stabilize the humeral head. The shoulder is abducted to approximately 80 to 100 degrees (4). In addition, during this phase, the elbow is flexed to approximately 80 to 100 degrees while the arm is pronating. Electromyographic analysis has shown that the wrist extensors (extensor carpi radialis, extensor carpi ulnaris, and extensor digitorum) exhibit moderately high levels of EMG activity (especially during late cocking).

During the late-cocking phase, the shoulder joint remains abducted approximately 80 to 100 degrees, while the arm externally rotates. Late cocking is characterized by the internal rotators acting eccentrically to control shoulder external rotation. The subscapularis exhibits high levels [99% maximum voluntary isometric contrac-

TABLE 45–1. *EMG analysis of the overhead throw*

	No. of pitchers	Windup	Early cocking	Late cocking	Acceleration	Deceleration	Follow-through
Scapular muscles							
Upper trapezius	11	18 ± 16	64 ± 53	37 ± 29	69 ± 31	53 ± 22	14 ± 12
Middle trapezius	11	7 ± 5	43 ± 22	51 ± 24	71 ± 32	35 ± 17	15 ± 14
Lower trapezius	13	13 ± 12	39 ± 30	38 ± 29	76 ± 55	78 ± 33	25 ± 15
Serratus anterior (sixth rib)	11	14 ± 13	44 ± 35	69 ± 32	60 ± 53	51 ± 30	32 ± 18
Serratus anterior (fourth rib)	10	20 ± 20	40 ± 22	106 ± 56	50 ± 46	34 ± 7	41 ± 24
Rhomboids	11	7 ± 8	35 ± 24	41 ± 26	71 ± 35	45 ± 28	14 ± 20
Levator scapula	11	6 ± 5	35 ± 14	72 ± 54	77 ± 28	33 ± 16	14 ± 13
Glenohumeral muscles							
Anterior deltoid	16	15 ± 12	40 ± 20	28 ± 30	27 ± 19	47 ± 34	21 ± 16
Middle deltoid	14	9 ± 8	44 ± 19	12 ± 17	36 ± 22	59 ± 19	16 ± 13
Posterior deltoid	18	6 ± 5	42 ± 26	28 ± 27	68 ± 66	60 ± 28	13 ± 11
Supraspinatus	16	13 ± 12	60 ± 31	49 ± 29	51 ± 46	39 ± 43	10 ± 9
Infraspinatus	16	11 ± 9	30 ± 18	74 ± 34	31 ± 28	37 ± 20	20 ± 16
Teres minor	12	5 ± 6	23 ± 15	71 ± 42	54 ± 50	84 ± 52	25 ± 21
Subscapularis (lower third)	11	7 ± 9	25 ± 22	62 ± 19	56 ± 31	41 ± 23	25 ± 18
Subscapularis (upper third)	11	7 ± 8	37 ± 26	99 ± 55	115 ± 82	60 ± 36	16 ± 15
Pectoralis major	14	6 ± 6	11 ± 13	56 ± 27	54 ± 24	29 ± 18	31 ± 21
Latissimus dorsi	13	12 ± 10	33 ± 33	50 ± 37	88 ± 53	59 ± 35	24 ± 18
Elbow and forearm muscles							
Triceps	13	4 ± 6	17 ± 17	37 ± 32	89 ± 40	54 ± 23	22 ± 18
Biceps	18	8 ± 9	22 ± 14	26 ± 20	20 ± 16	44 ± 32	16 ± 14
Brachialis	13	8 ± 5	17 ± 13	18 ± 26	20 ± 22	49 ± 29	13 ± 17
Brachioradialis	13	5 ± 5	35 ± 20	31 ± 24	16 ± 12	46 ± 24	22 ± 29
Pronator teres	14	14 ± 16	18 ± 15	39 ± 28	85 ± 39	51 ± 21	21 ± 21
Supinotor	13	9 ± 7	38 ± 20	54 ± 38	55 ± 31	59 ± 31	22 ± 19
Wrist and finger muscles							
Extensor carpi radialis longus	13	11 ± 8	53 ± 24	72 ± 37	30 ± 20	43 ± 24	22 ± 14
Extensor carpi radialis brevis	15	17 ± 17	47 ± 26	75 ± 41	55 ± 35	43 ± 28	24 ± 19
Extensor digitorum communis	14	21 ± 17	37 ± 25	59 ± 27	35 ± 35	47 ± 25	24 ± 18
Flexor carpi radialis	12	13 ± 9	24 ± 35	47 ± 33	120 ± 66	79 ± 36	35 ± 16
Flexor digitorum superficialis	11	16 ± 6	20 ± 23	47 ± 52	80 ± 66	71 ± 32	21 ± 11
Flexor carpi ulnaris	10	8 ± 5	27 ± 18	41 ± 25	112 ± 60	77 ± 42	24 ± 18

Means and standard deviations, expressed as a percentage of the maximal manual muscle test.

tion (MVIC)] of EMG activity, while the pectoralis major and latissimus dorsi exhibit moderately high (56% and 50% MVIC, respectively) EMG activity (see Table 45–1). Additionally, the serratus anterior exhibits extremely high muscular activity (106% MVIC), along with moderately high muscle activity of the levator scapula, middle trapezius, infraspinatus, and teres minor muscles. In addition, the internal rotators are elastically stretched to provide a stretch stimulus to the muscle spindle, provoking a powerful concentric contraction during the next phase of the throw, the acceleration phase. This type of stretch–shortening muscular contraction is referred to as a plyometric contraction. The throwing of a baseball is a classic example of a plyometric muscular contraction (5,6). It has been reported that, during late cocking, the arm externally rotates to a maximum of approximately 165 to 180 degrees (4). This excessive external rotation is the combination of scapular, thoracic, and lumbar spine motion. Nevertheless, for this motion to occur, the anterior glenohumeral joint capsule must exhibit significant laxity. During arm cocking, the shoulder joint angular velocity is approximately 1100°/s (4). Additionally, maximal anterior shear force is approximately 380 ± 90 N, and compressive forces of 660 ± 110 N (4). Thus approximately 85 ± 36 lb of force are acting at the glenohumeral joint, attempting to sublux the humeral head anteriorly, while approximately 145 ± 28 lb of force are compressing the humeral head within the glenoid. A maximal elbow-extensor torque of approximately 20 to 40 Newton-meters (Nm) has been noted during the arm-cocking phase (7). In addition, a significant varus torque of approximately 50 to 75 Nm, which resists a valgus force, occurs shortly before maximal shoulder external rotation (4,7).

The Acceleration Phase

Once the arm reaches maximal external rotation, the elbow joint begins to extend, and the shoulder joint rapidly internally rotates and adducts, initiating the acceleration phase of throwing. The acceleration phase of the overhead throw has been reported to be the fastest human motion recorded. During the acceleration phase, the maximal internal rotation/adduction velocity exceeds 7000 degree/s (4). This phase of the throw takes approximately 0.03 to 0.04 second. Regardless of what type of pitch is thrown, or the style of the pitcher (sidearm, overhead, three quarter, etc.), at ball release the shoulder joint is abducted between 90 and 100 degrees (8). The difference between the overhead and the sidearm throw is not the amount of shoulder abduction, but rather the degree of lateral tilt of the trunk. During the acceleration, the subscapularis, latissimus dorsi, and trapezius exhibit high levels of EMG activity (see Table 45–1).

During arm acceleration, the elbow begins to extend just before maximal shoulder external rotation; then shoulder internal rotation occurs. This sequence of integrated motions appears to enhance the velocity of internal rotation and thus arm speed, and is an example of the synchronicity of joint motions exhibited during the overhead throwing motion. Maximal elbow angular velocity is approximately 2100 to 2400°/s. During this phase of pitching, a valgus stress is imparted onto the elbow joint. Shoulder internal-rotation torque and elbow varus torque gradually decrease during the arm-acceleration phase as the arm begins rotating forward, and near ball release, low forces, and torques are generated at the elbow and shoulder joints (7,9,10). The wrist flexors (flexor carpi radialis, flexor carpi ulnaris, and flexor digitorum superficialis) exhibit significantly high EMG activity during this phase. It should be noted that the muscle that exhibits the highest EMG activity of any muscle in the body is the flexor carpi radialis (120% MVIC). During this phase, the elbow extends from approximately 85 degrees elbow flexion to 20 degrees elbow flexion (4). A maximal elbow compressive force of approximately 600 to 900 N is produced to prevent elbow-joint distraction. The elbow flexors act eccentrically to control elbow extension and also act to compress the elbow joint, contributing to joint stability. The mechanics of throwing a baseball and football are similar (11), with the most significant differences occurring at the elbow joint.

Additionally, the trunk contributes greatly to arm speed. As the elbow extends and the shoulder internally rotates, the trunk forward flexes from an extended position. Forward flexion by the trunk occurs at an angular velocity of approximately 300 to 450 degree/s and is accomplished by the action of the hip flexors and abdominal muscles (rectus abdominals and obliques) (12). This rapid and forceful forward trunk flexion contributes to the vertical force generated through the upper body, which contributes to arm speed.

The Deceleration/Follow-Through Phase

The arm deceleration/follow-through occurs from ball release to the termination of movement; this phase takes approximately 0.03 to 0.05 seconds to complete. After ball release, the arm continues to adduct horizontally, extend, and to a lesser extent internally rotate as the kinetic energy is gradually dissipated through the lower extremity. During arm deceleration, the forces at the glenohumeral joint reach relatively high levels. Maximal posterior shear force is approximately 400 ± 90 N, whereas the compressive force is approximately 1090 ± 110 N. This extremely high compressive force resists the distraction force generated at the glenohumeral joint. During deceleration, large eccentric muscle actions are needed at the shoulder and elbow joints. The teres minor exhibits significantly high EMG activity during this phase (84% MVIC); conversely, the infraspinatus exhibits relatively low musculature activity (37% MVIC). This discrepancy between the teres minor and infraspinatus during this phase suggests that the teres minor plays a more significant role in arm deceleration than does the infraspinatus muscle. Other muscles that exhibit significant EMG activity are the lower trapezius (78% MVIC), posterior deltoid (60% MVIC), and subscapularis (60% MVIC). At the elbow, wrist, and forearm, the muscles most active are the flexor carpi radialis (79% MVIC), flexor carpi ulnaris (77% MVIC), supinator (59% MVIC), and brachialis (49% MVIC). The elbow-extension motion terminates when the elbow is extended to approximately 15 to 25 degrees. The follow-through phase of the pitch is the continuation of the deceleration phase, during which the joint forces and muscular torques are gradually diminished.

The tremendous energy generated during the acceleration phase of throwing must be gradually dissipated after ball release, during the deceleration and follow-through phases. This dissipation usually occurs by the action of the larger body segments and muscles. To reduce the distraction forces generated during the deceleration phase, the thrower should exhibit a complete follow-through path of motion, allowing the energy and momentum to be dissipated over a longer period. Decelerating too quickly or abruptly will result in excessively high forces, which may lead to injury.

Consequently, the throwing shoulder and elbow-joint complexes are subjected to tremendous unnatural stresses. The thrower's shoulder joint must be loose enough to allow excessive motion, especially external rotation, yet maintain functional dynamic stability. Functional stability is provided by the integrated action of the joint capsule and surrounding musculature of the shoulder-joint complex. There are muscles that appear primarily responsible for arm acceleration, such as latissimus dorsi, pectoralis major, triceps brachii, and wrist flexors. Conversely, there appear to be muscles primarily responsible for providing dynamic joint stability; these muscles include the supraspinatus, infraspinatus, subscapularis, serratus anterior, biceps brachii, and rhomboids. Dynamic stability is accomplished by coactivation of the stabilizing muscles. Because of the tremendous forces occurring at extremely high angular velocities and the repetitive nature of throwing, the thrower becomes susceptible to a variety of shoulder and elbow-joint injuries. The most common shoulder-joint complex injuries include overuse tendinitis, capsular hyperlaxity (subluxation), posterior rotator-cuff impingement, undersurface tearing (fraying) of the rotator cuff, and glenoid labral lesions. The most common elbow-joint injuries include flexor/pronator tendinitis, ulnar collateral ligament (UCL) sprains, valgus extension overload syndromes, and posterior osteophyte formation. These injuries are discussed elsewhere in this book. It also is important to note that there are significant differences in muscular activity and kinetics in the amateur and professional thrower, as well as throwers with shoulder instability and a "normal" shoulder joint.

Gowan (13) compared the EMG activity of the shoulder musculature of amateur pitchers with that of professional pitchers. During arm cocking, the subscapularis muscle activity was approximately twice as great in the professional pitchers as that of the amateurs. Muscular activity of the biceps, serratus anterior, supraspinatus, and pectoralis major was approximately 50% greater in the amateur pitchers compared with that in the professional pitchers. During the acceleration phase, muscle activity of the infraspinatus, teres minor, supraspinatus, and biceps brachii was 2 to 3 times greater in the amateur pitchers. Conversely, the muscle activity of the subscapularis, serratus anterior, and latissimus dorsi was significantly greater in professional throwers. These findings suggest that the professional pitchers require less muscular activity of the stabilizing muscles because of improved throwing efficiency. During arm deceleration, the amateur throwers had more than twice the amount of muscle activity of the posterior deltoid and biceps brachii. This fact suggests that the less-skilled thrower requires greater muscular activity to perform the same task because of less efficient throwing biomechanics. This study may imply that the amateur pitcher may be more likely to sustain overuse tendinitis of the shoulder musculature compared with the highly skilled pitcher. Several investigators reported that the unskilled tennis player produces significantly greater EMG activity than the highly skilled player when performing the tennis service motion (14,15).

Gloussmann and colleagues (16) examined and compared the EMG activity of the shoulder musculature in individuals with glenohumeral instability with that of individuals without instability during the overhead pitching motion. The investigators reported a marked increase in EMG of the supraspinatus, infraspinatus, and biceps brachii muscles during the cocking and acceleration phases in the individuals with instability. Additionally, the subscapularis, pectoralis major, latissimus dorsi, and serratus anterior muscles exhibited a significant decrease in muscular activity during the cocking and acceleration phases. These findings may suggest a conscious or subconscious compensatory mechanism for shoulder instability, whereby the powerful accelerating muscles are inhibited, and the stabilizing muscles act to a greater degree.

THE ATHLETE

Because of the highly specific nature of throwing in baseball, it should be no surprise that much of the adaptation to training is focused on the shoulder and elbow.

The Thrower's Shoulder

On physical examination of the thrower's shoulder and elbow joint, a characteristic pattern becomes obvious.

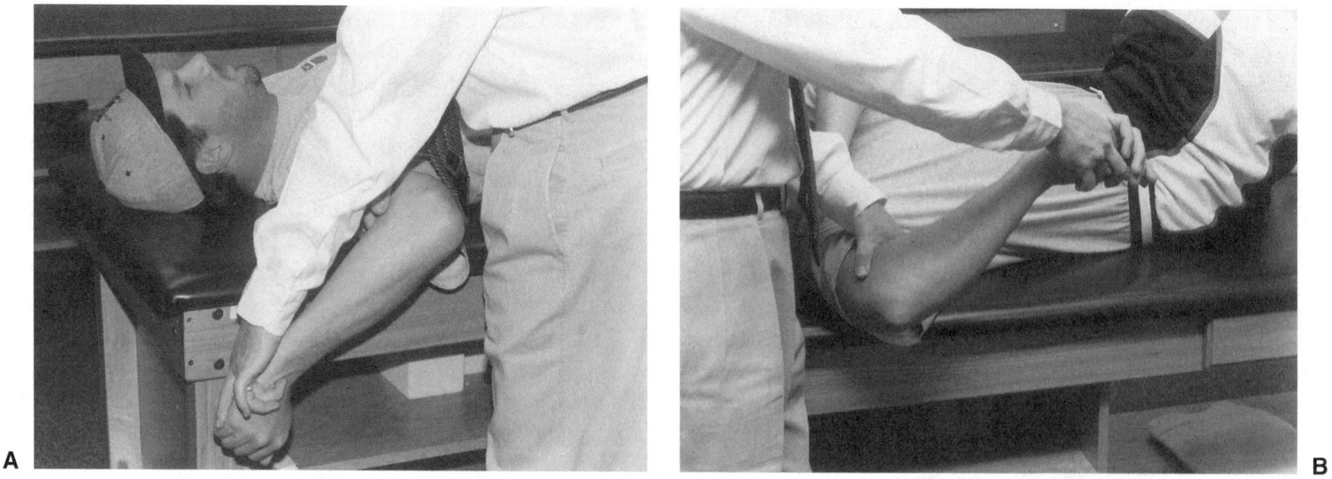

FIG. 45–4. The range of motion of the thrower's shoulder. **A**: External rotation to 138 degrees. **B**: Internal rotation to 50 degrees.

The professional baseball player's shoulder joint usually exhibits excessive external rotation (approximately 129 ± 9°) and a significant reduction in internal rotation (approximately 62 ± 9°; see Fig. 45–4). Additionally, the thrower's (particularly pitcher's) elbow joint usually exhibits a marked reduction in elbow extension; usually in the pitcher, a 5 to 20 degree flexion contracture is often present.

Several investigators examined the range of motion of the throwing shoulder in the pitcher as well as the position players. Brown and co-workers (17) examined the range of motion of 41 professional players and compared 18 pitchers' motions with those of 23 positional players. The investigators reported significant differences in range of motion of the dominant and nondominant arm for pitchers. Pitchers demonstrated 9 degrees more external rotation, 15 degrees less internal rotation, 11 degrees less horizontal abduction, and 6 degrees less elbow extension. Position players demonstrated 8 degrees more external rotation, a 14-degree loss of horizontal abduction, and 8 degrees loss of elbow extension. Additionally, pitchers exhibited 9 degrees more external rotation in the dominant arm than did position players.

Johnson (18) reported the range of motion of 26 collegiate baseball players from two universities. The players included 17 infielders and outfielders, and nine pitchers. The author reported that the pitchers' dominant arms exhibited 136 ± 14 degrees of external rotation; this was 8 degrees greater than the nondominant shoulder, 15 degrees greater than the outfielder's dominant shoulder, and 21 degrees greater than the infielder's dominant shoulder. The author reported that the pitcher's dominant shoulder exhibited greater internal rotation (111 degrees) than that of the infielders' (110 degrees) and outfielders' (106 degrees) shoulders. This result is a little surprising, as it has been my experience that the pitcher's shoulder usually exhibits significantly less internal rotation than reported by this study.

Recently Bigliani and associates (19) examined the range of motion of 148 professional baseball players: 72 pitchers and 76 position players. The average external rotation with the arm positioned in 90 degrees of abduction was statistically greater, and the average internal rotation was significantly less in the dominant shoulders that in the nondominant shoulders, both in pitchers and in position players. The authors reported that for pitchers, external rotation with the arm abducted to 90 degrees averaged 118 degrees (range, 95 to 145 degrees) on the dominant shoulder. Conversely, position players' dominant shoulders averaged 109 degrees (range, 80 to 150 degrees). In addition, the investigators noted that internal rotation was about the same for pitchers and for position players.

The Thrower's Elbow

Several investigators have reported a significant decrease in elbow extension in pitchers as well as position players (20–27). As previously mentioned, Brown and colleagues (17) reported elbow extension 6 degrees less in pitchers and 8 degrees less in position players when compared with the nondominant side. Other authors have noted a loss of elbow extension up to 15 to 20 degrees. King and associates (23) examined the radiographic changes at the elbow in professional baseball pitchers and found consistent evidence correlating these changes with decreased range of motion. Another possible cause of loss of elbow extension is soft-tissue trauma during the ball release to the deceleration phase of the throw. Additionally, as stated previously, during arm acceleration through deceleration, the elbow extends to an average of 20 degrees flexion and does not fully extend (4). This may represent adaptive changes at the elbow joint due to throwing.

Shoulder Laxity

Shoulder laxity is defined as the ability to translate the humeral head on the glenoid. One would expect the thrower's shoulder to exhibit significant laxity because of motion requirements necessary to throw a ball and the range of motion exhibited on clinical examination. Although this assumption appears obvious, few studies have documented shoulder laxity in the throwing athlete. Bigliani and co-workers (19) examined shoulder laxity in 72 professional baseball pitchers and 76 professional position players. The investigators noted a high degree of asymptomatic inferior glenohumeral joint laxity, with 61% of pitchers and 47% of position players exhibiting a sulcus sign on their dominant shoulders. Additionally, in the players who exhibited a positive sulcus sign on the dominant side, 54% of pitchers exhibited a sulcus sign on the nondominant shoulder; only 45% of position players exhibited this on the nondominant shoulder. The authors reported no correlation between laxity and players' age or length of professional baseball career in years.

Thus, it would appear from the findings of these studies and clinical observations that the following statements are true: (a) The thrower's shoulder exhibits excessive external rotation; (b) the pitcher's shoulder exhibits greater external rotation than that of position players; and (c) shoulder laxity is greater on the throwing shoulder than on the nonthrowing shoulder, but some throwers exhibit bilateral laxity.

The remaining question is whether these differences in range of motion and laxity are adaptive (i.e., a physiologic response to repetitive microtrauma) or selective (i.e., high-level athletes with inherent glenohumeral laxity), or a combination of the two. Some authors stated that these differences are adaptive (17,28). Certainly the presence of inferior laxity in the dominant shoulder of throwers can indicate an adaptive response to the repetitive throwing motion, particularly the higher degree of external rotation required during the late cocking and arm-acceleration phases of throwing. However, Bigliani and associates (19) reported that a significant number of players exhibited a positive bilateral sulcus sign. Thus I believe that, whereas some shoulder laxity may be the result of an adaptive response to repetitive throwing, preexisting inherent glenohumeral laxity may play a role in the selection of athletes who are able to succeed at a high level of competition.

Because of the excessive glenohumeral joint motion exhibited by the throwing athlete, most frequently the anterior and inferior aspect of the shoulder joint capsule is lax. This excessive laxity allows the excessive range of motion necessary to perform the throwing motion fluently. The hypermobility of the shoulder joint capsule can be appreciated during the stability assessment of the glenohumeral joint, particularly during the anterior drawer, anterior fulcrum, and sulcus tests (29). On clinical examination, the clinician will "feel" that the humeral head translates to a greater degree than does a nonthrowing shoulder. Additionally, the clinician should assess the end feel when performing these stability tests; this is an important variable to assess. The excessive laxity and increased motion is referred to as "thrower's laxity" in this chapter (30).

Muscular Strength and Performance

Several investigators have examined the muscular strength in the overhead throwing athlete (17,31–36), with varying results and conclusions. Alderink and Kuck (32) and Hinton (34) reported the external rotator strength being greater on the nonthrowing side compared with the throwing shoulder. Conversely, Brown and associates (17) reported that the throwing shoulder external rotators exhibited greater isokinetic strength. Cook and co-workers (33) reported that both shoulders were equal in strength. In the bilateral comparison of internal-rotation strength, Alderink and colleagues (32) and Cook and associates (33) reported the throwing and nonthrowing shoulder as being equal, whereas Brown and colleagues (17) and Hinton (34) noted that the throwing shoulders' internal rotation was significantly stronger. Additionally, these investigators published data regarding unilateral muscle ratios (ER/IR) of the shoulder (see Table 45–2).

Wilk and colleagues (35) reported the results of isokinetic muscular-performance testing in 150 professional baseball pitchers. The results of external-rotation

TABLE 45–2. *Unilateral muscle ratios (ER/IR)*

	Angular velocity (deg/s)						
	60	90	120	180	210	240	300
Alderink (32)							
D	—	66	68	—	71	—	70
ND	—	70	72	—	76	—	76
Brown (17)							
D	—	—	—	67	—	61	65
ND	—	—	—	71	—	66	65
Cook (33)							
D	—	—	—	70	—	—	70
ND	—	—	—	81	—	—	81
Hinton (35)							
D	—	69	—	—	—	71	—
ND	—	76	—	—	—	80	—
Wilk (35)							
D	—	—	—	65	—	—	61
ND	—	—	—	64	—	—	70

TABLE 45–3. *Data profile for the throwing athlete*

Velocity (deg/s)	Bilateral comparison			
	ER	IR	ABD	ADD
180	98–105	110–118	98–103	110–122
300	85–95	105–113	96–102	110–123
Velocity (deg/s)	**Unilateral muscle ratios**			
		ER/IR		ABD/ADD
180		65–75		78–84
300		61–71		88–94
Velocity (deg/s)	**Torque to body-weight ratios**			
	ER	IR	ABD	ADD
180	18–23	27–33	26–32	32–38
300	15–20	25–30	19–25	28–34

strength testing indicated that the dominant shoulder was weaker at 180 degree/s and bilaterally equal at 300°/s. The pitcher's internal-rotation strength was slightly stronger on the dominant side at both test speeds (180 and 300°/s). The unilateral muscle ratios for the ER/IR muscles are represented in Table 45–3. Additionally, peak torque-to–body weight ratios are illustrated in Table 45–3.

Wilk and co-workers (36) reported the abductor and adductor strength characteristics of professional baseball pitchers. The results indicated that shoulder abduction was approximately equal bilaterally; however, adduction was significantly stronger in the dominant shoulder. The abductor/adductor unilateral muscle ratios and peak torque-to–body weight ratios are represented in Table 45–3.

Often the question is raised, "Does a relationship between shoulder strength and the ability to throw exist?" Bartlett and colleagues (37) examined the relationship of shoulder strength and throwing speed in 11 professional pitchers and reported a positive statistical relationship between shoulder-adductor strength and throwing speed. In comparison, Pedegana and associates (31), in a similar research design of eight professional baseball pitchers, found no direct relationship between adductor muscular strength and throwing speed.

Additionally, it is not uncommon for the pitcher to exhibit significant muscular weakness of the throwing shoulder. Often muscular weakness can be noted of the supraspinatus and external rotators when compared with the contralateral shoulder. Magnusson and colleagues (38) compared static muscular strength in professional pitchers with that of an age-matched nonthrowing control group. The pitcher's dominant shoulder was weaker in external rotation and "isolated" supraspinatus muscle testing than that in the nondominant side and significantly weaker than that in the control group. This is a common observation and is often reconfirmed when the strength of a professional pitcher is tested by a trainer or clinician.

Scapular muscular strength also is very important for the overhead thrower. No published studies have documented the muscular strength of the scapular musculature in the overhead thrower. Scapular muscles of particular interest are the trapezius (upper, middle, and lower fibers), serratus anterior, rhomboids, and levator scapula. Scapular muscle strength is critical to the overhead athlete in establishing a stable base of support (foundation) from which the humerus and arm act (39–42). Additionally, trunk and leg musculature strength is very important to the throwing athlete.

Neuromuscular Control

Although muscular strength is an important physical attribute to the thrower's shoulder, perhaps as or more important are the neuromuscular control abilities exhibited by the athlete. As previously mentioned, the thrower's shoulder must be lax enough to throw but stable enough not to sublux. The dynamic stability required to prevent glenohumeral subluxation is accomplished through the combined actions of the glenohumeral joint capsule and surrounding musculature. The glenohumeral joint musculature must work in a synchronized fashion both to accelerate the arm and to stabilize the glenohumeral joint dynamically. The surrounding musculature of the glenohumeral joint must act to co-contract through coactivation to produce glenohumeral-joint compression, thus creating dynamic stability. Dynamic stability occurs through the combined actions of the neurologic system through afferent sensory input and the muscular actions (efferent response) to the sensory input. This is referred to as neuromuscular control and is a critical aspect to sports performance and particularly the overhead throw.

Proprioception refers to the conscious and unconscious appreciation of joint position (43). Kinesthesia is the sensation of joint motion or acceleration. The efferent (motor) response to sensory information is referred to as neuromuscular control (44). All three components play a vital role in dynamic stabilization of the thrower's shoulder. Although proprioception and neuromuscular control are critical components for dynamic stability, no published studies have tested these areas in the overhead athlete. However, two studies documented the effect of shoulder injury on proprioception (45,46).

Smith and Brunoli (45) were the first to investigate the effect of capsuloligamentous injury on proprioception in the shoulder. They reported that patients with unilateral, recurrent, traumatic anterior shoulder instability demonstrated proprioceptive sensory deficits. Lephart and colleagues (46) performed the first study comparing shoulder proprioception in groups of individuals with normal, unstable, and surgically repaired shoulders. The results revealed significant proprioceptive deficits in patients who have chronic, traumatic anterior shoulder instability and that surgical stabilization of such a shoulder normalizes proprioceptive sensibility. Voight and co-workers (47) examined the effects of muscular fatigue on shoulder-joint proprioception in individuals without shoulder pathology. The investigators noted that shoulder proprioception was diminished in the presence of muscular fatigue, suggesting that various muscular receptors contribute to proprioception.

Thus it would appear that proprioception and neuromuscular-control abilities play a significant role in effective injury-free throwing. Although a standardized proprioceptive test has not been established for the throwing athlete, I have clinically used a test maneuver to assess proprioception and neuromuscular control. The patient lies supine with eyes closed; the clinician passively moves the patient's arm through a proprioceptive neuromuscular facilitation (PNF) D_2 flexion/extension path (48) of motion twice; then the patient is asked to replicate that path of motion as closely as possible with the eyes remaining closed (Fig. 45–5). The patients are evaluated as to how closely they can replicate the exact movement without deviating from the path of motion. A deviation in motion of more than 3 inches has been treated as significant, and treatment would emphasize proprioceptive training to a greater extent than for the patient not exhibiting proprioception deficits. Recently, we have performed proprioception testing via joint repositioning in the throwing athlete. The results indicate no significant difference in proprioception between the throwing shoulder and the non-throwing shoulder.

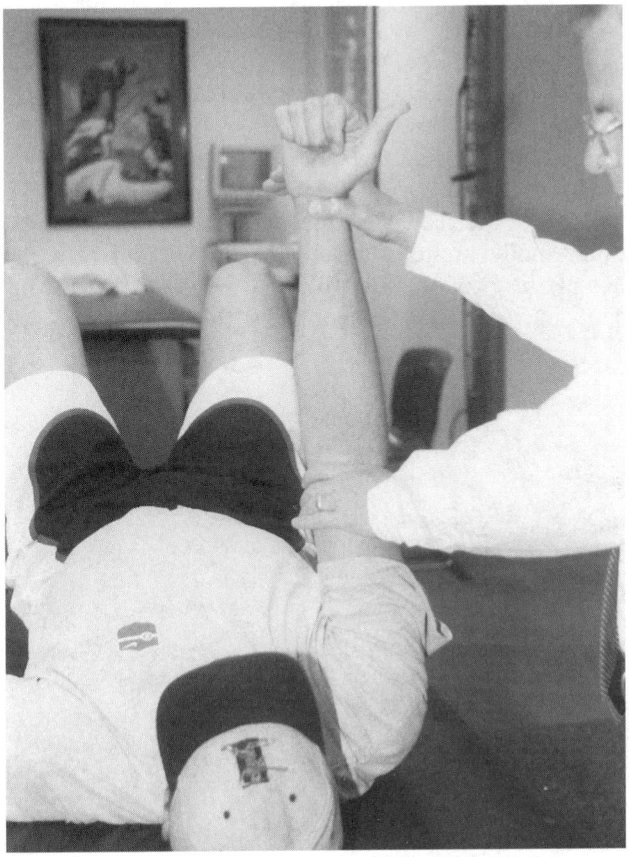

FIG. 45–5. Proprioceptive test for the overhead thrower. Initially, the patient's arm is passively taken though an arc of motion tracking a D_2 flexion/extension pattern; this is performed twice. Then the patient is asked to replicate the exact movement actively.

Thus the physiologic requirements of the overhead thrower are numerous. The requirements to throw effectively center around "the paradox of the thrower's shoulder"; the thrower's shoulder must be loose enough to be able to throw but exhibit enough stability to prevent glenohumeral joint subluxation. The thrower's shoulder appears to exhibit greater motion than the nondominant shoulder as a result of adaptive and inherent factors. Dynamic functional stability is accomplished through the combined efforts of the glenohumeral joint capsule and the neuromuscular systems. Muscular strength of the scapular region and the glenohumeral joint are important components in training or rehabilitating an overhead athlete. Additionally, proprioception and neuromuscular-control abilities are vital components and should also be included into the conditioning program.

TRAINING THE ATHLETE

When designing a training program for a throwing athlete, several questions must first be answered. What position does the athlete play? Pitcher or position player? What level is the athlete? Professional, collegiate, high school, and so on? Is the athlete recovering from an injury? Are there aspects of the rehabilitation program that must be integrated into the conditioning program? What type of pitcher is the athlete, finesse or overpowering? What type of program has the athlete used in the past? Was it effective?

After these questions have been thoroughly answered, then the conditioning program can be outlined. The professional baseball starting pitcher is usually limited to a specific number of pitches per game. The exact number varies slightly (each organization has different guidelines) but is usually between 110 and 125 pitches. Most starting pitchers pitch on a 4-day or 5-day rotation, so the pitcher will start a game every 4 to 5 days. Relief pitchers usually specialize, pitching either short relief (one to two innings) or middle relief (two to four innings). Collegiate pitchers usually pitch every 5 days.

Probably the most important pitching guidelines are for the adolescent players. Most Little League organizations limit the number of innings a pitcher can pitch per week. This number is usually limited to six to seven innings/week. Additionally, it is generally advocated that the adolescent pitcher not throw curveballs or sliders because of the excessively high stress applied to the elbow joint.

Sport-Specific Training

Optimal athletic performance requires three complementary abilities: skill, power, and motivation. All sports share these three elements. Skill is derived from the individual's own attributes (natural ability or God-given talent) and learned technical skill, as well as expertise. The learned portion of the skill equation takes years of training to develop. It requires hard work, determination, and guidance/direction from a qualified coach. One of the cornerstones of conditioning is the law of specificity, or the SAID principle, which states that the body will make specific adaptations to imposed demands.

Muscular power is derived from both natural ability and developed muscular characteristics. Power is a component of muscular strength but adds the additional element of time. Thus power is defined as total work divided by time; therefore power combines both strength and speed. Speed refers to the ability of the athlete rapidly to contract a muscle or muscle group; one component of speed is acceleration. Traditional weight training can develop strength, but another form of training is required to develop explosiveness or speed. Plyometrics is one form of exercise that can develop this type of explosive power and speed.

The third ingredient is motivation or desire. Motivation and desire come from many sources and experiences. For some athletes, it comes from within themselves. These athletes strive for greatness every day in training, practice, and games; they are self-motivated. On the other hand, there are athletes who are not self-motivated, and many times it is the coach or trainer who has to motivate the athlete. This situation is especially true with off-season conditioning programs, or rehabilitation from an injury. Thus the conditioning coach or trainer must learn ways to reach the athlete to motivate on the day that the athlete would rather skip the workout.

The major objectives of the conditioning program for the throwing athlete are injury prevention and performance enhancement. These two objectives are closely related to each other. A thorough, well-designed conditioning program will prevent injuries; a healthy athlete who trains properly should improve athletic performance and should experience a long, productive career. The conditioning program for the overhead throwing athlete should include the following components: strength, endurance, power, speed, flexibility, plyometrics, and neuromuscular and skill training. The athlete who trains or overemphasizes one component more than another, such as muscular strength, is prone to injury or diminished performance. The athlete cannot train at the same intensity or the same type of exercises throughout the year; rather the program must be specifically adjusted over the course of the year. The conditioning program should incorporate in-season and off-season goals and guidelines. These adjustments and modifications of the program throughout the year is referred to as the "periodization of training" (49).

Periodization

The concept of periodization refers to the year-round sequence and progression of weight-resistance training and skill training for the athlete. The periodization model specifies various phases during the year; most often, the program will use four specific and different training seasons during the calendar year. Table 45–3 illustrates a periodization model for the professional baseball player. This model can be modified to fit the collegiate player. These four phases are the competitive (in-season) phase, postcompetition phase, preparation phase, and the transition phase (49).

The periodization is based on controlling and adjusting three variables: volume of work, intensity of effort, and skill technique training (49). As illustrated in Fig. 45–5, volume and technique are inversely related, whereas intensity and technique are directly related. In some year-round sports, such as professional tennis, golf, or gymnastics, the periodization concept is difficult to implement. In these sports, often the athletes are expected to perform at a high level for 10 to 11 months of the year. This expectation is not realistic and cannot be accomplished for a long period or over a career. Usually the athlete will exhibit peaks and valleys in performance during the year and his or her career.

The conditioning program should change based on the time of the year. The objectives of using the periodization model are to (a) control peaking of athletic abilities at the proper time, (b) prevent the athlete from being untrained or undertrained at the beginning of the

TABLE 45–4. *Conditioning program for professional baseball player*

Phase I: Competition phase
In-season training
6 mo
April–September
Phase II: Postcompetition phase
Postseason (rest–recovery)
6–8 wk
October, November
Phase III: Preparation phase
Off-season conditioning
12 wk
Nov. 24–Feb. 15
Phase IV: Transitional phase
Spring training
6 wk
Feb. 16–Mar. 31

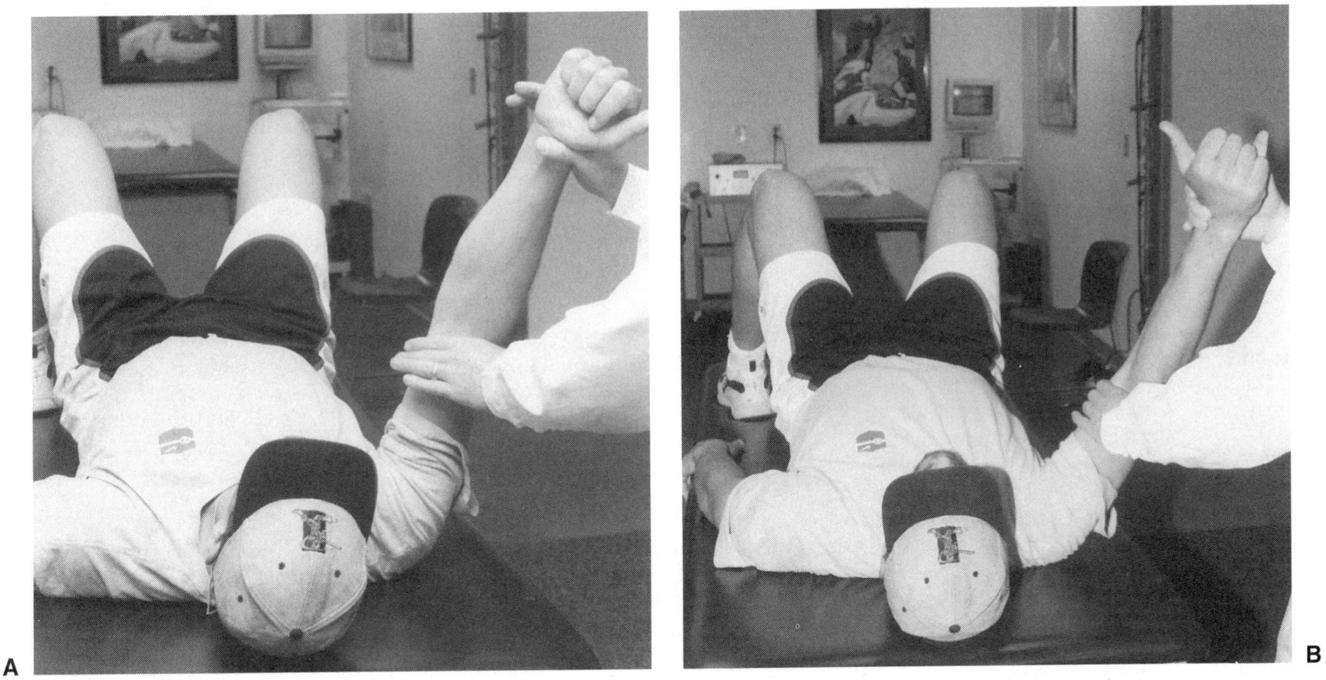

FIG. 45–6. Manual resistance is applied during a proprioceptive neuromuscular facilitation (PNF) D_2 flexion/extension pattern (**A** and **B**). Rhythm stabilization is performed at 105 degrees, with resistance applied during flexion and extension.

year, (c) prevent the athlete from overtraining, and (d) minimize boredom of training by adjusting and changing the program. All four of these scenarios can and often do lead to injuries or diminished athletic performance.

The concept of periodization has been applied to the conditioning program for a professional baseball pitcher (Table 45–4). The program is subdivided into four phases (seasons), each possessing its own goals as well as conditioning and skill exercises. This program can be modified for the collegiate or high school athlete.

During the off-season, there are three phases—two phases before the competitive season and one after the competitive season. For most professional baseball players, the competitive season usually ends approximately October 1. Immediately after the season, the phase is referred to as the postseason phase and lasts approximately 6 to 8 weeks. The goals during the phase are mental and physical recuperation, soft-tissue healing, and remaining physically active without baseball-related activities. During this phase, cardiovascular conditioning is emphasized with aerobic capacity training, and no skill training related to baseball is performed. We encourage athletes to perform low-intensity/long-duration conditioning activities, such as cycling, swimming, jogging, and walking, along with participation in recreational sports such as golf or tennis. The emphasis of this phase is aerobic capacity, general fitness, body-weight maintenance, and mental recuperation.

The preparation phase begins approximately the third

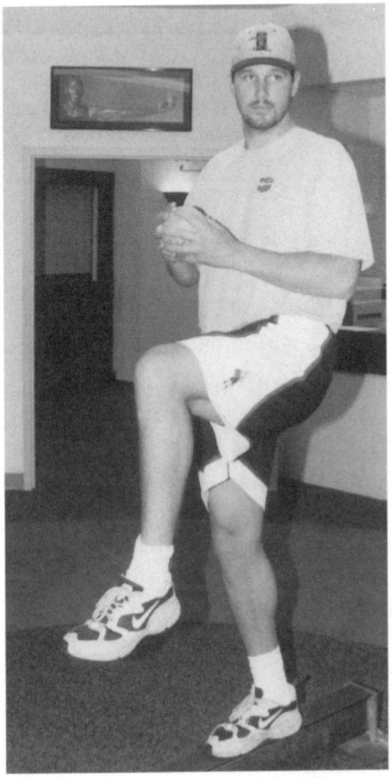

FIG. 45–7. A balance drill for the legs and trunk. The subject performs a "balance position" movement on a balance beam.

TABLE 45–5. *Concept of periodization in baseball*

	Goals	Conditioning exercises	Skill-training activities
In-season training "Competitive season" (6 mo)	Maintain strength, power, endurance to prevent arm injuries Prevent the breakdown of tissue Maintain cardiovascular endurance	Low weight/moderate number of repetitions per exercise; thrower's 10 exercise program Cardiovascular endurance 20–30 min daily to maintain fitness level/stamina training	Continue throwing activities to maintain proper throwing mechanics and refinement of pitches Throwing program is designed to emphasize the player's position Throwing/batting activities (volume) regulated by player's health status
Postseason training "Active-rest" (2 mo)	Mental and physical recuperation period Physical activity, but not baseball-type activities Allow tissues to heal Relaxation sports participation	Light conditioning program—bicycle, swimming, walking, jogging, aerobics Conditioning low intensity/long duration	No baseball-related drills Relaxation sports, such as golf, tennis, racquetball
Preparation phase "Off-season" (10–12 wk)	Gradually and progressively increase exercise demands—throwing exercises and drills Begin with light isotonic program; progress to eccentric and plyometric exercises Skill training is low to start with and throwing begins halfway through this phase *Ultimate goal* is be *in condition* for spring-training reporting date	Total body exercise program with emphasis on large muscle groups Moderate weight/moderate repetitive numbers to start with; isotonic concentric Progress program to eccentric program; progress to moderate weight/increase repetitions Cardiovascular training is emphasized—30 min daily to enhance fitness level Plyometric training drills initiated 2–3 wk before spring training	Initially no skill training 4–5 weeks into program, throwing program is initiated; interval long-toss program Batting practice initiated 4–5 weeks into phase
First transitional phase "Spring training" (4–6 wk)	Enhance conditioning level and enhance skill training (razor sharp) Initially high-volume conditioning, moderate-level skill training Then moderate-level conditioning, high-level skill training	Volume of conditioning drills is high at start of phase and sharply decreases halfway through Intensity of training and quality of movements is fine-tuned Plyometrics early phase, then discontinued Thrower's 10 program	Skill-technique training is emphasized Throwing/batting activities are emphasized; these skill activities are fine-tuned

week in November and lasts approximately 12 weeks. During this phase, the athlete begins to condition and prepare for sport-specific drills and spring training. In the beginning of this phase, the volume/quantity of exercise is high, whereas intensity is at a moderate level, and skill training is relatively low. The goals of this phase are to increase exercise demands gradually and progressively, beginning with light isotonic concentric work and progressing to isotonic eccentric, and eventually plyometrics. Baseball-related drills (skill training) are low at the start but gradually increase halfway through this phase.

The preparation phase may be subdivided into two stages of 6 weeks each. During the first stage, the emphasis is on total body conditioning and strengthening of the larger muscle groups, such as the latissimus dorsi, pectoralis major, subscapularis, deltoid, biceps/triceps, gluteal, quadriceps, hamstring, and gastrocsoleus muscles. The athlete will perform exercises such as rowing, pull-downs, push-ups, bench press, military press, squats, and lunges. Additionally, stabilization exercises are performed to enhance dynamic stabilization of the shoulder joint, stimulate co-contraction, and enhance proprioception (50,51). These exercises usually include PNF D_2 flexion/extension patterns (Fig. 45–6). Neuromuscular training drills are performed for the scapulothoracic joint. During this phase, the athlete must stretch to maintain flexibility and perform some type of cardiovascular exercise for at least 25 to 30 minutes. Core stability or balance are trained through balance drills on a balance board or balance beam. The pitcher is asked to maintain the "balance position" of the wind-up on the balance beam (Fig. 45–7). This drill has been beneficial for all levels of throwers.

Throwers Ten Exercise Program

The Throwers Ten Program is designed to exercise the major muscles necessary for throwing. The program's goal is to be an organized and concise exercise program. In addition, all exercises included are specific to the thrower and are designed to improve strength, power and endurance of the shoulder complex musculature.

1. A. **Diagonal Pattern D2 Extension:**
Involved hand will grip tubing handle overhead and out to the side. Pull tubing down and across your body to the opposite side of leg. During the motion lead with your thumb. Perform _______ sets of ____ repetitions ______ daily.

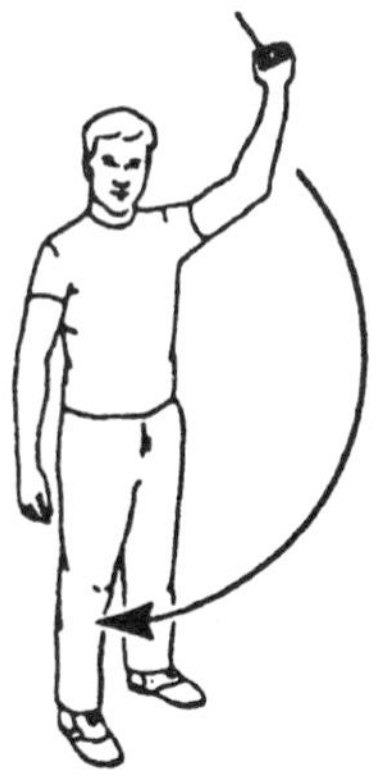

1. B. **Diagonal Pattern D2 Flexion:**
Gripping tubing handle in hand of involved arm, begin with arm out from side 45° and palm facing backward. After turning palm forward, proceed to flex elbow and bring arm up and over uninvolved shoulder. Turn palm down and reverse to take arm to starting position. Exercise should be performed in controlled manner. Perform _____ sets of ______ repetitions _____ daily.

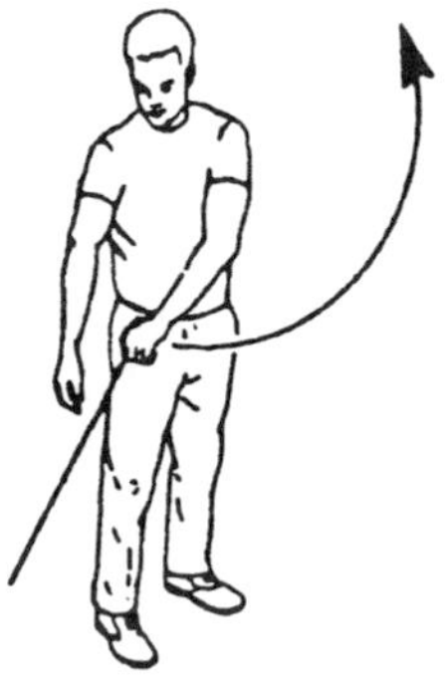

2. A. **External Rotation at 0° Abduction:**
Stand with involved elbow fixed at side, elbow at 90° and involved arm across front of body. Grip tubing handle while the other end of tubing is fixed. Pull out with arm, keeping elbow at side. Return tubing slowly and controlled. Perform ______ sets of ________ repetitions _____ times daily.

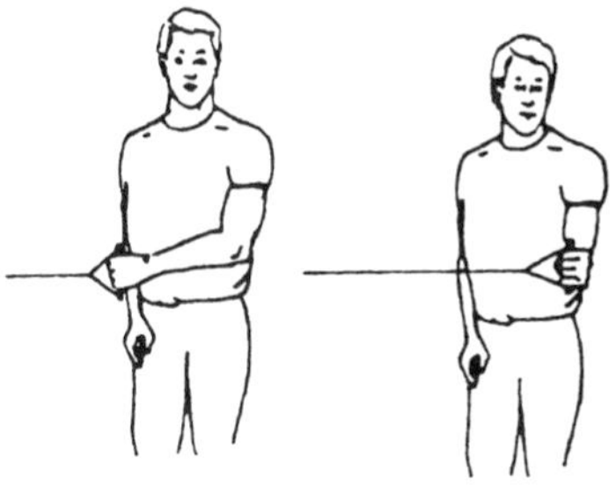

2. B. **Internal Rotation at 0° Abduction:**
Standing with elbow at side fixed at 90° and shoulder rotated out. Grip tubing handle while other end of tubing is fixed. Pull arm across body keeping elbow at side. Return tubing slowly and controlled. Perform _____ sets of _____ repetitions ______ times daily.

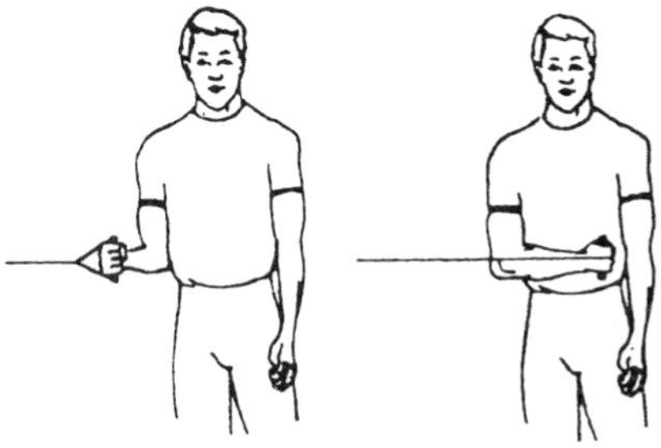

FIG. 45–8. The "thrower's ten" exercise program.

During the second stage of the preparation phase, the goals are to improve rotator-cuff strength and to initiate eccentric training, plyometric drills, and sport-specific drills (throwing and hitting). During this 6-week phase, the athlete is established on the "thrower's ten" exercise program (Fig. 45–8). This program was developed based on the collective EMG research of numerous investigators (52–56). Additional strengthening exercises can be added to this exercise program based on deficiencies or imbalances. Plyometric drills specific for the thrower can also be implemented at this time (Fig. 45–9). A throwing program also is initiated at the time,

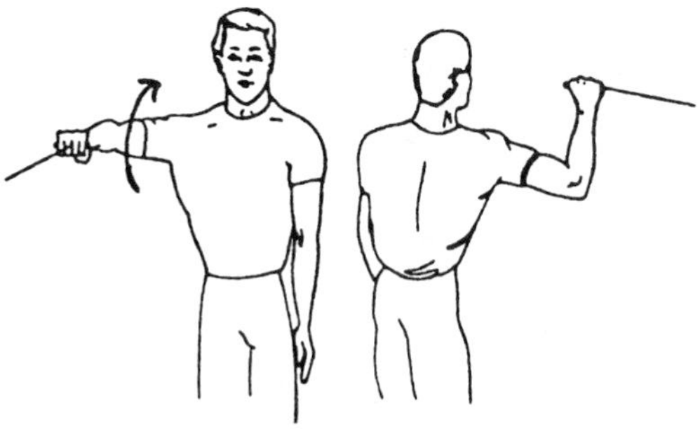

2. C. External Rotation at 90° Abduction:
Stand with shoulder abducted 90° and elbow flexed 90°. Grip tubing handle while the other end is fixed straight ahead, slightly lower than the shoulder. Keeping shoulder abducted, rotate shoulder back keeping elbow at 90°. Return tubing and hand to start position.

I. Slow Speed Sets: (Slow and Controlled): Perform _____ sets of _____ repetitions _____ times daily.

II. Fast Speed Sets: Perform _____ sets of _____ repetitions _____ times daily.

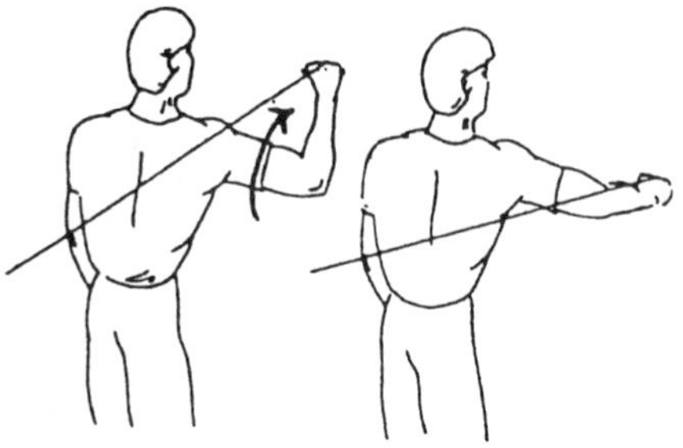

2. D Internal Rotation at 90° Abduction:
Stand with shoulder abducted to 90°, externally rotated 90° and elbow bent to 90°. Keeping shoulder abducted, rotate shoulder forward, keeping elbow bent at 90°. Return tubing and hand to start position.

I. Slow Speed Sets: (Slow and Controlled): Perform _____ sets of _____ repetitions _____ times daily.

II. Fast Speed Sets: Perform _____ sets of _____ repetitions _____ times daily.

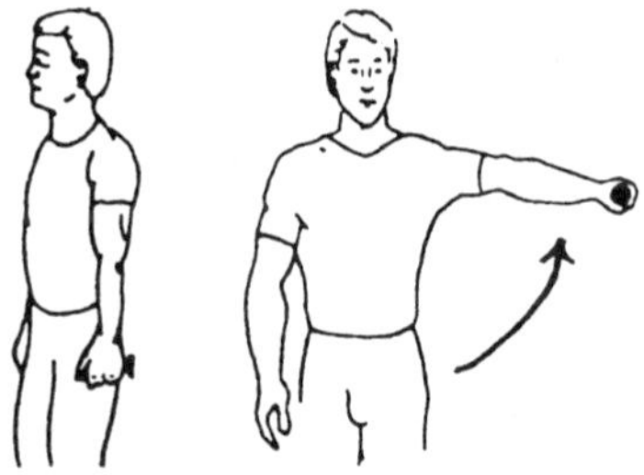

3. Shoulder Abduction to 90°:
Stand with arm at side, elbow straight, and palm against side. Raise arm to the side, palm down, until arm reaches 90° (shoulder level). Hold 2 seconds and lower slowly. Perform _____ sets of _____ repetitions ______ times daily.

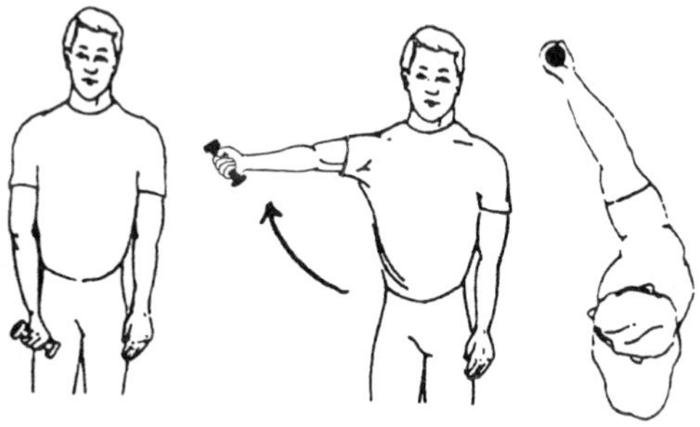

4. Scaption, Internal Rotation:
Stand with elbow straight and thumb up. Raise arm to shoulder level at 30° angle in front of body. Do not go above shoulder height. Hold 2 seconds and lower slowly. Perform _____ sets of _____ repetitions _____ times daily.

FIG. 45–8. *Continued*

5\. A. Prone Horizontal Abduction (Neutral):
Lie on table, face down, with involved arm hanging straight to the floor, and palm facing down. Raise arm out to the side, parallel to the floor. Hold 2 seconds and lower slowly. Perform ______ sets of _____ repetitions _____times daily.

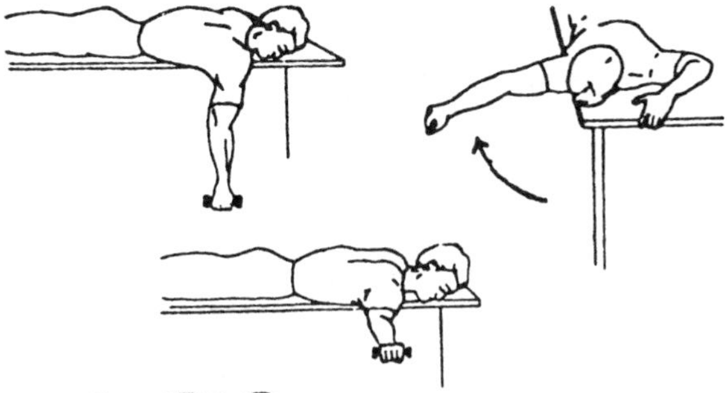

5\. B. Prone Horizontal Abduction Full ER, 100° ABD):
Lie on table, face down, with involved arm hanging straight to the floor, and thumb rotated up (hitchhiker). Raise arm out to the side with arm slightly in front of shoulder, parallel to the floor. Hold 2 seconds and lower slowly. Perform _____ sets of ______ repetitions _____ times daily.

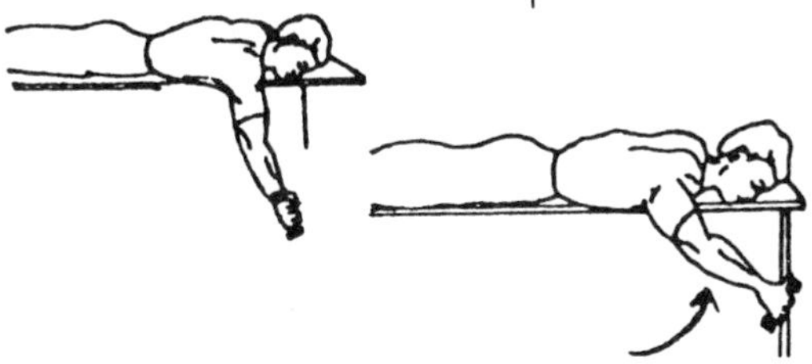

6\. Press-Ups:
Seated on a chair or on a table, place both hands firmly on the sides of the chair or table, palm down and fingers pointed outward. Hands should be placed equal with shoulders. Slowly push downward through the hands to elevate your body. Hold the elevated position for 2 seconds and lower body slowly. Perform _____ sets of _____ repetitions ______ times daily.

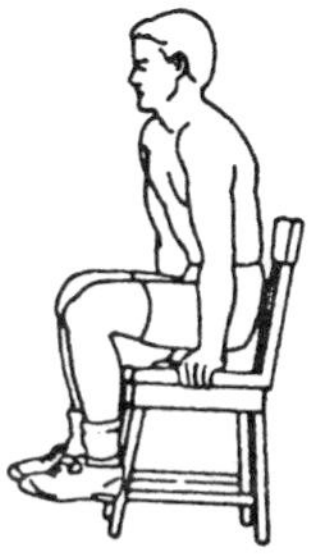

7\. Prone Rowing:
Lying on your stomach with your involved arm hanging over the side of the table, dumbbell in hand and elbow straight. Slowly raise arm, bending elbow, and bring dumbbell as high as possible. Hold at the top for 2 seconds, then slowly lower. Perform ______ sets of ______ repetitions _______ times daily.

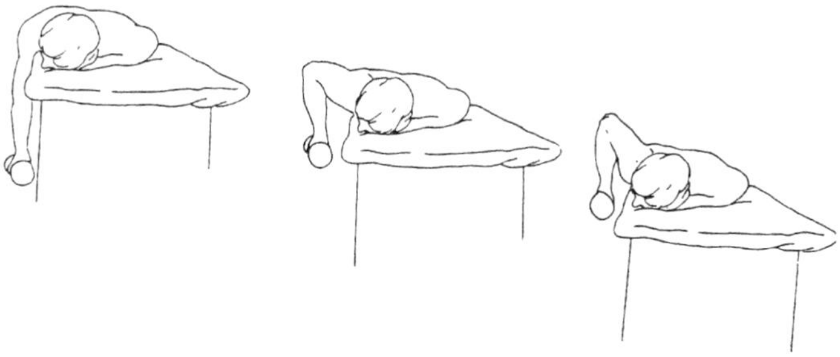

8\. Push-Ups:
Start in the down position with arms in a comfortable position. Place hands no more than shoulder width apart. Push up as high as possible, rolling shoulders forward after elbows are straight. Start with a push-up into wall.. Gradually progress to table top and evenutally to floor as tolerable. Perform ______ sets of ______ repetitions _______ times daily.

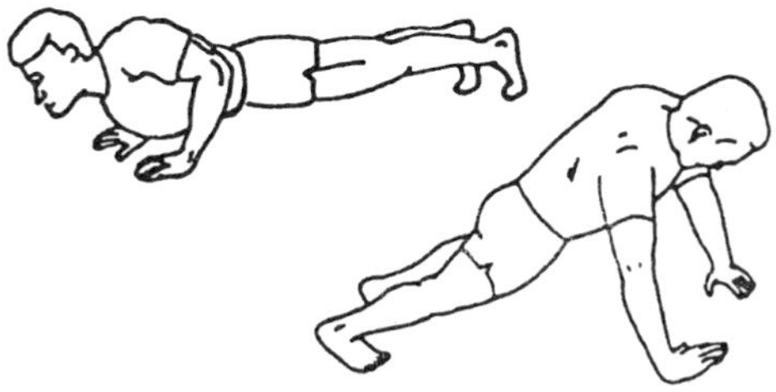

FIG. 45–8. *Continued*

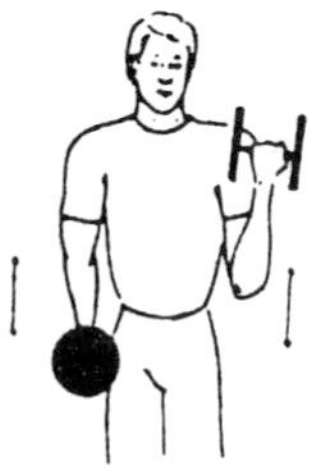

9. A. **Elbow Flexion:**
Standing with arm against side and palm facing inward, bend elbow upward turning palm up as you progress. Hold 2 seconds and lower slowly. Perform _____ sets of _____ repetitions _____ times daily.

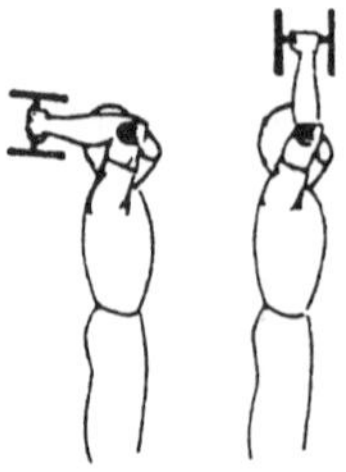

9. B. **Elbow Extension:**
Abduction:
Raise involved arm overhead. Provide support at elbow from uninvolved hand. Straighten arm overhead. Hold 2 seconds and lower slowly. Perform _____ sets of _____ repetitions ______ times daily.

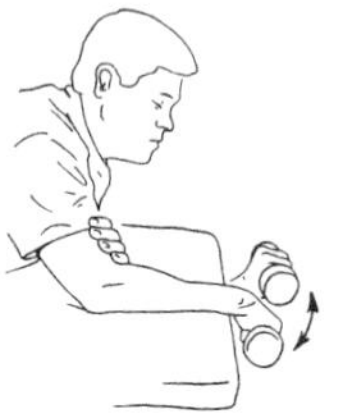

10. A. **Wrist Extension:**
Supporting the forearm and with palm facing downward, raise weight in hand as far as possible. Hold 2 seconds and lower slowly. Perform _____ sets of _____ repetitions ______ times daily.

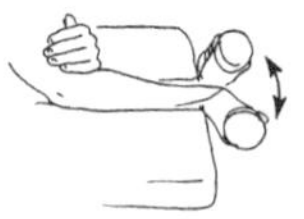

10. B. **Wrist Flexion:**
Supporting the forearm and with palm facing upward, lower a weight in hand as far as possible and then curl it up as high as possible. Hold for 2 seconds and lower slowly. Perform _____ sets of _____ repetitions _____ times daily.

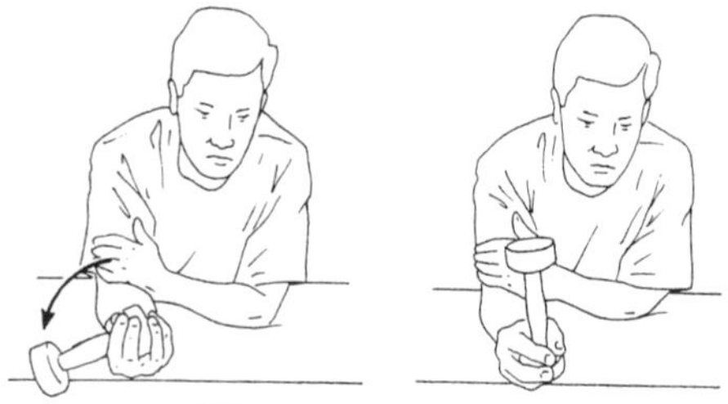

10. C. **Supination:**
Forearm supported on table with wrist in neutral position. Using a weight or hammer, roll wrist taking palm up. Hold for a 2 count and return to starting position. Perform ____ sets of _____ repetitions _____ times daily.

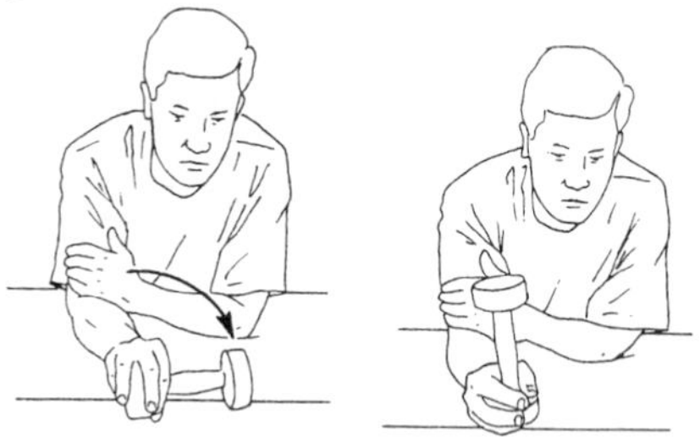

10. D. **Pronation:**
Forearm should be supported on a table with wrist in neutral position. Using a weight or hammer, roll wrist taking palm down. Hold for a 2 count and return to starting position. Perform ____ sets of ______ repetitions ____ times daily.

FIG. 45–8. *Continued*

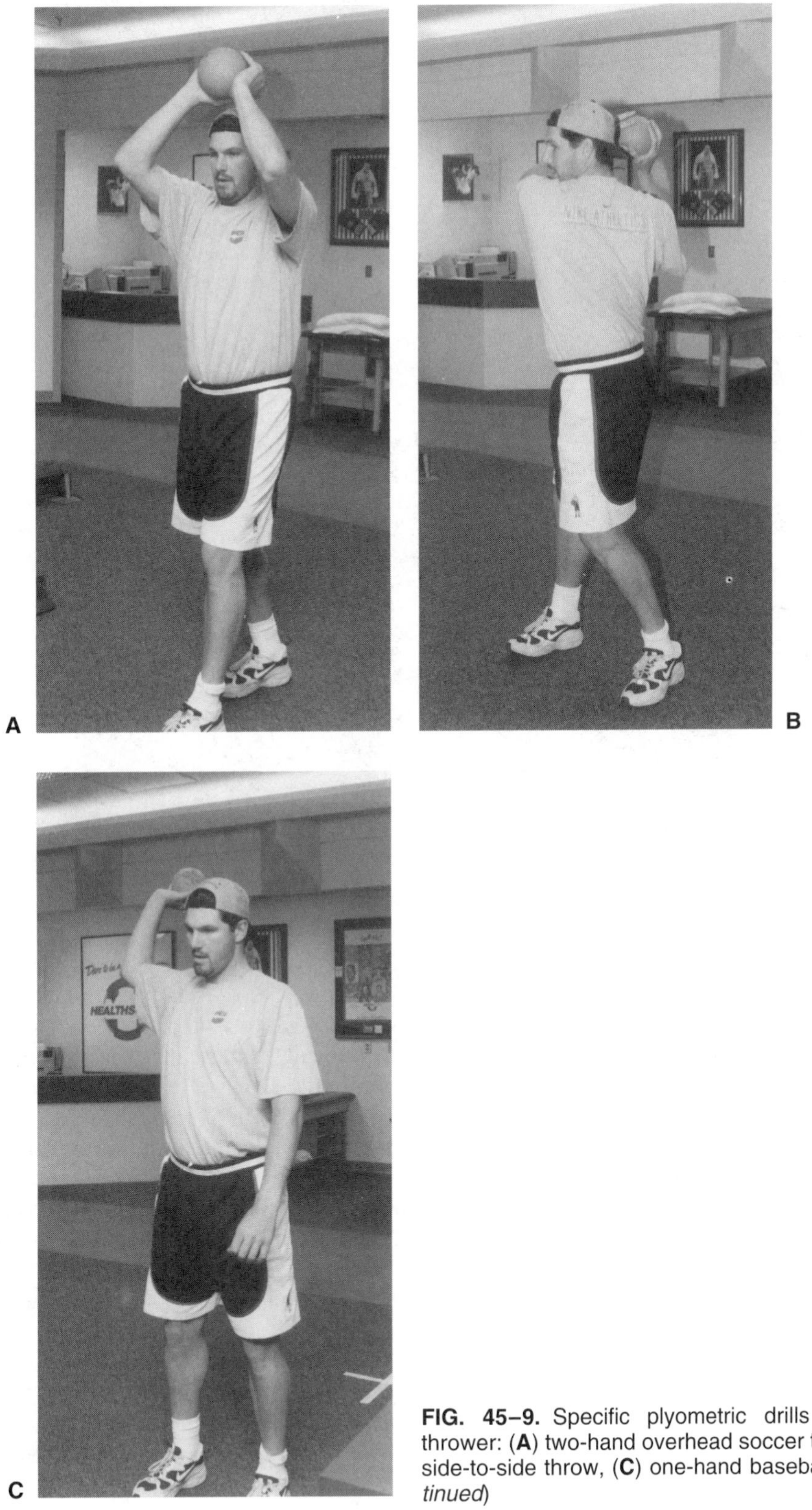

FIG. 45–9. Specific plyometric drills for the overhead thrower: (**A**) two-hand overhead soccer throw, (**B**) two-hand, side-to-side throw, (**C**) one-hand baseball-style throw. (*continued*)

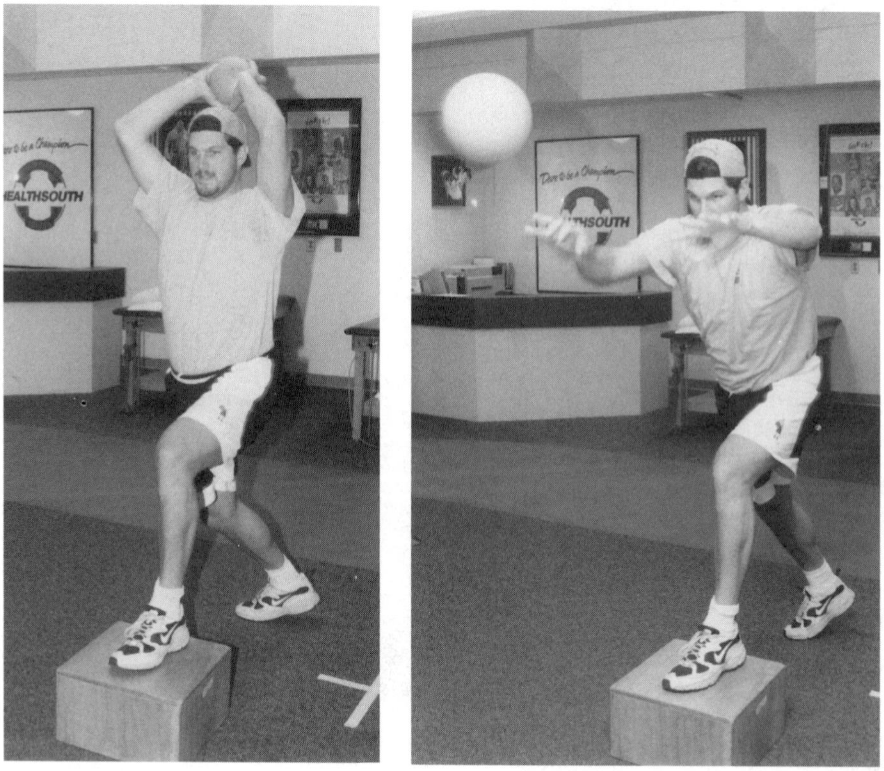

FIG. 45–9. *Continued.* (**D** and **E**) two-hand soccer throw with forward lunge and trunk flexion.

and usually begins with a long-toss program starting at 45 feet and progressing to 120 to 150 feet (Table 45–5) (56). Once the thrower can throw from 120 to 150 feet without soreness or pain, then the thrower can progress to a throwing program from the mound (Table 45–6). Another key component to training in this phase is endurance training. It has been shown that rotator-cuff fatigue results in the superior migration of the humeral head (57,58). This could contribute to rotator-cuff inflammation and injury. Thus endurance drills are critical for the overhead thrower. Numerous types of drills can be used to enhance endurance (Fig. 45–10). During this second stage, the intensity and skill-specific training aspects increase as the volume of exercise gradually decreases.

The next phase is the transitional phase, and in professional baseball this is spring training. This phase consists of 4 to 6 weeks of conditioning and skill training, preparing the player for the competitive season. The goals of this phase are to enhance the conditioning level and skill level of the athlete, along with sport-specific training to become mentally and physically prepared for the upcoming season. During this conditioning phase, the level of conditioning exercises is gradually decreased while the quality of work performed and the amount of skill training is rapidly increased, maintaining the inverse relation between volume and technique. Plyometric drills may be used early in this phase, but as the phase progresses these drills are gradually decreased.

The competitive season in professional baseball is long and physically demanding. The season lasts approximately 6 months. During the season, it is imperative to perform strengthening exercises to enhance and maintain muscular and connective tissue strength. The goals of this phase include (a) reaching peak performance; (b) maintaining achieved strength, power, and endurance to prevent injury; (c) preventing tissue breakdown (inflammation); and (d) maintaining cardiovascular endurance. The in-season exercise program is the thrower's 10 program, neuromuscular stabilization drills, stretching drills, and cardiovascular exercise. It must be explained to athletes that sport participation does not condition; rather, the athlete conditions to participate. During the competitive season, because of tissue breakdown, the athlete becomes susceptible to injury and diminishing performance if conditioning exercises are not performed to counteract this effect.

REHABILITATION OVERVIEW

The majority of injuries to the shoulder and elbow joint can be successfully treated nonoperatively with a thorough and comprehensive rehabilitation program. For

TABLE 45–6A. *Interval throwing program starting off the mound, phase I*

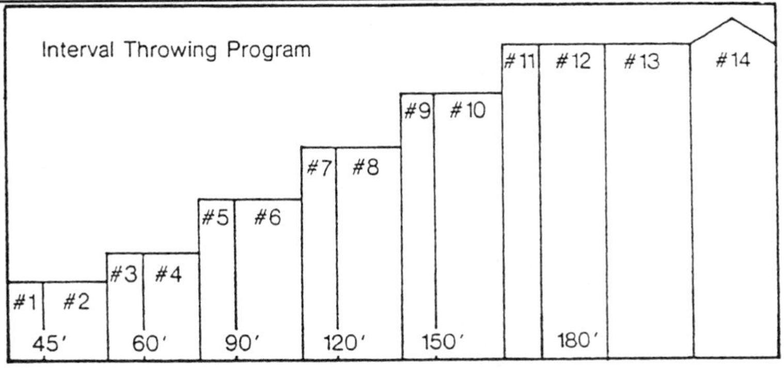

45' Phase

Step 1: A) Warm-up throwing
B) 45′ (25 throws)
C) Rest 15 minutes
D) Warm-up throwing
E) 45′ (25 throws)

Step 2: A) Warm-up throwing
B) 45′ (25 throws)
C) Rest 10 minutes
D) Warm-up throwing
E) 45′ (25 throws)
F) Rest 10 minutes
G) Warm-Up Throwing
H) 45′ (25 Throws)

60' Phase

Step 3: A) Warm-up throwing
B) 60′ (25 throws)
C) Rest 15 minutes
D) Warm-up throwing
E) 60′ (25 throws)

Step 4: A) Warm-up throwing
B) 60′ (25 throws)
C) Rest 10 minutes
D) Warm-up throwing
E) 60′ (25 throws)
F) Rest 10 minutes
G) Warm-Up Throwing
H) 60′ (25 Throws)

90' Phase

Step 5: A) Warm-up throwing
B) 90′ (25 throws)
C) Rest 15 minutes
D) Warm-up throwing
E) 90′ (25 throws)

Step 6: A) Warm-up throwing
B) 90′ (25 throws)
C) Rest 10 minutes
D) Warm-up throwing
E) 90′ (25 throws)
F) Rest 10 minutes
G) Warm-Up Throwing
H) 90′ (25 Throws)

120' Phase

Step 7: A) Warm-up throwing
B) 120′ (25 throws)
C) Rest 15 minutes
D) Warm-up throwing
E) 120′ (25 throws)

Step 8: A) Warm-up throwing
B) 120′ (25 throws)
C) Rest 10 minutes
D) Warm-up throwing
E) 120′ (25 throws)
F) Rest 10 minutes
G) Warm-Up Throwing
H) 120′ (25 Throws)

150' Phase

Step 9: A) Warm-up throwing
B) 150′ (25 throws)
C) Rest 15 minutes
D) Warm-up throwing
E) 150′ (25 throws)

Step 10: A) Warm-up throwing
B) 150′ (25 throws)
C) Rest 10 minutes
D) Warm-up throwing
E) 150′ (25 throws)
F) Rest 10 minutes
G) Warm-Up Throwing
H) 150′ (25 Throws)

180' Phase

Step 11: A) Warm-up throwing
B) 180′ (25 throws)
C) Rest 15 minutes
D) Warm-up throwing
E) 180′ (25 throws)

Step 12: A) Warm-up throwing
B) 180′ (25 throws)
C) Rest 10 minutes
D) Warm-up throwing
E) 180′ (25 throws)
F) Rest 10 minutes
G) Warm-Up Throwing
H) 180′ (25 Throws)

Step 13: A) Warm-up throwing
B) 180′ (25 throws)
C) Rest 15 minutes
D) Warm-up throwing
E) 180′ (25 throws)

Step 14: Begin throwing off the mound or return to respective position.

Throwing program should be performed every other day, unless otherwise specified by your physician or rehabilitation specialist.

the nonoperative program to be effective, the clinician must (a) identify the cause of the problem, (b) establish a differential diagnosis, and (c) identify all involved structures. The nonoperative rehabilitation program used for the overhead thrower involves a progressive and sequential multiphase approach. The specific goals of each of the four phases of the program are outlined in Table 45–6.

During the initial phase, one of the primary goals of the rehabilitation program is to normalize shoulder motion, particularly improving internal rotation and horizontal adduction. Thus specific stretches to address posterior rotator-cuff and capsular tightness should be performed. Another primary goal of the phase is to reestablish baseline dynamic stability as well as restoring proprioception and kinesthesia. Additionally, the patient's pain and inflammation is addressed and reduced through activity modifications, modalities, and gentle stretching.

In phase two of the rehabilitation program, the primary goals are to enhance dynamic stability and to facilitate neuromuscular control. Additionally, the program should emphasize the restoration of muscular balance at the glenohumeral and scapulothoracic joints. During this phase the patient is begun on an isotonic strengthening program and a plyometric exercise program.

Phase three primary goals are to enhance dynamic stabilization, improve reactive neuromuscular control, and improve power and endurance. Also during this phase, an interval throwing program can be initiated. The isotonic strengthening program and the thrower's ten program are continued, and manual resistance drills to enhance dynamic stability also are performed.

During phase four, the primary goals are a gradual return to throwing while maintaining the neuromuscular gains that have been established in the previous three phases. During this phase, isotonic, plyometric, and

TABLE 45–6B. *Interval throwing program starting off the mound, phase II*

Stage one: fastball only		
Step 1:	Interval throwing 15 Throws off mound 50%	(Use interval throwing to 120′ phase as warm-up)
Step 2:	Interval throwing 30 Throws off mound 50%	
Step 3:	Interval throwing 45 Throws off mound 50%	All throwing off the mound should be done in the presence of your pitching coach to stress proper throwing mechanics
Step 4:	Interval throwing 60 Throws off mound 50%	
Step 5:	Interval throwing 30 Throws off mound 50%	(Use speed gun to aid in effort control)
Step 6:	30 Throws off mound 75% 45 Throws off mound 50%	
Step 7:	45 Throws off mound 75% 15 Throws off mound 50%	
Step 8:	60 Throws off mound 75%	
Stage two: fastball only		
Step 9:	45 Throws off mound 75% 15 Throws in batting practice	
Step 10:	45 Throws off mound 75% 30 Throws in batting practice	
Step 11:	45 Throws off mound 75% 45 Throws in batting practice	
Stage three		
Step 11:	30 Throws off mound 75% warm-up 15 Throws off mound 50% breaking balls 45–60 Throws in batting practice (fastball only)	
Step 12:	30 Throws off mound 75% 30 Breaking balls 75% 30 Throws in batting practice	
Step 13:	30 Throws off mound 75% 60–90 Throws in batting practice 25% breaking balls	
Step 14:	Simulated game: progressing by 15 throws per work-out	

manual-resistance exercises are performed. Additionally, the interval throwing program is progressed. The interval throwing program is designed gradually to increase the number of throws and the distance, intensity, and types of throws to facilitate the restoration of normal biomechanics. The interval throwing program is organized into two phases: phase I, a long-toss program (from 45 to 180 ft); and phase II, an off-the-mound program for pitchers. The primary goal of the last phase is to enhance sport-specific techniques that reestablish proper biomechanics, thus reducing the chance of reinjury.

CONCLUSION

The thrower's shoulder and elbow joint are subjected to tremendous stresses and strains during the overhead throwing motion. Because of the excessive forces generated, significantly high muscular activity, and tremendously high angular velocities, the shoulder and elbow joints are susceptible to injury. Additionally, the hypermobility of the anterior glenohumeral joint capsule contributes significantly to some of the common pathomechanics. Through proper conditioning and training, some of these injuries can be avoided.

Optimal sports performance requires skill and power. The conditioning program should address the development of both entities and should motivate the athlete to strive for a higher level of performance. When designing a conditioning program for the overhead athlete, specific elements should include flexibility, strengthening, proprioception, kinesthesia, neuromuscular control, endurance, power, core stability, and the concepts of periodization. The conditioning program should be manageable, measurable, and motivational. Additionally, the elements of a rehabilitation program were discussed. The rehabilitation of the overhead athlete has dramatically changed in the past decade. The goals of the rehabilitation are muscular balance, proprioception, neuromuscular control, scapular strengthening, dynamic stabilization, and a gradual return to throwing activities. By using these principles and guidelines, athletes improve their chances to return to injury-free throwing.

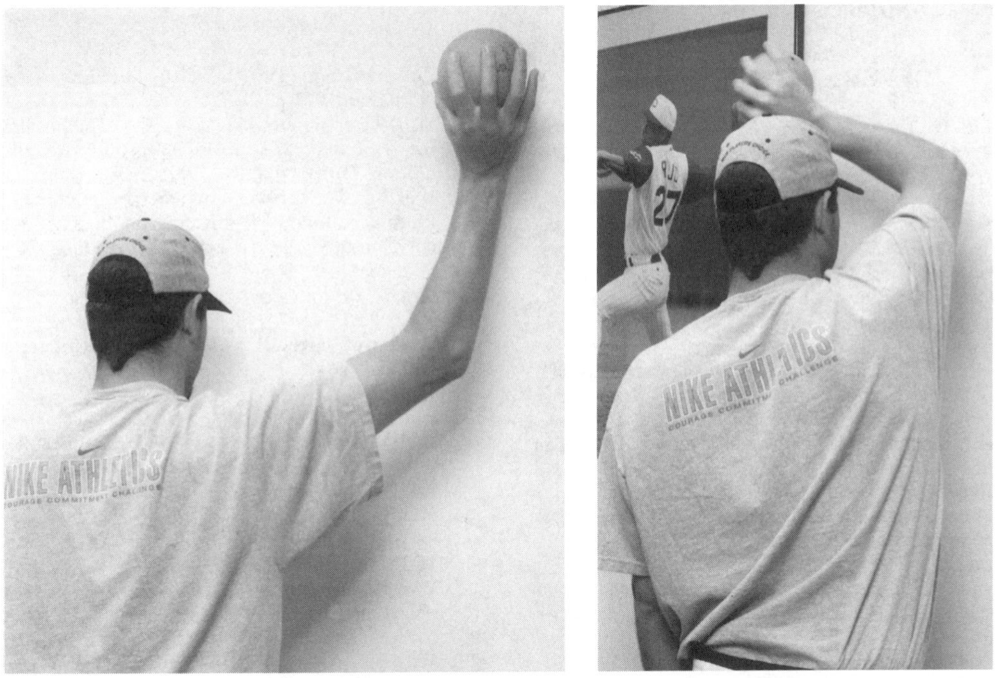

A B

FIG. 45–10. Endurance drills. Plyometric ball wall dribbling. The athlete uses a 2-lb plyoball (**A**) and dribbles it off a wall in a semicircular-movement pattern (**B**). This drill is usually performed for time, 30 seconds to 2 minutes.

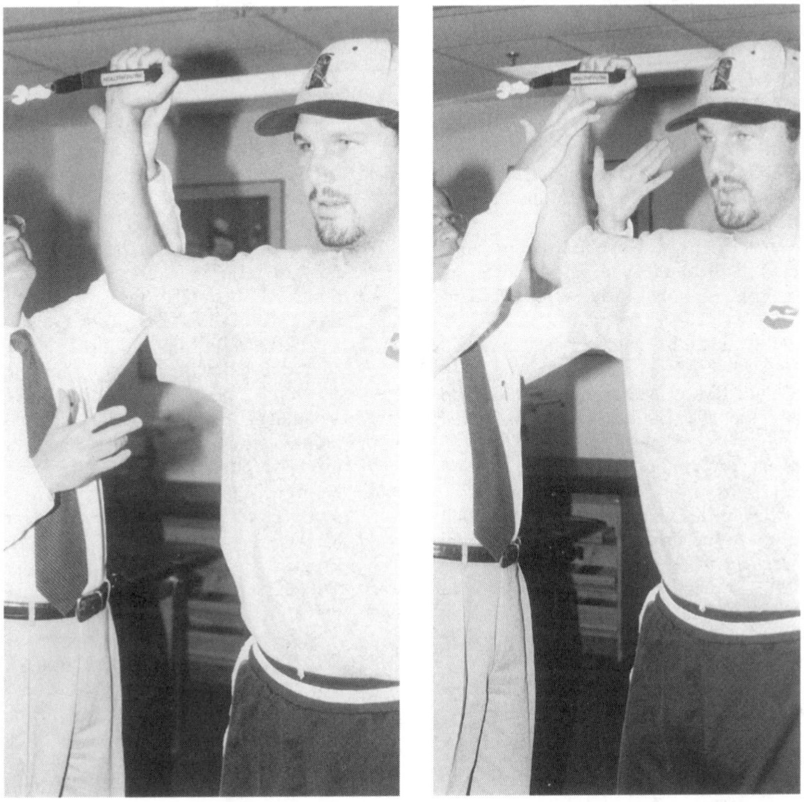

A B

FIG. 45–11. Rhythm-stabilization drills. **A**: The athlete externally rotates the arm against the resistance of the exercise tubing. **B**: Manual resistance is applied at end range, pushing into internal and external rotation.

REFERENCES

1. Jobe FW, Tibone JE, Jobe CM, et al. The shoulder in sports. In: Rockwood CA, Matsen FA, eds. *The shoulder.* Philadelphia: WB Saunders, 1990:961.
2. Toyoshima S, Hoshikawa T, Miyashita M, et al. Contribution of the body parts to throwing performance. In: Nelson RC, Morehouse CA, eds. *Biomechanics IV.* Baltimore: University Park Press, 1974:169–174.
3. DiGiovine NM, Jobe FW, Pink M, et al. An electromyographic analysis of the upper extremity in pitching. *J Shoulder Elbow Surg* 1992;1:15–24.
4. Fleisig GS, Andrews JR, Dillman CJ, et al. Kinetics of baseball pitching with implications about injury mechanisms. *Am J Sports Med* 1995;23:233–239.
5. Verkhoshanski Y. Perspectives in the improvement of speed-strength preparation for jumpers. *Yessis Rev Soviet Phys Educ Sports* 1969;4:28–35.
6. Wilk KE, Voight ML, Keirns MA, Gambetta V. Stretch-shortening drills for the upper extremity: theory and clinical application. *J Orthop Sports Phys Ther* 1993;17:225–239.
7. Werner SL, Dillman CJ, Escamilla RF, et al. Biomechanics of the elbow during baseball pitching. *J Orthop Sports Phys Ther* 1993;17:274–278.
8. Dillman CJ. Proper mechanics of pitching. *Sports Med Update* 1990;5:15–21.
9. Fleisig GS, Dillman CJ, Andrews JR. Biomechanics of the shoulder during throwing. In: Andrews JR, Wilk KE, eds. *The athlete's shoulder.* New York: Churchill Livingstone, 1994:355–368.
10. Fleisig GS, Dillman CJ, Andrews JR. Proper mechanics for baseball pitching. *Clin Sports Med* 1991;10:789–805.
11. Fleisig GS, Escamilla RF, Barrentine SW, et al. Kinematic and kinetic comparison between baseball pitching and football passing. *J Appl Biomech* 1996;12:207–224.
12. Moynes DR. Electromyography and motion analysis of the upper extremity in sports. *Phys Ther* 1986;66:1905–1911.
13. Gowan ID. Comparative electromyographic analysis of the shoulder during pitching. *J Sports Med* 1987;15:586–590.
14. Van Gheluwe B, Hebbelinck M. Muscle actions and ground reaction forces in tennis. *J Sport Biomech* 1986;2:88–93.
15. Miyashita M, Tsunoda T, Sakurai S, et al. Muscular activities in the tennis serve and overhead throwing. *Scand J Sports Sci* 1980;2:52–59.
16. Gloussman R, Jobe FW, Tibone JE, et al. Dynamic electromyographic analysis of the throwing shoulder with glenohumeral instability. *J Bone Joint Surg Am* 1988;70:220–226.
17. Brown LP, Niehues SL, Harrah A, et al. Upper extremity range of motion and isokinetic strength of the internal and external shoulder rotators in major league baseball players. *Am J Sports Med* 1988;16:577–585.
18. Johnson L. Patterns of shoulder flexibility among college baseball players. *J Athl Train* 1992;27:44–49.
19. Bigliani LU, Codd TP, Connor PM, et al. Shoulder motion and laxity in the professional baseball player. *Am J Sports Med* 1997;25:609–613.
20. Adams JE. Bone injuries in very young athletes. *Clin Orthop* 1968;58:129–140.
21. Albright JA, Jokl P, Shaw R, et al. Clinical study of baseball pitchers: correlation of injury to the throwing arm with method of delivery. *Am J Sports Med* 1978;6:15–21.
22. DeHaven KE, Evarts CM. Throwing injuries of the elbow in athletes. *Orthop Clin North Am* 1973;4:801–808.
23. King JW, Brelsford HJ, Tullos HS. Analysis of the pitching arm of the professional baseball pitcher. *Clin Orthop* 1969;67:116–123.
24. Slocum DB. Classification of elbow injuries from baseball pitching. *Texas Med* 1968;64:48–53.
25. Torg JS, Pollack H, Sweterlitsch P. The effects of competitive pitching on the shoulders and elbows of preadolescent baseball players. *Pediatrics* 1972;49:267–272.
26. Tullos HS, Erwin WD, Woods GW, et al. Unusual lesions of the pitching arm. *Clin Orthop* 1972;88:169–182.
27. Tullos HS, King JW. Lesions of the pitching arm in adolescents. *JAMA* 1972;220:264–271.
28. Tullos HS, King JW. Throwing mechanism in sports. *Orthop Clin North Am* 1973;4:709–720.
29. Wilk KE, Andrews JR, Arrigo CA. The physical examination of the glenohumeral joint: emphasis on the stabilizing structures. *J Orthop Sports Phys Ther* 1997;25:380–389.
30. Wilk KE. The thrower's shoulder; evaluation of common injuries. Presented at the 1997 Advances on the Knee & Shoulder. Cincinnati Sports Medicine Center, Hilton Head, SC: May 24, 1997.
31. Pedegana LR, Elsner RC, Roberts D, et al. The relationship of upper extremity strength to throwing speed. *Am J Sports Med* 1982;10:352–354.
32. Alderink GJ, Kuck DJ. Isokinetic shoulder strength of high school and college-aged pitchers. *J Orthop Sports Phys Ther* 1986; 7:163–172.
33. Cook EE, Gray VL, Savinar-Nogue E, et al. Shoulder antagonistic strength rations: a comparison between college-level baseball pitchers and non-pitchers. *J Orthop Sports Phys Ther* 1987; 8:451–461.
34. Hinton RY. Isokinetic evaluation of shoulder rotational strength in high school baseball pitchers. *Am J Sports Med* 1988; 16:274–279.
35. Wilk KE, Andrews JR, Arrigo CA, et al. The strength characteristics of internal and external rotator muscles in professional baseball pitchers. *Am J Sports Med* 1993;21:61–66.
36. Wilk KE, Andrews JR, Arrigo CA. The abductor and adductor strength characteristics of professional baseball pitchers. *Am J Sports Med* 1995;23:307–311.
37. Bartlett LR, Storey MD, Simons DB. Measurement of upper extremity torque production and its relationship to throwing speed in the competitive athlete. *Am J Sports Med* 1989;17:89–91.
38. Magnusson SP, Gleim GW, Nicholas JA. Shoulder weakness in professional baseball pitchers. *Med Sci Sports Exerc* 1994;26:5–9.
39. Kibler BW. The role of the scapula in the overhead throwing motion. *Contemp Orthop* 1991;22:525–531.
40. Paine RM. The role of the scapula in the shoulder. In: Andrews JR, Wilk KE, eds. *The athlete's shoulder.* New York: Churchill Livingstone, 1994:495–512.
41. Davies GJ, Dickoff-Hoffman SD. Neuromuscular testing and rehabilitation of the shoulder complex. *J Orthop Sports Phys Ther* 1993;18:449–456.
42. Moseley JB, Jobe FW, Pink M, et al. EMG analysis of the scapular muscles during a shoulder rehabilitation program. *Am J Sports Med* 1992;20:222–228.
43. Mooncastle VS. *Medical physiology.* 14th ed. St. Louis: Mosby, 1980.
44. Jonsson HJ, Karrholm J, Elmquist LG. Kinematics of active knee extensions after tear of the anterior cruciate ligament. *Am J Sports Med* 1989;17:796–802.
45. Smith RL, Brunoli J. Shoulder kinesthesia after anterior glenohumeral dislocation. *Phys Ther* 1989;69:106–112.
46. Lephart SM, Warner JJP, Borsa PA, Fu FH. Proprioception in the shoulder of healthy, unstable, and surgically repaired shoulders. *J Shoulder Elbow Surg* 1994;3:371–381.
47. Voight ML, Hardin JA, Blackburn TA, et al. The effects of muscle fatigue on and the relationship of arm dominance to shoulder proprioception. *J Sports Phys Ther* 1996;23:348–352.
48. Knott M, Voss D. *Proprioceptive neuromuscular facilitation.* New York: Hoeber Medical Division, Harper & Row, 1968:84–85.
49. Marveyev L. *Fundamentals of sports training.* Moscow, Russia: Progress Publishing, 1977.
50. Wilk KE, Arrigo CA. Current concepts in the rehabilitation of the athletic shoulder. *J Orthop Sports Phys Ther* 1993;18:365–378.
51. Wilk KE, Arrigo CA. An integrated approach to upper extremity exercises. *Orthop Phys Ther Clin North Am* 1992;9:337–360.
52. Townsend H, Jobe FW, Pink M, et al. EMG of the glenohumeral muscles during a baseball rehabilitation program. *Am J Sports Med* 1991;19:264–269.
53. Blackburn TA, McLeod WB, White B. EMG analysis of posterior rotator cuff exercises. *J Ath Train* 1990;25:40–45.
54. Jobe FW, Moynes DR. Delineation of diagnostic criteria and a rehabilitation program for rotator cuff injuries. *Am J Sports Med* 1982;10:336–342.

55. Pappas AM, Zawacki RM. Rehabilitation of the pitching shoulder. *Am J Sports Med* 1985;13:223–231.
56. Wilk KE, Andrews JR, Arrigo CA, et al. *Preventive and rehabilitative exercises for the shoulder and elbow.* 5th ed. Birmingham, AL: American Sports Medicine Institute, 1997.
57. Wickiewiez TH, Chen SK, Otis JC, et al. Glenohumeral kinematics in a muscle fatigue model: a radiographic study. Presented at the 1994 Specialty Day Meeting, American Orthopaedic Society for Sports Medicine, New Orleans: February 1994.
58. Gladstone J, Andrews JR, Wilk KE, et al. The effects of muscle fatigue on glenohumeral kinematics in the overhead professional baseball pitcher: a radiographic study. Presented at the American Sports Medicine Institute Fellows Research Day, July 12, 1996.

Exercise and Sport Science,
edited by William E. Garrett, Jr., and Donald T. Kirkendall.
Lippincott Williams & Wilkins, Philadelphia © 2000.

CHAPTER 46

Physiology of Basketball

Jay R. Hoffman and Carl M. Maresh

Basketball has attained an impressive level of international popularity. This is evident in the amount of fan support and media attention given to both male and female players at the professional and collegiate levels. Basketball has always been considered a game of precision, timing, accuracy, and agility. However, the changing character of the game and the improved athletic ability of players, from the high school to professional ranks, demands greater attention to player preparation. This review describes the game of basketball, discusses the physiologic demands of the game and the requirements it imposes on players, and addresses training considerations.

THE SPORT

Physical Requirements

The Game

The game of basketball is played with five players per team, on a court with an official length of 84 feet (25.6 m) for high school competitions and 94 feet (28.7 m) for collegiate and professional competitions. The width of the court is 45 feet (13.7 m) for all levels of competition. The length of time for a game varies depending on the league. Typical high school basketball games are played with four 8- or 10-minute quarters. Collegiate basketball games are played with two 20-minute halves, and professional games are played with four 12-minute quarters.

Basketball is played in a continuous flow of activity. The transition from offense to defense is performed without any discontinuation in play. Play is suspended only when there are rule infractions (fouls, violations) or time outs (a limited number), or at the end of each quarter or half. Substitutions are permitted freely, but only during a stoppage in play. There are no limitations on the number of times a player can enter or leave the game.

The intensity of the game is intermittent. Depending on the strategy or "philosophy" of the coach, the game can generally be played more "up-tempo" (i.e., a higher intensity of play) or "slowed down" (i.e., a lower intensity of play). Depending on the opponent or the circumstances in a game (e.g., point differential), however, the coach may decide to alter the team's style of play. In addition, several important factors concerning the team may influence the coach in determining the team's style of play. The athleticism, basketball skills, and physical condition of the players on the team affect the type of strategy the coach could successfully use in a game. Furthermore, the number of players that the coach believes could play within the team's system or style of play would affect the rotation of players (i.e., substitution pattern) into a game. Obviously, injuries also influence the rotation of players into the game. These factors have a large impact on the physiologic requirements of the basketball player; therefore the physiologic demand placed on the basketball player may be more specific to the style of play of each respective team.

Movement Patterns

The continuous flow of play, smooth transition from offense to defense, and shared responsibilities by the players (i.e., rebounding and shooting) in a basketball game require all players to perform similar movements on the basketball court. These movements range from runs (from a jog to a sprint) and shuffles (backwards and side), at various degrees of intensity, to jumps. The existing scientific literature concerning the physical demand and physiologic responses of basketball players is very limited, however. Only a recent study by McInnes

J. R. Hoffman: Knoll Pharmaceutical Company, Mt. Olive, New Jersey 07828.

C. M. Maresh: Department of Kinesiology, University of Connecticut, Storrs, Connecticut 06269-1110.

and colleagues (1) is known to have categorized the movement patterns of a basketball game. In that study the investigators separated the movement patterns into eight different categories (stand/walk, jog, run, stride/sprint, low, medium, or high shuffle, and jump). Their results illustrated the intermittent nature of basketball by demonstrating 997 ± 183 changes in movement during a 48-minute basketball game. This equated to a change of movement every 2 seconds (players averaged 36.3 minutes played per game). Shuffle movements (all intensities) were seen in 34.6% of the activity patterns of a basketball game, whereas running (intensities varying from a jog to a sprint) was observed in 31.2% of all movements. Jumps were reported to occur in 4.6% of all movements, whereas standing or walking was observed during 29.6% of the playing time. Movements characterized as high intensity were recorded once every 21 seconds of play. When considering both high-intensity shuffles and jumps, the investigators reported that only 15% of the actual playing time was spent engaged in high-intensity activity. Sixty-five percent of playing time was engaged in activities of greater intensity than walking. It appears that the majority of activity in a basketball game is performed at aerobic intensities. It should be noted, however, that the subjects in this study were Australian National League players; the style of their play may be quite different from that seen in other leagues (i.e., NCAA, NBA).

Physiologic Requirements

It is difficult to provide a precise assessment of the physiologic demands imposed during a competitive basketball contest, and limited data are available on the physiologic responses during game play. Furthermore, a direct comparison of variables between studies can be problematic because of differences in the level of play and individual differences in age, gender, and fitness level.

Heart Rate

Heart-rate responses measured during competition do provide some indication of the intensity of play. Most studies of heart rate during basketball have been conducted on female players and have shown heart rates ranging from 169 to 183 beats/min (1–3). Similar values have been reported in male players, with average heart rates of 170 beats/min (4). In a more recent study of elite Australian basketball players, McInnes and co-workers (1) reported heart rates during actual play of 169 ± 9 beats/min. These values corresponded to 89% ± 9% of the peak heart rate attained during laboratory testing. Furthermore, 75% of actual play occurred at a heart rate that was 85% of peak heart rate, whereas approximately 15% of play produced a heart rate greater than 95% of peak heart rate. In contrast, Beam and Merrill (2) found in female U.S. collegiate players that 61.8% of actual play occurred at a heart rate greater than 85% of maximal heart rate, and only 3.8% of actual play at greater than 95% of maximal heart rate. Differences in heart-rate responses between these male and female athletes are most likely due to differences in the level of play. There may be considerable variations in the heart-rate responses during game play between players. This may be due to the fitness level of players, the variation in actual time played, the intensity of the game, or different positions (1).

Oxygen Uptake

Based on heart-rate responses, McArdle and colleagues (3) estimated the average oxygen uptake during play in six female collegiate basketball players and reported a range from a low of 1.5 L/min to a high of 2.4 L/min. These authors also found no change in the maximal oxygen uptake (treadmill-walking protocol) of the players over the course of the basketball season, with values averaging 35.5 ± 4.1 mL/min/kg. Maresh and co-workers (5) also reported no change in the maximal oxygen uptake (46.9 ± 2.5 mL/min/kg, treadmill-running protocol) of female collegiate players before and after a 5-month basketball season, but exercise time to exhaustion increased ($p < .05$) from 6.0 ± 0.6 to 7.6 ± 0.5 minutes.

Blood Lactate

We are aware of only one study (1) of blood lactate concentrations during actual basketball competitions. In that study, mean lactate concentrations were 6.8 ± 2.8 m*M*. Blood lactate concentrations did not vary significantly between quarters of play. The mean maximal lactate concentration for all eight male subjects was 8.5 ± 3.1 m*M*, with the highest value for one player reaching 13.2 m*M*. Furthermore, significant correlations were found between the lactate concentration and both the percentage of time spent in high-intensity activity ($r = 0.64$; $p < .05$) and the mean percentage of peak heart rate ($r = 0.45$; $p < .05$). According to these authors, the wide range in lactate concentrations suggests that the glycolytic contribution may vary considerably between games as well as within each game, and it may be due to the varying intensity of the contest, the different physiologic characteristics of the players, and the amount of time played. Maresh and co-workers (5) found no differences in the maximal plasma lactate concentration (10.4 ± 0.5 m*M*) of female collegiate players, by treadmill testing, before and after a 5-month season.

Hydration and Factors Involved in the Regulation of Body Fluids

Hoffman and colleagues (6) examined the effect of water deprivation on anaerobic power and vertical jumping height in 10 male members (17.3 ± 0.9 years) of a regional youth basketball team. These players participated in two "two-on-two full court" basketball games. Water consumption was permitted in one game but not in the other, in a balanced crossover design. Players began each game euhydrated. Anaerobic power and jump tests were performed before at half-time, and immediately after each 40-minute game. It was concluded that the combination of high-intensity exercise and fluid restriction (−1.9% of body weight) did not cause significant decrements in vertical jump, anaerobic power, or basketball-shooting performance. However, several tendencies were observed that could have real practical significance, including a 19% decrement in anaerobic power and an 8% decrement in field-goal shooting percentage during the no-water trial compared with the water trial. Specifically, the contribution of high-intensity exercise and fluid restriction over a 40-minute athletic contest might be detrimental to performance.

The effect of a 5-month basketball season on plasma renin activity and hormones involved in the regulation of body fluids was examined in nine female collegiate basketball players (5). The study demonstrated that maximal exercise in these college women elicits increases in the secretion of plasma vasopressin, renin, and aldosterone. Furthermore, these responses were found to be quite consistent, being comparable in tests performed 5 months apart. There have been no studies examining these variables in response to basketball training in male players.

THE ATHLETE

A Physiologic Profile

The physiological profile of a sport describes the physical characteristics of an athlete, which can then be used to identify talent and develop sport-specific training programs. Unlike other sports (i.e. football) in which standard testing profiles (e.g. 40-yd sprint, 1 RM bench press) have been established and accepted, basketball has yet to become associated with any standard testing regimen. There has been much variation in the fitness testing of basketball players, which has made it difficult to establish specific standards. Latin and colleagues (7) have published the most comprehensive survey to date on the physical fitness and performance profile for Division I NCAA Men's College Basketball players. They reported a poor compliance rate (15.2% survey return), however, and a large inconsistency in how the fitness variables were reported. In this section we will discuss the existing literature concerning the physiological makeup of the basketball player. In addition, we will also discuss how specific fitness components relate to basketball performance.

Aerobic Capacity

Both laboratory measures and field tests common to athletic conditioning programs (i.e., 1.5-mile run or 12 minute run) have been used to describe the aerobic capacity of basketball players (8–16). Figure 46–1 depicts the maximal aerobic power ($\dot{V}O_2max$) of basketball players reported in the literature over the last 25 years in a chronologic fashion. The aerobic capacity of male basketball players appears to range from 42 mL/kg/min to 59 mL/kg/min. Studies that have used field tests to measure aerobic capacity have reported similar values (7,11). In comparing aerobic capacity between positions, the smaller players (guards) tend to have a greater aerobic capacity than either the forwards or centers in both college (17) and professional (15) basketball. This tendency did not reach statistical significance, however. There does not appear to be any pattern of improving or declining changes in aerobic capacity during the last 25 years. This is in contrast to Stone and Steingard (18), who suggested that aerobic capacities (in NBA players) have improved 20% within this similar time frame. However, no data were shown to substantiate that claim.

The maximal oxygen uptake values observed in basketball players encompass a wide range and are similar to values seen in sedentary individuals of comparable age and of athletes that participate in nonendurance events (19). The wide span in $\dot{V}O_2max$ values may reflect differences in playing styles and conditioning programs between basketball teams. In addition, these values also appear to reflect the reliance on both the aerobic and anaerobic energy systems for playing basketball. Although anaerobic metabolism has been suggested to be the primary energy source for playing basketball (20–23), there still appears to be an important aerobic component to basketball performance. Aerobic capacity may have more importance in the recovery processes (e.g., lactate clearance, cardiodeceleration patterns), rather than in providing a direct performance benefit. However, several indications suggest that there may be a limit to the benefits provided by a high aerobic capacity during recovery from an anaerobic activity (24,25). It appears that a certain threshold of aerobic capacity is needed; once this threshold is achieved, further improvement in aerobic capacity may not provide any additional advantage. A high aerobic capacity has been reported to have a negative relation with playing time in elite college basketball players (26).

Aerobic-capacity levels in female basketball players have been reported to range between 36 mL/kg/min to 51 mL/kg/min (3,16,27–30). In contrast to what has been reported in male basketball players, a significant differ-

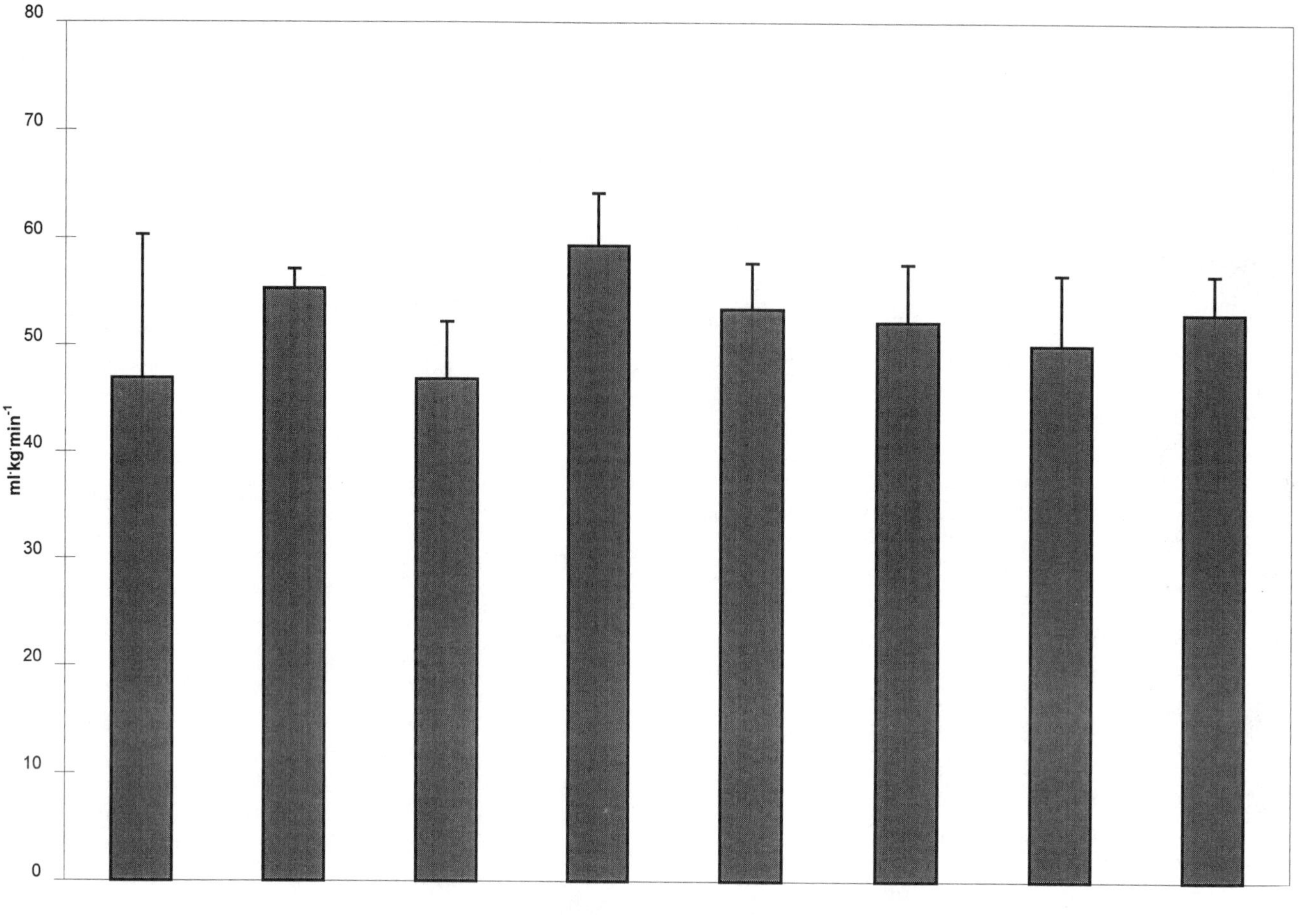

FIG. 46–1. Maximal oxygen consumption in male college basketball players. (From refs. 8–10, 12–14, 38, and 39.)

ence has been reported between guards (54.3 ± 4.9 mL/kg/min) and small forwards (47.0 ± 4.3 mL/kg/min) (30). No further significant differences between positions were noted, however. In addition, aerobic power is reported to be related to basketball performance in females and also discriminates between higher and lesser skilled female basketball players (31). This is in sharp contrast to what has been reported in male basketball players. The difference between the genders may be related to differences in style of play. The 14% difference observed between the genders in aerobic capacity is slightly less than previous reports of aerobic-capacity differences between male and female athletes (19).

Anaerobic Power

It has been suggested by a number of investigators that success in basketball appears to be more dependent on the athlete's anaerobic power and endurance rather than on aerobic power, per se (21,22,26). Although only 15% of the playing time in a basketball game has been described as high intensity (1), these actions are likely what determine the outcome of a contest. The quick change of direction and explosive speed needed to free oneself for an open shot or defend, the ability to jump quickly and repetitively, and the speed needed to reach loose balls and run a fast break, are examples of high-intensity activities common to basketball. Speed, vertical jump, and agility (activities anaerobic by nature) have been demonstrated to be strong predictors of playing time in college basketball players (26).

A wide range of tests has been used to assess anaerobic power and endurance in basketball players. Anaerobic power in basketball players has been determined from a Margaria–Kalman Power test (9), vertical jump using both the Lewis (7,23), and Harmon power formulas (13,29), vertical jump from a force mat (6,27), and the Wingate Anaerobic Power Test (24). The number of testing modalities has made it quite difficult to generate normative data for peak and mean anaerobic-power output levels for these athletes. The most frequent test used appears to be the vertical jump. This is a relatively simple test to perform and quite easy to interpret for both the player and coach. Latin and colleagues (7) reported that the mean vertical jump in NCAA Division I basketball players is 71.4 ± 10.4 cm (range, 25.4 to 105.4 cm). Vertical jump power (by using the Lewis formula) in these athletes was 1669.9 ± 209.7 W (range, 1073.1 to 2521.5 W). Significant differences were reported between positions. The vertical jump height for both guards (73.4 ± 9.6 cm) and forwards (71.4 ± 10.4 cm) was reported to be significantly greater than for centers (66.8 ± 10.7 cm) (7). Vertical jump power, however, has been reported to be significantly greater in both forwards (1749.3 ± 210.7 W) and centers (1784.6 ± 162.7 W) than in guards 1550.4 ± 161.7 W) (7).

Far fewer studies have been performed on the anaerobic power outputs in female basketball players. Recent studies reported vertical jump heights to be quite similar between NCAA Division I female basketball players (45.2 ± 2.7 cm) (29) and the Canadian National Women's Basketball team (44.7 ± 5.3 cm) (30). These were greater than the vertical jump heights previously reported in European female basketball players (26.3 ± 2.9 cm) (27). Smith and Thomas (30) reported significant differences between guards (48.9 ± 4.9 cm) and power forwards (40.5 ± 3.8 cm), but not between any other position comparisons in female basketball players.

Strength

Maximal strength in basketball players has been most often reported as the 1RM strength in the bench press, squat, and power clean exercises. These dynamic constant-resistance exercise tests are used to assess upper-body strength, lower-body strength, and explosive strength, respectively (32). These tests have strong test–retest reliability (11,32,33) and are familiar to athletic conditioning programs.

Lower-body strength (1RM squat) has been shown to be a strong predictor for playing time in NCAA Division I male basketball players' (26). Maximal strength for the squat exercise in these athletes is reported to range from 81.8 to 262.3 kg (152.2 ± 36.5 kg) (7,11,13,34). In a position-by-position analysis, collegiate forwards (161.9 ± 37.7 kg) were significantly stronger than centers (138.1 ± 32.1 kg), but not the guards (151.1 ± 35.5 kg) (7). When lower-body strength was expressed relative to body weight, centers were significantly weaker than both the guards and forwards (7). Lower-body strength is invaluable for "boxing-out" and positioning during a basketball game. In addition, the importance of leg strength to basketball players may be related to its positive relation to both speed and agility (32).

The power clean may be a more appropriate exercise than the squat for improving jumping height, speed, and agility. The explosive action of the power clean and its ability to integrate strength, explosive power, and neuromuscular coordination among several muscle groups suggests that strong performance in this exercise would correlate well with actions common to basketball players (32). Surprisingly, strength and conditioning coaches are not using the power clean as frequently as the squat or bench-press exercises in the testing of their players (7). Maximal strength in the power clean has been reported to be 99.2 ± 15.2 kg (range, 59.0 to 137.3 kg) in NCAA Division I male college basketball players (7). In comparisons between positions, forwards (105.1 ± 16.9 kg) were reported to be significantly stronger than guards (94.5 ± 13.0 kg), but not the centers (99.8 ± 13.7 kg) (7).

Maximal strength in the bench press appears to be the most frequent measure of strength reported in basketball players. Maximal strength for the bench-press exercise has been reported to range from 54.5 to 186.4 kg (102.7 ± 18.9) (7,12,13,23,35). Unfortunately, upper-body strength has been reported to be poorly correlated with playing time ($r = -0.04$ to 0.14) in male collegiate basketball players (26). Hoffman and associates (26) suggested that although the bench press may not be a determining factor in playing time, it is likely that certain positions such as power forward and center require more upper-body strength than other positions. However, Latin and co-workers (7) did not report any significant differences in maximal bench-press strength among collegiate guards (100.8 ± 17.6 kg), forwards (104.0 ± 21.5 kg), and centers (104.4 ± 17.0). Guards were seen to have a significantly greater relative strength than both forwards and centers. Of note is the greater upper-body strength measures seen in collegiate basketball players than that reported in 1978 in NBA players, by Parr and colleagues (15). They reported maximal strength values in the bench press to be 86.8 ± 15.0 kg, 101.3 ± 20.8 kg, and 70.0 ± 0.0 kg in NBA guards, forwards, and center, respectively. This difference appears to reflect the greater emphasis placed on strength training for basketball players in recent years (7).

Speed and Agility

Speed and agility have both been reported to be consistent predictors of playing time in NCAA Division I male basketball players (26). Speed has been generally determined by a timed 40- or 30-yard sprint. The 40-yard sprint may have greater popularity because of the familiarity with performance times associated with football players. However, the 30-yard sprint may be more specific for the basketball athlete because of the similarity between this distance and the length of the basketball court. Latin and colleagues (7) reported the mean 40- and 30-yard sprint times in collegiate basketball players to be 4.81 ± 0.26 seconds and 3.79 ± 0.19 seconds, respectively. Guards were observed to be significantly faster than centers in both 40-yard (4.68 ± 0.20 seconds versus 4.97 ± 0.21 seconds, respectively) and 30-yard (3.68 ± 0.14 seconds versus 3.97 ± 0.21 seconds, respectively) sprints. The times for forwards were 4.84 ± 0.29 seconds and 3.83 ± 0.16 seconds in the 40- and 30-yard sprints, respectively. These times were not significantly different from those of either guards or centers.

Agility is also considered an important component of basketball performance (26). This is not surprising considering the rapid changes in movement and direction during a game. There does not appear to be any widely accepted method of measuring agility in basketball players, however. This was reflected in the study of Latin and co-workers (7): only 7% of the NCAA Division I schools that responded to their survey reported agility performance scores. Although several tests are available to measure agility, the T-test may be the most appropriate for the basketball player. This drill uses the basic movements performed in a game: forward sprint, side shuffle, and backwards run (36). Latin and associates (7) reported no significant differences between positions in the T-test (8.95 ± 0.53 seconds). This was most likely due to the small sample size, considering that guards were 0.20 and 0.54 seconds faster than forwards and centers, respectively.

Flexibility

Flexibility is the ability to move muscles through their full range of motion about a joint. Flexibility is joint specific, however, and inference from one joint to another cannot be done without specifically measuring the flexibility of that particular joint. Most studies examining flexibility in the basketball player have reported on the sit-and-reach test. Hunter and colleagues (12,13) reported sit-and-reach score means ranging from 1.4 to 4.9 cm in two separate studies of collegiate basketball players. Parr and co-workers (15) reported slightly better scores in the sit-and-reach test (mean score ranges between positions, 6.7 to 7.4 cm) in NBA players. Flexibility should be considered an important component of basketball conditioning, not just for its role in performance enhancement (this has not been demonstrated) but also because of its role in injury prevention.

Body Mass and Body Composition

The body mass of Division I collegiate basketball players appears to be quite similar between teams (7). The range in body mass (84.5 to 97.9 kg) reported by Latin and colleagues (7) is consistent with the body mass reported in collegiate basketball players over the past 25 years (9–11,14,17,23,27,29,34,35,37,38). Significant differences between each position also were noted. Guards (82.9 ± 6.8 kg) are the lightest collegiate players, followed by forwards (95.1 ± 8.3 kg) and then centers (101.9 ± 9.7 kg) (7). A similar pattern of body-mass differences was reported in professional basketball players (15).

Several studies reporting on the body composition in college and professional basketball players observed body-fat percentages (BF%) ranging from 8.3% to 13.5% (7,8,12,13,15,17). This is consistent with the 9.4% ± 3.8% mean value recently reported in Division I collegiate basketball players (7). The mean BF% may be higher in players participating in lower-division colleges (i.e., Division II or III) (35) or in European players (10). Collegiate guards have a significantly lower BF% (8.4% ± 3.0%) than centers (11.2% ± 4.5%) but not forwards (9.7% ± 3.9%) (7). This may reflect the greater mass needed by centers to play the "low post" position, which involves much body contact during box-outs, picks, and rebounding. A reverse order of BF% has been observed in NBA players (15). Considering that this reversed order was described in only one study, however, it would be difficult to make any generalizations to the league as a whole.

The body mass of female basketball players has been reported to range from 61.5 to 68.3 kg (3,16,28–30), and BF% are reported to range from 19.5% to 26.2% (27,29). Women's basketball teams appear to have similar body-mass differences between positions as shown for male teams. Female guards are significantly lighter (67.3 ± 4.8 kg) than power forwards (77.1 ± 2.9 kg), small forwards (78.7 ± 5.7 kg) and centers (81.1 ± 7.2 kg) (30). No other significant differences were observed between positions. A similar pattern was observed in BF%. Smith and Thomas (30) reported that guards are the leanest athletes on a female basketball team (determined from the sum of six skinfolds) and were significantly leaner than both small forwards and centers. There were no other significant differences between positions.

TRAINING THE ATHLETE

Season Length and Contest Number

The length of a basketball season is dependent on both the league of play and the success of the team. The collegiate basketball season begins (official preseason practice) in mid-October and may continue, depending on the team's success, into March. Collegiate basketball teams are permitted to play 26 regular season games; with participation in both pre- and postseason tournaments, however, teams may play an additional 10 to 11 games. The high school basketball season varies depending on the state. Several states play fewer games than college teams, but high schools in other states may play a greater number of games. The men's professional basketball season is much longer (up to 9 months in duration) and encompasses a minimum of 82 regular season games. Depending on the success of a team, NBA players may play up to 25 additional games in the playoffs. In contrast, in women's professional basketball there are 32 regular season games, with the possibility of up to 11 additional playoff games.

Effect of the Season on the Physiologic Profile

Several studies have examined the effect of a basketball season on fitness parameters. It appears that basketball practice and games, without supplemental training, are a sufficient stimulus to maintain aerobic fitness throughout a basketball season (8,9,17,34,39). However, this may not necessarily be relevant for all players on the team. Caterisano and colleagues (39) showed that reserve members on a basketball team (those players playing less than 10 minutes per game) may not be able to maintain their aerobic fitness, and supplemental training may be appropriate for these team members.

Body mass also is maintained during the basketball season (7,9,17,34,39). Changes in body composition are not so consistent, however. Tavino and co-workers (17) and Hakkinen (10) reported significant increases in BF%, whereas Cabrera and associates (8) reported a significant decrease in BF%. Still others reported no change in BF% (39). Preseason BF% does not appear to be associated with any tendency for a directional change in BF%. The subjects in Hakkinen's study (10) had a high preseason BF% (14.9% ± 3.0%), yet still significantly increased BF% by season's end. In contrast, the subjects in Cabrera's study (8) significantly reduced their BF%, even when their preseason levels were in the low to normal range (9.2 ± 1.9%). Apparently the differences between these studies are related to specific differences in the training volume and intensity of their practices.

Anaerobic power has generally been shown to be maintained (17) or increased (9,27) during the basketball season. This is not surprising considering the highly anaerobic nature of practice and games. Hoffman and colleagues (11) reported significant decreases in both speed and vertical jump height within the competitive basketball season, however. These changes appeared to be related to some overreaching phenomenon, as vertical jump height returned to preseason levels by the season's conclusion. These fitness components (speed and vertical jump height) appear to be sensitive to changes in training volume and may serve as potential markers for predicting fatigue in basketball players.

The ability to maintain upper- and lower-body strength during a basketball season has met with conflicting results. It appears that maintenance of strength may be influenced to a large extent by the resistance-training experience of the athlete (34). Hoffman and co-workers (11) reported that both upper- and lower-body strength can be maintained during a season in players who have only 5 weeks of resistance-training experience, even when no in-season strength-training program was incorporated. It was suggested that the players did not achieve "full-fledged strength-training adaptations" during the 5-week preseason training program, and that the strength gains made were the result of only neural contributions. We did not examine whether strength increases could be maintained if there was no in-season resistance training program. In a later study (34), a 2 day/week in-season resistance-training program was shown to maintain strength levels in experienced resistance-trained basketball players and to improve upper-body strength in basketball players with minimal (5 weeks) resistance-training experience. In contrast, Caterisano and associates (39) were unable to confirm these results. Players in the earlier study (34) exercised at a higher intensity (5 to 8 RM) compared with the 10 repetitions at 70% of the player's 1RM in the latter study (39). Apparently the intensity of the in-season resistance-training program is an important variable in maintaining strength during a competitive basketball season.

Specific Training for Basketball

The initial question about an off-season training program is when to begin, and we are unaware of specific investigations that have examined ideal recovery times after a season. If the recovery time is not sufficient, however, there is an increased risk of overtraining the athlete (40). Empirically, 2 weeks of passive rest has appeared appropriate for collegiate basketball players, before they begin their off-season training program. Whether this is a sufficient recovery time for professional athletes, who compete in a season of greater duration, is not known.

The training program is based on the principles of *periodization*. Typically, periodization is a planned variation of acute training variables (i.e., intensity and volume) that brings an athlete to peak strength and power for a single competition (40). However, in contrast to a powerlifter or weightlifter, in whom the major competition culminates the year, the basketball players emphasize peak performance throughout the season and need to begin the season in peak condition. Furthermore, the basketball player needs to maintain this level of condition throughout the competitive year. Second, needs analysis of the basketball player demonstrates the importance of training multiple energy systems. Thus the athlete will concurrently perform various modes of training (e.g., strength, anaerobic, endurance). The training program should be developed with the understanding that concurrent training may influence maximal performance gains (41). Therefore, to maximize the training effect, a proper manipulation of these various stimuli must be performed.

There have been a number of recommendations and suggestions in the literature on conditioning for basketball (18,20,42,43). Typically, off-season training programs elicit significant increases (range, 8% to 17%) in both upper- and lower-body strength (13,29,34), but the magnitude of these increases appears related to the resistance-training experience of the athlete. Hunter and colleagues (13) reported significant increases in strength (24% and 32% in the 1RM bench press and 1RM squat exercises, respectively) during the 4-year playing career of Division I male college basketball players. These increases were similar to those reported after 4 years of training in female college basketball players (29). In both of these studies, the greatest strength increases were observed in the year between the athlete's freshman and sophomore seasons.

Off-season conditioning programs do not appear to cause any changes in the aerobic capacity of college basketball players (13,29). It appears that the aerobic component of the off-season training program is focused more on maintaining an aerobic base rather than on improving it and is consistent with the demonstrated relation between aerobic capacity and basketball performance.

There have been several conflicting reports concerning the effects of an off-season training program on agility, speed, and vertical jump height. Hunter and coworkers (13) and Petko and colleagues (29) reported significant improvements in vertical jump height (range, 8% to 12%) from the athlete's freshman to senior year. These improvements appear to have come during the initial years of training, however. As the athlete became more experienced, training improvements were remarkably lower. This may partly explain the results of Hoffman and associates (34) showing no improvement in sprint time and a less-than-one-percent improvement in both vertical jump height and T-test time after an off-season training program in experienced resistance-trained basketball players. In that same study, significant increases in 1RM bench press (17%) and 1RM squat (16%) were observed, suggesting that these athletes were closer to their full potential in speed, agility, and vertical jump than they were to their strength potential.

Resistance-Training Program

As mentioned previously in this chapter, strength appears to be an important component of the success of a basketball player. It also appears that of all the athletic components composing the basketball player, strength has the greatest potential to be developed. This is likely related to a lack of exposure of many basketball players to the weight room. Large increases of strength in basketball players appear to be related to only minor improvements in athletic skills (i.e., agility, speed, and vertical jump height). However, these minor improvements may have great practical significance in the success of the player.

The frequency of training is dependent on the resistance-training experience of the athlete (33). Several reports have recommended an off-season resistance-training program with a training frequency of 3 days/week (20,42,43). This may not be sufficient for all basketball players, however. Depending on the resistance-training experience of the athlete, a greater frequency of training may be more appropriate (33). Considering that team members with varying levels of resistance-training experience will train together, it may be prudent and more manageable to use a training program that will benefit both experienced and novice lifters. Therefore, the resistance-training program recommended is 4 days/week.

The resistance-training program can be divided into three phases. The initial phase is the off-season, followed by the preseason, and then the in-season (maintenance) phases. The off-season program is similar to that expected from a basic periodized training system (44). An example of a periodized off-season resistance-training program for basketball can be seen in Table 46–1. The first phase is the hypertrophy, or preparatory phase. This phase concentrates on developing muscle mass and building basic strength for the more complicated exercises in the strength and strength/power phases. The intensity of training is low (8 to 10 RM), volume of training is high, and the rest periods are short (about 1 minute) between exercises.

In the strength phase, additional multijoint structural exercises are added, whereas several of the assistance exercises used in the previous phase are eliminated. During this phase, more sport-specific and explosive power exercises, which better simulate the movement of a basketball player, are included. The push-press exercise simulates the movement of jumping for a rebound and shooting a jump shot. This exercise uses a slight countermovement before an explosive push upward. In addition, the lat pull-down, which is normally performed with the hands in a wide grip position, may be better performed with a closed and pronated grip while lowering the bar to the chest. This technique may better simulate the "rebound–grab" movement. During this phase, the volume of training is lower but intensity is increased. The rest period between sets may be increased to 2 to 3 minutes to promote maximal strength gains (44). Note that intensity remains slightly lower in the assistance exercises.

The strength/power phase is much shorter in duration (4 weeks) and precedes the preseason training. Intensity is even higher, whereas volume is lowered. The rest period between sets is similar to the previous macrocycle. Several assistance exercises can be eliminated during this phase. At the conclusion of each phase, a 1-week active recovery period should be included, in which the athlete does not perform any resistance training but will be active in training other fitness components.

The preseason for a collegiate basketball player may be defined as the time when the athlete returns from

TABLE 46–1. *Periodized off-season resistance training program for basketball players*

	Phase I (7 wk) Hypertrophy	Phase II (7 wk) Strength	Phase III (4 wk) Strength/Power
Days 1 and 3			
Power clean[a]	—	1 × 10, 4 × 4–6 RM	1 × 10, 4 × 3–5 RM
Push press[a]	—	1 × 10, 4 × 4–6 RM	1 × 10, 4 × 3–5 RM
Bench press[a]	1 × 10, 4 × 8–10 RM	1 × 10, 4 × 6–8 RM	1 × 10, 4 × 4–6 RM
Incline bench press	1 × 10, 3 × 8–10 RM	1 × 10, 3 × 6–8 RM	1 × 10, 3 × 4–6 RM
Incline dumbbell flys	3 × 8–10 RM	—	—
Shoulder press[a]	1 × 10, 3 × 8–10 RM	—	—
Upright row	1 × 10, 3 × 8–10 RM	—	—
Lateral raise	3 × 8–10 RM	—	—
Triceps pushdown	3 × 8–10 RM	3 × 8–10 RM	3 × 6–8 RM
Triceps dumbbell extension	3 × 8–10 RM	3 × 8–10 RM	—
Abdominal exercise	3 sets	3 sets	3 sets
Days 2 and 4			
Squat[a]	1 × 10, 4 × 8–10 RM	1 × 10, 4 × 6–8 RM	1 × 10, 4 × 4–6 RM
Leg extension	3 × 8–10 RM	3 × 8–10 RM	3 × 6–8 RM
Leg curl	3 × 8–10 RM	3 × 8–10 RM	3 × 6–8 RM
Standing calf raise	3 × 8–10 RM	3 × 8–10 RM	3 × 6–8 RM
Lat pulldown[a]	1 × 10, 3 × 8–10 RM	1 × 10, 3 × 6–8 RM	1 × 10, 3 × 6–8 RM
Seated row	1 × 10, 3 × 8–10 RM	1 × 10, 3 × 6–8 RM	1 × 10, 3 × 6–8 RM
Biceps exercise I	3 × 8–10 RM	3 × 8–10 RM	3 × 6–8 RM
Biceps exercise II	3 × 8–10 RM	3 × 8–10 RM	—
Abdominal exercise	3 sets	3 sets	3 sets

A 1-week active rest should precede phase II and III; see text for details. Biceps exercise I and II refers to any biceps exercise (i.e., standing or seated biceps dumbbell curls, barbell curls, hammer curls), which can be chosen at the discretion of the athlete.
[a] Core exercise.

summer vacation (end of August/beginning of September) until the start of official basketball practice (mid-October). This may differ slightly in other leagues. The resistance-training program during this time may comprise several different microcycles that may resemble the off-season training program. For example, a 6-week preseason resistance-training program may comprise a 2-week hypertrophy phase, a 2-week strength phase, and a 2-week strength/power phase. The exercises, and both the intensity and volume of training, will parallel the off-season resistance-training program. During this time, a greater emphasis on the conditioning program is devoted to anaerobic (e.g., intervals and sprint) and sport-specific (e.g., agility, plyometrics) training.

During the season, the primary concern is to maintain the strength gains achieved during the off-season. For first-year or inexperienced resistance-trained players, there is some evidence that supports the benefit of in-season resistance training for increasing strength during the season (34). The in-season training program is generally referred to as a maintenance program (44). An example of an in-season resistance-training program can be seen in Table 46–2.

Over the duration of the basketball season, the time available during practice sessions for supplemental training to enhance power may be limited. Brown and colleagues (45) examined the effect of plyometric training on the vertical jump ability of high school basketball players. For the players who performed plyometric training (three sets of 10 depth jumps, 3 days/week, for 12 weeks) in addition to their regular basketball training, there was a significant improvement in vertical jump, with arms assistance, compared with the control (basketball training only) group. It was determined that 57% of the vertical-jump gain was due to improved skill, and 43% was due to increased strength. They concluded that plyometric training appeared to enhance the coordination of arms with strength development of legs and provided a convenient in-season training method.

Endurance Program

It appears that once an aerobic base is reached (apparently a value between 42 mL/kg/min to 59 mL/kg/min

TABLE 46–2. *In-season resistance training program, 2 days/wk*

Power clean[a]	1 × 10, 3 × 4–6 RM
Push press[a]	1 × 10, 3 × 4–6 RM
Squat[a]	1 × 10, 3 × 6–8 RM
Bench press[a]	1 × 10, 3 × 6–8 RM
Lat pulldown	3 × 8–10 RM
Leg curl	3 × 8–10 RM
Triceps pushdown	3 × 8–10 RM
Biceps curl	3 × 8–10 RM
Abdominal exercise	3 sets

[a] Core exercise.

for male basketball players), any further increase in aerobic capacity may not provide any additional benefit to the basketball player (24). Therefore the goal of the endurance-training program should be to maintain aerobic capacity levels within this range. To maintain an aerobic base during the off-season training program, the basketball player should run at least 3 days/week for 20 to 30 minutes each session. Alternative means of aerobic training (i.e., cycling) may be a good training program variation for the athlete. The intensity for this exercise should be near 70% to 75% of age-predicted maximal heart rate. The coach or strength and conditioning specialist should be aware if the players are required to participate in "unsupervised" basketball scrimmages, which may run for 2 hours per day, 5 to 6 days/wk. If so, this may be a sufficient stimulus to maintain an aerobic base. If a goal of the off-season training program is to increase strength and body mass, then too much emphasis on an aerobic program (including the daily basketball scrimmages) may reduce the ability of these athletes to achieve maximal strength and body mass gains (41). If an athlete's primary goal is to reduce body fat, then a greater emphasis should be directed to increasing the aerobic component of the off-season training program.

Anaerobic Training

Specific conditioning of the anaerobic energy system is not initiated until the preseason training program begins. Until this phase, the athlete's conditioning program has focused on resistance training, maintaining an aerobic base, performing sport-specific drills (this may include both agility and speed development), and playing basketball (either scrimmages or in summer leagues). Anaerobic conditioning until this point was avoided to prevent any possible overtraining syndrome to occur during the season. The preseason (at the collegiate level) is approximately 6 weeks in duration. It is the goal of this phase of training to bring the athlete close to, but not necessarily at, peak condition. This last statement may seem unscientific, but the practicality of it will be explained. Once official basketball practice starts, the team will begin practicing with the basketball coaching staff. This period, before the competitive season begins, is also referred to as the "preseason" by the basketball coaching staff; however, for the strength and conditioning coach, this will be "preseason II." Depending on the specific situation involved, many basketball coaches will devote much of this time to conditioning drills. In this scenario, it may be prudent for the strength and conditioning specialist to leave some room for improvement during this period. A problem of fatigue or overreaching may develop if the athlete peaks too soon.

An example of a preseason anaerobic conditioning program can be seen in Table 46–3. This program is performed 4 days/week, with a progression in both intensity and volume. The work/rest ratio during the sprint training is manipulated to increase the intensity of exercise. The aim in reducing the work/rest ratio is to improve the recovery time from high-intensity activity during a basketball game. Interval or *fartlek* training also is used to simulate the energy demands experienced during competition. Interval training can be performed on an oval outdoor or indoor track. The athlete sprints the straight portion of the track (approximately 100 m) and jogs the turns (100 m). The required numbers of laps are performed continuously. *Fartlek* training, which is another method of anaerobic training that intersperses high-intensity sprints with lower-intensity running, can be substituted for any of the anaerobic conditioning activities shown.

TABLE 46–3. *Example of an anaerobic conditioning program*

	Exercise	Frequency	Work/rest ratio
Weeks 1–2			
Day 1	Intervals	3–4 laps	—
Day 2	400-m sprint	× 1	1:4
	100-m sprint	× 2	1:4
	30-m sprint	× 8	1:4
Day 3	Intervals	3–4 laps	—
Day 4	200-m sprint	× 4–5	1:4
Weeks 3–4			
Day 1	Intervals	4–5 laps	—
Day 2	400-m sprint	× 1	1:4
	100-m sprint	× 3–4	1:4
	30-m sprint	× 8–10	1:4
Day 3	Intervals	4–5 laps	—
Day 4	200-m sprint	× 5–6	1:4
Weeks 5–6			
Day 1	Intervals	5–6 laps	—
Day 2	400-m sprint	× 2	1:3
	100-m sprint	× 4–5	1:3
	30-m sprint	× 10–12	1:3
Day 3	Intervals	5–6 laps	—
Day 4	200-m sprint	× 6–7	1:3

Speed, Agility, and Basketball Skills Training

Specific speed and agility training is usually performed as a team during the preseason conditioning program. However, for individual athletes who show a deficiency in either running technique, sprint speed, agility, or quickness, further training can be performed during the off-season conditioning program. Many different exercises are available for improving agility in basketball players. Ideally, an exercise should be chosen that simulates movements and actions performed on the court. In addition, if agility will be tested, then the athlete should use that particular drill as part of the agility program (i.e., T-drill). Running-technique drills also can be performed during the off-season training program. Frequently these drills are part of the warm-up and flexibility routine of many teams. Examples of both agility and running-technique drills can be seen in Table 46–4. This is by no means a complete list of agility or running-technique drills; however, it should be able to provide a good starting point for agility training.

Basketball-specific drills should be performed throughout the training program. It is imperative that during the off-season resistance-training program, the athletes continue to shoot and play basketball. Those opposed to the use of resistance training for basketball players suggest that resistance training may harm the fine-motor sensitivity needed for shooting the basketball. If the player continues to shoot the basketball throughout the training program, however, he or she can apparently maintain shooting skills without any negative effects. Furthermore, the resistance-training program appears to enhance shooting skills by increasing the shooting range of the player, accelerating release time, and accelerating time to peak height during the vertical phase of the jump shot (42).

TABLE 46–4. *Examples of agility and running-technique drills*

Agility drills	
Side shuffle	Place two cones 5–7 m apart and side shuffle between cones for 10 s
Quick feet	Using the baseline of a basketball court, attempt to take small choppy steps over and under the baseline. The object is to stay as close to the line without touching, and to be as quick as possible
Four-corner drill	Place cones in a square (can possibly use foul lane extended) 5–7 m each side. Player initiates exercise by performing a backward run to the second cone; with a tight transition around cone, the player then performs a side shuffle from cone 2 to 3; as the player makes another tight transition around cone 3, the player then performs a karioki exercise (shuffle over, shuffle under) till cone 4; player then sprints back to cone 1
T-drill	Cones set in a T-formation. Player sprints from baseline to cone 1 (9 m), side shuffles to cone 2 (4.5 m), side shuffles back through cone 1 to cone 3, side shuffles back to cone 1 (4.5 m), and does a backward sprint to baseline
Jump rope	
Running-technique drills	
15-m knee to chest run	
15-m heels-to-butt run	
Striders	
Power skips	

Flexibility

The flexibility program should be performed before (as part of the warm-up) and after (as part of the cool-down) each workout. A number of exercises can be used for this program. It is not within the scope of this chapter to detail these exercises. Before performing flexibility exercises, it is recommended that the athlete perform 5 to 10 minutes of continuous aerobic exercise to increase blood flow to the active musculature, increase body and muscle temperature, and increase speed of neural conduction (46). It is hypothesized that this warm-up period before performing the flexibility exercises will prevent injuries (potential for muscle pulls or spasms) and enhance the adaptability of the muscles, tendons, and ligaments to the stretching exercise (19).

CONCLUSION

Basketball has attained an impressive level of international popularity. It is a game played with a continuous flow of activity, and several factors may affect the physiologic demands placed on the competitors. Few studies have examined specific physiologic requirements during actual basketball contests, but some assessments of heart rate, blood lactate, estimated oxygen uptake, and the importance of hydration have been made. Unlike some other sports, basketball is not associated with a standard testing regimen; laboratory and field tests of aerobic capacity, anaerobic power, strength, speed/agility, and flexibility are often used, however. An optimal training program for basketball is based on the principles of periodization. A true challenge, however, is for the player to begin the season in near-peak condition and maintain peak performance throughout the season. We have presented several recommendations on conditioning for basketball during both in-season and off-season cycles.

REFERENCES

1. McInnes SE, Carlson JS, Jones CJ, McKenna MJ. The physiological load imposed on basketball players during competition. *J Sport Sci* 1995;13:387–397.
2. Beam WC, Merrill TL. Analysis of heart rates recorded during female collegiate basketball [Abstract]. *Med Sci Sports Exerc* 1994;26:S66.
3. McArdle WD, Magel JR, Kyvallos LC. Aerobic capacity, heart rate and estimated energy cost during women's competitive basketball. *Res Q* 1971;42:178–186.
4. Ramsey JD, Ayoub MM, Dudek RA, Edgar HS. Heart rate recovery during a college basketball game. *Res Q* 1970;41:528–535.
5. Maresh CM, Wang BC, Goetz KL. Plasma vasopressin, renin activity, and aldosterone responses to maximal exercise in active college females. *Eur J Appl Physiol* 1985;54:398–403.

6. Hoffman JR, Stavsky H, Falk B. The effect of water restriction on anaerobic power and vertical jumping height in basketball players. *Int J Sports Med* 199516:214–218.
7. Latin RW, Berg K, Baechle T. Physical and performance characteristics of NCAA division. I male basketball players. *J Strength Cond Res* 1994;8:214–218.
8. Cabrera JM, Smith DP, Byrd RJ. Cardiovascular adaptations on Puerto Rican basketball players during a 14-week season. *J Sports Med* 1977;17:173–180.
9. Coleman AE, Kreuzer P, Friedrich DW, Juvenal JP. Aerobic and anaerobic responses of male college freshmen during a season of basketball. *J Sports Med* 1974;14:26–31.
10. Hakkinen K. Effects of the competitive season on physical fitness profile in elite basketball players. *J Hum Mov Stud* 1988; 15:119–128.
11. Hoffman JR, Fry AC, Howard R, Maresh CM, Kraemer WJ. Strength, speed and endurance changes during the course of a division I basketball season. *J Appl Sport Sci Res* 1991;5:144–149.
12. Hunter GR, Hilyer J. Evaluation of the University of Alabama at Birmingham men's basketball team. *NSCA J* 1989;11:14–15.
13. Hunter GR, Hilyer J, Forster MA. Changes in fitness during 4 years of intercollegiate basketball. *J Strength Cond Res* 1993; 7:26–29.
14. Parnat J, Viru A, Savi T, Nurmekivi A. Indices of aerobic work capacity and cardio-vascular response during exercise in athletes specializing in different events. *J Sports Med* 1975;15:100–105.
15. Parr RB, Hoover R, Wilmore JH, Bachman D, Kerlan RK. Professional basketball players: athletic profiles. *Physician Sportsmed* 1978;6:77–84.
16. Vaccaro P, Clarke DH, Wrenn JP. Physiological profiles of elite women basketball players. *J Sports Med* 1979;19:45–54.
17. Tavino LP, Bowers CJ, Archer CB. Effects of basketball on aerobic capacity, anaerobic capacity, and body composition of male college players. *J Strength Cond Res* 1995;9:75–77.
18. Stone WJ, Steingard PM. Year-round conditioning for basketball. *Clin Sports Med* 1993;2:173–191.
19. Wilmore JH, Costill DL. *Physiology of sport and exercise.* Champaign, IL: Human Kinetics, 1994.
20. Chandler J. Goals and activities for athletic conditioning for basketball. *NSCA J* 1986;8:52–55.
21. Fox EL. *Sports physiology.* 2nd ed. Philadelphia: WB Saunders, 19xx.
22. Gillam GM. Physiological basis of basketball bioenergetics. *NSCA J* 1985;6:44–71.
23. Gillam GM. Identification of anthropometric and physiological characteristics relative to participation in college basketball. *NSCA J* 1985;7:34–36.
24. Hoffman JR, Epstein S, Einbinder M, Weinstein I. The influence of aerobic capacity on recovery from high intensity exercise in basketball players. *J Strength Cond Res* 1999 (*in press*).
25. Hoffman JR. The relationship between aerobic fitness and recovery from high-intensity exercise in infantry soldiers. *Mil Med* 1997;162:484–488.
26. Hoffman JR, Tennenbaum G, Maresh CM, Kraemer WJ. Relationship between athletic performance tests and playing time in elite college basketball players. *J Strength Cond Res* 1996;10: 67–71.
27. Hakkinen K. Changes in physical fitness profile in female basketball players during the competitive season including explosive type strength training. *J Sports Med Phys Fitness* 1993;33:19–26.
28. Morrow JR, Hosler WW, Nelson JK. A comparison of women intercollegiate basketball players, volleyball players and non-athletes. *J Sports Med* 1980;20:435–440.
29. Petko M, Hunter GR. Four-year changes in strength, power, and aerobic fitness in women college basketball players. *Strength Cond* 1997;19:46–49.
30. Smith HK, Thomas SG. Physiological characteristics of elite female basketball players. *Can J Sport Sci* 1991;16:289–295.
31. Riezebos ML, Paterson DH, Hall CR, Yuhasz MS. Relationship of selected variables to performance in women's basketball. *Can J Appl Sport Sci* 1983;8:34–40.
32. Hoffman JR, Maresh CM, Armstrong LE. Isokinetic and dynamic constant resistance strength testing: implications for sport. *Phys Ther Pract* 1992;2:42–53.
33. Hoffman JR, Fry AC, Deschenes M, Kemp M, Kraemer WJ. The effects of self selection for frequency of training in a winter conditioning program for football. *J Appl Sport Sci Res* 1990; 4:76–82.
34. Hoffman JR, Maresh CM, Armstrong LE, Kraemer WJ. Effects of off-season and in-season resistance training programs on a collegiate male basketball team. *J Hum Muscle Perform* 1991; 1:48–55.
35. Groves BR. Gayle RC. Physiological changes in male basketball players in year-round. *J Strength Cond Res* 1993;7:30–33.
36. Seminick D. The T-test. *NSCA J* 1990;12:36–37.
37. Hakkinen K. Maximal force, explosive strength and speed in female volleyball and basketball players. *J Hum Mov Stud* 1989; 16:291–303.
38. Vaccaro P, Wrenn JP, Clarke DH. Selected aspects of pulmonary function and maximal oxygen uptake of elite college basketball players. *J Sports Med* 1980;20:103–108.
39. Caterisano A, Patrick BT, Edenfield WL, Batson MJ. The effects of a basketball season on aerobic and strength parameters among college men: starters vs. reserves. *J Strength Cond Res* 1997; 11:21–24.
40. Fry RW, Morton AR, Keast D. Overtraining in athletes. *Sports Med* 1991;12:32–65.
41. Dudley GA, Djamil R. Incompatibility of endurance- and strength-training modes of exercise. *J Appl Physiol* 1985;59:1446–1451.
42. Ball R. The basketball jump shot: a kinesiological analysis with recommendations for strength and conditioning programs. *NSCA J* 1989;11:4–12.
43. Hilyer J. A year-round strength development and conditioning program for men's basketball. *NSCA J* 1989;11:16–19.
44. Fleck SJ, Kraemer WJ. *Designing resistance training programs.* Champaign, IL: Human Kinetics, 1997.
45. Brown ME, Mayhew JL, Boleach LW. Effect of plyometric training on vertical jump performance in high school basketball players. *J Sports Med* 1986;26:1–4.
46. Alter MJ. *Sport stretch.* Champaign, IL: Human Kinetics, 1998.

Exercise and Sport Science,
edited by William E. Garrett, Jr., and Donald T. Kirkendall.
Lippincott Williams & Wilkins, Philadelphia © 2000.

CHAPTER 47

Physiology of Canoe Sport

Jay T. Kearney and Donald C. McKenzie

Indigenous cultures around the world have used canoes and kayaks, in their various evolutionary stages, as modes of transportation for exploration, commerce, and war. The identifiable origins of use of canoes and kayaks in sport is traceable to North America, and early accounts recall contests among the French voyageurs in their large freight canoes. The popularization of canoe sport (touring, sailing, and racing) can be traced to two books recounting romantic and legendary journeys by canoe, *A Thousand Miles in the ROB ROY Canoe on Twenty Rivers and Lakes in Europe* (1866) by John MacGregor and the *Voyage of the Paper Canoe* (1878) by Nathaneil Bishop. In 1880 the American Canoe Association, including Canada as one division, was founded. Sporting use of canoes and kayaks, both competitively and recreationally, flourished in the late 1800s and early 1900s in both Europe and North America.

In the 1920s Waldmar Von Brunt Claussen, a Dutch expatriate living in New York, along with a diverse group of western Europeans, met to establish what would evolve into the International Canoe Federation. Canoeing was a demonstration sport at the 1924 Olympic Games and became a full-medal sport in 1936. The original Olympic discipline was flatwater racing involving both sprint and distance, 10,000 m. Women first competed during the 1948 Games in London. The 10,000-m event was dropped and a 4 × 500-m relay added in Rome 1960. Slalom was added to the Olympic program in Munich (1972). Since the mid 1970s, a number of disciplines of canoeing, traditional cultural forms, and entirely new formats have established international competitions. These include dragon boats, Polynesian outriggers, marathon paddling, canoe polo, surf skis, and rodeo boating.

The purpose of this chapter is to synthesize and summarize the literature available on the applied physiology of canoe sport. The approach is to (a) develop a profile of competitive athletes including anthropometry, metabolic capacities, and muscular strength and power; (b) synthesize the literature describing and documenting training adaptations elicited, and (c) provide an overview of the training regimens used by each discipline. Within the literature we have had access to, primarily English, the vast majority of references discuss the Olympic disciplines—flatwater sprint paddling and slalom. Consequently, the sections on these disciplines are far more completely developed. The scientific literature available on marathon, dragon boat, and outrigger is reviewed in the last section of the chapter. We hope that readers will be able to generalize principles from the more thoroughly presented areas to disciplines in which a dearth of information still exists.

THE SPORT

Energetics of Paddling

An excellent treatise on the energy cost of human locomotion on land and in the water is provided by diPrampero (1). The simplest form of the equation describing the factors contributing to the velocity the athlete is capable of achieving is:

$$v = e \div c$$

where v is the velocity of the boat, e is the sum of the aerobic and anaerobic energy contributions, and c is the the energy cost per unit distance of paddling.

Canoe and kayak athletes at the internationally competitive level possess significant aerobic abilities, generally greater than 60 mL/kg/min in male athletes, and well-developed anaerobic capacities, as demonstrated

J. T. Kearney: Sport Science and Technology Division, United States Olympic Committee, Colorado Springs, Colorado 80909.

D. C. McKenzie: Allan McGaivin Sports Medicine Center, University of British Columbia, Vancouver, Canada.

TABLE 47–1. *Metabolic contributions simulated 200-, 500-, and 1000-m events*

	Kayak men			Kayak women			Canoe men		
Event	$\dot{V}O_2$ (L/min)	O_2 Eq (L/min)[a]	% Aerobic[b]	$\dot{V}O_2$ (L/min)	O_2 Eq (L/min)[a]	% Aerobic[b]	$\dot{V}O_2$ (L/min)	O_2 Eq (L/min)[a]	% Aerobic[b]
200 m	2.89	4.89	37.8	2.05	3.13	40.0	2.66	4.61	36.5
500 m	3.78	2.26	62.8	2.68	1.22	69.0	3.48	2.00	63.5
1000 m	4.25	0.94	82.2	2.76	0.46	86.0	3.98	0.70	84.5

[a] Calculated as the oxygen equivalent of the non–oxygen-dependent work output by using the Medbo procedure.
[b] Percentage of total work performed that can be attributed to $\dot{V}O_2$ uptake. Anaerobic contribution is assumed to be reciprocal.

by postrace lactates of 12 to 20 mmol/L. By using reasonable assumptions, this represents an available e of 200 to 250 kJ for a 500-m race. Byrnes and Kearney (2) presented data on the aerobic and anaerobic contribution to simulated competitive efforts comparable to the racing distances of 200, 500, and 1000 meters. Table 47–1 presents the mean data on the United States National Team before their selection in 1996.

The magnitude of c is significantly affected by velocity and hull design. The energy cost of paddling is relatively linear at the lowest speeds [8 to 13 km/h (3–6)]; however, as athletes approach competitive velocity, this energy cost begins to increase exponentially (5,7). Hull-design factors that influence drag include beam-to-length ratio, wetted surface area, rocker, prismatic coefficient, and total displacement. Each discipline maintains technical and design requirements within which boat designers attempt to optimize the performance characteristics of drag, maneuverability, stability, and seaworthiness. In a unique approach, Pendergast and colleagues (5) were able to determine the passive drag of the slalom kayak while a paddler sat passively in the boat ($Drag_N = 2.32\ V^{1.75}$), as well as the drag while the kayaker was paddling. These data revealed (a) a nonlinear increase in drag at higher speeds, (b) an increased drag with the athlete paddling, and (c) a significant difference between skilled and unskilled paddlers. The lower the skill of the paddler, the greater the increase in drag of the boat when the paddler is active. An excellent treatment of the interaction among hull design factors, drag components, mechanical power delivered by the paddler(s), and boat velocity is presented by Jackson (7).

In summary, to optimize boat velocity, the athlete or athletes in team boats need to (a) maximize the sum of aerobic and anaerobic or non–oxygen-dependent energy sources available for propulsion, (b) minimize the drag by selecting a boat of optimal design characteristics, (c) increase propulsive skill, and (d) carry the minimal required mass.

FLATWATER SPRINT

Flatwater sprint canoe/kayak races are contested on a buoyed, flat course, similar to a rowing course, at distances of 200, 500, and 1000 m. The boats used are single kayaks (K-1), single canoes (C-1), double kayaks (K-2), double canoes (C-2), and four-person kayaks (K-4). Women race in kayaks whereas men compete in both kayaks and canoes. An informative overview of flatwater paddling is provided by Toro (8).

The last thorough review of the applied physiology related to sprint or flatwater canoe/kayak racing was published by Shepherd in 1987 (6). Since then, a number of developments have occurred that affect applied physiology of flatwater sprint racing. Among these are (a) equipment changes, most notably, the introduction of the wing blade in 1985 and the associated change in technique; (b) the continued evolution of boat designs and materials; (c) the addition of 200-m events to the World Championship program, bringing the lower end of race durations down to a range of 35 seconds and, therefore, increasing the importance of absolute power output and anaerobic capacity in 200-m specialists; (d) the addition of 1000-m events for women and the segregation of the 10,000-m events away from the flatwater World Championships and into the marathon discipline; and (e) changes in the progression systems used (heat, reps, semis) that place an additional premium on performance in each race and limit the capacity of athletes to attempt to select their competition in the semifinals. These evolutionary changes and improvement in the overall physiologic capacity of the athletes led to a progressive increase in performances. In the 1996 Olympics, the "best time ever" was recorded in 7 of the 12 events on the course at Gainesville, Georgia (9). Although no official world records are maintained for the canoe/kayak distances (because of the constant potential for variability in water and wind conditions), establishing 7 of the 12 best-ever performances clearly indicates a progression of the competitive standard. Margins of victory in the 1996 Olympic Games were between 0.2% and 0.4%, further documenting the competitive standard.

The Elite Athlete

Anthropometric Characteristics

The 1987 review by Shepherd (6) concluded that canoe and kayak athletes, in general, were slightly above average height, were heavier, had a lower percentage of body fat, and had a higher-than-expected amount of lean mass. The data of Hirada, published in that review, were specific to flatwater sprint racers and indicated that the gold medalists from Montreal were heavier and taller than the less successful competitors in their respective events. The most extensive data on the anthropometry of paddlers was presented by Lindsey Carter (10–12). The somatotype of the male competitors at Montreal was 1.5 ± 0.45, 5.2 ± 0.83, 3.1 ± 0.95. Among this group of 12 paddlers, 58% were ectomorphic mesomorphs and 36% were balanced mesomorphs. The scale values for female competitors were 2.8 ± 0.26, 4.1 ± 0.78, and 2.9 ± 0.58; 37.5% balanced mesomorphs and 37% of a central somatotype. All of the paddlers had negative *z* scores on skin-fold measurements. There do not appear to have been well-organized studies on the anthropometric assessment of flatwater paddlers during the 1996 Olympic games, and therefore no current data are available.

Freeman (13,14), working with a group of four elite male sprinters from the Australian national team, reported somatotypes of 2.1, 5.8, and 2.2 for endomorphy, mesomorphy, and ectomorphy subscales, respectively. Fry and Morton (15) also used a group of Australian paddlers, including state team members and nationally competitive athletes, to evaluate the ability to differentiate among athletes on the basis of scientific data. The researchers were able to use anthropometric and physiologic characteristics to identify those individuals selected for the national team and those not selected. Of the 38 athletes involved in the project, the 7 selected were taller and had greater muscle mass, larger biceps, larger forearms, greater vital capacity, increased strength, and a higher $\dot{V}O_2$ in L/min. It is important to keep in mind that these factors differentiated between regional- and national-level athletes but may have limited generalizability to differentiating among elite athletes. In a comparable design, attempting to compare the anthropometric profile of 18 kayakers and 11 canoeists to the norm of the Yugoslavian population, Misigoj-Durakovic and Heimer (16) reported that the paddlers had the expected characteristics of lower subcutaneous fat, increased mass, increased upper-arm circumference and mass, above-average skeletal lengths especially in the upper body, increased sitting height, and greater forced vital capacity (FVC) and vital capacity (VC).

In summary, the profile of a flatwater paddler tends toward a mesomorphic somatotype, greater than average height, long limbs and body segments (especially upper body), well-developed upper-body musculature, and low body fat. It appears that the lack of contemporary information about the general anthropometric characteristics of international elite flatwater paddlers merits an investigation.

Muscular System

Information on the active muscles during canoe and kayak strokes has been acquired from (a) observation and intuitive analyses by coaches, (b) film-based biomechanical analysis (17,18), and (c) electromyographic (EMG) analysis on stationary ergometers (19,20) and on water (21). Given a choice of these techniques, recording of the EMG activity during on-water paddling is most desirable. EMG analysis is especially important because portions of strokes involve stabilization of joint segments that may not appear to require a significant muscular activity when using the motion or intuitive-analysis approaches. The most comprehensive EMG analysis of elite paddlers was completed by Capousek and Bruggemann by using one male and one female German National Team athlete (21). The anterior deltoids had the highest activation for the longest proportion of the stroke. The trapezius, triceps, and rectus abdominis also were active during most of the stroke phases but at a lower level relative to the deltoids. In contrast, the biceps, latissimus dorsi, and pectoralis major were active for only about 20% of the duration of the stroke. The abdominal obliques were not substantially active. This analysis was done just before the introduction of the wing blade; the new technique requires a greater involvement of trunk rotation and therefore undoubtedly places more reliance on the obliques. Capousek and Bruggemann did not use an EMG evaluation of the lower-body musculature; however, the work of Logan and Holt (19) indicated a significant involvement of the hip extensors, knee extensors, and ankle extensors. Although the range of motion of these lower-body extensor activities is limited, their contribution to the overall stroke is important for stabilization and transmission of force to the boat.

Gollnick and colleagues (22) and Bergh and colleagues (23) were among the first to perform muscle biopsies and fiber typing on canoeists. Gollnick reported a mean value of 63% slow twitch (ST) fibers. Bergh and associates fiber typed the gastrocnemius and vastus lateralis of six Swedish paddlers and reported a mean value of ST fibers of 60% with a range from 46% to 70%. Tesch and colleagues (24) reported that paddlers who were successful at 500 m had a higher percentage of fast twitch (FT) fibers (50% to 59%) than did 10,000-m specialists, with FT fibers 26% to 52%. Tesch and co-workers (25) performed muscle biopsies and typed fibers from the vastus lateralis and mid-deltoid of a group of European handball, ice hockey, kayak (n = 8), running, water skiing, and wrestling athletes. Fiber-type data on paddlers are presented in Table 47–2.

Among the groups of athletes, kayakers had the lowest percentage of ST fibers in the vastus lateralis and the highest percentage of ST fibers in the deltoids. The original authors speculated that, although genetics has an influence on fiber type, the data tended to support the concept of a transient change in fiber type. This speculation is now more controversial, especially in regard to interconversion between the FT and ST fibers.

Baker and Hardy (26) used a group of nine fit, adult,

TABLE 47–2. *Fiber type distributions in kayak paddlers*

Muscle	Fiber subtype		
	FTa	FTb	ST
Tesch et al., 1976			
Mid-deltoid	38 (26–44)		62 (56–74)
Tesch et al., 1982			
Vastus	30	29	41
Deltoid	7	20	73
Clarkson et al., 1982			
Vastus	39.7 ± 9.0	17.0 ± 9.2	43.3 ± 12.3
Biceps	42.1 ± 9.1	14.1 ± 7.9	43.9 ± 7.1

male physical education students exposed to 9 weeks of progressive, high-intensity training on a canoeing ergometer to evaluate the impact of training on fiber type and size. By using a fiber-typing scheme that reported only Type I (ST) and Type II (FT), the authors indicated a minimal change in the proportion of fiber types before and after training, well within the error of measurement. However, their data strongly supported the selective hypertrophy of the Type II fibers in the latissimus dorsi as a result of 9 weeks of training. The mean hypertrophy in the Type I fibers was 8%, whereas the Type II fibers hypertrophied by 82%. Paddlers demonstrated superior muscular endurance in their trained upper-body musculature when compared with other athletes or untrained controls on Thorstensson-type isokinetic tests. A portion of this quality is explained by the selective hypertrophy of active fibers and an increased total muscle mass (13,14,24,25,27–29).

Metabolic Characteristics

The majority of the extant publications profiling the metabolic characteristics of elite paddlers were in press before Shepherd's review in 1987. Paddling specific $\dot{V}O_2$ values tend to range between 4.5 and 6.0 L/min for men and between 2.5 and 4.5 L/min for women (3,15,30,31). Paddlers also consistently demonstrated the ability to use a consistently higher percentage of $\dot{V}O_2$max, cycle ergometer or treadmill, as $\dot{V}O_2$ peak during paddling-specific work. Furthermore, it is important to note that, in some cases, the in-boat $\dot{V}O_2$ is higher than the $\dot{V}O_2$ by using a paddling simulation or arm-crank procedure (4,32–34). The highest values recorded in this laboratory while monitoring American athletes, since 1987, is just over 70 mL/kg with an in-boat system.

Tesch and Karlsson (35) tested five Swedish kayak paddlers to compare the local metabolic demands of sprint paddling, 500-m or 2-minute effort, and marathon paddling, 10K or 45 minutes. As expected, peak heart rates were significantly different: 184 ± 9 beats/min at 500 m and 170 ± 8 beats/min at 45 minutes. Significant differences also were found in the traditional markers of energy demands at the cellular level. Comparing the 500-m with the 10K simulated effort, the creatine phosphate concentration was lower, glycogen depletion greater, lactate acid accumulation higher, blood glucose higher, glucose-6-phosphate (G-6-P) higher, and adenosine triphosphate (ATP) equal. The reliance on very high glycolytic rates is highlighted by comparing the rate of glycogen depletion: 10.0 m*M*/kg ww/min for the 500 and 1.4 m*M*/kg ww/min for the 10K. This rate of glycogen depletion is comparable to what is seen in 60 seconds of cycling at 150% of $\dot{V}O_2$max and causes an 80% depletion in one all-out effort.

The lactic acid or ventilatory threshold tends to be relatively high in well-conditioned paddlers. Typical values range from the very high 70% to the mid-80% of $\dot{V}O_2$max (36). These same paddlers concomitantly have very high peak lactate values. Some athletes may achieve postperformance values of greater than 20 mmol/L. Data collected in association with monitoring American paddlers ranged from peak post–World Championship race values as low as 11 mmol/L and as high as 18.6 mmol/L.

An increased level of documentation of the exceptional power-output capacity of trained flatwater paddlers has become available in the last 12 years (37,38). Ginn and Mackinnon (39) studied seven internationally ranked male kayakers from the 1988 Australian Olympic Team to evaluate the relation between power output at onset of blood lactic acid accumulation (OBLA), critical power (CP), and maximal lactic acid steady state (MLaSS). With these athletes, OBLA, defined as the work load equivalent to achieving a blood lactic acid concentration of 4.0 mmol/L, was obtained at 341 ± 104 W. CP was determined from maximal efforts at 600, 750, and 900 W and calculated to be 495 ± 24 W. MLaSS was determined by using a series of five maximal efforts ranging from 50 W below to 50 W above CP. In this group of athletes, CP and MLaSS were virtually the same, 496 versus 490 W. The important result of this study is the documentation of the exceptional power-output capacity of these highly trained paddlers. Fry and Morton (15) studied a group of kayakers to evaluate power-output capacity. The athletes included a broader range of individuals competing in an Australian state championship. Their anaerobic power output and capacity test was a 1-minute all-out performance on an air-braked kayak ergometer. The mean power output for their subjects was 363 W.

Freeman (13,14) also studied Australian national level paddlers to evaluate peak power-output capacity. The four elite male sprint kayakers reportedly were able to achieve a peak power output of 1150 ± 50 W in a 10-second all-out test on a kayaking ergometer. The peak value obtained at the beginning of a 60-second all-out test on the same equipment was not significantly different at 1100 W. These power-output capacities are truly exceptional for an upper body–oriented activity. In contrast to the exceptional power-output capabilities reported in the three previous studies, Clingeleffer and associates (40) studied a group of eight well-trained state and national kayakers from Tasmania in a project designed to evaluate critical power output on a K1 kayak ergometer. Their protocol involved determination of CP from a series of 90-, 240-, 600-, and 1200-second efforts. The statistical line of best fit for these particular subjects resulted in a mean critical power of 164 ± 29 W, less than 50% of the critical power values reported in the earlier studies.

Training Adaptations

In 1995 and 1996, Henderson (41) compiled data on the developmental profile of canoe/kayak athletes who have been either Olympic or World Championship medalists. One hundred medalists in the Olympic sprint events between 1980 and 1995 were identified and asked to complete a brief questionnaire. Based on an exceptional response, 85% of the target group from 15 nations, Henderson developed a profile of the mean age at critical milestones in an athlete's development. These data provide several important insights into the developmental and training process for canoe/kayak athletes: (a) the average paddler has been racing for 11 years before becoming a World or Olympic champion; (b) 74% of the respondents had competed in a World Championship or Olympic Games by age of 21; and (c) 85% of athletes who would become World or Olympic Champions had reached this benchmark by age 24 (Table 47–3). This study is especially important because it documents the time required to elicit the training adaptations necessary to be an elite flatwater paddler and how young an athlete should start training.

Increase in Upper Body Aerobic Capacity

The aerobic capacity of the trained upper body musculature of paddlers has been shown to be 1.5 (42) to 2.6 (43) times greater than the oxygen uptake per unit of fat-free volume in untrained muscles. The training adaptations assumed to be responsible for these physiologic capabilities are (a) increased mitochondrial density, (b) increased myoglobin concentration, (c) increased concentration of oxidative enzymes, (d) increased capillarization, (e) increased a-vo_2 difference, and (f) advantageous redistribution of blood flow to active musculature (44–46). Three studies (3,47,48) systematically monitored the changes in aerobic capacity of paddlers. Wojcieszak and colleagues (47) and Wojczuk and Wojcieszak (48) demonstrated an increased O_2 use during a 4-minute simulated competitive effort. In contrast, Bunc and Heller (3) reported a stable $\dot{V}O_2$ over a year of training with elite-level paddlers.

TABLE 47–3. *Mean age at critical development/training milestones in sprint paddlers*

Milestone	Age (yr)
First race	12.34
Junior Worlds	17.05
Senior World Start	20.41
Senior World Top 8	21.35
Senior World Top 3	22.20
Senior World Champion	23.15

Enhanced Power-Output Capacity

One of the primary objectives of training is to elicit an improvement in the ability to generate power. There is a high negative correlation, $r = -0.79$, between power in a 4-minute all-out test and the personal record for 1000 m (47).

During 3 months of training fit paddlers, 13 seniors had a $\dot{V}O_2$ of 5.1 ± 0.5 L/min, and 11 juniors had a $\dot{V}O_2$ of 4.7 ± 0.5 L/min. Wojcieszak and colleagues (47) demonstrated a 15% gain in power. Initially, the mean power output in a 4-minute test was 226 ± 17 W and increased to 260 ± 25 W. Gains were made in both increased maximal power and decreased rate of power fatigue.

Improved Lactate Kinetics and Threshold

Compared with sedentary controls, paddlers have an increased threshold for the release of lactate at the onset of work, lower lactates at any given absolute or relative submaximal load, higher power output at lactate threshold, increased rate of maximal lactate release, and the ability to generate high maximal lactate (31,35,42,49,50). Bunc and Heller (3) evaluated lactate threshold and associated physiologic parameters of 14 top canoeists during 2 years of training. The paddlers were repeatedly tested under field conditions, assessing both submaximal lactate and in-boat $\dot{V}O_2$ in the boat. Anaerobic threshold was evaluated from repeated submaximal efforts in the boat and confirmed with a threshold-verification trial. Velocity at anaerobic threshold increased 4.6%, lactate at anaerobic threshold decreased 11.7%, whereas $\dot{V}O_2max$ remained relatively stable. The lactate at anaerobic threshold ranged from 4.0 and 5.3 mmol/L and occurred between 79% and 82% of $\dot{V}O_2max$. The authors concluded that "adaptations are dependent on the qualitative content of the imposed training" (page 27).

Hypertrophy of the Active Musculature

The single training study that has sequentially followed the impact of canoe training on muscle fiber area and type was completed by Baker and Hardy (26). Their model used physical education students exposed to training on a canoeing ergometer 3 times a week for 9 weeks. The results indicated that although the muscle-fiber type in the latissimus dorsi remained unchanged, significant hypertrophy (82%) occurred in the type II fibers. Several comparative or cross-sectional studies (reviewed in earlier sections) documented the large upper body musculature and apparent hypertrophy in paddlers (14–16,24,27,50).

Lower Metabolic and Hormonal Responses to an Acute Exercise Challenge

The metabolic and hormonal responses to an acute exercise challenge by trained versus untrained individuals is as expected. Parameters specifically evaluated with paddlers include (a) a differentiation between seniors and juniors on the postexercise creatine kinase (CK) activity (49); (b) a reduction in uric acid concentration in plasma after an all-out 40-second arm-exercise bout; and (c) lower acute responses for growth hormone, adrenocorticotropic hormone (ACTH), and catecholamines with a concomitant increase in insulin and decreased adrenaline/noradrenaline excretion (51,52).

Left Ventricular Mass

Csanady and co-workers (53) had the opportunity to monitor serially the echocardiographic parameters of fifteen 13-year-old Hungarian boys who were beginning their competitive canoe-racing training. These data were compared with those of 17 boys of the same age, height, and mass. The authors found a preexisting difference in left ventricular mass between the two groups, which increased significantly during the 3-year training period. One interpretation of these data is that the genetic selectivity and prior exercise experience predisposed these young athletes to positive training adaptations.

Training Programs

The physiologic objectives of training programs for flatwater sprint paddlers are readily enumerated:

- Enhanced $\dot{V}O_2$, especially in liters per minute with upper body activity,
- Upper body muscular mass,
- High upper body power-output capacity with superior power endurance, and
- Maximized ability to produce, buffer, and tolerate lactic acid.

A number of distinct models of training programs are used internationally. The national approaches adopted by the top nations in flatwater paddling; Germany, Hungary, Russia, Sweden, and Norway are variant. Typically, programs follow a four-cycle, periodized training approach including active rest, general preparation, specific preparation, and varying phases of competition. The training volume used by elite paddlers is in the range of 3000 to 5000 km/year of paddling supplemented by resistance training and general cardiovascular development. Table 47–4 provides a basic outline of the training phases, time of the year, and objectives that are a reasonable representation across the various national approaches. Specific in-boat training sets used include (a) long, sustained paddles of 15 to 30 km at a Zone 1 to Zone 2 level; (b) classic lactate threshold workouts, 3 to 5 × 12 to 20 min at a velocity that elicits lactates near the individual lactate threshold or 4 mmol/L; (c) shorter high-intensity efforts such as 5 × 8 minutes, approaching a maximal lactate steady-state pace; (d) $\dot{V}O_2$-specific intervals such as 5 × 5 minutes at a pace that requires more than 95% $\dot{V}O_2max$; (e) many variations of short race-velocity pieces that allow the paddlers to do race pace–specific technique work and elicit specific metabolic-training stimuli; and (f) a small volume of work at above-race pace. A number of published texts discuss various training models for sprint paddling (8,54–58). One of the more interesting is a review of

TABLE 47–4. *Conceptual presentation of typical annual training plan for sprint canoe/kayak*

Phase	Dates	Training objectives
Active rest	9/1–10/15	Mental and physical restoration
General preparation	10/15–1/15	General cardiovascular work Develop muscle mass and power Establish paddling base
Specific preparation	1/15–4/15	Paddling-specific endurance Paddling-specific power Technique
Competition		
Early	4/15–5/15	Race experience
Mid	5/15–6/15	Speed endurance
Prime	7/1–9/1	Maximum speed Lactate tolerance

the training and preparation strategies used by Greg Barton, the American double gold medalist from Seoul (1988) in the K-1 1000-m and K-2 1000-m races (59).

One of the coaches' challenges in designing and administering a training program is to optimize the adaptive stimuli without eliciting overtraining or staleness. Traditional approaches focus on monitoring derivatives of volume, intensity and duration, resting heart rate, and blood chemistries. Recently Berglund and Safstrom (60) used the Profile of Mood States (POMS) and a subjective rating of training load to monitor and modulate training load in 14 world-class Swedish paddlers. The total mood-disturbance score of the POMS was initially stable, increased significantly during the period of heaviest training, and then recorded a statistically significant decrease during the tapering period. This pattern was tracked by the subjective rating of training load. The authors used elevated POMS scores, greater than 50%, as a criterion for determining if athletes were training excessively or developing staleness. This criterion was met by 12% of all of the weekly POMS assessments during the study, and intervention or titration of training stimulus was based on this diagnostic procedure. The authors concluded that psychological monitoring was an effective procedure because none of the paddlers developed signs of overtraining or staleness, and seven became medalists in Barcelona.

SLALOM

Slalom began to emerge on the racing scene in the late 1940s and early 1950s, held its first biannual World Championship in 1949, and grew slowly until its inclusion on the Olympic program in 1972. That inclusion in the Olympic Games and the subsequent high-profile television coverage provided a significant impetus for the international development of the sport. Regrettably, canoe/kayak slalom was not included in the 1976 to 1988 Olympic Games but was reintroduced in Barcelona in 1992. Slalom is not one of the required sports in the Summer Games but was hosted on the Occoe River in Tennessee in 1996 and will be contested at the 2000 Games in Sydney. In its present format, slalom is contested on a section of fast running water with naturally occurring or artificially engineered obstacles, drops, hydraulics, and complex wave structures. The gates that the athletes are required to pass through are arranged to require (a) speed on relatively flat sections, (b) skill and power to maneuver the boat, (c) ability to read currents and move the boat laterally or upstream, and (d) capacity to plan carefully the appropriate route through the gates.

Slalom boats belong in one of three classes. The kayak is a completely decked design with emphasis placed on maneuverability and low volume with absolute hull speed being compromised. It is paddled by both male (K-1) and female (K-1 W) athletes with a double-bladed paddle. The canoe (C-1), also fully decked, is paddled in a double, low-kneeling position with thigh straps securing the paddler to the boat. It is paddled with a single-bladed paddle that the athlete, only males in international competition, can use on either side of the boat. The third class of boat in Olympic and international competition is the double canoe (C-2), in which two individuals are in the canoeing position in the same boat with one slightly toward the bow and the other slightly toward the stern, with their positions being somewhat offset toward their paddling side in the boat. For all three classes of boats, a slalom race is scored on the time required to complete between 20 and 35 gates with penalties for touching or missing a gate. The latest version of the rules reduced the penalties for touching a gate. This puts an increased premium on the ability of the paddlers to negotiate the course as fast as possible. The typical competitive format is the best time on either of two runs through a 400- to 800-m long course (61,62).

The Elite Athlete

Physical and Anthropometric Characteristics

Sidney and Shephard (63) profiled 10 male and 2 female white-water paddlers, many of whom were candidates for selection to the 1972 Canadian Olympic Team. The distinguishing characteristics of their paddlers were (a) above-average height, (b) large lean body mass, (c) good muscular development, (d) above average but not outstanding $\dot{V}O_2$, and (e) a large oxygen debt capacity. The correlation coefficient between the coach's rating of athlete's ability and the overall score on the physiologic variables was $r = 0.87$. This relationship is stronger than expected and discounts the importance of experience and technical expertise in slalom racing.

Vaccaro and colleagues (64) evaluated 13 men from the United States National Slalom Team. At the time (1973), the United States was arguably the best slalom team in the world. The battery of tests used to evaluate the team included the Heath–Carter somatotype scale, hydrostatic weighing for body composition, and $\dot{V}O_2max$ on a treadmill and $\dot{V}O_2$ on a paddling ergometer. The somatotype of this group of athletes was endomorphy, 2.88 ± 0.57; mesomorphy, 5.21 ± 0.96; and ectomorphy, 2.42 ± 0.93. This describes an athlete with a strong expression of muscularity and balanced but relatively low on both the endomorphy and ectomorphy. The height of these subjects was 180 cm, with a body fatness of approximately 10%.

In 1994, Sklad and associates (65) profiled a group of elite rowers, flatwater kayakers, canoeists, and 10 male slalom kayakers, all members of the Polish National Team. The objective of this study was to determine the morphologic differences characterizing elite rowers and kayakers with the potential of determining selection criteria for these sports. A large battery of somatic traits was measured on each athlete, with the goal of establishing a set of five body-build factors that included length, skeletal breadth, skeletal robustness, muscularity, and a general body-size index. The slalom kayakers were characterized as being relatively close to a reference group of university students on most parameters. The distinguishing characteristics were relatively long arm span, 6 cm longer than standing height, and relative leanness, 10.4% body fat. Compared with the rowers, the slalom kayak men were shorter, had a lower sitting height, and had a mean mass of 14 kg less than the rowers and 8 kg less than the sprint kayakers. Of the five composite variables used to profile this group of athletes, the slalom kayakers were notable only on the muscularity factor. The authors summarized that the profile of the slalom kayakers reflected high muscular power associated with relatively low body weight and is affected by the character of their training and competition tasks.

The best recent information about the physical and anthropometric characteristic of female slalom racers comes from the work of Heller and co-workers (66). These investigators had the opportunity to profile four members of the Czech National White Water Team, three of whom were selected for the Olympic team in Barcelona, several times immediately before and after the 1992 Games. The descriptive data follow: height, 162 cm; mass, 54 kg; body mass index (BMI), 20.7 kg/m^2; body fat, 8.5%; lean body mass (LBM), 49.8 kg. With the exception of LBM, these values are lower than the mean of the Czech population and also lower than the elite flatwater female kayakers. The anthropometric data on slalom athletes are presented in Table 47–5.

In summary, the anthropometric characteristics of the contemporary slalom paddler are: slightly below-average height, relatively long arms, ectomorphic mesomorphic development, and low body fatness.

Active Musculature and Muscle Fiber Type

Although the nature of the paddling activity in slalom requires a significant acyclic component, especially in steering and bracing maneuvers, as well as the cyclic component involved in flatwater sprint racing, it can be assumed that similar musculature is used in both disciplines. The lower body is primarily involved in fixation and stabilization, whereas the upper body, including the trunk and musculature of the shoulder girdle, provides propulsion and maneuvering. Baker (67) verified the latissimus dorsi as one of the primarily active muscles in slalom kayaking. Clarkson and colleagues (27) fiber typed nine American national team members, including male and female athletes and flatwater and slalom paddlers; however, the data were not subdivided by discipline. Biopsies were performed on the biceps, the vastus lateralis, and latissimus dorsi of two male paddlers. The distribution of fiber subtypes was similar for the biceps and the vastus lateralis. The fiber-type data for the biceps were (ST) = 43.9 ± 7.1, (FTa) = 42.1 ± 9.1, and (FTb) = 14.1 ± 7.9. It appeared that the upper body–specific training led to a selective hypertrophy of the FT-fiber subtypes. The area of individual fibers and FT/ST area was significantly greater in the biceps but equal in the vastus. This training-specific hypertrophy is supported by the work of Baker and Hardy (26). See the section above on flatwater sprint for more details on fiber-type studies.

Metabolic Capacities

Analysis of the importance of the metabolic capacity of slalom paddlers requires a consideration of event duration, 1.5 to 3.0 minutes, and understanding of the technical requirements. Essentially, the slalom paddler must focus on the continuous execution of a series of technical or skill moves. These elements are linked by brief accelerations and full-speed paddling. The metabolic capacity must be optimized to support this combination of continuous power output and intermittent periods of maximal effort (68). The aerobic/anaerobic contributions in a simulated 140-second race staged by Heller and associates (66), with four Czech women, indicated a 48% and 52% contribution from the aerobic and anaerobic energy reserves, respectively. These authors reported, however, that the paddlers spend 50% to 70% of their training volume aimed at skill acquisition. This seems compatible with Endicott's (62) estimate that cardiorespiratory capability accounts for approximately 30% to 50% of the outcome in international slalom races.

TABLE 47–5. *Anthropometric data for slalom athletes*

Gender	Height (cm)	Mass (kg)	BMI (kg/m^2)	% Fat	Somatotype Endo	Somatotype Meso	Somatotype Ecto	Reference
M	180 ± 6.8	76 ± 6.1	23.5	10.4 ± 2.3	2.9 ± 0.57	5.2 ± 0.96	2.4 ± 0.93	Vaccara et al., 1984
M	178 ± 7.4	74 ± 6.0	23.4	10.4 ± 2.7				Sklad et al., 1994
F	162 ± 2.7	54 ± 2.1	20.7 ± 0.7	8.5 ± 1.6				Heller et al., 1994

The metabolic characteristics of the 13 United States national team slalom racers that Vaccaro and co-workers (64) profiled indicated an oxygen uptake of 4.70 ± 1.01 L/min, $\bar{x}$ = 60.1 ml/kg/min. On the arm-crank test, their oxygen-uptake capability was 86% of that demonstrated on the treadmill, with a $\dot{V}O_2$ of 4.0 ± .43 L/min or $\bar{x}$ = 54.2 ml/kg/min. Heller and colleagues (66) evaluated the paddlers on a progressive treadmill test as well as during an on-water assessment. Oxygen-uptake numbers were 2.72 L/min, 51.4 ml/kg/min, and 194.8 ml/kg$^{2/3}$/min. In an on-water race situation, the subjects of Heller and colleagues (66) were able to use 82% of their treadmill $\dot{V}O_2max$ or 2.38 L/min. These are comparable to other studies with paddlers (6,30). However, earlier studies with paddlers (69) and data from nonpaddlers suggest ratios of upper body to treadmill $\dot{V}O_2$ in the range of 50% to 70% (6,33,34,42).

The contribution of non–oxygen dependent or anaerobic resources to successful slalom paddling is well supported by the high post-race or post-maximal performance lactate values reported for paddlers. The values reported in the literature range from 10 to 18 mmol/L (6,26,63,66,67). The data available from post-race lactates in international competition are summarized in Table 47–6.

Training Programs

Construction of the ideal training program for a slalom racer must balance the requirement of skill and technical expertise with enhanced physiologic capacity. Endicott (61,62) has written two of the most extensive summaries of training for slalom racers. "Except for a very few of the world's top slalomists, physiologic considerations should never replace technical considerations" (62, p. 194). Endicott presented detailed analyses of the training systems used by the former DDR and Czech paddlers. These programs emphasized varying proportions of training time across in-boat work, resistance training, and ancillary cardiovascular training. In general, the focused training plan lasted 32 to 40 weeks and involved 500 to 700 h/year. Based on these historic data and his own experience, Endicott presents tenets of slalom training as follows:

- Maximize in-boat paddling time by workout design and year-round in-boat training.
- Resistance training, general cardiovascular conditioning, and other components of off-water training are only ancillary and should never replace in-boat training.
- Training must concomitantly develop technical or gate skills and speed.
- Gate training should be scored and timed during the specific preparation and competition phases.
- Training in groups provides motivation and objective performance data for athletes.
- Responses to training are highly specific, and workouts should be customized to elicit the intended responses.
- Training should be periodized into stress or loading cycles and recovery periods during a year and be individualized for different athletes.

Beyond these generalizations, specific types of workouts designed to elicit training adaptations in the slalomists' physiologic capacities are discussed in detail (61,62,68). Heller and co-workers (66) analyzed the acute physiologic responses to certain workouts and generally confirmed Endicott's suggestions.

In summary, the evolution of equipment, courses, and rules has had a significant impact on the applied physiology of the canoe/kayak slalom racer. Today's slalom racer may be characterized as an individual of average skeletal size, significant LBM, relatively low body fatness, an above-average oxygen uptake capability in general cardiovascular tasks, with a notably enhanced ability to use oxygen and generate power with the upper body, and a well-developed ability to produce and accumulate lactate. Additionally, the athlete who is successful on the international level will in all probability have been competing at a high level for a number of years and have acquired considerable technical expertise in reading the water and maneuvering the boat through the gates.

OTHER CANOEING DISCIPLINES

Although sprint and slalom canoeing are Olympic events, many other forms of canoeing are enjoyed at

TABLE 47–6. *Post-race lactate levels for slalom paddlers*

Class	Gender	*N*	La mmol/L	% HR max	Reference
K-1	M	5	16.2 ± 1.2	—	Baker, 1982
C-1	M	4	13.2 ± 1.7	—	
C-2	M	6	10.8 ± 1.7	—	
K-1	F	4	12.2 ± 1.8	—	
K-1	M	2	13.4 ± 4.7	93.0	Heller et al., 1994
K-1	F	2	10.8 ± 1.5	94.5	

both competitive and recreational levels. Long-distance competitions occur at National and International regattas, and a separate marathon World Championships is held. Long-distance competitions range from 10K to the classic marathon distance (42.2 km) and beyond, on to stage races that may take several days or weeks to complete (70,71). Competitive events also occur in canoe sailing, canoe polo, outrigger canoe, and dragon boats. There is very little detail on the physiology of these other disciplines. This is possibly because they are not Olympic events and therefore have failed to attract the interest of sport scientists. Certainly the popularity of events such as the marathon and dragon-boat racing is expanding, and the number of individuals who are introduced to the sport through these more recreational events also is increasing.

Marathon Canoe and Kayak Paddlers

Physical and Physiologic Characteristics

There have been very few reports on the physiologic demands of the marathon distance races; however, because the time required to complete these events is a minimum of 3 hours, a high aerobic capacity and fractional utilization of that $\dot{V}O_2$ capacity can be assumed to be a necessary prerequisite for success (72,73). As previously noted, typical training programs for elite flatwater paddlers involve periods of long-sustained paddling, 15 to 30 km, and therefore some of the data from these athletes also are applicable to marathon racing. In fact, it was not until the introduction of the 200-m event in the Flatwater Sprint World Championships race that specialization in competitive distances became evident. As recently as 1993, which was the last year for 10,000-m events at the World Canoeing Championships, several crews were competitive at the 500-m, 1000-m, and 10-km distances.

Hahn and colleagues (74) reported on the physiologic profiles of elite Australian marathon paddlers. Anthropometric and metabolic data were collected on seven kayakers (five men and two women) and three male canoeists. These athletes had a wide variability in height, weight, and sum of skinfolds. Values of maximal aerobic capacity were comparable to those reported previously in flatwater kayak paddlers and ranged from 3.25 to 5.09 L/min. The canoeists had lower values of $\dot{V}O_2$max than the male kayak paddlers, likely related to the lower muscle mass recruited during the laboratory simulations by using specific paddling ergometers. These authors also tested this group of marathon paddlers on an arm/leg ergometer and reported that the peak oxygen uptake on the canoe or kayak ergometer was 89% of that achieved on the combined arm/leg ergometer. This relationship has been used as an indicator of specific adaptation to the metabolic demands of paddling. Other researchers reported similar values (about 85%) of upper-body $\dot{V}O_2$ expressed as a percentage of treadmill values (24,50,64). In subjects who are unaccustomed to upper-body work, the percentage is closer to 70% (23).

Data obtained on Swedish 10,000-m paddlers confirmed the high aerobic capacities of these athletes. Tesch and co-workers (24) reported values of 4.2 to 4.7 L/min during stimulated races conducted in a swimming pool. Lutoslawska and colleagues (49) used graded arm exercise to study the aerobic capacity of six elite endurance-trained kayak paddlers. They reported very high values for $\dot{V}O_2$max (more than 5 L/min) and lower lactate accumulations, which they attributed to a positive adaptation to prolonged aerobic training.

Wash Riding

In addition to the physiologic requirements discussed earlier, there is a technical issue that pertains to marathon racing. A method known as "wash riding" is used by many competitors to reduce water resistance by riding on the wave produced by the lead paddler. Although this requires some technical skill, the returns, in terms of economy, are significant. Gray and associates (75) studied 10 male kayak paddlers from the Canadian National team under wash riding and non–wash riding conditions. By using a portable telemetric device, they measured the oxygen cost of steady exercise at a standardized 10,000-m race pace (3.7 m/s) in a single flatwater racing kayak under both conditions. Results demonstrated a decrease in oxygen consumption of 11% while using the wash-riding technique. Significant decreases also were found in minute ventilation (9.8%) and heart rate (4.8%). This is a competitive strategy, based on physiologic principles, that is used routinely in endurance events.

Race Response

There have been attempts to measure the physiologic response to long-distance racing. Tesch and colleagues (24) measured heart rate in two kayak paddlers during a 10,000-m World Championship event and discovered that the heart rates reached 189 beats/min, which represented 97% of maximal heart rate. Blood lactates at the end of a 10.000-m race were approximately 10.2 mmol/L, indicating a surprisingly high anaerobic contribution to the energy demands of this activity (this may have been related to a finishing sprint). In contrast, the American who won the 10,000-m race in the 1987 World Championships had a post-race lactate of 3.3 mmol/L.

The pattern of glycogen depletion from the deltoid muscle after a 10,000-m race indicated that the ST fibers were almost completely emptied and that only 10% of the FT fibers were glycogen depleted (24). This pattern is similar to that seen in the muscles of other athletes who participate in endurance events at a high percentage of their aerobic capacity. Tesch and Karlsson (35) confirmed the glycogen-depletion pattern from the deltoid muscles of elite Swedish paddlers after a simulated 10,000-m racing distance and also measured concentrations of muscle metabolites. They noted a significant decrease in creatine phosphate and G-6-P and a modest but significant increase in muscle lactate after the simulated 10,000-m event. These findings indicate that, similar to those in other endurance activities, muscle glycogen is an essential substrate; carbohydrate ingestion before (glycogen supercompensation), during, and after training or competition is an important nutritional consideration (70).

Lutoslawska and co-workers (76) described the hormonal changes associated with a 19- and 42-km paddling race. Blood samples was taken before the races, immediately after, and 18 hours after the races. Five elite male kayak paddlers completed a 19-km race and, 4 months later, participated in a longer 42-km marathon. Both races resulted in a elevation in the plasma cortisol level, indicating stimulation of the pituitary–adrenal axis. The values of plasma cortisol, obtained immediately after exercise, were significantly higher after the 42-km race in comparison to the values obtained after the 19-km race. Plasma testosterone values decreased after the race, although there were no differences between distances. The testosterone/cortisol ratio was reduced after both races, and this relationship was used to reflect the anabolic–catabolic state. This ratio had returned to basal levels by the next day, implying that adequate recovery had occurred.

By using four elite canoeists and eight male kayakers, Lutoslawska and Sendecki (77) studied the plasma biochemical changes after a 42-km race. There was a significant increase in hemoglobin and total protein concentration, coupled with a decrease in plasma volume: 13.6% and 10.9% for canoeists and kayakers, respectively, immediately after the race. The changes in hemoglobin and total protein were more pronounced in the canoeists, and the authors speculated that the high kneeling versus sitting position during paddling might influence body fluid redistribution. These authors noted that upper-body exercise results in more pronounced plasma volume changes in comparison to lower-body exercise. Plasma ammonia concentrations were elevated by 53% and 126% in canoeists and kayakers after the race, reflecting the intense physical demands of this activity. Plasma glucose was not affected by the race, but plasma glycerol concentration was elevated (164% and 138% in canoeists and kayakers, respectively) immediately after exercise; this is due to the significant lipolysis that occurs during the 42-km race. Plasma CK was elevated as expected, but the value the following day was more pronounced in the canoeists than in the kayak paddlers. The authors speculated that this might be due to a prolonged isometric technical component during paddling in the canoe competitor. It should be pointed out that the time taken to complete the 42-km distance is significantly longer for the canoeists, and thus some of these differences might be attributable to the longer duration of the race for this group.

Surf Ski and Dragon Boat Events

Noakes and colleagues (70) reported on the physiologic and biochemical changes associated with a 4-day, 244-km surf ski marathon in South Africa. They followed 30 participants and monitored sweat rates, rectal temperature, renal function, CK activity, and serum glucose and free fatty acids during the event. The subjects demonstrated low sweat rates and maintenance of rectal temperature. Renal function was unchanged, and CK increased, indicating muscle damage. Low blood glucose levels were observed in 27% of the athletes. To avoid hypoglycemia, the authors emphasized the need for a high-carbohydrate diet throughout the duration of the race and ingestion of carbohydrate-containing drinks and foods while paddling.

Singh and co-workers (78) described the physiologic profiles of Malaysian dragon boat paddlers. They determined maximal oxygen consumption and maximal work output in 28 dragon boat paddlers who exercised to exhaustion on an arm ergometer. The mean $\dot{V}O_2max$ was 2.75 L/min at a power output of 195.5 W.

No other data are available for comparison, but it should be noted that at the highest level of competition in the paddling sports of outrigger and dragon boat paddling, paddlers with elite flatwater training will be involved. [At the World Club Dragon-boat Championships (1998), the German team had two members of the German K-4 team from the Atlanta games: they won.] There is considerable overlap in the physiologic demands of the paddling sports, and the elite athlete will often participate in many or all of these events.

CONCLUSION

This chapter attempted to provide the reader with a comprehensive review of the applied physiology of the various disciplines of canoe sport. For flatwater and slalom racing, we provided anthropometric and physiologic profiles of elite athletes, synthesized the literature documenting training adaptations, and discussed the parameters of training programs used internationally. In the remaining disciplines, there is a dearth of published literature profiling or describing the physiology of these competitors. We have provided a synopsis of the data available and hope the reader can generalize from the more adequately presented sections.

REFERENCES

1. Di Prampero PE. The energy cost of human locomotion on land and in water. *Int J Sports Med* 1986;7:55–72.
2. Byrnes WC, Kearney JT. Aerobic and anaerobic contributions during simulated canoe/kayak events. *Med Sci Sports Exerc* 1997;29:S220.
3. Bunc V, Heller J. Changes of blood lactate concentration at anaerobic threshold during the year in trained athletes. *Acta Univ Carol Gymn* 1992;28:27–35.
4. Daniels J, Bales J. Arm and leg maximal and submaximal VO_2 among arm- and leg-trained athletes. In: Nagle FJ, Montoye HJ, eds. *Exercise in Health and Disease* Springfield, IL: Charles C Thomas, 1981:158–170.
5. Pendergast DR, Bushnell D, Wilson DW, Cerretelli P. Energetics of kayaking. *Eur J Appl Physiol* 1989;59:342–350.
6. Shephard RJ. Science and medicine of canoeing and kayaking. *Sports Med* 1987;4:19–33.
7. Jackson PS. Performance prediction for Olympic kayaks. *J Sports Sci* 1995;13:239–245.
8. Toro A. *Canoeing: an Olympic sport.* San Francisco: Olympian Graphics, 1986.
9. Lenz J. World top list of the racing discipline. *Canoeing Express* 1996;2:9–17.
10. Carter JEL. Age and body size of Olympic athletes. *Med Sport Sci* 1984;18:53–79.
11. Carter JEL. Somatotypes of Olympic athletes from 1948 to 1976. *Med Sport Sci* 1984;18:80–109.
12. Carter JEL, Ross WD, Aubry SP, Hebbelinck M, Borms J. Anthropometry of Montreal Olympic athletes. *Med Sport Sci* 1982;16:25–52.
13. Freeman PL. Physical and physiological characteristics of Australian canoeists. Presented to the Australian Sports Commission's Applied Sports Research Program, 1990.
14. Freeman PL, Chennells MHD, Sandstrom ER, Briggs CA. Specificity in performance: determination of the anthropometric and physiological characteristics of canoeists. Presented to the Applied Sports Research Program, Australian Sports Commission, 1987.
15. Fry RW, Morton AR. Physiological and kinanthropometric attributes of elite flatwater kayakists. *Med Sci Sports Exerc* 1991; 23:1297–1301.
16. Misigoj-Durakovic M, Heimer S. Characteristics of the morphological and functional status of kayakers and canoeists. *J Sports Med Phys Fitness* 1992;32:45–50.
17. Plagenhoef S. Biomechanical analysis of Olympic flatwater kayaking and canoeing. *Res Q* 1979;50:443–459.
18. Mann RV, Kearney JT. A biomechanical analysis of the Olympic-style flatwater kayak stroke. *Med Sci Sports Exerc* 1980; 12:183–188.
19. Logan SM, Holt LE. The flatwater kayak stroke. *NSCA J* 1985;7:4–11.
20. Pelham TW, Burke DG, Holt LE. The flatwater canoe stroke. *NSCA J* 1992;14:6–8, 88–90.
21. Capousek JB, Bruggemann P. Comparative electromyographic investigation of specific strength exercises and specific movement in kayak. In: Vrijens J, Verstuyft J, de Clercq D, eds. *International seminar on kayak-canoe coaching and sciences: strength training in kayak; a multidimensional concept.* Budapest: International Canoe Federation, 1990:69–82.
22. Gollnick PD, Armstrong RB, Saubert CW IV, Piehl K, Saltin B. Enzyme activity and fiber composition in skeletal muscle of untrained and trained men. *J Appl Physiol* 1972;33:312–319.
23. Bergh U, Thorstensson A, Sjödin B, Hulten B, Piehl K, Karlsson J. Maximal oxygen uptake and muscle fiber types in trained and untrained humans. *Med Sci Sports Exerc* 1978;10:151–154.
24. Tesch P, Piehl K, Wilson G, Karlsson J. Physiological investigations of Swedish elite canoe competitors. *Med Sci Sports* 1976;8:214–218.
25. Tesch P, Karlsson J, Sjödim B. Muscle fiber type distribution in trained and untrained muscles of athletes. In: Komi PV, Nelson RC, Morehouse CA, eds. *Exercise sport biology.* Champaign, Ill: Human Kinetics, 1982:79–83.
26. Baker SJ, Hardy L. Effects of high intensity canoeing training on fibre area and fibre type in the latissimus dorsi muscle. *Br J Sports Med* 1989;23:23–28.
27. Clarkson PM, Kroll W, Melchionda AM. Isokinetic strength, endurance, and fiber type composition in elite American paddlers. *Eur J Appl Physiol* 1982;48:67–76.
28. Wojcieszak I, Michael E, Lutoslawska G, Wojczuk J. Metabolic and power output changes as the signs of fatigue during short exercise on kayak ergometer. *Biol Sport* 1988;5:251–259.
29. Zinzen E, Cabri J, Vrijens J, Clarijs JP, Verstuyft J. Isokinetic strength and its relation to anthropometry and physiology in kayak. In: Vrijens J, Verstuyft J, de Clercq D, eds. *International seminar on kayak-canoe coaching and sciences: strength training in kayak; a multidimensional concept.* Budapest: International Canoe Federation, 1990:55–67.
30. Shapiro R, Kearney JT. Anatomical and physiological factors in elite female kayakers. In: Terauds J, ed. *Biomechanics in sports III & IV: proceedings of ISBS.* Del Mar, CA: Academic Publishers, 1987:129–137.
31. Tesch PA, Lindeberg S. Blood lactate accumulation during arm exercise in world class kayak paddlers and strength trained athletes. *Eur J Appl Physiol* 1984;52:441–445.
32. Bunc V, Heller J. Ventilatory threshold and work efficiency on a bicycle and paddling ergometer in top canoeists. *J Sports Med Phys Fitness* 1991;31:376–379.
33. Seals DR, Mullin JP. Vo_2 max in variable type exercise among well-trained upper body athletes. *Res Q Exerc Sport* 1982; 53:58–63.
34. Sawka MN, Foley ME, Pimental NA, Toner MM, Pandolf KB. Determination of maximal aerobic power during upper-body exercise. *J Appl Physiol* 1983;54:113–117.
35. Tesch PA, Karlsson J. Muscle metabolite accumulation following maximal exercise: a comparison between short-term and prolonged kayak performance. *Eur J Appl Physiol* 1984;52:243–246.
36. Bunc V, Heller J, Leso J, Sprynarova S, Zdanowicz R. Ventilatory threshold in various groups of highly trained athletes. *Int J Sports Med* 1987;8:275–280.
37. Wojczuk J, Wojcieszak I, Zdanowicz R. Anaerobic work capacity in athletes. *Biol Sport* 1984;1:119–130.
38. Wojcieszak I, Burke E, Danielewicz E, Trzaskoma Z, Wojczuk J. Steady-rate and all-out work on a kayak ergometer. *Biol Sport (Warsaw)* 1987;4:91–99.
39. Ginn EM, Mackinnon LT. The equivalence of onset of blood lactate accumulation, maximal lactate steady state and critical power during kayak ergometry: report to Department of Human Movement Studies. University of Queensland, Australia, 1988.
40. Clingeleffer A, Mc Naughton L, Davoren B. Critical power may be determined from two tests in elite kayakers. *Eur J Appl Physiol* 1994;68:36–40.
41. Henderson D. Competitive excellence study: world champion athlete tracking final report. United States Canoe and Kayak Team, 1996.
42. Pendergast D, Cerretelli P, Rennie DW. Aerobic and glycolytic metabolism in arm exercise. *J Appl Physiol* 1979;47:754–760.
43. Cerretelli P, Pendergast D, Paganelli WC, Rennie DW. Effects of specific muscle training on Vo_2 on-response and early blood lactate. *J Appl Physiol* 1979;47:761–769.
44. Clausen JP, Klausen K, Rasmussen B, Trap-Jensen J. Central and peripheral circulatory changes after training of the arms or legs. *Am J Physiol* 1973;225:675–682.
45. Klassen GA, Andrew GM, Becklake MR. Effect of training on total and regional blood flow and metabolism in paddlers. *J Appl Physiol* 1970;28:397–406.
46. Vrijens J, Hoekstra P, Bouckaert J, Van Uytvanck P. Effects of training on maximal working capacity and haemodynamic response during arm and leg-exercise in a group of paddlers. *Eur J Appl Physiol* 1975;34:113–119.
47. Wojcieszak I, Wojczuk J, Czapowska J, Posnik J. A specific test for determination of work capacity of kayak competitors. *Biol Sport* 1984;1:7–18.
48. Wojczuk J, Wojcieszak I. Effects of training specific work capacity in a group of junior kayakers. *Biol Sport (Warsaw)* 1984;1:209–220.
49. Lutoslawska G, Sitkowski D, Hübner-Wozniak E, Borkowski L, Klusiewicz A. Plasma glucose in elite wrestlers, swimmers and

kayakers subjected to exhausting laboratory exercise before and after the training season. *Biol Sport* 1994;11:171–180.
50. Tesch PA. Physiological characteristics of elite kayak paddlers. *Can J Appl Sport Sci* 1983;8:87–91.
51. Krogulski A, Wisniewska A, Lukaszewska J. Growth hormone response to standard exercise on arm ergometer as a criterion of adaptation in kayak competition. *Biol Sport* 1985;2:255–263.
52. Markowska L, Mickiewicz G, Wojczuk J, Sikorski W, Liwski G, Posnik J. Activity of sympathoadrenal system in athletes during a year's training cycle. *Biol Sport* 1987;4:109–119.
53. Csanády M, Forster T, Högye M, Gruber N, Móczó I. Three-year echocardiographic follow-up study on canoeist boys. *Acta Cardiol* 1986;41:413–425.
54. Cox RW. *The science of canoeing: a guide for competitors and coaches to understanding and improving performance in sprint and marathon kayaking.* Cheshire, England: Coxburn Press, 1992.
55. Szanto C. *Racing canoeing.* Budapest: International Canoe Federation, 1992.
56. Colli R, Faccini R, Schermi C, Intorini E, Dal Monte A. The training of canoeists. *Riv Cult Sport* 1991;2:10.
57. Dal Monte A, Leonardi LM. Functional evaluation of kayak paddlers from biomechanical and physiological viewpoints. In: Komi P, ed. *Biomechanics VB.* Baltimore: University Park Press, 1976:258–267.
58. Cermak J, Kuta I, Parizkova J. Some predispositions for top performance in speed canoeing and their changes during the whole year training program. *J Sports Med* 1975;15:243–251.
59. Endicott WT. *The Barton mold: a study in sprint kayaking.* Lake Placid, NY: United States Canoe Kayak Team, 1992.
60. Berglund B, Säfström H. Psychological monitoring and modulation of training load of world-class canoeists. *Med Sci Sports Exerc* 1994;26:1036–1040.
61. Endicott WT. *To win the worlds: a textbook for elite slalomists and their coaches.* Baltimore: Reese Press, 1980.
62. Endicott WT. *The ultimate run: canoe slalom at the highest levels.* Baltimore: Reese Press, 1983.
63. Sidney K, Shephard RJ. Physiological characteristics and performance of the white-water paddler. *Eur J Appl Physiol* 1973; 32:55–70.
64. Vaccaro P, Gray PR, Clarke DH, Morris AF. Physiological characteristics of world class white-water slalom paddlers. *Res Q Exerc Sport* 1984;55:206–210.
65. Sklad M, Krawczyk B, Majle B. Body build profiles of male and female rowers and kayakers. *Biol Sport* 1994;11:249–256.
66. Heller J, Bíl M, Pultera J, Sadilová M. Functional and energy demands of elite female kayak slalom: a comparison of training and competition performances. *Acta Univ Carol Kinanthropol* 1994;30:59–74.
67. Baker SJ. Post competition lactate levels in canoe slalomists. *Br J Sports Med* 1982;16:112–113.
68. Hofmann P, Peinhaupt G, Leitner H, Pokan R. Evaluation of heart rate threshold by means of lactate steady state and endurance tests in white water kayakers. In: Viitasalo J, Kujala U, eds. *The way to win, International Congress on Applied Research in Sports.* Helsinki: 1994:217–220.
69. Wakeling P, Saddler S. Aerobic capacities of some British slalom and wild-water racing kayak competitors of international status. *Res Papers Phys Ed* 1978;3:16–18.
70. Noakes TD, Nathan M, Irving RA, et al. Physiological and biochemical measurements during a 4-day surf-ski marathon. *SMAJ* 1985;76:212–216.
71. Paschke WS. *The world of marathon racing.* Budapest: International Canoe Federation 1987.
72. Kearney JT, Nance JE. The application of the principles of exercise physiology to downriver canoe racing. *KAHPER J* 1975; 12:19–20.
73. Lutoslawska G, Sitkowski D, Wojcieszak I, Sendecki W. Physiological response of marathon kayakers to graded arm exercise. *Biol Sport (Warsaw)* 1990;7:297–303.
74. Hahn AG, Pang PM, Tumilty DM, Telford RD. General and specific aerobic power of elite marathon kayakers and canoeists. *Excel* 1988;5:14–19.
75. Gray GL, Matheson GO, McKenzie DC. The metabolic cost of two kayaking techniques. *Int J Sports Med* 1995;16:250–254.
76. Lutoslawska G, Obminski Z, Krogulski A, Sendecki W. Plasma cortisol and testosterone following 19-km and 42-km kayak races. *J Sport Med Phys Fitness* 1991;31:538–542.
77. Lutoslawska G, Sendecki W. Plasma biochemical variables in response to 42-km kayak and canoe races. *J Sport Med Phys Fitness* 1990;30:406–411.
78. Singh R, Singh HJ, Sirisinghe RG. Physical and physiological profiles of Malaysian dragon boat rowers. *Br J Sports Med* 1995;29:13–15.

Exercise and Sport Science,
edited by William E. Garrett, Jr., and Donald T. Kirkendall.
Lippincott Williams & Wilkins, Philadelphia © 2000.

CHAPTER 48

Physiology of Cycling

Edmund R. Burke

THE SPORT

Physical Requirements

Competitive cycling, whether track or road, is physiologically demanding. Typically, races range from a 200-m sprint, lasting approximately 10 seconds, to the Tour de France, lasting 23 days and covering approximately 5000 km. Between these extremes, a whole range of individual, paired, and team events exists. This vast range of competitive distances has resulted in cyclists specializing in specific events that have similar metabolic energy demands. The racing cyclist typically has low body fat, a high maximal oxygen uptake, good anaerobic capacity, and strong lower-limb musculature.

Road racing requires the cyclist to have a substantial aerobic capacity for prolonged exertion and the anaerobic potential necessary for breakaways, hill climbing, and "all-out" sprints at the end of the race. Track racing requires a range of capabilities from sprint power to endurance speed. Both road and track cycling demand a specific knowledge of tactics, strategies, mastery of skills, and considerable courage.

Training procedures adopted by cyclists are those that simulate competitive conditions as closely as possible; attempts are often made to copy the training practices of champion cyclists. Emulation of champions, however, may be misguided because each individual possesses unique physical and physiological potentials.

During competition, the cyclist's oxygen-transport and energy-conversion systems often are taxed to their limits. Therefore a major portion of training is aimed toward the improvement of the oxygen-transport, oxygen-extraction, and specific energy-conversion systems. At the same time, tempo training is incorporated to enhance anaerobic capacity. Both road-racing and track cyclists aim to increase their exercise tolerance to be able to work at the highest possible percentage of maximal oxygen consumption.

Sprint events call on the use of the high-energy compounds adenosine triphosphate (ATP) and phosphocreatine (PC). Match sprints, which last approximately 10 seconds, rely heavily on the combined ATP–PC energy sources. Pursuit and kilometer races place high demands on both the ATP and PC energy resources as well as the glycolytic energy systems. Long-distance road racing relies heavily on the oxidative breakdown of carbohydrates and fats for energy, exploiting a large portion of aerobic capacity over long periods while minimizing excess lactate production.

Physiological Requirements

Energy Cost

Figure 48–1 demonstrates the energy cost of cycling at various speeds (1–3). The energy consumed increases gradually across body weights until about 20 mph, when energy consumption increases rapidly because of an increase in air resistance. The wind resistance is proportional to the square of the speed and is nearly proportional to a cyclist's frontal area. For larger body sizes, the frontal area increases at about two thirds of the power of weight; as could be expected, larger cyclists have larger frontal areas (4).

Body size also was shown to affect energy cost ($\dot{V}O_2$) while cycling. Swain and colleagues (1) found that the absolute oxygen consumption while cycling on a level road increases with body weight for any given speed. The increased oxygen cost was large enough for the authors to conclude that body size is an important factor in competitive cycling. Furthermore, it has been estimated that the difference in frontal area between large and small cyclists may account for up to 20% of the

E. R. Burke: Department of Biology, University of Colorado at Colorado Springs, Colorado Springs, Colorado 80933.

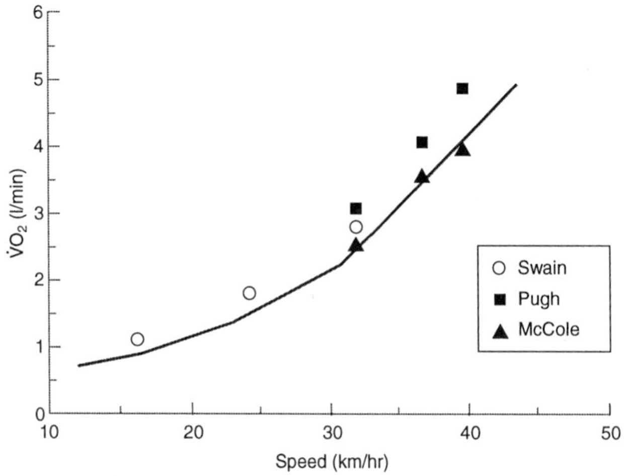

FIG. 48–1. Speed (km/min) versus $\dot{V}O_2$ (L/min) based on the following studies: ref. 1 (*open circles*); ref. 3 (*solid squares*); ref. 2 (*solid triangles*). From ref. 9, with permission.

resistive aerodynamic drag forces experienced in racing (6).

It should be mentioned that increasing body mass also increases power production, but it has less influence on frontal area and drag. This may be a major reason why cyclists who compete in the 100-km time trial and the pursuit events tend to be larger.

Although the large cyclist is at an advantage on level ground, cycling on hills is a different matter. The energy required for the vertical component of ascending a hill is dependent on the total weight of the bicycle and rider, not on the frontal area (7).

Furthermore, as the cyclist's speed is reduced during an ascent, the energy required to overcome air resistance is decreased markedly. Thus, hill climbing is a body weight–dependent activity and not a frontal area–dependent activity, and smaller cyclists should excel because of greater maximal $\dot{V}O_2$/body weight ratio (1).

McCole (2) showed a similar relationship among oxygen consumption, speed, and body weight. Results of his study demonstrated an 8% lower oxygen consumption at 32 km/h than those of Swain and colleagues. This may be because McCole's subjects were more experienced cyclists and may have been more efficient in pedaling technique and position on the bicycle than the subjects in Swain's study. An earlier study by Pugh (3) reported results that were about 7% higher than those of Swain's subjects. Kyle (8) suggested that this may have been due to the hillier course used in Pugh's study, which would have added to the energy cost.

Based on data from nearly 100 trials that were conducted under the same conditions, McCole and co-workers (2) derived an equation to predict the $\dot{V}O_2$ required for different riding speeds. In addition to riding speed, however, their analysis indicated that both rider weight and head/tailwinds further improve the predictive accuracy. Their analysis yielded the following equation:

$$\dot{V}O_2 = -4.50 + 0.17\,VR + 0.052\,VW + 0.22\,WR$$

where $\dot{V}O_2$ is in L/min, *VR* is the rider speed in km/h, *VW* is wind speed in km/h, and *WR* is the rider weight in kilograms. This equation accounted for more than 70% of the variability in $\dot{V}O_2$ observed among the different trials. Whereas this equation will not give a rider a precise value for $\dot{V}O_2$ under all conditions, it will provide a general estimate of a cyclist's energy expenditure, at least across the 32- to 40-km/h range of speeds used in the study (9).

Power Output

In 1986 it was reported that Eddy Merckx produced 450 watts (W) of power for 1 hour while on a bicycle ergometer (10). Recreational cyclists can hold this power output for only about 1 minute (11). At the other end of the scale, an Italian sprinter has produced 1644 W for 5 seconds (12). These same authors (10,11) showed that healthy individuals can produce more than 700 W for a short period, and about 180 W for 1 hour. The speed at which a bicycle will travel with a fixed power output is dependent on the resistance forces against the bicycle (8).

Acid–Base Balance

Competitive track cycling is a physiologically demanding sport, with events lasting from 10 to 12 seconds (200-m match sprints) to a 50-km points race lasting approximately 60 minutes. During a points race, there are sprints every few kilometers, during which the cyclists accumulate points. The cyclist with the most points wins the race. Races such as these place high demands on glycolytic energy production.

Craig and co-workers (13) showed that peak lactate reached 17.0 m*M* after a 1-km race that lasted approximately 70 seconds. Burke and associates (14) reported that blood lactate ranged from 12.1 m*M* for the team pursuit events to 13.7 m*M* for the match sprints, to 15.2 m*M* for the individual pursuit to 19.9 m*M* in the kilometer event. Craig and co-workers (13) showed mean peak lactates of 17.0 m*M* after a 1-km time trial in nine male elite track cyclists. They estimated that the energy mix for the kilometer was 30% aerobic and 70% anaerobic.

The high lactates seen after match sprints suggest that anaerobic glycogenolysis can take place in events lasting approximately 10 seconds. Muscle biopsies taken immediately after 10 and 30 seconds of supramaximal work during a Wingate test on a bicycle ergometer both in male and female healthy subjects averaged 36 and 61 mmol/kg dry weight after 10- and 30-second exercise bouts (15). Similar results were shown by Jones and coworkers (16) in which, after 10 seconds of isokinetic work on a bicycle ergometer, two subjects' muscle lactate increased to 17.2 and 15.1 mmol/kg at 140 rpm and to 14.3 and 14.2 mmol/kg at 60 rpm, demonstrating that glycogenolysis was activated very rapidly at both pedal speeds. In addition, the changes in glycolytic intermediates were consistent with the rate-limiting steps at the phosphofructokinase and pyruvate dehydrogenase reactions. The results of these two studies are evidence that pronounced lactate accumulation occurs during supramaximal exercise of 10-second duration, suggesting heavy reliance on that glycolysis in this time frame.

As expected, sprint cyclists generate significantly more power, about 20% more, during the first 40 seconds of such a test as compared with pursuit riders (17). In general, the maximal amount of power that a sprint-trained cyclist can generate in the first 5 seconds of such a test is fourfold higher than the athlete can generate at $\dot{V}O_2max$ (18), showing the large energy supply available from anaerobic energy sources.

Body Position and Oxygen Cost

The ability to sustain prolonged work is dependent on an adequate supply of oxygen to the active muscles. Faria (19) found that riding in the lowest position with standard dropped handlebars ("drops") resulted in significantly higher oxygen uptake, work output, and pulmonary ventilation, although no difference was found in heart rate from that while riding on the "tops" of the bars.

Johnson and Shultz (20) reported that there is no additional physiological cost to riding with aerodynamic clip-on handlebars. While riding a bicycle ergometer set up like their road bicycles, 15 highly trained cyclists worked at 80% of $\dot{V}O_2$ max for 10 minutes. The $\dot{V}O_2$ was 3.27 L/min while using standard "bull-horn" time-trial bars and 3.24 L/min when using clip-on bars. This strongly suggests that the aerodynamic enhancements afforded by these handlebars are obtained with no apparent physiologic costs.

Riding in the "aero" position does not impair physiologic responses to high-intensity exercise. Recently work by Origenes and associates (21) showed that moderately trained cyclists riding a cycle ergometer had absolute power outputs, ventilatory responses (as determined by respiratory pattern and timing), and metabolic cost; they were similar in an upright posture and aero-cycling posture.

A more important question arises as to how riding for long periods in a time trial in an aero position will alter muscle-fiber recruitment and fatigue in a long race. The rider's kinetics and kinematics on the bike, especially in the hip joint, are altered significantly while riding in this position.

Thermoregulation and Fluid Replacement

During competitive road racing, air flow over the skin surfaces increases heat loss through improved convective transfer and evaporation. This has been shown in research comparing both indoor and outdoor cycling. While riding indoors at a work load of 149 watts, net heat accumulation, temperature elevation, and fatigue caused a cyclist to quit riding after 30 minutes. However, peak performances in a 24-hour time trial can be analyzed by using wind-resistance and rolling-resistance data to show that 224 W is being expended at an average speed of 22 mph with no noticeable increase in thermal stress. It seems that exposure of the cyclist to moving air is principally responsible for the ability to ride continuously for long periods (22).

The effect of absorbed solar radiation and evaporative weight loss as a measure of absorbed thermal radiation on cycling also has been investigated in simulated cycling (23,24). The investigators studied the effect of "one-piece" skintight clothing on increased solar load and decreased moisture. Subjects wearing tight-fitting whole-body clothing were exposed to simulated solar-radiation intensities of 0, 190, 360, and 480 W/m^2. The subjects rested in a racing position on a bicycle in an environment of 27°C still air and constant humidity. The bicycle was placed on a sensitive recording balance that allowed the rate of weight loss to be constantly monitored. Steady-state sweat rates increased linearly with radiation intensity. It was shown that the color and weave of the clothing influenced the absorbed radiation. Berglund and colleagues (24) reported that aluminized fabric was superior to white and light-colored fabric. The aluminized fabric was superior in cooling to bare skin. The consequences of wearing one type of suit rather than another can be dramatic. A darker, tighter-weave suit may cause a projected increased water loss of 692 g over 4 hours of cycling compared with a lighter-colored suit with a looser weave (24). In other words, the selection of the right type and color of fabric can cut down on water losses in endurance cycling.

It is widely known that consuming fluids during prolonged exercise decreases hyperthermia and risk of heat illness. Until recently, the relation between the amount of fluid ingested during cycling and how it affected heat stress remained unclear.

Montain and Coyle (25) studied the effect of different amounts of dehydration on hyperthermia, heart rate, and stroke volume during prolonged cycling. On four separate occasions, trained endurance cyclists rode for 2 hours in a warm environment (33° dry bulb, 50% humidity) at 62% to 67% of their $\dot{V}O_2max$. During the rides, the cyclists randomly received either no fluid (NF), or drank small (SF, 300 mL/h), moderate (MF, 700 mL/h), or large (LF, 1200 mL/h) volumes of an energy drink containing 6% carbohydrate with electrolytes. These fluid volumes replaced approximately 20%, 50%, and 80%, respectively, of the fluid loss during the ride.

The fluid-replacement protocol allowed body-weight losses of 4%, 3%, 2%, and 1% during the NF, SF, MF, and LF trials. The increases in core temperature (both esophageal and rectal) during the 2-hour ride decreased correspondingly as more fluid was consumed. Core temperature, cardiac output, and heart-rate values also were directly related to the rate of fluid ingestion and thus to the degree of dehydration.

The authors noted that several cyclists were hardly able to complete 2 hours of cycling without fluids. Drinking increasingly larger volumes of fluid reduced the cyclists' rating of perceived exertion. No cyclist reported any gastrointestinal distress while drinking 1200 mL/h of fluid.

The loss of every kilogram of fluid (1000 mL) caused heart rate to be elevated by 8 beats/min and core temperature to increase by 0.3°C. In a separate study (26), it was noted that fluid ingestion attenuated hyperthermia by promoting a high skin blood flow and therefore a higher rate of heat loss. However, Mitchell and Voss (27) found that some cyclists ingesting 1200 mL/h fluid, and all subjects ingesting 1600 mL/h, were "visibly uncomfortable." Interestingly, 25% of the subjects developed diarrhea when ingesting 1600 mL/h, indicating that the rate of fluid ingestion exceeded the combined maximal rate of absorption of both the large and small intestines.

Fuel Depletion

Cyclists who ride continuously for 4 to 8 hours daily must consume large amounts of carbohydrate and additional calories daily to restore muscle glycogen and maintain energy balance. During repeated days of training or racing, the cyclist should consume 500 to 600 g of carbohydrate each day to replenish muscle glycogen. This corresponds to a carbohydrate intake of about 8 to 10 g/kg of body weight.

A practical problem for cyclists in long events, such as the Tour de France, is the difficulty they experience eating enough regular food to obtain the amount of carbohydrate needed for optimal performance (28). There are several reasons for this. The physical stress of such exercise can decrease appetite. Also, eating a large volume of food can cause gastrointestinal distress. Finally, the racing cyclist is spending so much time on the bicycle that there are not many hours available for energy replenishment.

A recent nutritional study found that Tour de France cyclists consumed an average of 850 g of carbohydrate (or about 60% of daily caloric intake; fat made up 23%) each day (29). Half of this was consumed during the race, mostly through carbohydrate beverages. The average caloric intake for the cyclists was 5900 Kcal/day.

Apart from the exercise-induced changes in appetite, during prolonged training and racing, cyclists must rely on easily digestible, high-energy foods that are low in fiber. Large volumes of conventional race foods, which are usually higher in fat, could interfere with adequate carbohydrate intake and may predispose one to dehydration if one does not drink enough.

In a study simulating the Tour de France, Brouns and co-workers (30) had cyclists consume a high-carbohydrate drink throughout exercise (20% solution: 85% maltodextrin, 15% fructose); subjects were able to ingest enough calories and carbohydrate to match their energy needs. However, cyclists who relied on conventional foods or high-fructose beverages (20% solution: 50% fructose, 50% maltodextrin) could not ingest enough calories or carbohydrate, and their performance deteriorated. In addition, the high-fructose drink was not palatable because it was too sweet and caused gastrointestinal distress.

THE ATHLETE

Body Composition

Excess body weight, particularly as superficial adipose tissue, does not contribute to work output in cycling. On the other hand, a high muscle-to-weight ratio is essential for hill-climbing efficiency, and a cyclist with a low percentage of body fat will have an advantage on hilly terrain. The estimated percentage of body fat for elite cyclists ranges from 6% to 9% for male road racers and 12% to 15% for elite female cyclists (31). Unpublished data from the U.S. Olympic Committee's Sports Physiology Laboratory showed that while these are means for elite cyclists, some elite cyclists have percentage body fats that are higher than these mean values.

White and co-workers (32) found that there were seasonal variations in body composition from January to July for male cyclists. In the road-race group, there was a clear trend toward body-weight reduction during the racing season (due to a decrease in body fat), along with somatotype modification (reduced endomorphy rather than changes in mesomorphy and ectomorphy). Percentage body fat decreased from 10.6% in January to 8.5% in July. The sprint cyclists (33) showed a trend toward a small increase in body weight during the racing season with a reduction in percentage body fat (12.2% to 10.8%). There was a decrease in endomorphy, along with a trend toward elevated mesomorphy and reduced ectomorphy. This is consistent with data on 10 members of the Czechoslovakian National Sprint Team, who also had a percentage of body fat of 10.8% (34).

Muscle-Fiber Composition

Studies on the muscle-fiber type distribution in male and female cyclists do not indicate a range of fiber compositions according to event specialty. Elite road-race (endurance) cyclists generally possess higher percentages of type I fibers (4,31,35). Work by Coyle (36) demonstrated that elite road cyclists (good time trialists) had 66% type I fibers. Mackova (34) showed that 10 track sprint cyclists on the Czechoslovakian National Team had 58% population of type I muscle fibers. However, there was a significant predominance of anaerobic structural (increased FT diameter) and metabolic conditions (increased anaerobic enzymes) in the skeletal muscle of elite sprint cyclists. They hypothesized that the nature of muscle-tissue adaptation in this group of sprint cyclists was evidence of the specific training adaptation. The sprint (anaerobic) and strength work completed by the sprint cyclists correlated with increased size of the FT fibers and the anaerobic enzyme activity seen in the muscle-tissue samples. In addition, many sprint and kilometer cyclists spend a significant amount of time completing high-resistance weight-training exercises. This could lead to further hypertrophy of the FT muscle fibers.

Mackova's (34) assumptions of increased anaerobic enzyme activity and FT-fiber hypertrophy may be correct because work by Ahlquist and colleagues (37) showed that higher pedal forces require more FT muscle-fiber recruitment. Their work showed that cycling at the same metabolic cost at 50 rpm resulted in a greater type II fiber glycogen depletion than that at 100 rpm. This was attributed to the increased muscle force required to meet the higher resistance per stroke at the lower pedal frequency, during starts and "jumps" on the velodrome. Coyle and co-workers (38) recently showed that while cycling at a cadence of 80 rpm, both gross and delta mechanical efficiency are highly correlated (i.e., about 0.75 to 0.85) with the percentage of type I muscle fibers within the vastus lateralis of well-trained cyclists. This observation in endurance-trained cyclists indicates that during relatively slow-velocity muscle contractions, type I muscle fibers appear to be the preferred fiber and are more efficient at converting chemical energy into mechanical work compared with type II muscle fibers.

Muscle Recruitment/Involvement

Gregor and others from the University of California (39,40) used surface electrodes (electromyogram; EMG) to observe leg muscle-activity patterns during cycling. There are, however, variations between riders in both timing and magnitude of activity. These patterns should, therefore, only be used as a guide. Recent work by Gregor and associates (40) indicates that the one-joint knee extensors [vastus medialis (VM), vastus lateralis (VL), and gluteus maximus (GM)] are temporally consistent across 18 experienced cyclists for a constant work load and cadence (250 W, 90 rpm). The two-joint rectus femoris (RF) muscle exhibits an activation pattern similar to the VL and VM during the early power phase (0 to 120 degrees) but displays an earlier onset of activity during recovery. Across riders, the biceps femoris (BF), semitendinosus (ST), and semimembranosus (SM), as a group, display more variability, with the BF being the most variable. The gastrocnemius (GA) and soleus (SOL) each display a consistent temporal pattern across riders, with SOL activity consistently beginning just before the GA activity. The single-joint tibialis anterior (TA) is usually active just before top dead center (TDC); however, the data of Gregor and associates (40) indicate that secondary bursts can occur in the first three quadrants (0 to 270 degrees).

Coyle and colleagues (36) compared a group of "elite-national class" (group 1) with "good-state class" (group 2) cyclists for power production during a simulated 40-km time trial on a stationary bicycle. Group 1 produced higher power outputs over the distance, and this was attributed to generating higher peak torques about the center of the crank by applying larger vertical forces to the crank arm during the cycling downstroke. Compared with group 2, group 1 also produced higher peak torques and vertical forces during the downstroke, even when cycling at the same absolute work rate as group 2. According to the authors, the higher power output was produced primarily by generating higher peak vertical forces and torque during the cycling downstroke and not by increasing the effectiveness of force application to the pedal. Factors possibly contributing to this ability may be a higher percentage of type I fibers and a 23% higher capillary density in group 1 compared with group 2.

Regarding the effects that changes in saddle height have on cycling mechanics, research conducted by Desipres (41) studied muscle-activity patterns (EMG) while changing saddle height and load. Three male cyclists rode their own bicycles at three different loads and two separate saddle heights. EMG measurements of eight muscles in the leg were sampled at 95% and 105% of leg-inseam length (measured from the ground to the crotch). The general conclusions were that as saddle height increased, the leg muscles were activated earlier in the pedal cycle and stayed active longer. The magnitude of muscle action did not appear larger. Rather muscles were active for a longer period. A complete review of biomechanics and pedaling-technique patterns in cycling is presented in the review articles presented by Gregor and others (40) and Kautz and co-workers (42), as well as in Chapter 35 in this volume.

Oxygen Uptake

The average values for maximal oxygen uptake for elite cyclists are among the highest levels recorded (14,32). The average maximal values for elite male subjects

TABLE 48–1. *Laboratory performance of groups 1 and 2*

	Laboratory 1-h cycling test			Progressive cycling test	
				Blood lactate threshold	
	Power (W)	$\dot{V}O_2$ (L/min)	Load (% $\dot{V}O_2$max)	$\dot{V}O_2$ (L/min)	% $\dot{V}O_2$max
Group 1	346[a]	4.54[a]	90[a]	4.0[a]	79.1[a]
Group 2	311	4.18	86	3.7	75.1
1 − 2	11%[a]	9%[a]	5%[a]	9%[a]	5%[a]

[a]$p < .05$ versus group 2. From ref. 36, with permission.

range from 67.1 to 77.4 ml/kg/min, and the mean for elite female cyclists is 61.1 ml/kg/min. Again, unpublished data from the laboratory at the U.S. Olympic Training Center show maximal values in the 80s for male and 70s for female subjects. These data suggest that high oxygen-uptake values are required for successful competition at the national and international levels. However, the importance of maintaining high oxygen-consumption levels relative to $\dot{V}O_2$max may have more relevance to success during endurance cycling events than does the absolute $\dot{V}O_2$max.

White and colleagues (32) examined seasonal variations in $\dot{V}O_2$max and found increases of about 5% during the preseason to peak-season periods, although differences in absolute $\dot{V}O_2$max values were observed between Olympic "select" and "nonselect" cyclists. The results corroborate those of Fagard and associates (43), who found that peak oxygen uptake increased 6% during the competitive season in competitive cyclists.

Krebs and co-workers (44) investigated numerous factors in an attempt to predict bicycle performance in an over-the-road 40-km time trial. Data from 35 competitive cyclists were reported. Competitive experience was found to be the single best predictor of bicycling performance. The physiological parameters of maximal oxygen consumption and body composition did not contribute to performance prediction. The data from this study suggest that the role of $\dot{V}O_2$max is less important than experience in competitive cycling.

Coyle and associates (36) found that in addition to needing a high maximal oxygen consumption for success in competition, "elite-national class" (group 1) time trialists (road cyclists) possessed a higher percentage of slow-twitch fiber and greater muscle capillary density than did "good-state class" (group 2) cyclists. Actual 40-km time-trial performance also was highly correlated with average absolute power output during a 1-hour laboratory performance test. They also found that 1-hour power output is highly related to the cyclist's $\dot{V}O_2$ at lactate threshold ($r = 0.93$).

What factors allowed group 1 to produce more force and perform better in competition? This is an interesting question because it begins specifically and directly to explain the superior performance of elite-national class cyclists. However, it is likely that there is no single factor but instead numerous factors that may vary in magnitude from one cyclist to another. Coyle (36) thought that cyclists with a high percentage of ST fibers have a distinct advantage because, at the same level of energy expenditure (oxygen consumed or ATP hydrolyzed), their muscles produce more force and power.

It also appears that the thigh muscles of cyclists in group 1 were less fatigable compared with those of group 2, which allowed them to maintain higher intensities (percentage $\dot{V}O_2$max) and to push down continually with more force. Indeed enzymes in the thigh muscles that are responsible for aerobic energy production were somewhat higher in group 1. Additionally, group 1 possessed more capillaries around each fiber, which effectively decreases the diffusion distance for oxygen to the active muscle fibers while also serving to flush lactic acid away from the exercising muscle and to reduce fatigue (Tables 48–1 and 48–2).

In many endurance sports, high performance is associated with the ability to sustain high work rates at a high percentage of maximal oxygen consumption. With this in mind, the number of years of training, having a high maximal oxygen consumption, and possessing a high percentage of type I muscle fibers and the ability to perform at a high percentage of $\dot{V}O_2$max at lactate threshold are several factors that may contribute to success in road and time-trial cycling.

TABLE 48–2. *Comparison of the vastus lateralis muscle in groups 1 and 2*

	Type I fibers (%)	Relative oxidative capacity	Capillary density (capillaries/mm^2 fiber area)
Group 1	67[a]	10[a]	464[a]
Group 2	53	8	377
1 − 2	26%[a]	20%[a]	5%[a]

[a]$p < .05$ versus group 2. From ref. 36, with permission.

TRAINING THE ATHLETE

Physical training and subsequent conditioning do not alter the energy expenditure required to perform a given level of work. Nevertheless, they do reduce the extent of cardiorespiratory changes necessary to achieve the required rate of oxygen consumption. The effects of training result in several broad metabolic and physical changes. At one extreme are the muscle fibers and metabolic changes that result from high-intensity exercise of short duration (e.g., anaerobic work including strength training). At the opposite end of the continuum are the long-term effects of prolonged exercise repeated many times at a submaximal level, which enhances central and peripheral aerobic functional capacity.

Specificity

Success in bicycle racing involves physical preparation in a long-term training program. Careful planning, keeping in mind the specificity of the sport and the varied distances, is essential, so that the elements of the training program should emulate competitive conditions as closely as possible.

Most cyclists use essentially three types of training intensities: (a) "over distance" training (involving long hours in the saddle) designed to improve aerobic or oxidative capacity; (b) "race pace" training designed to improve the body's lactic acid tolerance and use capacity, and (c) sprint training designed to improve efficiency and power of the ATP–PC energy system. Whereas it is impossible to cover all forms of training here, it is possible to outline some recent developments [e.g., "anaerobic threshold" or Onset of Blood Lactate Accumulation (OBLA) training].

Early-season training should be aimed toward building the stamina needed to endure the training and competition of the competitive season. A good aerobic foundation is essential, for it is the pivotal element of both performance of and recovery from hard exercise. Such training should be designed to stimulate optimal development of the oxygen-delivery system and of the oxygen-extraction processes at the cellular level.

Oxygen-Delivery Training

Elite cyclists are known to possess a high oxygen-uptake capability. During competition the cyclist's oxygen-transport (cardiac output) and uptake (cell enzymes) systems are often loaded maximally or almost maximally (80% to 85% $\dot{V}O_2$max). Therefore a major portion of the training program should aim to improve the determinants of oxygen transport and uptake.

Traditionally it was considered that all endurance training should be designed to improve the ability to consume oxygen, because cycling was considered primarily an event that lasted several hours on the road, with some track events lasting more than 4.5 min. Why cyclists spend so much time "getting in miles" and neglecting training for time-trial speed, "breakaway" speed, pursuiting, hill climbing, and so on remains obscure.

More recently a new concept of endurance training has been developed, recognizing that $\dot{V}O_2$max may not be the best predictor of endurance performance, and that the percentage of $\dot{V}O_2$max that can be maintained over periods of prolonged exercise is more important. Perhaps of greatest significance is the pace a cyclist can maintain without accumulating large amounts of lactate in the muscles and blood.

If the oxygen-transport and oxygen-use systems are to be trained, they must be overloaded. To achieve an overload, the training tempo has to be high. When the tempo is high for prolonged periods, muscle and blood lactate levels are likely to increase. Reduction in tempo is dictated by buildup of lactate. Reduced tempo relaxes the load on the heart, lungs, and energy-conversion systems. Alternating between hard and easy tempos will, to a certain extent, counteract blood lactate increases while overloading the oxygen-delivery and energy-conversion systems. Various forms of interval and continuous training may be used to this end.

Two basic training formats may be used. The first format attempts to load the metabolic systems at or just above the "anaerobic threshold." In the elite cyclist, the training intensity should be at 80% to 90% of $\dot{V}O_2$max. Short recovery periods between bouts of exercise should be included. For example, high-intensity cycling for periods lasting between 30 seconds and 2 minutes should prove to be an effective training stimulus. The training heart rate, in this example, should be close to the age-related maximal heart rate (220 − age in years), with a recovery rate of approximately 120 beats/min before beginning the next high-intensity cycling bout. As progress is made, the number and length of exercise periods should be increased while the recovery interval is shortened. The training volume and intensity should increase in a progressive manner. This type of interval training not only loads the whole of the aerobic system but also stresses the muscle cells' glycolytic system and results in significant lactate accumulation. Although the presence of excess lactate is distressing, a tolerance to it is built through repeated exposure. At the same time, the pathways of lactate removal are enhanced. This relatively high-intensity training has a secondary benefit of raising the red blood cells' 2,3-diphosphoglycerate (DPG) level. Because this compound binds loosely with subunits of the hemoglobin molecule, it reduces hemoglobin's affinity for oxygen, thereby increasing the availability of oxygen to the working tissues.

The objective of the second form of training is the enhancement of the cardiac output and oxidative capacity of muscle fibers. The expected outcome is an increased size, number, and density of muscle cells' mitochondria, enhanced aerobic enzyme activity, enhanced glycogen metabolism, and improved oxygen delivery. This form of training builds that essential foundation on which future endeavors rely. Training sessions may last 60 to 90 minutes, including the warm-up and warm-down. Effective recruitment of muscle fibers may be achieved through sustained pedalling at 90 to 110 rpm. The intensity of effort may be measured by using heart rate reserve (HRR) in which 70% to 85% of HRR is equivalent to about 57% to 78% of $\dot{V}O_2$max. Thus training intensity can be effectively monitored by using the heart rate as an indicator of percentage of $\dot{V}O_2$max during road cycling. Clifford and colleagues (45) found that there was no significant difference between the heart rate and oxygen consumption relation in the laboratory and on the road.

By using these two training formats, both the "anaerobic threshold" level and oxygen-consumption capacity should be enhanced. Changes in the "anaerobic threshold" as a result of endurance training are much larger than the concurrent changes in $\dot{V}O_2$max. Thus the anaerobic threshold is a more sensitive measure of training effects. The level of anaerobic threshold or percentage $\dot{V}O_2$max the cyclist is able to sustain without disturbing the balance between lactate entry into and exit from the plasma is a critical factor in the capacity for prolonged cycling. Benefits that result from physiologic adaptations to anaerobic training include decreases in the oxygen cost of ventilation, lower accumulation of lactate, and less reduction in glycogen at a given power output. The result is an increase in the intensity of effort that can be sustained aerobically.

The importance of anaerobic-threshold training to cycling has been illustrated by all the recent athletes who have used it as a major component of their training for the 1-hour world record achievement. Therefore it appears that this index of endurance capacity is important in most cycling events. In general, the type of training that improves anaerobic threshold seems to require reasonably long-distance sets with short recovery periods. Although this may not be new to cycling, the pace at which the cyclist rides may be; consequently it is important to establish this pace, which can be done in several ways.

On a cycle ergometer, the cyclist performs an incremental exercise test beginning at low intensity and increases the work load every 2 to 3 minutes until maximal work output is reached. The incremental work loads need to be ridden at a "steady state," during which time heart rate, $\dot{V}O_2$, and blood lactate sampled from fingertip or ear lobe are measured at the end of each increment. Road-training speed and effort can then be determined for the cyclist, based on the heart-rate equivalent of the anaerobic threshold, and monitoring of training intensity can be undertaken by using a portable heart-rate meter.

In summary, the goal of these forms of training is to increase the level of exercise at which aerobic energy production is supplemented by anaerobic mechanisms, that is, to cycle at a higher steady-state level without an increase in lactate and lactate/pyruvate ratio in muscle or arterial blood. For example, a cyclist with a maximal oxygen consumption of 72 mL/kg/min and an AT of 70% $\dot{V}O_2$max could cycle at steady-state oxygen uptake of 50 mL/kg/min. Increasing the AT to 80% steady-state oxygen uptake would increase the exercise intensity to a level corresponding to 57.6 mL/kg/min.

Anaerobic Training

Successful bicycle racing requires the cyclist to possess both speed and power. These performance factors are limited by the metabolic energy available from the high-energy compound ATP. If the cyclist intends to ride fast for any distance, the anaerobic energy-conversion systems must be highly trained. High anaerobic power represents the ability of the anaerobic systems (ATP–PC and lactate) to convert energy at a very high rate. The speed at which energy can be provided depends on the availability of ATP and its phosphate donor, creatine phosphate (CP), and the related enzymes. The cyclist needs a high anaerobic capacity for starts, acceleration, hill climbing, breakaways, sprints, and finishes. Therefore, some portion of the training schedule must address the short-term high-intensity cycling effort.

The purpose of such training is to recruit both type IIa and IIb muscle fibers. These fibers contract rapidly and fatigue somewhat faster than the slow-contracting type I fibers. The maximal involvement of these IIa and IIb fibers requires a training intensity greater than 90% $\dot{V}O_2$max. Because this intensity is difficult to sustain, interval training is the method recommended. High-intensity cycling periods of 8 to 30 seconds, interspersed with 20- to 30-second periods of active recovery, are advised. Results may be achieved with 8 to 12 repetitions and an active recovery interval that is twice the duration of the work period. Not more than two or three training sessions per week of this type of training are recommended. Level sprints and short uphill sprints with an easy return ride downhill are effective overload techniques. The intensity of the overload may be increased by reducing the duration of the recovery interval.

Blending the Systems

Long-distance or natural-interval training serves to balance a well-planned training program. This type of training, lasting 1 to 4 hours, is a blending of all the types of interval training previously discussed. Speed is kept high with increased tempo on uphill stretches. Energy must be delivered both aerobically and anaerobically.

The object is to exploit a large portion of aerobic capacity over longer periods. This type of training promotes technique, muscle-fiber function, the muscles' capability to use fatty acids, and the ability to reprocess and use lactate, all of which result in the sparing of liver and muscle glycogen stores.

Periodization of Training

The annual training cycle (*macrocycle*), in cycling, is conventionally divided into three main periods of training: preparation, competition, and transition (or active rest). Some cyclists refer to these intermediate or medium-length cycles as *mesocycles.* Within each of these periods, the athlete tries to direct the training volume, intensity, frequency, and skill training toward a peak performance.

Some periods are further divided into varying phases. We can divide each period into as many phases as necessary as long as these parts all lead to the main competition goal. In road cycling, competition usually lasts from March to October in the United States. This means that the general preparation phase will have to begin 4 to 5 months before the competition period. The transition period usually starts when the competition period is over, at about the beginning of October. Cyclists in other continents must adjust the months to fit their seasons of training and competition.

Preparation Period

The preparation period of the yearly program is the longest, lasting up to 6 months. Because of the length of the preparation period and the different tasks that must be accomplished in this period of the training program, it is divided into two phases. The first phase consists of the development of general conditioning through such activities as weight training, cyclo-cross, and cross-country skiing. The second phase marks specialized training on the bicycle in which the athlete (a) works on endurance, speed, and power and (b) begins racing.

General Preparation Phase

During this phase of the preparation period, the athlete should begin with relatively low intensity of effort and long duration with the activities chosen. In other words, training is low in effort but long in time, training 5 to 6 days per week, 3 to 4 hours each day.

Toward the end of general preparation phase, training intensity will continue to increase, and more and more miles will be put in on the bicycle.

In this phase, the athlete is engaging in activities that will build overall body conditioning. To build general endurance, for example, the athlete should go on long hilly hikes or cross-country ski for several hours. The intensity of these efforts should be in the 60% to 80% range of maximal heart rate effort for senior men, women, and junior cyclists. Keep the intensity below the anaerobic threshold for the majority of the workouts. Cross-country skiing, snowshoeing, running, hiking, and in-line skating are useful activities for developing endurance capacity.

Besides concentrating on general and resistant training exercises in this phase, it is necessary to start putting in miles on the bicycle during the months of December and January. During this time, on-the-bike training becomes more important, and supplemental training starts to taper off in January. Riding should consist of riding a road bike (both indoors and outdoors) and mountain bike during this phase. There is no such thing as a typical week during this time of the year because of weather and daylight considerations. Cycling may have to be done indoors but should be broken up into several sessions to relieve boredom. The following is a sample week of training during this general preparation phase.

Monday: Morning, 1 hour of easy endurance training; afternoon, resistance training.
Tuesday: Easy endurance training of 2 hours, one jump and one 3-minute effort at anaerobic threshold pace.
Wednesday: Resistance training, followed by 60 to 90 minutes of endurance training.
Thursday: Easy day of very little effort of 30 minutes or total rest day.
Friday: Morning, 1 to 3 hours of endurance training.
Saturday: Endurance training (other than bicycle) of 2 to 4 hours, with a few short efforts of 2 to 5 minutes at anaerobic threshold pace.
Sunday: Long bicycle ride of 2 to 3 hours, with one or two jumps.

Specialization Phase

At this point, racing starts to enter the program. General exercises in our example come to an end.

The physiologic requirements for this period increase in intensity. Work begins on intervals, power, sprints, and anaerobic threshold. Heart rate climbs at times to 85% to 95% of maximal heart rate or more. Adequate rest must be ensured between hard training or racing sessions. Short-stage races of 3 to 4 days can be added to the program.

The racing program during this phase must stay within the principles of the preparation period, the development of increased endurance, and the increasing speed and power work. Participation in races should be considered only when they do not interfere with the goals of the preparation period. In other words, the athlete does not want to compete in races that are too difficult: many races can also be ridden as "training races." Training races are ridden not necessarily to be won but to get in miles on the bike and occasionally to test oneself in breakaways and sprints.

Training intensities as well as duration increase steadily in this phase. The month of March will be the greatest in terms of both training and racing miles. The following is a sample week of training during this specialization phase. The specialization phase leads directly into the competition period. It is important for the athlete to be in top condition once the competition season begins. Maintaining the highest possible performance level is the main task of the competition period.

Monday: Easy, flat ride of 2 to 3 hours, heart rate 60% to 65% maximum.

Tuesday: After good warm-up, 2 hours of long intervals, heart rate up to 95% of maximum at the end of intervals. During this time of the year, use small gearing.

Wednesday: Two to 3 hours of jumps, sprints, and anaerobic threshold riding. Five to six long sprints of 400 to 500 yards, 20 to 30 minutes of anaerobic threshold pace, and two jumps of 150 to 200 yards.

Thursday: Two hours of mixed long intervals and one long climb of 20 to 40 minutes (heart rate ranging from 70% to 95%).

Friday: Easy ride of 1 hour, heart rate 60% to 65%. If really tired, take the day off.

Saturday: Club or team ride of 3 to 4 hours, heart rate no higher than 80% of maximal heart rate, or local road race.

Sunday: Club or team ride of 2 to 3 hours (60% to 95% maximal heart rate), one hill effort, and six to eight sprints or local road or criterium race.

Peaking in the Competition Period

Physical, mental, and tactical training must come to a peak during the competition period. The athlete's main concern during this period, besides producing results, is maintenance of racing performances as long as the competition period lasts. This is difficult to accomplish with a season that can last from May until the end of September. In this case, it is necessary that small rest or recovery phases be planned during the competition period.

If preparation is needed for a major event, such as the Regional or National Championships, it is advisable for the athlete to plan a short break in the training schedule of about 2 weeks without a competition. The 2-week period should start with 3 to 4 days of easy riding and then 9 to 10 days of peaking activities. This is specialized work in preparation for the event. For example, if the race will have a lot of climbing, the athlete needs to spend a few training sessions working on climbing technique and power.

The second phase of this short preparation period must be properly executed with special prerace scheduling. High-intensity and race-simulated intervals, sprints, motor pacing, and other exercises should be part of the program during this time. With 2 days to go before the race, the athlete should include only light training with low duration with two or three jumps each day and then prepare mentally and nutritionally for the competition.

Every cyclist needs competition to prepare properly for a major peak point in the season. We know that planned competitions cannot be replaced with just hard training; racing is necessary to reach top physical performance. The amount of competition needed for someone to reach top physical fitness, however, is different from cyclist to cyclist. The cyclist needs to be aware of that fact, especially if training and competing with other cyclists. They have to compete in the right amount of races and of the right caliber to ensure success. The cyclist may not be able to race as often as the strongest cyclist on the team. Entering lower-caliber races with a greater chance of success may be extremely useful for cyclists occasionally, especially if they find it hard to finish well for a period of time.

Most cyclists have heard about peaking, but many younger or less experienced athletes seem helpless when it comes to planning their yearly program. Peaking for a race does not just happen. It requires months, even years, of preparation for bigger events such as the World Championships. It requires setting goals. It requires discipline when establishing the priorities needed to achieve those goals.

This peaking concept need not be restricted to one season but can be approached on a much broader scale. For example, the cyclist may peak for a few regional events during the upcoming season. With the addition of longer events in the following year, the goal in the third year could be placing well in the age group at the National Championships.

Peaking is often difficult to plan because of the crowded race schedule and variety of races offered. It is one thing to peak at a specific event such as the district championships; it is another thing to peak for a series of races that may be spread out over 2 weeks. Include the National Championships, and you begin to appreciate the difficulty of scheduling peaks.

Most cyclists, coaches, and sport scientists say that one can peak only two or possibly three times per year. Athletes will need to leave a minimum of 6 to 8 weeks between events to perform well. For example, they may peak for a late spring event and then once again for a race in midsummer. A final peak could be established for the National Championships in the fall. Between the events, they will need to recover and rebuild and enter races for training and fine tuning.

The time before the event should allow the cyclists to cut down on distance work and add speed and last-minute technique training to the program. All hard training should end a few days before the event and be replaced with easy to moderate rides, with a few short bursts of speed when they feel good.

What has been outlined here is a systematized approach to planning peaking (and season) for important events. Remember that although the annals of cycling events are filled with stories of outstanding athletes who succeeded at big events, there are other stories of those who lined up at the starting line at the World or the National Championships as leading contenders, and failed. It should have been their moment, but they were not prepared to seize it because in many cases they had not properly peaked for the competition. Remember, the secret to success in any sporting event is being prepared for optimal performance at the right time.

Transition Period

The transition period is the end of the competitive season and serves as a transition time to the beginning of the general preparation period. After a competitive season and peaking for selected major competitions, the cyclist needs a period of reduced training to recover emotionally and physically.

This period is defined as active rest to maintain a specific performance level and training condition of medium to high fitness. It is important for the athlete to continue to exercise during this period because passive rest would make it difficult to start training properly in the general preparation phase.

The transition period should not be longer than 6 to 8 weeks. Cross-training in other activities should be included; if cyclists choose to race their bicycles in cyclocross or mountain-bike races during this period, the psychological pressure of performing should be as low as possible. This also is the time of the year to begin resistance training.

CONCLUSION

The core of fundamental research devoted to the sport of cycling is scattered in a variety of sources. This chapter attempts to synthesize, integrate, and apply the scientific knowledge pertaining to the physiology of cycling.

The physiologic determinants of success in cycling are as varied as the range of cycling disciplines covered by the sport. Only by special attention to the principle of specificity of training can the coach and competitor hope to attain realistic goals. A variety of sophisticated scientific techniques have been used to define a work-performance profile of the cyclist, and so to plan for training and competition. The evidence points to a range of physiological, biomechanical, and nutritional factors that must be used in the preparation of the competitive cyclist.

By using the techniques and protocols outlined, it is possible to evaluate the relative strengths and weaknesses of the cyclist, to determine improvements in the individual's performance, and, by use of training that simulates competitive conditions, to help the individual realize his or her potential.

REFERENCES

1. Swain DP, Coast JR, Clifford PS, Milliken MC, Gundersen JS. Influence of body size on oxygen consumption during cycling. *J Appl Physiol* 1987;62:668–672.
2. McCole SD, Claney K, Conte JC, Anderson R, Hagberg JM. Energy expenditure during bicycling. *J Appl Physiol* 1990;68: 748–853.
3. Pugh LGCE. The relation of oxygen intake and speed in competition cycling and comparative observations on the bicycle ergometer. *J Physiol (Lond)* 1974;241:795–808.
4. Sjogaard GB, Nielsen B, Mikkelsen F, Saltin B, Burke ER. *Physiology of cycling.* Ithaca: Movement Publications, 1982:33–37.
5. Swain DP, Coast JR, Milliken MC, Clifford PS, Vaughan R, Stray-Gundersen J. Is there an optimum body size for competitive cycling? In: Burke ER, Newsom MM, eds. *Medical and scientific aspects of cycling.* Champaign, IL: Human Kinetics, 1988:39–46.
6. Merrill EG. The B.C.C.S. physiological test program: British cycling coaching scheme. *Coaching News* 1980;Summer:13–25.
7. Di Prampero PE, Cortili G, Mognoni P, Saibene F. Equation of motion of a cyclist. *J Appl Physiol* 1979;47:201–206.
8. Kyle CR. Ergogenics for bicycling. In: Lamb DR, Williams W, eds. *Ergogenics: enhancement of performance in exercise and sport.* Indianapolis: Benchmark Press, 1991:373–413.
9. Hagberg JM, McCole MS. Energy expenditure during cycling. In: Burke ER, ed. *High tech cycling.* Champaign, IL: Human Kinetics, 1996:167–184.
10. Kyle CR, Caiozzo VJ. Experiments in human ergometry as applied to the design of human powered vehicles. *Int J Sport Biomech* 1986;2:6–19.
11. Whitt FR, Wilson DG. *Bicycling science.* Cambridge: MIT Press, 1982:29–67.
12. Dal Monte A, Faina AM. Human anaerobic power output. In: *UCI Congress on the medical and scientific aspects of cycling.* Abono Terme, Italy: 1989:19–21.
13. Craig NP, Pyke FS, Norton KI. Specificity of test duration when assessing the anaerobic lactic acid capacity of high-performance track cyclists. *Int J Sports Med* 1989;10:237–242.
14. Burke ER, Fleck S, Dickson T. Post-competition blood lactate concentrations in competitive track cyclists. *Br J Sports Med* 1981;15:242–245.
15. Jacobs R, Tesch PA, Bar-Or O, Karlsson J, Dotan R. Lactate in human skeletal muscle after 10 and 30 s of supramaximal exercise. *J Appl Physiol* 1983;55:365–367.
16. Jones NL, McCarthney N, Graham T, et al. Muscle performance and metabolism in maximal isokinetic cycling at slow and fast speeds. *J Appl Physiol* 1985;59:132–136.
17. Davies CTM. The physiology of cycling with reference to power output and muscularity. *Ann Physiol Anthropol* 1992;11:309–312.
18. Capelli C, di Prampero PE. Maximal explosive power and aerobic exercise in humans. *Schweiz Z Sportsmed* 1991;39:103–111.
19. Faria IE. Energy expenditure, aerodynamics and medical problems in cycling. *Sports Med* 1992;14:43–63.
20. Johnson S, Shultz B. The physiological effects of aerodynamic handlebars. *Cycling Sci* 1990;2:9–12.
21. Origenes MM, Blank SE, Schoene RB. Exercise ventilatory response to upright and aero-position cycling. *Med Sci Sports Exerc* 1993;25:608–612.
22. Whitt FR, Wilson DG. *Bicycling science.* Cambridge: MIT Press, 1982:71–80.
23. Berglund L, Fashena D, Su X, Gwosdow A. Absorbed solar radiation from measured sweat rate. In: *Proceedings of the Thirteenth Annual Northeast Bioengineering Conference.* Philadelphia: 1987: 507–510.

24. Berglund L, Fashena D, Su X. Evaporative weight loss as a measure of absorbed thermal radiation in the human. *8th Conference on Biometeorology and Aerobiology*. Boston: American Meteorologic Society, 1987:338–340.
25. Montain SJ, Coyle EF. The influence of graded dehydration on hyperthermia and cardiovascular drift during exercise. *J Appl Physiol* 1992;73:1340–1350.
26. Montain SJ, Coyle EF. Fluid ingestion during exercise increases skin blood flow independent of increases in blood volume. *J Appl Physiol* 1992;73:903–910.
27. Mitchell JB, Voss KW. The influence of volume on gastric emptying and fluid balance during prolonged exercise. *Med Sci Sports Exerc* 1991;23:314–319.
28. Brouns F, Saris WHM, Stroecken J, et al. Eating, drinking, and cycling, a controlled Tour de France simulation study: part 1. *Int J Sports Med* 1989;10:S32–S40.
29. Saris WHM, van Erp-Baart AMJ, Westerterp KR, ten Hoor F. Study on the food intake during extreme sustained exercise: the Tour de France. *Int J Sports Med* 1989;10:S26–S31.
30. Brouns F, Saris WHM, Stroecken J, et al. Eating, drinking, and cycling, a controlled Tour de France simulation study: part 2. *Int J Sports Med* 1989;10:S41–S48.
31. Burke ER. The physiological characteristics of competitive cyclists. *Physician Sportsmed* 1980;8:78–84.
32. White JA, Quinn G, Al-Dawalibi M, Nulhall J. Seasonal changes in cyclists' performance, part 1: the British Olympic road race squad. *Br J Sports Med* 1982;16:4–12.
33. White JA, Quinn G, Al-Dawalibi M, Nulhall J. Seasonal changes in cyclists' performance, part 2: the British Olympic track squad. *Br J Sports Med* 1982;16:13–21.
34. Mackova E, Melichna J, Placheta Z, Blahova D, Semiginovsky B. Skeletal muscle characteristics of sprint cyclists and nonathletes. *Int J Sports Med* 1986;7:295–297.
35. Burke ER, Cerny F, Costill D, Fink W. Characteristics of skeletal muscle in competitive cyclists. *Med Sci Sports Exerc* 1977;9:109–112.
36. Coyle EF, Feltner ME, Kautz SA, et al. Physiological and biomechanical factors associated with elite endurance cycling performance. *Med Sci Sports Exerc* 1991;23:93–107.
37. Ahlquist LE, Bassett DR, Sufit R, Nagle FJ, Thomas DP. The effect of pedaling frequency on glycogen depletion rates in type I and type II quadriceps muscle fibers during submaximal cycling exercise. *Eur J Appl Physiol* 1992;65:360–364.
38. Coyle EF, Sidossis LS, Horowitz JF, Beltz JD. Cycling efficiency is related to the percentage of type I muscle fibers. *Med Sci Sports Exerc* 1992;24:782–788.
39. Gregor RJ, Rugg SG. Effects of saddle height and pedaling cadence on power output and efficiency. In: Burke ER, ed. *Science of cycling*. Champaign, IL: Human Kinetics, 1986:69–90.
40. Gregor RJ, Broker JP, Ryan MM. The biomechanics of cycling. In: Holloszy JO, ed. *Exercise and sport science reviews*. Vol 19. Baltimore: Williams & Wilkins, 1991:127–169.
41. Desipres M. An electromyographic study of competitive road cycling conditions simulated on a treadmill. In: Nelson RC, Morehouse C, eds. *Biomechanics IV*. Baltimore: University Park Press, 1974:349–355.
42. Kautz SA, Feltner ME, Coyle EF, Baylor AM. The pedaling technique of elite endurance cyclists: changes with increasing workload at constant cadence. *Int J Sport Biomech* 1991;7:29–53.
43. Fagard R, Aubert A, Lysens R. Noninvasive assessment of seasonal variations in cardiac structure and function in cyclists. *Circulation* 1983;67:896–901.
44. Krebs PS, Zinkgraf S, Virgilio S. The effects of training variables, maximal aerobic capacities, and body composition upon cycling performance time. *Med Sci Sports Exerc* 1983;15:133.
45. Clifford PS, Coast JR, Swain DP. Heart rate/oxygen consumption relationship during cycling. *Med Sci Sports Exerc* 1986;18:S36.

Exercise and Sport Science,
edited by William E. Garrett, Jr., and Donald T. Kirkendall.
Lippincott Williams & Wilkins, Philadelphia © 2000.

CHAPTER 49

Physiology of Dance

Lynn A. Darby

THE SPORT

Dance is life . . . and life is dance.

Since the beginning of the ages, human movement has evolved, and so with dance. Dance as a form of human movement can be described by many different words: physical, rhythmic, aesthetic, or emotional. To define dance is to omit some unique forms of dance, but for the purpose of this chapter, two categories of dance will be used: (a) theatrical dance, and (b) aerobic dance exercise. These groupings reflect the difference in the intent of dance in each category, and most empiric studies concerning dance have described and quantified ballet and aerobic dance exercise.

According to Hardaker and Vander Woude (1), theatrical dance includes classic ballet, modern dance, ethnic dance, and various mixed forms of dance (e.g., Broadway, jazz, tap). Ballet represents a form of dance in which an aesthetic ideal is sought, whereas modern dance has its roots in freedom of expression (1). Aerobic dance exercise (ADE) is considered by many as a form of exercise, but various aerobic dance steps originated from the choreography of dance. Started in the late 1960s by Jackie Sorenson, ADE is calisthenics, steps, and movements to music performed to increase the physical fitness level of the participant (e.g., cardiorespiratory fitness, muscular strength, flexibility). Different types of ADE (e.g., jazzercise, funk, aerobic dance with hand-held weights, step aerobics) have evolved since the mid 1970s to vary the exercise intensity and to keep participants motivated to exercise.

Since the early 1980s there has been an identification of a specialty area in medicine for dance. This blending of the art and science of dance has been called *dance medicine* (2). This term was first used in 1979 and has evolved out of the need to find and disseminate information to treat and/or prevent dance injuries, to educate health-care providers about the special needs of dancers, and to study the training practices of dancers (2). Solomon and Micheli (3) noted that there are a number of risk factors for dance injury (e.g., deconditioning, improper warm-up, errors in training, technique flaws, and muscle-tendon imbalances). It has been postulated that dance injuries can be prevented through a proper understanding of kinesiology and how it applies to dance technique and training (3). Physiology is one portion of dance kinesiology, the study of the art and science of dance. The purpose of this chapter is to discuss the applied physiology of dance. Other exercise sciences (i.e., biomechanics, motor control, nutrition, sport psychology) have also been used to study dance and dance injuries, but a discussion of these is beyond the scope of this chapter.

L. A. Darby: Kinesiology Division, School of Human Movement, Sport and Leisure Studies, Bowling Green University, Bowling Green, Ohio 43403.

Physical Requirements

The physical requirements of dance are as varied as the steps and choreography that make up a dance routine or performance. Professional dancers today are asked to place extreme physical demands on their bodies (1). Most forms of dance require a combination of strength, power, flexibility, cardiorespiratory fitness, and neuromuscular coordination. The range of physical requirements necessary for dance is vast. For example, an elite professional ballet dancer performing a demi-plié, a modern dancer launching into a twisting jump, and a middle-aged woman completing a jog step in an aerobic dance class are all dancing, but they have vastly different physical requirements.

Theatrical Dance: Ballet

In Fig. 49–1, examples of some common ballet positions are shown (4). Many of these positions require "turn-

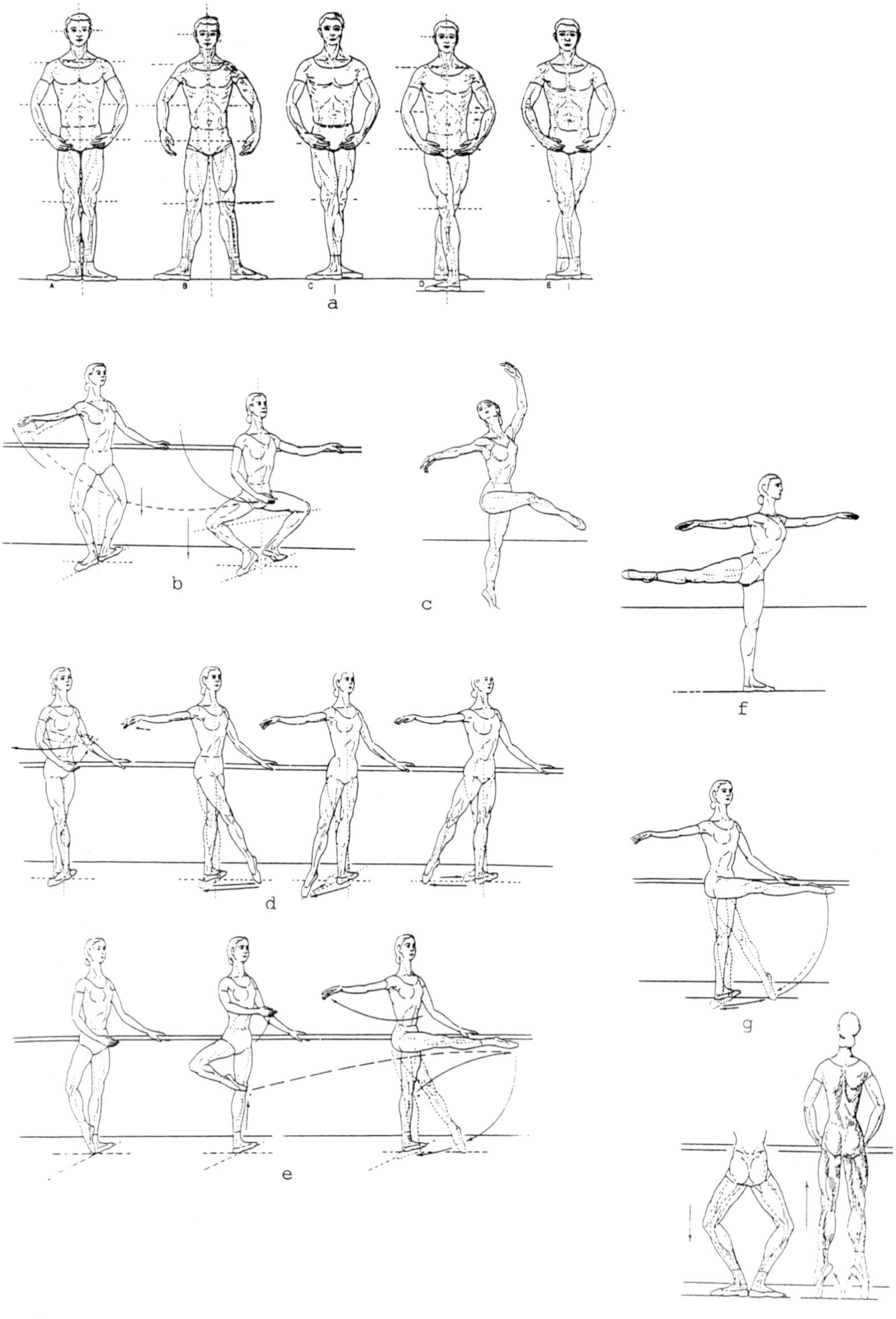

FIG. 49–1. Basic ballet positions. See text for details. (From ref. 4, with permission.)

out," which is external, outward rotation of the hip, knee, and ankle to 90 degrees. When the heels contact each other and form a line of 180 degrees and are flat on the floor, "perfect" turnout has been accomplished (5). Many ballet steps require excessive dorsiflexion or plantarflexion, and a great degree of flexibility in the gastrocnemius, hamstrings, and hip abductors. All ballet movements and poses emanate from the five fundamental positions, first through fifth, shown in Fig. 49–1*A* (4,5). Additional dance steps are shown in Figs. 49–1*B* through 49–1*H*. These steps are (*B*) grand plié, flexion of the knees while the lower leg is outwardly rotated; for the grand plié, the thigh is parallel to the floor at the lowest point; (*C*) attitude, a pose in which the leg is brought up to an angle of 90 degrees from the midline in front, back, or to the side of the torso, with the knee bent and the leg rotated outwardly; (*D*) battement tendu, pointing the foot to the front, back, or side; (*E*) developpé, unfolding of the leg as it is lifted into the air to full extension; (*F*) arabesque, various forms of extending one leg posteriorly while balancing on the supporting foot to make the longest line from the tip of the toe to the tip of the finger; (*G*) grand battement front, beating of one leg close to the other; in grand, the entire leg raises from the hip into the air; and (*H*) pointe, standing and moving on the points of the toes. From a functional standpoint, dancing on pointe is the most demanding ballet work, and the dancer's ability to do it correctly may be limited by anatomic make-up. Further definitions of commonly used dance terminology and movements inherent in all types of dance are given by Ryan and Stephens (5).

Unlike ballet, in which poses are imposed on the body, modern dance has its purpose in using the inherent characteristics of the human body to develop strong, skillful dancers (6). This dance form developed to contrast the linear, rigid fundamentals of ballet and emphasizes freedom of movement and artistic expression. In Fig. 49–2, a modern dance movement is shown.

The physical demands of dance encompass not only the execution of specific steps, but also the other physical requirements that make up a dancer's daily schedule. Chmelar and Fitt (7) have proposed a pyramid to describe the facets of dance training (Fig. 49–3). At the base of the pyramid, they describe dance training as composed of three areas: technique class, somatics, and conditioning. Above this, rehearsal would be that time in which all the components of training come together; finally, at the top of the pyramid is the dance performance, which represents the total integration of the rehearsal and training sessions. For ballet, a typical rehearsal workout begins with barre exercise and progresses to center floor work. The weekly number of hours for class work, rehearsal, and other activity for some professional dancers is shown in Table 49–1 (8–25). It is interesting to note that most female professional dancers begin at approximately age 7 years, with male students starting approximately 4 to 5 years later; by the time dancers of both genders are professionally employed, they have close to 15 to 20 years of dance experience (1,5).

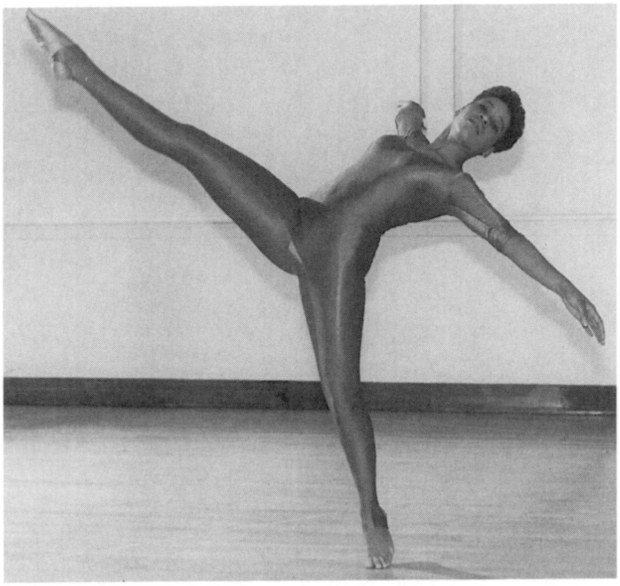

FIG. 49–2. A modern dance movement; note the diverse nonlinear axes that are created by the body lines of the appendages and torso. (Photo courtesy of Bowling Green State University, Dance Program.)

Aerobic Dance Exercise

The steps that can be choreographed into an aerobic dance routine can be varied by impact [i.e., high impact (HI; jumping, bouncing movements) versus low impact (LI; ADE during which one foot is kept in contact with the ground], cadence (i.e., beat of the music to which movements are timed), range of motion (i.e., full or partial movement through the arc of movement at a joint), muscle mass of the arms, legs, or a combination of both involved in the movement, position of arms (i.e., above and/or below shoulder/heart level), type of muscle contraction (i.e., isometric, dynamic; eccentric or concentric), and the addition of hand-held weights of varied weights. The arm position, isometric exercise, and use of hand-held weights are of particular importance because these may evoke the pressor response [i.e., an increase in heart rate (HR) and blood pressure due to the position or use of the arms or Valsalva maneuver].

ADE steps can usually be completed easily by participants of all ages and fitness levels. This is one of the unique characteristics of ADE in that the same step can be modified by the participant to meet the needs of his or her individual workout. For example, a step such as a low kick with one foot on the floor can be made more

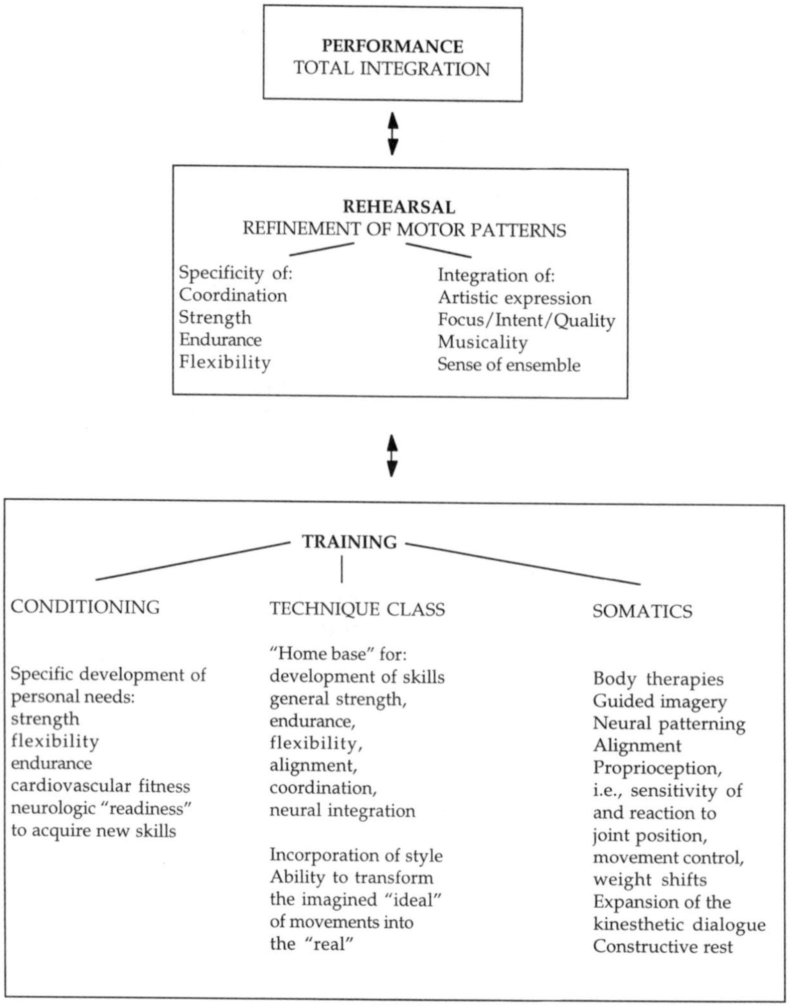

FIG. 49–3. The dance training pyramid. (From ref. 7, with permission.)

intense by increasing the height of the kick, and it can be made even more intense by completing a high kick with a jump on the nonkicking leg (26). Although this is good for individualizing exercise for the aerobic dancer, this variability in the execution of ADE steps makes measurement of the physiologic responses to ADE more difficult. In many previous studies, the steps have not been described in detail; therefore replication of the study or comparison with other studies may be impossible. Darby and colleagues (27) suggested that the methods sections in future studies should contain a detailed movement analysis of the ADE steps so that these comparisons may be made.

A typical ADE workout fulfills the cardiorespiratory training principles (i.e., frequency, intensity, duration, type of activity: continuous) and is similar to any cardiorespiratory workout (Table 49–2) (28–36). Classes begin with a warm-up of light activity and stretching exercises for 10 minutes, progress to the 20- to 30-minute workout phase, and then have a gradual cool-down period for 10 minutes: three parts of a typical 60-minute class. As Clippenger-Robertson (26) has stated, step sequences of ADE routines are a combination of basic locomotor movements. A number of steps have been defined: walk, run, skip, two-step, march, jog, jumping jack, step touches, heel touches, knee lifts, side kicks, knee curls, lunges, and touch backs (26). In addition, other ADE steps to improve cardiorespiratory fitness can be introduced by the instructor by adding traditional dance steps such as cha-cha, hustle, and polka (26). To improve muscular strength and endurance, exercises using elastic tubing and bench steps may be incorporated into the routines. Further descriptions of these commonly used steps can be found in "how to" ADE books or the *Aerobics Instructor Manual*, published by the American Council on Exercise (26).

Physiologic Requirements

Theatrical Dance

Physiologic measurements have been completed on various forms of dance and ADE (Tables 49–2 and 49–3)

TABLE 49–1. *Physiologic characteristics of ballet and modern dancers*

Author	Form	Level	Subj	Age (yr)	Ht (cm)	Wt (kg)	% fat	$\dot{V}O_2max$[d]	Other characteristics:
Abraham et al. (1982)	Ballet	Students in prof training	29F	17 (16–19)	160	47			Attending classes in local ballet schools previously 3–13 yr; 20 students reported secondary amenorrhea during the second 6 months of school
Calabrese et al. (1983)	Ballet	Prof	29F	22	167	53	16.9[a]		Age started dancing 7.5 ± 2.7
		Adv student	5F						Age turned professional 17.3 ± 2.5; 17 reported secondary amenorrhea; 11 had dance-related menstrual problems
Chatfield et al. (1990)	Modern	Beg	14F	25	163	56	23.7[a]	40.4	Dance subjects involved primarily in modern dance; Int/Adv also in some ballet and jazz
		Int	11F	23	162	54	20.9	42.5	
		Adv	8F	32	160	51	18.1	43.6	
Chemlar et al. (1988)	Ballet	Univ	10F	19	166	54	14.2[b]	47	Other physiologic variables were reported (e.g., lactate threshold, hamstring/quad isokinetic strength ratio
		Prof	9F	24	167	54	14.1	42	
	Modern	Univ	11F	27	163	54	14.7	48	
		Prof	9F	30	162	53	12.2	49	
Clarkson et al. (1985)	Ballet	Young	14F	15	161	48	16.4[a]	49	16.8 h/wk in class or rehearsal
Clarkson et al. (1989)	Ballet	Student							Unadv, Int, Adv, Prof
		Unadv	31F	15	161	48	Tall and slim		Yr. ballet training 4.6, 6.1, 5.5, 13.0
		Int	38F	16	164	50			Yr. on pointe 3.5, 5.0, 5.4, 13.3
		Adv	14F	17	166	51			Hrs/wk in class 12, 14.2, 13.1, 10.6
		Prof	15F	24	167	52			Hrs/wk in rehearsal 7.5, 10.4, 9.8, 28.6
Cohen et al. (1980)	Ballet	Prof	15F	23	165	50			↑ sinus bradycardia; ↑ sinus arrythmia in female dancers; ↑ third heart sound in male dancers; other heart changes comparable to athletes with similar training (isometric–isotonic demands)
			15M	24	177	67			
		Controls	8F	26	161	48			
			8M	30	175	70			
Crotts et al. (1996)	Varied	Univ	15F						Mean 14.9 ± 3.9 years of dance experience (10–24 yr range); 6 balance tests (Foam and Dome test); dancers had > balance than controls
		Controls	15F						
Dahlstrom et al. (1987)	Dancers	Univ	13F	24	167	57.4		Pre, 52.7	Females > % Type I (slow) fibers similar to end.-trained female runners or cross-country skiers; started at ages 4–8 yr; 15–20 h/wk training for 2.75 yr; detrained with 2–3 h/wk for 32 wk; no ΔBW after detraining
			8F					Post, 46.4	
Dolgener et al. (1980)	Ballet	Prof/Univ	19F	23	164	51	22[b]		Physiologic profile of dancers
		Modern	10F	25	164	53	22		
Fogelholm et al. (1996)	Ballet Netherlands	Prof/Stud	113F	(16–42)	167	52	18.3		Mean no. of years of dance 2 times > for ballet vs. modern dancers; mean starting age was 8.1 yr
Hergenroeder, et al. (1993)	Ballet		122F	15 (11–25)	159	45	20[c]		Formula to predict FFM in ballet dancers; can be calculated from BW due to homogeneity of ballet dancers
Karlsson et al. (1993)	Ballet	Prof	25F	36			18		Dancers had < fat and < BMI, but dancer's amount of lean body mass = controls; > BMD in lower extremities of female and hips of male dancers
		Prof	17M	40			11		
		Controls	25F	Age-, sex-matched			31		
		Controls	17M				19		
Kirkendall et al. (1984)	Ballet	Prof	14F	23.8	167	54			Dancers studied pre and peak season; > peak torque at 180°/s at peak season
			14M	24.6	178	68			
Kuno et al. (1995)	Ballet	Prof	18F	27	158	47	17		Ballet dancers had trained for 20 years. No other exercise training except dance training
	Controls Japanese	Sed	66F	24	159	51	24		
Micheli et al. (1984)	Ballet	Prof	9F	27	164	48	15.3		↑ level of flexibility in dancers
Mostardi (1986)	Ballet	Prof	11F	25	165	50	49		
			5M	28	175	64	59		
Novak et al. (1978)	Dancers	Students	12F	21	163	51	41.5		6–7 yr experience in dance programs; 10–15 h/wk; dancers lower BW, resting HR, DBP, and total body fat and > max $\dot{V}O_2$
		Controls	12F	24	167	55	36.5		

F, females; M, males.
[a]Underwater weighing.
[b]Skinfolds
[c]TOBEC (total body electrical conductivity).
[d](ml/kg/min).

TABLE 49–2. *Physiologic responses to various forms of dance*

Year	Author	Form	Subjects	Age (yr)	Wt (kg)	HR (beat/min)	$\dot{V}O_2$ (ml/kg^{-1}/min)	Other comments:
1994	Clapp, Little	LI	89F			165	32.4	No significant difference in $\dot{V}O_2$ due to type of exercise
		HI				162	33.9	
		Bench step				156	32.2	
1982	Cohen, Segal, Witriol, McArdle	Ballet	6F	25	50	Barre work / Center floor	Barre / Center floor	Ballet steps have large isometric component with high intensity, bursts of activity; $\dot{V}O_2$max similar to nonendurance athletes
			4M	24	68	117 / 137	16.5 / 20.1	
						134 / 153	18.5 / 26.3	
1982	Cohen, Segal, McArdle	Ballet	7F	24	49	Performance 169 (mean)		Performance 87% max HR
			6M	25	64	Allegro 184 (peak)		Allegro 94% max HR
						Class allegro 168 (mean), 179 (peak)		HR during ballet stage performance; HR for various ballet movements are reported
						Stage allegro (N = 4) 171 (mean), 183 (peak)		
1995	Darby et al.	Aerobic dance	16F Trained	23	58	LI (March) 155	29.86	
						LIA (Powerjack) 168	33.53	
						HI (Jog) 165	34.85	
						HIA (Jumping jack) 164	33.81	
1978	Haviland	Modern dance					48.2	
1975	Jette, Inglis	Western square	4F	37	55		17.6[a]	Energy cost of 3-h dancing: males, 425 kcal; females, 390 kcal
			4M	38	82		17.0[a]	
1982	Leger	Disco	7F	Univ students		135	28.1	
			7M			133	31.2	
1979	Noble, Howley	Tap	17F	17–26		Soft shoe	16.6	
						Slow buck	16.8	
1984	Shantz, Astrand	Ballet	7F	25	52	Barre	≈19.4 (36% $\dot{V}O_2$max)	Females $\dot{V}O_2$max 51
			6M	28	70	Center floor	≈23.2 (43% $\dot{V}O_2$max)	Males $\dot{V}O_2$max 57
						Center floor	≈25.8 (46% $\dot{V}O_2$max)	
						Choreographed dance	≈43.2 (80% $\dot{V}O_2$max)	
1980	Wigaeus, Kilbom	Folk	6M	27	69	172	37	
			6F	26	58	179	39	

LI, low-impact aerobic dance exercise (ADE) with arms below shoulder level; HI, high-impact ADE with arms below shoulder level; LIA, low-impact ADE with arms above shoulder level; HIA, high-impact ADE with arms above shoulder level.

[a] Net cost of dance + net cost of recovery.

(37–49). These studies focused primarily on the caloric cost (i.e., the $\dot{V}O_2$ of the dance). Pictures of data-collection procedures for ballet and ADE are shown in Figs. 49–4 and 49–5, respectively. It can be noted from Table 49–2 that the approximate energy cost for most forms of dance is ≈35 mL/kg/min, 10 METS, 2.28 L/min, or 11.4 kcal/min). All of these values are approximations and would be affected by physiologic attributes (e.g., body weight, percentage of fat, muscular strength) of the dancers.

As with many sports, the energy cost of dance can vary dependent on the fitness and skill levels of the participants. In theatrical dance, dance can be described as intermittent bursts of moderate to intense activity (50). Steps performed allegro last less than 30 seconds, and anaerobic sources [i.e., adenosine triphosphate–phosphocreatine (ATP–PC)] would be the predominant energy source (50). Most barre and center floor exercises last approximately 30 seconds to 1.5 minutes and rely on anaerobic glycolysis for energy production. In 1982, Cohen and colleagues (30) recorded HR responses during stage performance and rehearsal for ballet dancers. Mean HRs were 184 beats/min, which was 97% of maximal HR. The longest bout of continuous dance was approximately 4 minutes. Although most previous authors classified dance as primarily a short-term, high-intensity activity, some of the rehearsals or technique classes may be long enough and at a sufficient intensity to elicit moderate cardiorespiratory improvements. Rimmer and co-workers (51) monitored HR continuously during ballet classes and rehearsals. They reported that intensity levels were in the training zone (i.e., 60% to 90% maximal HR) 52% of the time during ballet class and 56% of the time during rehearsal. Rimmer and associates (51) noted that these dance training sessions were comparable to interval training. During rehearsals, periods of rest are usually part of the class because of need for directions and demonstration by the dance instructor.

Aerobic Dance Exercise

In contrast to theatrical dance, the intent of ADE is to increase cardiorespiratory fitness, and therefore ADE workouts focus primarily on improving aerobic capacity. In Table 49–3, the physiologic costs of various forms of ADE are shown. Since the 1970s, when two studies by Foster (52) and Igbanugo and Gutin (53) documented the energy cost of ADE, numerous studies have been completed concerning ADE (37–49). Because all of these studies could not be presented, the studies in Table 49–3 have been selected to represent factors that can be varied to affect ADE. For example, the studies by Blessing and colleagues (39), Milburn and Butts (44), and Williams and Morton (49) showed that significant cardiorespiratory training effects could be elicited from 8 or more weeks of ADE training. The studies by Bell and Bassey (37), Berry and colleagues (38), Parker and colleagues (45), and Perry and colleagues (46) specifically investigated the HR/$\dot{V}O_2$ relation. The fact that the HR/$\dot{V}O_2$ relation may not be linear for ADE was a concern, because if this linear relation did not exist then HR would not be representative of the $\dot{V}O_2$ of ADE. Results of other ADE studies are summarized in Table 49–3.

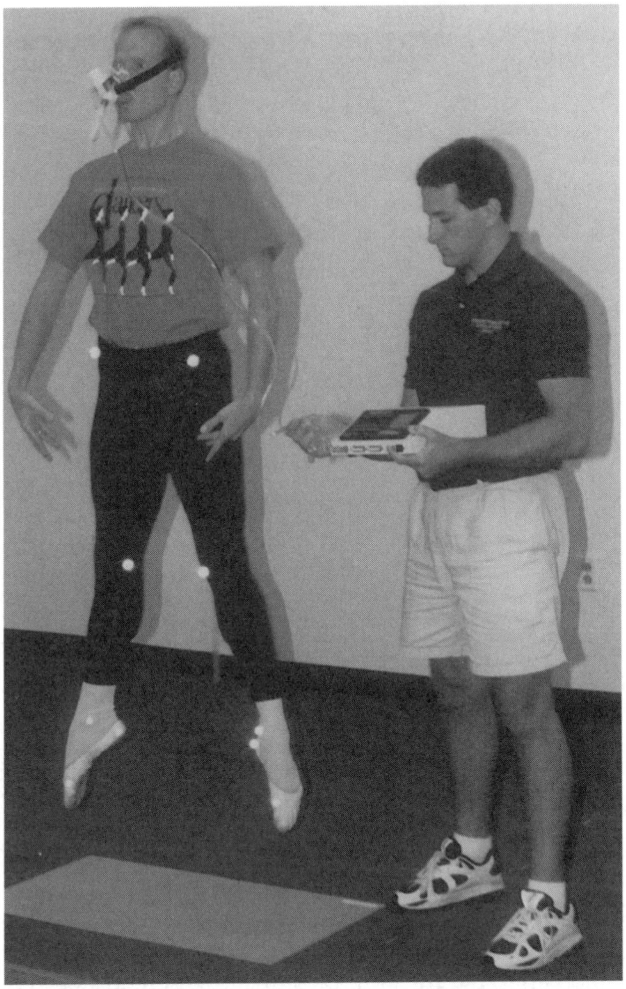

FIG. 49–4. Sauté (springing into the air) by a ballet dancer. Physiologic and biomechanical data being collected are (**A**) oxygen consumption by using the TEEM 100 (Aerosport, Ann Arbor, MI); (**B**) landing-force data by using the force platforms; and (**C**) kinematic data from filming (cameras not shown) and subsequent digitizing of body markers. (Photo courtesy of Bowling Green State University.)

THE ATHLETE

Theatrical Dance

As mentioned previously, ballet is the most studied form of theatrical dance. In Table 49–1, a summary of the physiologic profiles of male and female ballet and modern dancers is presented. As Clarkson and colleagues (13) have summarized, the body type of both adolescent and professional dancers usually consists of relatively small upper arms and large calves and ankles. Across the studies presented (8–25), it can be noted that the mean body weight and height of female ballet dancers is consistent (range, 47 to 52 kg; 103 to 114 lbs; 160 to 167 cm; 5 ft 2in. to 5 ft 5in.). For the two studies reporting on male ballet dancers (14,15), body weights were 64 and 70 kg (141 and 154 lbs), respectively. The body image of the ballet dancer requires a thin, slim, muscular physique able to perform movement requiring strength and flexibility without bulky musculature. For the few studies that included modern dancers, women were slightly heavier, with a range of 51 to 54 kg (112 to 119 lbs). No studies have been reported for male modern dancers.

In summary, it may be stated that ballet dancers are born, not made. If the physical attributes of the individual (i.e., body type, ability to rotate at the hip externally, to dorsiflex and plantarflex at the ankle, and to possess extensive isometric and dynamic muscular strength to attain the positions described in Fig. 49–1) do not meet or cannot meet the "ideal" of a ballet dancer, he or she will not have the ability to reach a high level of performance. These individuals may need to participate in another form of dance in which their physical attributes can form their own style of dance.

A number of studies have conducted muscular-strength testing on ballet and modern dancers; however, the results from these studies have not been consistent (Table 49–4). Chmelar and Fitt (7), in discussing the complexities of dance research, noted that this discrepancy may be because complex dance steps may be qualitatively and quantitatively different from isolation of a

TABLE 49–3. *Physiologic responses to various types of aerobic dance exercise*

Author (yr)	Subjects	Age (yr)	Wt (kg)	$\dot{V}O_2max$			HR (beats/min)		(HR_{max}) (%)	
Bell, Bassey	10F instructors	34	59				LI[a]	LIA[a]	HI[a]	HIA[a]
(1994)							135 (68)	155 (79)	160 (81)	174 (88)
Berry et al.	9F	26	62	47.3					Below	Above
(1992)									136 (72)	136 (72)
Blessing et				Pre	Post	Δ%				
al. (1987)	13F W			37.7	42.6	13				
	13F NW			36.5	41.9	15				
Bronstein et	18F	27	57				LI-NW	LI-W		
al. (1990)		17–40					163	170		
Carroll et al.	9F						Below-NW	Below-W		
(1991)	1M						146 (77)	153 (79)		
							Above-NW	Above-W		
							158 (81)	170 (86)		
Cearly et al.				Pre	Post	Δ%				
(1984)	7F 2d/wk	21	60	37	39	5				
	7F 3d/wk	20	59	40	45	13				
	7F Controls	23	59	30	35	17				
Clapp, Little	36F Instructors	30	58	52			165 (86)		162 (86)	
(1994)	53F Students	32	59	43						
Darby et al.	16F Trained	23	58	49.6			March	Power Jack	Jog	Jump Jack
(1995)							155 (80)	168 (87)	165 (86)	164 (85)
Milburn,				Pre	Post					
Butts	15F ADE		62	35	39					
(1983)	19F Joggers		64	36	39					
	12F Bowlers		59	37	38					
Parker et al.			Post	Pre	Post		ADE 180			ADE 24
(1989)	14F TR	19	55	34	38		TR 163			(62)
	10F Controls	23	63	38	37					TR 24 (63)
Perry et al.					Post		Interval training:			
(1988)	24 Interval	20	61		39.1		12 wk;	80–85%	7–10 routines of 3–5 min w/	
	24 Cont.	20	60		34.9			HR max	walk or jog relief of 3 min	
	24 Controls	20	62		32.7					
Scharff-Olson	11F	33	55	47.8				%HRmax	60 70 80 90	
et al.								ADE→ %$\dot{V}O_2max$	23 39 55 70	
(1992)								TR→ %$\dot{V}O_2max$	39 52 66 80	
Thomson,							HR	Level 1	Level 2	Level 3
Ballor	8F ADE Exp	27	55	42				135	149	162
(1991)	10F Trained	28	69	41				133	158	166
	9F Untrained	28	71	31				148	171	177
Williams,				Pre	Post	Δ%				
Morton	25F ADE	27	61	35.3	40.8	16				
(1986)	15F Controls	27	60	37.3	38.3	3				

[a] LI, low impact; LIA, low impact with arms; HI, high impact; HIA, high impact with arms.
[b] Above, ADE with arms used extensively above shoulder level; Below, ADE with arms kept below shoulder level.
[c] TR, treadmill running.
[d] NW, no handheld weights; W, handheld weights.
[e] Δ%, (Pre-Post/Post) · 100; calculated by author if not reported in original study.

single muscle or antagonist–agonist muscle group, for which isokinetic strength is measured. In Table 49–4, isokinetic strength measures are presented for female ballet dancers (10,21,23,24,54–57). Common speeds of measurement were 30°/s for muscular strength and 180°/s for muscular power. It is difficult to compare and contrast isokinetic strength-training results because muscle groups, speeds, and limb positions varied (10,54). Dorsiflexion and plantarflexion data from these dancers are comparable to those of female basketball players, however (58), and hamstring and quadriceps strength are comparable to those of nondisabled females (59). Kirkendall and colleagues (21) reported significantly greater peak torque curves of 180°/s at peak season as compared with preseason (i.e., December vs. August), but not at slower velocities. Data also were reported

TABLE 49–3. *(continued)*

$\dot{V}O_2$ (ml/kg^{-1}/min)		($\dot{V}O_2$max) (%)		Main factor investigated/conclusion:
LI[a]	LIA[a]	HI[a]	HIA[a]	HR to $\dot{V}O_2$ relation/no Δ due to impact or arm work
21.86	26.21	29.33	31.19	
		Below	Above	HR/$\dot{V}O_2$ relationship for LI vs TR; TR HR = 136; $\dot{V}O_2$ = 23.71 (50%); similar relationship for ADE and TR
		24.35 (52)	23.87 (51)	
				Effects of 8-wk ADE W and NW (1 lb); significant ↑ in $\dot{V}O_2$max for both groups; no sign. ↑ in energy cost due to handheld weights; ADE did not change % fat or BW
LI-NW	LI-W			LI by trained dancers W and NW; Addition of handheld weights (1 lb) did not significantly ↑ energy cost
34.72	37.40			
Below-NW	Below-W			Effects of .9-kg handheld wts and arm position; No change in $\dot{V}O_2$ due to arm position or handheld weights; HRs for Above-W sign > Below-W and -NW
23.6	25.8			
Above-NW	Above-W			
24.6	26.9			
				Training responses to ADE/Significantly greater ↑ in $\dot{V}O_2$ with 3 days/wk rather than 2 days/wk
32.41 (70)		33.95 (69)		Type of ADE: step vs. LI vs. HI, Step HR and $\dot{V}O_2$ NS diff from LI and HI; untrained dancers at > % $\dot{V}O_2$max (76%) than instructors (62%)
March	Power Jack	Jog	Jump Jack	Effects of impact and arm position; arm position × step type interaction; quantify steps in future studies
29.86 (60)	33.53 (68)	34.85 (71)	33.81 (68)	
				Training responses/7-wk training; 4-d/wk; 30 min/d; both groups ↑ $\dot{V}O_2$max
				Effects of 8-wk training and compare ADE and TR; ADE and TM at similar $\dot{V}O_2$s did not elicit the same HR
Continuous training: 30–35 min constant ADE				Interval vs. continuous workouts; 12 wk @80–85% max HR; both groups ↑ $\dot{V}O_2$max; ↓ % body fat; NS diff between groups; sign. ↑ anaerobic threshold, V_E max; O_2 pulse
				HR to $\dot{V}O_2$ relationship; HRs from TR do not represent ADE HRs
$\dot{V}O_2$	Level 1	Level 2	Level 3	Effects of level of ADE experience (exp) and $\dot{V}O_2$max at 3 workloads; less fit and less-exp. dancers worked at a > % max HR and % $\dot{V}O_2$max
	25	30	34	
	25	30	33	
	22	27	29	
				Training responses; 3-d/wk for 12 wk; sign. ↑ $\dot{V}O_2$max, max V_E, max HR, max O_2 pulse

for hamstring/quadriceps ratios (11,58) and muscular endurance (i.e., time to or number of repetitions for achieving half of the initial peak torque); however, these data have not identified specific muscular characteristics that identify ballet dancers. Physiologic profiling of dancers may need to be standardized in the future, similar to standardized screening procedures.

Aerobic Dance Exercise

There is no "typical" profile for aerobic dance exercisers; however, many of the previous ADE studies have been done on college-aged female subjects and ADE instructors. Individuals from varied backgrounds have participated in and have gained benefits from ADE:

FIG. 49–5. Metabolic data collection for aerobic dance exercise. (Photo courtesy of Bowling Green State University, Exercise Physiology Laboratory.)

TABLE 49–4. *Isometic muscular strength of ballet dancers for knee flexion and extension and ankle plantar and dorsiflexion*

Author	Velocity (deg)	Level of experience	Knee flexion	Knee extension	Plantar flexion	Dorsiflexion
Chatfield (1993)	30	Prof	59.6 ± 7.4	91.3 ± 12.1	57.4 ± 12.3	17.6 ± 4.4[a]
					48.1 10.0	15.9 2.3[b]
Chatfield et al. (1990)	30	Beg	56.7 ± 10.3	98.6 ± 6.23	48.9 ± 9.4	10.3 ± 2.9
		Int	54.9 ± 7.2	98.3 ± 19.7	51.3 ± 7.2	10.4 ± 2.4
		Adv	50.3 ± 9.5	85.4 ± 12.6	43.8 ± 11.1	9.1 ± 2.3
Micheli et al. (1984)	30	Prof	40.6 ± 6.3	69.8 ± 8.0	50.3 ± 13.3	8.3 ± 2.0
Mostardi (1986)	30	Prof	47.7 ± 2.7	79.4 ± 5.4		
Liederbach, Hiebert (1997)	30	Prof			62.0 ± 1.7[a]	12.9 ± 2.6[a]
					45.1 ± 3.2[b]	7.3 ± 0.8[b]
Liederbach, Hiebert (1997)	60	Prof			61.0 ± 4.0[a]	11.1 ± 1.43
					43.1 ± 3.6[b]	6.7 ± 0.8[b]
Hamilton (1992)	60	Prof	52.9 ± 7.5	95.1 ± 17.1	50.1 ± 8.9	11.4 ± 3.3
Kirkendall et al. (1984)	90	Prof		≈80		
		Prof Males		≈120		
Westblad et al. (1995)	90	Prof		118.9 ± 10.5[a]		
	90	Controls		98.2 ± 18.8[c]		
Chatfield (1993)	180	Prof	46.7 ± 9.9	56.6 ± 5.6	57.4 ± 12.3	17.6 ± 4.4
Chatfield et al. (1990)	180	Beg	40.7 ± 5.7	60.4 ± 11.5		
		Int	40.9 ± 4.4	61.0 ± 10.4		
		Adv	37.3 ± 5.0	50.7 ± 8.4		
Kirkendall et al. (1984)	180	Prof		≈60		
		Prof Males		≈90		
Micheli et al. (1984)	180	Prof	34.0 ± 3.5	44.7 ± 7.3		
	120				30.0 ± 1.1	6.0 ± 1.7
Mostardi (1986)	180	Prof	30.0 ± 1.1	79.4		

[a]Testing with knee extended.
[b]Testing with knee flexed.
[c]Values originally reported in other units were converted to ft·lbs.

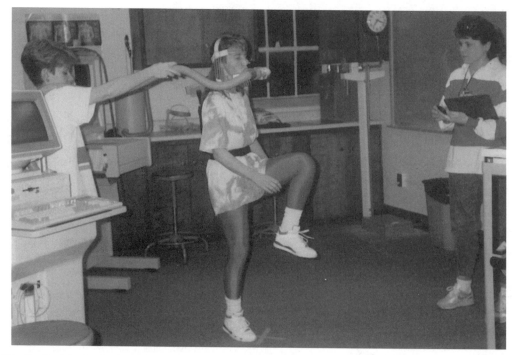

pregnant women (60), overweight women (61), elderly women (62), and men (64). As with all training programs, it is suggested that the participant work within her or his capabilities and that ADE be individualized. For the ADE instructor who is leading the class, it may be a challenge to individualize exercise for the entire class because classes may have 10 to 60 participants, and participants may be self-conscious about their ability to keep up with the other students in the class.

TRAINING THE ATHLETE

As mentioned previously, the dance-training pyramid encompasses the many facets of a dancer's training (see Fig. 49–3) (7). Of all sports, dance is probably one of the most steeped in mystique, with dancers training and performing under the tutelage of their dance masters with different styles and philosophies. It is important to study the training of dancers because, with improved conditioning regimens, dance performance and self-confidence may be enhanced, overtraining may be prevented, and the incidence of dance-related injuries may be reduced (3).

The Season

Theatrical Dance

Ryan and Stephens (2) have reported that the standard union contract for a dancer in the United States is approximately 32 weeks, typically involving three 10- to 12-week seasons. During the time between seasons, many dancers rehabilitate, rest, and prepare for the next season. Ryan (2) has listed risk factors associated with the incidence of dance injuries: inadequate warm-up, lack of training specificity, poor preseason conditioning, scheduling conflicts of rehearsals and performances, improper form and technique, muscle imbalances, and late starting age for ballet training. Some of these could be modified through proper attention to and/or implementation of conditioning principles (i.e., overload, progressive resistance, reversibility; frequency, intensity, duration, and type of exercise) and techniques.

Aerobic Dance Exercise

A typical ADE program would be scheduled similar to other aerobic programs designed to increase cardiorespiratory fitness. Programs lasting 8 to 12 weeks have been reported to evoke physiologic changes (i.e., ↑ $\dot{V}O_2max$, ↓ body weight and percentage of body fat; see Table 49–3) (39,42,46). These programs could be initiated at any time.

Sport-Specific Training

As shown in the dance-training pyramid (see Fig. 49–3) (7), sport-specific training for dance is the portion of the pyramid that includes rehearsal, technique, and somatics. Rehearsals and technique classes are specific to dance and the movements involved therein; however, rehearsal and technique alone may not provide the overload necessary to evoke some training responses.

Somatics may be defined as "bodily based access to information about the whole system and its interactive patterns" (64). Fitt (64) described eight leading somatic approaches that are popular with dancers: Pilates-based conditioning (i.e., exercises specific to dance movements and muscles), rolfing (i.e., ten 1-hour sessions of deep body massage), Feldenkrais (i.e., repetitive, low-intensity motion), Alexander technique (i.e., focus on increasing muscle efficiency and reducing the tension in everyday movements), ideokinesis (i.e., imagined action), body–mind centering, Bartenieff fundamentals, and Laban movement analysis (64). A number of other resources for dancers present the basic principles of conditioning and apply these specifically to dance; see Fitt (64), Berardi (65), Clippinger-Robertson (66), and Watkins and Clarkson (67).

Intuitively, it makes sense that dance-specific training would enhance dance performance. This has not been documented in the literature because of inherent research-design problems, however. As Chmelar and Fitt (7) have noted, research to document improvement in dance performance is difficult to complete because four conditioning variables (i.e., technique, conditioning, performance, and injuries) can vary and interact and therefore affect the research results. In addition, scientific research on dance training and medicine may have been impeded in the past because of the inherent aesthetic qualities of dance, and because dancers have traditionally viewed themselves as artists and not necessarily as athletes (68).

Aerobic Dance Exercise

It is easier to measure the outcomes of aerobic dance training compared with theatrical dance because ADE is a method of conditioning. Cardiorespiratory fitness, muscular strength, and other physiologic attributes can be quantified before and after training. As mentioned previously, ADE routines can be designed to exercise specific muscle groups and to elicit specific physiologic responses (27).

Supplemental Training

In many sports, progressive resistance training would be a necessity to compete at an advanced level. Previously, ballet dancers have been hesitant to do weight training, being afraid that they will develop large, bulky muscles. These training principles have been presented to and for the dance community (65,66,68); however, the extent to which supplemental weight training is used is not well documented. One study by Stalder (69) investigated the effects of a structured weight-training program on intermediate- and advanced-level university student dancers. Significant gains were reported for muscle strength during hip adduction, dorsiflexion, and knee extension at 150°/s, and time for endurance jumping. However, other measures of dance performance (e.g., ratings of dance performance, power measurements) were not significantly improved by weight training.

Periodization of Training

No systematic tapering programs have been described for dancers. From a physiologic standpoint, although this may be ideal, the realities of scheduling, performing, and cost make this impossible. Typically, dancers have limited time because of the cost of renting the theater before a performance to rehearse on the stage. Before the performance, therefore, the physical demands on the dancer increase rather than decrease (D. Tell and T. Veach, personal communication, 1997). The physical demands on the dancer can be extreme, if not exhaustive; coupled with the competition for a few dance positions, this can be a highly competitive, stressful occupation (5). Dancers may be performing one dance style while rehearsing or practicing for another (5). As Calabrese and Kirkendall (9) have stated, a further stress to the body is that most dancers achieve weight control and a lean body primarily from dietary restriction, in contrast to increasing caloric expenditure by completing aerobic exercise.

FUTURE RESEARCH

As Clarkson (68) has noted, there are many viable research areas for the future study of dance (i.e., biomechanical analysis of movement, ballet shoe design, supplemental forms of training, effects of heat stress, low body weight, overtraining, training techniques, and training for children and adolescents). In addition, future research questions are numerous concerning the nutritional habits of dancers (i.e., caloric restriction), the female athlete triad (i.e., osteoporosis, disordered eating, and amenorrhea) in dancers, and other topics in dance science and medicine.

CONCLUSION

Two groupings for forms of dance were used in this chapter to discuss the applied physiology of dance: (a) theatrical dance and (b) aerobic dance exercise. The physical requirements of and physiologic responses to specific forms of dance vary greatly depending on a multitude of factors that may include choreography, impact, cadence, range of motion of the limbs, quantity of muscle mass involved in the movement, position of arms, type of muscle contraction, and the addition of hand-held weights. Although some theatrical dancers may use supplemental training in addition to technique classes and rehearsals, few studies on supplemental training for dancers have been completed. Aerobic dance exercise is an activity that draws from the areas of dance and aerobic conditioning. Aerobic dance exercise has evolved since the mid 1970s and now encompasses many forms of calisthenics, exercises, and steps to music with the intent to increase physical fitness. Many potential areas of future research exist for the study of dance science and medicine.

REFERENCES

1. Hardaker WT, Vander Woude L. Dance medicine: an orthopaedist's view. *NCMJ* 1993;54:67–72.
2. Ryan AJ. Early history of dance medicine. *Dance Med Sci* 1997; 1:30–34.
3. Solomon RL, Micheli LJ. Applied research in dance medicine/science: presentation at the 1997 American College of Sports Medicine annual meeting, May 29, 1997.
4. Bachrach RM. A physician's primer of dance injuries. *Osteopath Med News* 1985;2:20–26.
5. Ryan AJ, Stephens RE. Glossary. In: Ryan AJ, Stephens RE, eds. *Dance medicine: a comprehensive guide.* Chicago: Pluribus Press, 1987:350–356.
6. Hay JF. *Modern dance: a biomechanical approach to teaching.* St Louis: Mosby, 1981.
7. Chmelar R, Fitt S. Conditioning for dance: the art of the science. *Kinesiol Med Dance* 1988;14:78–94.
8. Abraham SF, Beumont PJV, Fraser IS, Llewellyn-Jones D. Body weight, exercise and menstrual status among ballet dancers in training. *Br J Obstet Gynaecol* 1982;89:507–510.
9. Calabrese LH, Kirkendall DT. Nutritional and medical considerations in dancers. *Clin Sports Med* 1983;2:539–548.
10. Chatfield SJ, Byrnes WC, Lally DA, Rowe SE. Cross-sectional physiologic profiling of modern dancers. *Dance Res J* 1990; 22:13–20.
11. Chmelar RD, Shultz BB, Ruhling RO, Shepherd TA, Zupan MF, Fitt SS. A physiologic profile comparing levels and styles of female dancers. *Phys Sports Med* 1988;16:87–96.
12. Clarkson PM, Freedson PS, Keller B, Carney D, Skrinar M. Maximal oxygen uptake: nutritional patterns and body composition of adolescent female ballet dancers. *Res Q Exerc Sport* 1985; 56:180–184.
13. Clarkson PM, Freedson PS, Skrinar M, Keller B, Carney D. Anthropometric measurements of adolescent and professional classical ballet dancers. *J Sports Med Phys Fitness* 1989;29:157–162.
14. Cohen JL, Gupta PK, Lichstein E, Chadda KD. The heart of a dancer: noninvasive cardiac evaluation of professional ballet dancers. *Am J Cardiol* 1980;45:959–965.
15. Crotts D, Thompson B, Nahom M, Ryan S, Newton RA. Balance abilities of professional dancers on select balance tests. *J Orthop Sports Phys Ther* 1996;23:12–17.
16. Dahlström M, Esbjörnsson M, Jansson E, Kaijser L. Muscle fiber characteristics in female dancers during an active and an inactive period. *Int J Sports Med* 1987;8:84–87.
17. Dolgener F, Spasoff TC, St. John W. Body build and body composition of high ability female dancers. *Res Q Exerc Sport* 1980; 51:599–607.
18. Fogelholm M, Lichtenbelt WVM, Ottenheijm T, Westerterp K. Amenorrhea in ballet dancers in the Netherlands. *Med Sci Sports Exerc* 1996;28:545–550.
19. Hergenroeder AC, Brown B, Klish WJ. Anthropometric measurements and estimating body composition in ballet dancers. *Med Sci Sports Exerc* 1993;25:145–150.

20. Karlsson MK, Johnell O, Obrant KJ. Bone mineral density in professional ballet dancers. *Bone Miner* 1993;23:163–169.
21. Kirkendall DT, Bergfeld JA, Calabrese L, Lombardo JA, Street G, Weiker GG. Isokinetic characteristics of ballet dancers and the response to a season of ballet training. *J Occup Sports Phys Ther* 1984;5:207–211.
22. Kuno M, Fukunaga T, Hirano Y, Miyashita M. Anthropometric variables and muscle properties of Japanese female ballet dancers. *Int J Sports Med* 1996;18:100–105.
23. Micheli LJ, Gillespie WJ, Walaszek A. Physiologic profiles of female professional ballerinas. *Clin Sports Med* 1984;3:199–209.
24. Mostardi RA. Musculoskeletal and cardiopulmonary evaluation of professional ballet dancers. In: Shell CG, ed. *The dancer as athlete: the 1984 Olympic Scientific Congress Proceedings.* Vol 8. Champaign, IL: 1986:101–107.
25. Novak LP, Magill LA, Schutte JE. Maximal oxygen intake and body composition of female dancers. *Eur J Appl Physiol* 1978; 39:277–282.
26. Clippinger-Robertson K. Components of an aerobics class. In: Cotton RT, Goldstein RL, eds. *Aerobics instructor manual: the resource for group fitness instructors.* San Diego, CA: American Council on Exercise, 1997:197–241.
27. Darby LA, Browder KD, Reeves BD. The effects of cadence, impact, and step on physiological responses to aerobic dance exercise. *Res Q Exerc Sport* 1995;66:231–238.
28. Clapp JF, Little KD. The physiological response of instructors and participants to three aerobics regimens. *Med Sci Sports Exerc* 1994;26:1041–1046.
29. Cohen JL, Segal KR, Witriol I, McArdle WD. Cardiorespiratory responses to ballet exercise and the Vo_2max of elite ballet dancers. *Med Sci Sports Exerc* 1982;14:212–217.
30. Cohen JL, Segal KR, McArdle WD. Heart rate response to ballet stage performance. *Phys Sport Med* 1982;10:120–134.
31. Haviland WR. A physiological profile of modern dancers. Unpublished master's thesis, Ohio University, 1978.
32. Jette M, Inglis H. Energy cost of square dancing. *J Appl Physiol* 1975;38:44–45.
33. Leger LA. Energy cost of disco dancing. *Res Q Exerc Sport* 1982;53:46–49.
34. Noble RM, Howley ET. The energy requirement of selected tap dance routines. *Res Q Exerc Sport* 1979;50:438–442.
35. Shantz PG, Astrand P. Physiological characteristics of classical ballet. *Med Sci Sports Exerc* 1984;216:472–476.
36. Wigaeus E, Kilborn Å. Physical demands during folk dancing. *Eur J Appl Physiol* 1980;45:177–183.
37. Bell JM, Bassey EJ. A comparison of the relation between oxygen uptake and heart rate during different styles of aerobic dance and a traditional step test in women. *Eur J Appl Physiol* 1994;368:20–24.
38. Berry MJ, Cline CC, Berry CB, Davis M. A comparison between two forms of aerobic dance and treadmill running. *Med Sci Sports Exerc* 1992;24:946–951.
39. Blessing D, Wilson GD, Puckett JR, Ford HT. The physiologic effects of eight weeks of aerobic dance with and without handheld weights. *Am J Sports Med* 1987;15:508–510.
40. Bronstein M, Bishop P, Smith J, Conerly M, May E. Physiological response to low-impact aerobic dance by trained dancers with and without handheld weights. *Ann Sports Med* 1990;5:74–77.
41. Carroll MW, Otto RM, Wygand J. The metabolic cost of two ranges of arm position height with and without hand weight during low impact aerobic dance. *Res Q Exerc Sport* 1991;62:420–423.
42. Cearly M, Moffatt R, Knutzen K. The effects of two and three day-per-week aerobic dance programs on maximal oxygen uptake. *Res Q Exerc Sport* 1984;55:172–174.
43. Clapp JF, Little KD. The physiological response of instructors and participants to three aerobics regimens. *Med Sci Sports Exerc* 1994;26:1041–1046.
44. Milburn S, Butts K. A comparison of the training responses to aerobic dance and jogging in college females. *Med Sci Sports Exerc* 1983;15:510–513.
45. Parker SB, Hurley BF, Hanlon DP, Vaccaro P. Failure of target heart rate to accurately monitor intensity during aerobic dance. *Med Sci Sports Exerc* 1989;21:230–234.
46. Perry A, Mosher P, LaPerriere A, Roalstad M, Ostrovsky P. A comparison of training responses to interval versus continuous aerobic dance. *J Occup Sports Phys Ther* 1988;28:274–279.
47. Scharff-Olson M, Williford HN, Smith FH. The heart rate Vo_2 relationship of aerobic dance: a comparison of target heart rate methods. *J Sports Med Phys Fitness* 1992;32:372–377.
48. Thomsen D, Ballor DL. Physiological responses during aerobic dance of individuals grouped by aerobic capacity and dance experience. *Res Q Exerc Sport* 1991;62:68–72.
49. Williams LD, Morton AR. Changes in selected cardiorespiratory responses to exercise and in body composition following a 12-week aerobic dance programme. *J Sports Sci* 1986;4:189–199.
50. Clarkson PM. Energy production in dance. In: Clarkson PM, Skrinar M, eds. *Science of dance training.* Champaign, IL: Human Kinetics, 1988:31–44.
51. Rimmer JH, Jay D, Plowman SA. Physiological characteristics of trained dancers and intensity level of ballet class and rehearsal. *Impulse* 1994;2:97–105.
52. Foster C. Physiological requirements of aerobic dancing. *Res Q* 1975;46:120–122.
53. Igbanugo V, Gutin B. The energy cost of aerobic dancing. *Res Q* 1977;49:308–316.
54. Chatfield SJ. Electromyographic response of dancers to isokinetic work and select dance movements. *Kinesiol Med Dance* 1993/1994;16:60–82.
55. Liederbach M, Hiebert R. The relationship between eccentric and concentric measures of ankle strength and functional equinus in classical dancers. *J Dance Med Sci* 1997;1:55–61.
56. Hamilton WG, Hamilton LH, Marshall P, Molnar M. A profile of the musculoskeletal characteristics of elite professional ballet dancers. *Am J Sports Med* 1992;20:267–273.
57. Westblad P, Tsai-Felländer L, Johansson C. Eccentric and concentric knee extensor muscle performance in professional ballet dancers. *Clin J Sport Med* 1995;5:48–52.
58. Perrine DH. *Isokinetic exercise and assessment.* Champaign, IL: Human Kinetics, 1993.
59. Chmelar RD, Shultz BB, Ruhling RO, Fitt SS, Johnson MB. Isokinetic characteristics of the knee in female, professional and university, ballet and modern dancers. *J Occup Sports Phys Ther* 1988;9:410–418.
60. McMurray RG, Hackney AC, Guion WK, Katz VL. Metabolic and hormonal responses to low-impact aerobic dance during pregnancy. *Med Sci Sports Exerc* 1996:28:41–46.
61. Gillett PA, Eisenman PA. The effect of intensity controlled aerobic dance exercise on aerobic capacity of middle-aged, overweight women. *Res Nurs Health* 1987;10:383–390.
62. Hopkins DR, Murrah B, Hoeger WWK, Rhodes RC. Effect of low-impact aerobic dance on the functional fitness of elderly women. *Gerontology* 1990;30:189–192.
63. Hooper PL, Noland BJ. Aerobic dance program improves cardiovascular fitness in men. *Phys Sports Med* 1984;12:132–136.
64. Fitt SS. *Dance kinesiology.* 2nd ed. New York: Schirmer Books, 1996.
65. Berardi G. *Finding balance: fitness and training for a lifetime in dance.* Princeton, NJ: Dance horizons/Princeton Book Company, 1991.
66. Clippinger-Robertson K. Principles in dance training. In: Clarkson PM, Skrinar M, eds. *Science of dance training.* Champaign, IL: Human Kinetics, 1988:45–90.
67. Watkins A, Clarkson PM. *Dancing longer dancing stronger: a dancer's guide to improving technique and preventing injury.* Pennington, NJ: Princeton Book Company, 1990.
68. Clarkson PM. Science in dance. In: Clarkson PM, Skrinar M, eds. *Science of dance training.* Champaign, IL: Human Kinetics, 1988:17–22.
69. Stalder M. The effects of a supplemental weight training program on female ballet dancers. *Kinesiol Med Dance* 1987;10:9–11.

SUGGESTED READINGS

Garrick JG, Requa RK. Aerobic dance: a review. *Sports Med* 1988; 6:169–179.

Kirkendall DT, Calabrese LH. Physiological aspects of dance. *Clin Sports Med* 1983;2:525–537.

Solomon R, Solomon J. *Dance medicine & science bibliography.* Andover, NJ: J. Michael Ryan Publishing, 1996.
Williford HN, Scharff-Olson M, Blessing DL. The physiological effects of aerobic dance: a review. *Sports Med* 1989;8:335–345.
Dance Research Journal. New York: Committee on Research in Dance v.7 fall/winter 1974/75–present.
IDEA today. (ceased publication 1997).
Impulse. Champaign, IL: Human Kinetics Publishers, Inc. 1993–present.
Journal of Dance Medicine & Science. Andover, NJ: J. Michael Ryan Publishing, Inc. 1997–present.
Kinesiology and Medicine for Dance. Pennington, NJ: Princeton Periodicals, Inc.
Medecine des Arts. Montauban, France. 1992–present.

Exercise and Sport Science,
edited by William E. Garrett, Jr., and Donald T. Kirkendall.
Lippincott Williams & Wilkins, Philadelphia © 2000.

CHAPTER 50

Physiology of Figure Skating

Edward T. Mannix, Pieter Kollen, and Mark O. Farber

THE SPORT

Physical Requirements

Figure skating is a competitive sport that comprises three distinct events: singles freestyle for men and for women separately; pairs skating for female/male couples; and ice dancing for female/male couples. Competition in each of the three events is structured according to skill level, as indicated by successful completion of on-ice skills tests. In the United States, the levels of competition for men and women are preliminary, prejuvenile, juvenile, intermediate, novice, junior, and senior. The only ranking according to age is that through the juvenile level, in which a skater cannot be older than 12 years; however, a 10-year-old could compete as an intermediate or higher, as long as competency is displayed during formal examination (1). The national governing body that sets the rules and regulations for the sport and for all sanctioned competitions in the United States is the United States Figure Skating Association (USFSA), based in Colorado Springs. International competitions are sanctioned by The International Skating Union, based in Davos, Switzerland. Only three levels of competition are officially recognized for international competitions (i.e., novice, junior, and senior). The highest international level of competition in the sport occurs at the World Championships, which are held annually, and at the Winter Olympics, which are held every 4 years. For the World Championships, senior- and junior-level skaters are allowed to compete, but only senior-level skaters are allowed to compete in the Olympic Games.

Successful competition in singles freestyle skating is determined by scores attained during a short program and a long program (1). The length of the short program varies with competition level but not as a function of gender; juniors and seniors perform to music that cannot exceed 2 minutes and 40 seconds in length, novice skaters perform to music that cannot exceed 2 minutes and 15 seconds, and the music for intermediate-level skaters cannot exceed 2 minutes. A 10-second period immediately before and immediately after the music is allowed for on-ice performance. During the short program, each skater must perform required elements. For the men, there are eight such elements, including three jumps, three spins, and two footwork sequences performed while moving across the ice in either a circular, serpentine ("S" shaped), or straight-line pattern. For the women, the first seven elements are the same as described, but the eighth required element is unique. It is performed while the skater glides across the ice in a spiral-step sequence. During this movement the skater moves into several arabesque positions as she performs a series of lobes (curves) across the full surface of the rink (1).

On a separate day, a minimum of 24 hours after the short program, each skater performs the long program. A well-balanced senior long program for men must be performed to music not to exceed 4 minutes and 30 seconds and must contain jumps, jump combinations, spins, and stepwork. The number of double and triple jumps is optional, but no triple jump can be repeated. A minimum of one jump combination, defined as two jumps performed in sequence with an immediate takeoff from the end of the first jump into the beginning of the second jump, or at least one jump sequence, defined as two or more jumps with hops and/or small jumps between each major jump, must be performed. A minimum of four different spins must be included in a men's freestyle long program, one of which must be a spin

E. T. Mannix: Department of Medicine, Indiana University; The National Institute for Fitness and Sport, Indianapolis, Indiana 46202.

P. Kollen: Indiana/World Skating Academy, Indianapolis, Indiana 46202.

M. O. Farber: Department of Medicine, Indiana University; Veterans Administration Medical Center, Indianapolis, Indiana 46202.

combination. A flying spin, defined as a jump or lift of the body into the air in either a sit or camel (arabesque) position, also must be executed. The last prerequisite of a successful long program for men is the step sequence, so that two different sequences must be performed while the skater moves across the ice in a pattern of his own choice (e.g., serpentine, straight-line, or circle). Senior women competing in the long program skate to music not longer than 4 minutes in duration and must perform the same skills as the men, except that only one step sequence is mandatory, and a sequence of various spirals and/or a spiral-step sequence must be executed while the skater moves across the ice (1).

For the senior pairs competition, each pair must perform a short program; on a separate day, at least 24 hours later, they must perform a long program. The length of these programs in the various levels of competition is comparable to that previously cited for the men's singles freestyle event. Eight required elements compose the short program, including one overhead lift, a double-twist lift, one solo jump (either a double- or triple-spin jump performed by each skater while skating side by side), one pair spin combination, one death spiral, and one step sequence performed as the pair moves across the ice in either a straight-line, circular, or serpentine pattern (1).

Dance competition, also referred to as ice dancing, is the final event. This event is performed by a male/female couple and is made up of three separate disciplines [i.e., compulsory dance, an original set-pattern dance, and a free dance event (all performed on separate days, at least 24 hours apart)]. For seniors, each of the three disciplines is performed to music not to exceed 4 minutes, with the customary 10-second leeway at the beginning and end. The junior program is performed to music not to exceed 3 minutes, and the novice not to exceed 2 minutes and 30 seconds. The dance event requires that the couple move quickly in repetitive, set patterns by following specific dance rhythms, including the waltz, tango, fox-trot, paso doble, blues, and cha-cha. The skaters must maintain contact with each other except for brief moments during change in position. There are quick acceleration moves, quick stops and turns, full rotational moves, gliding moves while maintaining position, and various minilifts (the man's hands are not permitted to go above his shoulders), each of which are performed while the skaters move quickly across the ice surface. In addition, unprescribed dance steps are included in each performance; they must be creative and in character with the music (1).

Performance in all of the events described above is graded on technique, timing, and expression of movement. Since competition is performed to music, special attention is given to choreography, interpretation of music, intricate footwork, and speed. The entire ice surface should be used in an aesthetic fashion. Skaters are graded on a 6-point ordinal scale, with 0 the lowest and 6 the highest mark, with one-tenth point gradations. Each judge awards each skater a numeric score, which is translated into a rank (e.g., first, second, third), so that the cumulative ranking of the skaters for each event is computed, resulting in placement of each skater (from first place to last place) relative to all competitors (1). It is widely accepted that the grading scheme is often highly subjective and qualitative, with attention given by judges to past performances and reputations of the skaters. This is particularly true in national competitions, when each country is trying to select its best skaters for international competitions.

Physiologic Requirements

Successful competition in figure skating requires that participants possess high levels of flexibility, agility, and balance, along with the ability to perform skills consisting of repetitive bouts of explosive power and the generation and maintenance of high-speed movement across the ice. Sporting events with similar energy demands usually rely on a well-developed aerobic metabolic system, which serves as a foundation for all movement, and a well-developed anaerobic metabolic component, which supports short bursts of high-power-output exercise (2). Anecdotally, a striking difference often noted by coaches between figure skaters who score well at national and international competitions and those who do not is the greater on-ice speed of the former group.

The literature contains numerous reports describing physiologic requirements and performance characteristics of athletes who participate in on-ice sports, including speed skating (3–5) and ice hockey (6–8), whereas only two investigative reports describing the physiologic characteristics of figure skaters have been published (9,10). Whereas speed skaters and ice hockey players possess high levels of aerobic capacity (5,6,11) and anaerobic power (3,7,12), McMaster and co-workers (9) reported that figure skaters had average aerobic capacity (mean $\dot{V}O_2$max, 45 mL/kg/min; SD, not reported) when compared with age- and gender-matched untrained controls. Mannix and co-workers (10) confirmed the findings of McMaster's group, as they reported a $\dot{V}O_2$peak of 105% of predicted (47 ± 2 mL/kg/min) in a group of figure skaters (n = 15) who were training in a program sanctioned by the USFSA.

Each of the two investigative groups that reported average levels of aerobic capacity for figure skaters went on to study the effects of interval training on increasing various functional characteristics of their skaters. McMaster and colleagues (9) performed a 3-month training study that allowed their skaters to maintain their normal on-ice training schedule, with the addition of a vigorous 30-minute-per-day, 3-day-per-week on-ice interval training program. A 30-minute-per-day, 3-

day-per-week off-ice cross-training exercise program consisting of muscle-strengthening and flexibility exercises also was performed on alternate days. Results indicate that $\dot{V}O_2$max increased from 45 to 56 mL/kg/min, and the time of a 1/2 mile on-ice sprint decreased from 1:47.0 to 1:37.0 minutes. Other improvements also were reported, including attainment of higher speeds during freestyle routines and the sensation of less fatigue during the last minute of their on-ice skating routines.

Mannix and co-workers (10) performed a controlled training study with several predetermined goals. First, they sought to determine if on-ice training alone would improve aerobic capacity and supramaximal endurance times and if said training would manifest in an altered lactate and heart rate response to vigorous exercise on a cycle ergometer. Second, they sought to determine if the addition of a high-intensity, interval cycle training program performed 4 days per week for a period of 10 weeks would have a significant positive effect on criterion variables used to define aerobic and anaerobic power. The cross-training program was designed to elicit a power output equivalent to that attained at $\dot{V}O_2$peak, five separate times during a 33-minute exercise bout on a cycle ergometer. Results in the control group (group 1, $n = 8$), which performed on-ice training alone for 10 weeks, indicated lack of significant increases in $\dot{V}O_2$peak, maximal work rate, $\dot{V}O_2$ at anaerobic threshold, work rate at anaerobic threshold, and supramaximal endurance time (Table 50–1). Group 2 ($n = 7$), which performed interval cycle ergometer cross-training in addition to their on-ice training program, experienced significant improvements in all criterion variables, as listed in Table 50–1.

The blood lactate and heart-rate responses for each group of skaters in this study (10) are displayed in Figs 50–1 and 50–2, respectively. A training effect is noted by a lower blood lactate and/or heart rate (HR) at given, submaximal work rates (13,14). Figure 50–1 graphically represents venous blood lactate concentrations obtained at four target work rates for each group, before and after the 10-week training programs. The same absolute work rates for each subject were used for the pre- and posttraining sessions. Before training, group 1 (on-ice training only) experienced its first significant lactate increase at 75% of $\dot{V}O_2$peak. The lactate pattern observed in group 1 after the training period was similar, with the first significant increase observed at 75% of the original $\dot{V}O_2$peak. These data indicate that for the control group, the first significant lactate increase was not prolonged as a function of training. Repeated-measures analysis of variance did reveal an overall differ-

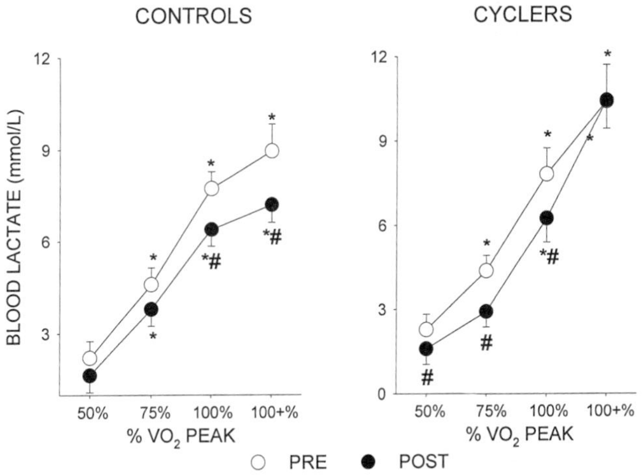

FIG. 50–1. Venous blood lactate concentrations of two groups of figure skaters before and after a 10-week training program. For the controls (on-ice training only), significant increases from 50% of $\dot{V}O_2$peak (*$p < .05$) occurred at all subsequent work rates before and after training. An adaptation to training was realized by the control group, as lactate levels were significantly reduced, relative to pretraining, at the 100% and 100+% levels after training ($^{\#}p < .05$). For the cyclers (on-ice plus cycle training), the first significant increase in lactate was prolonged after training, and circulating lactate was lower at 50%, 75%, and 100% of $\dot{V}O_2$peak, before versus after training. From ref. 10, with permission.

TABLE 50–1. *Effects of on-ice training and on-ice plus cycle training in two groups of figure skaters*

	Group 1 (n = 8)		Group 2 (n = 7)	
	Pre	Post	Pre	Post
$\dot{V}O_2$peak (L/min)	2.06 ± 0.15	1.94 ± 0.13	2.41 ± 0.17	2.68 ± 0.16[ab]
$\dot{V}O_2$peak (mL/kg/min)	44.2 ± 2.2	41.4 ± 1.6	50.7 ± 3.6	55.9 ± 3.3[ab]
Wattage at $\dot{V}O_2$peak	145 ± 9	144 ± 9	157 ± 10	182 ± 7[ab]
$\dot{V}O_2$peak (%pred)	100 ± 5	92 ± 4	110 ± 7	121 ± 6[ab]
AT (%$\dot{V}O_2$peak)	74 ± 3	73 ± 3	80 ± 2[b]	83 ± 2[ab]
Wattage at AT	97 ± 7	97 ± 7	114 ± 7	143 ± 7[ab]
SupMax Time (min)	0.87 ± 0.12	0.94 ± 0.12	1.31 ± 0.18[b]	2.69 ± 0.66[ab]

Values are expressed as mean ± SEM.
[a]$p < .05$ vs. pretraining value.
[b]$p < .05$ vs. Group 1 at same time point. From ref. 10, with permission.
Group 1, on-ice training only; Group 2, on-ice plus cycle training; PRE/POST, before/after training; AT, anaerobic threshold; SupMax Time, length of supramaximal exercise bout.

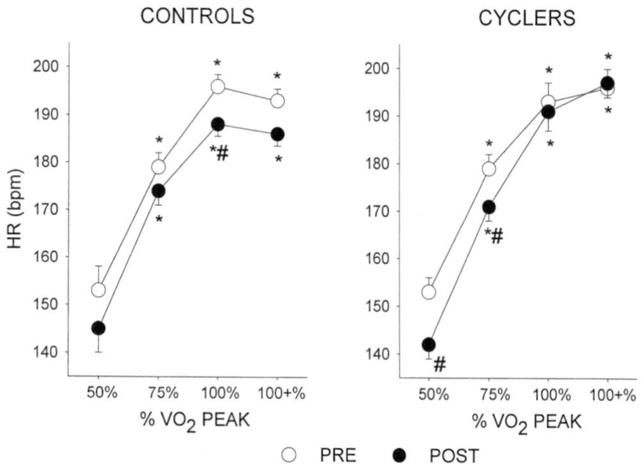

FIG. 50–2. Heart rates (HRs) of two groups of figure skaters before and after a 10-week training program. For the controls (on-ice training only), significant increases from 50% of V̇O₂peak (*$p < .05$) occurred at all subsequent work rates before and after training. An adaptation to training occurred in the control group, as HR was significantly reduced, relative to that before training, at the 100% level after training (#$p < .05$). For the cyclers (on-ice plus cycle training), HR was lower at 50% and 75% of V̇O_2peak, before versus after training. From ref. 10, with permission.

ence in the cumulative lactate response (all lactate data before training were compared with all lactate data obtained after training) in the control group, with lower lactate values measured after training. Specific points of difference occurred at V̇O_2peak and during supramaximal exercise, with lower posttraining lactate concentrations observed at those work rates. For the cycle trainers (group 2) before the 10-week training period, the first significant blood lactate increase was noted at 75% of V̇O_2peak. After training, the first significant increase was not detected until 100% of V̇O_2peak was reached, so that the first significant increase in circulating lactate was prolonged by the addition of cycle training to the on-ice training protocol. An overall statistical difference in the cumulative lactate responses also occurred in the cycle trainers, with lower values observed after training at 50%, 75%, and 100% of the original V̇O_2peak. An interesting secondary observation was that although no difference in circulating lactate was observed at the supramaximal level for group 2 before training versus after training, these skaters exercised significantly longer at the supramaximal level after training (Table 50–1), so theoretically they should have produced more lactate. The fact that they did not translates into an additional training adaptation, which was elicited by the combined training program.

Figure 50–2 depicts HR data gathered simultaneously with lactate data (10). Group 1 (on-ice training only) displayed progressive HR elevations through V̇O_2peak during both pretraining and posttraining testing. Further increases in HR did not occur from V̇O_2peak to the supramaximal level, either before or after training. An overall difference in the HR response to exercise, before versus after training, was observed in group 1, with the only specific point of difference observed at V̇O_2peak. The cycle trainers (group 2) also displayed progressive increases in HR through V̇O_2peak during pre- and posttraining testing. An overall difference in the HR response to exercise also was observed in this group, with lower exercise HRs after 10 weeks of cycle plus on-ice training, and a significant difference noted at 50% and 75% of original V̇O_2peak. Taken together, these findings indicate that although gas-exchange parameters did not indicate that a training adaptation had occurred in the on-ice–only group, the lactate and HR data indicate that this group did exhibit a training benefit. It is quite apparent, however, that the magnitude of the lactate and HR adaptations experienced by the on-ice-plus-cycle trainers, along with the numerous physiologic adaptations that also occurred in this group (as evidenced by the changes observed in the gas-exchange parameters), indicate that the addition of the cycle-training protocol produced skaters with increased potential to perform vigorous on-ice routines.

Another observation worthy of mention is that the two figure skaters in the study described above (10) who experienced the smallest increases in V̇O_2peak after the cycle plus on-ice training (3% and 7% increases) experienced the largest increases in supramaximal endurance time on the cycle ergometer (181% and 237%, respectively). The fact that these skaters possessed the highest V̇O_2peak before the study indicates that they may have been near the limit of their aerobic capacity potential. The fact that these two skaters were able to improve their supramaximal endurance by such a large amount of time indicates that their anaerobic metabolic machinery still had significant potential for improvement. The intense nature of the cycle-training regimen implemented during the study apparently delivered a stimulus that resulted in significant improvements of anaerobic energy metabolism while having little effect on the aerobic capacity of those with the highest pretraining V̇O_2peak.

The previous reports cited in this section have described several physiologic factors that appear to play roles in limiting a figure skater's performance. Two recent reports indicate that a pathophysiologic factor is apparently operative in a significant number of figure skaters, a factor that may pose a significant threat to the performance status of any individual afflicted with the disorder (i.e., the development of asthma symptoms during or immediately after exercise). Exercise-induced bronchospasm (EIB), or exercise-induced asthma, is a common condition in the general population (15) and in highly trained athletes. The United States Olympic Committee reported that 67 of 597 (11.2%) American athletes who competed in the 1984 Summer Games had EIB (16).

Exercise-induced bronchospasm is defined as a decrease in lung function, usually greater than a 10% decrease in forced expiratory volume in one second (FEV_1), occurring within 15 minutes after completion of vigorous exercise at power outputs that elicit at least 85% of maximal O_2 consumption for 4- to 10-minute periods (16–18). The bronchospasm usually reaches detectable levels 1 to 15 minutes after exercise, with spontaneous resolution to preexercise levels usually occurring no later than 45 to 60 minutes after exercise (16). The causative factor for EIB is thought to be evaporative water loss from the airway mucosa (17), resulting in local airway hyperosmolality, triggering bronchospasm in susceptible individuals. Airway cooling also is known to play a precipitating role (19), as reports indicate that cold-air inhalation can exacerbate bronchospastic episodes in individuals with documented cases of asthma (17). In figure skaters, the additive effect of repetitive bouts of extremely vigorous exercise (where HRs may reach 100% of predicted maximum during the first minute), which are performed in cold air (7°C to 10°C) and which may last 4 to 5 minutes during their long program and for longer periods during training), may put this group of athletes at increased risk for EIB.

Provost-Craig's investigative team (20) tested for the presence of EIB in a group of 100 male and female figure skaters (aged 7 to 25 years; mean age, 14.6 years) who were enrolled in sanctioned, coach-supervised training programs and ranged in skill level from juvenile to elite national, international, and Olympic-caliber skaters. Pulmonary-function testing was performed on the skaters immediately before and after a strenuous 4-minute on-ice exercise bout. Criteria for the presence of EIB were a decrease in FEV_1 of 10% or greater, which suggests the presence of hyperactivity, bronchospasm, and increased airway resistance of the large airways and/or a decrease in midmaximal flows (FEF_{25-75}) of 20% or greater, suggesting bronchospasm of the middle and small airways (20). Results indicated that 30 skaters (30% of the group) tested positive for EIB. Of further interest, when the group was partitioned into three subgroups by age, the younger skaters had a higher incidence of EIB, as 13 of 39 (33%) of the 7- to 12-year-olds were positive for EIB; 17 of 50 (34%) of 13- to 18-year-olds tested positive; and 0 of 11 of the 19- to 25-year-olds experienced EIB. The fact that the younger skaters were affected to a larger degree than the older skaters may have a basis in clinical medicine. It has been reported that as many as 41% of all children will be adversely affected by stimuli known to cause EIB; of these susceptible children, approximately 90% will experience EIB. Pierson (21) indicated that childhood asthmatics often outgrow their disease within 7 years of its onset, so that the older skaters in the Provost-Craig study may have simply experienced a spontaneous resolution of this disorder.

Mannix and colleagues (22) sought to determine the incidence of EIB in 124 figure skaters (11 to 30 years) who were enrolled in sanctioned, coach-supervised training programs and who ranged in skill level from juvenile to elite national, international, and Olympic-caliber skaters. Rink-side spirometry (temperature, 8°C; humidity, 60%) was used to assess lung function immediately before and at 1, 5, 10, and 15 minutes after a simulated long program (4 to 5 minutes of high-intensity skating). EIB was documented by a decline in FEV_1 of at least 10% from preexercise values. Results indicate that 43 of 124 (35%) experienced EIB. The timing of the exercise-induced changes in airflow indicates two time points when skaters experienced their greatest decline in FEV_1: the 0-to-1-minute and 15-minute postexercise time points. The 0-to-1-minute decline is earlier than one might expect, as others reported that the greatest decline in airflow occurs 5 to 25 minutes after exercise (15). Perhaps the more rapid onset of bronchospasm in these skaters is related to an additive effect of vigorous exercise plus the cold ambient conditions, two factors that can independently cause bronchospasm (17,19).

A few last notes concerning EIB in figure skaters as a detractor from performance. First, in the reports of both Provost-Craig and co-workers (20) and Mannix (22), the skaters who had previously been diagnosed with asthma continued taking their prescribed, metered-dose medication during the experimental trials. Provost-Craig and colleagues (20) reported that four of 13 with previously diagnosed asthma experienced EIB during their testing, whereas all eight asthmatics in Mannix's study (22) experienced EIB after the on-ice exercise bout. It is apparent from these findings that the prescribed treatment regimens were less than universally successful in controlling this disorder. Review of questionnaires in one of the studies (22) indicated that none of the previously diagnosed asthmatics used their medication routinely at least 15 min before heavy exercise, and most did not use their medication regularly during training sessions. The athletes incorrectly believed that if they used inhaled medication 2 to 5 minutes before exercise, this would achieve adequate airway protection. As long as beliefs similar to these are held by asthmatic figure skaters, EIB in this population will continue to be a significant detriment to performance. Second, one might wonder why EIB would limit performance, as it is known to occur after, not during, strenuous physical activities. The fact is that during a typical training session, a skater performs many high-intensity bouts of exercise of sufficient duration, in a susceptible individual, to cause EIB. This being the case, the skater might adjust his or her skating intensity during training in a downward fashion to avoid EIB. This decrease in training intensity would potentially have significant negative effects on the state of conditioning of the athlete, perhaps precluding attainment of a higher level of performance.

THE ATHLETE

Competitive, championship-level figure skating is generally considered a sport for young people, ranging in age from approximately 5 years for preliminary and prejuvenile levels to the early teens and into the twenties or even early thirties for senior-level skaters.

Table 50–2 contains demographic data of a typical cohort of skaters (n = 52; 35 female and 17 male skaters) who participated in a USFSA-sanctioned training camp in the early to mid-1990s. Each of these skaters was under the tutelage of a coach and was training to compete at the national and international level. Data indicated a normal progression in height and weight according to age for each of the subgroups. The body mass index (BMI, weight in kg/height in m^2) is included to allow comparison of the stature of these skaters with that of the population at large. Although no consistent BMI ranges are accepted by all investigators, a reasonable set of guidelines has been established, with normal BMI for adults considered to be within a range of 18.5 to 25.0 kg/m^2 (23). For children aged 11 to 13 years, the lowest normal value is 15.0 kg/m^2; for children aged 14 to 17 years, the lowest normal value is 16.5 kg/m^2 (24). By using these standards, it is apparent that all subgroups displayed in Table 50–2 fall into the lower portion of the normal range, as stated earlier.

The BMI data presented in Table 50–2 are in conceptual agreement with the findings of Slemenda and Johnston (25), who assessed body composition in a group (n = 22) of young (11- to 23-year-old) female figure skaters, including international-caliber competitors. A group (n = 22) of healthy, sedentary young female subjects (11 to 23 years old) was used as controls. These investigators found the skaters to be significantly leaner than age- and gender-matched controls, as indicated by determination of body-fat percentage by dual energy x-ray absorptiometry: skaters (body fat, 18.7% ± 5.4%); and controls (body fat, 24.3% ± 6.0%). Another important finding was that the skaters had similar skeletal densities at upper-body sites (spine, arm, ribs) but significantly greater bone densities in the pelvis and legs. The younger skaters of the group did not exhibit increased bone density in the weight-bearing, lower extremities. These findings suggest that a training adaptation has occurred over time in these skaters (i.e., increased bone density in the lower extremities), which apparently better equips them to deal with the high weight-bearing loads inherent in the sport.

Table 50–3 contains demographic data of gold, silver, and bronze medalists (first, second, and third place) for men's and women's freestyle competition at the United States National Championships for the years 1973 through 1996 (demographic data provided by USFSA, Colorado Springs). No clear differences appear for any of the four criterion variables when comparisons are made among gold, silver, and bronze medal winners. Other than the expected size differences, comparisons across gender indicate that the men are, on average, approximately 2 to 3 years older than the women. When one examines the height, weight, and BMI data for all gold medalists over the three decades of data displayed, it appears that the changes in training techniques that began in the early 1990s, which emphasized enhancement of both upper- and lower-body strength, resulted in skaters with more mass per height. Note that the average weight of the skaters from the 1970s to the 1980s is relatively stable (an increase of 0.1 kg for the men and an increase of 0.6 kg for the women). The weight from the 1970s to the 1990s, however, increased 4.3 kg for the men and 2.0 kg for the women. One might argue that each group is taller in the 1990s versus the 1970s, but the increase in height for each group of 0.03 m should have been accompanied

TABLE 50–2. *Demographic data of a typical cohort of skaters*

	Height (m)	Weight (kg)	BMI (kg/m^2)
Female skaters			
Age 9–12 yr n = 17	1.45 ± 0.10	36.8 ± 6.9	17.5 ± 1.7
Age 13–16 yr n = 18	1.62 ± 0.05	51.4 ± 6.6	19.6 ± 2.0
Male skaters			
Age 12–16 yr n = 7	1.60 ± 0.12	53.0 ± 8.9	20.8 ± 2.7
Age 17–22 yr n = 10	1.72 ± 0.09	66.0 ± 6.0	22.3 ± 2.2

Data presented as mean ± SD.
BMI, body mass index. (Unpublished data.)

TABLE 50–3. *Demographic data of National Championship medalists: 1973–1996*

	Male skaters				Female skaters			
	Age (yr)	Ht (m)	Wt (kg)	BMI (kg/m²)	Age (yr)	Ht (m)	Wt (kg)	BMI (kg/m²)
1st, 2nd, 3rd places (all years)	22.4 ± 2.7	1.72 ± 0.07	63.3 ± 6.2	21.3 ± 0.9	19.0 ± 2.2	1.60 ± 0.06	49.1 ± 5.0	19.0 ± 0.9
1st place (all years)	23.0 ± 2.2	1.71 ± 0.08	63.3 ± 7.5	21.6 ± 1.1	19.5 ± 2.2	1.60 ± 0.04	48.5 ± 3.8	19.1 ± 0.9
2nd place (all years)	22.3 ± 3.2	1.74 ± 0.07	64.6 ± 5.5	21.2 ± 0.8	18.6 ± 2.3	1.60 ± 0.07	48.2 ± 6.2	18.7 ± 1.1
3rd place (all years)	22.0 ± 2.4	1.71 ± 0.07	61.9 ± 5.9	21.2 ± 1.0	19.0 ± 2.3	1.60 ± 0.07	50.5 ± 5.0	19.2 ± 1.0
1st place (1973–1979)	22.4 ± 2.6	1.69 ± 0.06	62.0 ± 3.9	21.6 ± 0.4	18.7 ± 1.1	1.57 ± 0.03	47.7 ± 3.7	19.2 ± 1.1
1st place (1980–1989)	24.1 ± 1.7	1.71 ± 0.10	62.1 ± 10.6	21.0 ± 1.3	19.1 ± 1.5	1.61 ± 0.05	48.3 ± 3.6	18.7 ± 0.7
1st place (1990–1996)	22.1 ± 2.3	1.72 ± 0.07	66.3 ± 4.3	22.4 ± 0.5	21.0 ± 3.2	1.60 ± 0.05	49.7 ± 4.6	19.5 ± 0.7

Data presented as mean ± SD.
BMI, body mass index. (Data provided by USFSA.)

by only a 1.0-kg increase for the men and a 1.2-kg increase for the women (26).

TRAINING THE ATHLETE

The sport of competitive figure skating has undergone a series of gradual changes since the early 1970s, which has taken it from a two-season sport to, in all practicality, a sport that runs the entire year except for a small break in midspring. For the purpose of fostering a more complete understanding of the state of today's figure skater and the training and competitive seasons that help mold these athletes into highly trained performers, a brief description of the long-standing "traditional" training and competitive season, sport-specific training, and supplemental training is offered, followed by a description of the state of affairs as they presently exist.

The Season

In the mid-1950s through the early 1970s, a typical training year for a competitive figure skater consisted of a summer season, which began in mid-June and ran through Labor Day, and a winter season, which ran from October through March. The summer season was dedicated to training and preparation for the upcoming winter competitions. In the United States, the format of these competitions is, to this day, based on geographic location, so that there are three sections (East Coast, Midwest, Pacific Coast), each of which is made up of three regions. The competitive schedule began each year during the winter season (for non-Olympic years) with the regional figure-skating qualifying competitions. These events were typically held in late October or early November. Skaters who qualified at the regional level moved on to compete in their sectional figure-skating competitions, which were held in early December. Successful qualification at the sectional competitions resulted in an invitation to the National Figure Skating Championships, which were held at least 4 weeks later, but in some cases may have been held up to 9 weeks after the sectionals. The World Figure Skating Championship was then held 4 weeks later, with successful competitors from national championships from all over the world vying for the coveted crown of world champion. Every 4 years, the season was modified to accommodate the Olympic Games, which were, and still are, typically held in early February. The only change in the competitive season was to move the date of the National Championships so that they were completed 4 weeks before the beginning of the Olympic Games. Thus, the winter season ended in mid-March, and training did not resume again until the summer season. For the skaters who performed in the World and/or Olympic Championships, this "off-season" period was usually a time for a European tour and ice shows back in the United States. The skaters who failed to reach this level of competition remained at home, continuing their on-ice workouts and refinement of their routines. The ensuing summer season was structured around a series of nonqualifying competitive events held in venues across the country and continued training.

As mentioned previously, the modern training and competitive seasons now run virtually the entire year, with only a small break occurring in midspring. The winter season follows the same "traditional" schedule listed above. The two major differences between today's year-round schedule and the one of the past are the structure and content of the summer season; there are more nonqualifying competitions in the summer season, and the season is longer by approximately 2 months, beginning in mid-April and running through September.

In addition, nonqualifying international competitions start as early as August in this system, which allows competitors to perform before international judges and audiences in preparation for World and Olympic Championships.

Sport-Specific Training

The traditional figure-skating training regimen consisted almost entirely of on-ice activities, with the only off-ice activity being a minimal number of stretching exercises performed on an occasional basis (personal communication). Skaters from successful programs of the 1950s and 1960s trained 6 days per week. A typical day might include one, two, or three patch sessions each day, during which time compulsory figures (various patterns that the skater would follow on the ice while skating on one foot; e.g., a figure-8 pattern) were practiced, with emphasis placed on proper technique and style. Patch sessions are not very physically demanding, producing HRs of 105 to 120 beats/min for 60 minutes per session (10). Two hours of freestyle skating would be performed, during which skaters would intermittently skate laps with an occasional jump, jump sequence, spin, or multiple spin moves interspersed throughout, or sometimes a number of laps would be skated without the inclusion of jumps or spins. Lap skating, especially when performed at moderate to high intensity and when interspersed with jumps, is the most strenuous activity skaters perform. It is not uncommon for maximal HRs to be achieved within the first minute of such an exercise (10). Freestyle skating time also includes periods in which skaters may perform run-throughs of their short and long programs. If these are performed without rest periods so that 3- or 4-minute bouts of skating are performed with the execution of various jumps, the activity is quite strenuous, placing stress on both the O_2-delivery system and aerobic metabolism, as well as a large demand being placed on the anaerobic metabolic machinery (i.e., anaerobic glycolysis). For ice dancing specialists, a daily 1-hour dance session would be performed by a couple, during which time specific parts of programs are practiced, or entire 3- and 4-minute programs are performed *in toto*. Advanced pairs and dance couples would often substitute additional time with their partners for patch time, with perhaps as much as 2 to 3 hours spent each day skating pairs routines. The primary goal of the training program was for each participant to learn to execute the various components of the short and long programs effectively and to learn how to execute the movement patterns successfully in a well-choreographed pattern in an aesthetically pleasing manner. Perhaps of equal or greater import was a secondary goal of the training program, to deliver each participant to a level of fitness that would allow a performance perceived as "easy to perform," so that the skater could concentrate on presentation rather than on execution and technique.

Modern training is quite different from the traditional model. Early in the skater's training, an emphasis is placed on developing general athleticism before starting sport-specific training (for details, see the section below on Supplemental Training).

An example of a typical on-ice training regimen used by a training facility sanctioned by the USFSA is presented for review. This particular program is initiated in late spring each year and usually runs through most of the summer. It is a bit more intense than programs that run through the competition session, as it is designed to raise the skaters to their maximal level of strength and endurance in preparation for competition. On-ice training is typically performed 5 or 6 days a week and consists of the following (10): a minimum of a 10- to 20-minute stretching session immediately preceding and immediately following on-ice work; 10 to 15 minutes of on-ice aerobic warm-up in which skaters practice turns and changes in speed while moving across the entire surface of the ice; two, three, or sometimes four 45-minute freestyle sessions during which the skaters practice their jumps/spins/routines on the ice (HR range, 120 to 200 beats/min); and power-stroking routines for 10 to 20 minutes per session, during which the skaters speed around the ice as rapidly as possible with two or three built-in active recovery periods (interval-type training; HR range, 185 to 205 beats/min).

During the competitive season, less time is spent on the power-stroking portion of the workouts, and more time is dedicated to skating and perfecting the routines that will be executed in competitions.

Supplemental Training

Supplemental training in the traditional skate-training program simply did not exist. For years coaches looked at training programs of successful skaters and designed programs as carbon copies. This mentality led to a long history of designing training programs empirically from anecdotal evidence or hearsay, rather than using scientific findings gathered from other sports and applying them to figure skaters. This mode of training was still in place until perhaps the late 1980s and early 1990s, when cross-training methods started to be tested and incorporated into skate-training programs.

Modern training uses extensive cross-training modalities to improve the athleticism of figure skaters. This is often accomplished by weight training to improve strength and muscular endurance, plyometric jump training to improve explosive power development, and gymnastics, ballet, and/or jazz training to improve grace and movement skills. A comprehensive modern training regimen also includes stretching routines performed before and after on-ice workouts to improve and maintain flexibility and quite often includes off-ice exercise designed to improve cardiovascular fitness and aerobic capacity.

One such program, initiated at a facility sanctioned by the USFSA, was the source of a controlled experiment designed to test the efficacy of a high-intensity interval-training program performed on a cycle ergometer (10). The main goal of the training program was to introduce a training stimulus that would stress the aerobic and anaerobic metabolic systems to produce significant increases in aerobic capacity and supramaximal endurance time, while avoiding high-impact stress to the lower extremities. A key component of the program was that it had to be of short duration, so as to not significantly curtail the time devoted to on-ice training exercises.

For this, a high-intensity interval-type cycle ergometer workout was implemented, which was fashioned after a training protocol established by Hickson and colleagues (27). This off-ice cycle-ergometer training regimen was performed 4 days each week for 10 successive weeks in one group of skaters. Subjects exercised for 33 consecutive minutes a day by using five 5-minute intervals, each separated by 2 minutes of active recovery at 25 W. During each of the 5-minute intervals, the ergometer was set at a work rate that elicited 25% of each subject's previously determined $\dot{V}O_2$peak during minute 1, 50% of $\dot{V}O_2$peak during minute 2, 75% of $\dot{V}O_2$peak during minute 3, and 100% of $\dot{V}O_2$peak during minutes 4 and 5. To account for the increase in work capacity that is known to occur during training (23), increases in target maximal work rates (and therefore increases in the absolute work rates needed to elicit the various percentages of $\dot{V}O_2$peak) were built into the protocol. This was accomplished by adding a 10% increase in wattage for weeks 3 and 4, an additional 5% increase for weeks 5 through 7, and a final 5% increase for weeks 8 through 10, so that a 20% increase in the maximal power output originally attained in the laboratory was accomplished by the end of the 10-week training period. Compliance was maintained by investigators and by ongoing recording of training sessions in a daily log book. A second group of skaters was used as a control group, which maintained its regular on-ice workouts over the same period without the addition of cycle training. An effort was made to ensure that both groups of skaters trained the same total amount of time each day; accordingly, the cycle-ergometer skaters decreased on-ice time by approximately 30 minutes on the days they exercised on the ergometer.

After completion of the aforementioned study, the facility at which it was conducted implemented the high-intensity interval-type cycle-ergometer training regimen each year during the summer season, to increase the aerobic capacity and anaerobic power output of their skaters. Anecdotal evidence indicates that other training facilities have encouraged their skaters to participate in vigorous off-ice cross-training protocols. The widespread belief in the skating community is that such training has great potential to improve the overall fitness of their skaters, thus enabling them to execute their routines without displaying signs of fatigue or physical strain.

REFERENCES

1. *The 1997 Official United States Figure Skating Association Rule Book.* Colorado Springs: United States Figure Skating Association. 1997.
2. McArdle WD, Katch FI, Katch VL. *Exercise physiology: energy, nutrition, and human performance*, 4th ed. Baltimore: Williams & Wilkins, 1996:121–138, 167–180.
3. Foster C, Snyder AC, Thompson NN, Kuettel KK, Conway MJ. Cycle ergometry during training for speed skating. *J Appl Sport Sci Res* 1989;3:79–84.
4. van Ingen Schenau GJ, de Grout G. Differences in oxygen consumption and external power between male and female skaters during supramaximal cycling. *Eur J Appl Physiol* 1983;51:337–345.
5. van Ingen Schenau GJ, de Groot G, Hollander AP. Some technical, physiological and anthropological aspects of speed skating. *Eur J Appl Physiol* 1983;50:343–354.
6. Daub WB, Green HJ, Houston ME, Thomson JA, Fraser IG, Ranney DA. Specificity of physiologic adaptations resulting from ice-hockey training. *Med Sci Sports Exerc* 1983;15:290–294.
7. Green HJ, Houston ME. Effect of a season of ice hockey on energy capacities and associated functions. *Med Sci Sports Exerc* 1975;7:299–303.
8. Green HJ, Thompson JA, Daub WB, Houston ME, Ranney DA. Fiber composition: fiber size and enzyme activities in vastus lateralis of elite athletes involved in high intensity exercise. *Eur J Appl Physiol* 1979;41:109–117.
9. McMaster WC, Liddle S, Walsh J. Conditioning program for competitive figure skating. *Am J Sports Med* 1979;7:43–47.
10. Mannix ET, Healey A, Farber MO. Aerobic power and supramaximal endurance of competitive figure skaters. *J Sports Med Phys Fitness* 1996;36:161–168.
11. Maksud MG, Farrel P, Foster C, et al. VO_2, ventilation and heart rate of Olympic speed skating candidates. *J Sports Med Phys Fitness* 1982;22:217–223.
12. Geijsel J, Bomhoff G, Van Velzen J, de Groot G, van Ingen Schenau GJ. Bicycle ergometry and speed skating performance. *Int J Sports Med* 1984;5:241–245.
13. Ekblom B, Astrand P-O, Saltin B, Stenberg J, Wallstrom B. Effect of training on circulatory response to exercise. *J Appl Physiol* 1968;24:518–528.
14. Donovan CM, Brooks GA. Endurance training affects lactate clearance, not lactate production. *Am J Physiol* 1983;244:E83–E92.
15. Roberts JA. Exercise-induced asthma in athletes. *Sports Med* 1988;6:193–196.
16. Voy RO. The US Olympic Committee experience with exercise-induced bronchospasm, 1984. *Med Sci Sports Exerc* 1986;18:328–330.
17. Anderson SD, Schoeffel RE, Black JL, Daviskas E. Airway cooling as a stimulus to exercise induced asthma: a reevaluation. *Eur J Respir Dis* 1985;67:20–25.
18. Anderson DA. Exercise-induced asthma. In: Middleton E, Reed CE, Ellis EF, Adkinson NF, Yunginger JW, Busse WW, eds. *Allergy: principles and practice.* Vol II. St. Louis: Mosby, 1993:1343–1367.
19. Strauss RH, McFadden ER, Ingram RH, Jaeger JJ. Enhancement of exercise induced asthma by cold air. *N Engl J Med* 1977;297:734–747.
20. Provost-Craig MA, Arbour KS, Sestili DC, Chabalko JJ, Ekinci E.

The incidence of exercise-induced bronchospasm in competitive figure skaters. *J Asthma* 1996;33:67–71.
21. Pierson WE. Exercise-induced bronchospasm in clinical practice. *Clin Rev Allergy* 1988;6:443–452.
22. Mannix ET, Farber MO, Palange P, Galassetti P, Manfredi F. Exercise-induced asthma in figure skaters. *Chest* 1996;109:312–314.
23. Heymsfield SB, Tighe A, Wang Z. Nutritional assessment by anthropometric and biochemical methods. In: Shils ME, Olson JA, Shike M, eds. *Modern nutrition in health and disease*. 8th ed. Philadelphia: Lea & Febiger, 1994:812–841.
24. Torun B, Chew F. Protein-energy malnutrition. In: Shils ME, Olson JA, Shike M, eds. *Modern nutrition in health and disease*. 8th ed. Philadelphia: Lea & Febiger, 1994:950–976.
25. Slemenda CW, Johnston CC. High intensity activities in young women: site specific bone mass effects among female figure skaters. *Bone Miner* 1993;20:125–132.
26. Russell RM, McGandy RB, Jelliffe D. Reference weights: practical considerations. *Am J Med* 1984;76:767–769.
27. Hickson RC, Bomze HA, Holloszy JO. Linear increase in aerobic power by a strenuous program of endurance exercise. *J Appl Physiol* 1977;42:372–376.

Exercise and Sport Science,
edited by William E. Garrett, Jr., and Donald T. Kirkendall.
Lippincott Williams & Wilkins, Philadelphia © 2000.

CHAPTER 51

Physiology of American Football

William J. Kraemer and Lincoln A. Gotshalk

THE SPORT

Football is one of the most popular sports in the United States, with organized participation from youth to professional leagues. The sport is played almost solely by boys and men; some girls and women do play football, however, and some semiprofessional leagues have been made up solely of women football players. Paradoxically, although American football is one of the major revenue sports in the world today, our scientific understanding of the sport is typically related to descriptive studies of players, medical aspects of injury treatment, and techniques of training used to condition the players for the sport. In fact, we know very little about the physiologic demands and stresses of the actual competition of a football game. As a society, we are impressed with the collisions or "hits" observed on the field, and this appears to be part of the attraction of the game. With players getting bigger and faster each year, the physical impact of each collision continues to become more dramatic in both magnitude and physical impact. The ability to tolerate the intensity of the game has continued to demand a higher and higher price on players at the elite levels of competition. To understand this concept, read the comments below by former Atlanta Falcon football player and now author/sports commentator Tim Green on various aspects of what it feels like to play in the highest level of competition, the National Football League (NFL) (1).

> The best way to describe the feeling of a player's first moments of an NFL game is to compare it to stepping suddenly out into the middle of a busy interstate. The bodies moving past you are immense, like pickups, sports cars, motor cycles, dump trucks. The speed at which they travel is frightening. You didn't know something with those kinds of mass could move so fast, or if you did, it seems somehow so much more impressive to watch them moving up close. Suddenly you get hit. You reel. You stagger. You try to avoid getting hit again, but once they've got you spinning you can't recover. . . . Pain and football are inseparable. . . . Pain is when the physical damage is so extreme that the jolting messages sent from the injured area to the brain are just too much to be ignored, even during a game when your entire focus is on doing your job and winning.

Basic Rules of the Game

By understanding the basics of the football game, one can start to gain insights into the demands placed on the various players on the field. The game is played with great physical intensity and psychological arousal to gain the advantage against an opponent. Ultimately, it is one team's players beating another team's players in many one-on-one battles in the complex plays designed for offensive and defensive teams.

The football game is broken up into four quarters (a quarter is typically 12 to 15 minutes of play, depending on the level of play). The winner is the team that has the most points by the end of the game. Football is one of the most intricate team sports. Various specialty teams are also used to perform specific plays such as punts, extra points, and field goals, and there are kickoff and receiving teams. Each football team has offensive, defensive, and special teams, with some players at some levels (e.g., high school) playing on more than one team. Eleven players (some high schools have eight-man teams) make up each of the opposing teams on the field at any one time. Each position is governed by sets of specific rules, and each has specific duties in a specific offensive, defensive, or special-teams scheme (play) that

W. J. Kraemer: Human Performance Laboratory, Graduate and Undergraduate Programs in Exercise Science, Ball State University, Muncie, Indiana 47306.
L. A. Gotshalk: College of Osteopathic Medicine, Ohio University, Athens, Ohio, 45701.

starts at the movement (e.g., snap) of the ball from a specific formation.

Figure 51–1 shows a starting formation for a play from the line of scrimmage once the ball has been put into play after a kickoff, punt, fumble recovery, or interception. The offensive center snaps the ball, and the offensive team tries to perform a specific play; meanwhile, the defensive team reacts and attempts to stop the play by tackling the ball carrier to the ground. The offensive team tries to run or pass the ball down the field (which consists of 100 yards total) to score by advancing the ball as far as it can in four plays (i.e., running or passing plays). This requires proper blocking to shield the defensive team from getting to the ball carrier or quarterback, who is attempting to pass the ball down the field to a receiver. If the offensive team moves the ball 10 yards or more in a series of four plays, a "first down" is awarded, and four more plays are given for the team to move the ball 10 more yards or to score. If, on its fourth try (or "fourth down"), the offensive team has too far to go to cover the 10 yards, it can decide to punt, or kick, the ball to the other team; this puts the other team farther from the goal line it is defending. If the offensive team is close enough to the opponent's goal line, however, it may opt to attempt to kick a field goal.

The aim of the offensive team is to move the ball down the field and score points (it hopes) with a touchdown (6 points, with 1 or 2 points for extra points afterwards), but it also can attempt to kick a field goal (3 points) through the goalposts. The defensive team tries to match up with the offensive team's formation, and its strategies are formulated to stop the offensive team's forward movement of the ball. The primary defensive goal is to stop the offensive team from moving the ball down the field and scoring. The defensive team can score by intercepting a pass or picking up a fumble (dropped ball) and running for a touchdown, or it can tackle an offensive ball carrier who is behind his goal line for a

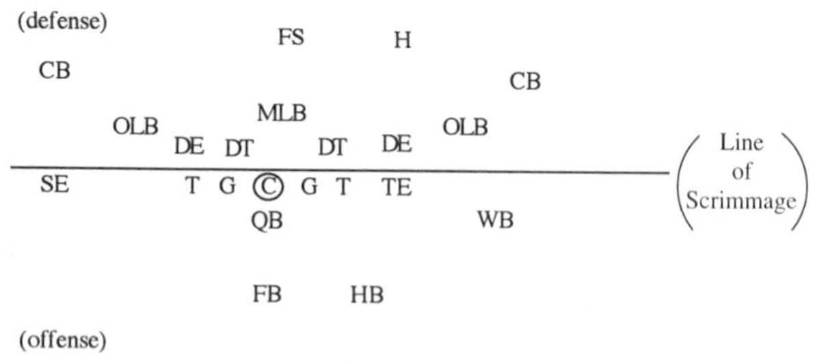

FIG. 51–1. One example of a vast multitude of offensive (strong right, split T) and defensive (4-3) formations used in American football. Offense: *T*, tackle; *G*, guard; *C*, center; *TE*, tight end; *WB*, wingback; *QB*, quarterback; *SE*, split end, *FB*, fullback; *HB*, halfback. Defense (*top*): *DE*, defensive end; *DT*, defensive tackle; *MLB*, middle linebacker; *OLB*, outside linebacker; *CB*, cornerback; *FS*, free safety; *H*, halfback.

"safety" (2 points). Thus, as many great football coaches have said, "Success in this game is about who blocks and tackles the best" (2,3).

Physiologic Requirements

Physical Attributes of Major College and Professional Football Players

In general, each position on the football team has different physiologic and biomechanical demands related to the position-specific jobs required. Ultimately, this has led to position-specific variations in body size, body composition, speed, strength, power, and cardiovascular endurance (4,5). In general, often various positions can be separated into different groups by such physical parameters. These different biomechanical and physiologic position demands tend to separate into distinct categories according to physical attributes. In general, offensive and defensive linemen can be grouped together because these players today tend to be taller and larger, have higher levels of body fat, are relatively slower, and have greater absolute strength and power than do the other positions (4–6). Linemen can be subcategorized into offensive linemen and defensive linemen. Offensive linemen, typically, are slower, stronger, larger, and heavier than the defensive linemen, who typically are quicker and more powerful. Such opposing physical capabilities are related to the fundamental fact that the offensive players know where the play (or the ball) is going, and the defensive players do not and must react to the ball or defend a specific area on the field. In addition, offensive styles have developed in which large offensive linemen just have to shield the running back from the defensive players, and thus the amount of movement for success is defined by only a couple of yards.

Thus, a type of physical evolution of the player's physical abilities by position has occurred over the years because of the genetics of each subsequent generation and strategies/rules of the game. With higher levels of competition, player sizes have been dramatically affected by rule changes. For example, short offensive linemen are very rare on major college and professional teams because the rules have now made "chop blocks" and "spear blocks" below the waist illegal to reduce injury, primarily protecting the player's knees. Taking such an effective violent physical weapon away from shorter offensive linemen resulted in dramatic changes in the average height of linemen. In general, offensive backs, wide receivers, and defensive backs tend to have the lowest levels of body fat, fastest sprint times, quickest reaction times, and highest relative $\dot{V}O_2max$ values (6–8). These players must typically survive or evade "hits" by the larger players. Inside linebackers and tight ends tend to form a group next to the linemen in body size, strength, and power, whereas outside linebackers and fullbacks form the group between the small backs and the inside linebackers and tight ends (6–8). These players need speed and quickness but also the strength, body size, and power to take on the linemen during a game. Table 51–1 gives some examples of data on the physical abilities of major college football players.

The position-specific tasks required of football players tend to determine the characteristics the players possess. Body size, body composition, strength, power, quickness, reaction time, speed, and endurance again all add up to determine distinct player groupings, as discussed above. In 1987, Berg and colleagues (5) analyzed the data from 41 NCAA Division I college football teams, including many top-20 teams. In comparing ranked versus unranked teams, they found that the mean scores in strength, power, and speed tests for the ranked teams were much higher than those of the unranked teams. Vertical jump height, vertical jump power, and the bench press/weight scores were significantly higher in ranked teams. Berg and colleagues (5) found that the only variable significantly related to rank among the 17 ranked teams was "power" measured from the vertical jump. Therefore, although strength appears to be important for success in football, it is in fact the ability to generate a rapid rate of force development in the lower body that appears to distinguish top teams as a whole. Thus, training for power appears to be a key element in the physical development of football players. Power not only differentiated ranked and unranked teams, but it also determined the order of the ranked teams. This supported the general contention of Wilmore and associates (9) that power distinguishes the best from the lesser football players at all positions.

Again, there are subtle factors in the game of football that affect changes in the anatomic and physiologic abilities of positions. Whereas the differences between players' size and speed over the years are relative, another example of how rule changes affect stereotypical physical characteristics is seen in the positions of defensive backs and wide receivers. In the 1960s and the early 1970s, defensive backs and linebackers could make contact with a wide receiver not possessing the ball, anywhere on the field. The strategy was to have large defensive backs disrupt pass routes by being able to apply continuous bumps to control the wide receivers. Wide receivers had to be quick and shifty, needing to avoid or deflect the contact to get free on a pass route. Prime examples in the 1960s were wide receiver Lance Alworth of the San Diego Chargers and defensive back Johnny Sample of the New York Jets. Alworth was small, extremely fast, and quick, relying on his ability to deflect contact and streak downfield, skills that allowed him to average more than 20 yards a catch and more than 100 yards a game through much of his career. Sample was large and tough, relying on contact skills rather than the speed and quickness of his shadowing skills to defend the routes of top wide receivers and decrease their effectiveness. In the 1970s, rule changes allowed defensive contact on the receiver without the ball to be made only within 5 yards of the line of scrimmage. Shortly thereafter, wide receivers became taller, big enough to fend off an initial "bump," and faster runners (for example, the San Francisco 49er's Jerry Rice). In response, defensive backs generally became smaller and less bulky, but also quicker and faster (for example, the Washington Redskin's Darrell Green and the Dallas Cowboy's Deion Sanders), relying now on shadowing, quickness, and speed to recover rather than route disruption and more contact downfield to defend against the passing game. Imagine if the size of a standard football field was changed to be 150 yards wide and 200 yards long: player sizes, endurance capabilities, and team strategies might change as well. It is the fan who ultimately sets the stage for what "sells," however, and big fast men playing a hard-hitting game have captured society's fancy and made football a top revenue sport; the Super Bowl to determine the top team in the NFL, which takes place every January, has become one of the biggest annual events in the country.

TABLE 51–1. *Descriptive strength characteristics of NCAA Division I football players*

1 RM bench press (lb) (*n* = 283)	319 ± 58
1 RM squat (lb) (*n* = 115)	425 ± 82
1 RM power clean (lb) (*n* = 166)	271 ± 39
40-yard sprint (s) (*n* = 281)	4.88 ± 0.27
Maximal vertical jump (inch) (*n* = 193)	28.6 ± 3.6

Defensive tackles, offensive guards, offensive tackles, defensive linesmen, offensive running backs, offensive wide receivers, defensive cornerbacks, and defensive safeties. From ref. 4, with permission.

Bioenergetics of Football

Fox and Matthews (10) and Gleim and colleagues (8) have theorized that the anaerobic energy systems provide almost all of the body's energy during a football game, with the phosphocreatine (PCr) system providing 90% of the energy production, and glycolysis (lactic acid system) providing the remaining 10%. Lactate production has been seen to play a greater role in repetitive short maximal bursts of activity (2 to 5 seconds) followed by brief periods of recovery (15 to 60 seconds) (6,11). We observed (unpublished data) that college plays averaged 5.49 seconds (1.87 to 12.88 seconds), whereas rest between plays (of a continuous series) averaged 32.67 seconds; professional plays averaged 5.05 seconds (1.99 to 12.31 seconds), and rest between plays averaged 38.46 seconds. This pattern reflects the repetitive nature of a football game, with series ranging from 3 to 20 plays, with 25 seconds or so between plays (12). A limited number of studies (6,11) have measured the response of blood variables to the stress of a football game, and only one study has examined American football (13). It was shown that the game of football increases blood lactate concentrations of players three- to fivefold above resting levels, with blood glucose levels not significantly affected, indicating moderate stress on the glycolytic pathway. It appears plausible that the influence of television breaks and delayed clock starts between plays on the major college and professional levels have reduced the physiologic stress on the lactic acid system, making the phosphogens [adenosine triphosphate–phosphocreatine (ATP-PCr)] system the dominant system challenged (8,10).

Takahashi and co-workers (12) demonstrated that the time required to restore intramuscular PCr in trained muscles after isolated exercise may require 55 to 90 seconds. With the football rest periods significantly less than this, the repeated bouts of high intensity may rely on the glycolytic system more highly than previously theorized. During the course of a game, the resynthesis of ATP by way of anaerobic glycolysis may increase under conditions of fatigue and PCr depletion (6,8). Smith and Jackson (13) observed that prepractice lactate values for Division III small-college football players were within normal ranges, with prepractice concentrations of 1.41 mmol/L and pregame concentrations of 1.67 mmol/L. In the game, by halftime these values increased to 4.39 mmol/L, and they increased to 5.08 mmol/L by the end of the game. Lactate during practice was 2.54 mmol/L for unit position drills, but after conditioning drills at the end of practice increased to 5.46 mmol/L. It was concluded that football conditioning drills but not football unit position drills provide a metabolic stimulus for lactate production similar to game conditions. Although not excessively high, the game of football does demand a significant source of energy from anaerobic glycolysis, and only conditioning drills appear to prepare the player for such game demands. Thus unit and team practice do not prepare football players for the physiologic demands of the game, and only the conditioning drills and "in-season" weight workouts maintain physiologic fitness for the game. The battle between unit coaches for time and the conditioning demands of the player continues to be an uneasy interface of player sport-fitness development and maintenance and injury prevention over the season and during spring football (college Divisions I, IAA to II).

Cardiovascular Fitness

Although football is primarily a high-intensity anaerobic sport with intervals of high-intensity activity and short rests, there is a cardiovascular component to football as well. The importance of the cardiovascular system may be related to the overall stress a game can place on the body's systems, especially under conditions of extreme environmental heat stress. Cardiovascular endurance can play an important role in determining the efficiency of a player's performance and recovery ability (8,9,14). However, many larger players are generally in low to average aerobic condition when specifically compared with aerobically trained athletes (14). In addition, the physiologic strain is greater for players who play "both ways" (both offensive and defensive teams), and this requires greater cardiovascular fitness. Typically "two-way" players are seen more often at the high school or in some cases small-college levels of play. A fatigued player may also be at a greater risk for injury. Gleim and associates (14) observed that most game injuries occurred during the late second and fourth quarters. This is the time when a player is most fatigued and when a player with inadequate aerobic training may be most susceptible to injury (14).

Cardiovascular fitness also may be a factor for safety and survival in football games or practices in "high heat" conditions, as cardiovascular fitness is the first line of defense against heat illness (15,16). Summer camp and early season performance and safety may rely heavily on the cardiovascular system, because death in football has been attributed to acute hyperthermia and dehydration (17). As the thermal load increases, stress to the cardiovascular system becomes greater because of the large increases in cutaneous blood flow to dissipate heat. Football players typically wear up to 9 kg of protective equipment, including a helmet, during much of summer and fall practices, making them susceptible to hyperthermia, especially if they are hypohydrated or dehydrated or if they practice when heat and humidity are at dangerous levels. Many teams also travel great distances to play opponents in very different thermal conditions and require heat acclimatization before the game. Whereas initial adaptations are seen within the first 3 days of an acclimatization, significant adaptations to the heat typically require 14 days for more complete physiologic adjustments to take place (17). Thus many players are physiologically challenged from a cardiovascular-fitness perspective when faced with a "hot" game, if they are not adequately exposed to the higher temperature and humidity conditions observed in many competitive venues. In addition, more continuous exercise (typically of the endurance type) that maintains an elevated core temperature also is more effective in helping the body gain the initial adaptations for heat tolerance. Thus a higher level of cardiovascular fitness is one important factor in the prevention of heat illness, to which less cardiovascularly fit, heavier linemen appear to be the most vulnerable (16,17).

THE ATHLETE

Body Size and Composition

A general finding on size and force-production capabilities among NCAA Division I football players was reported in a study in 1990 by Berg and colleagues (5). The average player is relatively large (n = 880; the average player height, 6 ft 1 in.; body mass, 230 pounds). They also showed that interior linemen are characterized by larger size (average, 6 ft 4 in., 272 pounds) and great strength (one repetition maximal squat, 534 pounds) while having greater body fatness (average, 17.1%) than those playing in speed positions such as offensive and defensive backs and wide receivers. Linebackers and tight ends were in between on these attributes. Offensive backs were larger than defensive backs, which is a trend that continues today, but were similar with regard to speed, strength, and power abilities. Offensive linemen were heavier, fatter, and greater in "absolute" strength than the defensive linemen. However, defensive lineman were faster and also had the same relative strength and power to body mass as offensive linemen (5).

To observe how much change occurs in the body mass of football players over a longitudinal period, we analyzed the rosters of Pennsylvania State University football players for height and body mass over a 30-year period (i.e., 1967, 1977, 1987, and 1997 teams). Comparisons of the body weights by position groupings are presented in Figs. 51–2 and 51–3. For major colleges, the move toward offensive and defensive players averaging 300 or more pounds each is closer each decade, and many NFL teams have already achieved it. It is interesting to note that the largest athletes in our sample, such as the offensive linemen, made the most significant gains in body mass over the 3 decades, whereas the smallest athletes, such as the defensive backs and running backs, essentially made no changes at all in body mass. With all of the recent attention to the larger fullbacks who block and are tackled by bigger people, we noted the same trend in our data, as the middle-sized athletes (the fullbacks and linebackers) made significant weight gains only over the last 10 years. The size differences among players has been a classic finding over the years, with only the magnitude being different (15). This was brought out in a study by Olson and Hunter (18), who compared the size, plus strength and speed, of 13 teams in 1974 and 1984 Division I. They demonstrated that, for almost all of the positions, the 1984 players were taller and heavier, as well as stronger and faster. No doubt the size of the field in American football has affected both the size and cardiovascular requirements for players. The Canadian game is characterized by a larger playing field (110 by 65 yards), 25-yard end zones, three downs, and only 20 seconds to put the ball into play; this promotes longer movements, the passing game, and the need for the ability to recover more quickly (19). Increases in body size reflect a combination of factors in football today, including rule changes, better conditioning, improved nutrition, and ultimately improved genetics (20). Thus recruitment or drafting of top players by both college and professional teams remains the most important factor in the success on the football field.

In recent studies Snow and co-workers (21) and Clark and colleagues (22) reported that professional football players and Division I collegiate players are heavier and fatter than previous collegiate and professional football players, especially linemen. The body fat of professional linemen and offensive backs, as reported by Snow and co-workers (21), was higher than the body fat in the data presented by Wilmore (15), which were often used as reference sources for the size and body composition of professional football players. Even the lightest average offensive line in 1994 was 13% heavier than the older reference body weight for an offensive line (15). Snow and co-workers (21) determined that the majority of the additional weight was due to higher fat mass, and although it is possible that body fat could be useful in absorbing force and producing momentum, excess fat may adversely affect performance by creating a higher metabolic workload involved with moving of such body mass around the field and decreasing the associated power and velocity of movements with fatigue. With the current success of some undersized (all less than 300 pounds) offensive line—who have been able to dominate larger defensive lines in the NFL because of more power, mobility, and greater local muscular endurance—the need for megasized linemen, even on the professional level, continues to be debated. In addition, more important than body mass is height, which provides the needed leverage in today's "above the waist" blocking game. Linemen shorter than 6 ft 3 in. are now a much more rare occurrence than in the 1980s and before. After a career, concerns for increasing cardiovascular problems (e.g., hypertension, coronary artery disease) because of the high body-mass and body-fat profiles and altered eating behaviors of larger players cannot be easily dismissed by medical professionals (1). These concerns have been raised for quite some time, yet for the most part such concerns have gone unnoticed by professional team owners or athletic administrations and the NCAA on the collegiate level (23). Unlike previous decades, players now appear to put more time into physical conditioning than ever before, and this may help offset some of the concerns for large body sizes; the impact of aberrant eating behaviors on long-term health and body-size characteristics is still unclear, however.

With the increasing size of the players, the impacts and frequencies of injury, especially concussions, remain troubling aspects of the game. It is vital that one attempts to better understand the exact physiologic changes at the cell level that occur from playing the game, the extent and amount of damage after a game, and the time course of the recovery process of various tissues so as to better deal with the implications for enhanced medical care, physical training, and equip-

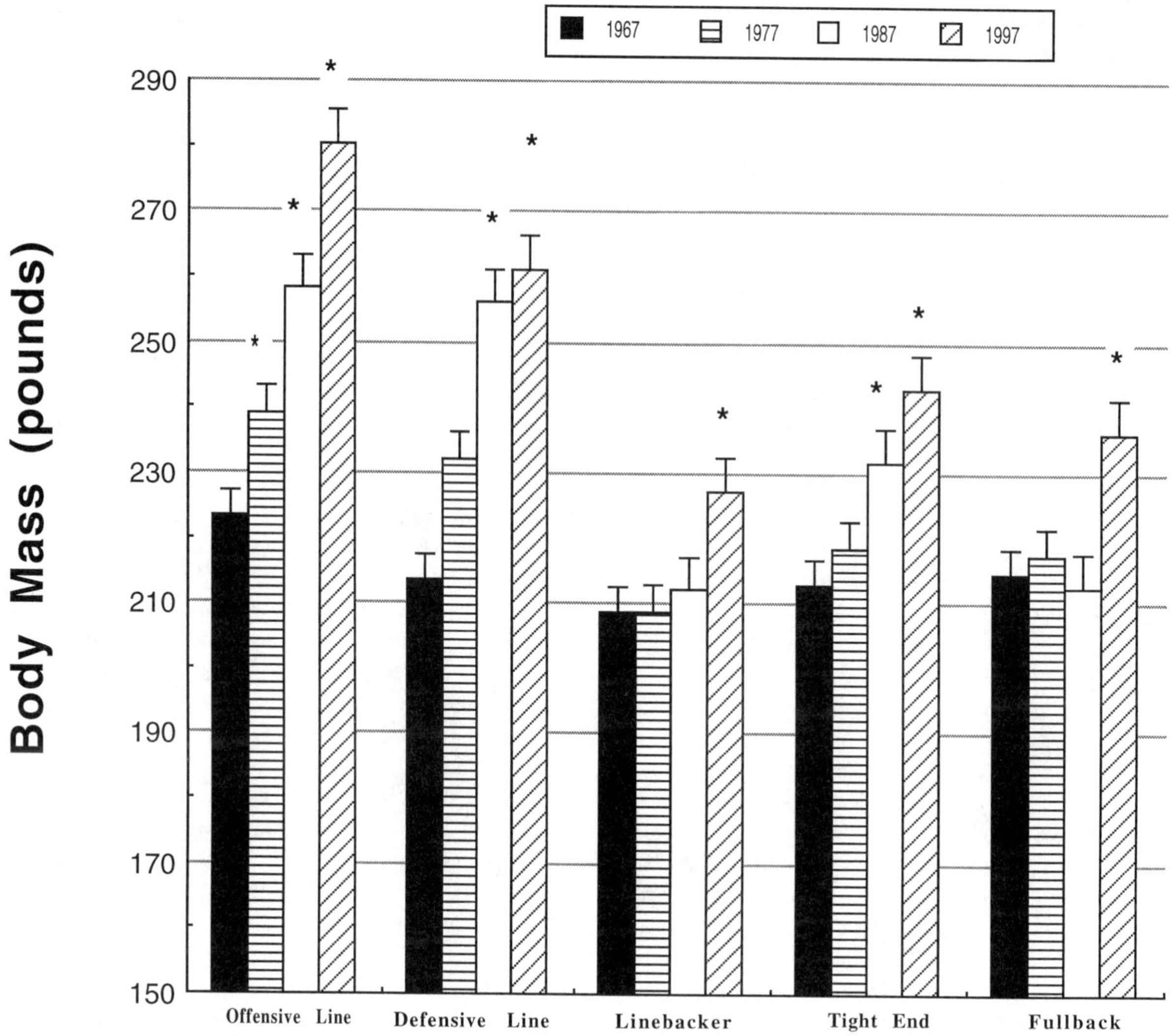

FIG. 51–2. Changes in body mass for Pennsylvania State football teams by position over 30 years. $^*p < .05$ from the corresponding 1967 value.

ment modifications. New frontiers in medical diagnostic testing [e.g., magnetic resonance imaging (MRI) scans of functional brain activity and damage] to evaluate player health, new equipment designs to offset impact forces (e.g., ProCap, a soft shell placed over or possibly integrated into normal helmet design), and better tools in physical training to allow the body to produce more force and help to develop tissues to be more resistant to damage (e.g., the Plyometrics Power system with computerized weight equipment to allow higher close kinetic-chain power movements without eccentric damage from landing) have all been pushed by the ever-changing face of the game. Our understanding of the impact of football on the physiologic system of the body remains speculative at best.

Speed and Quickness

Probably one of the biggest factors that separates level of play between high school and small college and major college and professional ranks is the speed of the game (1,4). The 40-yard (36.6-m) sprint has been the traditional "gold standard" of assessing speed in football players, although few players ever run this distance in a game. This is especially true for linemen. This distance is probably most important for many special team players, who routinely cover 40 to 60 yards on punts and kickoffs. As with many traditional beliefs in football, almost all professional scouts and most professional, collegiate, and high-school teams have used this test as a marker of football speed. In addition, it has been

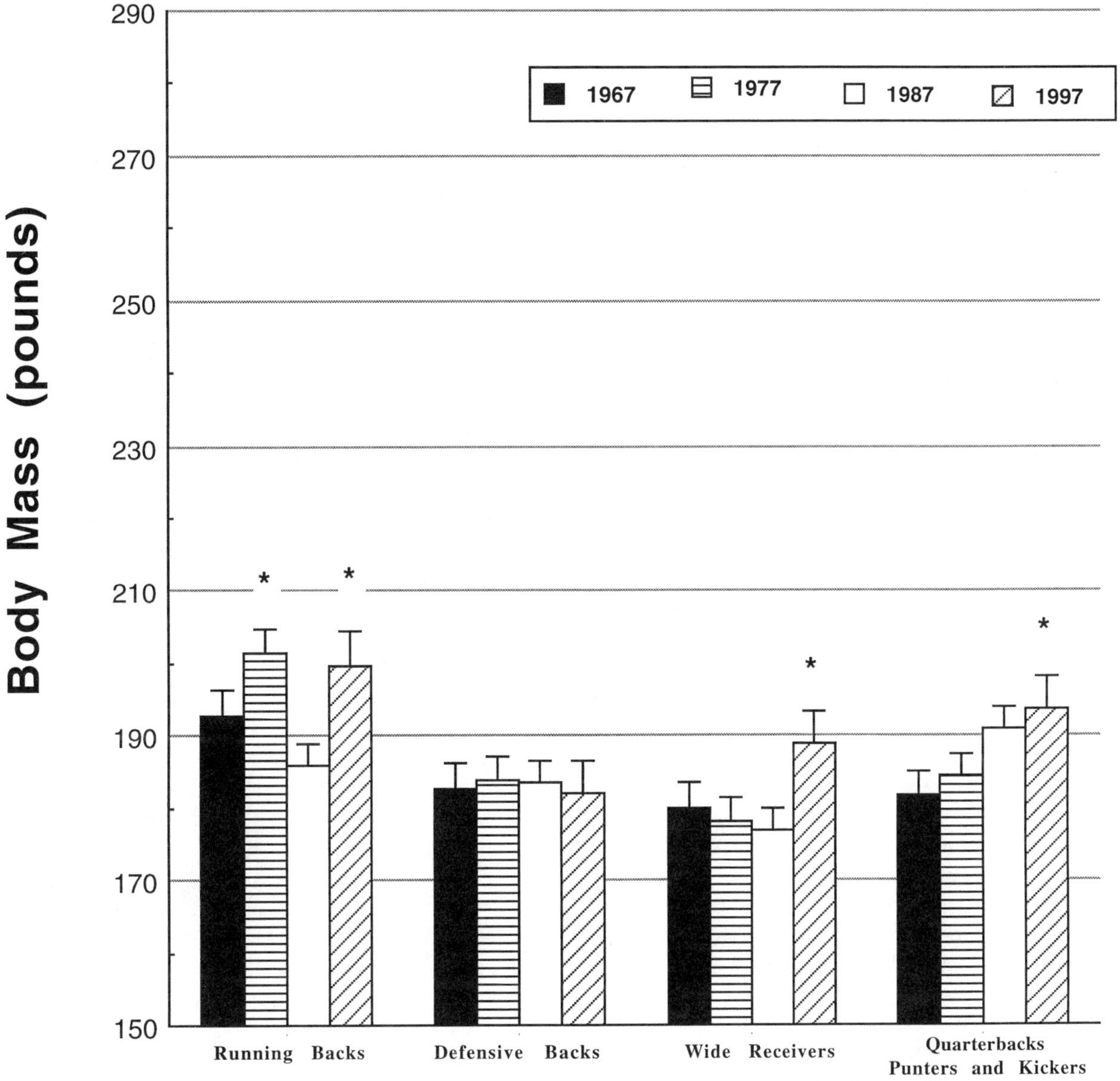

FIG. 51–3. Changes in body mass for Pennsylvania State football teams by position over 30 years. $*p < .05$ from the corresponding 1967 value.

assumed by many that it tests for quickness (i.e., reaction time). This concept was first studied in the late 1970s by Crews and Meadors (24), who investigated the relation among the 5-, 15-, and 40-yard sprints and reaction time. They discovered that there was only a low correlation between reaction time and 5-, 15-, and 40-yard sprint time, indicating that the physical abilities exhibited by performance in the 5-, 15-, and 40-yard sprints were not very dependent on reaction time. However, the 40-yard sprint time correlated highly with the 5- and 15-yard sprint times. The authors concluded that the 40-yard sprint time is representative of a football player's sprinting speed across various distances germane to football but that it was not an indication of the player's reaction time or quickness. This finding was later confirmed by Gotshalk (25), who electronically timed 129 football players for reaction time and 10-, 20-, 30-, and 40-yard sprint times and found that there was no significant correlation between reaction time and 40-yard sprint time. Only a moderate correlation between reaction time and 10-yard sprint time was observed. Gotshalk also found that there was about an 0.18-second difference between an electronically timed 40-yard sprint and the typical hand-held stopwatch times of 27 professional scouts of eight football players, with the electronic times being slower.

In a classic study, Manolis (26) also showed a low

negative correlation between sprinting speed and blocking ability (as determined by two types of scouting ratings), further separating the ability to sprint from the ability to block. Later, McDavid (27) concurred that blocking ability is influenced more by variables such as size, strength, agility, and power than by speed. The concept of quickness (rate of force development or power) of a skilled movement became a crucial factor in the success of a player to produce a more effective block and to gain the position advantage over the defensive opponent.

Strength and Power Capabilities In Football

In general, Fry and Kraemer (4) showed a general low-to-high continuum for various measures of power, strength, and speed in college football players from NCAA Division III to Division II to Division I. All teams studied (19 teams) performed similar conditioning programs by using standard lifts in the sport-conditioning process to make such analyses possible. The maximal performance in the power clean, bench press, and vertical jump differentiated most effectively between the divisions of play and playing ability on a specific team. The 40-yard sprint differentiated fairly well between playing ability (starter and nonstarter) but not well between divisions. The back squat differentiated poorly between playing ability and also divisions of play. These trends again appear to reflect the general recruiting trends, scholarship awards, conditioning emphasis, and competitive level of the team.

Gotshalk (25) observed that over a 10-year period, the second- and third-team players actually had a significantly higher mean bench press one-repetition maximum (1 RM) than the starters at all positions but showed slightly less strength in the 1-RM squat and significantly less in the maximal power clean, standing long jump, and standing vertical jump, along with the 40-yard sprint and reaction time. In combination, these findings point to the need for high speed and power to be successful in a team or in a league. Many of the conditioning strategies focused on these speed and power capabilities to prepare the football player's physical capabilities for performance on the field (4,20,28–34). Predicting football player success has been more complicated, however (4,35).

It is important to note that the development of power for football requires the use of exercises that promote closed-kinetic-chain mullet-joint power generation. In a study by Newton and colleagues (34), the use of "speed reps" in exercises in which the lifter holds on to the bar (bench press) or remains in contact with the mass (seated knee extensions) as it accelerates through the range of motion was shown to be ineffective, as the body protects a joint(s) by actually decelerating the mass through more than 40% of the range of motion, with a concomitant reduction in power generation and reduced activation of the agonists and increased activation of the antagonists. Thus, one must attempt to choose exercises that do not involve protective mechanisms for a joint(s) when trying to develop power. That is why exercises like plyometrics jumping and medicine-ball routines have gained greater popularity, along with the use of whole-body Olympic-style lifts (e.g., hang cleans from the knees) and other specialized resistance equipment that does not allow mass acceleration (e.g., isokinetic and pneumatic devices) and does not engage any of the

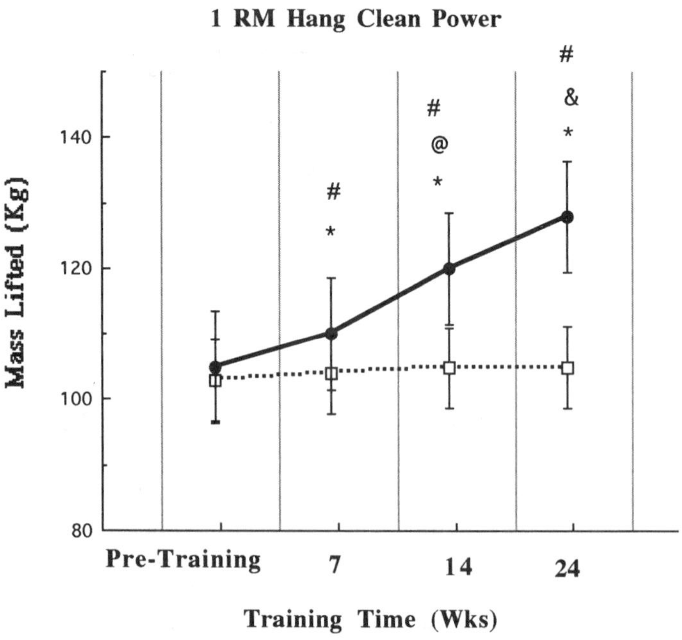

FIG. 51–4. Hang-clean power changes in mass lifted (mean ± SD) with two type of training in previously trained football players experienced in the test lift. *Boxes,* players who used a low-volume isolated-joint training program without explosive exercise movements; *solid circles,* players who used a periodized multijoint training program that included power cleans, pulls, and plyometrics. This study demonstrated the needed specificity for loaded power development in previously trained football players. No significant changes were observed for the players (*boxes*) who did not train with explosive methods and for the *solid circle* group. *$p < .05$ from corresponding pretraining value; @$p < .05$ from corresponding week 7 value; &$p < .05$ from corresponding week 14 value; #$p < .05$ from the corresponding value for the other training group. Data redrawn from ref. 20, with permission.

protective mechanisms used by the body to slow an accelerating mass to protect the joint(s) (34). Thus, the choice of exercises for strength versus power are quite different, and one cannot just lighten the weight and try to move the bar faster unless the exercise is appropriate (33).

Another striking fact about power in football is that many times the effective expression of muscle force is relegated to fractions of a second. Enhancement of the slow-velocity 1 RM strength is important for other physiologic adaptations and can contribute to the production of power, but it is only one part of the power equation. The time factor and distance factor must also be given consideration (31). The "rate of force development" becomes a very important factor for performance, and heavy slow lifting alone will not promote this improvement in the early phase of the force–time curve (31,33). In addition, using only isolated joint exercises (knee extensions, leg curls) will not result in power development in total body movements. In a study by Kraemer (20) (Fig. 51–4), it was shown that low-volume training using primarily isolated, open-chain, single-joint exercises did not contribute to whole-body power production in a closed-kinetic-chain hang pull movement over 6 months in already trained football players. Although strength is an important component of a program directed at improving the football player's physical abilities, the lack of inclusion of whole-body power exercises performed by using the closed kinetic chain (power cleans, pulls, etc.) can be detrimental to whole-body power development (20). Because power development is so vital for football success, the myth of just developing strength and then practicing the sport is not going to optimize the physical abilities of players to meet the ever-increasing demands for strength, speed, and power on the field.

TRAINING THE ATHLETE

Periodization of Strength and Conditioning for Football

Periodization of training was a concept originally developed in the former Soviet Union and Eastern Bloc countries and has been adapted by strength and conditioning specialists for American sports, including football (20,33). The beauty of this concept is that no one workout has to be the same, and systematic variation can be used to provide rest and recovery from the training stresses. The programs outlined in this chapter allow one to see a basic framework of a program adapted to the scheduling of an American university football team and should be viewed as a starting point for ideas to be crafted by professional and factual judgments of one's own situation. The needs of the game are reflected in the development of the (a) choice of exercises, (b) order of exercises, (c) rest periods used, (d) number of sets, and (e) resistance used in the exercise (33).

Obviously the use of a physical-conditioning program in football is essential to the optimal development of the physical capabilities needed to compete. The need for communication and interaction among "strength coaches" was realized in the early 1970s, not only for football but also for all other sports. In 1978 the National Strength and Conditioning (then Coaches) Association (NSCA) was founded in Lincoln, Nebraska. This organization has from the start been dedicated to "bridging the gap" between the scientist and the strength coach practitioner in the field. Nevertheless, the science of conditioning and sport have many times been uneasy companions because of the superstition, mythology, corporate influences, and coaching pressures to win, which have ignored the facts involved with the development of scientific approaches to conditioning football players (20). The importance of a solid strength and conditioning program to success at the highest level of play can be seen in the statements by Tim Green (1).

> I had the opportunity to train under Mike [Woicik] during my four years as a player at Syracuse University. During that time, Mike turned me from a two-hundred-and twenty-five pound high school kid into a two hundred and fifty pound first round draft choice. My time in the forty-yard dash went dropped [sic] from 4.85 to 4.58 . That's how I ended up in the first round. My bench press went from 325 to 425. My squat went from 450 to 700. My vertical jump went from 27 to 34 inches. All these physical gains enabled me to get more quarterback sacks than anyone in the NCAA history with the exception of Hugh Green from Pittsburgh. Woicik made it happen for me. He made it happen for our team at Syracuse, then he made it happen for the Cowboys. . . . People used to think Mike was crazy. Gruff and grumbling, he had more in common with a Soviet scientist than an NFL weight coach. In fact he used all the Soviet's latest training methods in making his football players the best they could be. He is as zealous in his commitment to plyometrics training, a series of jumping exercises used to increase explosiveness. . . . Mike is, and always was adamant in his stance against the use of any kind of performance drugs, most especially steroids. He figured a way to make incredible physical gains without the use of dangerous substances so many other weight coaches were pushing in the 1980's. . . . Because football is and always will be a game of strength, speed, and explosiveness, that move [to keep Woicik] was more important to the Cowboys organization than signing Deion Sanders.

The primary purpose of the basic design for a football strength and conditioning program is to increase overall physical capabilities of football players along with reducing the potential for injuries. It is important to understand that in training football players, the "pretraining" status of the players will affect the amount of development that can be expected with just short-term training. Thus mistakes in exercise prescription can lead to little or no changes (20). Individualized and periodized training is vital for development, as noted above. Zemper (32) has shown that injuries in the weight room are very low despite the use of many advanced forms of lifting (e.g., squats, power cleans). In football, too often coaches are not schooled in the science of strength and conditioning and thus can be convinced of the efficacy of a particular system based on factors other than physical development. Yet resistance training is capable of training only four specific characteristics of skeletal muscle: (a) strength (maximal dynamic or static force produced by a muscle or muscle group), (b) power (rate of force development) under different load conditions, (c) local muscular endurance (the ability to produce repetitive muscle actions under different load conditions), and (d) hypertrophy (the increase in muscle size). In addition, periodization of conditioning programs is essential to provide rest and recovery from exercise stress (20,33). The biggest difference in the various NCAA divisions of competition is the presence or lack of "spring practice." Division III schools, despite having a distinct recruiting disadvantage, have had a distinct advantage for physical development of their players because they have no interruptions in physical-conditioning programs or injuries due to spring football drills and scrimmages. Another recent rule change by the NCAA placed limitations on supervised training time in the weight room. This has put undue pressures on conditioning coaches because of the desires of the unit coaches to have more time for practice. Thus, many times "systems" have promoted conditioning concepts and programs that are not based on scientific facts but rather on posturing of "time economy" for needed training effects.

Information accrued from position coaches on a player's strengths and weaknesses at his position, athletic trainers overviewing injury problems, and strength and conditioning testing data are all important pieces of information for the year-to-year development of the overall program and for subtle program-design changes of an individual player's program. Ultimately each program must be individualized, as that is the ultimate program for a player. A chart (paper or computer file) should be kept for each player, with the general program design and the player's personal specifications detailed, along with the charting of the actual performances. Today it is easy to keep information on computer that can profile in detail all of the collected information on a particular player.

The prespring and preseason training programs are essentially identical in design, because the preseason (or summer) training program many times is unsupervised; only the players who stay on campus or in the area have supervision over the summer. Thus, a detailed day-to-day program is given to all players when they leave for the summer. The players should be educated as to the nature and reasoning behind the strength and conditioning programs used over the year. Each player should be able to keep training charts during the summer and should have strength and conditioning staff periodically review the charts and give feedback and encouragement. During the year, workouts are supervised

The yearly training schedule macrocycle can be divided into two similar mesocycles, the first beginning after the first week of the year and terminating when spring practice ends at the end of April. Preliminary testing of power, strength, aerobic and anaerobic fitness, anthropometry, and flexibility is conducted before the mesocycle starts, and posttesting is conducted during the four days before spring practice. The second mesocycle begins after the second week in May and ends at the start of the season in late August. Testing for the parameters listed above should be again conducted during the 4 days before fall camp practice, begun after the first week in August.

Each mesocycle is divided into four microcycles and ends with two microcycles. The first microcycle is a 3-week preparation cycle, reintroducing the athletes to training protocol and exercise techniques. The second microcycle is a 4-week hypertrophy cycle, its prime goal being increase in muscular cross-sectional area and basic strength. The third microcycle is a 3-week strength cycle, incorporating the use of heavier resistance. The fourth microcycle is a 3-week power cycle, focusing on Olympic-style lifts and attempted quick movements against resistance. After the power cycle is completed, there is a week of recovery in which the major muscle groups are trained but only with very light weights. Testing is usually performed during the latter part of this week. The next 2 or 3 weeks consist of in-season spring-practice maintenance training to keep strength and power increased with a minimal amount of time and effort.

Program Design: Strength and Conditioning Program for Football

The program design shown here was developed for a college football team. As shown in Tables 51–2 through 51–13, the general program design through all cycles is set up to emphasize lower-body training on Monday and Thursday and upper-body training on Tuesday and Friday. Speed and plyometrics training are conducted on Wednesday. Also shown in Tables 51–2 through 51–6 is a subtle differentiation between the general program for running backs, linebackers, wide receivers, and defensive backs, as compared with offensive linemen, defensive linemen, and tight ends, predicated on the task of the position (Tables 51–7 through 51–13). Although a general program can be followed, close monitoring and changes in the program should be made for the needs of each individual athlete as he develops, and strengths and weaknesses are analyzed. Each year the physical abilities of each athlete should be tested, and goals should be formulated according to the athlete's needs

TABLE 51–2. *Three-week preparation cycle*

Monday	Tuesday	Wednesday	Thursday	Friday
Squat 3 × 8	Bench press 3 × 8	Plyometric program	Hang-pull clean 4 × 5	Incline bench press 3 × 8
Straight leg deadlift 3 × 12	Front pull-down 3 × 12		Front squat 3 × 8	Chin-up 3 × 12
Leg extension 3 × 12	Push press 3 × 8		Straight leg deadlift 3 × 12	Dumbbell press 3 × 8
Leg curl 3 × 12	DB row 3 × 12		Heel raise 3 × 15	Seated row 3 × 12
Heel raise 3 × 15	Parallel bar dip 3 × 10–20		Medicine ball sit-up 3 × 15	Overhead dumbbell triceps extension 3 × 12
Alternating sit-ups 3 × 20	Curl 3 × 12		Alternating crunch 2 × 20	Preacher curl 3 × 12
Crunch 1 × 20	Neck 4-way 3 × 10		Stretch routine	Neck 4-way 3 × 10
Stretch routine	Stretch routine			Humeral rotation, med./lat. 3 × 10
				Stretch routine

Football winter training program: running backs, linebackers, wide receivers, and defensive backs.

TABLE 51–3. *Four-week hypertrophy cycle*

Monday	Tuesday	Wednesday	Thursday	Friday
Squat 4 × 5	Bench press 4 × 5	Plyometric program	Hang-pull clean 4 × 5	Dumbbell bench press 3 × 5
Straight leg deadlift 3 × 12	Towel chin-up 3 × 8+		Front squat 3 × 8	Lat pull-down 3 × 8
Dumbbell lunge 3 × 8	Press 3 × 5		Romanian abs deadlift 3 × 8	Dumbbell press 3 × 5
Leg curl 3 × 10	DB row 3 × 8		Heel raise 3 × 12	Seated row 3 × 8
Heel raise 3 × 12	Parallel bar dip 3 × 10–20		Medicine ball sit-up 3 × 15	Overhead dumbbell triceps extension 3 × 8
Weighted sit-ups 3 × 10	Curl 3 × 8		Alternating crunch 2 × 25	Preacher curl 3 × 8
Crunch 2 × 30	Neck 4-way 3 × 10		Stretch routine	Neck 4-way 3 × 10
Stretch routine	Stretch routine			Humeral rotation, med./lat. 3 × 10
				Stretch routine

Football winter training program: running backs, linebackers, wide receivers, and defensive backs.

TABLE 51–4. *Three-week strength cycle*

Monday	Tuesday	Wednesday	Thursday	Friday
Hanging power clean 4 × 3	Bench press 4 × 3	Plyometric program	Power clean 4 × 3	Bench press 3 × 5
Squat 4 × 3	Towel chin-up 3 × 8+		Hanging snatch 3 × 5	Towel chin-up 3 × 8+
Push jerk 3 × 5	DB row 3 × 5		Dumbbell step-up squat 3 × 5	Dumbbell press 3 × 5
Romanian deadlift 3 × 5	Upright row 3 × 8		Dumbbell oblique lunge 3 × 5	Seated row 3 × 8
Dumbbell lunge 3 × 5	Narrow grip bench press 3 × 5		Medicine ball abdominal 3 × 20	Overhead dumbbell triceps extension 3 × 8
Weighted sit-ups 3 × 10	Curl 3 × 5		Crunch 1 × 50	Preacher curl 3 × 8
Crunch 2 × 50	Neck 4-way 3 × 8		Stretch routine	Humeral rotation, med./lat. 3 × 10
Stretch routine	Humeral rotation, med./lat. 3 × 10			Neck 4-way 3 × 8
	Stretch routine			Stretch routine

Football winter training program: running backs, linebackers, wide receivers, and defensive backs.

TABLE 51–5. *Three-week power cycle*

Monday	Tuesday	Wednesday	Thursday	Friday
Power clean pull 5 × 3 Dumbbell step-up 3 × 5 Weighted back extension 3 × 8 Medicine ball sit and throw 3 × 10 Alternating crunch 3 × 20 Stretch routine	Push jerk 5 × 3 Dumbbell bench 3 × 5 Towel chin-up 3 × 10+ Dumbbell upright 3 × 8 Dumbbell row 3 × 8 Triceps pushdown 3 × 5 Curl 3 × 5 Neck 4-way 3 × 6 Stretch routine	Plyometric program	Hanging snatch 5 × 3 Hanging power clean pull 3 × 3 Dumbbell oblique lunge 3 × 5 Medicine ball twist 3 × 10 Crunch 3 × 20 Stretch routine	Dumbbell incline 3 × 5 Decline pull-down 3 × 8 Weighted dip 3 × 5 Dumbbell upright row 3 × 5 Curl 3 × 5 Neck 4-way 3 × 6 Stretch routine

Football winter training program: running backs, linebackers, wide receivers, and defensive backs.

TABLE 51–6. *One-week unload cycle*

Monday	Tuesday	Wednesday	Thursday	Friday
Squat 2 × 5 Romanian deadlift 2 × 5 Weighted sit-up 2 × 15 Stretch routine	Bench press 2 × 5 Seated row 2 × 8 Dumbbell press 2 × 5 Pull-down 2 × 8 Stretch routine	Stretch routine	Squat 2 × 8 Leg extension 2 × 8 Leg curl 2 × 8 Alternating crunch 2 × 25 Stretch routine	Incline press 2 × 8 Decline pull-down 2 × 8 Dip 2 × 10 Curl 2 × 10 Stretch routine

Football winter training program: running backs, linebackers, wide receivers, and defensive backs.

TABLE 51–7. *Two-week spring football in-season cycle*

Monday	Tuesday	Wednesday	Thursday	Friday
Hanging clean 3 × 3 Dumbbell step-up 3 × 5 Weighted back extension 3 × 5 Crunch 3 × 25 Stretch routine	Dumbbell bench press 3 × 5 Dumbbell row 3 × 5 Upright row 3 × 5 Overhead dumbbell triceps extension 3 × 8 Stretch routine		Hanging snatch 3 × 3 Dumbbell lunge 3 × 5 Medicine ball seated twist 3 × 15 Stretch routine	Dumbbell press 3 × 5 Towel chin-up 3 × 8+ Dip 3 × 10 Preacher curl 3 × 8 Stretch routine

Football training program: running backs, linebackers, wide receivers, and defensive backs.

TABLE 51–8. *Three-week preparation cycle*

Monday	Tuesday	Wednesday	Thursday	Friday
Full squat 3 × 8 Straight leg deadlift 3 × 12 Leg extension 3 × 12 Leg curl 3 × 12 Heel raise 3 × 15 Alternating sit-ups 3 × 20 Crunch 1 × 20 Stretch routine	Bench press 3 × 8 Front pulldown 3 × 12 Press 3 × 8 DB row 3 × 12 Parallel bar dip 3 × 10–20 Curl 3 × 12 Neck 4-way 3 × 10 Stretch routine	Plyometric program	Hanging power clean 4 × 5 Front squat 3 × 8 Straight leg deadlift 3 × 12 Heel raise 3 × 15 Medicine ball sit-up 3 × 15 Alternating crunch 2 × 20 Stretch routine	Incline bench press 3 × 8 Chin-up 3 × 12 Dumbbell press 3 × 8 Seated row 3 × 12 Overhead dumbbell triceps extension 3 × 12 Preacher curl 3 × 12 Neck 4-way 3 × 10 Humeral rotation, med./lat. 3 × 10 Stretch routine

Football winter training program: offensive linemen, defensive linemen, tight ends.

TABLE 51–9. *Four-week hypertrophy cycle*

Monday	Tuesday	Wednesday	Thursday	Friday
Power squat 4 × 5 High full extension pull 3 × 5 Dumbbell lunge 3 × 8 Leg curl 3 × 10 Heel raise 3 × 12 Weighted sit-ups 3 × 10 Crunch 2 × 30 Stretch routine	Bench press 4 × 5 Front pull-down 3 × 8 Press 3 × 5 DB row 3 × 8 Parallel bar dip 3 × 10 Curl 3 × 8 Neck 4-way 3 × 10 Stretch routine	Plyometric program	Hanging power clean 4 × 5 Frong squat 3 × 8 Romanian deadlift 3 × 8 Heel raise 3 × 12 Medicine ball sit-up 3 × 15 Alternating crunch 2 × 25 Stretch routine	Narrow bench press 3 × 5 Lat pulldown 3 × 8 Push press 3 × 5 Seated row 3 × 8 Triceps pushdown extension 3 × 8 Curl 3 × 8 Neck 4-way 3 × 10 Humeral rotation, med./lat. 3 × 10 Stretch routine

Football winter training program: offensive linemen, defensive linemen, tight ends.

TABLE 51–10. *Three-week strength cycle*

Monday	Tuesday	Wednesday	Thursday	Friday
Hanging power clean 4 × 3 Power squat 4 × 3 Romanian deadlift 3 × 5 Dumbbell lunge 3 × 5 Weighted sit-ups 3 × 10 Abdominal 3 × 20 Stretch routine	Bench press 4 × 3 Front pull-down 3 × 8 Push jerk 3 × 5 DB row 3 × 5 Upright row 3 × 8 Triceps extension bench press 3 × 5 Curl 3 × 5 Lat. 3 × 10 Humeral rotation, med./lat. 3 × 10 Stretch routine	Plyometric program	Power clean 4 × 3 Hanging snatch 3 × 5 Dumbbell step-up squat 3 × 5 Dumbbell oblique lunge 3 × 5 Medicine ball Crunch 1 × 50 Stretch routine	Narrow bench press 3 × 5 Decline pull-down 3 × 8 Dumbbell press 3 × 5 Seated row 3 × 8 Overhead dumbbell triceps extension 3 × 8 Preacher curl 3 × 8 Neck 4-way 3 × 8 Humeral rotation, med./lat. 3 × 10 Crunch 2 × 50 Neck 4-way 3 × 8 Stretch routine

Football winter training program: offensive linemen, defensive linemen, tight ends.

TABLE 51–11. *Three-week power cycle*

Monday	Tuesday	Wednesday	Thursday	Friday
Power clean pull 5 × 3 Dumbbell step-up 3 × 5 Weighted back extension 3 × 8 Medicine ball sit and throw 3 × 10 Alternating crunch 3 × 20 Stretch routine	Push jerk 5 × 3 Dumbbell bench 3 × 5 Towel chin-up 3 × 10+ Dumbbell upright 3 × 8 Dumbbell row 3 × 8 Triceps push-down 3 × 5 Curl 3 × 5 Neck 4-way 3 × 6 Stretch routine	Plyometric program	Hanging snatch 5 × 3 Hanging power clean pull 3 × 3 Dumbbell oblique lunge 3 × 5 Medicine ball twist 3 × 10 Crunch 3 × 20 Stretch routine	Dumbbell incline 3 × 5 Decline pull-down 3 × 8 Weighted dip 3 × 5 Dumbbell upright row 3 × 5 Curl 3 × 5 Neck 4-way 3 × 6 Stretch routine

Football winter training program: offensive linemen, defensive linemen, tight ends.

TABLE 51–12. *One-week unload cycle*

Monday	Tuesday	Wednesday	Thursday	Friday
Squat 2 × 5 Romanian deadlift 2 × 5 Weighted sit-up 2 × 15 Stretch routine	Bench press 2 × 5 Seated row 2 × 8 Dumbbell press 2 × 5 Pull-down 2 × 8 Stretch routine	Stretch routine	Squat 2 × 8 Leg extension 2 × 8 Leg curl 2 × 8 Alternating crunch 2 × 25 Stretch routine	Incline press 2 × 8 Decline pull-down 2 × 8 Dip 2 × 10 Curl 2 × 10 Stretch routine

Football winter training program: offensive linemen, defensive linemen, tight ends.

on the playing field. The needs for "priority attention" of training should be determined. For example, athletes who had developed great hip and leg strength in the squat but were lacking in comparative hip and leg power should shift in emphasis to the Olympic-style lifts and a deemphasis of the squat. Athletes with reasonable upper-body strength and power but lacking in lower-body strength and power would have a shift in emphasis in their programs as well. Training priorities should be used and testing should be conducted to determine whether the program is successful. Programs that do not test have no real facts or data on which to base changes in the program, and they cannot individualize any conditioning protocols.

Exercise Emphasis

The core exercises of all cycles and all training days should be large muscle group, multijoint free-weight exercises to benefit from synergistic muscle-group incorporation and neuromuscular demands that free-weight exercises require. Free-weight multijoint exercises should be emphasized over machine training, and closed-kinetic-chain exercises emphasized over open-kinetic-chain exercises. Any machine exercise should be used for "isolation" of specific body parts. Dumbbells and unilateral exercises such as lunges should be incorporated to make sure that the players are strong and powerful, with the use of single limbs, as many football skills are dependent on a single-limb support or contact. Besides the core strength exercises such as the squat and bench press, and the core power exercises such as the Olympic-style lifts, the program should incorporate myriad "antagonistic" exercises such as chin-ups, rows, pull-downs, curls, and abdominal exercises, to train opposing muscle groups to develop and maintain joint balance, flexibility, and suppleness. The prime purpose of the abdominal exercises, humeral rotation exercises, and neck exercises is to increase resistance to and reduce the probability of injury.

Resistance, Repetitions, and Rest

Training volume and intensity can be continuously manipulated by the shifting of amount of resistance, number of sets, repetitions, and rest periods between sets. Each cycle's volume and intensity depend on the resistance, sets, and repetitions. The classic cycles for a program are as follows (33).

Preparation Cycle

The preparation cycle represents a high-volume, low-intensity cycle. The core exercises of the preparation cycle are performed for eight repetitions with 70% of the one repetition maximum (1 RM). Secondary exercises are generally performed for 12 repetitions, with some exceptions. Two-minute rests are taken between sets and exercises. Warm-up exercises are performed in

TABLE 51–13. *Two-week spring football in-season cycle*

Monday	Tuesday	Wednesday	Thursday	Friday
Hanging clean 3 × 3 Power squat 3 × 5 Romanian deadlift 3 × 5 Crunch 3 × 25 Stretch routine	Narrow bench bench 3 × 5 Dumbbell row 3 × 5 Upright row 3 × 5 Overhead dumbell triceps extension 3 × 8 Stretch routine		Hanging snatch 3 × 3 Dumbbell lunge 3 × 5 Medicine ball seated twist 3 × 15 Stretch routine	Bench press 3 × 5 Pull-down 3 × 5 Dumbbell press 3 × 10 Preacher curl 3 × 8 Stretch routine

Football winter training program: offensive linemen, defensive linemen, tight ends.

the core exercises, with the last warm-up performed with 80% of the first main set. The heaviest main set is performed first, and 5 pounds (sometimes 10, with strong athletes) dropped from each of the ensuing two sets. Usually no weight is dropped from the secondary exercises.

Hypertrophy Cycle

This cycle represents a medium-volume, medium-intensity cycle. The core exercises are performed for five repetitions with about 85% of maximum. Secondary exercises are generally performed for eight repetitions, again with exceptions. Ninety-second rest periods are used between sets and exercises. The last warm-up for the core exercises is performed with 85% of the first main set. The heaviest main set is performed first, and 5 pounds (sometimes 10, with strong athletes) dropped from each of the ensuing two sets. Usually no weight is dropped from the secondary exercises.

Strength Cycle

This cycle represents medium-low volume and medium-high intensity. The core exercises are performed for three repetitions with about 95% to 100% of the previous maximum (depending on the individual athlete's progress). Secondary exercises are generally performed for five repetitions. Three minutes of rest are taken between sets and exercises, with the exception of secondary truly antagonistic exercises (such as the overhead dumbbell triceps extension/preacher curl exercises), which are supersetted (alternated) with the first exercise and repeated 3 minutes apart.

Power Cycle

This cycle represents a low-volume, high-intensity cycle. The Olympic-style exercises are performed for three repetitions with an attempt at 3 RM for each set. Four minutes of rest are taken between sets of the Olympic-style exercises. For the rest of the workout, five repetitions for the core sets and eight repetitions (with exceptions) for the secondary exercises are supersetted, with the first exercise repeated 3 minutes apart. The mindset for most of the exercises should be that of "power," with the athletes attempting to complete each repetition as quickly as possible. It is important to note that recent findings have shown that "speed reps" cannot be performed by using exercises in which the athlete builds up momentum and has to stop at the end or the range of motion (e.g., bench press, knee extension), as these types of exercises do not build power. In such movements, medicine-ball exercises in which the mass can be released at the end of the range of motion are superior for power development (34).

Unload Week

The exercises are performed with 67% of maximum and with 90-second rest periods. Often testing would commence on the Saturday of this week, and so Wednesday, Thursday, and Friday would be used as rest days.

Spring-Practice Weeks

The exercises are performed with about 80% of maximum for three repetitions for the core exercises and five repetitions for the secondary exercises, with 2 minutes of rest between sets. The workout is usually performed early in the day, preceding the practice by half the day, and is completed in less than 30 minutes.

Football Preseason Conditioning (Non–Weight-Training Activities) Program

The running program begins 10 weeks before the preseason camp and is conducted concurrently with the strength, power, and flexibility training. It is important that the running program mimic the game but not be a long-distance training program, as this can negatively affect power and speed development (36–39). The concept of an "aerobic base" also is not related to the facts, as one can develop aerobic capabilities by using interval-type training programs, and there are low relationships between aerobic and anaerobic fitness levels (16,30). The running program is periodized, with the first 2 weeks introducing the players to general cardiovascular conditioning and slow striding; the next 2 weeks introducing long strides and plyometrics; and, in the fifth week, introducing the pride drill, an anaerobic workout consisting of a series of all-out sprints with a 30-second rest period (mimicking a game situation) between each sprint. Agility drills are included to provide the athletes with exercises for balance, quickness of foot, response to visual stimuli, and coordination. The last few weeks before camp accentuate the pride drill, the plyometrics program, and the agility drills. The pride drill is used in camp to test the athlete's aerobic/anaerobic capacities. The performance is scored by the overall time of completion of the drill. Rest time between sprints is determined by the time necessary for an athlete's heart rate to return to 120 beats/min, the point at which the athlete starts the next sprint. An athlete who does not reach the prescribed time (by position) or less of any sprint must repeat that particular sprint. Speed development must be looked at over a longer period than just 7 to 10 weeks, as players who are already trained do not see dramatic changes with short-term programs (40).

Plyometrics

Plyometrics (stretch–shortening cycle movements) are drills designed to combine power, speed, and strength

TABLE 51–14. *Example conditioning program*

Weeks 1–2

Mon. and Fri. Distance run

Warmup; Jog $\frac{1}{4}$ mile

10 strides, 40 yards, $\frac{2}{3}$ speed

Stretch routine

Distance run: run 1.5 miles with the following goals:

OL,DL	12:00 min
K,P	11:00 min
QB,ILB	10:30 min
OLB,FB,TE	10:00 min
DB,RB	9:30 min
WR	9:00 min

Striders: 10 × 10 yd, $\frac{1}{2}$ to $\frac{2}{3}$ speed

Postexercise cool down: $\frac{1}{4}$ mile walk–jog

Stretch routine

Wed. Interval striders

Warmup; Jog $\frac{1}{4}$ mile

10 strides, 40 yards, $\frac{2}{3}$ speed

Stretch routine

Interval running: 12 × 110 yd at $\frac{3}{4}$ speed (on track, 30-s walk between striders) Postexercise cool down: $\frac{1}{4}$ mile walk–jog. Stretch routine

Weeks 3–4

Mon. and Fri. Long sprint training

Warmup; Jog $\frac{1}{4}$ mile

10 strides, 40 yards, $\frac{2}{3}$ speed

Stretch routine

Running drill: Long sprints (30-s walk between sprints)

5 × 220 yd

4 × 160 yd

3 × 100 yd

Agility:

6	40-yd carioca
5	30-s 5-yd lateral reaction drill (wave drill)
5	20-yd backward sprint

Thur. Short spring training

Warmup; Jog $\frac{1}{4}$ mile

10 strides, 40 yards, $\frac{2}{3}$ speed

Stretch routine

Full-speed sprint: 10 sprints, 40 yd, alternated with 10 sprints, 20 yd (30-s walk between sprints)

Postexercise cool down: $\frac{1}{4}$ mile walk–jog

Stretch routine

Wed. Plyometrics drills

OL,DL,ILB,TE

1. Single knees	4 × 20 yd (15-sec. rest)
2. Single heels	4 × 20 yd (15-sec. rest)
3. Double high knees	3 × 10 reps (1-min. rest)
4. Double high heels	3 × 10 reps (1-min. rest)
5. Squat jumps	2 × 10 reps (1-min. rest)
6. Lunge walks	2 × 20 yd (30-sec. rest)

DB,WR,RB,OLB,QB,K,P

1. Single knees	4 × 20 yd (15-s rest)
2. Single heels	4 × 20 yd (15-s rest)
3. Single leg hops	3 × 30 yd (2-min rest)
4. Double leg hops	3 × 30 yd (2-min rest)
5. Lateral jump	2 × 10 reps (1-min rest)
6. Russian hops	2 × 10 reps (1-min rest)

Weeks 5–7

Mon. and Fri. Sprint training

Warmup; jog $\frac{1}{4}$ mile

10 strides, 40 yards, $\frac{2}{3}$ speed

Stretch routine

TABLE 51–14. *Continued*

- Running drill: pride drill (30-s walk between sprints)

Sets	Distance	DB,WR,RB	QB,K,TE,LB	OL,DL
8	100 yd	14–16 s	15–17 s	16–18 s
6	80	10–12	11–13	12–14
5	60	8–10	9–11	10–12
4	40	6–7	7–8	8–9

- Agility
  - 5 20-yd carioca
  - 4 30-s 5-yd lateral reaction drill (wave drill)
  - 4 20-yd backward sprint
  - 5 10-yd starts
- Postexercise cool down: $\frac{1}{4}$ mile walk–jog
- Stretch routine

Tue. and Thur. Stadium fartlek
- Warmup; jog $\frac{1}{4}$ mile
  - 10 strides, 40 yards, $\frac{2}{3}$ speed
  - Stretch routine
- Stadium fartlek: 30 min of slow jogging on the horizontal surfaces and declining steps, and all-out sprinting up the inclining steps (two steps at a time)
- Postexercise cool down: $\frac{1}{4}$ mile walk–jog
  - Stretch routine

Wed. Plyometrics drills
- OL,DL,ILB,TE
  1. Single knees — 4 × 20 yd (15-s rest)
  2. Single heels — 4 × 20 yd (15-s rest)
  3. Double high knees — 3 × 10 reps (1-min rest)
  4. Double high heels — 3 × 10 reps (1-min rest)
  5. Squat jumps — 2 × 10 reps (1-min rest)
  6. Lujnge walks — 2 × 20 yd (30-s rest)
- DB,WR,RB,OLB,QB,K,P
  1. Single knees — 4 × 20 yd (15-s rest)
  2. Single heels — 4 × 20 yd (15-s rest)
  3. Single leg hops — 3 × 30 yd (2-min rest)
  4. Double leg hops — 3 × 30 yd (2-min rest)
  5. Lateral jump — 2 × 10 reps (1-min. rest)
  6. Russian hops — 2 × 10 reps (1-min rest)

Weeks 8–10

Mon., Wed., Fri. Sprint training
- Warmup; jog $\frac{1}{4}$ mile
  - 10 strides, 40 yards, $\frac{2}{3}$ speed
  - Stretch routine
- Running drill: pride drill (30-s walk between sprints)

Sets	Distance	DB,WR,RB	QB,K,TE,LB	OL,DL
10	100 yd	14–16 s	15–17 s	16–18 s
8	80	10–12	11–13	12–14
6	60	8–10	9–11	10–12
4	40	6–7	7–8	8–9

- Agility:
  - 6 20-yd carioca
  - 5 30-s 5-yd lateral reaction drill (wave drill)
  - 4 20-yd backward sprint
- Postexercise cool down: $\frac{1}{4}$ mile walk–jog
  - Stretch routine

Thur. Plyometrics drills
- OL,DL,ILB,TE
  1. Single knees — 4 × 20 yd (15-s rest)
  2. Single heels — 4 × 20 yd (15-s rest)
  3. Double high knees — 3 × 10 reps (1-min rest)
  4. Double high heels — 3 × 10 reps (1-min rest)
  5. Squat jumps — 2 × 10 reps (1-min rest)
  6. Lunge walks — 2 × 20 yd (30-s rest)
- DB,WR,RB,OLB,QB,K,P
  1. Single knees — 4 × 20 yd (15-s rest)
  2. Single heels — 4 × 20 yd (15-s rest)
  3. Single leg hops — 3 × 30 yd (2-min rest)
  4. Double leg hops — 3 × 30 yd (2-min rest)
  5. Lateral jump — 2 × 10 reps (1-min rest)
  6. Russian hops — 2 × 10 reps (1-min rest)

OL, offensive linesman; DL, defensive linesman; K, kicker; P, punter; QB, quarterback; ILB, inside linebacker; OLB, outside linebacker; FB, fullback; TE, tight end; DB, defensive back; RB, running back; WR, wide receiver.

to produce an explosive–reactive movement. Important points to consider are the following:

1. Progress from simple movements to more complex ones.
2. Use the proper rest intervals that are given for each exercise.
3. Perform on a soft surface (grass is preferred to Astroturf).
4. To prevent injury, never perform plyometrics in a fatigued state, because each repetition requires maximal force.
5. Do not do plyometrics on consecutive days.
6. Use proper technique and maximal output with each repetition.
7. Wear proper, stable footwear with a good arch support and no lateral give.
8. Do only the prescribed number of sets and repetitions: quality, not quantity.
9. Walk or stretch out during the rest interval to speed the recovery process.
10. Do plyometrics before running or other large-muscle-group activities.

The following is an explanation of specific plyometrics exercises:

1. Single knees: A warm-up drill. Pick knees up one at a time as high as possible and as rapidly as possible, with a coordinated pumping action of the arms.
2. Single heels: A warm-up drill. Heels are kicked to the buttocks one at a time as rapidly as possible while the knees stay down, with a coordinated pumping action of the arms.
3. Double high knees: Both knees are tucked up to the chest while jumping as high as possible. As soon as the feet touch the ground, explode back up into the next jump tucking the knees up to the chest again. The arms swing upward with each jump.

CONCLUSION

The game of football in the United States continues to grow in popularity as a spectator sport. In addition, players are becoming bigger, stronger, faster, and more powerful. The physiologic demands of the game have been highly influenced by official rule changes and football strategies to gain competitive advantages on the field. Our understanding of the game itself and its effects on the body are limited at times to speculation, as no studies have looked at cellular and tissue damage after a game or at the recovery processes involved. Player health, both from the demands of the game and after a player ends his career, are of concern and continue to dominate sports medicine challenges. We are using more information today in sports medicine and sports science to deal with these ever-increasing demands to treat football players positively and to help the game of football to be a safe sport. Our understanding of the methods of physical conditioning has dramatically improved over the years, but use of such factual data has many times been hampered by the misunderstanding of basic strength and conditioning science by football coaches, time constraints, and influence of corporate marketing to sell products. The use of individualized, periodized training programs, which are the future of strength and conditioning programs, and group programs such as the one presented in this chapter allow only a theoretical starting point for the sport. The hope for greater study of American football in the future will help to ensure a greater understanding of the game and ultimately help sport medical and sport science professionals make better decisions for the good of the player.

ACKNOWLEDGMENT

The writing of this chapter was supported in part by the Robert F. and Sandra M. Leitzinger Research Fund in Sports Medicine at the Pennsylvania State University.

REFERENCES

1. Green T. *My life in the NFL: the dark side of the game.* New York: Warner Books, 1996.
2. Allen G, Weiskopf D. *Handbook of winning football.* Boston: Allyn & Bacon, 1975.
3. Lombardi V, Flynn GIL, eds. *Vince Lombardi on football.* Vols 1 and 2. Greenwich, CT: New York Graphic Society, 1973.
4. Fry AC, Kraemer WJ. Physical performance characteristics of American collegiate football players. *J Appl Sport Sci Res* 1991;5:126–138.
5. Berg K, Latin RW, Baechle T. Physical and performance characteristics of NCAA Division I football players. *Res Q Exerc Sport* 1990;61:395–401.
6. Pincivero DM, Bompa TO. A physiological review of American football. *Sports Med* 1997;23:241–260.
7. Black W, Roundy E. Comparisons of size, strength, speed and power in NCAA division I-A football players. *J Strength Cond Res* 1994;8:80–85.
8. Gleim GW. The profiling of professional football players. *Clin Sports Med* 1984;3:185–197.
9. Wilmore JH, Parr RB, Haskell WL, Costill DL, Milburn LJ, Kerlan RK. Football pros' strengths—and CV weakness—charted. *Physician Sportsmed* 1976;4:45–54.
10. Fox EL, Matthews D. *Interval training: conditioning for sports and general fitness.* Orlando: Saunders College/Harcourt Brace Jovanovich, 1974.
11. Zapiec C, Taylor AW. Muscle fiber composition and energy utilization in CFL football players. *Can J Appl Sport Sci* 1979; 4:140–142.
12. Takahashi H, Inaki M, Fujimoto K. Control of the rate of phosphocreatine resynthesis after exercise in trained and untrained human quadriceps muscles. *Eur J Appl Physiol* 1995;71:396–404.
13. Smith ME, Jackson CGR. Lactate response of college football players to practices and a game [Abstract]. *J Appl Sport Sci Res* 1991;5:163.
14. Gleim GW, Witman PA, Nicholas JA. Indirect assessment of cardiovascular "demands" using telemetry on professional football players. *Am J Sports Med* 1981;9:178–183.
15. Wilmore JH, Haskell WL. Body composition and endurance capacity of professional football players. *J Appl Physiol* 1972; 33:564–567.

16. Astrand PO, Rodahl K. *Textbook of work physiology.* New York: McGraw-Hill Book Co., 1977.
17. Van Handel PV, Blosser T, Butts N. A method of heat stress prevention for football players. *Am Correct Ther J* 1973; 27:180–183.
18. Olson JR, Hunter GR. Comparison of 1974 and 1984 player sizes, and maximal strength and speed efforts for Division I NCAA universities. *Natl Strength Cond Assoc J* 1985;6:26–28.
19. Schneider V, Arnold B, Martin K, Bell D, Crocker P. Detraining effects in college football players during the competitive season. *J Strength Cond Res* 1998;12:42–45.
20. Kraemer WJ. A series of studies: the physiological basis for strength training in American football: fact over philosophy. *J Strength Cond Res* 1997;11:131–142.
21. Snow TK, Millard-Stafford M, Rosskopf LB. Body composition profile of NFL football players. *J Strength Cond Res* 1998; 12(3):146–149.
22. Clark RR, Kuta JM, Sullivan JC. Cross-validation of methods to predict body fat in African-American and Caucasian collegiate football players. *Res Q Exerc Sport* 1994;65:255–262.
23. Kraemer WJ. Detraining the "bulked-up" athlete: prospects for lifetime health and fitness. *Natl Strength Cond Assoc J* 1983; 5:10–12.
24. Crews TR, Meadors WJ. Analysis of reaction time, speed, and body composition of college football players. *J Sports Med* 1978; 18:169–174.
25. Gotshalk LA. *Temple University football data: 1978–1990.* Unpublished. Philadelphia, PA: Temple University Athletics.
26. Manolis GG. Relation of charging time to blocking performance in football. *Res Q* 1955;26:170–178.
27. McDavid RF. Predicting potential in football players. *Res Q* 1977;48:98–104.
28. Barker M, Wyatt TJ, Johnson RL, et al. Performance factors, psychological assessment, physical characteristics, and football playing ability. *J Strength Cond Res* 1993;7:224–233.
29. Bale P, Colley E, Mayhew JL, Piper FC, Ware JS. Anthropometric and somatotype variables related to strength in American football players. *J Sports Med Phys Fitness* 1994;34:383–389.
30. Koziris LP, Kraemer WJ, Patton JF, et al. Relationship of aerobic power to anaerobic performance indices. *J Strength Cond Res* 1996;10:35–39.
31. Newton RU, Kraemer WJ. Developing explosive muscular power: implications for a mixed methods training strategy. *J Strength Cond Res* 1994;16:20–31.
32. Zemper ED. Four-year study of weightroom injuries in a national sample of college football teams. *Natl Strength Cond Assoc J* 1990;12:32–34.
33. Fleck SJ, Kraemer WJ. *Designing resistance training programs.* 2nd ed. Champaign, IL: Human Kinetics, 1997.
34. Newton RU, Kraemer WJ, Häkkinen K, Humphries BJ, Murphy AJ. Kinematics, kinetics, and muscle activation during explosive upper body movements: implications for power development. *J Appl Biomech* 1996;12:31–43.
35. Daus AT, Wilson J, Freeman WA. Predicting success in football. *J Sports Med Phys Fitness* 1989;29:209–212.
36. Plisk SS, Gambetta V. Tactical metabolic training. *Strength Cond* 1997;19:44–53.
37. Seiler S, Taylor M, Diana R, Layer J, Newton P, Brown B. Assessing anaerobic power in collegiate football players. *J Appl Sport Res* 1990;4:9–15.
38. Shields CL, Whitney FE, Zomar VD. Exercise performance of professional football players. *Am J Sports Med* 1984:12:455–459.
39. Kraemer WJ, Patton J, Gordon SE, et al. Compatibility of high intensity strength and endurance training on hormonal and skeletal muscle adaptations. *J Appl Physiol* 1995;78:976–989.
40. Hoffman JR, Kraemer WJ, Fry AC, Deschenes M, Kemp M. The effects of self-selection for frequency of training in a winter conditioning program for football. *J Appl Sport Sci Res* 1990: 4:76–82.

Exercise and Sport Science,
edited by William E. Garrett, Jr., and Donald T. Kirkendall.
Lippincott Williams & Wilkins, Philadelphia © 2000.

CHAPTER 52

Physiology of Ice Hockey

David L. Montgomery

THE SPORT

Physical Requirements

Ice hockey is characterized by high-intensity intermittent skating and rapid changes in direction and velocity, as well as frequent body contact. Elite skaters are able to exceed a velocity of 8 m/s after only four strides (1). Forward propulsion is impeded by the frictional resistance of the ice, air resistance, drag, and contact from opponents. High-speed collisions with other players and the boards produce injuries.

Skills of passing, shooting, and stick handling must be executed at high tempo. The anaerobic nature of the game creates fatigue, resulting in a deterioration in skating and the fundamental skills. The challenge for the coach from the bioenergetics and physiologic perspectives is to maintain the player's energy and skill levels throughout the game by using short shifts to avoid fatigue, providing adequate recovery time between shifts, and maximizing potential with physical training and nutritional supplements.

The bioenergetics and physiology of ice hockey have been examined in five articles (2–6). These reviews help to establish the physiologic profile for the elite male player. There are few data on female ice hockey players, with only one abstract (18) describing the elite female player.

Depending on the level of the game, teams participate with 18 to 20 players. The players are categorized as forwards (n = 11 or 12), defense (n = 5 or 6), and goalies (n = 7).

Time–Motion Analysis

Games are 60 minutes in duration and consist of three 20-minute periods. In addition, there is a 15-minute intermission between each period. With frequent stops of play for various infractions of the rules, games extend for 150 to 170 minutes. The typical player performs for 15 to 20 minutes; however, star players could have 30 to 35 minutes of ice time.

Skating is the most important skill and task during a hockey game. Time–motion analysis has been used to estimate skating activity. Players from the Czechoslovakian national team averaged 5160 m (range, 4860 to 5620 m) during a game (8). During 24 minutes of playing time, university players skated 5553 m (9) with an average velocity of 227 m/min. Whereas skating velocity represents a major component of work intensity, its singular use underestimates energy expenditure. Changing acceleration and frequent turning, shooting, and checking are activities that add to exercise intensity but are not evident from velocity analysis. Compared with forwards, the defensemen skate at a lower average velocity, with one investigation reporting a 61.6% lower velocity (9).

The National Hockey League (NHL) funds a central scouting bureau whose mandate is to evaluate amateur prospects for the annual NHL entry draft. Players are assessed by scouts on 10 task requirements: (a) skating, (b) shooting/scoring, (c) positional play, (d) checking, (e) puck control, (f) passing, (g) hockey sense, (h) desire/attitude, (i) aggressiveness/toughness, and (j) size/strength. Renger (10) asked 16 scouts to rank these task requirements and to assign relative importance to the tasks by using a 100-point distribution. The task requirement of skating ranked first for both forwards and defensemen, with relative weighting of 22.5 for the forwards and 20.5 for the defensemen. The results revealed that not all skills and tasks are of equal importance to forwards and defense. The task of shooting/scoring was weighted significantly higher for forwards than for defensemen. In contrast, checking, size/strength, and positional play were weighted more heavily for defensemen than for forwards. Thus the tasks necessary for success in professional hockey vary as a function of position.

An analysis of the task of skating by hockey scouts

D. L. Montgomery: Department of Physical Education, McGill University, Montreal, Quebec, Canada.

(10) identified components that were both common and unique to the positions of forward and defense. Common elements included quickness, starts/stops, balance, speed, acceleration, turns, agility, and pivots. The components of stride and power were identified as unique for the position of forwards only. The components of backward skating and mobility were unique elements for the defense. These components of skating should be considered when developing on-ice and off-ice programs.

Data from time–motion studies reveal that variables such as the ratio of bench time to on-ice time and playing time per shift are a function of the level of play and the number of players per team. Recreational teams tend to play with only enough players to form two forward lines, whereas junior, university, and professional teams use three or four forward lines. The ratio between bench time and playing time was 1.20 for Old Timers (11), 1.43 for young players (12), 2.25 for junior players (13), 2.52 for university players (14), and more recently 3.81 for university players (15). From these studies, playing time per shift averaged 58 and 62 seconds for the university players, 87 seconds for the junior players, 95 seconds for the youth players, and 139 seconds for the Old Timers.

Compared with forwards, the defense has a longer playing time, a greater number of shifts, a longer playing time per shift, and less recovery time between shifts (9,14). Leger (13) summarized data on observations of 80 junior and 170 midget players. Because the defense spent less time on the bench between shifts, the ratio of bench time to on-ice time was higher for forwards (2.3 ratio) than defense (2.1 ratio).

Within a shift, there are typically five to seven bursts of maximal skating, with the bursts ranging in duration from 2.0 to 3.5 seconds. Total burst time per game averages 4 to 6 minutes. The period of coasting between bursts may be a key factor in partial restoration of adenosine triphosphate (ATP) and creatine phosphokinase (CP) concentrations in muscle. The effect of this strategy is to minimize anaerobic glycolysis while maximizing the aerobic contribution (3). Forwards display more anaerobic activity than does the defense (16). During a shift, there are two to three stops in play for rule infractions averaging 20 to 30 seconds per stop (9,11,13,14).

Given the short intense nature of each shift and the variability among shifts, both aerobic and anaerobic metabolism contribute to energy expenditure. The proportion of energy from each system will depend on the characteristics of the shift.

Physiologic Requirements

Heart-Rate Telemetry

Heart rate (HR) has been used to estimate the aerobic demands of playing hockey. The average on-ice intensity is estimated at 70% to 90% of $\dot{V}O_2$max (11,12,15). Ice hockey is a high-intensity activity with peak HRs in excess of 90% of maximum and average on-ice values about 85% of maximum (4). Forwards and defense have similar on-ice HRs during games, with the average intensity equal to 82.5% of HRmax. (15). The HRs of goaltenders also have been monitored during adult recreational games, with average rates of 143 beats/min or 64% intensity (17).

Heart-rate telemetry, like other techniques used to assess the aerobic demands of ice hockey, has limitations that should be recognized when interpreting the results. In hockey, HR may be influenced by conditions that do not increase oxygen cost such as (a) the emotional nature of the game, (b) upper-body static contractions, (c) the intermittent nature of play, and (d) elevation of core temperature because hockey equipment may limit heat dissipation (4).

Muscle Glycogen

The muscle-biopsy technique has been used to examine the demands that are placed on the muscles' fuel storage. Muscle glycogen depletion has been associated with a decrease in physical performance. Because the vastus lateralis is active during intense intermittent skating, it is selected as the muscle for examination during biopsy studies.

During a hockey game as well as during skating tasks to simulate the game, glycogen is used from type I, IIa, and IIb fibers, with the greatest depletion from the type I fibers (14,18–21). The involvement of all fiber types in the vastus lateralis would be expected because of the explosive nature of the skating movements in hockey. Compared with pregame levels, type I fibers are depleted by about 80% after a hockey game (21). With ice time averaging less than 16 minutes for elite players (2) and because there are significant quantities of glycogen remaining in the type II fibers (14), it is difficult to conceive that glycogen depletion could be the cause of fatigue.

Glycogen-depletion patterns have been examined during continuous and intermittent ice skating (22). The intermittent skating consisted of 10 bouts of high-intensity work corresponding to 120% of $\dot{V}O_2$max. Each bout consisted of 1 minute of skating followed by 5 minutes of recovery. This regimen was selected to represent the most extreme example of play during a hockey game. The continuous skating was performed at 55% of $\dot{V}O_2$max for 60 minutes. Muscle biopsies were taken at the start of each skate and after 30 minutes (five work bouts) and 60 minutes (10 work bouts).

During continuous skating, there was a 29% reduction in muscle glycogen, with a greater loss from the type I fibers. During the intermittent skating condition, there was a twofold depletion of muscle glycogen (70%), with a preferential loss from the type II fibers, particularly the type IIb fibers. In the intermittent condition, anaerobic energy production was evident, with a high concentration of muscle lactate (26.4 mmol/L). The muscle's potential to sustain work output is reduced with either a high concentration of lactate or an excessive reduction of glycogen in type IIb fibers (23).

Back-to-back games on consecutive days are common in ice hockey. Muscle biopsies have shown that glycogen has not been replenished before the second game with an ad libitum diet between games (24). Back-to-back games may reduce muscle and liver glycogen levels. During the second game, blood glucose levels were lower after each period of play. Coaches should provide guidance on diet between games because glycogen levels may be reduced to the point where performance is impaired.

The effects of carbohydrate (CHO) intake on blood and muscle energy substrates before (100 g of glucose) and during (20 g of glucose) an ice hockey game have been examined (25). After CHO feeding, the hockey players skated 10.2% more at a slightly faster average velocity. CHO feeding maintained blood glucose level and reduced glycogen use by 10.3%.

Lactate Accumulation

Blood lactate has been measured by using fingerprick and venous samples to assess the anaerobic energy contribution from glycolysis. Lactate accumulation depends on fitness level, state of training, active muscle mass, muscle-fiber composition, nutritional status, blood flow, and fatigue (2). No studies have reported lactate levels during ice hockey games among professional players.

The highest postgame lactate values were reported for European players (9 to 11 mmol/L). For Canadian university players, blood lactate values were highest after the first (8.7 mmol/L) and second (7.3 mmol/L) periods and then declined during the third period (4.9 mmol/L), with a similar response for the forwards and defense (9). In a follow-up study, Green and colleagues (14) reported values of 5.5 mmol/L for the forwards and only 2.9 mmol/L for the defense. The lower lactates were attributed to shorter shift duration.

One explanation for the relatively low lactate values during a hockey game has to do with the frequent play stops during each shift. With an average of 2 play stops per shift, there is about 30 seconds for recovery. This pause provides sufficient time for 60% to 65% of the PC to be resynthesized and available for the next phase of the shift (22). A typical shift is interspersed with short bursts of high-intensity skating followed by longer periods of coasting. Elite players have learned to optimize the high-intensity bursts to avoid lactate accumulation that would interfere with the execution of hockey skills.

Two studies (26,27) have examined muscular fatigue in hockey players over a 6-day cycle of practices and games. Fatigue was measured isometrically during knee extension by using a maximal voluntary contraction. After an initial hockey practice, muscle-force output was impaired and remained impaired throughout the cycle of practices and games. The onset and persistence of fatigue affected muscular-force output and was associated with lactic acidosis.

Coaches should use short shifts in hockey. Long shifts of high intensity result in accumulation of muscle lactate and a rapid reduction in muscle glycogen, particularly from the fast-twitch (FT) fibers (28). If high concentrations of lactic acid are produced, the muscle acidity causes metabolic and contractile disturbances that result in decreased work performance (22). Short shifts reduce muscle lactate and allow more time for restoring the high-energy phosphagens. The recovery period can be used to reload myoglobin stores and resynthesize PC. As a consequence of shorter shifts, there is a larger contribution of PC and oxidative phosphorylation to ATP turnover. With a reduced contribution from anaerobic glycolysis, glycogen reserves are depleted at a slower rate.

After a high-intensity shift, hockey players sit passively for 4 to 6 minutes on the bench waiting for their next on-ice shift. Active recovery enhances lactate removal. Two studies used skating regimens to elevate lactate levels and then compared lactate removal with active and passive recovery. Bench stepping and skating were superior to passive recovery for removal of lactate (29). By using the Repeat Sprint Skate (RSS) test to simulate the high intensity of a hockey shift, Kaczynski (30) elevated blood lactate values to 11 mmol/L after six shifts of the RSS test. Between repetitions, players were randomly assigned to three modes of recovery: (a) cycling at 40% of $\dot{V}O_2max$ on a modified ergometer while wearing skates, (b) skating at a self-selected pace, and (c) sitting passively on the bench. The anaerobic endurance index of the RSS test for the six shifts is graphed in Fig. 52–1. After six shifts, the anaerobic endurance index was 62.02 ± 2.47 seconds, 62.52 ± 2.21 seconds, and 64.63 ± 2.69 seconds, respectively, for the three modes of recovery. Cycling was superior to passive recovery for removal of lactate, and both cycling and skating recovery enhanced performance in the anaerobic endurance index of the RSS test.

Some NHL teams have players cycle at 130 W for about 20 minutes after a game (2). The purpose of this exercise is to promote lactate clearance. Because the half-life for removal of lactate is about 9.5 minutes (31), and given that there is no requirement for repeated maximal performance after the game, this practice is questionable.

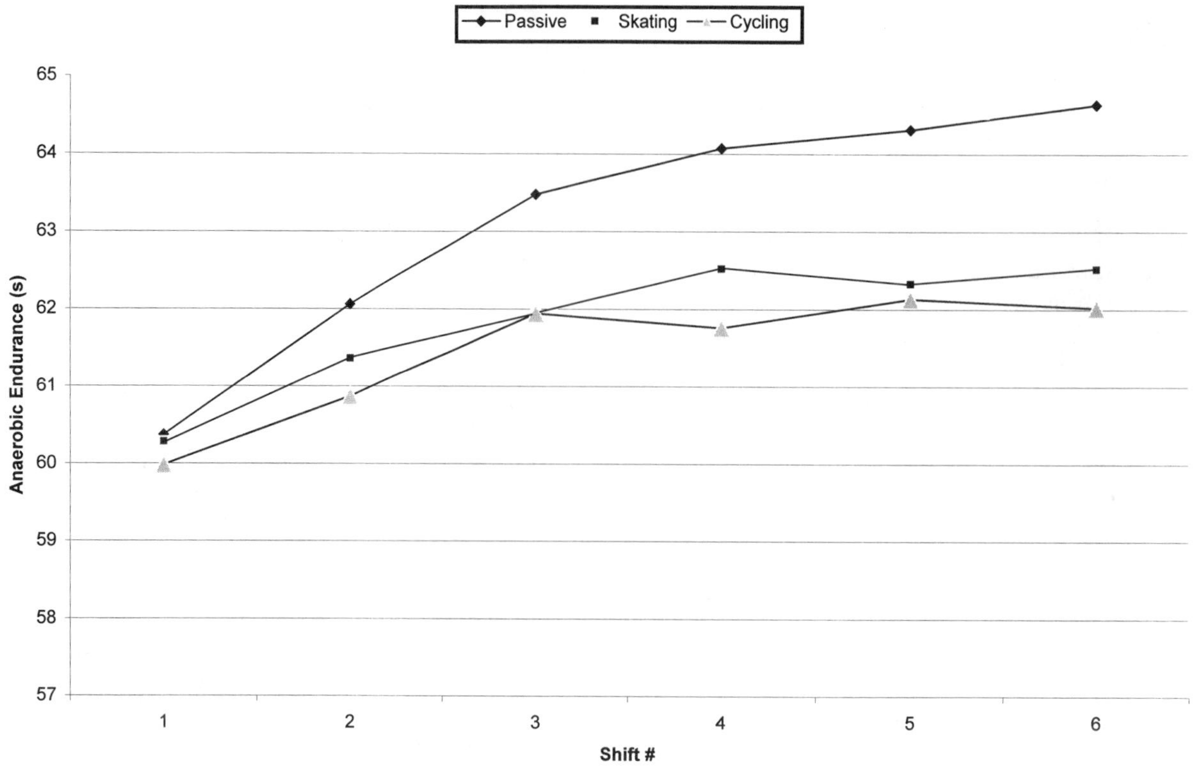

FIG. 52–1. Effect of recovery mode on skating.

THE ATHLETE

Vickers (33) developed a knowledge structures approach to help hockey coaches and scientists identify and evaluate the skills and abilities needed for successful performance. From approximately 400 skills, abilities, and concepts, Vickers identified five building blocks in the knowledge structure of ice hockey: background knowledge, philosophy of the game, physiologic training, psychomotor skills, and psychological concepts. This review is concerned with only the physiologic components.

Physiologic assessment of the hockey player can be used to identify (a) strengths and weaknesses of the individual, (b) physiologic potential, (c) injuries, (d) when the player is ready to return to action after an injury, and (e) responses to a training regimen (2). Physiologic testing not only provides precise information to develop potential but also offers a motivational basis for training and allows the establishment of objective, measurable goals. A testing program also can be used as an educational process by which the athlete gains a better understanding of the physiologic demands of the sport (34).

Beginning in 1993, the NHL initiated physiologic testing for entry draft players. The sport-specific test battery for hockey players (35) included assessment of:

- Physical characteristics
- Aerobic power
- Anaerobic power and capacity (Wingate test)
- Strength and muscular endurance
- Flexibility

Some data pertaining to each of these measurements are presented in the following sections. In addition, muscle-fiber composition is also an important characteristics.

Physical Characteristics and Added Mass

At the elite level, players range in age from 20 to 35 years, with team averages in the mid-20s. The body mass, stature, and fatness of elite players were previously described (2,4,6,36–38). Since the late 1970s, body mass and height have progressively increased. In general, players are about 5 cm taller and carry an extra mass of 5 kg. Team averages in the NHL now exceed 185 cm for height and 90 kg for mass.

Cox and colleagues (39) compared physiologic data from 170 players on five NHL teams between 1980 and 1991. In 1980, 40% of the players weighed less than 85 kg, and 71% were shorter than 180 cm. By 1991, only 26% of the players weighed less than 85 kg, whereas 85% were taller than 180 cm. During this same period, the body-fat content remained constant at 13% (2). Within a team, the defensemen are taller and heavier than forwards (6,40–46).

The body composition of hockey players is usually estimated from skin-fold thickness. Mean adipose levels range from 10% to 14% (2,4). Some of the variability can be attributed to the different equations used to estimate percentage of body fat. Because hockey is a contact game, fat mass may offer some protection during collisions with boards and opponents. Fat mass also may be beneficial when body checking, as it will add to the inertial mass.

Hockey players carry excess mass in the form of adipose tissue and equipment. The effect of added mass on skating performance has been examined with the RSS test (47). With a weighted vest, added mass was secured to the waist and shoulders in a manner not to impede skating movements. Added mass caused a significantly slower performance on both the speed and anaerobic endurance components of the RSS test. With 5% excess mass, anaerobic endurance time increased by 4%. Excess body mass increases the energy required to skate at a particular velocity, so that energy systems are challenged at a slower velocity; it also reduces the time that a player can maintain the pace. Elite players should be encouraged to decrease body-fat mass and to wear as light a uniform as possible without sacrificing protection.

The effect of experimental alterations in skate weight on performance in the RSS test were investigated (48). During the added skate-weight conditions, there was a significant increase in performance, resulting in slower performance on both the speed and anaerobic-endurance components of the RSS test. When purchasing skates and other protection equipment, players should use mass as an important selection criterion.

Hockey equipment serves to protect the player, but it also increases energy expenditure. The effect of equipment weight (7.3 kg) on $\dot{V}O_2max$ and skating performance was examined during a 20-m shuttle-skating test (49). Hockey players performed the test with and without equipment. Whereas $\dot{V}O_2max$ was similar in both trials, the duration of the test was reduced by 20%. Final skating speed decreased by 7 m/min (2.9%) when skaters performed the test wearing hockey equipment. Calculation of mechanical-efficiency ratios indicated a 4.8% additional energy cost of skating while wearing hockey equipment.

Aerobic Endurance

Table 52–1 summarizes the $\dot{V}O_2max$ results for elite players at the university, junior, national, and professional levels by using cycle ergometer, treadmill, and skating protocols. On the cycle ergometer, team means for both forwards and defense ranged from 52 to 63 mL/kg/min, with one exception. One of the highest team means reported was from the data on 55 players recruited for Team Canada in the 1991 Canada Cup. For this elite group, $\dot{V}O_2max$ averaged 62.4 mL/kg/min.

On the treadmill, team means ranged from 52 to 66 mL/kg/min (see Table 52–1). Measurement of $\dot{V}O_2max$ by using skating protocols was performed only with university players. Hockey players appear to have the same $\dot{V}O_2max$ when tested on ice and on the treadmill (49,66–68).

As the mean weight of the hockey team increases, the $\dot{V}O_2max$ expressed as mL/kg/min decreases. Within a team, positional comparisons support this trend. The defensemen are usually taller and heavier than the forwards, so it is expected that the defense will have a lower $\dot{V}O_2max$ (mL/kg/min).

There also appears to be an upward shift in aerobic endurance. Cox and co-workers (39) examined $\dot{V}O_2max$ data from 170 players on five NHL teams between 1980 and 1991. In 1980, 58% of the players had a $\dot{V}O_2max$ less than 55 mL/kg/min. In contrast, only 15% were below this value in 1991. The improvements in aerobic power were independent of an increase in body mass, suggesting that conditioning methods had been effective in improving aerobic power (2).

Anaerobic Power and Endurance

Anaerobic power and endurance are important attributes for a hockey player. Cycling tests are generally preferred over other ergometers when evaluating hockey players. Research has indicated that the patterns of glycogen depletion and recruitment of muscles when cycling are similar to those used in skating (14,69,70).

Laboratory test results with a cycling test have been compared with on-ice maximal skating performance by using the RSS test (71,72). Correlation coefficients of $r = -0.87$ for peak power on the cycling test and speed index on the RSS test, and $r = -0.78$ between mean power on the cycling test and total time for the RSS test provide support to the establishment of validity. The cycling test discriminated among hockey players at three levels: varsity, junior varsity, and nonvarsity players.

The most common test to assess anaerobic qualities in hockey players has been the Wingate test. Table 52–2 summarizes some results for the Wingate tests. Caution is warranted when comparing results across studies because of (a) lack of standardization with respect to the type of cycle ergometer, (b) variance in test duration from 30 to 60 seconds, (c) variance in loading from 70 to 100 g/kg of body mass, (d) stabilization of the ergometer, and (e) the presence or lack of toe clips on the pedals.

When peak power and mean power are expressed relative to body mass, forwards and defense have similar scores. Because the defensemen tend to be heavier than

TABLE 52–1. *Maximal oxygen uptake of elite teams*

Group	*n*	Weight (kg)	$\dot{V}O_2max$	Reference
Treadmill				
USA Olympic 1976	22		58.7	Enos et al. (1976)
University	8	70.5	58.1	Montpetit et al. (1979)
University	10	72.8	61.4	Leger et al. (1979)
Swedish national	24	75.8	57.0	Forsberg et al. (1974)
Junior	18	76.4	56.4	Green & Houston (1975)
Finnish national	13	77.3	61.5	Rusko et al. (1978)
University	19	77.4	58.9	Green et al. (1978a)
University	19	77.6	58.9	Green et al. (1979b)
NHL goalies	4	77.7	53.1	Agre et al. (1988)
Junior	9	78.7	55.4	Green et al. (1979b)
Swedish national 1971	24	78.1	56.3	Wilson & Hedberg (1976)
Junior	44	78.2	55.4	Houston & Green (1976)
University	11	79.5	56.4	Montgomery (1982)
NHL goalies 1985–1986	8	79.2	49.1	Rhodes et al. (1986)
Swedish national 1966	24	80.0	53.6	Wilson & Hedberg (1976)
University	9	80.9	56.3	Hutchinson et al. (1979)
Swedish professional (DIF)	22	81.4	62.4	Tegelman et al. (1992)
Swedish professional (SSK)	21	82.4	65.8	Tegelman et al. (1992)
NHL forwards	15	86.1	54.2	Agre et al. (1988)
Professional		86.4	53.6	Wilmore (1979)
NHL forwards	26	87.0	56.3	Cox et al. (1988)
NHL forwards 1985–1986	27	87.1	57.4	Rhodes et al. (1986)
NHL defense	8	88.5	52.2	Agre et al. (1988)
NHL defense	21	91.0	53.4	Cox et al. (1988)
NHL defense 1985–1986	40	90.3	54.8	Rhodes et al. (1986)
Junior and varsity	8	94.1	58.4	Watson & Hanley (1986)
Cycle ergometer				
Quebec Nordiques 1972–1973	12	75.9	54.1	Bouchard et al. (1974)
University	15	76.9	54.5	Thoden & Jette (1975)
Junior	24	77.0	58.4	Bouchard et al. (1974)
University	9	77.1	53.2	Hermiston (1975)
University	18	78.1	55.2	Romet et al. (1978)
Canadian national	34	78.5	53.4	Coyne (1975)
Czechoslovakian national	13	79.1	54.6	Seliger et al. (1972)
NHL goalies 1985–1986	8	79.2	44.1	Rhodes et al. (1986)
University	5	79.5	54.3	Daub et al. (1983)
University	21	79.8	58.4	Krotee et al. (1979)
Canadian national	23	81.1	54.0	Smith et al. (1982)
Finnish national	27	81.1	52.0	Vainikka et al. (1982)
Professional	38	82.3	43.5	Romet et al. (1978)
Junior	9	82.4	52.6	Green et al. (1979b)
NHL players 1980	38	85.3	54.0	Cox et al. (1993)
Montreal Canadiens 1982–1983	29	86.8	51.9	Montgomery & Dallaire (1986)
NHL forwards 1985–1986	27	87.1	53.3	Rhodes et al. (1986)
NHL players 1984	38	88.2	54.4	Cox et al. (1993)
NHL players 1991	75	88.4	60.2	Cox et al. (1993)
Team Canada 1991	55	89.3	62.4	Cox et al. (1993)
NHL players	22	90.0	51.4	Cox et al. (1988)
NHL defense 1985–1986	40	90.3	51.6	Rhodes et al. (1986)
NHL players 1988	23	91.2	57.8	Cox et al. (1993)
Professional players	28		54.2	Wygand et al. (1987)
Skating				
University	10	72.8	62.1	Leger et al. (1979)
University	17	73.7	55.0	Ferguson et al. (1969)
University	8	78.7	52.8	Green (1978)
University	5	79.5	52.1	Daub et al. (1983)

TABLE 52–2. *Wingate test results of elite hockey teams*

Group	*n*	Peak power	Mean power	Reference
Forwards				
Canadian Olympic team 1980	15	11.7 ± 1.0	9.6 ± 0.6	Smith et al. (1982)
NHL players	40	12.0 ± 1.2	9.1 ± 5.5[a]	Cox et al. (1988)
Montreal Canadiens	6	10.3 ± 0.4	8.7 ± 0.7	Montgomery & Dallaire (1986)
NHL players	24	10.6	9.1	Quinney et al. (1982)
NHL players	31	13.4 ± 1.2	10.3 ± 1.3	Twist & Rhodes (1993)
NHL players	42	12.0	9.1	Rhodes et al. (1987)
NHL players	105	12.3 ± 0.1	8.6 ± 0.6[a]	Cox et al. (1993)
Defense				
Canadian Olympic team 1980	6	11.5 ± 0.4	9.6 ± 0.9	Smith et al. (1982)
NHL players	27	12.0 ± 1.5	9.5 ± 1.0[a]	Cox et al. (1988)
Montreal Canadiens	12	9.8 ± 1.1	8.2 ± 0.3	Montgomery & Dallaire (1986)
NHL players	24	10.4	8.6	Quinney et al. (1982)
NHL players	31	13.1 ± 1.5	10.2 ± 0.9	Twist & Rhodes (1993)
NHL players	30	12.1	9.5	Rhodes et al. (1987)
NHL players	57	12.3 ± 0.1	8.5 ± 0.1	Cox et al. (1993)
Goalies				
NHL players	8	11.4 ± 1.1	8.6 ± 5.2[a]	Cox et al. (1988)
Montreal Canadiens	3	10.6 ± 1.0	8.3 ± 0.1	Montgomery & Dallaire (1986)
NHL players	24	10.6	8.2	Quinney et al. (1982)
NHL players	31	12.7 ± 1.1	9.5 ± 1.6	Twist & Rhodes (1993)
NHL players	8	11.4	8.6	Rhodes et al. (1987)
NHL players	19	11.9 ± 0.2	8.3 ± 0.2[a]	Cox et al. (1993)
Entire Team				
Montreal Canadiens 1981–1982	27	9.9 ± 0.7	8.3 ± 0.3	Montgomery & Dallaire (1986)
Montreal Canadiens 1982–1983	30	10.4 ± 1.1	8.7 ± 0.8	Montgomery & Dallaire (1986)
University and junior	24	10.1 ± 1.0	7.7 ± 1.0	Watson & Sargeant (1986)
University	17	11.5 ± 0.6	9.2 ± 0.5	Gamble (1986)
University	17	11.5 ± 0.8	9.0 ± 0.7	Brayne (1985)

[a]45-s test.
Data expressed as watts per kilogram (mean ± SD).

the forwards, their absolute scores are higher on cycle-ergometer tests.

NHL players have significantly higher power outputs (W and W/kg) than minor-league players. By using games played at the NHL level to establish two groups, differences in peak power, mean power, and minimum power on a 45-second Wingate test were able to be seen between NHL players and minor-league players (67a). Figure 52–2 compares the results for the NHL players with those of the minor-league players over three seasons.

There is some dispute about what constitutes an anaerobic capacity test (79). Jacobs and associates (80) concluded that a 30-second Wingate test is too short to quantify glycolytic anaerobic capacity. Bouchard and colleagues (81) recommended that an anaerobic capacity test requires a maximal effort for 60 to 90 seconds. Hence, Table 52–2 uses mean power as the label rather than anaerobic capacity. Blood lactate levels for the 30-second Wingate test are high, with mean values of 15.1, 14.9 and 14.9 mmol/L reported for forwards, defense, and goalies, respectively (74). These values suggest that hockey players have good anaerobic lactate capacity even though the test duration was shorter than recommended for an anaerobic capacity test. Finnish national team players performed two 60-second all-out cycling tests separated by a 3-minute recovery period. Blood lactate concentration increased from 13.8 after test 1 to 17.6 mmol/L after test 2.

Another anaerobic test that has been used to assess hockey players has been a treadmill run at 8.0 mph (12.8 km/h) and 20% grade. A pre- to postseason comparison demonstrated that a season of hockey improves anaerobic fitness, with treadmill run time increasing from 64.3 to 74.8 seconds (43). Maximal blood lactate after the test increased from 11.9 to 13.3 mmol/L. University and junior hockey players have similar anaerobic run times and peak blood lactate levels (53).

Muscle Strength and Endurance

Muscular strength is one of the factors that discriminates between professional and amateur players (82). A comparison of 54 professional and 94 junior players on 11 strength measures revealed that the professional players were significantly stronger on six of the tests.

A hand grip test is frequently used to measure grip and forearm strength, because they are important as-

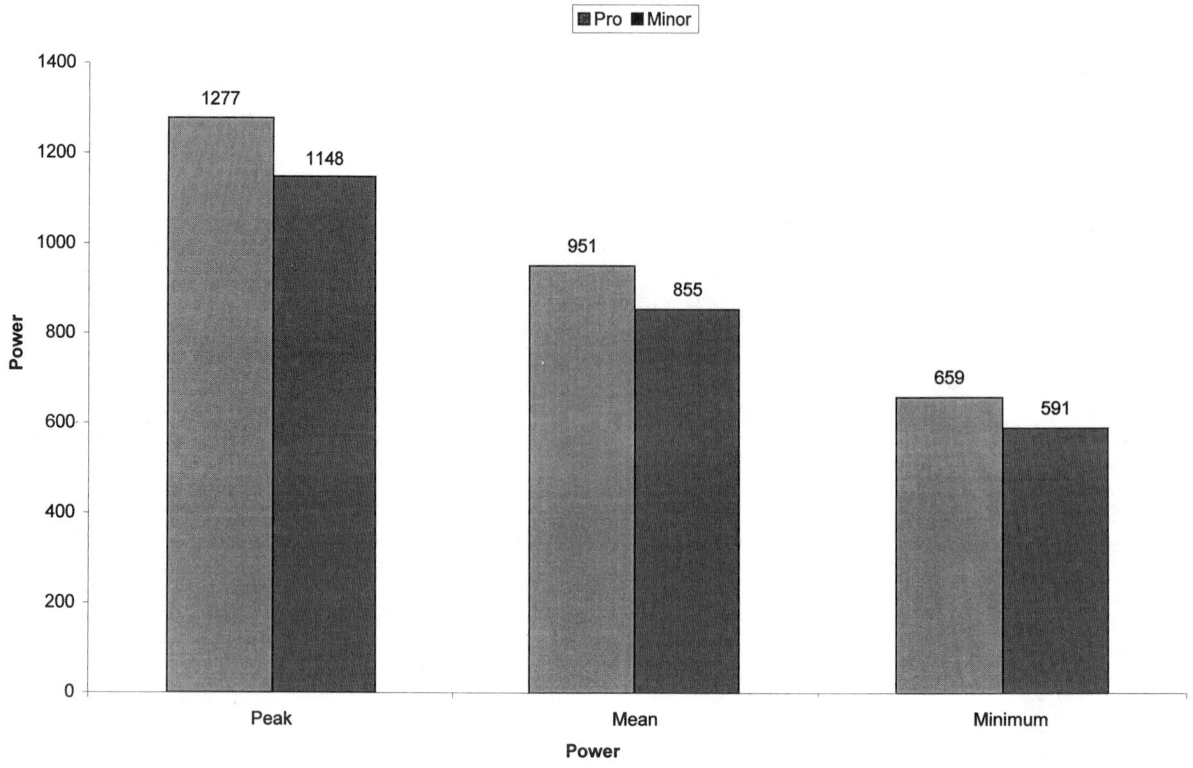

FIG. 52–2. Wingate results for professional ice hockey players.

pects that contribute to shot velocity. Elite hockey players have high values compared with other athletic teams (36). Table 52–3 summarizes mean values from some elite teams. Professional players have higher hand-grip strength than university or junior players. Forwards and defensemen have higher values than goaltenders. As players at the elite level become bigger and stronger, grip strength increases. In 1980, 40% of the players had combined grip strength scores less than 120 kg, whereas only 20% were below this standard by 1991 (2). There also is a trend for right-grip-strength scores to be higher than left-grip-strength scores, which is unrelated to shooting "handedness" (76a).

Assessment of the upper-body strength and endurance of hockey players is made using the bench press. Team average strength for one professional team was 98.1 ± 18.3 kg, which was 13% greater than their body mass (44). Primarily for safety reasons, most teams now measure the number of repetitions with 150 pounds instead of the 1 RM. Some data for this test are illustrated in Table 52–4. Players drafted by the NHL at age 17 to 18 years average 9.9 reps on the bench-press test. By age 20 years, the players have increased their strength to about 18 reps. For players in the NHL, the averages for one team ranged between 25.6 to 27.0 over a 3-year period.

Data from Twist and Rhodes (6) on the number of bench-press repetitions with 200 pounds indicate that the forwards (12.0 ± 3.0 reps) and defensemen (14.0 ± 3.3 reps) are stronger than goaltenders (4.3 ± 2.1 reps). Defensemen were stronger than forwards on the 1 RM bench-press test when expressed as an absolute score; when the results were adjusted for differences in body weight, however, the scores were similar (44).

Abdominal muscular endurance of hockey players is commonly assessed with curl-ups at a rate of 25 repetitions per minute with a maximum of 100 repetitions (86). Professional hockey players (n = 117) averaged 49.7 ± 23.7 reps, with scores ranging from 15 to 100. Only 11% of the players were able to achieve 100 repetitions. The average score for NHL draft picks (n = 306) between 1994 and 1997 was only 26.1 curl-ups (87). Table 52–5 summarizes mean values from some elite teams.

Flexibility

Flexibility aids the hockey player in the execution of skills, in the performance of explosive skating movements by extending the range of motion, and by decreasing injuries. Although flexibility is important for hockey players, few data exist for comparison purposes. Trunk flexion is measured by many teams and is included as part of the fitness-assessment protocol for NHL entry draft players. The average score for NHL draft picks (n = 305) between 1994 and 1997 was 38.1 ± 8.6 cm (87). Positional comparisons indicate that goaltenders

TABLE 52–3. *Hand-grip values for some elite ice hockey teams*

Group	*n*	Right + left grip (kg)	Reference
Czechoslovakian elite	11	115.7	Chovanova (1976)
Canadian Olympic team	23	130.1	Smith et al. (1982)
NHL defense 1985–1986	27	135.7	Cox et al. (1988)
NHL forwards 1985–1986	40	132.0	Cox et al. (1988)
NHL goaltenders 1985–1986	8	110.2	Cox et al. (1988)
Edmonton 1980–1981	20	123.2	Smith et al. (1981a)
University	17	107.7	Song & Reid (1979)
Professional	52	116.2	Gauthier et al. (1979)
Junor	87	113.9	Gauthier et al. (1979)
Midget (mean, 16 yr)	18	102.4	Lariviere et al. (1976)
University	18	64.5 ± 6.4[a]	Romet et al. (1978)
Team Canada 1974	36	71.0 ± 8.2[a]	Romet et al. (1978)
Montreal Canadiens 1981–1982	27	66.6 ± 5.8[a]	Montgomery & Dallaire (1986)
Montreal Canadiens 1982–1983	30	67.6 ± 7.8[a]	Montgomery & Dallaire (1986)
NHL forwards	31	142.4 ± 8.6	Twist & Rhodes (1993)
NHL defensemen		138.1 ± 9.4	Twist & Rhodes (1993)
NHL goaltenders		121.5 ± 8.4	Twist & Rhodes (1993)
NHL players 1980	38	123.3 ± 1.9	Cox et al. (1993)
NHL players 1984	30	131.9 ± 4.9	Cox et al. (1993)
NHL players 1988	23	130.4 ± 2.5	Cox et al. (1993)
NHL players 1991	72	130.9 ± 1.8	Cox et al. (1993)
Team Canada 1991	55	115.6 ± 1.5[b]	Cox et al. (1993)

[a]Dominant hand.
[b]Hydraulic dynamometer vs. spring-loaded dynamometer.

TABLE 52–4. *Maximal repetitions of bench press (150 pounds)*

Group	*n*	Age (yr)	Body mass (pounds)	Bench press (reps)	(Reps × 150 lb)/mass (lb/lb of body mass)
NHL draft picks					
1994–1997	310	17.8	190.4	9.9	7.7
Minor professionals					
1995	35	20	195.3	16.0	12.2
1996	34	20	192.2	18.9	14.6
1997	40	20.3	193.3	18.7	14.5
NHL players					
1995	31	25	196.1	25.6	19.2
1996	25	25	203.9	27.0	19.6
1997	25	26.8	204.0	26.7	19.6

TABLE 52–5. *Abdominal endurance of elite ice hockey teams*

Level	*n*	Repetitions	Reference
Feet unsupported			
Professional	117	49.7 ± 23.7	Quinney et al. (1984)
NHL defensemen	27	43.7 ± 15.1	Rhodes et al. (1986)
NHL forwards	40	38.5 ± 15.1	Rhodes et al. (1986)
NHL goaltenders	8	37.5 ± 13.3	Rhodes et al. (1986)
Feet stabilized			
Montreal Canadiens 1981–1982	27	54.2 ± 26.9	Montgomery & Dallaire (1986)
Montreal Canadiens 1982–1983	30	70.8 ± 22.5	Montgomery & Dallaire (1986)
NHL forwards	31[a]	59.0 ± 21.0	Twist & Rhodes (1993)
NHL defensemen		72.0 ± 16.0	Twist & Rhodes (1993)
NHL goaltenders		58.0 ± 8.2	Twist & Rhodes (1993)

Data expressed as mean ± SD.
[a]Total group.

have the best flexibility (37,44). Forwards and defense have similar scores for trunk flexion, trunk extension, and shoulder extension.

Many hockey players experience significant injuries that can be detected as musculoskeletal and/or flexibility abnormalities. Agre and co-workers (7) identified specific deficits in 37% of professional players ($n = 27$) that had gone unnoticed. Poor flexibility in the groin and hamstring muscles and tightness in the low-back extensor muscles may be predisposing factors leading to injury.

The flexibility of university hockey players has been compared with that of other university athletes (basketball, baseball, football, shot put and discus throwers, swimming, and wrestling) on 10 joint actions (83). Except for the swimmers, hockey players exceeded the other teams on wrist, hip, knee, and ankle flexibility. The hockey players had lower values for neck rotation, shoulder movements, elbow radial–ulnar actions, trunk extension-flexibility, and lateral flexion.

Muscle-Fiber Type and Area

Athletes who specialize in sprinting activities tend to have a predominance of FT fibers in their leg muscles, whereas athletes involved in endurance activities display a predominance of ST fibers. Hockey players display a wide range of fiber composition (20% to 71% ST fibers in the vastus lateralis), reflecting the requirements of the game (87a). This range should be expected because ice hockey involves skating at maximal velocity and requires distribution of energy over 2.5 hours.

Muscle biopsies from the vastus lateralis of 48 Canadian hockey players revealed no differences in the type I fiber distribution of university (47.8% ± 2.5%), junior (50.2% ± 2.9%), and professional (50.1% ± 3.2%) players (14). Goalies, forwards, and defense had similar ST-fiber percentages. European players may have a higher percentage of ST fibers. The Finnish national team averaged 61% ± 12% ST fibers in the vastus lateralis muscle (52).

Prolonged endurance activity decreases the proportion of type IIb fibers and increases the proportion of type IIa fibers. Hockey training brings about interconversions in the FT metabolic profile (87a) and increases the size of both the FTa (22%) and FTb (28%) fibers. In this study, there was no change in the slow-twitch (ST) fiber area.

On-Ice Evaluation

Ice-skating performance tests measure both physiologic fitness and skill (5). The more complex the skill component in an on-ice hockey test, the greater the differences between competitive and recreational youth players (88). A test that contains primarily forward skating is better for measurement of the fitness component. Tests that contain elements of puck control and agility are better suited to measure the skill component (88). Based on skating patterns of elite players in game situations, a skating-agility test has been developed that contains both aerobic and anaerobic components (89).

The RSS test is a popular forward-skating test that has been validated as an on-ice test of hockey fitness (82). The RSS test consists of six repetitions of maximal velocity skating for 91.4 m (300 feet). Repeats are initiated every 30 seconds. From this test, four variables are recorded. The time to skate one length of the ice (54 m or 180 feet) is designated the speed index. The total time for the six repetitions is the anaerobic endurance component. A drop-off index is calculated as the difference between the slowest and fastest repetitions. Heart rates are recorded immediately on completion of the test, and at 3 and 5 minutes after exercise. Recovery is calculated as the difference between the exercise and postexercise heart rates. Typical results (4,30,46,47,76–78) for university and professional players are:

Speed Index, 7.0 to 7.7 seconds
Anaerobic Endurance Index, 88 to 94 seconds
Drop-off Index, 1.5 to 3.5 seconds
HR Recovery at 3 minutes, 40 to 60 beats/min

A modified version (four repetitions) of the RSS test is recommended for use with young hockey players (90,91).

Other on-ice tests include a 40-lap skate around a figure-8 course (92) and an 8-minute skate for assessment of aerobic endurance (93). In the latter test, players skate as many laps as possible around a 140-m oval course. Norms are available for minor-league players (94–96).

The Canadian National female hockey team uses three on-ice skating tests to monitor the development of players (97). The tests measure acceleration (6.1 m), sprinting speed (56.4 m), aerobic power (20 laps), and anaerobic capacity.

The latter test requires the player to skate maximally six times forward and backward (total of 12 skates) at 18.3 m per repetition. The time to complete the 12 skates is the measure of anaerobic capacity.

TRAINING THE ATHLETE

The Season

At the elite level, training camps open in early September. Professional and junior players compete in 70 to 82 games during the regular season, beginning on October 1 and ending in mid-April. In addition, the play-off schedule could include as many as another 28 games and extend the competitive season until late June. Typically, teams play three games per week.

College and university players have a reduced schedule with two games per week for a schedule of 30 to 40 games. The season for these players begins in October and usually ends in March.

Sport-Specific Training

During the competitive season, most teams will practice on a daily basis. On-ice training is used to develop skill, team tactics, and some aspects of hockey fitness. Speed, power, and anaerobic endurance are developed in skating drills by varying the duration of the exercise and recovery to develop hockey-specific anaerobic fitness. Indeed, a season of hockey play has been shown to improve anaerobic fitness but not aerobic fitness when $\dot{V}O_2max$ was expressed in mL/kg/min (43,98).

The nature of the practices probably does not provide enough high-intensity stress of sufficient duration to increase aerobic power of elite hockey players (2,24,61,73). Telemetry monitoring of heart rate during practice supports this argument (15). The on-ice intensity during games is high (82% of HRmax); however, the average intensity during practices is significantly lower (69% of HRmax). During practices, heart rates seldom approach maximal levels (2,15,59). Players in these studies rarely skated at high velocity for longer than 10 seconds.

Supplemental Training

During the competitive season, hockey players supplement their on-ice training with additional dry-land sessions specifically designed to maintain aerobic fitness, muscular strength, and power. Aerobic endurance is maintained with two high-intensity sessions of cycling or running with the duration between 20 and 30 minutes. During summer training, some players add in-line skating or StairMaster exercise as part of the aerobic-training program (99).

Can hockey players improve their hockey fitness during the competitive season? The magnitude of change in fitness depends partly on the player's initial fitness level. Players with low and moderate levels of aerobic endurance such as "Old Timers" and recreational players will improve $\dot{V}O_2max$ when participating in a hockey program (100). For hockey players already at a high level of fitness, the exercise intensity is the key to improvement. Intensity is often monitored with heart rate or occasionally with lactate threshold (42). One program brought about changes in the magnitude of 7% for $\dot{V}O_2max$ and 25% for leg power, which are clearly physiologically significant improvements for elite players (42).

Two studies with professional players have shown that improvements in $\dot{V}O_2max$ are possible during the competitive season if training is appropriate (42,101). Based on minutes of ice time during game situations, frequency of training was established from 2 to 4 times per week and intensity set at the individual's lactate threshold. For 24 professional hockey players, lactate threshold during cycling exercise occurred at 352.7 ± 9.9 W, corresponding to 89.5% of HRmax or 82.5% of $\dot{V}O_2max$. The necessity for individual programs was evident because the range extended from 73% to 92% of $\dot{V}O_2max$ (2).

One of the major objectives of an ice-hockey training program is the development of skating speed by means of weight training, plyometrics, and on-ice skating intervals. The weight-training program is designed to develop lower-body strength and power. Elite players have about 12 weeks during the summer months to focus on aerobic training and weight training. One model for the weight-training program is to spend the first 4 weeks on muscular endurance, 4 weeks on muscular strength, and the final 4 weeks on muscular power. The latter phase usually incorporates plyometrics training. The summer weight-training program is typically 4 days per week. During the competitive season, strength and power can be maintained with two sessions per week.

Periodization of Training

The calendar year for the hockey player is divided into four or five phases. The length of each phase for elite players is typically:

- Summer training, 8 to 16 weeks
- Preseason, 4 weeks
- Competitive season, 28 weeks
- Play-offs (peaking), 1 to 9 weeks
- Recovery phase, 3 weeks

The length of the summer training program will depend on the success of the team during the play-offs.

The summer training program is designed to improve muscular strength and power, and aerobic fitness. Summer training programs specifically designed for ice hockey have been shown to develop $\dot{V}O_2max$, lean-body mass, vertical jump, on-ice endurance, and sprinting speed (54,102,103).

The preseason phase is a training-camp environment that is used to select the team. About 60 to 70 players are invited to the training camp to compete for 20 positions. Emphasis is placed on the assessment of talent. Many teams do their medical and physiologic evaluations during the start of this phase.

During the competitive season, anaerobic power and endurance are developed during the daily on-ice practices. A typical week will include three hockey games. The challenge for the fitness specialist is to schedule additional dry-land workouts aimed at maintaining aerobic fitness and muscular strength while providing adequate recovery time to reduce fatigue before games. The goal is to include two sessions per week for weight training and two sessions per week for aerobic fitness.

Sometimes it is necessary to schedule these workouts immediately after games to provide 48 hours of recovery before the next game.

Teams aim to peak during the play-offs. It is important that the players have adequate recovery time during this period. During this phase, the total volume of training is reduced. The duration of on-ice practices and dry-land workouts is reduced. In the past, too frequently ice hockey players have complained of "heavy legs" late in the season. Overtraining should be avoided during the peaking phase.

The emotional and physical stresses during the peaking phase result in the expenditure of much energy. After the play-offs, the player should take about 3 weeks for recovery. In this phase, relaxation is the goal. The physical activities are recreational, such as golf and swimming.

The demands of ice hockey at the elite level necessitate an annual training program. Dry-land training programs during the competitive season and summer training programs specifically geared for ice hockey fitness are developing better athletes. In the words of Wayne Gretzky, "For a better conditioned athlete, there is less chance of injury, and conditioning promotes career longevity" (104).

In summary, physiological attributes of the ice hockey player will define the style of play and the potential for success. Developing players need to be educated on the importance of each fitness component.

REFERENCES

1. Lariviere G. Relationship between skating velocity and length of stride, angle of forward inclination and angle of propulsion. Master's thesis, University of Oregon, 1968.
2. Cox MH, Miles DS, Verde TJ, Rhodes EC. Applied physiology of ice hockey. *Sports Med* 1995;19:184–201.
3. Green HJ. Bioenergetics of ice hockey: considerations for fatigue. *J Sports Sci* 1987;5:305–317.
4. Montgomery DL. Physiology of ice hockey. *Sports Med* 1988; 5:99–126.
5. Shephard RJ. Physiological factors limiting the ice hockey player. In: Tornquist C, ed. *Proceedings of the Third International Conference on the Coaching Aspects of Ice Hockey.* Gothenberg, Sweden: International Ice Hockey Federation, 1981:1–32.
6. Twist P, Rhodes T. A physiological analysis of ice hockey positions. *Natl Strength Cond Assoc J* 1993;15:44–46.
7. Agre JC, Baxter TL, Casal DC, Leon AS, McNally MC, Serfass RC. Musculoskeletal characteristics of professional ice-hockey players. *Can J Sport Sci* 1987;12:202–206.
8. Seliger V, Kostka V, Grusova D, et al. Energy expenditure and physical fitness of ice hockey players. *Int Z Angewandte Physiol* 1972;30:283–291.
9. Green HJ, Bishop P, Houston M, McKillop R, Norman R, Stothart P. Time-motion and physiological assessments of ice hockey performance. *J Appl Physiol* 1976;40:159–163.
10. Renger R. Identifying the task requirements essential to the success of a professional ice hockey player: a scout's perspective. *J Teach Phys Educ* 1994;13:180–195.
11. Montgomery DL, Vartzbedian B. Duration and intensity of play in adult recreational hockey games. In: Terauds J, Gros HJ, eds. *Sciences in skiing, skating and hockey.* Del Mar, CA: Academic Publishers, 1979:193–200.
12. Paterson DH. Respiratory and cardiovascular aspects of intermittent exercise with regard to ice hockey. *Can J Appl Sport Sci* 199;4:22–28.
13. Léger L. Le hockey sur glace. In: Nadeau CH, Peronnet F, eds. *Physiologie appliqué de l'activité physique.* Quebec: Edisem, St-Hyacinthe, 1980:115–129.
14. Green HJ, Daub BD, Painter DC, Thomson JA. Glycogen depletion patterns during ice hockey performance. *Med Sci Sports Exerc* 1978;10:289–293.
15. Peddie DL. Time motion analysis and heart rate telemetry of ice hockey play. Unpublished master's thesis, McGill University, Montreal, 1995.
16. Thoden JS, Jetté M. Aerobic and anaerobic activity patterns in junior and professional hockey. *Mouvement* 1975;2:145–153.
17. Montgomery DL. Characteristics of "old timer" hockey play. *Can J Appl Sport Sci* 1979;4:39–42.
18. Green HJ. Glycogen depletion patterns during continuous and intermittent ice skating. *Med Sci Sports Exerc* 1978;10:183–187.
19. Luetsolo S. Ice hockey and the energy of muscles. In: Almstedt J, ed. *Proceedings of the International Coaches Symposium.* Ottawa: Canadian Amateur Hockey Association, 1976:53–56.
20. Montpetit RR, Binette P, Taylor AW. Glycogen depletion in a game-simulated hockey task. *Can J Appl Sport Sci* 1979;4:43–45.
21. Wilson G, Hedberg A. *Physiology of ice-hockey: a report.* Ottawa: Canadian Amateur Hockey Association, 1976.
22. Green HJ. Metabolic aspects of intermittent work with specific regard to ice hockey. *Can J Appl Sport Sci* 1979;4:29–34.
23. Tesch P, Sjodin B, Karlsson J. Relationship between lactate accumulation, LDH activity, LDH isozyme and fibre type distribution in human skeletal muscle. *Acta Physiol Scand* 1978; 103:40–46.
24. Green HJ, Houston ME, Thomson JA. Inter- and intragame alterations in selected blood parameters during ice hockey performance. In: Landry F, Orban WAR, eds. *Ice hockey.* Miami: Symposia Specialists, 1978:37–46.
25. Simard C, Tremblay A, Jobin M. Effects of carbohydrate intake before and during an ice hockey game on blood and energy substrates. *Res Q Exerc Sport* 1988;59:144–147.
26. Jones S, Green HJ. Human muscle fatigue during and following high intensity intermittent exercise. *Can J Appl Sport Sci* 1984; 9:9P.
27. Jones S, Green HJ, Houston M, Frank J. Fatigue patterns in ice hockey players. *Can J Appl Sport Sci* 1983;8:211.
28. Thomson JA, Green HJ, Houston ME. Muscle glycogen depletion patterns in fast twitch fibre subgroups of man during submaximal and supramaximal exercise. *Pflugers Arch* 1979;379: 105–108.
29. Watson RC, Hanley RD. Application of active recovery techniques for a simulated ice hockey task. *Can J Appl Sport Sci* 1986;11:82–87.
30. Kaczynski M. The effects of active and passive recovery on blood lactate concentration and performance in a simulated ice hockey task. Unpublished master's thesis, McGill University, Montreal, 1989.
31. Sahli K, Harris RC, Nylind B, Hultman E. Lactate content and pH in muscle samples obtained after dynamic exercise. *Pflugers Arch* 1976;367:143–149.
32. Reference deleted in proofs.
33. Vickers J. *Instructional design for teaching physical activities: a knowledge structures approach.* Champaign, IL: Human Kinetics, 1990.
34. MacDougall JD, Wenger HA. The purpose of physiological testing. In: MacDougall JD, Wenger HA, Green HJ, eds. *Physiological testing of the high-performance athlete.* Champaign, IL: Human Kinetics, 1991:1–5.
35. Gledhill N, Jamnik V. *Detailed fitness and medical assessment protocols for NHL entry draft players.* Toronto: York University, 1994.
36. Chovanova E. The physique of the Czechoslovak top ice-hockey players. *Acta Facultatis Rerum Naturalium Universitatis Comenianae Anthropologia* 1976;22:115–118.
37. Rhodes EC, Cox MH, Quinney HA. Physiological monitoring of National Hockey League regulars during the 1985-1986 season. *Can J Appl Sport Sci* 1986;11:36P.

38. Smith DJ, Quinney HA, Wenger HA, Steadward RD, Sexsmith JR. Isokinetic torque outputs of professional and elite amateur ice hockey players. *J Orthop Sports Phys Ther* 1981;3:42–47.
39. Cox MH, Miles DS, Verde TJ, Levine AR. Physical and physiological characteristics of NHL players over the last decade. *Med Sci Sports Exerc* 1993;25:S169.
40. Agre JC, Casal DC, Leon AS, McNally MC, Baxter TL, Serfass RC. Professional ice hockey players: physiologic, anthropometric, and musculoskeletal characteristics. *Arch Phys Med Rehabil* 1988;69:188–192.
41. Chovanova E. Somatotypes of ice hockey forwards, backs and goal-keepers. *Acta Facultatis Rerum Naturalium Universitatis Comenianae Anthropologia* 1976;23:141–146.
42. Cox MH, Rhodes EC, Thomas S, Quinney HA. Fitness testing of elite hockey players. *Can Athl Ther J* 1988;1(2):6–13.
43. Green HJ, Houston ME. Effect of a season of ice hockey on energy capacities and associated functions. *Med Sci Sports* 1975;7:299–303.
44. Montgomery DL, Dallaire JA. Physiological characteristics of elite ice hockey players over two consecutive years. In: Broekhoft J, Ellis MJ, Tripps DG, et al. eds. *Sport and elite performers*. Champaign, IL: Human Kinetics, 1986:133–141.
45. Quinney HA. Sport on ice. In: Reilly T, Secher R, Sevell P, eds. *Physiology of sports*. London: E and FW Spon, 1990:311–336.
46. Smith DJ, Quinney HA, Steadward RD, Wenger HA, Sexsmith JR. Physiological profiles of the Canadian Olympic Hockey Team. *Can J Appl Sport Sci* 1982;7:142–146.
47. Montgomery DL. The effect of added weight on ice hockey performance. *Physician Sportsmed* 1982;10:91–99.
48. Chomay J, Montgomery DL, Hoshizaki TB, Brayne SP. The effect of added state weight on performance in an ice hockey fitness test. *Can J Appl Sport Sci* 1982;7:240.
49. Léger L, Seliger V, Brassard L. Comparisons among VO_{2max} values for hockey players and runners. *Can J Appl Sport Sci* 1979;4:18–21.
50. Enos E, Hoerner EF, Ryan J, Sellers W, Smith M. Recommendations for "pre and in-training" for United States World Hockey Team. *AHAUS* 1976;May:14–15.
51. Forsberg A, Hubten B, Wilson G, Karlsson J. Ishockey idrottsfysiologi ratport no. 14. *Trygg-hansa forlagsverksamheten*. Sweden, 1974.
52. Rusko H, Havu M, Karvinen Esko. Aerobic performance capacity in athletes. *Eur J Appl Phys Occup Physiol* 1978;38:151–159.
53. Houston ME, Green HJ. Physiological and anthropometric characteristics of elite Canadian ice hockey players. *J Sports Med Phys Fitness* 1976;16:123–128.
54. Hutchinson WW, Maas GM, Murdoch AJ. Effect of dry land training on aerobic capacity of college hockey players. *J Sports Med Phys Fitness* 1979;19:271–276.
55. Tegelman R, Åberg T, Poussette Å, Carlstrom K. Effects of a diet regimen on pituitary and steroid hormones in male ice hockey players. *Int J Sports Med* 1992;13:424–430.
56. Wilmore JA. The application of science to sport: physiological profiles of male and female athletes. *Can J Appl Sport Sci* 1979;4:103–115.
57. Bouchard C, Landry F, Leblanc C. Quelques-unes des caracteristiques physiques et physiologiques des joueurs de hockey et leurs relation avec la performance. *Mouvement* 1974;9:95–110.
58. Hermiston R. Ice hockey. In: Taylor AW, ed. *The scientific aspects of sports training*. Springfield, IL: Charles C Thomas, 1975:222–229.
59. Romet TT, Goode RC, Watt T, et al. Possible discriminating factors between amateur and professional hockey players in Canada. In: Landry F, Orban WAR, eds. *Ice hockey*. Vol 10. Miami: Symposia Specialists, 1978:75–80.
60. Coyne L. Cited by Marcotte G, and Hermiston R. Ice hockey. In: Taylor AW, ed. *The scientific aspects of sports training*. Springfield, IL: Charles C Thomas, 1975:222–224.
61. Daub WB, Green HJ, Houston ME, Thomson JA, Fraser IG, Ranney DA. Specificity of physiologic adaptations resulting from ice-hockey training. *Med Sci Sports Exerc* 1983;15:290–294.
62. Krotee ML, Alexander JF, Chien IH, LaPoint JD, Brooks H. The psychophysiological characteristics of university ice hockey players. In: Terauds J, Gros HJ, eds. *Science in skiing, skating and hockey*. Del Mar, CA: Academic Publishers, 1979:159–171.
63. Vainikka P, Rahkila P, Rusko H. Physical performance characteristics of the Finnish national hockey team. In: Komi PU, ed. *Exercise and sport biology*. Champaign, IL: Human Kinetics, 1982:158–165.
64. Wygand JW, Luchsinger E, Otto R, Perez HR, Kamimukai C. Position related characteristics of professional ice hockey players. *Med Sci Sports Exerc* 1987;19(suppl):S46.
65. Ferguson RJ, Marcotte GG, Montpetit RR. A maximal oxygen uptake test during ice skating. *Med Sci Sports* 1969;1:207–211.
66. Lariviere G. Comparison of the efficiency of six different patterns of intermittent ice hockey skating. Ph.D. thesis, Miami, Florida State University, 1972.
67. Riby SG. Skating economy of ice players. Unpublished master's thesis, McGill University, Montreal, 1993.
67a. Montgomery DL, Lacroix VJ, Lefebvre G. Relationship among variables in the Wingate test in professional hockey players over three years. *Med Sci Sports Exerc* 1998;30(suppl):S256.
68. Simard P. Epreuve progressive et intermittente de consommation d'oxygène maximale chez les hockeyeurs lors du patinage sur glace. Master's thesis. Montreal: Université de Montréal, 1975.
69. Geisel JSM. Training and testing in marathon speed skating. *J Sports Med Phys Fitness* 1979;19:277–282.
70. Geisel JSM. The endurance time on a bicycle ergometer as a test for marathon speed skaters. *J Sports Med Phys Fitness* 1980;20:333–340.
71. Gamble F, Montgomery DL. A cycling test of anaerobic endurance for ice hockey players. *Can J Appl Sport Sci* 1986;11:14P.
72. Montgomery DL, Turcotte R, Gamble W, Ladouceur G. Validation of a cycling test of anaerobic endurance for ice hockey players. *Sports Train Med Rehabil* 1990;2:11–22.
73. Quinney HA, Belcastro A, Steadward RD. Seasonal fitness variations and pre-playoff blood analysis in NHL players. *Can J Appl Sport Sci* 1982;7:237.
74. Twist P, Rhodes T. The bioenergetic and physiological demands of ice hockey. *Natl Strength Cond Assoc J* 1993;15:68–70.
75. Rhodes EC, Cox MH, Quinney HA. Comparison of National Hockey League regular players on selected physiological parameters. *Med Sci Sports Exerc* 1987;19(suppl):S46.
76a. Reed AT, Cotton C, Hansen H, Gauthier R. Upper body strength and handedness-shooting characteristics of junior and professional hockey players. In: Terauds J, Gros HJ, eds. *Science in skiing, skating and hockey*. Del Mar, CA: Academic Publishers, 1979:127–131.
77. Watson RC, Sargeant TLC. Laboratory and on-ice test comparisons of anaerobic power of ice hockey players. *Can J Appl Sport Sci* 1986;11:218–224.
77. Gamble F. A laboratory test of anaerobic endurance for ice hockey players. master's thesis, Montreal, McGill University, 1986.
78. Brayne SP. A comparison of on ice and laboratory tests of hockey fitness. Unpublished master's thesis, McGill University, Montreal, 1985.
79. Goslin BR, Graham TE. A comparison of "anaerobic" components of O_2 debt and the Wingate test. *Can J Appl Sport Sci* 1985;10:134–140.
80. Jacobs I, Bar-Or O, Karlsson J, et al. Changes in muscle metabolites in females with 30-s exhaustive exercise. *Med Sci Sports Exerc* 1982;14:457–460.
81. Bouchard C, Taylor AW, Dulac S. Testing maximal anaerobic power and capacity. In: MacDougall JD, Wenger HA, Green HJ, eds. *Physiological testing of the elite athlete*. Ithaca, NY: Mouvement, 1982:61–73.
82. Reed A, Hansen H, Cotton C, et al. Development and validation of an on-ice hockey fitness test. *Can J Appl Sport Sci* 1979;4:245.
83. Song TMK. Flexibility of ice hockey players and comparison with other groups. In: Terauds J, Gros HG, eds. *Science in skiing, skating and hockey*. Del Mar, CA: Academic Publishers, 1979:117–225.
84. Gauthier R, Cotton C, Reed A, Hansen H. A comparison of upper body and leg strength between professional and major junior A hockey ice hockey players. In: Terauds J, Gros HG, eds.

Science in skiing, skating and hockey. Del Mar, CA: Academic Publishers, 1979:133–138.
85. Lariviere G, LaVallee H, Shephard RJ. A simple skating test for ice hockey players. *Can J Appl Sport Sci* 1976;1:223–228.
86. Quinney HA, Smith DJ, Wenger HA. A field test for the assessment of abdominal muscular endurance in professional ice hockey players. *J Orthop Sports Phys Ther* 1984;6:30–33.
87. Trépanier A. Physiological characteristics of NHL entry draft players and performance. Unpublished master's thesis, McGill University, Montreal, 1998.
87a. Green HJ, Thomson JA, Daub WD, Houston ME, Ranney DA. Fiber composition, fiber size and enzyme activities in vastus lateralis of elite athletes involved in high intensity exercise. *Eur J Appl Physiol Occupat Physiol* 1979;41:109–117.
88. MacNab RBJ. A longitudinal study of ice hockey in boys aged 8-12. *Can J Appl Sport Sci* 1979;4:11–17.
89. Chouinard N, Reardon F. Development of a skating agility test for ice hockey players. *Can J Appl Sport Sci* 1984;9:18P.
90. Adrian OK, Rhodes EC. Comparison of anaerobic capacity of elite prepubertal ice hockey players between their eighth and ninth year. *Can J Appl Sport Sci* 1986;11:2P.
91. Rhodes EC, Potts JE, Benicky DE. Prediction of anaerobic capacity in eight year old ice hockey players. *Can J Appl Sport Sci* 1985;10:26P.
92. Rhodes EC, Twist P. *The physiology of ice hockey*. 1st ed. Vancouver: University of British Columbia, 1989.
93. Montpetit RR, Ferguson RJ, Marcotte G. Détermination indirecte de la consommation d'oxygène maximale à partir de la vitesse de patinage sur glace. *Kinanthropologie* 1971;3:97–109.
94. Dulac S, Lariviere G, Boulay M. Relations entre diverses mesures physiologiques et la performance a des tests de patinage. In: Landry F, Orban WAR, eds. *Ice hockey*. Vol 10. Miami: Symposia Specialists, 1978:55–63.
94a. Song TMK, Reid R. Relationship of lower limb flexibility, strength and anthropometric measures to skating speed. In: Terauds J, Gros HJ, eds. *Science in skiing, skating and hockey*. Del Mar, CA: Academic Publishers, 1979:83–98.
95. Lariviere G. Tests de performance visant à mesurer l'efficacité technique et la condition physique des joueurs de hockey. *Mouvement* 1974;9:77–82.
96. Lariviere G, Godbout P. *Mesure de la condition physique et de l'efficacité technique des joueurs de hockey sur glace*. Quebec City: Editions de Pelican, 1976.
97. Doyle-Baker PK, Fagan CD, Wagner OT. On-ice testing and monitoring of twenty national female ice hockey players. *Can J Sports Sci* 1997;22:13P.
98. Minkoff J. Evaluating parameters of a professional hockey team. *Am J Sports Med* 1982;10:285–292.
99. Carroll TR, Bacharach D, Kelly J, Rudrud E, Karns P. Metabolic cost of ice and in-line skating in Division I collegiate ice hockey players. *Can J Appl Physiol* 1993;18:255–262.
100. Montgomery DL. Hockey programs as a fitness vehicle for adult men. *CAHPER J* 1981;48:9–12.
101. Quinney HA, Petersen SR, Drake CJ, Tubman LA, Bell GJ, Wenger HA. The effects of a power training mini-cycle for ice hockey. *Can J Sports Sci* 1987;12:19P.
102. Blatherwick J, Knoblauch S. The effects of a dry-land interval training program on various components of fitness in college hockey players. *Med Sci Sports Exerc* 1983;15:101.
103. Greer N, Serfass R, Picconatto W. The effects of a hockey-specific training program on performance of bantam players. *Can J Sports Sci* 1992;17:65–69.
104. Twist P. *Complete conditioning for ice hockey*. Champaign, IL: Human Kinetics, 1997.

Exercise and Sport Science,
edited by William E. Garrett, Jr., and Donald T. Kirkendall.
Lippincott Williams & Wilkins, Philadelphia © 2000.

CHAPTER 53

Physiology of Cross-Country Skiing

Martin D. Hoffman, Philip S. Clifford, and Steven E. Gaskill

Cross-country skiing has undergone dramatic evolution from its origins as a utilitarian mode of travel more than 4000 years ago. Since the mid 1980s, the sport has undergone revolutionary changes with the development of the ski-skating techniques. The contemporary world of cross-country skiing includes ultralight composite skis, graphite and aramid fiber (Kevlar) poles, sophisticated boot/binding systems, and a multitude of expensive chemicals applied to the base of the skis (Fig. 53–1).

The competitive sports of biathlon and Nordic combined also include cross-country skiing. Biathlon is a sport involving cross-country skiing while carrying a .22-caliber rifle and periods of rifle marksmanship interrupting the skiing. Nordic combined is a sport that involves separate competitions in cross-country skiing and ski jumping. This chapter focuses on the physiologic demands and training issues associated with cross-country skiing and also includes a limited discussion on the unique physiologic requirements associated with biathlon. The issues associated with Nordic ski jumping are not addressed in this chapter.

THE SPORT

Cross-country skiing takes its origins from northern Europe and Scandinavia more than 4000 years ago, where it was initially used for travel, hunting, and fighting. The oldest known reference to skiing is a petroglyph from

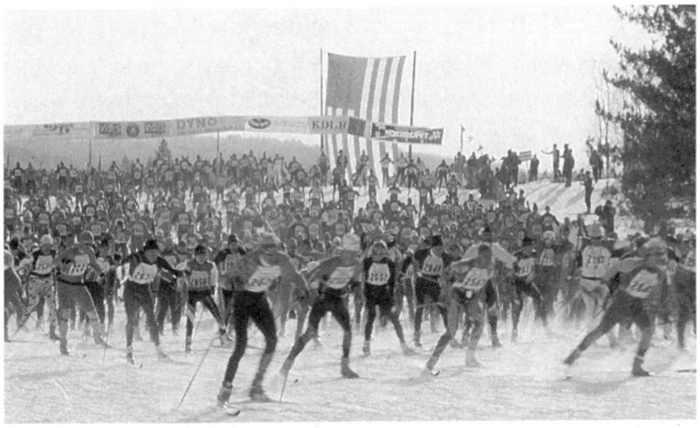

FIG. 53–1. Competitors near the start of the American Birkebeiner ski race showing modern freestyle cross-country skiing techniques. The American Birkebeiner ski race is the largest race in North America. Photo courtesy of the American Birkebeiner Ski Foundation.

about 2000 B.C. discovered in a Norwegian cave. This petroglyph shows two stick figures riding long skis in pursuit of elk. The oldest ski yet discovered is estimated to be from around 2500 B.C. The first competitions in skiing and biathlon were held in the 1760s in the Norwegian military. However, it was the latter part of the nineteenth century before skiing became more than just a Scandinavian sport. Cross-country skiing and biathlon were included as events in the first Winter Olympic Games in 1924.

For thousands of years, skis were made from a single piece of wood. Some of the early pairs of skis had one short, wide, kicking ski, and one long, narrow, gliding ski. In some cases, the short ski had an animal hide secured to its bottom to provide grip. Laminated wooden skis appeared in 1891 and were recently replaced by synthetic materials. It is thought that in the early years of skiing, no poles were used and that hunters carried only their spears, bows, and other hunting equipment. Some time later, a single pole was used. This practice was continued until the end of the nineteenth

M. D. Hoffman: Sports Performance and Technology Laboratory, Department of Physical Medicine and Rehabilitation, The Medical College of Wisconsin; and the Veterans' Affairs Medical Center, Milwaukee, Wisconsin 53295.

P. S. Clifford: Sports Performance and Technology Laboratory, Departments of Anesthesiology and Physiology, The Medical College of Wisconsin; Department of Anesthesia Research, Veterans Affairs Medical Center, Milwaukee, Wisconsin 53295.

S. E. Gaskill: School of Kinesiology and Leisure Studies, University of Minnesota, Minneapolis, Minnesota 55455.

century, when it was found that two poles were faster for competition. Early skis were attached to the boot with only a toe strap. The development of the osier binding by Sondre Nordheim in the 1850s significantly advanced the evolution of cross-country skiing. This binding held the heel in place with twisted birch roots and allowed greater maneuverability with the skis.

The cross-country ski racer of today makes use of dramatic technologic advances that have taken place in recent years. Skis are now made of modern composites, often weighing less than 500 g per ski and with lengths generally on the order of 170 to 210 cm. Poles are made of graphite and Kevlar and are extremely light and rigid. The boot and binding systems allow flexion within the binding rather than forcing the boot or forefoot to bend, and they provide significant lateral control. The skis are made faster by various base-preparation techniques and the application of expensive chemicals. Yet with all the technologic advances that have occurred, the process that accompanies selection of the base-preparation technique and wax for a given race condition continues to be shrouded in mysticism.

Perhaps the most dramatic changes in cross-country skiing occurred since the mid 1980s, as a result of the development of new skiing styles collectively referred to as "skating" because of their similarity in movement patterns to ice and roller skating. Since the initial use of ski skating, there has been an exciting evolution of more advanced techniques, accompanied by changes in skiing equipment and trail-preparation methods.

Prior to the 1980s, cross-country skiers primarily used what are now referred to as the classic techniques of diagonal striding, double poling, and kick double poling. Although Scandinavian skiers had occasionally used a form of skating during long ski marathons, the widespread use of the skating techniques really began soon after a form of ski skating was used by the American skier Bill Koch in winning the cross-country skiing World Cup in 1982. By 1985, skating had been universally accepted by international competitors. All medals at the cross-country World Championships that year were won by skiers who applied only glide wax to the skis and skated the entire race.

Some people in the international skiing community were concerned that skating techniques might completely replace conventional cross-country skiing. Out of this concern, the official governing body of international ski racing, the Federation Internationale de Ski (FIS), ruled in 1985 that half of all World Cup cross-country ski races would be "classical," with the allowance of skating only on corners, and the remaining races would be "freestyle," with any technique being allowed. In contrast to the approach taken by cross-country skiing, no restrictions on technique have been placed on competitors in Nordic combined and biathlon. Because the ski skating techniques allow cross-country ski races to be completed 10% to 30% faster than the classic techniques (1,2), these competitors now use skating techniques exclusively during their races.

Physical Requirements

The Competitive Events

Race Lengths and Format

Cross-country ski races vary in length from 5 to 50 km in International World Cup, Olympic Games, and World Championship competitions. However, citizen races vary from 1-km sprints to grueling endurance events of more than 100 km. The largest citizen races may have 8000 to 15,000 participants. In international World Cup events, women race 5-, 10-, 15-, and 30-km individual races, and men race 10-, 15-, 30-, and 50-km races using both freestyle and classic techniques. In addition to individual races, relays are popular events. In World Championships and Olympic Games, the relays include four skiers, with the first two skiers required to use classic technique, and the final two skiers using freestyle techniques. In international competitions, men ski 10 km for each relay leg, and women ski 5 km.

In recent years there have been attempts by some competitors to specialize in one technique or in races of specific lengths. World Cup rules, however, require skiers to compete using both techniques and over multiple race lengths to score adequate points to remain in contention. It is not uncommon for top individuals to compete effectively in both techniques and at all lengths.

Elite cross-country skiing events are generally run in two different formats, individual start and pursuit start. With the individual start format, skiers start racing one at a time at 30-second intervals. In 1988, the pursuit format was added to the World Cup circuit. The pursuit format combines two races. The first race is an individual start race, generally using classic technique. The following day, a freestyle race is held, with the winner of the previous day starting first, and each subsequent skier starting behind the first skier based on their finishing time behind the leader the previous day. The pursuit format is more exciting for spectators, as the skier who crosses the finish line first is the combined two-race, overall winner. In citizen and many marathon races, a mass start format is used. In these races, all skiers begin at the same time.

Course Design

Cross-country ski courses are in principle expected to be designed to include one-third uphill skiing (grades between 9% and 11%, with some short, steeper climbs), one-third downhill, and one-third gentle rolling, undulating terrain. In practice, however, since the mid 1980s courses have been increasing in total climb, lengthening the time spent on uphills and reducing the time on easier sections. International course rules include minimum and maximum total and individual climbs. For example, during a 30-km race, the total climb is expected to be between 800 and 1200 m, with individual climbs not allowed to exceed 100 m without at least a 200-m break. In addition, the high point of a course must not exceed 1800 m in altitude.

World Records and Racing Velocities

Because of the variations in course contour and snow conditions, establishing world records in cross-country skiing is impractical. Yet cross-country skiing results are commonly compared by average speed or by the average time required per kilometer. These data demonstrate that average race velocities have increased steadily since the early days of cross-country skiing (Fig. 53–2). Major increases in race velocities were evident in the 1960s with the advent of improved track preparation by using mechanized means, in the 1970s with the development of technologically superior synthetic ski bases and lighter synthetic skis, and in the 1980s with the development of the ski-skating techniques. Continued increases in speed reflect improvements in skiing techniques, advances in training methods, and the development of chemicals used on the ski bases to reduce drag. During the 1996 to 1997 season, the average winning time for men over a variety of freestyle race lengths was about 6.6 m/s or 151 seconds (2:31) per kilometer. Women average about 10% to 12% slower than men on similar courses. Downhill speeds of more than 51 km/h (14 m/s) have been recorded in some cross-country ski races.

Biathlon

Biathlon is a sport that combines cross-country skiing and rifle marksmanship. In competitions, biathletes typically ski races of 7.5 to 30 km, with the skiing interrupted at regular intervals for shooting. Races usually include two to four visits to the shooting range interspersed with skiing loops of 3 to 7 km. Biathlon has no restrictions on the skiing techniques that may be used, so skating techniques are always used by elite competitors because these techniques are faster. The shooting is performed in the prone and standing positions, with the position alternating for each visit to the shooting range. While at the shooting range, the biathlete fires a specialized .22-caliber rifle, attempting to hit five targets. The targets are 50 m from the firing line, with the prone targets being 40 mm in diameter and the standing targets being 110 mm in diameter. A penalty, either of added skiing distance or time, is assessed for each missed target. The rifle must weigh at least 3.5 kg and is carried on the biathlete's back while skiing. Courses for biathlon races have similar requirements to those in cross-country skiing, but the total climb during the race is about one third less.

Nordic Combined

Competitions in Nordic combined are scored by combining the results in cross-country ski racing with the scores from Nordic ski jumping, in which the best jumps will average about 80 to 90 m in length. Competitions in Nordic combined are freestyle and use a pursuit-style format, with the winner of the jumping event starting first. The remaining competitors start in order of their finish in the ski-jumping event, with each point they finished behind the winner of the jumping being converted to a 9-second handicap. The Nordic combined competitor who reaches the finish line first in the cross-country race wins the overall event. Nordic combined skiers race both a 15-km individual race and a team-relay event, with each skier racing 10 km. The relay uses a pursuit format based on jumping results for the team of four competitors.

Description of the Classic Techniques

Classic cross-country skiing generally involves maintaining the skis parallel with each other, and forward

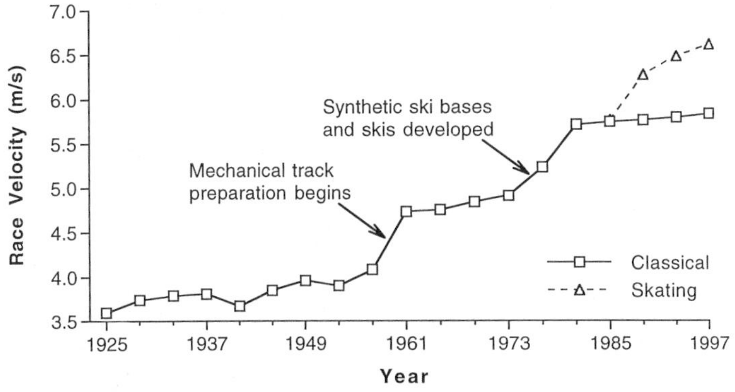

FIG. 53–2. Cross-country ski-racing velocities since 1925 averaging available data over a variety of race lengths. All data are for men, as very few data are available for women prior to 1965.

progression is assisted by the horizontal forces from a posteriorly and downward directed "kick" through the skis. The ski is at a standstill roughly 300 milliseconds or less during the application of the kick, and the vertical force can reach 2 to 3 times body weight (3–9). Transferring this kick into forward movement along the track is dependent on the amount of grip between the snow and ski that results from compression of the midsection of the ski, where grip wax has been applied.

Classic skiing primarily involves four techniques (Fig. 53–3). The diagonal stride uses a movement pattern similar to those of walking and running, characterized by alternate thrusts with each pole as the opposite leg applies a kick. With the kick double-pole technique, the poling is performed simultaneously with both poles after the kick. The double-pole technique is performed without a kick and relies entirely on the upper body providing propulsive forces through the poles. On steep uphills when a kick can no longer be obtained, the skis are placed obliquely, and a walking or running movement termed the "herringbone" technique is used.

Description of the Skating Techniques

The ski-skating techniques require that at least one ski be placed at an angle to the direction of travel. Forward progression is assisted by the posteriorly directed component of force applied to the obliquely directed skating ski. The propulsive forces are transmitted through a continuously moving ski, so grip wax is not used with skating. Because the body position is more upright at the beginning of pole plant with the skating techniques, pole lengths are 10 to 15 cm longer compared with those used in the classic techniques.

Several different skating techniques are currently used (Fig. 53–4). The earliest form of skating is now known as the *marathon skate* technique and is characterized by one ski remaining in the track while the other ski performs the skating motion. Thrusts are applied

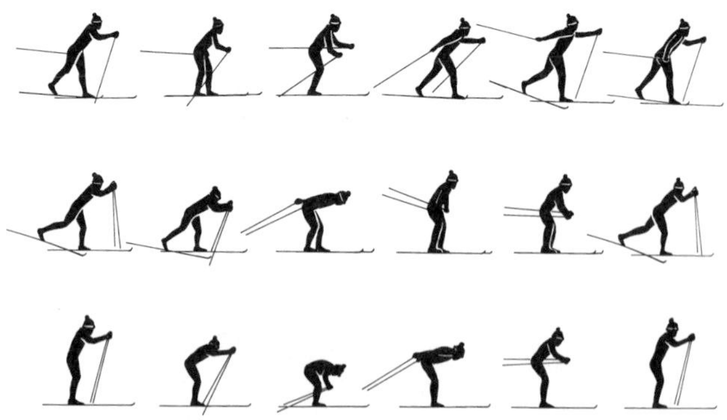

FIG. 53–3. Classical cross-country skiing techniques. **Top:** The diagonal-stride technique. **Middle:** The kick double pole technique. **Bottom:** The double pole technique.

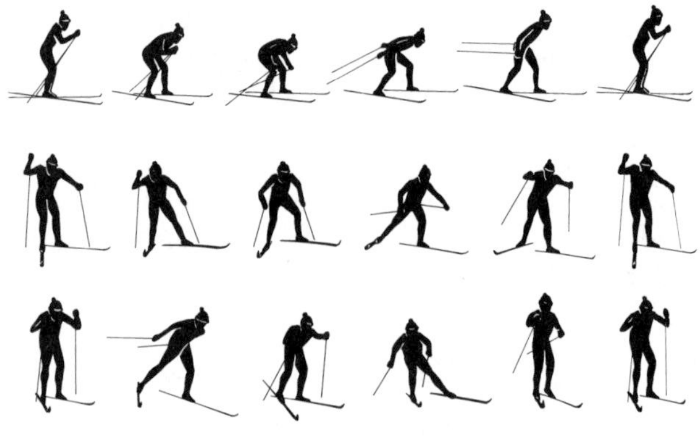

FIG. 53–4. Some freestyle cross-country skiing techniques. **Top**: The marathon skate technique. **Middle**: The V1 skate technique. **Bottom**: The V2 skate technique.

simultaneously with both poles, while weight is transferred to the skating ski. Numerous variations have evolved from this early form of skating. The *V1 skate* (offset) technique is distinguished by skating to both sides and slightly asynchronous and asymmetric thrusts with both poles occurring as weight is shifted to one ski. As weight is transferred to the other ski, the arms swing forward and prepare for the next poling motion; thus poling occurs on only one side. The *V2 skate* (one-skate) technique involves symmetric poling with both poles concurrent with the skating motion to each side, so that two pole thrusts occur per cycle. The *V2 alternate* (Gunde or two-skate) technique is similar in timing and movement pattern to the V2 skate, except that the poling is performed on only one side. Other variations include the *diagonal V-skate* technique, which is like the herringbone but is performed with the skis gliding while weighted and is used on steep uphills. *Skating without poles* is another technique that is used primarily at high skiing speeds.

Physiologic Requirements

The duration of cross-country ski competitions generally ranges from several minutes for 5-km events to hours for ski marathons. The duration of these events suggests that aerobic processes account for at least 85% of the total energy metabolism in cross-country ski racing (10–12). Nevertheless, competitions are performed at very high intensities. Metabolic measurements have suggested that skiers maintain approximately 88% to 93% of their maximal oxygen uptake ($\dot{V}O_2max$) during 20- to 50-minute races (13,14) and 82% of their $\dot{V}O_2max$ during 2.5-hour ski races (15). From heart-rate data during 10-km and 20-km races, Bergh (11) reached a similar conclusion that elite skiers are seldom operating at less than 85% of their $\dot{V}O_2max$.

Compared with aerobic metabolism, anaerobic metabolism plays a small role in cross-country ski racing. The importance of anaerobic capacity in cross-country skiing should not be completely disregarded, however. It is clear that there is an important anaerobic contribution during uphill sections of races and even in the later portions of long races. Indirect assessment of anaerobic metabolism by measurements of blood lactate concentration after races of various distances has shown that, after races of 13 to 30 km, there are relatively high plasma lactate concentrations suggestive of an important anaerobic contribution during the later portions of the race (11,14,16). Shorter races induce even higher postrace lactate levels. Because the race times for a given distance are faster with the skating techniques, anaerobic capacity is likely to play an even more important role now than it did prior to the early 1980s. Thus, when the top finishers are separated by only a few seconds, anaerobic power can play a decisive role in the final results of a race.

The muscular contractions in cross-country skiing are dynamic in nature and generally reach only a small proportion of maximal strength. Nevertheless, there are certain competitive situations, such as the sprint at the end of a race, in which the force requirements become greater, so muscular strength and power can be important factors.

Technique-Specific Requirements

Competitive success in cross-country skiing requires skill in the use of the various skiing techniques. Besides the differences in movement patterns requiring the development of skills that are unique to each technique, the physiologic demands of classic and freestyle cross-country skiing also are somewhat different.

An important distinction between the skating techniques and classic techniques of diagonal stride and kick double pole is the way in which propulsive forces are applied through the skis. The classic techniques use a downward and posteriorly directed "kick" to drive the skier forward. During the application of this kick in classic skiing, the ski must momentarily come to a complete stop. As skiing velocity is increased, the speed of muscle contraction that is required to apply the kick must increase, and at some point it can become a limiting factor to further increases in skiing velocity. Therefore maximal velocity of the classic techniques under some conditions is limited by speed of muscle contraction rather than by the physiologic energy-delivery system. In contrast, with the skating techniques, the ski forces are applied over a significantly longer time (17), and speed of muscle contraction does not appear to be a limiting factor. Because speed of muscle contraction is thought to affect muscular efficiency, the differences in application of ski forces between the classic and skating techniques are important with regard to relative energy costs and maximal velocities with the different techniques.

Several investigations (18–26) compared the oxygen cost of different cross-country skiing techniques. At a given velocity over flat or varying terrain, the diagonal stride technique requires a higher oxygen consumption than does ski skating (Fig. 53–5). The oxygen cost for the kick double pole technique is similar to that for the marathon and V1 skate techniques. Most interestingly, double poling has a lower oxygen cost than the diagonal stride and kick double pole techniques for skiing at a given velocity on flat terrain. Furthermore, double poling has been shown to have greater economy than the skating techniques on flat terrain. There is probably a requirement for greater anaerobic metabolism with double poling, however, making this technique less desirable for extended use. Additionally, the greater economy of double poling compared with diagonal striding is lost when going up steep hills (22). Nevertheless, some ski racers have experimented with double poling during races. It is conceivable that the added glide that would be achieved from not applying grip wax could allow double poling to be effectively used in classic races on relatively flat courses.

The greater economy with the double pole technique is probably due largely to the biomechanical properties of the technique, of which the most important factor is the direction of force application. With double poling, a greater proportion of the forces is directed horizontally along the line of travel rather than being "wasted" in a lateral or inferior direction. This is enhanced by the large amount of trunk and hip flexion that occurs during double poling, causing the poles to be placed at a more acute angle with the ground. This trunk and hip flexion

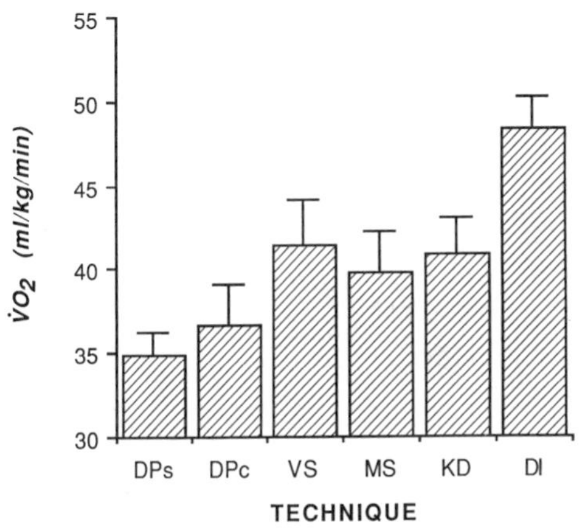

FIG. 53–5. Oxygen uptake ($\dot{V}O_2$) for skiing on flat snow at the same velocity with various cross-country skiing techniques. *DPs*, double pole on skating skis; *DPc*, double pole on classic skis; *VS*, V1 skate; *MS*, marathon skate; *KD*, kick double pole; *DI*, diagonal stride. Brackets represent 1 SEM. Reprinted from ref. 18, with permission.

also produces a lower average air resistance with the double pole technique. Additionally, the absence of laterally directed forces through the skis and a more even distribution of weight on the skis probably results in lower average ski forces and snow drag with the double pole technique compared with the skating techniques.

The various cross-country skiing techniques differ in regard to the poling forces required. The peak forces transmitted though the poles with the diagonal stride technique are on the order of about 10% to 20% of body weight (8). In contrast, the peak poling forces with the skating techniques have been found to be 20% to 30% of body weight in some studies (27,28), and as high as 45% to 60% in other studies (29,30). The duration of poling force application is also considerably longer for skating as a result of greater trunk flexion during the poling thrust and the use of longer poles. Therefore the average poling force per cycle is considerably greater for the skating techniques compared with diagonal striding. Of considerable importance is that more than half of the total propulsive forces for the V1 skate technique are generated through the poles (31). Because of the importance of the poling forces with ski skating, more emphasis has been placed on training the upper body. In addition, technology has been directed at developing stiffer poles. Some have also suggested that modification of the form of the pole grip might allow an increase in peak poling forces, but it is unlikely that skiing economy can be improved through modification of the pole grip (20).

One other interesting difference among the various skiing techniques is the amount of time that the two skis are simultaneously on the ground. With the V1 and V2 skate techniques, double support accounts for less than 20% to 30% of the cycle (9,17,32). In contrast, double support occurs during about 50% to 80% of the cycle for the kick double pole and diagonal stride techniques (5,9). Thus better balance and equipment that provides greater stability are important with the skating techniques. The evolution of ski skating has been accompanied by the development of skis with better tracking ability, above-the-ankle boots with greater lateral support and more torsionally rigid soles, and binding systems that provide greater control.

Unique Physiologic Demands of Biathlon

The intense physical exertion of cross-country skiing and the requirement for precision rifle marksmanship give rise to a unique set of physiologic demands for the sport of biathlon. The competitor must ski fast and shoot quickly because the fastest time wins the race. Yet the shooting must be performed well because the biathlete is penalized by skiing a penalty loop or by having penalty time added to the skiing time for each target that is missed.

Adding to the demands of the sport is the requirement that, while skiing, the biathlete must carry a rifle that weighs a minimum of 3.5 kg, but more typically weighs 4 to 5 kg. From energy-cost calculations, it has been estimated that carriage of the rifle accounts for approximately 7% of the energy expenditure during skiing with the V2 skating technique (33). Biathletes seem to prefer the V2 skating technique, possibly because the technique minimizes the additional energy cost associated with carriage of the rifle.

Examination of heart rate profiles, in conjunction with timing of the procedures at the shooting range, has given some insight into the demands of the biathlon (34). From these evaluations, it is evident that biathletes work at very high intensities during competitions. Heart rates during the skiing portion of the competition have been found to be about 90% of maximum (Fig. 53–6). This intensity may be slightly lower than intensities ob-

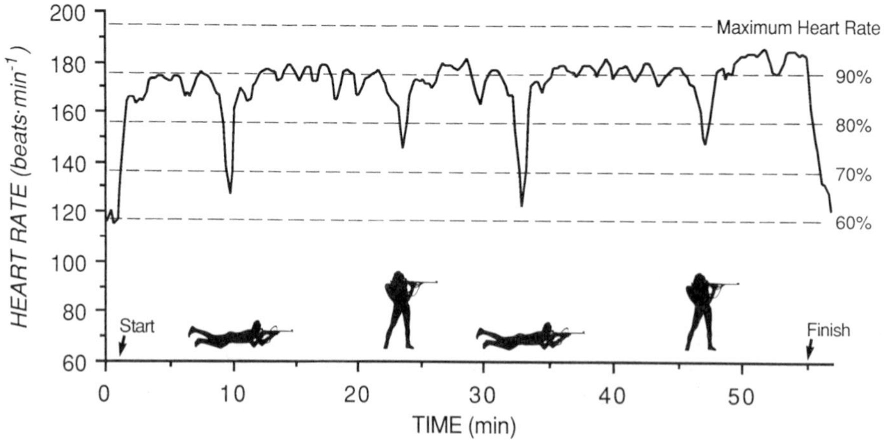

FIG. 53–6. Representative heart rate profile during a national level biathlon competition demonstrating the high heart rates maintained during skiing and the decrease in heart rate during each period of shooting. Reprinted from ref. 34, with permission.

served during cross-country ski racing, probably because of the demands for precision marksmanship placed on the biathlete. Biathletes typically reduce their skiing intensity for approximately 50 to 60 seconds as they approach the firing range and spend less than 60 seconds at the range. As a result, heart rate typically drops 10 to 12 beats/min to 85% to 87% of maximum before arrival at the firing line and is at 60% to 70% of maximum at the completion of shooting. There is evidence that the intensity of the preceding exercise influences shooting ability, particularly for the standing shooting position (35,36). This may explain why biathletes seem to reduce the intensity of skiing as they are approaching the firing line for a longer time before standing shooting compared with prone shooting (36).

THE ATHLETE

Aerobic Capacity

Because aerobic processes account for most of the energy metabolism in cross-country ski racing (10–12), it should not be surprising that successful cross-country skiers have some of the highest $\dot{V}O_2$max values of all athletes. It is not uncommon for elite male cross-country skiers to have $\dot{V}O_2$max values greater than 80 mL/min/kg (10,37–42). Maximal aerobic power has been identified as one of the main factors predicting success in cross-country ski racing at the elite (37,39), intercollegiate (43), and citizen racer (44) levels. Whereas $\dot{V}O_2$max values are usually expressed in the units of mL/min/kg, expression in the units of mL/min/kg$^{2/3}$ appears to provide a better predictor of success (37,39). Bergh's data (37) suggest that winning a world-class championship requires a minimal aerobic capacity of about 350 mL/min/kg$^{2/3}$ for men and 290 mL/min/kg$^{2/3}$ for women.

Because of the high aerobic demands of cross-country skiing, the muscles of elite competitors are characterized by high oxidative enzyme activity (11,40,45–48). Interestingly, Rusko and co-workers (40) found lower succinate dehydrogenase activity in the leg muscles of cross-country skiers compared with that in long-distance runners. They suggested that local factors of aerobic performance are stressed when a relatively small muscle mass is activated as in running, whereas greater demands are placed on central factors when a larger muscle mass is used, as in cross-country skiing. This hypothesis is supported by evidence that the central circulatory system becomes the important limiting factor when the exercising muscle mass is increased (49–51) and may be an important factor in the development of the high $\dot{V}O_2$max values in cross-country skiers. In addition, the nature of the sport requiring maximal or near-maximal efforts on uphills and relative rests on downhills (11) may promote a greater adaptation in $\dot{V}O_2$max (52).

Competitive cross-country skiers have also generally been characterized by muscle-fiber compositions of at least 60% slow-twitch fibers (11,46,53,54). Some preliminary data of Stray-Gunderson and colleagues (48) suggest that elite American cross-country skiers may have a preponderance of fast-twitch fibers in the rectus femoris and triceps muscles, however. A high percentage of fast-twitch fibers may be advantageous for the power requirements of the sport, and sufficient oxidative capacity may still be possible, as recent data suggest that fast-twitch fibers can develop very high oxidative capacity with endurance training (55).

As is discussed below, the skating techniques require the generation of greater propulsive forces from the upper body than does the diagonal stride technique. This has resulted in a greater emphasis on aerobic training and testing of the upper body. A number of studies have shown a good association between upper-body aerobic power-output tests and ski or biathlon racing performance (56–58). Untrained individuals can seldom achieve oxygen uptakes with their upper bodies of more than 70% of their leg values, whereas highly trained cross-country skiers and biathletes may achieve values of 80% to 95% (42,56,58,59).

Although a high $\dot{V}O_2$max is necessary for elite-level competition, it does not necessarily guarantee success at this level. The successful cross-country skier must also be able to sustain a high proportion of his or her $\dot{V}O_2$max throughout the duration of the race. The proportion of $\dot{V}O_2$max that an individual can sustain has been characterized by a measure commonly referred to as the "aerobic threshold." This term was coined by Wasserman and McIlroy (60) to describe the oxygen uptake above which blood lactate concentration begins to increase. Much debate has ensued among scientists about both the concept and the terminology of an anaerobic threshold, as well as whether the increase in blood lactate concentration is due to increased production or reduced clearance of lactate. For a thorough review of this topic, the reader is referred to the jointly published articles by Davis (61) and Brooks (62). Nevertheless, there appears to be a relation between the experimentally determined values for the anaerobic threshold and the metabolic rate that be maintained over an extended period.

Sedentary subjects generally have anaerobic thresholds at 50% to 60% of their $\dot{V}O_2$max (63,64). In contrast, anaerobic thresholds have been reported to be at 80% to 92% of $\dot{V}O_2$max among United States National cross-country team members (42), at 86% of $\dot{V}O_2$max among top young Finnish female skiers (54), and average 81% to 89% of $\dot{V}O_2$max among female United States National biathlon team members (57). Because cross-country skiers have been found to race at 82% to 93% of their $\dot{V}O_2$max (11,13–15), they are functioning very near their anaerobic thresholds during competitions. Further importance of the anaerobic threshold as a determinant of performance in cross-country skiing has been provided by Droghetti and colleagues (65) with their finding of a strong correlation between a noninvasive measure of anaerobic threshold and average racing velocity for Italian National team members. Similar studies in runners have also shown that race times had a higher correlation with the oxygen uptake at the anaerobic threshold than with $\dot{V}O_2max$ (66–68).

Anaerobic Capacity

Because anaerobic metabolism plays a relatively small role in cross-country ski racing compared with aerobic metabolism, comparison of cross-country skiers with untrained individuals shows that the skiers' oxidative enzyme activity is substantially more elevated than the glycolytic enzyme activity (46).

In assessing a number of different athletic populations, Komi and co-workers (53) found cross-country skiers to rate relatively low in anaerobic performance capacity. Their measures of anaerobic capacity included the Margaria vertical velocity test, maximal isometric strength, and capillary blood lactate concentration after maximal exercise. Haymes and Dickinson (69) also found cross-country skiers to rate low in anaerobic power scores compared with alpine skiers, based on results of the Margaria vertical velocity and vertical jump tests. By using the Wingate test, Patton and Duggan (70) found that elite British biathletes possessed a greater capacity for anaerobic exercise in both the upper and lower body compared with control subjects when the power outputs were expressed relative to body mass.

Muscular Strength and Power

Cross-country skiing requires dynamic muscular contractions that are generally at only a fraction of maximal strength. Nevertheless, there are certain competitive situations in which strength and power become important. Furthermore, the greater poling forces with skating compared with the diagonal stride technique (8,30,31) suggest that upper-body strength may be more important with the skating techniques. Therefore it is not too surprising that upper-body and quadriceps strength were found to be significantly correlated with 10-km race results by Ng and co-workers (44) in their stepwise regression analysis evaluating determinants of cross-country ski racing performance among citizen racers.

Although the importance of muscular strength in competitive cross-country skiing is now recognized, relatively little emphasis has previously been placed on the evaluation or training of muscular strength in cross-country skiers. Haymes and Dickinson (69) found cross-country skiers to have lower isometric strength of the quadriceps than alpine skiers, even after the strength measures were adjusted for body mass. Komi and colleagues (53) also found cross-country skiers to have lower relative isometric quadriceps strength than alpine skiers, but the cross-country skiers were stronger than 800-m runners and speed skaters. Davies and colleagues (71) reported isokinetic strength data of various muscle groups of United States National cross-country skiing team members, but comparable strength measures in other populations were unfortunately not reported.

In recent years, maximal upper-body power output has become a common physiologic measurement used in testing cross-country skiers and biathletes (58,59). Maximal upper-body power adjusted for body mass has been found to be a better predictor of race performance than $\dot{V}O_2$ max or oxygen uptake at anaerobic threshold in both junior members of an Olympic development program and experienced master skiers (72). From testing of a large group of high school athletes, it was found that the cross-country skiers with the best race results were able to develop more than twice the upper-body power as the slower skiers, and they had four times greater upper-body power compared with cross-country runners who did not cross-country ski (Gaskill, unpublished results).

Anthropometric Characteristics

Body size, shape, and composition have an obvious influence on performance in many sports. With the exception of body composition, however, the impact of these factors in cross-country skiing is not obvious. Because cross-country skiing requires the transport of body mass, it would stand to reason that the best competitors would be lean. Indeed, elite Nordic skiers have a low percentage of body fat, and the best skiers tend to have the lowest percentage of body fat. Typical percentages of body fat range from about 5% to 12% for elite men and 10% to 22% for elite women (57,58,73). Among intercollegiate ski racers, percentage of body fat has been found to be one of the main predictive factors of 5- to 15-km race performance (43).

Orvanova (73) recently presented a thorough review of the body characteristics of various winter sports athletes. Male cross-country skiers were classified as ectomorphic mesomorphs, whereas female skiers were characterized as endomorphic mesomorphs. In general, the strongest competitors placed highest on the mesomorphy axis. Interestingly, the best skiers also were found to have longer limb segments and greater limb girths (74).

The influence of body mass in cross-country skiing was examined by Bergh (37). He performed a theoretical analysis comparing the effect of body mass on physical capacity with its effect on the power costs of skiing. This analysis suggests that the larger, heavier skier has the advantage on downhills, flats, and low-grade uphills, whereas the lighter skier has the advantage on steep uphills. Hoffman and colleagues (75) subsequently pro-

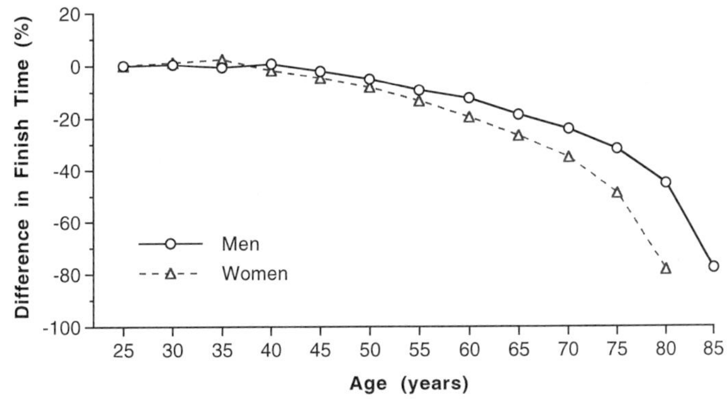

FIG. 53–7. Effect of age on racing results in the 1993 to 1996 American Birkebeiner. Average finish times for the top 10% of competitors in each 5-year age group are compared with the times for the 20- to 24-year age group. The data are plotted at the oldest age of each age group. Of interest is the maintenance of high speed through the 35- to 39-year age group for men and the 30- to 34-year age group for women. These results are probably due to the best 20- to 30-year-old skiers participating in World Cup and other events and not in citizen races like the American Birkebeiner until they become master skiers at age 30 or older. If 20- to 29-year-old World Cup skiers participated in the American Birkebeiner, it is likely that the speeds for the 20- to 24- and 25- to 29-year age groups would be higher. The drop-off of speed at older than age 50, and especially in the older age groups, may also be skewed because of declining numbers of racers. Modified from ref. 76, with permission.

vided experimental evidence supporting this theoretic analysis by demonstrating that heavier skiers have a lower oxygen consumption per unit body mass than lighter skiers for roller skiing on flat terrain. Nonetheless, because the distribution of flats, uphills, and downhills in race courses varies, competitive skiers may be of quite different body weights. This is supported by the data presented by Bergh (37) showing a body-weight range of 30 kg for elite world-class male skiers.

Age

The physiologic factors that allow peak performances in cross-country skiing are at their height when skiers are in their twenties and thirties (42). By this age, those who will become elite competitors have already mastered the techniques and have the necessary experience. Thus, these are the years in which physical capacity and skill are optimal. As should be expected, race performances appear to be best between the ages of 20 and 30 years, after which there is a gradual deterioration until 50 to 60 years, when a more rapid effect of aging is observed (2,76). Figure 53–7 displays a cross-sectional examination of performance in the American Birkebeiner as a function of age.

TRAINING THE ATHLETE

The Season

The international World Cup season extends from December through the end of March and spans the entire northern hemisphere. Races are awarded annually to sites around the world as diverse as Canada, central Asia, Japan, and the United States, including Alaska, the midwest states, and New England. The majority of races are still held in Western Europe and Scandinavia, however. A few sites, such as the Holmenkollen events in Oslo, Norway, the Salpausselka Games in Lahti, Finland, and the Swedish Ski Games in Falun, Sweden, are annual events. The season is normally divided into three blocks of races. Three to four weekends of races usually precede a Christmas break. Four weekends of racing in January are followed by a break for National Championships. The spring series of five to six weekends typically lasts from the middle of February through March.

World Cup events typically account for about 15 races each competition season for top competitors and include races with both techniques and at all standard distances. In addition to the World Cup events, most elite racers will compete in national, club, and promotional races. The typical number of races for elite international racers often exceeds 35 to 40 races in a season spanning December through April.

Olympic and World Championship events present a special challenge to the cross-country skiing competitor. Both men and women may race in up to five races during a 10- to 12-day period, racing nearly every second day over a wide variety of distances and using both classic and freestyle techniques. The physical demands on these athletes is tremendous, and every effort is made to improve recovery between events. These measures typically include efforts to replenish glycogen stores and normalize fluid balance. It also is common for skiers to use other measures, which lack rigorous scientific support, such as massage and nutritional aids. Many methods have been used to attempt to quantify recovery and fitness for racing, including measurements of resting and submaximal exercise heart rates, blood lactate concentrations, and testosterone-to-cortisol ratios.

One of the biggest challenges for cross-country skiers is maintaining health over the extended race season. During a single season, an elite skier may ski more than 4000 to 7000 km and race more than 1000 km. Travel may continue over a 3- to 5-month period, including multiple airline flights and changes in time zones. With the added stress from regular exposure to dry air and cold temperatures, it is understandable that many athletes suffer from upper respiratory problems and symptoms of overtraining.

In addition to the demands of the competitive season, serious athletes train all year. Each country has differing methods and schedules for training their athletes, but nearly all include regularly scheduled camps for group training. These camps generally take two forms: (a) dryland camps for physical training and instruction including roller skiing, running, hiking, strength work, physiologic testing, technique work, and other group activities, and (b) summer snow camps that may require travel either to a glacier or to the southern hemisphere. Because of the nature of summer snow, skiing in the northern hemisphere often takes place at relatively high altitudes of 1500 to 3200 m, although a few locations with lower elevations can be used in the early summer. During summer snow camps, teams will generally focus on technique with long-distance, low-intensity skiing. Athletes will often live at much lower elevations than where they ski, and they do their speed training at these lower elevations on foot or roller skis. This arrangement is dictated by the location and availability of snow. Some countries report as many as 100 days a year spent at training camps by national team athletes.

Altitude training has become an accepted portion of most training plans. Recent research (77,78) has demonstrated the benefits of living at high elevation and training at low elevations. This approach provides the athlete the high altitude–associated benefits of increased oxygen-carrying capacity without sacrificing the ability to train at higher intensities. Several countries now have hypobaric houses allowing athletes to live under conditions simulating high altitude for specific periods with the intent to improve peak performance.

Sport-Specific Training

An understanding of the physiologic demands of cross-country skiing makes it obvious that certain areas must be emphasized in training for the sport. Inducing the central and peripheral adaptations from aerobic training sets the foundation for the training program because a high aerobic capacity is essential for successful competition in the sport. Development of muscular strength and power, economy of movement, and technical skills are other important components of the training program. The general training principles for endurance athletes can be learned from other sources. The primary mission of this section is to concentrate on the training issues specific to cross-country skiing that have become evident in recent years.

Skating Versus Classic Skiing

The development of the skating techniques has resulted in considerable confusion among some skiers and coaches about how best to integrate classic and freestyle skiing into training programs. Soon after the advent of ski skating, training programs that incorporated a limited amount of classic skiing were accused of being responsible for decreased fitness and performance levels among some elite skiers. There was apparently concern that ski skating might not have the same capacity to develop and maintain aerobic fitness, because of either lower aerobic demands or greater anaerobic demands. Obviously, for those skiers competing in both disciplines, some training time must be spent with both classic and freestyle skiing. Biathletes and Nordic combined skiers do not use classic techniques in their competitions, however. It has still been questioned whether there is any rationale for these skiers to use classic skiing in their training.

Whereas some coaches and skiers still express opinions that a certain proportion of training should be with classic skiing, research has not provided a rationale for believing that one discipline would induce greater aerobic training benefits than the other. Scientific investigations have shown that for a maximal or specific submaximal level of perceived effort, similar oxygen uptakes, heart rates, and blood lactate concentrations are induced with classic and freestyle skiing (79,80). In other words, the two cross-country skiing disciplines should produce comparable physiologic stimuli for cardiorespiratory adaptations. Therefore, the proportion of training time devoted to a given cross-country skiing technique should not affect cardiorespiratory fitness. Determination of the relative amounts of training with the two cross-country skiing disciplines probably should be made on the bases of training specificity, overuse injuries, and training variety for psychological purposes.

Upper-Body Training

Upper-body strength and endurance training seem to have greater importance in the present era of cross-country skiing. The forces generated through the poles are greater with the skating techniques compared with the diagonal stride technique. In addition, a greater proportion of the propulsive forces is generated through the poles with the skating techniques. Incorporation of double poling workouts is one approach that would seem to be of value for competitive cross-country skiers. Furthermore, greater emphasis on training of the upper body will improve the oxidative capacity of these muscle groups and may allow increased use of the double pole technique in competitions where its greater economy under some conditions may be advantageous.

Whereas double poling may be a valuable method of increasing upper-body muscular strength and endurance, the technique has less potential for inducing desirable cardiorespiratory adaptations. Anaerobic metabolism plays a greater role with double poling, and exercising at a given oxygen-uptake level requires a greater perceived effort compared with other techniques (18,20,22,23,25,26,81). This is probably due to the smaller muscle mass used with this technique. The practical implication is that the greater anaerobic demand and greater relative perceived effort make it difficult to use double poling at adequate oxygen-uptake levels for development of central cardiovascular training adaptations.

Dry-Land Training

Few cross-country skiers have available snow for year-around training. As a result, much of the training by cross-country skiers involves activities other than on-snow skiing. This off-snow training has been termed *dry-land* training. Typical dry-land training includes roller skiing, running, running while simultaneously using poles (pole running), cycling, kayaking, canoeing, swimming, and strength-training activities. The greatest training specificity of the various dry-land training techniques is achieved with roller skiing. The importance of training specificity achieved through roller skiing may be even greater now with the advent of the skating techniques because these techniques cannot be simulated as well as the diagonal stride technique by pole running.

Questions have recently been raised about the optimization of training specificity from roller skiing. Improved technology and the lack of necessity to include a ratchet system in roller skis used for the skating techniques have resulted in the availability of faster wheels and bearings. As a result, many commercial roller skis now have rolling resistances that are much lower than on-snow resistances. Besides allowing skiers to travel at speeds that may be unsafe in some training environments, it was thought that low-resistance roller skis were responsible for a decline in fitness levels among some elite cross-country skiers (82,83). It was thought that skiers might not naturally travel faster on the lower-resistance roller skis to induce comparable aerobic demands as with slower roller skis. Recent work (21,84), however, has demonstrated that the relation of oxygen uptake with rating of perceived exertion is not affected by roller-ski rolling resistance. On the other hand, average poling forces across the cycle were found to be higher for the same perceived effort when using high-resistance roller skis (84). Therefore, it would seem that differences in roller ski rolling resistance should have no effect on the cardiovascular training adaptations that result from roller skiing, but higher-resistance roller skis are likely to induce greater upper-body aerobic adaptations than are lower-resistance roller skis.

In general, the physiological differences as well as the biomechanical differences for roller skiing compared with on-snow skiing can probably be reduced by using wheels and bearings that produce drag forces similar to those present with on-snow skiing. In this way, it should be possible to improve the ski-specific training that can result from roller skiing.

In-line skates have recently become popular among recreational athletes and also are frequently used by cross-country skiers for simulating ski skating. These skates have several aligned wheels that are attached to an above-the-ankle boot. The design prevents ankle plantarflexion to the extent that occurs with the ski-skating techniques on snow or roller skis. For this reason, in-line skates probably do not simulate the biomechanics of on-snow skiing technique as well as roller skis. In terms of the cardiorespiratory demands, however, it probably does not matter whether in-line skates or roller skis are used. The goal of most in-line skate manufacturers appears to be to produce skates with minimal rolling resistance. As in the selection of roller skis, the competitive cross-country skier who uses in-line skates for cardiorespiratory training should choose in-line skates with a frictional resistance comparable to that of on-snow skis.

Supplemental Training

Cross-country skiers continue to use a wide variety of training techniques. Little research is available to support the range of training activities or to correlate activities to race results. Nevertheless, there seems to be general agreement among coaches that a varied set of activities is necessary to maintain muscular balance during a year-round training program. Most competitive cross-country skiers participate in a wide range of aerobic and skill sports including swimming, cycling, kayaking, hiking, mountaineering, running, and orienteering. Many of the activities that are not ski specific are done at a very low intensity and are performed as active recovery. Some cross-country skiers compete at high levels in cycling, running, and orienteering, however, and many junior cross-country skiers also compete in swimming, soccer, and other sports.

No conclusive literature is available on the effectiveness of resistance training for cross-country skiers, and the use of resistance training varies from country to country and within countries. With the increasing demands on upper-body power brought on by the ski skating techniques, there seems to be a move to include more upper-body training during the off season, although methods of training vary widely; most include the more traditional circuit training (low resistance, high repetition) and skiing-specific strength training (maximal-effort skiing, roller skiing, and hill bounding for durations of 10 to 15 seconds).

Periodization of Training

No controlled studies have been done to support the concept of periodization of training, but observational studies (39,72) and training reports at international coaching seminars have reported that athletes who vary their training on an annual basis, with a significant detraining period after the competitive season, seem to be able to demonstrate greater improvements during the following competitive season.

Several authors (11,72,85,86) have published training theories outlining multiple layers of periodization. These are generally referred to as macrocycles, mesocycles, and microcycles. In a more practical sense, these cycles can be thought of as multiyear training variations (macrocycles), annual and monthly variations (mesocycles), and weekly cycling (microcycles) of training. These cycles are all designed to enhance performance by varying training method, load, and recovery.

Multiyear cycles may be used by mature athletes to allow a focus on the Olympic Games and World Championships, and by developing athletes to optimize training with physiological development. During nonchampionship years, elite athletes may increase volume and decrease intensity of training with the goal of increasing aerobic capacity and anaerobic threshold. These nonchampionship years may also prove to be effective for increasing strength. During championship years, the total volume and amount of low-intensity training is decreased, and the amount of high-intensity training may be doubled to improve performance in mature athletes (72).

Annual training is generally divided into four major components:

1. A nonspecific detraining period of 1 to 2 months follows the competitive season. This period involves low-intensity and low-volume activities that are not skiing-specific in nature. This results in a decrease in $\dot{V}O_2$max, and anaerobic threshold may drop to as low as 65% to 80% of $\dot{V}O_2$max.
2. A basic endurance period lasting 3 to 4 months then follows. This period is characterized by an increasing volume of low-intensity training. Athletes may increase training to between 30 and 40 hours during an average week. During this period, there is also increasing use of strength training with high-resistance and low-repetition programs. The $\dot{V}O_2$max and the oxygen uptake at anaerobic threshold should begin to increase, and blood lactate concentrations at submaximal work rates generally decrease.
3. A precompetition period of 2 to 3 months precedes the important competitions and generally includes early season warm-up races. This period is characterized initially by high training volume with increasing amounts of high-intensity training. Resistance training shifts to focus on power and ski-specific strengthening through the use of lower resistances and more repetitions. During the later portion of this period, total training volume is decreased.
4. The competitive season is characterized by greatly reduced total volume of both endurance and resistance training with a focus on speed and technique. Over the long duration of the competitive season, most athletes find it necessary to maintain periods with higher volume and lower intensity. Many athletes will maintain at least one or more long (2- to 3-hour) low-intensity workout each week.

Monthly cycles are loosely defined to mean a period consisting of 3 to 5 weeks. Conceptually, within each "monthly cycle," the weeks are varied so that each week will have a varied load and recovery. In a 3-week cycle, for example, the first week might involve a high training volume at low intensities, the second week might involve a low training volume but be performed at a high intensity, and the third week might be a recovery week with a low volume of training performed at a low intensity. The actual load and intensity of each week also is adjusted relative to the larger cycles.

Weekly cycles reflect the daily cycle of training. Most coaches use a 7-day-week cycle, as it fits the life cycle of the athletes and works best during the competitive season. Within each week, the training is planned so that the athlete gets periods of high stress followed by recovery. It is recognized that both high-volume and high-intensity training can be stressful, and that each athlete may respond differently to specific training programs. Therefore, coaches individualize the training program of each athlete to attempt to best help him or her optimally balance the necessary training stimulus with an adequate recovery.

Thus, it is through a combination of scientifically based methods and observational insight that attempts are made to optimally prepare the cross-country ski racer for competition.

REFERENCES

1. Frederick EC, Street GM. Nordic ski racing: biomedical and technical improvements in cross-country skiing. *Sci Am* 1988;258: T20–T22.
2. Pinchak AC, Hagen JF, Hall FB, Hancock DE. Factors affecting

performance of cross-country skiers. In: Rekow ED, Thacker JG, Erdman AG, eds. *Biomechanics in sport: a 1987 update.* New York: The American Society of Mechanical Engineers, 1987: 55–60.

3. Bauman W. The mechanics of the roller ski and its influence on technique in cross country skiing. In: Perren SM, Schneider E, eds. *Biomechanics: current interdisciplinary research.* Dordrecht, Netherlands: Martinus Nijhoff, 1985:711–716.
4. Dal Monte A, Fucci S, Leonardi LM, Trozzi V. An evaluation of the diagonal stride technique in cross country skiing. In: Matsui H, Kobayashi K, eds. *Biomechanics VIII-B.* Champaign, IL: Human Kinetics, 1983:851–855.
5. Ekstrom H. Force interplay in cross-country skiing. *Scand J Sports Sci* 1981;3:69–76.
6. Komi PV. Ground reaction forces in cross-country skiing. In: Winter D, Norman RW, Wells RP, Hagyes KC, Patla AE, eds. *Biomechanics IX-B.* Champaign, IL: Human Kinetics, 1985: 185–190.
7. Komi PV. Force measurements during cross-country skiing. *Int J Sport Biomech* 1987;3:370–381.
8. Pierce JC, Pope MH, Renstrom P, Johnson RJ, Dufek J, Dillman C. Force measurement in cross-country skiing. *Int J Sport Biomech* 1987;3:382–391.
9. Pinchak AC, Hancock DE, Hagen JF, Hall FB. Biomechanical differences between cross country snow skiing and roller skiing: analysis of some kinematic measurements. In: Rekow ED, Thacker JG, Erdman AG, eds. *Biomechanics in sport: a 1987 update.* New York: The American Society of Mechanical Engineers, 1987:69–76.
10. Astrand PO, Rodah K. *Textbook of work physiology.* New York: McGraw-Hill, 1986.
11. Bergh U. *Physiology of cross-country ski racing.* Champaign, IL: Human Kinetics, 1982.
12. Karlsson J. Profiles of cross-country and alpine skiers. *Clin Sports Med* 1984;3:245–271.
13. Jette M, Thoden JS, Spence J. The energy expenditure of a 5 km cross-country ski run. *J Appl Physiol* 1976;20:425–431.
14. Mygind E, Andersen LB, Rasmussen B. Blood lactate and respiratory variables in elite cross-country skiing at racing speeds. *Scand J Med Sci Sports* 1994;4:243–251.
15. Hedman R. The available glycogen in man and the connection between rate of oxygen intake and carbohydrate usage. *Acta Physiol Scand* 1957;40:305–321.
16. Astrand PO, Hallback I, Hedman R, Saltin B. Blood lactate after prolonged severe exercise. *J Appl Physiol* 1963;18:619–622.
17. Street GM. Kinetic analysis of the V1 skating technique during roller skiing. Doctoral dissertation. University Park: Pennsylvania State University, 1988.
18. Hoffman MD, Clifford PS. Physiological responses to different cross country skiing techniques on level terrain. *Med Sci Sports Exerc* 1990;22:841–848.
19. Hoffman MD, Clifford PS, Foley PJ, Brice AG. Physiological responses during different roller skiing techniques. *Med Sci Sports Exerc* 1990;22:391–396.
20. Hoffman MD, Clifford PS, Jones GM, Mandli M, Bota B. Effects of technique and pole grip on physiological demands of roller skiing on level terrain. *Int J Sports Med* 1991;12:468–473.
21. Hoffman MD, Clifford PS, Snyder AC, et al. Physiological effects of technique and rolling resistance in uphill roller skiing. *Med Sci Sports Exerc* 1998;30:311–317.
22. Hoffman MD, Clifford PS, Watts PB, et al. Physiological comparison of uphill roller skiing: diagonal stride versus double pole. *Med Sci Sports Exerc* 1994;26:1284–1289.
23. Hoffman MD, Jones GM, Bota B, Mandli M, Clifford PS. In-line skating: physiological responses and comparison with roller skiing. *Int J Sports Med* 1992;13:137–144.
24. MacDougall JD, Hughson R, Sutton JR, Moroz JR. The energy cost of cross-country skiing among elite competitors. *Med Sci Sports* 1979;11:270–273.
25. Rusko H. Oxygen uptake and blood lactate concentration during diagonal skiing and double poling in cross-country skiers. *Proceedings of the First IOC World Congress on Sport Sciences*, Colorado Springs, CO: US Olympic Committee, 1989:108–109.
26. Saibene F, Cortili G, Roi G, Colombini A. The energy cost of level cross-country skiing and the effect of the friction of the ski. *Eur J Appl Physiol* 1989;58:791–795.
27. Millet GY, Hoffman MD, Candau RB, Clifford PS. Poling forces during roller skiing: effects of technique and speed. *Med Sci Sports Exerc* 1998;30:1645–1653.
28. Millet GY, Hoffman MD, Candau RB, Clifford PS. Poling forces during roller skiing: effects of grade. *Med Sci Sports Exerc* 1998: 30:1637–1644.
29. Smith GA. Biomechanics of crosscountry skiing. *Sports Med* 1990; 9:273–285.
30. Street GM. Kinetic analysis of the V1 skate technique during roller skiing. *Med Sci Sports Exerc* 1989;21:S79.
31. Smith GA. Kinetic analysis of the V1 skate in cross country skiing. *Proceedings of the First IOC World Congress on Sport Sciences*, Colorado Springs, CO: US Olympic Committee, 1989:281–282.
32. Smith GA, McNitt-Gray J, Nelson RC. Kinematic analysis of alternate stride skating in cross-country skiing. *Int J Sport Biomech* 1988;4:49–58.
33. Frederick EC. Estimates of the energy cost of rifle carriage in biathlon ski skating. *Int J Sport Biomech* 1987;3:392–403.
34. Hoffman MD, Street GM. Characterization of the heart rate response during biathlon. *Int J Sports Med* 1992;13:390–394.
35. Groslambert A, Gillot G, Davenne D, Rouillon JD. Influence de l'exercice physique sur la qualite du tir en biathlon. *Sci Sport* 1995;10:47–48.
36. Hoffman MD, Gilson PM, Westenburg TM, Spencer WA. Biathlon shooting performance after exercise of different intensities. *Int J Sports Med* 1992;13:270–273.
37. Bergh U. The influence of body mass in cross-country skiing. *Med Sci Sports Exerc* 1987;19:324–331.
38. Hanson JS. Maximal exercise performance in members of the US nordic ski team. *J Appl Physiol* 1973;35:592–595.
39. Ingjer F. Maximal oxygen uptake as a predictor of performance ability in women and men elite cross-country skiers. *Scand J Med Sci Sports* 1991;1:25–30.
40. Rusko H, Havu M, Karvinen E. Aerobic performance capacity in athletes. *Eur J Appl Physiol* 1978;38:151–159.
41. Saltin B, Astrand PO. Maximal oxygen uptake in athletes. *J Appl Physiol* 1967;23:353–358.
42. Sharkey BJ. *Training for cross-country ski racing.* Champaign, IL: Human Kinetics, 1984.
43. Niinimaa V, Dyon M, Shephard RJ. Performance and efficiency of intercollegiate cross-country skiers. *Med Sci Sports Exerc* 1978; 10:91–93.
44. Ng AV, Demment RB, Bassett DR, et al. Characteristics and performance of male citizen cross-country ski racers. *Int J Sports Med* 1988;9:205–209.
45. Mackova EV, Bass A, Sprynarova S, Teisinger J, Vondra K, Bojanovsky I. Enzyme activity patterns of energy metabolism in skiers of different performance levels (m. quadriceps femoris). *Eur J Appl Physiol* 1982;48:315–322.
46. Mackova EV, Melichna J, Sprynarova S, et al. Muscle enzyme activities and fiber composition (m. vastus lateralis) and efficiency of the cardiorespiratory system in cross-country skiers. *Physiol Bohemoslov* 1983;32:272–280.
47. Sprynarova S, Bass A, Mackova E, et al. Changes in maximal aerobic power, aerobic capacity, and muscle enzyme activities at two stages of the annual training cycle in ski-runners. *Eur J Appl Physiol* 1980;44:17–23.
48. Stray-Gundersen J, Parsons D, Moore RL. Fiber type subclasses and biochemical properties of the muscles of young elite cross-country skiers. *Med Sci Sports Exerc* 1984;16:46.
49. Bergh U, Kanstrup I-L, Ekblom B. Maximal oxygen uptake during exercise with various combinations of arm and leg work. *J Appl Physiol* 1976;41:191–196.
50. Secher NH, Ruberg-Larsen N, Binkhorst RA, Bonde-Petersen F. Maximal oxygen uptake during arm cranking and combined arm plus leg exercise. *J Appl Physiol* 1974;36:515–518.
51. Shephard RJ, Bouhlel E, Vandewalle H, Monod H. Muscle mass as a factor limiting physical work. *J Appl Physiol* 1988;64:1472–1479.
52. Rusko H. The effect of training on aerobic power characteristics of young cross-country skiers. *J Sports Sci* 1987;5:273–286.

53. Komi PV, Rusko H, Vos J, Vihko V. Anaerobic performance capacity in athletes. *Acta Physiol Scand* 1977;100:107–114.
54. Rusko H, Rahkila P, Karvinen E. Anaerobic threshold, skeletal muscle enzymes and fiber composition in young female cross-country skiers. *Acta Physiol Scand* 1980;108:263–268.
55. Gollnick PD, Matoba H. The muscle fiber composition of skeletal muscle as a predictor of athletic success: an overview. *Am J Sports Med* 1984;12:212–217.
56. Mygind E, Larsson B, Klausen T. Evaluation of a specific test in cross-country skiing. *J Sports Sci* 1991;9:249–257.
57. Rundell KW. Treadmill roller ski test predicts biathlon roller ski race results of elite US biathlon women. *Med Sci Sports Exerc* 1995;27:1677–1685.
58. Rundell KW, Bacharach DW. Physiological characteristics and performance of top US biathletes. *Med Sci Sports Exerc* 1995; 27:1302–1310.
59. Bilodeau B, Roy B, Boulay MR. Upper-body testing of cross-country skiers. *Med Sci Sports Exerc* 1995;27:1557–1562.
60. Wasserman K, McIlroy MB. Detecting the threshold of anaerobic metabolism in cardiac patients during exercise. *Am J Cardiol* 1964;14:844–852.
61. Davis JA. Anaerobic threshold: review of the concept and directions for future research. *Med Sci Sports Exerc* 1985;17:6–18.
62. Brooks GA. Anaerobic threshold: review of the concept and directions for future research. *Med Sci Sports Exerc* 1985;17:22–31.
63. Davis JA, Frank MH, Whipp BJ, Wasserman K. Anaerobic threshold alterations caused by endurance training in middle-aged men. *J Appl Physiol* 1979;46:1039–1046.
64. Davis JA, Vodak P, Wilmore JH, Vodak J, Kurtz P. Anaerobic threshold and maximal aerobic power for three modes of exercise. *J Appl Physiol* 1976;41:544–550.
65. Droghetti P, Borsetto C, Casoni I, et al. Noninvasive determination of the anaerobic threshold in canoeing, cross-country skiing, cycling, roller and ice skating, rowing, and walking. *Eur J Appl Physiol* 1985;53:299–303.
66. Farrell PA, Wilmore JH, Coyle EF, Billings JE, Costill DL. Plasma lactate accumulation and distance running performance. *Med Sci Sports* 1979;11:338–344.
67. Kumagai S, Tanaka K, Matsura Y, Mutsuzaka A, Hirakoba K, Asano K. Relationships of the anaerobic threshold with the 5 km, 10 km, and 10 mile races. *Eur J Appl Physiol* 1982;49:13–23.
68. Powers SK, Dodd S, Deadson R, Byrd R, McKnight T. Ventilatory threshold, running economy, and distance running performance of trained athletes. *Res Q Exerc Sport* 1983;54:179–182.
69. Haymes EM, Dickinson A. Characteristics of elite male and female ski racers. *Med Sci Sports* 1980;12:153–158.
70. Patton JF, Duggan A. Upper and lower body anaerobic power: comparison between biathletes and control subjects. *Int J Sports Med* 1987;8:94–98.
71. Davies GJ, Halbach JW, Carpenter MA, et al. A descriptive muscular power analysis of the United States cross country ski team. *Med Sci Sports Exerc* 1980;12:141.
72. Gaskill SE, Serfass RA, Bacharach WD, Kelly JM. Responses to training in cross-country skiers. *Med Sci Sports Exerc* 1999; 31:1211–1217.
73. Orvanova E. Physical structure of winter sports athletes. *J Sports Sci* 1987;5:197–248.
74. Chovanova E. Body structure of elite ice hockey players and skiers. Doctoral dissertation. Bratislava, Czechoslovakia: Comenius University, 1976.
75. Hoffman MD, Clifford PS, Bota B, Mandli M, Jones GM. Influence of body mass on energy cost of roller skiing. *Int J Sports Biomech* 1990;6:374–385.
76. Gaskill SE. *Fitness cross country skiing.* Champaign, IL: Human Kinetics, 1997.
77. Levine BD, Stray-Gundersen J. A practical approach to altitude training: where to live and train for optimal performance enhancement. *Int J Sports Med* 1992;13(suppl 1):S209–212.
78. Rusko HR. New aspects of altitude training. *Am J Sports Med* 1996;24:S48–S52.
79. Bilodeau B, Roy B, Boulay MR. A comparison of three skating techniques and the diagonal stride on heart rate responses and speed in cross-country skiing. *Int J Sports Med* 1991;12:71–76.
80. Karvonen J, Kubica R, Wilk B, Wnorowski J, Krasicki S, Kalli S. Effects of skating and diagonal skiing techniques on results and some physiological variables. *Can J Sports Sci* 1989;14:117–121.
81. Mittelstadt SW, Hoffman MD, Watts PB, et al. Lactate response to uphill roller skiing with the diagonal stride and double pole techniques. *Med Sci Sports Exerc* 1995;27:1563–1568.
82. Berg R, Forsberg A. Effective roller skiing. *Am Ski Coach* 1991; 14:21–22.
83. Taylor D. Traditional technique and skating: what we know now. *Prof Skier* 1988;1:9–10.
84. Millet GY, Hoffman MD, Candau RB, Buckwalter JB, Clifford PS. Effect of rolling resistance on poling forces and metabolic demands of roller skiing. *Med Sci Sports Exerc* 1998;30:755–762.
85. Bompa TO. *Theory and methodology of training: the key to athletic success.* Dubuque, IA: Kendall Hunt, 1983.
86. Karlsen T. *How to, when to, why to, a Norwegian model; training guide and programs for cross-country skiers.* Salt Lake City, UT: Nordic Equipment Inc, 1992.

Exercise and Sport Science,
edited by William E. Garrett, Jr., and Donald T. Kirkendall.
Lippincott Williams & Wilkins, Philadelphia © 2000.

CHAPTER 54

Physiology of Competitive Rowing

Fredrick C. Hagerman

Although the sport of rowing was among those introduced at the modern revival of the Olympic Games in 1896, there is no record of its existence as a sport of the ancient Games. Rowing, in some form, was important to early seafarers, and human power was often harnessed for Norsemen's small ocean crafts or the large Roman galleys. It is not known whether ancient mariners may have engaged in friendly competition when they were not trading, fishing, ferrying, exploring, or at war. However, the modern sport of rowing was developed by English tradesmen in the early eighteenth century when, after carrying goods and people on their Thames River barges, they would race one another in these same boats after work hours or on weekends (1). Many city and university rowing clubs were established in Europe in the nineteenth century, and this growth was reflected in the rapid development of school-boy and club rowing in Great Britain and the inaugural Cambridge–Oxford boat race, which began as an annual event in 1829. The oldest and most traditional rowing regatta, the famous Royal Henley Regatta, was introduced in 1839. Successful attempts at organizing international rowing came to fruition when the first international sports federation of its kind, the Fédération Internationale des Sociétés d'Aviron (International Rowing Federation), was founded in 1892.

The sport began growing in the United States with this country's immigrant explosion of the nineteenth and early twentieth centuries. Several early rowing (boat) clubs were established in Boston, New York City, and Philadelphia, with simultaneous growth in some older American universities prompting the first annual Harvard–Yale boat race in 1852. Unfortunately, for many years rowing was largely a sport for the privileged; with the exception of a few professional rowers, it was strongly segregated, as were golf and tennis at that time. The growth of our industrial complex and increased technology during and after World War II not only increased the population of the larger eastern cities in the United States, which were already rowing strongholds, but it also had a profound effect on cities of the west coast, where more suitable weather conditions and an abundance of water permitted year-round rowing. The post–World War II years saw not only major urban growth where rowing was routinely practiced but also leisure time for everyone, and interest in physical fitness increased. All of these factors contributed to the popularity of rowing and other sports. Although the sport of rowing is initially a very expensive sport, increased membership in rowing clubs and university rowing programs is on the rise. Today, many college and university varsity club and city club rowing programs are thriving. With the order by the National Collegiate Athletic Association (NCAA) to colleges and universities to fulfill Title IX requirements for sport equality between men's and women's athletic programs, varsity rowing programs for women are being added at an extraordinary rate; in 1997, the first NCAA national rowing championships for women were held in Sacramento, California. Although women first competed in the European Championships in 1954, it was not until 20 years later that they were allowed to row in World Championship competition; two years after that women rowers competed at their first Olympic Games (1976).

Rowing has been an Olympic sport since the inaugural Olympic Games of the modern era and is now second only to Track and Field (Athletics) in the total number of athletes competing in one sport. World Rowing Championships are conducted annually. For many years U.S. Olympic rowing teams competed successfully and won almost every eight-oared gold medal until 1968. Rowing teams of the German Democratic Republic were the most successful in the 1970s and early 1980s,

F. C. Hagerman: Department of Biomedical Sciences, Ohio University, Athens, Ohio 45701.

and now a united Germany competes successfully for World Championship and Olympic medals against strong competition from Australia, Belarus, Canada, France, Great Britain, Italy, Romania, Russia, and a resurgent U.S. national program. International rowing has gained in universality; more than 45 countries and 500 athletes competed at the centennial Olympic Games in Atlanta, and 52 countries and more than 1500 rowers participated in the 1997 World Rowing Championships, which have been conducted each year since 1962.

THE SPORT

Physical Requirements

The sport of rowing is divided into two distinct categories, sweep rowing and sculling. Sweep rowing requires competitors to row with a single long oar (3.8 m; 12.5 ft) on one side of the boat, either port (left) or starboard (right), whereas sculling boats require that each sculler use two shorter oars (3.0 m; 9 ft 9 in), pulling on them simultaneously to propel the boat. Previously all sweep and sculling oars were constructed of light wood but now they are made of carbon fiber and are hollow to reduce weight. The current blade design (end of oar placed in the water) has been enlarged and shaped like the head of a hatchet or axe so that a greater amount of water may be displaced with each stroke. Blade design has changed several times over the years and has helped to add speed to each event (Fig. 54–1). Before 1970, both sweep and sculling boats (shells) were made of wood and were produced by shaping thinly layered steamed wood around a wooden skeletal frame (Fig. 54–2). These older wooden boats resemble works of art due to the handiwork and careful preparation that went into making the boats. Only a small number of wooden boats are produced today, replaced instead by narrow (60 to 62 cm; 23.6 to 24.4 in) sleek hydrodynamically and computer-designed lightweight boats made of synthetic polymers (Fig. 54–3). Single sculls are 8.2 m (27 ft) long and weigh between 10 and 15 kg (24-33 lbs); larger eight-oared boats range in weight from 88 to 98 kg (194 to 216 lbs) and are 19.9 m (62 ft) long. The weights and lengths of the other sweep and sculling boats measure between these. Sweep-boat competition may involve as few as two rowers or as many as eight, excluding the coxswain, who steers the boat, implements racing strategy, including stroke rating or cadence, and encourages the crew members to do their best. Coxswains usually sit low in the stern (back) of the boat but also are permitted to sit in the bow (front) of the boat. Although many university, high school, and club crews train and compete on bays, lakes, and rivers and at varying racing distances throughout the world, the standard competitive distance for international and national rowing regattas is 2000 m with no water current.

Rowing competition at annual world championships includes five sweep-boat classes in the men's open division: Pair (two rowers) without coxswain, pair (two rowers) with coxswain, four (four rowers) without coxswain, four (four rowers) with coxswain, and eight (eight rowers) with coxswain. For women at world championships, sweep competition includes pair without coxswain, four without coxswain, and the eight-oared crew with coxswain. Sculling events for men and women are the same: single scull, double scull, and quadruple scull. None of the sculling boats uses a coxswain. Steering for all boats without coxswain is assigned to one of the rowers, who performs this task with assistance from a special rotatable foot plate connected to the rudder. All of the sweep- and sculling-boat classes described previously are open events for men and women without restrictions of age or body weight. Descriptions of these boat classes appear as silhouettes in Fig. 54–4. Because of the recent

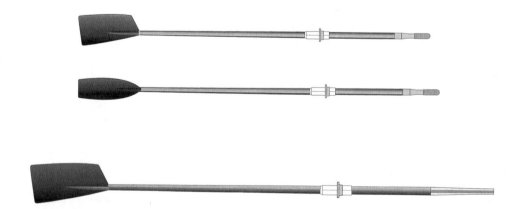

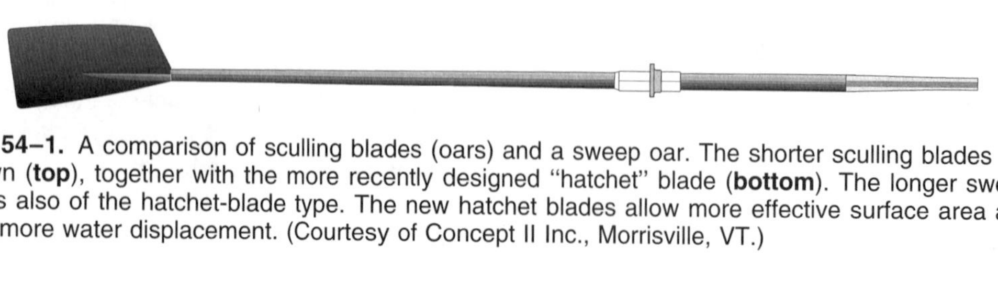

FIG. 54–1. A comparison of sculling blades (oars) and a sweep oar. The shorter sculling blades are shown (**top**), together with the more recently designed "hatchet" blade (**bottom**). The longer sweep oar is also of the hatchet-blade type. The new hatchet blades allow more effective surface area and thus more water displacement. (Courtesy of Concept II Inc., Morrisville, VT.)

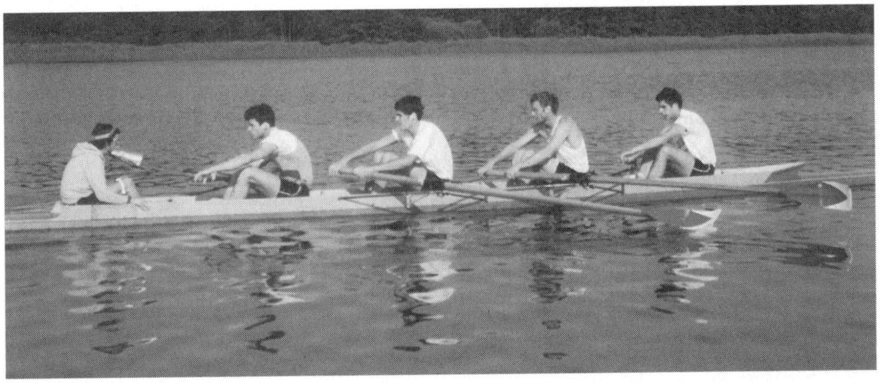

FIG. 54–2. Wooden-hulled racing boat (shell) used almost exclusively prior to 1972 (four with coxswain).

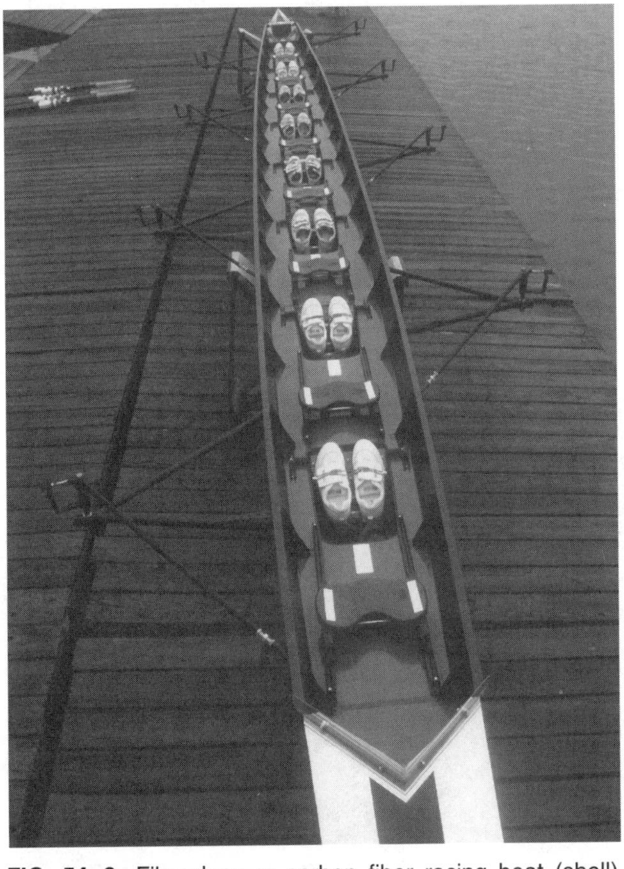

FIG. 54–3. Fiberglass or carbon fiber racing boat (shell). (Courtesy of Vespoli USA, New Haven, CT.)

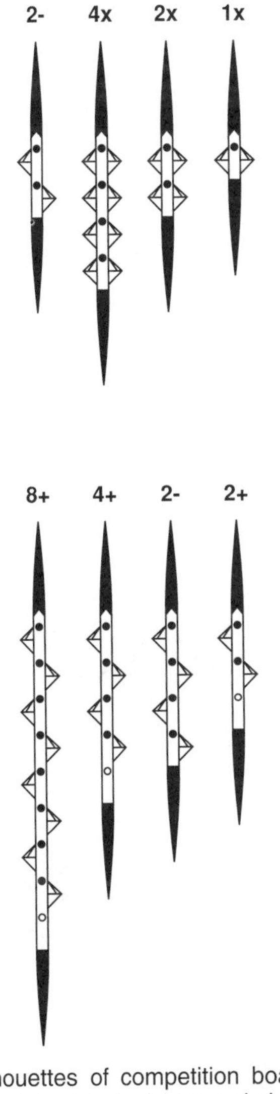

FIG. 54–4. Silhouettes of competition boat classes (coxswains are indicated with *single open circles*).

decision by the International Olympic Committee (IOC) to reduce the number of athletes competing in each Olympic sport, the open men's coxed pair and coxed four events have been eliminated from Olympic regattas only. Changes also were made in women's Olympic competition, where the pair without coxswain and double sculls were eliminated. Four lightweight events, men's coxless four and double sculls and women's coxless pair and double sculls, replaced the four Olympic open events eliminated. There is also an abbreviated racing schedule for younger rowers (younger than 19 years), and an annual junior world championship is conducted separately from the open world championship. There is also a weight-restricted competition referred to as lightweight rowing in which, for men's competition, athletes cannot weigh more than 72.5 kg and the average of the whole crew cannot exceed 70 kg (single sculler can weigh no more than 72.5 kg). Lightweight women cannot weigh more than 59 kg, and the average weight of the crew cannot exceed 57 kg (single sculler can weigh no more than 59 kg). Lightweight world championship events, with some exceptions, are similar to open events. In addition, coxswain's minimal weight for open men's events cannot be less than 55 kg, and for women, the lowest weight limit is 45 kg. For junior men's events, the minimal weight limit for coxswains is 50 kg, and for junior women's events, 45 kg. If a coxswain does not meet the minimal weight requirements, then artificial weight is added and carried next to the coxswain's seat.

For the reader who is unfamiliar with the sport of rowing, it may appear to be primarily an upper-body activity. On closer examination, however, it is evident that boat propulsion is dependent on leg-extension power produced by vigorous and sustained contractions of the quadriceps femoris and gluteus maximus muscles. This is because the boats are equipped with sliding seats. Rowing differs from other aerobic activities as it is performed in a sitting position and, with the exception of the coxswain, all athletes are sitting with their backs to the bow of the boat or the direction that the boat is moving. Each rower is assigned a seat in multiple-oared sweep and sculling boats, and seat assignments are critical to producing optimal power in a boat. Probably the most important strategic decision a rowing coach must make is the selection of seat order of the crew or "boating" of the athletes. Seat numbers are ordered from number one beginning at the bow (front) of the boat to the "stroke," who sits nearest the stern (back). The stroke is often the most highly skilled athlete in the boat; he or she sets the pace and establishes the rhythm and is usually the most competitive and tenacious crew member. The "middle" of the boat (e.g., seats 3, 4, 5, and 6 in 8-oared crews) is considered the "engine room" or major power unit in the boat (Fig. 54–5). Unlike those in many other aerobic sports, almost every major muscle group is used during rowing. It has been estimated that the most successful elite rowers produce about 75% to 80% of their power with their legs and 20% to 25% with their arms.

Biomechanically, the competitive rowing stroke can be divided into four phases (Fig. 54–6*A–F*). During the initial "catch" or "entry" phase of the rowing stroke, when the blade is placed in the water, the muscles of the arms and back perform static contractions and are severely loaded; the rower has achieved maximal reach. There should be no body lift while placing the blade in the water; only the hands should lift the oar handle to put the blade in the water. The speed of entry into the water is critical so as not to lose length. The efficiency

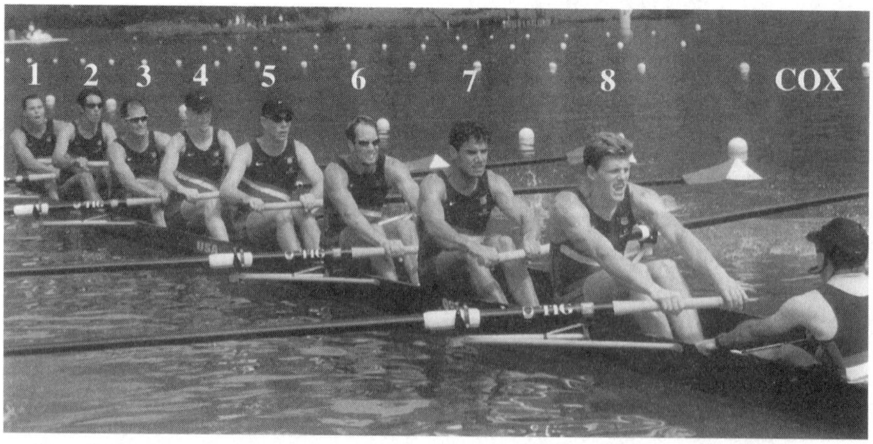

FIG. 54–5. 1997 World Champion U.S. eight-oared crew: numbers indicate individual positions in boat. (Courtesy of Vespoli USA, New Haven, CT.)

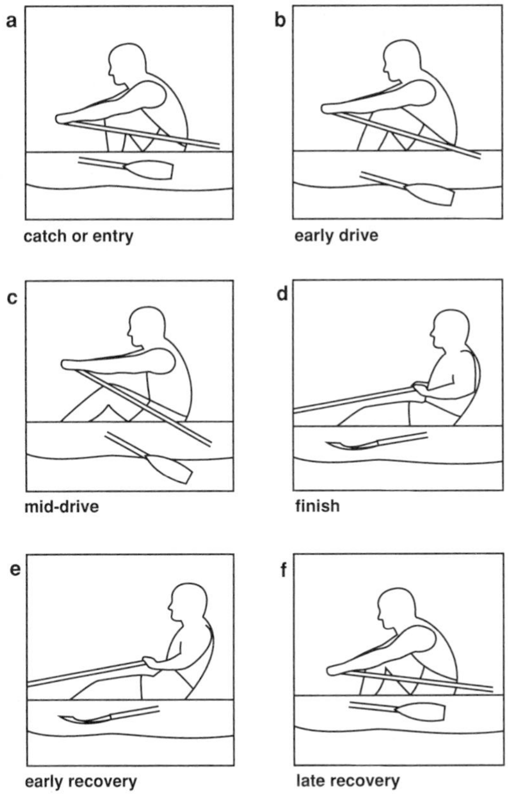

FIG. 54–6. A–F: Phases of rowing stroke. See text for details.

of the next phase, the leg drive, is lost if the blade is not buried in the water. At the same time, the body is placed in a compressed position with maximal knee flexion and knees drawn to the chest (Fig. 54–6*A*). After the entry of the blade into the water, the body weight is transmitted to the footstretchers by using the force of the legs. The legs first, then followed quickly by the back, are forcibly extended during the early and middle parts of the "drive" or power phase (Figs. 54–6*B* and *C*), accompanied by vigorous shoulder-joint extension and elbow flexion, causing the blade to sweep through the water. Power is sustained during the "finish" or "release" phase (Fig. 54–6*D*) or follow-through of the stroke, and this is accomplished by completing leg extension, extending the back slightly beyond the vertical plane, and quickly drawing the hands (enclosed on the blade handle) toward the chest. Legs and back finish their work almost simultaneously, while keeping the body in a tall position about 10 degrees past vertical; the hands and chest should be behind the oar handles (no slouching). Semicircular motion of release occurs in front of the body without touching it. The "recovery" phase (Fig. 54–6*E* and *F*) involves "rolling up" the body quickly on the sliding seat toward the stern of the boat, again achieving the initial compacted position. This is accomplished by maintaining the outside shoulder slightly higher than the inside shoulder (outside shoulder is the side on which athlete is rowing (port or starboard). The outside arm is totally outstretched as hands go over the knees; the inside arm is slightly bent. The hand and upper-body movement, all in a backward fluid sequence, compose the initial part of the recovery phase. The final part of the recovery phase brings the rower to the rolled-up compacted position in preparation for the catch or entry, and the sequence is then repeated.

Rowing differs from other types of human locomotion because, unlike the alternate force application of the limbs during running and cycling, the limbs are used simultaneously during rowing. Rowing is unique also because it is the only predominantly aerobic sport in which, for all events except the single scull, there are multiple participants. Thus a specific boat and its crew's competitive effort are only as good as the weakest human link.

International races for men in the open division usually last between 5.5 and 7.2 minutes, whereas those for women last between 5.7 and 7.4 minutes. These time differences are affected by the number of rowers in a specific boat, the presence or absence of a coxswain, and by environmental conditions, including wind, temperature, humidity, and water depth. Despite the year-to-year differences in environmental conditions, competitive results over the years have improved, on an average, by about 0.7 s/year (2,3). More recent performance times have improved at a more rapid rate, however (Table 54–1). The average improvement in four common men's Olympic events from 1956 to 1997 was about 0.5% per year, with the pair without coxswain showing the most improvement during this 41-year period. Although women have been competing in the 2000-m since 1986 (primarily at World Championships), Olympic competition for this distance has been conducted only three times (Table 54–1), and the four-oared without coxswain event was not introduced until 1992. The average improvement for the women in four events from 1988 to 1997 was almost 20 seconds; single sculls and pair-oared without coxswain showed the greatest improvements. Because there are very few comparative Olympic data between men and women, it is difficult to explain the apparent gender-related differences. Gender comparisons with absolute data for other aerobic sports indicate certain anatomic and physiologic advantages for men, but when relative values based on body weight and fat-free mass are considered, competitive efforts for men and women are almost equal (4,5). It is clear from Table 54–1 that women improved performances substantially from 1988 to 1996. For the events summarized in Table 54–1, the men were, on an average, almost 50 seconds faster than the women in 1988, but this difference had been reduced to 40 seconds faster in 1996; the one exception was the eight-oared event,

TABLE 54–1. *A comparison of 2000-m times for selected boat classes of U.S. National and Olympic Teams; 1956–1997*

	Event			
Years	Single scull	Double sculls	Pair-oared without coxswain	Eight-oared with coxswain
Men				
1956	8:03	7:24	7:55	6:35
1960[a]	7:14	6:48	7:02	5:57
1964	8:23	7:11	7:33	6:18
1968	7:48	6:52	7:27	6:07
1972	7:10	7:02	6:53	6:09
1976	7:29	7:13	7:23	5:58
1980	7:10	6:24	6:48	5:49
1984	7:00	6:36	6:45	5:41
1988	6:50	6:21	6:37	5:46
1992	6:51	6:17	6:28	5:29
1996	6:45	6:17	6:20	5:42
1997	6:45	6:13	6:28	5:27
Women				
1976[b]	4:06	3:44	4:01	3:33
1980[b]	3:41	3:48	3:31	3:03
1984[b]	3:41	3:27	3:32	3:00
1988	7:47	7:01	7:28	6:15
1992	7:26	6:49	7:06	6:03
1996	7:32	6:57	No competition in 1996	6:19
1997	7:29	6:51	7:08	6:02

[a]Racing distance short of 2000 m.
[b]1000 m.

in which the men showed more improvement between 1988 and 1996. Faster 2000-m times for both men and women over the years have been a result of better equipment, better and more experienced athletes, and improved training programs. It does appear that women are now improving at a faster rate than men, and this can be accounted for by the attraction of better athletes to the sport and the accumulation of more experience at the 2000-m distance (prior to 1988, women competed over 1000 m). It is evident that as women continue to train and race over the longer distance, performance times will continue to improve.

Physiologic Requirements

The physiology of rowing was previously reviewed by Törner (6), Secher (7,8), Hagerman (9), Körner and Schwanitz (10), Steinacker (11), Zsidegh (12), and more recently again by Secher (13) and Hagerman (14). Thus far, most of the physiologic data have been reported for oarsmen, as it has only been more recently that women's rowing was added to the Olympic and World Championship programs.

Muscle Strength and Power

Muscular forces generated during competitive rowing are not so high when compared with other sports; however, considerable average force must be maintained for a total of about 200 strokes to compete successfully over the 2000-m distance. Although isometric and isokinetic strength have been found to correlate highly with rowing ergometer performance (15,16), others have reported very poor correlations between strength and rowing performance (17–19).

High-velocity strength training in one study did increase peak force during high-velocity resistance testing, just as low-velocity training improved peak force produced during low-velocity testing; however, neither mode of strength training improved rowing power (20). In a previous study by Hagerman and colleagues (21), two groups of elite rowers were assigned to one of two groups for 16 weeks of off-season training; one used a more traditional combination of resistance and rowing ergometer training, whereas the other group trained on the ergometer only. Performances, as measured on the ergometer and during actual rowing, including 2000-m time and various metabolic responses, both favored the ergometer-trained-only subjects. No differences were observed in muscle structure or histochemistry of pre- and posttraining biopsies or in muscular strength and power. These studies seem to illustrate a high degree of training specificity for rowing. Although both training groups showed significant fiber-type conversion from IIB to IIA, type I fiber proportions remained unchanged, and all other intramuscular changes were similar for both groups. Fiber diameters also increased significantly for both groups, but they also were similar.

Because muscular strength and power in nonrowing circumstances seem to have little value when applied to rowing, it was suggested in 1977 that only strength training involving the rowing motion be recommended for rowers (22); our recent data appear to confirm this recommendation. Because leg extension during the drive or power phase is the major source of power, developing force and increasing velocity of contraction in the quadriceps femoris and gluteal muscle groups become primary goals. However, rowers, unlike most other elite endurance athletes, produce force by using both legs; thus force and power development correspond to the sum of their combined efforts (19,23).

Isokinetic strength of elite rowers is comparable to that of other elite athletes (24–26). Peak isokinetic strength for the knee extensors of oarsmen was recorded at 0.5 rad/s and averaged 319 Nm (25). Clarkson and coworkers (24) tested female rowers at 0 rad/s (isometric contraction) and observed a peak strength of 220 Nm for the knee extensors. Muscle strength–velocity curves representing some endurance-trained elite athletes are illustrated in Fig. 54–7 (9); with the exception of the two fastest velocities, 4.2 and 5.3 rad/s, oarsmen exhibited the highest isokinetic strength. Lowered strength responses for oarsmen at the faster velocities may be accounted for, at least in part, by the differences in muscle-fiber type proportions found in the quadriceps femoris of these athletes. The presence of an unusually high proportion of slow-twitch (type I) fibers in rowers may be responsible for the reduced torque at faster velocities. The highest absolute strength values for oarsmen, on the other hand, probably reflect their larger muscle masses. With the exception of some swimmers, the data depicted in Fig. 54–7 represented athletes who were shorter in stature and possessed much less muscle mass than elite rowers. Absolute strength for oarswomen was lower at all test velocities than that of their male counterparts (see Fig. 54–7). Leg strength per kilogram of fat-free mass (FFM; i.e., relative strength) for the oarswomen was equal to or greater than that calculated for their male counterparts, however. This finding was consistent with relative-leg-strength data reported previously for untrained men and women by Wilmore (27) and for elite alpine and cross-country skiers (28). Muscular power (W) was measured isokinetically for the knee extensors and flexors of oarsmen for 1 minute at 3.2 rad/s (25). This velocity was used because the velocity of leg extension during the drive phase of the rowing stroke was estimated at or slightly above 3.2 rad/s (29). Oarsmen achieved an average power output of 660 W, whereas other elite male athletes we studied averaged 550 W. Relative values for power did favor the smaller and lighter elite road cyclists (7.59 W/kg), with oarsmen only slightly lower at 7.3 W/kg. The relative leg power values for canoeists and swimmers were 7.25 and 7.11 W/kg, respectively.

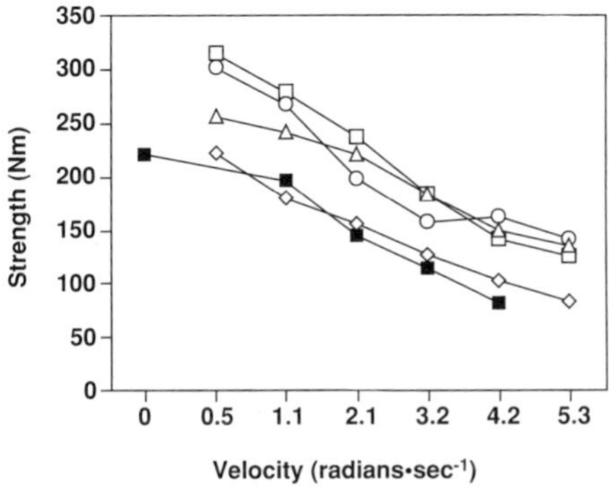

FIG. 54–7. A comparison of isokinetic strength responses among elite athletes.

Ishiko (30) measured peak power between 700 and 900 W in elite oarsmen during rowing at racing speeds, whereas women rowers have produced peak power outputs of about 500 W during ergometric rowing and also at racing speeds (31). Although we observed similar peak-power values for short periods during ergometric rowing, it is more important that average power output be maintained at very high levels throughout the 2000 m if an athlete and/or crew are to be successful. If male rowers intend to be competitive in the open events, then they must be able to generate an average power output of about 500 W during ergometric rowing for 2000 m. The most successful female rowers average about 350 W for 2000 m, and lightweight men and women about 420 W and 310 W, respectively, for this same distance (14).

Although the ability to maintain high muscular forces for a 5- to 7-minute competitive effort is absolutely crucial, it appears that enhancing muscular strength and power is not so important to rowing performance as are the development of better rowing technique for each crew member, the improvement of aerobic and anaerobic capacities, and the process of molding the efforts of individual crew members into a highly coordinated cohesive unit (32).

Aerobic Metabolism

Aerobic Capacity

It is well known that absolute maximal oxygen consumption of elite rowers is among the highest recorded (7–

TABLE 54–2. *A comparison of peak physiologic responses of 1992 U.S. Olympic Team rowers and 1997 U.S. National Team rowers*

	N	Power (watts)	HR (beats/min)	$\dot{V}_E$ (L/min)	$\dot{V}O_2$ (L/min)	$\dot{V}O_2$ (mL/kg/min)	LA (mmol/L)
1992							
Men	35	467 (± 18.1)	189 (± 6.10)	212.7 (± 11.33)	6.25 (± 0.26)	70.9 (± 2.12)	17.4 (± 2.06)
Women	25	310 (± 19.2)	190 (± 9.19)	153.1 (± 10.91)	4.31 (± 0.46)	58.6 (± 3.65)	13.1 (± 1.73)
1997							
Men	35	476 (± 17.1)	191 (± 5.82)	213.3 (± 12.10)	6.40 (± 0.49)	68.9 (± 3.03)	22.4 (± 3.19)
Women	25	331 (± 18.0)	192 (± 6.10)	155.6 (± 11.52)	4.41 (± 0.61)	57.8 (± 4.21)	14.6 (± 1.90)

HR, heart rate; $\dot{V}_E$, minute ventilation; $\dot{V}O_2$, absolute and relative oxygen consumption; LA, lactic acid.

9,13,14,26,33–51). We recorded absolute peak $\dot{V}O_2$ values exceeding 7 L/min in several elite oarsmen, the highest being 7.5 L/min, and more than 5.5 L/min in a number of female rowers. These results translate into relative values higher than 80 mL/kg/min for men and more than 70 mL/kg/min for women. A comparison of recent peak physiologic responses is shown in Table 54–2, and these data indicate a high degree of similarity in both groups in the physiologic capacities of 1992 U.S. Olympic and 1997 National Team rowers. After more than 30 years of testing elite rowers, which included more than 4000 men and 500 women, it is usually not possible to achieve international success in competitive rowing consistently unless men can consume O_2 in excess of 6 L/min, and women, 4.5 L/min. Successful lightweight rowers attain absolute $\dot{V}O_2$ values that are 500 to 1000 mL/min less than their open-class counterparts; however, because of their significantly lower body weights, they exhibit higher relative values as high as 85 to 88 mL/kg/min for men and 70 to 75 mL/kg/min for women. Absolute aerobic capacity may be more important than relative values in the assessment of a rower's aerobic power because body weight is supported in a seated position.

For the most part, early measurements of oxygen consumption of rowers were conducted during cycle ergometry or while exercising on a treadmill (15,47–50,52–65). Hagerman and Howie (66), Hagerman and Lee (67), and Hagerman and associates (38,39,41) introduced measurement of aerobic capacity during rowing ergometry, and these studies were followed by other studies (29,51,63,64,68–77). Similar measurements also were made during sculling (78,79). Oxygen consumption was first measured during tank rowing by Hagerman and Lee (67) and by DiPrampero and colleagues (35), followed by a similar study of Asami and co-workers (80). Rowing tanks are special indoor training facilities, similar in many respects to modern swimming flumes, which rowers use to improve skill and conditioning. Oxygen consumption also was measured on the water during actual rowing by DiPrampero and associates (35), Hagerman and co-workers (38,39,41), Jackson and Secher (46), and Strømme and colleagues (65).

Aerobic Testing

Although the recent development of solid-state portable measurement equipment has afforded the opportunity to determine aerobic capacity during actual rowing on the water, performing these measurements in the boat still presents several logistical problems and is extremely time-consuming. Instead, we have developed a testing protocol that we believe provides an abundance of pertinent data in the shortest time possible.

The design of the U.S. National and/or Olympic Team selection process that seems to have produced our best results gives coaches very little time to choose their competitors, and as a result, time is at a premium. Although the current design involves several athletes training regularly at one site full time, it also provides college or university rowers an equal chance to be considered as serious team candidates after their commitment to their respective college or university programs in the spring. Because most of the student rowers will not arrive at national team camps until early June, the coaches must make their selection and decide their boatings (teams) rather quickly and begin training; world championships and/or Olympic Games are usually only 8 to 10 weeks away. As a result of the time constraints but yet not to compromise the useful information physiologic testing may provide, it was decided as early as 1966 to use a simulated 2000-m rowing ergometer test not only as the basis for aerobic evaluation but also to provide some important anaerobic information. Because of the simulated exercise protocol, the highest oxygen consumption achieved during the usual 6- to 7-minute exercise was labeled *peak* $\dot{V}O_2$ (as opposed to $\dot{V}O_2$max, which is recorded during an exercise of increasing work intensity). With the exception of our earlier studies, we used this term consistently to report a rower's upper aerobic limits. Although several studies have measured $\dot{V}O_2$max for rowers, including our own (29), these values tend to be lower than the peak $\dot{V}O_2$ measurements we have reported (9,36,38,39,41,42,66,81–83). Peak $\dot{V}O_2$ measurements during simulated maximal 2000-m ergometric efforts are about 6% to 8% higher than $\dot{V}O_2$max observed during a standard rowing-ergometer exercise of increasing intensity (e.g., peak $\dot{V}O_2$ averaged 6.6 L/min for the 1976 U.S. Men's Olympic Team, whereas $\dot{V}O_2$max averaged 6.2 L/min). Foster and associates (84) reported similar observations with elite speed skaters, cyclists, and triathletes. The difference between peak and maximal $\dot{V}O_2$ values is probably a function of task specificity, and that is precisely why the test preference is a 2000-m simulated rowing-ergometer test. It is well known that skeletal muscle and its transport systems respond specifically to type, duration, and intensity of exercise; therefore the difference in the relative recruitment of muscle-fiber types between the two exercises and differing demands placed on the cardiovascular and respiratory systems could account for the differences in $\dot{V}O_2$ responses. The $\dot{V}O_2$ measurements made during ergometric rowing tests tend to agree with estimates of oxygen cost during actual rowing (7,40,41,46,85). Because the simulated testing provides as accurate as possible an evaluation of the athlete's individual response to "racing" without being on the water, it is possible to determine moment-to-moment changes throughout the 2000-m ergometric exercise. Rowers are accustomed to initiating a 2000-m competitive effort with a vigorous start in which the highest power outputs and stroke ratings are produced (Fig. 54–8). Stroke ratings may reach as high as 50 strokes/min, and this intensity may last for 30 to 45 seconds during the start. This response is necessary to overcome inertia and to increase boat velocity to racing speed. After this explosive start, power output is reduced only slightly, and stroke rating continues to be high, with between 35 and 40 strokes/min. With the exception of brief strategic increases in power and stroke rating to ensure competitiveness, power output and stroke rating remain relatively constant for about the next 3.5 to 4 minutes. The final 45 to 60 seconds of the race involve an all-out sprint to the finish, during which power and stroke rating (40 strokes/min or greater) are increased significantly. A typical 2000-m international race, if divided into four 500-m segments, would show that the first 500-m segment is the fastest phase of the race, with each 500-m segment of the middle 1000 m being about 2 to 4 seconds slower than the first 500 m. Although the boat will usually not reach the speed of the first 500 m during the sprint to the finish because of rower fatigue, the final 500 m is usually the second fastest and is about 1 to 2 seconds slower than the first 500 m. Because simulated competitive efforts on the rowing ergometer mimic this pacing pattern, the $\dot{V}O_2$ responses reflect this somewhat unique pattern of racing strategy. If the curve representing oxygen uptake during a simulated competitive effort is examined carefully (Fig. 54–9), the data indicate that with the exception of the first and last minutes of exercise, oarsmen perform near their peak aerobic capacities for almost the entire duration of the exercise and often achieve peak $\dot{V}O_2$ between the second and fifth minutes

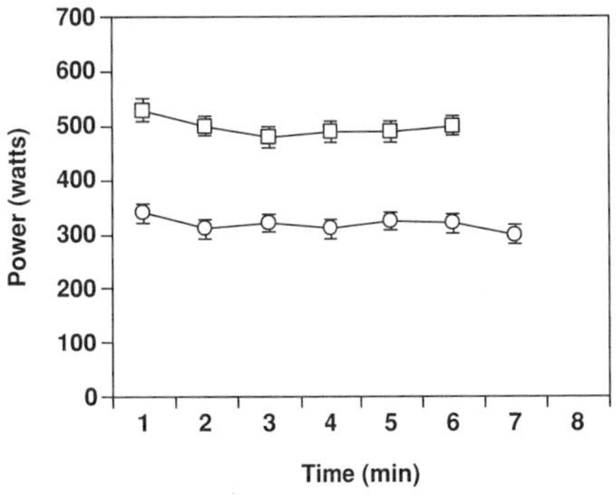

FIG. 54–8. Representative power curves for men and women during a 2000-m simulated competitive effort on a Concept II rowing ergometer.

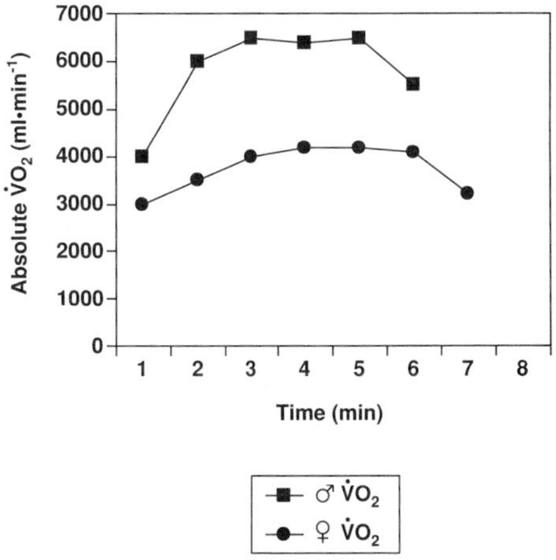

FIG. 54–9. Representative oxygen-consumption curves for men and women during a 2000-m simulated competitive effort on a Concept II rowing ergometer.

of the simulated exercise and almost never during the final minute. Although rowers exhibit rapid aerobic adjustment during the first minute of exercise, oxygen use and transport adaptations require time and thus a lag in the aerobic response. Because of fatigue and the more prominent role of anaerobiosis, $\dot{V}O_2$ decreases significantly during the last minute of the ergometer exercise.

The power output and $\dot{V}O_2$ curves for women (Figs. 54–8 and 54–9) are slightly different from the men's, probably because of the additional 1 to 1:30 min necessary to row 2000 m. The more gradual increase in $\dot{V}O_2$ is most likely a result of a lower power output because of a smaller muscle mass and decreased cardiorespiratory response. With the exception of the first and last minutes of the 2000-m effort, when anaerobiosis is more important, the absolute aerobic power of male rowers is 40% to 50% higher than that of female rowers. Relative $\dot{V}O_2$, based on body weight, results in reducing this difference to 21%; if lean body mass or FFM is considered, male rowers have only a 10% to 12% higher aerobic capacity than female rowers.

In most aerobic sports, $\dot{V}O_2max$ is often considered the most important limitation to or predictor of competitive performance. However, aerobic data accumulated for rowers over a 30-year period in our laboratory demonstrated that average $\dot{V}O_2$ measured during the simulated 2000-m ergometer effort is far more important in predicting rowing performance on the water than is peak $\dot{V}O_2$ or $\dot{V}O_2max$. Although rowers have achieved outstanding absolute peak and maximal $\dot{V}O_2$ values, their single most impressive attribute seems to be their ability to sustain an extremely high percentage of absolute peak $\dot{V}O_2$, even after they have exceeded their anaerobic threshold (AT) levels (14,29,42,86). After excluding $\dot{V}O_2$ measured during the first minute of exercise because of significant transient metabolic responses, and the last minute because of increased dependence on anaerobic metabolism, oxygen consumption is then averaged for about the middle four minutes of work. This average is then divided by peak $\dot{V}O_2$. Correlations exceeding +0.95 have been calculated between average $\dot{V}O_2$ and competitive rowing performance, whereas correlations of less than +0.85 were obtained between both peak and maximal $\dot{V}O_2$ and performance. The highest correlation for average $\dot{V}O_2$ as opposed to peak and maximal $\dot{V}O_2$ is probably due to the importance of sustaining such a high power output for a 5- to 7-minute period to be successful. Thus the major physiologic criterion used in predicting successful rowing performances at the international level is the ability of the rower to sustain an average $\dot{V}O_2$ that is between 95% and 98% of peak $\dot{V}O_2$ measured during the simulated rowing test. This criterion is especially impressive because it demonstrates that exercise intensities eliciting near-maximal metabolic responses can be maintained for 2000-m. Foster and colleagues (84) obtained similar results for simulated competitive efforts of other elite aerobic athletes.

The emphasis on the use of our data for the purposes of team selection and monitoring and modification of training programs has been a strong motivational factor over the years for athletes to perform at their highest level and, in the process, to provide valid and reliable data. Furthermore, physiologic testing has provided an open forum among coaches, athletes, and scientists for the discussion of physiologic definitions and explanations, training principles, injury and overtraining prevention, nutrition, and other topics pertinent to improving training and competitive efforts.

It is now standard protocol for U.S. National Team testing to follow the simulated competitive ergometer test with a series of 5-minute sequential submaximal rowing ergometer tests based on peak power output achieved 16 to 20 hours earlier. Each rower is required to row three 5-minute submaximal ergometric bouts, the first at 60% of peak power output recorded the previous day, followed by bouts of 70% and 80% of peak power output. Heart rate is recorded at the end of each minute of exercise, and a 1- to 2-minute recovery period separates each of the 5-minute exercise bouts. During each recovery period, a capillary blood sample is removed from the fingertip for lactic acid analysis. Submaximal heart rate and lactate data are used to assist in monitoring training effects and have proved effective in planning optimal training programs, charting an athlete's progress, and making specific recommendations for changes or modifications in training. The combination of the simulated competitive 2000-m ergometer test followed by submaximal testing has now been used consistently for more than 10 years to evaluate our national and Olympic team candidates. The accumulative data for submaximal testing have permitted the development of a set of norms that are currently used to indicate responses to training. These norms appear in Table 54–3, and it should be noted that these values are optimal and should indicate when the athlete is in the best physiologically trained state (e.g., just before World

TABLE 54–3. *Optimal heart rate and lactic acid responses for sequential submaximal rowing ergometer testing*

Test (% average 2000-m power)	HR (beats/min)	LA (mmol/L)
60	130–145	1–2
70	146–160	2.1–3
80	161–175	3.1–4

HR, heart rate; LA, lactic acid.

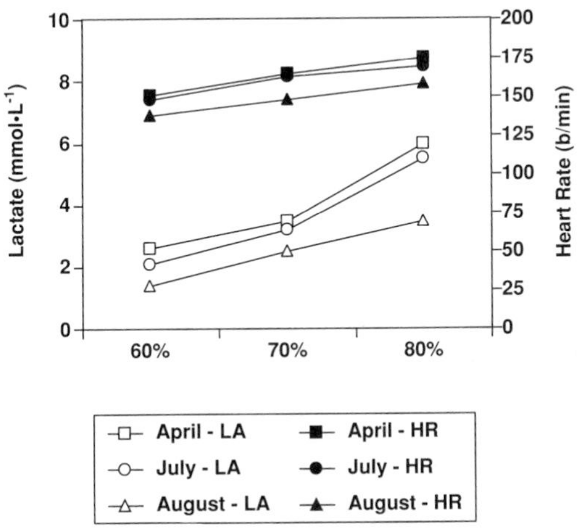

FIG. 54–10. Average submaximal heart rate (*HR*) and lactic acid (*LA*) responses of the 1997 World Champion U.S. eight-oared crew for three precompetition tests before the World Championship.

Championships or Olympic Games). Because of the progressive nature of optimal training programs, a quantitative shift to the right of the submaximal heart rate and lactate curves will be expected; representative curves for the 1997 World Championship gold medal U.S. Men's eight-oared crew are shown in Fig. 54–10. Submaximal test results were less than optimal after initial testing in April 1997 (see Table 54–3 and Fig. 54–10). It must be noted that, at the time, subjects had been rowing on the water for only a short time after an indoor winter training program, and, based on previous results for this period of testing, these results were expected. The results of the July testing should have indicated better adaptations (shift of HR and LA curves to the right) because intensity, frequency, and duration of training sessions were designed to elicit this type of response. Therefore modifications in the training program were recommended so that optimal responses were achieved by the August testing (see Fig. 54–10). It is important to note that the final submaximal test in the sequence (80% of peak power) is performed at or near AT for rowers, depending on the date of testing. Specific training sessions designed to improve AT are increased as training progresses; as a result, effort for most rowers during the 80% test in December will be achieved at a level above AT, whereas in August this same effort should be below AT. The AT for elite rowers has been determined to be 85% to 95% of $\dot{V}O_2max$ (29).

To provide comprehensive testing of our national and/or Olympic team candidates, physiologic testing is conducted according to the following schedule:

1. December 15: combination simulated ergometer 2000-m test; submaximal testing of permanent training group at site of national training center (currently Princeton University);
2. April 15: submaximal testing only of permanent training group and combination testing of any new candidates joining permanent training group;
3. July 1: follow-up combination testing of permanent training group who participated in December and April testing and first combination testing of college and university rowers who have recently arrived at training center; and
4. August 1: submaximal testing only of remaining national or Olympic team candidates (World Championships will be conducted in 5 weeks).

This testing schedule has permitted adequate evaluation of all team candidates relating to their physiologic capabilities and responses to training. In addition, the final evaluation provides enough time for coaches and athletes to make important adjustments in training to assist in athletes' peaking at the designated time.

This testing program has evolved over several years of study of the best U.S. rowers and from discussions with coaches and athletes. Because of its simplicity, applicability, and minimal time commitment, test results have provided valuable information for the athletes and coaches. Application of results of this testing program should not be overemphasized, however; they are not used as the primary source for team selection or designing training programs. Instead, test results can help to distinguish the extremes in athletes' physiologic capacities and competitive efforts, and repeated submaximal data can help in training-program design and assist in charting its progress. It also is important to note that over the years this basic testing program involving elite rowers has been the foundation for several definitive research studies. The results of these studies have contributed important data to understanding the upper limits of human performance.

Anaerobic Metabolism

The relative contribution of anaerobic metabolism to a competitive rowing effort has been estimated by using a variety of methods, including measurements of O_2 deficit, O_2 debt, and the energy equivalent of postexercise blood lactic acid concentrations (35,36,40–43,71,74, 80,81,87–89). A study of lightweight oarsmen showed no significant correlation between aerobic endurance measured by average aerobic–anaerobic thresholds and performances in anaerobic tests (90). It was concluded that use of anaerobic tests may be of little value for prediction of performance in rowing. Koutedakis and Sharp (91) developed a modified Wingate test for determining anaerobic power in rowers and reported unusually high anaerobic capacities.

O_2 Deficit

Although O_2 deficit would probably be the best noninvasive estimate of anaerobic metabolism's contribution during maximal exercise, the difficulties involved with its accurate determination discourage its use by most investigators. It has been suggested that the difference between the O_2 demand and O_2 uptake accumulating during high-intensity exercise is considered a valid estimate of anaerobic metabolism (92,93). However, other studies have reported that there was no relationship between accumulated O_2 deficit and estimates of anaerobic capacity in elite or highly trained athletes (94,95). Because oarsmen maintain a relatively high metabolic steady state during actual competition and during the simulated rowing-ergometry testing discussed earlier (see Fig. 54–9), we compared accumulated O_2 deficit calculated during ergometry by using the high steady-state portion of the $\dot{V}O_2$ curve and the increase of $\dot{V}O_2$ during exercise (43,89) with the $\dot{V}O_2$ power-regression method of O_2-deficit estimation (92,96) and calculated O_2 deficits exceeding 12 L. Secher and co-workers (97) reported somewhat lower values. Roth and associates (71) and Steinacker and colleagues (74) also reported lower values that ranged between 300 and 400 mL for a 7- to 13-minute ergometer exercise. For rowers, relative O_2 deficits of 88 to 97 mL/kg/min have been determined (42,89,98), and this range compares with 52 to 90 mL/kg/min measured for runners during treadmill running (96). Bangsbo and colleagues (92) compared indirect O_2-deficit and O_2-debt measurements with anaerobic energy yield in isolated human muscle during exhaustive exercise and discovered that O_2 deficit represented an accurate estimation of anaerobic energy contribution to a specific exercise. An estimated pulmonary oxygen deficit during submaximal exercise probably does not account for total anaerobic energy produced during whole-body exercise, however.

O2 Debt

"O_2 debt" is, of course, an outdated term, originally described by A.V. Hill, that has acquired a variety of contemporary descriptions; prominent among them is *excess postexercise oxygen consumption* (EPOC). This recovery O_2 consumption has been used to estimate anaerobic capacity of rowers; however, it has been suggested that some of this excess O_2 is used for functions not strictly associated with anaerobiosis, and thus EPOC is probably not an accurate estimate of the role of anaerobic metabolism during exercise. We observed maximal or peak O_2 debts as high as 20 L measured over a 30-minute recovery period after a simulated 2000-m ergometer exercise with an average of 13.5 L for international-caliber oarsmen (42). Secher and co-workers (97) reported a maximal value of 33 L. The O_2 debts calculated for oarswomen and lightweight men were 10 L and 12 L, respectively (42,81).

Blood Lactate

Extremely high venous lactic acid concentrations have been reported after maximal actual and simulated rowing (14). Earlier reports of maximal lactate concentrations in elite oarsmen ranged from 14 to 18 mmol/L after a 6-minute simulated rowing exercise (42). Vaage (99) measured average team values of 11 mmol/L immediately after rowing competition at the national level, 15 mmol/L for oarsmen after running on a treadmill, and 17 mmol/L after international competition. We have consistently measured lactates ranging from 10 to 20 mmol/L in oarsmen after simulated 2000-m efforts on a rowing ergometer; women's values for the same exercise were slightly lower (9,82,83,100). Average lactate values for the 1997 U.S. eight-oared crew, who were world champions, after a simulated 2000-m ergometer exercise exceeded 22 mmol/L (101). Lactic acid concentrations were measured immediately after several competitive efforts of different boat classes at the 1987 World Rowing Championships (100), the first such measurements for any elite aerobic athletes either during or after world championship competition. Lactate concentrations for men ranged between 16 and 28 mmol/L, the latter value being the highest our group has thus far observed; women's lactate concentrations after similar competitive efforts ranged from 10 to 20 mmol/L. It is clear that rowers show significant increases in blood lactate during exercise; furthermore, plasma bicarbonate tends to be lower after rowing than after running or arm cranking (102–104). The excessive lactate values reported after maximal actual and simulated rowing indicate that the anaerobic capacities of these athletes are extremely high; when expressed as O_2 deficit, they may be equivalent to 100 mL O_2/kg body weight (98).

The appearance of lactic acid concentrations in excess of 20 mmol/L in venous and capillary blood of both men and women after exhaustive actual and simulated rowing seems to indicate extraordinary anaerobic capacity, increased lactate tolerance, and probably enhanced cellular, blood, and respiratory buffering capacity. Venous blood lactate levels in our studies have been measured after exercise, however; despite extensive muscle biopsy sampling, we have, heretofore, not analyzed muscle samples for pH or cell-buffering power. We had hypothesized even in our earlier studies that perhaps the venous or capillary lactate responses were not an accurate representation of maximal production and/or clearance of lactate. This prompted us to determine the intensity and duration of exercise at which rowers produce the highest lactate concentrations. Because it is impossible to row at high intensities with an indwelling venous catheter in either an arm or a leg, we asked 33 U.S. Olympic Team candidates during the 1976 testing and team-selection process to perform two simulated 2000-m competitive efforts on a rowing ergometer on separate days with a 5-day rest between the tests. Both tests were designated as providing important data for team selection. During the second test, however, rowers were stopped randomly at minutes 1, 2, 3, 4, or 5, or were allowed to complete the exercise. Venous blood was withdrawn after a 5-minute recovery period, which has been standard procedure after simulated 2000-m ergometer tests since 1966. All 33 subjects were naive to the random procedures and, after completing the second test, were requested not to reveal the changes in procedure until all subjects had finished testing; they provided full cooperation. When the lactate results of the interrupted tests were compared with lactate data analyzed for all subjects after completion of the first test (entire 2000 m), the comparisons revealed that significant amounts of lactate were formed during the first minute of the simulated rowing exercise, and that lactate reaches its peak in 2 minutes, decreasing slightly during work but still remaining relatively high (Fig. 54–11). Minute analysis of lactates clearly show that rowers, after producing significant lactate concentrations very early in the simulated exercise, must maintain a high tolerance to lactate throughout the remainder of the exercise. This procedure was repeated in 1989 (also see Fig. 54–11) for U.S. National Team candidates, but this time it included both men and women, and, with the exception of slightly higher values in 1989, the shapes of the two curves for the men were similar. When one considers the pacing pattern of a 2000-m competitive effort by men and compatible energy system use, it may not seem surprising that these high lactate levels are observed in the first 2 minutes of exercise. The increase in lactate values for women is more gradual and reaches a peak during the final minutes of exercise (see Fig. 54–11). This response, in contrast to that of the men, probably reflects anatomic and physiologic differences associated with decreased muscle mass and heart and lung size among women and resulting functional characteristics such as lower anaerobic capacity and power output related to these differences.

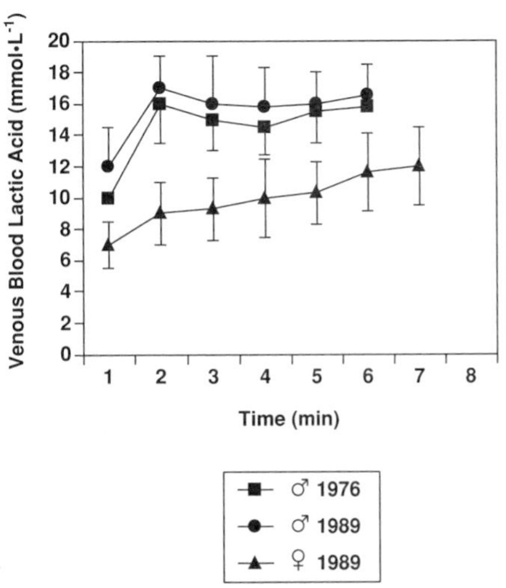

FIG. 54–11. A comparison of blood lactate curves for men and women during a 2000-m simulated competitive effort on a Concept II rowing ergometer.

Lactic acid accumulation in both men and women after actual or simulated rowing that we have measured over the years may not represent the quantity of lactate produced during these high-intensity exercises, especially in view of the recent identification in skeletal muscle fibers of mammalian lactic acid transporters (105) and the possibility of increased cellular and systemic buffering power. Rowers have greater than normal buffering capacity in skeletal muscle, especially in the critical vastus lateralis (106). Induced alkalosis through bicarbonate ingestion does not seem to improve rowing performance, however (107). The most successful rowers produce significantly less lactate at standard submaximal exercise intensities (82,83,101, 108). Whether these transporters are more abundant or more active in muscles of elite rowers is unknown; however, the pattern of lactic acid accumulation after simulated rowing (see Fig. 54–11) indicates that there may be some resynthesis of lactate as exercise continues, especially between minutes 2 and 4. It may be that rowers are capable of "clearing" lactate at a greater rate. As will be more thoroughly described, rowers possess almost exclusively oxidative muscle-fiber types in the major power muscles of rowing with type I (SO) fibers exceeding 70% of the total fiber population. Because type I fibers have been shown to have a greater lactate–proton transport capacity than type IIB (FG) fibers (109–112), this may provide at least part of the explanation of increased lactate efflux. In addition, the very-high-intensity training practices of elite rowers may increase lactate–proton transporter capacity.

Measurement of lactates during recovery from exercise has been used extensively to characterize rowing training intensities and to monitor effects of training (59,79,82,83,101,113,114). Assistance has been afforded to coaches and athletes in planning and modification of training programs as a result of combining heart rate and lactate measurements. These measurements have been used more accurately to distinguish between relative aerobic and relative anaerobic training efforts. At present, however, there are no valid invasive or noninvasive analytic techniques that permit an accurate representation of the anaerobic energy system's production of adenosine triphosphate (ATP) during rowing.

Energy Expenditure and Mechanical Efficiency

Metabolic Cost

It has been estimated from O_2 consumption and lactate data and more recently by using O_2 deficit during actual and simulated rowing that the relative contributions of aerobic and anaerobic metabolic pathways are approximately 70% to 80% and 20% to 30%, respectively (8,9,13, 14,42,87,115). These data were generated during and after rowing ergometry under simulated competitive conditions. Connors (87) estimated the relative energy contributions of the phosphagens [adenosine triphosphate (ATP)–phosphocreatine (PCr) system], anaerobic glycolysis (lactic acid system), and aerobic energy production (the O_2 system). The aerobic component was calculated from net exercise $\dot{V}O_2$ measured during rowing ergometry and was reported to be 77.8% of the total energy input. Postexercise venous lactates were converted to glycolytic energy equivalents by using Margaria's formula (116,117), and this calculation produced an energy contribution of 13.8% of the total. This value is comparable to 14% attributed to glycolysis proposed by Secher (7). More recent calculations by our group of anaerobic energy contribution to simulated rowing by using the accumulative O_2 deficit method proposed by Medbø and associates (96) estimated the total anaerobic component to represent almost 26% of the total energy contributed to simulated rowing. In an earlier study, the contribution of the phosphagens as determined by using Fox's equation was estimated to be 5% to 7% (81). These proposed relative energy contributions are only estimates, as it is not possible to calculate accurately the net exergonic energy released aerobically and anaerobically by indirect means, and this is especially the case concerning the energy currency produced by anaerobiosis. By using older definitions of relative anaerobic components, Roth and co-workers (71) reported a lactic component of 10% during a simulated 2000-m effort. Hagerman and colleagues (42), by using exercise $\dot{V}O_2$ and O_2 debt, estimated an aerobic-to-anaerobic ratio of energy contribution of 70:30, which is similar to that reported previously (98) and in more recent studies in our laboratory (37). Because many of the earlier simulated rowing studies used a maximum of 6 minutes of exercise and because some rowing events (small boats) last longer than 6 minutes, Secher suggested that the relative proportion of aerobic metabolism to actual rowing may be higher than that determined during the 6-minute test (8). Competitive times for all boat classes continue to improve, and it has been estimated that metabolic cost increases proportionately with faster and more powerful crews. Secher (7) suggested that the O_2 cost of race rowing has increased about 0.2 L/min per decade; however, our more recent metabolic and performance data suggest that this value has almost doubled in the last 10 years (100,101). In addition to the improvement of rower's metabolic capacities over the years, skill levels have also improved, and boat and oar designs have been enhanced. An oxygen cost of 5.1 L/min reported in 1919 had increased to 6.4 L/min by 1979 (7). As early as 1925, Henderson and Haggard (52) estimated the O_2 cost of rowing a competitive race to be about 6.1 L/min (i.e., approximately 30 kcal/min). Current estimations of O_2 cost during ergometric rowing range from 6.7 to 7.0 L/min (85). We recently measured an average peak absolute oxygen consumption of 6.40 L/min for heavyweight men and 5.77 L/min for lightweight men, which when converted relative to body weight, were 69 and 73 mL/kg/min, respectively.

The metabolic cost of rowing also is influenced by the drag force on the boat, and at least three mathematical models have been described comparing the metabolic capacity of rowers and the energy cost of rowing (118–120). Secher and Vaage (120) reported that race results from international regattas have been predicted with an $r = 0.99$ from these models. The body weight of rowers also influences metabolic cost, and the basis for these models has been the assumption that aerobic capacity and boat resistance increase with the weight of the oarsmen to the second power. It is obvious, however, that having bigger and more fat-free rowers in shorter races would be advantageous because of the importance of anaerobic muscular power required for successful performance. Several studies have attempted measurement of O_2 cost during actual rowing (35,45,46). Secher (7,8) and Törner (6) reported that the metabolic cost of rowing increases with the speed of the boat to the 2.4 power, which is somewhat less than to the 3.0 power needed to overcome the drag force on the boat (7). These differences in actual versus theoretic metabolic-cost models could possibly be attributed to the "checking" effects of rowers moving forward and backward on sliding seats, thereby affecting boat acceleration and deceleration. Unfortunately, the extent to which movement on the seat influences the metabolic cost is not known (8).

The relative contributions of aerobic and anaerobic metabolism to a 2000-m competitive rowing performance are not unique; other studies have reported similar contributions during other simulated sport activities of about the same duration (121–124). What is unusual is the manner in which the energy systems are recruited and the extreme maximal capacities of these systems displayed by elite rowers (9,14,42,81,101,125). The standard practice of rowers producing peak power in the initial 30 to 40 seconds followed by a high steady-state and finally an all-out sprint to the finish seems a very uneconomic approach to energy use or "pacing." Other elite athletes competing in events of similar duration do not follow a similar exercise pattern. There seem to be at least two possible reasons for emphasis on high velocities at the onset of rowing competition. One is the need to overcome the inertia of the boat to bring it up to racing speed. The other possible reason relates to the competitive attitude of crews; that is, regardless of its potential overall speed, each crew insists on keeping close contact with other crews in the race.

It is difficult to estimate the energy expenditure in a sport accurately by using simulated exercise or training efforts. This was emphasized recently when we measured capillary lactate and heart-rate responses of rowers during and after World Championship and Olympic competitions and discovered responses clearly different from those recorded during simulated competitive efforts or during actual rowing competitions of lesser significance. We are certain that what we have measured as maximal or peak physiologic responses have been specific to the relative competitive conditions. It appears that highly competitive elite rowers have another exercise "gear" and are thus able to elevate their physiologic capacities for special or more important competitive efforts (100). The accumulation of energy-cost data from more than 30 years of studies conducted with elite rowers has permitted us to build on the energy continuum originally described by Åstrand and Rodahl (54). Figure 54–12 displays energy-cost comparisons at different exercise intensities for several different endurance sports and indicates that the power outputs and energy costs of rowing are among the highest recorded and represent the upper limits of human exercise capacity (14,88).

Power and Mechanical Efficiency

Secher (7) estimated power generated at racing speed in the pair-oared with coxswain boat at about 400 W in the direction of the boat and, considering work done in a transverse direction because of the biomechanics of the rowing stroke, a total power output of about 470 W was estimated. By using estimated power output and metabolic cost of rowing at racing speed, he calculated mechanical efficiency at approximately 22%. We measured average power outputs in excess of 500 W during simulated rowing. As described earlier, the highest or peak power output during a simulated 2000-m effort occurs early in the exercise. Typical power curves are shown in Fig. 54–8. It is interesting to note that peak power is observed simultaneous with or followed closely by peak lactic acid values and peak $\dot{V}O_2$ (Figs. 54–9 and 54–11). All three values appear to follow closely the energy demands and the time limitations placed on the energy systems during a competitive effort. As expected, power data during simulated rowing closely resembles the same strategy of pacing used during actual rowing, with the highest power outputs achieved during the vigorous start, followed by a slightly lower, almost metabolic steady state, and ending with an increase in power output at the finish. Power outputs during simulated rowing of the 1992 U.S. Olympic Team rowers were compared with those of the 1997 U.S. National Team, and, as illustrated in Table 54–2, a power output for the 1997 rowers was about 12% higher than that recorded in 1992. The higher power outputs were produced at an aerobic cost of between 25 and 35 kcal/min (see Fig. 54–12). Mechanical efficiencies averaged between 19% and 21% for the 1992 competitors and increased slightly to 20% to 22% for the 1997 group. Our power and efficiency observations compare favorably with those estimated by Secher (7). Mechanical

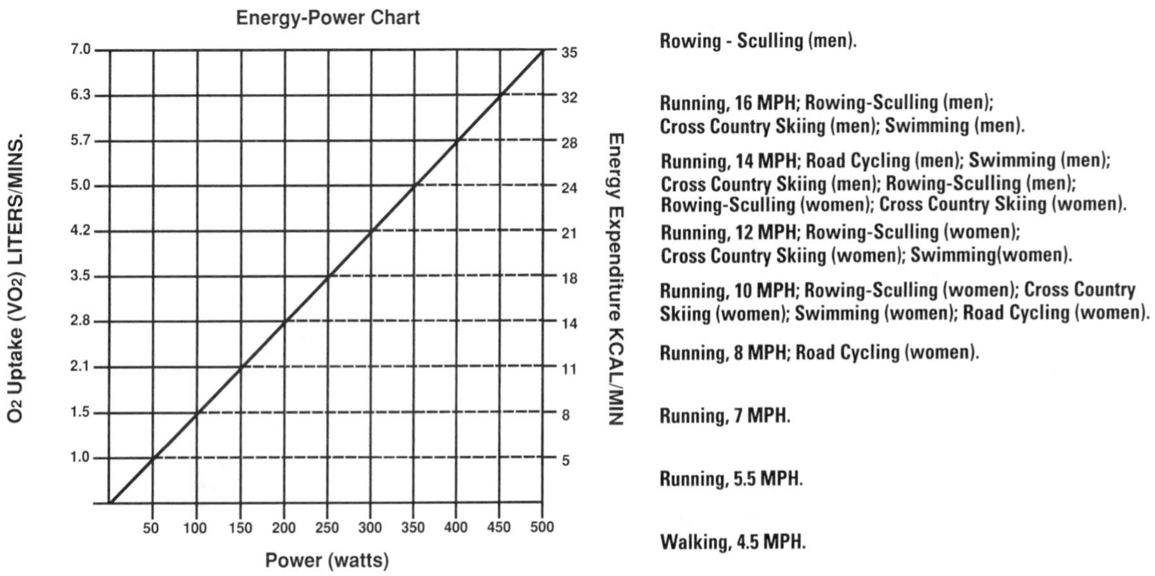

FIG. 54–12. Comparisons for oxygen consumption and energy expenditure at increasing exercise intensity for various activities. Rowing data based on more than 4000 rowers.

efficiency measured during simulated competitive rowing efforts has ranged from 10% to 25% (7,35,42,43, 46,69,71,74,87,126). Our earlier work produced low mechanical efficiencies (12% to 16%); however, these results were obtained by using the Gamut–Stanford ergometer. Although it probably simulates the sweep-rowing stroke better than the other, more frequently used rowing ergometers, Concept II and Gjessing-Ergorow, it offers a heavier resistance compared with these other ergometers and actual rowing and thus a reduction in mechanical efficiency. The mechanically braked Gamut–Stanford ergometer used in our earlier studies was described by Hagerman and colleagues (42), and its use and value were discussed in earlier reports (127,128) (Fig. 54–13). More recently, the mechanically braked and fixed-resistance Gjessing-Ergorow and variable resistance Concept II ergometers have been identified as more closely simulating actual rowing, especially the Concept II ergometer, which is probably the most widely used for indoor rowing today (129,130); athletes and coaches alike suggest that the Concept II ergometer simulates actual rowing better than any other ergometer. The Concept II and Gjessing-Ergorow ergometers are shown in Figs. 54–14 and 54–15. More accurate simulation of actual rowing has led to improved mechanical-efficiency measurements. Roth and co-workers (71) calculated mean efficiency values of 26% (ranging from 17% to 41%) during simulated rowing. Our more recent mechanical-efficiency calculations for simulated rowing using the Concept II ergometer have ranged between 18% and 24%, and these data compare favorably with mechanical efficiencies estimated during actual rowing (7,35,69,128). Because of the similarity of efficiency data between simulated and actual rowing, it appears that more recent ergometric efforts and compatible data may be used adequately to represent the task of rowing. Because rowing is a noncontinuous acceleration–deceleration activity and also inserts an implement (oar) between the athlete and the exercise medium (water), estimates of mechanical efficiency will not match those of continuous, constant-acceleration aerobic activities such as cycling and running.

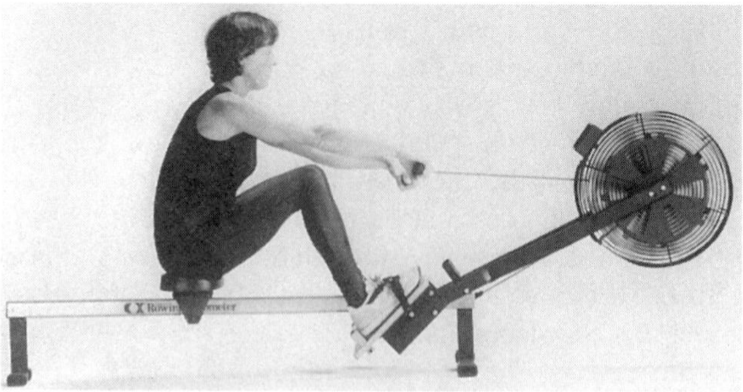

FIG. 54–14. Concept II rowing ergometer. (Courtesy of Concept II Inc., Morrisville, VT.)

In addition to having the aerobic capacity to maintain between 95% and 98% of peak $\dot{V}O_2$ during most of a 2000-m competitive effort, successful international rowers exhibit a consistent increase in mechanical efficiency as they continue to train and compete at the elite level (9). We have longitudinal data for 12 oarsmen who were candidates for the U.S. National and Olympic teams for 8 consecutive years. Although some of these rowers were teammates, others competed consecutively but at different periods during my 30-year study of rowers. The average mechanical efficiencies for each year of

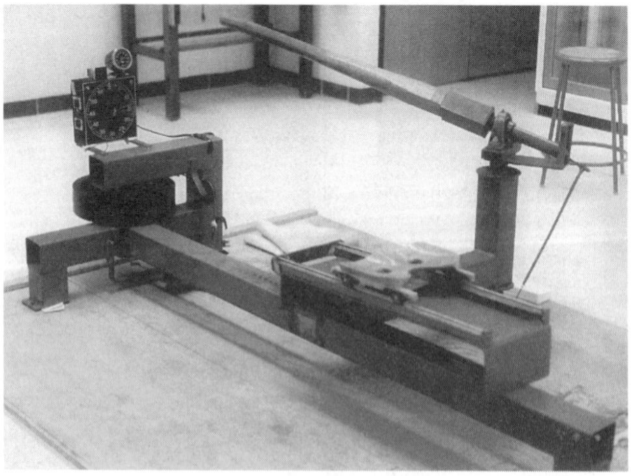

FIG. 54–13. Gamut–Stanford rowing ergometer.

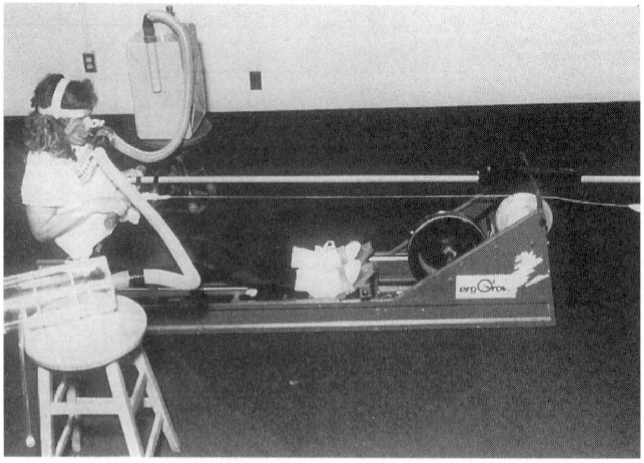

FIG. 54–15. Gjessing-Ergorow rowing ergometer.

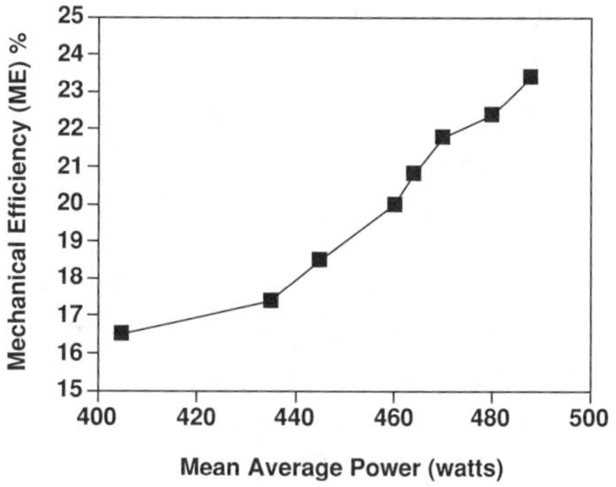

FIG. 54–16. Average mechanical efficiency over an 8-year period of 12 elite oarsmen calculated by using $\dot{V}O_2$ and power-output data recorded during a 2000-m simulated competitive effort on a Concept II rowing ergometer.

their candidacies are shown in Figure 54–16. All were outstanding college oarsmen during the first two to three years of their candidacies for the U.S. National and Olympic teams; however, they did not become successful candidates until they were able to achieve mechanical efficiencies at or above 20%. Although probably favored genetically, these athletes gradually improved important physiologic responses necessary to increase mechanical efficiency, and I view this factor as being the single most important criterion for predicting rowing performance. These changes in efficiency can be attributed to several factors, including specific and consistent training programs, accumulative effects of training, rowing with more skilled, experienced, and highly trained teammates, better coaching, and better equipment.

Anaerobic Threshold: Lactate Threshold

Both of these concepts have prompted significant controversy among exercise scientists, and although it has been suggested that they can be equated, opposing views to this relation have confused athletes and coaches (131,132). Lactate threshold (LT) is considered by many to be a good indicator of an athlete's capacity to perform endurance exercise and is usually defined as that point at which venous blood lactate begins to accumulate above resting levels during exercise of increasing intensity. LT is suggested as a transition point between less dependence on aerobic energy systems and more dependence on anaerobic metabolism, and a compatible increase in lactic acid. The validity of this measurement is questionable because skeletal muscle begins to produce lactate before LT, and at the same time lactate is cleared by other tissues including skeletal muscle (105). The accuracy of this measurement is therefore confounded by both rate of lactate production and rate of clearance, and the difference between the two processes is really what is measured; it may not be necessarily a true indication of a significant onset of anaerobiosis. We successfully measured major break points in lactate and responses of elite rowers during continuous rowing-ergometer exercise of increasing intensity and have found LT to range between 80% and 90% of $\dot{V}O_2$max (100,101). We have used LT to assist in determining intensities of work sessions and as a guide to training effects in both rowing and in other aerobically based sports. The increase in clearance of lactate, increases in both the quantitative and qualitative responses of key enzymes, and a shift in metabolic substrate help to increase (improve) LT in a highly trained rower.

The first reference to AT was made by Wassermann and McIlroy in 1964 (133) and was supposed to indicate when a significant increase in blood lactate and the lactate/pyruvate ratio occurred because of an ever-decreasing PO_2 in exercising muscle (134). AT is often expressed as a percentage of maximal power output, heart rate, or $\dot{V}O_2$. Although we have been able to satisfactorily equate AT with LT in most elite rowers, some consistently do not exhibit a characteristic ventilatory break point. This is in spite of accurately measuring ventilatory equivalents for both O_2 and CO_2. There is a linear relation between $\dot{V}O_2$, $\dot{V}CO_2$, and V_E at low exercise intensities during an incremental exercise test on the rowing ergometer. The first major departure of the curves for V_E and $\dot{V}CO_2$ from a linear relation with $\dot{V}O_2$ as the rowing intensity increases has been designated the AT (Fig. 54–17). Anaerobic thresholds of 85% to 95% of $\dot{V}O_2$max (29,86,135–137) attest to the very high aerobic capacities of rowers reported earlier in this chapter, and this increased oxygen use coupled with high anaerobic thresholds may suggest an endurance athlete's ability to use lactic acid as a fuel during exercise (138,139). The oxidation of lactic acid by skeletal and cardiac muscle during exercise could help elevate the AT of rowers, and it then may seem reasonable that lactate clearance and oxidation occur during the high steady-state phase of a 2000-m race (see Fig. 54–11).

Increased capacity of AT and peak $\dot{V}O_2$ in rowers are due, in part, to the specificity of training. Because rowing for both men and women is primarily an aerobic event, more than 85% of training time is devoted to aerobic conditioning. Furthermore, rowing training induces increases in maximal cardiac output, pulmonary ventilation, diffusion capacity for oxygen, mean arteriovenous oxygen difference (a-vO_2 diff), and a delay in the rapid increase in the ventilation equivalent for oxygen ($V_E/\dot{V}O_2$), the latter response suggesting that AT adapts to rowing training. AT has been found to be 70% to 75% of $\dot{V}O_2$max for rowers during the off season but 85% to 95% of $\dot{V}O_2$max during the competitive season (25,29,82,83,86). Average AT data from these studies

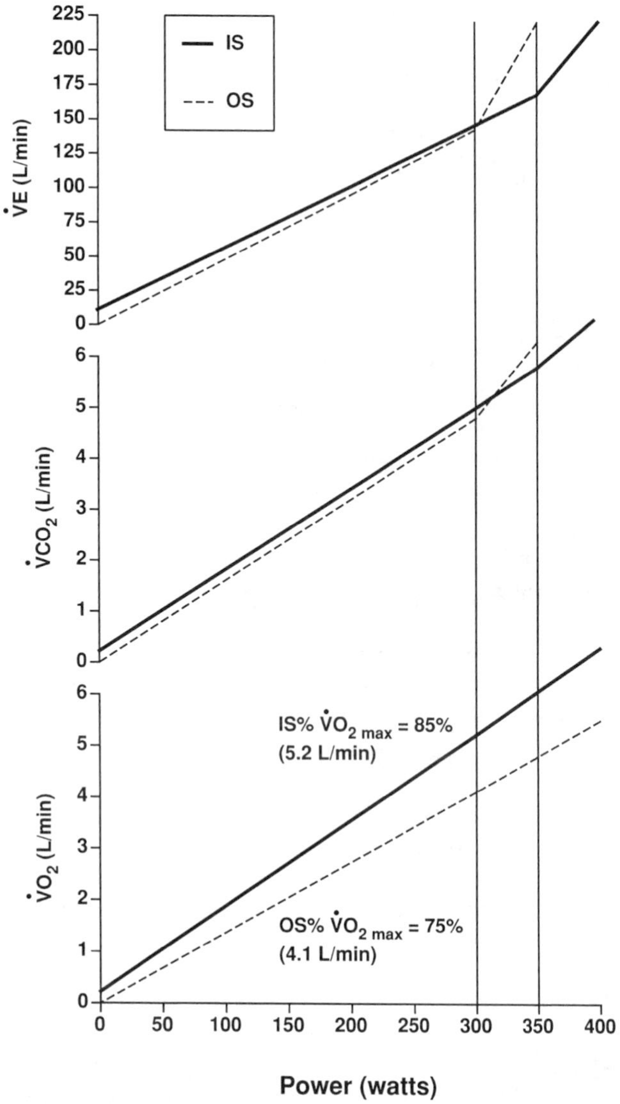

FIG. 54–17. A comparison of off-season (*OS*) and in-season (*IS*) anaerobic thresholds of 1983 Men's National Rowing Team based on V_E, $\dot{V}O_2$, and $\dot{V}CO_2$ responses during exercise of progressive intensity on a Concept II rowing ergometer.

are shown in Fig. 54–17 and confirm the transitory character of AT among elite rowers.

Cardiopulmonary

Pulmonary Ventilation

We have recorded several maximal or peak V_E values in excess of 240 L/min at body temperature and ambient pressure, saturated with water vapor (BTPS) during simulated rowing, the highest being 270 L/min BTPS. Excluding the transitory effects during the first minute of a 2000-m simulated exercise, most elite oarsmen average more than 200 L/min BTPS throughout the exercise. We also measured V_E values exceeding 200 L/min BTPS in some women rowers, and it is common for oarswomen to sustain an average V_E greater than 170 L/min BTPS for an exhaustive 2000-m ergometric effort. Peak minute ventilations in our simulated studies have always exceeded V_{Emax} recorded during standard incremental rowing protocols, and these responses parallel similar metabolic responses described earlier (see comparison of peak $\dot{V}O_2$ and $\dot{V}O_2$max values). Similar responses were observed by Foster and colleagues (84) in studies of other elite aerobic athletes. The large ventilatory volumes of rowers are a result, at least in part, of their large body masses and surface areas. They tend to have very large vital capacities, with some men exceeding 9 L (7,40). Biersteker and Biersteker (140) and Biersteker and associates (141) measured pulmonary function in rowers and suggested that increases in intrathoracic pressure during rowing, especially in the catch position (body compressed and early Valsalva response), should limit lung elasticity. This phenomenon was found in female rowers only, however, and there seemed to be no explanation for why male rowers do not exhibit this response because they develop very high intrathoracic pressures during exercise. Some rowers have exhibited comparatively low ventilation equivalents for oxygen ($V_E/\dot{V}O_2$) during exercise (7,142,143), presumably because the rower assumes a compressed body position during the initial or catch phase of the stroke, thus theoretically (not measured) impairing normal excursion of the diaphragm (69). We have shown that ventilatory equivalents for oxygen of rowers equal or exceed those of most other endurance athletes (9,14,36,38–41,101). Hyperventilation during rowing is more pronounced than during cycling and is accomplished with a higher breathing frequency accompanied by a relatively lower tidal volume (144). Peak breathing frequencies in our simulated rowing studies have ranged from 60 to 90 breaths/min, and tidal volumes of greater than 3 L have been observed. Some studies have reported that breathing rate and depth are entrained with the rowing stroke (38–41,142,143). Typically, a rower will have one rather long respiratory cycle during the drive phase of the stroke followed by a more brief cycle during the recovery phase. Steinacker and co-workers (145) investigated ventilatory responses in elite rowers during an incremental simulated rowing exercise and observed two distinct breathing patterns: type 1, with one expiration during the drive phase of the stroke and one inspiration during recovery, and type 2, with one complete breath during the drive phase and a complete breath during recovery; type 2 is similar to entrainment patterns identified by Hagerman and colleagues (38–41,142,143).

Exhaustive rowing has been associated with marked hypoxia. Despite significant exercise hyperpnea, arterial P_{O_2} was shown to decline from 105 mm Hg at rest to 88 mm Hg during the last minute of maximal simulated rowing (146). Hemoglobin saturation was reduced to 91% and arterial pH decreased to 6.8 (103) during rowing, and Chance and associates (147) revealed significant hemoglobin desaturation during severe simulated ergometric rowing. This hypoxia could be accompanied by a reduction in blood bicarbonate to a point at which it may be temporarily eliminated from the blood. The decrease in arterial P_{O_2} during intense rowing also may indicate a diffusion limitation for oxygen at the liquid–gaseous interface as the brevity of erythrocyte presence in the pulmonary capillaries is exaggerated when cardiac outputs for rowers reach extraordinary levels.

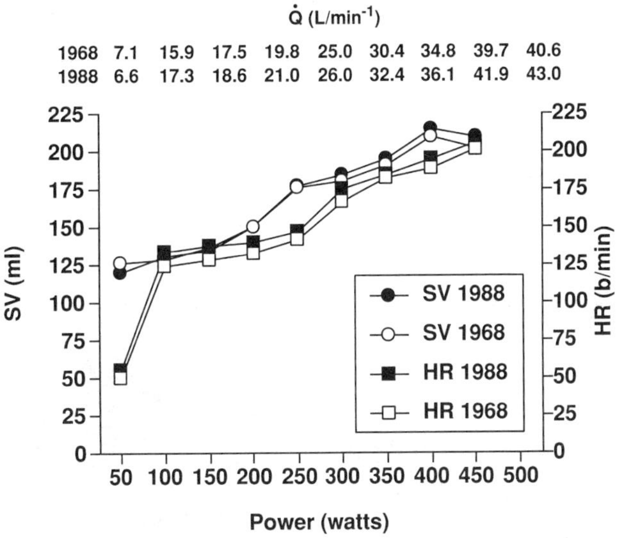

FIG. 54–18. A comparison of average cardiac responses to cycle-ergometer exercise of increasing intensity; 1968 versus 1988 U.S. Olympic rowing teams. *SV*, stroke volume; *HR*, heart rate.

Heart Rate, Stroke Volume, and Cardiac Output

An increase in heart rate was probably one of the first physiologic responses observed during rowing (148), and this same study also reported an abnormal increase in pulse pressure. Maximal and peak heart rates ranging widely between 165 and 220 beats/min have been observed during both actual and simulated rowing (7–9,13,37–39,42,43,46,51,61,66,67,69,74,78,83,97,125,136, 149). These studies also reported rowers' ability to maintain very high heart rates throughout actual and simulated rowing.

Measurement of cardiac output of rowers was first reported by Liljestrand and Lindhard (53) during actual rowing, and they recorded a value of 17 L/min. Later, during a rowing ergometer exercise of low intensity, an attempt was made again to measure cardiac output, but because the subjects were not elite athletes and the exercise was submaximal ($\dot{V}O_2$, 2.4 L/min), prediction of cardiac output by regression analysis resulted in values of less than 7 L/min (150), which were similar to values recorded or predicted for other aerobic activities of submaximal intensity (7). We first measured cardiac output in 1968 in U.S. Olympic oarsmen by using the dye-dilution technique and then again in 1988 with Doppler echocardiography, obtaining measurements both at rest and during an incremental cycle-ergometer exercise test to exhaustion (accurate measurements during rowing were not possible). Maximal cardiac outputs ranged from 29 to 40 L/min, with the highest values achieved by those rowers who met the following criteria: height exceeded 199 cm, weight did not exceed 90 kg, body fat did not exceed 9%, peak $\dot{V}O_2$ was higher than 6.7 L/min, average $\dot{V}O_2$ was at least 98% of peak $\dot{V}O_2$ during a 2000-m simulated rowing effort on a Concept II ergometer, and average power output for this effort was greater than 500 W. A summary of our cardiac data is depicted in Fig. 54–18; these data, plotted as averages for each power output, indicate the extraordinary cardiac adaptations of elite oarsmen, especially at extreme exercise intensities. Similar responses have been reported for other outstanding elite endurance athletes (121). Saltin (151) suggested that maximal stroke volume is the most important distinguishing difference between elite endurance athletes and nonelite endurance-trained subjects; our cardiac functional data tend to support this observation. We recorded resting heart rates of rowers in the sitting position as low as 26 beats/min. Such low rates seem to indicate an influence of very high stroke volumes. The O_2 pulse ($\dot{V}O_2$/heart rate) is an indirect estimate of stroke volume, and we have calculated an O_2 pulse as high as 39.4 mL O_2/beat during a simulated competitive ergometer effort or in a rower whose peak $\dot{V}O_2$ was 7.1 L/min and whose peak heart rate was 180 beats/min (9).

In addition to increasing end-diastolic volume, decreasing end-systolic volume, facilitating sympathetic stimulation and control, and increasing elasticity and contractility, elite endurance athletes exhibit a larger cardiac mass than normal (152,153). Several studies have reported large internal diameters and wall thicknesses of the left myocardium of oarsmen (154–157), further evidence of significant exercise adaptation and the capacity to deliver very large stroke volumes. Cardiac mass measurements of oarsmen are apparently similar to those of weightlifters, who routinely show selective hypertrophy of myocardial tissue (158).

TABLE 54–4. *A summary of physical characteristics of U.S. men's elite eight-oared crews (National or Olympic teams) reported every 5 years between 1972 and 1997*

	Age (yr)	Height (cm)	Weight (kg)	Body fat (%)
1972	23.8 ± 1.45	189.4 ± 2.9	87.4 ± 6.1	12.3 ± 2.3
1977	21.4 ± 2.5	193.1 ± 3.0	91.2 ± 4.8	11.5 ± 2.0
1982	22.8 ± 2.1	194.3 ± 4.3	90.2 ± 4.3	9.3 ± 1.6
1987	23.1 ± 3.3	195.0 ± 5.5	88.2 ± 3.7	8.5 ± 1.2
1992	24.2 ± 3.1	195.8 ± 5.1	92.0 ± 2.9	8.6 ± 1.1
1997	23.1 ± 3.4	196.3 ± 3.0	94.1 ± 2.7	8.9 ± 0.7
Change between 1972 and 1997 (%)		3.6	7.7	−27.6

THE ATHLETE

Body Composition and Anthropometry

Elite rowers tend to be tall, muscular, and lean (159–162). Physical data accumulated for more than 4000 of our subjects since 1966 have shown that open division or heavyweight oarsmen average 192 cm in height and 87 kg in weight. Women competing in the open division averaged 180 cm in height and 76 kg in weight. Percentage body fat has steadily decreased for both men and women since earlier investigations, so that men now average about 8% to 10% body fat, whereas women average about 15% to 17% body fat. Table 54–4 summarizes changes in anthropometric measurements of men's elite eight-oared crews every 5 years between 1972 and 1997 and substantiates the trend toward taller, heavier, and leaner rowers competing in this boat class.

As discussed previously, the lightweight rowing category restricts a men's crew to no more than an average of 70 kg and a women's crew can weigh no more than an average of 57 kg. Lightweight men and women are not only lighter but are shorter (men, 178 cm; women, 172 cm) and leaner (men, 6% to 8% body fat; women, 12% to 14%). This weight-limited category of competitors, much like wrestling and boxing, presents some potentially serious problems relating to "cutting" or "making" weight. Consequently, information appears regularly in national and international rowing publications describing the short-term effects of severe dehydration and fasting and the long-term effects of these physical insults, especially concerning women and their susceptibility to "female athlete's triad."

Skeletal Muscle Qualities

Several recent studies revealed that highly trained elite rowers, both men and women, have a preponderance of slow-twitch or type I muscle fibers in the major power muscles of rowing (14,25,26,29,71,163,164). Although it is not unique for an endurance athlete to show a predominance of oxidative fibers (165,166), results of our biopsy studies were most interesting. Competitive rowing has been identified as primarily dependent on aerobic energy sources for successful efforts over 2000 m, so the appearance of a predominance of oxidative fibers was no surprise, but to discover that the most highly representative fiber type is slow twitch (SO) or type I instead of type IIA (FOG) was not expected. Because rowing is a high power–endurance activity, we hypothesized the presence of a greater proportion of the normally larger type IIA fibers in the vastus lateralis muscle of rowers. Instead, we found type I fibers of unusually large diameters as the dominant fiber type in these muscles (14,25). Mean percentages of 70% to 75% for type I fibers have been consistently observed in the vastus lateralis of rowers as opposed to controls, who normally have about 40% type I fibers. Figure 54–19 shows that

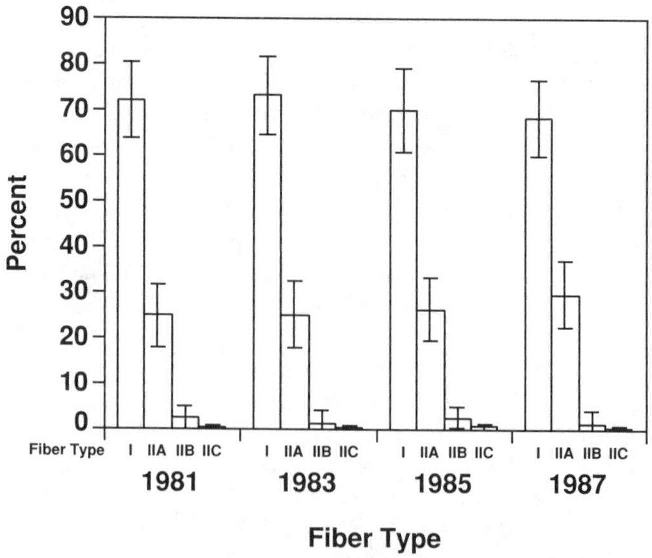

FIG. 54–19. A comparison of average proportions of major skeletal muscle fiber types in the vastus lateralis muscle of U.S. National Team oarsmen measured between 1981 and 1987. Some data represent longitudinal observations, but most are cross-sectional.

type IIA fibers have accounted for 20% to 25% of the fibers in the vastus lateralis of oarsmen, whereas fast-twitch IIB (FG) fibers are almost nonexistent. The average representation of type IIB fibers in rowers is somewhat misleading, because most elite oarsmen do not have any of these fiber types (Table 54–5). The mean value for IIB fibers was strongly influenced by a few subjects having 2% to 10% of these fibers.

Larsson and Forsberg (26) and Roth and colleagues (71) observed similar proportions of fast versus slow fibers in oarsmen's leg muscles. These groups also reported percentages of type I fibers ranging from 73% to 76% in deltoid muscles of elite oarsmen. It is noteworthy that results of serial biopsy data accumulated for 15 oarsmen over an 8-year period and for four oarsmen over a 12-year period showed consistent fiber proportion responses (see Fig. 54–19). Most of these subjects were initially sampled at age 20 or younger and, with no exception, displayed the same fiber-type proportions throughout the test periods. Despite changes in training and possible cumulative effects of training over these periods, fiber-type proportions remained stable. This is in contrast to similar studies conducted with elite cyclists who exhibited changes in fiber-type proportions with time, most of which favored an increase in oxidative fiber types (167). We are not certain what accounts for the differences in the adaptive responses between these elite athletes. However, it may be possible that rowing training simply elicits a more rapid and complete adaptive response early in an elite oarsman's exposure to training. Because most elite rowers are not exposed to their sport until age 18, it is possible that the transition from IIB to IIA fibers has been completed by the time we test them as national or Olympic team candidates. Because there is very little or no evidence to indicate that type I fibers are prone to changes, heredity may have the most significant influence on the relative presence of these fiber types in rowers.

TABLE 54–5. *A comparison of individual athlete skeletal muscle fiber–type proportions for 1987 World Champion U.S. men's crew.*

Subject	Fiber type (%)			
	I	IIA	IIB	IIC
1	67.5	32.5	0.0	0.0
2	70.1	29.2	0.0	0.7
3	55.0	43.4	1.0	0.6
4	55.9	44.1	0.0	0.0
5	80.7	19.2	0.0	0.1
6	74.6	25.4	0.0	0.0
7	73.1	26.0	0.0	0.9
8	69.8	26.6	2.1	1.5
9	81.3	17.5	0.8	0.4
10	61.1	34.0	4.9	0.0
11	64.1	35.9	0.0	0.0
12	67.9	31.6	0.5	0.0
13	55.2	32.8	10.0	2.0
14	75.1	24.1	0.0	0.8
15	74.5	24.5	0.0	1.0
$\bar{X}$	68.4	29.8	1.4	0.4
SD	8.36	7.45	2.80	0.60

Only limited biopsy sampling has been conducted with female rowers. Clarkson and co-workers (24) found the ratio of slow- to fast-twitch fibers in the vastus lateralis to be about 60:40, whereas a 55:45 ratio favoring slow-twitch fibers was reported in the biceps brachii. An earlier study reported slightly higher type I/type II ratios in these same muscles [i.e., 68:30 for the vastus lateralis and 60:40 for the biceps brachii (168)].

In one of our recent studies, type I fibers composed about 64% of all fibers in the vastus lateralis of elite male rowers, type IIA fibers were about 30%, and IIB fibers were only about 1%. The capacity to identify hybrid transitional fibers, subtypes IC, IIC, and IIAB, provided a collective representation of about 5%, with IIAB being the dominant type of this subgrouping. Type IIC representation also is shown in Table 54–5 and Fig. 54–18 and indicates only a small population of fibers among rowers. A higher proportion of IIA fibers than IIB fibers in active muscles of highly trained subjects correlates well with training intensity (169–171).

We also observed significantly greater mitochondrial size and density and increased activities of oxidative enzymes in muscles of rowers, especially type I fibers, when compared with untrained subjects and muscles of elite power lifters (25). These findings perhaps help explain the extraordinary aerobic capacities of elite rowers. Bergh and colleagues (172) showed a positive relation between high aerobic capacity and an abundance of type I fibers in muscles of elite endurance athletes. Secher (7) suggested that the absence of fast-twitch fibers in oarsmen may be due to the specificity of the exercise. He suggested that the cyclic power-recovery technique of a typical rowing stroke permits adequate time for type I fibers to generate maximal force, thus placing major contractile responsibility on these oxidative muscle fibers. Increased oxidative capacity in the muscles of oarsmen also was observed by Larsson and Forsberg (25), who reported capillary densities in trained rowers' muscles that nearly doubled those observed for the same muscles in untrained subjects (173,174).

A simple muscle-tissue spectrophotometer has been adapted to measure recovery time (T_R) for hemoglobin/myoglobin (Hb/Mb) desaturation in the capillary bed of exercising muscle (175). This technique was applied to the study of the quadriceps femoris muscle in elite male and female rowers during two separate exhaustive 2000-m rowing ergometer efforts (147). Because T_R reflects the balance of localized O_2 delivery and O_2 demand in the muscles, T_R can be interpreted as a measure of the time for mitochondrial repayment of O_2 and energy deficits accumulated during intense exercise. An analysis of T_R after submaximal and high-intensity exercise in conjunction with plasma lactate, power output, and oxygen uptake may lead to suggestions for improving performance. Magnetic resonance imaging techniques applied to muscles of highly trained rowers reflected the trained state of muscles by indicating smaller exercise-induced decreases in pH and smaller increases in ratios of free phosphate (Pi) to creatine phosphate (PCr) than those observed for untrained subjects (176,177). Elite rowers normalized their Pi/PCr ratios more rapidly after exercise than did the controls.

Both type I and type II fibers in rowers show abnormally large cross-sectional areas when compared with the same fiber types in other endurance athletes (25,26). Type I fibers are larger in diameter than are those reported for other athletes and controls (178). We measured fiber areas in excess of 8000 μm^2 for type I fibers and 11,000 μm^2 for IIA fibers in elite oarsmen. Elite oarswomen's fibers are somewhat smaller, with some type I and IIA fibers measured in excess of 7000 μm^2. Type IIB fibers in rowers are the smallest in both men and women, ranging between 5000 and 8000 μm^2.

The combination of the dominance of type I fibers and their large cross-sectional areas seem to represent both hereditary and specific adaptive responses in elite rowers. The power muscles of rowing in these athletes seem to be dominated by a "super" type I muscle fiber with little or no presence of IIB fibers, some of which have probably been previously converted to IIA fiber types.

Aging of Elite Oarsmen

We recently reported the results of a 20-year longitudinal study of members of the 1972 U.S. Men's Olympic eight-oared crew (silver medal) who were studied before the Olympic Games and again 10 and 20 years later (179). Peak power, metabolic responses, and heart rate were recorded during 6 minutes of rowing ergometry; blood lactate was measured after exercise, and anthropometric measurements, including percentage body fat, were recorded for each test session. These tests also were repeated in 1982 and 1997 and thus, with the exception of 1977, these former successful Olympic oarsmen have been studied every 5 years since their pre-Olympic testing. The average change among measurements from 1972 to 1997 was about 40% (Table 54–6). As expected, the most significant changes occurred during the first post-Olympic decade, when most subjects ceased high-intensity, long-duration training. The most significant change from 1972 to 1997 was a decrease in peak blood lactate (74%). Decreases in peak power and peak oxygen consumption were similar (30%) and averaged about a 1% decline per year. This is similar to a 1% per year decline of $\dot{V}O_2max$ after the third decade of life of normal untrained subjects (179). Percentage body fat also increased significantly over the 25-year period, with the largest increase (33%) coming during the first decade after Olympic competition. Although peak exercise heart rate declined over the 25-year period, it seemed to be affected the least (13% decline) by aging and less activity. The magnitude of decline in aerobic capacity and rapidity of diminished anaerobic capacity in these subjects cannot be explained by the aging process alone. These former elite athletes were once adapted to high-intensity, long-duration, and frequent training sessions, and when these training stimuli were eliminated, the adaptive responses began a rapid decline. Most of the aging rowers in this study continued to exercise at light to moderate levels, however; despite the significant reductions in their physiologic capacities since 1972, they still exhibited fitness levels and physical attributes far exceeding other men of similar ages.

TRAINING THE ATHLETE

The Season

The competitive or racing months in the northern hemisphere extend from mid-March to late October. College and university crews will usually race weekly from April

TABLE 54–6. *A longitudinal study of physiologic responses of the 1972 Olympic silver medal eight-oared crew*

	Age (yr)	Height (cm)	Weight (kg)	Body fat (%)	Erg time (min)	Peak power (watts)	Peak HR (beats/min)	Peak V_E (L/min)	Peak $\dot{V}O_2$ (L/min)	Peak $\dot{V}O_2$ (ml/kg/min)	Lactate (mmol/L)
1972	23.5 ± 1.49	189.4 ± 2.92	87.4 ± 6.25	12.3 ± 2.44	6:00	472 ± 30.1	190 ± 4.9	188 ± 14.9	5.72 ± 1.16	65.5 ± 5.98	14.4
1982	34.4 ± 1.19	189.4 ± 2.92	91.1 ± 12.16	16.8 ± 6.99	6:00	419 ± 28.8	182 ± 6.1	161 ± 24.0	4.69 ± 1.31	51.5 ± 9.89	11.5
1987	39.3 ± 1.28	189.4 ± 2.89	91.3 ± 11.4	15.6 ± 6.31	6:00	374 ± 27.6	176 ± 5.7	146 ± 26.3	4.42 ± 1.25	49.0 ± 8.31	8.8
1992	44.2 ± 1.32	189.2 ± 2.88	93.8 ± 10.62	15.6 ± 6.18	6:00	339 ± 24.1	175 ± 5.4	143 ± 24.9	4.39 ± 0.89	46.8 ± 7.63	7.0
1997	49.1 ± 1.36	189.3 ± 2.64	93.9 ± 10.29	16.4 ± 5.13	6:00	325 ± 23.9	165 ± 7.1	140 ± 13.1	4.25 ± 0.47	45.7 ± 6.68	3.8

to June, culminating in conference, regional, and national collegiate championship regattas in May and June. Club rowers will race in various club and open regattas also beginning in April and then complete the racing season with open national championships in July or August. Several club regattas are conducted in North America and Europe over the summer, with some racing going on as late as early November. For National and Olympic teams, regattas for elite rowers usually begin in late May and are held about one per month, culminating in either the World Rowing Championships (early September) or, in the case of an Olympic year, at various times depending on the geographic location of the Games. Countries competing at World Championships have different team-selection processes; however, the United States maintains a year-round training center for elite rowers and then accepts additional candidates for National and Olympic teams from colleges, universities, and clubs at the end of June. Periods of training for elite rowers (the names and durations of the training periods may differ among coaches and athletes), including specific months, are as follows:

Early preparation period: October through December, off-season
Late preparation period: January through March, off-season
Precompetition period: April through June, in-season
Competition period: July through September, in-season

Sport-Specific Training

There have been some scientific investigations of rowing training (17,25,82,83,100,180,181). Hagerman and Staron (25) compared off-season (OS) and in-season (IS) physiologic data for nine members of the U.S. Men's Olympic Rowing Team. No changes were noted for body composition or maximal heart rate; however, V_{Emax}, $\dot{V}O_2max$, and maximal rowing-ergometer power increased from OS to IS. Isokinetic leg strength increased at six different velocities from OS to IS, especially at the lower velocities. Based on these comparisons, it was suggested that oarsmen should attempt to maintain higher aerobic capacity during the OS so that there is less decrement to overcome as the season begins. It appears that during the OS, rowers should deemphasize resistance training at low velocities and emphasize power development at higher velocities (i.e., train more specifically for the types and velocities of movements used in the rowing technique and at speeds necessary to mimic the competitive pace). Results of the 1983 study by Hagerman and Staron (25) prompted a recent comparison of the effects of normal weight training of rowers versus no weight training during the OS on muscular strength and power, muscle fiber proportions and cross-sectional areas, ergometric power, and metabolic responses of elite male and female rowers (14). The rowers who underwent OS weight training significantly reduced their aerobic capacity and did not improve their ergometer performance; more important, the OS weight training may have detracted from IS rowing performance. Accordingly, it appears that elite rowers would benefit more from performing only simulated or actual rowing training during the OS rather than including resistance training during this period. These specific training recommendations were substantiated by not only significantly better IS competitive performance by the OS non–weight-training group, but this group also showed no differences in specific fiber types and diameters or muscular strength and power when compared with the OS weight-training–only group. It appears that task-specificity training has the greatest influence on important physiologic responses of elite rowers.

Periodization of Training and Training Intensity and Volume

Beginning in the early 1970s, international competitive rowing was dominated by Germany, first the German Democratic Republic, and more recently a unified Germany. Between 1985 and 1988, several successful elite German male rowers were studied during training with an emphasis on heart rate and lactate measurements during and after training sessions of varying intensities and durations (113). The specific training intensities were divided into four categories based on postexercise venous blood lactate responses: category I, greater than 8 mmol/L; category II, 4 to 8 mmol/L; category III, 2 to 4 mmol/L; and category IV, less than 2 mmol/L. These categories were determined as a result of careful observations of lactate responses during submaximal exercise (182–188). A lactate concentration of 8.0 mmol/L was considered by these investigators to be the transition value between exercises of moderate and high intensity, whereas a lactate level of 12 mmol/L or more represented exhaustive work. By using the four intensity categories and closely monitoring lactates of the elite oarsmen over a 3-year period, it was possible to determine not only the relative proportion of each intensity to the total amount of training but also to calculate how each training intensity related to the periodization of training (Table 54–7). Throughout the total training period, excluding competition, the use of the lower-intensity aerobic-training regimens (categories III and IV) represented more than 90% of total training time. Category IV decreased to about 74% during the competitive period, whereas category III increased to about 18% for the same period. The greater emphasis on low-intensity aerobic training for rowing is somewhat surprising because other recommendations suggested a

TABLE 54–7. *Training intensities as recommended and used by DDR Ruderverband*

	Categories [total amount of training (%)]				
Training period	IV	III	IV + III	II	I
Preparation period					
Autumn/winter	90–94	5–8	98–99	1	0–1
Winter/spring	86–88	5–9	93–95	4	1–3
Competition period	70–77	15–22	92–93	6	2

greater proportion of high-intensity training (189–194), especially during the competitive period. This training regimen proved to be very successful for crews from the German Democratic Republic.

Previous work suggested that endurance training for rowing is effective only if it is done at a blood lactate concentration between 2.5 mmol/L and 3.5 mmol/L (195–198) or 4 mmol/L (198). However, Hartmann and colleagues (113) found that athletes they observed subjectively chose steady-state training intensities at which exertion could be maintained with very little increase in lactate (category IV; see Table 54–7). It was very difficult for rowers to exercise for 45 minutes at an intensity corresponding to a lactate concentration of 3.5 mmol/L; even higher intensities were found to lead more quickly to fatigue (113). Thus it appears that training for endurance improvement in rowing at lactate levels of 4 mmol/L or higher is not advisable. It is interesting to note that a lactate concentration of 4 mmol/L has been proposed as a common reference point at which exertion begins to depend more on anaerobic metabolism to supply energy (59,187,188) and was the basis for developing the concept of *onset of blood lactate* (OBLA) as a possible break point for transition between aerobic and anaerobic energy production.

Contrary to the results of the German studies, our lactate measurements during training suggest that lactate values proposed by Hartmann and colleagues (113) may underestimate an elite rower's lactate tolerance. Based on training heart rates and lactates of U.S. rowers, we developed a training-intensity continuum that was modified from one originally proposed by Nilsen and colleagues (199,200). By using several years of observations of training heart rates and lactates and the collation of national coaches' and rowers' training diaries, we produced a more specific description and comparison of rowing training intensities (Table 54–8). The major categories of training intensities are anaerobic, transportation, anaerobic threshold, and utilization. Anaerobic training emphasizes the phosphagen and glycolytic energy systems, whereas transportation training is designed to provide a maximal stimulus to the cardiovascular and respiratory systems. The anaerobic-threshold training represents a transition stimulus between aerobic and anaerobic training, and finally, utilization training is designed to improve the transport of O_2 to skeletal muscle and its uptake by the fibers. Although not precise, the categories offer the coach and athlete a relatively easy continuum to understand and a set of exercise recipes from which to choose, and provide useful data to identify and monitor specific training sessions more

TABLE 54–8. *Training intensity continuum with physiologic and metabolic equivalents*

Training intensity	Optimal time	Max effort (%)	HR max (%)[a]	HR range[a]	Lactate range (mmol/L)	Energy systems
Anaerobic 1 (AN_1)	10–30 s	≥100	100	191±	Small amounts	ATP-PCr
Anaerobic 2 (AN_2)	30–90 s	95–100	95–100	181–190	Maximal values (10–25)	LA
Transportation (TR)	90 s–10 min	90–95	90–95	171–180	6–10	LA (most) O_2 (some)
Anaerobic threshold (AT)	10–20 min	85–90	85–90	161–170	4–6	LA-O_2 (about equal)
Utilization 1 (U_1)	10–40 min	75–85	75–85	141–160	2–4	O_2 (most) LA (some)
Utilization 2 (U_2)	30–120 min	65–75	65–75	126–140	≤2	O_2 (more than U_1) LA (less than U_1)
Utilization 3 (U_3)	30–120 min	55–65	55–65	105–125	Small amounts	O_2 (almost all) LA (little-none)

ATP-PC, energy derived primarily from adenosine triphosphate and phosphocreatine; LA, energy derived primarily from anaerobic glycolysis; O_2, energy derived primarily from oxidative sources.

[a]Based on a maximal heart rate of 190 beats/min.

accurately. As indicated in Table 54–8, a wider range of lactate responses is presented for each training intensity than that presented by Hartmann and associates (113) (see Table 54–7), with our upper limits being slightly higher. It has been one of our observations that rowers can train at relatively high exercise intensities before producing significant concentrations of blood lactate and, contrary to the observations of Hartmann and coworkers (113), rowers can tolerate lactate concentrations of 4 mmol/L for relatively long periods of continuous rowing. Most of the training by U.S. rowers takes place at intensities U_1 and U_2. As the competition period begins, a great proportion of training includes anaerobic threshold, transportation, and anaerobic 1 and 2 intensities.

A complete discussion of training for competitive rowing is beyond the scope of this chapter. Although competitive rowing efforts last only 5 to 8 minutes, the elite rower generally trains twice daily, with each training session usually lasting 60 to 120 minutes. Total training time thus seems extraordinary, considering the duration of the races. Perception of success at the international level dictates such an imbalance between training time and competition time, however, that consideration of reduction of training time for an international-caliber crew is untested and untried. An acceptable minimal/maximal limit of training duration, frequency, and intensity has evolved over the years in the sport of rowing and, with the exception of a few modifications, mostly subtle innovations, training has changed very little since the 1970s and 1980s. Because the sport of rowing requires a unique mixture of skill, aerobic and anaerobic capacity, and muscular power, each of these factors must be given special attention. The optimal extent and timing of this attention during off season and in season are difficult to assess, especially because most rowers begin training rather late (age 18 to 20 years) because of few or no opportunities to row in high school.

Although the majority of elite rowers train twice daily throughout the year, knowledgeable coaches and athletes will include strategic and needed rest days on a regular basis, resulting in an average of about 10 to 12 training sessions per week. Rowing training emphasizes improving aerobic capacity during the early and late preparation period (October through March). By using the exercise intensities in Table 54–8 as a guide, specific training recommendations can be made for periodization planning. For the early preparation period (October through December), about 75% of the training time should be devoted to utilization 2 (U_2) and 20% to utilization 1 (U_1), and by late November most North American rowers have moved indoors for ergometric rowing. The remaining 5% of training time should include at least one workout each per week for maintenance by using anaerobic threshold (AT), transportation (TR), and anaerobic 2 (AN_2). The bulk of the training time should continue to be aerobic during the late preparation period (January through March); however, the proportion of U_1 training is gradually increased and U_2 decreased so that a balance is achieved between these two intensities. AT and TR training increase slightly. April begins the precompetition period and represents an important transition period from indoor training to rowing on the water again as weather improves. Again, more than 90% of training is aerobic, but now U_1 accounts for about 60% of training time versus 40% for U_2. A gradual increase in training time for AT, TR, and AN_2 should also occur at this time by using an ever-increasing amount of interval training. The competitive season should signal a reduction of aerobic training to 80% to 85% of total training time, with most devoted to U_1 intensity. Contributions of AT, TR, and AN_2 should dramatically increase, with limited attention to AN_1. Increasing the intensity of training during this period is critical, especially during the 6 to 8 weeks before a major competition, because it is during this portion of the competitive period that the crews must become completely adapted to higher work intensities and racing paces. It is important to note that increasing training intensity too early in the training process may cause the athletes to "peak" too soon, and in many cases it can lead to overtraining syndrome, whereas not raising the intensity level at the optimal time will often cause the athletes to fall short of their competitive potentials (201). Because of the narrow window of competition at World Championships and Olympic Games, it is difficult for a crew to be at its best on the target date, and thus the athlete and coach must carefully use a mixture of science and art to meet the challenges of this small window of opportunity.

The Coaches' Development Program of the Fédération Internationale des Sociétés d'Aviron (International Federation of Rowing), Nilsen and associates (181,199,200), and Hagerman and Falkel (181) have emphasized the importance of training the aerobic metabolic system because this system provides about 70% to 80% of the total energy during a rowing race. The following recommendations were presented by these authors:

1. To improve oxygen use in the muscle, continuous long-distance training should be used at a heart rate of 130 to 160 beats/min and below the anaerobic threshold.
2. To increase oxygen delivery to the exercising muscle and build tolerance to lactate, discontinuous or interval training should be used so that the heart rate ranges between 180 and 190 beats/min and above the anaerobic threshold.

Two major objectives of training are to improve a rower's ability to compete at a greater percentage of maximal oxygen consumption without producing significant lactate accumulation and to improve the rower's ability to tolerate and clear lactate. The type of training that most effectively addresses the first objective is training at or above anaerobic threshold; interval training at high intensities with sufficient rest periods to remove most accumulated lactate improves the athlete's ability to tolerate accumulated lactate. Maximal aerobic capacity decreases quite rapidly in the elite endurance athlete who discontinues regular training; for example, inability to train for 1 week results in a significant decline in aerobic capacity (202). It is therefore very important that aerobic capacity be maintained at high levels, even during the off season.

Supplemental Training

About 1964, rowing coaches and athletes could not afford to perform supplemental weight or resistance training; today they cannot afford not to. This statement has nothing to do with economics. Instead, it has everything to do with imitative training, because it was once thought that resistance training developed tight muscles, increased unnecessary bulk, decreased flexibility, and resulted in injury. Today many rowing coaches and athletes continue an intensive weight program because other sports appear to benefit from this type of supplemental training, and no coach wants to lose the competitive or training "edge" with his or her peers. There is a fear that rowing performances will decline unless traditional weight training is performed every year, and besides, "my competitors are doing it"; thus, imitative training. As indicated in a description of our recent studies concerning supplemental weight training, the rowing exercise is an inherently weight-training exercise, and results of our studies have clearly demonstrated this phenomenon, as using traditional supplemental weight training had no beneficial effect on rowing performance. I am not suggesting eliminating all resistance training. If an athlete with significant potential enters a rowing program and exhibits considerable muscular weakness and lacks the ability to generate power, then an individually prescribed resistance-training program emphasizing the specific muscle actions involved in the rowing technique, and using light to moderate resistance and moderate to high repetitions, should be recommended. An analysis of the most successful university and college rowing programs in the United States and the U.S. National Team training programs indicates a deemphasis on supplemental weight training and its complete elimination during the competitive season. I am convinced that using extra time more productively on the water or ergometer is more valuable than results obtained from the methods of weight training used in most boat houses today.

Supplemental aerobic training for rowing, however, is both popular and beneficial. Many elite rowers will engage in distance running, cycling, swimming, and cross-country skiing during the preparation periods or off season. The nonspecific aerobic activities offer the opportunity for rowers to get away from their sport for a while yet to maintain reasonable fitness levels. Whether it be for psychological relief or injury rehabilitation, cross-training during the off season can be an important diversion and benefit.

CONCLUSION

Rowers are tall and lean athletes who train for long durations and compete at extremely high intensities. Ventilatory, metabolic, and cardiovascular responses to exercise in elite rowers are at the upper limits of human capacity, as is the power they can generate during rowing. It is rather extraordinary that aerobic metabolism contributes such a large share of the total energy for the 2000-m effort, as rowing competition is of such short duration compared with most aerobic events. Rowers possess an abundance of slow-twitch (type I) muscle fibers in the power muscles of rowing and demonstrate their extreme adaptation to exercise specificity by exhibiting very large muscle-fiber diameters. Rowers also use a racing pace that seems metabolically uneconomic and counterproductive, as the very intense initial sprint at the start of a race creates a significant O_2 deficit and possible early fatigue unparalleled when compared with other aerobic events. Rowers must tolerate a significant lactate load throughout the race and then call on their remaining aerobic and anaerobic energy resources to sprint to the finish. The physiology of rowing represents the extremes of skeletal muscle adaptations to exercise and the supporting roles of the transport systems.

ACKNOWLEDGMENTS

Our rowing studies have been supported by the United States Rowing Association, United States Olympic Committee, the New Zealand Amateur Rowing Association, Fédération Internationale des Sociétés d'Aviron (International Federation of Rowing), and the Ohio University Foundation. I am especially grateful to Randall Jablonic, Kris Korzeniowski, Harry Parker, Michael Teti, Curtis Jordan, and the other coaches of past U.S. National and Olympic teams for their encouragement and cooperation. I also thank all of those oarsmen and oarswomen who participated in our studies from 1966 to the present. We have gathered a wealth of data over the years; this would not have been possible without the extraordinary efforts and excellent science of Janice Gault, Marjorie Hagerman, Thomas Murray, and Kumika Toma, and Drs. Gary Dudley, Jeffrey Falkel, Gene Hagerman, Robert Hikida, Timothy Mickelson, William Polinski, Kerry Ragg, and Robert Staron. I also appreciate the work of the many graduate and undergraduate students from Ohio University, who over the years provided valuable assistance in our rowing studies.

REFERENCES

1. Gardner EN. *Athletics of the ancient world.* Oxford: Oxford University Press, 1965.
2. Schwanitz P. Applying biomechanics to improve rowing performance. *FISA Coach* 1991;2:1–7.
3. Secher NH. Development of results in international rowing championships, 1893-1971. *Med Sci Sports* 1973;5:195–199.
4. Pate RR, Sparling PB, Wilson GE, Cureton KJ, Miller BJ. Cardiorespiratory and metabolic responses to submaximal and maximal exercise in elite women distance runners. *Int J Sports Med* 1987;8:91–95.
5. Pollock ML. Submaximal and maximal working capacity of elite distance runners. Part I: cardiorespiratory aspects. *Ann N Y Acad Sci* 1977;301:310–322.
6. Törner W. *Biologische Grundlagen den Leiberziehung.* Bonn: Dummer, 1959:459.
7. Secher NH. The physiology of rowing. *J Sports Sci* 1983;1:23–53.
8. Secher NH. Rowing. In: Reilly T, Secher N, Snell P, Williams C, eds. *Physiology of sports.* London: E & FN Spon, 1990:259–285.
9. Hagerman FC. Applied physiology of rowing. *Sports Med* 1984; 1:303–326.
10. Körner T, Schwanitz P. *Rudern.* Berlin: Sports Verlag, 1985.
11. Steinacker JM, ed. *Rudern: Sportmedizinische und sportwissenschaftliche Aspehte.* Berlin: Springer Verlag, 1987.
12. Zsidegh M. A survey of the physiological and biomechanical investigations made into kayaking, canoeing, and rowing. *Hungarian Rev Sports Med* 1981;22:97–116.
13. Secher NH. Physiological and biomechanical aspects of rowing. *Sports Med* 1993;15:24–42.
14. Hagerman FC. Physiology and nutrition for rowing. In: Lamb DR, Knuttgen HG, Murray R, eds. *Perspectives in exercise science and sports medicine.* Vol 7. Carmel, IN: Cooper, 1994:221–302.
15. Yamakawa J, Ishiko T. Standardization of physical fitness test for oarsmen. In: Kato K, ed. *Proceedings of International Congress of Sports Sciences.* Tokyo: Japanese Union of Sports Sciences, 1966:435–436.
16. Pyke FS, Minikin BR, Woodman LR, Roberts AD, Wright TG. Isokinetic strength and maximal oxygen uptake. *Can J Appl Sports Sci* 1979;4:277–279.
17. Bloomfield J, Roberts AD. A correlation and trend analysis of strength and aerobic power and scores in the prediction of rowing performance. *Aust J Sports Med* 1972;4:25–36.
18. Kramer JF, Leger A, Morrow A. Oarside and nonoarside knee extensor strength measures and their relationship to rowing ergometer performance. *J Orthop Sports Phys Ther* 1991;14: 213–219.
19. Secher NH. Isometric rowing strength of experienced and inexperienced oarsmen. *Med Sci Sports* 1975;7:280–283.
20. Bell GJ, Petersen SR, Quinney HA, Wenger HA. The effect of velocity-specific strength training on peak torque and anaerobic rowing power. *J Sports Sci* 1989;7:205–214.
21. Hagerman FC, Staron RS, Murray TF, Hikida RS, Grant S. A comparison of the effects of traditional and non-traditional resistance training programs on rowing performance and muscle metabolism. Sports Medicine Symposium, USRA. Los Angeles, 1992.
22. Bompa TO, Roaf WA. Some characteristics of strength development for rowing. *Can J Appl Sports Sci* 1977;2:142–148.
23. Secher NH, Rube N, Elers J. Strength of two and one leg extension in man. *Acta Physiol Scand* 1988;134:333–339.
24. Clarkson PM, Graves J, Melchionda AM, Johnson J. Isokinetic strength and endurance and muscle fiber type of elite oarswomen. *Can J Appl Sports Sci* 1984;9:127–132.
25. Hagerman FC, Staron RS. Seasonal variations among physiological variables in elite rowers. *Can J Appl Sport Sci* 1983;83: 143–148.
26. Larsson L. Forsberg A. Morphological muscle characteristics in rowers. *Can J Appl Sports Sci* 1980;5:239–244.
27. Wilmore JH. Alterations in strength, body composition, and anthropometric measurements consequent to a 10-week weight training program. *Med Sci Sports* 1974;6:133–138.
28. Haymes EM, Dickinson AL. Characteristics of elite male and female ski racers. *Med Sci Sports Exerc* 1980;12:153–158.
29. Mickelson TC, Hagerman FC. Anaerobic threshold measurements of elite oarsmen. *Med Sci Sports Exerc* 1982;14:440–444.
30. Ishiko T. Application of telemetry to sports activities. In: Wartenweiler J, et al, eds. *Biomechanics I.* Basel: Karger, 1968:138–145.
31. Mason BR, Shakespear P, Doherty P. The use of biomechanical analysis in rowing to monitor the effect of training. *Excel* 1988;4:7–11.
32. Rodriquez RJ, Rodriguez RP, Cook SD, Sandbom PM. Electromyographic analysis of rowing stroke biomechanics. *J Sports Med Phys Fitness* 1990;30:103–108.
33. Celentano F, Cortili G, DiPrampero PE, Cerretelli P. Mechanical aspects of rowing. *J Appl Physiol* 1974;36:642–647.
34. Clark JM, Hagerman FC, Gelfand R. Breathing patterns during submaximal and maximal exercise in elite oarsmen. *J Appl Physiol* 1983;55:440–446.
35. DiPrampero PE, Cortilli G, Celentano F, Cerretelli P. Physiological aspects of rowing. *J Appl Physiol* 1971;31:853–857.
36. Hagerman FC. Teamwork in the hardest pull in sports. *Phys Sports Med* 1975;3:39–44.
37. Hagerman FC, Hagerman MT. A comparison of energy output and input among elite rowers. *FISA Coach* 1990;1:5–8.
38. Hagerman FC, Addington WW, Gaensler EA. A comparison of selected physiological variables among outstanding competitive oarsmen. *J Sports Med Phys Fitness* 1972;12:12–22.
39. Hagerman FC, Addington WW, Gaensler EA. Severe steady state exercise at sea level and altitude in Olympic oarsmen. *Med Sci Sports* 1975;7:275–279.
40. Hagerman FC, Gault JA, Connors MF, Hagerman GR. A summary of physiological testing at the 1974 U.S. National Rowing Camp. *Oarsman* 1975;7:34–37.
41. Hagerman FC, McKirnan MD, Pompei JA. Maximal oxygen consumption of conditioned and unconditioned oarsmen. *J Sports Med* 1975;15:43–48.
42. Hagerman FC, Connors MC, Gault JA, Hagerman GR, Polinski WJ. Energy expenditure during simulated rowing. *J Appl Physiol* 1978;45:87–93.
43. Hagerman FC, Hagerman GR, Mickelson TC. Physiological profiles of elite rowers. *Phys Sports Med* 1979;7:74–81.
44. Mahler DA, Nelson WN, Hagerman FC. Mechanical and physiological evaluation of exercise performance in elite national rowers. *JAMA* 1984;252:496–499.
45. Jackson RC, Secher NH. The metabolic cost of rowing and physiological characteristics of world class oarsmen [Abstract]. *Med Sci Sports* 1973;5:65.
46. Jackson RC, Secher NH. The aerobic demands of rowing in two Olympic rowers. *Med Sci Sports* 1976;8:168–170.
47. Nowacki PE, Krause R, Adam K. Maximal oxygen uptake by the rowing crew winning the Olympic gold medal 1968. *Pflugers Arch* 1969;312:R66–R67.
48. Nowacki PE, Krause R, Adam K, Rulieffs M. Über die cardiopulmonale leistungsfäkigkeit des Deutschland: Achters vor seinein Olympiasieg 1968. *Sportarzt Sportmed* 1971;10:227–229.

49. Nowacki PE, Adam K, Krause R, Ritter V. Die spiroergometrie in neuen untersuch-ungs-system für den spitzensport. *Trainer-Journal Rudersport* 1971;26:I–VI.
50. Saltin B, Åstrand PO. Maximal oxygen uptake in athletes. *J Appl Physiol* 1967;23:353–358.
51. Secher NH, Vaage O, Jackson RC. Rowing performance and maximal aerobic power in oarsmen. *Scand J Sports Sci* 1982; 4:9–11.
52. Henderson JY, Haggard HW. The maximum of human power and its fuel. *Am J Physiol* 1925;72:264–282.
53. Liljestrand G, Lindhard J. Zur physiologie des ruderns. *Skand Arch Physiol* 1920;39:215–235.
54. Åstrand PO, Rodahl K. *Textbook of work physiology.* 3rd ed. New York: McGraw-Hill, 1986.
55. DePauw D, Vrijens J. Untersuchungen bei Elite-Ruderern in Belgien. *Sportarzt Sportmed* 1971;22:176–179.
56. Hamby EJ, Thomas V. Comparison of rowing and cycling work capacity tests using heart rate as the parameter. *J Physiol* 1969;203:80P–81P.
57. Hay JG. Rowing: an analysis of the New Zealand Olympic selection tests. *NZ J Health Phys Ed Rec* 1968;1:83–90.
58. Ishiko T. Aerobic capacity and external criteria of performance. *Can Med Assoc* 1967;26:746–749.
59. Mader A, Hollmann W. Zur bedeutung der stoffwechselleistungsfähigkeit des eliteruderers in training and welt kampf. *Beiheft Leistungssport* 1977;9:8–62.
60. Mellerowicz H, Hansen G. Sauerstaff kapazität und andere spiroergometrische maximal werte der ruder-Olympiasieger im viser mit st. vom Berliner Ruderclub. *Sportarzt Sportmed* 1965;5: 188.
61. Niu H, Ito K, Takagi K, Ito M. A study of the development of cardio-respiratory function of the oarsmen. In: Kato K, ed. *Proceedings of International Congress of Sport Sciences.* Tokyo: Japanese Union of Sport Sciences, 1966:360–361.
62. Scharschmidt F, Pieper KS. Die aerobe leistungsfähigkeit junger rudersportler beiderlei geschlechts. *Med Sport* 1984;24:43–48.
63. Secher NH, Vaage O, Jensen K, Jackson RC. Maximal aerobic power in oarsmen. *Eur J Appl Physiol* 1983;51:155–162.
64. Steinacker JM, Marx TR, Fiegenbaum FA, Wodick RE. Die rudenspiroergometrie als eine methode der sportartspezifischen leistungsdiagnostik. *Dtsch Z Sportmed* 1983;34:333–342.
65. Strömme SB, Ingjer F, Meen HD. Assessment of maximal aerobic power in specifically trained athletes. *J Appl Physiol* 1977; 42:933–937.
66. Hagerman FC, Howie GA. Use of certain physiological variables in the selection of the 1967 New Zealand crew. *Res Q* 1971; 42:264–273.
67. Hagerman FC, Lee WD. Measurement of oxygen consumption, heart rate, and work output during rowing. *Med Sci Sports* 1971;3:155–160.
68. Carey P, Stensland M, Hartley LH. Comparison of oxygen uptake during maximal work on the treadmill and the rowing ergometer. *Med Sci Sports* 1974;6:101–103.
69. Cunningham DA, Goode PB, Critz JB. Cardiorespiratory response to exercise on a rowing and bicycle ergometer. *Med Sci Sports* 1975;7:37–43.
70. Koutedakis Y. The role of physiological assessment in team selection with special reference to rowing. *Br J Sports Med* 1982;23:51–55.
71. Roth W, Hasart E, Wolf W, Pansold B. Untersuchungen zur synamik der energiebereitstellung während maximaler mittel zeitausdauerbelastung. *Med Sport* 1983;23:107–114.
72. Steinacker JM, Marx TR, Thiel U. A rowing ergometer test with stepwise increased workloads. In: Bachl N, Prokop L, Suckert R. *Current topics in sports medicine.* München: Urban and Schwarzenberg, 1984:175–187.
73. Steinacker JM, Marx TR, Wodich RE. The oxygen consumption for rowing. *Pflugers Arch* 1984;400(suppl):1R61.
74. Steinacker JM, Marx TR, Marx U, Lormes W. Oxygen consumption and metabolic strain in rowing ergometer exercise. *Eur J Appl Physiol* 1986;55:240–247.
75. Steinacker JM, Hübner C, Berger A, Röcker A, Stauch M. Modified rowing ergometry in upper body exercise testing compared to supine bicycle ergometry in surgical patients [Abstract]. *Int J Sports Med* 1991;12:131.
76. Steinacker JM, Lormes W, Stauch M. Sport specific testing in rowing. In: Bachl N, Graham TE, Löllgen H, eds. *Advances in ergometry.* Berlin: Springer Verlag, 1991:S443–S454.
77. Williams LRT. Prediction of high-level rowing ability. *J Sports Med* 1978;18:11–17.
78. Hagerman FC, Lawrence RA, Mansfield MC. A comparison of energy expenditure during rowing and cycling ergometry. *Med Sci Sports Exerc* 1988;20:479–488.
79. Hartmann U, Mader A, Hollmann W. Querschnittuntersuchungen an leistungs-ruderern mit einem zweisterfigen test auf einem Gjessing-ruderergometer. In: Riechert H, ed. *Sportsmedizine-Kursbestimmung.* Berlin: Springer Verlag, 1987:16–22.
80. Asami T, Aduchi N, Yamamoto K, Ikuta K, Takahashi K. Biomechanical analysis of rowing skill. In: Assmussen E, Jorgensen K, eds. *Biomechanics VI-B.* Baltimore: University Park Press, 1978:109–114.
81. Hagerman FC. Metabolic responses of women rowers during ergometric rowing [Abstract]. *Med Sci Sports* 1974;6:87.
82. Hagerman FC, Korzeniowski K. Applied rowing ergometer testing. *FISA Colloque Entraineurs* 1989;19:115–133.
83. Korzeniowski K, Hagerman FC. Monitoring training of elite rowers [Abstract]. *Med Sci Sports Exerc* 1991;23:632.
84. Foster C, Green MA, Snyder AC, Thompson NN. Physiological responses during simulated competition. *Med Sci Sports Exerc* 1993;25:877–882.
85. Droghetti P, Jensen K, Nielsen TS. The total estimated metabolic cost of rowing. *FISA Coach* 1991;2:1–4.
86. Hagerman FC, Mickelson TC. A task specificity comparison of anaerobic thresholds among competitive oarsmen [Abstract]. *Med Sci Sports Exerc* 1981;13:17–20.
87. Connors MC. An energetic analysis of rowing. Unpublished doctoral dissertation. Athens, Ohio: Ohio University, 1974.
88. Hagerman FC. Energy metabolism and fuel utilization. *Med Sci Sports Exerc* 1992;24:S309–S314.
89. Polinski WJ. Indirect determination of oxygen deficit during maximal ergometric rowing. Master's thesis. Athens, Ohio: Ohio University, 1976.
90. Lormes W, Debatin HJ, Grünert-Fuchs M, Müller T, Steinacker JM, Stauch M. Anaerobic rowing tests: test design, application, and interpretation. In: Backl N, Graham TE, Löllgen H, eds. *Advances in ergometry.* Berlin: Springer, 1991:S477–S482.
91. Koutedakis Y, Sharp NCC. A modified Wingate test for measuring anaerobic work of the upper body in junior rowers. *Br J Sports Med* 1986;20:153–156.
92. Bangsbo J, Gollnick PD, Graham TE, et al. Anaerobic energy production and O_2 deficit-debt relationship during exhaustive exercise in humans. *J Physiol* 1990;422:539–559.
93. Medbö JI, Tabata I. Anaerobic energy release in working muscle during 30 s to 3 min of exhausting bicycling. *J Appl Physiol* 1993;75:1654–1660.
94. Bangsbo J, Michalski L, Petersen A. Accumulated O_2 deficit during intense exercise and muscle characteristics of elite athletes. *Int J Sports Med* 1993;14:207–213.
95. Green S, Dawson BT, Goodman C, Carey MF. Anaerobic ATP production and accumulated O_2 deficit in cyclists. *Med Sci Sports Exerc* 1996;28:315–321.
96. Medbö JI, Mohn A-C, Tabata I, Bahr R, Vaage O, Sejersted OM. Anaerobic capacity determined by maximal accumulated O_2 deficit. *J Appl Physiol* 1988;64:50–60.
97. Secher NH, Espersen M, Brinkhorst RA, Andersen PA, Rube N. Aerobic power at the onset of maximal exercise. *Scand J Sports Sci* 1982;4:12.
98. Szögy A, Cherebetiu G. Physical work capacity testing in male performance rowers with practical conclusions for their training process. *J Sports Med* 1974;14:218–223.
99. Vaage O. Table 14-2. In: Åstrand PO, Rodahl K, eds. *Textbook of work physiology.* New York: McGraw-Hill, 1986:673.
100. Hagerman FC, Falkel JE, Korzeniowski K, O'Leary K, Proctor D. Lactic acid responses of elite rowers following heavy training,

tapering, competitive and simulated rowing. *Proc Seoul Olympic Sci Congr* 1989;1:13–16.
101. Hagerman FC, Toma K, Hostler D, et al. Physiological responses of 1997 men's national rowing team. Sports Medicine Symposium USRA, Hartford, 1997:3–6.
102. Haber P, Ferlitsch A. Vergleichende einschätzung des trainingszustandes mittels spiroergometrischer untersuchungen am ruder-und fahrradergometer bei ruderern. *Schweiz Z Sportsmed* 1979;27:53–59.
103. Rasmussen J, Hanel B, Diamant B, Secher NH. Muscle mass effect on arterial desaturation after maximal exercise. *Med Sci Sports Exerc* 1991;23:1349–1352.
104. Secher NH, Ruberg-Larsen N, Brinkhorst RA, Bonde-Peterson F. Maximum oxygen uptake during arm cranking and combined arm plus leg exercise. *J Appl Physiol* 1974;36:515–518.
105. Juel C. Lactate-proton cotransport in skeletal muscle. *Physiol Rev* 1997;77:321–358.
106. Parkhouse WS, McKenzie DC, Hochachka PW, Ovalle WK. Buffering capacity of deproteinized human vastus lateralis muscle. *J Appl Physiol* 1985;58:14–17.
107. Brien DM, McKenzie DC. The effect of induced alkalosis and acidosis on plasma lactate and work output in elite oarsmen. *Eur J Appl Physiol* 1989;58:797–802.
108. Steinacker JM, Marx U, Grünert M, Lormes W, Wodick E. Vergleichsuntersuchungen über den zweistufentest und den mehrstufentest bei der ruderergometrie. *Leistungssport* 1985;6:47–51.
109. Vanheel B, De Hemptinne A. Facilitated diffusion of L-lactate and pyruvate across red and white skeletal muscle cell membranes of the mouse [Abstract]. *Arch Int Physiol Biochim* 1986;94:72.
110. Juel C, Honig A, Pilegaard H. Muscle lactate transport studied in sarcolemmal giant vesicles: dependence on fibre type and age. *Acta Physiol Scand* 1991;143:361–365.
111. Pilegaard H, Bangsbo J, Richter EA, Juel C. Lactate transport studied in sarcolemmal giant vesicles from human muscle biopsies: relation to training status. *J Appl Physiol* 1994;77:1858–1862.
112. Pilegaard H, Juel C. Lactate transport studied in sarcolemmal giant vesicles from rat skeletal muscle: effect of denervation. *Am J Physiol* 1995;269:E679–E682.
113. Hartmann U, Mader A, Hollmann W. Heart rate and lactate during endurance training programs in rowing and its relation to the duration of exercise by top flight rowers. *FISA Coach* 1990;1:1–4.
114. Koutedakis Y, Sharp NCC. Lactic acid removal and heart rate frequencies during recovery after strenuous rowing exercise. *Br J Sports Med* 1985;19:199–202.
115. Grujic N. The long-term follow up of the physical working capacity of rowers. In: Karvonen MJ, ed. *The physiological follow up methods of sports training.* Helsinki: Varala, 1989:20–37.
116. Margaria R, Cerretelli P, DiPrampero PE, Massari PE, Torelli G. Kinetics and mechanisms of oxygen debt contraction in men. *J Appl Physiol* 1963;18:371–377.
117. Margaria R, Cerretelli P, Mangili F. Balance and kinetics of anaerobic energy release during strenuous exercise in man. *J Appl Physiol* 1964;19:623–628.
118. McMahon TA. Rowing: a similarity analysis. *Science* 1971; 173:349–351.
119. Sanderson B, Martindale W. Towards optimizing rowing technique. *Med Sci Sports Exerc* 1986;18:454–468.
120. Secher NH, Vaage O. Rowing performance: a mathematical model based on body dimensions as exemplified by body weight. *Eur J Appl Physiol* 1983;52:88–93.
121. Ekblom B, Hermansen L. Cardiac output in athletes. *J Appl Physiol* 1968;25:619–625.
122. Gollnick PD, Hermansen L. Biochemical adaptations to exercise: anaerobic metabolism. In: Wilmore J, ed. *Exercise and sport sciences reviews.* New York: Academic Press, 1973:1–43.
123. Hansen G. Vergleichende untersuchungen über dem verhältnis der aeroben zur anaeroben kapazität bei maximaler ergometrischen belstung. *Schweiz Z Sportsmed* 1967;15:68–75.
124. Lundin A, Saltin B. Oxygen demands of swimming. II Medico-Scientific Conference of FINA. Dublin, Ireland, 1971.
125. Hagerman FC, Falkel JE, Murray TF, Korzeniowski K, O'Leary L, Proctor D. A comparison of maximal absolute and relative metabolic responses between elite men and women rowers [Abstract]. *Med Sci Sports Exerc* 1987;19:549.
126. Fukunaga T, Matsuo A, Yamamoto K, Asami T. Mechanical efficiency in rowing. *Eur J Appl Physiol* 1986;55:471–475.
127. Harrison JY. A constant torque-brake for use in bicycle and other ergometers. *J Appl Physiol* 1967;23:482–483.
128. Harrison JY. Maximizing human power output by suitable selection of motion cycle and load. *Hum Factors* 1970;12:315–329.
129. Hahn AG, Tumilty D, Sheakespear P, Telford RD. Physiological testing of oarswomen on Gjessing and Concept II rowing ergometers. *Excel* 1988;5:19–25.
130. Tumility D, Hahn A, Telford R. Effect of test protocol: ergometer type and state of training on peak oxygen uptake in rowers. *Excel* 1987;3:12–14.
131. Brooks GA. Anaerobic threshold: review of the concept and directions for future research. *Med Sci Sports Exerc* 1985; 17:22–31.
132. Davis JA, Vodak P, Wilmore JH, Vodak J, Kurtz P. Anaerobic threshold and maximal aerobic power for three modes of exercise. *J Appl Physiol* 1976;41:544–550.
133. Wasserman K, McIlroy MB. Detecting the threshold of anaerobic metabolism in cardiac patients during exercise. *Am J Cardiol* 1964;14:844–852.
134. Wasserman K, Whipp BJ, Casaburi R, Golden M, Beaver WL. Anaerobic threshold and respiratory gas exhange during exercise. *J Appl Physiol* 1973;35:236–243.
135. Mahler DA, Andresen DC, Parker HW, Mitchell WS, Hagerman FC. Physiological comparison of rowing performance between national and collegiate women rowers [Abstract]. *Med Sci Sports Exerc* 1983;15:157.
136. Droghetti P. Determination of the anaerobic threshold on a rowing ergometer by the relationship between work output and the heart rate. *Scand J Sports Sci* 1986;8:59—62.
137. Droghetti P, Borsetto C, Casoni I, et al. Noninvasive determination of the anaerobic threshold in canoeing, cross-country skiing, cycling, roller- and ice-skating, rowing, and walking. *Eur J Appl Physiol* 1985;53:299–303.
138. Orfeldt L. Metabolism of 1(+)-lactate in human skeletal muscle during exercise. *Acta Physiol Scand* 1970;338:1–66.
139. Spitzer JJ. Effect of lactate infusion of canine myocardial free fatty acid metabolism *in vivo*. *Am J Physiol* 1974;226:213–217.
140. Biersteker MWA, Biersteker PA. Vital capacity in trained and untrained healthy young adults in the Netherlands. *Eur J Appl Physiol* 1985;54:46–53.
141. Biersteker MWA, Biersteker PA, Schreurs AJM. Reduction of lung elasticity due to training and expiratory flow limitation during exercise in competitive female rowers. *Int J Sports Med* 1986;7:73–79.
142. Mahler DA, Shuhart CR, Brew E, Stukel TA. Ventilatory responses and entrainment of breathing during rowing. *Med Sci Sports Exerc* 1991;23:186–192.
143. Mahler DA, Andrea BE, Andresen DC. Comparison of six-minute "all-out" and incremental exercise tests in elite oarsmen. *Med Sci Sports Exerc* 1984;16:567–571.
144. Szal SE, Schoene RB. Ventilatory response to rowing and cycling in elite oarsmen. *J Appl Physiol* 1989;67:264–269.
145. Steinacker JM, Both M, Whipp BJ. Pulmonary mechanics and the entrainment of respiratory and stroke frequencies during rowing [Abstract]. *Med Sci Sports Exerc* 1992;24:S165.
146. Clifford PS, Hanel B, Secher NH. Arterial blood gases during exhaustive exercise. *Med Sci Sports Exerc* 1990;22:S99.
147. Chance B, Dait MT, Zhang C, Hamaoka T, Hagerman FC. Recovery from exercise-induced desaturation in the quadriceps muscles of elite competitive rowers. *Am J Physiol* 1992; 262:C766–C775.
148. Fraser TR. The effect on the circulation as shown by examina-

tion with the sphygmograph. *J Anat Physiol* 1868-1869;3:127–130.
149. Williams LRT. Work output and heart rate response of top level New Zealand oarsmen. *Res Q* 1976;47:506–512.
150. Rosiello RA, Mahler DA, Ward JL. Cardiovascular responses to rowing. *Med Sci Sports Exerc* 1987;19:239–245.
151. Saltin B. Physiological effects of physical conditioning. *Med Sci Sports* 1969;1:50–59.
152. Seals DR, Hagberg JM, Spina RJ, Rogers MA, Schechtman KB, Ehsani AA. Enhanced left ventricular performance in endurance trained older men. *Circulation* 1994;89:198–205.
153. Pelliccia A, Maron BJ, Spataro A, Proschan M, Spirito P. Cardiac hypertrophy in highly trained athletes. *N Engl J Med* 1991; 324:295–301.
154. Chignon JC, Distel R. Vector cardiographic criteria of ventricular hypertrophy in a population of athletes. *Arch Mal Coeur* 1981; 74:1099–1105.
155. Dickhuth HH, Simon G, Kindermann W, Wildenberg A, Keul J. Echocardiographic studies on athletes of various sports types and non-athletic persons. *Z Kardiol* 1979;68:449–453.
156. Jensen K, Secher NH, Fiskestrand Ä, Christensen NJ, Lund JO. Influence of body weight on physiologic variables measured during maximal dynamic exercise [Abstract]. *Acta Physiol Scand* 1986;121:39A.
157. Weiling W, Borghols EA, Hollander AP, Darner SA, Dunning AJ. Echocardiographic dimensions and maximal oxygen uptake in oarsmen during training. *Br Heart J* 1981;46:190–195.
158. Howald H, Marie R, Heierli B, Follath F. Echokardiographische befunde bei trainierten sportlern. *Schweiz Med Wochenshr* 1977;107:1662–1666.
159. deGaray AL, Levine L, Carter JEL. *Genetic and anthropological studies of Olympic athletes.* New York: Academic Press, 1974.
160. DeRose EH, Crawford SM, Kerr DA, Ward R, Ross WD. Physique characteristics of Pan American Games lightweight rowers. *Int J Sports Med* 1989;10:292–297.
161. Hebbellinck M, Ross WD, Carter JEL, Boems J. Anthropometric characteristics of female Olympic rowers. *Can J Appl Sports Sci* 1980;5:255–262.
162. Khosla T. Sports for tall. *Br Med J* 1983;287:736–738.
163. Bonde-Peterson F, Gollnick PD, Hansen TI, Kristensen N, Secher NH, Secher O. Glycogen depletion pattern in human muscle fiber during work under curarization (*d*-tubocurarine). In: Howald H, Poortmans JR, eds. *Metabolic adaptation to prolonged physical exercise.* Basel: Birkhauser Verlag, 1975:422–430.
164. Secher NH, Rube N, Molbech S. The voluntary muscle contraction pattern in man. In: DePotter, ed. *Adapted physical activities.* Bruxelles: Editions de L'Université de Bruxelles, 1981:225–236.
165. Costill DL, Fink WJ, Pollock M. Muscle fiber composition and enzyme activities of elite distance runners. *Med Sci Sports* 1976;8:96–100.
166. Saltin B, Henriksson J, Nygaard E, Anderson P, Jansson E. Fiber types and metabolic potentials of skeletal muscle in sedentary man and endurance runners. *Ann N Y Acad Sci* 1977;302:3–29.
167. Coyle EF, Sidossis LS, Horowitz JF, Beltz JD. Cycling efficiency is related to the percentage of type I muscle fibers. *Med Sci Sports Exerc* 1992;24:782–788.
168. Pohlentz H. *Physiological evaluation of rowers in the German Democratic Republic.* Rome, Italy: Abstract at FISA Coach's Conference, 1980;4:5–8.
169. Staron RS, Malicky ES, Leonardi MJ, Falkel JE, Hagerman FC, Dudley GA. Muscle hypertrophy and fast fiber type conversions in heavy resistance-trained women. *Eur J Appl Physiol* 1989; 60:71–79.
170. Staron RS, Leonardi MJ, Karapondo DL, et al. Strength and skeletal muscle adaptations in heavy-resistance-trained women after detraining and retraining. *J Appl Physiol* 1991;70:631–640.
171. Staron R, Walsh S, Hikida R, Hagerman F, Gilders R, Murray T. Muscular adaptations in elderly men following a 16-week high-intensity resistance training program. *Med Sci Sports Exerc* 1996;28:S115.
172. Bergh U, Thorstensson A, Sjodin B, Hulten B, Riehl K, Karlsson J. Maximal oxygen uptake and muscle fiber types in trained and untrained humans. *Med Sci Sports* 1975;7:37–43.
173. Anderson P. Capillary density in skeletal muscle of man. *Acta Physiol Scand* 1975;95:203–205.
174. Ingjer F. Effects of endurance training on muscle fibre ATPase activity, capillary supply and mitochondrial content in man. *J Physiol* 1979;294:419–432.
175. Chance B, Nioka S, Kent J, et al. Time-resolved spectroscopy of hemoglobin and myoglobin in resting and ischemic muscle. *Anal Biochem* 1988;174:698–707.
176. Fountain MR, McCully RR. A new approach to exercise testing and training evaluation. *Am Rowing* 1988;20:42–43.
177. McCully KK, Boden BP, Tuchler M, Fountain MR, Chance B. Wrist flexor muscles of elite rowers measured with magnetic resonance spectroscopy. *J Appl Physiol* 1989;67:926–932.
178. Prince RP, Hikida RS, Hagerman FC. Human muscle fiber types in power lifters, distance runners, and untrained subjects. *Pflugers Arch* 1976;363:19–26.
179. Hagerman FC, Fielding RA, Fiatarone MA, et al. A 20-year longitudinal study of Olympic oarsmen. *Med Sci Sports Exerc* 1996;28:1150–1156.
180. Grujic N, Bajic M, Vukovic B, Jakovijevic D. Energy demand of competitive rowing [Abstract]. Seventh Balkan Congress of Sports Medicine 1987;112.
181. Hagerman FC, Falkel JE. Training the energy systems. *Am Rowing* 1987;18:40–43.
182. Hartmann U. *Querschnittuntersuchungen an leistungsruderern in Flackland and längschnittuntersuchungen an elite-rudern in der höhe mittels eines zwistufigen tests auf einem Gjessing-ruderergometer.* Konstanz: Hartung-Gorre Verlag, 1987.
183. Heck H, Hess G, Mader A. Vergleichende untersuchungen zu verschiedenen lakat-schwellenkonzepten. *Dtsch Z Sportmed* 1985;36:1–2.
184. Heck H, Mader A, Hess G, Muecke S, Muller R, Hollmann W. Justification of the 4 mmol/L lactate threshold. *J Sports Med* 1985;6:117.
185. Hollmann W, Hettinger T. *Sportmedizin-arbeits-und Trainingsgrundlagen.* Stuttgart: Schattauer, 1980.
186. Jacobs I, Sjoedin B, Kaiser P, Karlsson J. Onset of blood lactate exercise accumulation after prolonged exercise. *Acta Physiol Scand* 1981;114:461.
187. Mader A, Heck H. A theory of the metabolic origin of "anaerobic threshold." *Int J Sports Med* 1986;7:45.
188. Mader A, Liesen H, Heck H, Phillipe H, Schuerch PM, Hollmann W. Zur beurteilung der sportartspezifischen ausdauerleistungsfaehigkeit im Tabor. *Sportarzt Sportmed* 1976;27:80, 109.
189. Fritsch W. Zur entwicklung der speziellen ausdauer in rudern. In: *Information zun training: rudern.* Frankfort: DSB, Bundesausschuss teistung sport, 1981:S26.
190. Fritsch W. Trainingssteuerung im rudern. *Rudersport* 1985; 35:80.
191. Fritsch W. Die letzten wochen vor dem finale. *Rudersport* 1986; 36:82.
192. Marx U, Steinacker JM. Ruderspiroergometrische längsschnittuntersuchungen über 2 jahre bei zwei weltmeisterschaftsteilnehmern. In: Steinacker JM, ed. *Rudern.* Berlin: Springer-Verlag, 1988:83–89.
193. Nolte V. Trainingssteuerung-Woraussetzungen, Anwendung, Grenzen. *Leistungssport* 1986;16:39.
194. Nolte V. Trainingsprotokollierung-Fuer wen? Und wie? Welche konsequenzen werden daraus gezogen? In: Steinacker JM, ed. *Rudern.* Berlin: Springer-Verlag, 1988:218–222.
195. Lormes W, Michalsky RJW, Gruenert-Fuchs M, Steinacker JM. Belastung und beanspruchungsempfinden in rudern. In: Steinacker JM, ed. *Rudern.* Berlin: Springer-Verlag, 1988:332–336.
196. Steinacker JM. Methoden für die leistungsdiagnostik und trainingssteuerung im rudern und ihre anwendung. In: Steinacker JM, ed. *Rudern.* Berlin: Springer Verlag, 1988:39–54.
197. Urhausen A, Mueller M, Foerester HJ, Weiler B, Kindermann W. Trainingssteuerung im rudern. *Dtsch Z Sportmed* 1986; 37:340.

198. Hirsch L. Trainingsformen zur Verbesserung der aeroben Kapazitaet. In: *Information zum training: ausdauertraining, staffwechselgrundlegen und steuerungsansatze.* Frankfurt: DSB, Bunderausschuss Leistungssport, 1977 (Suppl 9).
199. Nilsen T, Daigneault T, Smith M, eds. *The FISA coaching development programme course.* Sui: Level 1 Handbook Oberhoffen, 1987.
200. Nilsen T, Daigneault T, Smith M, eds. *The FISA coaching development programme course, Level 2.* Sui: Handbook Oberhoffen, 1987.
201. Hagerman FC. Failing to adapt to training. *FISA Coach* 1992;3:1–4.
202. Costill DL, Fink WJ, Hargreaves M, King DS, Thomas R, Fielding R. Metabolic characteristics of skeletal muscle during detraining from competitive swimming. *Med Sci Sports Exerc* 1985;17:339–343.

Exercise and Sport Science,
edited by William E. Garrett, Jr., and Donald T. Kirkendall.
Lippincott Williams & Wilkins, Philadelphia © 2000.

CHAPTER 55

Physiology of Soccer

Donald T. Kirkendall

The organized participation in the sport of soccer probably dwarfs that of the other sports discussed in this section. It is estimated that there are more than 60 million registered soccer players worldwide, with another 60 million unregistered players. Depending on the political climate of the world, the Federation International de Football (FIFA) has equal or more member nations than does the United Nations. It was estimated that more than 2 billion people watched the 1998 World Cup final match. Given this kind of exposure and participation, it is indeed remarkable to find that investigations into the science of soccer lag far behind those of many other sports.

All sports involve the interaction of sport-specific fitness, technique (skill), and tactics (strategy). It is beyond the scope of this chapter to discuss the latter two aspects. Therefore physiologic aspects as they relate to the required fitness to play soccer are discussed. Because of the limited nature of the literature, the chapter focuses mostly on the male elite/professional players.

THE SPORT

Soccer is a game that involves two teams of 11 players each: 10 outfield players and one goalkeeper. At the most basic level, the division of positions is defenders, midfielders, and forwards (strikers). Depending of the playing system, the number of players at each line can be nearly any combination of arrangements to total 10 players. The size of the field is routinely up to 105 m long and 68 m wide. The game is nominally two 45-minute halves with a 15-minute pause. Field and ball size, as well as game length, are reduced for younger players. Smaller-sided teams, shorter games, and smaller fields are frequently contested in special settings like tournaments for younger age players or for lesser competitive settings (e.g., "masters" leagues). No time-outs are allowed, the clock is stopped only at the referee's discretion (e.g., injuries in which a player needs to be removed from the field), and substitution rules vary by league from very lenient (free substitution) to highly restrictive (maximum of two outfield players and one goalkeeper with no reentry).

Physical Requirements

The time limits of the adult game (90 minutes) and the lack of time-outs suggest that the game is one of constant running with no stoppages of play. Studies of soccer suggest that the ball is "in play" for only about 60 minutes of the full 90 minutes, however. The "lost" time is due to the ball's being out of bounds, injuries, fouls, and so on. This in-play time also is affected by environmental conditions like heat, humidity, and altitude. In one game played at altitude in hot conditions during the 1986 World Cup in Mexico, the ball was in play for only 45 minutes. Reductions in high-intensity running, especially in the second half, are routinely seen when temperatures are above 30°C.

It is tempting to describe soccer as a monumental physical effort. However, the total distance covered averages about 10 km in 90 minutes, which is 6.6 km/h (4 mph), and many people can cover the same distance in that duration by walking. The physical demands of the game have been described by using time–motion analysis with either real-time paper–pencil note taking, audio or video recording, or computer-aided data reduction. Most of the work has been confined to professional male players in Europe and Japan, but there are data on the South American game as well. The professional player typically covers around 10 km during the course of a game (1,2). The South American player covers around 10% to 15% less (3). The intensities, first described in

D. T. Kirkendall: Department of Orthopaedics, University of North Carolina, Chapel Hill, North Carolina 27599-7055.

1976 by Reilly and Thomas (4), are usually listed as walking (25% of the total distance), jogging (37%), sprinting (11%), backing (6%), and cruising ("running with manifest purpose and effort," 20%). These percentages seem to have been fairly consistent over the years since the original description. Each sprint is between 10 and 40 m, accumulating about 800 to 1000 m. There are about 850 to 1000 distinct activities, which corresponds to about one change in direction or intensity about every 5 to 6 seconds (5,6). A player sprints about once every 90 seconds and works at the higher intensities of sprinting/cruising about once every 30 seconds (5). About two thirds of the distance in a game is covered at a walk or a jog (1,2,4). More than half the total distance is covered in the first half (1,2,6–8). It is the rare player who covers more distance in the second half. The intermittent nature of the game argues against the use of constant-speed running as an appropriate training stimulus when one is trying to obtain sport-specific fitness during a competitive season. Therefore the time–motion data support the use of the ball in an intermittent pattern of running, consistent with the competitive game.

The pattern of possession is also of interest when describing the game. It has been determined that about 40% of all possessions of the ball begin and end without a completed pass and that 90% of all possessions are of three completed passes or fewer (9,10). Not all possessions lead to a shooting opportunity, and shooting opportunities sometimes depend on where possession of the ball was obtained. Unpublished observations from the 1996 U.S. Women's Olympic champion team showed that if the ball was obtained in the offensive third of the field, the play usually involves two players and one pass. If possession is obtained in the defensive third of the field, however, four or five players and four or five passes are involved. Despite the methodical build-up and the attractiveness of long possessions, more than three fourths of the shots and goals in soccer are a result of a quick, controlled strike once possession has been obtained (11).

Averaged out over many games, a team will have possession of the ball about 240 times during a game, with 180 possessions per goal scored (12). Part of the art of coaching is the attempt to improve those odds. These patterns of movement and possession seem to be independent of level of play. The volume and intensity of activity seem to decrease as the level of play and commitment decrease. Players tackle about 15 to 20 times per game with 10 to 15 heading opportunities per game. There is a fairly constant ratio of 10 shots per goal scored (4,8). The most intense aspect of the game involves dribbling the ball. It is estimated that the increase in energy expenditure while dribbling is about 15% (13). Thus, to increase the intensity of soccer-specific training, coaches will frequently modify games to increase the number of opportunities to dribble.

It can be concluded that soccer is a game of intermittent activity containing high- and low-intensity activities with a very low level of success (goals) per possession. Professional players typically cover 10 km per game at a higher intensity than those at lower divisions of the game.

Physiologic Requirements

The physiologic responses to play reflect the physical demands of the game. The nature of the game makes direct recording of anything but heart rate problematic.

Aerobic Requirement

Heart rate has been measured during game conditions on numerous occasions in both male and female soccer players. Typically, heart rate is consistently greater than 150 beats/min, with rates above 85% of maximum for up to two thirds of the game (1,2,14). Given the nature of the game, this corresponds to an aerobic requirement of more than 80% of $\dot{V}O_2$max (15,16). This demand seems to hold regardless of the professional division (highest to lowest) or gender. Rectal temperature also is related to $\dot{V}O_2$max and can be easily taken during half-time and at the end of a game to estimate aerobic demand. Core temperature of 39°C to 40°C are the norm. Should the ambient temperature be high (20°C to 22°C or more), rectal temperatures of 40°C are not unexpected (16). Whereas intermittent exercise can give a higher temperature because of the high anaerobic yield, it is safe to say that this method confirms the heart rate estimate of around 80% of $\dot{V}O_2$max.

Anaerobic Requirement

The anaerobic requirement is harder to estimate. The most common marker of anaerobic demand is the use of blood lactate measurements. The higher level and intensity of play should result in higher lactate responses, especially in the first half (Table 55–1, ref. 15). Lactate results should be interpreted with caution, considering the timing of the sampling in relation to the last high-intensity bout of activity during the game.

TABLE 55–1. *Blood lactate levels by half and by professional division*

	1st half (mmol/L)	2nd half (mmol/L)
Division I	9.5	7.0
Division II	8.0	6.0
Division III	5.5	4.5
Division IV	4.5	4.0

Data estimated from Fig. 2 of ref. 15, with permission.

Although the levels depicted are fairly impressive, they are probably an underestimate of the actual anaerobic contribution. The chapter on intermittent exercise (Chapter 5) contains a more detailed description of the energetics.

Fuel Requirements

Because soccer has both high- and low-intensity aspects, a fuel mixture of fats and carbohydrates should be expected. Muscle glycogen use has been reported in only a limited number of players, but three trends are clear: First, the pregame levels are lower than the levels reported in other trained athletes; second, there is significant glycogen depletion in the first half; and third, players finish the game nearly devoid of muscle glycogen. About 67% of the total muscle glycogen is depleted in the first half, with a total of 85% or more depleted by game's end (17). This is further evidence of the anaerobic demand of the game. It is probably reasonable to assume that the low intensities of walking and jogging are powered by a fuel mixture higher in fat.

Blood glucose levels increase in response to hepatic liberation of its stores. It is known that glucose ingestion increases performance in intermittent exercise. In fact, when it was ingested over multiple games, teams ingesting a glucose syrup scored more and conceded fewer goals. Ingestion of a glucose polymer before a game and during half-time resulted in greater distance covered at the high intensities during the second half (18). In either case, such acute support of blood glucose should be beneficial.

Dehydration

Most of the published data on soccer come from northern Europe, so it is not surprising that little on dehydration from soccer has been reported. From 1 to 2.5 kg of water loss is typical in temperate climates, with 4 to 5 kg reported in challenging conditions in Africa (19). Performance must be impaired in such instances. Perhaps the excessive heat and humidity at so many of the sites during the 1994 World Cup in the United States will spark some interest in this topic.

Other Aspects

Serum enzymes like creatine kinase (CK), a marker of muscle damage, are difficult to document in soccer because the time delay to peak CK response is masked by successive practices and the frequency of games. Players typically have higher than clinically normal levels (because of repetitive exercise) and can expect about a threefold increase as a result of controlled practice, with no differences to type of surface (natural grass or artificial turf) (20). Unpublished observations of muscle strength (isokinetically) before and after soccer indicate no decrements; however, it should be intuitive that local muscle endurance is affected by game play and the resulting fatigue.

THE ATHLETE

The wide participation in soccer indicates that the game is within the reach of an enormous fraction of the population. Specific genetic gifts, necessary for some activities (e.g., stature for basketball, mass for American football, high slow-twitch muscle fiber population for purely endurance events) seem to be of minor importance in soccer. The data presented below reinforce this concept because few characteristics would be considered exceptional.

Stature and Mass

Table 55–2 lists some results, by year, of stature and mass for elite soccer players (5). The data indicate that the soccer player is of rather ordinary size. What one might notice is the trend toward the taller, heavier, and leaner player. Percentage-of-fat measurements typically average 8% to 12%, with the goalkeeper carrying the most fat (21). Size does not appear to be a good predictor of success (first team vs. reserve), as only about 25% of the information necessary to predict success is due to size, with an added 10% due to body density (21). Yet there will always be the "old-timer" who can predict soccer success by various aspects of size (foot size, "bow" legs, quadriceps size and shape).

Aerobic Power

The high demands of the game do not result in high $\dot{V}O_2$max of soccer players. Table 55–2 also lists aerobic power by year. The $\dot{V}O_2$max of 55 to 65 mL/kg/min seems to be the expected range, which is far below the 70s and 80s of world-class runners, cross-country skiers, and cyclists. Level of play and the resulting differences in training emphasis also are reflected in $\dot{V}O_2$max, with

TABLE 55–2. *Size and aerobic power of soccer players by year*

Year	Height (cm)	Weight (kg)	%Fat	$\dot{V}O_2$ (ml/kg/min)
1973	174.6	69.4	12.4	57.8
1975	176.3	71.3	14.9	62.0
1976	176.3	75.7	9.6	56.1
1978	178.3	72.3	9.4	61.8
1984	177.3	74.5	10.0	57.4
1991	180.4	75.0	10.0	62.0

Data are summarized from various studies and do not reflect individual players or teams.

TABLE 55–3. *Aerobic power by level of play*

National team	63.0
Professional	69.2
Elite youth	68.8
2nd division	52.1
Regional amateur	50.0
Youth	48.4

Values expressed as ml/kg/min.
Data from ref. 45.

amateur players being far below their more elite counterparts (Table 55–3). Whereas the levels necessary for soccer are rather moderate in the athletic range of values, they are, nonetheless, high when considering the population as a whole. There are few published data to suggest that improving $\dot{V}O_2max$ or anaerobic threshold will improve game running performance. Furthermore, there are only scant data to suggest that improving endurance will result in better on-field results like goals for/goals against, points per game (3 for a win, 1 for a tie, 0 for a loss) (22–24). There are just too many variables (e.g., surface, environment, opponents, and own "style") in the game to make such a claim at this point. But, intuitively, the greater the endurance, the more work performed, the more goal-scoring opportunities and eventually goals, especially in the second half. From eastern Europe, data suggest that the final ranking of teams after a competitive season was similar to the $\dot{V}O_2max$ of the team, with the league champions having the highest average aerobic power (22).

Players are notorious for their disdain for "the lab" and would prefer to have their fitness measured "on the field." A popular method of determining endurance fitness is the 12-minute run. Professionals and other elite players routinely average nearly 2 miles in 12 minutes and probably should be able to maintain a 6:00/mile pace as evidence of adequate endurance fitness to play the professional or collegiate game (21). Other field methods can be designed around the demands of the game and involve running a circuit mimicking running patterns described earlier. Such circuits usually use the whole field, may or may not involve the ball, and take 10 to 15 minutes to complete (1,2,16). Repeated testing can confirm training adequacy or appropriate fitness to return to play after an injury.

Recently the 20-m shuttle runs, popularized by the Canadians for mass screening of fitness, have been modified for games, soccer included. An intermittent test has been widely used in this country and Europe. The test (1) involves running back and forth on a 20-m course, paced by an audiotape. After each run is a 10-second pause. The speed increases until the player is unable to keep up with the pace. Results for this task across age groups are listed in Table 55–4. Although no single field

TABLE 55–4. *Average performance on field tests of fitness by gender and level of play*

Player level	Speed[a] (m/s)	Vert jump[b] (cm)	Illinois agility (s)	300-meter shuttle (s)	Yo-Yo intermittent recovery test (m)
Females					
U12	5.64	40.26		76.26	528
U13	5.59	40.84	18.71	78.36	530
U14	5.97	42.82	19.11	75.64	586
U15	5.82	44.89	17.79	73.88	756
U16	6.07	45.54	18.62	75.81	624
U17	6.13	49.56	18.59	74.08	634
U18	5.97	43.05	19.22	75.17	634
U20 national	7.21	52.39	16.44	64.65	1554
Males					
U13	5.89	47.24	17.59	75.25	644
U14	6.65	53.80	17.52	73.25	907
U15	6.24	61.00	17.86	68.56	868
U16	7.03	65.20	16.38	66.22	982
U16 national	7.55	61.00	15.06	63.46	1420
U17 national	7.78	65.28	15.00	61.28	485[c]
U20 national	8.77	66.34	14.78	62.94	644[c]
U23 national	9.54	70.36	15.30	64.40	720[c]

Data from the youth teams based on an average of 15 players per team. The youth teams train about 2 times per week and play two to three games per week. Data from national teams were from training camps at various times of their training cycle. Most national teams had 25 or more players at the time of testing.

[a]Based on a 40-yard (36.58 m) dash. All tests on national team players were with a running start.

[b]One-step approach.

[c]Level 2 of test; all others are level 1.

test has been "adopted" by the soccer community, these shuttle tests are becoming more and more widely used.

Anaerobic Power

There are a variety of tests to estimate anaerobic power. The alactacid component can be estimated by the standard vertical jump. Between 50 and 65 cm are values recorded for collegiate, professional, and national team players (5; see Table 55–4). The Margaria–Kalamen stair-climbing test has been used for various aged American national team members with results of 170 to 180 kgm/s recorded (5). According to published norms, these values are average for their age group. A timed reciprocal jumping task (to estimate lactacid capacity) resulted in values of 21 to 23 W/kg in American professional and collegiate players (25), which was consistent for other volleyball, basketball, and physical education students. A 300-m shuttle run (see Table 55–4) is another option for testing a player's lactacid capacity. By using a cycle-ergometer sprint test (lacking the use of elastic recoil seen in repetitive jumping tests), power outputs of 13 to 14 W/kg (+10% of untrained controls) have been determined. Treadmill sprints to exhaustion (26) result in lactates greater than 14 mmol/L, which is not different from those in other endurance athletes or untrained controls.

These results suggest that the soccer player possesses some ability to buffer the lactate produced, but their buffering capacity is not exceptional when compared with athletes who compete in very-high-intensity events like the 400-m sprint. Their alactacid capacity also is consistent with that of other athletes.

Strength

There are so many different ways to measure strength (grip strength, maximal voluntary contraction, isokinetically, eccentrically), and no method has been performed enough to draw a clear picture of the soccer player. Of the limited data available, goalkeepers and defenders seem to possess greater quadriceps strength, and soccer players overall possess a greater hamstring/quadriceps ratio (isokinetically) than do controls (5,27–30). Team physicians expect that a torque/mass ratio at 30 to 60 degree/s (in ft lbs/lb) should exceed 1.0 for adequate protection against knee injuries, and soccer players satisfy this criterion. Other measures of balance between and within legs are within clinically normal limits. High-velocity torque production seems to correlate with kick velocity and distance (27,28).

Flexibility

Soccer players tend to be less flexible than other athletic counterparts (29). Whether this is due to training or other factors is open for discussion. Screening for hip, low-back, and hamstring flexibility (Wells sit-and-reach) shows results of 25 to 35 cm (5). What was demonstrated is that a prophylactic program that included flexibility training reduced the injury incidence (29).

Agility

The "controlled ability to change position and direction rapidly and accurately" would seem to be a characteristic needed to play soccer or any team sport. Whereas there are numerous agility tests available, few data have been reported. In small samples, soccer players routinely score in the 99th percentile (Illinois Agility Run; 21). It should be noted that the norms are not based on athletic populations, and numerous other athletes, especially team sport athletes, should also score as well. Table 55–4 lists results for the Illinois Agility Run across a range of ages and abilities.

The 20-yard Pro Agility Drill has been used across age groups, without much discrimination between ages and levels of play. The Illinois Agility Run, a longer run, has been substituted, and some trends are more evident. Players of national caliber are extremely agile, and this may be a feature that distinguishes soccer players from other athletes. It is likely that most team-sport athletes (e.g., basketball, lacrosse, football) would score equally well.

Fiber Composition

Considering the demands of the game, a predominance of one fiber type over the other would not be required. The game demands both endurance and high power output. Thus the reporting of fiber compositions of 45% to 60% (30,31) fast twitch should not be surprising.

Glycogen Repletion

One of the unique aspects of the game involves the scheduling of practices and games coupled with the nutritional requirements for adequate glycogen levels. The manipulation of training and diet around the schedule of games is important so that a player enters a glycogen-depleting game with as great a reserve of glycogen as possible to delay fatigue further into the second half (32). As already mentioned, soccer players do not show the levels of glycogen usually seen in other top-class athletes (17). Is this the result of their training or of poor nutrition? About two thirds of their glycogen is depleted by half-time, and most of the remaining is used in the second half (17). As expected, the distance run in the first half is greater and more intense than that in the second half (2,4,6,8,15,18), and scoring is reflected in this, with a gradual increase in the number of goals scored as the game progresses (6). Dietary repletion over the hours and days after has been shown to be inadequate, with low carbohydrate intake (less than 50%, about 250 to 300 g/24 h) (30) far below the 500 to 600 g/24 h usually suggested (33). The diet of the player results in low pregame muscle glycogen. When pregame glycogen levels were manipulated, those with low glycogen ran less and walked more than those with "normal" glycogen levels (7). The timing of food intake also is critical. Players should try to eat about 50 or more grams of carbohydrate in the first 2 hours after play because glycogen repletion occurs at the fastest rate when carbohydrates are consumed immediately after exercise (34). Then chose high-carbohydrate foods over the rest of the 24-hour period, trying to reach the 500- to 600-g/24 h recommendation. Done routinely, this should improve the level of muscle glycogen to a level more consistent with that of other athletes.

Injuries

A more detailed treatment of soccer injuries can be found in other reviews (e.g., 29,35). Any survey of the literature will show that injury incidence is the main academic topic in soccer. It should be rather obvious that the primary site of injuries in soccer is the leg. Contusions and abrasions are the most frequent of injuries. Muscle strains (quads, adductors, hamstrings), ligamentous sprains (lateral ankle, knee collaterals, and cruciates), and broken bones (tibia, fibula) follow the more common injuries. Concussions are rare and usually result from collisions with other players or goal posts (36). In a study of elite collegiate players over a two-season period, the incidence of concussions was about one per team per year (37). If a male player keeps playing competitively for 10 years, the odds are about 50:50 that he will have one concussion. The odds for women are about 25:75 (36). Obviously, the goalkeeper has more hand, wrist, and finger injuries than do outfield players. Severe traumatic injuries are rare.

TRAINING THE ATHLETE

The Season

The competitive season varies according to age, level of play, climate, country, and continent. Youth leagues (players younger than 12 years) in the United States typically have a fall and a spring season and play about 10 games each season. These games are usually shorter and may be divided into quarters rather than halves, on smaller fields, with an age-appropriate sized ball. Coeducational teams at this age are common. In some leagues, the number of players may be reduced to as few as five (four plus a goalkeeper) on each team. School-aged players (12 to 18 years) also have a fall and spring season. Their school may sponsor a team, however, so the player could compete on the school team in one season and the club team in the other season. Although it is not a nationwide trend, the school season for high-school age boys is the fall and for girls is the spring. The number of games varies considerably, but 15 to 20 full-sided games is not unusual. The length of a game may be 80 to 90 minutes. In college, the length of the season is dictated by the governing body of the school. The National Collegiate Athletic Association (NCAA) dictates the starting date (usually the middle of August) and the maximum number of games (20, not including conference or national championship tournaments). Professional leagues have their league season plus "cup" tournaments that are contested throughout the season. In Europe, the season begins in the fall and lasts into late spring, with a winter break. Over a full year, a professional soccer player can play more than 60 games. In South America, the season is around 10 months long, and a club could be scheduled for 80 games. Players for each club are rotated so that no one player competes in all scheduled games.

Sport-Specific Training

Optimal preparation of the competitive soccer player is very challenging because the player must be technically advanced, tactically sound, and of sufficient fitness to carry out the skills and strategies of the game.

Philosophies of training vary with the tradition, history, and playing style of each country. There are also varied training seasons depending on the climate of the county. Professional soccer leagues in northern Europe tend to take a winter break between the fall and spring sessions, whereas Brazil, for example, has a continuous 10- to 10.5-month season. In the United States, the professional season begins in March and lasts until October, whereas collegiate soccer is a very compact season, beginning in August and concluding in late November or early December. Training schedules will reflect the local competitive season.

Training is a manipulation of the work volume and intensity as well as an emphasis on technique. This is dealt with in detail in the chapter on periodization (Chapter 34) and the chapter on weight training (Chapter 39). In brief, during preparation for a season, the volume of work is high and intensity is low. This is gradually reversed throughout training until competition, when the volume and intensity are decreased, and sport-specific aspects (situations like corner kicks, throw-ins, other restarts) are stressed.

The American model taught in the coaching schools focuses on the economic use of time by combining training emphasis. Each training activity should require some combination of fitness, technique, and tactics. For example, a technical game might be six versus six, and each controlling touch (trap) should be with the weak foot. A tactical game might emphasize wing play by requiring the ball to pass through some gate (by passing or dribbling) near either sideline in the offensive third of the field before shooting. A fitness game might require that each player sprint 10 m in any direction after passing the ball. Economic training might combine two restrictions into one activity: all traps with the weak foot, and emphasize wing play.

There is some debate over the best training methods. In Europe, much of the training time is spent with the ball. In South America, many teams have a physical trainer who will oversee distance running and interval training, and ball work is directed toward technical and tactical refinements. Teams from both continents have been successful internationally, so the debate will continue.

Bangsbo (38,39) breaks training into anaerobic, aerobic, strength, and flexibility training. These factors are broken down further (Fig. 55–1). Recovery training is 40% to 80% of maximal heart rate, low-intensity training is 65% to 90% of maximal heart rate, and high-intensity training is 80% to 100% of maximal heart rate.

A training example is offered to illustrate the use of these training intensities and how a game can be organized to work all three intensities. Place 2 full-size goals about 30 m on either side of the center line, facing away from each other. Divide the players into equal teams of six to eight players. For recovery training, there are no restrictions, but just free play. For low-intensity training, limit midfield play to three passes. This will force players to run harder to get open to receive a pass and move to the other end of the field quickly. For high-intensity training, play the game to 6 points. If one team gets a score with all their players on the open side of the goal before the other opponents get all their players on the open side of the goal, 2 points are awarded.

Bangsbo (38,39) divides anaerobic training into speed training and speed endurance training (see Fig. 55–1). To improve speed, training schemes should be of maximal intensity for 2 to 10 seconds, with a rest period of around 5 times the work duration (e.g., 5 seconds of work and 25 seconds of rest). These work/rest bouts should number two to 10 repetitions. For speed endurance training, there are two phases: production (near-maximal work for short durations) and maintenance

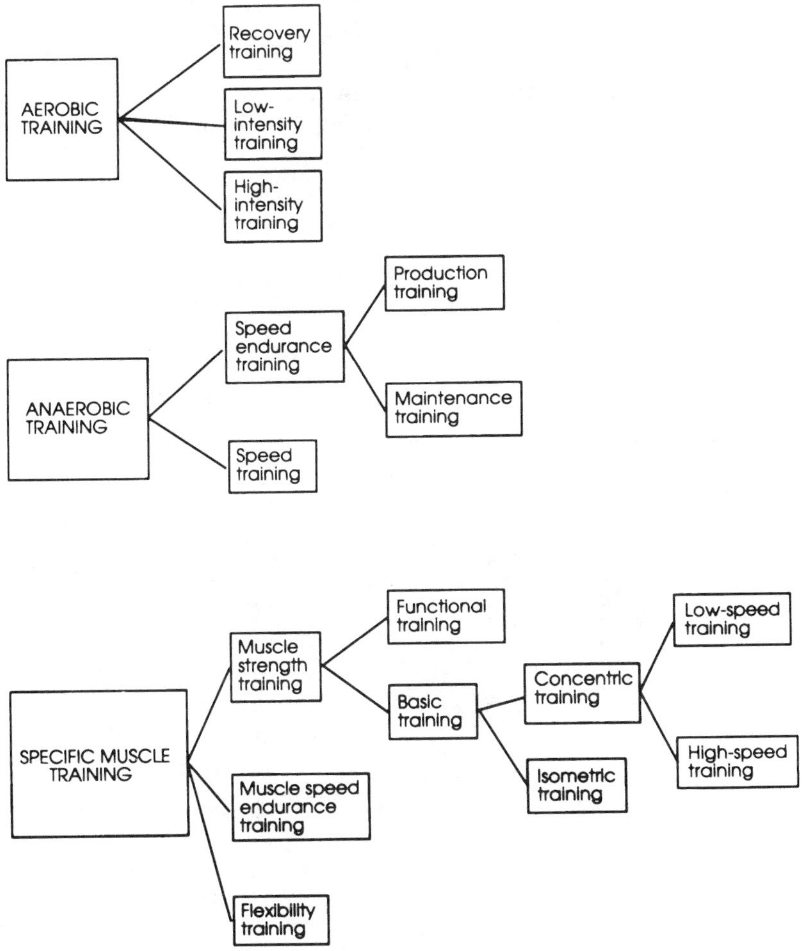

FIG. 55–1. Components in fitness training in soccer. From ref. 38, with permission.

(near-maximal work for longer periods). During production training, the exercise duration should be 20 to 40 seconds, at near-maximal intensity, with a rest period that is greater than 5 times the length of the work period. Two to 10 repetitions are sufficient. For maintenance training, the work duration might be 30 to 90 seconds with less recovery and a slightly lower intensity. Again, 2 to 10 repetitions are appropriate.

The following is an example: Play in one fourth of a full field. Use cones to set up six randomly placed goals in the area. Two teams of five, using man-to-man marking, play with one ball. The goal is to pass the ball through the cones to a teammate for a point. Very rapid, ballistic, well-timed movements are necessary to get away from the marking opponent. The game can be played for 1 to 2 minutes with 30-second rest periods. Another example is to put two players off to the side of the field about 40 m from the goal. The coach passes the ball toward the goal, and both give chase. The first player to the ball is on offense, and the other defends. The offensive player is encouraged to dribble directly at the goal and the goalkeeper. This forces both players to play at high speed to either score or defend. The activity lasts only a few seconds, and with three or four groups of two, should get sufficient recovery.

The question about training frequency for youth players is often asked. There are no definitive guidelines, but the more competitive the league and the older the player, the more frequent the training session (2). The recreational league player will practice probably once per week and may hold true regardless of age. As the youth player gets older and participates in more select or competitive leagues (e.g., middle-school age), training sessions may increase to two or three per week. Only the most competitive settings (high school and college-age teams and players) train daily. It must be remembered that age is a poor criterion for determining training sessions, as there can be drastic differences in physical maturation during puberty.

Supplemental Training

The use of weight training has gained much attention. Traditionally, weight training was not a part of soccer training because it was thought that the hypertrophy would hinder skill development and execution. However, many people are realizing that weight training is a valuable adjunct to training so as to limit injuries (1,2). In soccer, the current trend is toward a generalized program that addresses all major muscle groups. A more complete discussion of weight training is found in Chapter 39 of this volume.

Of interest is whether weight training has any effect on soccer skills (27,28,40–42). Cabri and colleagues (28) showed that a supplemental weight-training program had little affect on kicking distance, and Poulmedis (27) failed to find any improvement in shooting velocity with weight training. Thus, although weight training is very valuable at limiting some injuries, it has little influence on skill performance.

The earlier data of Ekstrand (29) showed the specific areas in which soccer players were deficient in flexibility and made definite recommendations. Special emphasis should be directed to the hamstrings and adductor groups; areas that have been linked to risk of muscle-strain injury. The peculiar "athletic pubalgia" frequently seen in soccer players is related to the adductor muscle group and sports medicine physicians think increased flexibility may be prophylactic for this injury. The lack of flexibility about the ankle has been noted in Scandinavian (29), English (8), and Japanese (43) players and may be an adaptive response improving ankle stability (38).

Periodization of Training

The seasonal planning of a program has not been discussed in much detail. Early work by Thomas and Reilly

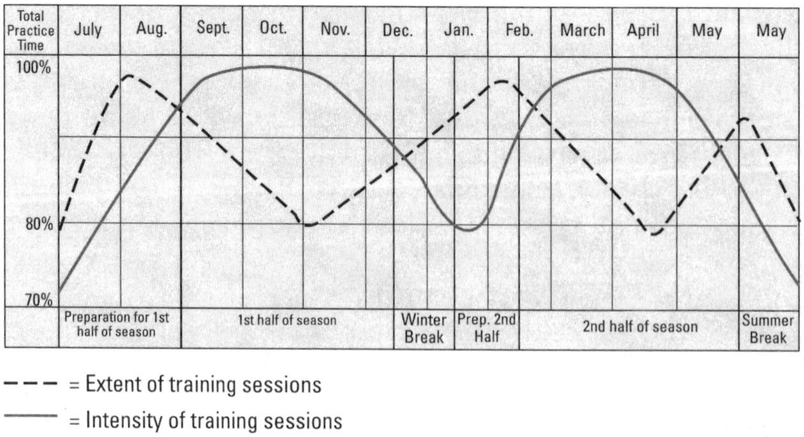

FIG. 55–2. Overview of a training calendar. From ref. 2, with permission.

TABLE 55–5. *Priority of fitness training through a year*

	Off-season				Season							
Aerobic training												
Low-intensity	3344	4445	5555	4433	4343	4343	4343	4343	4343	4343	4343	4343
High-intensity	2223	3234	4445	4555	5545	5545	5545	5545	5545	5545	5545	5444
Anaerobic training												
Speed endurance	1111	1111	2234	4555	4353	4353	4353	4353	4353	4353	4353	3453
Speed	1111	1111	2234	4555	5555	5555	5555	5555	5555	5555	5555	5554
Muscle strength training												
Basic	3334	5555	5543	2222	2222	2222	2222	2222	2222	2222	2222	2222
Functional	2222	3333	3344	4343	4343	4343	4343	4343	4343	4343	4343	4322
Muscle speed training	1111	1112	3333	3333	3333	3333	3333	3333	3333	3333	3333	3333
Flexibility training	3232	3434	4444	4444	4444	4444	4444	4444	4444	4444	4444	4444

Each single number represents a week. For practical purposes, each month is given 4 weeks. The values represent the following priorities: 1, very low priority; 2, low priority; 3, moderate priority; 4, high priority; 5, very high priority.

(44) demonstrated that most fitness is developed in the first third of the season and then maintained throughout the rest of the season. The Dutch model illustrates the interaction of volume and intensity (Fig. 55–2) as well as the relation of general to soccer-specific training over the professional season. The Scandinavian model (Table 55–5) shows the emphasis placed on each of the components in the off-season and in-season. In South America, the season is so long that there is little "off-season" training. Therefore, they go through a brief period of general running under the direction of the physical trainer and then go to the field and soccer-specific training. Typically, the South American player will reach maintenance levels around one third of the way into the season (T. Barros, 1997), like their European counterpart. In each case, the goal is to develop fitness to a high level and maintain that fitness throughout the entire season.

Many coaching books focus on training games, but the development of training from off-season to preseason through the competitive season is not well discussed.

CONCLUSION

When comparing soccer players with the general public, their physiologic profile is above the norm. When comparing soccer players with the athletic population, their profile is basically average. No one characteristic stands out from the other or from other sports. Agility has been shown to be exceptional, but until more data on an athletic population are reported, there is no way to tell if this is indeed exceptional. This means that the game is accessible to a large variety of people, not discriminating against people of average abilities. Part of the joy of the game is having the fitness necessary to perform the difficult and sometimes artistic skills in rapidly changing tactical situations.

ACKNOWLEDGMENTS

Data presented in this chapter were collected with the support of a grant from Nike, Inc.

REFERENCES

1. Bangsbo J. *Fitness training in football: a scientific approach.* Bagsvaerd, Denmark: HO+Storm, 1994.
2. Verheijen R. *Conditioning for soccer.* Spring City, PA: Reedswain, 1998.
3. Barros TL, Valquer M, Santa'Anna M, Barbosa AR. Motion patterns of Brazilian professional soccer players. *Med Sci Sport Exerc* 1998;30(suppl 5):S31.
4. Reilly T, Thomas VR. Time motion analysis of work rate in different positional roles in professional football. *J Hum Mov Stud* 1976;2:87–97.
5. Kirkendall DT. The applied sports science of soccer. *Phys Sportsmed* 1985;13:53–59.
6. Reilly T. Motion analysis and physiological demands. In: Reilly T, ed. *Science and soccer.* New York: E & FN Spon, 1994:65–81.
7. Saltin B. Metabolic fundamental of exercise. *Med Sci Sports Exerc* 1973;5:137–146.
8. Reilly T. *What research tells the coach about soccer.* Reston, VA: American Alliance for Health, Physical Education, Recreation and Dance, 1979.
9. Reep C, Benjamin B. Skill and chance in association football. *J R Stat Soc (A)* 1968;131:581–585.
10. Bate R. Football chance: tactics and strategy. In: Reilly T, Lees A, Davids K, Murphy WJ, eds. *Science and football.* New York: E & FN Spon, 1988:293–301.
11. Olsen E. An analysis of goal scoring strategies in the world championships in Mexico, 1986. In: Reilly T, Lees A, Davids K, Murphy WJ, eds. *Science and football.* New York: E & FN Spon, 1988: 373–376.
12. Lanham N. Figures do not cease to exist because they are not counted. In: Reilly T, Clarys J, Stibbe A, eds. *Science and football II.* New York: E & FN Spon, 1993:180–185.
13. Reilly T, Ball D. The net physiological cost of dribbling a soccer ball. *Res Q Exerc Sport* 1984;55:267–271.
14. Kirkendall DT, Marchak PM, Lohnes J, Garrett WE. Heart rate responses to training and competition in women soccer players. IOC Conference on Sports Medicine, Atlanta, Georgia, 1996.
15. Ekblom B, ed. The applied physiology of soccer. *Sports Med* 1986;3:50–60.
16. Ekblom B. *Football (soccer).* London: Blackwell Scientific, 1994.
17. Agnevik G. *Football. Indroftsfysiologi: Rapport Nr 7.* Stockholm: Trugg-Hansa, 1970.

18. Kirkendall DT, Foster C, Dean JA, Grogan J, Thompson NN. Effect of glucose polymer supplementation on performance in soccer. In: Reilly T, Lees A, Davids K, Murphy WJ, eds. *Science and football.* New York: E & FN Spon, 1988:33–41.
19. Mustafa KY, Mahmoud EDA. Evaporative water loss in African soccer players. *J Sports Med Phys Fitness* 1979;19:181–183.
20. Kirkendall DT, Kasa M. Serum creatine kinase responses to physical activity on natural and artificial surfaces. In: Reilly T, Lees A, Davids K, Murphy WJ, eds. *Science and football.* New York: E & FN Spon, 1988.
21. Raven PB, Gettman LR, Pollack ML. A physiological evaluation of professional soccer players. *Br J Sports Med* 1976;100:209–216.
22. Apor P. Successful formula for fitness training. In: Reilly T, Lees A, Davids K, Murphy WJ, eds. *Science and football.* New York: E & FN Spon, 1988:95–107.
23. Wisloff U, Helgerud J, Hoff J. Strength and endurance of elite soccer players. *Med Sci Sport Exerc* 1998;30:462–467.
24. Nowaki PE, Cai DY, Buhl C, Krummelbein U. Biological performance of German soccer players (professional and juniors) tested by special ergometry and treadmill methods. In: Reilly T, Lees A, Davids K, Murphy WJ, eds. *Science and football.* New York: E & FN Spon, 1988:145–157.
25. Kirkendall DT, Street GM. Mechanical jumping power in athletes. *Br J Sports Med* 1986;20:163–164.
26. Holmyard DJ, Cheetham ME, Lakomy LKA, Williams C. Effect of recovery duration on performance during multiple treadmill sprints. In: Reilly T, Lees A, Davids K, Murphy WJ, eds. *Science and football.* New York: E & FN Spon, 1988:134–144.
27. Poulmedis P. Isokinetic maximal torque power of Greek elite soccer players. *J Orthop Sports Phys Ther* 1985;5:293–295.
28. Cabri J, DeProft E, Dufour W, Clarys JP. The relation between muscular strength and kick performance. In: Reilly T, Lees A, Davids K, Murphy WJ, eds. *Science and football.* New York: E & FN Spon, 1988:186–193.
29. Ekstrand J. *Soccer injuries and their prevention.* Linkoping, Sweden: Linkoping University, 1982.
29. Torgari H, Ohasi J, Ohgushi T. Isokinetic muscle strength of soccer players. In: Reilly T, Lees A, Davids K, Murphy WJ, eds. *Science and football.* New York: E & FN Spon, 1988:181–185.
30. Jacobs I, Westlin N, Karlsson J, Rasmusson M, Houghton B. Muscle glycogen and diet in elite soccer players. *Eur J Appl Physiol* 1982;48:297–302.
31. Ingemann-Hansen T, Halkjaer-Kristensen J. Force-velocity relationships in the human quadriceps muscles. *Scand J Rehabil Med* 1979;11:85–89.
32. Kirkendall DT. Nutrition and performance in soccer. *Med Sci Sports Exerc* 1993;25:1370–1374.
33. Sherman WM, Costill DL. The marathon: dietary manipulation to optimize performance. *Am J Sports Med* 1984;12:44–51.
34. Ivy JL, Katz AL, Cutler CL, Sherman WM, Coyle EF. Muscle glycogen synthesis after exercise: effect of time of carbohydrate ingestion. *J Appl Physiol* 1988;64:1480–1485.
35. Garrett WE Jr, Kirkendall DT, Contiguglia RS, eds. *The US soccer book of sports medicine.* Media, PA: Williams & Wilkins, 1996.
36. Barnes BC, Cooper L, Kirkendall DT, et al. Concussion history in elite male and female soccer players. *Am J Sports Med* 1998;26:433–438.
37. Boden B, Kirkendall DT, Garrett WE. Concussion incidence in elite college soccer players. *Am J Sports Med* 1998;26:238–241.
38. Bangsbo J. Physiology of training. In: Reilly T, ed. *Science and soccer.* London: E & FN Spon, 1996:51–64.
39. Bangsbo J. Physical conditioning. In: Ekblom B, ed. *Football (soccer).* Cambridge, MA: Blackwell Scientific, 1994:124–139.
40. Taiana F, Grehainge JF, Cometti G. Influence of maximal strength training of lower limbs of soccer players on their physical and kick performance. In: Reilly T, Clarys J, Stibbe A. *Science and football II.* New York: E & FN Spon, 1993:98–103.
41. Trolle M, Aagaard P, Simonsen EB, Bangsbo J, Klausen K. Effects of strength training on kicking performance in soccer. In: Reilly T, Clarys J, Stibbe A. *Science and football II.* New York: E & FN Spon, 1993:95–97.
42. Mognon P, Narici MC, Sirtori MD, Lorenzelli F. Isokinetic torques and kicking maximal velocity in young soccer players. *J Sports Med Phys Fitness* 1994;34:357–361.
43. Haltori K, Ohta S. Ankle joint flexibility in college soccer players. *J Hum Ergol* 1986;15:85–89.
44. Thomas V, Reilly T. Fitness assessment of English league soccer players through the competitive season. *Br J Sports Med* 1979;13:103–109.
45. Nowacki PE, Cai DY, Bihl C, Krummelbein U. Biological performance of German soccer players (professional and juniors) tested by special ergometry and treadmill methods. In: Reilly T, Lees A, Davidsk, Murphy WJ, eds. *Science and Football.* New York: E & FN Spon, 1988: 145–157.

Exercise and Sport Science,
edited by William E. Garrett, Jr., and Donald T. Kirkendall.
Lippincott Williams & Wilkins, Philadelphia © 2000.

CHAPTER 56

Physiology of Speed Skating

Carl Foster, Jos J. deKoning, Kenneth W. Rundell, and Ann C. Snyder

THE SPORT

Physical Requirements

Speed skating is a group of related competitive events contested on either specialized ice skates or on specialized roller skates. The nucleus event is long-track (or metric-style) ice speed skating. This is the traditionally popular event contested in the Olympic Winter Games and associated with widely recognizable athletic personalities such as Eric Heiden, Dan Jansen, and Bonnie Blair. In long-track speed skating each athlete races against the clock in seeded pairs over a variety of distances ranging from 500 to 10,000 m (5000 m for women). During these events, the goal is to reach the finish in minimal time. Accordingly, the competitors are pacing themselves for best possible performance without immediate concern for the tactics of their pair. The races are contested on tracks of 400-m length. There are special rules regarding crossing over from inner track to outer track, so that each athlete skates exactly the required distance. Olympic events, except for the 500 m beginning in 1998, are contested as a single run. The 500 m is an average of two runs. In world all-around championship competition, each athlete compiles four events over a 3-day period (men: 500 m, 1500 m, 5000 m, 10,000 m; women: 500 m, 1500 m, 3000 m, 5000 m) with a score (Samalog) for each event arrived at by dividing the time required to complete the event by the number of 500-m segments in the event; the skater with the smallest combined score is the champion. There are separate world sprint championships (2 × 500 m + 2 × 1000 m), world single distance championships, and World Cup competitions. Because of the historical importance of the world all-around championships, as well as the substantial importance of skating technique to performance, skating performance is less event specialized than many other energy demand sports (running, cycling, skiing). The world's best 1500-m skater may also be in the top 10 in the world in the 500 m and the 10,000 m. Probably less than 10% of elite speed skaters are truly sprint specialists or distance specialists. World records at the beginning of the 1997–1998 competitive season are shown in Table 56–1.

In developmental competition, pack-style events similar to cycle races are relatively common. During these events, time is relatively unimportant since finish order determines the competitive result. As a result there is considerable use of drafting and tactical maneuvering with the intent of disrupting the race plan of one's competitors. These races may range from as short as 200 m to quite long distances (≥42 km). In the Netherlands, which is not only the point of origin of modern speed skating but also the country where speed skating is most

TABLE 56–1. *World records in speed skating at the beginning of the 1997–1998 season*

Distance (m)	Men	Women
500	35.39	37.90
1,000	1:10.42	1:15.43
1,500	1:49.07	1:57.63
3,000	3:53.06[a]	4:09.32
5,000	6:34.96	7:03.26
10,000	13:30.55	14:22.00[a]

[a]Not contested in Olympic or world championship competition.

C. Foster: Department of Exercise and Sport Science, University of Wisconsin–LaCrosse, LaCrosse, Wisconsin 54601.
J. J. deKoning: Faculty of Human Movement Sciences, Vrije Universiteit, Amsterdam, The Netherlands.
K. W. Rundell: Sport Science and Technology Division, U.S. Olympic Committee, Lake Placid, NY 12946.
A. C. Snyder: Department of Human Kinetics, University of Wisconsin–Milwaukee, Milwaukee, Wisconsin 53201.

popular, there is a unique pack-style skating event, the Elfstedentocht, or 11-cities tour. This event, which in some respects is the most important speed skating event in the world, is conducted only in years when weather conditions in the northeast of the Netherlands allow for natural ice on the canals connecting the 11 cities. The race is ~200 km is length and is conducted pack style. Beyond the approximately 200 serious competitors, there is a tour that admits only 10,000 starters. It is estimated that 13 million of the 15 million people in the Netherlands watch the event either live on or television.

There is also Olympic competition in short-track ice speed skating. The venue for this competition is inside an Olympic-size hockey rink, with a track length of 109 m. In Olympic competition, individual events are conducted pack style in the 500 and 1000 m and in relays of 3000 m (women) and 5000 m (men). There are typically a series of elimination races designed to reduce the final race to six competitors, or four teams for the relays. In world championship competition, individual events include 500, 1000, 1500, 3000 (women), and 5000 (men) m. World championship competition usually involves some sort of cumulative point value representing placings in both elimination and final events, with the world champion being the skater with the most points. As with pack-style long-track speed skating events, drafting and tactical maneuvering are very important during short-track races. Short-track speed skating is usually more popular with the nonskating public since the competition is head to head and there are frequent spectacular crashes. In national-level competitions, there is often a 1000-m time trial, similar to metric-style events, designed to serve as a first level of elimination. Because of the necessity of competing in heats and finals and in multiple events, a short-track speed skater may compete in 10 or more races during a given day of competition, versus a maximum of two during long-track speed skating.

In recent years competitive events on in-line roller skates have become quite popular. Although not contested in Olympic competition, in-line races are contested at the Pan American Games and in world championship competition. Races may be contested either on a track (with distances as short as 300 m) or on the road (with distances as long as 100 km). Road races, often in the general range of 10 km, are quite popular even with recreational-level competitors. In terms of tactics and overall "feel," these races are very similar to cycling competitions of approximately the same length, with drafting, tactical maneuvering, and team tactics being very important. Still important at the developmental level are races held indoors in roller skating rinks. These races are generally quite short, usually contested as a certain number of laps. Since the size of indoor roller rinks is poorly standardized, a 10-lap race may vary from 1000 to 1800 m. For the most part, in-line races are very similar to pack-style long-track ice speed skating events.

Ice speed skating events are traditionally contested during the winter months. This means that unique problems with cold weather are important to both training and competition. Since the mid-1980s a number of indoor 400-m ovals have been developed around the world, which have lengthened the training year (often to 365 days) and, more important, have allowed for more stable conditions during competition. Although there are rules regarding how often the ice is resurfaced during competition, changing weather conditions during the course of a competition could often drastically change ice conditions and, accordingly, the competitive result. This was a problem as recently as the 1992 Olympic Winter Games in Albertville where unexpectedly warm conditions and sunlight on a portion of the track created generally unfavorable, and widely varying, conditions for the competitors. Given the number of enclosed ovals in the world, it seems unlikely that many major competitions will be contested outdoors in the future. Since pack-style races are contested "head to head," unfavorable weather conditions are unlikely to immediately affect the competitive result. Accordingly, these events will remain important with developmental skaters and for the longer-distance events. Major in-line roller skating events are usually contested during the warmer months of the year, or during the winter months in warm climates. Day-to-day and moment-to-moment weather conditions can vary greatly. Since the competition is head to head, however, the effect on competitive result is not large.

Physiologic Requirements

The physiologic requirements of a given speed skating race are primarily influenced by the length of the race and by the type of competition (against the clock versus pack style). Although direct measures of physiologic responses during speed skating competitions have been made only infrequently, there are enough data from a variety of sources and from laboratory simulations to construct a fairly reasonable estimate of the physiology of competition, at least during solo competition such as that which takes place during Olympic long-track events. Other data obtained during pack-style skating competitions, cycling races, laboratory simulations, and fundamental studies of interval training allow for a reasonable reconstruction of physiologic responses during pack-style competition.

$\dot{V}O_2$

$\dot{V}O_2$ increases rapidly at the beginning of an event, probably achieving the skating specific $\dot{V}O_2$max during races longer than 1000 m. Since only the longest event for men (10,000 m) takes much more than 7 minutes, it is probable that the skating-specific $\dot{V}O_2$max is reached and sustained during the majority of events. It should be pointed out that $\dot{V}O_2$max during skating is only about 85% to 90% of that achieved during cycling or running, however. This is probably attributable both to a somewhat smaller active muscle mass during skating and to restriction of muscle blood flow during skating. The lower the skating position, the greater the reduction in $\dot{V}O_2$max during skating. This is consistent with a reduction in muscle blood flow secondary to high intramuscular forces during skating.

During submaximal skating, $\dot{V}O_2$ increases with the square of velocity because the primary resisting force is air friction. The actual $\dot{V}O_2$ for a given individual at a certain speed is much more variable than, for example, the aerobic requirements of running. It varies depending on skating posture (i.e., the frontal area presented to the resisting air), the local barometric pressure, the characteristics of the surface over which the athlete is skating (ice friction, rolling resistance of in-line skates), and the skill of the skater. There is a considerable effect attributable to drafting behind other skaters (Fig. 56–1), which is of definitive importance during pack-style competitions.

Pulmonary Ventilation

Pulmonary ventilation generally tracks quite well with $\dot{V}O_2$ during skating. Thus, given the slightly reduced $\dot{V}O_2$max during skating, the slight reduction in observed

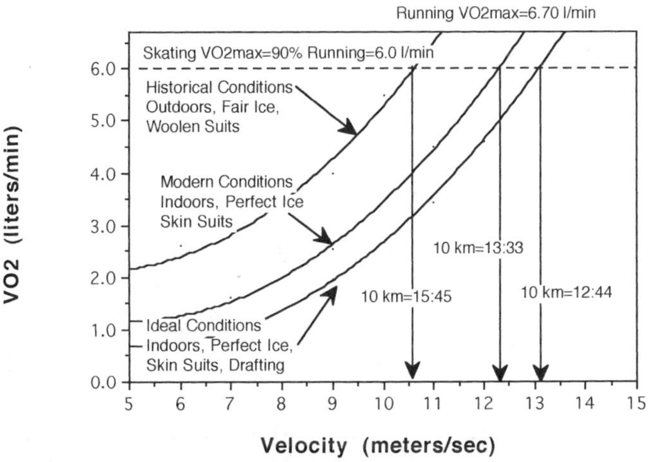

FIG. 56–1. Comparative aerobic requirements of skating under a variety of circumstances. Note that the aerobic requirements increase in a nonlinear fashion (because air is the primary resisting element). Aerodynamic suits and the good ice available at contemporary indoor venues act to shift the curve to the right and allow faster times. If drafting is allowed, skating times can be even faster. Although not accounted for in the figure, the use of klap skates could move the middle "contemporary" curve to the right by about 25 seconds.

$\dot{V}_E$max is expected. There is some evidence that the $\dot{V}_E/\dot{V}O_2$ during skating may be slightly higher than during cycling, probably secondary to the accelerated lactate accumulation during skating.

Heart Rate

Heart rate (HR) during skating also generally follows $\dot{V}O_2$, and accordingly accelerates very rapidly at the beginning of competition. HRmax during skating is similar to that achieved during either cycling or running; thus, the maximal O_2 pulse during skating is somewhat reduced. There is some evidence that HR may be disproportionately high during skating compared to the $\dot{V}O_2$. However, not all studies support this finding. Recent data suggest that the %HRmax tracks quite well with the mode-specific %$\dot{V}O_2$max for the activity. Thus, if the skating $\dot{V}O_2$max is reduced, a given absolute $\dot{V}O_2$ represents a disproportionately high %$\dot{V}O_2$max. Thus, a slight increase in HR is to be expected.

Stroke Volume and Cardiac Output

Cardiac output increases in the same general pattern during skating as during cycling. There is some evidence that at a given $\dot{V}O_2$, cycling versus skating, the cardiac output is slightly lower and the atrioventricular (A-V) O_2 difference slightly wider during skating. This is consistent with the concept that muscle blood flow is somewhat impaired during skating because the high forces within the muscle act to crimp the smaller arterioles and make muscle blood flow more difficult. At maximal exercise, the maximal cardiac output is significantly less during skating than cycling, more or less in proportion to the reduced $\dot{V}O_2$max during skating.

Muscle Oxygenation

During skating, particularly in the low position characteristic of metric style skating, there is a rapid and profound desaturation of hemoglobin/myoglobin in the active muscles (Fig. 56–2). Similar desaturation has also been noted during short-track skating. These results are consistent with a reduction in muscle blood flow secondary to mechanical occlusion of the blood vessels in the active muscles. The magnitude of desaturation during maximal skating is significantly greater than during cycling. During skating in a more upright position, such as during in-line racing, there is a desaturation pattern substantially similar to that observed during cycling, although at maximal exercise the magnitude of desaturation during skating is somewhat greater than during cycling. Studies of muscle desaturation during static exercise in the skating position, using either one or two legs, are consistent with the concept that high

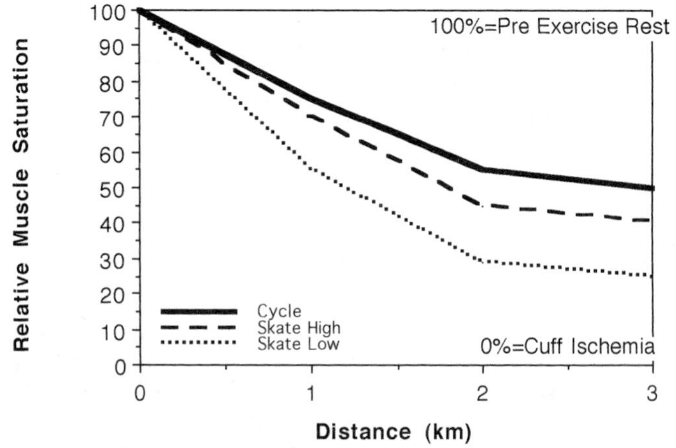

FIG. 56–2. Schematic pattern of muscle desaturation during a 3000-m skating effort, just below competitive intensities. Note that during skating in the low position, the magnitude of desaturation is not only greater than during cycling or skating in the high position, but that it also occurs earlier in the event. During maximal effort skating in the low position, muscle saturation may approximate that achieved during cuff ischemia.

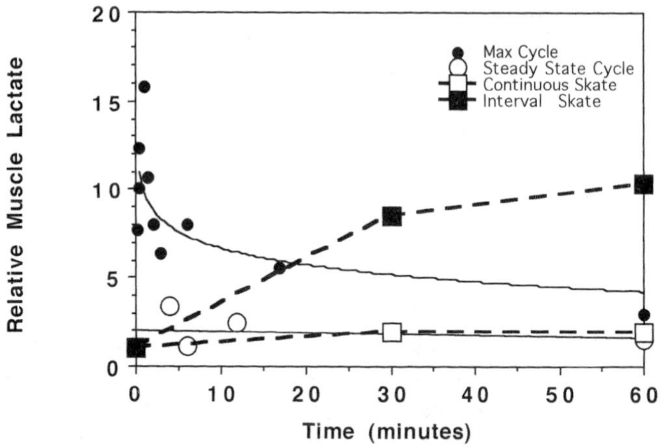

FIG. 56–3. Schematic increases in muscle lactate during cycling and skating in relation to the duration of effort, normalized to the resting muscle lactate observed in the same study. The cycling data are collected from a number of studies in the literature of either exhaustive exercise or steady-state exercise. The skating data are from a single study comparing interval skating and continuous skating for 1 hour, with an intermediate measurement after 30 minutes. In this regard, the skating data are probably most comparable to the steady-state cycling data. Muscle lactate concentrations during exhaustive speed skating have never been measured, but must greatly exceed those observed during exhaustive cycling of similar duration.

intramuscular forces during skating lead to muscle desaturation.

Lactate Accumulation

Direct measures of muscle lactate accumulation have never been performed during speed skating. Studies comparing muscle lactate accumulation during intermittent high-velocity skating on hockey skates (low position) versus continuous moderate-intensity skating (high position) have demonstrated profound levels of muscle lactate accumulation during skating in the low position. The magnitude of muscle lactate concentration during these studies is somewhat more profound than during similar levels of exercise during cycling (Fig. 56–3). An analysis of the relationship between muscle and blood lactate during cycling suggests that the generally accelerated blood lactate accumulation (even relative to $\%\dot{V}O_2max$) that is observed during skating is attributable to a generally increased level of muscle lactate accumulation (Fig. 56–4). Postcompetition blood lactate values during speed skating are among the highest reported in the literature, routinely exceeding 20 $mmol{\cdot}L^{-1}$. The highest postcompetition blood lactate values are observed in 1000- and 1500-m events. Studies using the technique of broken competition (i.e., having the athlete skate several segments of the entire race at the pace associated with the full competition), supported by laboratory cycling studies, suggest that lactate accumulation during competition is fundamentally linear following an early increase. There is some evidence that

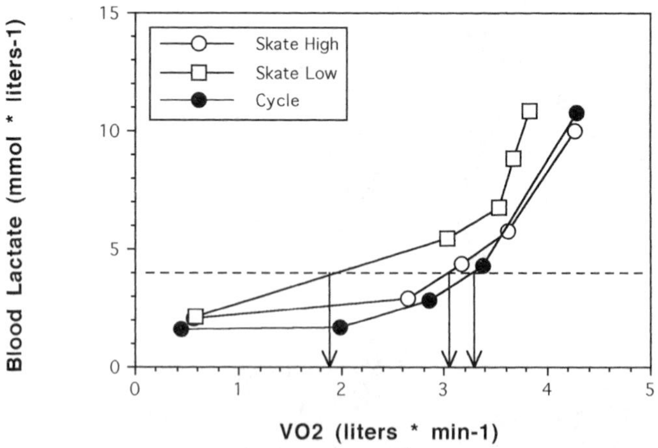

FIG. 56–4. Accumulation of blood lactate during incremental exercise cycling, and during skating in the low and high position. Note the accelerated rate of lactate accumulation during skating in the low position (probably due to desaturation attributable to restricted muscle blood flow) and the left shift of standard indices of lactate accumulation (such as the $\dot{V}O_2$ at 4 $mmol{\cdot}L^{-1}$).

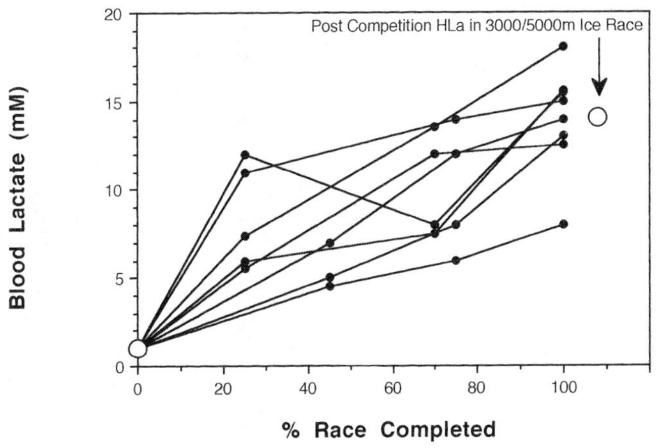

FIG. 56–5. Lactate accumulation during an in-line time trial designed to mimic an ice speed skating race of 3000/5000 m. For this study we used the technique of broken competition, recording the pace of the full effort as well as the lactate at the conclusion of the full effort. Then, subsequent efforts represent fractions of the whole distance, but with the pace controlled to match that observed during the full effort. Note the wide variations in blood lactate in a few athletes, which seem to be attributable to variations in pace in these athletes. The final values of blood lactate match reasonably well with actual postcompetition lactates in these same athletes.

the rate of lactate accumulation follows momentary variations in pace (Fig. 56–5).

THE ATHLETE

The majority of studies describing speed skaters have been conducted with metric-style ice speed skaters. In general speed skaters can be described as comparatively small, muscular athletes. It is rare for an elite male metric style speed skater to be more than 1.90 m in height or 90 kg in weight. Compared to elite athletes in many popular American team sports (football, basketball, baseball), the size of speed skaters is very modest. As a general principle, short-track speed skaters are somewhat smaller than metric-style skaters. The comparatively small size of speed skaters is probably attributable both to the fact that larger athletes are often recruited to play ice hockey and to the disadvantages of trying to overcome centrifigual force during cornering. In-line speed skaters are probably less physically specialized than ice speed skaters since the sport is not as developed. As a general principle, it is probably fair to say that in-liners are leaner and less muscular than metric-style skaters, since higher body weight would be a significant disadvantage during uphill segments.

Speed skaters are generally fairly lean, although not to the degree observed in elite runners or cyclists. Like many athletes, speed skaters demonstrate a striking degree of sport-specific muscular hypertrophy. For speed skaters this hypertrophy is located in the hip and knee extensors. In particular, there is great hypertrophy of the vastus medialis, the gluteus maximus, and the erector spinae. There is also a minor degree of selection for skaters with relatively short legs compared to height, and for a relatively small thigh to shank ratio. This anatomic selection reduces the forces on the hip extensors during the push off. It also accentuates the impression of large legs for which speed skaters are famous.

There have been a number of descriptive physiologic studies of elite metric-style speed skaters. With the exception of an early study from Sweden, speed skaters have usually returned unremarkable values for $\dot{V}O_2max$ normalized for body weight, with groups of elite skaters averaging about 65 to 70 and 55 to 60 $mL \cdot min^{-1} \cdot kg^{-1}$ for males and females, respectively. In recent years, using simulated time trials on the cycle in the laboratory, we have noted substantially higher values of $\dot{V}O_2max$ than were previously reported with incremental cycle ergometry, with the elite U.S. all-arounders routinely averaging in excess of 80 $mL \cdot min^{-1} \cdot kg^{-1}$ during a 5-km time trial. The highest value which we have recorded is 93 $mL \cdot min \cdot kg^{-1}$ in a seven-time member of the U.S. World Championships Team (with a best finish of fifth in the world championships). During 5- and 3-km cycle time trials, the mean power output will be about 6.5 and 5.5 $W \cdot kg^{-1}$ for males and females, respectively. A similar pattern of observations has been observed in the Netherlands with the use of simulated 4-km time trials. Values for sustainable exercise tolerance based on measures of lactate accumulation are comparatively ordinary in elite speed skaters, with the power output at a blood lactate concentration of 5 $mmol \cdot L^{-1}$ of about 4.5 and 3.5 $W \cdot kg^{-1}$ in males and females, respectively (at the conclusion of the preparatory season). Peak power outputs, however, are rather remarkably high among athletes, with values over 1 to 2 seconds frequently exceeding 20 and 17 $W \cdot kg^{-1}$ in elite males and females, respectively. Lastly, as might be expected from their sport and their training, speed skaters are rather strong, at least in the hip and knee extensors. It is not unusual to observe a mature elite male skater doing five repetition sets of full squats with 2.5 × body weight. Isokinetic studies have demonstrated that, not only are speed skaters capable of producing high values for muscle torque, but they can create high values for torque at locations within the range of motion where most people are very weak (e.g., at the joint angles associated with the beginning of the push-off).

TRAINING THE ATHLETE

The Season

The competitive season depends on the type of speed skating event in which the athlete participates. Longtrack speed skating typically begins with local competitions in October, the beginning of the World Cup circuit in early November, national championships in late December or early January, world championships in late February or early March, and the ending of the World Cup events by late March or early April. The competitive season has only recently been lengthened to this extent because of the availability of indoor 400-m ovals that allow competition even when weather conditions do not allow for maintenance of adequate ice conditions. The short-track season is more or less parallel to the long-track season. The in-line roller skating season continues to some degree throughout the entire year, because of the feasibility of competing in warm weather venues even during the winter months in the Northern Hemisphere. However, the main season in Europe, North America and much of the world takes place from May to October, with world championships usually taking place during the early fall.

Using long-track skating as a general model, the training year is divided into three broad periods. First is a period of recovery following completion of the major championships, generally in the months of April and May. Most elite skaters take 2 to 3 weeks off entirely, then participate in recreational-level activities for fun prior to the resumption of formal training. Second is a preparatory period prior to competition, generally in the months of June through October. During this period, the training load is progressively increased from 5 to 10 hours per week during June, frequently to 30 hours per week during September in elite skaters. The mixture of training changes progressively from more general training to more specific training across the course of this general phase of training. Third is the competitive period, which ranges from November through the end of the season. During this period, the overall training load is generally decreased and the amount of nonspecific training progressively decreased so that the athlete reaches peak performance capacity in February/March. A few elite long-track skaters will compete seriously in in-line roller skating events during the summer. However, the demands of both long-track and in-line racing schedules are large enough that few athletes can sustain the demands for high-level performance for two extensive periods of the year.

Sports-Specific Training

Sports-specific training can be divided into two basic varieties. The first is skating itself. The other is dry-land training drills designed to mimic certain aspects of the skating stroke. There are some subtle biomechanical differences between in-line roller skating and ice speed skating, which means that elite competitors in one discipline often have difficulty using one type of skating to train for the other. In particular, the better "grip" provided in ice speed skating allows a somewhat more forceful pushoff, which causes slipping when attempted on in-line skates. Likewise, ice skates allow a use of edges that is not possible during in-line skating. Thus, there is less crossover between in-line and ice speed skating than one might expect. Given this important difference, skating of any variety is still recognized as the best form of training for skating, and most elite skaters train frequently using other disciplines of skating. The same problem exists to a smaller degree for short-track versus long-track ice speed skaters. In former times, the technical differences were thought to be critical. However, the great overall similarity makes skating training of any variety still the best way to train for skating.

Skating training varies widely ranging from continuous training to a wide combination of interval exercises similar to those used in running or cycling. For metric-style ice speed skaters, intervals tend to focus on learning how to skate at the requisite speed to meet the year's competitive goals, then building endurance to allow sustaining of the speed through the duration of the race. Because of the tendency to accumulate lactate during skating, many repetitions of shorter intervals are often chosen over fewer repetitions of longer repetitions. Much of the continuous training done by skaters is performed as comparatively brief timed sets (e.g., 10 minutes) at velocities or heart rates associated with the maximal lactate steady state. There is comparatively little truly prolonged training such as the several-hour duration bouts undertaken by runners, cyclists, or nordic skiers. Occasionally marathon skaters will do training that is fundamentally similar to that undertaken by cyclists (long continuous efforts with many changes in effort), but this is uncommon in metric style or short-track ice speed skating. In-line skaters tend to train much like cyclists and marathon skaters. Much of their specifically focused training is related to practicing tactical situations (passing, blocking, drafting). To some degree this is also true for short-track ice speed skaters.

Supplemental Training

The supplemental training of speed skaters is extraordinarily varied (Fig. 56–6). Using the model of metric-style ice speed skaters (about which there are more data available), training can be divided into several different basic types, including strength, explosiveness, tolerance for the down position, anaerobic power, aerobic power, and general endurance. Additionally, some of the training exercises are intended to allow practice of various aspects of technique. During the first portion of the preparation season (May to July), supplemental training probably forms the bulk of the training load. Beginning in August, there is a progressive reduction in the volume of supplemental training as more specific training is added. Many coaches advocate continuing a certain

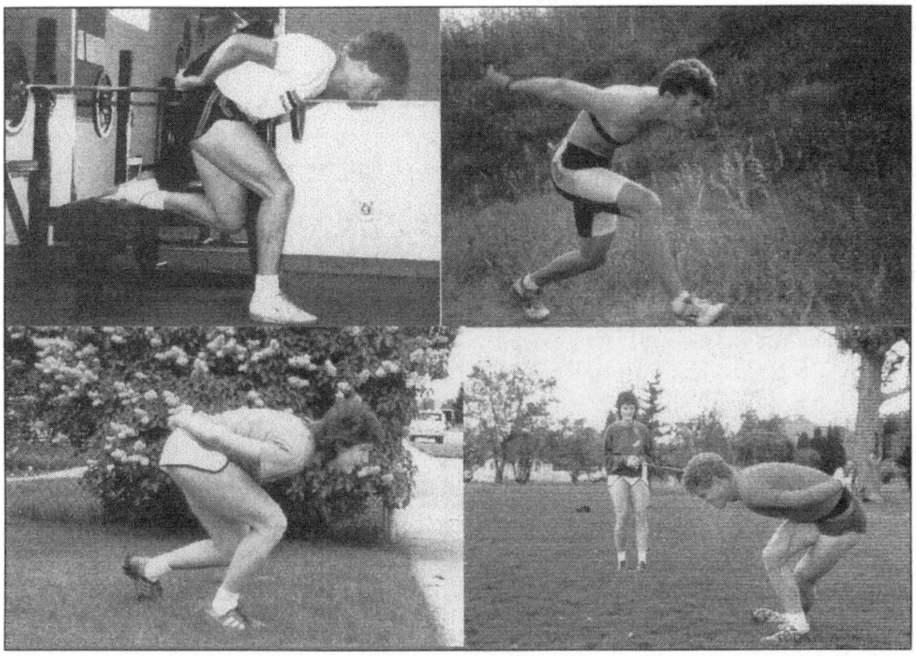

FIG. 56–6. Depiction of a few of the wide variety of sports-specific dry-land exercises routinely performed by speed skaters with the intent of improving tolerance for the "down" position as well as working on some elements of technique. They are, clockwise from the **upper left**, one leg squats (often with a barbell plate held on the back); low walks, often conducted up hills for durations ranging from 30 seconds to 5 minutes; turn cable, in which one athlete wears a belt attached to rubber tubing held by another athlete, and the first athlete then moves to the left using the turn technique while being resisted by the other skater; and dry skating, in which the athlete stays in one position and skates in place.

amount of supplemental training throughout the competitive year, however.

Resistance training is divided into two basic types. First is general strength training, designed to allow the athlete to stabilize the hips during the push-off and have generally good muscular power. This includes a large amount of "core" exercises (squats, power cleans, abdominal exercises) as well as general body strengthening exercises. Second are exercises designed to increase the power of the push-off. Given the fairly high joint opening velocities of the push-off (~700 degrees/sec) and the poor transfer of strength training from slow to faster exercise, the only effective way to train is by jumping exercises. Since the early part of the push-off is particularly important, skaters tend to focus on jumps from a deep position that mimic the beginning of the skating stroke. One interesting variation that has been well received in the United States is to do skating-specific jumps immediately following a conventional resistance exercise (e.g., squats). This is designed to teach athletes to recruit all of their muscle fibers even when fatigued. Skating jumps also may be done with a sandbag or weight vest to provide resistance. Many skaters, particularly during the developmental part of their careers, have trouble making the early part of the push-off explosive. They are just not strong enough in the deep position to be explosive. By wearing a climber's belt attached to a garage-door spring, they can effectively reduce their weight and practice the velocity-specific characteristics from the position desired. As athletes become stronger, they can gradually reduce the amount of support, so long as the velocity of the jump does not deteriorate. This may also be accomplished by using two-legged jumps instead of one-legged jumps, although the biomechanics are somewhat different. Lastly, skaters frequently perform one-legged squats, often with either a barbell plate or sandbag on the back to develop local endurance in the hip and thigh extensors. Typically they start with 20 seconds on, 40 seconds off, continued for 10 minutes or more, alternating legs from 1 minute to the next. By the end of the preparation period, they may be performing 50 seconds on, 10 seconds off, continuing for 40 minutes or more. Fairly high blood lactate concentrations, typical of those observed during 5- and 10-km races, are frequently observed during this type of training.

Because the crouched position, which is necessary for an effective push-off, interferes with blood flow, there is a great need to build tolerance to the "down" position. This may be accomplished by a variety of skating drills that mimic some aspects of skating and force the athlete to spend much time in the skating position. These exercises often have somewhat unusual names, such as dry skating, low walks, and cross-backs. Whether the acquired tolerance for the down position is attributable to improved blood flow in the muscle (improved capillarization) or to better buffering of the metabolites of anaerobic metabolism remains to be determined.

Because of the need for high muscular power outputs during skating, there is considerable effort given to trying to develop anaerobic power and to develop tolerance for lactate. This is usually accomplished during cycling or running. These bouts may vary from several brief bursts (often only 5 to 6 seconds in duration), to more sustained efforts that are usually accomplished as "tempos" or efforts where the muscular power output is maximal from the beginning and allowed to decay during the course of the effort. The most common type is the "hill tempo": a steep hill is run for a specified time, ranging from 30 to 90 sec, with the athlete moving at maximal speed from the very beginning. Often there is a 5- to 10-minute recovery following each effort, and rarely are more than four repetitions accomplished during a given training session. We have noted very high blood lactate concentrations during training sessions of this type (>25 $mmol \cdot L^{-1}$).

Lastly, conventional aerobic training is performed using both cycling and running. Because of the common reliance on the hip and knee extensors as well as the negative influence of high thigh masses on running performance, cycling is usually much more important to skaters. Indeed, it is not uncommon for elite skaters to compete fairly successfully in cycling events either during the preparation period or after their skating career is over.

Periodization of Training

We have developed a method of quantifying training load based on multiplying the duration of training by a global rating of perceived exertion (RPE) for the entire training session. This method has been useful not only in gaining an appreciation of the magnitude of the training load in skaters, but also in identifying factors that might be related to maladaptation to training, as well as allowing comparison of the pattern of the training program. As a general plan, most skaters are on a 4-week periodization plan, with either progressively harder or progressively easier weeks of training for 3 weeks, then a week of comparative rest (Fig. 56–7). The total training load usually peaks during September, when the specific training really begins in earnest and the amount of supplemental training is still substantial.

Future Issues

Historically, speed skating has been a very untechnical sport. Compared to many contemporary sports, the basic equipment in skating has remained largely unchanged for most of this century. Until the last season, the last technical innovation in speed skating was the use of the aerodynamic "skin suit" first introduced around

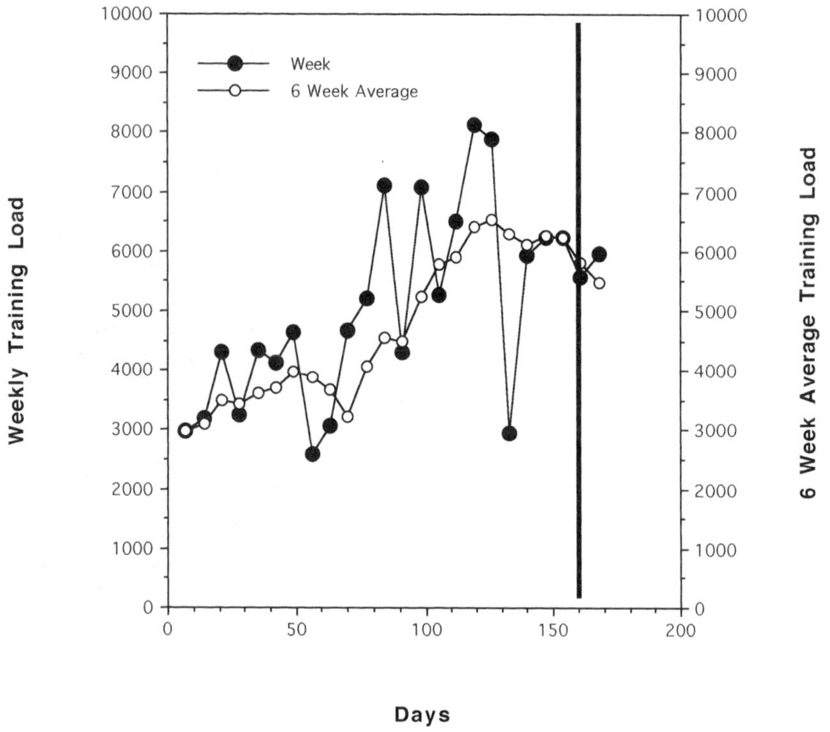

FIG. 56–7. Schematic presentation of the weekly training load undertaken by an elite skater, leading up to major selection trials (*heavy vertical line*). The load is calculated using our session rating of perceived exertion method in which the athlete rates the effort for each training session using the Borg scale, then multiplies this value by the duration of the training session. The weekly value is the summation of all training conducted during that week. Note the week-to-week variation in the training load and the gradual increase across the training period, with a decrease in the training load as the athlete freshens up prior to the selection trials. The 6-week average is a rolling average of the immediately preceding 6 weeks, which may represent the momentary fitness of the athlete.

1976. Since 1996, on the basis of an idea that dates back to the turn of the twentieth century, a new skate design has become accepted by the skating community. The skate is hinged at the toe, with the blade held in place by a spring. These skates are widely referred to as "klap" skates, after the sound the blade makes when the spring returns it to the neutral position prior to gliding on that foot. If the athlete pushes hard enough, the spring may be overcome and the skate unhinges. This allows the skater to use plantar flexion and to extend the stroke, without the tip of the skate blade digging into the ice and increasing gliding friction. The use of the new skate seems to provide primarily a biomechanical advantage, allowing a longer stroke and higher velocities at the same metabolic power production. Although experience with the skate is still evolving, it appears to be about 1 second per lap faster than conventional speed skates. Needless to say, the world record list has been extensively rewritten during the last few seasons. Although there are only a few acute physiologic studies available, it appears that the fundamental physiologic issues in speed skating are unchanged; skating is just more efficient with the klap skates.

SUGGESTED READINGS

Beneke R, Boldte F, Meller W, Behn C. Maximal lactate steady state in speed skating. *Leistungsdiagnostik-Trainingssteuerung* 1991; 10:766–767.

Broshears C, Matiasek M, Hill HR, et al. Knee angle and Hb/Mb O_2 desaturation in the vastus lateralis of speed skaters. *Med Sci Sports Exerc* 1997;29:S262(abst).

Daines E, Rundell K, Goodwin GT, Foster C. Comparative heart rate relationships during walking, low walking, and slideboard exercise. *Med Sci Sports Exerc* 1995;27:S597(abst).

deBoer RW, Ettema GJC, Faessen BGM, et al. Specific characteristics of speed skating: implications for summer training. *Med Sci Sports Exerc* 1987;19:504–510.

deBoer RW, Cabri J, Vaes W, et al. Moments of force, power and muscle coordination in speed skating. *Int J Sports Med* 1987; 8:371–378.

deGroot G, Hollander AP, Sargeant AJ, van Ingen Schenau GJ. Applied physiology of speed skating. *J Sports Sci* 1987;5:249–259.

diPrampero PE, Cortili G, Mognoni P, Saibene F. Energy cost of speed skating and efficiency of work against air resistance. *J Appl Physiol* 1976;40:584–591.

Diamant B, Karlsson J. Muscle tissue lactate after maximal exercise in man. *Acta Physiol Scand* 1968;72:383–384.

Ekblom B, Hermansen L, Saltin B. *Hastighetskinng pa Skridsko: Idrotsfysiology rapport,* no. 5. Stockholm: Trygg-Hansa, 1967.

Fedel FJ, Keteyian SJ, Brawner CA, Marks CRC, Hakim MJ, Katoka T. Cardiorespiratory responses during exercise in competitive in-line skaters. *Med Sci Sports Exerc* 1995;27:682–687.

Foster C, Green MA, Snyder AC, Thompson NN. Physiological responses during simulated competition. *Med Sci Sports Exerc* 1993;25:877–882.

Foster C, Snyder AC, Thompson NN, Green MA, Foley M, Schrager M. Effect of pacing strategy on cycle time trial performance. *Med Sci Sports Exerc* 1993;25:383–388.

Foster C. *Physiological perspectives in speed skating*. Milwaukee, WI: Sinai Samaritan Medical Center, 1996.

Foster C, Kemkers G, Matiasek M, et al. Restricted muscle blood flow during skating. *Med Sci Sports Exerc* 1997;29:S284(abst).

Foster C. Monitoring training in athletes with reference to overtraining syndrome. *Med Sci Sports Exerc* 1998;30:1164–1168.

Green HJ. Glycogen depletion patterns during continuous and intermittent ice skating. *Med Sci Sports* 1978;10:183–187.

Jacobs I, Tesch PA, Bar-Or, Karlsson J, Dotan R. Lactate in human skeletal muscle after 10 and 30 s of supramaximal exercise. *J Appl Physiol* 1983;55:365–367.

Jorfeldt L, Juhlin-Dannfelt A, Karlsson J. Lactate release in relation to tissue lactate in human skeletal muscle during exercise. *J Appl Physiol* 1978;44:350–352.

Karlsson J. Lactate and phosphagen concentrations in working muscle of man. *Acta Physiol Scand* 1971;suppl 358.

deKoning JJ, deGroot G, van Ingen Schenau GJ. A power equation for the print in speed skating. *J Biomechanics* 1992;25:573–580.

deKoning JJ, deGroot G, van Ingen Schenau GJ. Coordination of leg muscles in speed skating. *J Biomech* 1991;24:137–146.

deKoning JJ, Bakker FC, deGroot G, van Ingen Schenau GJ. Longitudinal development of young talented speed skaters: physiological and anthropometric aspects. *J Appl Physiol* 1994;77:2311–2317.

deKoning JJ, deHaan E, Stam R, deGroot G, van Ingen Schenau GJ. Speed skating on skates that allow plantar flexion improves mechanical efficiency. *Med Sci Sports Exerc* 1997;28:S262(abst).

Nemoto I, Iwaoka K, Funato K, Yoshioka N, Miyashita M. Aerobic threshold, anaerobic threshold and maximal oxygen uptake of Japanese speed skaters. *Int J Sports Med* 1988;9:433–437.

Pollock ML, Pels AE, Foster C, Holum D. Comparison of male and female Olympic speed skating candidates. In: Landers DM, ed. *Sport and elite performers*. Champaign, IL: Human Kinetics, 1984.

Rajala GM, Neumann DA, Foster C, Jensen RH. Quadriceps muscle performance in male speed skaters. *J Strength Conditioning Res* 1994;8:48–52.

Rundell KW. Compromised oxygen uptake in speed skaters during treadmill in-line skating. *Med Sci Sports Exerc* 1996;28:120–127.

Rundell KW, Nioka S, Chance B. Hemoglobin/myoglobin desaturation during speed skating. *Med Sci Sports Exerc.* 1997;29:248–258.

Rundell KW, Osbeck JS, Amico VJ. Effects of drafting during short track speed skating. *Med Sci Sports Exerc* 1996;28:765–771.

Snyder AC, O'Hagen KP, Clifford PS, Hoffman MD, Foster C. Exercise responses to in-line skating: comparisons to running and cycling. *Int J Sports Med* 1993;14:38–42.

van Ingen Schenau GJ. Influence of air friction in speed skating. *J Biomech* 1982;15:449–458.

van Ingen Schenau GJ, deKoning JJ, deGroot G. A simulation of speed skating performances based on a power equation. *Med Sci Sports Exerc* 1990;22:718–728.

van Ingen Schenau GJ, deGroot G. Differences in oxygen consumption and external power between male and female speed skaters during supramaximal cycling. *Eur J Appl Physiol* 1983;51:337–345.

van Ingen Schenau GJ, deKoning JJ, deGroot G. The distribution of anaerobic energy in 1000 and 4000 meter cycling bouts. *Int J Sports Med* 1992;13:447–451.

van Ingen Schenau GJ, deGroot G, Scheurs AW, Meester H, deKoning JJ. A new skate allowing powerful plantar flexions improves performance. *Med Sci Sports Exerc* 1996;28:531–535.

Wallick ME, Porcari JP, Wallick SB, Berg KM, Brice GA, Arimond GR. Physiological responses to in-line skating compared to treadmill running. *Med Sci Sports Exerc* 1995;27:242–248.

Withers RT, Sherman WM, Clark DG, et al. Muscle metabolism during 30, 60 and 90 s of maximal cycling. *Eur J Appl Physiol* 1991;63:354–362.

Exercise and Sport Science,
edited by William E. Garrett, Jr., and Donald T. Kirkendall.
Lippincott Williams & Wilkins, Philadelphia © 2000.

CHAPTER 57

Physiology of Swimming

Rick L. Sharp

Understanding the physiologic responses to and determinants of swimming performance is most simply approached by comparison with other forms of exercise. Competitive swimming events range in duration from about 20 seconds (50-m freestyle) to about 15 minutes (1500-m freestyle). Based on the traditional view of an energy continuum, swimming events should be energetically equivalent to middle-distance track running. Thus, swimming athletes require elements of both speed and endurance to reach their performance potential. However, the fact that this activity is performed in the water instead of on land poses unique challenges to our understanding of the specific physiologic demands placed on these athletes. Included among these problems is the significantly greater resistance of water than air and the difficulty in applying propulsion in a fluid medium. Because of these constraints, the swimmer's skill in reducing water resistance and in effectively applying propulsive forces may be more important in dictating the physiologic demands of swimming than a simple analysis of race duration would reveal.

THE SPORT

The four strokes contested in competitive swimming are butterfly, backstroke, breaststroke, and freestyle. Arm and leg motions of the first three are specified by the rules of the governing body sponsoring the competition [National Collegiate Athletic Association (NCAA), La Fédération Internationale de Natation Amateur (FINA), high school association, etc.]. In freestyle, however, the swimmer may use any stroking style, but nearly all competitors use the front crawl because it is the fastest means of propulsion. For a more detailed description of these strokes, refer to Chapter 41. Distances contested vary by stroke; 100- and 200-m (or yard) distances are contested for all strokes. In freestyle, however, distances of 50, 400 m or 500 yards, 800 m or 1000 yards, and 1500 m or 1650 yards are also swum. The other two events are the 200 and 400 individual medley, which consist of equal lengths of all four strokes swum in order of butterfly, backstroke, breaststroke, and freestyle. Team relays are also included in many competitive meets and are of various distances (200 to 800 m) and are swum either as freestyle or medley (consisting of a backstroke leg, breaststroke, butterfly, and freestyle). Current world records for both men and women in all events are shown in Table 57–1.

Physical Requirements

The work of swimming involves generating enough propulsive force to overcome the water resistance acting on the body to impede forward progress. In addition, energy is expended to minimize the amount of this resistance the body experiences while trying to move forward. Energy expenditure has been shown to increase exponentially with an increase in swimming velocity due to an exponential increase in resistance (drag) (1). At any given velocity of swimming, there appears to be a great deal of variability in the amount of drag between individuals, and among the four swimming strokes used in competition (freestyle or front crawl, backstroke, breaststroke, and butterfly). Among individuals, the variability in drag seems to be accounted for by differences in body morphology and degree of skill of the swimmer.

By measuring oxygen uptake while swimming at standardized speeds in a swimming flume, Holmer (2) showed that energy expenditure during butterfly and breaststroke swimming is roughly twice as high as when using either backstroke or freestyle swimming. These differences can be attributed to the increase in form drag during butterfly and breaststroke as dictated by

R. L. Sharp: Department of Health and Human Performance, Iowa State University, Ames, Iowa 50011.

TABLE 57–1. *Men's and women's world long-course (50-m pool) swimming records as of May 1999*

Event (m)	Women	Men
50 freestyle	24.51 Le, CHN 1994	21.81 Jager, USA 1990
100 freestyle	54.01 Le, CHN 1994	48.21 Popov, RUS 1994
200 freestyle	1:56.78 van Almsick, GER 1994	1:46.69 Lamberti, ITA 1989
400 freestyle	4:03.85 Evans, USA 1989	3:43.80 Perkins, AUS 1994
800 freestyle	8:16.22 Evans, USA 1989	7:46.00 Perkins, AUS 1994
1500 freestyle	15:52.10 Evans, USA 1989	14:41.66 Perkins, AUS 1994
100 backstroke	1:00.16 He, CHN 1994	53.86 Rouse, USA 1992
200 backstroke	2:06.62 Egerszegi, HUN 1991	1:56.57 Zubero, ESP 1991
100 breaststroke	1:07.02 Heyns, RSA 1996	1:00.60 deBurghgraeve, BEL 1996
200 breatstroke	2:24.76 Brown, AUS 1994	2:10.16 Barrowman, USA 1992
100 butterfly	57.93 Meagher, USA 1981	52.15 Klim, AUS 1997
200 butterfly	2:05.96 Meagher, USA 1981	1:55.22 Pankratov, RUS 1995
200 individual medley	2:09.72 Wu, CHN 1997	1:58.16 Sievinen, FIN 1994
400 individual medley	4:34.79 Chen, CHN 1997	4:12.30 Dolan, USA 1994

AUS, Australia; BEL, Belgium; CHN, China; ESP, Spain; GER, Germany; HUN, Hungary; ITA, Italy; RSA, Republic of South Africa; RUS, Russia; USA, United States.

the mechanics of these strokes. Thus, physiologic responses to swimming are largely dependent on the amount of drag a swimmer experiences at any given speed, and they are not nearly as constant as in running or cycling when subjects perform at a given velocity.

In comparing energy expenditure among swimmers of varied ability or skill levels, Holmer (3,4) discovered that when swimming at the same speed and using the same stroke, more accomplished competitive swimmers had significantly lower energy expenditure than noncompetitive swimmers. For example, at a swimming velocity of 0.8 m/s, observed $\dot{V}O_2$ was 4.1 L/min for the recreational swimmers, 2.6 L/min for the good swimmer, and 2.0 L/min for the elite swimmer.

In a similar study, Van Handel and colleagues (5) measured energy expenditure at a velocity of 1.2 m/s for male and female world-class swimmers using freestyle. The women had an average oxygen uptake of 28 mL/kg/min while the mean $\dot{V}O_2$ for the men was 36 mL/kg/min. Furthermore, it was noted that the range of $\dot{V}O_2$ between the most economical and least economical swimmers was 20 mL/kg/min, or from 25 to 40 mL/kg/min while swimming at the same velocity. When these swimmers' submaximal $\dot{V}O_2$ (economy) was correlated with their best 400 m competitive performance, a correlation of $r = 0.67$ was observed. Considering that these were all elite athletes and likely were very homogeneous with respect to performance, the relatively high correlation between economy and performance is remarkable. However, $\dot{V}O_2$max was also significantly correlated with their 400-m performance time, but when the analysis was conducted separately for men and women there was no correlation between $\dot{V}O_2$max and performance.

Several other studies have also examined the relationship between swimming economy and performance and generally have shown that economy is associated with better performance ability, especially in middle distance swimming (6–10). In the study by Klentrou and Montpetit (8), 25 male Canadian swimmers aged 16.8 ± 2.2 years (standard deviation) were tested for both $\dot{V}O_2$max and swimming economy while swimming in a 25-m pool. $\dot{V}O_2$ measurements were obtained during the first 20 seconds of recovery following each swim (2 × 250 m + 1 × 400 m maximal swim). Economy was calculated as the $\dot{V}O_2$ required to swim at 1.3 m/s. Twelve of the swimmers regularly trained and competed at the 100-m freestyle distance while the other 13 specialized in the 400-m freestyle. The two groups had similar $\dot{V}O_2$max

(100 m: 4.76 ± 0.6 L/min; 400 m: 4.68 ± 0.6 L/min) and economy at 1.3 m/s (100 m: 3.26 ± 0.5 L/min; 400 m: 3.38 ± 0.5 L/min). Using a forward stepwise multiple regression analysis to determine which of several physiologic and physical variables significantly contribute to performance, the authors showed that the combination of maximal stroking rate, power, arm span, and height provided the best prediction of 100-m performance time ($R = 0.84$). Performance in 400-m freestyle was best predicted using a combination of economy, height, and maximal stroking rate ($R = 0.82$). In both regression models, it should be noted that maximal stroking rate was negatively related to performance, meaning that slower stroke rates were associated with better performance. By inference, therefore, better performance ability was associated with longer distance per stroke, in agreement with several other studies (11–13).

These studies provide evidence that an essential determinant of swimming performance is the skill with which the athlete can provide needed propulsion in the most economical manner possible. These findings also underscore the notion that swimming physiology is largely a function of the mechanical aspects of both propulsion and drag reduction. Efforts to reduce the amount of active drag experienced by the swimmer, therefore, should return great performance benefits by reducing the physiologic work associated with maintaining any given speed. Further evidence of this was obtained in a study that examined the physiologic effects of shaving exposed body hair, a practice common among swimmers in preparation for championship competition (14). In this study, nine male competitive swimmers aged 19 to 23 years were tested for submaximal responses to standardized swimming speeds before and immediately after shaving the exposed hair from their body. Four other swimmers were used as controls and did the same testing as the experimental group, but they did not shave. Before and after shaving, each swimmer performed a 366-m breaststroke swim at 90% of his best practice time-trial for that distance. Speeds were controlled using pacing lights placed on the bottom of the pool. Heart rate was measured throughout the swim by telemetry, and oxygen uptake was measured during the first 20 seconds of recovery as in the study by Klentrou and Montpetit (8). In addition to performing the submaximal 366-m swim, each swimmer also was tested for oxygen uptake and heart rate responses to three submaximal loads during tethered swimming. Finally, all swimmers performed a push-off and glide test in which the swimmer performed an underwater push-off and glide from the side of the pool while velocities were measured using a nonelastic wire attached to the swimmer and pulled from a reel that was modified to produce a voltage proportional to velocity. Shaving body hair resulted in 12% increase in distance per stroke, a 9% decrease in $\dot{V}O_2$, and a 20% decrease in the blood lactate accumulation (Fig. 57–1). In contrast, the control group experienced no significant changes in any of these variables. To eliminate the possibility that shaving might somehow result in improved ability to generate propulsive force, the swimmers also were tested in tethered swimming where body drag is not a factor in determining the energy cost of a given speed. In tethered swimming, there were no pre–post differences in any of the physiologic responses for either the experimental or control groups. In the push-off and glide test, shaving significantly reduced the amount of deceleration after the push-off in the experimental subjects by an average of 12%.

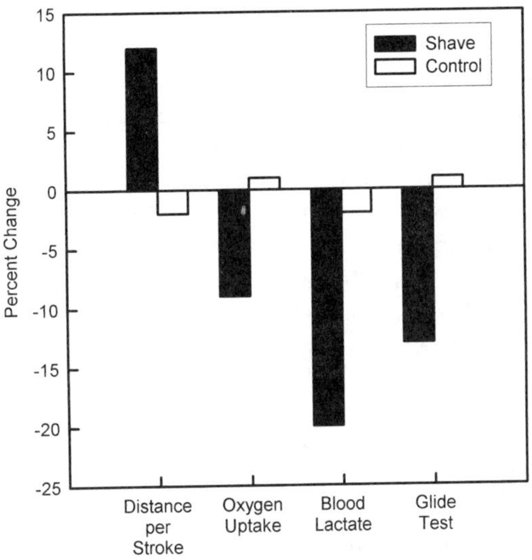

FIG. 57–1. Effects of shaving body hair on physiologic response to standard swimming speed. (Adapted from ref. 14.)

Physiologic Requirements

Swimmers commonly train twice per day in the pool, covering up to 16,000 m per day, 6 days per week. Much of this training is done at submaximal speeds for purposes of developing aerobic adaptations and swimming mechanics, and is mixed with some supramaximal interval training to develop speed and physiologic capacities specific to the race distances the swimmer will compete in. Studies of the energy requirements of swimming training have confirmed the expected enormous energy demand that this kind of training schedule requires.

Sherman and Maglischo (15) estimated the total energy demand of swimming training at 4016 to 5402 kcal/day for male swimmers and 3394 to 4016 kcal/day for female swimmers training for about 4 hours per day. A recent study by Trappe and colleagues (16) used the double-labeled water method to assess total energy expenditure during swim training in a group of national-caliber female swimmers. These swimmers were participating in twice per day training lasting about 5 to 6 hours a day and covering 17,500 m/day during the 5-day period they were monitored. During this time, total energy expenditure averaged 23.4 ± 2.1 megajoules (MJ)/day. Energy intake was estimated from diet records collected during the same period in which total energy expenditure was measured. Based on these records, the authors estimated that the swimmers maintained a negative energy balance of approximately 43% during the study period.

Costill and colleagues (17) examined energy metabolism of 12 male collegiate swimmers before and at the end of 10 days of training in which training volume was suddenly increased from 4266 m/day to 8970 m/day. During this 10-day period of increased training, intensity was maintained at an average of 94% $\dot{V}O_2max$. The combined effect of the increased volume and maintained intensity resulted in an energy cost of training that increased from 1192 kcal/day during the lower volume training to 2293 kcal/day during the higher volume training. Coupled with estimated resting energy expenditure of 2374 kcal/day (32 kcal/kg/day), total energy expenditure was 3516 kcal/day in lower-volume training, and 4667 kcal/day during higher-volume training. The authors noted that four of the subjects failed to increase their energy intake to match the larger energy demand of the higher-volume training. These four remained in a negative energy balance that amounted to about 1000 kcal/day. As a consequence of this negative energy balance, these subjects reported difficulty in performing the training. Furthermore, muscle glycogen concentration in this subgroup fell from 106 mmol/kg at the beginning of the increased training to 80 mmol/kg by the end of the high-volume training. This was in contrast to the other eight men whose muscle glycogen concentration dropped from 130 mmol/kg at the beginning of training to 110 mmol/kg at day 11. The subjective fatigue and chronic muscle glycogen depletion of these swimmers was also associated with a 10% decline in distance per stroke that was not observed in the swimmers who adjusted their energy intake to match the metabolic demand of the increased training.

These findings help to provide clues as to possible causes of the overtraining state that many swimmers seem to experience at some time during their competitive careers. The data reviewed above suggest that some swimmers may fail to adjust their energy intake to the training demands. These swimmers are therefore more likely to experience chronic muscle glycogen depletion as a consequence of the inadequate intake of dietary carbohydrate. If this pattern is maintained for more than a few days, swimmers may start to experience performance decrements in both training and competition, biomechanical changes resulting from muscle fatigue, disturbances of mood state, sleep disturbance, and altered hormonal profiles.

THE ATHLETE

It stands to reason that competitive swimmers who are tall, lean, have large upper body power, and possess good endurance would have an advantage in this sport. Khosla (18) showed that height was related to better swimming performance in an analysis of the physical characteristics of female swimmers at the 1976 Olympic Games. Lavoie and Montpetit (19) report that sprint freestyle and backstroke specialists tend to be the tallest among competitive swimmers. Although there are few published data on the physical characteristics of recent elite swimmers, these assumptions are generally confirmed. Bradley and colleagues (20) reported average height of members of the 1984 United States Olympic team as 183.1 cm for males (n = 18) and 172.7 cm for females (n = 20). In a later study of male swimmers who had placed in the finals of the U.S. National Championships, average height was reported as 186.9 cm and body weight of 79.4 kg (n = 20) (21). Percent fat of swimmers on the U.S. Olympic Team was reported as 12% ± 4% for males and 20% ± 3% for females (22).

In an effort to determine the relative importance of anthropometric characteristics and physiologic capacities in swimming, Klentrou and Montpetit (8) examined the relationships among height, weight, arm span, maximum oxygen uptake, economy during submaximal swimming, and performance in 100-m and 400-m freestyle. Using data obtained on 25 male Canadian age-group swimmers (mean age = 16.8 years), these authors found that the single best predictor of success in the 100-m freestyle was height (r = −0.60, height vs. time to complete 100 m). In the 400-m event, maximum stroke rate was the best predictor of success (r = −0.70, maximum stroke rate vs. time to complete 400 m). When all the variables were entered into a stepwise multiple regression model, however, the combination of height, arm power, maximum stroke rate, and arm span yielded the best prediction model [R = 0.84, standard error of estimate (SEE) = 1.03] for the 100-m freestyle. For the 400-m freestyle, the best prediction model consisted of economy at 1.3 m/s, height, and maximum stroke rate (R = 0.82, SEE = 3.40). These findings confirm the hypothesis that taller swimmers should have an advantage, but only if height is also coupled with high physiologic capacities specific to the event in which the swimmer competes.

TRAINING THE ATHLETE

Sport-Specific Training

A typical training day for a top-level swimmer often consists of two water workouts, one in the morning and another in the afternoon, each lasting about 2 hours. In addition, there may also be some dry-land work involving strength/power training, flexibility exercises, and/or cross-training for development of endurance. During a single training session in the pool, the practice usually consists of a series of warmup swims, one to three main training sets, sets to concentrate on some particular stroke or kicking drill, and some cool-down swimming. The main training sets are usually designed to target a particular adaptation such as aerobic endurance, lactate tolerance, or speed. A sample training session is shown in Table 57–2.

Endurance Adaptations During Swimming Training

Because competitive swimmers spend so much of their training time in developing endurance, both laboratory tests and field tests of aerobic endurance have been used to determine if physiologic measures of endurance are related to performance and to characterize changes in endurance during training. In part, changes in endurance capacities during training have been examined to determine if competitive swimmers' long periods of endurance training provide them with continued improvement throughout their competitive season. Another purpose of these investigations is to develop "field tests" of endurance capacities that coaches can use for monitoring the effectiveness of the training and for avoiding overtraining.

Considering the large amount of training done by competitive swimmers, it is not at all surprising to find that competitive swimmers have very high aerobic power when measured as maximum oxygen uptake during swimming (3,4). In his review of the literature on aerobic power of competitive swimmers, Holmer (4) reported that swimmers had a $\dot{V}O_2$max comparable to other endurance athletes such as distance runners and cyclists. In addition, he pointed out that in the 20 years prior to his review, there did not seem to be much change in the aerobic power of elite swimmers despite the continued improvement in performance times. Studies done since Holmer's review in 1978 have obtained similar results, confirming the high aerobic power of these athletes that does not seem to be much different from the period before 1978.

Besides finding that aerobic power has not changed much for elite swimmers in recent years, investigators have also addressed the question of whether aerobic power changes during a season of training. A study by Montpetit and colleagues (23) tested swimming $\dot{V}O_2$max of 11 male and five female members of the French National Team at four times through a 64-day period within a season of training. $\dot{V}O_2$max of the male swimmers did not change significantly among the four testing times (4.60 L/min at T1, 4.51 L/min at T2, 4.81 L/min at T3, and 4.77 L/min at T4) (Fig. 57–2). Likewise, the females also did not experience significant changes in $\dot{V}O_2$max during the season (3.54 L/min at T1, 3.51 L/min at T2, 3.55 L/min at T3, and 3.51 L/min at T4). The lack of change in aerobic power during the season may be due in part to the timing of the experiment. The first test was conducted in May, a time of year when most swimmers have already done much of their preparatory training progression. If this is the case with these swimmers, then earlier testing at the time when the swimmers began training may have shown lower $\dot{V}O_2$max. Nevertheless, the findings indicate that little change in aerobic power occurs during the latter part of a training period in elite swimmers.

Possible changes in economy during swimming training have been studied by several investigators using both direct ($\dot{V}O_2$ at standardized speeds) and indirect measures (blood lactate, heart rate at standardized speeds) of swimming economy. Ryan and colleagues

TABLE 57–2. *Sample training session*

Warmup	Swim 300 m
	Pull 300 m
	Swim 4 × 50 m in 1 minute
Main set	Swim 6 × 50 m on 3 minutes
	Swim easy 150 m between each 50 m
Stroke drill	Swim 10 × 100 m in 2 minutes
	(25 m right arm, 25 m left arm, 50 m both arms)
Main set	Swim 2 × 1000 m in 12 minutes
Kick set	Kick 6 × 200 m in 4 minutes
Main set	Swim 8 × 200 m in 2 minutes, 45 seconds
Cool down	Swim 4 × 200 m in 2 minutes, 45 seconds (progressively slower until recovered)
Total = 8450 m	

Adapted from ref. 17.

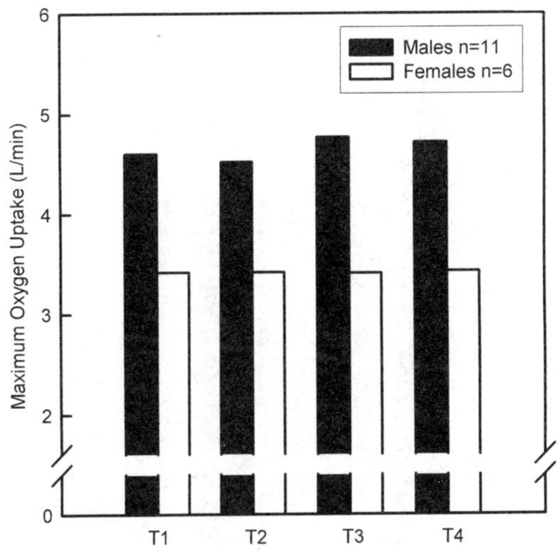

FIG. 57–2. Maximum oxygen uptake during season of training in international level swimmers. (Adapted from ref. 23.)

(24) evaluated changes in the velocity at which 4 mM blood lactate concentration is reached (V4) in 14 female elite swimmers during a season of training. The first testing was done in September after the first 2 weeks of training. Subsequent tests were done every 2 weeks during the training until mid-February. Velocity at 4 mM blood lactate concentration increased from 1.32 m/s to 1.52 m/s when the training volume was increased from 6400 m/day to 8229 m/day in the 2 weeks between the first and second testing date (Fig. 57–3). Thereafter, the velocity at 4 mM remained constant at 1.52 to 1.55 m/s while training volume fluctuated from approximately 6096 m/day to 10,973 m/day. The authors concluded that further adaptation of blood lactate profiles cannot be used as a rationale for training volumes above about 44,000 m/wk.

When training volume was increased from 4200 to 8200 m/day in the study by Costill and colleagues (17), blood lactate response to a standardized speed decreased significantly within only 5 days (Fig. 57–4). These investigators reported that the blood lactate dropped from 7.5 mM while training 4200 m/day to 4.9 mM 5 days after starting 8200 m/day and to 4.0 mM 10 days into the increased training. The large decline in blood lactate concentration with increased training volume was attributed to possible chronic muscle glycogen depletion, improved mechanisms of lactate clearance, or enhanced oxidative capacity of the muscle. These results are similar to those of Ryan and colleagues (24), who showed significant changes in velocity at 4 mM blood lactate concentration when training was increased from 6400 to 8229 m/day.

Another study that has shown economy-related changes during swimming training measured blood lactate and heart rate-velocity profiles during a season of

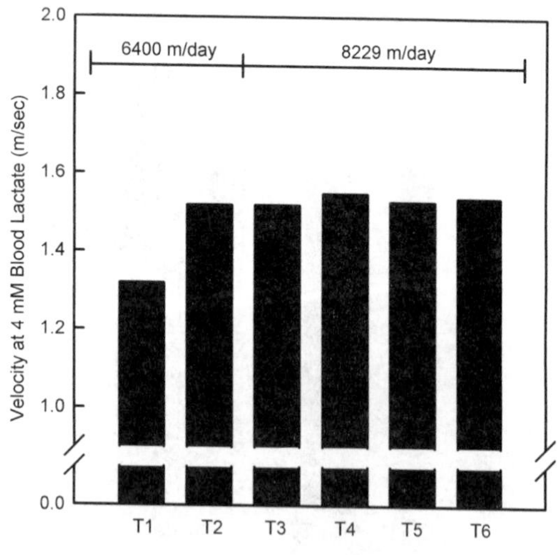

FIG. 57–3. Blood lactate economy during a season of training in elite female swimmers. (Adapted from ref. 24.)

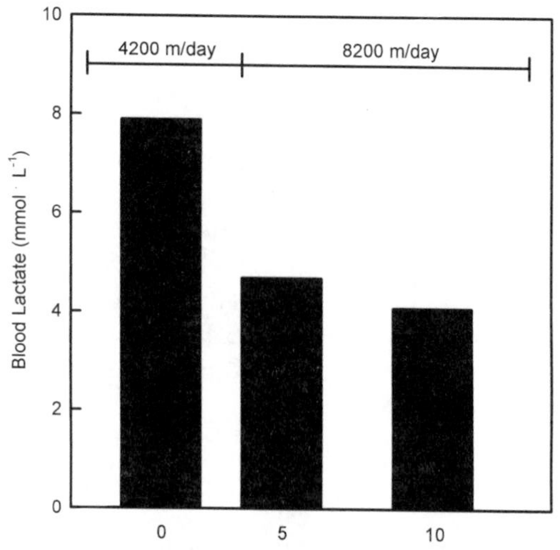

FIG. 57–4. Changes in blood lactate response to standard swimming speed during 10 days of increased training volume. (Adapted from ref. 17.)

training in male collegiate swimmers (25). To construct the profiles, the swimmers in this study swam two 200-yard freestyle swims with blood sampling and heart rate measurements after each swim. The first swim was performed at a submaximal intensity (~80% effort) and the second was swum with maximal effort. Testing periods were the beginning of season (T1), 8 weeks into the season (T2), and 16 weeks into the season (T3). Blood was sampled at 5 minutes postexercise for measurement of lactate concentration. Heart rate was measured at 15, 45, and 90 seconds after each swim. Both blood lactate and recovery heart rate were plotted as functions of mean swimming velocity. Blood lactate concentration at a standardized speed of 1.50 m/s significantly decreased throughout the season (T1: 10.7 mM; T2: 7.4 mM; T3: 6.2 mM) (Fig. 57–5). A similar result was found for average recovery heart rate (T1: 139 beats/min; T2: 125 beats/min; T3: 122 beats/min). The authors concluded that the adaptations responsible for reduced blood lactate response and reduced heart rate response occur to the greatest extent during the first part of a season of training. They also proposed that the similar findings for both heart rate and lactate indicate that heart rate profiles can be used as a simple and objective way for coaches to monitor their athletes' training progress during a season or across several seasons of training.

Both aerobic power and economy are related to performance ability in competitive swimming and both seem to respond to swimming training, especially at the beginning of a training period or season. Neither aerobic power nor economy seem to change much after the first 8 weeks or so of training, however, based on the studies reviewed earlier in this chapter. Thereafter, the focus of training typically starts to change to incorporate more

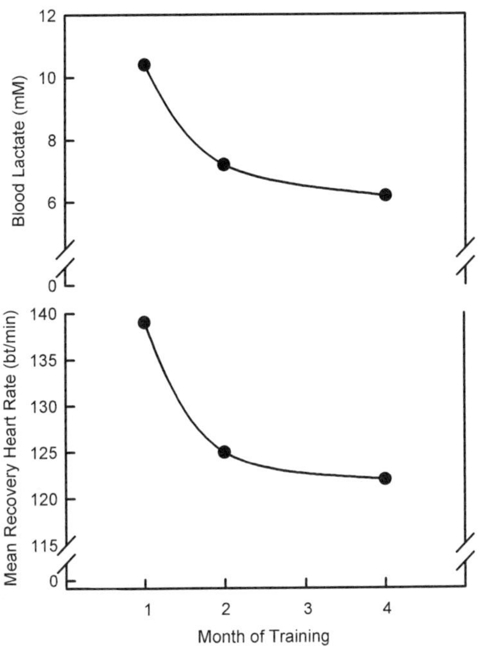

FIG. 57–5. Changes in blood lactate and recovery heart rate responses to standard swimming speed during a season of training. (Adapted from ref. 25.)

high-intensity training designed to develop specific physiologic characteristics thought to be necessary for success in competition, such as anaerobic power, lactate tolerance, and speed-specific economy. Although this basic training model may seem to follow a logical physiologic progression, there is a great risk of developing an overtraining state if the training load is not adjusted to accommodate the extra physiologic stress incurred when high-intensity training bouts are added to the program.

Figure 57–6 shows the training design of a typical college swimming season. According to this model of training, the early-season focus is progressively increasing training volume for development of endurance abilities followed by a shift in training emphasis toward more high-intensity race-specific training. Most coaches will acknowledge that once this change in emphasis is made, the volume of endurance training is reduced but not by a great deal. The reason usually cited by coaches for maintaining a relatively high volume of endurance training during the competitive phase of the season is to maintain the aerobic adaptations created earlier in the season. However, coaches should carefully consider the total physiologic stress placed on the athlete during this part of the training when high-intensity training is added to the endurance training. If training volume is not reduced in proportion to the added stress of high-intensity work, the total training stress may not change, or, at worst, may increase. The combined effect of many weeks of heavy training with little variation in training stress, inclusion of the high-intensity work, and the stresses of frequent competition undoubtedly places these athletes a great risk of developing an overtraining state.

Muscle Strength and Power

Because most competitive swimming races are less than 2 minutes in duration, the ability to generate large amounts of propulsive force and power is generally thought to provide these competitors a performance advantage. Consequently, most competitive swimmers older than about 15 years participate in some kind of resistance training program concurrently with their swimming training. Various modes of resistance training are typically used and include free weights, isokinetic machines, surgical tubing, and even swimming against

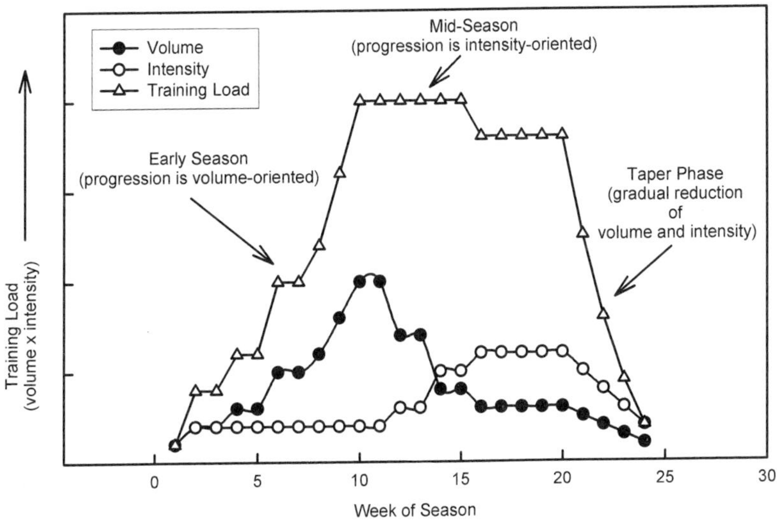

FIG. 57–6. Typical training plan during 24-week season for competitive swimmers. Training load is shown in arbitrary units as product of volume and intensity.

resistance. Often, swimmers use a variety of these modes throughout their season for injury prevention and for performance enhancement.

Research has confirmed that the ability to generate power in a movement-specific manner is closely related to sprint swimming performance (26–30), and that seasonal fluctuations in performances are linked to changes in power abilities (30–35). In 1979 Miyashita and Kaneshisa (28) reported that peak torque of the arm musculature during a simulated swimming arm-pull was significantly related to arms-only performance in the 100-m freestyle. Correlations between peak torque and performance were $r = 0.73$ for males and $r = 0.52$ for females. The swimmers in this study ranged in age from 11 to 21 years and were widely distributed in terms of both strength and performance ability.

We hypothesized that Miyashita and Kaneshisa's findings may have underestimated the role of strength in sprint swimming by using 100-m performance as the dependent variable and by defining strength as peak torque. We felt that sprint swimming performance would be better measured using a shorter time-trial distance and that power might be a more appropriate measure of muscle function than torque for these athletes. With these thoughts in mind, we designed a study similar to Miyashita and Kaneshisa's to define the relationship between upper-body power measured in a movement-specific manner and performance in 22.9-m freestyle (~12 s). Maximal upper-body power was measured during a single double-arm pull mimicking the swimmer's underwater pull. The measurements were made on dry land using a variable-resistance device commonly used by swimmers in their resistance training programs. Like Miyashita and Kaneshisa's study, this study used a heterogeneous sample of swimmers ranging in age from 12 to 20 years. The correlation between sprint performance and maximal arm power was $r = 0.90$. This result was taken as evidence that swimmers are justified in participating in resistance training programs designed to improve maximum power output (29).

Part of the explanation for such high correlations between strength and sprint swimming performance is likely the heterogeneous nature of the subjects used in the studies by Miyashita and Kaneshisa and Sharp and colleagues (29). By using swimmers ranging in age from 12 to 20 years old, any real dependence of sprint performance on strength could be obscured by the fact that older swimmers are more physically mature and tend to have better sprint performance simply because of their physical maturity and longer time in the sport. Logically, one would expect the more mature swimmers to have higher strength and power scores than their younger counterparts. For this reason, the Miyashita and Sharp results are probably biased in favor of high correlations.

Recognizing the potential bias inherent in studies using a heterogeneous population of swimmers, we extended our studies to include elite swimmers participating at the U.S. National Championships in 1982 (30). Because entry time-standards are enforced for qualifying to swim in this meet, the swimmers are relatively homogeneous with respect to their performance. Maximal power was determined on 382 swimmers competing at this meet and correlated with their competitive performances during the meet. No significant correlations were obtained between power and performance in any event for either males or females. However, sprinters (50 to 100 m) were most powerful, middle-distance swimmers (200 to 400 m) were intermediate in power, and distance swimmers (1500 m) were least powerful (Fig. 57–7). These findings confirmed that among a homogeneous population of elite swimmers, dry-land measures of maximum power cannot discriminate among the varied performance abilities.

These studies indicate that the ability to generate power in a movement-specific manner seems to be necessary for top performance. At the elite level, however, power no longer acts as an independent variable in determining one's performance. Perhaps at the elite level, factors such as the ability to apply power to propulsion in the most efficient and effective manner are more related to performance. It is also possible that the power requirements are markedly different among elite swimmers according to the amount of active drag they experience when swimming at competitive speeds. For example, an elite swimmer with a relatively larger active drag would have need for greater power than the swimmer with low active drag just to reach and maintain the same speed. If this is correct, then the ability to measure active drag and improve it would be imperative for our

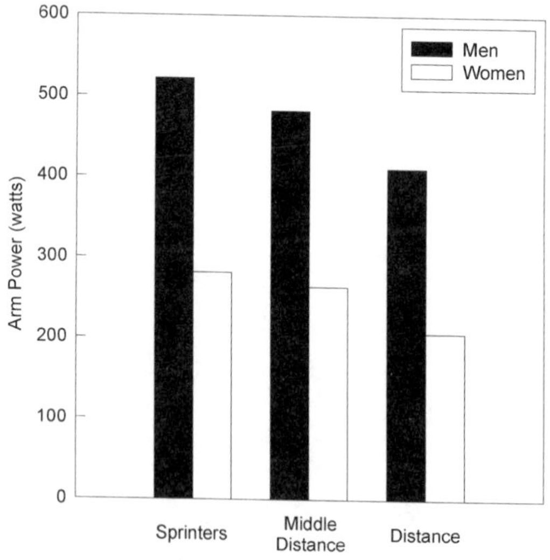

FIG. 57–7. Maximal arm power of competitors at 1982 U.S. National Swimming Championships measured on a Biokinetic Swim Bench. (Adapted from ref. 30.)

understanding the specific training needs of individual swimmers striving to compete at the elite level.

Studies have confirmed that the ability to apply upper-body power during swimming may be more important to performance than either dry-land power or strength. In a study by Costill and colleagues (26), 76 swimmers were tested for dry-land power on a Biokinetic Swim Bench (Biokenetics, Inc., Albany, CA), for maximum sprint speed during 22.9-m freestyle sprint, and for in-water maximum power. The in-water measure of power output was made by tethering the swimmers to a Biokinetic apparatus that measured power output as the swimmer pulled the cable out from the spool while swimming away from the apparatus. The correlation between dry-land power and sprint performance was $r = 0.24$, while the correlation between swimming power and sprint performance was $r = 0.84$. The relatively low correlation between dry-land power and performance was attributed to the fact that the subjects of this study were more homogeneous with respect to power and performance than the subjects used in the earlier studies. More important, the test of swimming power was highly related to performance even in a relatively homogeneous subject population. This finding lends credence to the idea that once some level of performance ability is reached, the ability to apply power to propulsion becomes the more important factor in determining performance.

Changes in Power During Training

The need to develop and maintain the strength and power of swimmers has driven swimming coaches to incorporate resistance training programs throughout the training season. Thus, swimmers train concurrently for endurance and power. Besides the obvious problem of finding the time for all this training, there is the possibility of interference between these two types of training (36). According to this hypothesis, athletes engaged in both resistance training and endurance training may not be able to achieve maximal adaptations in both. Several studies support this contention by providing evidence that power typically declines during periods of heavy swimming training, even when resistance training is continued (17,30,31,37).

We reported that dry-land measures of power output decreased during a season of training in male collegiate swimmers (30). Every 2 weeks throughout one competitive season, the swimmers were tested for maximal power output using a single double-arm pull on the Biokinetic Swim Bench. The largest improvement in power output occurred during the first 6 weeks of the season, as the swimmers gradually increased the volume and intensity of both the swimming training and resistance training. In the next 14 weeks of training, power output gradually decreased by approximately 10% compared with the early-season peak. At this point, the swimmers began a 3-week taper in preparation for their championship competition at the end of the season. The taper phase was characterized by a gradual reduction in both swimming and resistance training. No resistance training was done during the final week of this taper phase. By the end of the 3-week taper phase, the swimmers experienced a significant increase in power output that exceeded even the early-season peak. Interference from endurance training or chronic training fatigue were cited as possible causes of the mid-season slump in power output. The subsequent normalization and supercompensation of power during the taper phase was attributed to recovery from the negative effects of the heavy training load maintained throughout the season.

Using a test of swimming power described earlier in this chapter, Costill and colleagues (32) observed a loss of power and decline in sprinting performance during a 6-week period of training in which swim training volume was increased to approximately 10,000 m/day from 5,000 m/day. Both sprint performance and swimming power were subsequently normalized during the taper period.

The study by Fitts and colleagues (37) provides evidence that the mechanism for the mid-season loss of power output and sprint ability is related to changes in the contractile properties of the muscle. He obtained biopsies from the deltoid muscles of male collegiate swimmers during a 10-day period in which training volume was increased from 4266 to 8200 m/day. The authors noted that the 10 days of intensified training caused a significant reduction in type II muscle fiber size and a significant reduction in the contraction velocity of the type II fibers.

Seasonal fluctuations in muscle power and contractile properties help explain the variations in performance. The improved performance during the following taper period also seems to be related to a recovery and possible supercompensation of these characteristics. The role of shaving body hair and the psychologic effects of taper in enhancing performance after a taper also must be considered, however. Whether the mid-season depression of muscular performance brought about by the heavy swim training (see Fig. 57–6) is necessary to maximize the performance-enhancing effects of the taper is not yet clear. Answering this question will require studies in which coaches allow the training of their swimmers to be manipulated in such a way that strength-endurance interference is avoided and the consequent effects on seasonal variations in performance are measured. Until then, we cannot know if the taper phenomenon is truly a supercompensation or simply a normalization of performance abilities.

CONCLUSION

Competitive swimming performance is a skill-oriented and physiologically challenging sport that requires a careful balance of muscular strength/power and endurance training to achieve optimal results. The large volume of training performed by these athletes seems to have multiple purposes: (a) development of economy, (b) development of aerobic endurance and aerobic power, and (c) development of power. In attempting to maximize each of these capacities, competitive swimmers face an unfortunate training paradox: if they overemphasize one aspect of training, skill and other physiologic capacities needed for optimal performance are sacrificed. Furthermore, the ideal combination of training modes, volume, and intensities is likely quite different among individuals. This point is illustrated by the example of some swimmers whose power output needs to be greater than others just to achieve the same velocity. While scientists continue their quest to gain a clearer understanding of the specific training needs of swimmers, coaches bear the burden of orchestrating the development of these divergent physiologic capacities for the benefit of each individual athlete.

REFERENCES

1. Pendergast DR, DiPrampero P, Craig AB Jr, Rennie DW. Quantitative analysis of the front crawl in men and women. *J Appl Physiol* 1977;43:475–479.
2. Holmer I. Energy cost of arm stroke, leg kick, and the whole stroke in competitive swimming. *Eur J Appl Physiol* 1974;33:105–118.
3. Holmer I. Oxygen uptake during swimming in man. *J Appl Physiol* 1972;33: 502–509.
4. Holmer I. Physiology of swimming man. *Exerc Sports Sci Rev* 1979;7:87–124.
5. Van Handel PJ, Katz A, Morrow JR, Troup JP, Daniels JT, Bradley PW. Aerobic economy and competitive swimming performance of elite U.S. swimmers. In: Ungerechts BE, Wilkie K, Reischle K, eds. *Swimming science*. International series on sports science, vol 18. Champaign, IL: Human Kinetics, 1988:295–303.
6. Chatard J-C, Collomp C, Maglischo E, Maglischo C. Swimming skill and stroking characteristics of front crawl swimmers. *Int J Sports Med* 1990;11:206–211.
7. Costill DL, Kovaleski J, Porter D, Kirwan J, Fielding R, King D. Energy expenditure during crawl swimming: predicting success in middle distance events. *Int J Sports Med* 1985;6:266–270.
8. Klentrou PP, Montpetit RR. Physiologic and physical correlates of swimming performance. *J Swim Res* 1991;7:13–18.
9. Montpetit RR, Lavoie J-M, Cazorla GA. Aerobic energy cost of swimming the front crawl at high velocity in international class and adolescent swimmers. In: Hollander AP, Huijing PA, DeGroot G, eds. *Biomechanics and medicine in swimming*. International series on sports sciences, vol. 14. Champaign, IL: Human Kinetics, 1983:228–234.
10. Smith HK, Montpetit RR, Perrault H. The aerobic demand of backstroke swimming and its relation to body size, stroke technique, and performance. *Eur J Appl Physiol* 1988;58:182–188.
11. Craig AB, Skehan PL, Powelcyzk JA, Boomer WL. Velocity, stroke rate, and distance per stroke during elite swimming competition. *Med Sci Sports Exerc* 1985;17:625–634.
12. Toussaint HM. Differences in propelling efficiency between competitive and triathlon swimmers. *Med Sci Sports Exerc* 1990;22:409–415.
13. Toussaint HM, Van der Helm FCT, Elzerman JR, Hollander AP, DeGroot G, Van Ingen Schenau GJ. A power balance applied to swimming. In: Hollander AP, Huijing PA, DeGroot G, eds. *Biomechanics and medicine in swimming*. International series on sports sciences, vol 14. Champaign, IL: Human Kinetics, 1983:165–172.
14. Sharp RL, Costill DL. Influence of body hair removal on physiological responses during breaststroke swimming. *Med Sci Sports Exerc* 1989;21:576–580.
15. Sherman WM, Maglischo EW. Minimizing athletic fatigue among swimmers: special emphasis on nutrition. In: *Sports science exchange*, vol 4. Barrington, IL: Gatorade Sports Science Institute, 1992:35–39.
16. Trappe TA, Gastaldelli A, Joszi AC, Troup JP, Wolfe RR. Energy expenditure of swimmers during high volume training. *Med Sci Sports Exerc* 1997;29:950–954.
17. Costill DL, Flynn MG, Kirwan JP, et al. Effects of repeated days of intensified training on muscle glycogen and swimming performance. *Med Sci Sports Exerc* 1988;20:249–254.
18. Khosla T. Physique of female swimmers and divers from the 1976 Montreal Olympics. *JAMA* 1984;252:536–537.
19. Lavoie JM, Montpetit RR. Applied physiology of swimming. *Sports Med* 1986;3:165–189.
20. Bradley PW, Troup J, Van Handel P. Pulmonary function measurements in U.S. elite swimmers. *J Swim Res* 1985;1:23–26.
21. Cavanaugh DJ, Musch KI. Arm and leg power of elite swimmers increases after taper as measured by Biokinetic variable resistance machines. *J Swim Res* 1989;5:7–10.
22. Fleck SJ. Body composition of elite American athletes. *Am J Sports Med* 1983;6:398–403.
23. Montpetit RR, Duvallet A, Cazorla G, Smith H. The relative stability of maximal aerobic power in elite swimmers and its relation to training performance. *J Swim Res* 1987;3:15–18.
24. Ryan R, Coyle EF, Quick RW. Blood lactate profile throughout a training season in elite female swimmers. *J Swim Res* 1990;6:5–100.
25. Sharp RL, Vitelli CA, Costill DL. Comparison between blood lactate and heart rate profiles during a season of competitive swim training. *J Swim Res* 1984;1:17–20.
26. Costill DL, Rayfield R, Kirwan J, Thomas R. A computer based system for the measurement of force and power during front crawl swimming. *J Swim Res* 1986;2:16–19.
27. Hawley JA, Williams MM, Vickovic MM, Handcock PJ. Muscle power predicts freestyle swimming performance. *Br J Sports Med* 1992;26:151–155.
28. Miyashita M, Kaneshisa H. Dynamic peak torque related to age, sex, and performance. *Res Q Exerc Sport* 1979;50:249–255.
29. Sharp RL, Troup JP, Costill DL. Relationship between power and sprint freestyle swimming. *Med Sci Sports Exerc* 1982;14:53–56.
30. Sharp RL. Muscle strength and power as related to competitive swimming. *J Swim Res* 1986;2:5–10.
31. Cavanaugh DJ, Musch KI. Arm and leg power of elite swimmers increase after taper as measured by Biokinetic variable resistance machines. *J Swim Res* 1989;5:7–10.
32. Costill DL, Thomas R, Robergs RA, et al. Adaptations to swim training: influence of training volume. *Med Sci Sports Exerc* 1991;23:371–377.
33. Hooper S, MacKinnon L, Wilson B. Biomechanical responses of elite swimmers to staleness and recovery. *Aust J Sci Med Sport* 1995;27:9–13.
34. Houmard JA, Johns RA. Effects of taper on swim performance. Practical implications. *Sports Med* 1994;17:224–232.
35. Johns RA, Houmard JA, Kobe RW, et al. Effects of taper on swim power, stroke distance, and performance. *Med Sci Sports Exerc* 1992;24:1141–1146.
36. Hickson RC. Interference of strength development by simultaneously training for strength and endurance. *Eur J Appl Physiol* 1980;45:255–263.
37. Fitts RH, Costill DL, Gardetto PR. Effect of swim exercise training on human muscle fiber function. *J Appl Physiol* 1989; 66:465–475.

Exercise and Sport Science,
edited by William E. Garrett, Jr., and Donald T. Kirkendall.
Lippincott Williams & Wilkins, Philadelphia © 2000.

CHAPTER 58

Physiology of Racquet Sports

T. Jeff Chandler

Racquet sports are popular around the world. Tennis, squash, racquetball, table tennis, and badminton account for a majority of racquet sports participants. Although more research has been performed on tennis, there are some general similarities among racquet sports. By evaluating the sport-specific demands of each sport and by comparing the demands to research that has been performed on racquet sports, the reader can apply the information in this chapter to specific racquet sports.

Tennis is the most popular of all racquet sports. It is a sport that can be enjoyed by athletes and recreational players of all ages and abilities. Tennis is different from many other competitive sports in that players can continue to compete as they get older, and they can find competition at their level. In the United States, organized tennis begins at a very young age and progresses by age divisions through the entire life span. This chapter discusses racquet sports, primarily tennis, focusing on the physical characteristics of the sport, the physiologic adaptations of the athlete, and the training of the athlete.

The widespread popularity of tennis has also made it a popular sport for analysis by sports scientists. Because tennis, like most racquet sports, is an individual sport, research can focus on specific movement characteristics and metabolic requirements for an individual player. Several organizations, such as the International Tennis Federation, the United States Tennis Association (USTA), and the United States Professional Tennis Registry, have emphasized understanding the biomechanics and physiology of tennis. From this research, we can gather information both on competitive players regarding improving performance, and recreational players regarding the health benefits of playing tennis and other racquet sports.

T. J. Chandler: Department of Exercise Science, Sports, and Recreation, Marshall University, Huntington, West Virginia 25755-2450.

THE SPORT

Tennis is a sport characterized by a variety of demands on the human body, all depending on the level of play, the style of play, and the conditions of play. Tennis, similarly to most racquet sports, requires coordination, agility, speed, quickness, cardiorespiratory endurance, local muscle endurance, strength, and power. Each aspect becomes more important at higher levels of play. Professional players need specific combinations of physical characteristics, while recreational players require some of the same characteristics at different levels.

The physical characteristics of tennis players along with skill levels are the primary determining factors of their ability to play tennis. Other potential factors include strategy and mental toughness. Thus, this chapter discusses aspects of the sport related to the highly competitive tennis player as well as to the recreational tennis player.

The competitive tennis player includes professional tennis players; college tennis players; junior tennis players playing for a state, regional, or national ranking; and other players who regularly play intense competitive tennis, usually for a ranking. The main focus of the competitive tennis player is performance. Competitive tennis players play each point with intensity, play through what they consider to be minor injuries, and perform additional training to improve their fitness level and on court performance. They continue to train to improve tennis performance, even in the face of fatigue and injury.

The recreational tennis player may play tennis either regularly or sporadically and may occasionally play a competitive tournament. Recreational players can still be competitive with their desire to win the matches they play, but they do not focus primarily on competitive tournaments and rankings. Their main focus is to play the game for fun. Both tennis play and additional training are directed more toward improving health rather than enhancing performance. Competition and winning can still be an important part of the game, but the primary benefit of participation is for the health of the individual tennis player.

Even though we refer to several classifications of tennis players, in reality there is a continuum from the professional tennis player to the recreational tennis player, and an individual player can fall anywhere on this continuum. This continuum could also be compared to the ranking of the National Tennis Rating Program (NTRP), where tennis players of all abilities are rated on a scale of 2.0 to 7.0, depending on their playing ability and consistency in hitting specific strokes. This ranking is one method tennis players use to choose opponents at their skill level.

Both competitive and recreational tennis players should be aware of the physical adaptations to repetitive activity, and the potential for repetitive use injuries associated with those adaptations. Just as we are concerned with improving performance, we are also aware of the risks and benefits of tennis play in recreational tennis players. The health and well-being of many racquet sports participants are enhanced by regular participation in that sport.

Physical Requirements

Table 58–1 presents the results of a time study analysis performed on the 1988 U.S. Open's men's and women's final matches (1). These results indicate that a large majority of the points in tennis at the U.S. Open, on a hard surface, were of relatively short duration. Since 1988, points have likely become shorter rather than longer due to several factors. New racquet technology has likely increased service velocity, thus causing an increased incidence of nonreturnable or weak returns of serve. This holds true for both the professional and the recreational players. Also, the serve and volley style of play remains popular, as players like Pete Sampras, Goran Ivanisevic, Richard Krajicek, and Patrick Rafter rise to the top of the sport. As tennis continues to recruit taller and better athletes, point durations will likely remain short unless there are rule changes to the game.

Work/rest intervals in recreational tennis players were reported by Kibler and Chandler (2). In recreational players, there is likely to be a larger variation in work/rest intervals, particularly related to the skill levels of the participants. In the accomplished recreational player, work/rest intervals on clay averaged 15.8/33.6 seconds in females and 16.7/29.2 seconds in males. On a hard court surface, the average work/rest ratio was 14.2/32.5 seconds in females and 12.7/28.4 seconds in males.

TABLE 58–1. *Work/rest intervals measured during the 1988 U.S. Open men's and women's final matches*

Lendl vs. Wilander—men's finals	
Average point	12.2 sec.
Rest between points	28.3 sec.
Rest on out/net serves	12.1 sec.
Rest between games	
With court change	128.2 sec.
Without court change	42.3 sec.
Total points	325
Match time	294 min. (4 hr., 54 min.)
Work/rest interval within games	1:2.3
Overall work/rest interval	1:3.4
Men's finals—summary of point durations	
<10 sec.	59%
10–20 sec.	22%
>20 sec.	19%
Graf vs. Sabatini—women's finals	
Average point	10.8 sec.
Rest between points	16.2 sec.
Rest on out/net serves	10.7 sec.
Rest between games	
With court change	100.1 sec.
Without court change	24.1 sec.
Total points	151
Match time	101 min. (1 hr., 41 min.)
Work/rest interval within games	1:1.5
Overall work/rest interval	1:2.7
Women's finals—summary of point durations	
<10 sec.	62%
10–20 sec.	25%
>20 sec.	13%

Physiologic Requirements

The metabolic demands of the sport of tennis have long been characterized as being approximately 70% alactic anaerobic, 20% lactic anaerobic, and 10% aerobic (3), which varies with the level of play, the length of the points, and the intensity of play. Since tennis play is intermittent, the metabolic pathway of energy production varies depending on specifically what the player is doing at a given moment. Recovery from anaerobic work is performed aerobically, so both aerobic and anaerobic energy systems are a factor in energy production. By evaluating the work/rest interval data, the actual points are generally anaerobic in nature. For the first 10 to 15 seconds of activity, energy is produced using the alactic anaerobic system. From 30 seconds to 2 minutes, energy is produced primarily using the lactic anaerobic system. At approximately 2 minutes, a majority of the energy is produced from aerobic metabolism. Of the three primary energy systems, tennis uses primarily the alactic anaerobic energy system.

Researchers have reported that accomplished tennis players exhibit an aerobic capacity above that of an average individual. Keul and colleagues (4) determined the heart size, oxygen pulse, maximum oxygen uptake, and lactate levels of 44 top-class tennis players using both cycle and treadmill ergometry. Compared to average persons, male tennis players and young male and female tennis players demonstrated increased aerobic capacity and endurance performance. Female tennis players showed insufficient training adaptations and were not different from average females. Kibler and colleagues (5) reported that junior tennis players had increased aerobic capacities above those of average youths, but they did not report sufficient aerobic training to produce that effect. These changes were apparently a result of tennis practice and play rather than aerobic conditioning. Both sprint and interval training have been shown to improve aerobic fitness parameters (6). The sport of tennis can apparently provide an aerobic fitness stimulus if the intensity is high enough and the rest periods remain relatively short.

Another factor to consider in the case of the individual athlete is the difference between playing a doubles match and a singles match. While it is possible that an intensely competitive doubles match could be as strenuous as a singles match, on average singles play is seen to be more intense than doubles play. This is generally true of singles versus doubles play in other racquet sports as well.

Specific physiologic adaptations to racquet sports have been reported in a number of research studies. Undoubtedly, a majority of the research involves tennis, but may be applicable to other racquet sports. Research on the physiologic adaptations of tennis players covers a wide range of variables. One problem in collecting such physiologic data is in simulating competitive match play and allowing for testing without interrupting play.

Vergauwen and colleagues (7) developed a method of evaluating stroke performance in tennis. Match-like physiologic conditions were simulated by using a ball machine to hit balls to unpredictable areas of the court. The player was required to return the ball to the right or left side of the court as determined by a lighted sign. The test consisted of 350 strokes grouped in five "games" of 10 rallies. Quality of play was evaluated by scoring the percentage of errors and by measurements of ball velocity and stroke accuracy.

The effects of age on heart rate (HR) response during a strenuous tennis match have been reported in the literature (8). Ten young women players (age range 15 to 30 years) and 10 veteran players (age range 40 to 51 years) were studied. HRmax, $\dot{V}O_2$ max, and blood lactate at exhaustion were measured in the laboratory. The young players demonstrated significantly higher values on all three laboratory measurements. On the tennis court, heart rate remained steady in the young players, but continued to increase in the veteran players. Six of the veteran women maintained an HR greater than 90% of HRmax obtained in the laboratory for more than 30 minutes. Blood lactate accumulation was low, and could not explain the fatigue.

Hormonal and metabolic changes during a strenuous tennis match were studied by Therminarias and colleagues (9). Nine young female players, mean age 21.2 years, were compared to 10 veteran women players, mean age 46.5 years, all of equal tennis playing ability. Heart rate remained steady in young players but continued to increase during the match in older players, reaching a very high level at the end of the match. Results of all subjects over time indicated there were no changes in plasma lactate and electrolyte concentrations, a large increase in free fatty acids, no increase in epinephrine, a moderate increase in norepinephrine, and large increases in plasma rennin activity and arginine vasopressin concentration. Both age groups lost a similar amount of weight during the matches, but only the veteran players experienced a loss of plasma volume. In this study, it appears that aging was related to changes in plasma volume, which could partially explain the differences in heart rate.

Bergeron and colleagues (10) evaluated the metabolic response of simulated singles tennis play in 10 male Division I players. HR averaged 144.6 beats per minute during 85 minutes of play. Plasma lactate increased 50% during play from a post–warm-up value of 1.6 mmol/L. Blood glucose decreased slightly (8%) during a 10-minute warm-up. After 30 minutes, there was 23% rise in blood glucose, where it remained steady during the remainder of the activity. Plasma cortisol rose significantly (9%) during warm-up, followed by a 40% decrease during the activity. Plasma testosterone rose 22% from preexercise to recovery.

The effect of combined sprint and endurance training on performance on the USTA sport science testing protocol has been reported. Bulbullian and colleagues (11) evaluated the maximal oxygen consumption increased in both the sprint- (43.6 to 45.4 mL/kg/min) and endurance- (45.4 to 49.8 mL/kg/min) trained groups. Treadmill time to exhaustion increased significantly in only the sprint-trained group (sprint, 13.91 to 15.03 minutes; endurance, 15.02 to 15.01 minutes). Isokinetic peak torque demonstrated a trend for improvement at the high testing speed (300 degree/second), suggesting improvement in muscular power specific to the speed of sprint training.

While the recreational tennis player is concerned with performance, it is perhaps more important that tennis provide a training effect and therefore some degree of protection from cardiorespiratory disease. It is likely that tennis does train the cardiorespiratory system to the point where health benefits are received by the participant. This depends to some degree on the fitness level of the player prior to the activity and the intensity of play. In players with high cardiorespiratory fitness, tennis may help to maintain that level, but will not likely improve it. In players with low levels of cardiorespiratory fitness, tennis may improve that level if the intensity of play meets a threshold level.

Bernardi and colleagues (12) measured cardiorespiratory values in middle-level nonprofessional tennis players chosen based on their style of play. Two players were categorized as baseline players, two as attacking players (serve and volley), and three subjects who used both styles of play were categorized as whole-court players. Attacking players attained a mean heart rate of 190 beats/min, baseline players 200 beats/min, and whole-court players 192 beats/min. Attacking players exhibited the highest $\dot{V}O_2max$, expressed in liters per minute, at 5.09 L/min, followed by whole-court players 4.62 L/min, and baseline players 4.55 L/min. Attacking players also demonstrated the highest $\dot{V}O_2max$, expressed in milliliters per kilogram per minute, of 67 mL/kg/min, followed by baseline players at 66 mL/kg/min, and whole-court players at 62 mL/kg/min. The small number of subjects in each group limits any firm conclusions that may be drawn from this study.

The effect of tennis on lipid metabolism and cardiovascular risk was studied by Ferrauti and colleagues (13). In the first phase of the study, eight male and eight female adult recreational tennis players were randomly exposed to both technical tennis training and a running intensive tennis training program. It was determined that the running intensive tennis training program caused a higher cardiopulmonary demand and an increased lypolytic activity and was better accepted by the training subjects. For the second phase of the study, a 6-week training program compared the running intensive tennis program to a control group consisting of 16 non–tennis players (eight men and eight women). Subjects consisted of 22 recreational tennis players—11 males and 11 females. After the 6-week training program, there was a significant decrease in body fat, a significant improvement in anaerobic threshold, and nonsignificant but positive changes in blood lipids. It was concluded that the running intensive tennis training program can be used as an attractive alternative to other health enhancement programs.

Ferrauti and colleagues (14) compared the physiologic profiles of senior golfers to senior tennis players. During cycle ergometry performed on both golf and tennis players prior to the study, tennis players reached a significantly higher power output, and exhibited a higher anaerobic threshold. Age-related norms were not attained by golfers, but were exceeded by 9% in tennis players. Eighteen tennis players, mean age 59.1 years, played singles tennis for 2 hours with approximately 24 minutes of actual playing time. Twenty-one golfers, mean age 60.0 years, played 18 holes of golf in approximately 255 minutes. The net walking time for golf was approximately 90 minutes. Significant differences were found between the physiologic responses to tennis and those to golf. Heart rate, monitored at 15-second intervals, was significantly higher in singles tennis, 137 beats/min compared to a mean heart rate in golf of 103 beats/min. Both lactate (2.3 mmol/L for tennis compared to 1.5 mmol/L for golf) and $\dot{V}O_2$ (60% $\dot{V}O_2$ in tennis compared to 35% $\dot{V}O_2$ for golf) were significantly higher in tennis. Energy consumption per unit of time in golf (0.052 kcal/kg/min) was half the value found in tennis (0.104 kcal/kg/min).

Substrate utilization for performance in tennis is primarily carbohydrate, as is indicated by the work/rest intervals of competitive play. However, there is some evidence that very long, intense, competitive play may cause protein to be used as an energy substrate. Struder and colleagues (15) evaluated amino acid metabolism in tennis. Eight nationally ranked players played under tournament conditions for 4 hours. Branched-chain amino acids decreased by 28% during tennis play. It was determined that branched-chain amino acids are used as energy substrates in long tennis matches. This has important implications for competitive tennis players. Proper nutrition to provide all the amino acids necessary for growth and repair of body tissue is essential.

Bergeron and colleagues (16) studied fluid and electrolyte loss during tennis play in the heat. A majority of the heat generated during tennis play is lost through evaporation. During hot, humid conditions, fluid loss can lead to impairment of cardiovascular and thermoregulatory functions. A player can develop a dangerously high core body temperature and premature fatigue, leading to decreased performance. Extended tennis play in the heat may lead to a net loss of sodium and chloride ions. Under severe conditions, sodium and chloride should be included in the fluid replacement beverage of tennis players.

The physiologic demands of squash were reviewed by Sharp (17). The durations of squash matches were reported to range from 6 minutes to 2 hours and 45 minutes. Rallies ranged from 1.5 seconds minimum to 10 minutes maximum with an approximate 7-second rest period between rallies. Heart rate increased to 80% to 90% of maximum within the first few minutes of play, where it remained throughout the match. Body temperature rose approximately 2° during the first 40 minutes, then more slowly. Blood pressure response was similar to most intermittent physical activities, with an increase in systolic during the first 5 minutes followed by a slow return to preactivity levels during the following 30 to 40 minutes. Diastolic blood pressure fell approximately 10 mm Hg during the same period. Oxygen consumption during squash averaged 32 mL/kg/min for women and 40 mL/kg/min for males. Maximum $\dot{V}O_2$ for top male players is reported in the mid-60s or higher (mL/kg/min), with body fat percentages ranging from 7% to 12%. Maximum $\dot{V}O_2$s for top female squash players were reported in the low to mid-50s (mL/kg/min), with body fat percentages ranging from 18% to 27%. Lactic acid levels for men averaged 3.5 to 10 mmol/L, and less for women.

Sharp proposed "shadow training" or "ghosting" for training squash players. This involves simulating the on-court movements by completing a number of "sets" at 90% maximum intensity with a jogging recovery period between sets. Using this method, training blood lactates approximated the blood lactates seen in the actual squash matches.

Brown and colleagues (18) reported maximum oxygen uptake values in squash players. Values were reported for junior men and women and senior men and women. Senior men (mean age 24.9 years) demonstrated the highest O_2 utilization in liters/minute (4.86 L/min), followed by junior men (mean age 17.7 years) (4.43 L/min), senior women (mean age 25.6 years) (3.50 L/min), and junior women (mean age 16.7 years) (3.14 L/min). The data demonstrate an increased $\dot{V}O_2max$ in senior squash players compared to junior players.

THE ATHLETE

The musculoskeletal system and resultant profile of tennis athletes undergo adaptations primarily based on the frequency and intensity of play. These changes include decreased range of motion (ROM), increased muscle strength, and muscle strength imbalances. A number of studies have measured shoulder ROM in internal and external rotation in tennis. Most studies test in the supine position with 90 degrees of shoulder abduction.

One study measured ROM at the glenohumeral joint of 113 male and 90 female tennis players, ages 11 to 17 (19). Subjects were measured bilaterally in internal and external rotation at 90 degrees of abduction in a supine position. The methodology attempted to isolate glenohumeral motion while minimizing scapulothoracic motion. Results demonstrated a significant decrease in ROM in the dominant arm in internal rotation (males: 45.4 degrees dominant vs. 56.3 degrees nondominant; females: 52.2 degrees dominant vs. 60.3 degrees nondominant) and in total rotation (males: 149.1 degrees dominant vs. 158.2 degrees nondominant; females: 157.4 degrees dominant vs. 164.4 degrees nondominant).

A similar study measured shoulder ROM goniometrically in internal rotation/external rotation (IR/ER) on 86 tennis players and compared the measurements to 139 non–tennis-playing athletes (20). Tennis players were significantly tighter in sit and reach (+2.3 to +6.2 cm), dominant shoulder internal rotation (65 to 74 degrees), and nondominant shoulder internal rotation (76 to 82 degrees). Tennis players were significantly more flexible in dominant shoulder external rotation (110 to 96 degrees) and nondominant shoulder external rotation (103 to 94 degrees). The muscular adaptations that did occur suggest sport-specific ROM adaptations do occur in tennis players, and that flexibility programs should address these adaptations to promote maximum performance and help prevent ROM-related injuries.

Kibler and colleagues (21) reported on the effect of age and years of tournament play on shoulder rotation in 39 elite tennis players who were members of the USTA National Team or touring professional program. Dominant shoulder internal rotation ROM declined with both age and years of tournament play. The under-16 age group was measured with 45.5 degrees of internal rotation ROM compared to 42.3 degrees for the 16- to 18-year-old age group, and 40.3 degrees for the over-18 age group. Dominant shoulder internal rotation with less than 6 years of tournament experience was 50.2 degrees compared to 39.0 degrees in the group with 6 to 9 years of tournament play, and 41.8 degrees in the group with over 9 years of tournament play. The difference between the ROM in the dominant and nondominant shoulder also increased with age and years of tournament play. The loss of internal rotation was determined to be predominant in the dominant shoulder and was primarily related to intense use.

The effect of a conditioning program on several ROM variables was determined in a group of 51 tennis players ranked at the state level or above (22). Baseline ROM measurements were obtained prior to the study, at 1 year, and at 2 years into the study. Subjects were prescribed standard flexibility exercises and recorded their compliance in exercise logs. Mean changes in the ROM in most anatomic areas improved after 1 year of training, with minimal improvements in the second year. Except for forearm supination, there were no differences between high compliers and low compliers. Significant improvement compared to a control group was seen in sit and reach, dominant shoulder internal rotation, nondominant gastrocnemius, dominant and nondominant shoulder external rotation, dominant iliotibial band, dominant and nondominant hip internal rotation, dominant and nondominant hip external rotation, and dominant and nondominant forearm pronation. It was concluded that this particular conditioning program specifically directed toward flexibility was effective in increasing joint ROM in these specific areas.

The strength of the shoulder in internal/external rotation is important to both performance and injury risk of the tennis player. Most published studies use isokinetic dynomometry to measure strength, power, and endurance of the muscles that internally and externally rotate the shoulder. In general, muscle strength imbalances have been found that indicate a relative weakness of the external rotator muscle group of the dominant shoulder compared to the internal rotator muscle group of the dominant shoulder.

Chandler and colleagues (23) studied the concentric

isokinetic strength, power, and endurance in college tennis players. Subjects were significantly stronger at 60 (29.9 to 23.8 foot-pounds) and 300 (20.6 to 16.0 foot-pounds) degrees per second in the dominant arm compared to the nondominant arm. Subjects produced more power in internal rotation at 60 (30.9 to 26.0 foot-pounds) and 300 (99.1 to 80 foot-pounds) degrees per second in the dominant arm. No significant differences were found in external rotation at 60 degrees per second. Ratios of ER/IR muscle balance were significantly different in both peak torque (60.5:70.3) and power (59.5:65.8) at 60 degrees per second but not at 300 degrees per second. By significantly increasing strength in internal rotation without subsequently increasing strength in external rotation, a muscle strength imbalance may occur in the dominant arm with the internal rotators becoming proportionally stronger than the external rotators. This imbalance could be one of the factors that increase the risk of overuse injuries to the shoulder of tennis players.

Ellenbecker (24) studied isokinetic rotator cuff strength in 22 male highly competitive tennis players. Tests were conducted bilaterally for shoulder internal/external rotation, flexion/extension, forearm pronation/supination, and wrist flexion/extension using a Cybex II isokinetic dynamometer. Significantly greater strength ($p < .05$) was found in the dominant arm in shoulder internal rotation, shoulder flexion, wrist flexion, and forearm pronation. Service velocity was measured by a radar gun and with high-speed video. Mean ball velocity on the serve (107.8 mph by radar gun, 117.3 mph by video digitizing) did not correlate with any pattern of isokinetic strength.

Not all isokinetic studies of tennis players indicate muscle imbalances. Codine and colleagues (25) reported on the influence of sports discipline on the balance of rotator cuff muscle capacity measured isokinetically. Tests were performed on seated subjects, with 45 degrees of humeral abduction with movement in the scapular plane at 60, 180, and 300 degrees per second. Strength ratios for nonathletes and runners ranged from 1.3 to 1.5. Tennis players averaged close to 1.5, and baseball players ranged from 1.6 to 2.2. There were no side-to-side differences reported in tennis players in this study. All athletes were said to be "regular competitors in their sport." The level and intensity of play may be the reason no muscle strength imbalance was found.

Strength and endurance of the lower body are important in upper-body activities (26), with the lower body serving as an important part of the kinetic link system. Upper-body activities, as many racquet sports are classified, involve a series of links in the kinetic chain beginning with ground reaction forces. The lower body is an important link, even in upper body sports, and is primarily responsible for the initiation of force development and deceleration of the body. Lower body strength and power measurements, then, are important to racquet sports.

Lower-body isokinetic values have been obtained on junior tennis players (27) for knee flexion/extension. Eighty-seven elite junior players (62 males and 25 females) were tested at speeds of 180 and 300 degrees per second for males and 300 degrees per second for females on a Cybex isokinetic dynamometer. Peak torque and single repetition work were evaluated. No significant differences between the dominant and nondominant extremities were found in either knee flexion or knee extension in males or females. This study determined that, in contrast to the upper body, the lower body exhibits muscular balance in tennis players on side-to-side measures of muscular strength.

General profiling of athletes can be related to performance. Roetert and colleagues (28) attempted to correlate scores on a fitness test with tennis performance in 8- to 12-year-old male and female junior tennis players. The tennis stroke ratings of the tennis players were compared to both the individual players' fitness score and national and/or sectional USTA ranking; 48% of the shared variance in national ranking was explained by the forehand tennis stroke rating. Both sectional and national rankings were positively correlated with stroke ratings (r = 0.57 to 0.68), but the scores for physical tests were not as predictive. Agility was the only physical performance parameter to correlate significantly with rankings, $r = 0.23$, in the players studied.

Kraemer and colleagues (29) reported a sports medicine "profile" of women collegiate tennis players. Thirty-eight non–resistance-trained women from National Collegiate Athletic Association (NCAA) Divisions I and II performed tests including dynamic, isometric, and isokinetic strength; joint laxity and flexibility; speed, agility, power, and power endurance; oxygen consumption; body composition; and ball velocity of the serve, forehand, and backhand. No single measurement correlated strongly with performance. Knee flexion and knee extension, both isometric and isokinetic, were most highly correlated with ball velocity ($r = 0.88$). Isometric measures of shoulder internal and external rotation were moderately correlated to ball velocity ($r = 0.54$). Finally, the military press was moderately correlated to ball velocity ($r = 0.69$). Muscle strength imbalances were reported between the dominant and nondominant shoulders in internal rotation, with the dominant shoulder being 38% stronger than the nondominant shoulder in internal rotation. Isometric strength imbalances at the elbow were reported in both elbow flexion and extension between the dominant and nondominant arms. Grip strength was significantly different between the dominant (33.0 kg) and nondominant (26.4 kg) hands.

Bone mass is another physical characteristic that can be modified with participation in sports. The bone mass in the dominant arm of female tennis and squash players was related to the age of starting physical activity in a study by Kannus and colleagues (30). The dominant to nondominant side difference in bone density was significantly greater in players compared to controls in all anatomic sites measured. The dominant side demonstrated increased bone density ranging from 8.5% to 16.2% in players compared to 3.2% to 4.6% in controls. Girls who began playing before menarche demonstrated at least two times greater increases in bone density than players who began after menarche. This study demonstrates the importance of physical activity at a young age, and that both tennis and squash at a young age have a positive effect on bone density.

To study sport-specific demands of and physical adaptations to tennis, a systematic musculoskeletal evaluation program should be employed (31). By continuing to evaluate these musculoskeletal adaptations to repetitive intense use, we can better understand the role these adaptations play in injury risk. Due to the nature of the sport, it is relatively easy to study strength and ROM in the sport of tennis. Future studies should analyze this information in terms of injuries and other health-related parameters.

Musculoskeletal Adaptations and Injury Risk

Tennis and other racquet sports place the participant at a high risk of overuse injury as a result of the physiologic musculoskeletal adaptations that occur with regular intense tennis participation. Many studies define injury in terms of days lost to practice or competition. In tennis and other racquet sports, participants often continue to play or practice despite an injury that alters play. It is important, therefore, that injury studies in racquet sports consider overuse injuries that do not necessarily cause a cessation of play.

The musculoskeletal adaptations seen in the competitive tennis player may be factors that lead to this type of injury. Kibler and colleagues (32) reported injury incidence and the results of fitness testing in junior elite players. Injury was defined as a condition that arose from playing tennis, caused an alteration in playing level or performance, or caused a cessation of playing that lasted 5 or more days. A large majority of the injuries were of the overload variety (61 overload, 29 traumatic). The percentage of injuries related to overuse did not differ between males (32 overload injuries, 15 traumatic injuries) and females (29 overload injuries, 14 traumatic injuries). Furthermore, in evaluating injuries to the upper body (shoulder, elbow, and wrist), 20 of 21 injuries were related to overuse. More male tennis players scored poorly on the flexibility tests (sit and reach and goniometric ROM testing), and more female athletes scored poorly on the strength and power tests (vertical jump, sit-ups, push-ups, and grip strength).

Winge and colleagues (33) studied the incidence of injuries in 104 randomly chosen competitive elite tennis players. The definition of injury included all injuries that bothered the athlete, not just those seen by a physician. Injuries were self-reported on a standardized form. There were 2.3 injuries/player/1000 hours of participation; 67% of the injuries were classified as overuse injuries. Males (0.64 injuries/player/season) were injured more frequently than females (0.20 injuries/player/season).

Injury data presented in the USTA's "Complete Conditioning for Tennis" (34) indicate that a majority of injuries to intensely trained junior players occur in the back (24%) and the shoulder (21%). Injuries were equally well distributed in other anatomic locations (foot, 19%; knee, 15%; ankle, 12%; and elbow, 12%). In professional players, the USTA reports that the elbow was the number one area of complaint from players at the 1995 U.S. Open tennis championship.

One of the major goals of the conditioning program for tennis players should be to prevent or lessen the severity of common overuse tennis injuries. Currently, the popular belief is that this can be accomplished by correcting the musculoskeletal deficits in strength and ROM, and by building a good general strength, flexibility, and power base in the tennis athlete. For more information on injuries to participants in racquet sports, the reader is referred to Chapter 38.

Nutritional Aspects and Ergogenic Aids in Tennis Play

Nutritional substances and ergogenic aids could logically be used to improve performance in racquet sports. Recent studies have been reported using caffeine and carbohydrate drinks. Since the sport of tennis involves high-intensity work, strength, and power, anabolic steroids could potentially be used to improve performance by building strength and power or aiding in recovery.

Ferrauti and Weber (35) reported on the metabolic responses of caffeine ingestion relative to tennis performance. Caffeine may increase the availability of glycogen by increasing the oxidation of lipids. This could improve performance, particularly in a fatigued state, since the nervous system depends on carbohydrate for fuel. In tennis, this could improve hitting accuracy, running speed/agility, and overall playing success. In men players, compared to a placebo condition, games won and hitting accuracy did not improve with a 150-mL solution every 15 minutes containing 130 mg caffeine per liter. Women players on the caffeine condition, consisting of 100 mL of the same beverage taken every 15 minutes, won more games and achieved a better hitting accuracy compared to the placebo condition. The women players also reported a higher "energetic drive" during the last hour of play under the caffeine condition. There were no significant differences between men and women on blood glucose concentrations in the placebo versus caffeine conditions. After 180 minutes of tennis play, subjects were given a 30-minute break. During this break, the blood glucose in the caffeine condition recovered to a significantly higher level and was maintained at a higher level throughout the remainder of the test (270 minutes).

One tennis study evaluated the effect of a carbohydrate beverage on performance and fluid balance during prolonged competitive play (36). Twelve competitive players performed 2- to 3-hour matches after ingesting either a 7.5-g, 100-mL carbohydrate solution or a water placebo. Performance measurements obtained before and after each match included service velocity and a 183-m shuttle run. Blood samples were taken and analyzed for plasma volume and blood glucose. Carbohydrate ingestion led to a significantly increased blood glucose level but no significant changes in plasma volume. Therefore, carbohydrate is effective in maintaining blood glucose but has no effect on plasma volume. Although blood glucose was increased, there was no significant effect on either service velocity or shuttle run time.

In a recent study on tennis performance, Vergauwen and colleagues (37) reported on the effect of carbohydrate supplementation and carbohydrate-caffeine supplementation on stroke performance and anaerobic performance. Well-trained tennis players were tested using the Leuven Tennis Performance Test and a shuttle run both before and after a 2-hour strenuous training session. Subjects were tested on three occasions, where they were provided, in a double-blind manner, either a placebo drink, a carbohydrate (CHO) drink [0.7g CHO/kg body weight (BW)/h], or a carbohydrate plus caffeine (5 mg/kg BW) drink. Pretest scores were similar in the placebo and carbohydrate conditions. During the placebo condition, significantly decreased performance scores were obtained on first serves, strokes during defensive rallies, and the shuttle run. Comparing the carbohydrate condition to the placebo condition, the decrease in performance of the first serve was significantly less using the carbohydrate drink. Shuttle run performance was improved in the carbohydrate condition. Stroke performance and shuttle run times were similar for the carbohydrate and carbohydrate plus caffeine conditions.

The effect of carbohydrate ingestion on shot accuracy in squash has also been investigated (38). Eight club-level players accustomed to high levels of exertion served as subjects for the study. Participants played three simulated games of squash while consuming calibrated amounts of a commercially available glucose polymer energy beverage. The first accuracy test was performed after a 5-minute warm-up. The second was performed immediately after simulated game 3. Tests were performed blindly relative to placebo and carbohydrate conditions. Mean scores for the carbohydrate trials were 62.6 for the pretest and 60.6 for the posttest. Mean scores for the placebo trial were 59.1 for the pretest and 47.6 for the posttest. Mean heart rate scores were nonsignificant for both placebo and carbohydrate trials, with a trend toward increasing heart rates with an increasing number of games in both conditions. These results suggest that the glucose polymer beverage was effective in improving accuracy scores after three simulated games of squash.

Anabolic steroid medications could possibly be used in racquet sports to enhance performance. Although no studies to date have been published in this area, there are two primary mechanisms by which performance enhancement could occur. The first is by increasing the ability of the athlete to produce power. Second, anabolic steroids could allow the athlete to train harder by facilitating recovery, and possibly by increasing aggression. These medications are illegal when used to enhance performance, and their use is discouraged. Drug testing has been implemented at different levels of performance to discourage their use. Two over-the-counter substances that are related to increasing testosterone levels are dehydroepiandrosterone (DHEA) and androstenedione. These substances are precursor hormones either once removed (androstenedione) or twice removed (DHEA) from testosterone. Both substances can be converted by the liver to testosterone, androstenedione more readily than DHEA. While these substances might have a positive effect on performance in tennis, they are an artificial means of doing so. Also, the safety of either drug over the long term has not been established.

TRAINING THE ATHLETE

There are a number of published articles and books on conditioning for racquet sports (34,39–43). Each of these publications adds specific information to the literature regarding training for racquet sports. Here, the training plan for the tennis athlete will be to defined in terms of a yearly plan. The theoretical concept of periodization states that maximum performance is cyclical; by manipulating the volume and intensity of training, we can promote maximum performance at the appropriate time.

The Season

One problem in planning training programs for tennis players is the lack of a defined off-season. Tennis is a sport without seasons at most levels of play. When planning conditioning programs for tennis players, seasonal variation must be built into the program for maximum results to occur. The season for elite tennis players depends on the level of play and individual strengths or weaknesses.

For the top professional tennis players, the season is generally built around the four major grand slam tournaments. These tournaments are in January, May, June, and September. Most professional players want to peak physically at these times. Young professionals without a high ranking may plan their schedule to peak at some of the less important tournaments. A top-20 professional would have a different plan for conditioning than a satellite player. As players improve, they can choose to peak for the more important tournaments.

At the college level, both fall and spring seasons occur in most divisions. The fall season is often considered an "indoor" season. At the NCAA Division I level, the fall season ends with an indoor championship, and the spring season ends with an outdoor championship. Collegiate tennis players may choose to have two major peaks in their schedule to coincide with the fall and spring seasons. This is an important difference in the plan for the collegiate athlete and the professional athlete. College players will play two 3-month seasons, and will peak for the last 3 weeks of both seasons. Professional players in our sample program peak for 2 to 3 weeks around each of the four major tournaments.

Elite junior tennis players play tennis year round, with a major emphasis on summer tournaments. The most important junior tournament is played between Christmas and New Year's Day, however. The scheduling of tournaments plays a large role in the periodization plan for the individual athlete. Often athletes' schedules change, depending on how well they do in qualifying tournaments.

The in-season for tennis players is the time when on-court play is high. The time available for a conditioning program during the in-season phase is short. A training plan must be developed that can be integrated with this high demand for court time without overtraining the athlete. This is usually accomplished by performing a majority of the conditioning exercises in the early part of the season, devoting the in-season to skill and maintenance of conditioning.

Sport-Specific Training

Sport-specific training for tennis is important in two distinctive areas: musculoskeletal training and metabolic training. Sport-specific training for the musculoskeletal system should be directed toward general strength and flexibility training for the demands of the sport, as well as specific anatomic areas that have been determined through research to be under high stress in the sport of tennis. Research studies mentioned previously point to specific anatomic areas that should be included in the conditioning program both in terms of ROM and strength.

Training the metabolic system for tennis involves building an adequate base of cardiorespiratory fitness, then gradually moving toward interval training using sport-specific work/rest intervals at sport-specific intensities. It should be noted that the cardiorespiratory fitness base can be built by using purely interval training, which is more sport specific for tennis athletes. At the same time, for variety, long, slow, distance training can be a part of the early training program. Long, slow, distance training should be limited to the earliest phases of training, as it is not mechanically or metabolically specific to actual tennis play and it may interfere with strength and power development (29). Long, slow, distance training has a place, even in training for tennis, but it should generally be limited to athletes in the preparatory phase of training, athletes with a poor aerobic base, or athletes who need to lose body fat.

Supplemental Training

Supplemental training for the individual tennis player should be based on specific deficiencies in the musculoskeletal base of the individual athlete as determined by a preparticipation evaluation of strength and ROM. A good preparticipation evaluation will focus on the musculoskeletal areas that are under high load during practice and play. A history of previous injuries is also important to consider in planning supplemental training. An athlete with a muscle strength imbalance in IR/ER should perform isolated strengthening exercises to correct this imbalance. The player with significantly decreased ROM in dominant internal rotation should spend time working to normalize that deficiency. This type of supplemental training is performed mostly in the in-season, as that is when these maladaptations occur and perhaps worsen. That is also when the athlete is at the highest risk of injury and decreased performance related to these specific maladaptations.

Periodization of Training

Periodization of training for tennis players and other racquet sports participants depends on the individual player's needs and level of play. Sample periodization programs will be presented for the professional player, the elite junior player, and the competitive recreational player. Periodization is simply a plan for conditioning. Periodized training manipulates the variables of intensity and volume to promote maximum benefits from training and to increase the chances that athletes will reach their maximum level of performance at the appropriate time.

Periodization programs are generally divided into four parts: the preparatory phase, the precompetitive phase, the competitive phase, and active rest. Each phase has specific characteristics, and the racquet sport athlete will work on different aspects of conditioning as well as have different goals for on-court training. It is important to periodize the on-court time as well, since it is the total volume of physical activity that must be controlled to prevent possible overtraining. For racquet sports, it is most logical to periodize for a 1-year block of time, or macrocycle.

A sample periodization macrocycle is presented in Table 58–2 for a professional tennis player, a junior elite tennis player, and a competitive recreational player. The actual program for these athletes would vary depending on the individual needs of the player. The professional

TABLE 58–2. *Sample periodization macrocycle for professional tennis player, elite junior tennis player, and recreational tennis player*

Week no.	Professional	Elite junior	Recreational
1	Precompetitive	Active rest	Precompetitive
2	Competitive	Active rest	(Precomp) League
3	(Comp) Australian Open	Active rest	(Precomp) League
4	(Comp) Australian Open	Active rest	(Precomp) League
5	Active rest	Preparation	(Precomp) League
6	Active rest	Preparation	(Precomp) League
7	Preparation	Preparation	(Precomp) League
8	Preparation	Preparation	(Precomp) League
9	Preparation	Preparation	(Precomp) League
10	Preparation	Preparation	(Comp) League
11	Preparation	Preparation	(Comp) League
12	Preparation	Preparation	Active rest
13	Prepreparation	(Prep) Easter Bowl	Active rest
14	Prepreparation	Preparation	Preparation
15	Prepreparation	Precompetitive	Preparation
16	Prepreparation	Precompetitive	Preparation
17	Prepreparation	Precompetitive	Preparation
18	Competitive	Precompetitive	Precompetitive
19	(Comp) French Open	Precompetitive	Precompetitive
20	(Comp) French Open	Precompetitive	Precompetitive
21	Prepreparation	Competitive	Competitive
22	Prepreparation	(Comp) State Closed	(Comp) Club Tournament
23	Competitive	Prepreparation	Precompetitive
24	(Comp) Wimbledon	Competitive	Precompetitive
25	(Comp) Wimbledon	(Comp) Sectionals	Precompetitive
26	Active rest	Prepreparation	(Comp) Tournament
27	Preparation	Competitive	Precompetitive
28	Preparation	(Comp) State Open	Precompetitive
29	Preparation	Active rest	Precompetitive
30	Preparation	Preparation	Precompetitive
31	Prepreparation	Preparation	(Comp) Tournament
32	Prepreparation	Preparation	Precompetitive
33	Prepreparation	Preparation	Precompetitive
34	Prepreparation	Preparation	Precompetitive
35	Competitive	Preparation	Competitive
36	(Comp) U.S. Open	Precompetitive	(Comp) Club Tournament
37	(Comp) U.S. Open	Precompetitive	Active rest
38	Active rest	Precompetitive	Active rest
39	Active rest	Precompetitive	Active rest
40	Active rest	Precompetitive	Active rest
41	Active rest	Precompetitive	Active rest
42	Preparation	Precompetitive	Active rest
43	Preparation	Precompetitive	Preparation
44	Preparation	Precompetitive	Preparation
45	Preparation	Precompetitive	Preparation
46	Preparation	Precompetitive	Preparation
47	Preparation	Precompetitive	Active rest
48	Prepreparation	Precompetitive	Preparation
49	Prepreparation	Precompetitive	Preparation
50	Prepreparation	Competitive	Preparation
51	Prepreparation	Competitive	Preparation
52	Prepreparation	(Comp) Orange Bowl	Preparation

Note: Additional tennis tournaments will be included based on the individual player's schedule, but the training program should not be modified for those tournaments.

tennis player in this sample program wants to peak at the four major grand slam tournaments.

The junior player in this sample program is spending the first 3 months of the year in a preparation phase. Young athletes may need an extended preparation phase to build a good strength and endurance base. The player may choose to play in some tournaments during the early part of the year, but the conditioning program will not change for the tournaments. This is a situation that will be faced often in junior tennis players. The question the athlete is faced with is, "Where do I need to be physically 3 to 5 years from now?" By placing an emphasis on physical training during a portion of the yearly plan, it is hoped the athlete will be a better tennis player 3 to 5 years down the road.

The recreational adult player in our sample program plays in a 10-week winter league, two club tournaments, and a couple of other tournaments during the summer. Since one of the primary goals of the recreational player is general health and fitness, this player is scheduled for additional weeks of "active rest," which for this player means cross-training using other activities to improve health and fitness.

Preparation Phase

In the preparation phase, the athlete should build a general fitness base including the aerobic base, the strength base, and general flexibility. The athlete has several choices on how to build the aerobic base for racquet sports, including interval training. The length of the preparation phase depends on the needs of the individual athlete, but it should last a minimum of 4 weeks for the proper adaptations to occur. A young athlete who is in the developmental stages of strength and aerobic conditioning may spend 8 to 12 weeks in the preparation phase. The advanced athlete may spend 4 weeks. In one macrocycle, the athlete may use two or more preparation phases depending on the number of mezocycles the athlete will go through during the year. Resistance training consisting of high-volume moderate-intensity training does build an anaerobic base. On-court practice sessions during the preparation phase should concentrate on hitting basic strokes and making changes in stroke mechanics. It would also be appropriate to develop new shots during this phase. General movement and footwork drills are appropriate. Because the volume and intensity of off-court training is moderately high, the volume and intensity of on-court training should be moderate as well.

Precompetitive Phase

The precompetitive phase is a time for the conditioning exercises to become more sport-specific. Aerobic training should move toward anaerobic training, which would include interval training in sport-specific work/rest intervals and intensities. Movement speed may increase during strength training, since the movement speeds are high in most racquet sports. The general intensity of resistance training increases, causing an increase in power output. Sport-specific movement and footwork drills are used. Plyometric exercises are incorporated into the training program. On-court drills during the precompetitive phase are at a high volume and include practice matches and simulated points to prepare the athlete for competition. During the precompetitive phase, sport-specific musculoskeletal adaptations are likely to occur due to the high volume of on-court training.

Competitive (Peaking) Phase

The competitive phase should be reserved for major competitions where athletes wants to perform at their best. True physiologic peaks can only be maintained for 2 to 3 weeks. By using various microcycle training routines, the athlete may be able to sustain a peak for longer periods of time. During the competitive phase, athletes generally perform only a very low volume of weight training, movement training, and plyometric training. The training that is performed is high intensity but very low volume. On-court training consists primarily of short-duration high-intensity tennis play.

Active Rest Phase

The active rest phase is a time for the intensely competitive player to take a break from playing tennis while remaining physically active. It is important to remain active during this phase to prevent detraining. The player may perform resistance training at low volumes and intensities. The player may choose to cross-train using such activities as jogging, soccer, basketball, and golf. In most cases, the active rest phase will range from 1 to 3 weeks, but this may vary depending on the individual needs of the athlete. It is possible that an athlete who is tired and exhibiting signs of overtraining could benefit from a 3-to 5-day period of active rest during another phase of training. The recreational player can use the active rest phase as a time to rest from tennis and train using other modes of exercise with health-related benefits.

The Professional Tennis Player

The professional tennis player (Table 58–3) has 12 weeks in the competitive or peaking phase, compared to 9 for the elite junior player (Table 58–4) and 9 for the recreational adult player (Table 58–5). Keep in mind that the stated length of the competitive phase is the goal, assuming the player continues to win in tourna-

TABLE 58–3. *Professional tennis player*

Active rest—jog, play golf, play soccer, light resistance training
Preparation phase—resistance training 3 × wk, 3–5 sets of strengthening exercises, abdominal exercises, movement training/plyometrics—20–30 minutes training 3 × wk, interval running 3 × wk
Precompetitive phase—resistance training 3 × wk, 2–3 sets, movement training/plyometrics—15 minutes 2–3 × wk, sprint running 2 × wk, general flexibility exercises 6 × wk, sport-specific supplemental strength and flexibility training 5 × wk
Competitive phase—very short high-intensity on-court training, resistance training, movement/plyometric training

TABLE 58–4. *Junior elite tennis player*

Active rest—jog, play soccer, light resistance training
Preparation phase—resistance training 3 × wk, 3–5 sets of free weight or machine strengthening exercises, abdominal exercises, movement training/plyometrics—20–30 minutes training 3 × wk, interval running 3 × wk
Precompetitive phase—resistance training 3 × wk, 2–3 sets, movement training/plyometrics—15 minutes 2–3 × wk, sprint running 2 × wk
Competitive phase—very short high-intensity on-court training, resistance training, movement/plyometric training

TABLE 58–5. *Competitive recreational tennis player*

Active rest—jog, play golf, play basketball
Preparation phase—resistance training 3 × wk, 3–5 sets of moderate-intensity strengthening exercises, abdominal exercises, 3 × 8, movement training—15 minutes interval movement training 3 × wk.
Precompetitive phase—resistance training 3 × wk, 2–3 sets, sprint training with footwork, 10 minutes 2 × wk
Competitive phase—general and sport-specific flexibility training; little or no resistance training

ments. When the player is eliminated from a tournament, then a decision should be made about the training schedule for the remainder of the week. The player may need to go into a short (2- to 3-day) active rest phase or may begin the training cycle for the following week early.

The Junior Elite Tennis Player

Junior tennis players deal with perhaps more variables than the professional players. They are growing, and their strokes are still developing in terms of tennis skill. Many times, the most important decision to make with the junior player is whether to focus on tournament play and winning, or whether to focus on developing solid strokes and a solid fitness base. In many cases, developing a solid base should be the main goal, but it is surpassed for the sake of "winning now." Note that in the sample program in Table 58–2, the player is playing in an Easter tournament but is not changing his training schedule to do so.

The Recreational Tennis Player

The primary focus of the recreational tennis player is improving health and having fun. Tennis is an excellent sport to accomplish both goals. In the periodization plan, recreational tennis players are recommended to spend additional weeks in the active rest phase, which is simply another way of stating they should cross-train with other enjoyable activities.

CONCLUSION

Tennis is an excellent sport for a lifetime of fitness, competition, and enjoyment. Tennis is a relatively easy sport to research, since it is an individual sport. Physiologic adaptations to tennis are easier to track than in team sports, where the adaptations may depend on the position of the player, among other factors. With proper training, tennis can provide an individual with positive physiologic adaptations that improve general fitness as well as the quality of life. However, playing tennis for too long a time or without adequate preparation can cause negative physiologic adaptations, primarily to the musculoskeletal system. These adaptations may increase the risk of musculoskeletal overuse injuries in tennis players. So the general recommendation should be, "Get fit for tennis, then use tennis to stay fit, or move to the next level of fitness."

Other racquet sports have been studied, but generally not to the same extent as tennis. In many cases, the results of studies on tennis players can be extrapolated to other racquet sports athletes. This depends, of course, on how specific the sport is to tennis, both mechanically and metabolically. Many of the positive health adaptations noted in tennis players apply to other racquet sports athletes. In the instances where mechanical and metabolic specificity is not specific to tennis, additional research on those racquet sports may be required.

REFERENCES

1. Chandler TJ. Work/rest intervals in world class tennis. *Tennis Pro* 1991;3:4.
2. Kibler WB, Chandler TJ. *Racquet sports.* Baltimore: Williams and Wilkins, 1995:531–550.
3. Fox EL, Mathews DK. *Interval training.* Philadelphia: WB Saunders, 1974.
4. Keul J, Berg G, Huber A, et al. Circulatory and metabolic adaptation of tennis players, *Herz Kreislauf* 1982;7:373–381.
5. Kibler WB, McQueen C, Uhl T. Fitness evaluations and fitness findings in competitive junior tennis players. *Clin Sports Med* 1988;7:403–416.

6. Bulbullian R, Chandler J, Amos M. The effect of sprint and endurance supplemental training on aerobic and anaerobic measures of fitness. *J Strength Conditioning Res* 1996;10:51–55.
7. Vergauwen L, Spaepen J, Lefevre J, Hespel P. Evaluation of stroke performance in tennis. *Med Sci Sports Exerc* 1998;30:1281–1288.
8. Therminarias A, Dansou P, Chirpaz-Oddou M-F, Quirion A. Effects of age on heart rate response during a strenuous match of tennis. *J Sports Med Phys Fitness* 1990;30:389–396.
9. Therminarias A, Danson P, Chirpaz-Oddou M-F, Gharib C, Quirion A. Hormonal and metabolic changes during a strenuous tennis match. Effect of aging. *Int J Sports Med* 1991;12:10–16.
10. Bergeron MF, Maresh CM, Kraemer WJ, Abraham A, Conroy B, Gabaree C. Tennis: physiological profile during match play. *Int J Sports Med* 1991;12:474–479.
11. Bulbullian R, Chandler J, Amos M. The effect of sprint and endurance supplemental training on aerobic and anaerobic measures of fitness. *J Strength Conditioning Res* 1996;10:51–55.
12. Bernardi M, De Vito G, Falvo ME, et al. Cardiorespiratory adjustment in middle-level tennis players: are long term cardiovascular adjustments possible? In: Lees A, Maynard I, Hughes M, Reilly T, eds. *Science and racket sports,* vol 2. London: E & F Spon, 1998:20–26.
13. Ferrauti A, Weber K, Struder HK. Effects of tennis training on lipid metabolism and lipoprotein in recreational players. *Br J Sports Med* 1997;31:322–327.
14. Ferrauti A, Weber K, Struder HK, Predel G, Rost R. Tennis versus golf: profile of demands and physical performance in senior players. In: Lees A, Maynard I, Hughes M, Reilly T, eds. *Science and racket sports,* vol 2. London: E & F Spon, 1998:27–33.
15. Struder HK, Hollman W, Duperly MD, Weber K. Amino acid metabolism in tennis and its possible influence on the neuroendocrine system. *Br J Sports Med* 1995;29:28–30.
16. Bergeron MF, Armstrong LE, Maresh CM. Fluid and electrolyte losses during tennis in the heat. *Clin Sports Med* 1995;14:23–31.
17. Sharp NCC. Physiological demands and fitness for squash. Science and Racket Sports II. 1998. Lees, A, Maynard, ,I, Hughes, M, Reilly, T, E & F Spon, London, 3–13.
18. Brown, D, Weigand, DA, Winter, EM. Maximum oxygen uptake in junior and senior elite squash players. In: Lees A, Maynard I, Hughes M, Reilly T, eds. *Science and racket sports,* vol 2. London: E & F Spon, 1998:14–19.
19. Ellenbecker TS, Roetert EP, Piorkowski PA, Schultz DA. Glenohumeral joint internal and external rotation range of motion in elite junior tennis players. *J Sports Phys Ther* 1996;24:336–341.
20. Chandler TJ, Kibler WB, Uhl TL, et al. Flexibility comparisons of junior elite tennis players to other athletes. *Am J Sports Med* 1990;18:134–135.
21. Kibler WB, Chandler TJ, Livingston BP, et al. Shoulder range of motion in elite tennis players, effect of age and years of tournament play. *Am J Sports Med* 1996;24:1–7.
22. Kibler WB, Chandler TJ. Changes in range of motion in junior tennis players participating in an injury risk modification conditioning program. *Am J Sports Med*
23. Chandler TJ, Kibler WB, Stracener EC, et al. Shoulder strength, power, and endurance in college tennis players. *Am J Sports Med* 1992;20:455–458.
24. Ellenbecker TS. A total arm strength isokinetic profile of highly skilled tennis players. *Isokinet Exerc Sci* 1991;1:9–21.
25. Codine P, Bernard PL, Pocholle, et al. Influence of sports discipline on shoulder rotator cuff balance. *Med Sci Sports Exerc* 1997;29:1400–1405.
26. Kibler WB, Chandler TJ. Baseball and tennis. In: Hunter-Griffin L, ed. *The Knee.*
27. Ellenbecker TS, Roetert EP. Concentric isokinetic quadricep and hamstring strength in elite junior tennis players. *Isokinet Exerc Sci* 1995;5:3–5.
28. Roetert EP, Garrett GE, Brown, et al. Performance profiles of nationally ranked junior tennis players. *J Appl Sports Sci Res* 1992;6:225–231.
29. Kraemer WJ, Triplett NT, Fry, et al. An in-depth sports medicine profile of women college tennis players. *J Sports Rehabil* 1995;4:79–98.
30. Kannus P, Haapasalo H, Sankelo M, et al. Effect of starting age of physical activity on bone mass in the dominant arm of tennis and squash players. *Ann Intern Med* 1995;123:27–31.
31. Kibler WB, Chandler TJ, Uhl TL, et al. A musculoskeletal approach to the preparticipation physical examination. Preventing injury and improving performance. *J Sports Med* 1989;17:525–531.
32. Kibler WB, McQueen C, Uhl T. Fitness evaluations and fitness findings in competitive junior tennis players. *Clin Sports Med* 1988;7:403–416.
33. Winge S, Jorgensen U, Lassen Nielsen A. Epidemiology of injuries in Danish championship tennis. *Int J Sports Med* 1989;10:368–371.
34. United States Tennis Association. *Complete conditioning for tennis.* Champaign, IL: Human Kinetics, 1998.
35. Ferrauti A, Weber K. Metabolic responses and performance in tennis after caffeine ingestion. In: Lees A, Maynard I, Hughes M, Reilly T, eds. *Science and racket sports,* vol 2. London: E & F Spon, 1998.
36. Mitchell JB, Cole KJ, Grandjean PW, et al. The effect of a carbohydrate beverage on tennis performance and fluid balance during prolonged tennis play. *J Appl Sport Sci Res* 1992;6:96–102.
37. Vergauwen L, Brouns F, Hespel P. Carbohydrate supplementation improves stroke performance in tennis. *Med Sci Sports Exerc* 1998;30:1289–1295.
38. Graydon J, Taylor S, Smith M. The effect of carbohydrate ingestion on shot accuracy during a conditioned squash match. In: Lees A, Maynard I, Hughes M, Reilly T, eds. *Science and racket sports,* vol 2. London: E & F Spon, 1998:68–76.
39. Chandler TJ. Exercise training for tennis. *Clin Sports Med* 1995;14:33–46.
40. Chandler TJ, Conditioning for tennis. In: Lees A, Maynard I, Hughes M, Reilly T, eds. *Science and racket sports,* vol 2. London: E & F Spon, 1998:77–85.
41. Chu D. *Power training for tennis.* Champaign, IL: Human Kinetics.
42. Kibler WB, Chandler TJ. Sport specific conditioning. *Am J Sports Med* 1994;22:424–432.
43. Lees A, Maynard I, Hughes M, Reilly T, eds. *Science and racket sports,* vol 2. London: E & F Spon, 1998.

Exercise and Sport Science,
edited by William E. Garrett, Jr., and Donald T. Kirkendall.
Lippincott Williams & Wilkins, Philadelphia © 2000.

CHAPTER 59

Physiology of Triathlon

David S. Rowlands and Brendon Downey

A triathlon is an event composed of the continuous and sequential completion of three endurance disciplines. Diverse orders and combinations of sports have been used. In snow-bound regions, the winter triathlon involves skiing or snow-shoeing, mountain-biking, and running. Where suitable water bodies and terrain exist, events including paddling, cycling, and mountain running attract a sizable following. The most popular and widely recognized triathlon combines swimming, cycling, and running.

This chapter focuses on the swim-cycle-run triathlon (referred hereafter as triathlon), which originated in San Diego in 1974 (1). Today, triathlon events typically range in duration from around 20 minutes up to several days (Canadian Ultraman). We will concentrate on two subgroups of triathlon—the short-course triathlon, comprising a 1.5-km swim, 40-km cycle, and a 10-km run, and the long-course (Ironman) triathlon, comprising a swim of approximately 4.0-km, an 180-km cycle, and a 42.2-km run. In recognition of the growing popularity and status of triathlon, the short-course event has recently been included in the Olympics.

While much of the information in this chapter is applicable to recreational triathletes, the focus is on the physical and physiologic characteristics, the racing and training of the modern elite triathlete, and the main factors that determine triathlon performance (Fig. 59–1).

THE SPORT

Participants in a triathlon must sequentially complete a swim, a cycle, and a run. Most events have all competitors start at the same time, with the first competitor to cross the finish line being the winner. Triathlon swim racing involves bunch swimming. When swimming, triathletes create a bow wave and a water flow in the direction they are swimming. Other athletes can take advantage of this by positioning themselves either directly behind a leading swimmer, gaining an estimated 16% to 23% reduction in drag (2), or by swimming on the bow wave. The start of the swim is often contested ferociously as competitors scramble for the best positions.

At the completion of the swim, triathletes exit the water and run to the transition area. There are two transitions in triathlon—the swim to cycle and the cycle to run. Both take less than 1 minute to complete in short-course and around 1 to 3 minutes in long-course events. The swim to bike transition involves removal of the wetsuit (when permitted) and collection of cycle, helmet, shoes, and other items (e.g., food, drink, and sunglasses) required on the cycle. The cycle to run transition requires the athletes to dismount their cycle and replace their cycling shoes, which are usually left attached to the pedal, with running shoes.

In most triathlons, it is illegal to gain benefits by riding in the "slipstream" (drafting) of another competitor in the cycle section. Recently in some short-course triathlons drafting has been legalized, however. The rule change has made a significant impact on tactics, times (Table 59–1), and training for draft-legal World Cup and championship events. It is usual for triathletes to settle into a strong steady pace after the initial few kilometers on the cycle. In draft-legal events, the pace is governed by the triathlete's position in the field at the end of the swim, by collective speed of the bunch, and by tactical movements (e.g., attacks). A slow-swimming triathlete will have to cycle faster at the start of the cycle to catch the leading group in order to be in serious contention during the run. In long-course events, most of the eating in the event is done during the cycle section. In most events, the final placing in a triathlon is decided during the run section. The run sections in short-course events are commonly contested in large

D. S. Rowlands: School of Physical Education, University of Otago, Dunedin, New Zealand.
B. Downey: Performance Lab, Berkenhead, Auckland, New Zealand.

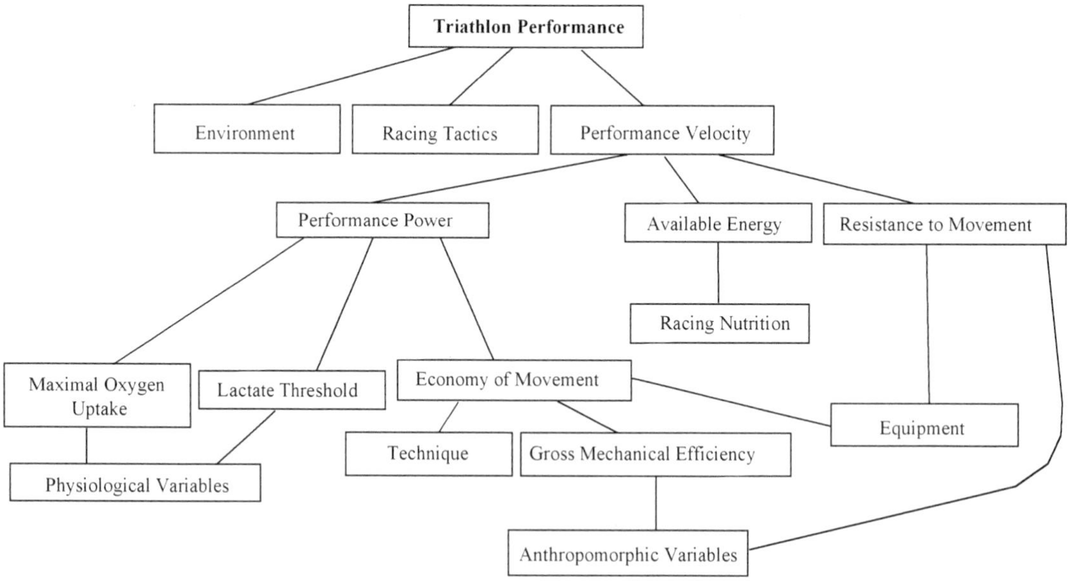

FIG. 59–1. Interrelationship between the major factors determining triathlon performance.

packs, with the final outcome coming down to a sprint or surges near the finish.

We have pooled data from the Hawaiian long-course and recent draft-legal and older draft-illegal short-course world championship events to provide information about the relative contribution of each leg of the triathlon to overall finish time and the impact of the cycling draft rule change in the short-course events (see Table 59–1). In both short- and long-course events, the greatest amount of time is spent on the cycle, followed by the run and the swim. Overall, the legalization of drafting appears to have had little effect on swim times. Cycle and run times, however, appear to have decreased by several minutes for both men and women (see Table 59–1). These conclusions should be viewed with caution because of the variability of terrain and environmental conditions between events.

To establish an idea of the relative importance of each leg of the triathlon to overall finishing time, we ran a Pearson's regression analysis on the swim, cycle, and run times with overall time on the top ten finishers at recent short- and long-course world championship events. The resulting correlations are presented in Table 59–2.

In all events except short-course draft-illegal, swim time has the lowest correlation to final time, suggesting that swim time may contribute the least to overall performance in a triathlon. The legalization of drafting appears to have reduced the importance of the cycle section, while increasing the importance of the run section to overall finishing time in short-course events. The relationships in short-course events are similar between male and female athletes.

We found a strong correlation between women's long-

TABLE 59–1. *Average splits and percent contribution of swim, cycle, and run sections to total time in elite triathlon*

Event	Swim (min)	Percent contribution	Cycle (min)	Percent contribution	Run (min)	Percent contribution	Total
Short-course draft-illegal, 1990–94							
Men	18.9 (1.0)	16.9	58.1 (2.8)	51.8	33.3 (1.1)	29.7	112.1 (2.1)
Women	21.9 (1.2)	17.4	65.6 (3.1)	52.1	38.1 (1.7)	30.2	126.0 (2.6)
Short-course draft-legal, 1995–97							
Men	20.3 (1.6)	19.0	54.2 (3.7)	50.7	31.3 (1.6)	29.3	106.9 (4.4)
Women	22.5 (2.2)	18.7	60.1 (4.3)	50.0	35.8 (1.7)	29.8	120.2 (5.8)
Long-course, 1995–97							
Men	53.4 (1.9)	10.4	286.1 (9.5)	55.8	172.9 (5.5)	33.7	512.7 (11.0)
Women	58.2 (5.9)	10.0	323.7 (13.7)	55.5	205.6 (11.7)	35.2	583.5 (19.5)

Note: Short-course events are the International Triathlon Union World Championship and long-course events are the Hawaiian Ironman. Times are the average of the top ten finishers, with standard deviations in parentheses. Swim, cycle, and run splits exclude transitions. From refs. 119 and 120.

TABLE 59–2. *Pearson correlation of swim, cycle, and run split times with overall time in world championship triathlon*

Event	Swim *r* value	Bike *r* value	Run *r* value
Short-course draft-illegal, 1990–94			
Men	0.62	0.62	0.55
Women	0.33	0.71	0.61
Short-course draft-legal, 1995–97			
Men	0.31	0.17	0.83
Women	−0.11	0.29	0.89
Long-course, 1995–97			
Men	0.33	0.56	0.69
Women	0.46	0.82	0.47

See Table 59–1 for data source. Correlation strength: weak, $r < 0.3$; moderate, $r = 0.3–0.7$; strong, $r > 0.7$.

course cycle time and final time. This relationship could be influenced by two factors relating to the environment and the nature of the Hawaiian Ironman event: women can cycle with subelite men, thereby gaining benefit from the "rolling bunch effect," which assists pace judgment and probably decreases air resistance; and a faster cyclist gains a considerable advantage by avoiding the strong headwinds that develop as the day progresses. Bike time for the top women at Hawaii is closely related to the final finish time.

THE ATHLETE

Although success in sports is dependent on the sum of interactions among genetic, physiologic, psychologic, social-cultural, biomechanical, and technologic factors, there is little doubt of an important link between physique and optimum performance (3–6). Elite single-sport athletes are characterized by morphologic characteristics unique to their sport (3). Since triathlon involves training for high performance in swimming, cycling, and running, the physiologic profile of a triathlete is a blend of the physiques found in swimmers, cyclists, and runners.

Physical Characteristics

Age

Similar to most endurance athletes, triathletes reach peak performance in their mid- to late 20s (5). For elite short-course triathletes, the mean reported age is 25.1 years for men and 27.1 years for women. Long-course

TABLE 59–3. *Anthropometric characteristics in elite male and female single-sport athletes: distance swimmers (800–1500 m); cyclist (road, long-distance track and time trial); runners (5,000 m—marathon), and in short- and long-course triathletes*

Population	*N*	Age (years)	Height (cm)	Mass (kg)	Reference	Body fat (%)	Reference
Men							
Single-sport athletes							
Elite swimmers	—	20.5	184.5 (3.4)	78.9 (2.3)	3–5, 28, 41, 95, 121–122	6.8 (1.4)	5, 121
Elite cyclists	—	23.8 (0.9)	181.6 (2.4)	72.3 (2.9)	6, 11, 31, 40, 123, 124	7.3 (1.4)	11, 40, 121
Elite runners	—	26.6 (3.9)	177.0 (1.2)	63.5 (1.1)	3, 39, 125–128	5.8 (1.2)	39, 126
Triathletes							
Recreational	286	33	179.3 (176.4–185.5)	74.6 (66.6–90.9)	12–16, 19–22, 37, 58	11.1 (7.4–12.5)	17, 130
Sub-elite	104	28.5	178.8 (175–182.9)	72.6 (68.9–73.8)	13, 17, 45, 46, 129–131	10.3 (8.6–12.3)	12, 19, 20, 22, 39
Elite short-course	43	25.1	178.9 (176–181.3)	71.1 (69–72.7)	4, 12, 13, 42	7.2 (7.2–7.4)	4, 129
Elite juniors	30	17.8	177.8	67.2		8.2	18
Average all long-course	317	28.9	180.1 (176.5–181.9)	67.2 (69.4–76.6)	3, 4, 8, 9, 12, 43, 52	9.0	4, 9, 12, 43, 63
Eite long-course	50	25.8	178 (176.5–180.1)	71 (69.4–74.1)	4, 12, 43, 63	9.0	4, 43, 63
Women							
Single-sport athletes							
Elite swimmers	—	17.6 (2.4)	169.8 (3.4)	62. (1.6)	3, 121, 132, 135	17.1	132
Elite cyclists	—	26	168.9 (1.7)	60.8 (0.9)	3, 6, 11, 40	13.7 (1.75)	11, 40
Elite runners	—	27.4 (2.4)	163.6 (2.8)	50.2 (3.2)	3, 125, 132	16.1 (0.9)	132, 135
Triathletes							
Recreational	52	29.1 (21–32)	166.5 (162.9–168.9)	58.8 (56.3–63.1)	21, 22, 58, 133	19.8 (19–22.7)	21, 22
Sub-elite	41	31.1 (26.2–35.7)	165 (162.1–169.1)	57.8 (55.2–63.4)	12, 23–25	18.8 (17.7–20)	12, 31
Elite short-course	10	27.1	167	56.4	25	17.3	25
Elite juniors	21	17.5 (17.1–17.8)	168.4 (168–169)	58.2 (57.1–58.8)	18, 134	10.4	18
Average all long-course	—	29.8 (28–35.7)	168.2 (166–171)	59.3 (57.3–61)	1, 8, 9, 12	17.1 (12.6–22.7)	1, 8, 9, 12
Elite long-course	8	30.5 (28–31.3)	169.1 (168.5–171)	60.5 (60.3–61)	8, 12	15.2	8, 12

Note: Values for single-sport athletes are means of reported means, while values for triathletes are sample-size weighted means (see text for explanation). Population variance is shown in parentheses as standard deviations for single-sport athletes and ranges of the reported means for triathletes. N = sum of the sample size for each study. Mean values for single-sport athletes were obtained largely from review articles and textbooks in which sample size values were not reported.

triathletes appear marginally older than short-course triathletes. Elite triathletes are older than most groups of elite swimmers and cyclists previously studied, but they are of similar age to that of elite distance runners (Table 59–3).

Roalstad (7) suggested that the older age of triathletes (compared to swimmers and cyclists) may be due to the later age in which athletes take up triathlon following years of competition in a single sport and the recent development of the sport. Alternatively, one of the reasons for the older age of elite triathlon performers may be that triathlon is not a collegiate sport, and many successful triathletes graduate to triathlons after specializing in single sports (8). The similarity in the age of elite triathletes and elite runners may reflect the time required for training adaptations to amass to a level required for elite running performance. The onset of physical maturity may also be important in determining the age for elite performance.

Height and Weight

To best summarize the available information, anthropometric means for each triathlete population were generated by taking a mean of the reported means weighted against the sample size reported in each study, using the following equation of Sleivert and Rowlands (9):

$$X = ({}^{P}{}_{i}\,(n_i{\cdot}x_i))/N$$

where X = mean of the means, ${}^{P}{}_{i}$ = sum of sample size weighted means, n_i = sample number in each study, x_i = mean value for each study, N = sum of n_i for all studies. While it is recognized there can be considerable variation of anthropometric measurements within a population, the means of a population provide information from which generalizations can be made.

Triathletes are on average 1 to 3 cm taller than individuals of the same age from the general population (Fig. 59–2*A,B*). All categories of male triathletes appear similar in height, the only difference being that elite male long-course triathletes are marginally shorter than both elite short-course and the average long-course competitor (see Fig. 59–2*A,B*). In female triathletes, long-course competitors are reported to be taller than short-course triathletes. The limited research available suggests there may be a trend for elite female triathletes to be taller than nonelite (see Fig. 59–2*A*), which requires clarifying in future research.

Previous reports of studies on triathletes from the mid- to late 1980s suggested that both male and female triathletes were similar in height to specialist cyclists (1,9,10). Combining the data previously reported with more recent data (11–16) suggests the average height of triathletes lies between the average for specialist runners and cyclists (see Fig. 59–2*A,B*).

Body Mass and Body Composition

Triathletes are on average 3 to 7 kg lighter than individuals of comparative age from the normal population. Compared to elite single-sport athletes, triathletes are similar in weight to elite cyclists. Recreational and subelite triathletes are heavier than elite triathletes (see Table 59–3; Fig. 59–2*C,D*).

The majority of triathlon research has used the two-compartment anatomic model (5) to estimate body composition in triathletes (4,7,8,12,17–25). The dual compartmental model is based on linear equations and measurements of body mass and skinfolds. It divides the components of the body into *fat mass* and *fat-free mass*, with assumptions regarding the density of various tissues (5). Triathletes are typical of endurance athletes, having estimated body fat percentages of around half that seen in the average individual of comparable age (see Table 59–3). Male triathletes typically have 6% to 11% body fat, whereas female triathletes have 10% to 20% body fat. Elite triathletes have less fat mass than subelite and recreational triathletes, and have comparable levels to elite single-sport athletes (see Table 59–3). Body fat mass influences performance in swimming, cycling, and running differently. In swimming, there appears to be little effect of body fat percentage on performance (26). In running and cycling (especially up hills), excess fatness is likely to be detrimental because it adds mass to the body without the additional capacity to produce force.

Since total body mass is related to both body height and body composition (3), making a correction for the influence of body height on body mass allows the relationship between body mass and performance to be viewed more clearly. Assuming a linear relationship between body height and mass in a normal population, the body mass of athletes can be expressed relative to the body mass expected for an individual of a given height using equations based on a normal population. For women, $y = 0.6x - 39.2$, and for men, $y = 0.8x - 69.6$, where x = the individual's height, y = expected weight for an individual of x height (3). The relative body mass (RBM) for the average elite female cyclist was calculate from body height and mass values (see Table 59–3) as follows:

$$\text{Expected Body Mass } (y) = 0.6\,(168.9) - 39.2 = 62.14$$

$$\text{RBM} = \text{Actual Mass/Expected Mass} = 60.8/62.14 = 0.978$$

The average individual has a RBM of 1.0. A relative body composition index (RBCI) can be derived from the product of RBM and estimated dual-component values of fat and fat-free mass. The RBCI standardizes body composition to a population norm (effectively correcting for height), making it easier to view the contribu-

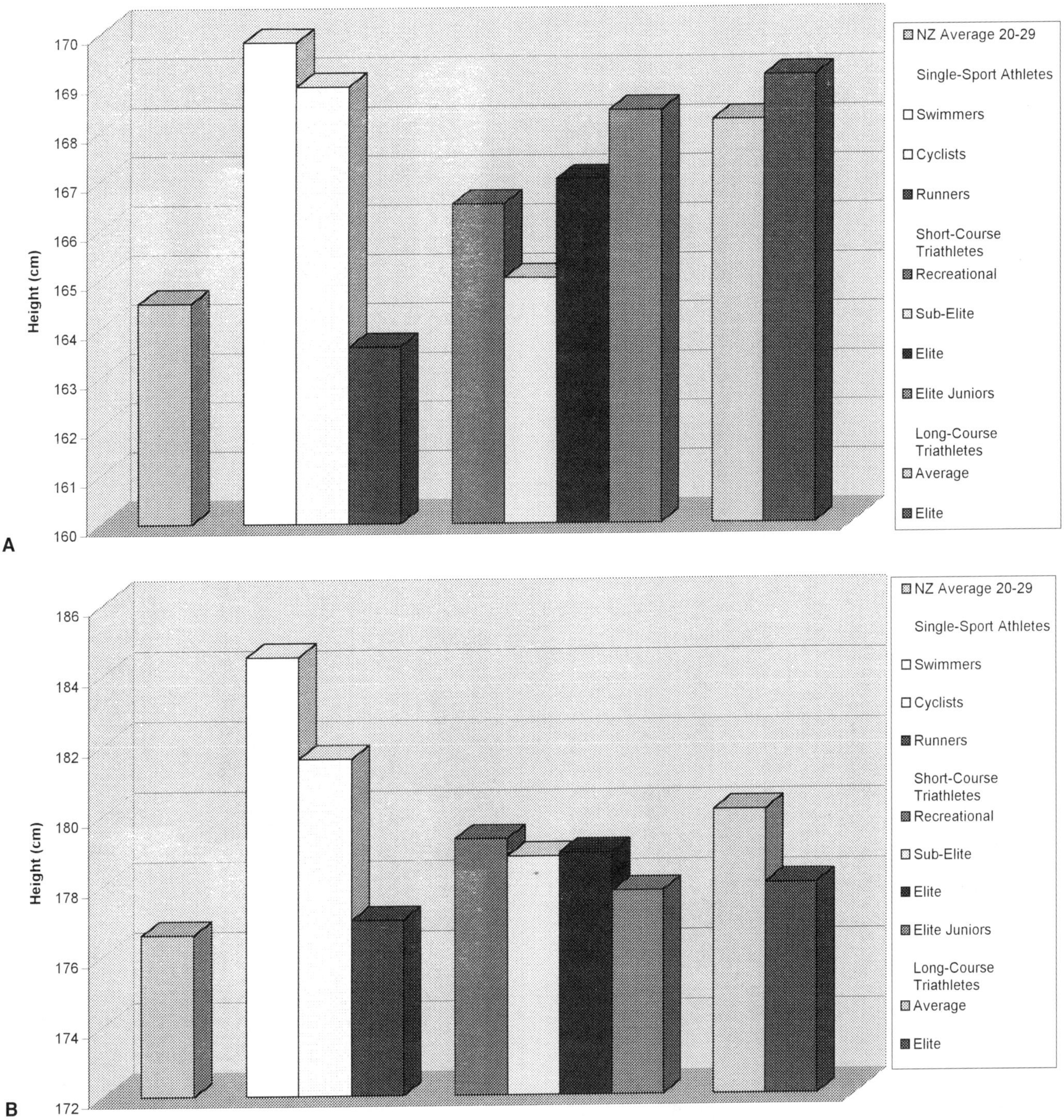

FIG. 59–2. Anthropometric values for the normal population, elite single-sport endurance athletes, and groups of triathletes. Mean body height: females (**A**), males (**B**). (*continued*)

tions of fat and fat-free mass to body mass in athlete populations (Fig. 59–3).

In endurance athletes, the lowest RBM values are found in athletes in whom the greatest form of resistance to movement for an extended period of time is gravity. The best example is seen in distance runners. Typical values for finalists in the 1988 Olympic 10,000 m ranged from 0.815 to 0.898 in men and 0.73 to 0.836 in women (3). During swimming, body mass is almost fully compensated against gravity. The major force to overcome in swimming is drag associated with propulsion through the water (27). Consequently, strength can be increased

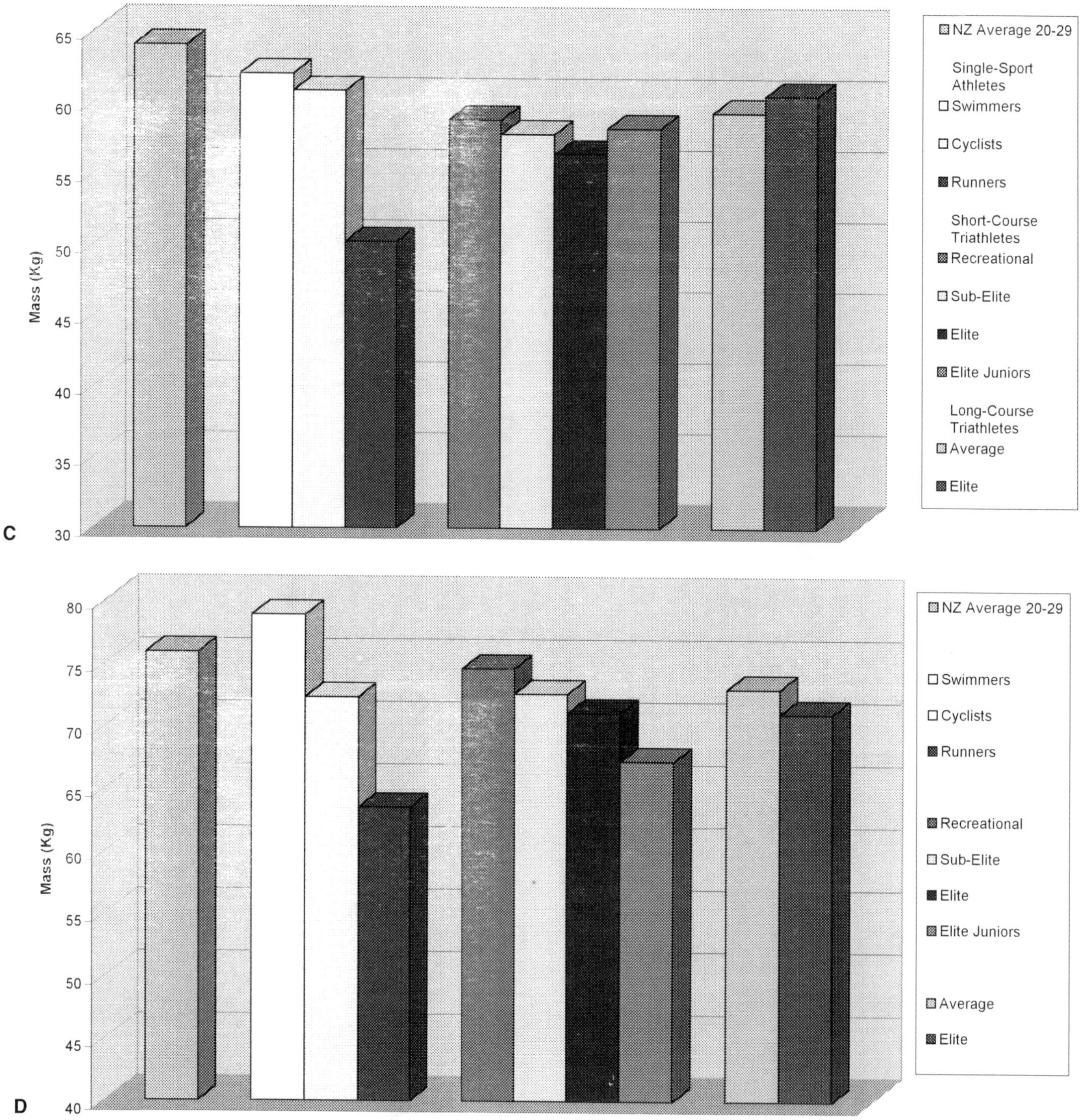

FIG. 59–2. *Continued.* Mean body mass: females (**C**), males (**D**). (Figures prepared from data presented in Table 59–3 and ref. 10.)

in swimmers by increasing muscle mass without incurring significant additions to resistance, as would be the case in runners. The RBM of the 1988 Olympic swim finalists ranged from 0.92 to 1.026 for men in the 1500 m and from 0.745 to 1.017 for women in the 800 m (3). The RBM of cyclists is a combination of (a) added muscle mass giving greater absolute strength (higher RBM) on the flat, where resistance against gravity is partially compensated and the primary form of resistance is drag generated from movement through the air; and (b) of moderate muscle mass (lower RBM) for climbing where the primary form of resistance is gravity. Elite runners of both sexes have a lower fat-free (lean) mass than elite cyclists and swimmers (see Fig. 59–3).

All categories of triathletes have a similar fat-free component (i.e., lean body mass), but the difference in

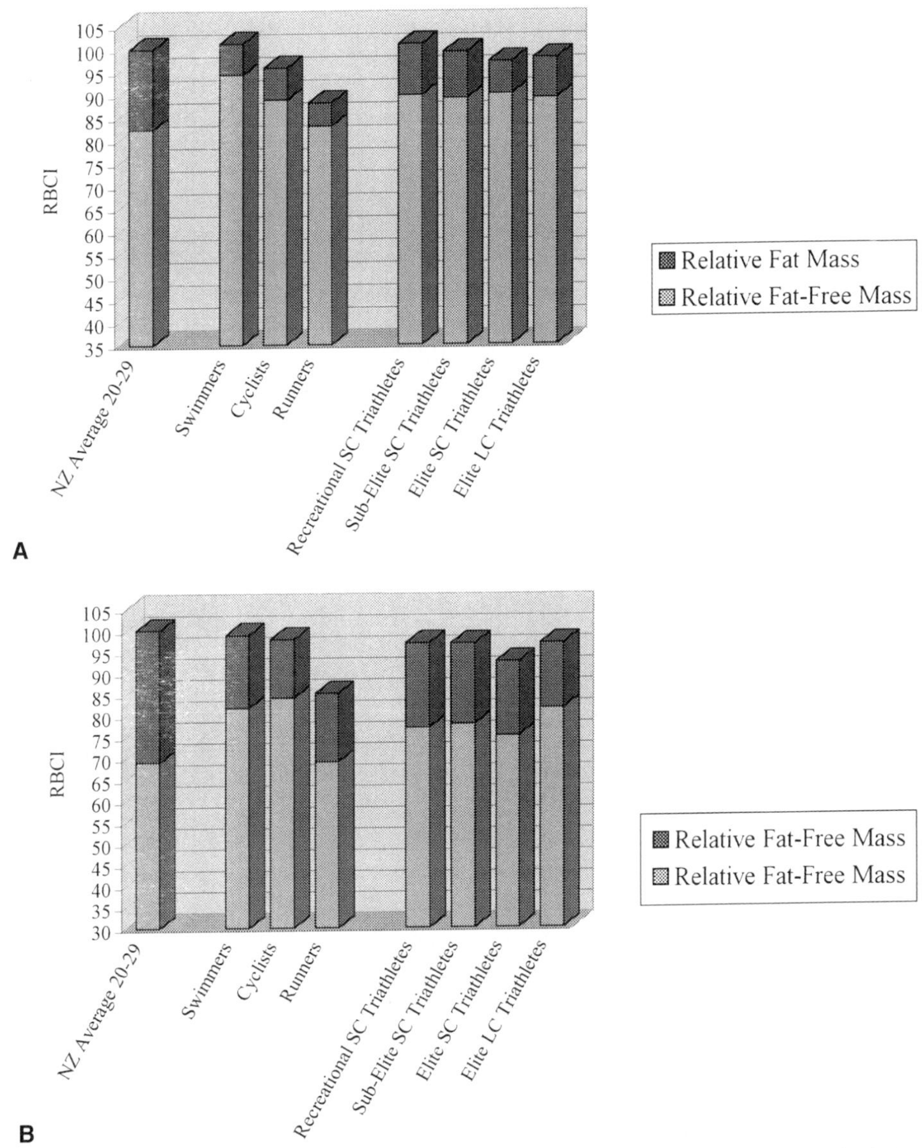

FIG. 59–3. Relative body composition index in male (**A**) and female (**B**) normal, elite single-sport and triathlete populations. *SC*, short course; *LC*, long course. (See text for derivation of index.)

RBM among elite, subelite, and recreational triathletes appears to be accounted for by a greater fat mass in the nonelite. The average fat-free component of triathletes is greater than that of elite runners, less than that of elite swimmers, but similar to that of elite cyclists (see Fig. 59–3).

Linear regression analysis is another method of predicting the "ideal" body mass for a given height. Sample-size weighted regression analysis of our own and reported data (see Table 59–3) indicates a strong relationship between body height and body weight in elite male short-course ($r = 0.89$, $y = 0.72x - 57.91$) and in elite male long-course ($r = 0.86$, $y = 0.915x - 91.81$) triathletes. Combining elite populations resulted in a regression equation for all elite male triathletes ($r = 0.847$, $y = 0.774x - 67.05$) (Fig. 59–4*A*). Slope comparisons suggest the relationship between height and weight is similar to that in the normal population, and therefore anthropometric predictions based on the normal population would seem valid for the elite male triathlete. At the time of this writing, the data were insufficient for regression analysis of elite female triathletes.

Hypothetical Elite Triathlete

Because of the functional link between physique and performance in swimming, cycling, and running (3), the ideal triathlete physique should be a combination of the physiques of elite swimmers, cyclists, and runners.

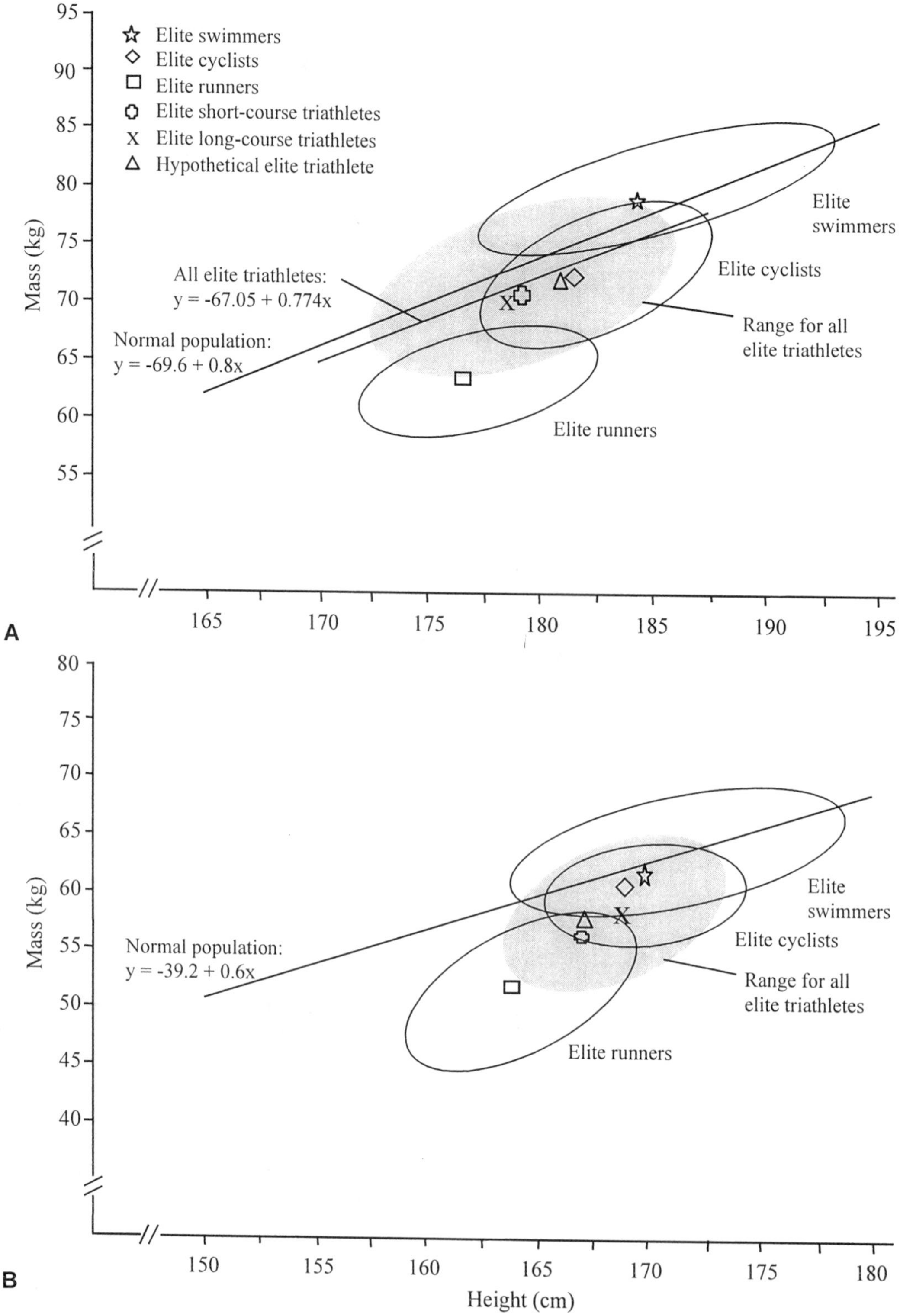

FIG. 59–4. Body height and mass relationships in elite male (**A**) and elite female (**B**) swimmers, cyclists, runners, and triathletes. Regression lines for the correlation of height with weight for all elite triathletes, that is, short- and long-course, and the normal population are shown. *Oblongs* represent the area enclosed by approximately one standard deviation from the range of means for each population reported (Table 59–3). *Large symbols* represent the reported means for single-sport athletes, and the sample-size weighted means for short- and long-course triathletes and the hypothetical elite triathlete.

Taking the average of body height and mass means for elite single-sport athletes (see Table 59–3) provides a value for a hypothetical elite triathlete (HET). For males the values are 181.0 cm and 71.6 kg and for females 167.4 cm and 57.7 kg (see Fig. 59–4).

Strong linear relationships between body height and body mass suggest that RBM changes little in groups of endurance athletes. Since RBM characterizes successful endurance performers well, RBM can be used to predict an "ideal" elite body mass in an athlete for a given body height. For female HET, RBM can be derived as follows:

$$\text{Expected Mass} = 0.6\,(167.4) - 39.2 = 61.24$$

$$\text{RBM} = \text{Actual Mass/Expected Mass} = 57.7/61.24 = 0.942$$

Similarly, for male HET:

$$\text{Expected Mass} = 0.8\,(181) - 69.6 = 75.2$$

$$\text{RBM} = \text{Actual Mass/Expected Mass} = 71.6/75.2 = 0.952$$

Using RBM for the HET, an ideal elite target racing weight can be estimated for a triathlete of a given height. For example, the ideal target weight for an 183-cm elite male triathlete is:

$$\text{Expected Mass HET RBM} = 0.8\,(183) - 69.6 = 76.8$$

$$\text{Ideal Mass} = 76.8\,(0.952) = 73.1$$

The model assumes the height/weight relationship in elite triathletes resembles the normal population. Relative body mass, like most values we ascribe to an individual's physique, will not predict a winning triathlon performance since many other factors are obviously involved (see Fig. 59–1).

A similar model could be derived using elite single-sport means for biathletes and for triathletes specializing in events involving cross-country skiing, paddling, or any other multiple combination of sports.

Within a population of triathletes, taller triathletes may have a physical advantage over shorter triathletes during the swim because of the greater leverage provided by longer limbs. Assuming a constant applied force, longer levers allow a larger amplitude of movement (i.e., distance covered per stroke), but also require a lower frequency (i.e., stroke rate) for movement economy (3). Conversely, too much height in triathletes may be a disadvantage because of a greater body mass, volume, and surface area ratio. Force production relative to body mass increases as body mass decreases. That is, smaller endurance athletes (both shorter and lighter) have a greater ratio of power to volume and mass. A low power-to-mass ratio is of particular advantage during distance running and uphill cycling, reducing the energy required to overcome gravity. Lower muscle cross-sectional area (volume) reduces the blood-tissue diffusion distance, enhancing oxygen delivery and metabolite removal (28).

Taller cyclists have an advantage on the flat, where gravitational resistance accounts for less than 10% of total resistance. While cycling on the flat, the greatest proportion (80% to 90%) of work is done overcoming air resistance (29). With an appropriate bicycle setup, larger cyclists can obtain a frontal surface area only marginally greater than smaller cyclists, giving the larger cyclists a greater power-to-frontal surface area ratio. The advantages a larger triathlete has over a smaller triathlete on a flat cycle course are somewhat attenuated when the drafting effects of bunch riding are taken into consideration. In a group of four riders, air resistance relative to the first rider is decreased by 51% for the second and 36% for the fourth rider in the pace line relative to the rider in front. At 41 km/h, the fourth rider in the pace line would be producing about 54% less power to keep with the group than if he were riding alone. Air resistance in a large group of cyclists at race pace is only 30% to 35% of riding alone (6,29). In running, around 7.5% of total energy is used to overcome air resistance. About 80% of air resistance can be eliminated by shielding behind another runner (30).

The range of body height, mass, and composition in successful triathletes may reflect a morphologic link between stature, body composition, and the relative importance of the swim, cycle, and run sections of the triathlon to overall performance (see Fig. 59–4). For example, elite male long-distance triathletes display anthropometric characteristics close to that of elite cyclists and runners (see Fig. 59–2*B,D*), and cycling and running performance appear important determinants of success in long-distance triathlon in males (see Table 59–2).

The legalization of drafting on the bike in 1995 in preparation for the introduction of triathlon into the Olympics (Sydney 2000) may alter the average physique of elite triathletes competing in short-course events. The elite triathlete competing in draft-legal events may adopt morphologic features more characteristic of an elite distance runner (for example, reduced RBM, low fat mass, and reduced lean mass), but still retain sufficient characteristics of swimmers (for example, shoulder breadth, body height, arm and leg-length) (3,4) and of cyclists (for example, upper leg circumference) (31), to remain competitive in the swim and cycle sections preceding the run. The successful athlete competing in nondraft events, however, may retain a more even balance of the morphology components found in swimmers, cyclists, and runners, similar to that suggested by the hypothetical elite triathlete model below. Shorter triathletes (i.e., resembling runners) may have a morphologic advantage over taller triathletes in draft-legal triathlon.

PHYSIOLOGIC CHARACTERISTICS

Prolonged exercise performance is limited by the capacity of the aerobic energy systems to provide a continuous supply of energy to the contracting muscle. This requires that there be adequate supply of fuels, the physiologic capacity to deliver oxygen and fuels efficiently, and the effective removal of metabolic end products (28,32,70).

Exercise physiologists have identified at least five physiologic variables that relate significantly to endurance swimming (33), cycling (29,31,32), and running (34,35) performance:

1. Maximal aerobic power
2. Blood lactate threshold
3. Economy of motion
4. Fractional utilization of maximal aerobic power
5. Fuel supply

Since the competitive demands of triathlon are similar to the component single sports, it is reasonable to assume that the physiologic variables most important to endurance swimming, cycling, and running success have a similar influence in determining success in the triathlon. The physiologic demands of sequential swimming, cycling, and running are unique, however, and specific physiologic acclimations are likely present in triathletes to accommodate the unique demands of triathlon competition.

The physiologic profile of triathletes and the factors associated with success in triathlon have been extensively reviewed (1,7,9,36) and are summarized in the following paragraphs.

Maximal Aerobic Power

Maximal aerobic power ($\dot{V}O_2max$) is the greatest rate of aerobic energy production, and in a sense, sets the ceiling for endurance work output. Maximal aerobic power is thought to be limited by one or more central and peripheral factors. The most important central factor is cardiac output (heart rate × stroke volume), while influential peripheral factors include muscle capillary density, oxidative enzyme activities, and muscle fiber type (32,37,38). Several lines of evidence indicate that $\dot{V}O_2max$ is a key determinant of endurance performance. For example, $\dot{V}O_2max$ in elite performing male runners, cyclists, and triathletes usually exceeds 70 mL/kg/min (9,37,39,40), and is greater than in groups of good (subelite) and slower (recreational) athletes (Table 59–4) (9,36,37). $\dot{V}O_2max$ positively correlates with performance velocity (9,28,32,34,36,41).

Most triathletes display the greatest $\dot{V}O_2max$ values during running, followed by cycling and swimming. Treadmill and cycle ergometry $\dot{V}O_2max$ values in elite male triathletes have been reported to range from 69.4 to 84.5, with means of around 71 to 73 mL/kg/min (8,9,36,42,43). The means for triathletes are marginally lower, but within a similar range to that reported for elite runners and cyclists (see Table 59–4).

Treadmill $\dot{V}O_2max$ values in elite female triathletes are reported to lie between 54.2 and 80.0 mL/kg/min (8,9,25). Mean values of 63.6 (44) and 65.6 mL/kg/min (25) for short-course, and 65.9 mL/kg/min for long-course elite female triathletes have been reported (8). Subelite female triathletes average 60.4 for running and

TABLE 59–4. *Sample size weighted mean maximal oxygen uptake (mL/kg/min) values in elite single-sport athletes and triathletes in tethered swimming (TS), cycle ergometry (CE), and treadmill running (TR)*

	TS	CE	TR	Reference
Men				
Swimmers	67.4 (60–76)		68.6	1, 3, 41, 95, 136, 137
Cyclists		74.8 (73.5–78)		3, 6, 11, 28, 31, 40, 123, 124
Runners			77.6 (71.7–78.8)	4, 5, 8, 28, 34, 35, 39, 41, 95, 125, 138
Triathletes				
Recreational		53 (43.6–60.1)		19, 22, 46, 130, 131
Subelite	54.3 (51–59.4)	63.6 (60.5–64.3)	66.9 (63.7–69.9)	17, 20, 37, 42, 45, 48
Elite			71.7 (71.3–72)	42, 43
Juniors			70.0 (67.9–78.7)	18, 134
Women				
Swimmers	54.9 (48.9–60)		58	1, 28, 41, 95, 136, 137
Cyclists		61 (57.4–65)		3, 6, 11, 40, 95
Runners			70.2 (65–77)	3, 5, 8, 34, 41, 125
Triathletes				
Recreational	38.1	51.1	51.4	46
Subelite		56.9	60.3 (58.7–61)	7, 25, 43
Elite			65 (63.6–65.9)	8, 16, 25, 44, 92, 139
Juniors			58.6 (56.1–62.6)	18, 134

Values in parentheses represent the range of reported means.

60.3 mL/kg/min for cycling. As a comparison, elite female runners and cyclists average 70.2 and 61.0 mL/kg/min, respectively (see Table 59–4).

In groups of recreational and subelite male triathletes (20,45–47), average $\dot{V}O_2$max during tethered swimming ranged between 49.9 and 59.4 mL/kg/min, which is 11% to 35% less than the average for elite swimmers (67 mL/kg/min) (9). In recreational triathletes, Sleivert and Wenger (46) found average tethered swim $\dot{V}O_2$max to be around 25% lower than cycle and run values (see Table 59–4). Elite triathletes may have similar swim $\dot{V}O_2$max to elite swimmers since the percentage difference between recreational and subelite triathletes and elite swimmers is similar to the difference seen in these triathlete groups during cycle ergometry and treadmill running (see Table 59–4). Technical discrepancies, however, may result in the velocity at maximal and submaximal oxygen uptakes in elite triathletes being less than that of elite swimmers (27). Further work into swimming physiology in triathletes is required.

The literature up to 1995 investigating the relationship between $\dot{V}O_2$max and triathlon performance is extensively reviewed in Sleivert and Rowlands (9) and O'Toole and Douglas (36). Briefly, in groups of recreational and subelite short-course and half-Ironman triathletes, there appears to be weak or moderate-level correlations between cycle and run $\dot{V}O_2$max and cycle and run performance, but there is little evidence of a relationship for swimming (9,16,21,46–48). O'Toole and colleagues (8) found little evidence of a relationship in well-trained long-course triathletes, with tactical factors and physiologic factors associated with fuel stores, fluid, and electrolyte homeostasis being cited as more important determinants of success in these events (9,36). More results from elite short-course triathletes are required before correlations can be made on $\dot{V}O_2$max and performance in this group.

Lactate Threshold and Factional Utilization of $\dot{V}O_2$max

The fastest pace an athlete can sustain during an endurance event is strongly related to the rate of aerobic energy production approximating the threshold of blood lactate accumulation (LT), or the onset of hyperventilation (ventilatory threshold, VT) (32,49). Both LT and VT have been termed the *anaerobic threshold,* based on a common misunderstanding that the onset of lactic acid production in the muscle, and hence appearance in the blood, is caused by insufficient oxygen in the contracting muscle (41,50). The LT and VT appear closely linked but may not be physiologically coupled (49). Regardless of physiology or terminology, exercise above LT and VT cannot be maintained indefinitely due to factors related to accelerated glycogen depletion, reduced fat oxidation, and metabolic acidosis (9,32,49).

The ventilatory and lactate thresholds reported in triathletes are similar or slightly lower than those reported in elite single-sport athletes (11,9,32–34,51). Average LT expressed as a percentage of sport-specific $\dot{V}O_2$max appears to be greater during running than cycling (52). In recreational and subelite triathletes, VT occurred at 72% to 75% of swim $\dot{V}O_2$max, 63% to 82% of cycle $\dot{V}O_2$max, and 74% to 75% of run $\dot{V}O_2$max (9). Similarly, LT (defined at 4 mmol/L) was reported to occur at 72% to 88% of bike $\dot{V}O_2$max and 80% to 85% of run $\dot{V}O_2$max (36). Energy output at VT or LT would appear to be the lowest in swimming followed by cycling and running.

In a group of international-caliber short-course triathletes, relative run VT was lowered on average from 84.6% to 74.3% $\dot{V}O_2$max after the swim and cycle sections of a triathlon, indicating the loss of efficiency and physiologic capacity over the duration of a triathlon (42).

Factors associated with LT limit the fractional utilization of maximal aerobic capacity that can be sustained during endurance exercise. In cyclists with similar $\dot{V}O_2$max values, time to fatigue was more than double for the athletes whose LT occurred at 81% of $\dot{V}O_2$max, compared to a group whose LT occurred at 66% $\dot{V}O_2$max (32). In well-trained runners and cyclists with differing $\dot{V}O_2$max values, strong positive correlations between performance and velocity at LT have been reported (1,32,34,49). Lactate thresholds, expressed as a percent of $\dot{V}O_2$max, are reported to be greater in elite compared to moderately trained runners (34,37).

Lactate thresholds have become a popular means of assessing fitness. Over the course of a triathlon season, LT was found to increase by 6% in cycling and by 10% in running (52). Since velocity at LT is strongly related to endurance performance, training methods aimed at increasing LT in should also improve triathlon performance—in cycling and running in particular (31,32,34).

Exercise Efficiency and Economy

Exercise efficiency is the relationship between energy expenditure and mechanical output. Individuals with greater efficiency produce higher speed with less energy and oxygen use. The energy efficiency of running and cycling is between 20% and 30%, but only 5% to 10% during swimming (36). Efficiency and cycling performance has been recently found to be strongly related to percent of type I (slow-twitch, high-oxidative) muscle fibers (32). Heat and friction account for most of the energy not converted into useful work (28).

Economy, defined as the oxygen uptake required to produce a specific rate of power output or velocity of movement, has been shown to account for the large variation in performance times of elite runners with similar $\dot{V}O_2$max values (53). Other groups have shown significant relationships between economy and cycling

(32) and swimming performances (54), sports that likely require greater technical proficiency. As with $\dot{V}O_2max$, however, within a group of runners with similar performance times, economy and performance are not highly correlated (37). Exercise economy is governed by a combination of (a) muscular efficiency; (b) technical factors, for example, muscle recruitment area related to pedaling technique in cycling and stroke mechanics in swimming; (c) psychologic (relaxation) factors; (d) equipment; and (e) environmental conditions.

In a group of long-course triathletes, submaximal swimming, cycling, and running economy were all found to be positively correlated with swim, cycle, and run performance (47). Laureson and colleagues (25) found elite female triathletes were significantly more economical at 15 km/h (51.2 mL/kg/min) than subelite female triathletes (53.8 mL/kg/min). The elite women were also exercising at a lower fraction of their $\dot{V}O_2max$ (78.2% vs. 89.2%) and had lower heart rate and lactate values at submaximal running velocity (9). In a group of well-trained male triathletes, Miura and colleagues (16) found cycle and run, but not swim, economy to be significantly correlated with finishing time. Economy is likely to be an important factor in determining triathlon success.

Toussaint (27) found a group of elite swimmers had a greater propelling efficiency than a group of elite triathletes. Swimmers, compared to triathletes, had a greater mean swimming velocity for a given power output (1.17 vs. 0.95 m/s) and covered a greater distance per stroke (1.23 vs. 0.92 m). The difference in swimming speed was explained by the findings that the swimmers used a higher proportion of their power output to overcome drag (49 vs. 35 W) and expended less power moving water backward (32 vs. 45 W). Overall mean propelling efficiency for swimmers was 61% but only 44% for triathletes. These findings indicate triathletes could benefit from improvements in swimming technique.

Triathletes may also benefit from technique training in running and cycling. Longer stride lengths during running have been shown to be more economical in terms of oxygen uptake and blood lactate measurement, but any major derivations from an individuals' optimum results in reduced economy (55). In cycling, an effective pedaling technique may result in the distribution of load across a greater muscle mass. This may increase economy (32) and decrease time to fatigue in isolated muscle groups.

Equipment factors must also be taken into consideration for improvements in economy. Wetsuits during swimming raise the body out of the water and thereby reduce drag (56). Cycling economy can be affected by bike setup and equipment selection (29).

There is likely to be a decline in economy through the course of a triathlon (57). Kreider and colleagues (58) found that a triathlon run required a higher $\dot{V}O_2$, ventilation, and heart rates, and resulted in a lower stroke volume and mean arterial pressure, when compared to a control run. Guezennec and colleagues (59) and Hausswirth and colleagues (15) found a mean increase of around 7% to 8% in the oxygen cost of a triathlon run compared to a control run, which was related to a greater loss of body mass (0.9 kg). Maintaining hydration status during competition has been suggested to be important in minimizing detrimental changes in economy (1,9,45,58).

Fuel Stores

The triathlete has three principal fuel substrates available for use as energy during exercise: glucose, fatty acids, and amino acids. These fuels can be made available for oxidation in the mitochondria from endogenous stores (i.e., muscle and liver glycogen, muscle and adipose triglycerides, tissue protein), and exogenous sources (i.e., feeding). Evidence suggests the rate-limiting fuel store is glycogen during prolonged exercise (60).

Classic Swedish studies in the 1960s established that a high-carbohydrate diet in the final days before an exhaustive exercise bout improved endurance (61,62). In response to these findings, endurance athletes, including triathletes, have been told to consume a high-carbohydrate diet (i.e., 60% to 70% by energy; 8 to 10 g/kg/day) during training and before racing (63,64). The assumption underlying this dietary regime is that by maintaining full glycogen stores, the athlete will perform better in training and therefore perform better in racing. While a high-carbohydrate diet will indeed maintain high-glycogen stores (64), it may not, however, provide optimal conditions for endurance training adaptations in the muscle of an endurance athlete. Indeed, a number of studies show that endurance athletes prefer to eat moderate carbohydrate diets in the range of 43% to 55% (64,65), and do not receive any more benefit from increasing carbohydrate intakes to 60% to 70% (50,66–68). Despite the trends seen in single-sport endurance athletes (64,65), three studies found triathletes follow a moderate- to high-carbohydrate diet (55% to 60%) (43,63,69).

By engaging in high volumes of training, endurance athletes expose the exercising muscle to low glycogen levels, forcing a greater use of fatty acids as a fuel. By doing so, the capacity to burn fat and spare and store glycogen is increased, which may improve endurance (34,70). These training adaptations, however, may be impeded by the consumption of very high carbohydrate diets, since the presence of continuously high-levels of muscle glycogen result in the suppression of fat oxidation and the downregulation of enzymatic processes responsible for the breakdown of fats to energy (71–74).

If muscle glycogen depletion indeed limits endurance

performance, triathletes, particularly those competing in Ironman events, may benefit from a period of training on a carbohydrate-restricted diet, which might in turn promote muscular and hepatic adaptations to further increase the capacity to burn fat (60,71,72,75–79). Similarly, training (but not racing) in the postabsorptive state may also have benefit to muscular metabolism for endurance exercise, since fasting increases fat availability and oxidation (76). Glycogen utilization may also be decreased and performance enhanced in some situations by the use of caffeine, and the ingestion of a mixed composition or high-fat pre-exercise meals and exercise supplements (76,77,80). Sports nutrition is a rapidly advancing field, and in time we may see triathletes periodizing their nutrition to manipulate metabolism so as to enhance performance. Interested readers are referred elsewhere for discussion of the role of nutrition and energy stores on performance in endurance athletes (50,60,64,65,67,74,76,77,81,93).

Application of Exercise Physiology to Elite Triathletes

We are unable to find a literature source for the physiologic data on the population of elite triathletes of the late 1990s. The pace at which the most successful male triathletes now complete the 10-km run portion of a standard short-course triathlon (30 to 32 minutes) is similar to the world-record marathon pace. Since the short-course triathlon is of similar duration to a marathon, elite male triathletes are likely to have a physiologic profile similar to the best distance runners.

Based on the oxygen cost for a 10-km run split approximating the world-record marathon pace of around 4.7 L/min (82), we have calculated the relative oxygen cost to be around 67 mL/kg/min for a triathlete with average running economy (53). The true cost could be up to 10% greater, with a number of studies demonstrating reduced running economy after prior swimming and cycling (14,15,42,52). Since top 10-km performers can sustain an oxygen consumption of around 85% to 90% of their $\dot{V}O_2$max for the distance (34), elite male short-course triathletes may require run $\dot{V}O_2$max values in the vicinity of 80 to 85 mL/kg/min during competition. High economy, however, could reduce O_2 cost by some 7 to 13 mL/kg/min in the most efficient triathletes based on studies in runners (30,53). A high $\dot{V}O_2$max will gain an elite triathlete membership into the elite group, but economy may be a more important determinant of success within a field of elite triathletes.

TRAINING THE ATHLETE

Numerous accounts of the training practices and programs for triathletes have now been published in the popular (83–88) and scientific (13,63,7,89) literature. Training programs and practices for triathlon are as diverse and varied as those found for single sports, but in most programs the basic established principles of specificity and periodization, overload, recovery, tapering, and peaking are followed (37,83,86,90). This section provides an overview of the basic training strategies used in triathlon. Much of the information is descriptive and derived from both the scientific and popular literature, and from the practical coaching and training experience of the authors. We believe the optimal way to train for the triathlon is by blending endurance, technique, specific strength, and speed work into a comprehensive program that neither neglects nor overemphasizes a particular training component.

Sport-Specific Training

High training volume appears to be an important determinant of triathlon success (4,13,17,20,43,89). Holly and colleagues (43) reported four top-15 male finishers at the 1982 Hawaii Ironman averaged 19-km swimming, 590-km cycling, and 95-km running per week in the month leading up to the event. Similarly, average training distance in seven elite triathletes ranked in the world top-20 in 1985 was reported to be 18.7, 611, and 100 km per week for swimming, cycling, and running, respectively (4).

The best short-course male triathletes cover somewhat less distance than their long-course counterparts. Average training volumes of around 10- to 20-km swimming, 200- to 400-km cycling, and 40- to 70-km running have been reported (13,17,20,91). Average weekly training volume in a group of New Zealand representative male triathletes was 16-km swimming, 195-km of cycling, and 72-km running. These elite triathletes had maximal weeks averaging 24-km swimming, 290-km cycling, and 100-km running (12). Two studies suggest elite short-course females may cover some 20% to 30% less distance in training (25,92). The longest training sessions a short-course triathlete typically undertakes are 5-km swim, 120-km cycle, 30-km run, while long-course triathletes may train up to 6-km swim, 180-km cycle, and 40-km run. Average sessions are usually more moderate, for example, 2- to 4-km swim, 30- to 60-km cycle, and 10- to 15-km run for short course, and 3-to 4-km swim, 60-to 90-km cycle, and 10- to 20-km run for long course (83,86,89).

Top triathletes train over shorter distances in a particular discipline than single sport athletes, but overall, total training hours are usually higher than those of elite athletes specializing in swimming, cycling, or running (34,40,82–87,89,90,94).

Training Methods for Triathlon

Training sessions for endurance sports are often prescribed on the basis of measured or perceived metabolic intensity. The terms most commonly used are endurance or long steady (or slow) distance training, up tempo or threshold training, speed work, and strength or power training (37,82,84,86). In this chapter the terms described by Ackland (83) are used where the triathlete periodizes training moving through the components from easy to load to speed. Using this scheme, most training components are utilized in 1 week, with the emphasis shifting from low-intensity, low-volume training at the beginning of the buildup phase to moderate-intensity, -strength, and high-volume emphases at the end of the buildup, moving finally to a high-intensity, moderate-volume phase during the specific/speed preparatory phase of the buildup (Table 59–5, Fig. 59–5).

Endurance

Endurance training constitutes a major fraction of the triathlete's training load. Intensity is generally low to moderate and the volume high. The benefits of endurance training manifest in an improved endurance capacity and ability to recover (82). Adaptations to endurance training include:

1. Improved cardiovascular function apparent in an increased (a) $\dot{V}O_2max$, (b) cardiac output, (c) capillary density and networking, and (d) plasma and blood volume.
2. Increased oxidative capacity of the exercising muscle (i.e., more mitochondria and altered composition of mitochondria).

TABLE 59–5. *Summary of training techniques for triathlon and presumed benefits*

Training component	Swimming	Cycling	Running	AMI	ML	Purpose	Physiologic responses (7, 9, 72, 117)
Endurance	Easy–moderate	Easy–moderate	Easy–moderate	50–70	40–60	Establish fitness base	See text
Load	Small pads; feet tied	Hills in low gear	Hill running with normal stride length and rate; soft sand	50–65	60–70	Introduce resistance training, for strength development	Recruitment of motor pattern associated with the full range of movement in each discipline; increased motor unit recruitment, altered firing rates and synchronization Conditioning of type II fibers Muscle hypertrophy Increased maximal force-generating capacity Endurance training acclimations
High load	Large pads; tethered-swimming; swim bench	Hills and flat in high gear (low cadence)	Bounding or strideouts on hills	65–75	75–95	Increase strength	Progression from load training
Load speed	Small pads; approx. 3000-m pace	Ironman race-pace in high gear	Exaggerated strides on flat intervals up gradual incline	60–70	65–75	Strength transfer to event-specific speed; develop power	
Low speed	Intervals; approx. 3000-m pace	Long intervals at Ironman race pace	Long intervals at Marathon race pace	75–80	70–75	Ironman race-specific training; preparation for short-course race pace training	Introduced competition specific neuromuscular recruitment patterns Increased mitochondrial material
High speed	4-min intervals; approx. 1500-m pace	5-min intervals; approx. 40-km pace; motor pacing	1-km intervals; approx. 10-km pace	85–95	85–95	Race-specific training for short course	Increase lactate threshold, glycolytic capacity, and $\dot{V}O_2max$ Competition-specific neuromuscular recruitment patterns Psychologic conditioning for racing
Sprint	50-m intervals	Sprints: 10–90 sec	100–400 m intervals	85–100	85–100	Anaerobic conditioning for short-course events	Recruitment and hypertrophy of type II fibers Increased activity of glycolytic and glycogenolytic enzyme Increase muscular contraction speed
Over speed	25-m intervals	Motor pacing; downhill spinning sprints	Strideouts down 1–3% hill; leg turnover drills	50–60	50–60	Make high leg turnover more comfortable	Increase muscular contraction speed

Aerobic metabolic intensity (AMI) = % $\dot{V}O_2max$. Muscular load (ML) = % of maximal muscular effort for the exercise task.

3. Increased capacity to mobilize fatty acids from the adipose and utilize fatty acids in the mitochondria.
4. Increased capacity to store intramuscular fuels (glycogen and triglycerides).
5. Enhanced thermoregulatory function.
6. Development of supporting tendons and musculature (increase movement economy).
7. Conditioning of the mind to deal with the demands of prolonged exercise.
8. Decreased fat mass (see refs. 28,37,38,82,95).

Endurance training adaptations are a general response to exercise. Several endurance adaptation will occur also in response to load and speed training sessions (see Table 59–5).

Load Training

Load training is a form of resistance training often referred to as strength-endurance training. The load training phase is introduced after a period of early-season low- to moderate-intensity endurance training and could last anywhere from 2 to 8 weeks (83). Load training is basically an increase in the resistance during an endurance training session. The resistance and muscular load progresses from low to high during the load training phase. During run training, for example, the triathlete may move from simple continuous hill running to bounding and striding out up moderate to steep slopes, while during cycle training increasingly larger gears up hill and on the flat can be used (see Table 59–5).

From our practical coaching experience, load training appears to be a particularly beneficial form of training for the triathlete. Load training may stress the neuromuscular system and trigger similar motor unit recruitment patterns to those experienced in racing, but without inducing equivalently elevated general stress and cardiovascular responses associated with race-pace speed training. Load training can also be done in the gym using high-repetition, low-resistance weights, but it can be difficult to replicate the specific movement patterns involved in swimming, cycling, and running. Strength training for the triathlon may therefore be more effective when done in the field, adding resistance to swimming, cycling, or running. Load training may help the triathlete by improving economy of movement (96) and peak muscular strength, and increasing the power or velocity at the lactate threshold (37).

Speed Training

Speed training is introduced nearing the end of the buildup phase of a training macrocycle (Fig. 59–5). The intensity and volume of speed training and racing increases during the speed phase, while total training volume decreases. Speed sessions move from an up-tempo pace early in the phase to a race pace or faster closer

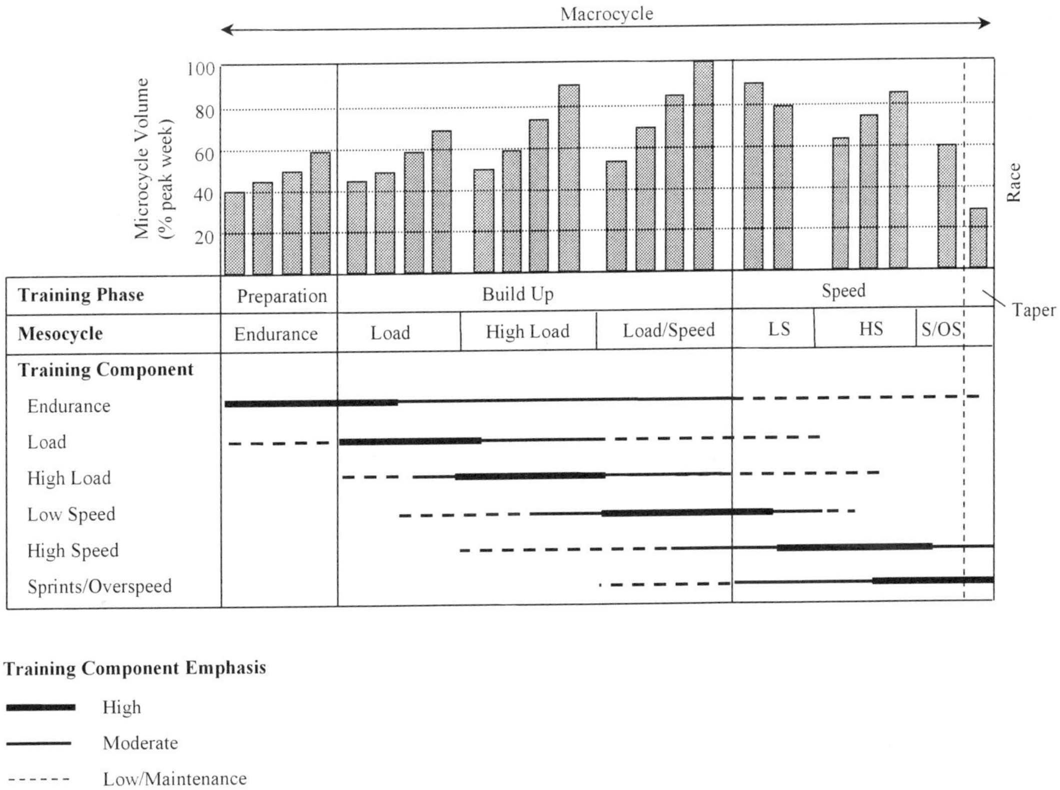

FIG. 59–5. Periodization distribution of training cycles for the triathlon. (Adapted from ref. 83.)

to the race (83,86). Elite short-course triathletes may incorporate some sprinting or overspeed training (see Table 59–5) to increase anaerobic capacity and muscular contraction in preparation for the mass start swim, attacks, and chasing breaks on the cycle, and for a sprint to the line on the run (37,83,97). During the speed phase there is an increased emphasis on racing and race-simulation training (85,86). After speed training, triathletes will usually gain considerable confidence in their competitive ability.

Taper

Short-course triathletes typically reduce training volume to 20% to 30% in the last week prior to an event (83–88). An element of race-specific, high-intensity training is maintained (86). Ironman triathletes reduce training volume from as much as 2 weeks out from racing (83,85,86).

Technique

Technique training is likely to be important for triathletes, particularly in swimming and cycling (27,29,30, 83,85,94). Triathletes begin technique training in the buildup phase, and maintain what was developed through the speed phase. Many triathletes lack the cycling skills of bunch riding, descending, and cornering, and they may benefit from developing a strong, smooth pedal technique (85). Some triathletes could benefit from modified running action and technical drills used by sprinters. A common error seen in triathletes is overstriding, which brakes the forward motion by planting the foot in front of the center of gravity (85).

Transition Training

Transition training is likely to benefit performance by minimizing the time between stages and by acclimatizing the triathlete to the physiologic and psychologic demands of sequential exercise. The rapid changing of equipment requires practice. Triathletes can gain or lose as much as 10 to 20 seconds during transitions in short races, and 1 to 2 minutes during Ironman events compared with other competitors.

PERIODIZATION

Many training programs for triathlon are prescribed in a cyclic format with a buildup toward a peak. The overall training cycle is termed a macrocycle. Within each macrocycle, periods of easy and hard weeks are grouped into mesocycles. Each training week is termed a microcycle. An example of a periodized triathlon training program is presented in Fig. 59–5.

Triathletes train specifically anywhere from 12 weeks to 10 months for a major competition (83,89). The preparation phase (macrocycle) is generally split into an initial base or buildup phase lasting at least 4 weeks, where the emphasis is on developing a sound endurance fitness base, technique, and increasing strength. The buildup is followed by a more event-specific, higher-intensity phase of around 5 to 8 weeks (83–86). Macrocycle completion is followed by several weeks of active recovery (83,86). Training can be scheduled so that macrocycle work load and fitness develop progressively over a number of years toward a career peak such as the world championship or the Olympics. Although mesocycling training has become popular in the lay training literature, there is little experimental evidence to suggest the structured programming of hard/easy training weeks to be any better than a steady increase in training load toward a peak (82,90).

Weekly Organization of Training

Triathletes generally train in all sports four to six times per week (microcycle). Recovery is taken as either 1 day off per week or 1 day of easy swimming only (83–86,89). Within a weekly microcycle, triathlon training appears most effective when following a hard/easy/hard/easy pattern, and when workouts of a similar nature are kept apart (83,86). For example high-intensity workouts and long duration training for the different sports are set as far as possible each week (Table 59–6).

Triathletes generally train different disciplines on alternate days during a microcycle to allow the muscle groups used in the previous workout to be rested while training continues in the other two disciplines. To satisfy the need for specificity, however, triathletes incorporate continuous swim-cycle-run sessions on at least 1 day of the week during the buildup phase, and up to 3 days per week during the specific phase in the final weeks

TABLE 59–6. *Example of a weekly training schedule for a short-course triathlete*

	Mon	Tue	Wed	Thurs	Fri	Sat	Sun
Swim	3 k		4 k, strength		4-k intervals	2 k	
Bike		50 k, speed		45 k, hills		25 k	80 k, long
Run	17 k, hills		25 k, long	12 k		16 k, speed	

before their target event (83–86). Research supports the inclusion of race-specific back-to-back sessions with benefits being obtained in physiologic and biomechanical variables and in metabolic efficiency (14,42,58,59). Psychologic benefits are also likely to be gained from back-to-back sessions (85,86).

Racing and Tactical Considerations

Tactics can have a considerable influence on triathlon performance. Some of the more important tactical considerations are positioning in the field and pace judgment.

As mentioned earlier, it is advantageous in terms of energy cost for a triathlete to swim in the wake of another. It is a useful tactic, therefore, to swim near the front of the pack among the faster swimmers. Triathlon swims are usually conducted in open water, and as a result it is useful for triathletes to have an understanding of water movement and the effect of wind and the tide. Triathletes benefit from finding course markers such as buoys on the swim.

Tactics can have a considerable influence on the cycle section of a draft-legal triathlon. Hills, for example, provide an excellent opportunity for attacks to break up a bunch or to establish a winning break. Triathletes are likely to benefit from some cycle racing, training, and practice in bridging and making breaks. The fastest approach for riding a hilly course during a short-course event is to ride harder than average up the hill, holding the effort over the crest, then recover and establish an aerodynamic posture on the downhill. During a long-course event, however, a more economical, even-paced strategy could be preferable. Even-pace riding requires the triathlete to climb using a similar work output to the flat. By doing so, energy reserves are used at a more economical rate and are conserved for later in the race. Many triathletes use heart rate monitors to optimize pace judgment (98).

It can take several kilometers to adjust to the change in locomotion when running after cycling. A commonly employed strategy to lose the "rubbery" feeling is to start the run using a short stride before moving into normal running rhythm. An even pace should then be maintained to the finish. The highly trained triathlete may employ surges to break up packs, and finish with a powerful sprint to the line.

Equipment

In most events, when water temperature is below 21°C (70°F), wetsuits are permitted. Wetsuits improve swimming performance by about 5% through increased buoyancy and reduced drag, allowing more energy to be directed into forward propulsion (56). Wetsuits appear to make changes to swimming technique (56), so some regular training in a wetsuit is useful.

Several of the recent technologic innovations in bicycle equipment have originated from the triathlon, the most important being the aerodynamic handlebar. Aerobars can make as much as 3 minutes' difference in a 40-km time trial (29,86). An aerodynamically shaped helmet and high-quality tires can save between 15 and 30 seconds each. Bladed spokes can save another 20 and 60 seconds. Lycra clothing creates less drag than wool or polypropylene (29). Mechanical advantage can also be gained by reductions in weight of certain areas of cycle equipment, for example, reducing rotating weight in wheel rims and pedals. Durability must be considered when lighter equipment is chosen, as equipment failure during cycling can put a triathlete out of contention. Carbon fiber, alloy, and titanium components are now common.

On the run, shoe weight and cushioning affects running economy (99,100) and Velcro closures or elastic laces can shorten transition time. Clothing can make a difference to heat dissipation (86). Gloves and thermal garments help reduce heat loss in cold conditions.

Racing Nutrition

Water, carbohydrate, and sodium replacement are the most important nutritional concerns for a triathlete during competition. Loss of body fluid, resulting largely from a mismatch between sweating and fluid consumption, can result in dehydration, which can reduce plasma volume, and impair cardiovascular and thermoregulatory function (101). Dehydration of as little as 1% of body weight can cause increased heart rate, core temperature, and perceived exertion, and can reduce endurance performance (101,102). Mental performance also deteriorates, and death can occur in extreme cases of heat exposure and dehydration (101). Readers are referred elsewhere for reviews on the physiologic and psychologic responses to dehydration during endurance exercise (101–105).

Rates of fluid loss will vary depending on a number of factors, including the intensity and duration of the triathlon, the fitness and (climatic) acclimation state of the triathlete, and the environmental conditions (36,101,102,106). Carbohydrate requirements are governed by numerous factors: (a) the length and nature of the event; (b) the fitness, dietary, and training practices of the triathlete, which determine the rate of glycogen utilization and hepatic glucose production (75,107); and (c) the quality and quantity of food consumed in the week and hours before the event (64,74,98). Sodium requirements will be influenced mostly by heat acclimation and training status (64). Due to a large number of contributing factors, it is difficult to prescribe the "ideal" fluid-carbohydrate-electrolyte strategy for triathletes. We recommend that triathletes take some time to educate themselves on issues relating to race-day nutrition and formulate their own nutrition strategy based on trials during training and recommendations from the literature, experienced athletes, and sports nutrition specialists. Generally, triathletes can ingest at least 10 mL/h/kg body weight (500 to 900 mL/h) of fluid without discomfort (64,106,108). In hot environments such as Hawaii, triathletes can expect to lose between 1000 and 2500 mL of fluid per hour (36,64,108,109). The rate of fluid loss is likely to be greater on the run than on the cycle because of reduced convective cooling and early afternoon heat. While some dehydration may be acceptable (e.g., 1% to 3% body weight), the closer the balance between sweat rate and fluid consumption, the better the performance and athlete safety will be.

In short-course triathlons (<2 hours), little or no carbohydrate may be required as sufficient glycogen stores are available in the rested triathlete (64,74,81,102,108). Recent studies however have demonstrated that carbohydrate supplementation improves 1-hour cycle performance (98,110–112), suggesting that short-course triathletes could therefore benefit from the ingestion of 4% to 8% carbohydrate solutions in shorter events. The effect, however, may be largely placebo (140). In longer events, fluid intake is complicated by the need to also ensure adequate carbohydrate intake. Typically, triathletes will deplete their muscle glycogen prior to the completion of long-course events. Carbohydrate ingestion, therefore, is required to maintain blood sugar levels and muscle carbohydrate oxidation rates for the completion of the event. Research suggests that the peak rate of ingested carbohydrate is in the range of 0.7 to 1.0 g/min (113) and the ingestion of 30 to 60 g/h, in 4% to 10% solutions, will generally be sufficient to maintain blood glucose oxidation late in exercise (108). Elite long-course triathletes could benefit from carbohydrate intakes as high as 100 g/h, similar to that used by Tour de France cyclists (113). Some athletes, however, experience problems when gastric carbohydrate concentrations are high (above 10%); this may be a result of insufficient fluid intake.

Long-course triathletes generally use a mix of sports drinks and solids (e.g., fruit or sports bars). Large particles (solids) may be preferred over solutions when fluid requirements are low (e.g., cool climate, slower athletes) because of osmotic influences (114). Readers are referred elsewhere for useful information regarding the formulation of fluid and carbohydrate drinks (108,115). It is recommended that triathletes practice drinking and eating the type and quantities of fluid and food they are expecting to require during an event (114). The addition of salt to rehydration beverages increases fluid retention, which could assist recovery (98).

In recent long-distance triathlon and ultra-running events there have been several cases of athletes being treated by medical staff for hyponatremia (blood sodium levels <135 mEq/L) (116,117). The incidence of hyponatremia in the triathlon has been reported to be proportional to race distance (109) and is more prevalent in recreational triathletes and in triathletes unacclimatized to the heat (117). It is thought to be associated with excessive loss of sodium in the sweat combined with fluid overload (117), but it can occur in association with dehydration (109,116), making correct diagnosis important for appropriate medical treatment (36,116,117,118). Symptoms associated with low blood sodium include malaise, disorientation, nausea, fatigue, seizures, and collapse (116). Triathletes competing in long-course events are recommended to take some salt (e.g., NaCl, 1 g/h) (116) during the event, most easily accomplished by the use of commercially prepared carbohydrate-electrolyte solutions. To reduce the chance of hyponatremia and to improve performance in the heat, triathletes who live in cool climates should spend several weeks acclimatizing and should salt their food or otherwise increase their salt intake by 10 to 25 g/day during the acclimatization period (116).

ACKNOWLEDGMENTS

The authors would like to acknowledge the assistance of Jonathan Peak, Annemarie Jutel, Jon Ackland, and Val Burke in the proofreading of the chapter.

REFERENCES

1. O'Toole, Douglas PS, Hiller WDB. Applied physiology of triathlon. *Sports Med* 1989;8:201–225.
2. Chatard J-C, Chollet D, Millet G. Effects of draft swimming on performance and drag. In: *8th International Symposium on Biomechanics and Medicine in Swimming.* Hong Kong: Hong Kong Olympic Academy, 1998:46.
3. Tittel K, Wutsherk H. Anatomical and anthropometric fundamentals of endurance. In: Shephard RJ, Astrand P-O, eds. *Endurance in sport.* Oxford: Blackwell, 1992:35–45.
4. Travill AL, Carter JEL, Dolan KP. Anthropometric characteristics of elite male triathletes. In: Bell FI, Van Gyn GH, eds. *Proceedings of the 10th Commonwealth and International Scientific Congress. Access to active living.* Victoria, Canada: University of Victoria, 1994:340–343.
5. Wilmore JH. Body Composition and body energy stores. In: Shephard RJ, Astrand P-O, eds. *Endurance in sport.* Oxford: Blackwell, 1992:244–255.
6. Neumann G. Cycling. In: Shephard RJ, Astrand P-O, eds. *Endurance in sport.* Oxford: Blackwell, 1992:582–596.
7. Roalstad MS. Physiologic testing of the ultraendurance triathlete. *Med Sci Sports Exerc* 1989;21:S200–S204.
8. O'Toole ML, Hiller WDB, Crosby L, Douglas PS. The ultraendurance triathlete: a physiological profile. *Med Sci Sports Exerc* 1987;19:45–50.
9. Sleivert GG, Rowlands DS. Physical and physiological factors associated with success in triathlon. *Sports Med* 1996;22:8–18.
10. Wilson N, Russell D, Wilson B. *Body composition of New Zealanders. Life in New Zealand activity and health research unit.* Otage, New Zealand: University of Otago, 1993.
11. Wilber RL, Zawadzki KM, Kearney JT, Shannon MP, Disalvo D. Physiological profiles of elite off-road and road cyclists. *Med Sci Sports Exerc* 1997;29:1090–1094.

12. Ackland J, Downey B. Unpublished data 1998, Performance Lab, Auckland.
13. Vleck VE, Garbutt G. Injury and training characteristics of male elite, development squad, and club triathletes. *Int J Sports Med* 1998;19:38–42.
14. Hue O, Le Gallais D, Chollet D, Boussana A, Prefaut C. The influence of prior cycling on biomechanical and cardiorespiratory response profiles during running in triathletes. *Eur J Appl Physiol* 1998;77:98–105.
15. Hausswirth C, Bigard AX, Guezennex CY. Relationships between running mechanics and energy cost of running at the end of a triathlon and a marathon. *Int J Sports Med* 1997;18:330–339.
16. Miura H, Kitagawa K, Ishiko T. Economy during a simulated laboratory test triathlon is highly related to Olympic distance triathlon. *Int J Sports Med* 1997;18:276–280.
17. Deitrick RW. Physiological responses of typical versus heavy weight triathletes to treadmill and bicycle exercise. *J Sports Med Phys Fitness* 1991;31:367–375.
18. Bunc V, Heller J, Horcic J, Novotny J. Physiological profile of best Czech male and female young triathletes. *J Sports Med Phys Fitness* 1996;36:265–270.
19. Delistraty DA, Noble BJ, Wilkinson JG. Treadmill and swim bench ergometry in triathletes, runners and swimmers. *J Appl Sport Sci Res* 1990;4:31–36.
20. Millard-Stafford M, Sparling PB, Rosskopf LB. Differences in peak physiological responses during running, cycling and swimming. *J Appl Sport Sci Res* 1991;5:213–218.
21. Butts NK, Henry BA, McLean D. Correlations between $\dot{V}O_2$max and performance times of recreational triathletes. *J Sports Med Phys Fit* 1991;31:339–344.
22. Albrecht TJ, Foster UL, Dickinson AL. Triathletes: exercise parameters measured during bicycle, swim bench, and treadmill testing. *Med Sci Sports Exerc* 1986;18:S86.
23. O'Toole ML, Douglas PS, Hiller WD. Lactate, oxygen uptake, and cycling performance in triathletes. *Int J Sports Med* 1989;10:413–418.
24. Leake CN, Carter JEL. Comparison of body composition and somatotype of trained female triathletes. *J Sports Sci* 1991; 9:125–135.
25. Laureson NM, Fulcher KY, Korkia P. Physiological characteristics of elite and club level female triathletes during running. *Int J Sports Med* 1993;14:455–459.
26. Stager JM, Cordain L. Relationship of body composition to swimming performance in female swimmers. *J Swim Res* 1984;1:21–26.
27. Toussaint HM. Differences in propelling efficiency between competitive and triathlon swimmers. *Med Sci Sports Exerc* 1990;22:409–415.
28. Astrand P-O, Rodahl K. *Textbook of work physiology: physiological bases of exercise,* 3rd ed. New York: McGraw-Hill, 1986.
29. Faria IE. Energy expenditure, aerodynamics and medical problems in cycling. *Sports Med* 1992;14:43–63.
30. Daniels J. A physiologists view of running economy. *Med Sci Sport Exerc* 1985;17:332–338.
31. Coyle EF, Feltner MA, Kautz SA, et al. Physiological and biomechanical factors associated with elite endurance cycling performance. *Med Sci Sports Exerc* 1991;23:93–107.
32. Coyle EF. Integration of the physiological factors determining endurance performance ability. *Exerc Sport Sci Rev* 1995; 23:25–63.
33. Lavoie JM, Montpetit RR. Applied physiology of swimming. *Sports Med* 1986;3:165–189.
34. Sjoden B, Svendenhag J. Applied physiology of marathon running. *Sports Med* 1985;2:83–99.
35. Daniels J. Physiological characteristics of champion male athletes. *Res Q* 1974;43:342–348.
36. O'Toole ML, Douglas PS. Applied physiology of triathlon. *Sports Med* 1995;19:251–267.
37. Wells CL, Pate RR. Training for performance of prolonged exercise. In: Lamb D, Murry R, eds. *Perspectives in exercise science and sports medicine, vol 1: prolonged exercise.* Indianapolis, Indiana: Benchmark Press, 1988:357–391.
38. Clausen JP. Effects of physical training on cardiovascular adjustments to exercise in man. *Physiol Rev* 1977;57:779–815.
39. Pollack ML. Characteristics of elite class distance runners. *Ann NY Acad Sci* 1977;301:278–282.
40. Burke ER. Physiological characteristics of competitive cyclists. *Phys Sports Med* 1980;8:79–64.
41. Powers SK, Howley ET. *Exercise physiology: theory and application to fitness and performance.* Dubuque, IA: Brown WC Pub, 1990.
42. De Vito G, Bernardi M, Sproiero E, Figura F. Decrease in endurance performance during Olympic triathlon. *Int J Sports Med* 1995;16:24–28.
43. Holly RG, Barnard RJ, Rosenthal M, Applegate E, Pritikin N. Triathlete characterisation and response to prolonged strenuous competition. *Med Sci Sports Exerc* 1986;18:123–127.
44. Schneider DA, Pollack J. Ventilatory threshold and maximal oxygen uptake during cycling and running in female triathletes. *Int J Sports Med* 1991;12:379–383.
45. Kreider RB, Cundiff DE, Hammett JB. Effects of cycling on running performance in triathletes. *Ann Sports Med* 1988; 3:220–225.
46. Sleivert GS, Wenger HA. Physiological predictors of short-coarse triathlon performance. *Med Sci Sports Exerc* 1993;25:871–876.
47. Dengel DR, Flynn MG, Costill DL, Kirwin JP. Determinants of success during triathlon competition. *Res Q Exerc Sport* 1989;60:234–238.
48. Kohrt WM, Morgan DW, Bates B, Skinner JS. Physiological responses of triathletes to maximal swimming, cycling and running. *Med Sci Sports Exerc* 1987;1991:51–55.
49. Spurway NC. Aerobic exercise, anaerobic exercise and the lactate threshold. *Br Med Bull* 1992;48:569–591.
50. Noakes TD. 1996 J.B. Wolfe Memorial Lecture. Challenging beliefs: ex Africa semper aliquid novi. *Med Sci Sports Exerc* 1997;29:571–590.
51. Martin DE, Vroon DH, May DF, Plibeam SP. Physiological changes in elite male distance runners training. *Phys Sports Med* 1986;14:152–171.
52. Kohrt WM, O'Conner JS, Skinner JS. Longitudinal assessment of responses by triathletes to swimming, cycling and running. *Med Sci Sports Exerc* 1989;21:569–575.
53. Conley DL, Krahanbuhl GS. Running economy and distance running performance of highly trained athletes. *Med Sci Sports Exerc* 1980;12:357–360.
54. Montpetit RR, Smith H, Boie G. Swimming economy: how to standardize the data to compare swimming proficiency. *J Swim Res* 1988;4:5–8.
55. Shields SL. The effects of varying lengths of stride on performance during submaximal treadmill testing. *J Sports Med Phys Fitness* 1982;22:66–72.
56. Toussaint HM, Bruinunk L, Coster R, et al. Effect of a triathlon wet suit on drag during swimming. *Med Sci Sports Exerc* 1989;21:325–328.
57. Hausswirth C, Bigard AX, Berthelot M, Thomaidis M, Tuezennec CY. Variability in energy cost of running at the end of a triathlon and a marathon. *Int J Sports Med* 1996;17:572–579.
58. Kreider RB, Boone T, Thompson WR, Burkes S, Cortes CW. Cardiovascular and thermal responses of triathlon performance. *Med Sci Sports Exerc* 1988;20:385–390.
59. Guezennec CY, Vallier JM, Bigard, Durey A. Increase in energy cost of running at the end of a triathlon. *Eur J Appl Physiol* 1996;73:440–445.
60. Conlee RK. Muscle glycogen and exercise endurance: a twenty-year perspective. *Exerc Sport Sci Rev* 1987;15:1–28.
61. Bergstrom J, Hermansen L, Hultman E, Saltin B. Diet, muscle glucose and physical performance. *Acta Physiol Scand* 1967; 71:140–150.
62. Hermansen L, Hultman E, Saltin B. Muscle glycogen during prolonged severe exercise. *Acta Physiol Scand* 1967;71:129–139.
63. Burke LM, Read RSD. Diet patterns of elite Australian male triathletes. *Phys Sports Med* 1987;15:140–155.
64. Shearman WM, Lamb DR. Nutrition and prolonged exercise. In: Lamb D, Murry R, eds. *Perspectives in exercise science and sports medicine, vol 1: prolonged exercise.* Benchmark Press, 1988:213–280.
65. Hawley JA, Dennis SC, Lindsay FH, Noakes TD. Nutritional

practices of athletes: are they sub-optimal? *J Sports Sci* 1995;13:S75–S87.
66. Lamb DR, Rinehardt KF, Bartels RL, Sherman WM, Snook JT. Dietary carbohydrates and intensity of interval swim training. *Am J Clin Nutr* 1990;52:1058–1063.
67. Shearman WM, Wilmer GS. Insufficient dietary carbohydrate during training: does it impair performance? *Int J Sports Med* 1991;1:28–44.
68. Simonsen JC, Sherman WM, Lamb DR, Dernbach JA, Doyle JA, Strauss R. Dietary carbohydrate, muscle glycogen, and power output during rowing training. *J Appl Physiol* 1991;70:1500–1505.
69. Khoo CS, Rawson NE, Robinson ML. Nutrient intake and eating habits of triathletes. *Ann Sports Med* 1987;3:144–150.
70. Gollnick PD. Metabolism of substrates: energy substrate metabolism during exercise and as modified by training. *Fed Proc* 1985;44:353–357.
71. Lambert EV, Speechly DP, Dennis SC, Noakes TD. Enhanced endurance in trained cyclists during moderate intensity exercise following two weeks adaptation to a high fat diet. *Eur J Appl Physiol* 1994;69:287–293.
72. Simi B, Sempore B, Mayet M, Favier RJ. Additive effects of training and high-fat diet on energy metabolism during exercise. *J Appl Physiol* 1991;71:197–203.
73. Fisher EC, Evans WJ, Phinney SD, Blackburn GL, Bistrian BR, Young VR. Changes in skeletal muscle metabolism induced by a eucaloric ketogenic diet. In: Knuttgen HG, Vogel JA, Poortsmans J, eds. *Biochemistry of Exercise: International Series of Sports Sciences,* Champaign, IL: Human Kinetics, 1983:13: 497–501.
74. Coggan AR, Mendenhall MA. Effect of diet on substrate metabolism during exercise. In: Lamb D, Murry R, eds. *Perspectives in exercise science and sports medicine, vol 1: prolonged exercise.* Indianapolis: Benchmark Press, 1988.
75. Coggan AR. Plasma glucose metabolism during exercise: effect of endurance training in humans. *Med Sci Sports Exerc* 1997;29:620–627.
76. Hawley JA, Brouns F, Jeukendrup A. Strategies to enhance fat utilization during exercise. *Sports Med* 1998;24:241–257.
77. Lambert EV. Hawley JA. Goedecke J. Noakes TD. Dennis SC. Nutritional strategies for promoting fat utilization and delaying the onset of fatigue during prolonged exercise. *J Sports Sci* 1997;15:315–324.
78. Conlee RK, Hammer RL, Winder WW, Bracken ML, Nelson AG, Barnett DW. Glycogen repletion and exercise endurance in rats adapted to a high fat diet. *Metabolism* 1990;39:289–294.
79. Miller WC, Bryce GR, Conlee RK. Adaptations to a high-fat diet that increase exercise endurance in male rats. *J Appl Physiol* 1984;56:78–83.
80. Vukovich MD, Costill DL, Hickey MS Trappe SW, Cole KJ, Fink WJ. Effect of fat emulsion infusion and fat feeding on muscle glycogen utilization during exercise. *J Appl Physiol* 1993;75:1513–1518.
81. Williams C. Macronutrients and performance. *J Sports Sci* 1995;13:S1–S10.
82. Noakes TD. *Lore of running.* Oxford University Press, Oxford 1985.
83. Ackland J. *Precision training.* Auckland: Reed, 1998.
84. Sleamaker R, Browning R. *Serious training for endurance athletes,* 2nd ed. Champaign, IL: Human Kinetics, 1996.
85. Cedaro R. Triathlon: achieving your personal best. Sydney, Australia: Murrychild, 1993.
86. Hellemans J. *Triathlon: a complete guide for training and racing.* Auckland: Reed. 1993.
87. Maffetone P. *Training for endurance.* Stamford, NY: David Barmore, 1996.
88. Niles R, Niles R, Smyers K. *Time-saving training for multisport athletes.* Champaign. IL: Human Kinetics, 1997.
89. O'Toole M. Training for ultraendurance triathlons. *Med Sci Sports Exerc* 1989;21:S209–S213.
90. Hopkins WG. New guidelines for hard training. *NZ Coach* 1993;2:16–20.
91. Wells CL, Stern JR, Kohrt WM, Campbell KD. Fluid shifts with successive running and bicycling performance. *Med Sci Sports Exerc* 1987;19:137–142.
92. Schneider DA, Pollack J. Ventilatory threshold and maximal oxygen uptake during cycling and running in female triathletes. *Int J Sports Med* 1991;12:379–383.
93. Hawley JA, Hopkins WG. Aerobic glycolytic and lipolytic powers systems: A new paradigm with implications for endurance and ultraendurance events. *Sports Med* 1995;19:240–250.
94. Lydiard A, Gilmore G. *Running with Lydiard way.* Auckland: Hdder and Stoughton, 1983.
95. Shepard RJ. Maximal oxygen intake. In: Shephard RJ, Astrand P-O, eds. *Endurance in sport.* Oxford: Blackwell, 1992:192–200.
96. Svedenhag J, Sjodin B. Endurance conditioning. In: Shepard RJ, Astrand P-O, eds. *Endurance in sport.* Oxford: Blackwell, 1992:294–295.
97. Westgarth-Taylor C, Hawley JA, Rickard S, Myburgh KH, Noakes TD, Dennis SC. Metabolic and performance adaptations to interval training in endurance-trained cyclists. *Eur J Appl Physiol Occup Physiol* 1997;75:298–304.
98. Hawley J, Burke L. *Peak performance: training and nutritional strategies for sport.* St. Leonards, Australia: Allen and Unwin, 1998.
99. Catlin ME, Dressendorfer DH. Effect of shoe weight on the energy cost of running. *Med Sci Sports* 1979;11:80.
100. Frederick EC, Clarke TE, Larsen JL, Cooper LB. The effects of shoe cushioning on the oxygen demands of running. In: Nigg B, Kerr B, eds. *Biomechanical aspects of sports shoes and playing surfaces.* Calgary: University of Calgary, 1983:107–114.
101. Murray R. Fluid needs in hot and cold environments. *Int J Sports Nutr* 1995;5:S62–S73.
102. Buskirk ER, Puhl S. Nutritional beverages: exercise and sport. In: Hickson JF, Wolinsky I, eds. *Nutrition in exercise and sport.* Boca Raton, FL:CRC Press, 1989.
103. Murray R. Nutrition for the marathon and other endurance sports: environmental stress and dehydration. *Med Sci Sports Exerc* 1992;24:S319–S323.
104. Sawka MN. Physiological consequences of dehydration: exercise performance and theromregulation. *Med Sci Sports Exerc* 1992;24:657–670.
105. Gopinathan PM, Pichan G, Sharma VM. Role of dehydration in heat stress-induced variations in mental performance. *Arch Environ Health* 1988;43:15–17.
106. Schedl HP, Maughan RJ, Gisolfi CV. Intestinal absorption during rest and exercise: Implications for formulating an oral rehydration solution. *Med Sci Sports Exerc* 1994;26:267–280.
107. Coggan AR, Swanson SC, Mendenhall LA, Habash DL, Kien CL. Effect of endurance training on hepatic glycogenolysis and gluconeogenesis during prolonged exercise in men. *Am J Physiol* 1995;268(3 pt 1):E375–E383.
108. Coyle EF, Montain SJ. Benefits of fluid replacement with carbohydrate during exercise. *Med Sci Sports Exerc* 1992;24:S324–S330.
109. Hiller WDB, O'Toole ML, Fortess EE, Laird RH, Imbert PC, Sisk TD. Medical and physiological considerations in triathlon. *Am J Sports Med* 1987;15:164–167.
110. Jeukendrup A, Brouns F, Wagenmakers AJ, Saris WH. Carbohydrate-electrolyte feedings improve 1 h time trial cycling performance. *Int J Sports Med* 1997;18:125–129.
111. el-Sayed MS, Balmer J, Rattu AJ. Carbohydrate ingestion improves endurance performance during a 1 hr simulated cycling time trial. *J Sports Sci* 1997;15:223–230.
112. Below PR, Mora-Rodriguez R, Gonzalez-Alonso J, Coyle EF. Fluid and carbohydrate ingestion independently improve performance during 1-hr of intense exercise. *Med Sci Sports Exerc* 1995;27:200–210.
113. Hawley JA, Dennis SC, Noakes TD. Oxidation of carbohydrate ingested during prolonged endurance exercise. *Sports Med* 1992;14:27–42.
114. Rehrer NJ. Factors influencing fluid bioavailability. *Aust J Nutr Dietetics* 1996;53:S8–S11.
115. Gisolfi CV, Duchman SM. Guidelines for optimal replacement beverages for different athletic events. *Med Sci Sports Exerc* 1992;24:679–687.
116. Douglas W, Hiller B. Dehydration and hyponatremia during triathlons. *Med Sci Sports Exerc* 1989;21:S219–S212.

117. Noakes TD. The hyponatremia of exercise. *Int J Sports Med* 1992;2:205–208.
118. Holtzhausen LM, Noakes TD. Collapsed ultraendurance athlete: proposed mechanisms and an approach to management. *Clin J Sport Med* 1997;7:292–301.
119. International triathlon database. http://aspra9.informatik.uni-leipzig.de/triathlon.htm.
120. Ironman World Championships. http://www.ironmantri.com/results.html.
121. Spurgeon JH, Sargent RG. *Measures of physique and nutrition on outstanding male swimmers.* Report. College of Health and Physical Education, University of South Carolina, Columbia, 1977.
122. Pyne DB, Baker MS, Fricker PA, McDonald WA, Telford RD, Weidemann MJ. Effects of an intensive 12-wk training program by elite swimmers on neutrophil oxidative activity. *Med Sci Sports Exerc* 1995;27:536–542.
123. Foley JP, Bird SR, White JA. Anthropometric comparison of cyclists from different events. *Br J Sports Med* 1989;23:30–33.
124. Hagburg JM, Mullin JP, Bahrake M, Limburg J. Physiological profiles and selected psychological characteristics of national class American cyclists. *J Sports Med* 1979;19:341–346.
125. Davies CTM, Thompson MW. Aerobic performance of female marathon and male ultramarathon athletes. *J Appl Physiol* 1979;41:233–245.
126. Sprynarova S, Parizkova J. Functional capacity and body composition in top weightlifters, swimmers, runners and skiers. *Int Z Angew Physiol* 1971;29:184–194.
127. Costill DL, Bowers R, Krammer WF. Skinfold estimates of body fat among marathon runners. *Med Sci Sports* 1970;2:93–95.
128. Hetland ML, Haarbo J, Christiansen C. Regional body composition determined by dual-energy X-ray absorptiometry. Relation to training, sex hormones, and serum lipids in male long-distance runners. *Scand J Med Sci Sports* 1998;8:102–108.
129. McNaughton LR. Plasma volume responses associated with a sprint triathlon in novice triathletes. *Int J Sports Med* 1989;10:161–164.
130. Loftin M, Warren BL, Zingraf SA. Peak physiological function and performance of recreational triathletes. *J Sports Med Phys Fitness* 1988;28:330–335.
131. Zingraf SA, Jones CJ, Warren B. An empirical investigation of triathlon performance. *J Sports Med Phys Fitness* 1986; 26:350–356.
132. Wilmore C, Brown H, Davies JA. Body physique and composition of the female distance runner. *Ann NY Acad Sci* 1977;301:765–776.
133. Korkia PK, Tunstall-Pedoe DS, Maffulli N. An epidemiological investigation of training and injury patterns in British triathletes. *Br J Sports Med* 1994;28:191–196.
134. Pickard R. Unpublished data,1995, Triathlon Australia.
135. Wilmore JH, Brown CH. Physiological profiles of women distance runners. *Med Sci Sports* 1974;6:178–181.
136. Holmer I, Lundin A, Eriksson BO. Maximal oxygen uptake in swimming and running by elite swimmers. *J Appl Physiol* 1974; 36:711–714.
137. Holmer I. Oxygen uptake during swimming in man. *J Appl Physiol* 1972;33:502–509.
138. Conley DL, Krahanbuhl GS. Running economy and distance running performance of highly trained athletes. *Med Sci Sports Exerc* 1980;12:357–360.
139. Horrell SA. *An investigation into the physiological responses of triathletes during running and cycling.* Master's dissertation. Otago, New Zealand: University of Otago, 1989.
140. Clark VR, Hopkins WG, Hawley JA, Burk LM. The size of the placebo effect of a sports drink in endurance cycling performance. *Med Sci Sports Exerc* 1998;30(5):S61.

Exercise and Sport Science,
edited by William E. Garrett, Jr., and Donald T. Kirkendall.
Lippincott Williams & Wilkins, Philadelphia © 2000.

CHAPTER 60

Physiology of Weightlifting

Michael H. Stone and Kenton B. Kirksey

THE SPORT

Historical records of tests of maximum strength and training for improved strength can be traced as far back as illustrations of weightlifting and strength movements on the tomb of the Egyptian prince Baghti dating from approximately 2040 B.C. and writings from Lu's annals in China dating from 551 B.C. (1). Although contests of strength were not included in the ancient Greek Olympics, ancient writings indicate that training with weights and contests of strength were popular in ancient Greece at least as early as 557 B.C. and that these contest were likely included in other Panhellenic games (1). The modern sport of weightlifting requires great strength, power, and speed of movement, and it can trace its beginnings to the mid-1800s when several clubs devoted to weightlifting and general strength training began to spring up in Europe, particularly in Austria and Germany. As a part of track and field, men's weightlifting was included in the first modern Olympics in 1896. Weightlifting formed its own international federation in 1905 and was recognized by the International Olympic Committee (IOC) in 1914. Women's weightlifting gained popularity in the early 1980s; the first women's world championships were held in Daytona Beach, Florida, in 1987 and women will be included in weightlifting at the Olympics for the first time in the 2000 Olympic games in Sydney, Australia. Weightlifting includes both junior (12 to 20 years) and senior men's and women's competitions at the local, regional, national, and international level.

Weightlifting competition in the Olympics and world championships included both one- and two-arm lifts from 1896 until 1925, when an IOC congress decided to limit competition to the two-hand press, snatch, and clean and jerk (1). Three lifts were contested from 1925 until 1972, when the press was dropped from competition. The two lifts contested in modern weightlifting are the snatch and clean and jerk. Currently, weightlifting is contested in approximately 160 countries, and, by number of countries participating, is one of the seven largest events in the Olympics. Each country has its own governing body. In the United States the governing body is USA Weightlifting (USAW) based at the Olympic training center in Colorado Springs. Worldwide, the governing body is the International Weightlifting Federation (IWF), in Budapest, Hungary.

Physical Requirements

The performance of competitive weightlifting movements depends primarily upon leg and hip strength and power (2). In the snatch, the bar is raised from the floor to an overhead position in one motion and the lifter either splits or squats under the bar, then stands erect Fig. 60–1). The second lift contested is the clean and jerk. The bar (weight) is first cleaned by lifting it from the floor to the shoulders (in front of the neck), and the lifter either splits or squats under the bar, and then stands erect. After cleaning the bar, it is driven overhead by the legs and caught on straight arms, and the lifter either splits or squats under the bar and again stands erect (Fig. 60–2).

It is obvious that weightlifters possess great strength and power. The amount of weight lifted is partially related to body mass; however, larger weightlifters have a lower mass lifted/body mass ratio than smaller weightlifters (Table 60–1). This difference between large and smaller athletes results from the relationship between muscle force capabilities and the cross-sectional area, which is related to the square of linear body dimensions. However, muscle mass is proportional to its volume, which is related to the cube of linear body dimensions (3). Therefore, body mass increases at a faster rate than

M. H. Stone: Department of Sports Science, Edinburgh University, Edinburgh, Scotland.
K. B. Kirksey: Department of Exercise Science, Appalachian State University, Boone, North Carolina 28608.

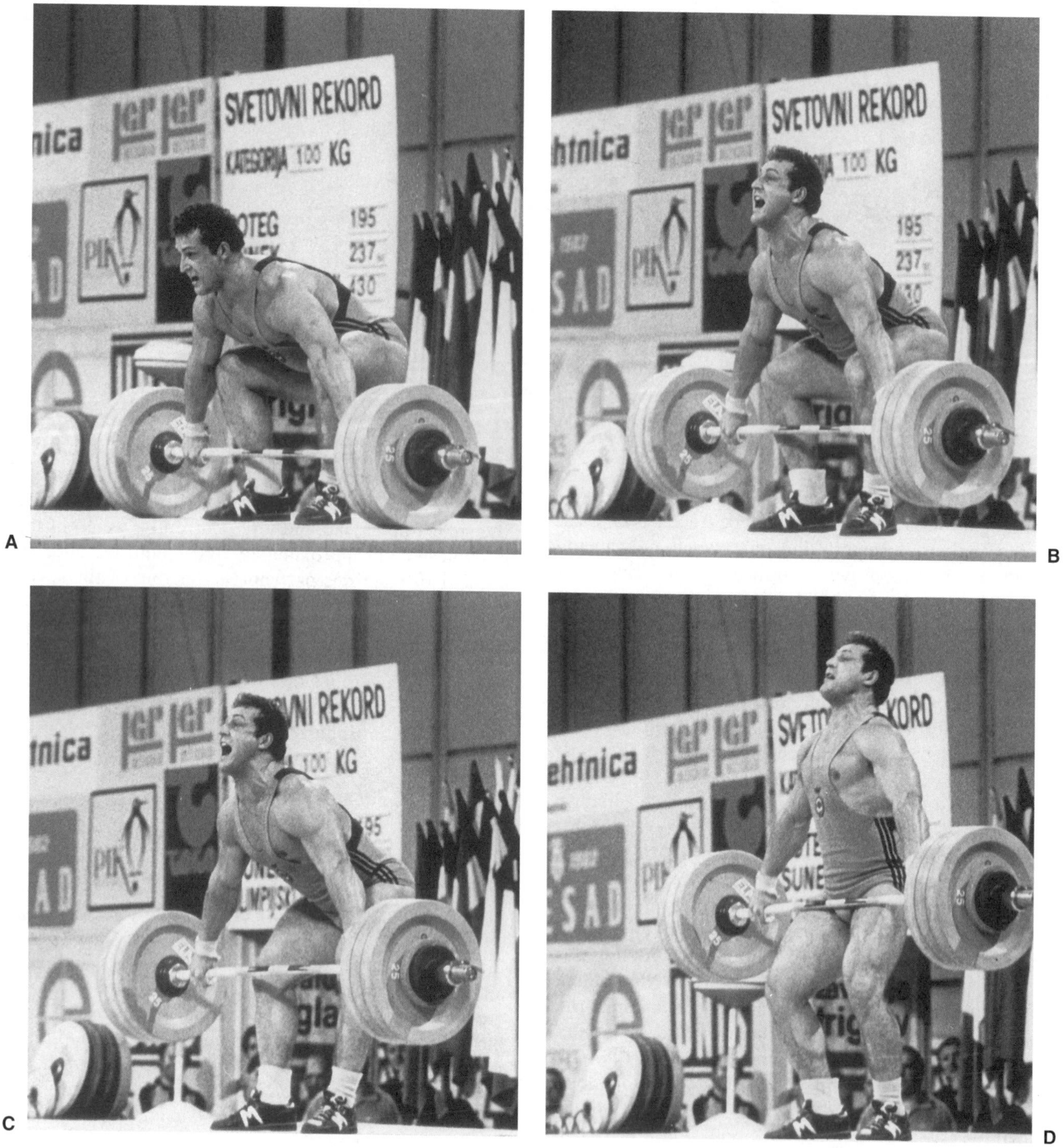

FIG. 60–1. The snatch (squat technique). (Courtesy of Bruce Klemens.) **A, B:** Initiation of the lift with leg extensors. Back is flat or arched (lordodic), arms are straight. **C:** Bar at knee; center of pressure has moved back toward the heel of the foot. **D:** "Double knee bend" position; knees have re-bent slightly, center of pressure has moved back toward the ball of the feet, feet are flat on the floor. (*continues*)

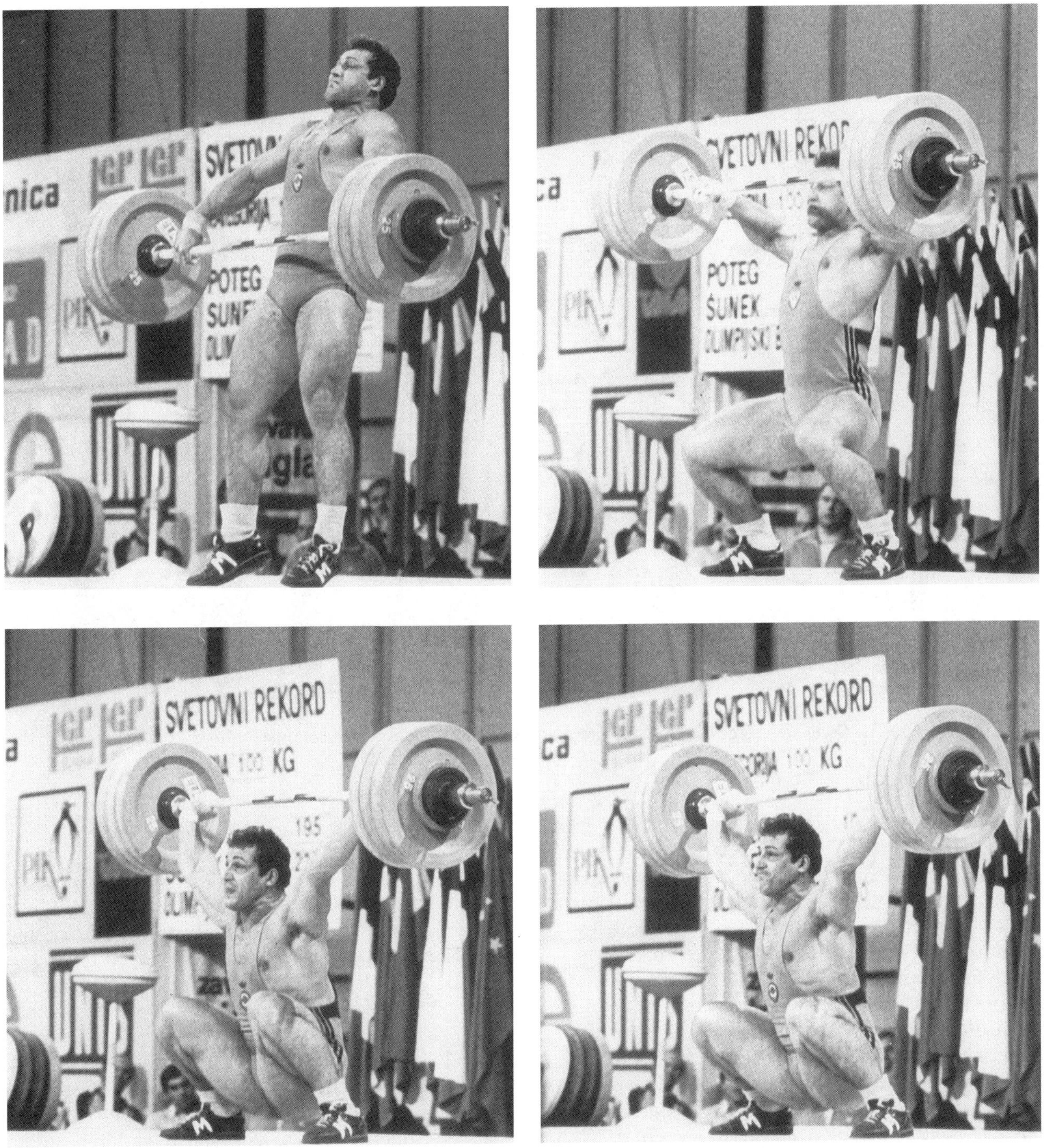

E F G H

FIG. 60–1. *Continued.* **E:** Full extension (from double knee bend position); note arms are straight until the lifter begins to move under the bar. This is the most explosive position and allows the lifter to generate maximum power. **F, G, H:** Overhead catch; lifter rapidly drops under the bar and "catches" it overhead on straight arms. (*continues*)

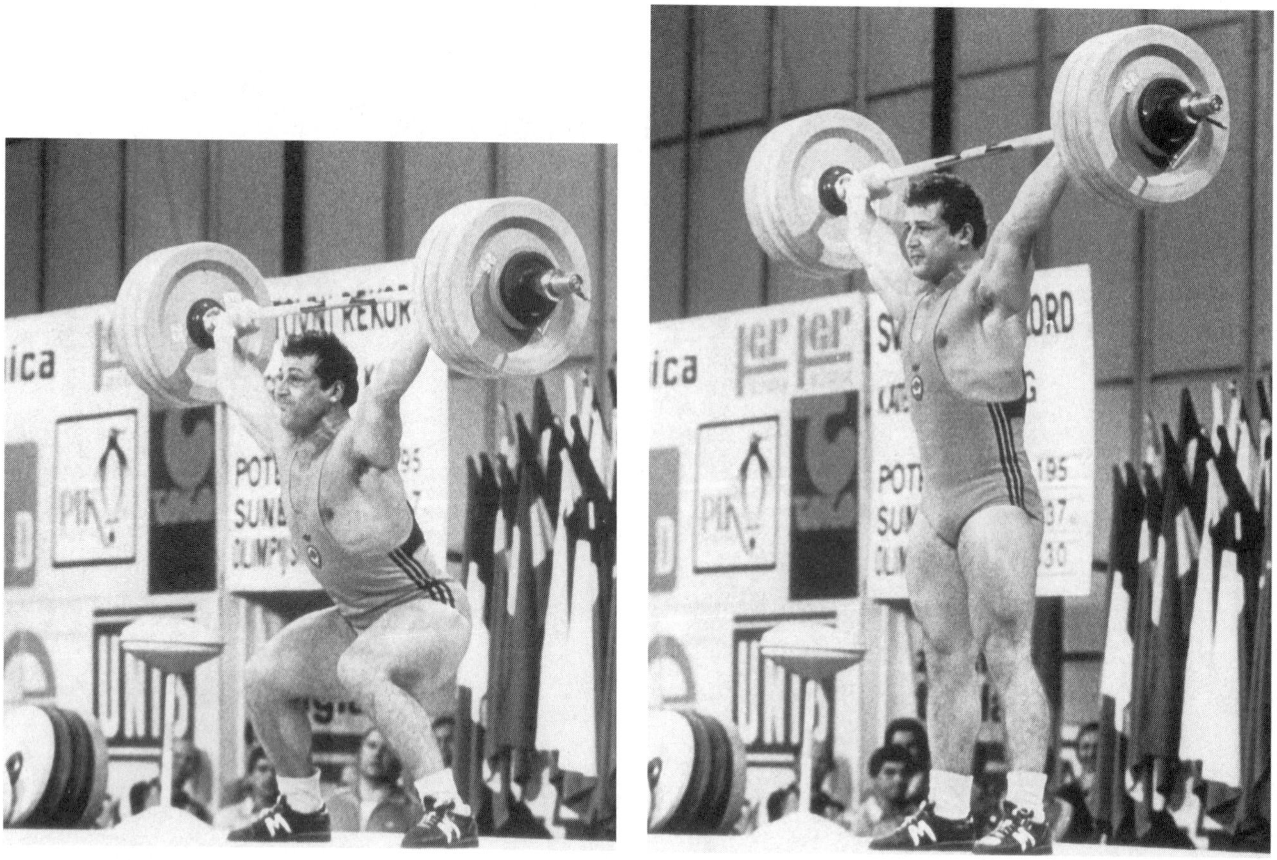

I J

FIG. 60–1. *Continued.* **I, J:** Lifter stands erect and moves feet into a parallel position.

strength. Given constant body proportions, smaller athletes are typically stronger on a per kilogram of body mass basis (strength/mass ratio) than larger athletes.

Comparisons between athletes of different sizes may provide an index as to which athlete is actually the better performer (Table 60–1). However, dividing the absolute weight lifted by body mass biases the results in favor of the smaller athlete because it does not take into account the expected decrease in the strength/mass ratio with increasing body size. Dividing the weight lifted by body mass$^{2/3}$ attempts to obviate differences in size, but apparently biases result in favor of middle-sized athletes (4,5). A number of different models for comparison of athletes of different body mass have been developed for both powerlifting and weightlifting (4,5). The comparison model most commonly used in weightlifting is the Sinclair formula (6). Table 60–1*B* shows the results of the 1996 Atlanta Olympic games; while there is a steady decrease in the total divided by body mass, this pattern is not readily apparent using the Sinclair formula.

Body weight classes have changed several times over the years. These changes result from differences in the number of athletes entering various weight classes from year to year and differences in the average weight lifted in each class at continental and world championships (7). The body weight categories have been revised for the sixth time and beginning in January 1998 are, for men, 56, 62, 69, 77, 94, 105, 105+ kg, and for women, 48, 53, 59, 63, 75, 75+ kg.

Tests of speed and power consistently show weightlifters to be among the most powerful of athletes (8–10). Tables 60–2 and 60–3 show the relative power outputs derived from the vertical jump for weightlifters and for various other male and female athletes. The superior power output of weightlifters may be partially genetic, but it more likely stems from specific training programs (2,10–12). Evidence suggests that training at high power outputs, as occurs with weightlifting training, can result in superior power performances (10,12–14).

Physiologic Requirements

The training programs used by weightlifters have been shown to markedly increase strength and power (13). It should be noted that, in terms of a whole-body move-

Text continues on page 950.

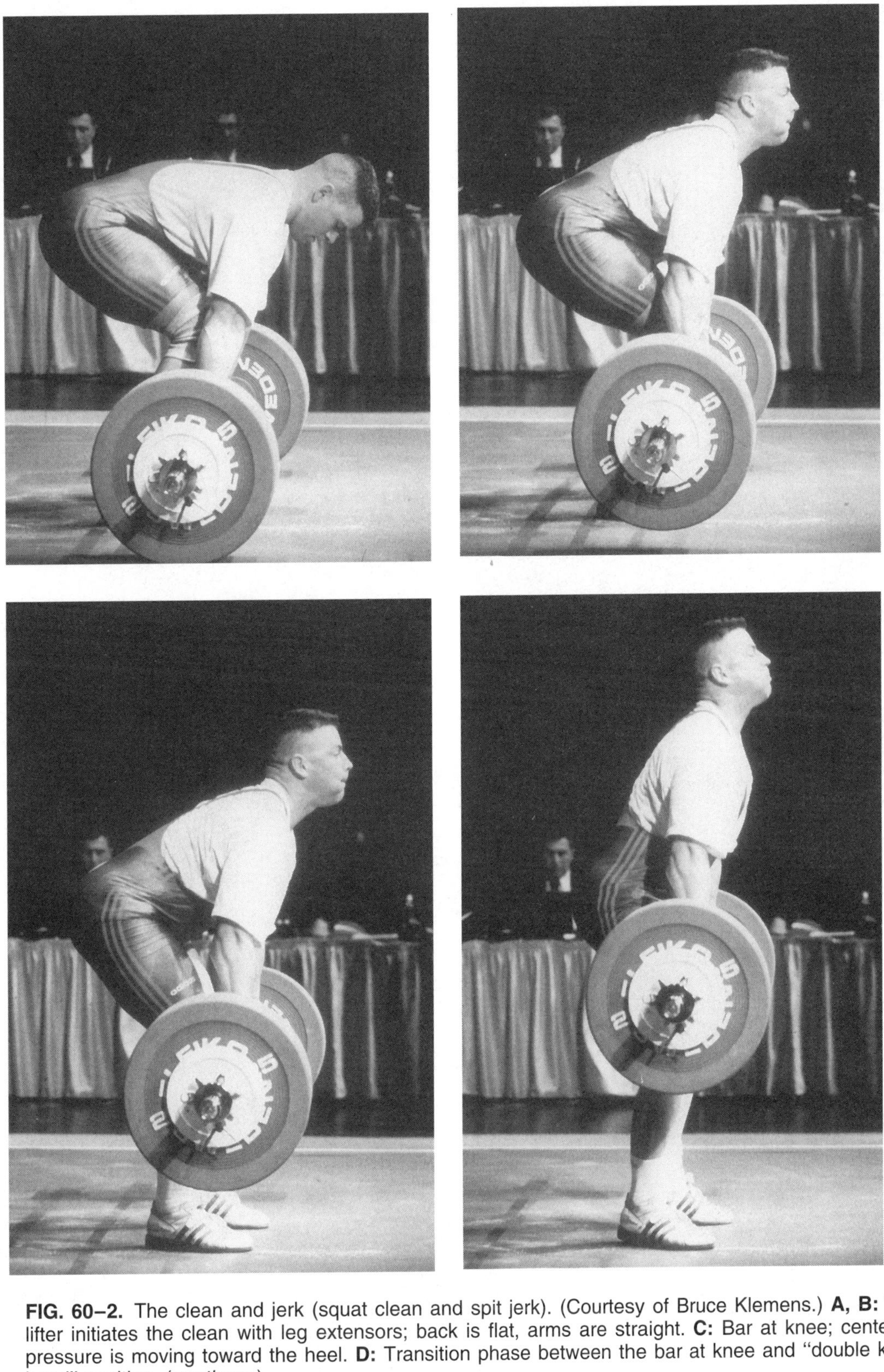

A B C D

FIG. 60–2. The clean and jerk (squat clean and spit jerk). (Courtesy of Bruce Klemens.) **A, B:** The lifter initiates the clean with leg extensors; back is flat, arms are straight. **C:** Bar at knee; center of pressure is moving toward the heel. **D:** Transition phase between the bar at knee and "double knee bend" position. (*continues*)

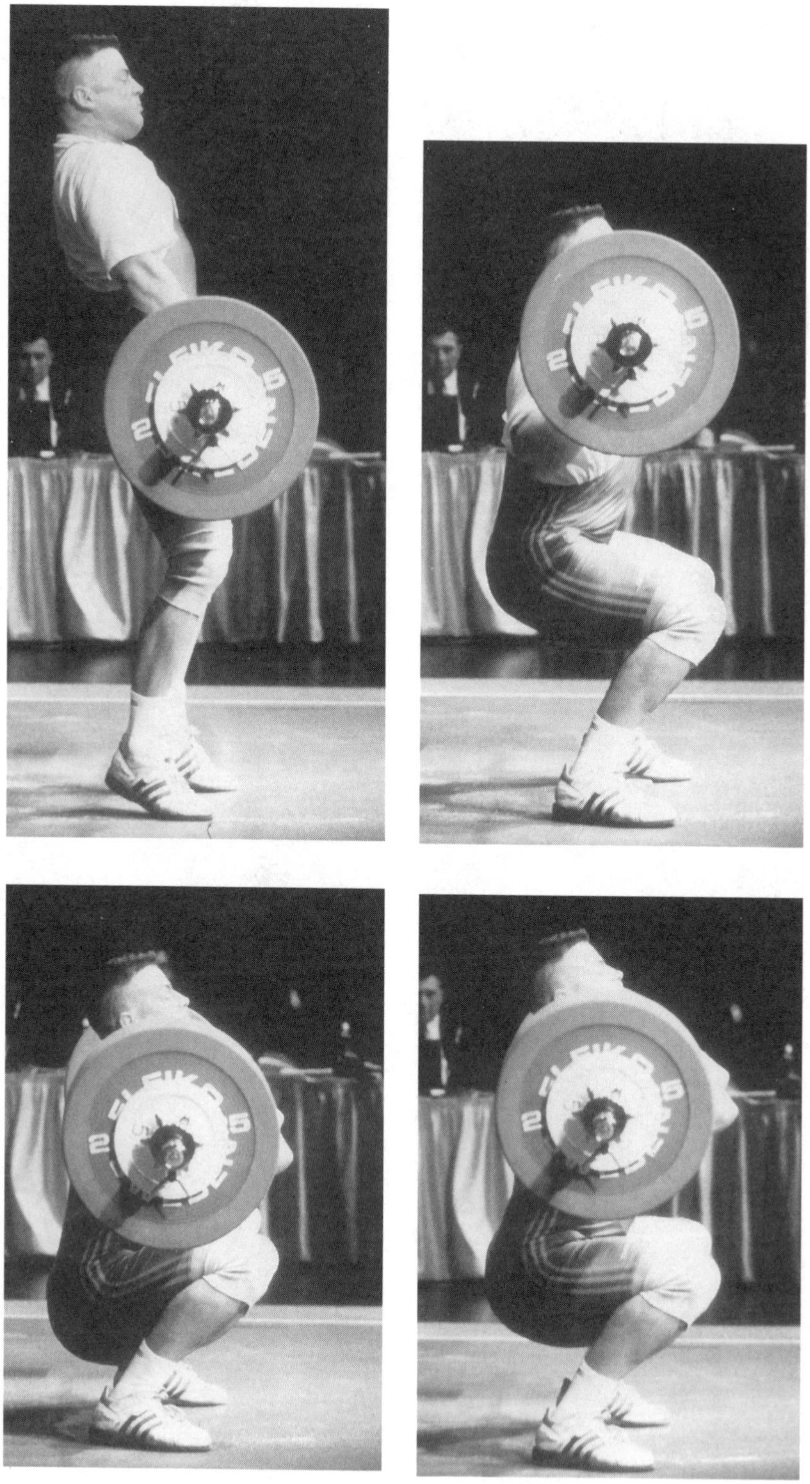

FIG. 60–2. *Continued.* **E:** Extension (from double knee bend position). **F, G, H:** Lifter rapidly moves under the bar, catching the weight on the shoulders. (*continues*)

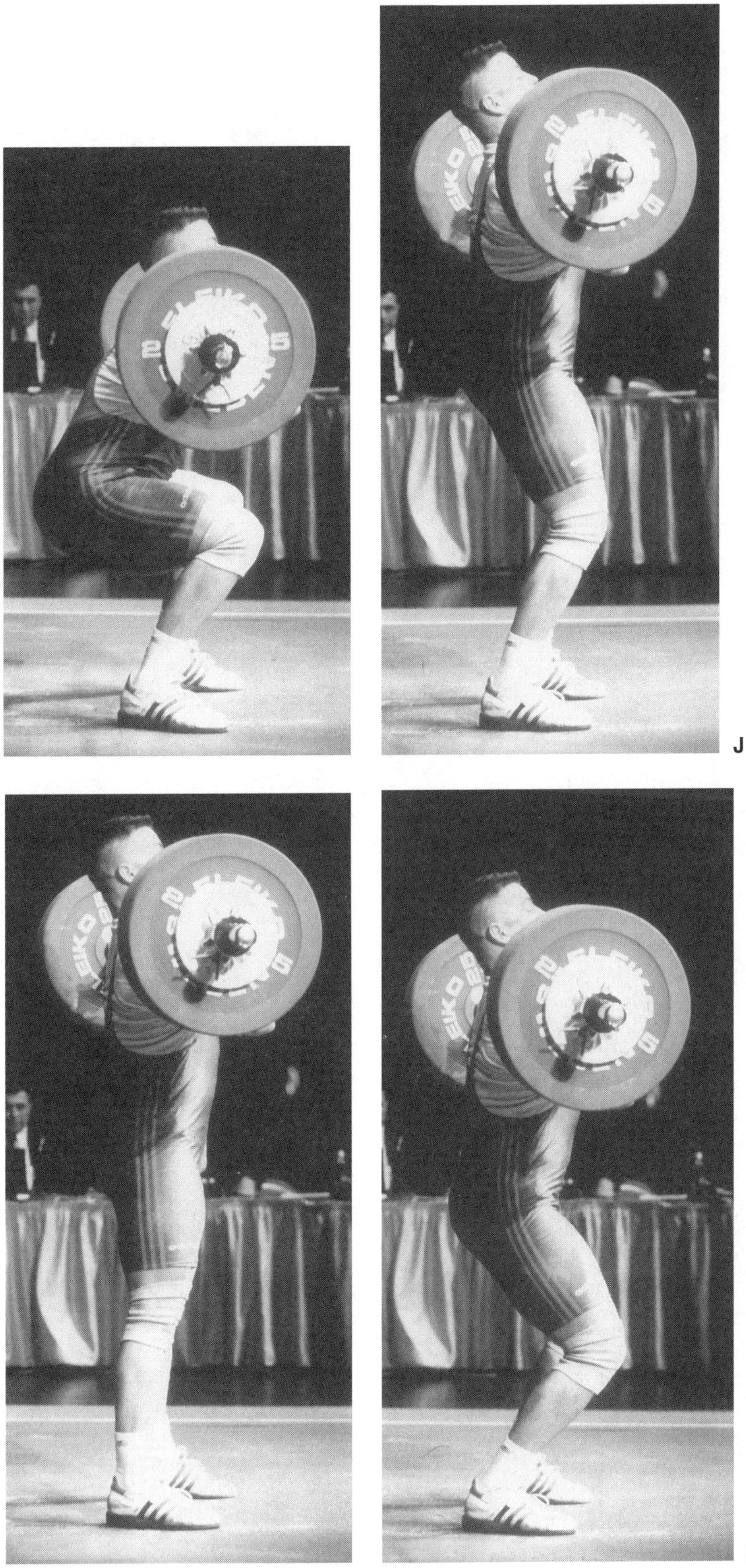

FIG. 60–2. *Continued.* **I, J, K:** Lifter stands erect, completing the clean. **L:** The dip for the jerk; initiated by eccentric action of the leg and hip extensors. (*continues*)

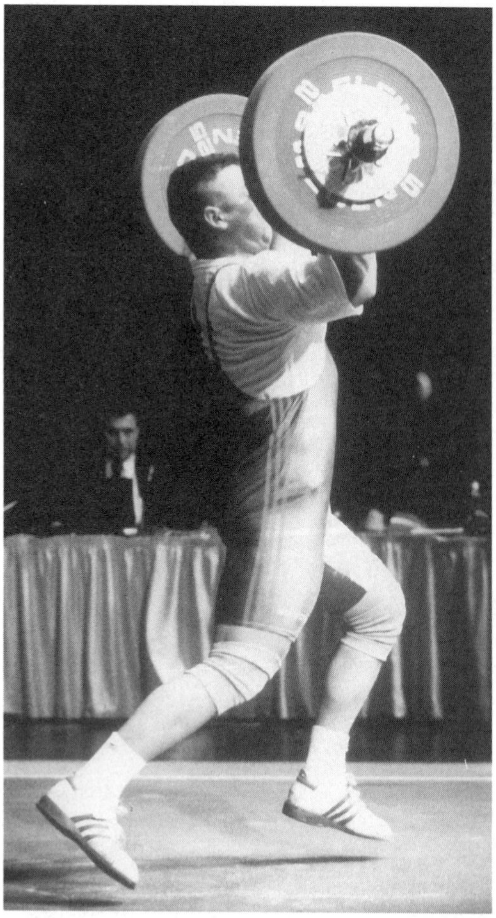

M

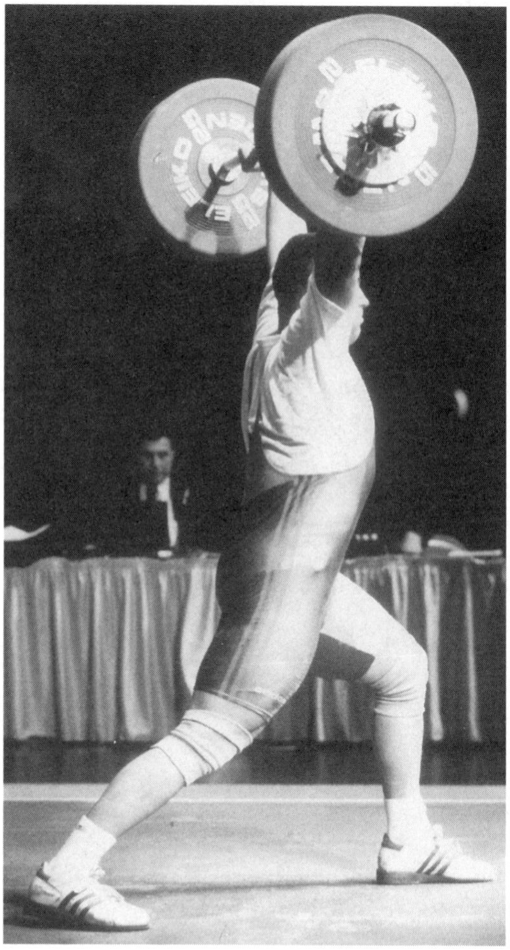

N

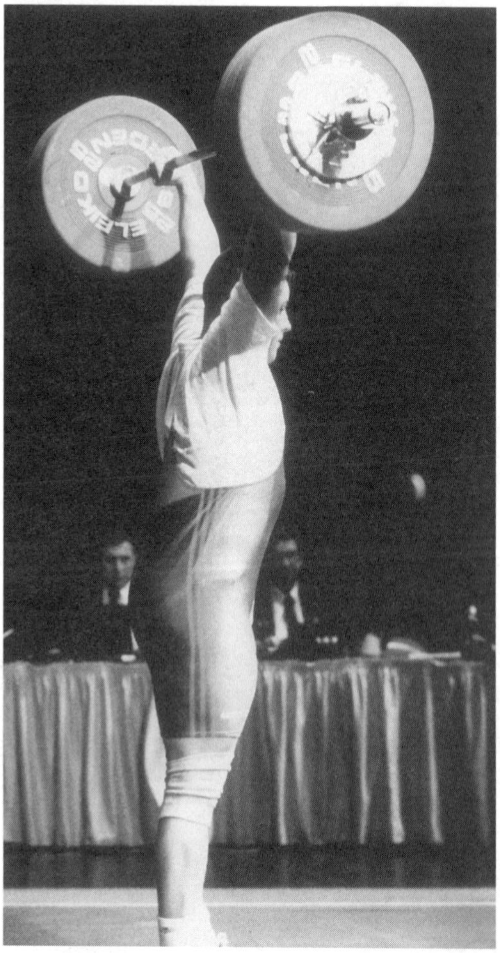

O

FIG. 60–2. *Continued.* **M, N:** The lifter thrusts upward using the leg extensors and splits (feet fore and aft), catching the bar overhead. **O:** Lifter stands erect with the feet parallel.

TABLE 60–1A. *Body height (BH), body mass (BM), and performance (1986)*

Class	Body height (cm)	Body mass	BM/BH (kg/cm)	Total (kg)	Total/BM (kg/kg)
52	156.3	51.7	0.33	292.5	5.66
56	158.0	55.8	0.35	300.0	5.38
60	157.0	59.5	0.38	335.0	5.63
67.5	163.1	66.9	0.41	355.0	5.31
75	167.5	74.4	0.44	377.5	5.07
82.5	170.1	80.8	0.48	405.0	5.01
90	176.4	88.9	0.50	422.5	4.75
100	177.7	97.7	0.55	440.0	4.50
110	180.0	105.3	0.59	447.5	4.25
>110	183.5	129.6	0.71	472.5	3.65

Modified from Tittle K, Wutscherk H. Anthropometric factors. In: Komi PV, ed. *Strength and power in sport,* London: Blackwell, 1992:186.

TABLE 60–1B. *Body mass and performance: 1996 Olympics*

Class	Body mass	Snatch	Clean and jerk	Total	T/kg	Sinclair
54	53.91	132.5	155.0	287.5	5.33	475.66
59	58.61	137.5	170.0	307.5	5.25	465.41
64	63.90	147.5	187.5	335.0	5.24	466.61
70	69.98	162.5	195.0	357.5	5.11	460.84
76	75.91	162.5	205.0	367.5	4.84	418.38
83	82.06	180.0	212.5	392.5	4.78	452.93
91	90.89	187.5	215.0	402.5	4.43	439.96
99	96.78	185.0	235.0	420.0	4.34	446.82
108	107.32	195.0	235.0	430.0	4.01	442.28
108+	165.47	197.5	260.0	457.5	2.76	457.5[a]

[a]Sinclair number listed as 1.0000 after 150.0 kg.

TABLE 60–2. *Vertical jump and power index for various male athletes*

Group	VJ (cm)	Power index (kg-m × s^{-1})	Body mass
FB OLDL (*n* = 21)*	58.4 ± 6.5	190 ± 27	115.0 ± 11.9
FB BLBTW (*n* = 36)*	68.1 ± 5.9	155 ± 18	86.7 ± 10.8
BSKB (*n* = 13)*	68.2 ± 7.2	169 ± 15	93.2 ± 9.1
TSJHT (*n* = 21)*	68.4 ± 8.7	140 ± 20	76.8 ± 12.2
EL (*n* = 17)**	75.4 ± 9.1	166 ± 30	86.8 ± 18.0
M + 1 (*n* = 10)**	67.7 ± 7.5	154 ± 40	84.9 ± 21.6
C2< (*n* = 16)**	61.7 ± 7.3	149 ± 30	85.7 ± 20.0
UT (*n* = 30)**	53.0 ± 10.3	126 ± 26	78.1 ± 11.5

FB OLDL, offensive and defensive linemen; FB BLBTW, backs, linebackers, tight ends, and wide receivers; BSKB, basketball; TSJHT, track and field, sprinters, jumpers, hurdlers, and throwers; EL, elite weightlifters; M + 1, master and 1st class; C2<, class 2 and below; UT, untrained.

*Data collected at Appalachian State University, 1988.

**Data collected at the United States Olympics Committee (USOC), Colorado Springs, 1990–1994.

TABLE 60–3. *Vertical jump and power index for various female athletes*

Group	VJ (cm)	Power index (kg-m × s^{-1})	Body mass
TSJHT (*n* = 19)*	50.5 ± 5.3	101 ± 25	64.9 ± 16.5
TDR (*n* = 8)*	42.4 ± 5.6	77 ± 11	53.6 ± 5.9
VB (*n* = 8)*	44.7 ± 4.7	91 ± 10	61.5 ± 3.9
FH (*n* = 8)*	37.1 ± 2.8	77 ± 10	56.6 ± 6.3
WL (*n* = 14)**	50.0 ± 8.0	94 ± 24	61.3 ± 11.5
UT (*n* = 11)**	32.4 ± 7.5	80 ± 12	61.1 ± 9.9

TSJHT, track and field, sprinters, jumpers, hurdlers, and throwers; TDR, track, distance runners; VB, volleyball; FH, field hockey; WL, elite weightlifters; UT, untrained.

*Data collected at Appalachian State University, 1988.

**Data from 1987 women's world championships.

TABLE 60–4. *Power outputs of different exercises*

Exercise	Absolute power (W) 100-kg male	75-kg female
Bench press	300	
Squat	1100	
Dead lift	1100	
Snatch*	3000	1750
2nd pull**	5500	2900
Clean*	2950	1750
2nd pull**	5500	2650
Jerk	5400	2600

*Total pull—lift off until maximum vertical velocity.
**2nd pull—transition until maximum vertical velocity.
Modified from ref. 2.

TABLE 60–5. *Caloric expenditure and consumption of sports activities*

Activity	Expenditure (kcal × kg^{-1} × d^{-1})	Consumption (kcal × d^{-1})
Untrained	≤40	2000–3000
Marathon	50–80	2500–6000
Basketball	55–70	5000–6000
Sprinting (track)	55–65	4300–6000
Judo	55–65	3000–6000
Throwing (field)	60–65	6000–8000
Weightlifting	55–75	3000–10,000

Modified from ref. 28.

ment, the snatch and clean and jerk afford the highest power outputs ever recorded in athletics (2,11). Examples of the power outputs from various weight training lifts are shown in Table 60–4. Logical arguments and evidence from objective studies indicate that training at high power outputs will result in superior increases in power compared to typical resistance training methods. Evidence indicates that once a reasonable strength base has been attained, weight training at high power outputs is superior in development of various movements requiring high speed and power outputs to other forms of training (14,15).

Metabolic Considerations

The energy cost of various forms of weight training, and particularly weightlifting, are often underestimated by coaches and athletes. It is not uncommon for elite weightlifters to lift 25,000 to 50,000 kg per week, not including warm-ups. Studies of energy cost suggest that during the preparation phase of weightlifting, energy expenditure may be a high as 600 kcal per hour and 3000 or more kcal per week (16,17,28). During the competition phase, energy cost is somewhat lower. Much of the energy expenditure that occurs as a result of weight training and weightlifting occurs during recovery (18,19). Furthermore, the magnitude of energy expenditure during recovery appears to be dependent on the volume of training (19). Considering the relatively large energy total expenditure, caloric intake (food) can be quite high, especially among the larger weight classes (Table 60–5).

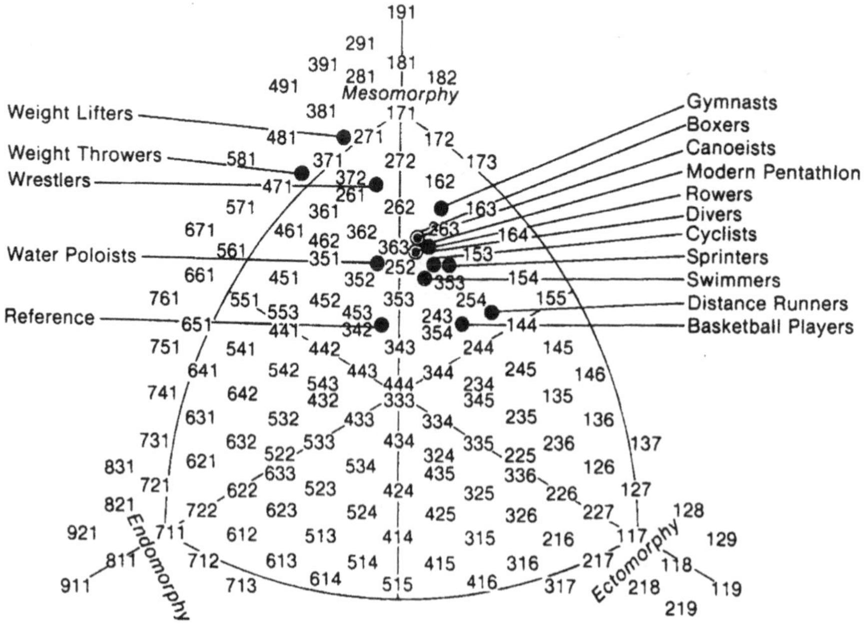

FIG. 60–3. Somatotype of various athletes. (Modified from ref. 29, with permission.)

TABLE 60–6A. *Size of weightlifters in the 1986 European championships*

Category no. (kg)	Body mass (kg)	Body height (cm)	Lengths		Diameters			Circumferences		BM/BH (g/cm)	Relative BM (%)	ST	Muscle mass (%)	Fat (%)	Bone mass (%)
			Arm (cm)	Leg (cm)	Shoulder (cm)	Chest (transv.) (cm)	Chest (sag.) (cm)	Chest (cm)	Epicond. (cm)						
East Germany															
2 (56.0)	59.0	156.0	66.9	81.8	37.5	29.0	19.7	88.5	28.2	378	107.3	D5	55.1	8.5	15.8
3 (60.0)	61.0	157.0	67.4	82.8	37.8	29.3	17.8	92.5	28.3	389	109.3	E4	54.6	6.9	15.4
3 (60.0)	63.5	157.5	66.0	82.3	38.8	29.9	17.7	94.0	29.1	403	113.0	E6	54.3	7.7	15.7
4 (67.5)	67.3	164.4	73.3	88.0	37.6	29.1	19.0	100.5	29.3	409	108.7	E6	53.7	8.4	15.8
4 (67.5)	70.0	163.1	69.8	87.8	40.8	31.5	18.0	102.0	30.3	429	115.3	E7	53.2	9.6	16.0
6 (82.5)	81.6	176.2	77.4	95.9	40.3	30.9	18.6	104.0	30.1	463	114.7	F7	54.5	11.0	14.7
7 (90.0)	90.8	178.6	76.3	91.3	40.0	29.4	20.3	103.5	32.0	508	124.2	F8	53.7	11.0	15.1
8 (100.0)	100.8	178.7	78.5	96.1	43.6	32.1	22.5	113.0	32.5	564	137.8	$D9_{oc}$	53.2	15.2	14.1
10 (>110.0)	128.3	179.8	84.2	96.8	46.0	35.7	26.2	131.0	34.7	714	173.4	$_{oc}A9$	47.4	17.0	12.6
France															
1 (<52.0)	53.0	161.5	69.0	81.7	38.3	25.7	15.7	83.0	27.2	309	89.2	H5	53.0	8.9	17.2
2 (56.0)	59.2	161.2	70.5	85.0	36.9	26.5	17.1	94.0	29.5	365	100.0	G5	51.8	9.7	16.6
4 (67.5)	66.7	172.6	74.9	91.4	38.5	29.2	19.5	96.0	28.4	386	97.7	F6	53.1	8.6	15.6
6 (82.5)	83.9	176.3	76.3	92.3	41.9	30.9	19.8	101.0	30.0	476	117.8	F8	48.7	11.1	14.2
7 (90.0)	87.8	168.9	73.6	88.5	41.9	27.3	20.9	103.0	32.6	520	134.4	F6	55.2	11.4	15.4
7 (90.0)	90.5	182.0	79.2	96.5	43.5	31.0	19.1	100.5	30.9	497	119.1	$G9_{oc}$	54.9	9.5	14.4
8 (100.0)	96.0	178.6	82.3	94.5	44.1	31.1	22.3	111.0	33.4	538	131.3	$E9_{oc}$	54.2	12.2	15.5
9 (110.0)	102.2	174.6	76.7	92.0	43.0	33.1	21.5	117.5	33.1	585	146.2	$D9_{oc}$	50.3	18.5	14.0
Bulgaria															
1 (52.0)	56.0	150.0	57.1	75.8	38.3	28.2	18.3	93.0	27.7	373	111.6	D5	46.8	11.6	15.4
2 (56.0)	60.0	155.5	69.2	83.1	37.8	29.1	19.7	97.0	28.5	386	109.9	C6	49.8	10.6	15.8
3 (60.0)	59.6	150.0	62.5	75.1	38.3	30.5	16.3	93.0	29.6	397	118.7	D6	51.9	10.4	16.6
4 (67.5)	70.0	161.2	70.8	87.4	38.8	29.5	20.5	98.0	28.9	434	118.2	C7	51.3	9.8	14.4
5 (75.0)	74.5	159.6	72.4	84.4	42.1	29.4	18.4	97.0	30.4	467	128.7	E9	55.7	10.2	14.9
5 (75.0)	74.5	169.5	73.9	88.0	39.5	28.7	18.2	101.0	30.9	439	113.2	E8	54.4	12.0	16.2
6 (82.5)	82.0	171.2	77.9	93.0	40.6	31.0	19.2	101.0	31.4	479	122.0	E8	51.1	11.1	15.5

BH, body height; BM, body mass; sag., sagittal; ST, somatotype; transv., transverse; $_{oc}$, outside the coordinate system.

TABLE 60–6B. *Physical characteristics of U.S. male weightlifters*

Number	Age (years)	Body mass (kg)	% fat	LBM (kg)	Height (cm)
EL ($n = 14$)	24 ± 3	89.1 ± 18.0	10.1 ± 4.0	80.1 ± 13.0	171.0 ± 9.5
M + 1 ($n = 7$)	26 ± 4	84.9 ± 20.9	11.7 ± 5.0	74.1 ± 14.9	173.5 ± 11.0
C2 < ($n = 13$)	24 ± 4	86.2 ± 18.2	12.4 ± 6.9	75.4 ± 15.2	172.5 ± 13.0
UT ($n = 7$)	20 ± 3	90.1 ± 5.4	18.2 ± 7.4	74.0 ± 9.6	179.0 ± 3.5

EL, elite; M + 1, master and 1st class; C2<, class 2 and below; UT, untrained males (group match statistically on physical characteristics).
LBM, lean body mass.
Body composition—skin folds.

TABLE 60–7. *Physical characteristics of elite world- and national-class female weightlifters*

Number	Age (years)	Body mass (kg)	% fat	LBM (kg)	Height (cm)
WL ($n = 14$)	27 ± 5	61.3 ± 11.5	20.4 ± 3.9	49.0 ± 12.2	161.6 ± 8.6
UT ($n = 13$)	26 ± 7	61.1 ± 9.9	27.0 ± 7.4	44.6 ± 16.8	164.2 ± 8.6

WL, elite weightlifters; UT, untrained females (group match statistically on physical characteristics); LBM, lean body mass.
Body composition—skin folds.

THE ATHLETE

Physical Characteristics

Elite weightlifters' physical characteristics are somewhat similar to those of wrestlers and throwers in track and field (Fig. 60–3). With the exception of the largest weight class, weightlifters generally have a relatively low body fat and a relatively high body mass/height ratio (20). Based on classification of weightlifters, Table 60–6 shows some of the physical characteristics of male

TABLE 60–8. *Physical characteristics of various male athletes*

Number	Age (years)	Body mass (kg)	% fat	LBM (kg)	Height (cm)
FB OLDL (n = 21)*	20 ± 3	115.0 ± 11.9	22.8 ± 5.5	88.5 ± 7.9	188.5 ± 4.7
FB BLBTW (n = 36)*	20 ± 3	86.6 ± 10.8	11.4 ± 5.8	75.8 ± 7.5	180.3 ± 4.4
BSKB (n = 13)*	20 ± 3	93.2 ± 9.1	15.3 ± 4.8	78.6 ± 5.3	194.5 ± 8.9
TSJHT (n = 21)*	20 ± 3	76.8 ± 12.2	11.8 ± 3.3	67.7 ± 7.8	178.6 ± 8.0
EL (n = 14)**	24 ± 3	89.1 ± 18.0	10.1 ± 4.0	80.1 ± 13.0	171.0 ± 9.5
UT (n = 7)**	20 ± 3	90.1 ± 5.4	18.2 ± 7.4	74.0 ± 9.6	179.0 ± 3.5

FB OLDL, offensive and defensive linemen; FB BLBTW, backs, linebackers, tight ends, and wide receivers; BSKB, basketball; TSJHT, track and field, sprinters, jumpers, hurdlers, and throwers; EL, elite weightlifters; UT, untrained.

*Data collected at Appalachian State University, 1988.

**Data collected at the USOC, Colorado Springs, 1988–1994.

TABLE 60–9. *Physical characteristics of various female athletes*

Number	Age (years)	Body mass (kg)	% fat	LBM (kg)	Height (cm)
TSJHT (n = 15)*	20 ± 3	64.9 ± 6.5	19.3 ± 3.9	52.1 ± 5.3	167.9 ± 7.0
TDR (n = 8)*	19 ± 3	53.6 ± 5.9	18.0 ± 2.1	44.9 ± 4.3	165.9 ± 18.0
VB (n = 8)*	19 ± 2	61.5 ± 3.9	19.5 ± 4.4	48.6 ± 2.7	NA
FH (n = 8)*	19 ± 4	56.6 ± 6.3	22.1 ± 5.8	42.9 ± 3.4	NA
WL (n = 14)**	27 ± 5	61.3 ± 11.5	20.4 ± 3.9	49.0 ± 12.2	161.6 ± 8.6
UT (n = 13)**	26 ± 7	61.1 ± 9.9	27.0 ± 7.4	44.6 ± 16.8	164.2 ± 8.6

TSJHT, track and field, sprinters, jumpers, hurdlers, and throwers; TDR, track, distance runners; VB, volleyball; FH, field hockey; WL, elite weightlifters; UT, untrained.

*Data collected at Appalachian State University, 1988.

**Data from 1987 women's world championships.

weightlifters of different abilities. Note that percent fat tends to decrease with the level of athlete. The same characteristics of female weightlifters are shown in Table 60–7. These characteristics can be compared to the characteristics of high-level football players, basketball players, and track and field participants (Table 60–8). Comparisons of female lifters' physical characteristics are shown in Table 60–9.

The high body mass/height ratio compared to untrained subjects and other athletic groups is advantageous because it can provide a force production advantage. This advantage is associated with the strong positive relationship between muscle cross-sectional area and maximum muscle force generating capabilities. If two athletes of different heights and different limb lengths have the same muscle mass and volume, the shorter athlete will have the greatest muscle cross section and therefore a greater muscle generating force. The relatively low body fats and high lean body mass among elite weightlifters can be associated with the extensive training programs used (19,21).

TRAINING THE ATHLETE

Sport-Specific Training

Two overhead lifts have been contested since 1972. The training programs for competition are based on general training principles (22). These principles are:

1. Overload of volume and intensity
2. Variation
3. Specificity

The overload principle relates to stressing the biologic system beyond the norm. Thus, over a period of years, in order to provide a continued stimulus, the training volume and training intensity will increase. Volume of training is typically estimated as the volume load (repetitions × mass lifted), and training intensity is estimated by the average weight of the bar per week, per month, and so on. The volume load can be related to the total work accomplished, and the training intensity can be related to the rate at which training proceeds. Training intensity should be differentiated from exercise intensity, which is the power output of a movement (22). Relative intensity is the percentage of the 1 repetition maximum (RM) for a given exercise (lift). Weights equal to approximately 30% to 50% of the maximum isometric capabilities usually produce the highest exercise intensity (i.e., power outputs). This would be equal to about 70% to 85% of the 1 RM snatch and clean and jerk (4; MH Stone, unpublished data, 1996), a relative intensity at which most training takes place (23).

Variation relates to the changes in the composition of the training program. These changes can include alterations in volume, training intensity, and exercise intensity, as well as exercise selection. Variation is extremely important so as to avoid the maladaptations associated with various forms of overtraining (24). Variation of training volume and intensity can be used to achieve desired goals; for example, high-volume, low-intensity exercise may be used to enhance high-intensity exercise endurance and beneficially alter body composition, while high-intensity, low-volume training may emphasize increases in maximum strength. Exercise variation would include the use of different exercises as well as variations of the same exercise.

Specificity relates to stressing the appropriate bioenergetic system and using appropriate mechanics. The specificity principle implies that the greatest training effects will occur if the training lifts are similar to the snatch and clean and jerk. This mechanical similarity includes peak force, rates of force development, velocity, and movement patterns.

Periodization

The concept of periodization appears to be the most effective method of applying the principles of training to most sports including weightlifting. A periodized program is divided into specific phases, each of which relates to variation in volume, intensity, and exercise selection. A period or macrocycle is the largest time division, typically lasting 1 year. A mesocyle or middle-length cycle typically last a few months. Microcycles relate to day-to-day variation and are typically a week long. Summated microcycles relate to the week-to-week variation in volume and intensity and are typically 4 weeks long. Figure 60–4 shows a typical macrocycle for weightlifting. Note that within the macrocycle or period, training volume begins high and decreases prior to the most important meets. Training intensity begins relatively low and increases across the macrocyle. Several mesocycles can be embedded within the macrocycle. Each mesocycle takes the same general form as the macrocycle (i.e., high volume to low volume; low intensity to high intensity).

Of considerable importance is the variation in exercise selection. An important tenet of periodization is the concept of moving from general to specific. This means that as the macrocycle and mesocycle progress, there is an increasing emphasis on specificity as it relates to the performance characteristics of the sport. Thus, in weightlifting as each mesocycle progresses, more emphasis is placed on the complete squat snatch and complete clean and jerk as well as speed of movement. In this respect there is greater emphasis placed on technique training as the mesocycle progresses.

Based on the variation of volume, intensity, and exercise selection, each mesocycle can be divided into preparation, competition, and active rest phases. The preparation phase is used to prepare the athlete to better handle the high training and exercise intensity that comes later in the mesocycle. The competition phase emphasizes increasing the training intensity and the mechanical specificity (i.e., technique work). Active rest is necessary

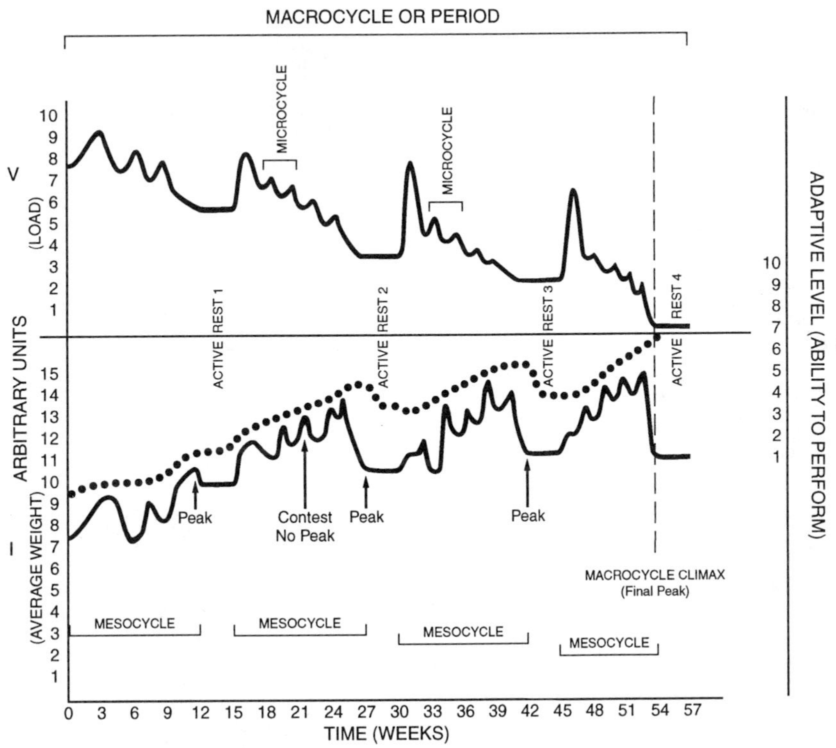

FIG. 60–4. Periodization model.

to recover properly from the rigors of training and preparing for competition (e.g., microtrauma, emotional strain, etc.). Active rest typically requires the athlete to train at low volumes and low to moderate intensities (see Fig. 60–4). Active rest is important because complete rest results in a great deal of detraining.

Although most coaches use some variation of the periodization concept, there is no universal agreement on the details, especially in the United States. For example, during the preparation phase, some coaches increase the number of repetitions per set and others increase the number of sets in order to increase the volume of training. Other differences may include the number and timing of complete lifts (i.e., squat snatch and squat clean and jerk) or the number of lifts performed at various relative intensities during a mesocycle.

While ballistic movements such as those used in weightlifting have been criticized as producing excessive injuries (25), little objective evidence has been offered to substantiate this claim. Reviews and studies of injuries and injury rates associated with weight training and weightlifting indicate that neither rates nor severity of injuries are excessive, and the incidence is less than that associated with sports such as American football, rugby, basketball, and gymnastics (26,27).

CONCLUSION

1. Physical attributes of weightlifters resemble those of wrestler's and throwers.
2. The height/weight ratio of weightlifters is smaller than for most athletes.
3. The weight lifted in competition is partially related to body mass.
4. Smaller lifters have a higher mass lifted/body mass ratio.
5. Weightlifters are among the most powerful of all athletic groups.
6. Weightlifting training typically follows a periodized program.
7. The metabolic cost of weightlifting training is often underestimated.

ACKNOWLEDGMENT

A special thanks goes to Mr. Lyn Jones, USA Weightlifting coaching director, for his help and patience in the preparation of this manuscript.

REFERENCES

1. Schodl G. *The lost past.* Budapest: International Weightlifting Federation, 1992.
2. Garhammer JJ. Power production by Olympic weightlifters. *Med Sci Sports Exerc* 1980;12:54–60.
3. Harman E. Biomechanical factors in human strength. *Strength Conditioning* 1994;16:46–53.
4. Hester D, Hunter G, Shuleva K, et al. Review and evaluation of relative strength-handicapping models. *Natl Strength Conditioning Assoc J* 1990;12:54–57.
5. Hunter G, Hester D, Snyder S, et al. Rationale and methods for evaluating relative strength-handicapping models. *Natl Strength Conditioning Assoc J* 1990;12:47–57.
6. Sinclair RG. Normalizing the performances of athletes in Olympic weightlifting. *Can J Appl Sports Sci* 1985;10:94–98.
7. Virvidakis K. The new categories. *World Weightlifting* 1997;1:37.
8. Baker D. Improving vertical jump performance through general, special and specific strength training: a brief review. *J Strength Conditioning Res* 1996;10:131–136.
9. Stone MH. Physical and physiological preparation for weightlifting. In: Chandler J, Stone M, eds. *USWF safety manual.* Colorado Springs, CO: USWF, 1991:70–101.
10. Stone MH. NSCA position stance literature review: explosive exercise. *Natl Strength Conditioning Assoc J* 1993;15:7–15.
11. Garhammer JJ. A comparison of maximal power outputs between elite male and female weightlifters in competition. *Int J Sport Biomech* 1991;7:3–11.
12. Hakkinen K. Neuromuscular adaptation during strength training, aging, detraining and immobilization. *Crit Rev Phys Rehabil Med* 1994;6:161–198.
13. Stone MH, Byrd R, Tew J, Wood M. Relationship between anaerobic power and Olympic weightlifting performance. *J Sports Med Phys Fitness* 1980;20:99–102..
14. Wilson GJ, Newton RU, Murphy AJ, Humphries BJ. The optimal training load for the development of dynamic athletic performance. *Med Sci Sport Exerc* 1993;25:1279–1286.
15. Harris G, Stone M, O'Bryant H, et al. Effects of three different weight training programs on measures of athletic performance: maximum strength, power, speed and agility. Paper presented at the NSCA National Convention, Atlanta, June 1996.
16. Scala D, McMillan J, Blessing D, et al. Metabolic cost of a preparatory phase of training in weightlifting. A practical observation. *J Appl Sports Sci Res* 1987;1:48–52.
17. Laritcheva KA, Valovarya NI, Shybin NI, Smirnov, SA, et al. Study of energy expenditure and protein needs of top weightlifters. In: Parizkova J, Rogozkin V, eds. *Nutrition, physical fitness, and health. International series on sport sciences*, vol 7. Baltimore: University Park Press, 1978:53–68.
18. Burleson MA, O'Bryant HS, Stone MH, Collins M, Triplett-McBride T. Effect of weight training exercise and treadmill exercise on post-exercise oxygen consumption. *Med Sci Sport Exerc* 1998;30:518–522.
19. Melby CC, Scholl G, Edwards G, Bullough R. Effect of acute resistance exercise on post-exercise energy expenditure and resting metabolic rate. *J Appl Physiol* 1993;75:1847–1853.
20. Tittle K, Wutscherk H. Anthropometric factors. In: Komi PV, ed. *Strength and power in sport.* London: Blackwell Scientific, 1992;180–196.
21. McMillan JL, Stone MH, Sartain J, et al. 20-hour physiological responses to a single weight training session. *J Strength Conditioning Res* 1993;7:9–21.
22. Stone MH, O'Bryant HS. *Weight training: a scientific approach.* Minneapolis: Burgess International, 1987.
23. Zatsiorsky VM. *Science and practice of strength training.* Champaign, IL: Human Kinetics, 1995.
24. Stone MH, Keith R, Kearney JT, Wilson GD, Fleck J. Overtraining: a review of the signs and symptoms of overtraining. *J Appl Sports Sci Res* 1991;5:3550.
25. Brzycki M. Speed of movement an explosive issue. *Nautilus* 1994;Spring:8–11.
26. Hamill BP. Relative safety of weightlifting and weight training. *J Strength Conditioning Res* 1994;8:5357.
27. Stone MH, Fry AC, Ritchie M, Stoessel Ross L, Marsit JL. Injury potential and safety aspects of weightlifting movements. *Strength Conditioning* 1994;16:1524.
28. Stone MH. Weight gain and loss. In: Baechle T, ed. *Essentials of strength and conditioning.* Champaign, IL: Human Kinetics, 1994;231–237.
29. Fox EL, Bowers RW, Foss ML. *Physiological basis of physical education and athletics,* 4th ed. Philadelphia: WB Saunders, 1988:561.

Exercise and Sport Science,
edited by William E. Garrett, Jr., and Donald T. Kirkendall.
Lippincott Williams & Wilkins, Philadelphia © 2000.

CHAPTER 61

Physiology of Wrestling

Craig A. Horswill

This chapter summarizes the applied physiology of wrestling as it pertains to competition at the international level (Pan American Games, Common Wealth Games, World Cup, World Games, and Olympics) and at the scholastic and intercollegiate levels in the United States. The objective in all these levels is identical: to pin the opponent's back (scapulae) to the ground (mat). The duration that defines this objective, which is called a *fall*, varies depending on the level of competition. If a fall does not occur, a scoring system has been established for each level of competition to determine the winner based on points earned for obtaining degrees of control over the opponent. The scoring systems for the three levels of competition presented in this chapter are listed Table 61–1. The chapter also discusses the physical requirements for the sport, the physiologic profile of the wrestler, and the training protocols that wrestlers use to prepare for competition. Within the preparatory protocols, we identify physical conditioning and the nutrition and weight loss practices used by wrestlers.

THE SPORT

Physical Requirements

Wrestling can be described as a high-intensity sport in which an athlete attempts to maintain superior, direct physical control over an opponent. The sport is contested without an intermediary device (such as a ball), and opponents are matched for body mass. A multitude of styles of wrestling exist around the world, each being unique to the culture where it is played. Overall, though, due to the relative brevity of the match and for other reasons detailed within this chapter, power is a critical element in success among all styles.

C.A. Horswill: Department of Research and Development, Gatorade Exercise Physiology Laboratory, The Quaker Oats Co., Barrington, Illinois 60010.

The Arena: The Mat

With wrestling being a high-contact sport, the most important piece of equipment for injury prevention is the mat. Depending on the level of competition, the size requirements will vary, but universally mats are about 10 cm in depth.

In international competition for freestyle and Greco-Roman wrestling, the surface of the mat has an inner circle (9-m diameter) for the active wrestling area and an outer ring, called the zone, which is 1 m in width beyond the inner circle. The zone provides a visual warning to the wrestlers that they are moving off the mat into an area in which action will be stopped by the official. Beyond the zone is the out-of-bounds area, which merely protects the wrestlers when the momentum of their action carries them off the mat. Although control points may be awarded when the wrestlers land out of bounds, movement into the out-of-bounds area will eventually stop the match.

The mat used at the scholastic and collegiate levels are similar to each other, and differ from the international mat only in that there is no zone and there is one pair of parallel lines at the center of the mat. The parallel lines are the starting lines that are used when there is a break in the action at a point when one wrestler is in control of the opponent. This may occur after wrestlers have gone out of bounds or at the beginning of a new period of the match. The position that employs the starting lines on the mat is called the referee's position or the optional start (international style). The size of the wrestling areas of the mat for scholastic and collegiate competition are 58 m^2 and 76 m^2, respectively. A minimum of 1.5 m of mat is the out-of-bounds area.

Match Duration

Matches are relatively short and high in intensity. The general trend in recent history, has been to decrease

TABLE 61–1. *Scoring system for wrestling*

Execution	Definition	Score: International	Score: Collegiate	Score: Scholastic
Takedown	Obtaining control of opponent from a neutral start	Depends whether control is gained with opponent on: Knees, stomach—1 pt Back—2 or 3 pts	2 pts	2 pts
Escape	Reestablishing neutral position, after starting under the control of the opponent (defensive position)	0 pt	1 pt	1 pt
Reversal	Obtaining control from defensive position	1 pt, depending on degree on control obtained (like takedown)	2 pts	2 pts
Near fall	Opponent is turned onto his back	Opponent's back is: Momentarily exposed at 90-degree angle—1 pt Exposed at 45-degree angle—2 pts Held for up to 5 sec—3 pts	Opponent on back for: 1–4 sec—2 pts ≥5 sec—3 pts	Opponent on back for: 1–4 sec—2 pts >5 sec—3 pts
Fall	Opponent's scapulae, or area between are held to mat; immediately ends match and determines victor regardless of score to that point	Momentary (less than 1 sec)	1 sec	2 sec

the match duration. A description of the match is given at each level of competition.

Internationally, matches are a continuous 5 minutes in duration. There is no break in the action unless the match is stopped by the official for an injury, an out-of-bounds call, or a situation in which one wrestler is penalized for avoiding activity (stalling). The 5-minute duration is a digression from the 9-minute match of the mid-1970s and the 15-minute match of the 1950s.

At the collegiate level, matches consistent of three periods of wrestling: a 3-minute first period, followed by 2-minute second and third periods, for a total of 7 minutes. This is a reduction in total time from 8 minutes (2 minutes, 3 minutes, and 3 minutes for the three periods, respectively), which was used in collegiate matches in the 1950s through the 1970s.

At the scholastic level, matches are 6 minutes in length, consisting of three 2-minute periods.

Weight Classes and Weigh-In

Like few other sports, wrestling attempts to match competitors by body mass, so that power and strength are evenly matched, and skill, among other factors, becomes the major determinant of success. In addition, matching opponents for equal body mass may help reduce the risks of injury to the participants. To ensure that opponents are of equal mass, a weigh-in is conducted by an objective party (official) prior to the competition. At this time each wrestler must weigh exactly the mass of the weight class or less in order to be eligible to compete. Failure to meet this requirement will cause the wrestler to default victory to the opponent.

In international competition the weigh-ins are conducted the evening or afternoon before competition is initiated. Thus, some 20 hours may pass before the athletes actually wrestle. This recovery period, which has important implications for the nutritional preparation for competition (see below), has been lengthened from the 3 hours allowed in previous eras of the sport (before the 1980s). As a consequence of the deaths caused by drastic weight reduction in three collegiate wrestlers in 1997, collegiate weigh-ins are held 2 hours before competition.

The weight classes for international and collegiate competition have changed sporadically over the years (Table 61–2). Interested readers can consult the sport-governing bodies (SGBs), such as USA Wrestling or the National Collegiate Athletic Association (NCAA) for the most current weight classifications (1–3). The change in 1997 reduced the number of international weight classes from 10 to 8, and discriminates against wrestlers in the lightest weight classes, which previously included the 48- and 52-kg classes.

At the scholastic level, the weight classes span a broader range and contain more classes to encourage more participation. The scholastic classes (presented in Table 61–2) have also changed over the years in an attempt to maximize fairness and offer maximum opportunity in accordance with the frequency distribution of

TABLE 61–2. *Weight classifications for wrestling*

International		U.S. Collegiate,	Scholastic,
kg	lb	lb	lb
54	119	125	103
58	127.75	133	112
63	138.75	141	119
69	152	149	125
76	167.5	157	130
85	187.25	165	135
97	213.75	174	140
97–125	213.75–275.5	184	145
		197	152
		197–285	160
			171
			189
			≤275

Data from refs. 1 (Collegiate), 2 (Scholastic), and 3 (International).

body mass for adolescent males in the United States. Weigh-ins are held 30 minutes to 1 hour prior to competition, although this may lengthen to several hours at the time of major tournament competition. One state (Michigan) has even allowed weigh-ins to be conducted the day prior to competition for the final state tournament championship. Unlike collegiate and international competition, many of the SGBs at the scholastic level will grant an additional 1 or 2 pounds for the weight class over the course of a season to accommodate the growth of the young athletes.

Equipment

Because competition is based on the direct contact between opponents, there are few requirements for the equipment at any level of competition. At all levels, wrestlers must wear high-cut shoes, historically required to prevent a wrestler from purposely kicking off a shoe so to obtain a rest while the shoe is refitted. Wrestlers must also wear a standard singlet for competition. At the international level, one wrestler wears a blue singlet while the other wears red. This is required to facilitate the scoring during a match: the officials, who may not speak a common language, wear a blue band on one wrist and a red band on the opposite wrist. Fingers for the appropriate hand can be raised to signify the number of points scored for the wrestler in the corresponding color. At the scholastic and collegiate levels, wrestlers wear qualified uniforms that signify their school colors; ankle bands of red or green color may be used to assist in assigning points scored during the match.

At the scholastic and collegiate levels, the only other requirement is the wearing of head gear to protect the ears from contusions and permanent scarring (called cauliflower ear). The cauliflower ear is often a trademark of those who have persisted in the sport beyond the college years into international competition, where head gear is not permitted.

The Official

One last element on the match of competition is the official or referee. Typically only one is present at each match to help facilitate the flow of action, prevent injury and unfair maneuvers, and award control points from an objective perspective. At higher levels of competition, such as the state and collegiate championships, two or more may be present per match. Internationally, three officials—the referee, the mat judge, and the mat chairman—are required; two of the three must agree on the points before any scores are awarded to a wrestler who has performed a maneuver for control.

Physiologic Requirements

Wrestling has been described as an intermediary sport, one that makes demands on both the aerobic and anaerobic energy systems. The priority for physiologic requirements is complicated because a match may last as short as 10 seconds or as long as 9 minutes (into sudden-death overtime), possibly stressing explosiveness of the lower body or endurance in the upper body. The average rate of energy expenditure in wrestling has been estimated to be 54 to 59 $kJ \cdot min^{-1}$ (13 to 14 $kcal \cdot min^{-1}$) (4,5), giving wrestling one of the highest rates of expenditure among other sports (4). Recently, we reported a figure of about 560 kcal per hour during a wrestling practice (6). Considering that rest periods and efforts of only mild to moderate intensity are used during practice drills, our estimates for a 2-hour training session are not inconsistent with literature estimates for the full-effort activity. At such intensities that may last for nearly 9 minutes, well-developed physiologic capacities at both the peripheral and central levels are critical. In the following sections, the demands on peripheral and central physiologic capacities are presented.

Peripheral Fitness

The substrate used to supply the energy during wrestling appears to be a mixture of fat and carbohydrate, with carbohydrate becoming more critical as intensity increases. For example, muscle glycogen levels in the vastus lateralis were reduced by 21.5% as a result of a 6-minute Olympic-style match (7). The reduction was consistent across all muscle fiber types; hence, wrestling places similar demands on slow-twitch (oxidative) fibers, and fast-twitch (glycolytic) fibers (7). At first, these findings appear to conflict with recent data showing no change in muscle glycogen of wrestlers competing in four matches during a tournament (8). However, the more recent study did not account for carbohydrate intake between matches (8); thus, muscle glycogen could have been resynthesized and restored during the recovery periods between matches, creating the appearance that glycogen was not an important source of fuel. High lactate levels in the subjects (8), in the range of 9 to 14 mmol/L in blood drawn 4 minutes after the match, suggest carbohydrate, either muscle glycogen or blood glucose, is an important substrate. Similarly, Houston and colleagues (7) reported an almost 10-fold increase in blood lactate levels (10.5 ± 1.4 mmol·L^{-1}) and an average blood pH level of 7.06.

Limited aerobic capacity of the skeletal muscle of wrestlers, as suggested by the activity of succinate dehydrogenase in elite wrestlers at the international level (9), may require greater contributions from anaerobic metabolism and tolerance to lactate accumulation during a wrestling match. In support of the importance of a high capacity for anaerobic metabolism in wrestling, the activity of phosphofructokinase (PFK), a glycolytic enzyme, was reported to be an average of 34.5 mmol·g^{-1}·min^{-1} (9) in wrestlers. This value is relatively high compared to that of weightlifters (24.7 mmol·g^{-1}·min^{-1}), cyclists (23.9 mmol·g^{-1}·min^{-1}), and hockey players (approximately 25.5 mmol·g^{-1}·min^{-1}) (10). Nevertheless, lactate levels at the end of a match are not extraordinarily high. Average values of 10.5 mmol/L and 11.6 mmol/L have been reported following 6-minute (two 3-minute periods with a 1-minute rest between) freestyle matches under experimental conditions (7) and 5-minute continuous matches at the European freestyle championships (11).

An area in which future research might focus is the contribution of acid-buffering capacity to delay fatigue in wrestlers. The accumulation of hydrogen ions (H^+) from lactate production is the significant limiting factor, physiologically, in sustained or repeated efforts of high intensity, such as those exerted during a wrestling match. Both energy metabolism (12) and the contractile processes (12,13) are disrupted as a consequence of the decrease in muscle pH. Studies have not been conducted on the buffering capacity in wrestlers, yet such work is warranted based on Sharratt's (14) observations that elite Olympic-level wrestlers had maximum minute ventilation values that were low relative to peak $\dot{V}O_2$ values and lactate levels. Sharratt suggested that the Olympic-level wrestlers may hypoventilate during maximum exercise as a result of becoming conditioned to years of restricted breathing during self-generated isometric contractions or physical restrictions imposed by the opponent. The idea that successful wrestlers may be more tolerant of lactic acid accumulation compared to the less-successful wrestler is supported by the observation that wrestlers who were successful in earning a spot on an Olympic team had greater dynamic endurance (maximum number of repetitions of bench press performed with a free weight of 22.7 kg) than did the runners-up for the final team (15). Studies might examine, then, the muscle-buffering capacity of wrestlers before and after a period of weeks of wrestling-specific training. In addition, it might be of value to use indirect measures of blood bicarbonate buffering capacity to determine the extent to which peripheral and central fitness contribute to training adaptations in wrestlers.

Central Fitness

A commonly used index of central fitness in athletes is peak oxygen uptake (peak $\dot{V}O_2$). Most studies of the peak $\dot{V}O_2$ values for running on the treadmill in wrestlers were conducted between the late 1960s and the mid-1980s (9,15–19). The data from these studies indicate peak $\dot{V}O_2$ values between 50 and 62 mL·kg^{-1}·min^{-1} for scholastic age to Olympic-caliber wrestlers (10).

Clinicians or scientists who may use these data in profiling wrestlers are cautioned for two reasons. First, since the time of these studies, rule changes have shortened the duration of matches and encouraged the use power maneuvers (explosiveness) to score points (10). Thus, the conditioning for the sport or the selection of the type of athlete in the sport may have changed to reflected the rule changes. Second, because of the specificity of training, treadmill running is not likely to discriminate between successful and less successful wrestlers, as the available data on Olympic, collegiate, and scholastic wrestlers indicate (15,18,20). Instead, peak $\dot{V}O_2$ for body-specific segments may be more useful (10,21). Ergometry, particularly the arm crank, simulates movements that are more similar to those of wrestling, isolates efforts to a specific area of the body as wrestling frequently does, and provides an index of physical performance (work rate or power) at the point when the physiologic measure (peak $\dot{V}O_2$) is achieved.

Besides peak $\dot{V}O_2$, specific myocardial characteristics may be an important attribute for participation in the sport. Morganroth and colleagues (22), Cohen and Segal (23), and Pelliccia's group (24,25) reported that the mass of the wall and septum of the left ventricle were greater in wrestlers compared to nonathletes or endurance athletes. Wrestlers had left-ventricular (LV) end-diastolic volumes that were less than those of endurance-trained athletes but similar to those of nonathletes. One might conclude that the greater LV mass is a prerequisite for the sport. Recently, though, Smith and colleagues (26) showed that training-induced hypertrophy is likely an adaptation to the increased afterload placed on the heart during wrestling-specific training, an adaptation that others have hypothesized (22,24). Interestingly, weight loss by the wrestlers did not dampen the adaptation; hence, the training stimulus appears to be quite great and is not overridden by potential nutritional deficiencies that may occur with restricted food intake to reach the weight limit. Physiologically, this adaptation may be a necessary feature to allow blood flow to continue to the muscle despite the vascular resistance that is generated during maximal isometric contractions executed in wrestling training and competition.

THE ATHLETE

The ability to control the opponent physically is critical for success in the sport. This can be accomplished several ways: (a) by having greater absolute power or strength than the opponent; (b) by acquiring greater relative power or strength through the selection of the weight class; (c) by greater endurance, provided that the wrestler can withstand the power of the opponent; and (d) by developing superior technical skills, which allow the wrestler to outmaneuver a potentially stronger opponent, or allow the wrestler to maximize leverage. Obviously, the combination of all of these would be the optimal approach to maximizes one's chances of success in wrestling. We will address what the research shows about each of these. To this point, no systematic research has been conducted on all methods at one time.

Power and Strength

In reviewing these attributes, where available, the data for elite and nonelite wrestlers will be compared. Also, data across levels of competition will be presented. Much of the research suggests that having greater strength is advantageous in wrestling. Cisar and colleagues (27) showed that in scholastic wrestlers, a combination of isokinetic strength measurements distinguished the successful wrestler from the least successful. Similarly, a tendency for greater isokinetic strength appeared to exist in successful collegiate wrestlers, particularly in the upper body, compared to less successful collegiate wrestlers in the same tournament (18). Although isometric strength does not appear to differentiate between the successful and less successful (15,28), it still may be an important trait needed to participate in the sport.

Anaerobic power appears to be of critical value to success in the sport. At the scholastic level, peak anaerobic power and mean power (anaerobic capacity) in both the upper and lower body of elite junior wrestlers measured using the Wingate test exceeded those of nonelite counterparts by about 13% ($p < .05$) (20). The differences might be due to differences in the relative amount of muscle or to differences in neuromuscular recruitment, but age, body weight, and wrestling training experience were similar between groups (20). It is not known whether anaerobic power distinguishes successful from less successful wrestlers at the collegiate and international level. The interested reader can consult prior reviews for comparisons of power and strength among wrestlers at various levels of competition.

Power and Strength Relative to Weight Class

Wrestlers can increase relative strength by two means: by training, which may increase absolute strength, and by changing a weight class, usually achieved through weight reduction to reach a classification at a lower than normal body weight. In this section, we focus on the latter, as the debate continues over whether weight loss can in fact increase relative strength.

Among the studies investigating physical performance of wrestlers, few if any demonstrate a change in short-duration (less than 30 seconds) intense performance (e.g., anaerobic power or strength) after rapid weight loss (29–36). These findings are derived from studies in which the subjects were wrestlers who were accustomed to undergoing weight loss and were psychologically prepared to perform at maximal level (37). Physiologic explanations for the lack of a decrement in performance after weight loss include the muscle's self-containment during short-duration maximal efforts, and temporary independence of blood-borne nutrients such as glucose or oxygen. For a single short exertion, there appears to be normal amounts of adenosine triphosphate (ATP) and phosphocreatine stores even when glycogen has been severely reduced (36), and with the presence of some myoglobin, the lack of oxygen would not be a limitation. Also, it appears that in the dehydrated state the motor unit can still "fire" when recruited, despite having lost electrolytes. Maintenance of the muscle's excitability despite imbalances in the mineral and water content in the dehydrated state have been confirmed (38). Because of the apparent lack of a reduction in short-duration, high-intensity power efforts after weight loss, in theory weight loss might enhance performance relative to the weight class. Presently, though, there is only one study showing a tendency for increased power relative to the lower body weight (30), but there are no data to support an improvement relative to the lower weight class in which the wrestler would now compete. The distinction between body weight and weight class appears subtle, but high-power performance relative to the weight class should be the focus of future research in this area.

Recent investigations have attempted to determine whether a relationship exists between weight variation and success on the mat (39,40). Such an association would support the contention that weight loss may enhance strength and power relative to the weight class in which the wrestler wants to compete. In these studies, the practice of weight gain following the weigh-in but prior to competition was presumed to reflect weight loss to make the competitive weight class. No relationship was observed for likelihood of defeating the opponent or placing in the collegiate national tournament in conjunction with weight gain or being heavier than the opponent at the time of competition (39). The high degree of prevalence of weight gain among all competitors likely negates any plausible benefits of such a practice (40). The question remains whether a wrestler would be at a disadvantage relative to his weight class if he did not reduce body weight to a lower classification.

Endurance

The ability of the wrestler to maintain high power performance throughout practice or across all matches within a 1- to 3-day tournament encompasses the endurance requirements of the wrestler. A wrestler with high aerobic capacity can be as successful as the powerful wrestler who has less endurance. The style or technical execution and strategies used by the endurance wrestler vary from that of the more powerful wrestler. This is exemplified in the overall trend of a high maximum oxygen uptake (about 60 $mL \cdot kg^{-1} \cdot min^{-1}$) at least in elite wrestlers in the Western nations in the 1970s and 1980s. Those familiar with international competition in that era know that wrestlers from such nations appeared to lack power but relied on stamina to win matches in the third period of the match.

When the efforts are sustained or repeated at near-maximal levels for more than 30 seconds (41–44) or are prolonged submaximal efforts (45–47), endurance capacity is diminished after rapid weight loss in the wrestler. Reduced muscle blood flow in the dehydrated state may slow nutrient exchange, waste removal, and heat dissipation from the muscle during the relaxation period between contractions and thereby impede the muscle's ability to recover. Also, following rapid weight loss of between 6% and 8% of body weight, wrestlers may experience nearly a 50% reduction in muscle glycogen (8,36), which could adversely affect sustained efforts. The glycogen reduction appears consistent for the fibers in the upper (8) and lower (36) body. Buffering capacity of the muscle and blood may also be compromised with rapid weight loss. In previous research (42), the blood base excess at rest was significantly lower after weight loss than before weight loss; the reduced buffering capacity was dependent on the type of diet used during weight loss, with a high-carbohydrate diet tending to preserve blood base excess. The only other investigation on blood buffering capacity of wrestlers does not corroborate this depression following weight loss, however (48). In summary, the weight-reduced wrestler may not be able to recover completely after a flurry of high-power efforts, and subsequent or sustained physical performance may be diminished.

Nutrition components will also have a major bearing on a wrestler's endurance, regardless of the strategic style of the wrestler. Wrestlers will alter training patterns (i.e., increase the volume of training) and their diet plans (i.e., decrease energy and fluid intake) to reduce body weight to reach the weight limit for competition. Consequently, their nutritional preparedness for competition can be severely compromised and could greatly influence their endurance capacity. With a period of up to 20 hours between the weigh-in and competition for international matches, wrestlers have the opportunity to make a substantial recovery. One recommendation for maximizing the speed of replenishing muscle glycogen is to consume approximately 50 g of carbohydrate (e.g., the amount in 2.5 medium-sized apples or 2.5 cups of unsweetened oatmeal) every 2 hours for 20 hours (49). A minimum of about 4.5 g carbohydrate per kilogram per day of training appears to prevent a loss of high-power muscular performance (42,50). Fluid intake that restores body weight to normal level and fluids that contain sodium to restore plasma and total body water are recommended. Fluids that contain carbohydrate are ideal for helping recovery from dehydration as well as from reduced glycogen stores. The benefit of such carbohydrate intake on performance after only 5 hours of recovery was recently demonstrated by Rankin and colleagues (48). The effect of longer-term diet treatments on optimizing glycogen levels in muscle, particularly in regard to fiber type in wrestlers, has yet to be investigated.

Technical Skills

Little information exists on how wrestling effectiveness is influenced by biomechanical factors. Most coaches and experienced wrestlers agree that regardless of the physiologic capacities, the ability to execute technical skills is the greatest factor determining success on the mat. As a tribute to this, the majority of the training time in supervised practices, particularly in the early portion of the season, is spent learning new techniques, drilling, refining familiar skills, and wrestling at 100% effort against a partner. Superior wrestlers are often described as being extremely strong by their opponents and training partners; yet, strength discrepancies do not stand out in the literature as a distinction between successful and less successful wrestlers. This is possibly explained by the fact that laboratory methodologies do not include the technical skill component of wrestling when strength is assessed in the lab. The most successful wrestlers are likely to utilize an economy of movement that allows them to exert a minimum of energy and optimal force, power, or torque in order to score points on the opponent.

Unfortunately, little research has been conducted on any aspect of technical skill performance in wrestlers in the Western world. In contrast, applied research was the mainstay of the former Communist countries (Harold Tunnemann, personal communication); however, the results of such research were seldom published due to the confidential nature and desire to keep the information within their own programs. In an earlier effort to account for technical skills as well as reaction-movement time, Taylor and colleagues (16) developed a battery of tests specifically for wrestling. Because of the small sample size of eight in this initial study, and because all the wrestlers were of high caliber, it was not possible to correlate technical speed with success on the mat. Unfortunately, other researchers of the sport have not used the test protocol. More recently, Utter and colleagues (51) developed a performance test specific for wrestlers. The series of tests such as those of Utter and colleagues or Taylor and colleagues could be a promising way to profile champion wrestlers and to monitor technical training in future research, but these novel tests must be linked to objective measures of torque, force production, or power to make the assessment truly beneficial to studying the relationship between technical execution and the chances of success.

A final point should be made about the integration of training programs for optimizing physiologic capacities with technical skill development. Often, the coach will develop in his mind the ideal physiologic profile of a wrestler and will proceed to train his individual wrestlers to conform to the profile. However, because the genetic potential of the individuals on a team is so diverse, it might be better to adapt technical skills and mat strategies that optimize the existing physiologic strengths of each individual. The goal of this approach would be to allow each wrestler the opportunity to emphasize his physiologic strengths on the mat and minimize the exposure of his physiologic weaknesses during competition.

TRAINING THE ATHLETE

The Season

Training plans are developed around the course and length of the season, which is dependent on the level of competition. For example, international competition is nearly year-round. Elite wrestlers and coaches identify the key competition for any particular year (Olympics every 4 years; World Games every year except Olympic years; Pan Am games every other year and in non-Olympic years), and prepare their training accordingly. No limits are set on the amount of training or exposure to the coach at this level. At the scholastic and collegiate levels, more limitations are placed on the season length and amount of coach-supervised training. Scholastically, the seasons typically run for 4 months, beginning with a mixture of dual meets and culminating with the state championships. The collegiate season follows a similar format except that it runs about 1 month longer and ends with national, rather than state, championships. State or national governing bodies, in conjunction with the academic institutions, regulate the length of season, the number of competitions (dual meets and tournaments), and the amount and time of practices controlled by the coach of the athletes. For both of these levels, there are off-season competitions outside of academic regulatory bodies (i.e., the international style conducted at the club level).

With the season and competitive schedule in mind (i.e., dual meets and lesser competitions first, followed by the significant championship tournaments), the training programs are developed to meet the following four objectives:

- maximize conditioning—strength, power, and muscular endurance—specific to wrestling;
- optimize technical skill execution, and refine and possibly expand the repertoire of skills (moves);
- foster competitive attitudes and mental toughness;
- adapt strategies and physiologic capacities to achieve goals (win matches and tournaments, or beat specific opponents).

A number of studies have tested wrestlers for physical performance and fitness before and at the end of the competitive season, but it is difficult to interpret the training effects from such descriptions because the studies are confounded by weight loss, diet restrictions, and lack of accounting for the type of training that wrestlers undergo (31,52–54). The importance of accounting for the training is underscored by the revelation in one study that peak torque measurements decreased in wrestlers who gained weight during the season (54). Because experimental research has compared systematic methods of training for wrestling, the information presented herein is based on historical perspectives (10,55), the recommendations from SGBs in the United States (56), and theoretical considerations of the physiology of wrestling (57).

Sport-Specific Training

Obviously, the most specific and best method of training for the sport is to wrestle. Most coaches use a systematic approach, rather than a haphazard approach of just throwing two teammates together. Initially, as the season begins, the athletes might not have the stamina to wrestling at a 100% effort for a duration that stimulates training adaptations. This is particularly true for novice wrestlers and those returning from a long break in training. Hence, the coach will start with drills and fundamentals, including the seven basic skills of stance, motion, changing levels, penetration, lifting, back step, and the high arch (58). This provides a minimum fitness base as well as coordination and skill acquisition (10). In a matter of several days, the coach will introduce live wrestling for short periods of time. The coach may also have the athletes wrestle abbreviated matches, for example a match composed of three 1-minute periods. After several weeks, the coach will introduce full-length matches into practice session. This provides further sport-specific training and meets the four objectives identified on page 961. Not only do the matches condition the participants for upcoming competition, the practice matches also prepare the wrestlers for challenge matches, or wrestler-offs, used to determine the team's starting lineup.

Once the team is selected and the inter-team competition starts, the live wrestling portion of practice sessions focuses on maximizing both the peripheral and central fitness of each wrestler. To accomplish this, interval training is often used in practice. Intervals may take several different forms, as discussed below.

Round-Robin

In this case, three wrestlers are grouped together. Wrestlers A and B wrestle while C rests. After the preestablished interval time expires, wrestler C replaces wrestler A. Again, after wrestlers C and A have competed for the established time, wrestlers B and C will compete. In this way, a fatigued wrestler is forced to wrestle against a fresher opponent. As a variation to this, four wrestlers may be grouped. Wrestler A will wrestle, in order, wrestlers B, C, and D, each for the appropriate interval duration. Wrestler A then rests while wrestler B starts down the list of C, D, and finally A, who has now recovered. Either approach to intervals allows self-regulation within the group (wrestlers who are resting keep track of the time), so that the coach may observe the wrestlers for skill execution. The disadvantage of this approach is that the ratio of work to rest is fixed; the rest period cannot be lengthened or shortened relative to the duration of wrestling.

Timed Intervals

In this case, the coach is responsible for timing the intervals. At the end of each interval, wrestlers pair up with a new teammate for the next interval. To provide greater challenges to a wrestler, pairing may be with a teammate who competes in the next higher weight class. A 119-pound wrestler may wrestle the 126-pound wrestler. At the next interval the 119 pounder may meet the 112 pounder, while the 126-pound wrestler competes against the 132 pounder. This approach restricts the coach's opportunity to observe his athletes, but it allows for modifications in the ratio of work to rest.

Timed Intervals with Progressively Reduced Recovery Time

This approach is often used to train the starting lineup at the time of the season when the focus is on preparing the first-string wrestlers for key competition. Each varsity wrestler takes a position on the mat. A second-string teammate steps up for the first interval. At the completion of the interval, the varsity wrestler receives a preestablished rest, for example, 1 minute. Following the rest, a new second- or third-string teammate steps up against the varsity wrestler. A total of 20 intervals may proceed. This would be conducted every other day in practice; since dual meet and tournament competition occur at the end of the week, however, only two practice sessions with intervals occur per week. The following week, intervals are conducted again; however, the rest periods are then only 50 seconds in duration. Each week the recovery period between intervals is reduced so that after 6 weeks there is just enough time to find a new partner before the next interval starts. This strategy is very effective for sport-specific conditioning, and it has proven to be particularly efficient when limited time is available for wrestling practice sessions.

It should be noted that this approach was used effectively during the 1970s at the University of Northern Iowa and the University of Wisconsin. In retrospect, though, it may have been more appropriate to increase the duration of the rest period between wrestling intervals during the 6-week period (59). Research on swimming, a sport not unlike wrestling in terms of upper body effort and total body conditioning, indicates that the longer rest interval allows the athletes to recover and push harder during subsequent intervals. This further taxes the anaerobic energy systems for the potentially greater optimization of training adaptations (60). In contrast, the short rest intervals require the swimmers to pace themselves and rely more on aerobic metabolism. The goal would be to instill attitudes of going all out, rather than pacing, to maximize fitness gains in wrestlers (57). Future research should investigate the optimal training programs and, specifically, the effect of varying the interval recovery period on fitness development in wrestlers.

Supplemental Training

Supplemental training during the season includes specific resistance training exercises, exercises to simulate wrestling movements with a teammate of equal mass, and running, cycling, and rope skipping to develop endurance and lose weight (calorie expenditure and sweat production). Specific examples of such drills can be found elsewhere (55). The purpose of using such exercises is to provide an overload stimulus for training adaptations and also offer variety in training, as a part of the periodization of training (see below). Because wrestlers are concerned about maintaining body weight and not increasing it, supplemental training during the season is usually limited to those exercises that promote muscular endurance. Heavy resistance training that may increase muscle mass is typically avoided during the season.

Supplemental training occurs in pre- and postseason training. For the most part, training during these off-season periods consists of resistance training to increase strength, power, and possibly muscle mass. Historically, resistance training has been less likely to occur during the season for fear of gaining weight and because of restraints on training time during the schedule of numerous competitive events. Although recommendations have been made for wrestlers to train for strength advancement during the off-season (57,61), no systematic research has been done to determine which programs optimize strength gains.

In addition, postseason may be a time when interscholastic and intercollegiate wrestlers experiment with new maneuvers and with the international styles of wrestling, namely Greco-Roman and freestyle. The more relaxed atmosphere at this time of the season helps add new skills to the base of fundamentals learned during the competitive season.

Training in the postseason is recommended to minimize the gain in body fat often seen in wrestlers following the season (62,63). Perhaps the postseason training should provide a debriefing period as wrestlers resume their normal diet, which in essence is a hypercaloric diet relative to that consumed during the season. For this reason, some aerobic or endurance training may also be warranted to minimize fat accretion, particularly in the upper body (63).

Periodization of Training

Periodization can help the athlete focus on different aspects of fitness and performance as each aspect becomes most important during the season (e.g., starting the season with a good aerobic base and adequate strength, for injury prevention; developing the anaerobic capacity and muscular endurance in the middle of the season; and finally, developing speed and refining technique while maintaining endurance at the end, or peak, of the season) (10,56). Wrestlers are susceptible to overtraining due to the rigorous and demanding training schedule, with frequent matches during the scholastic and collegiate season; the lack of time off or taper during the season because of the rigid restrictions on maintaining body weight; and the self-imposed diet restrictions that may contribute to compromised nutritional status (8,36,64–70). Periodization brings variety to the practice sessions, some degree of tapering, and definite but limited number of times to peak during the season. In this way a training program that employs periodization and peaking avoids or at least reduces the risk of becoming overtrained.

Unfortunately, wrestling has never been used as a model to study overtraining, nor has anyone investigated how to prevent overtraining in the sport.

CONCLUSION

Wrestling is an extremely physically demanding sport. The scoring system, which allows for the end of the competition before the allotted time of a match, emphasizes power as a key attribute. Although the match length is short relative to many other athletic events, endurance is also required in the wrestler due to the possibility of overtime and multiple matches in a day tournament. The physiologic profile of the wrestlers at various levels of development has been assessed, but there is a lack of integration of this information in biomechanical studies on technical skill execution and training studies to determine optimal conditioning methods.

REFERENCES

1. NCAA Wrestling Committee, Nelson M. *1997 NCAA wrestling rules and interpretations.* Overland Park, KS: NCAA, 1996:3–79.
2. National Federation Wrestling Rules Committee. *1996–97 high school wrestling rules book.* Kansas City: NFSHSA, 1996:7–76.
3. *FILA bureau international rules for wrestling.* Lausanne, Switzerland: FILA, 1992.
4. American Association for Health, Physical Education, and Recreation. *Nutrition for athletics: a handbook for coaches.* Washington, DC: AAHPER, 1971:26.
5. Wilmore JH, Costill DL. *Training for sport and activity.* Dubuque: Wm. C. Brown, 1988.
6. Horswill CA, Curby DG, Bartoli WP, Murray R. Rate of CO_2 production ($RaCO_2$) and estimates of energy expenditure (EE) in wrestling practice. *Med Sci Sports Exerc* 1997;29:S47(abst).
7. Houston ME, Sharratt MT, Bruce RW. Glycogen depletion and lactate responses in freestyle wrestling. *Can J Appl Sports Sci* 1983;8:79–82.
8. Tarnopolsky MA, Cipriano N, Woodcroft C, et al. Effects of rapid weight loss and wrestling on muscle glycogen concentration. *Clin J Sport Med* 1996;6:78–84.
9. Sharratt MT, Taylor AW, Song TMK. A physiological profile of elite Canadian freestyle wrestlers. *Can J Appl Sports Sci* 1986;11:100–115.
10. Horswill CA. Physiology and nutrition for wrestling. In: Lamb DR, Knuttgen HG, Murray R, eds. *Perspectives in exercise science and sports medicine: physiology and nutrition for competitive sport.* Indianapolis: Benchmark, 1994:131–179.
11. Cinar G, Tamer K. Lactate profiles of wrestlers who participated in 32nd European free-style wrestling championship in 1898. *J Sports Med Phys Fitness* 1994;34:156–160.
12. Hermansen L. Effect of metabolic changes on force production in skeletal muscle during maximal exercise. In: Porter R, Whelan J, eds. *Human muscle fatigue: physiological measurements.* London: Pittman, 1981:72–88.
13. Fabiato A, Fabiato F. Effects of pH on the myofilaments and the sarcoplasmic reticulum of skinned cells from cardiac and skeletal muscles. *J Physiol* 1978;276:233–255.
14. Sharratt MT. Wrestling profile. *Clin Sports Med* 1984;3:273–289.
15. Nagle FJ, Morgan WP, Hellickson RO, Serfass RC, Alexander JF. Spotting success traits in Olympic contenders. *Phys Sports Med* 1975;3:31–34.
16. Taylor AW, Brassard L, Proteau RD. A physiological profile of Canadian Greco-Roman wrestlers. *Can J Appl Sports Sci* 1979;4:131–134.
17. Seals DR, Mullin JP. $\dot{V}O_2$max in variable type exercise and among well-trained upper body athletes. *Res Q Exerc Sport* 1982;53:58–63.
18. Stine G, Ratliff R, Shierman G, Grana WA. Physical profile of the wrestlers at the 1977 NCAA championships. *Phys Sports Med* 1979;7:98–105.

19. Horswill CA, Scott J, Galea P, Park SH. Physiological profile of elite junior wrestlers. *Res Q Exerc Sport* 1988;59:257–261.
20. Horswill CA, Scott JA, Galea P. Comparison of maximum aerobic power, maximum anaerobic power, and skinfold thickness of elite and nonelite junior wrestlers. *Int J Sports Med* 1989;10:165–168.
21. Horswill CA, Miller JE, Scott JR, Smith CM, Welk G, Van Handel P. Anerobic and aerobic power in arms and legs of elite senior wrestlers. *Int J Sports Med* 1992;13:558–561.
22. Morganroth J, Maron BJ, Henry WL, Epstein SE. Comparative left ventricular dimensions in trained athletes. *Ann Internal Med* 1975;82:521–524.
23. Cohen JL, Segal KR. Left ventricular hypertrophy in athletes: an exercise-echocardiographic study. *Med Sci Sports* 1985;17: 695–700.
24. Spirito P, Pelliccia A, Proschan MA, et al. Morphology of the "athlete's heart" assessed by echocardiography in 947 elite athletes representing 27 sports. *Am J Cardiol* 1994;74:802–806.
25. Pelliccia A, Spataro A, Caselli G, Maron BJ. Absence of left ventricular wall thickening in athletes engaged in intense power training. *Am J Cardiol* 1993;72:1048–1054.
26. Smith SA, Humphrey RH, Wohlford JC, Flint DL. Myocardial adaptation and weight fluctuation in college wrestlers. *Int J Sports Med* 1994;15:70–73.
27. Cisar CJ, Johnson GO, Fry AC, Housh TJ, Hughes RA. Preseason body competition, build, and strength as predictors of high school wrestling success. *J Appl Sports Sci Res* 1987;1:66–70.
28. Silva JM, Schultz BB, Haslam RW, Murray D. A physiological assessment of elite wrestlers. *Res Q Exerc Sport* 1981;52:348–358.
29. Ahlman K, Karvoner MJ. Weight reduction by sweating in wrestlers, and its effects on physical fitness. *J Sports Med* 1961;1:58–62.
30. Jacobs I. The effects of thermal dehydration on performance on the Wingate anaerobic test. *Int J Sports Med* 1980;1:21–24.
31. Park SH, Roemmich JN, Horswill CA. A season of wrestling and weight loss by adolescent wrestlers: effect on anaerobic arm power. *J Appl Sport Sci Res* 1990;4:1–4.
32. Serfass RC, Stull GA, Alexander JF, Ewing JL. The effects of rapid weight loss and attempted rehydration on strength and endurance of the handgripping muscle in college wrestlers. *Res Q Exerc Sport* 1984;55:46–52.
33. Singer RN, Weiss SA. Effects of weight reduction on selected anthropometric, physical, and performance measures of wrestlers. *Res Q* 1968;39:361–369.
34. Widerman PM, Hagen RD. Bodyweight loss in a wrestler preparing for competition: a case report. *Med Sci Sports Exerc* 1982;14:413–418.
35. Roemmich JN, Sinning WE. Sport-seasonal changes in body composition, growth, power and strength of adolescent wrestlers. *Int J Sports Med* 1996;17:92–99.
36. Houston ME, Marin DA, Green HJ, Thomson JA. The effect of rapid weight loss on physiological function in wrestlers. *Phys Sports Med* 1981;9:73–78.
37. Horswill CA. Does rapid weight loss by dehydration adversely affect high-power performance? *Sports Sci Exchange* 1991;3:1–4.
38. Costill DL, Cote R, Fink W. Muscle water and electrolytes following varied levels of dehydration in man. *J Appl Physiol* 1976;40:6–11.
39. Horswill CA, Scott JA, Dick RW, Hayes J. Influence of rapid weight gain after the weigh-in on success in collegiate wrestlers. *Med Sci Sports Exerc* 1994;26:1290–1294.
40. Scott JR, Horswill CA, Dick RW. Acute weight gain in collegiate wrestlers following a tournament weigh-in. *Med Sci Sports Exerc* 1994;26:1181–1185.
41. Hickner RC, Horswill C, Welker J, Scott JR, Costill DL. Test development for study of physical performance in wrestlers following weight loss. *Int J Sports Med* 1991;12:557–562.
42. Horswill CA, Hickner RC, Scott JR, Costill DL, Gould D. Weight loss, dietary carbohydrate modification and high intensity, physical performance. *Med Sci Sports Exerc* 1990;22:470–476.
43. Klinzing JE, Karpowicz W. The effects of rapid weight loss and rehydration on a wrestling performance test. *J Sports Med* 1986;26:149–156.
44. Webster S, Rutt R, Weltman A. Physiological effects of a weight loss regimen practiced by college wrestlers. *Med Sci Sports Exerc* 1990;22:229–234.
45. Caldwell JE, Ahonen E, Nousiainen U. Different effects of sauna-, diuretic-, and exercise-induced hypohydration. *J Appl Physiol* 1984;57:1018–1023.
46. Herbert WG, Ribisl PM. Effects of dehydration upon physical working capacity of wrestlers under competitive conditions. *Res Q* 1972;43:416–422.
47. Ribisl PM, Herbert WG. Effects of rapid weight reduction and subsequent rehydration upon the physical working capacity of wrestlers. *Res Q* 1970;41:536–541.
48. Rankin JW, Ocel JV, Craft LL. Effect of weight loss and refeeding diet composition on anaerobic performance in wrestlers. *Med Sci Sports Exerc* 1996;28:1292–1299.
49. Coyle EF, Coyle E. Carbohydrates that speed recovery from training. *Phys Sports Med* 1993;21:111–123.
50. Mourier A, Bigard AX, deKerviler E, Roger B, Legrand H, Guezennec CY. Combined effects of caloric restriction and branched-chain amino acid supplementation on body composition and exercise performance in elite wrestlers. *Int J Sports Med* 1997;18:47–55.
51. Utter A, Goss F, DaSilva S, et al. Development of a wrestling-specific performance test. *J Strength Conditioning Res* 1997;11:88–91.
52. Kelly JM, Gorney BA, Kalm KK. The effects of a collegiate wrestlers on body composition, cardiovascular fitness and muscle strength and endurance. *Med Sci Sports* 1978;10:119–124.
53. Song TMK, Cipriano N. Effects of seasonal training on physical and physiological function on elite varsity wrestlers. *J Sports Med* 1984;24:123–130.
54. Eckerson JM, Housh DJ, Housh TJ, Johnson GO. Seasonal changes in body composition, strength, and muscular power in high school wrestlers. *Pediatr Exerc Sci* 1994;6:39–52.
55. Jefferies SC. *Sport physiology course: American coaching effectiveness program,* level 2. Champaign, IL: Human Kinetics, 1986.
56. *USA wrestling coach's guide to excellence.* Carmel, IN: Cooper, 1995.
57. Johnson GO, Cisar CJ. Basic conditioning principles for high school wrestlers. *Phys Sports Med* 1987;15:153–159.
58. Combs S, Frank C. *Winning wrestling.* Chicago: Contemporary Books, 1980:1–127.
59. Horswill CA. Interval training for wrestlers. *Wrestling USA* 1997;28:7–9.
60. Beltz JD, Costill DL, Thomas R, Fink WJ, Kirwan JP. Energy demands for interval training for competitive swimming. *J Swimming Res* 1988;4:5–9.
61. Horswill CA. Post season weight training. *Wrestling USA* 1992;27:42–43.
62. Sinning WE, Wilensky NF, Meyers EJ. Post-season body composition changes and weight estimation in high-school wrestlers. In: Brockhoff J, ed. *Physical education sports and the sciences.* Eugene, OR: Microform, 1976:137–153.
63. McCargar LJ, Crawford SM. Metabolic and anthropometric changes with weight cycling in wrestlers. *Med Sci Sports Exerc* 1992;24:1270–1275.
64. Horswill C, Park S, Roemmich J. Changes in the protein nutritional status of adolescent wrestlers. *Med Sci Sports Exerc* 1990;22:599–604.
65. Fogelholm M, Koskinen R, Laakso J, Rankinen J, Ruokonen I. Gradual and rapid weight loss: effects on nutrition and performance in males athletes. *Med Sci Sports Exerc* 1993;25:371–377.
66. Roemmich JN, Sinning WE. Weight loss and wrestling training: effects on nutrition, growth, maturation, body composition, and strength. *J Appl Physiol* 1997;82:1751–1759.
67. Roemmich JN, Sinning WE. Weight loss and wrestling training: effects on growth-related hormones. *J Appl Physiol* 1997;82:1760–1764.
68. Strauss RH, Lanese RR, Malarkey WB. Weight loss in amateur wrestlers and its effect on serum testosterone levels. *JAMA* 1985;254:3337–3338.
69. Melby CL, Schmidt WD, Corrigan D. Resting metabolic rate in weight-cycling collegiate wrestlers compared with physically active, noncycling and control subjects. *Am J Clin Nutr* 1990;52:409–414.
70. McMurray RG, Proctor CR, Wilson WL. Effect of the caloric deficit and dietary manipulation on aerobic and anaerobic exercise. *Int J Sports Med* 1991;12(2):167–172.

Subject Index

Subject Index

Page references for figures are followed by an *f*, and page references for tables are followed by a *t*.

Exercise and Sport Science

Exercise and Sport Science

Editors

WILLIAM E. GARRETT, JR., MD, PhD
Frank C. Wilson Professor and Chairman
Department of Orthopaedics
University of North Carolina School of Medicine
Chapel Hill, North Carolina

DONALD T. KIRKENDALL, PhD
Clinical Assistant Professor
Department of Orthopaedics
University of North Carolina School of Medicine
Chapel Hill, North Carolina

Illustrator
Marsha Dohrmann

LIPPINCOTT WILLIAMS & WILKINS
A Wolters Kluwer Company
Philadelphia • Baltimore • New York • London
Buenos Aires • Hong Kong • Sydney • Tokyo

Acquisitions Editor: Danette Knopp
Developmental Editors: Tanya Lazar; Sonya L. Seigafuse
Production Editor: Sally M. Scott
Manufacturing Manager: Tim Reynolds
Cover Designer: Catherine Lau Hunt
Compositor: Bi-Comp/PRD Group
Printer: Maple Press

227 East Washington Square
Philadelphia, PA 19106-3780 USA
LWW.com

Printed in the USA

Library of Congress Cataloging-in-Publication Data

Exercise and sport science / editors, William E. Garrett, Jr., Donald Kirkendall ; illustrator, Marsha Dohrmann.
p. cm.
Includes bibliographical references and index.
ISBN 0-683-03421-9
1. Sports—Physiological aspects. 2. Exercise—Physiological aspects. 3. Human mechanics. I. Garrett, William E. II. Kirkendall, Don T.
RC1235.E94 1999
612′.044—dc21 99-038884
CIP

---

10 9 8 7 6 5 4 3 2 1